T0200031

PROFESSIONAL
GUIDE TO
DISEASES

ELEVENTH EDITION

PROFESSIONAL
GUIDE TO
DISEASES

ELEVENTH EDITION

CLINICAL EDITOR
LAURA M. WILLIS, DNP, APRN-CNP, CMSRN
Family Nurse Practitioner
Mercy Health—Urbana Family Medicine and Pediatrics
Urbana, Ohio

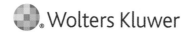

Philadelphia • Baltimore • New York • London
Buenos Aires • Hong Kong • Sydney • Tokyo

Acquisitions Editor: Nicole Dernoski
Development Editor: Maria M. McAvey
Editorial Coordinator: Lindsay Ries
Production Project Manager: Marian Bellus
Design Coordinator: Holly Reid McLaughlin
Manufacturing Coordinator: Kathleen Brown
Marketing Manager: Linda Wetmore
Prepress Vendor: S4Carlisle Publishing Services

Eleventh edition

9 8 7 6 5 4 3 2 1

Printed in China

Library of Congress Cataloging-in-Publication Data

Names: Willis, Laura M., 1969- editor. | Lippincott Williams & Wilkins,
   issuing body.
Title: Professional guide to diseases / clinical editor, Dr. Laura M. Willis,
   DNP, APRN-CNP, CMSRN, Family Nurse Practitioner Urbana Family Medicine and
   Pediatrics, Urbana, Ohio.
Description: Eleventh edition. | Philadelphia: Wolters Kluwer, [2020] |
   Includes bibliographical references and index.
Identifiers: LCCN 2018056438 | ISBN 9781975107727
Subjects: LCSH: Clinical medicine—Handbooks, manuals, etc. |
   Diseases—Handbooks, manuals, etc. | Nursing—Handbooks, manuals, etc.
Classification: LCC RT65 .P69 2020 | DDC 616—dc23
LC record available at https://lccn.loc.gov/2018056438

*To my teachers and mentors, past and present,
and to those patients who have truly touched
my life with a difficult diagnosis or a tough
conversation—this work is for you.*

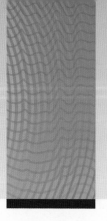

CONTRIBUTORS

Samuel A. Borchers, OD
Optometrist
Northern Arizona VA Health System
Prescott, Arizona

Melanie N. DeGonzague, MSN, APRN, AGPCNP-BC
Certified Nurses Practitioner
The Christ Hospital Physicians—Primary Care
Cincinnati, Ohio

Kathryn Dinh, MSN, APRN, AGPCNP-BC
Nurse Practitioner
The Christ Hospital
Cincinnati, Ohio

Ellie Franges, DNP, CRNP, CNRN
Neurological Surgery
Chestmont Neurosurgery
Main Line Healthcare
Paoli, Pennsylvania

Bridget A. Howard, MSN, CNP
Department of Gastroenterology
Mayo Clinic
Scottsdale, Arizona

Katrin Moskowitz, DNP, FNP
Assistant Clinical Director
Community Health and Wellness Center of
  Greater Torrington
Torrington, Connecticut

Susan Raymond, MSN, RN, CCRN
Deputy Commander for Nursing
Weed Army Hospital
Fort Irwin, California

Cherie R. Rebar, PhD, MBA, RN, COI
Vice President for Communication and
  Marketing
Connect: RN2ED
Beavercreek, Ohio
Faculty, Division of Nursing
Wittenberg University
Springfield, Ohio

Michael J. Rebar, DO
Internal Medicine Specialist
Dayton, Ohio

Amy Slusher, MSN, APRN, ANP-C
Nurse Practitioner
Optum
Miamisburg, Ohio

Stefanie Nelson Tyler, DNP, WHNP, RN
Nurse Practitioner
The Centre for Reproductive and Genetic Health
London, United Kingdom

Daniel T. Vetrosky, PhD, PA-C, DFAAPA
Professor and Director of Didactic Education
University of South Alabama
Mobile, Alabama

Amy Weaver, DNP, FNP-BC
Family Nurse Practitioner
Greeneville, Tennessee

Alisha H. Wilkes, DNP, CNM, ARNP
Nurse-Midwife
Three Moons Midwifery
Renton, Washington

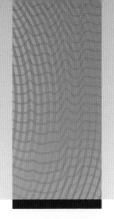

PREVIOUS EDITION CONTRIBUTORS

Deborah Hutchinson Allen, MSN, RN

Charles L. Bevins, MD, PHD

Donna C. Bond, DNP, RN-BC, CCNS, AE-C

Vicki L. Brinsko, RN, BS, CIC

Raymond A. Costabile, MD

Ellie Z. Franges, MSN, ANP-BC, CNRN

Bridget Howard, MSN, APRN, BC

Seanra J. Kalil, PA-C

Joshua F. Knox, PA-C

Wanda M. Martinez, MD, PHD

E. Ann Myers, MD, FACP, FACE

Diana Noller, MSPT, MMS, PA-C

Jody Ralph, PHD, BSc, BSN, MSc, RN

Sundaram V. Ramanan, MD, MS, FRCP, FACP

Susan M. Raymond, MSN, RN, CCRN

Christie L. Rogers, MS, RD, CNSC

Christopher R. A. Sim, MPAS, PA-C

Dominique A. Thuriere, MD

Daniel T. Vetrosky, PA-C, PHD

Benita Walton-Moss, DNS, FNP-BC

Linda Weinberg, PHD, FNP-C, RN, ET

Lei Xi, MD

FOREWORD

How can health care providers respond to the new model of consumerism in medicine, in which patients are encouraged to question everything, are bombarded with health care information in the media, and are targeted by direct advertising campaigns marketing everything from weight loss programs to therapies for erectile dysfunction? In today's information- and technology-driven environment, staying on the leading edge of ever-changing medical information can be overwhelming. The reality of contemporary medical economics and regulation of medical practice is driving many clinicians to see greater numbers of patients each day, each with more complex illnesses. This has resulted in less time spent with the patient, less time to perform detailed literature searches for complex conditions, and more time devoted to medical record completion, negotiating with medical insurance companies and other administrative representatives and justifying the medical necessity for many orders. In this environment there's a need for a well-organized and comprehensive summary of a wide variety of illnesses to help the busy clinician.

This 11th edition of *Professional Guide to Diseases* features well-organized chapters coordinated around disease clusters. The data in this edition are accurate, updated in terms of original research and practice guidelines, and designed to provide a brief yet comprehensive overview of a large array of disease processes and new sections for a quick pathophysiology review. Readers ranging from the trainee preparing for a board certification examination to the senior faculty member or other health care provider needing a ready reference will find that this book provides a clear and concise overview of hundreds of diseases and conditions.

This edition features improved sections focused on health promotion, disease prevention, and special focuses on elderly patients. Additionally, there is an updated section on bioterrorism and a new section on approaches to care of LGBTQ individuals—topics that have been receiving added emphasis in health care circles in recent years. Complications associated with different diseases are also included. This edition also updates information on many conditions for which a variety of clinical treatment guidelines have been published recently by major professional medical and surgical organizations. The content of clinical practice guidelines typically includes a detailed review of the literature for the specific topic.

For the variety of health care providers for whom this book has been created, the organizational format allows the option of reviewing an entire topic, such as clinical genetics and genomics, or narrowing the focus to one aspect of disease, such as the details of treatment or special considerations of emerging illnesses. The text is written clearly and includes graphic data displays that make it useful as a quick reference, but it also contains comprehensive material that allows for more complete coverage of a group of similar disease entities. In this edition of the book are artwork and figures that illustrate the pathophysiology of many conditions in a full-color format. These images can not only be used to better understand the topic on a professional level, but can also be leveraged for patient teaching while in the office or hospital. This book continues to feature information on efficient health care delivery for routine conditions seen almost daily, as well as cultural considerations in patient care, information on potential bioterrorism agents, updates on rare diseases, and a revised section discussing complementary and alternative therapies for specific conditions.

As the practice of medicine continues to evolve, providers must face the challenges of achieving correct diagnoses using more targeted and cost-effective testing in a more constricted time frame. The 11th edition of *Professional Guide to Diseases* offers a strong background of successful editions combined with the latest updates and recommendations that will help you provide accurate information to your patients.

Enjoy this book!

Laura M. Willis, DNP, APRN-CNP, CMSRN
Family Nurse Practitioner
Mercy Health—Urbana Family
Medicine and Pediatrics
Urbana, Ohio

CONTENTS

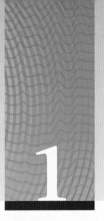

CARDIOVASCULAR DISORDERS

Introduction

The cardiovascular system begins its activity when the fetus is barely a month old and is the last body system to cease activity at the end of life. This system is so vital that its activity defines the presence of life.

LIFE-GIVING TRANSPORT SYSTEM

The heart, arteries, veins, and lymphatics form the cardiovascular network that serves as the body's transport system, bringing life-supporting oxygen and nutrients to cells, removing metabolic waste products, and carrying hormones from one part of the body to another. Often called the *circulatory system*, it may be divided into two branches: *pulmonary circulation*, in which blood picks up new oxygen and liberates the waste product carbon dioxide; and *systemic circulation* (including coronary circulation), in which blood carries oxygen and nutrients to all active cells while transporting waste products to the kidneys, liver, and skin for excretion.

Circulation requires normal functioning of the heart, which propels blood through the system by continuous rhythmic contractions. Located behind the sternum, the heart is a muscular organ the size of a man's fist. It has three layers: the *endocardium*—the smooth inner layer; the *myocardium*—the thick, muscular middle layer that contracts in rhythmic beats; and the *epicardium*—the thin, serous membrane, or outer surface of the heart. Covering the entire heart is a saclike membrane called the *pericardium*, which has two layers: a *visceral* layer

that's in contact with the heart and a *parietal*, or outer, layer. To prevent irritation when the heart moves against this layer during contraction, fluid lubricates the parietal pericardium.

The heart has four chambers: two thin-walled chambers called *atria* and two thick-walled chambers called *ventricles*. The atria serve as reservoirs during ventricular contraction (systole) and as booster pumps during ventricular relaxation (diastole). The left ventricle propels blood through the systemic circulation. The right ventricle, which forces blood through the pulmonary circulation, is much thinner than the left because it meets only one sixth the resistance.

ELDER TIP *As a person's body ages, the ventricular and aortic walls stiffen, decreasing the heart's pumping action.*

HEART VALVES

Two kinds of valves work inside the heart: *atrioventricular* (AV) and *semilunar*. The AV valve between the right atrium and the ventricle has three leaflets, or cusps, and three papillary muscles; hence, it's called the *tricuspid valve*. The AV valve between the left atrium and the ventricle consists of two cusps shaped like a bishop's hat, or miter, and two papillary muscles and is called the *mitral valve*. The tricuspid and mitral valves prevent blood backflow from the ventricles to the atria during ventricular contraction. The leaflets of both valves are attached to the ventricles' papillary muscles by thin, fibrous bands called *chordae tendineae*; the leaflets separate and descend funnel-like into the ventricles during diastole and are pushed upward and together during systole to occlude the mitral and tricuspid orifices. The valves' action isn't entirely passive because papillary muscles contract during systole and prevent the leaflets from prolapsing into the atria during ventricular contraction.

The two semilunar valves, which resemble half-moons, prevent blood backflow from the aorta and pulmonary arteries into the ventricles when those chambers relax and fill with blood from the atria. They're referred to as the *aortic valve* and *pulmonic valve* for their respective arteries.

⬡ **ELDER TIP** *In elderly people, fibrotic and sclerotic changes thicken heart valves and reduce their flexibility. These changes lead to rigidity and incomplete closure of the valves, which may result in systolic or diastolic murmurs.*

THE CARDIAC CYCLE

Diastole is the phase of ventricular relaxation and filling. As diastole begins, ventricular pressure falls below arterial pressure, and the aortic and pulmonic valves close. As ventricular pressure continues to fall below atrial pressure, the mitral and tricuspid valves open, and blood flows rapidly into the ventricles. Atrial contraction then increases the volume of ventricular filling by pumping 15% to 25% more blood into the ventricles. When *systole* begins, the ventricular muscle contracts, raising ventricular pressure above atrial pressure and closing the mitral and tricuspid valves. When ventricular pressure finally becomes greater than that in the aorta and pulmonary artery, the aortic and pulmonic valves open, and the ventricles eject blood. Ventricular pressure continues to rise as blood is expelled from the heart. As systole ends, the ventricles relax and stop ejecting blood, and ventricular pressure falls, closing both valves.

S_1 (the first heart sound) is heard as the ventricles contract and the AV valves close. S_1 is loudest at the heart's apex, over the mitral area. S_2 (the second heart sound), which is normally rapid and sharp, occurs when the aortic and pulmonic valves close. S_2 is loudest at the heart's base (second intercostal space [ICS] on both sides of the sternum).

Ventricular distention during diastole, which can occur in systolic heart failure, creates low-frequency vibrations that may be heard as a third heart sound (S_3), or ventricular gallop. An atrial gallop (S_4) may appear at the end of diastole, just before S_1, if atrial filling is forced into a ventricle that has become less compliant or overdistended or has a decreased ability to contract. A pressure rise and ventricular vibrations cause this sound.

CARDIAC CONDUCTION

The heart's conduction system is composed of specialized cells capable of generating and conducting rhythmic electrical impulses to stimulate heart contraction. This system includes the sinoatrial (SA) node, the AV junction, the bundle of His and its bundle branches, and the ventricular conduction tissue and Purkinje fibers.

Normally, the SA node controls the heart rate and rhythm at 60 to 100 beats/minute. Because the SA node has the lowest resting potential, it's the heart's pacemaker. If it defaults, another part of the system takes over. The AV junction may emerge at 40 to 60 beats/minute; the bundle of His and bundle branches at 30 to 40 beats/minute; and ventricular conduction tissue at 20 to 30 beats/minute.

⬡ **ELDER TIP** *As the myocardium of the aging heart becomes more irritable, extrasystoles may occur along with sinus arrhythmias and sinus bradycardias. In addition, increased fibrous tissue infiltrates the SA nodes and internodal atrial tracts, which may cause atrial fibrillation and flutter.*

CARDIAC OUTPUT

Cardiac output—the amount of blood pumped by the left ventricle into the aorta each minute—is calculated by multiplying the *stroke volume* (the amount of blood the left ventricle ejects during each contraction) by the *heart rate* (number of beats/minute). When cellular demands increase, stroke volume or heart rate must increase.

Many factors affect the heart rate, including exercise, pregnancy, and stress. When the sympathetic nervous system releases norepinephrine, the heart rate increases; when the parasympathetic system releases acetylcholine, it slows. As a person ages, the heart rate takes longer to normalize after exercise.

Stroke volume depends on the ventricular blood volume and pressure at the end of diastole (preload), resistance to ejection (afterload), and the myocardium's contractile strength (inotropy). Changes in preload, afterload, or inotropic state can alter the stroke volume.

⬡ **ELDER TIP** *Exercise cardiac output declines slightly with age. A decrease in maximum heart rate and contractility may cause this change.*

CIRCULATION AND PULSES

Blood circulates through three types of vessels: *arteries, veins,* and *capillaries.* The sturdy, pliable walls of the arteries adjust to the volume of blood leaving the heart. The major artery branching out of the left ventricle is the aorta.

Its segments and subbranches ultimately divide into minute, thin-walled (one-cell thick) capillaries. Capillaries pass the blood to the veins, which return it to the heart. In the veins, valves prevent blood backflow.

ELDER TIP *Aging contributes to arterial and venous insufficiency as the strength and elasticity of blood vessels decrease.*

Pulses are felt best wherever an artery runs near the skin and over a hard structure. (See *Pulse points.*) Easily found pulses are:

♦ *radial artery*—anterolateral aspect of the wrist
♦ *temporal artery*—in front of the ear, above and lateral to the eye
♦ *common carotid artery*—neck (side)
♦ *femoral artery*—groin

Pulse points

Peripheral pulse rhythm should correspond exactly to the auscultatory heart rhythm. The pulse's character may offer useful information. For example, *pulsus alternans*, a strong beat followed by a weak one, can mean myocardial weakness. A *water-hammer* (or *Corrigan*) *pulse*, a forceful bounding pulse best felt in the carotid arteries or in the forearm, accompanies increased pulse pressure— commonly with capillary pulsations of the fingernails (*Quincke sign*). This pulse usually indicates aortic valve regurgitation.

Pulsus bisferiens, a double peripheral pulse for every apical beat, can signal aortic regurgitation or hypertrophic obstructive cardiomyopathy. *Pulsus bigeminus* is a coupled rhythm; you feel its beat in pairs. *Pulsus paradoxus* is exaggerated waxing and waning of the arterial pressure (≥15 mm Hg decrease in systolic blood pressure during inspiration), often seen in cardiac tamponade.

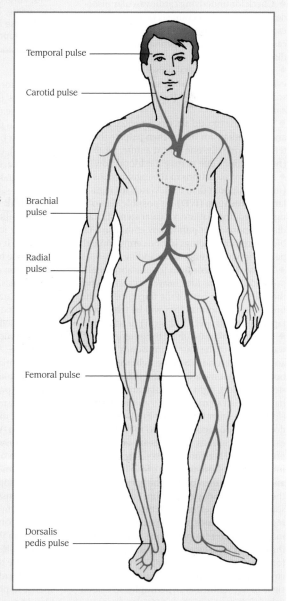

Temporal pulse

Carotid pulse

Brachial pulse

Radial pulse

Femoral pulse

Dorsalis pedis pulse

The lymphatic system also plays a role in the cardiovascular network. Originating in tissue spaces, the lymphatic system drains fluid and other plasma components that build up in extravascular spaces and reroutes them back to the circulatory system as lymph, a plasmalike fluid. Lymphatics also extract bacteria and foreign bodies.

CARDIOVASCULAR ASSESSMENT

Physical assessment provides vital information about cardiovascular status.

◆ Check for underlying cardiovascular disorders, such as central cyanosis (impaired gas exchange), edema (heart failure or valvular disease), and clubbing (congenital cardiovascular disease).

◆ Palpate the peripheral pulses bilaterally and evaluate their rate, equality, and quality on a scale of 0 (absent) to +4 (bounding). (See *Pulse amplitude scale.*)

◆ Inspect the carotid arteries for equal appearance. Auscultate for bruits; then palpate the arteries individually, one side at a time, for *thrills* (fine vibrations due to irregular blood flow).

◆ Check for pulsations in the jugular veins (more easily seen than felt). Watch for jugular vein distention (JVD)—a possible sign of right-sided heart failure, valvular stenosis, cardiac tamponade, or pulmonary embolism. Take blood pressure readings in both arms while the patient is lying, sitting, and standing.

◆ Palpate the precordium for any abnormal pulsations, such as lifts, heaves, or thrills. Use the palms (at the base of the fingertips) or the fingertips. The normal apex will be felt as a light tap and extends over 1" (2.5 cm) or less.

◆ Systematically auscultate the anterior chest wall for each of the four heart sounds in the aortic area (second ICS at the right sternal border), pulmonic area (second ICS at the left sternal border), right ventricular area (lower half of the left sternal border), and mitral area (fifth ICS at the midclavicular line). However, don't limit your auscultation to these four areas. Valvular sounds may be heard all over the precordium. Therefore, inch your stethoscope in a Z pattern, from the base of the heart across and down and then over to the apex, or start at the apex and work your way up. For low-pitched sounds, use the bell of the stethoscope; for high-pitched sounds, the diaphragm. Carefully inspect each area for pulsations, and palpate for thrills. Check the location of apical pulsation for deviations in normal size ($^3/_8$" to $^3/_4$" [1 to 2 cm]) and position (in the mitral area)—possible signs of left ventricular hypertrophy, left-sided valvular disease, or right ventricular disease.

◆ Listen for the vibrating sound of turbulent blood flow through a stenotic or incompetent valve. Time the murmur to determine where it occurs in the cardiac cycle—between S_1 and S_2 (systolic), between S_2 and the following S_1 (diastolic), or throughout systole (holosystolic). Finally, listen for the scratching or squeaking of a pericardial friction rub.

SPECIAL CARDIOVASCULAR TESTS

Electrocardiography (ECG) measures electrical activity by recording currents transmitted by the heart. It can detect ischemia, injury, necrosis, bundle branch blocks, fascicular blocks, conduction delay, chamber enlargement, and arrhythmias. In Holter monitoring, a tape recording tracks as many as 100,000 cardiac cycles over a 12- or 24-hour period. This test may be used to assess the effectiveness of antiarrhythmic drugs or to evaluate arrhythmia symptoms. A signal-averaged ECG will identify afterpotentials, which are associated with a risk of ventricular arrhythmias. (See *Positioning chest electrodes,* page 5.)

Chest X-rays may reveal cardiac enlargement and aortic dilation. They also assess pulmonary circulation. When pulmonary venous and arterial pressures rise, characteristic changes appear, such as dilation of the pulmonary venous shadows. When pulmonary venous pressure exceeds oncotic pressure of the blood, capillary fluid leaks into lung tissues, causing pulmonary edema. This fluid may settle in the alveoli, producing a butterfly pattern, or the lungs may appear cloudy or hazy; in the interlobular septa, sharp linear densities (Kerley lines) may appear.

Exercise testing intra-aortic balloon pump (IABP) treadmill determines the heart's response to physical stress. This test measures blood pressure and ECG changes during

Positioning chest electrodes

To record the 12-lead electrocardiogram, place electrodes on the patient's arms and legs (with the ground lead on the patient's right leg). The three standard limb leads (I, II, III) and the three augmented leads (aV_R, aV_L, aV_F) are recorded using these electrodes.

To record the precordial (chest) leads, place the electrodes as follows:

♦ V_1—fourth ICS, right sternal border
♦ V_2—fourth ICS, left sternal border
♦ V_3—midway between V_2 and V_4
♦ V_4—fifth ICS, left midclavicular line
♦ V_5—fifth ICS, left anterior axillary line
♦ V_6—fifth ICS, left midaxillary line

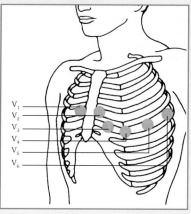

increasingly rigorous exercises. Myocardial ischemia, abnormal blood pressure response, or arrhythmias indicate the circulatory system's failure to adapt to exercise.

Cardiac catheterization evaluates chest pain, the need for coronary artery surgery or angioplasty, congenital heart defects, and valvular heart disease and determines the extent of heart failure. Right-sided catheterization involves threading a pulmonary artery thermodilution catheter, which can measure cardiac output, through a vein into the right side of the heart, pulmonary artery, and its branches in the lungs to measure right atrial, right ventricular, pulmonary artery, and pulmonary artery wedge pressures (PAWPs). Left-sided catheterization entails retrograde catheterization of the left ventricle or transseptal catheterization of the left atrium. Ventriculography during left-sided catheterization involves injecting radiopaque dye into the left ventricle to measure ejection fraction and to disclose abnormal heart wall motion or mitral valve incompetence.

In coronary angiography, radiopaque material injected into coronary arteries allows cineangiographic visualization of coronary arterial narrowing or occlusion.

Echocardiography uses echoes from pulsed high-frequency sound waves (ultrasound) to evaluate cardiac structures. Two-dimensional echocardiography (most common), in which an ultrasound beam rapidly sweeps through an arc, produces a cross-sectional or fan-shaped view of cardiac structures. Contrast agents may be used for image enhancement. Doppler echocardiography records blood flow within the cardiovascular system. Color Doppler echocardiography shows the direction of blood flow, which provides information about the degree of valvular insufficiency. Transesophageal echocardiography combines ultrasound with endoscopy to better view the heart's structures. This procedure allows images to be taken from the heart's posterior aspect.

Echocardiography provides information about valve leaflets, size and dimensions of heart chambers, and thickness and motion of the septum and the ventricular walls. It can also reveal intracardiac masses, detect pericardial effusion, diagnose hypertrophic cardiomyopathy, and estimate cardiac output and ejection fraction. This test can also evaluate possible aortic dissection when it involves the ascending aorta.

In multiple-gated acquisition scanning (MUGA), a radioactive isotope in the intravascular compartment allows measurement of stroke volume, wall motion, and ventricular ejection fraction. Myocardial imaging uses a radioactive isotope to detect abnormalities in myocardial perfusion. This agent concentrates in normally perfused areas of the myocardium but not in ischemic areas ("cold spots"), which may be permanent (scar tissue) or temporary (from transient ischemia). These tests can be done as exercise studies or can be combined with drugs (nuclear stress test), in patients unable to exercise.

Peripheral arteriography consists of a fluoroscopic X-ray after arterial injection of a contrast medium. Similarly, phlebography defines the venous system after injection of a contrast medium into a vein.

Doppler ultrasonography evaluates the peripheral vascular system and assesses peripheral artery disease (PAD) when combined with sequential systolic blood pressure readings.

Endomyocardial biopsy can detect cardiomyopathy, infiltrative myocardial diseases, and, most often, transplant rejection.

Electrophysiologic studies help diagnose conduction system disease and serious arrhythmias. Electronic induction and termination of arrhythmias aid drug selection. Endocardial mapping detects an arrhythmia's focus using a finger electrode. Epicardial mapping uses a computer and a device containing electrodes that's slipped over the heart to detect arrhythmias.

Magnetic resonance imaging (MRI) can investigate cardiac structure and function. Positron emission tomography and magnetic resonance spectroscopy are used to assess myocardial metabolism.

Electron-beam computed tomography, also known as ultrafast computed tomography, is used to detect microcalcifications in the coronary arteries and can give a coronary calcium score. This test is useful for identifying early coronary artery disease (CAD).

Blood tests

Cardiac enzymes (cellular proteins released into blood after cell membrane injury) confirm acute myocardial infarction (MI) or severe cardiac trauma. All cardiac enzymes—creatine kinase (CK), lactate dehydrogenase, and aspartate aminotransferase, for example—are also found in other cells. Fractionation of enzymes can determine the source of damaged cells. For example, three fractions of CK are isolated, one of which (an isoenzyme called *CK-MB*) is found only in cardiac cells. CK-MB in the blood indicates injury to myocardial cells.

Measurement of a cardiac protein called *troponin* is the most precise way to determine whether a patient has experienced an MI. Some 6 hours after an MI, a blood test can detect two forms of troponin: T and I. Troponin T levels peak about 2 days after an MI and return to normal about 16 days later. Troponin I levels reach their peak in less than 1 day after an MI and return to normal in about 7 days.

MANAGING CARDIOVASCULAR DISEASE

Patients with cardiovascular disease pose a tremendous challenge. Their sheer numbers alone compel a thorough understanding of cardiovascular anatomy, physiology, and pathophysiology. Anticipate a high anxiety level in cardiac patients, and provide support and reassurance, especially during procedures such as cardiac catheterization.

Cardiac rehabilitation programs are widely prescribed and offer education and support along with exercise instruction. Rehabilitation programs begin in healthcare facilities and continue on an outpatient basis. Helping the patient resume a satisfying lifestyle requires planning and comprehensive teaching. Inform the patient about healthcare facilities and organizations that offer cardiac rehabilitation programs.

Congenital acyanotic defects

VENTRICULAR SEPTAL DEFECT

Causes and incidence

In ventricular septal defect (VSD), the most common congenital heart disorder, an opening in the septum between the ventricles allows blood to shunt between the left and the right ventricles. This disease accounts for up to 30% of all congenital heart defects. Although most children with congenital heart defects are otherwise normal, in some, VSD coexists with additional birth defects, especially Down syndrome and other autosomal trisomies, renal anomalies, and such cardiac defects as patent ductus arteriosus (PDA) and coarctation of the aorta. VSDs are located in the membranous or muscular portion of the ventricular septum and vary in size. Some defects close spontaneously; in other defects, the entire septum is absent, creating a single ventricle. The prognosis is good for defects that close spontaneously or are correctable surgically but poor for untreated defects, which are sometimes fatal by age 1, usually from secondary complications. Less than 1% of neonates are born with VSD. In 80% to 90% of neonates who are born with this disorder, the hole is small and will usually close spontaneously. In the remaining 10% to 20% of neonates, surgery is needed to close the hole. (See *Understanding ventricular septal defect*, page 7.)

Pathophysiology

In neonates with VSD, the ventricular septum fails to close completely by the eighth week of gestation, as it would normally.

VSD isn't readily apparent at birth, because right and left ventricular pressures are about equal, so blood doesn't shunt through the defect. As the pulmonary vasculature gradually relaxes, 4 to 8 weeks after birth, right ventricular

Understanding ventricular septal defect

A ventricular septal defect (VSD), the most common type of congenital disorder, is an abnormal opening between the right and left ventricles that allows blood to shunt between them. Not always readily apparent at birth, the defect can be small and may close spontaneously. The septum may be entirely absent, resulting in a single ventricle. A large, untreated defect can cause right ventricular hypertrophy, pulmonary hypertension, and heart failure. VSD is classified as an increased pulmonary blood flow defect.

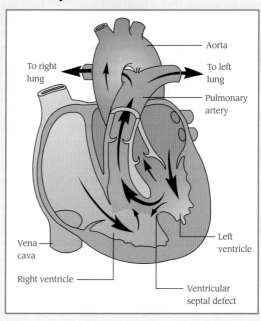

pressure decreases, allowing blood to shunt from the left to the right ventricle. In small or restrictive defects, right ventricle pressure is only slightly elevated, while pulmonary artery pressures (PAPs) and peripheral vascular resistance (PVR) remain normal. In moderate defects, the size of the defect determines the magnitude of the shunt. When right ventricular pressure decreases, the left atrium and ventricle may become fluid overloaded. Because large defects do not meet a lot of flow resistance, the pressure of the ventricles is equal at first. As PVR decreases, volume increases to the pulmonary system, in turn increasing the volume of the left ventricle. This, in turn, can create left ventricular dilation, followed by increased left atrial pressure and pulmonary venous pressure.

Complications
◆ Right arterial and ventricular hypertrophy
◆ Heart failure
◆ Pulmonary hypertension

Signs and symptoms
Clinical features of VSD vary with the defect's size, the shunting's effect on the pulmonary vasculature, and the infant's age. In a small VSD, shunting is minimal, and PAP and heart

size remain normal. Such defects may eventually close spontaneously without ever causing symptoms.

Initially, large VSD shunts cause left atrial and left ventricular hypertrophy. Later, an uncorrected VSD will cause right ventricular hypertrophy due to increasing pulmonary vascular resistance. Eventually, biventricular heart failure and cyanosis (from reversal of shunt direction) occur. Resulting cardiac hypertrophy may make the anterior chest wall prominent. A large VSD increases the risk of pneumonia.

Infants with large VSDs are thin and small and gain weight slowly. They may develop heart failure with dusky skin; liver, heart, and spleen enlargement because of systemic venous congestion; diaphoresis; feeding difficulties; rapid, grunting respirations; and increased heart rate. They may also develop severe pulmonary hypertension. Fixed pulmonary hypertension may occur much later in life with right-to-left shunt (Eisenmenger syndrome), causing cyanosis and clubbing of the nail beds.

The typical murmur associated with a VSD is blowing or rumbling and varies in frequency. In the neonate, a moderately loud early systolic murmur may be heard along the lower left sternal border. About the second or third day after birth, the murmur may become louder and longer. In infants, the murmur may be loudest near the heart's base and may suggest pulmonary stenosis (PS). A small VSD may produce a functional murmur or a characteristic loud, harsh systolic murmur. Larger VSDs produce audible murmurs (at least a grade 3 pansystolic), loudest at the fourth ICS, usually with a thrill; however, a large VSD with minimal pressure gradient may have no audible murmur. In addition, the pulmonic component of S_2 sounds loud and is widely split. Palpation reveals displacement of the point of maximal impulse to the left. When fixed pulmonary hypertension is present, a diastolic murmur may be audible on auscultation, the systolic murmur becomes quieter, and S_2 is greatly accentuated.

Diagnosis

Diagnostic findings include:
◆ Chest X-ray is normal in small defects; in large VSDs, it shows cardiomegaly, left atrial and left ventricular enlargement, and prominent pulmonary vascular markings.
◆ ECG is normal in children with small VSDs; in large VSDs, it shows left and right ventricular hypertrophy, suggesting pulmonary hypertension.
◆ Echocardiography may detect a large VSD and its location in the septum, estimate the size of a left-to-right shunt, suggest pulmonary hypertension, and identify associated lesions and complications.

℞ **CONFIRMING DIAGNOSIS** *Cardiac catheterization determines the VSD's size and exact location, calculates the degree of shunting by comparing the blood oxygen saturation in each ventricle, determines the extent of pulmonary hypertension, and detects associated defects.*

Treatment

In mild cases, no treatment is needed, although the infant should be closely followed to make sure that the hole closes properly as the infant grows. Large defects usually require early surgical correction before heart failure and irreversible pulmonary vascular disease develop.

For small defects, surgery consists of simple suture closure. Moderate to large defects require insertion of a patch graft, using cardiopulmonary bypass. In patients with heart failure, digoxin and diuretics may be prescribed to control symptoms. In patients who develop increased pulmonary resistance and irreversible pulmonary vascular changes that produce a reversible right-to-left shunt (Eisenmenger syndrome), a heart–lung transplant may be required.

If the child has other defects and will benefit from delaying surgery, pulmonary artery banding normalizes pressures and flow distal to the band and prevents pulmonary vascular disease, allowing postponement of surgery. (Pulmonary artery banding is done only when the child has other complications.) A rare complication of VSD repair is complete heart block from interference with the bundle of His during surgery. (Heart block may require temporary or permanent pacemaker implantation.)

Before surgery, treatment consists of:
◆ digoxin, sodium restriction, and diuretics to prevent heart failure
◆ careful monitoring by physical examination, X-ray, and ECG to detect increased pulmonary hypertension, which indicates a need for early surgery
◆ measures to prevent infection (prophylactic antibiotics, e.g., to prevent infective endocarditis)

Generally, postoperative treatment includes a brief period of mechanical ventilation. The patient will need analgesics and may also require diuretics to increase urine output, continuous infusions of nitroprusside or adrenergic agents to regulate blood pressure and cardiac output and, in rare cases, a temporary pacemaker.

Special considerations

Although the parents of an infant with VSD often suspect something is wrong with their child before diagnosis, they need psychological support to help them accept the reality of a serious cardiac disorder. Because surgery may take place months after diagnosis, parent teaching is vital to prevent complications until the child is scheduled for surgery or the defect closes. Thorough explanations of all tests are also essential.
◆ Instruct parents to watch for signs of heart failure, such as poor feeding, sweating, and heavy breathing.
◆ If the child is receiving digoxin or other medications, tell the parents how to give it and how to recognize adverse effects. Caution them to keep medications out of the reach of all children.
◆ Teach parents to recognize and report early signs of infection and to avoid exposing the child to people with obvious infections.
◆ Encourage parents to let the child engage in normal activities.
◆ Tell parents to follow up with their pediatrician. Also tell them that child life therapy may be appropriate if their child displays delayed growth and development or failure to thrive.
◆ Stress the importance of prophylactic antibiotics before and after surgery.

After surgery to correct VSD:
◆ Monitor vital signs and intake and output. Maintain the infant's body temperature with an overbed warmer. Give catecholamines, nitroprusside, and diuretics, as ordered; analgesics as needed.
◆ Monitor central venous pressure (CVP), intra-arterial blood pressure, and left atrial or PAP readings. Assess heart rate and rhythm for signs of conduction block.
◆ Check oxygenation, particularly in a child who requires mechanical ventilation. Suction to maintain a patent airway and to prevent atelectasis and pneumonia, as needed.
◆ Monitor pacemaker effectiveness if needed. Watch for signs of failure, such as bradycardia and hypotension.
◆ Reassure parents and allow them to participate in their child's care.

ATRIAL SEPTAL DEFECT
Causes and incidence
In an atrial septal defect (ASD), an opening between the left and the right atria allows shunting of blood between the chambers. *Ostium secundum defect* (most common) occurs in the region of the fossa ovalis and occasionally extends inferiorly, close to the vena cava; *sinus venosus defect* occurs in the superior–posterior portion of the atrial septum, sometimes extending into the vena cava, and is almost always associated with abnormal drainage of pulmonary veins into the right atrium; *ostium primum defect* occurs in the inferior portion of the septum primum and is usually associated with AV valve abnormalities (cleft mitral valve) and conduction defects. The cause of ASD is unknown.

ASD accounts for about 6% to 8% of congenital heart defects and appears almost twice as often in females as in males, with a strong familial tendency. Although ASD is usually a benign defect during infancy and childhood, delayed development of symptoms and complications makes it one of the most common congenital heart defects diagnosed in adults. ASD is present in 4 of every 100,000 people. Symptoms usually develop before age 30. When no other congenital defect exists, the patient—especially if a child—may be asymptomatic. The prognosis is excellent in asymptomatic patients but poor in those with cyanosis caused by large, untreated defects. (See *Understanding atrial septal defect.*)

Understanding atrial septal defect

An atrial septal defect (ASD) is an abnormal opening between the left and the right atria. A small opening may cause few symptoms. However, if the opening is large, higher pressure in the left atrium can shunt large amounts of blood into the right atrium, which can result in right heart volume overload, right atrial and ventricular enlargement, and pulmonary hypertension. ASD is classified as an increased pulmonary blood flow defect and is one of the most common congenital heart defects.

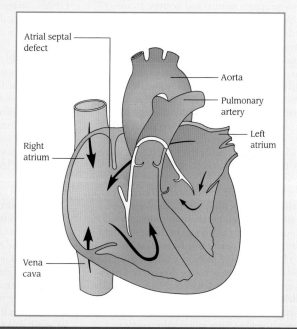

Pathophysiology

In this condition, blood shunts from left to right because left atrial pressure normally is slightly higher than right atrial pressure; this pressure difference forces large amounts of blood through a defect. The left-to-right shunt results in right heart volume overload, affecting the right atrium, right ventricle, and pulmonary arteries. Eventually, the right atrium enlarges, and the right ventricle dilates to accommodate the increased blood volume. If pulmonary artery hypertension develops because of the shunt (rare in children), increased pulmonary vascular resistance and right ventricular hypertrophy will follow. In some adult patients, irreversible (fixed) pulmonary artery hypertension causes reversal of the shunt direction, which results in unoxygenated blood entering the systemic circulation, causing cyanosis.

Complications

- Unoxygenated blood in systemic circulation
- Right and left ventricular hypertrophy
- Atrial arrhythmias
- Heart failure
- Emboli

Signs and symptoms

ASD commonly goes undetected in preschoolers; such children may complain about feeling tired only after extreme exertion and may have frequent respiratory tract infections but otherwise appear normal and healthy. However, children with large shunts may show growth retardation. Children with ASD seldom develop heart failure, pulmonary hypertension, infective endocarditis, or other complications. However, as adults, they usually manifest pronounced symptoms, such as fatigability and dyspnea on exertion, frequently to the point of severe limitation of activity (especially after age 40).

In children, auscultation reveals an early to midsystolic murmur, superficial in quality, heard at the second or third left ICS. In patients with large shunts (resulting from increased tricuspid valve flow), a low-pitched diastolic murmur is heard at the lower left sternal border, which becomes more pronounced on inspiration. Although the murmur's intensity is a rough indicator of the size of the left-to-right shunt, its low pitch sometimes makes it difficult to hear and, if the pressure gradient is relatively low, a murmur may not be detectable. Other signs include a fixed, widely split S_2, caused by delayed closure of the pulmonic valve, and a systolic click or late systolic murmur at the apex, resulting from mitral valve prolapse (MVP), which occasionally affects older children with ASD.

In older patients with large, uncorrected defects and fixed pulmonary artery hypertension, auscultation reveals an accentuated S_2. A pulmonary ejection click and an audible S_4 may also be present. Clubbing and cyanosis become evident; syncope and hemoptysis may occur with severe pulmonary vascular disease.

Diagnosis

A history of increasing fatigue and characteristic physical features suggest ASD. The following findings confirm it:

- Chest X-ray shows an enlarged right atrium and right ventricle, a prominent pulmonary artery, and increased pulmonary vascular markings.
- ECG may be normal but usually shows right axis deviation, prolonged PR interval, varying degrees of right bundle branch block, right ventricular hypertrophy, atrial fibrillation (particularly in severe cases after age 30) and, in ostium primum defect, left axis deviation.
- Echocardiography measures right ventricular enlargement, may locate the defect, and shows volume overload in the right side of the heart. (Other causes of right ventricular enlargement must be ruled out.)

℞ **CONFIRMING DIAGNOSIS** *Two-dimensional echocardiography with color Doppler flow, contrast echocardiography, or both have supplanted cardiac catheterization as the confirming tests for ASD. Cardiac catheterization is used if inconsistencies exist in the clinical data or if significant pulmonary hypertension is suspected.*

Treatment

Operative repair is advised for all patients with uncomplicated ASD with evidence of significant left-to-right shunting. Ideally, this is performed when the patient is between ages 2 and 4. Operative treatment shouldn't be performed in patients with small defects and trivial left-to-right shunts. Because ASD seldom produces complications in infants and toddlers, surgery can be delayed until they reach preschool or early school age. A large defect may need immediate surgical closure with sutures or a patch graft.

Physicians have developed a new procedure, referred to as catheter closure or transcatheter closure of the ASD, that uses wires or catheters to close ASD without surgery. In this procedure, the surgeon makes a tiny incision in the groin to introduce the catheters, then advances the catheters into the heart, and places the closure device across the ASD. This procedure may not be applicable to all patients.

Special considerations

◆ Before cardiac catheterization, explain pretest and posttest procedures to the child and her parents. If possible, use drawings or other visual aids to explain it to the child.

◆ As needed, teach the patient about prophylactic antibiotics to prevent infective endocarditis. (They may be administered before dental or other invasive procedures.)

◆ If surgery is scheduled, teach the child and his or her parents about the intensive care unit (ICU) and introduce them to the staff. Show parents where they can wait during the operation. Explain postoperative procedures, tubes, dressings, and monitoring equipment.

◆ After surgery, closely monitor the patient's vital signs, central venous and intra-arterial pressures, and intake and output. Watch for atrial arrhythmias, which may remain uncorrected.

COARCTATION OF THE AORTA

Causes and incidence

Coarctation is a narrowing of the aorta, usually just below the left subclavian artery, near the site where the ligamentum arteriosum (the remnant of the ductus arteriosus, a fetal blood vessel) joins the pulmonary artery to the aorta. Coarctation may occur with aortic valve stenosis (usually of a bicuspid aortic valve) and with severe cases of hypoplasia of the aortic arch, PDA, and VSD. This is typically sporadic and without clear cause before this condition induces severe systemic hypertension or degenerative changes in the aorta. (See *Understanding coarctation of the aorta.*)

Coarctation of the aorta occurs in 4 of every 10,000 people born each year in the United States and is usually diagnosed in children or adults younger than age 40. It accounts for about 4% to 6% of all congenital heart defects in children and is twice as common in males as in females. When it occurs in females, it's commonly associated with Turner syndrome, a chromosomal disorder that causes ovarian dysgenesis. Generally, the prognosis for coarctation of the aorta depends on the severity of associated cardiac anomalies; the prognosis for isolated coarctation is good if corrective surgery is performed.

Pathophysiology

Coarctation of the aorta may develop as a result of spasm and constriction of the smooth muscle in the ductus arteriosus as it closes. Possibly, this contractile tissue extends into the aortic wall, causing narrowing. The obstructive process causes hypertension in the aortic branches

Understanding coarctation of the aorta

Coarctation is a narrowing of the aorta, usually just below the left subclavian artery, near the site where the ligamentum arteriosum joins the pulmonary artery to the aorta. It can result from spasm and constriction of the smooth muscle in the ductus arteriosus as it closes. Restricted blood flow through the narrow aorta increases the pressure load on the left ventricle, resulting in dilation of the proximal aorta, left ventricular hypertrophy, elevated upper body blood pressures, and diminished blood flow to the lower body. The ductus arteriosus may be open or closed. Coarctation of the aorta is more common in boys and is the leading cause of heart failure in the first few months of life. It's classified as an obstruction to blood flow leaving the heart.

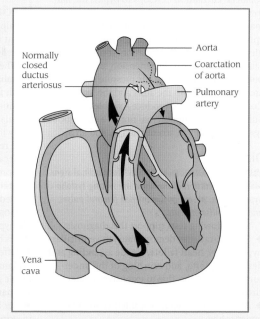

above the constriction (arteries that supply the arms, neck, and head) and diminished pressure in the vessels below the constriction.

Restricted blood flow through the narrowed aorta increases the pressure load on the left ventricle and causes dilation of the proximal aorta and ventricular hypertrophy. Untreated, this condition may lead to left-sided heart failure and, rarely, to cerebral hemorrhage and aortic rupture. If VSD accompanies coarctation, blood shunts left to right, straining the right side of the heart. This leads to pulmonary hypertension and, eventually, right-sided heart hypertrophy and failure.

Complications

◆ Infective endocarditis
◆ Pulmonary hypertension
◆ Right ventricular hypertrophy
◆ Right-sided heart failure

Signs and symptoms

Clinical features vary with age. During the first year of life, when aortic coarctation may cause heart failure, the infant displays tachypnea, dyspnea, pulmonary edema, pallor, tachycardia, failure to thrive, cardiomegaly, and hepatomegaly. In most cases, heart sounds are normal unless a coexisting cardiac defect is present. Femoral pulses are absent or diminished.

If coarctation is asymptomatic in infancy, it usually remains so throughout adolescence, as collateral circulation develops to bypass the narrowed segment. During adolescence, this defect may produce dyspnea, claudication, headaches, epistaxis, and hypertension in the upper extremities despite collateral circulation. It commonly causes resting systolic hypertension and wide pulse pressure; high diastolic pressure readings are the same in both the arms and the legs. Coarctation may also produce a visible aortic pulsation in the suprasternal notch, a continuous systolic murmur, an accentuated S_2, and an S_4.

Diagnosis

℞ CONFIRMING DIAGNOSIS *The cardinal signs of coarctation of the aorta are resting systolic hypertension, absent or diminished femoral pulses, and wide pulse pressure.*

The following tests support this diagnosis:
◆ Chest X-ray may demonstrate left ventricular hypertrophy, heart failure, a wide ascending and descending aorta, and notching of the undersurfaces of the ribs, due to extensive collateral circulation.
◆ ECG may eventually reveal left ventricular hypertrophy.

◆ Echocardiography may show increased left ventricular muscle thickness, coexisting aortic valve abnormalities, and the coarctation site.
◆ Doppler ultrasound and cardiac catheterization evaluate collateral circulation and measure pressure in the right and left ventricles and in the ascending and descending aortas (on both sides of the obstruction).
◆ MRI enables assessment of the anatomy and function of aortic abnormalities.

Treatment

For an infant with heart failure caused by coarctation of the aorta, treatment consists of medical management with digoxin, diuretics, oxygen, and sedatives. If medical management fails, surgery may be needed.

The child's condition usually determines the timing of surgery. Signs of heart failure or hypertension may call for early surgery. If these signs don't appear, surgery usually occurs during the preschool years.

Before the operation, the child may require endocarditis prophylaxis or, if he or she is older and has previously undetected coarctation, antihypertensive therapy. During surgery, the surgeon uses a flap of the left subclavian artery to reconstruct an unobstructed aorta.

Balloon angioplasty with possible stent placement may also be indicated for some patients as an alternative to surgical repair. It uses a technique similar to that used to open the coronary arteries, but is performed on the aorta.

Special considerations

◆ Palpate the pulses in the legs in newborns and at well-baby visits to detect absent or diminished pulses.
◆ When coarctation in an infant requires rapid digitalization, monitor vital signs closely and watch for digoxin toxicity (poor feeding and vomiting).
◆ Balance intake and output carefully, especially if the infant is receiving diuretics with fluid restriction.
◆ Because the infant may not be able to maintain proper body temperature, regulate environmental temperature with an overbed warmer if needed.
◆ Monitor blood glucose levels to detect possible hypoglycemia, which may occur as glycogen stores become depleted.
◆ Offer the parents emotional support and an explanation of the disorder. Also explain diagnostic procedures, surgery, and drug therapy. Tell parents what to expect postoperatively.
◆ For an older child, assess the blood pressure in extremities regularly, explain any exercise

restrictions, stress the need to take medications properly and to watch for adverse effects, and teach about tests and other procedures.

After corrective surgery:

♦ Monitor blood pressure closely, using an intra-arterial line. Measure blood pressure in arms and legs. Monitor intake and output.

♦ If the patient develops hypertension and requires a medication such as nitroprusside, administer it, as ordered, using an infusion pump. Watch for severe hypotension and regulate the dosage carefully.

♦ Provide pain relief and encourage a gradual increase in activity.

♦ Promote adequate respiratory functioning through turning, coughing, and deep breathing.

♦ Watch for abdominal pain or rigidity and signs of gastrointestinal (GI) or urinary bleeding.

♦ If an older child needs to continue antihypertensives after surgery, teach the patient and his parents about them.

♦ Stress the importance of continued endocarditis prophylaxis as appropriate.

PATENT DUCTUS ARTERIOSUS
Causes and incidence

The ductus arteriosus is a fetal blood vessel that connects the pulmonary artery to the descending aorta. In PDA, the lumen of the ductus remains open after birth. This creates a left-to-right shunt of blood from the aorta to the pulmonary artery and results in recirculation of arterial blood through the lungs. Normally, the ductus closes within days to weeks after birth. Failure to close is most prevalent in premature neonates, probably as a result of abnormalities in oxygenation or the relaxant action of prostaglandin E, which prevents ductal spasm and contracture necessary for closure. However, most of the time, the cause of this condition is unknown. PDA commonly accompanies rubella syndrome and may be associated with other congenital defects, such as coarctation of the aorta, VSD, and pulmonary and aortic stenoses.

Initially, PDA may produce no clinical effects, but in time it can precipitate pulmonary vascular disease, causing symptoms to appear by age 40. PDA is found in 1 of every 2,000 infants and is the most common congenital heart defect found in adults. It affects twice as many females as males. Additionally, babies born at above 10,000 feet in altitude are more affected.

The prognosis is good if the shunt is small or surgical repair is effective. Otherwise, PDA may advance to intractable heart failure, which may be fatal. (See *Understanding patent ductus arteriosus.*)

Understanding patent ductus arteriosus

The ductus arteriosus is a fetal blood vessel that connects the pulmonary artery to the descending aorta. Normally, the ductus closes within weeks after birth. However, with patent ductus arteriosus (PDA), it remains open, creating a left-to-right shunt of blood from the aorta to the pulmonary artery and resulting in recirculation of arterial blood through the lungs. PDA is classified as an increased pulmonary blood flow defect.

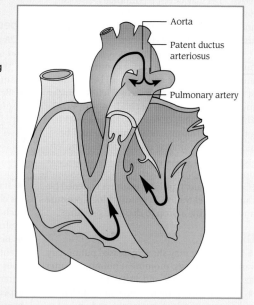

Pathophysiology

In PDA, relative resistances in pulmonary and systemic vasculature and the size of the ductus determine the amount of left-to-right shunting. The left atrium and left ventricle must accommodate the increased pulmonary venous return, in turn increasing filling pressure and workload on the left side of the heart and possibly causing heart failure. In the final stages of untreated PDA, the left-to-right shunt leads to chronic pulmonary artery hypertension that becomes fixed and unreactive. This causes the shunt to reverse; unoxygenated blood thus enters systemic circulation, causing cyanosis.

Complications

◆ Left-sided heart failure
◆ Pulmonary artery hypertension
◆ Respiratory distress (children)

Signs and symptoms

In neonates, especially those who are premature, a large PDA usually produces respiratory distress, with signs of heart failure due to the tremendous volume of blood shunted to the lungs through a patent ductus and the increased workload on the left side of the heart. Other characteristic features may include heightened susceptibility to respiratory tract infections, slow motor development, and failure to thrive. Most children with PDA have no symptoms except cardiac ones. Others may exhibit signs of heart disease, such as physical underdevelopment, fatigability, and frequent respiratory tract infections. Adults with undetected PDA may develop pulmonary vascular disease and, by age 40, may display fatigability and dyspnea on exertion. About 10% of them also develop infective endocarditis.

Auscultation reveals the classic machinery murmur (Gibson murmur): a continuous murmur (during systole and diastole) best heard at the heart's base, at the second left ICS under the left clavicle in 85% of children with PDA. This murmur may obscure S_2. However, with a right-to-left shunt, such a murmur may be absent. Palpation may reveal a thrill at the left sternal border and a prominent left ventricular impulse. Peripheral arterial pulses are bounding (Corrigan pulse); pulse pressure is widened because of an elevation in systolic blood pressure and, primarily, a drop in diastolic pressure.

Diagnosis

◆ Chest X-ray may show increased pulmonary vascular markings, prominent pulmonary arteries, and left ventricle and aorta enlargement.
◆ ECG may be normal or may indicate left atrial or ventricular hypertrophy and, in pulmonary vascular disease, biventricular hypertrophy.
◆ Echocardiography confirms the diagnosis, detecting and helping to estimate the size of a PDA. It also reveals an enlarged left atrium and left ventricle or right ventricular hypertrophy from pulmonary vascular disease.

℞ **CONFIRMING DIAGNOSIS** *Cardiac catheterization can also be performed and shows pulmonary arterial oxygen content higher than right ventricular content because of the influx of aortic blood. Increased PAP indicates a large shunt or, if it exceeds systemic arterial pressure, severe pulmonary vascular disease. Catheterization allows calculation of blood volume crossing the ductus and can rule out associated cardiac defects. Dye injection definitively demonstrates PDA.*

Treatment

Asymptomatic infants with PDA require no immediate treatment. Those with heart failure require fluid restriction, diuretics, and cardiac glycosides to minimize or control symptoms. If these measures can't control heart failure, surgery is necessary to ligate the ductus. If symptoms are mild, surgical correction is usually delayed until the infant is between ages 6 months and 3 years, unless problems develop. Before surgery, children with PDA require antibiotics to protect against infective endocarditis.

Other forms of therapy include cardiac catheterization to deposit a plug or coil in the ductus to stop shunting or administration of indomethacin I.V. (a prostaglandin inhibitor that's an alternative to surgery in premature neonates) to induce ductus spasm and closure.

Special considerations

PDA necessitates careful monitoring, patient and family teaching, and emotional support.
◆ Watch carefully for signs of PDA in all premature neonates.
◆ Be alert for respiratory distress symptoms resulting from heart failure, which may develop rapidly in a premature neonate. Frequently assess vital signs, ECG, electrolyte levels, and intake and output. Record response to diuretics and other therapy. Watch for signs of digoxin toxicity (poor feeding and vomiting).
◆ If the infant receives indomethacin for ductus closure, watch for possible adverse effects, such as diarrhea, jaundice, bleeding, and renal dysfunction.
◆ Before surgery, carefully explain all treatments and tests to parents. Include the child in your explanations. Arrange for the child and her parents to meet the ICU staff. Tell them about expected I.V. lines, monitoring equipment, and postoperative procedures.

◆ Immediately after surgery, the child may have a CVP catheter and an arterial line in place. Carefully assess vital signs, intake and output, and arterial and venous pressures. Provide pain relief as needed.

◆ Before discharge, review instructions to the parents about activity restrictions based on the child's tolerance and energy levels. Advise parents not to become overprotective as their child's tolerance for physical activity increases.

◆ Stress the need for regular follow-up examinations. Advise parents to inform any practitioner who treats their child about the history of surgery for PDA—even if the child is being treated for an unrelated medical problem.

Congenital cyanotic defects

TETRALOGY OF FALLOT

Causes and incidence

Tetralogy of Fallot is a combination of four cardiac defects: VSD, right ventricular outflow tract obstruction (PS), right ventricular hypertrophy, and dextroposition of the aorta, with overriding of the VSD. Blood shunts right to left through the VSD, permitting unoxygenated blood to mix with oxygenated blood, resulting in cyanosis. Tetralogy of Fallot sometimes coexists with other congenital heart defects, such as PDA or ASD.

The cause of tetralogy of Fallot is unknown, but it results from embryologic hypoplasia of the outflow tract of the right ventricle. Multiple factors, such as Down syndrome, have been associated with its presence. Prenatal risk factors include maternal rubella or other viral illnesses, poor prenatal nutrition, maternal alcoholism, mother older than age 40, and diabetes.

Tetralogy of Fallot occurs in about 5 of every 10,000 infants and accounts for about 10% of all congenital heart diseases. It occurs equally in boys and girls. Before surgical advances made correction possible, about one third of these children died in infancy.

Pathophysiology

Tetralogy of Fallot is present at birth.

Pathophysiology depends on the degree of right ventricular outflow obstruction. A mild obstruction may result in a net left-to-right shunt through the VSD; a severe obstruction causes a right-to-left shunt, resulting in low systemic arterial saturation (cyanosis) that is unresponsive to supplemental oxygen.

Each patient may have a varying degree of defect.

Complications

◆ Cerebral abscess
◆ Pulmonary thrombosis
◆ Venous thrombosis
◆ Cerebral embolism
◆ Infective endocarditis

Signs and symptoms

Generally, the hallmark of the disorder is cyanosis, which usually becomes evident within several months after birth but may be present at birth if the neonate has severe PS. Between ages 2 months and 2 years, children with tetralogy of Fallot may experience cyanotic or "tet" spells. Such spells result from increased right-to-left shunting, possibly caused by spasm of the right ventricular outflow tract, increased systemic venous return, or decreased systemic arterial resistance.

Exercise, crying, straining, infection, or fever can precipitate blue spells. Blue spells are characterized by dyspnea; deep, sighing respirations; bradycardia; fainting; seizures; and loss of consciousness. Older children may also develop other signs of poor oxygenation, such as clubbing, diminished exercise tolerance, increasing dyspnea on exertion, growth retardation, and eating difficulties. These children habitually squat when they feel short of breath; this is thought to decrease venous return of unoxygenated blood from the legs and increase systemic arterial resistance.

Children with tetralogy of Fallot also risk developing cerebral abscesses, pulmonary thrombosis, venous thrombosis or cerebral embolism, and infective endocarditis.

In females with tetralogy of Fallot who live to childbearing age, the incidence of spontaneous abortion, premature births, and low birth weight rises.

Diagnosis

In a patient with tetralogy of Fallot, auscultation detects a loud systolic heart murmur (best heard along the left sternal border), which may diminish or obscure the pulmonic component of S_2. In a patient with a large PDA, the continuous murmur of the ductus obscures the systolic murmur. Palpation may reveal a cardiac thrill at the left sternal border and an obvious right ventricular impulse. The inferior sternum appears prominent.

The results of special tests also support the diagnosis:

◆ Chest X-ray may demonstrate decreased pulmonary vascular marking, depending on the pulmonary obstruction's severity, and a boot-shaped cardiac silhouette.

◆ ECG shows right ventricular hypertrophy, right axis deviation, and, possibly, right atrial hypertrophy.

◆ Echocardiography identifies septal overriding of the aorta, the VSD, and PS and detects the hypertrophied walls of the right ventricle.

◆ Pulse oximetry shows a decrease in oxygen saturation.

R CONFIRMING DIAGNOSIS *Cardiac catheterization confirms the diagnosis by visualizing PS, the VSD, and the overriding aorta and ruling out other cyanotic heart defects. This test also measures the degree of oxygen saturation in aortic blood.*

Treatment

Effective management of tetralogy of Fallot necessitates prevention and treatment of complications, measures to relieve cyanosis, and palliative or corrective surgery. During cyanotic spells, the knee–chest position and administration of oxygen and morphine improve oxygenation. Propranolol (a beta-adrenergic blocking agent) may prevent blue spells.

Palliative surgery is performed in infants with potentially fatal hypoxic spells or occasionally needed prior to final correction. The goal of surgery is to enhance blood flow to the lungs to reduce hypoxia; this is often accomplished by joining the subclavian artery to the pulmonary artery (modified Blalock–Taussig procedure). Supportive measures include prophylactic antibiotics to prevent infective endocarditis or cerebral abscess administered before, during, and after bowel, bladder, or any other surgery or dental treatments. Management may also include phlebotomy in children with polycythemia.

Complete corrective surgery to relieve PS and close the VSD, directing left ventricular outflow to the aorta, requires cardiopulmonary bypass with hypothermia to decrease oxygen utilization during surgery, especially in young children. An infant may have this corrective surgery without prior palliative surgery. It's usually done when progressive hypoxia and polycythemia impair the quality of life, rather than at a specific age. However, most children require surgery, some as young as 6 months old as long as oxygen levels remain adequate.

Special considerations

◆ Explain tetralogy of Fallot to the parents. Inform them that their child will set their own exercise limits and will know when to rest. Make sure they understand that their child can engage in physical activity, and advise them not to be overprotective.

◆ Teach the parents to recognize serious hypoxic spells, which can dramatically increase cyanosis; deep, sighing respirations; and loss of consciousness. Tell them to place their child in the knee–chest position and to report such spells immediately. Emergency treatment may be necessary.

◆ Instruct the parents on ways to prevent overexerting their child, such as feeding slowly and providing smaller and more frequent meals. Tell them that remaining calm may decrease anxiety and that anticipating needs may minimize crying. Encourage the parents to recruit other family members in the care of the child to help prevent their own exhaustion.

◆ To prevent infective endocarditis and other infections, warn the parents to keep their child away from people with infections. Urge them to encourage good dental hygiene, and tell them to watch for ear, nose, and throat infections and dental caries, all of which necessitate immediate treatment. When dental care, infections, or surgery requires prophylactic antibiotics, tell the parents to make sure the child completes the prescribed regimen.

◆ If the child requires medical attention for an unrelated problem, advise the parents to inform the practitioner immediately of the child's history of tetralogy of Fallot because any treatment must take this serious heart defect into consideration.

◆ During hospitalization, alert the staff to the child's condition. Because of the right-to-left shunt through the VSD, treat I.V. lines like arterial lines. A clot dislodged from a catheter tip in a vein can cross the VSD and cause cerebral embolism. The same thing can happen if air enters the venous lines.

After palliative surgery:

◆ Monitor oxygenation and arterial blood gas (ABG) values closely in the ICU.

◆ If the child has undergone the modified Blalock–Taussig procedure, don't use the arm on the operative side for measuring blood pressure, inserting I.V. lines, or drawing blood samples, because blood perfusion on this side diminishes greatly until collateral circulation develops. Note this on the child's chart and at the bedside.

After corrective surgery:

◆ Watch for right bundle branch block or more serious disturbances of AV conduction and for ventricular ectopic beats.

◆ Be alert for other postoperative complications, such as bleeding, right-sided heart failure, and respiratory failure. After surgery, transient heart failure is common and may require treatment with digoxin and diuretics.

◆ Monitor left atrial pressure directly. A pulmonary artery catheter may also be used to check central venous and PAPs.

◆ Frequently check color and vital signs. Obtain ABG measurements regularly to assess oxygenation. Suction to prevent atelectasis and pneumonia, as needed. Monitor mechanical ventilation.

◆ Monitor and record intake and output accurately.

◆ If AV block develops with a low heart rate, a temporary external pacemaker may be necessary.

◆ If blood pressure or cardiac output is inadequate, catecholamines may be ordered by continuous I.V. infusion. To decrease left ventricular workload, administer nitroprusside, if ordered, and provide analgesics, as needed.

◆ Keep the parents informed about their child's progress. After discharge, the child may require digoxin, diuretics, and other drugs. Stress the importance of complying with the prescribed regimen, and make sure the parents know how and when to administer these medications. Teach the parents to watch for signs of digoxin toxicity (anorexia, nausea, and vomiting). Prophylactic antibiotics to prevent infective endocarditis will still be required. Advise the parents to avoid becoming overprotective as the child's tolerance for physical activity rises.

TRANSPOSITION OF THE GREAT ARTERIES

Causes and incidence

In this congenital heart defect, the great arteries are reversed: the aorta arises from the right ventricle and the pulmonary artery from the left ventricle, producing two noncommunicating circulatory systems (pulmonary and systemic). Transposition accounts for about 3% of all congenital heart defects and often coexists with other congenital heart defects, such as VSD, VSD with PS, ASD, and PDA. It affects two to three times more males than females. Transposition of the great arteries results from faulty embryonic development, but the cause of such development is unknown. Transposition of the great arteries occurs in about 30 of every 100,000 infants.

Pathophysiology

In transposition, oxygenated blood returning to the left side of the heart is carried back to the lungs by a transposed pulmonary artery; unoxygenated blood returning to the right side of the heart is carried to the systemic circulation by a transposed aorta.

Communication between the pulmonary and systemic circulations is necessary for survival. In infants with isolated transposition, blood mixes only at the patent foramen ovale and at the PDA, resulting in slight mixing of unoxygenated systemic blood and oxygenated pulmonary blood. In infants with concurrent cardiac defects, greater mixing of blood occurs.

Complications

◆ Chronic heart failure
◆ Poor oxygenation
◆ Arrhythmias
◆ Right-sided heart failure

Signs and symptoms

Within the first few hours after birth, neonates with transposition of the great arteries and no other heart defects generally show cyanosis and tachypnea, which worsen with crying. After several days or weeks, such neonates usually develop signs of heart failure (gallop rhythm, tachycardia, dyspnea, hepatomegaly, and cardiomegaly). S_2 is louder than normal because the anteriorly transposed aorta is directly behind the sternum; in many cases, however, no murmur can be heard during the first few days of life. Associated defects (ASD, VSD, or PDA) cause their typical murmurs and may minimize cyanosis but may also cause other complications (especially severe heart failure). VSD with PS produces a characteristic murmur and severe cyanosis.

As infants with this defect grow older, cyanosis is their most prominent abnormality. However, they also develop diminished exercise tolerance, fatigability, coughing, clubbing, and more pronounced murmurs if ASD, VSD, PDA, or PS is present.

Diagnosis

◆ Chest X-rays are normal in the first days of life. Within days to weeks, right atrial and right ventricular enlargement characteristically cause the heart to appear oblong. X-rays also show increased pulmonary vascular markings, except when PS coexists.

◆ ECG typically reveals right axis deviation and right ventricular hypertrophy but may be normal in a neonate.

℞ **CONFIRMING DIAGNOSIS** *Echocardiography demonstrates the reversed position of the aorta and pulmonary artery and records echoes from both semilunar valves simultaneously, due to aortic valve displacement. It also detects other cardiac defects. Cardiac catheterization reveals decreased oxygen saturation in left ventricular blood and aortic blood; increased right atrial, right ventricular, and pulmonary artery oxygen saturation; and right ventricular systolic pressure equal to systemic pressure. Dye injection reveals the transposed vessels and the presence of any other cardiac defects.*

◆ ABG measurements indicate hypoxia and secondary metabolic acidosis.

Treatment

An infant with transposition may undergo atrial balloon septostomy (Rashkind procedure) during cardiac catheterization. This procedure enlarges the patent foramen ovale, which improves oxygenation by allowing greater mixing of the pulmonary and systemic circulations. Atrial balloon septostomy requires passage of a balloon-tipped catheter through the foramen ovale and subsequent inflation and withdrawal across the atrial septum. This procedure alleviates hypoxia to a certain degree. Afterward, digoxin and diuretics can lessen heart failure until the infant is ready to withstand corrective surgery (usually by 1 to 2 weeks of age).

One of three surgical procedures can correct transposition, depending on the defect's physiology. The Mustard procedure replaces the atrial septum with a Dacron or pericardial partition that allows systemic venous blood to be channeled to the pulmonary artery—which carries the blood to the lungs for oxygenation—and oxygenated blood returning to the heart to be channeled from the pulmonary veins into the aorta. The Senning procedure accomplishes the same result, using the atrial septum to create partitions to redirect blood flow. In the arterial switch, or Jantene procedure, transposed arteries are surgically anastomosed to the correct ventricle. For this procedure to be successful, the left ventricle must be used to pump at systemic pressure, as it does in neonates or in children with a left ventricular outflow obstruction or a large VSD. The Jantene procedure is the procedure of choice; however, the Mustard and Senning procedures may be used when specific anatomic conditions exist.

Special considerations

◆ Explain cardiac catheterization and all necessary procedures to the parents. Offer emotional support.
◆ Monitor vital signs, ABG values, urine output, and CVP, watching for signs of heart failure. Give digoxin and I.V. fluids, being careful to avoid fluid overload.
◆ Teach the parents to recognize signs of heart failure and digoxin toxicity (poor feeding and vomiting). Stress the importance of regular checkups to monitor cardiovascular status.
◆ Teach the parents to protect their infant from infection and to give antibiotics.
◆ Tell the parents to let their child develop normally. They need not restrict activities; let the child set his or her own limits.
◆ If the patient is scheduled for surgery, explain the procedure to the parents and child, if old enough. Teach them about the ICU and introduce them to the staff. Also explain postoperative care.

◆ Preoperatively, monitor ABG values, acid–base balance, intake and output, and vital signs.

After corrective surgery:
◆ Monitor cardiac output by checking blood pressure, skin color, heart rate, urine output, central venous and left atrial pressures, and level of consciousness (LOC). Report abnormalities or changes.
◆ Carefully monitor ABG levels and report changes in trends.
◆ To detect supraventricular conduction blocks and arrhythmias, monitor the patient closely. Watch for signs of AV blocks, atrial arrhythmias, and faulty SA function.
◆ After the Mustard or Senning procedure, watch for signs of baffle obstruction such as marked facial edema.
◆ Encourage parents to help their child assume new activity levels and independence. Teach them about postoperative antibiotic prophylaxis for endocarditis.

Acquired inflammatory heart disease

MYOCARDITIS
Causes and incidence
Myocarditis is focal or diffuse inflammation of the cardiac muscle (myocardium). It may be acute or chronic and can occur at any age. In many cases, myocarditis fails to produce specific cardiovascular symptoms or electrocardiogram (ECG) abnormalities, and recovery is usually spontaneous, without residual defects. Occasionally, myocarditis is complicated by heart failure; in rare cases, it leads to cardiomyopathy.

Myocarditis may result from:
◆ bacterial infections—diphtheria; tuberculosis; typhoid fever; tetanus; and staphylococcal, pneumococcal, and gonococcal infections
◆ chemical poisons—such as chronic alcoholism
◆ helminthic infections—such as trichinosis
◆ hypersensitive immune reactions—acute rheumatic fever and postcardiotomy syndrome
◆ parasitic infections—especially South American trypanosomiasis (Chagas disease) in infants and immunosuppressed adults; also toxoplasmosis
◆ radiation therapy—large doses of radiation to the chest in treating lung or breast cancer
◆ viral infections (most common cause in the United States and Western Europe)—coxsackievirus A and B strains and, possibly, poliomyelitis, influenza, rubeola, rubella, and adenoviruses and echoviruses

Myocarditis occurs in 1 to 10 of every 100,000 people in the United States. The median age for this disorder is 42, and incidence is equal between males and females. Children, especially neonates, and persons who are immunocompromised or pregnant (especially pregnant black women) are at higher risk for developing this disorder.

Pathophysiology

The pathophysiology of myocarditis is still being researched, but it is usually caused by a virus, as already mentioned. It results in necrosis of myocardial cells either through direct injury or as a result of an autoimmune reaction of an infectious or toxic process. The extent of the involvement depends on the magnitude of the insult; if it extends to the pericardium, myopericarditis occurs.

Complications

◆ Arrhythmias
◆ Thromboembolism
◆ Chronic valvulitis (when disease results from rheumatic fever)
◆ Recurrence of disease
◆ Left-sided heart failure (occasional)
◆ Cardiomyopathy (rare)

Signs and symptoms

Myocarditis usually causes nonspecific symptoms—such as fatigue, dyspnea, palpitations, and fever—that reflect the accompanying systemic infection. Occasionally, it may produce mild, continuous pressure or soreness in the chest (unlike the recurring, stress-related pain of angina pectoris). Although myocarditis is usually self-limiting, it may induce myofibril degeneration that results in right- and left-sided heart failure, with cardiomegaly, JVD, dyspnea, persistent fever with resting or exertional tachycardia disproportionate to the degree of fever, and supraventricular and ventricular arrhythmias. Sometimes myocarditis recurs or produces chronic valvulitis (when it results from rheumatic fever), cardiomyopathy, arrhythmias, and thromboembolism.

Diagnosis

Patient history commonly reveals recent febrile upper respiratory tract infection, viral pharyngitis, or tonsillitis. Physical examination shows supraventricular and ventricular arrhythmias, S_3 and S_4 gallops, a faint S_1, possibly a murmur of mitral insufficiency (from papillary muscle dysfunction) and, if pericarditis is present, a pericardial friction rub.

Laboratory tests can't unequivocally confirm myocarditis, but the following findings support this diagnosis:
◆ cardiac enzymes: elevated CK, CK-MB, aspartate aminotransferase, and lactate dehydrogenase levels
◆ increased white blood cell count and erythrocyte sedimentation rate
◆ elevated antibody titers (such as antistreptolysin-O titer in rheumatic fever)

℞ CONFIRMING DIAGNOSIS *Endomyocardial biopsy is rarely performed to diagnose myocarditis; the procedure is invasive and costly. A negative biopsy doesn't exclude the diagnosis, and a repeat biopsy may be needed.*

ECG typically shows diffuse ST-segment and T-wave abnormalities as in pericarditis, conduction defects (prolonged PR interval), and other supraventricular arrhythmias. Echocardiography demonstrates some degree of left ventricular dysfunction, and radionuclide scanning may identify inflammatory and necrotic changes characteristic of myocarditis.

Stool and throat cultures may identify bacteria.

Treatment

While myositis is usually self-limiting, treatment may include antibiotics for bacterial infection, modified bed rest to decrease cardiac workload, and careful management of complications. Inotropic support of cardiac function with amrinone, dopamine, or dobutamine may be needed. Heart failure requires restriction of activity to minimize myocardial oxygen consumption, supplemental oxygen therapy, sodium restriction, diuretics to decrease fluid retention, and cardiac glycosides to increase myocardial contractility. However, cardiac glycosides should be administered cautiously because some patients with myocarditis may show a paradoxical sensitivity to even small doses. Arrhythmias necessitate prompt but cautious administration of antiarrhythmics because these drugs depress myocardial contractility. Thromboembolism requires anticoagulation therapy. Treatment with corticosteroids or other immunosuppressants may be used to reduce inflammation, but they haven't been shown to change the progression of myocarditis. Nonsteroidal anti-inflammatory drugs are contraindicated during the acute phase (first 2 weeks) because they increase myocardial damage.

Surgical treatment may include left ventricular assistive devices and extracorporeal membrane oxygenation for support of cardiogenic shock. Cardiac transplantation has been beneficial for giant cell myocarditis.

Special considerations

◆ Assess cardiovascular status frequently, watching for signs of heart failure, such as dyspnea, hypotension, and tachycardia. Check for changes in cardiac rhythm or conduction.

◆ Observe for signs of digoxin toxicity (anorexia, nausea, vomiting, blurred vision, and cardiac arrhythmias) and for complicating factors that may potentiate toxicity, such as electrolyte imbalance or hypoxia.

◆ Stress the importance of bed rest. Assist with bathing, as necessary; provide a bedside commode because this stresses the heart less than using a bedpan. Reassure the patient that activity limitations are temporary. Offer diversional activities that are physically undemanding.

◆ During recovery, recommend that the patient resume normal activities slowly and avoid competitive sports.

▦ PREVENTION
◆ *Instruct patient to obtain prompt treatment of causative disorders.*
◆ *Instruct patient to practice good hygiene, including thorough handwashing.*
◆ *Tell patient to thoroughly wash and cook food.*

ENDOCARDITIS
Causes and incidence

Endocarditis (also known as *infective* or *bacterial endocarditis*) is an infection of the endocardium, heart valves, or cardiac prostheses resulting from bacterial or fungal invasion. Most cases of endocarditis occur in I.V. drug abusers, patients with prosthetic heart valves, and those with MVP (especially males with a systolic murmur). These conditions have surpassed rheumatic heart disease as the leading risk factor. Other predisposing conditions include coarctation of the aorta, tetralogy of Fallot, subaortic and valvular aortic stenosis, VSDs, PS, Marfan syndrome, degenerative heart disease (especially calcific aortic stenosis), and, rarely, syphilitic aortic valve. However, some patients with endocarditis have no underlying heart disease. In the United States, endocarditis affects 2 to 6 people out of every 100,000. Males are twice as likely as females to acquire this infection, and the mean age of onset is 50. Mortality is associated with increased age, infection of the aortic valve, heart failure and underlying heart disease, and central nervous system complications; mortality rates vary with the infecting organism. Untreated endocarditis is usually fatal, but with proper treatment, 70% of patients recover. The prognosis is worst when endocarditis causes severe valvular damage, leading to insufficiency and heart failure, or when it involves a prosthetic valve.

Degenerative changes in endocarditis

This illustration shows typical vegetations on the endocardium produced by fibrin and platelet deposits on infection sites.

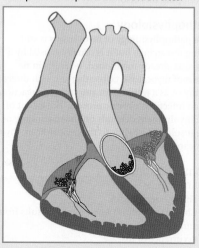

Pathophysiology

The invasion of bacteria or fungi produces vegetative growths on the heart valves, endocardial lining of a heart chamber, or endothelium of a blood vessel that may embolize to the spleen, kidneys, central nervous system, and lungs. In endocarditis, fibrin and platelets aggregate on the valve tissue and engulf circulating bacteria or fungi that flourish and produce friable verrucous vegetations. (See *Degenerative changes in endocarditis.*) Such vegetations may cover the valve surfaces, causing ulceration and necrosis; they may also extend to the chordae tendineae, leading to their rupture and subsequent valvular insufficiency.

Infecting organisms differ depending on the cause of endocarditis. In patients with native valve endocarditis who aren't I.V. drug abusers, causative organisms usually include—in the order of frequency—streptococci (especially *Streptococcus viridans*), staphylococci, or enterococci. Although many other bacteria occasionally cause the disorder, fungal causes are rare in this group. The mitral valve is involved most commonly, followed by the aortic valve.

In patients who are I.V. drug abusers, *Staphylococcus aureus* is the most common infecting organism. Less commonly, streptococci, enterococci, gram-negative bacilli, or fungi cause the disorder. The tricuspid valve is involved most commonly, followed by the aortic and then the mitral valve.

In patients with prosthetic valve endocarditis, early cases (those that develop within 60 days of valve insertion) are usually due to staphylococcal infection. However, gram-negative aerobic organisms, fungi, streptococci, enterococci, or diphtheroids may also cause the disorder. The course is usually fulminant and is associated with a high mortality. Late cases (occurring after 60 days) present similar to native valve endocarditis.

Complications
◆ Left-sided heart failure
◆ Valvular stenosis or insufficiency
◆ Myocardial erosion

Signs and symptoms
Early clinical features of endocarditis are usually nonspecific and include malaise, weakness, fatigue, weight loss, anorexia, arthralgia, night sweats, chills, valvular insufficiency and, in 90% of patients, an intermittent fever that may recur for weeks. A more acute onset is associated with organisms of high pathogenicity such as *S. aureus*. Endocarditis commonly causes a loud, regurgitant murmur typical of the underlying heart lesion. A suddenly changing murmur or the discovery of a new murmur in the presence of fever is a classic physical sign of endocarditis.

In about 30% of patients, embolization from vegetating lesions or diseased valvular tissue may produce typical features of splenic, renal, cerebral, or pulmonary infarction or of peripheral vascular occlusion:
◆ splenic infarction—pain in the left upper quadrant, radiating to the left shoulder, and abdominal rigidity
◆ renal infarction—hematuria, pyuria, flank pain, and decreased urine output
◆ cerebral infarction—hemiparesis, aphasia, or other neurologic deficits
◆ pulmonary infarction (most common in right-sided endocarditis, which commonly occurs among I.V. drug abusers and after cardiac surgery)—cough, pleuritic pain, pleural friction rub, dyspnea, and hemoptysis
◆ peripheral vascular occlusion—numbness and tingling in an arm, leg, finger, or toe, or signs of impending peripheral gangrene

Other signs may include splenomegaly; petechiae of the skin (especially common on the upper anterior trunk) and the buccal, pharyngeal, or conjunctival mucosa; and splinter hemorrhages under the nails. Rarely, endocarditis produces Osler nodes (tender, raised, subcutaneous lesions on the fingers or toes), Roth spots (hemorrhagic areas with white centers on the retina), and Janeway lesions (purplish macules on the palms or soles).

Diagnosis
R̟x **CONFIRMING DIAGNOSIS** *Three or more blood cultures in a 24- to 48-hour period (each from a separate venipuncture) identify the causative organism in up to 90% of patients. Blood cultures should be drawn from three different sites with 1 hour between each draw.*

The remaining 10% may have negative blood cultures, possibly suggesting fungal infection or infections that are difficult to diagnose, such as *Haemophilus parainfluenzae*.

Other abnormal but nonspecific laboratory test results include:
◆ normal or elevated white blood cell count
◆ abnormal histiocytes (macrophages)
◆ elevated erythrocyte sedimentation rate
◆ normocytic, normochromic anemia (in 70% to 90% of patients)
◆ proteinuria and microscopic hematuria (in about 50% of patients)
◆ positive serum rheumatoid factor (in about 50% of patients after endocarditis is present for 3 to 6 weeks)

Echocardiography (particularly, transesophageal) may identify valvular damage; ECG may show atrial fibrillation and other arrhythmias that accompany valvular disease.

Treatment
The goal of treatment is to eradicate the infecting organism with appropriate antimicrobial therapy, which should start promptly and continue over 4 to 6 weeks. Selection of an antibiotic is based on identification of the infecting organism and on sensitivity studies. While awaiting results, or if blood cultures are negative, empiric antimicrobial therapy is based on the likely infecting organism.

Supportive treatment includes bed rest, aspirin for fever and aches, and sufficient fluid intake. Severe valvular damage, especially aortic or mitral insufficiency, may require corrective surgery if refractory heart failure develops, or in cases requiring that an infected prosthetic valve be replaced.

Special considerations
◆ Before giving antibiotics, obtain a patient history of allergies. Administer antibiotics on time to maintain consistent antibiotic blood levels.
◆ Observe for signs of infiltration or inflammation at the venipuncture site, possible

complications of long-term I.V. drug administration. To reduce the risk of these complications, rotate venous access sites.

◆ Watch for signs of embolization (hematuria, pleuritic chest pain, left upper quadrant pain, or paresis), a common occurrence during the first 3 months of treatment. Tell the patient to watch for and report these signs, which may indicate impending peripheral vascular occlusion or splenic, renal, cerebral, or pulmonary infarction.

◆ Monitor the patient's renal status (blood urea nitrogen [BUN] levels, creatinine clearance, and urine output) to check for signs of renal emboli or evidence of drug toxicity.

◆ Observe for signs of heart failure, such as dyspnea, tachypnea, tachycardia, crackles, JVD, edema, and weight gain.

◆ Provide reassurance by teaching the patient and family about this disease and the need for prolonged treatment. Tell them to watch closely for fever, anorexia, and other signs of relapse about 2 weeks after treatment stops. Suggest quiet diversionary activities to prevent excessive physical exertion.

◆ Make sure susceptible patients understand the need for prophylactic antibiotics before, during, and after dental work, childbirth, and genitourinary, GI, or gynecologic procedures.

◆ Teach patients how to recognize symptoms of endocarditis and tell them to notify the practitioner at once if such symptoms occur. (See *Preventing endocarditis*.)

PERICARDITIS
Causes and incidence
Pericarditis is an inflammation of the pericardium, the fibroserous sac that envelops,

supports, and protects the heart. Common causes of this disease include:

◆ bacterial, fungal, or viral infection (infectious pericarditis)

◆ neoplasms (primary or metastatic from lungs, breasts, or other organs)

◆ high-dose radiation to the chest

◆ uremia

◆ hypersensitivity or autoimmune disease, such as acute rheumatic fever (most common cause of pericarditis in children), systemic lupus erythematosus (SLE), and rheumatoid arthritis

◆ postcardiac injury such as MI, which later causes an autoimmune reaction (Dressler syndrome) in the pericardium; trauma; or surgery that leaves the pericardium intact but causes blood to leak into the pericardial cavity

◆ drugs, such as hydralazine or procainamide

◆ idiopathic factors (most common in acute pericarditis)

Less common causes include aortic aneurysm with pericardial leakage and myxedema with cholesterol deposits in the pericardium.

Pericarditis most commonly affects men 20 to 50 years old, but it can also occur in children after infection with an adenovirus or coxsackievirus.

The prognosis depends on the underlying cause but is generally good in acute pericarditis, unless constriction occurs.

Pathophysiology
The pericardium protects the heart mechanically and reduces friction of the surrounding structures through a small amount of pericardial fluid (25 to 50 mL). Inflammation of the layers of the pericardium leads to an increase in the production of this fluid in the form of exudate. Pericarditis occurs in both acute

and chronic forms. Acute pericarditis can be fibrinous or effusive, with purulent serous or hemorrhagic exudate; chronic constrictive pericarditis is characterized by dense fibrous pericardial thickening.

Complications
◆ Pericardial effusion
◆ Cardiac tamponade
◆ Shock
◆ Cardiovascular collapse
◆ Death

Signs and symptoms
Acute pericarditis typically produces a sharp and often sudden pain that usually starts over the sternum and radiates to the neck, shoulders, back, and arms. However, unlike the pain of MI, pericardial pain is often pleuritic, increasing with deep inspiration and decreasing when the patient sits up and leans forward, pulling the heart away from the diaphragmatic pleurae of the lungs.

Pericardial effusion, the major complication of acute pericarditis, may produce effects of heart failure (such as dyspnea, orthopnea, and tachycardia), ill-defined substernal chest pain, and a feeling of fullness in the chest. (See *Patterns of cardiac pain.*)

⚠ **ALERT** *If the fluid accumulates rapidly, cardiac tamponade may occur, resulting in pallor, clammy skin, hypotension, pulsus paradoxus (a decrease in systolic blood pressure of 15 mm Hg or more during slow inspiration), JVD and, eventually, cardiovascular collapse and death.*

Chronic constrictive pericarditis causes a gradual increase in systemic venous pressure and produces symptoms similar to those of chronic right-sided heart failure (fluid retention, ascites, and hepatomegaly).

Diagnosis
Because pericarditis commonly coexists with other conditions, the diagnosis of acute pericarditis depends on typical clinical features and elimination of other possible causes.

Patterns of cardiac pain

Although pain perception is individualistic, specific characteristics are associated with different types of cardiac pain, as shown below.

Pericarditis	*Angina*	*Myocardial infarction*
Onset and duration ◆ Sudden onset; continuous pain lasting for days; residual soreness	**Onset and duration** ◆ Gradual or sudden onset; pain usually lasts <15 minutes and not >30 minutes (average: 3 minutes)	**Onset and duration** ◆ Sudden onset; pain lasts 30 minutes to 2 hours; waxes and wanes; residual soreness 1 to 3 days
Location and radiation ◆ Substernal pain to left of midline; radiation to back or subclavicular area	**Location and radiation** ◆ Substernal or anterior chest pain, not sharply localized; radiation to back, neck, arms, jaws, even upper abdomen or fingers	**Location and radiation** ◆ Substernal, midline, or anterior chest pain; radiation to jaws, neck, back, shoulders, or one or both arms
Quality and intensity ◆ Mild ache to severe pain, deep or superficial; "stabbing," "knifelike"	**Quality and intensity** ◆ Mild-to-moderate pressure; deep sensation; varied pattern of attacks; "tightness," "squeezing," "crushing," "pressure"	**Quality and intensity** ◆ Persistent, severe pressure; deep sensation; "crushing," "squeezing," "heavy," "oppressive"
Signs and symptoms ◆ Precordial friction rub; increased pain with movement, inspiration, laughing, coughing; decreased pain with sitting or leaning forward (sitting up pulls heart away from diaphragm)	**Signs and symptoms** ◆ Dyspnea, diaphoresis, nausea, desire to void, belching, apprehension	**Signs and symptoms** ◆ Nausea, vomiting, apprehension, dyspnea, diaphoresis, increased or decreased blood pressure; gallop heart sound, "sensation of impending doom"
Precipitating factors ◆ Myocardial infarction or upper respiratory tract infection; invasive cardiac trauma	**Precipitating factors** ◆ Exertion, stress, eating, cold or hot and humid weather	**Precipitating factors** ◆ Occurrence at rest or during physical exertion or emotional stress

The pericardial friction rub, a classic symptom, is a grating sound heard as the heart moves. It can usually be auscultated best during forced expiration, while the patient leans forward or is on hands and knees in bed. It may have up to three components, corresponding to the timing of atrial systole, ventricular systole, and the rapid-filling phase of ventricular diastole. Occasionally, this friction rub is heard only briefly or not at all. Nevertheless, its presence, together with other characteristic features, is diagnostic of acute pericarditis. In addition, if acute pericarditis has caused very large pericardial effusions, physical examination reveals increased cardiac dullness and diminished or absent apical impulse and distant heart sounds.

Chest X-ray, echocardiogram, chest MRI, heart MRI, heart computed tomography scan, and radionuclide scanning can detect fluid that has accumulated in the pericardial sac. They may also show enlargement of the heart and signs of inflammation or scarring, depending on the cause of pericarditis.

In patients with chronic pericarditis, acute inflammation or effusions don't occur—only restricted cardiac filling.

Laboratory results reflect inflammation and may identify its cause:
♦ normal or elevated white blood cell count, especially in infectious pericarditis
♦ elevated erythrocyte sedimentation rate
♦ slightly elevated cardiac enzyme levels with associated myocarditis
♦ culture of pericardial fluid obtained by open surgical drainage or cardiocentesis (sometimes identifies a causative organism in bacterial or fungal pericarditis)
♦ ECG showing the following changes in acute pericarditis: elevation of ST segments in the standard limb leads and most precordial leads without the significant changes in QRS morphology that occur with MI, atrial ectopic rhythms such as atrial fibrillation and, in pericardial effusion, diminished QRS voltage

Other pertinent laboratory data include BUN levels to check for uremia, antistreptolysin-O titers to detect rheumatic fever, and a purified protein derivative skin test to check for tuberculosis. In pericardial effusion, echocardiography is diagnostic when it shows an echo-free space between the ventricular wall and the pericardium.

Treatment
The goal of treatment is to relieve symptoms and manage the underlying systemic disease. In acute idiopathic pericarditis and postthoracotomy pericarditis, treatment consists of bed rest as long as fever and pain persist,

and nonsteroidal drugs, such as aspirin and indomethacin, to relieve pain and reduce inflammation. Post-MI patients should avoid nonsteroidal anti-inflammatory drugs and steroids because they may interfere with myocardial scar formation. If these drugs fail to relieve symptoms, corticosteroids may be used. Although corticosteroids produce rapid and effective relief, they must be used cautiously because episodes may recur when therapy is discontinued.

Infectious pericarditis that results from disease of the left pleural space, mediastinal abscesses, or septicemia requires antibiotics (possibly by direct pericardial injection), surgical drainage, or both. Cardiac tamponade may require pericardiocentesis. Signs of tamponade include pulsus paradoxus, JVD, dyspnea, and shock.

Recurrent pericarditis may necessitate partial pericardectomy, which creates a "window" that allows fluid to drain into the pleural space. In constrictive pericarditis, total pericardectomy to permit adequate filling and contraction of the heart may be necessary. Treatment must also include management of rheumatic fever, uremia, tuberculosis, and other underlying disorders.

Special considerations
A patient with pericarditis needs complete bed rest. In addition, healthcare includes:
♦ assessing pain in relation to respiration and body position to distinguish pericardial pain from myocardial ischemic pain
♦ placing the patient in an upright position to relieve dyspnea and chest pain; providing analgesics and oxygen; and reassuring the patient with acute pericarditis that the condition is temporary and treatable
♦ monitoring for signs of cardiac compression or cardiac tamponade, possible complications of pericardial effusion (Signs include decreased blood pressure, increased CVP, and pulsus paradoxus. Because cardiac tamponade requires immediate treatment, keep a pericardiocentesis set handy whenever pericardial effusion is suspected.)
♦ explaining tests and treatments to the patient (If surgery is necessary, the patient should learn deep breathing and coughing exercises beforehand. Postoperative care is similar to that given after cardiothoracic surgery.)

RHEUMATIC FEVER AND RHEUMATIC HEART DISEASE
Causes and incidence
Acute rheumatic fever is a systemic inflammatory disease of childhood, in many cases recurrent, that follows a group A beta-hemolytic

streptococcal infection. Rheumatic heart disease refers to the cardiac manifestations of rheumatic fever and includes pancarditis (myocarditis, pericarditis, and endocarditis) during the early acute phase and chronic valvular disease later. Although rheumatic fever tends to be familial, this may merely reflect contributing environmental factors. For example, in lower socioeconomic groups, incidence is highest in children between 5 and 15 years old, probably as a result of malnutrition and crowded living conditions. This disease strikes generally during cool, damp weather in the winter and early spring. In the United States, it's most common in the northern states. Long-term antibiotic therapy can minimize the recurrence of rheumatic fever, reducing the risk of permanent cardiac damage and eventual valvular deformity. However, severe pancarditis occasionally produces fatal heart failure during the acute phase. Of the patients who survive this complication, about 20% die within 10 years.

Pathophysiology

Rheumatic fever appears to be a hypersensitivity reaction to a group A beta-hemolytic streptococcal infection, in which antibodies manufactured to combat streptococci react and produce characteristic lesions at specific tissue sites, especially in the heart and joints. Because very few persons (0.3%) with streptococcal infections ever contract rheumatic fever, altered host resistance must be involved in its development or recurrence.

Complications

◆ Destruction of mitral and aortic valves
◆ Severe pancarditis
◆ Pericardial effusion
◆ Fatal heart failure

Signs and symptoms

In 95% of patients, rheumatic fever characteristically follows a streptococcal infection that appeared a few days to 6 weeks earlier. A temperature of at least 100.4° F (38° C) occurs, and most patients complain of migratory joint pain or polyarthritis. Swelling, redness, and signs of effusion usually accompany such pain, which most commonly affects the knees, ankles, elbows, or hips. In 5% of patients (generally those with carditis), rheumatic fever causes skin lesions such as erythema marginatum, a nonpruritic, macular, transient rash that gives rise to red lesions with blanched centers. Rheumatic fever may also produce firm, movable, nontender, subcutaneous

nodules about 3 mm to 2 cm in diameter, usually near tendons or bony prominences of joints (especially the elbows, knuckles, wrists, and knees) and less often on the scalp and backs of the hands. These nodules persist for a few days to several weeks and, like erythema marginatum, often accompany carditis.

Later, rheumatic fever may cause transient chorea, which develops up to 6 months after the original streptococcal infection. Mild chorea may produce hyperirritability, a deterioration in handwriting, or an inability to concentrate. Severe chorea (Sydenham chorea) causes purposeless, nonrepetitive, involuntary muscle spasms; poor muscle coordination; and weakness. Chorea always resolves without residual neurologic damage.

The most destructive effect of rheumatic fever is carditis, which develops in up to 50% of patients and may affect the endocardium, myocardium, pericardium, or the heart valves. Pericarditis causes a pericardial friction rub and, occasionally, pain and effusion. Myocarditis produces characteristic lesions called Aschoff bodies (in the acute stages) and cellular swelling and fragmentation of interstitial collagen, leading to the formation of a progressively fibrotic nodule and interstitial scars. Endocarditis causes valve leaflet swelling; erosion along the lines of leaflet closure; and blood, platelet, and fibrin deposits, which form beadlike vegetations. Endocarditis affects the mitral valve most often in females and the aortic valve most often in males. In both females and males, endocarditis affects the tricuspid valves occasionally and the pulmonic valve only rarely.

Severe rheumatic carditis may cause heart failure with dyspnea; right upper quadrant pain; tachycardia; tachypnea; a hacking, nonproductive cough; edema; and significant mitral and aortic murmurs. The most common of such murmurs include:
◆ a systolic murmur of mitral insufficiency (high-pitched, blowing, holosystolic, loudest at apex, possibly radiating to the anterior axillary line)
◆ a midsystolic murmur due to stiffening and swelling of the mitral leaflet
◆ occasionally, a diastolic murmur of aortic insufficiency (low-pitched, rumbling, almost inaudible). Valvular disease may eventually result in chronic valvular stenosis and insufficiency, including mitral stenosis and insufficiency, and aortic insufficiency. In children, mitral insufficiency remains the major sequela of rheumatic heart disease.

Diagnosis

Diagnosis depends on recognition of one or more of the classic symptoms (carditis, rheumatic fever without carditis, polyarthritis, chorea, erythema marginatum, or subcutaneous nodules) and a detailed patient history. Laboratory data support the diagnosis:

◆ White blood cell count and erythrocyte sedimentation rate may be elevated (during the acute phase); blood studies show slight anemia due to suppressed erythropoiesis during inflammation.

◆ C-reactive protein is positive (especially during the acute phase).

◆ Cardiac enzyme levels may be increased in severe carditis.

◆ Antistreptolysin-O titer is elevated in 95% of patients within 2 months of onset.

◆ Electrocardiogram changes aren't diagnostic, but PR interval is prolonged in 20% of patients.

◆ Chest X-rays show normal heart size (except with myocarditis, heart failure, or pericardial effusion).

◆ Echocardiography helps evaluate valvular damage, chamber size, and ventricular function.

◆ Cardiac catheterization evaluates valvular damage and left ventricular function in severe cardiac dysfunction.

Treatment

Effective management eradicates the streptococcal infection, relieves symptoms, and prevents recurrence, reducing the chance of permanent cardiac damage. During the acute phase, treatment includes penicillin, sulfadiazine, or erythromycin. Salicylates such as aspirin relieve fever and minimize joint swelling and pain; if carditis is present or salicylates fail to relieve pain and inflammation, corticosteroids may be used. Supportive treatment requires strict bed rest for about 5 weeks during the acute phase with active carditis, followed by a progressive increase in physical activity, depending on clinical and laboratory findings and the response to treatment.

After the acute phase subsides, low-dose antibiotics may be used to prevent recurrence. Such preventive treatment usually continues for 5 years or until age 21 (whichever is longer). Heart failure necessitates continued bed rest and diuretics. Severe mitral or aortic valve dysfunction that causes persistent heart failure requires corrective valvular surgery, including commissurotomy (separation of the adherent, thickened leaflets of the mitral valve), valvuloplasty (inflation of a balloon within a valve), or valve replacement (with prosthetic valve). Such surgery is seldom necessary before late adolescence.

Special considerations

Because rheumatic fever and rheumatic heart disease require prolonged treatment, the care plan should include comprehensive patient teaching to promote compliance with the prescribed therapy.

◆ Before giving penicillin, ask the patient or parents if the patient has ever had a hypersensitivity reaction to it. If not, warn that such a reaction is possible. Tell them to stop the drug and call the practitioner immediately if the patient develops a rash, fever, chills, or other signs of allergy *at any time* during penicillin therapy.

◆ Instruct the patient and family to watch for and report early signs of heart failure, such as dyspnea and a hacking, nonproductive cough.

◆ Stress the need for bed rest during the acute phase, and suggest appropriate, physically undemanding diversions. After the acute phase, encourage family and friends to spend as much time as possible with the patient to minimize boredom. Advise parents to secure tutorial services to help the child keep up with schoolwork during the long convalescence.

◆ Help the child's parents overcome any guilt feelings they may have about the illness. Tell them that failure to seek treatment for streptococcal infection is common because this illness often seems no worse than a cold. Encourage the child and his or her parents to vent their frustrations during the long, tedious recovery. If the child has severe carditis, help them prepare for permanent changes in lifestyle.

◆ Teach the patient and his or her family about this disease and its treatment. Warn parents to watch for and immediately report signs of recurrent streptococcal infection—sudden sore throat, diffuse throat redness and oropharyngeal exudate, swollen and tender cervical lymph glands, pain on swallowing, temperature of 101° to 104° F (38.3° to 40° C), headache, and nausea. Urge them to keep the child away from people with respiratory tract infections.

◆ Promote good dental hygiene to prevent gingival infection. Make sure the patient and his or her family understand the need to comply with prolonged antibiotic therapy and follow-up care and the need for additional antibiotics during dental surgery or procedures. Arrange for a home health nurse to oversee home care if necessary.

◆ Teach the patient to follow current recommendations of the American Heart Association for prevention of bacterial endocarditis. Antibiotic regimens used to prevent recurrence of acute rheumatic fever are inadequate for preventing bacterial endocarditis.

Valve disorders

VALVULAR HEART DISEASE

Causes and incidence

More than 5 million people in the United States are diagnosed with some form of valvular disease each year. The mitral and aortic valves are most commonly affected. Common causes of each type can be found in *Types of valvular heart disease.*

Pathophysiology

In valvular heart disease, three types of mechanical disruption can occur: stenosis, or narrowing, of the valve opening; incomplete closure of the valve; and prolapse of the valve. A combination of these three in the same valve may also occur. They can result from such disorders as endocarditis (most common), congenital defects, and inflammation, and they can lead to heart failure.

Valvular heart disease occurs in varying forms, described in the following.

◆ Mitral insufficiency: In this form, blood from the left ventricle flows back into the left atrium during systole, causing the atrium to enlarge to accommodate the backflow. As a result, the left ventricle also dilates to accommodate the increased volume of blood from the atrium and to compensate for diminishing cardiac output. Ventricular hypertrophy and increased end-diastolic pressure result in increased PAP, eventually leading to left- and right-sided heart failure.

◆ Mitral stenosis: Narrowing of the valve by valvular abnormalities, fibrosis, or calcification obstructs blood flow from the left atrium to the left ventricle. Consequently, left atrial volume and pressure rise and the chamber dilates. Greater resistance to blood flow causes pulmonary hypertension, right ventricular hypertrophy, and right-sided heart failure. Also, inadequate filling of the left ventricle produces low cardiac output.

◆ Mitral valve prolapse: One or both valve leaflets protrude into the left atrium. *MVP* is the term used when the anatomic prolapse is accompanied by signs and symptoms unrelated to the valvular abnormality.

◆ Aortic insufficiency: Blood flows back into the left ventricle during diastole, causing fluid overload in the ventricle, which dilates and hypertrophies. The excess volume causes fluid overload in the left atrium, and, finally, the pulmonary system. Left-sided heart failure and pulmonary edema eventually result.

◆ Aortic stenosis: Increased left ventricular pressure tries to overcome the resistance of the narrowed valvular opening. The added workload increases the demand for oxygen, whereas diminished cardiac output causes poor coronary artery perfusion, ischemia of the left ventricle, and left-sided heart failure.

◆ Pulmonic insufficiency: Blood ejected into the pulmonary artery during systole flows back into the right ventricle during diastole, causing fluid overload in the ventricle, ventricular hypertrophy and, finally, right-sided heart failure.

◆ Pulmonic stenosis: Obstructed right ventricular outflow causes right ventricular hypertrophy, eventually resulting in right-sided heart failure.

◆ Tricuspid insufficiency: Blood flows back into the right atrium during systole, decreasing blood flow to the lungs and the left side of the heart. Cardiac output also lessens. Fluid overload in the right side of the heart can eventually lead to right-sided heart failure.

◆ Tricuspid stenosis: Obstructed blood flow from the right atrium to the right ventricle causes the right atrium to dilate and hypertrophy. Eventually, this leads to right-sided heart failure and increases pressure in the vena cava.

Treatment

Treatment depends on the nature and severity of associated symptoms. For example, heart failure requires diuretics, a sodium-restricted diet and, in acute cases, oxygen. Other measures may include anticoagulant therapy or antiplatelet medications to prevent thrombus formation around diseased or replaced valves, prophylactic antibiotics before and after surgery, and valvuloplasty. An IABP may be used temporarily to reduce backflow by enhancing forward blood flow into the aorta.

If the patient has severe signs and symptoms that can't be managed medically, open heart surgery using cardiopulmonary bypass for valve repair or replacement is indicated. Newer procedures are available, such as transcatheter aortic valve replacement, and may be an option, as well. This is a minimally invasive procedure that wedges a replacement valve in the position of the old valve. This valve begins to take over the duties of the old valve while pushing the leaflets of the old valve away.

Special considerations

◆ Watch closely for signs of heart failure or pulmonary edema and for adverse effects of drug therapy.

◆ Teach the patient about diet restrictions, medications, and the importance of consistent follow-up care.

◆ If the patient undergoes surgery, watch for hypotension, arrhythmias, and thrombus

Types of valvular heart disease

Causes and incidence	Signs and symptoms	Diagnostic measures
Aortic insufficiency		
◆ Results from rheumatic fever, syphilis, hypertension, endocarditis, or may be idiopathic ◆ Associated with Marfan syndrome ◆ Most common in males ◆ Associated with ventricular septal defect, even after surgical closure	◆ Dyspnea, cough, fatigue, palpitations, angina, syncope ◆ Pulmonary venous congestion, heart failure, pulmonary edema (left-sided heart failure), "pulsating" nail beds ◆ Rapidly rising and collapsing pulses (pulsus bisferiens), cardiac arrhythmias, wide pulse pressure in severe insufficiency ◆ Auscultation: reveals S_3 and diastolic blowing murmur at left sternal border ◆ Palpation and visualization of apical impulse in chronic disease	◆ Cardiac catheterization: reduction in arterial diastolic pressures, aortic insufficiency, other valvular abnormalities, and increased left ventricular end-diastolic pressure ◆ X-ray: left ventricular enlargement, pulmonary vein congestion ◆ Echocardiography: left ventricular enlargement, alterations in mitral valve movement (indirect indication of aortic valve disease), and mitral thickening ◆ Electrocardiography (ECG): sinus tachycardia, left ventricular hypertrophy, and left atrial hypertrophy in severe disease
Aortic stenosis		
◆ Results from congenital aortic bicuspid valve (associated with coarctation of the aorta), congenital stenosis of valve cusps, rheumatic fever, or atherosclerosis in elderly persons ◆ Most common in males	◆ Dyspnea on exertion, paroxysmal nocturnal dyspnea, fatigue, syncope, angina, palpitations ◆ Pulmonary venous congestion, heart failure, pulmonary edema ◆ Diminished carotid pulses, decreased cardiac output, cardiac arrhythmias; may have pulsus alternans ◆ Auscultation: reveals systolic murmur at base or in carotids and, possibly, S_4	◆ Cardiac catheterization: pressure gradient across valve (indicating obstruction), increased left ventricular end-diastolic pressures ◆ X-ray: valvular calcification, left ventricular enlargement, and pulmonary venous congestion ◆ Echocardiography: thickened aortic valve and left ventricular wall ◆ ECG: left ventricular hypertrophy
Mitral insufficiency		
◆ Results from rheumatic fever, hypertrophic cardiomyopathy, mitral valve prolapse, myocardial infarction, severe left-sided heart failure, or ruptured chordae tendineae ◆ Associated with other congenital anomalies such as transposition of the great arteries ◆ Rare in children without other congenital anomalies	◆ Orthopnea, dyspnea, fatigue, angina, palpitations ◆ Peripheral edema, jugular vein distention (JVD), hepatomegaly (right-sided heart failure) ◆ Tachycardia, crackles, pulmonary edema ◆ Auscultation: reveals holosystolic murmur at apex, possible split S_2, and S_3	◆ Cardiac catheterization: mitral insufficiency with increased left ventricular end-diastolic volume and pressure, increased atrial pressure and pulmonary artery wedge pressure (PAWP); and decreased cardiac output ◆ X-ray: left atrial and ventricular enlargement, pulmonary venous congestion ◆ Echocardiography: abnormal valve leaflet motion, left atrial enlargement ◆ ECG: left atrial and ventricular hypertrophy, sinus tachycardia, and atrial fibrillation

Types of valvular heart disease (*continued*)

Causes and incidence	Signs and symptoms	Diagnostic measures
Mitral stenosis		
♦ Results from rheumatic fever (most common cause) ♦ Most common in females ♦ May be associated with other congenital anomalies	♦ Dyspnea on exertion, paroxysmal nocturnal dyspnea, orthopnea, weakness, fatigue, palpitations ♦ Peripheral edema, JVD, ascites, hepatomegaly (right-sided heart failure in severe pulmonary hypertension) ♦ Crackles, cardiac arrhythmias (atrial fibrillation), signs of systemic emboli ♦ Auscultation: reveals loud S_1 or opening snap and diastolic murmur at apex	♦ Cardiac catheterization: diastolic pressure gradient across valve; elevated left atrial pressure and PAWP (>15 mm Hg) with severe pulmonary hypertension and pulmonary artery pressures (PAPs); elevated right-sided heart pressure; decreased cardiac output; and abnormal contraction of the left ventricle ♦ X-ray: left atrial and ventricular enlargement, enlarged pulmonary arteries, and mitral valve calcification ♦ Echocardiography: thickened mitral valve leaflets, left atrial enlargement ♦ ECG: left atrial hypertrophy, atrial fibrillation, right ventricular hypertrophy, and right axis deviation
Mitral valve prolapse syndrome		
♦ Can be genetic or associated with conditions such as Ehlers–Danlos syndrome, Marfan syndrome, Graves disease, and muscular dystrophy ♦ Most commonly affects young women but may occur in both sexes and in all age groups	♦ May produce no signs ♦ Chest pain, palpitations, headache, fatigue, exercise intolerance, dyspnea, light-headedness, syncope, mood swings, anxiety, panic attacks ♦ Auscultation: typically reveals mobile, midsystolic click, with or without mid-to-late systolic murmur	♦ Two-dimensional echocardiography: prolapse of mitral valve leaflets into left atrium ♦ Color-flow Doppler studies: mitral insufficiency ♦ Resting ECG: ST-segment changes, biphasic or inverted T waves in leads II, III, or AV ♦ Exercise ECG: evaluates chest pain and arrhythmias
Pulmonic insufficiency		
♦ May be congenital or may result from pulmonary hypertension ♦ May rarely result from prolonged use of pressure-monitoring catheter in the pulmonary artery	♦ Dyspnea, weakness, fatigue, chest pain ♦ Peripheral edema, JVD, hepatomegaly (right-sided heart failure) ♦ Auscultation: reveals diastolic murmur in pulmonic area	♦ Cardiac catheterization: pulmonic insufficiency, increased right ventricular pressure, and associated cardiac defects ♦ X-ray: right ventricular and pulmonary arterial enlargement ♦ ECG: right ventricular or right atrial enlargement
Pulmonic stenosis		
♦ Results from congenital stenosis of valve cusp or rheumatic heart disease (infrequent) ♦ Associated with other congenital heart defects such as tetralogy of Fallot	♦ Asymptomatic or symptomatic with dyspnea on exertion, fatigue, chest pain, syncope ♦ May lead to peripheral edema, JVD, hepatomegaly (right-sided heart failure) ♦ Auscultation: reveals systolic murmur at left sternal border, split S_2 with delayed or absent pulmonic component	♦ Cardiac catheterization: increased right ventricular pressure, decreased PAP, and abnormal valve orifice ♦ ECG: may show right ventricular hypertrophy, right axis deviation, right atrial hypertrophy, and atrial fibrillation

(continued)

Types of valvular heart disease (*continued*)

Causes and incidence	Signs and symptoms	Diagnostic measures
Tricuspid insufficiency		
♦ Results from right-sided heart failure, rheumatic fever and, rarely, trauma and endocarditis ♦ Associated with congenital disorders ♦ Associated with I.V. drug abuse and infective endocarditis manifesting as tricuspid valve disease	♦ Dyspnea and fatigue ♦ May lead to peripheral edema, JVD, hepatomegaly, and ascites (right-sided heart failure) ♦ Auscultation: reveals possible S_3 and systolic murmur at lower left sternal border that increases with inspiration	♦ Right-sided heart catheterization: high atrial pressure, tricuspid insufficiency, decreased or normal cardiac output ♦ X-ray: right atrial dilation, right ventricular enlargement ♦ Echocardiography: shows systolic prolapse of tricuspid valve, right atrial enlargement ♦ ECG: right atrial or right ventricular hypertrophy, atrial fibrillation
Tricuspid stenosis		
♦ Results from rheumatic fever ♦ May be congenital ♦ Associated with mitral or aortic valve disease ♦ Most common in women	♦ May be symptomatic with dyspnea, fatigue, syncope ♦ Possibly peripheral edema, JVD, hepatomegaly, and ascites (right-sided heart failure) ♦ Auscultation: reveals diastolic murmur at lower left sternal border that increases with inspiration	♦ Cardiac catheterization: increased pressure gradient across valve, increased right atrial pressure, decreased cardiac output ♦ X-ray: right atrial enlargement ♦ Echocardiography: leaflet abnormality, right atrial enlargement ♦ ECG: right atrial hypertrophy, right or left ventricular hypertrophy, and atrial fibrillation

formation. Monitor vital signs, ABG values, intake, output, daily weight, blood chemistries, chest X-rays, and pulmonary artery catheter readings.

Degenerative cardiovascular disorders

HYPERTENSION

Causes and incidence

Hypertension, an intermittent or sustained elevation in diastolic or systolic blood pressure, occurs as two major types: essential (idiopathic) hypertension, the most common, and secondary hypertension, which results from renal disease or another identifiable cause. Malignant hypertension is a severe, fulminant form of hypertension common to both types. Hypertension is a major cause of stroke, cardiac disease, and renal failure. Hypertension affects 25% of adults in the United States. If untreated, it carries a high mortality. Risk factors for hypertension include family history, race (most

common in blacks), stress, obesity, a diet high in saturated fats or sodium, tobacco use, sedentary lifestyle, and aging.

Secondary hypertension may result from renal vascular disease; pheochromocytoma; primary hyperaldosteronism; Cushing syndrome; thyroid, pituitary, or parathyroid dysfunction; coarctation of the aorta; pregnancy; neurologic disorders; and use of hormonal contraceptives or other drugs, such as cocaine, epoetin alfa (erythropoietin), and cyclosporine.

The prognosis is good if this disorder is detected early and treatment begins before complications develop. Severely elevated blood pressure (hypertensive crisis) may be fatal. (See *What happens in a hypertensive crisis*, page 31.)

Pathophysiology

Cardiac output and PVR determine blood pressure. Increased blood volume, cardiac rate, and stroke volume as well as arteriolar vasoconstriction can raise blood pressure. The link to sustained hypertension, however, is unclear.

PATHOPHYSIOLOGY
What happens in a hypertensive crisis

Hypertensive crisis is a severe rise in arterial blood pressure caused by a disturbance in one or more of the regulating mechanisms. If left untreated, hypertensive crisis may result in renal, cardiac, or cerebral complications and, possibly, death.

Causes of hypertensive crisis

- Abnormal renal function
- Hypertensive encephalopathy
- Intracerebral hemorrhage
- Heart failure

- Withdrawal of antihypertensive drugs (abrupt)
- Myocardial ischemia

- Eclampsia
- Pheochromocytoma
- Monoamine oxidase inhibitor interactions

↓

Prolonged hypertension

↓

Inflammation and necrosis of arterioles

↓

Narrowing of blood vessels

↓

Restriction of blood flow to major organs

↓

Organ damage

↓ ↓ ↓

Renal
- Decreased renal perfusion
- Progressive deterioration of nephrons
- Decreased ability to concentrate urine
- Increased serum creatinine and blood urea nitrogen levels
- Increased renal tubule permeability with protein leakage into tubules
- Renal insufficiency
- Uremia
- Renal failure

Cardiac
- Decreased cardiac perfusion
- Coronary artery disease
- Angina or myocardial infarction
- Increased cardiac workload
- Left ventricular hypertrophy
- Heart failure

Cerebral
- Decreased cerebral perfusion
- Increased stress on vessel wall
- Arterial spasm
- Ischemia
- Transient ischemic attacks
- Weakening of vessel intima
- Aneurysm formation
- Intracranial hemorrhage

Hypertension may also result from failure of intrinsic regulatory mechanisms:

♦ Renal hypoperfusion causes release of renin, which is converted by angiotensinogen, a liver enzyme, to angiotensin I. Angiotensin I is converted to angiotensin II, a powerful vasoconstrictor. The resulting vasoconstriction increases afterload. Angiotensin II stimulates adrenal secretion of aldosterone, which increases sodium reabsorption. Hypertonic-stimulated release of antidiuretic hormone from the pituitary gland follows, increasing water reabsorption, plasma volume, cardiac output, and blood pressure.

♦ Autoregulation changes an artery's diameter to maintain perfusion despite fluctuations in systemic blood pressure. The intrinsic mechanisms responsible include stress relaxation (vessels gradually dilate when blood pressure rises to reduce peripheral resistance) and capillary fluid shift (plasma moves between vessels and extravascular spaces to maintain intravascular volume).

♦ When the blood pressure drops, baroreceptors in the aortic arch and carotid sinuses decrease their inhibition of the medulla's vasomotor center, which increases sympathetic stimulation of the heart by norepinephrine. This, in turn, increases cardiac output by strengthening the contractile force, increasing the heart rate, and augmenting peripheral resistance by vasoconstriction. Stress can also stimulate the sympathetic nervous system to increase cardiac output and PVR.

Complications
♦ Stroke
♦ Coronary artery disease
♦ Angina
♦ Myocardial infarction
♦ Heart failure
♦ Arrhythmias
♦ Sudden death
♦ Cerebral infarction
♦ Hypertensive encephalopathy
♦ Hypertensive retinopathy
♦ Renal failure

Signs and symptoms
Hypertension usually doesn't produce clinical effects until vascular changes in the heart, brain, or kidneys occur. Severely elevated blood pressure damages the intima of small vessels, resulting in fibrin accumulation in the vessels, development of local edema and, possibly, intravascular clotting. Symptoms produced by this process depend on the location of the damaged vessels:

♦ brain—stroke
♦ retina—blindness
♦ heart—myocardial infarction
♦ kidneys—proteinuria, edema, and, eventually, renal failure

Hypertension increases the heart's workload, causing left ventricular hypertrophy and, later, left- and right-sided heart failure and pulmonary edema.

Classifying blood pressure readings

The Eighth Joint National Committee (JNC8) released updated guidelines in 2014 for classifying and treating hypertension.

The following categories are based on the average of two or more readings taken on separate visits after an initial screening. They apply to adults 18 years old and older.

Normal blood pressure with respect to cardiovascular risk is a systolic reading below 120 mm Hg and a diastolic reading below 80 mm Hg. Historically, hypertension was defined as a systolic blood pressure of 140 mm Hg or higher or a diastolic pressure above 90 mm Hg. The latest guidelines, however, classify hypertension as a systolic reading of 130 mm Hg or higher, or a diastolic pressure above 90 mm Hg.

In addition to classifying stages of hypertension based on average blood pressure readings, clinicians should also take note of target organ disease and any additional risk factors.

Category	Systolic (mm Hg)		Diastolic (mm Hg)
Normal	<120	and	<80
Elevated	120 to 129	and	<80
Hypertension			
Stage 1	130 to 139	or	80 to 89
Stage 2	≥140	or	≥90
Hypertensive crisis	≥180	and/or	≥120

Diagnosis

Serial blood pressure measurements are obtained and compared to previous readings and trends to reveal an increase in diastolic and systolic pressures. (See *Classifying blood pressure readings*, page 32.)

Auscultation may reveal bruits over the abdominal aorta and the carotid, renal, and femoral arteries; ophthalmoscopy reveals arteriovenous nicking and, in hypertensive encephalopathy, papilledema. Patient history and the following additional tests may show predisposing factors and help identify an underlying cause such as renal disease:

♦ Urinalysis: Protein levels and red and white blood cell counts may indicate glomerulonephritis.

♦ Excretory urography: Renal atrophy indicates chronic renal disease; one kidney more than $5/8''$ (1.5 cm) shorter than the other suggests unilateral renal disease.

♦ Serum potassium: Levels less than 3.5 mEq/L may indicate adrenal dysfunction (primary hyperaldosteronism).

♦ BUN and serum creatinine: BUN level that's normal or elevated to more than 20 mg/dL and serum creatinine level that's normal or elevated to more than 1.5 mg/dL suggest renal disease.

Other tests help detect cardiovascular damage and other complications:

♦ ECG may show left ventricular hypertrophy or ischemia.

♦ Chest X-ray may show cardiomegaly.

♦ Echocardiography may show left ventricular hypertrophy.

Treatment

The JNC8 recommends the following approach for treating primary hypertension:

♦ First, help the patient start needed lifestyle modifications, including weight reduction, moderation of alcohol intake, regular physical exercise, reduction in sodium intake, and smoking cessation.

♦ If the patient fails to achieve the desired blood pressure or make significant progress, continue lifestyle modifications and begin drug therapy.

♦ Pharmacologic therapy should begin when blood pressure is 140/90 in patients less than 60, and 150/90 in those 60 and older.

♦ If the patient has comorbid conditions such as diabetes mellitus or chronic kidney disease (CKD), the goal should be to achieve blood pressure less than 140/90 regardless of age.

♦ In nonblack patients without CKD, consider using a thiazide diuretic, an angiotensin-converting enzyme (ACE) inhibitor, an angiotensin receptor blocker (ARB), or a calcium channel blocker (CCB), alone or in combination.

♦ In black patients without CKD, consider using a thiazide diuretic or a CCB, alone or in combination.

♦ In all patients with CKD, consider initiating an ACE or ARB, alone or in combination with another class.

♦ If the patient has one or more compelling indications, base drug treatment on benefits from outcome studies or existing clinical guidelines. Treatment may include the following, depending on indication:

  ♦ Heart failure—ACE/ARB + beta-adrenergic blocker (BB) + diuretic + spironolactone

  ♦ CAD—ACE, BB, diuretic, CCB

  ♦ Diabetes—ACE/ARB, CCB, diuretic

  ♦ CKD—ACE inhibitor or ARB

  ♦ Postmyocardial infarction/clinical CAD—ACE/ARB + BB

  ♦ Recurrent stroke prevention—ACE, diuretic

  ♦ Pregnancy—labetalol (first line), nifedipine, methyldopa

  Give other antihypertensive drugs as needed.

♦ If the patient fails to achieve the desired blood pressure, continue lifestyle modifications and optimize drug dosages or add drugs until the goal blood pressure is achieved. Also, consider consultation with a hypertension specialist.

Treatment of secondary hypertension focuses on correcting the underlying cause and controlling hypertensive effects.

Typically, hypertensive emergencies require parenteral administration of a vasodilator or an adrenergic inhibitor. Oral administration of a selected drug, such as nicardipine, hydralazine, or esmolol to rapidly reduces blood pressure. The initial goal is to reduce mean arterial blood pressure by no more than 25% (within minutes to hours) and then to 160/110 mm Hg within 2 hours while avoiding excessive falls in blood pressure that can precipitate renal, cerebral, or myocardial ischemia.

Examples of hypertensive emergencies include hypertensive encephalopathy, intracranial hemorrhage, acute left-sided heart failure with pulmonary edema, and dissecting aortic aneurysm. Hypertensive emergencies are also associated with eclampsia or severe gestational hypertension, unstable angina, and acute MI.

Hypertension without accompanying symptoms or target organ disease seldom requires emergency drug therapy.

Special considerations

◆ To encourage adherence to antihypertensive therapy, suggest that the patient establish a daily routine for taking medication. Warn that uncontrolled hypertension may cause stroke and heart attack. Tell the patient to report adverse drug effects. Also, advise the patient to avoid high-sodium antacids and over-the-counter cold and sinus medications, which contain harmful vasoconstrictors.

◆ Encourage a change in dietary habits. Help the obese patient plan a weight-reduction diet; tell the patient to avoid high-sodium foods (pickles, potato chips, canned soups, and cold cuts) and table salt.

◆ Help the patient examine and modify lifestyle (e.g., by reducing stress and exercising regularly).

◆ If a patient is hospitalized with hypertension, find out if the patient was taking his or her prescribed medication. If not, ask why. If the patient can't afford the medication, refer to appropriate social service agencies. Tell the patient and family to keep a record of drugs used in the past, noting especially those that were or weren't effective. Suggest that the patient record this information on a card and show it to his or her practitioner.

◆ When routine blood pressure screening reveals elevated pressure, first make sure the cuff size is appropriate for the patient's upper arm circumference. Take the pressure in both arms in lying, sitting, and standing positions. Ask the patient if he or she smoked, drank a beverage containing caffeine, or was emotionally upset before the test. Advise the patient to return for

---

PREVENTION
Preventing hypertension

Certain risk factors for hypertension can't be changed, such as family history, race, and aging, but lifestyle modifications can help prevent hypertension. Based on American Heart Association recommendations, advise your patient to do the following:

Maintain a healthy weight
Maintain a normal weight or lose weight if overweight. Weight loss lowers blood pressure.

Reduce salt
Salt intake should be reduced to about 1.5 g/day. Reducing salt intake can lower blood pressure in individuals with and without hypertension.

Increase potassium
Patients should eat 8 to 10 servings of fruits and vegetables per day to increase potassium intake. Potassium reduces blood pressure in individuals with and without hypertension. Those with kidney disease or heart failure should contact their practitioner before increasing their potassium intake.

Limit alcohol intake
Studies have shown a correlation between alcohol intake and increased blood pressure, especially in individuals who drink >2 drinks/day.

Include exercise
Regular physical activity is defined by the American Heart Association as

moderate-intensity exercise such as brisk walking for 150 minutes each week. A lack of physical activity can lead to obesity and increase the risk of hypertension, heart attack, and stroke.

Manage stress
Stress can lead to increased alcohol consumption, smoking, overeating, and other activities that increase the risk of heart attack or stroke. Daily relaxation for short periods during the workday and on weekends can also lower blood pressure.

Stop smoking
Smoking even filtered and light or ultra cigarettes can lead to atherosclerosis. Quitting or not starting is the only way to prevent this major risk factor for heart attack and stroke.

Follow the DASH diet
The Dietary Approaches to Stop Hypertension (DASH) diet encourages vegetables, fruits, and low-fat dairy as well as whole grains, fish, poultry, and nuts. Discourage the eating of fats, red meat, sweets, and sugar-containing beverages. However, individuals with reduced kidney function should always consult their practitioners before starting this diet; it's rich in potassium, which isn't recommended for individuals with these disorders.

blood pressure testing at frequent and regular intervals.

◆ To help identify hypertension and prevent untreated hypertension, participate in public education programs dealing with hypertension and ways to reduce risk factors. Encourage public participation in blood pressure screening programs. Routinely screen all patients, especially those at risk (blacks and people with family histories of hypertension, stroke, or heart attack). (See *Preventing hypertension*, page 34.)

CORONARY ARTERY DISEASE
Causes and incidence
CAD occurs when the arteries that supply blood to the heart muscle harden and narrow, usually as a result of atherosclerosis. The result is the loss of oxygen and nutrients to myocardial tissue because of diminished coronary blood flow. This reduction in blood flow can also lead to coronary syndrome (angina or MI). (See *Understanding coronary artery disease*.)

CAD has been linked to many risk factors: family history, male gender, age (risk increased in those 65 years old or older), hypertension, obesity, smoking, diabetes mellitus, stress, sedentary lifestyle, high serum cholesterol (particularly high low-density lipoprotein cholesterol) or triglyceride levels, low high-density lipoprotein cholesterol levels, high blood homocysteine levels, menopause and, possibly, infections producing inflammatory responses in the artery walls.

Uncommon causes of reduced coronary artery blood flow include dissecting aneurysms, infectious vasculitis, syphilis, and congenital defects in the coronary vascular system. Coronary artery spasms may also impede blood flow. (See *Coronary artery spasm*, page 36.)

CAD is the leading cause of death in the United States. According to the American Heart Association, 1 in 3 deaths is due to cardiovascular disease, and someone dies from such an event about every 40 seconds.

Pathophysiology
In atherosclerosis, a form of arteriosclerosis, fatty, fibrous plaques, possibly including calcium deposits, narrow the lumen of the coronary arteries and reduce the volume of blood that can flow through them, and leading to myocardial ischemia. Plaque formation also predisposes to thrombosis, which can provoke MI.

Atherosclerosis usually develops in high-flow, high-pressure arteries, such as those in the heart, brain, kidneys, and in the aorta, especially at bifurcation points.

Signs and symptoms
The classic symptom of CAD is angina, the direct result of inadequate oxygen flow to the myocardium. Anginal pain is usually described as a burning, squeezing, or tight feeling in the substernal or precordial chest that may radiate to the left arm, neck, jaw, or shoulder blade. Typically, the patient clenches a fist over his chest or rubs the left arm when describing the pain, which may be accompanied by nausea, vomiting, fainting, sweating, and cool extremities. Anginal episodes most often follow physical exertion but may also follow emotional excitement, exposure to cold, or a large meal. Some patients, particularly those with diabetes, may not experience typical anginal pain but

Understanding coronary artery disease

Coronary artery disease (CAD) results as atherosclerotic plaque fills the lumens of the coronary arteries and obstructs blood flow. The primary effect of CAD is a diminished supply of oxygen and nutrients to myocardial tissues.

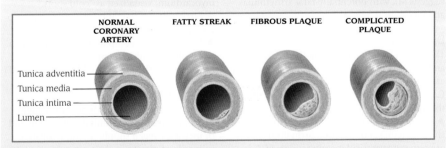

NORMAL CORONARY ARTERY   FATTY STREAK   FIBROUS PLAQUE   COMPLICATED PLAQUE

Tunica adventitia
Tunica media
Tunica intima
Lumen

Coronary artery spasm

In coronary artery spasm, a spontaneous, sustained contraction of one or more coronary arteries causes ischemia and dysfunction of the heart muscle. This disorder also causes Prinzmetal angina and even myocardial infarction in patients with unoccluded coronary arteries. Its cause is unknown but possible contributing factors include:

♦ altered flow of calcium into the cell
♦ intimal hemorrhage into the medial layer of the blood vessel
♦ hyperventilation
♦ elevated catecholamine levels
♦ fatty buildup in lumen

Signs and symptoms

The major symptom of coronary artery spasm is angina. However, unlike classic angina, this pain often occurs spontaneously and may not be related to physical exertion or emotional stress; it's also more severe, usually lasts longer, and may be cyclic, frequently recurring every day at the same time. Such ischemic episodes may cause arrhythmias, altered heart rate, lower blood pressure and, occasionally, fainting due to diminished cardiac output. Spasm in the left coronary artery may result in mitral insufficiency, producing a loud systolic murmur and, possibly, pulmonary edema, with dyspnea, crackles, hemoptysis, or sudden death.

Treatment

After diagnosis by coronary angiography and electrocardiography (ECG), the patient may receive calcium channel blockers (CCBs; verapamil, nifedipine, or diltiazem) to reduce coronary artery spasm and vascular resistance and nitrates (nitroglycerin or isosorbide dinitrate) to relieve chest pain.

When caring for a patient with coronary artery spasm, explain all necessary procedures and teach them how to take medications safely. For CCB therapy, monitor blood pressure, pulse rate, and ECG patterns to detect arrhythmias. In patients receiving nifedipine and verapamil along with digoxin, monitor digoxin levels and check for signs of digoxin toxicity. Because nifedipine may cause peripheral and periorbital edema, watch for fluid retention.

Because coronary artery spasm is commonly associated with atherosclerotic disease, advise the patient to stop smoking, avoid overeating, maintain a low-fat diet, use alcohol sparingly, and maintain a balance between exercise and rest.

---

may have dyspnea, fatigue, diaphoresis, or more vague symptoms.

Angina has four major forms: *stable* (pain is predictable in frequency and duration and can be relieved with nitrates and rest), *unstable* (pain increases in frequency and duration and is more easily induced), *Prinzmetal* or *variant* (from unpredictable coronary artery spasm), and *microvascular* (in which impairment of vasodilator reserve causes angina-like chest pain in a patient with normal coronary arteries). Severe and prolonged anginal pain generally suggests MI, with potentially fatal arrhythmias and mechanical failure.

Diagnosis

The patient history—including the frequency and duration of angina and the presence of associated risk factors—is crucial in evaluating CAD. Additional diagnostic measures include the following:

♦ Electrocardiogram (ECG) during angina may show ischemia and, possibly, arrhythmias such as premature ventricular contractions. ECG is apt to be normal when the patient is pain-free. Arrhythmias may occur without infarction, secondary to ischemia.

♦ Treadmill or exercise stress test may provoke chest pain and ECG signs of myocardial ischemia.

♦ Coronary angiography reveals coronary artery stenosis or obstruction, possible collateral circulation, and the arteries' condition beyond the narrowing.

♦ Myocardial perfusion imaging with thallium-201, Cardiolite, or Myoview during treadmill exercise detects ischemic areas of the myocardium, visualized as "cold spots."

♦ Stress echocardiography may show wall motion abnormalities.

♦ Electron-beam computed tomography identifies calcium within arterial plaque; the more calcium seen, the higher the likelihood of CAD.

Treatment

The goal of treatment in patients with angina is to either reduce myocardial oxygen demand or increase oxygen supply. Therapy consists primarily of nitrates such as nitroglycerin (given sublingually, orally, transdermally, or topically in ointment form) to dilate coronary arteries and improve blood supply to the heart. Glycoprotein IIb to IIIa inhibitors and antithrombin drugs may be used to reduce the risk of blood clots. BBs may be used to decrease heart rate and lower the heart's oxygen use. CCBs may be used to relax the coronary arteries and all systemic arteries, reducing the heart's workload. ACE inhibitors, diuretics, or other medications may be used to lower blood pressure.

Percutaneous transluminal coronary angioplasty (PTCA) may be performed during cardiac catheterization to compress fatty deposits and relieve occlusion in patients with no calcification and partial occlusion. PTCA carries a certain risk, but the morbidity associated with it is lower than that for surgery. (See *Relieving occlusions with angioplasty*, pages 38 and 39.)

PTCA is an alternative to grafting in elderly patients or others who can't tolerate cardiac surgery. However, patients who have a left main coronary artery occlusion, lesions in extremely tortuous vessels, or occlusions older than 3 months aren't candidates for PTCA.

PTCA can be done along with coronary stenting, or stents may be placed alone. Stents provide a framework to hold an artery open by securing the flaps of the tunica media against an artery wall. Intravascular coronary artery stenting is done to reduce the incidence of restenosis. Prosthetic cylindrical stents made of stainless steel coil are positioned at the site of occlusion. Drug-eluting stents have proven to be safe and effective and have a lower rate of restenosis when compared with bare-metal stents.

Laser angioplasty corrects occlusion by vaporizing fatty deposits with the excimer, or hot-tipped laser device. Percutaneous myocardial revascularization uses a laser to create channels in the heart muscle to improve perfusion to the myocardium. A carbon dioxide laser is used to create transmural channels from the epicardium to the myocardium, extending into the left ventricle. This technique is also known as transmyocardial revascularization and appears to be effective for severe symptoms. In addition, a stent may be placed in the artery to act as a scaffold to hold the artery open. Obstructive lesions may necessitate coronary artery bypass graft (CABG) surgery and the use of vein grafts.

A surgical technique available as an alternative to traditional CABG surgery is minimally invasive coronary artery bypass surgery, also known as *laparoscopic surgery*. This procedure requires a shorter recovery period and has fewer postoperative complications. Instead of sawing open the patient's sternum and spreading the ribs apart, several small cuts are made in the torso through which small surgical instruments and fiber-optic cameras are inserted. This procedure was initially designed to correct blockages in just one or two easily reached arteries; it may not be suitable for more complicated cases.

Coronary brachytherapy, which involves delivering beta or gamma radiation into the coronary arteries, may be used in patients who've undergone stent implantation in a coronary artery but then developed such problems as diffuse in-stent restenosis. Brachytherapy is a promising technique, but its use is restricted to the treatment of stent-related problems because of complications and the unknown long-term effects of the radiation. However, in some facilities, brachytherapy is being studied as a first-line treatment of CAD.

▦ **PREVENTION** *Because CAD is so widespread, prevention is of great importance. Encourage dietary restrictions aimed at reducing intake of calories (in obesity) and salt, saturated fats, and cholesterol, in order to minimize the risk, especially when supplemented with regular exercise. Also, encourage the patient to stop smoking and to reduce stress. Other preventive actions to encourage include control of hypertension, control of elevated serum cholesterol or triglyceride levels (with antilipemics), and measures to minimize platelet aggregation and the danger of blood clots (with aspirin or other antiplatelet drugs).*

Special considerations
◆ During anginal episodes, monitor blood pressure and heart rate. Take an ECG during anginal episodes and before administering nitroglycerin or other nitrates. Record duration of pain, amount of medication required to relieve it, and accompanying symptoms.
◆ Keep nitroglycerin available for immediate use. Instruct the patient to call immediately whenever feeling chest, arm, or neck pain.
◆ Before cardiac catheterization, explain the procedure to the patient. Make sure the patient knows why it's necessary, understands the risks, and realizes that it may indicate a need for surgery.
◆ After catheterization, review the expected course of treatment with the patient and family. Monitor the catheter site for bleeding. Also, check for distal pulses. To counter the dye's diuretic effect, make sure the patient drinks plenty of fluids. Assess potassium levels.
◆ If the patient is scheduled for surgery, explain the procedure to the patient and family. Give them a tour of the ICU and introduce them to the staff.

Relieving occlusions with angioplasty

Percutaneous transluminal coronary angioplasty can open an occluded coronary artery without opening the chest—an important advantage over bypass surgery. First, coronary angiography must confirm the presence and location of the arterial occlusion. Then, the physician threads a guide catheter through the patient's femoral or radial artery into the coronary artery under fluoroscopic guidance, as shown at right.

When angiography shows the guide catheter positioned at the occlusion site, the physician carefully inserts a smaller double-lumen balloon catheter through the guide catheter and directs the balloon through the occlusion (opposite page, left). A marked pressure gradient will be obvious.

The physician alternately inflates and deflates the balloon until an angiogram verifies successful arterial dilation (opposite page, right) and the pressure gradient has decreased.

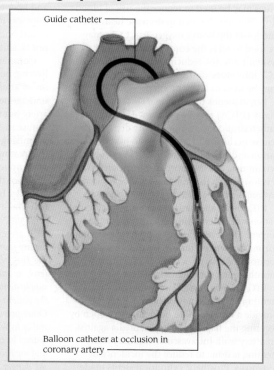

Guide catheter

Balloon catheter at occlusion in coronary artery

♦ After surgery, monitor blood pressure, intake and output, breath sounds, chest tube drainage, and ECG, watching for signs of ischemia and arrhythmias. Also, observe for and treat chest pain and possible dye reactions. Give vigorous chest physiotherapy and guide the patient in removal of secretions through deep breathing, coughing, and expectoration of mucus.

♦ Before discharge, stress the need to follow the prescribed drug regimen (e.g., antihypertensives, nitrates, and antilipemics), exercise program, and diet. Encourage regular, moderate exercise. Refer the patient to a self-help program to stop smoking.

MYOCARDIAL INFARCTION
Causes and incidence

MI, commonly known as a *heart attack* and part of a broader category of disease known as *acute coronary syndrome*, results from prolonged myocardial ischemia due to reduced blood flow through one of the coronary arteries. (See *Tissue destruction in myocardial infarction*, page 40.) In cardiovascular disease, the leading cause of death in the United States and Western Europe, death usually results from the cardiac damage

or complications of MI. (See *Complications of myocardial infarction*, page 41.)

Incidence is high: About 1 million patients visit the hospital each year with an MI, and another 120,000 people die from MI-related complications without seeking medical care. Men and postmenopausal women are more susceptible to MI than premenopausal women, although incidence is rising among females, especially those who smoke and take hormonal contraceptives.

Mortality is high when treatment is delayed, and almost one half of sudden deaths due to an MI occur before hospitalization, within 1 hour of the onset of symptoms. The prognosis improves if vigorous treatment begins immediately.

Predisposing risk factors include:
♦ diabetes mellitus
♦ drug use, especially cocaine
♦ elevated serum triglyceride, total cholesterol, and low-density lipoprotein levels
♦ hypertension
♦ obesity or excessive intake of saturated fats, carbohydrates, or salt
♦ positive family history
♦ sedentary lifestyle

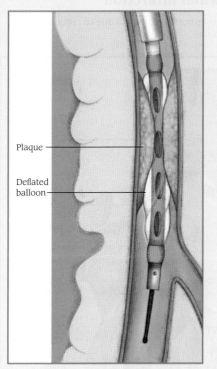

Plaque

Deflated balloon

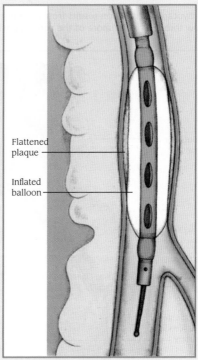

Flattened plaque

Inflated balloon

- ◆ smoking
- ◆ stress or a type A personality

Pathophysiology

The site of the MI depends on the vessels involved. Occlusion of the circumflex branch of the left coronary artery causes a lateral wall infarction; occlusion of the anterior descending branch of the left coronary artery, an anterior wall infarction. True posterior or inferior wall infarctions generally result from occlusion of the right coronary artery or one of its branches. Right ventricular infarctions can also result from right coronary artery occlusion, can accompany inferior infarctions, and may cause right-sided heart failure.

Signs and symptoms

The cardinal symptom of MI is persistent, crushing substernal pain that may radiate to the left arm, jaw, neck, or shoulder blades. Such pain is usually described as heavy, squeezing, or crushing, and may persist for 12 hours or more. However, in some MI patients—particularly elderly people or those with diabetes—pain may not occur at all; in others, it may be mild and confused with indigestion. In patients with

CAD, angina of increasing frequency, severity, or duration (especially if not provoked by exertion, a heavy meal, or cold and wind) may signal impending infarction.

Other clinical effects include a feeling of impending doom, fatigue, nausea, vomiting, and shortness of breath. Some patients may have no symptoms. The patient may experience catecholamine responses, such as coolness in extremities, perspiration, anxiety, and restlessness. Fever is unusual at the onset of an MI, but a low-grade temperature elevation may develop during the next few days. Blood pressure varies; hypotension or hypertension may be present.

The most common post-MI complications include recurrent or persistent chest pain, arrhythmias, left-sided heart failure (resulting in heart failure or acute pulmonary edema), and cardiogenic shock. Unusual but potentially lethal complications that may develop soon after infarction include thromboembolism; papillary muscle dysfunction or rupture, causing mitral insufficiency; rupture of the ventricular septum, causing VSD; rupture of the myocardium; and ventricular aneurysm. Up to several months after infarction, Dressler syndrome (pericarditis, pericardial

Tissue destruction in myocardial infarction

A myocardial infarction results from prolonged myocardial ischemia due to reduced blood flow through one or more of the coronary arteries.

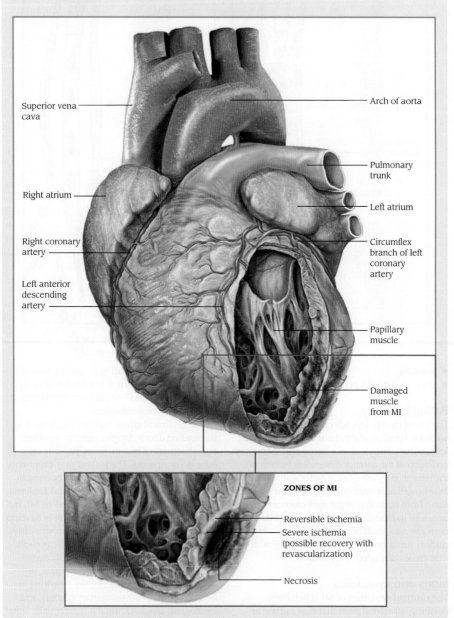

Superior vena cava

Arch of aorta

Pulmonary trunk

Right atrium

Left atrium

Right coronary artery

Circumflex branch of left coronary artery

Left anterior descending artery

Papillary muscle

Damaged muscle from MI

ZONES OF MI

Reversible ischemia

Severe ischemia (possible recovery with revascularization)

Necrosis

Complications of myocardial infarction

Complication	Diagnosis	Treatment
Arrhythmias	◆ Electrocardiogram (ECG) shows premature ventricular contractions, ventricular tachycardia, or ventricular fibrillation; in inferior wall myocardial infarction (MI), bradycardia and junctional rhythms or atrioventricular block; in anterior wall MI, tachycardia or heart block	◆ Antiarrhythmics, atropine, and pacemaker; cardioversion for tachycardia
Heart failure	◆ In left-sided heart failure, chest X-rays show venous congestion, cardiomegaly, and Kerley B lines ◆ Catheterization shows increased pulmonary artery pressure (PAP) and central venous pressure	◆ Diuretics, angiotensin-converting enzyme inhibitors, vasodilators, inotropic agents, cardiac glycosides, and beta-adrenergic blockers
Cardiogenic shock	◆ Catheterization shows decreased cardiac output and increased PAP and pulmonary artery wedge pressure (PAWP) ◆ Signs include hypertension, tachycardia, S_3, S_4, decreased levels of consciousness, decreased urine output, jugular vein distention, and cool, pale skin	◆ I.V. fluids, vasodilators, diuretics, cardiac glycosides, intra-aortic balloon pump (IABP), and beta-adrenergic stimulants
Rupture of left ventricular papillary muscle	◆ Auscultation reveals an apical holosystolic murmur. Inspection of jugular vein pulse or hemodynamic monitoring shows increased v waves ◆ Dyspnea is prominent ◆ Color-flow and Doppler echocardiogram show mitral insufficiency. Pulmonary artery catheterization shows increased PAP and PAWP	◆ Nitroprusside (Nitropress) ◆ IABP ◆ Surgical replacement of the mitral valve with possible concomitant myocardial revascularization (in patients with significant coronary artery disease)
Ventricular septal rupture	◆ In left-to-right shunt, auscultation reveals a holosystolic murmur and thrill ◆ Catheterization shows increased PAP and PAWP ◆ Confirmation is by increased oxygen saturation of the right ventricle and pulmonary artery	◆ Surgical correction, IABP, nitroglycerin, nitroprusside, low-dose inotropic agents, or pacemaker
Pericarditis or Dressler syndrome	◆ Auscultation reveals a friction rub ◆ Chest pain is relieved by sitting up	◆ Aspirin or NSAIDs
	◆ Chest X-ray may show cardiomegaly ◆ ECG may show arrhythmias and persistent ST-segment elevation ◆ Left ventriculography shows altered or paradoxical left ventricular motion	◆ Cardioversion, defibrillation, antiarrhythmics, vasodilators, anticoagulants, cardiac glycosides, and diuretics (if conservative treatment fails, surgical resection is necessary)
Thromboembolism	◆ Severe dyspnea and chest pain or neurologic changes ◆ Nuclear scan shows ventilation–perfusion mismatch ◆ Angiography shows arterial blockage	◆ Oxygen and heparin

friction rub, chest pain, fever, leukocytosis and, possibly, pleurisy or pneumonitis) may develop.

Diagnosis

℞ **CONFIRMING DIAGNOSIS** *Persistent chest pain, elevated ST segment on ECG, and elevated total CK and CK-MB levels over a 72-hour period are consistent with ST-elevation MI (STEMI). Troponin T or troponin I is also used in the diagnosis because both are specific to cardiac necrosis, and levels rise 6 to 8 hours after onset of ischemia. These labs are also useful when no ST-segment elevation occurs, as in non–ST elevation MI (NSTEMI).*

Auscultation may reveal diminished heart sounds, gallops, and, in papillary dysfunction, the apical systolic murmur of mitral insufficiency over the mitral valve area.

When clinical features are equivocal, assume that the patient had an MI until tests rule it out. Diagnostic laboratory results include:

♦ serial 12-lead ECG—ECG abnormalities may be absent or inconclusive during the first few hours after an MI. When present, characteristic abnormalities include serial ST-segment depression NSTEMI and STEMI.

♦ serial serum enzyme levels—CK levels are elevated, specifically, the CK-MB isoenzyme.

♦ echocardiography—may show ventricular wall motion abnormalities.

♦ nuclear ventriculography scans (MUGA or radionuclide ventriculography)—using I.V. radioactive substance, can identify acutely damaged muscle by picking up radioactive nucleotide, which appears as a "hot spot" on the film; useful in localizing a recent MI.

Treatment

The goals of treatment are to relieve chest pain, stabilize heart rhythm, reduce cardiac workload, revascularize the coronary artery, and preserve myocardial tissue. Arrhythmias, the predominant problem during the first 48 hours after the infarction, may require antiarrhythmics, possibly a pacemaker, and, rarely, cardioversion. Arrhythmias are best detected using a 12-lead ECG.

To preserve myocardial tissue is primary percutaneous coronary intervention (PCI) (mechanical reperfusion). PCI has been shown in many studies to be superior to fibrinolysis in the combined end points of death, stroke, and reinfarction when it is performed within 90 minutes of patient arrival. When primary PCI cannot be performed within 90 minutes, thrombolysis is the treatment of choice in STEMI. (See *Comparing thrombolytics,* page 43.)

Other treatments consist of:

♦ lidocaine, vasopressin, or amiodarone for ventricular arrhythmias, or other drugs, such as procainamide, quinidine, or disopyramide

♦ antiplatelet therapy with glycoprotein IIb to IIIa inhibitors, such as clopidogrel for non-STEMI

♦ atropine I.V. or a temporary pacemaker for heart block or bradycardia

♦ nitroglycerin (sublingual, topical, transdermal, or I.V.); CCBs, such as nifedipine, verapamil, or diltiazem (sublingual, oral, or I.V.); or isosorbide dinitrate (sublingual, oral, or I.V.) to relieve pain by redistributing blood to ischemic areas of the myocardium, increasing cardiac output, and reducing myocardial workload

♦ heparin I.V. (usually follows thrombolytic therapy)

♦ morphine I.V. for pain and sedation

♦ bed rest with bedside commode to decrease cardiac workload

♦ oxygen administration at a modest flow rate for 2 to 3 hours (a lower concentration is necessary if the patient has chronic obstructive pulmonary disease)

♦ ACE inhibitors for patients with large anterior wall MIs and for those with an MI and a left ventricular ejection fraction less than 40%

♦ drugs to increase myocardial contractility or blood pressure

♦ BBs, such as carvedilol or atenolol, after acute MI to help prevent reinfarction by reducing the heart's workload

♦ aspirin to inhibit platelet aggregation (should be initiated immediately and continued for years)

♦ pulmonary artery catheterization to detect left- or right-sided heart failure and to monitor the patient's response to treatment.

Special considerations

Care for patients who have suffered an MI is directed toward detecting complications; preventing further myocardial damage; and promoting comfort, rest, and emotional well-being. Most MI patients receive treatment in the ICU or on a telemetry unit, where they're under constant observation for complications.

♦ On admission, monitor and record the patient's ECG, blood pressure, temperature, and heart and breath sounds.

♦ Assess and record the severity and duration of pain, and administer analgesics. Avoid I.M. injections; absorption from the muscle is unpredictable, and bleeding is likely if the patient is receiving thrombolytic therapy.

♦ Check the patient's blood pressure after giving nitroglycerin, especially the first dose.

♦ Frequently monitor the ECG to detect rate changes or arrhythmias. Place rhythm strips in the patient's chart periodically for evaluation.

♦ During episodes of chest pain, obtain 12-lead ECG (before and after nitroglycerin

Comparing thrombolytics

If your patient has suffered a myocardial infarction (MI), you must intervene promptly to minimize cardiac damage and avert death. If appropriate, prepare the patient for thrombolytic therapy as ordered.

Thrombolytic drugs enhance the body's natural ability to dispose of blood clots. To lyse (dissolve) fibrin, the essential component of a clot, tissue activators convert plasminogen to plasmin. A nonspecific protease, plasmin, degrades fibrin, fibrinogen, and procoagulant factors (such as factors V, VII, and XII).

Candidates for thrombolytic therapy include patients with acute ST-segment elevation and chest pain that has lasted no more than 6 hours and who have no access to cardiac catheterization. Timely use of thrombolytic agents can restore myocardial perfusion and prevent further injury. When effective, thrombolytic agents relieve chest pain, restore the ST segment to baseline, and induce reperfusion arrhythmias within 30 to 45 minutes.

Contraindications to thrombolytic therapy include surgery within the past 2 months, active bleeding, a history of stroke, intracranial neoplasm, arteriovenous malformation, aneurysm, or uncontrolled hypertension.

Here's how selected thrombolytics open occluded coronary arteries in patients with an acute MI.

Alteplase (Activase)

This naturally occurring enzyme has been cloned and produced as a drug, alteplase (tissue plasminogen activator). Binding to plasminogen, it catalyzes the conversion of plasminogen to plasmin in the presence of fibrin. Because of its strong affinity for fibrin, alteplase concentrates at the clot site, resulting in a minimal decrease in the fibrinogen level.

This thrombolytic has a half-life of 5 minutes, so maintaining coronary artery patency depends on continued anticoagulation with heparin. Alteplase doesn't induce antigenic responses; doses may be repeated at any time.

Reteplase (Retavase)

Reteplase, recombinant plasminogen activator, has a half-life of 13 to 16 minutes. Its longer half-life allows it to be administered as a bolus. Two boluses are required.

Streptokinase (Streptase)

Streptokinase, a thrombolytic, is a bacterial protein that binds to circulating plasminogen and catalyzes plasmin formation. Its low specificity for fibrin induces a systemic lytic state and increases the risk of bleeding.

The half-life is ~20 minutes. Like anistreplase, streptokinase is antigenic.

Tenecteplase (TNKase)

Tenecteplase is a modified form of human tissue plasminogen activator that binds to fibrin and converts plasminogen to plasmin. It's given as a single bolus dose.

Urokinase (Abbokinase)

Naturally produced by the human kidney, urokinase promotes thrombolysis by directly activating the conversion of plasminogen to plasmin.

With a serum half-life of 10 to 20 minutes, urokinase is rapidly cleared by the kidneys and liver. Unlike streptokinase, it doesn't induce an antigenic response. Urokinase isn't given through a peripheral I.V. line to treat an acute MI, but patients who undergo cardiac catheterization may receive it directly in a coronary artery.

---

therapy as well), blood pressure, and pulmonary artery catheter measurements, and monitor them for changes.

◆ Watch for signs and symptoms of fluid retention (crackles, cough, tachypnea, and edema), which may indicate impending heart failure. Carefully monitor daily weight, intake and output, respirations, serum enzyme levels, and blood pressure. Auscultate for adventitious breath sounds periodically (patients on bed rest frequently have atelectatic crackles, which disappear after coughing), for S_3 or S_4 gallops, and for new-onset heart murmurs.

◆ Organize patient care and activities to maximize periods of uninterrupted rest.

◆ Initiate a cardiac rehabilitation program. This usually includes education regarding heart disease, exercise, and emotional support for the patient and family.

◆ Ask the dietary department to provide a clear liquid diet until nausea subsides. A low-cholesterol, low-sodium, low-fat, high-fiber diet may be prescribed.

◆ Provide a stool softener to prevent straining during defecation, because this causes vagal stimulation and may slow the heart rate. Allow use of a bedside commode and provide as much privacy as possible.

◆ Assist with range-of-motion exercises. If the patient is completely immobilized by a severe

MI, turn often. Antiembolism stockings help prevent venostasis and thrombophlebitis.
◆ Provide emotional support and help reduce stress and anxiety. Explain procedures and answer questions. Explaining the ICU environment and routine can ease anxiety. Involve the patient's family in the care as much as possible.

To prepare the patient for discharge:
◆ Thoroughly explain dosages and therapy to promote compliance with the prescribed medication regimen and other treatment measures. Warn about drug adverse effects, and advise the patient to watch for and report signs of toxicity (anorexia, nausea, vomiting, and yellow vision, e.g., if the patient is receiving digoxin).
◆ Review dietary restrictions with the patient. If the patient must follow a low-sodium or low-fat and low-cholesterol diet, provide a list of foods that the patient should avoid. Ask the dietitian to speak to the patient and family.

PATHOPHYSIOLOGY
What happens in heart failure

Heart failure occurs when cardiac output is inadequate to meet the body's needs. The pathophysiology of heart failure is shown in the flow chart below.

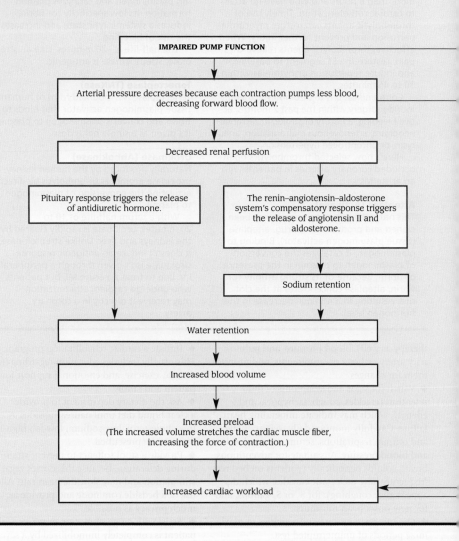

◆ Counsel the patient to resume sexual activity progressively.

◆ Advise the patient to report typical or atypical chest pain. Postinfarction syndrome may develop, producing chest pain that must be differentiated from recurrent MI, pulmonary infarct, or heart failure.

◆ If the patient has a Holter monitor in place, explain its purpose and use.

◆ Stress the need to stop smoking.

◆ Encourage participation in a cardiac rehabilitation program.

◆ Review follow-up procedures and office visits with the patient.

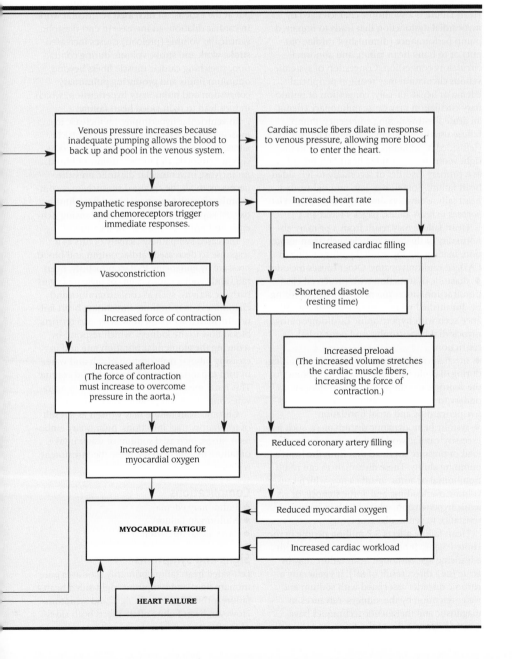

◆ *Instruct patient to practice heart-healthy living, with a heart-healthy diet, regular exercise, stress reduction and preventive care, maintenance of a healthy weight, smoking cessation, and abstinence from alcohol and illegal drugs, especially cocaine.*
◆ *Suggest a daily aspirin regimen for patients with CAD or history of an MI.*

HEART FAILURE

Causes and incidence

Heart failure is a syndrome characterized by myocardial dysfunction that leads to impaired pump performance (diminished cardiac output) or to frank heart failure and abnormal circulatory congestion. Congestion of systemic venous circulation may result in peripheral edema or hepatomegaly; congestion of pulmonary circulation may cause pulmonary edema, an acute life-threatening emergency. Pump failure usually occurs in a damaged left ventricle (left-sided heart failure) but may occur in the right ventricle (right-sided heart failure) either as a primary disorder or secondary to left-sided heart failure. Sometimes, left- and right-sided heart failure develop simultaneously. (See *What happens in heart failure*, pages 44 and 45.)

Heart failure may result from a primary abnormality of the heart muscle such as an infarction, inadequate myocardial perfusion due to CAD, or cardiomyopathy. Other causes include:
◆ diastolic dysfunction with preserved ejection fraction, impairment of ventricular filling by diminished relaxation or reduced compliance seen with hypertrophic cardiomyopathy, myocardial hypertrophy, and pericardial restriction
◆ mechanical disturbances in ventricular filling during diastole when there's too little blood for the ventricle to pump, as in mitral stenosis secondary to rheumatic heart disease or constrictive pericarditis and atrial fibrillation
◆ systolic hemodynamic disturbances, such as excessive cardiac workload due to volume overload or pressure overload that limit the heart's pumping ability. These disturbances can result from mitral or aortic insufficiency, which causes volume overloading, and aortic stenosis or systemic hypertension, which result in increased resistance to ventricular emptying.

Heart failure affects 5.7 million people in the United States. It becomes more common with advancing age. Although heart failure may be acute (as a direct result of MI), it's generally a chronic disorder associated with sodium and water retention by the kidneys. Advances in diagnostic and therapeutic techniques have greatly improved the outlook for patients with heart failure, but the prognosis still depends on the underlying cause and its response to treatment. Fifty percent will diet within 5 years of diagnosis.

Pathophysiology

Reduced cardiac output triggers compensatory mechanisms, such as ventricular dilation, hypertrophy, increased sympathetic activity, and activation of the renin–angiotensin–aldosterone system. These mechanisms improve cardiac output at the expense of increased ventricular work. In cardiac dilation, an increase in end-diastolic ventricular volume (preload) causes increased stroke work and stroke volume during contraction, stretching cardiac muscle fibers beyond optimum limits and producing pulmonary congestion and pulmonary hypertension, which in turn lead to right-sided heart failure.

In ventricular hypertrophy, an increase in muscle mass or diameter of the left ventricle allows the heart to pump against increased resistance (impedance) to the outflow of blood. An increase in ventricular diastolic pressure necessary to fill the enlarged ventricle may compromise diastolic coronary blood flow, limiting oxygen supply to the ventricle and causing ischemia and impaired muscle contractility.

Increased sympathetic activity occurs as a response to decreased cardiac output and blood pressure by enhancing PVR, contractility, heart rate, and venous return. Signs of increased sympathetic activity, such as cool extremities and clamminess, may indicate impending heart failure. Increased sympathetic activity also restricts blood flow to the kidneys, which respond by reducing the glomerular filtration rate and increasing tubular reabsorption of salt and water, in turn expanding the circulating blood volume. This renal mechanism, if unchecked, can aggravate congestion and produce overt edema.

Chronic heart failure may worsen as a result of respiratory tract infections, pulmonary embolism, stress, increased sodium or water intake, or failure to adhere to the prescribed treatment regimen.

Complications
◆ Pulmonary edema
◆ Multiorgan failure
◆ Myocardial infarction

Signs and symptoms

Left-sided heart failure primarily produces pulmonary signs and symptoms; right-sided heart failure, primarily systemic signs and symptoms. However, heart failure often affects both sides of the heart.

Clinical signs of left-sided heart failure include dyspnea, orthopnea, crackles, possibly wheezing, hypoxia, respiratory acidosis, cough, cyanosis or pallor, palpitations, arrhythmias, elevated blood pressure, and pulsus alternans.

Clinical signs of right-sided heart failure include dependent peripheral edema, hepatomegaly, splenomegaly, JVD, ascites, slow weight gain, arrhythmias, positive hepatojugular reflex, abdominal distention, nausea, vomiting, anorexia, weakness, fatigue, dizziness, and syncope.

ALERT *Excessive fluid can accumulate in the pericardium, requiring removal through pericardiocentesis.*

Diagnosis

◆ ECG may reflect heart strain or enlargement, ischemia, or old MI. It may also reveal atrial enlargement, tachycardia, and extrasystoles.

◆ Chest X-ray shows increased pulmonary vascular markings, interstitial edema, or pleural effusion and cardiomegaly.

◆ PAP monitoring typically demonstrates elevated pulmonary artery and PAWPs elevated; left ventricular end-diastolic pressure in left-sided heart failure; and elevated right atrial pressure or CVP in right-sided heart failure.

◆ B-type natriuretic peptide (BNP) is a neurohormone produced predominantly by the ventricles and released in response to blood volume expansion or pressure overload. Blood concentrations greater than 100 pg/mL can be an accurate predictor of acute heart failure.

◆ Echocardiogram may demonstrate wall motion abnormalities and chamber dilation.

Other tests that may also demonstrate enlargement of the heart or decreased functioning include chest computed tomography scan, cardiac MRI, or nuclear scans, such as MUGA and radionuclide ventriculography.

Treatment

The goal of therapy is to improve pump function by reversing the compensatory mechanisms producing the clinical effects, underlying disorders, and precipitating factors. Heart failure can be quickly controlled by treatment consisting of:

◆ ACE inhibitors to decrease PVR

◆ antiembolism stockings to reduce the risk of venostasis and thromboembolus formation

◆ bed rest for acute heart failure

◆ carvedilol, a nonselective BB with alpha-receptor blockade to reduce mortality and improve quality of life

◆ digoxin or dopamine to strengthen myocardial contractility

◆ diuresis to reduce total blood volume and circulatory congestion

◆ inotropic agents, such as dobutamine and milrinone, given I.V. to improve the heart's ability to pump

◆ nesiritide, a recombinant form of endogenous human BNP, to reduce sodium through its diuretic action

◆ vasodilators to increase cardiac output by reducing the impedance to ventricular outflow (afterload).

Excess fluid can be removed through dialysis if necessary. Circulatory assistance can be provided by implanted devices, such as the IABP and the left ventricular assist device (LVAD), but they're only temporary solutions.

A LVAD may be an option for those with refractory heart failure who are not eligible for transplant. This procedure may increase the patient's quality of life.

Watch for and treat complications, which typically may include pulmonary edema (See *Pulmonary edema: How to intervene*, pages 48 and 49); venostasis, with predisposition to thromboembolism (associated primarily with prolonged bed rest); cerebral insufficiency; and renal insufficiency, with severe electrolyte imbalance.

Special considerations

During the acute phase of heart failure:

◆ Give supplemental oxygen to help make breathing easier.

◆ Weigh the patient daily and check for peripheral edema. Carefully monitor I.V. intake and urine output, vital signs, and mental status. Auscultate the heart for abnormal sounds (S_3 gallop) and the lungs for crackles or rhonchi. Report changes at once.

◆ Give the patient a fluid restriction of less than 2 L/day from all sources.

◆ Frequently monitor BUN, creatinine, and serum potassium, sodium, chloride, and magnesium levels.

◆ Make sure the patient has continuous cardiac monitoring during acute and advanced stages to identify and treat arrhythmias promptly.

◆ To reduce the risk of deep vein thrombosis (DVT) due to vascular congestion, assist the patient with range-of-motion exercises. Enforce bed rest and apply antiembolism stockings.

◆ Allow adequate rest periods.

To prepare the patient for discharge:

◆ Advise the patient to avoid foods high in sodium, such as canned or commercially prepared foods and dairy products, to curb fluid overload.

◆ Encourage participation in an outpatient cardiac rehabilitation program.

Pulmonary edema: How to intervene

Obtain the patient history; assist with diagnostic tests; and assess respiratory, mental, and cardiovascular status.

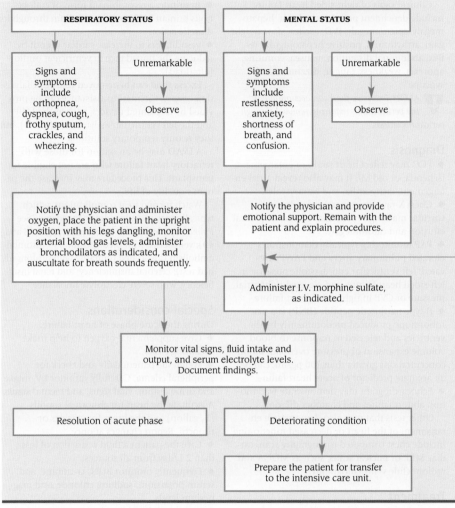

◆ Explain to the patient that the potassium lost through diuretic therapy may need to be replaced by taking a prescribed potassium supplement and eating high-potassium foods, such as bananas and apricots.

◆ Stress the need for regular checkups.

◆ Stress the importance of taking digoxin exactly as prescribed. Tell the patient to watch for and immediately report signs of toxicity, such as anorexia, vomiting, and yellow vision.

◆ Tell the patient to notify the practitioner promptly if his or her pulse is unusually irregular or measures less than 60 beats/minute; if experiencing dizziness, blurred vision, shortness

of breath, a persistent dry cough, palpitations, increased fatigue, paroxysmal nocturnal dyspnea, swollen ankles, or decreased urine output; or if he notices rapid weight gain (3 to 5 lb [1.4 to 2.3 kg] in 1 week).

▚▚▚▚▚ **PREVENTION**

◆ *Instruct patient to make lifestyle modifications, including regular exercise, weight loss, smoking cessation, stress reduction, and reduced sodium, alcohol, and fat intake.*

◆ *Instruct patient to practice compliance with and timely administration of maintenance doses of diuretics and cardiac drugs.*

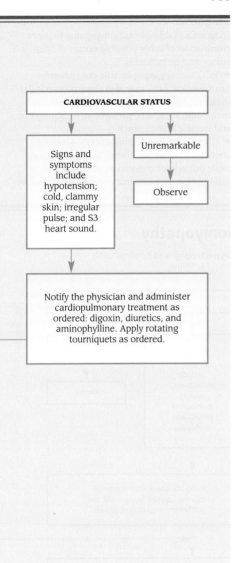

The cause of most cardiomyopathies is unknown. Occasionally, dilated cardiomyopathy results from myocardial destruction by toxic, infectious, or metabolic agents, such as certain viruses, endocrine and electrolyte disorders, nutritional deficiencies, and certain cardiotoxic anticancer drugs (e.g., doxorubicin). Other causes include muscle disorders (myasthenia gravis, progressive muscular dystrophy, and myotonic dystrophy), infiltrative disorders (hemochromatosis and amyloidosis), and sarcoidosis.

Cardiomyopathy may also be a complication of alcoholism. In such cases, it may improve with abstinence from alcohol but recurs when the patient resumes drinking.

Dilated cardiomyopathy occurs in 1 in 2,500 people and affects all ages and both sexes. It's most common in adult men between the ages of 30 and 40.

Pathophysiology

How viruses induce cardiomyopathy is unclear, but researchers suspect a link between viral myocarditis and subsequent dilated cardiomyopathy, especially after infection with poliovirus, coxsackievirus B, influenza virus, or human immunodeficiency virus.

Metabolic cardiomyopathies are related to endocrine and electrolyte disorders and nutritional deficiencies. Thus, dilated cardiomyopathy may develop in patients with hyperthyroidism, pheochromocytoma, beriberi (thiamine deficiency), or kwashiorkor (protein deficiency). Cardiomyopathy may also result from rheumatic fever, especially among children with myocarditis.

Antepartal or postpartal cardiomyopathy may develop during the last trimester or within months after delivery. Its cause is unknown, but it occurs most frequently in multiparous women older than 30, particularly those with malnutrition or preeclampsia. In these patients, cardiomegaly and heart failure may reverse with treatment, allowing a subsequent normal pregnancy. If cardiomegaly persists despite treatment, the prognosis is poor.

Complications

◆ Heart failure
◆ Arrhythmias
◆ Emboli
◆ Ventricular arrhythmias
◆ Syncope
◆ Sudden death

Signs and symptoms

In dilated cardiomyopathy, the heart ejects blood less efficiently than normal. Consequently, a large volume of blood remains in the left

DILATED CARDIOMYOPATHY
Causes and incidence

Dilated cardiomyopathy results from extensively damaged myocardial muscle fibers. It is the most common type of cardiomyopathy. This disorder interferes with myocardial metabolism and grossly dilates all four chambers of the heart, giving the heart a globular appearance and shape. In this disorder, hypertrophy may be present. Dilated cardiomyopathy leads to intractable heart failure, arrhythmias, and emboli. Because this disease isn't usually diagnosed until it's in the advanced stages, the patient's prognosis is generally poor.

ventricle after systole, causing signs of heart failure—both left-sided (shortness of breath, orthopnea, dyspnea on exertion, paroxysmal nocturnal dyspnea, fatigue, and an irritating dry cough at night) and right-sided (edema, liver engorgement, and JVD). Dilated cardiomyopathy also produces peripheral cyanosis and sinus tachycardia or atrial fibrillation at rest in some patients secondary to low cardiac output. Auscultation reveals diffuse apical impulses, pansystolic murmur (mitral and tricuspid insufficiency secondary to cardiomegaly and weak papillary muscles), and S_3 and S_4 gallop rhythms.

Diagnosis

Diagnosis of dilated cardiomyopathy requires elimination of other possible causes of heart failure and arrhythmias.

◆ ECG and angiography rule out ischemic heart disease; ECG may also show biventricular hypertrophy, sinus tachycardia, atrial enlargement, and, in 20% of patients, atrial fibrillation and bundle branch block.

◆ Chest X-ray shows cardiomegaly—usually affecting all heart chambers—and may demonstrate pulmonary congestion, pleural or pericardial effusion, or pulmonary venous hypertension.

Looking at hypertrophic cardiomyopathy

1. The left ventricle and interventricular septum hypertrophy and become stiff, noncompliant, and unable to relax during ventricular filling.

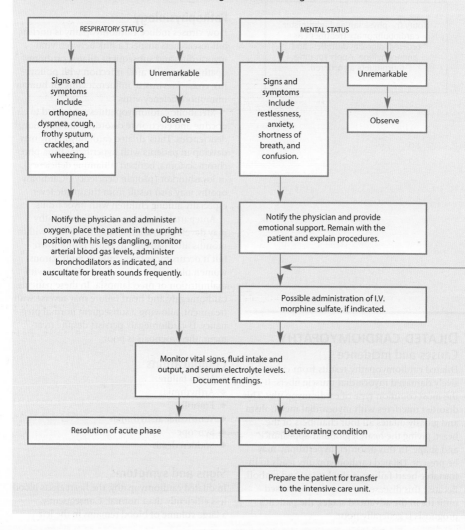

◆ Chest computed tomography scan or echocardiography identifies left ventricular thrombi, global hypokinesia, and degree of left ventricular dilation.

◆ Nuclear heart scans, such as MUGA and ventriculography, show heart enlargement, lung congestion, heart failure, and decreased movement or functioning of the heart.

Treatment

Therapeutic goals include correcting the underlying causes and improving the heart's pumping ability with digoxin, diuretics, oxygen, and a

sodium-restricted diet. Other options include an ACE inhibitor or ARB, a beta-blocker, aspirin, and, potentially, other blood-thinning medications. Vasodilators reduce preload and afterload, thereby decreasing congestion and increasing cardiac output. Acute heart failure requires vasodilation with nitroprusside or nitroglycerin I.V.

When these treatments fail, therapy may require pacemakers, implantable cardiac defibrillations, LVADs, or, as a last resort, a heart transplant for carefully selected patients.

Special considerations

In the patient with acute failure:

◆ Monitor for signs of progressive failure (increasing crackles and dyspnea and increased JVD) and compromised renal perfusion (oliguria, elevated BUN and creatinine levels, and electrolyte imbalances). Weigh the patient daily.

◆ If the patient is receiving vasodilators, check blood pressure and heart rate. If the patient becomes hypotensive, stop the infusion and place in a supine position, with legs elevated to increase venous return and to ensure cerebral blood flow.

◆ If the patient is receiving diuretics, monitor for signs of resolving congestion (decreased crackles and dyspnea) or too-vigorous diuresis. Check serum potassium level for hypokalemia, especially if therapy includes digoxin.

◆ Therapeutic restrictions and an uncertain prognosis usually cause profound anxiety and depression, so offer support and let the patient express his or her feelings. Be flexible with visiting hours.

◆ Before discharge, teach the patient about their illness and its treatment. Emphasize the need to avoid alcohol and smoking, to restrict sodium intake, to watch for weight gain (a weight gain of 3 lb [1.4 kg] over 1 to 2 days indicates fluid accumulation), and to take digoxin as prescribed, watching for its adverse effects (anorexia, nausea, vomiting, and yellow vision).

◆ Encourage family members to learn cardiopulmonary resuscitation (CPR).

HYPERTROPHIC CARDIOMYOPATHY

Causes and incidence

This primary disease of cardiac muscle, also called *idiopathic hypertrophic subaortic stenosis*, is characterized by disproportionate, asymmetrical thickening of the interventricular septum, particularly in the left ventricle's free wall. In hypertrophic cardiomyopathy, cardiac output may be low, normal, or high, depending on whether the stenosis is obstructive or nonobstructive.

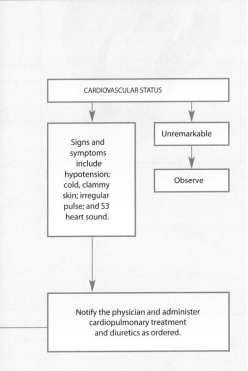

(continued on next page)

Looking at hypertrophic cardiomyopathy (*continued*)

2. As the ventricle's ability to fill decreases, the pressure increases, and left atrial and pulmonary venous pressures rise.

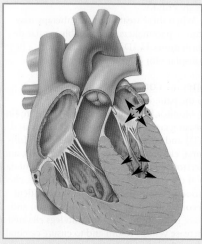

3. The left ventricle forcefully contracts but can't sufficiently relax.

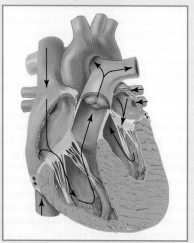

4. The anterior leaflet of the mitral valve is drawn toward the interventricular septum as the blood is forcefully ejected. Early closure of the outflow tract results because of the decreasing ejection fraction.

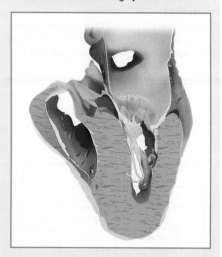

If cardiac output is normal or high, the disorder may go undetected for years; but low cardiac output may lead to potentially fatal heart failure. The disease course varies; some patients progressively deteriorate; others remain stable for years. (See *Looking at hypertrophic cardiomyopathy*, pages 50 to 52.)

This disorder affects 1 in 500 people and is more common in men than in women and more so in blacks than in whites. It is also usually the cause of sudden death, particularly in otherwise healthy athletes.

Pathophysiology

Despite being designated as idiopathic, hypertrophic cardiomyopathy may be inherited as a non–sex-linked autosomal dominant trait in almost all cases. Most patients have obstructive disease, resulting from effects of ventricular septal hypertrophy and the movement of the anterior mitral valve leaflet into the outflow tract during systole. Eventually, left ventricular dysfunction, from rigidity and decreased compliance, causes pump failure.

Complications
◆ Pulmonary hypertension
◆ Heart failure
◆ Ventricular arrhythmias
◆ Sudden death

Signs and symptoms
Clinical features of the disorder may not appear until it's well advanced, when atrial dilation and, possibly, atrial fibrillation abruptly reduce blood flow to the left ventricle. Reduced inflow and subsequent low output may produce angina pectoris, arrhythmias, dyspnea, orthopnea, syncope, heart failure, and death. Auscultation reveals a medium-pitched systolic ejection murmur along the left sternal border and at the apex; palpation reveals a peripheral pulse with a characteristic double impulse (pulsus bisferiens) and, with atrial fibrillation, an irregular pulse.

Diagnosis
Diagnosis depends on typical clinical findings and these test results:
◆ Echocardiography (most useful) shows increased thickness of the intraventricular septum and abnormal motion of the anterior mitral leaflet during systole, occluding left ventricular outflow in obstructive disease.
◆ Cardiac catheterization reveals elevated left ventricular end-diastolic pressure and, possibly, mitral insufficiency.
◆ ECG usually shows left ventricular hypertrophy, T-wave inversion, left anterior hemiblock, Q waves in precordial and inferior leads, ventricular arrhythmias, and, possibly, atrial fibrillation.
◆ Auscultation confirms an early systolic murmur.

Treatment
The goals of treatment are to relax the ventricle and to relieve outflow tract obstruction. Agents such as metoprolol, a BB, slow heart rate and increase ventricular filling by relaxing the obstructing muscle, thereby reducing angina, syncope, dyspnea, and arrhythmias. Atrial fibrillation necessitates cardioversion to treat the arrhythmia and, because of the high risk of systemic embolism, anticoagulant therapy until

fibrillation subsides. Because vasodilators such as nitroglycerin reduce venous return by permitting pooling of blood in the periphery, decreasing ventricular volume and chamber size, and may cause further obstruction, they're contraindicated in patients with hypertrophic cardiomyopathy. Also contraindicated are ACE inhibitors and ARBs because they can also worsen the obstruction. Disopyramide is preferred because of its negative inotropic properties. Patients with potentially lethal arrhythmias may need an implantable cardioverter–defibrillator to prevent sudden death.

If drug therapy fails, surgery is indicated. Septal myectomy reduces the thickness of the septum through removal of a portion of the proximal septum. This can be performed alone or in combination with mitral valve replacement, which may ease outflow tract obstruction and relieve symptoms. However, complications, such as complete heart block and VSD, can occur, requiring pacemaker implantation.

Special considerations
◆ Because syncope or sudden death may follow well-tolerated exercise, warn such patients against strenuous physical activity such as running.
◆ Administer medications as prescribed. *Caution:* Avoid nitroglycerin, digoxin, and diuretics because they can worsen obstruction. Warn the patient not to stop taking their beta-blocker abruptly, because doing so may increase myocardial demands. To determine the patient's tolerance for an increased dosage of the beta-blocker, take his or her pulse to check for bradycardia. Also take a blood pressure reading while the patient is supine and while standing (a drop in blood pressure [>10 mm Hg] when standing may indicate orthostatic hypotension).
◆ Before dental work or surgery, tell the patient to discuss prophylaxis for subacute infective endocarditis with his or her healthcare provider.
◆ Provide psychological support. If the patient is hospitalized for a long time, be flexible with visiting hours and encourage occasional weekends away from the hospital, if possible. Refer the patient for psychosocial counseling to help the patient and family accept restricted lifestyle and poor prognosis.
◆ If the patient is a child, have the parents arrange for them to continue school work or studies in the healthcare facility.
◆ Because sudden cardiac arrest is possible, urge the patient's family to learn cardiopulmonary resuscitation.

Cardiac complications

HYPOVOLEMIC SHOCK

Causes and incidence

In hypovolemic shock, reduced intravascular blood volume causes circulatory dysfunction and inadequate tissue perfusion. Without sufficient blood or fluid replacement, hypovolemic shock syndrome may lead to irreversible cerebral and renal damage, cardiac arrest, and, ultimately, death. Hypovolemic shock requires early recognition of signs and symptoms and prompt, aggressive treatment to improve the prognosis. (See *What happens in hypovolemic shock*, page 55.)

Hypovolemic shock usually results from acute blood loss—about one fifth of total volume. Such massive blood loss may result from GI bleeding, internal hemorrhage (hemothorax and hemoperitoneum), external hemorrhage (accidental or surgical trauma), or from any condition that reduces circulating intravascular plasma volume or other body fluids such as in severe burns. Other underlying causes of hypovolemic shock include intestinal obstruction, peritonitis, acute pancreatitis, ascites and dehydration from excessive perspiration, severe diarrhea or protracted vomiting, diabetes insipidus, diuresis, or inadequate fluid intake.

Pathophysiology

Hypovolemic shock occurs when there is not enough intravascular volume to maintain tissue perfusion. At first, the body responds by stimulating thirst and reducing the amount of fluid filtered through the kidneys. Additionally, heart rate becomes elevated to increase cardiac output, contractility increases to maintain stroke volume, and increased systemic vascular resistance shunts blood away from the periphery and toward the heart and central nervous system. Hypotension is a late sign since blood pressure can be maintained initially through compensatory vasoconstriction, which decreases tissue perfusion. Cardiac arrest may occur soon after.

Complications

- Acute respiratory distress syndrome
- Acute tubular necrosis
- Disseminated intravascular coagulation (DIC)
- Multiple-organ-dysfunction syndrome

Signs and symptoms

Hypovolemic shock produces a syndrome of hypotension, with narrowing pulse pressure; decreased sensorium; tachycardia; rapid, shallow respirations; reduced urine output (<25 mL/hour); and cold, pale, clammy skin. Metabolic acidosis with an accumulation of lactic acid develops as a result of tissue anoxia, as cellular metabolism shifts from aerobic to anaerobic pathways. DIC is a possible complication of hypovolemic shock.

Diagnosis

No single symptom or diagnostic test establishes the diagnosis or severity of shock. Characteristic laboratory findings include:

- elevated potassium, serum lactate, and BUN levels
- increased urine specific gravity (>1.020) and urine osmolality
- decreased blood pH and partial pressure of arterial oxygen and increased partial pressure of arterial carbon dioxide.

In addition, gastroscopy, aspiration of gastric contents through a nasogastric (NG) tube, computed tomography scan, and X-rays identify internal bleeding sites; coagulation studies may detect coagulopathy from DIC. Echocardiography or right heart catheterization can help differentiate between hypovolemic and cardiogenic shock.

Treatment

Emergency treatment measures must include prompt and adequate blood and fluid replacement to restore intravascular volume and raise blood pressure. Saline solution or lactated Ringer solution, then possibly plasma proteins (albumin) or other plasma expanders, may produce adequate volume expansion until whole blood can be matched. A rapid solution infusion system of 1 to 2 L of isotonic crystalloids can be used and continued if hypotension persists. Measuring CVP can assist in directing therapy. Treatment may also include oxygen administration, identification of bleeding site, control of bleeding by direct measures (such as application of pressure and elevation of a limb) and, possibly, surgery.

Special considerations

Management of hypovolemic shock necessitates prompt, aggressive supportive measures and careful assessment and monitoring of vital signs. Follow these priorities:

- Check for a patent airway and adequate circulation. If blood pressure and heart rate are absent, start CPR.
- Record blood pressure, pulse rate, peripheral pulses, respiratory rate, and other vital signs every 15 minutes and the electrocardiograph

PATHOPHYSIOLOGY

What happens in hypovolemic shock

In hypovolemic shock, vascular fluid volume loss causes extreme tissue hypoperfusion. Internal fluid losses can result from hemorrhage or third-space fluid shifting. External fluid loss can result from severe bleeding or from severe diarrhea, diuresis, or vomiting. Inadequate vascular volume leads to decreased venous return and cardiac output. The resulting drop in arterial blood pressure activates the body's compensatory mechanisms in an attempt to increase vascular volume. If compensation is unsuccessful, decompensation and death may occur.

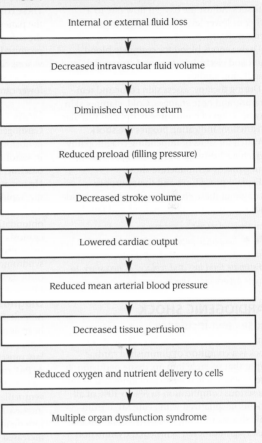

Internal or external fluid loss

↓

Decreased intravascular fluid volume

↓

Diminished venous return

↓

Reduced preload (filling pressure)

↓

Decreased stroke volume

↓

Lowered cardiac output

↓

Reduced mean arterial blood pressure

↓

Decreased tissue perfusion

↓

Reduced oxygen and nutrient delivery to cells

↓

Multiple organ dysfunction syndrome

---

continuously. Systolic blood pressure lower than 80 mm Hg usually results in inadequate coronary artery blood flow, cardiac ischemia, arrhythmias, and further complications of low cardiac output. When blood pressure drops below 80 mm Hg, increase the oxygen flow rate and notify the practitioner immediately. A progressive drop in blood pressure, accompanied by a thready pulse, generally signals inadequate cardiac output from reduced intravascular volume. Notify the practitioner and increase the infusion rate.

◆ Start I.V. lines with normal saline or lactated Ringer solution, using a large-bore catheter (14G), which allows easier administration of later blood transfusions. (*Caution:* Don't start

I.V. lines in the legs of a patient in shock who has suffered abdominal trauma, because infused fluid may escape through the ruptured vessel into the abdomen.)

◆ An indwelling urinary catheter may be inserted to measure hourly urine output. If output is less than 30 mL/hour in adults, increase the fluid infusion rate, but watch for signs of fluid overload such as an increase in PAWP. Notify the practitioner if urine output doesn't improve. An osmotic diuretic such as mannitol may be ordered to increase renal blood flow and urine output. Determine how much fluid to give by checking blood pressure, urine output, CVP, or PAWP. (To increase accuracy, CVP should be measured at the level of the right atrium, using the same reference point on the chest each time.)

◆ Draw an arterial blood sample to measure blood gas levels. Administer oxygen by face mask or airway to ensure adequate oxygenation of tissues. Adjust the oxygen flow rate to a higher or lower level, as blood gas measurements indicate.

◆ Draw venous blood for complete blood count and electrolyte, type and crossmatch, and coagulation studies.

◆ During therapy, assess skin color and temperature, and note changes. Cold, clammy skin may be a sign of continuing peripheral vascular constriction, indicating progressive shock.

◆ Watch for signs of impending coagulopathy (petechiae, bruising, and bleeding or oozing from gums or venipuncture sites).

◆ Explain procedures and their purpose. Throughout these emergency measures, provide emotional support to the patient and family.

⁞⁞⁞⁞⁞ PREVENTION
◆ *Recognize patients with conditions that reduce blood volume as at-risk patients.*
◆ *Estimate fluid loss and replace, as necessary, to prevent hypovolemic shock.*

CARDIOGENIC SHOCK
Causes and incidence
Sometimes called *pump failure,* cardiogenic shock is a condition of diminished cardiac output that severely impairs tissue perfusion. It reflects severe left-sided heart failure and occurs as a serious complication in 5% to 10% of all patients hospitalized with acute MI. Cardiogenic shock can result from any condition that causes significant left ventricular dysfunction with reduced cardiac output, such as MI (most common), myocardial ischemia, papillary muscle dysfunction, or end-stage cardiomyopathy. The incidence of cardiogenic shock is higher those with an elevated body mass index, and also higher in men than in women because of their higher incidence of CAD. Historically, mortality for cardiogenic shock had been 80% to 90%, but recent studies indicate that the rate has dropped to 40% to 50% due to improved interventional procedures and better therapies. Mortality is expected to decline even further.

Pathophysiology
Regardless of the underlying cause, left ventricular dysfunction sets into motion a series of compensatory mechanisms that attempt to increase cardiac output and, in turn, maintain vital organ function. (See *What happens in cardiogenic shock,* page 57.) As cardiac output falls

in left ventricular dysfunction, aortic and carotid baroreceptors initiate sympathetic nervous responses, which increase heart rate, left ventricular filling pressure, and peripheral resistance to flow, to enhance venous return to the heart. These compensatory responses initially stabilize the patient but later cause deterioration with the rising oxygen demands of the already compromised myocardium. These events comprise a vicious circle of low cardiac output, sympathetic compensation, myocardial ischemia, and even lower cardiac output.

Signs and symptoms
Cardiogenic shock produces signs of poor tissue perfusion: cold, pale, clammy skin; a decrease in systolic blood pressure to 30 mm Hg below baseline, or a sustained reading below 80 mm Hg not attributable to medication; tachycardia; rapid, shallow respirations; oliguria (<20 mL/hour); restlessness; mental confusion and obtundation; narrowing pulse pressure; and cyanosis. Although many of these clinical features also occur in heart failure and other shock syndromes, they're usually more profound in cardiogenic shock.

Diagnosis
Auscultation may detect gallop rhythm, faint heart sounds, and, possibly, if the shock results from rupture of the ventricular septum or papillary muscles, a holosystolic murmur.

◆ PAP monitoring may show increased PAP and increased PAWP, reflecting a rise in left ventricular end-diastolic pressure (preload) and increased resistance to left ventricular emptying (afterload) due to ineffective pumping and increased PVR. Thermodilution technique measures decreased cardiac output.

◆ Invasive arterial pressure monitoring may indicate hypotension due to impaired ventricular ejection.

◆ ABG analysis may show metabolic acidosis and hypoxia.

◆ ECG may show possible evidence of acute MI, ischemia, or ventricular aneurysm.

◆ Echocardiography can determine left ventricular function and reveal valvular abnormalities.

◆ Enzyme levels may show elevated CK, lactate dehydrogenase, aspartate aminotransferase, and alanine aminotransferase, which point to MI or ischemia and suggest heart failure or shock. Troponin I, troponin T, and CK may confirm acute MI.

Additional tests determine other conditions that can lead to pump dysfunction and failure, such as cardiac arrhythmias, cardiac tamponade, papillary muscle infarct or rupture, ventricular

PATHOPHYSIOLOGY
What happens in cardiogenic shock

When the myocardium can't contract sufficiently to maintain adequate cardiac output, stroke volume decreases, and the heart can't eject an adequate volume of blood with each contraction. The blood backs up behind the weakened left ventricle, increasing preload and causing pulmonary congestion. In addition, to compensate for the drop in stroke volume, the heart rate increases in an attempt to maintain cardiac output. As a result of the diminished stroke volume, coronary artery perfusion and collateral blood flow decrease. All of these mechanisms increase the heart's workload and enhance left-sided heart failure. The result is myocardial hypoxia, further decreased cardiac output, and a triggering of compensatory mechanisms to prevent decompensation and death.

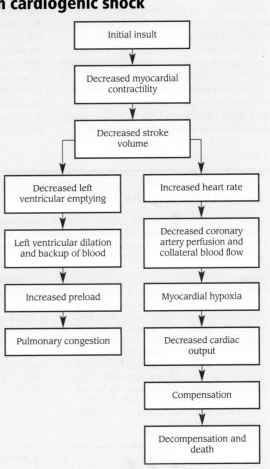

septal rupture, pulmonary emboli, venous pooling (associated with vasodilators and continuous intermittent positive-pressure breathing), and hypovolemia.

Treatment

The aim of treatment is to enhance cardiovascular status by increasing cardiac output, improving myocardial perfusion, and decreasing cardiac workload with combinations of various cardiovascular drugs and mechanical-assist techniques. Myocardial reperfusion can be accomplished by PTCA, stents, thrombolytic therapy, or bypass grafting. Drug therapy may include dopamine I.V., a vasopressor that increases cardiac output, blood pressure, and renal blood

flow; milrinone or dobutamine I.V., inotropic agents that increase myocardial contractility; norepinephrine, when a more potent vasoconstrictor is necessary; and nitroprusside I.V., a vasodilator that may be used with a vasopressor to further improve cardiac output by decreasing PVR (afterload) and reducing left ventricular end-diastolic pressure (preload). However, the patient's blood pressure must be adequate to support nitroprusside therapy and must be monitored closely.

The IABP is a mechanical-assist device that attempts to improve coronary artery perfusion and decrease cardiac workload. (See *Understanding the IABP*, page 58.) The inflatable balloon pump is percutaneously or surgically inserted through the femoral artery into the descending thoracic aorta. The balloon inflates during diastole to increase coronary artery perfusion pressure and deflates before systole (before the aortic valve opens) to reduce resistance to ejection (afterload) and reduce cardiac workload. Improved ventricular ejection, which significantly improves cardiac output, and a subsequent vasodilation in the peripheral vasculature lead to lower preload volume.

When drug therapy and IABP insertion fail, treatment may require the use of a ventricular assist device. This device (which may be either temporary or permanent) diverts systemic blood flow from a diseased ventricle into a centrifugal pump. It assists the heart's pumping action rather than replacing it.

Special considerations

◆ At the first sign of cardiogenic shock, check the patient's blood pressure and heart rate. If the patient is hypotensive or is having difficulty breathing, ensure a patent I.V. line and a patent airway, and provide oxygen to promote tissue oxygenation. Notify the practitioner immediately.

◆ Monitor ABG values to measure oxygenation and detect acidosis from poor tissue perfusion.

Understanding the IABP

An intra-aortic balloon pump (IABP) consists of a polyurethane balloon attached to an external pump console by means of a large-lumen catheter. It is inserted percutaneously through the femoral artery and positioned in the descending aorta, just distal to the left subclavian artery and above the renal arteries.

Push. . .

This external pump works in precise counterpoint to the left ventricle, inflating the balloon with helium early in diastole and deflating it just before systole. As the balloon inflates, it forces blood toward the aortic valve, thereby raising pressure in the aortic root and augmenting diastolic pressure to improve coronary perfusion. It also improves peripheral circulation by forcing blood through the brachiocephalic, common carotid, and subclavian arteries arising from the aortic trunk.

. . .and Pull

The balloon deflates rapidly at the end of diastole, creating a vacuum in the aorta. This reduces aortic volume and pressure, thereby decreasing the resistance to left ventricular ejection (afterload). This decreased workload, in turn, reduces the heart's oxygen requirements and, combined with the improved myocardial perfusion, helps prevent or diminish myocardial ischemia.

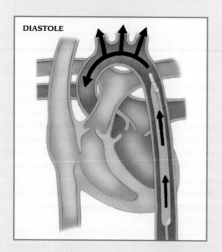

DIASTOLE

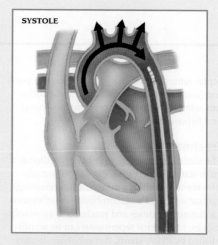

SYSTOLE

Increase oxygen delivery as indicated. Check complete blood count and electrolyte levels.

◆ After diagnosis, monitor cardiac rhythm continuously and assess skin color, temperature, and other vital signs often. Watch for a drop in systolic blood pressure to less than 80 mm Hg (usually compromising cardiac output further). Report hypotension immediately.

◆ An indwelling urinary catheter may be inserted to measure urine output. Notify the practitioner if output drops below 30 mL/hour.

◆ Using a pulmonary artery catheter, closely monitor PAP, PAWP, and, if equipment is available, cardiac output. A high PAWP indicates heart failure and should be reported.

◆ When a patient is on the IABP, reposition the patient often and perform passive range-of-motion exercises to prevent skin breakdown. However, don't flex the patient's "ballooned" leg at the hip because this may displace or fracture the catheter. Assess pedal pulses and skin temperature and color to make sure circulation to the leg is adequate. Check the dressing on the insertion site frequently for bleeding, and change it according to facility protocol. Also, check the site for hematoma or signs of infection, and culture any drainage.

◆ After the patient becomes hemodynamically stable, the frequency of balloon inflation is gradually reduced to wean from the IABP. During weaning, carefully watch for monitor changes, chest pain, and other signs of recurring cardiac ischemia and shock.

◆ Provide psychological support and reassurance because the patient and family may be anxious about the ICU, IABP, and other tubes and devices. To ease emotional stress, plan your care to allow frequent rest periods, and provide as much privacy as possible.

:::::: PREVENTION *Emphasize the fact that prevention requires timely, thorough, and aggressive identification and treatment of causative disorders.*

VENTRICULAR ANEURYSM
Causes and incidence
A ventricular aneurysm is an outpouching, almost always of the left ventricle, that produces ventricular wall dysfunction in about 25% of patients after MI. Ventricular aneurysm may develop within weeks after MI. Untreated ventricular aneurysm can lead to arrhythmias, systemic embolization, or heart failure and may cause sudden death. Resection improves the prognosis in patients with heart failure or refractory patients who have developed ventricular arrhythmias.

Pathophysiology
When MI destroys a large muscular section of the left ventricle, necrosis reduces the ventricular wall to a thin sheath of fibrous tissue. Under intracardiac pressure, this thin layer stretches and forms a separate noncontractile sac (aneurysm). Abnormal muscular wall movement accompanies ventricular aneurysm and includes akinesia (lack of movement), dyskinesia (paradoxical movement), asynergia (decreased and inadequate movement), and asynchrony (uncoordinated movement). During systolic ejection, the abnormal muscular wall movements associated with the aneurysm cause the remaining normally functioning myocardial fibers to increase the force of contraction to maintain stroke volume and cardiac output. At the same time, a portion of the stroke volume is lost to passive distention of the noncontractile sac.

Complications
◆ Ventricular arrhythmias
◆ Cerebral embolism
◆ Heart failure
◆ Death

Signs and symptoms
Ventricular aneurysm may cause arrhythmias—such as premature ventricular contractions or ventricular tachycardia—palpitations, signs of cardiac dysfunction (weakness on exertion, fatigue, and angina) and, occasionally, a visible or palpable systolic precordial bulge. This condition may also lead to left ventricular dysfunction, with chronic heart failure (dyspnea, fatigue, edema, crackles, gallop rhythm, and JVD); pulmonary edema; systemic embolization; and, with left-sided heart failure, pulsus alternans. Ventricular aneurysms enlarge but seldom rupture.

Diagnosis
Persistent ventricular arrhythmias, onset of heart failure, or systemic embolization in a patient with left-sided heart failure and a history of MI strongly suggest ventricular aneurysm. Indicative tests include the following:

◆ Left ventriculography during catheterization reveals left ventricular enlargement, with an area of akinesia or dyskinesia and diminished cardiac function.

◆ ECG may show persistent ST–T wave elevations after infarction.

◆ Chest X-ray may demonstrate an abnormal bulge distorting the heart's contour if the aneurysm is large; the X-ray may be normal if the aneurysm is small.

♦ Noninvasive nuclear cardiology scan may indicate the site of infarction and suggest the area of aneurysm.

♦ Echocardiography shows abnormal motion in the left ventricular wall.

♦ MRI gives excellent visualization of the heart's apex.

Treatment

Depending on the aneurysm's size and the complications, treatment may necessitate only routine medical examination to follow the patient's condition or aggressive measures for intractable ventricular arrhythmias, heart failure, and emboli.

Emergency treatment of ventricular arrhythmia includes antiarrhythmics I.V. or cardioversion. Preventive treatment continues with medications that decrease afterload to increase left ventricular function such as ACE inhibitors, anti-ischemic medications for angina, and anticoagulation if thrombus formation.

Emergency treatment for heart failure with pulmonary edema includes oxygen, cardiac glycosides I.V., furosemide I.V., morphine I.V., and, when necessary, nitroprusside I.V. and intubation. Maintenance therapy may include nitrates, prazosin, and oral hydralazine. Systemic embolization requires anticoagulation therapy or embolectomy. Refractory ventricular tachycardia, heart failure, recurrent arterial embolization, and persistent angina with coronary artery occlusion may necessitate surgery, of which the most effective procedure is aneurysmectomy with myocardial revascularization.

Special considerations

♦ If ventricular tachycardia occurs, administer a prescribed antiarrhythmic such as lidocaine. Monitor blood pressure and heart rate. If cardiac arrest develops, initiate CPR and call for assistance, resuscitative equipment, and medication.

♦ In a patient with heart failure, closely monitor vital signs, heart sounds, intake and output, fluid and electrolyte balances, and BUN and creatinine levels. Because of the threat of systemic embolization, frequently check peripheral pulses and the color and temperature of extremities. Be alert for sudden changes in sensorium that indicate cerebral embolization and for any signs that suggest renal failure or progressive MI.

If the patient is scheduled to undergo resection:

♦ Before surgery, explain expected postoperative care in the ICU (including use of such things as endotracheal [ET] tube, ventilator, hemodynamic monitoring, chest tubes, and drainage bottle).

♦ After surgery, monitor vital signs, intake and output, heart sounds, and pulmonary artery catheter. Watch for signs of infection, such as fever and drainage.

To prepare the patient for discharge:

♦ Teach how to check for pulse irregularity and rate changes. Encourage the patient to follow the prescribed medication regimen—even during the night—and to watch for adverse effects.

♦ Because arrhythmias can cause sudden death, refer the family to a community-based CPR training program.

♦ Provide psychological support for the patient and family.

CARDIAC TAMPONADE

Causes and incidence

In cardiac tamponade, a rapid, unchecked rise in intrapericardial pressure impairs diastolic filling of the heart. The rise in pressure usually results from blood or fluid accumulation in the pericardial sac. If fluid accumulates rapidly, this condition requires emergency lifesaving measures to prevent death. A slow accumulation and rise in pressure, as in pericardial effusion associated with malignant tumors, may not produce immediate symptoms, because the fibrous wall of the pericardial sac can gradually stretch to accommodate as much as 1 to 2 L of fluid.

Increased intrapericardial pressure and cardiac tamponade may be idiopathic (Dressler syndrome) or may result from:

♦ effusion (in cancer, bacterial infections, tuberculosis, and, rarely, acute rheumatic fever)

♦ hemorrhage from trauma (such as gunshot or stab wounds of the chest and perforation by catheter during cardiac or central venous catheterization or postcardiac surgery)

♦ hemorrhage from nontraumatic causes (such as rupture of the heart or great vessels or anticoagulant therapy in a patient with pericarditis)

♦ acute MI

♦ end-stage lung cancer

♦ heart tumors

♦ radiation therapy

♦ hypothyroidism

♦ systemic lupus erythematosus

♦ uremia.

Cardiac tamponade occurs in 2 of every 10,000 people.

Pathophysiology

Increased fluid in the pericardial space leads to increased pressure. The right ventricle is unable to expand adequately, and so pressure shifts

Normal cardiac conduction

The conduction system of the heart begins with the heart's pacemaker: the sinoatrial (SA) node. When an impulse leaves the SA node, it travels through the atria along the Bachmann bundle and the internodal tracts on its way to the atrioventricular (AV) node. After the impulse passes through the AV node, it travels to the ventricles, first down the bundle of His, then along the bundle branches and, finally, down the Purkinje fibers.

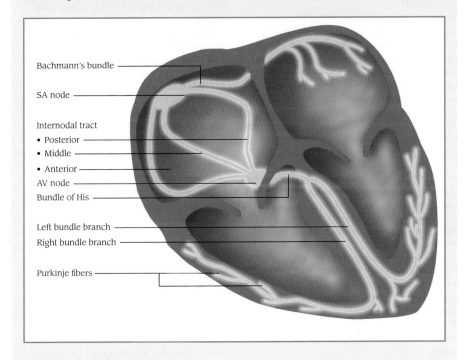

Bachmann's bundle

SA node

Internodal tract
• Posterior
• Middle
• Anterior
AV node
Bundle of His

Left bundle branch
Right bundle branch

Purkinje fibers

the interventricular septum to the left. This decreases the left ventricle end-diastolic volume, resulting in decreased cardiac output and hypotension.

Complications
◆ Cardiogenic shock
◆ Death

Signs and symptoms
Cardiac tamponade classically produces increased venous pressure with JVD, reduced arterial blood pressure, muffled heart sounds on auscultation, and pulsus paradoxus (an abnormal inspiratory drop in systemic blood pressure >15 mm Hg). The absence of a preexisting pericardial friction rub may suggest an increase in fluid in the pericardial space. These classic symptoms represent failure of physiologic compensatory mechanisms to override the effects of rapidly rising pericardial pressure, which limits

diastolic filling of the ventricles and reduces stroke volume to a critically low level. Generally, ventricular end-systolic volume may drop because of inadequate preload. The increasing pericardial pressure is transmitted equally across the heart cavities, producing a matching rise in intracardiac pressure, especially atrial and end-diastolic ventricular pressures. Cardiac tamponade may also cause dyspnea, diaphoresis, pallor or cyanosis, anxiety, tachycardia, narrow pulse pressure, restlessness, and hepatomegaly, but the lung fields will be clear. The patient typically sits upright and leans forward.

Diagnosis
◆ Chest X-ray shows slightly widened mediastinum and cardiomegaly.
◆ ECG is rarely diagnostic of tamponade but is useful in ruling out other cardiac disorders. It may reveal changes produced by acute pericarditis.

◆ Pulmonary artery catheterization detects increased right atrial pressure, right ventricular diastolic pressure, and CVP.
◆ Echocardiography, computed tomography scan, or MRI shows pericardial effusion with signs of right ventricular and atrial compression.

Treatment

The goal of treatment is to relieve intrapericardial pressure and cardiac compression by removing accumulated blood or fluid. Pericardiocentesis (needle aspiration of the pericardial cavity) or surgical creation of an opening (pericardiectomy or pericardial window) dramatically improves systemic arterial pressure and cardiac output with aspiration of as little as 25 mL of fluid. Such treatment necessitates continuous hemodynamic and ECG monitoring in the ICU. Trial volume loading with temporary I.V. normal saline solution and perhaps an inotropic drug, such as isoproterenol or dopamine, may be necessary in the hypotensive patient to maintain cardiac output. Although these drugs normally improve myocardial function, they may further compromise an ischemic myocardium after MI.

Depending on the cause of tamponade, additional treatment may include:
◆ in traumatic injury—blood transfusion or a thoracotomy to drain reaccumulating fluid or to repair bleeding sites
◆ in heparin-induced tamponade (not often used)—the heparin antagonist protamine sulfate
◆ in warfarin-induced tamponade—vitamin K.

Resection of a portion or all of the pericardium to allow full communication with the pleura may be needed if repeated pericardiocentesis fails to prevent recurrence.

Special considerations

If the patient needs pericardiocentesis:
◆ Explain the procedure to him. Keep a pericardial aspiration needle attached to a 50-mL syringe by a three-way stopcock, an ECG machine, and an emergency cart with a defibrillator at the bedside. Make sure the equipment is turned on and ready for immediate use. Position the patient at a 45- to 60-degree angle. Connect the precordial ECG lead to the hub of the aspiration needle with an alligator clamp and connecting wire, and assist with fluid aspiration. When the needle touches the myocardium, you'll see an ST-segment elevation or premature ventricular contractions.
◆ Monitor blood pressure and CVP during and after pericardiocentesis. Infuse I.V. solutions, as

prescribed, to maintain blood pressure. Watch for a decrease in CVP and a concomitant rise in blood pressure, which indicate relief of cardiac compression.
◆ Watch for complications of pericardiocentesis, such as ventricular fibrillation, vasovagal response, or coronary artery or cardiac chamber puncture. Closely monitor ECG changes, blood pressure, pulse rate, LOC, and urine output.

If the patient needs thoracotomy:
◆ Explain the procedure to him. Tell the patient what to expect postoperatively (chest tubes, drainage bottles, and oxygen administration). Teach the patient how to turn, deep breathe, and cough.
◆ Give antibiotics, protamine sulfate, or vitamin K, as ordered.
◆ Postoperatively, monitor critical parameters, such as vital signs and ABG values, and assess heart and breath sounds. Give pain medication as ordered. Maintain the chest drainage system and be alert for complications, such as hemorrhage and arrhythmias.

▓▓▓ PREVENTION *Instruct patient to practice heart-healthy living, with a heart-healthy diet, stress reduction, regular exercise and preventive care, maintenance of a healthy weight, smoking cessation, and abstinence from alcohol.*

CARDIAC ARRHYTHMIAS

Causes and incidence

Arrhythmias may be congenital or may result from one of several factors, including myocardial ischemia, MI, or organic heart disease. Drug ingestion (cocaine, amphetamines, caffeine, BBs, psychotropics, sympathomimetics), drug toxicity, or degeneration of the conductive tissue necessary to maintain normal heart rhythm (sick sinus syndrome) can sometimes precipitate arrhythmias. People with imbalances of blood chemistries or those with a history of cardiac conditions (CAD or heart valve disorders) are at higher risk for developing arrhythmias.

Pathophysiology

In cardiac arrhythmias (sometimes called *cardiac dysrhythmias*), abnormal electrical conduction or automaticity changes heart rate and rhythm. (See *Normal cardiac conduction*, page 61.) Arrhythmias vary in severity, from those that are mild, asymptomatic, and require no treatment (such as sinus arrhythmia, in which heart rate increases and decreases with respiration) to catastrophic ventricular fibrillation, which necessitates immediate resuscitation. Arrhythmias are generally classified according to their origin (ventricular or supraventricular). Their effect on cardiac output and blood pressure, partially influenced by the site of origin, determines their clinical significance. (See *Types of cardiac arrhythmias*, pages 65 to 71.)

Complications
◆ Impaired cardiac output

Signs and symptoms
Signs and symptoms of cardiac arrhythmias include palpitations, fainting, light-headedness, dizziness, chest pain, shortness of breath, changes in pulse patterns, paleness, and the temporary absence of breathing. However, the patient with a cardiac arrhythmia may be asymptomatic until the development of sudden cardiac arrest.

Diagnosis
Diagnosis is made by tests that reveal the arrhythmia, such as 12-lead ECG. Ambulatory cardiac monitoring (Holter monitoring), echocardiography, electrophysiology studies, and coronary angiography may also confirm or rule out suspected causes of arrhythmias and help determine treatment.

Special considerations
◆ Assess an unmonitored patient for rhythm disturbances.
◆ If the patient's pulse is abnormally rapid, slow, or irregular, watch for signs of hypoperfusion, such as altered LOC, hypotension, and diminished urine output.
◆ Document arrhythmias in a monitored patient, and assess for possible causes and effects.
◆ When life-threatening arrhythmias develop, rapidly assess LOC, respirations, and pulse rate.
◆ Initiate CPR if indicated.
◆ Evaluate the patient for altered cardiac output resulting from arrhythmias.
◆ Administer medications as ordered and prepare to assist with medical procedures (e.g., cardioversion), if indicated.
◆ Monitor patient for predisposing factors— such as fluid and electrolyte imbalance—and signs of drug toxicity, especially with digoxin. If you suspect drug toxicity, report such signs to the practitioner immediately and withhold the next dose.
◆ To prevent arrhythmias in a postoperative cardiac patient, provide adequate oxygen and reduce the heart's workload while carefully maintaining metabolic, neurologic, respiratory, and hemodynamic status.
◆ Consider sedation for transcutaneous pacing if appropriate.

◆ To avoid temporary pacemaker malfunction, install a fresh battery before each insertion. Carefully secure the external catheter wires and the pacemaker box. Assess the threshold daily. Watch closely for premature contractions, a sign of myocardial irritation.
◆ To avert permanent pacemaker malfunction, restrict the patient's activity after insertion as ordered. Monitor the pulse rate regularly and watch for signs of decreased cardiac output.
◆ If the patient has a permanent pacemaker, warn about environmental hazards, as indicated by the pacemaker manufacturer. Although hazards may not present a problem, in doubtful situations, 24-hour Holter monitoring may be helpful. Tell the patient to report light-headedness or syncope, and stress the importance of regular checkups.
◆ Compare the patient's cardiac status (pulse, blood pressure, and cardiac output) with the cardiac rhythm before and after treatments.

▓▓▓ **PREVENTION**
◆ *Maintain adequate oxygenation.*
◆ *Maintain normal fluid, acid–base, and electrolyte (especially potassium, magnesium, and calcium) balance.*
◆ *Maintain normal drug levels.*

Vascular disorders

THORACIC AORTIC ANEURYSM
Causes and incidence
Thoracic aortic aneurysm is an abnormal widening of the ascending, transverse, or descending part of the aorta. Aneurysm of the ascending aorta is the most common type and has the highest mortality. Aneurysms may be *dissecting*, a hemorrhagic separation in the aortic wall, usually within the medial layer; *saccular*, an outpouching of the arterial wall, with a narrow neck; or *fusiform*, a spindle-shaped enlargement encompassing the entire aortic circumference. (See *Types of aortic aneurysms*, page 64.) Some aneurysms progress to serious and, eventually, lethal complications, such as rupture of an untreated thoracic dissecting aneurysm into the pericardium, with resulting tamponade.

Thoracic aortic aneurysms commonly result from atherosclerosis, which weakens the aortic wall and gradually distends the lumen. An intimal tear in the ascending aorta initiates dissecting aneurysm in about 65% of patients. Regardless of causation, these aneurysms affect 6 out of every 100,000 people.

⬡ **ELDER TIP** *Ascending aortic aneurysms, the most common type, are usually seen in hypertensive men younger than 60 years old. Descending*

Types of aortic aneurysms

Dissecting aneurysm
A hemorrhagic separation of the medial layer of the vessel wall, which creates a false lumen

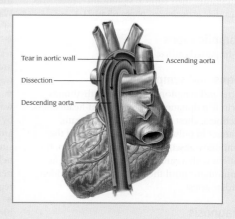

Tear in aortic wall
Dissection
Descending aorta
Ascending aorta

Saccular aneurysm
Unilateral pouchlike bulge with a narrow neck

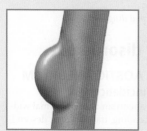

Fusiform aneurysm
A spindle-shaped bulge encompassing the vessel's entire diameter

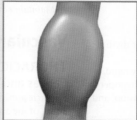

False aneurysm
A pulsating hematoma resulting from trauma; usually seen in the femoral artery after catheterization

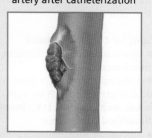

aortic aneurysms, usually found just below the origin of the subclavian artery, are most common in elderly men who are hypertensive.

Descending aortic aneurysms are also seen in younger patients with a history of traumatic chest injury less often in those with infection. Transverse aortic aneurysms are the least common type.

Other causes include:
♦ fungal infection (mycotic aneurysms) of the aortic arch and descending segments
♦ congenital disorders, such as coarctation of the aorta and Marfan syndrome
♦ trauma, usually of the descending thoracic aorta, from an accident that shears the aorta transversely (acceleration–deceleration injuries)

♦ syphilis, usually of the ascending aorta (uncommon because of antibiotics)
♦ hypertension (in dissecting aneurysm).

Pathophysiology
Most aneurysms result from changes to the vascular wall of arteries caused by failure of important proteins, elastin and collagen, leading to dilation. This eventually affects the structural stability and strength of the vessel. The location of the aneurysm, its diameter, the cause, and its morphology all assist in determining rate of expansion per year. Saccular aneurysms are thought to rupture more readily than other types, such as fusiform.

Types of cardiac arrhythmias

This chart reviews many common cardiac arrhythmias and outlines their features, causes, and treatments. Use a normal electrocardiogram strip, if available, to compare normal cardiac rhythm configurations with the rhythm strips below. Characteristics of normal rhythm include:

♦ ventricular and atrial rates of 60 to 100 beats/minute
♦ regular and uniform QRS complexes and P waves
♦ PR interval of 0.12 to 0.2 second
♦ QRS duration <0.12 second
♦ identical atrial and ventricular rates, with constant PR interval.

Arrhythmia and features	Causes	Treatment
Sinus arrhythmia 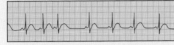 ♦ Irregular atrial and ventricular rhythms ♦ Normal P wave preceding each QRS complex	♦ A normal variation of normal sinus rhythm in athletes, children, and elderly people ♦ Also seen in digoxin toxicity and inferior wall myocardial infarction (MI)	♦ Atropine if rate decreases below 40 beats/minute and patient is symptomatic (e.g., has hypotension)
Sinus tachycardia 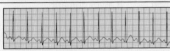 ♦ Atrial and ventricular rhythms regular ♦ Rate > 100 beats/minute; rarely, >160 beats/minute ♦ Normal P wave preceding each QRS complex	♦ Normal physiologic response to fever, exercise, anxiety, pain, dehydration; may also accompany shock, left-sided heart failure, cardiac tamponade, hyperthyroidism, anemia, hypovolemia, pulmonary embolism, and anterior wall MI ♦ May also occur with atropine, epinephrine, isoproterenol, quinidine, caffeine, alcohol, and nicotine use	♦ Correction of underlying cause ♦ Beta-adrenergic blockers or calcium channel blockers for symptomatic patients
Sinus bradycardia 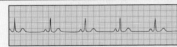 ♦ Regular atrial and ventricular rhythms ♦ Rate < 60 beats/minute ♦ Normal P wave preceding each QRS complex	♦ Normal in well-conditioned heart, as in an athlete ♦ Increased intracranial pressure; increased vagal tone due to straining during defecation, vomiting, intubation, mechanical ventilation; sick sinus syndrome; hypothyroidism; inferior wall MI ♦ May also occur with anticholinesterase, beta-adrenergic blocker, digoxin, and morphine use	♦ For low cardiac output, dizziness, weakness, altered level of consciousness, or low blood pressure: follow advanced cardiac life support (ACLS) protocol for administration of atropine ♦ Temporary pacemaker; may need to be evaluated for permanent pacemaker at a later time

(continued)

Types of cardiac arrhythmias (*continued*)

Arrhythmia and features	Causes	Treatment
Sinoatrial (SA) arrest or block (sinus arrest)		

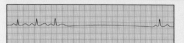

Arrhythmia and features	Causes	Treatment
◆ Atrial and ventricular rhythms normal except for missing complex ◆ Normal P wave preceding each QRS complex ◆ Pause not equal to a multiple of the previous sinus rhythm	◆ Acute infection ◆ Coronary artery disease, degenerative heart disease, and acute inferior wall MI ◆ Vagal stimulation, Valsalva maneuver, or carotid sinus massage ◆ Digoxin, quinidine, or salicylate toxicity ◆ Pesticide poisoning ◆ Pharyngeal irritation caused by endotracheal (ET) intubation ◆ Sick sinus syndrome	◆ Treat symptoms with atropine I.V. ◆ Temporary pacemaker; consider permanent pacemaker for repeated episodes
Wandering atrial pacemaker		

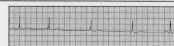

Arrhythmia and features	Causes	Treatment
◆ Atrial and ventricular rhythms vary slightly ◆ Irregular PR interval ◆ P waves irregular with changing configuration, indicating that they aren't all from SA node or single atrial focus; may appear after the QRS complex ◆ QRS complexes uniform in shape but irregular in rhythm	◆ Rheumatic carditis due to inflammation involving the SA node ◆ Digoxin toxicity ◆ Sick sinus syndrome	◆ No treatment if patient is asymptomatic ◆ Treatment of underlying cause if patient is symptomatic
Premature atrial contraction (PAC)		

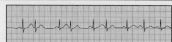

Arrhythmia and features	Causes	Treatment
◆ Premature, abnormal-looking P waves that differ in configuration from normal P waves ◆ QRS complexes after P waves, except in very early or blocked PACs ◆ P wave often buried in the preceding T wave or identified in the preceding T wave	◆ Coronary or valvular heart disease, atrial ischemia, coronary atherosclerosis, heart failure, acute respiratory failure, chronic obstructive pulmonary disease (COPD), electrolyte imbalance, and hypoxia ◆ Digoxin toxicity; use of aminophylline, adrenergics, or caffeine ◆ Anxiety	◆ Usually no treatment needed ◆ Treatment of underlying cause if patient is symptomatic

Types of cardiac arrhythmias (*continued*)

Arrhythmia and features	Causes	Treatment

Paroxysmal supraventricular tachycardia

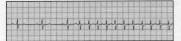

♦ Atrial and ventricular rhythms regular
♦ Heart rate >160 beats/minute; rarely exceeds 250 beats/minute
♦ P waves regular but aberrant; difficult to differentiate from preceding T wave
♦ P wave preceding each QRS complex
♦ Sudden onset and termination of arrhythmia
♦ When a normal P wave is present, it's called *paroxysmal atrial tachycardia*; when a normal P wave isn't present, it's called *paroxysmal junctional tachycardia*

♦ Intrinsic abnormality of atrioventricular (AV) conduction system
♦ Physical or psychological stress, hypoxia, hypokalemia, cardiomyopathy, congenital heart disease, MI, valvular disease, Wolff–Parkinson–White syndrome, cor pulmonale, hyperthyroidism, and systemic hypertension
♦ Digoxin toxicity; use of caffeine, marijuana, or central nervous system stimulants

♦ If patient is unstable, prepare for immediate cardioversion
♦ If patient is stable, vagal stimulation, Valsalva maneuver, or carotid sinus massage
♦ Adenosine by rapid I.V. bolus injection to rapidly convert arrhythmia
♦ If patient has a normal ejection fraction, consider calcium channel blockers, beta-adrenergic blockers, or amiodarone
♦ If patient has an ejection fraction <40%, consider amiodarone

Atrial flutter

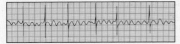

♦ Atrial rhythm regular; rate, 250 to 400 beats/minute
♦ Ventricular rate variable, depending on degree of AV block (usually 60 to 100 beats/minute)
♦ Sawtooth P-wave configuration possible (F waves)
♦ QRS complexes uniform in shape but often irregular in rate

♦ Heart failure, tricuspid or mitral valve disease, pulmonary embolism, cor pulmonale, inferior wall MI, and carditis
♦ Digoxin toxicity

♦ If patient is unstable with a ventricular rate >150 beats/minute, prepare for immediate cardioversion
♦ If patient is stable, drug therapy may include calcium channel blockers, beta-adrenergic blockers, or antiarrhythmics
♦ Anticoagulation therapy may be necessary
♦ Catheter ablation using radiofrequency energy to eliminate cardiac tissue causing the rapid heartbeat

Atrial fibrillation

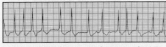

♦ Atrial rhythm grossly irregular; rate >400 beats/minute
♦ Ventricular rhythm grossly irregular
♦ QRS complexes of uniform configuration and duration
♦ PR interval indiscernible
♦ No P waves, or P waves that appear as erratic, irregular, baseline fibrillatory waves

♦ Heart failure, COPD, thyrotoxicosis, constrictive pericarditis, ischemic heart disease, sepsis, pulmonary embolus, rheumatic heart disease, hypertension, mitral stenosis, and atrial irritation; complication of coronary bypass or valve replacement surgery

♦ If patient is unstable with a ventricular rate >150 beats/minute, prepare for immediate cardioversion
♦ If patient is stable, drug therapy may include calcium channel blockers, beta-adrenergic blockers, digoxin, procainamide, quinidine, ibutilide, or amiodarone
♦ Consider anticoagulation to prevent emboli
♦ Dual-chamber atrial pacing, implantable atrial pacemaker, or surgical maze procedure may also be used
♦ Catheter ablation

(continued)

Types of cardiac arrhythmias (*continued*)

Arrhythmia and features	Causes	Treatment
Junctional rhythm		
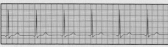 ♦ Atrial and ventricular rhythms regular ♦ Atrial rate 40 to 60 beats/minute ♦ Ventricular rate usually 40 to 60 beats/minute (60 to 100 beats/minute is accelerated junctional rhythm) ♦ P waves preceding, hidden within (absent), or after QRS complex; usually inverted if visible ♦ PR interval (when present) <0.12 second ♦ QRS complex configuration and duration normal, except in aberrant conduction	♦ Inferior wall MI or ischemia, hypoxia, vagal stimulation, and sick sinus syndrome ♦ Acute rheumatic fever ♦ Valve surgery ♦ Digoxin toxicity	♦ Correction of underlying cause ♦ Atropine for symptomatic slow rate ♦ Pacemaker insertion if patient is refractory to drugs ♦ Discontinuation of digoxin if appropriate
Premature junctional contractions		
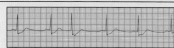 ♦ Atrial and ventricular rhythms irregular ♦ P waves inverted; may precede, be hidden within, or follow QRS complex ♦ PR interval <0.12 second if P wave precedes QRS complex ♦ QRS complex configuration and duration normal	♦ MI or ischemia ♦ Digoxin toxicity and excessive caffeine or amphetamine use	♦ Correction of underlying cause ♦ Discontinuation of digoxin if appropriate
Junctional tachycardia		
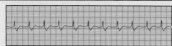 ♦ Atrial rate >100 beats/minute; however, P wave may be absent, hidden in QRS complex, or preceding T wave ♦ Ventricular rate >100 beats/minute ♦ P wave inverted ♦ QRS complex configuration and duration normal ♦ Onset of rhythm often sudden, occurring in bursts	♦ Myocarditis, cardiomyopathy, inferior wall MI or ischemia, and acute rheumatic fever; complication of valve replacement surgery ♦ Digoxin toxicity	♦ Cardioversion if ventricular rate is >150 beats/minute or if patient is symptomatic ♦ Amiodarone, beta-adrenergic blockers, or calcium channel blockers if patient is stable ♦ Discontinuation of digoxin if appropriate

Types of cardiac arrhythmias (*continued*)

Arrhythmia and features	Causes	Treatment
First-degree AV block		
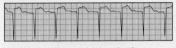 ♦ Atrial and ventricular rhythms regular ♦ PR interval >0.20 second ♦ P wave preceding each QRS complex ♦ QRS complex normal	♦ Inferior wall MI or ischemia or infarction, hypothyroidism, hypokalemia, and hyperkalemia ♦ Digoxin toxicity; use of quinidine, procainamide, beta-adrenergic blockers, calcium channel blockers, or amiodarone	♦ Correction of underlying cause ♦ No treatment is typically required
Second-degree AV block Mobitz I (Wenckebach)		
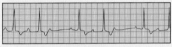 ♦ Atrial rhythm regular ♦ Ventricular rhythm irregular ♦ Atrial rate exceeds ventricular rate ♦ PR interval progressively, but only slightly, longer with each cycle until QRS complex disappears (dropped beat); PR interval shorter after dropped beat	♦ Inferior wall MI, cardiac surgery, acute rheumatic fever, and vagal stimulation ♦ Digoxin toxicity; use of propranolol, quinidine, or procainamide	♦ No specific treatment is required if asymptomatic ♦ Treatment of underlying cause ♦ Atropine or temporary pacemaker for symptomatic bradycardia ♦ Discontinuation of digoxin if appropriate
Second-degree AV block Mobitz II		
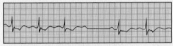 ♦ Atrial rhythm regular ♦ Ventricular rhythm regular or irregular, with varying degree of block ♦ P-P interval constant ♦ QRS complexes periodically absent	♦ Severe coronary artery disease, anterior wall MI, and acute myocarditis ♦ Digoxin toxicity	♦ Atropine, for symptomatic bradycardia ♦ Dopamine for hypotension ♦ Dobutamine for heart failure symptoms ♦ Temporary or permanent pacemaker for symptomatic bradycardia ♦ Discontinuation of digoxin if appropriate
Third-degree AV block (complete heart block)		
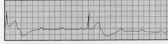 ♦ Atrial rhythm regular ♦ Ventricular rhythm regular and rate slower than atrial rate ♦ No relation between P waves and QRS complexes ♦ No constant PR interval ♦ QRS interval normal (nodal pacemaker) or wide and bizarre (ventricular pacemaker)	♦ Inferior or anterior wall MI, congenital abnormality, rheumatic fever, hypoxia, postoperative complication of mitral valve replacement, Lev disease (fibrosis and calcification that spreads from cardiac structures to the conductive tissue), and Lenegre disease (conductive tissue fibrosis) ♦ Digoxin toxicity	♦ Atropine, for symptomatic bradycardia ♦ Dopamine for hypotension ♦ Dobutamine for heart failure symptoms ♦ Temporary or permanent pacemaker for symptomatic bradycardia

(*continued*)

Types of cardiac arrhythmias (*continued*)

Arrhythmia and features	*Causes*	*Treatment*
Premature ventricular contraction (PVC)		

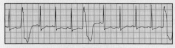

Arrhythmia and features	*Causes*	*Treatment*
♦ Atrial rhythm regular ♦ Ventricular rhythm irregular ♦ QRS complex premature, usually followed by a complete compensatory pause ♦ QRS complex wide and distorted, usually >0.14 second ♦ Premature QRS complexes occurring singly, in pairs, or in threes; alternating with normal beats; focus from one or more sites ♦ Ominous when clustered, multifocal, with R wave on T pattern	♦ Heart failure; old or acute myocardial ischemia, infarction, or contusion; myocardial irritation by ventricular catheter such as a pacemaker; hypercapnia; hypokalemia; and hypocalcemia ♦ Drug toxicity (cardiac glycosides, aminophylline, tricyclic antidepressants, beta-adrenergics [isoproterenol or dopamine]) ♦ Caffeine, tobacco, or alcohol use ♦ Psychological stress, anxiety, pain, exercise	♦ Treatment of underlying cause ♦ Discontinuation of drug causing toxicity ♦ Correction of electrolyte imbalances ♦ Beta-blockers, calcium channel blockers, or antiarrhythmics may be used to treat symptoms
Ventricular tachycardia (VT)		

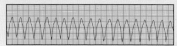

Arrhythmia and features	*Causes*	*Treatment*
♦ Ventricular rate 140 to 220 beats/minute, regular or irregular ♦ QRS complexes wide, bizarre, and independent of P waves ♦ P waves not discernible ♦ May start and stop suddenly	♦ Myocardial ischemia, infarction, or aneurysm; coronary artery disease; rheumatic heart disease; mitral valve prolapse; heart failure; cardiomyopathy; ventricular catheters; hypokalemia; hypercalcemia; and pulmonary embolism ♦ Digoxin, procainamide, epinephrine, or quinidine toxicity ♦ Anxiety	♦ Pulseless: Initiate cardiopulmonary resuscitation (CPR); follow ACLS protocol for defibrillation, ET intubation, and administration of epinephrine by amiodarone or lidocaine; if ineffective, consider magnesium sulfate ♦ With pulse: If hemodynamically stable, follow ACLS protocol for administration of amiodarone; if ineffective, initiate synchronized cardioversion ♦ If polymorphic VT, consult an expert in arrhythmia management
Ventricular fibrillation		

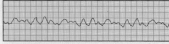

Arrhythmia and features	*Causes*	*Treatment*
♦ Ventricular rhythm and rate rapid and chaotic ♦ QRS complexes wide and irregular; no visible P waves	♦ Myocardial ischemia or infarction, R-on-T phenomenon, untreated ventricular tachycardia, hypokalemia, hyperkalemia, hypercalcemia, alkalosis, electric shock, and hypothermia ♦ Digoxin, epinephrine, or quinidine toxicity	♦ Pulseless: Start CPR; follow ACLS protocol for defibrillation, ET intubation, and administration of epinephrine, lidocaine, or amiodarone; if ineffective, consider magnesium sulfate

Types of cardiac arrhythmias (*continued*)

Arrhythmia and features	Causes	Treatment
Asystole 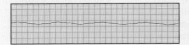 ♦ No atrial or ventricular rate or rhythm ♦ No discernible P waves, QRS complexes, or T waves	♦ Myocardial ischemia or infarction, aortic valve disease, heart failure, hypoxemia, hypokalemia, severe acidosis, electric shock, ventricular arrhythmias, AV block, pulmonary embolism, heart rupture, cardiac tamponade, hyperkalemia, and electromechanical dissociation ♦ Cocaine overdose	♦ Start CPR; follow ACLS protocol for ET intubation, transcutaneous pacing, and administration of epinephrine

Complications
♦ Rupture into pericardium
♦ Cardiac tamponade

Signs and symptoms
The most common symptom of thoracic aortic aneurysm is pain. With ascending aneurysm, the pain is described as severe, boring, and ripping and extends to the neck, shoulders, lower back, or abdomen but seldom radiates to the jaw and arms. Pain is more severe on the right side.

Other signs of ascending aneurysm may include bradycardia, aortic insufficiency, pericardial friction rub caused by a hemopericardium, unequal intensities of the right carotid and left radial pulses, and a difference in blood pressure between the right and the left arms. These signs are absent in descending aneurysm. If dissection involves the carotids, an abrupt onset of neurologic deficits may occur.

With descending aneurysm, pain usually starts suddenly between the shoulder blades and may radiate to the chest; it's described as sharp and tearing. Transverse aneurysm causes a sudden, sharp, tearing pain radiating to the shoulders. It may also cause hoarseness, dyspnea, dysphagia, and a dry cough because of compression of surrounding structures in this area. (See *Clinical characteristics of thoracic dissection*, page 72.)

Diagnosis
Diagnosis relies on patient history, clinical features, and appropriate tests. In an asymptomatic patient, diagnosis often occurs accidentally when chest X-rays show widening of the aorta. Other tests help confirm aneurysm:
♦ Aortography can show the lumen of the aneurysm, its size and location, and the false lumen in dissecting aneurysm.
♦ ECG helps distinguish thoracic aneurysm from MI.
♦ Echocardiography may help identify dissecting aneurysm of the aortic root.
♦ Hemoglobin levels may be normal or low, due to blood loss from a leaking aneurysm.
♦ Computed tomography scan is considered the gold standard and can confirm and locate the aneurysm and may be used to monitor its progression.
♦ MRI may aid diagnosis.
♦ Transesophageal echocardiography is used to diagnose and size an aneurysm in either the ascending or the descending aorta.
♦ Ultrasound is frequently used for screening purposes in high-risk patients.

Treatment
Dissecting aortic aneurysm is an emergency that requires prompt surgery and stabilizing measures: antihypertensives such as nitroprusside; negative inotropic agents that decrease contractility force such as propranolol; oxygen for respiratory distress; opioids for pain; I.V. fluids and, possibly, whole blood transfusions.

Surgery consists of resecting the aneurysm, restoring normal blood flow through a graft replacement, and, with aortic valve insufficiency, replacing the aortic valve. Groin catheter placement may be used for aortic stenting.

Clinical characteristics of thoracic dissection

Ascending aorta	Descending aorta	Transverse aorta
Character of pain		
Severe, boring, ripping; extending to neck, shoulders, lower back, or abdomen (rarely to jaw and arms); more severe on right side	Sudden onset; sharp, tearing; usually between the shoulder blades; may radiate to the chest; most diagnostic feature	Sudden onset; sharp, boring, tearing; radiates to shoulders
Other symptoms and effects		
If dissection involves carotids, abrupt onset of neurologic deficit (usually intermittent); bradycardia, aortic insufficiency, and hemopericardium detected by pericardial friction rub; unequal intensity of right and left carotid pulses and radial pulses; difference in blood pressure, especially systolic, between right and left arms	Aortic insufficiency without murmur, hemopericardium, or pleural friction rub; carotid and radial pulses and blood pressure in both arms tend to stay equal	Hoarseness, dyspnea, pain, dysphagia, and dry cough resulting from compression of surrounding structures
Diagnostic features		
Chest X-ray		
Best diagnostic tool; shows widening of mediastinum, enlargement of ascending aorta	Shows widening of mediastinum, descending aorta larger than ascending	Shows widening of mediastinum, descending aorta larger than ascending, widened transverse arch
Computerized tomography		
Shows false lumen; narrowing of lumen of aorta in ascending section. Also good for visualizing anatomic details to help determine the extent of the aneurysm, and to assist in preparing for repair	Shows false lumen; narrowing of lumen of aorta in descending section. Also good for visualizing anatomic details to help determine the extent of the aneurysm, and to assist in preparing for repair	Shows false lumen, narrowing of lumen of aorta in transverse arch. Also good for visualizing anatomic details to help determine the extent of the aneurysm, and to assist in preparing for repair
Treatment		
This is a medical emergency requiring immediate, aggressive treatment to reduce blood pressure (usually with labetalol or verapamil). Nitroprusside may be required if there is persistent hypertension. Surgical repair is also required	Surgical repair is required but less urgent than for the ascending dissection	Immediate surgical repair (mortality as high as 50%) and control of hypertension are required

This procedure, which may be used for aneurysms of the descending aorta, eliminates the need for a chest incision.

Postoperative measures include careful monitoring and continuous assessment in the ICU, antibiotics, placement of ET and chest tubes, ECG monitoring, and pulmonary artery catheterization.

Long-term management includes treatment of underlying conditions, such as heart disease and diabetes.

Special considerations

◆ Monitor blood pressure, PAWP, and CVP. Assess pain; breathing; and carotid, radial, and femoral pulses.

◆ Make sure laboratory tests include complete blood count, differential, electrolyte levels, type and crossmatching for whole blood, ABG studies, and urinalysis.

◆ Insert an indwelling urinary catheter. Administer dextrose 5% in water or lactated Ringer solution, and antibiotics, as ordered. Carefully monitor nitroprusside I.V., if ordered; use a separate I.V. line for infusion. Adjust the dose by slowly increasing the infusion rate. Meanwhile, check blood pressure every 5 minutes until it stabilizes. With suspected bleeding from aneurysm, give whole blood transfusion.

◆ Explain diagnostic tests. If surgery is scheduled, explain the procedure and expected postoperative care (I.V. lines, ET and drainage tubes, cardiac monitoring, and ventilation).

After repair of thoracic aneurysm:

◆ Assess LOC. Monitor vital signs; PAP, PAWP, and CVP; pulse rate; urine output; and pain.

◆ Check respiratory function. Carefully observe and record type and amount of chest tube drainage, and frequently assess heart and breath sounds.

◆ Monitor I.V. therapy.

◆ Give medications as appropriate.

◆ Watch for signs of infection, especially fever, and excessive wound drainage.

◆ Assist with range-of-motion exercises of legs to prevent thromboembolic phenomenon due to venostasis during prolonged bed rest.

◆ After stabilization of vital signs and respiration, encourage and assist the patient in turning, coughing, and deep breathing. If necessary, provide intermittent positive-pressure breathing to promote lung expansion. Help the patient walk as soon as he or she is able.

◆ Before discharge, ensure compliance with antihypertensive therapy by explaining the need for such drugs and the expected adverse effects. Teach the patient how to monitor blood pressure. Refer to community agencies for continued support and assistance, as needed.

◆ Throughout hospitalization, offer the patient and family psychological support. Answer all of their questions honestly and provide reassurance.

ABDOMINAL ANEURYSM
Causes and incidence

Abdominal aneurysm, an abnormal dilation in the arterial wall, generally occurs in the aorta between the renal arteries and the iliac branches. Rupture—in which the aneurysm breaks open, resulting in profuse bleeding—is a common complication that occurs in larger aneurysms. Dissection occurs when the artery's lining tears, and blood leaks into the walls.

Abdominal aortic aneurysms (AAAs) result from arteriosclerosis, hypertension, congenital weakening, cystic medial necrosis, trauma, syphilis, and other infections. In children, this disorder can result from blunt abdominal injury or Marfan syndrome.

This disorder is four times more common in men than in women and is most prevalent in whites 40 to 70 years old. It is especially prevalent in male smokers who are 65 and older. Less than 50% of people with a ruptured AAA survive.

Pathophysiology

These aneurysms develop slowly. First, a focal weakness in the muscular layer of the aorta (tunica media), due to degenerative changes, allows the inner layer (tunica intima) and outer layer (tunica adventitia) to stretch outward. Blood pressure within the aorta progressively weakens the vessel walls and enlarges the aneurysm.

Complications

◆ Rupture

◆ Hemorrhage

◆ Shock

Signs and symptoms

Although abdominal aneurysms usually don't produce symptoms, most are evident (unless the patient is obese) as a pulsating mass in the periumbilical area, accompanied by a systolic bruit over the aorta. Some tenderness may be present on deep palpation. A large aneurysm may produce symptoms that mimic renal calculi, lumbar disk disease, and duodenal compression. Abdominal aneurysms rarely cause diminished peripheral pulses or claudication, unless embolization occurs.

Lumbar pain that radiates to the flank and groin from pressure on lumbar nerves may signify enlargement and imminent rupture. A rare but recognized symptom is unrelenting testicular pain with no other cause. If the aneurysm ruptures into the peritoneal cavity, it causes severe, persistent abdominal and back pain, mimicking renal or ureteral colic. Signs of hemorrhage—such as weakness, sweating, tachycardia, and hypotension—may be subtle because rupture into the retroperitoneal space produces a tamponade effect that prevents continued hemorrhage. Patients with such rupture may remain stable for hours before shock and death occur, although 20% die immediately.

Diagnosis

Because abdominal aneurysms seldom produce symptoms, they're commonly detected accidentally as the result of an X-ray or a routine physical examination.

CONFIRMING DIAGNOSIS *Several tests can confirm a suspected abdominal aneurysm. Serial ultrasound (sonography) can accurately determine the aneurysm's size, shape, and location. Anteroposterior and lateral X-rays of the abdomen can detect aortic calcification, which outlines the mass, at least 75% of the time. Aortography shows the condition of vessels proximal and distal to the aneurysm and the aneurysm's extent but may underestimate aneurysm diameter because it visualizes only the flow channel and not the surrounding clot. Computed tomography scan is used to diagnose and size the aneurysm. MRI can be used as an alternative to aortography.*

Treatment

Usually, abdominal aneurysm requires resection of the aneurysm and replacement of the damaged aortic section with a Dacron graft. (See *Abdominal aneurysms: Before and after surgery,* page 75. Also see *Endovascular grafting for repair of an AAA,* page 76.) If the aneurysm is small and asymptomatic, surgery may be delayed, and the aneurysm may be followed and allowed to expand to a certain size because of possible surgical complications; however, small aneurysms may also rupture. Because of this risk, surgical repair or replacement is recommended for symptomatic patients or for patients with aneurysms greater than 5 cm in diameter.

Stenting is also a treatment option. It can be performed without an abdominal incision by introducing the catheters through arteries in the groin. However, not all patients with AAAs are candidates for this treatment.

Regular physical examination and ultrasound checks are necessary to detect enlargement, which may forewarn rupture. Large aneurysms or those that produce symptoms pose a significant risk of rupture and necessitate immediate repair. In patients with poor distal runoff, external grafting may be done.

Risk factor modification is fundamental in the medical management of abdominal aneurysm, including control of hypocholesterolemia and hypertension. BBs are commonly prescribed to reduce the risk of aneurysm expansion and rupture.

Special considerations

Abdominal aneurysm requires meticulous preoperative and postoperative care, psychological support, and comprehensive patient teaching. Following diagnosis, if rupture isn't imminent, elective surgery allows time for additional preoperative tests to evaluate the patient's clinical status.

◆ Monitor vital signs, and type and crossmatch blood.

◆ Use only gentle abdominal palpation.

◆ As ordered, obtain renal function tests (BUN, creatinine, and electrolyte levels), blood samples (complete blood count with differential), electrocardiogram and cardiac evaluation, baseline pulmonary function tests, and ABG analysis.

◆ Be alert for signs of rupture, which may be immediately fatal. Watch closely for signs of acute blood loss (decreasing blood pressure; increasing pulse and respiratory rate; cool, clammy skin; restlessness; and decreased sensorium).

◆ If rupture does occur, the first priority is to get the patient to surgery immediately. Surgery allows direct compression of the aorta to control hemorrhage. Large amounts of blood may be needed during the resuscitative period to replace blood loss. In such a patient, renal failure caused by ischemia is a major postoperative complication, possibly requiring hemodialysis.

◆ Before elective surgery, weigh the patient, insert an indwelling urinary catheter and an I.V. line, and assist with insertion of an arterial line and pulmonary artery catheter to monitor fluid and hemodynamic balance. Give prophylactic antibiotics as ordered.

◆ Explain the surgical procedure and the expected postoperative care in the ICU for patients undergoing complex abdominal surgery (I.V. lines, ET and NG intubation, and mechanical ventilation).

◆ After surgery, in the ICU, closely monitor vital signs, intake and hourly output, neurologic status (LOC, pupil size, and sensation in arms and legs), and ABG values. Assess the depth, rate, and character of respirations and breath sounds at least every hour.

◆ Watch for signs of bleeding (increased pulse and respiratory rates and hypotension) and back pain, which may indicate that the graft is

Abdominal aneurysms: Before and after surgery

During surgery, a prosthetic graft replaces or encloses the weakened area.

Before surgery
Aneurysm below renal arteries and above bifurcation

After surgery
The prosthesis extends distal to the renal arteries to above the aortic bifurcation.

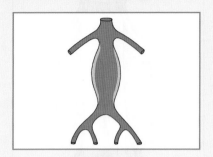

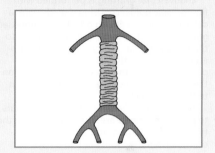

Before surgery
Aneurysm below renal arteries involving the iliac branches

After surgery
The prosthesis extends to the common femoral arteries.

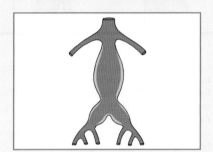

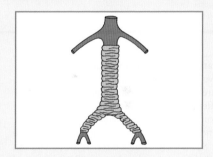

Before surgery
Small aneurysm in a patient with poor distal runoff (poor risk)

After surgery
The external prosthesis encircles the aneurysm and is held in place with sutures.

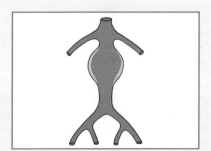

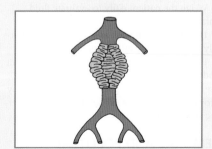

Endovascular grafting for repair of an AAA

Endovascular grafting is a minimally invasive procedure for the repair of an abdominal aortic aneurysm (AAA). This procedure reinforces the walls of the aorta to prevent rupture and prevent expansion of the aneurysm.

Endovascular grafting is performed with fluoroscopic guidance: Using a guide wire, a delivery catheter with an attached compressed graft is inserted through a small incision into the femoral or iliac artery. The delivery catheter is advanced into the aorta, where it's positioned across the aneurysm. A balloon on the catheter expands the graft and affixes it to the vessel wall.

The procedure generally takes 2 to 3 hours to perform. Patients are instructed to walk the first day after surgery and are generally discharged from the facility in 1 to 3 days.

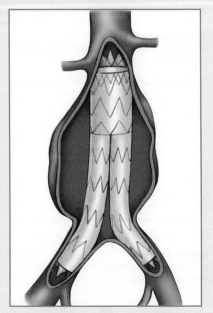

tearing. Check abdominal dressings for excessive bleeding or drainage. Be alert for temperature elevations and other signs of infection. After NG intubation for intestinal decompression, irrigate the tube frequently to ensure patency. Record the amount and type of drainage.

◆ Suction the ET tube often. If the patient can breathe unassisted and has good breath sounds and adequate ABG values, tidal volume, and vital capacity 24 hours after surgery, it is likely he or she will be extubated and will require oxygen by mask.

◆ Weigh the patient daily to evaluate fluid balance.

◆ Help the patient walk as soon as able (generally the second day after surgery).

◆ Provide psychological support for the patient and family. Help ease their fears about the ICU, the threat of impending rupture, and surgery by providing appropriate explanations and answering all questions.

FEMORAL AND POPLITEAL ANEURYSMS

Causes and incidence

Femoral and popliteal aneurysms (sometimes called *peripheral arterial aneurysms*) are the end result of progressive atherosclerotic changes occurring in the walls (medial layer) of these major peripheral arteries. These aneurysmal formations may be *fusiform* (spindle-shaped) or *saccular* (pouchlike); the fusiform type is three times more common. They may be singular or multiple segmental lesions, often affecting both legs, and may accompany other arterial aneurysms located in the abdominal aorta or iliac arteries.

Femoral and popliteal aneurysms are usually secondary to atherosclerosis. Rarely, they result from congenital weakness in the arterial wall. They may also result from trauma (blunt or penetrating), bacterial infection, or peripheral vascular reconstructive surgery (which causes "suture line" aneurysms, or false aneurysms, in which a blood clot forms a second lumen).

This condition occurs most frequently in men older than 50. The clinical course is usually progressive, eventually ending in thrombosis, embolization, and gangrene. Elective surgery before complications arise greatly improves the prognosis.

Pathophysiology

As with other aneurysms, a weakening of the vessel wall caused by inflammation, proteolysis, and changes in the matrix result in the outpouching seen in this condition.

Complications
◆ Amputation of thrombosis
◆ Emboli
◆ Gangrene

Signs and symptoms
Popliteal aneurysms may cause pain in the popliteal space when they're large enough to compress the medial popliteal nerve and edema and venous distention if the vein is compressed. Femoral and popliteal aneurysms can produce symptoms of severe ischemia in the leg or foot due to acute thrombosis within the aneurysmal sac, embolization of mural thrombus fragments and, rarely, rupture. Symptoms of acute aneurysmal thrombosis include severe pain, loss of pulse and color, coldness in the affected leg or foot, and gangrene. Distal petechial hemorrhages may develop from aneurysmal emboli.

Diagnosis
Diagnosis is usually confirmed by bilateral palpation that reveals a pulsating mass above or below the inguinal ligament in femoral aneurysm. When thrombosis has occurred, palpation detects a firm, nonpulsating mass. Arteriography or ultrasound may be indicated in doubtful situations. Arteriography may also detect associated aneurysms, especially those in the abdominal aorta and the iliac arteries. Ultrasound may be helpful in determining the size of the popliteal or femoral artery.

Treatment
Femoral and popliteal aneurysms require surgical bypass and reconstruction of the artery, usually with an autogenous saphenous vein graft replacement. Arterial occlusion that causes severe ischemia and gangrene may require leg amputation.

Special considerations
Before corrective surgery:
◆ Assess and record circulatory status, noting the location and quality of peripheral pulses in the affected arm or leg.
◆ Administer prophylactic antibiotics or anticoagulants, as ordered.
◆ Discuss postoperative procedures and review the explanation of the surgery.
After arterial surgery:
◆ Monitor carefully for early signs of thrombosis or graft occlusion (loss of pulse, decreased skin temperature and sensation, and severe pain) and infection (fever).
◆ Palpate distal pulses at least every hour for the first 24 hours and then as frequently as ordered. Correlate these findings with preoperative circulatory assessment. Mark the sites on the patient's skin where pulses are palpable to facilitate repeated checks.
◆ Help the patient walk soon after surgery to prevent venostasis and possible thrombus formation.
To prepare the patient for discharge:
◆ Tell the patient to immediately report any recurrence of symptoms because the saphenous vein graft replacement can fail or another aneurysm may develop.
◆ Explain to the patient with popliteal artery resection that swelling may persist for some time. If antiembolism stockings are ordered, make sure they fit properly and teach the patient how to apply them. Warn against wearing constrictive apparel.
◆ If the patient is receiving anticoagulants, suggest measures to prevent bleeding, such as using an electric razor. Tell the patient to report any signs of bleeding (bleeding gums, tarry stools, and easy bruising) immediately. Explain the importance of follow-up blood studies to monitor anticoagulant therapy. Warn the patient to avoid trauma, tobacco, and aspirin.

THROMBOPHLEBITIS
Causes and incidence
An acute condition characterized by inflammation and thrombus formation, thrombophlebitis may occur in deep (intermuscular or intramuscular) or superficial (subcutaneous) veins. DVT or thrombophlebitis affects small veins, such as the soleal venous sinuses, or large veins, such as the vena cava and the femoral, iliac, and subclavian veins, causing venous insufficiency. (See *Chronic venous insufficiency*, page 78.) This disorder is typically progressive, leading to pulmonary embolism, a potentially lethal complication. Superficial thrombophlebitis is usually self-limiting and seldom leads to pulmonary embolism. Thrombophlebitis often begins with localized inflammation alone (phlebitis), but such inflammation rapidly provokes thrombus formation. Rarely, venous thrombosis develops without associated inflammation of the vein (phlebothrombosis).

DVT may be idiopathic, but it usually results from endothelial damage, accelerated blood clotting, and reduced blood flow, known as the *Virchow triad*. Predisposing factors are prolonged bed rest, trauma, surgery, childbirth, and use of hormonal contraceptives such as estrogens. It occurs in about 80 of every 100,000 people; 1 of every 20 persons is affected at some point during their lifetime. Males are at slightly greater risk than females. People older than 40 are also at increased risk.

Chronic venous insufficiency

Chronic venous insufficiency results from the valvular destruction of deep vein thrombophlebitis, usually in the iliac and femoral veins, and occasionally the saphenous veins. It's often accompanied by incompetence of the communicating veins at the ankle, causing increased venous pressure and fluid migration into the interstitial tissue. Clinical effects include chronic swelling of the affected leg from edema, leading to tissue fibrosis, and induration; skin discoloration from extravasation of blood in subcutaneous tissue; and stasis ulcers around the ankle.

Treatment of small ulcers includes bed rest, elevation of the legs, warm soaks, and antimicrobial therapy for infection. Treatment to counteract increased venous pressure, the result of reflux from the deep venous system to surface veins, may include compression dressings, such as a sponge rubber pressure dressing or a zinc gelatin boot (Unna boot). This therapy begins after massive swelling subsides with leg elevation and bed rest.

Large stasis ulcers unresponsive to conservative treatment may require excision and skin grafting. Patient care includes daily inspection to assess healing. Other care measures are the same as for varicose veins.

Causes of superficial thrombophlebitis include trauma, infection, I.V. drug abuse, and chemical irritation due to extensive use of the I.V. route for medications and diagnostic tests.

Pathophysiology

A thrombus occurs when an alteration in the epithelial lining causes platelet aggregation and consequent fibrin entrapment of red and white blood cells and additional platelets. Thrombus formation is more rapid in areas where blood flow is slower, due to greater contact between platelet and thrombin accumulation. The rapidly expanding thrombus initiates a chemical inflammatory process in the vessel epithelium, which leads to fibrosis. The enlarging clot may occlude the vessel lumen partially or totally, or it may detach and embolize to lodge elsewhere in the systemic circulation.

Complications

◆ Pulmonary embolism
◆ Chronic venous insufficiency

Signs and symptoms

In both types of thrombophlebitis, clinical features vary with the site and length of the affected vein. Although DVT may occur asymptomatically, it may also produce severe pain, fever, chills, malaise and, possibly, swelling and cyanosis of the affected arm or leg. Superficial thrombophlebitis produces visible and palpable signs, such as heat, pain, swelling, rubor, tenderness, and induration along the length of the affected vein. Varicose veins may also be present. (See *Varicose veins,* page 79.) Extensive vein involvement may cause lymphadenitis.

Diagnosis

Findings are usually nonspecific and are not reliable for making the diagnosis of DVT. Essential laboratory tests include:
◆ Duplex Doppler is most commonly performed; this makes it possible to noninvasively examine the major veins (but not calf veins).

CONFIRMING DIAGNOSIS *Compression ultrasonography with Doppler is the diagnostic test of choice in the evaluation of DVT.*

Diagnosis must also rule out PAD, lymphangitis, cellulitis, and myositis.

Diagnosis of superficial thrombophlebitis is based on physical examination (redness and warmth over the affected area, palpable vein, and pain during palpation or compression).

Treatment

The goals of treatment are to control thrombus development, prevent complications, relieve pain, and prevent recurrence of the disorder. Symptomatic measures include bed rest, with elevation of the affected arm or leg; warm, moist soaks to the affected area; and analgesics. After the acute episode of DVT subsides, the patient may resume activity while wearing antiembolism stockings that were applied before getting out of bed.

Treatment also includes anticoagulants to prolong clotting time. While warfarin is still an option for the treatment of DVT, new medications are now available that are safer, as effective, and do not require monitoring of blood levels through frequent lab draws. These medications are called direct factor Xa inhibitors and include rivaroxaban and apixaban. If the patient is not a candidate for these novel medications,

Varicose veins

Varicose veins are dilated, tortuous veins, usually affecting the subcutaneous leg veins—the saphenous veins and their branches. They can result from congenital weakness of the valves or venous wall, diseases of the venous system such as deep vein thrombophlebitis, conditions that produce prolonged venostasis such as pregnancy, or occupations that necessitate standing for an extended period.

Varicose veins may be asymptomatic or may produce mild to severe leg symptoms, including a feeling of heaviness; cramps at night; diffuse, dull aching after prolonged standing or walking; aching during menses; fatigability; palpable nodules, and, with deep vein incompetency, orthostatic edema and stasis pigmentation of the calves and ankles.

Treatment

In mild-to-moderate varicose veins, anti-embolism stockings or elastic bandages counteract pedal and ankle swelling by supporting the veins and improving circulation. An exercise program such as walking promotes muscular contraction and forces blood through the veins, thereby minimizing venous pooling. Severe varicose veins may necessitate stripping and ligation or, as an alternative to surgery, injection of a sclerosing agent into small affected vein segments.

To promote comfort and minimize worsening of varicosities:
♦ Discourage the patient from wearing constrictive clothing.
♦ Advise the patient to elevate the legs above heart level whenever possible and to avoid prolonged standing or sitting.

After stripping and ligation or after injection of a sclerosing agent:
♦ To relieve pain, administer analgesics as ordered.
♦ Frequently check circulation in toes (color and temperature) and observe elastic bandages for bleeding. When ordered, rewrap bandages at least once a shift, wrapping from toe to thigh, with the leg elevated.
♦ Watch for signs of complications, such as sensory loss in the leg (which could indicate saphenous nerve damage), calf pain (thrombophlebitis), and fever (infection).

---

low-molecular-weight (LMW) heparin has been shown to be effective in treating DVT or can be used as bridge therapy until a therapeutic level of warfarin is achieved. Although LMW heparin is more expensive, it doesn't require monitoring for its anticoagulant effect, either. Full anticoagulant doses must be discontinued during any operative period because of the risk of hemorrhage. After some types of surgery, especially major abdominal or pelvic operations, prophylactic doses of anticoagulants may reduce the risk of DVT and pulmonary embolism. For lysis of acute, extensive DVT, treatment may include thrombolysis with or without thrombectomy. Rarely, DVT may cause complete venous occlusion, which necessitates venous interruption through simple ligation to vein plication, or clipping. Embolectomy and insertion of a vena caval umbrella or filter may also be done.

Therapy for severe superficial thrombophlebitis may include an anti-inflammatory drug such as indomethacin, antiembolism stockings, warm soaks, and elevation of the leg.

Special considerations

Patient teaching, identification of high-risk patients, and measures to prevent venostasis can prevent DVT; close monitoring of anticoagulant therapy can prevent serious complications such as internal hemorrhage.

♦ Enforce bed rest as ordered, and elevate the patient's affected arm or leg. If you plan to use pillows for elevating the leg, place them so they support the entire length of the affected extremity to prevent possible compression of the popliteal space.
♦ Apply warm soaks to increase circulation to the affected area and to relieve pain and inflammation. Give analgesics to relieve pain, as ordered.
♦ Measure and record the affected arm or leg's circumference daily, and compare this measurement to the other arm or leg. To ensure accuracy and consistency of serial measurements, mark the skin over the area and measure at the same spot daily.
♦ Administer heparin I.V., as ordered, with an infusion monitor or pump to control the flow rate if necessary. Remember that this medication is not being used as often with the growing popularity of direct factor Xa inhibitors.
♦ Measure partial thromboplastin time regularly for the patient on heparin therapy; prothrombin time and international normalized ratio (INR) for the patient on warfarin (therapeutic anticoagulation values are $1\frac{1}{2}$ to 2

Preventing thrombophlebitis

To prevent thrombophlebitis in a high-risk patient, perform range-of-motion exercise while the patient is on bed rest, use intermittent pneumatic calf massage during lengthy surgical or diagnostic procedures, apply antiembolism stockings postoperatively, and encourage early ambulation.

After some types of surgery, especially major abdominal or pelvic operations, prophylactic doses of anticoagulants may reduce the risk of deep vein thrombosis and pulmonary embolism.

times control values for prothrombin time and an INR of 2 to 3). Watch for signs and symptoms of bleeding, such as dark, tarry stools; coffee-ground vomitus; and ecchymosis. Encourage the patient to use an electric razor and to avoid medications that contain aspirin.

◆ Be alert for signs of pulmonary emboli (crackles, dyspnea, hemoptysis, sudden changes in mental status, restlessness, and hypotension).

To prepare the patient with thrombophlebitis for discharge:

◆ Emphasize the importance of follow-up blood studies to monitor anticoagulant therapy, if necessary.

◆ If the patient is being discharged on heparin therapy, teach the patient or family how to give subcutaneous injections. If the patient requires further assistance, arrange for a home health nurse.

◆ Tell the patient to avoid prolonged sitting or standing to help prevent recurrence.

◆ Teach the patient how to properly apply and use antiembolism stockings. Tell the patient to report any complications such as cold, blue toes. (See *Preventing thrombophlebitis*.)

RAYNAUD DISEASE
Causes and incidence
Raynaud disease is one of several primary arteriospastic disorders characterized by episodic vasospasm in the small peripheral arteries and arterioles, precipitated by exposure to cold or stress. This condition occurs bilaterally and usually affects the hands or, less often, the feet. Raynaud disease is most prevalent in females, particularly those between puberty and 40 years old. It's a benign condition, requiring no specific treatment and causing no serious sequelae.

Although the cause is unknown, several theories account for the reduced digital blood flow: intrinsic vascular wall hyperactivity to cold, increased vasomotor tone due to sympathetic stimulation, and antigen–antibody immune

response (the most likely theory because abnormal immunologic test results accompany Raynaud phenomenon). Risk factors include associated diseases (Buerger disease, atherosclerosis, rheumatoid arthritis, scleroderma, and SLE) and smoking.

This disorder affects females more often than males.

Raynaud phenomenon, however, a condition commonly associated with several connective tissue disorders—such as scleroderma, SLE, or polymyositis—has a progressive course, leading to ischemia, gangrene, and amputation. Distinguishing between the two disorders is difficult because some patients who experience mild symptoms of Raynaud disease for several years may later develop overt connective tissue disease—especially scleroderma.

Pathophysiology
Complications
◆ Ischemia
◆ Gangrene
◆ Amputation

Signs and symptoms
After exposure to cold or stress, the skin on the fingers typically blanches and then becomes cyanotic before changing to red and before changing from cold to normal temperature. Numbness and tingling may also occur. These symptoms are relieved by warmth. In long-standing disease, trophic changes, such as sclerodactyly, ulcerations, or chronic paronychia, may result. Although it's extremely uncommon, minimal cutaneous gangrene necessitates amputation of one or more phalanges.

Diagnosis
Clinical criteria that establish Raynaud disease include skin color changes induced by cold or stress; bilateral involvement; absence of gangrene or, if present, minimal cutaneous

Types of peripheral artery disease

Site of occlusion	*Signs and symptoms*
Carotid arterial system	
Internal carotids External carotids	♦ Absent or decreased pulsation with an auscultatory bruit over the affected vessels ♦ Neurologic dysfunction: transient ischemic attacks (TIAs) due to reduced cerebral circulation producing unilateral sensory or motor dysfunction (transient monocular blindness, hemiparesis), possible aphasia or dysarthria, confusion, decreased mentation, and headache (These are recurrent features that usually last 5 to 10 minutes but may persist up to 24 hours and may herald a stroke)
Vertebrobasilar system	
Vertebral arteries Basilar arteries	♦ Neurologic dysfunction: TIAs of the brainstem and cerebellum producing binocular vision disturbances, vertigo, dysarthria, and "drop attacks" (falling down without loss of consciousness); less common than carotid TIA
Innominate	
Brachiocephalic artery	♦ Indications of ischemia (claudication) of the right arm ♦ Neurologic dysfunction: signs and symptoms of vertebrobasilar occlusion ♦ Possible bruit over the right side of the neck
Subclavian artery	
	♦ Clinical effects of vertebrobasilar occlusion and exercise-induced arm claudication ♦ Subclavian steal syndrome (characterized by the backflow of blood from the brain through the vertebral artery on the same side as the occlusion, into the subclavian artery distal to the occlusion) ♦ Possibly gangrene (usually limited to the digits)
Mesenteric artery	
Superior (most commonly affected) Celiac axis Inferior	♦ Bowel ischemia, infarct necrosis, and gangrene ♦ Diarrhea ♦ Leukocytosis ♦ Nausea and vomiting ♦ Shock due to massive intraluminal fluid and plasma loss ♦ Sudden, acute abdominal pain
Aortic bifurcation	
(Saddle block occlusion, a medical emergency associated with cardiac embolization)	♦ Sensory and motor deficits (muscle weakness, numbness, paresthesias, and paralysis) in both legs ♦ Signs of ischemia (sudden pain and cold, pale legs with decreased or absent peripheral pulses) in both legs
Iliac artery	
(Leriche syndrome)	♦ Absent or reduced femoral or distal pulses ♦ Impotence ♦ Intermittent claudication of the lower back, buttocks, and thighs, relieved by rest ♦ Possible bruit over femoral arteries
Femoral and popliteal artery	
(Associated with aneurysm formation)	♦ Gangrene ♦ Intermittent claudication of the calves on exertion ♦ Ischemic pain in feet ♦ Leg pallor and coolness; blanching of the feet on elevation ♦ No palpable pulses in the ankles and feet ♦ Pretrophic pain (heralds necrosis and ulceration)

gangrene; normal arterial pulses; and patient history of clinical symptoms of longer than 2 years' duration. Diagnosis must also rule out secondary disease processes, such as chronic arterial occlusive or connective tissue disease.

Treatment

Initially, treatment consists of avoidance of cold, mechanical, or chemical injury; cessation of smoking; and reassurance that symptoms are benign. Because adverse drug effects, especially from vasodilators, may be more bothersome than the disease itself, drug therapy is reserved for unusually severe symptoms. Such therapy may include low doses of nifedipine. Sympathectomy may be helpful when conservative modalities fail to prevent ischemic ulcers and becomes necessary in less than 25% of patients.

Special considerations

◆ Warn the patient against exposure to the cold. Tell the patient to wear mittens or gloves in cold weather or when handling cold items or defrosting the freezer.
◆ Advise the patient to avoid stressful situations and to stop smoking.
◆ Instruct the patient to inspect the skin frequently and to seek immediate care for signs of skin breakdown or infection.
◆ Teach the patient about drugs, their use, and their adverse effects.
◆ Provide psychological support and reassurance to allay the patient's fear of amputation and disfigurement.

BUERGER DISEASE
Causes and incidence

Buerger disease (sometimes called *thromboangiitis obliterans*)—an inflammatory, nonatheromatous occlusive condition—causes segmental lesions and subsequent thrombus formation in the small and medium arteries (and sometimes the veins), resulting in decreased blood flow to the feet and legs. This disorder may produce ulceration and, eventually, gangrene.

Buerger disease is caused by vasculitis, an inflammation of blood vessels, primarily of the hands and feet. The vessels become constricted or totally blocked, reducing blood flow to the tissues and resulting in pain and, eventually, damage.

This disorder occurs in 12 to 20 of every 100,000 people. Incidence is highest among males 20 to 40 years old who have a history of smoking or chewing tobacco. It may be associated with a history of Raynaud disease and may occur in people with autoimmune disease.

Pathophysiology

The pathophysiology of Buerger disease is not well understood. In the acute phase, occlusive thrombi develop in arteries and veins of distal extremities. Next, thrombi start to organize into larger vessels. Over time, inflammation resides but fibrosis and organized thrombi remain.

There is also evidence that dysfunction of the endothelial layer of the vessels occurs, as well as the possibility of issues with prothrombin.

Complications
◆ Gangrene
◆ Muscle atrophy
◆ Ulceration

Signs and symptoms

Buerger disease typically produces intermittent claudication of the instep, which is aggravated by exercise and relieved by rest. During exposure to low temperature, the feet initially become cold, cyanotic, and numb; later, they redden, become hot, and tingle. Occasionally, Buerger disease also affects the hands, possibly resulting in painful fingertip ulcerations. Associated signs and symptoms may include impaired peripheral pulses, migratory superficial thrombophlebitis and, in later stages, ulceration, muscle atrophy, and gangrene.

Diagnosis

Patient history and physical examination strongly suggest Buerger disease. Supportive diagnostic tests include:
◆ Doppler ultrasonography to show diminished circulation in the peripheral vessels
◆ angiography or arteriography to locate lesions and rule out atherosclerosis.

Treatment

The primary goals of treatment are to relieve symptoms and prevent complications. Such therapy may include an exercise program that uses gravity to fill and drain the blood vessels or, in severe disease, a lumbar sympathectomy to increase blood supply to the skin. Aspirin and vasodilators may also be used. Amputation may be necessary for nonhealing ulcers, intractable pain, or gangrene.

Special considerations

◆ Strongly urge the patient to stop smoking to enhance the treatment's effectiveness. Symptoms may disappear if the patient stops tobacco use. If necessary, refer the patient to a self-help group to stop smoking.

◆ Warn the patient to avoid precipitating factors, such as emotional stress, exposure to extreme temperatures, and trauma.

◆ Teach the patient proper foot care, especially the importance of wearing well-fitting shoes and cotton or wool socks. Show the patient how to inspect feet daily for cuts, abrasions, and signs of skin breakdown, such as redness and soreness. Remind the patient to seek medical attention at once after any trauma.

◆ If the patient has ulcers and gangrene, enforce bed rest and use a padded footboard or bed cradle to prevent pressure from bed linens. Protect the feet with soft padding. Wash them gently with a mild soap and tepid water, rinse thoroughly, and pat dry with a soft towel.

◆ Provide emotional support. If necessary, refer the patient for psychological counseling to help the patient cope with restrictions imposed by this chronic disease. If the patient has undergone amputation, assess rehabilitative needs, especially regarding changes in body image. Refer the patient to physical therapists, occupational therapists, and social service agencies, as needed.

PERIPHERAL ARTERY DISEASE
Causes and incidence
PAD, referred to as *arterial occlusive disease*, is the obstruction or narrowing of the lumen of the aorta and its major branches, causing an interruption of blood flow, usually to the legs and feet. PAD may affect the carotid, vertebral, innominate, subclavian, mesenteric, and celiac arteries. Occlusions may be acute or chronic and commonly cause severe ischemia, skin ulceration, and gangrene.

The prognosis depends on the occlusion's location, the development of collateral circulation to counteract reduced blood flow, and, in acute disease, the time elapsed between occlusion and its removal.

Predisposing factors include smoking; aging; such conditions as hypertension, hyperlipidemia, and diabetes; and a family history of vascular disorders, MI, or stroke. PAD has no racial predilection. Men older than 50 are at increased risk for intermittent claudication, a common sign of PAD.

Pathophysiology
PAD is a common complication of atherosclerosis. The occlusive mechanism may be endogenous, due to emboli formation or thrombosis, or exogenous, due to trauma or fracture.

Complications
◆ Severe ischemia
◆ Skin ulceration
◆ Gangrene
◆ Limb loss

Signs and symptoms
The signs and symptoms of PAD depend on the site of the occlusion. (See *Types of peripheral artery disease*, page 81.)

Diagnosis
Diagnosis of PAD is usually indicated by patient history and physical examination.

Pertinent supportive diagnostic tests include the following:

◆ Arteriography demonstrates the type (thrombus or embolus), location, and degree of obstruction and the collateral circulation. It's particularly useful in chronic disease or for evaluating candidates for reconstructive surgery.

◆ Doppler ultrasonography and plethysmography are noninvasive tests that show decreased blood flow distal to the occlusion in acute disease.

◆ EEG and computed tomography scan may be necessary to rule out brain lesions.

◆ Ankle-brachial indices compare the systolic blood pressures between the upper and lower extremities and have been shown to be sensitive in detecting PAD.

Treatment
Treatment depends on the obstruction's cause, location, and size. For mild chronic disease, supportive measures include elimination of smoking, hypertension control, and walking exercise. For carotid artery occlusion, antiplatelet therapy may begin with clopidogrel and aspirin. For intermittent claudication of chronic occlusive disease, cilostazol may improve blood flow through the capillaries, particularly for patients who are poor candidates for surgery. Statin medications are used frequently, as well, to lessen the progression of atherosclerosis.

Acute PAD usually requires surgery to restore circulation to the affected area, for example:

◆ Atherectomy—Excision of plaque using a drill or slicing mechanism.

◆ Balloon angioplasty—Compression of the obstruction using balloon inflation.

◆ Bypass graft—Blood flow is diverted through an anastomosed autogenous or Dacron graft past the thrombosed segment.

◆ Combined therapy—Concomitant use of any of the above treatments.

◆ Embolectomy—A balloon-tipped Fogarty catheter is used to remove thrombotic material from the artery. Embolectomy is used mainly for mesenteric, femoral, or popliteal artery occlusion.

◆ Laser angioplasty—Use of excision and hot-tipped lasers to vaporize the obstruction.

◆ Lumbar sympathectomy—An adjunct to surgery, depending on the sympathetic nervous system's condition.

◆ Patch grafting—Removal of the thrombosed arterial segment and replacement with an autogenous vein or Dacron graft.

◆ Stents—Insertion of a mesh of wires that stretch and mold to the arterial wall to prevent reocclusion. This follows laser angioplasty or atherectomy.

◆ Thromboendarterectomy—Opening of the occluded artery and direct removal of the obstructing thrombus and the medial layer of the arterial wall; usually performed after angiography and commonly used with autogenous vein or Dacron bypass surgery (femoral-popliteal or aortofemoral).

◆ Thrombolytic therapy—Lysis of any clot around or in the plaque by urokinase, streptokinase, or alteplase.

Amputation becomes necessary with failure of arterial reconstructive surgery or with the development of gangrene, persistent infection, or intractable pain.

Other therapy includes heparin to prevent emboli (for embolic occlusion) and bowel resection after restoration of blood flow (for mesenteric artery occlusion).

Special considerations

◆ Provide comprehensive patient teaching, including proper foot care. Explain diagnostic tests and procedures. Advise the patient to stop smoking and to follow the prescribed medical regimen.

Preoperatively, during an acute episode:

◆ Assess the patient's circulatory status by checking for the most distal pulses and by inspecting skin color and temperature.

◆ Provide pain relief as needed.

◆ Administer heparin by continuous I.V. drip as ordered. Use an infusion monitor or pump to ensure the proper flow rate.

◆ Wrap the patient's affected foot in soft cotton batting, and reposition it frequently to prevent pressure on any one area. Strictly avoid elevating or applying heat to the affected leg.

◆ Watch for signs of fluid and electrolyte imbalance, and monitor intake and output for signs of renal failure (urine output <30 mL/ hour).

◆ If the patient has carotid, innominate, vertebral, or subclavian artery occlusion, monitor for signs of stroke, such as numbness in an arm or leg and intermittent blindness.

Postoperatively:

◆ Monitor the patient's vital signs. Continuously assess circulatory function by inspecting skin color and temperature and by checking for distal pulses. In charting, compare earlier assessments and observations. Watch closely for signs of hemorrhage (tachycardia and hypotension) and check dressings for excessive bleeding.

◆ In carotid, innominate, vertebral, or subclavian artery occlusion, assess neurologic status frequently for changes in LOC or muscle strength and pupil size.

◆ In mesenteric artery occlusion, connect the NG tube to low intermittent suction. Monitor intake and output (low urine output may indicate damage to renal arteries during surgery). Check bowel sounds for return of peristalsis. Increasing abdominal distention and tenderness may indicate extension of bowel ischemia with resulting gangrene, necessitating further excision, or it may indicate peritonitis.

◆ In saddle block occlusion, check distal pulses for adequate circulation. Watch for signs of renal failure and mesenteric artery occlusion (severe abdominal pain), and for cardiac arrhythmias, which may precipitate embolus formation.

◆ In iliac artery occlusion, monitor urine output for signs of renal failure from decreased perfusion to the kidneys as a result of surgery. Provide meticulous catheter care.

◆ In both femoral and popliteal artery occlusions, assist with early ambulation, but discourage prolonged sitting.

◆ After amputation, check the patient's stump carefully for drainage; record the color and amount of damage, and the time. Elevate the stump as ordered, and administer adequate analgesic medication. Because phantom limb pain is common, explain this phenomenon to the patient.

◆ When preparing the patient for discharge, instruct the patient to watch for signs of recurrence (pain, pallor, numbness, paralysis, and absence of pulse) that can result from graft occlusion or occlusion at another site. Warn the patient against wearing constrictive clothing.

SELECTED REFERENCES

American Heart Association. (2018). *Changes you can make to manage high blood pressure.* Retrieved from http://www .heart.org/HEARTORG/Conditions/HighBloodPressure/ MakeChangesThatMatter/Changes-You-Can-Make-to-Manage-High-Blood-Pressure_UCM_002054_Article. jsp#.Wv9rG8gvzIU

American Heart Association. (2018). *What is TAVR?* Retrieved from http://www.heart.org/HEARTORG/ Conditions/More/HeartValveProblemsandDisease/ What-is-TAVR_UCM_450827_Article.jsp#.Wv9fOcgvzIU

Baldor, R., et al. (2009). *The 5-minute clinical consult 2010* (18th ed.). Philadelphia: Lippincott Williams & Wilkins.

Black, J., III, Greene, C., & Woo, J. (2017). Epidemiology, risk factors, pathogenesis, and natural history of thoracic aortic aneurysm. In K. Collins (Ed.), *UpToDate*. Retrieved from https://www.uptodate.com/contents/epidemiology-risk-factors-pathogenesis-and-natural-history-of-thoracic-aortic-aneurysm

Centers for Disease Control and Prevention. (2018). *Facts about dextro-transposition of the great arteries*. Retrieved from https://www.cdc.gov/ncbddd/heartdefects/d-tga.html

Cleveland Clinic. (2018). *Hypertrophic cardiomyopathy*. Retrieved from https://my.clevelandclinic.org/health/diseases/17116-hypertrophic-cardiomyopathy

Doyle, T., & Kavanaugh-McHugh, A. (2018). Pathophysiology, clinical features, and diagnosis of tetralogy of Fallot. In C. Armsby (Ed.), *UpToDate*. Retrieved from https://www.uptodate.com/contents/pathophysiology-clinical-features-and-diagnosis-of-tetralogy-of-fallot

Fulton, D., & Saleeb, S. (2016). Pathophysiology and clinical features of isolated ventricular septal defects in infants and children. In C. Armsby (Ed.), *UpToDate*. Retrieved from https://www.uptodate.com/contents/pathophysiology-and-clinical-features-of-isolated-ventricular-septal-defects-in-infants-and-children

Ghosh, N., & Haddad, H. (2011). Recent progress in genetics of cardiomyopathy and its role in clinical evaluation of patients with cardiomyopathy. *Current Opinion in Cardiology, 26*(2), 155–164.

Guzman, R., & Lo, R. (2017). Femoral artery aneurysm. In K. Collins (Ed.), *UpToDate*. Retrieved from https://www.uptodate.com/contents/femoral-artery-aneurysm

Helbing, W. A., et al. (2010). Cardiac stress testing after surgery for congenital heart disease. *Current Opinion in Pediatrics, 22*(5), 579–586.

Imazio, M. (2011). Pericarditis: Pathophysiology, diagnosis, and management. *Current Infectious Disease Reports, 13*(4), 308–316. doi:10.1007/S11908-011-0189-5

James, P., et al. (2014). 2014 Evidence-based guideline for the management of high blood pressure in adults. *Journal of the American Medical Association, 311*(5), 507–520. doi:10.1001/jama.2013.284427

Longo, D., et al., eds. (2011). *Harrison's principles of internal medicine* (18th ed.). New York: McGraw-Hill.

Mayo Clinic. (2018). *Mitral valve prolapse*. Retrieved from https://www.mayoclinic.org/diseases-conditions/mitral-valve-prolapse/symptoms-causes/syc-20355446

Mayo Clinic. (2018). *Patent ductus arteriosus (PDA)*. Retrieved from https://www.mayoclinic.org/diseases-conditions/patent-ductus-arteriosus/symptoms-causes/syc-20376145

Merck Manual. (2018). *Myocarditis*. Retrieved from https://www.merckmanuals.com/professional/cardiovascular-disorders/myocarditis-and-pericarditis/myocarditis

Miller, L. (2016). Cardiogenic shock in acute myocardial infarction. *Journal of American College of Cardiology, 67*(16), 1881–1884.

Morise, A. (2011). Exercise testing in nonatherosclerotic heart disease: Hypertrophic cardiomyopathy, valvular heart disease, and arrhythmias. *Circulation, 123*(2), 216–225.

Olin, J. (2017). Thromboangiitis obliterans (Buerger's disease). In K. Collins (Ed.), *UpToDate*. Retrieved from https://www.uptodate.com/contents/thromboangiitis-obliterans-buergers-disease

Pathway Medicine. (2017). *Cardiac tamponade*. Retrieved from http://pathwaymedicine.org/cardiac-tamponade

Phoenix Children's Heart Center. (2018). *Atrial septal defect (ASD) in children*. Retrieved from http://phoenixchildrens.staywellsolutionsonline.com/Search/90,P01766

Pomerantz, W., & Roback, M. (2018). Hypovolemic shock in children: Initial evaluation and management. In J. Wiley (Ed.), *UpToDate*. Retrieved from https://www.uptodate.com/contents/hypovolemic-shock-in-children-initial-evaluation-and-management

Rafiq, I., et al. (2011). Breathlessness and ascending aortic aneurysms: Getting to the root of the problem. *Journal of Cardiovascular Medicine, 12*(3), 201–202.

Sauer, W. (2017). Second degree atrioventricular block: Mobitz type II. In B. Downey (Ed.), *UpToDate*. Retrieved from https://www.uptodate.com/contents/second-degree-atrioventricular-block-mobitz-type-ii

Stanford Children's Health. (2018). *Coarctation of the aorta*. Retrieved from http://www.stanfordchildrens.org/en/topic/default?id=coarctation-of-the-aorta-90-P01770

Wigley, F. (2018). Pathogenesis of Raynaud phenomenon. In M. Curtis (Ed.), *UpToDate*. Retrieved from https://www.uptodate.com/contents/pathogenesis-of-the-raynaud-phenomenon

Woods, S. L., et al., eds. (2009). *Cardiac nursing* (6th ed.). Philadelphia: Lippincott Williams & Wilkins.

2

RESPIRATORY DISORDERS

Introduction

The respiratory system distributes air to the alveoli, where gas exchange—the addition of oxygen (O_2) and the removal of carbon dioxide (CO_2) from pulmonary capillary blood—takes place. Certain specialized structures within this system play a vital role in preparing air for use by the body. The nose, for example, contains vestibular hairs that filter the air and an extensive vascular network that warms it. The nose also contains a layer of goblet cells and a moist mucosal surface; water vapor enters the airstream from this mucosal surface to saturate inspired air as it's warmed in the upper airways. Ciliated mucosa in the posterior portion of the nose and nasopharynx as well as major portions of the tracheobronchial tree propel particles deposited by impaction or gravity to the oropharynx, where the particles are swallowed.

EXTERNAL RESPIRATION

The external component of respiration—ventilation or breathing—delivers inspired air to the lower respiratory tract and alveoli. Contraction and relaxation of the respiratory muscles move air into and out of the lungs. Ventilation begins with the contraction of the inspiratory muscles: the diaphragm (the major muscle of respiration) descends, while external intercostal muscles move the rib cage upward and outward.

Air then enters the lungs in response to the pressure gradient between the atmosphere and the lungs. The lungs adhere to the chest wall and diaphragm because of the vacuum created within the pleural space. As the thorax expands, negative pressure is created in the intrapleural space, causing the lungs to also expand and draw in the warmed, humidified air. The accessory muscles of inspiration, which include the scalene and sternocleidomastoid muscles, raise the clavicles, upper ribs, and sternum. The accessory muscles aren't used in normal inspiration but may be used in some pathologic conditions.

Normal expiration is passive; the inspiratory muscles cease to contract, the diaphragm rises, and the elastic recoil of the lungs causes the lungs to contract. These actions raise the pressure within the lungs above atmospheric pressure, moving air from the lungs to the atmosphere. Active expiration causes pleural pressure to become less negative. (See *Mechanics of ventilation*, page 87.)

An adult lung contains an estimated 300 million alveoli; each alveolus is supplied by many capillaries. To reach the capillary lumen, O_2 must cross the alveolocapillary membrane, which consists of an alveolar epithelial cell, a thin interstitial space, the capillary basement membrane, and the capillary endothelial cell membrane. The O_2 tension of air entering the respiratory tract is approximately 150 mm Hg. In the alveoli, inspired air mixes with CO_2 and water vapor, lowering the O_2 pressure to approximately 100 mm Hg. Because alveolar partial pressure of O_2 is higher than that present in mixed venous blood entering the pulmonary capillaries (~40 mm Hg), O_2 diffuses across the alveolocapillary membrane into the blood.

Mechanics of ventilation

Breathing results from differences between atmospheric and intrapulmonary pressures, as described below.

Before inspiration, intrapulmonary pressure equals atmospheric pressure (~760 mm Hg). Intrapleural pressure is 756 mm Hg.

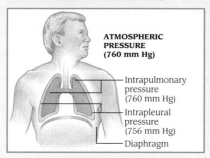

During inspiration, the diaphragm and external intercostal muscles contract, enlarging the thorax vertically and horizontally. As the thorax expands, intrapleural pressure decreases and the lungs expand to fill the enlarging thoracic cavity.

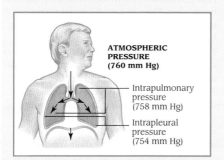

The intrapulmonary atmospheric pressure gradient pulls air into the lungs until the two pressures are equal.

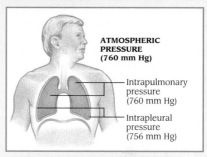

During normal expiration, the diaphragm slowly relaxes and the lungs and thorax passively return to resting size and position. During deep or forced expiration, contraction of internal intercostal and abdominal muscles reduces thoracic volume. Lung and thorax compression raises intrapulmonary pressure above atmospheric pressure.

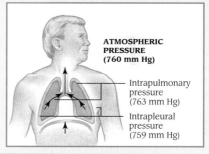

O_2 AND CO_2 TRANSPORT AND INTERNAL RESPIRATION

Circulating blood delivers O_2 to the cells of the body for metabolism and transports metabolic wastes and CO_2 from the tissues back to the lungs. When oxygenated arterial blood reaches tissue capillaries, O_2 diffuses from the blood into the cells because of the O_2 tension gradient. The amount of O_2 available is determined by the concentration of hemoglobin (Hb; the principal carrier of O_2), the percentage of O_2 saturation of the Hb, regional blood flow, arterial O_2 content, and cardiac output.

Internal (cellular) respiration occurs as a part of cellular metabolism, which can take place

with O_2 (aerobic) or without O_2 (anaerobic). The most efficient method for providing fuel (high-energy compounds such as adenosine triphosphate [ATP]) for cellular reactions is aerobic metabolism, which produces CO_2 and water in addition to ATP. Anaerobic metabolism is less efficient because a cell produces only a limited amount of ATP and yields lactic acid as well as CO_2 as a metabolic by-product.

Because circulation is continuous, CO_2 doesn't normally accumulate in tissues. CO_2 produced during cellular respiration diffuses from tissues into regional capillaries and is transported by systemic venous circulation. When CO_2 reaches the alveolar capillaries, it diffuses into the alveoli, where the partial pressure of CO_2 is lower; CO_2 is removed from the alveoli during exhalation.

MECHANISMS OF CONTROL

The central nervous system's (CNS) control of respiration lies in the respiratory center, located in the lateral medulla oblongata of the brainstem. Impulses travel down the phrenic nerves to the diaphragm, and down the intercostal nerves to the intercostal muscles, where the impulses change the rate and depth of respiration. The inspiratory and expiratory centers, located in the posterior medulla, establish the involuntary rhythm of the breathing pattern.

Apneustic and pneumotaxic centers in the pons influence the pattern of breathing. Stimulation of the lower pontine apneustic center (e.g., by trauma, tumor, or stroke) produces forceful inspiratory gasps alternating with weak expiration. The apneustic center continually excites the medullary inspiratory center and thus facilitates inspiration. Signals from the pneumotaxic center as well as afferent impulses from the vagus nerve inhibit the apneustic center and "turn off" inspiration. The apneustic pattern doesn't occur if the vagus nerves are intact.

Partial pressure of arterial oxygen (PaO_2), pH, and pH of cerebrospinal fluid (CSF) influence output from the respiratory center. When CO_2 enters the CSF, the pH of CSF falls, stimulating central chemoreceptors to increase ventilation.

The respiratory center also receives information from peripheral chemoreceptors in the carotid and aortic bodies. These chemoreceptors respond primarily to decreased PaO_2 but also to decreased pH. The peripheral chemoreceptors have little control over respirations until the PaO_2 is less than 60 mm Hg.

During exercise, stretch receptors in lung tissue and the diaphragm prevent overexpansion of the lungs. During swallowing, the cortex can interrupt automatic control of ventilation. During sleep, respiratory drive may fluctuate, producing hypoventilation and periods of apnea. External sensations, drugs, chronic hypercapnia, and changes in body temperature can also alter the respiratory pattern.

DIAGNOSTIC TESTS

Diagnostic tests evaluate physiologic characteristics and pathologic states within the respiratory tract.

Noninvasive tests include:

◆ Chest X-ray shows such conditions as atelectasis, pleural effusion, infiltrates, pneumothorax, lesions, mediastinal shifts, pulmonary edema, and chronic obstructive pulmonary disease (COPD).

◆ Computed tomography (or CT) scan provides a three-dimensional picture that's 100 times more sensitive than a chest X-ray.

◆ Magnetic resonance imaging identifies obstructed arteries and tissue perfusion, but movement of the heart and lungs reduces the image's clarity.

◆ Sputum specimen analysis assesses sputum quantity, color, viscosity, and odor; microbiological stains and culture of sputum can identify infectious organisms; and cytologic preparations can detect respiratory tract neoplasms. Sensitivity tests determine antibiotic sensitivity and resistance.

◆ Pulmonary function tests (or PFTs) measure lung volume, flow rates, and compliance. Normal values, individualized by body stature, ethnicity, and age, are reported in percentage of the normal predicted value. Static measurements are volume measurements that include tidal volume, volume of air contained in a normal breath; functional residual capacity, volume of air remaining in the lungs after normal expiration; vital capacity, volume of air that can be exhaled after maximal inspiration; residual volume, air remaining in the lungs after maximal expiration; and total lung capacity (TLC), volume of air in the lungs after maximal inspiration. Dynamic measurements characterize the movement of air into and out of the lungs and show changes in lung mechanics. They include measurement of forced expiratory volume in 1 second (FEV_1), maximum volume of air that can be expired in 1 second from TLC; maximal voluntary ventilation, volume of air that can be expired in 1 minute with the patient's maximum voluntary effort; and forced vital capacity (FVC), maximal volume of air that the patient can exhale from TLC. (Peak flow rate, which can be obtained at the bedside, is also a dynamic measurement of pulmonary function.)

◆ Methacholine challenge is one method of assessing airway responsiveness and is used to determine a diagnosis of asthma.

◆ Exercise stress test evaluates the ability to transport O_2 and remove CO_2 with increasing metabolic demands.

◆ Polysomnography can diagnose sleep disorders.

◆ Lung scan (ventilation–perfusion or scintiphotography scan) demonstrates ventilation and perfusion patterns. It's used primarily to evaluate pulmonary embolus.

◆ Arterial blood gas (ABG) analysis assesses gas exchange. Decreased PaO_2 may indicate hypoventilation, ventilation–perfusion mismatch, or shunting of blood away from gas exchange sites. Increased partial pressure of arterial carbon dioxide ($PaCO_2$) reflects marked ventilation–perfusion mismatch or hypoventilation; decreased $PaCO_2$ reflects increased alveolar ventilation. Changes in pH may reflect metabolic or respiratory dysfunction.

◆ Pulse oximetry is a noninvasive assessment of arterial oxygen saturation.

◆ Capnography may be used either transcutaneously or in ventilator circuit to determine $PaCO_2$ trends.

Invasive tests include:

◆ Bronchoscopy permits direct visualization of the trachea and mainstem, lobar, segmental, and subsegmental bronchi. It may be used to localize the site of lung hemorrhage, visualize masses in these airways, and collect respiratory tract secretions. Brush biopsy may be used to obtain specimens from the lungs for microbiological stains, culture, and cytology. Lesion biopsies may be performed by using small forceps under direct visualization (when present in the proximal airways) or with the aid of fluoroscopy (when present distal to regions of direct visualization). Bronchoscopy can also be used to clear secretions and remove foreign bodies.

◆ Thoracentesis permits removal of pleural fluid for analysis.

◆ Pleural biopsy obtains pleural tissue for histologic examination and culture.

◆ Pulmonary artery angiography, the injection of dye into the pulmonary artery, can locate pulmonary embolism. This is considered the gold standard for diagnosing pulmonary emboli.

◆ Positron emission tomography scan uses a short-life radionuclide. Increased uptake of the substance is seen in malignant cells.

ASSESSMENT

Assessment of the respiratory system begins with a thorough patient history. Ask the patient to describe his or her respiratory problem. How long has he or she had it? How long does each attack last? Does one attack differ from another? Does any activity in particular bring on an attack or make it worse? What relieves the symptoms? Always ask whether the patient was or is a smoker, what and how often he or she smoked or smokes, and how long he or she smoked or has been smoking. Record this information in *pack years*—the number of packs of cigarettes per day multiplied by the number of smoking years. Remember to ask about the patient's occupation, hobbies, and travel; some of these activities may involve exposure to toxic or allergenic substances.

If the patient has dyspnea, ask if it occurs during activity or at rest. What position is the patient in when dyspnea occurs? How far can he or she walk? How many flights of stairs can he or she climb? Has his or her exercise tolerance been decreasing? Can he or she relate dyspnea to allergies or environmental conditions? Does it occur only at night, during sleep? If the patient has a cough, ask about its severity, persistence, and duration; ask if it produces sputum and, if so, how much and what kind. Have the patient's cough habits and character of sputum changed recently?

PHYSICAL EXAMINATION

Use inspection skills to check for clues to respiratory disease, beginning with the patient's general appearance. If he or she is frail or cachectic, he or she may have a chronic disease that has impaired his or her appetite. If he or she is diaphoretic, restless, or irritable or protective of a painful body part, he or she may be in acute distress. Also, look for behavior changes that may indicate hypoxemia or hypercapnia. Confusion, lethargy, bizarre behavior, or quiet sleep from which the patient can't be aroused may point to hypercapnia. Watch for marked cyanosis, indicated by bluish or ashen skin (usually best seen on the lips, tongue, earlobes, and nail beds), which may be due to hypoxemia or poor tissue perfusion.

Assess chest shape and symmetry at rest and during ventilation. Increased anteroposterior diameter ("barrel chest") characterizes emphysema. Kyphoscoliosis also alters chest configuration, which in turn restricts breathing. Assess respiratory excursion and observe for accessory muscle use during breathing. The use of upper chest and neck muscles is normal only during physical stress.

Observe the rate and pattern of breathing because certain disorders produce characteristic changes in breathing patterns. For example, an acute respiratory disorder can produce tachypnea (rapid, shallow breathing) or hyperpnea (increased rate and depth of breathing); intracranial lesions can produce Cheyne–Stokes and Biot's respirations; increased intracranial pressure can result in central hyperventilation and apneustic or ataxic breathing; metabolic disorders can cause Kussmaul's respirations; and airway obstruction can lead to prolonged forceful expiration and pursed-lip breathing.

Also observe posture and carriage. A patient with COPD, for example, usually supports rib cage movement by placing his or her arms on the sides of a chair to increase expansion and lean forward during exhalation to help expel air.

Palpation of the chest wall detects areas of tenderness, masses, changes in fremitus (palpable vocal vibrations), or crepitus (air in subcutaneous tissues). To assess chest excursion and symmetry, place your hands in a horizontal position, bilaterally on the posterior chest, with your thumbs pressed lightly against the spine, creating folds in the skin. As the patient takes a deep breath, your thumbs should move quickly and equally away from the spine. Repeat this with your hands placed anteriorly, at the costal margins (lower lobes) and clavicles (apices). Unequal movement indicates differences in expansion, seen in atelectasis, diaphragm or chest wall muscle disease, or splinting due to pain.

Percussion should detect resonance over lung fields that aren't covered by bony structures or the heart. A dull sound on percussion may mean consolidation or pleural disease. (See *Characterizing and interpreting percussion sounds*.)

Auscultation normally detects soft, vesicular breath sounds throughout most of the lung fields. Absent or adventitious breath sounds may indicate fluid in small airways or interstitial lung disease (crackles), secretions in moderate and large airways (rhonchi), and airflow obstruction (wheezes).

SPECIAL RESPIRATORY CARE
The hospitalized patient with respiratory disease may require an artificial upper airway, chest tubes, chest physiotherapy, and supervision of mechanical ventilation. In cardiopulmonary arrest, establishing an airway always takes precedence. In a patient with this condition, airway obstruction usually results when the tongue slides back and blocks the posterior pharynx. The head-tilt method or, in suspected or confirmed cervical fracture or arthritis, the jaw-thrust maneuver can immediately push the tongue forward, relieving such obstruction. Endotracheal (ET) intubation and, sometimes, a tracheotomy may be necessary.

Characterizing and interpreting percussion sounds

Percussion may produce several kinds of sounds. Known as flat, dull, resonant, hyperresonant, or tympanic, these sounds indicate the location and density of various structures. During percussion, determining other tonal characteristics, such as pitch, intensity, and quality, also will help identify respiratory structure. Use this chart as a guide to interpreting percussion sounds.

Characteristic

Sound	Pitch	Intensity	Quality	Implications
Flatness	High	Soft	Extremely dull	These sounds are normal over the sternum. Over the lung, they may indicate atelectasis or pleural effusion.
Dullness	Medium	Medium	Thudlike	Normal over the liver, heart, and diaphragm, these sounds over the lung may point to pneumonia, tumor, atelectasis, or pleural effusion.
Resonance	Low	Moderate to loud	Hollow	When percussed over the lung, these sounds are normal.
Hyperresonance	Lower than resonance	Very loud	Booming	These are normal findings with percussion over a child's lung. Over an adult's lung, these findings may indicate emphysema, chronic bronchitis, asthma, or pneumothorax.
Tympany	High	Loud	Musical, drumlike	Over the stomach, these are normal findings; over the lung, they suggest tension pneumothorax.

CHEST TUBES

An important procedure in patients with respiratory disease is chest tube drainage, which removes air or fluid from the pleural space. This allows the collapsed lung to re-expand to fill the evacuated pleural space. Chest drainage also allows removal of pleural fluid for culture. Chest tubes are commonly used after thoracic surgery, penetrating chest wounds, pleural effusion, and empyema. They're also used for evacuation of pneumothorax, hydrothorax, or hemothorax. Sometimes chest tubes are used to instill sclerosing drugs into the pleural space to prevent recurrent malignant pleural effusions.

Commonly, the chest tube is placed in the sixth or seventh intercostal space, in the axillary region. Occasionally, in pneumothorax, the tube is placed in the second or third intercostal space, in the midclavicular region.

Follow these guidelines when caring for a patient with a chest tube:
◆ Monitor changes in suction pressure.
◆ Make sure that all connections in the system are tight and secured with tape.
◆ Never clamp the chest tube unless checking for air leaks or changing the drainage system.
◆ Record the amount, color, and consistency of drainage. Watch for signs of shock, such as tachycardia and hypotension, if drainage is excessive.
◆ Encourage the patient to cough and breathe deeply every hour to enhance lung expansion.

Additionally, if a water seal–wet suction system is in place:
◆ Check for fluctuation in the water-seal chamber as the patient breathes. Normal fluctuations of 2″ to 4″ (about 5 to 10 cm) reflect pressure changes in the pleural space during respiration.
◆ Watch for intermittent bubbling in the water-seal chamber. This bubbling occurs normally when the system is removing air from the pleural cavity. Absence of bubbling indicates that the pleural space has sealed.
◆ Check the water level in the suction-control chamber. If necessary, add sterile water to bring the level to the ordered level.
◆ Check for gentle bubbling in the suction-control chamber, which indicates that the proper suction level has been reached.

If a dry-suction system is in place, check that the rotary dry-suction control dial is turned to the ordered suction mark and verify that the appropriate indicator is present, indicating that the desired amount of suction is applied.

VENTILATOR METHODS

Mechanical ventilators are typically used for CNS problems, hypoxemia, or failure of the normal bellows action provided by the diaphragm and rib cage. Positive-pressure ventilators cause inspiration while increasing tidal volume (V_T). The inspiratory cycles of these ventilators may vary in volume, pressure, time, or frequency. For example, a volume-cycled ventilator—the type most commonly used—delivers a preset volume of air each time, regardless of the amount of lung resistance. A pressure-cycled ventilator generates flow until the machine reaches a preset pressure regardless of the volume delivered or the time required to achieve the pressure. A time-cycled ventilator generates flow for a preset amount of time. A high-frequency ventilator uses high respiratory rates and low V_T to maintain alveolar ventilation. Positive end-expiratory pressure (PEEP) is used to retain a certain amount of pressure in the lungs at the end of expiration. By keeping small airways and alveoli open with this method, functional residual capacity is increased and oxygenation is improved.

Implement strategies to prevent ventilator-associated pneumonia (VAP) and plan to remove the patient from ventilator support as soon as the cause of respiratory failure has resolved. (See *Preventing ventilator-associated pneumonia*, page 92.) Several weaning methods are used. The patient may be taken off the ventilator and supplied with a T-piece (ET tube O_2 adapter) that provides O_2 and humidification. The patient then breathes spontaneously without the ventilator for gradually increasing periods.

With intermittent mandatory ventilation, the ventilator provides a specific number of breaths, and the patient is able to breathe spontaneously between ventilator breaths. The frequency of ventilator breaths is gradually decreased until the patient can breathe on his or her own. Pressure support ventilation, in which the patient receives a preset pressure boost with each spontaneous breath, has proved effective. Vital signs, ABG levels, physical findings, and subjective symptoms should be monitored periodically during weaning to assess respiratory status.

Chest physiotherapy

In respiratory conditions marked by excessive accumulation of secretions in the lungs, chest physiotherapy may enhance removal of secretions. Chest physiotherapy includes chest assessment, effective breathing and coughing exercises, postural drainage, percussion, vibration, and evaluation of the therapy's effectiveness. Before initiating treatment, review X-rays and physical assessment findings to locate areas of secretions.
◆ Deep breathing maintains diaphragm use, increases negative intrathoracic pressure, and

Preventing ventilator-associated pneumonia

Ventilator-associated pneumonia (VAP) is the leading cause of death among all hospital-acquired infections. VAP also prolongs time spent on the ventilator, length of critical care unit (CCU) stay, and length of hospital stay after discharge from the CCU. Research has shown that the mortality rate due to VAP can be reduced by early recognition of pneumonia and consistent application of evidence-based practices. The Ventilator Bundle is a group of interventions related to ventilator care that, when implemented together, achieve significantly better outcomes than when implemented individually. The key components of the Ventilator Bundle include:

♦ elevating the head of the bed 30 to 45 degrees
♦ interrupting sedation daily and assessing the readiness to extubate
♦ instituting peptic ulcer disease prophylaxis
♦ instituting deep vein thrombosis prophylaxis
♦ providing daily oral care with chlorhexidine

Various other best practices can be combined with the bundle to prevent VAP. They include:

♦ adhering to Centers for Disease Control and Prevention or World Health Organization hand hygiene guidelines to prevent the spread of infection
♦ using noninvasive ventilatory support, such as bilevel positive-airway ventilation instead of endotracheal (ET) intubation and mechanical ventilation, to eliminate the risk of VAP
♦ using the oral route instead of the nasal route for ET intubation to prevent sinusitis
♦ maintaining ET tube cuff pressure at 20 cm or more to prevent aspiration
♦ using a cuffed ET tube with in-line and subglottic suctioning to prevent secretion aspiration
♦ avoiding gastric distention to reduce the risk for aspiration
♦ avoiding unexplained extubation and reintubation to prevent secretion aspiration
♦ minimizing equipment contamination (by removing condensate from ventilator circuits, keeping the circuit closed during removal, changing the ventilator circuit only when visibly soiled or malfunctioning, and disinfecting and storing respiratory equipment properly) to prevent airway contamination
♦ teaching the patient and family about measures to prevent VAP and involving them in monitoring

promotes venous return; it's especially important when pain or dressings restrict chest movement. An incentive spirometer can provide positive visual reinforcement to promote deep breathing.

♦ Pursed-lip breathing is used primarily in obstructive disease to slow expiration and prevent small airway collapse. Such breathing slows air through smaller bronchi, maintaining positive pressure and preventing collapse of small airways and resultant air trapping.

♦ Segmental breathing or lateral costal breathing is used after lung resection and for localized disorders. Place your hand over the lung area on the affected side. Instruct the patient to try to push that portion of the chest against your hand on deep inspiration. You should be able to feel this with your hand.

♦ Coughing that's controlled and staged gradually increases intrathoracic pressure, reducing pain and bronchospasm of explosive coughing. When wound pain prevents effective coughing, splint the wound with a pillow, towel, or your hand during coughing exercises.

♦ Postural drainage uses gravity to drain secretions into larger airways, where they can be expectorated. This technique is used in the patient with copious or tenacious secretions. Before performing postural drainage, auscultate the patient's chest and review chest X-rays to determine the best position for maximum drainage. To prevent vomiting, schedule postural drainage at least 1 hour after meals.

♦ Percussion moves air against the chest wall, enhancing the effectiveness of postural drainage by loosening lung secretions. Percussion is contraindicated in severe pain, extreme obesity, cancer that has metastasized to the ribs, crushing chest injuries, bleeding disorders, spontaneous pneumothorax, spinal compression fractures, and in patients with temporary pacemakers.

♦ Vibration can be used with percussion or alone when percussion is contraindicated.

♦ PEEP therapy maintains positive pressure in airways, preventing small airway collapse.

Before and after chest physiotherapy, auscultate the patient's lung fields and assess for sputum production to evaluate the effectiveness of therapy.

Congenital and pediatric disorders

RESPIRATORY DISTRESS SYNDROME

Respiratory distress syndrome (RDS), also called *hyaline membrane disease*, is the most common cause of neonatal mortality. In the United States alone, it kills 40,000 neonates every year. RDS occurs in premature neonates and, if untreated, is fatal within 72 hours of birth in up to 14% of neonates weighing less than 5½ lb (2.5 kg). Aggressive management using mechanical ventilation can improve the prognosis, but some surviving neonates may develop some degree of bronchopulmonary dysplasia (BPD).

Causes and incidence

Although airways and alveoli of a neonate's respiratory system are present by 27 weeks' gestation, the intercostal muscles are weak, and the alveolar capillary system is immature. The preterm neonate with RDS develops widespread alveolar collapse because of a lack of surfactant, a lipoprotein present in alveoli and respiratory bronchioles. The surfactant lowers surface tension and helps prevent alveolar collapse. This surfactant deficiency results in widespread atelectasis, which leads to inadequate alveolar ventilation with shunting of blood through collapsed areas of lung, causing hypoxemia and acidosis.

RDS occurs almost exclusively in neonates born before 37 weeks' gestation (in 60% of those born before the 28th week). The incidence is greatest in those with birth weights of 1,000 to 1,500 g. Infants of diabetic mothers, those born by cesarean delivery, second-born twins, infants with perinatal asphyxia, and those delivered suddenly after antepartum hemorrhage are more commonly affected.

Pathophysiology

The lack of surfactant coating the alveoli reduces the available pulmonary surface and decreases the area for gas exchange. Worsening hypercapnia and hypoxia cause metabolic and respiratory acidosis leading to pulmonary vasoconstriction and peripheral vasodilation. Damage to the endothelial and alveolar cells results from the ongoing hypoxia. The subsequent vascular disruption leads to plasma leakage into the alveolar spaces, layering of fibrin and necrotic cells creating hyaline membranes. These membranes impede the exchange of gases across the alveolar surface.

Complications

- ◆ Pneumothorax
- ◆ Pneumomediastinum
- ◆ Pneumopericardium
- ◆ BPD
- ◆ Intraventricular bleed
- ◆ Hemorrhage into lungs after surfactant use
- ◆ Retinopathy of prematurity (or ROP)
- ◆ Delayed mental development or mental retardation

Signs and symptoms

Although a neonate with RDS may breathe normally at first, they usually develop rapid, shallow respirations within minutes or hours of birth, with intercostal, subcostal, or sternal retractions; nasal flaring; and audible expiratory grunting. This grunting is a natural compensatory mechanism designed to produce PEEP and prevent further alveolar collapse.

Severe disease is marked by apnea, bradycardia, and cyanosis (from hypoxemia, left-to-right shunting through the foramen ovale, or right-to-left intrapulmonary shunting through atelectatic regions of the lung). Other clinical features include pallor, frothy sputum, and low body temperature as a result of an immature nervous system and the absence of subcutaneous fat.

Diagnosis

℞ CONFIRMING DIAGNOSIS *Signs of respiratory distress in a premature neonate during the first few hours of life strongly suggest RDS, but a chest X-ray and ABG analysis are needed to confirm the diagnosis.*

- ◆ Chest X-ray may be normal for the first 6 to 12 hours (in 50% of neonates with RDS), but 24 hours after birth it will show the characteristic ground-glass appearance and air bronchograms.
- ◆ ABG analysis shows decreased PaO₂; normal, decreased, or increased PaCO₂; and decreased pH (from respiratory or metabolic acidosis or both).
- ◆ Chest auscultation reveals normal or diminished air entry and crackles (rare in early stages).

When a cesarean birth is necessary before 36 weeks' gestation, amniocentesis enables the determination of the lecithin/sphingomyelin (L/S) ratio and the presence of phosphatidylglycerol. An L/S ratio of more than 2:1 and the presence of phosphatidylglycerol decrease the likelihood of RDS.

Treatment

Treatment of an infant with RDS requires vigorous respiratory support. Warm, humidified, oxygen-enriched gases are administered by oxygen hood or, if such treatment fails, by mechanical ventilation. Severe cases may require mechanical ventilation with PEEP or continuous positive-airway pressure (CPAP), administered by nasal prongs or, when necessary, ET intubation. Special ventilation techniques are now used on the patient's refractory to conventional mechanical ventilation. These include high-frequency jet ventilation and high-frequency oscillatory ventilation. Extracorporeal membrane oxygenation is the last choice for ventilation and is only available in certain specialized facilities. Treatment of RDS also includes:

◆ a radiant warmer or isolette for thermoregulation

◆ I.V. fluids and sodium bicarbonate to control acidosis and maintain fluid and electrolyte balance

◆ tube feedings or total parenteral nutrition if the neonate is too weak to eat

◆ administration of surfactant by an ET tube (Studies show that this treatment can prevent or improve the course of RDS as well as reduce mortality.)

Special considerations

◆ Neonates with RDS require continual assessment and monitoring in an intensive care nursery.

◆ Closely monitor ABGs as well as fluid intake and output. If the neonate has an umbilical catheter (arterial or venous), check for arterial hypotension or abnormal central venous pressure. Watch for complications, such as infection, thrombosis, or decreased circulation to the legs. If the neonate has a transcutaneous oxygen monitor, change the site of the lead placement every 2 to 4 hours.

◆ To evaluate progress, assess skin color, rate and depth of respirations, severity of retractions, nostril flaring, frequency of expiratory grunting, frothing at the lips, and restlessness.

◆ Regularly assess the effectiveness of oxygen or ventilator therapy. Evaluate every change in fraction of inspired oxygen and PEEP or CPAP by monitoring arterial oxygen saturation or ABG levels. Adjust the PEEP or CPAP as indicated, on the basis of findings.

◆ Mechanical ventilation in neonates is usually done in a pressure-limited mode rather than in the volume-limited mode used in adults.

◆ When the neonate is on mechanical ventilation, watch carefully for signs of barotrauma (an increase in respiratory distress and subcutaneous emphysema) and accidental disconnection from the ventilator. Check ventilator settings frequently. Be alert for signs of complications of PEEP or CPAP therapy, such as decreased cardiac output, pneumothorax, and pneumomediastinum. Mechanical ventilation

increases the risk of infection in the preterm neonate, so preventive measures are essential.

◆ As needed, arrange for follow-up care with a neonatal ophthalmologist to check for retinal damage. Preterm neonates in an oxygen-rich environment are at increased risk for developing ROP.

◆ Teach the parents about their neonate's condition and, if possible, let them participate in their care (using sterile technique), to encourage normal parent–infant bonding. Advise parents that full recovery may take up to 12 months. When the prognosis is poor, prepare the parents for the neonate's impending death and offer emotional support.

◆ Help reduce mortality in the neonate with RDS by detecting respiratory distress early. Recognize intercostal retractions and grunting, especially in a premature neonate, as signs of RDS; make sure the neonate receives immediate treatment.

:::::::: **PREVENTION**
◆ *Prenatal care can help prevent prematurity.*
◆ *Give corticosteroids to the mother 2 to 3 days before delivery to help the infant's lungs mature in preterm deliveries.*

SUDDEN INFANT DEATH SYNDROME

A medical mystery of early infancy, sudden infant death syndrome (SIDS), also called *crib death*, is the unexpected, sudden death of an infant or child younger than age 1 year. Reasons for the death remain unexplained even after an autopsy. Typically, parents put the infant to bed and later find him or her dead, commonly with no indications of a struggle or distress of any kind. Incidence has decreased with the practice of teaching parents to place an infant on their back to sleep.

Causes and incidence

SIDS is the third leading cause of death in infants between 1 month and 1 year old. It occurs more commonly in winter months. The incidence is higher in males, preterm neonates, and those who sleep on their stomachs or in cribs with soft bedding. Incidence is also higher among neonates born in conditions of poverty and to those who were one of a single multiple birth, such as twins and triplets, and to mothers who smoke, take drugs, or failed to seek prenatal care until late in the pregnancy. SIDS may also result from an abnormality in the control of ventilation that allows CO_2 to build up in the blood, thereby causing prolonged apneic periods with profound hypoxemia and serious cardiac arrhythmias. It's also thought to be associated with problems in sleep arousal.

Pathophysiology

Although the exact pathophysiology of SIDS is not known, there is a common theory. Abnormalities of the autoimmune nervous system and brainstem cause dysfunctions of breathing. Episodes of hypoxia contribute to delaying the arousal response when oxygen availability is decreased and potentially leading to death.

Signs and symptoms

Although parents find some victims wedged in crib corners or with blankets wrapped around their heads, autopsies rule out suffocation as the cause of death. Autopsy shows a patent airway, so aspiration of vomitus isn't the cause of death. Typically, SIDS babies don't cry out and show no signs of having been disturbed in their sleep. However, their positions or tangled blankets may suggest movement just before death, perhaps due to terminal spasm.

Depending on how long the infant has been dead, a SIDS baby may have a mottled complexion with extreme cyanosis of the lips and fingertips or pooling of blood in the legs and feet that may be mistaken for bruises. Pulse and respirations are absent, and the diaper is wet and full of stool.

Diagnosis

Diagnosis of SIDS requires an autopsy to rule out other causes of death. Characteristic histologic findings on autopsy include small or normal adrenal glands and petechiae over the visceral surfaces of the pleura, within the thymus, and in the epicardium. Autopsy also reveals extremely well-preserved lymphoid structures and certain pathologic characteristics that suggest chronic hypoxemia such as increased pulmonary artery smooth muscle. Examination also shows edematous, congestive lungs fully expanded in the pleural cavities, liquid (not clotted) blood in the heart, and curd from the stomach inside the trachea.

Treatment

If the parents bring the infant to the emergency department (ED), the physician will decide whether to try to resuscitate him. An "aborted SIDS" infant is one who's found apneic and is successfully resuscitated. Such an infant, or any infant who had a sibling stricken by SIDS, should be tested for infantile apnea. If tests are positive, a home apnea monitor may be recommended. Because the infant usually can't be resuscitated, however, treatment focuses on providing emotional support for the family.

Special considerations

◆ Make sure that parents are present when the child's death is announced. They may lash out at ED personnel, the babysitter, or anyone else involved in the child's care—even each other. Stay calm and let them express their feelings. Reassure them that they weren't to blame.

◆ Let the parents see the baby in a private room. Allow them to express their grief in their own way. Stay in the room with them if appropriate. Offer to call clergy, friends, or relatives.

◆ After the parents and family have recovered from their initial shock, explain the necessity for an autopsy to confirm the diagnosis of SIDS (in some states, this is mandatory). At this time, provide the family with some basic facts about SIDS and encourage them to give their consent for the autopsy. Make sure that they receive the autopsy report promptly.

◆ Find out whether your community has a local counseling and information program for SIDS parents. Participants in such a program will contact the parents, ensure that they receive the autopsy report promptly, put them in touch with a professional counselor, and maintain supportive telephone contact. Also, find out whether there's a local SIDS parent group; such a group can provide significant emotional support. Contact the National Sudden Infant Death Foundation for information about such local groups.

◆ If your facility's policy is to assign a public health nurse to the family, they will provide the continuing reassurance and assistance the parents will need.

◆ If the parents decide to have another child, they'll need information and counseling to help them through the pregnancy and the first year of the new infant's life.

◆ Infants at high risk for SIDS may be placed on apnea monitoring at home.

◆ All new parents should be informed of the American Academy of Pediatrics' recommendation that infants be positioned on their back, not on their stomach or side, for sleeping.

> ::::::: **PREVENTION**
> ◆ *Tell parents to place infants on their backs to sleep.*
> ◆ *Tell parents infants should sleep on a firm mattress and shouldn't have soft objects in the crib; like stuffed toys and blankets.*
> ◆ *Tell parents infants shouldn't sleep in the same bed as their parents.*
> ◆ *Tell parents to give infants pacifiers at bedtime.*
> ◆ *Tell parents infants shouldn't be exposed to secondhand smoke.*

CROUP

Croup is a severe inflammation and obstruction of the upper airway, occurring as acute laryngotracheobronchitis (most common), laryngitis, and acute spasmodic laryngitis; it must always be distinguished from epiglottitis. It's derived from an old German word for "voice box" and refers to swelling around the larynx or vocal cords. Recovery is usually complete.

Causes and incidence

Croup usually results from a viral infection but can also be caused by bacteria, allergens, and inhaled irritants. Parainfluenza viruses cause 75% of such infections; adenoviruses, respiratory syncytial virus (RSV), influenza, and measles viruses account for the rest.

Croup is a childhood disease affecting more boys than girls (typically between 3 months and 5 years old) that usually occurs during the winter. Up to 15% of patients have a strong family history of croup.

Pathophysiology

Infection of the laryngeal mucosa leads to edema and inflammation of the epiglottal area. This swelling leads to a narrowing of the airway and increasingly deep respirations. The ongoing effort to breath as the narrowing progresses becomes more difficult and the air flowing through the upper airway becomes turbulent. During inspiration, the flexible chest wall caves in slightly and causing paradoxical breathing.

Complications

◆ Respiratory distress
◆ Respiratory arrest
◆ Epiglottitis
◆ Bacterial tracheitis
◆ Atelectasis
◆ Dehydration

Signs and symptoms

The onset of croup usually follows an upper respiratory tract infection. Clinical features include inspiratory stridor, hoarse or muffled vocal sounds, varying degrees of laryngeal obstruction and respiratory distress, and a characteristic sharp, barking, seal-like cough. These symptoms may last only a few hours or persist for a day or two. As it progresses, croup causes inflammatory edema and, possibly, spasm, which can obstruct the upper airway and severely compromise ventilation. (See *How croup affects the upper airway*.)

PATHOPHYSIOLOGY
How croup affects the upper airway

In croup, inflammatory swelling and spasms constrict the larynx, thereby reducing airflow. This cross-sectional drawing (from chin to chest) shows the upper airway changes caused by croup. Inflammatory changes almost completely obstruct the larynx (which includes the epiglottis) and significantly narrow the trachea.

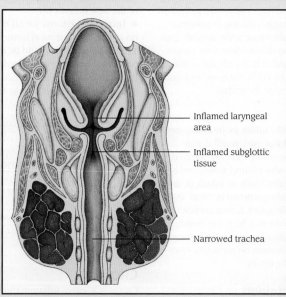

Inflamed laryngeal area

Inflamed subglottic tissue

Narrowed trachea

Each form of croup has additional characteristics:

In *laryngotracheobronchitis*, the symptoms seem to worsen at night. Inflammation causes edema of the bronchi and bronchioles as well as increasingly difficult expiration that frightens the child. Other characteristic features include fever, diffusely decreased breath sounds, expiratory rhonchi, and scattered crackles.

Laryngitis, which results from vocal cord edema, is usually mild and produces no respiratory distress except in infants. Early signs include a sore throat and cough, which, rarely, may progress to marked hoarseness, suprasternal and intercostal retractions, inspiratory stridor, dyspnea, diminished breath sounds, restlessness and, in later stages, severe dyspnea and exhaustion.

Acute spasmodic laryngitis affects a child between 1 and 3 years old, particularly one with allergies and a family history of croup. It typically begins with mild to moderate hoarseness and nasal discharge, followed by the characteristic cough and noisy inspiration (that usually awaken the child at night), labored breathing with retractions, rapid pulse, and clammy skin. The child understandably becomes anxious, which may lead to increasing dyspnea and transient cyanosis. These severe symptoms diminish after several hours but reappear in a milder form on the next one or two nights.

Diagnosis

The clinical picture is very characteristic, so the diagnosis should be suspected immediately. When bacterial infection is the cause, throat cultures may identify the organisms and their sensitivity to antibiotics and rule out diphtheria. On a posterior–anterior X-ray of the chest, narrowing of the upper airway ("steeple sign") may be apparent. Laryngoscopy may reveal inflammation and obstruction in epiglottal and laryngeal areas. In evaluating the patient, assess for foreign body obstruction (a common cause of crouplike cough in a young child) as well as masses and cysts.

Treatment

For most children with croup, home care with rest, cool mist humidification during sleep, and antipyretics, such as acetaminophen, relieve symptoms. However, respiratory distress that's severe or interferes with oral hydration requires hospitalization and parenteral fluid replacement to prevent dehydration. If bacterial infection is the cause, antibiotic therapy is necessary. Oxygen therapy may also be required.

Increasing obstruction of the airway requires intubation and mechanical ventilation.

Inhaled racemic epinephrine and corticosteroids may be used to alleviate respiratory distress.

Special considerations

Monitor and support respiration, and control fever. Because croup is so frightening to the child and family, you must also provide support and reassurance.

◆ Carefully monitor cough and breath sounds, hoarseness, severity of retractions, inspiratory stridor, cyanosis, respiratory rate and character (especially prolonged and labored respirations), restlessness, fever, and cardiac rate.

◆ Keep the child as quiet as possible. However, avoid sedation because it may depress respiration. If the patient is an infant, position them in an infant seat or propped up with a pillow; place an older child in Fowler's position. If an older child requires a cool mist tent to help them breathe, explain why it's needed.

◆ Isolate patients suspected of having RSV and parainfluenza infections if possible. Wash your hands carefully before leaving the room, to avoid transmission to other children, particularly infants. Instruct parents and others involved in the care of these children to take similar precautions.

◆ Control fever with sponge baths and antipyretics. Keep a hypothermia blanket on hand for temperatures above 102° F (38.9° C). Watch for seizures in infants and young children with high fevers. Give I.V. antibiotics as ordered.

◆ Relieve sore throat with soothing, water-based ices, such as fruit sherbet and ice pops. Avoid thicker, milk-based fluids if the child is producing heavy mucus or has great difficulty in swallowing. Apply petroleum jelly or another ointment around the nose and lips to soothe irritation from nasal discharge and mouth breathing.

◆ Maintain a calm, quiet environment and offer reassurance. Explain all procedures and answer any questions.

When croup doesn't require hospitalization:

◆ Teach the parents effective home care. Suggest the use of a cool mist humidifier (vaporizer). To relieve croupy spells, tell parents to carry the child into the bathroom, shut the door, and turn on the hot water. Breathing in warm, moist air quickly eases an acute spell of croup.

◆ Warn parents that ear infections and pneumonia are complications of croup, which may appear about 5 days after recovery. Stress the importance of immediately reporting earache, productive cough, high fever, or increased shortness of breath.

::::::: **PREVENTION**
◆ *Perform hand hygiene frequently to prevent a respiratory infection.*
◆ *Give diphtheria, tetanus, and pertussis (DpT); Haemophilus influenzae B (Hib); and measles, mumps, and rubella (MMR) vaccines to children.*

EPIGLOTTITIS

Acute epiglottitis is an acute inflammation of the epiglottis that tends to cause airway obstruction. A critical emergency, epiglottitis can prove fatal unless it's recognized and treated promptly.

Causes and incidence

Epiglottitis usually results from infection with Hib and, occasionally, pneumococci and group A streptococci. It typically strikes children between 2 and 6 years old. (However, immunosuppression can predispose adults to epiglottitis.) Since the advent of the Hib vaccine, epiglottitis is becoming more rare.

Pathophysiology

The causative bacteria invade the mucosa and into the bloodstream causing bacteremia and infection of the epiglottis as well as surrounding tissues. Acute inflammation and edema begin in the epiglottic area and progressing to the epiglottic folds, arytenoids, and entire supraglottic larynx. The aggressive swelling and edema greatly reduces the available airway and quickly increasing the risk for a respiratory crisis.

Complications

◆ Respiratory failure
◆ Pneumonia
◆ Meningitis
◆ Death
◆ Pericarditis

Signs and symptoms

Sometimes preceded by an upper respiratory infection, epiglottitis may rapidly progress to complete upper airway obstruction within 2 to 5 hours. Laryngeal obstruction results from inflammation and edema of the epiglottis. Accompanying symptoms include high fever, stridor, sore throat, dysphagia, irritability, restlessness, and drooling. To relieve severe respiratory distress, the child with epiglottitis may hyperextend his or her neck, sit up, and lean forward with his or her mouth open, tongue protruding, and nostrils flaring as he or she tries to breathe. The child may develop inspiratory retractions and rhonchi.

Diagnosis

In acute epiglottitis, throat examination reveals a large, edematous, bright red epiglottis. Such examination should follow lateral neck X-rays and, generally, *shouldn't* be performed if the suspected obstruction is great. Special equipment (laryngoscope and ET tubes) should be available because a tongue blade can cause sudden complete airway obstruction. Trained personnel (such as an anesthesiologist) should be on hand during the throat examination to secure an emergency airway. On the lateral soft-tissue X-ray of the neck, a large, thick but indistinct ("thumbprint") epiglottis will be seen. Blood or throat culture may show *H. influenzae* or other bacteria.

Treatment

A child with acute epiglottitis and airway obstruction requires emergency hospitalization; the child may need emergency ET intubation or a tracheotomy with subsequent monitoring in an intensive care unit. Respiratory distress that interferes with swallowing necessitates parenteral fluid administration to prevent dehydration. A patient with acute epiglottitis should always receive a complete course of parenteral antibiotics—usually a second- or third-generation cephalosporin. (If the child is allergic to penicillin, a quinolone or sulfa drug may be substituted.) Corticosteroids should be used to decrease swelling of the throat.

Special considerations

◆ Keep equipment available in case of sudden complete airway obstruction to secure an airway. Be prepared to assist with intubation or tracheotomy, as necessary.

⚠ ALERT *Watch for increasing restlessness, rising cardiac rate, fever, dyspnea, and retractions, which may indicate the need for an emergency tracheotomy. Monitor blood gases for hypoxemia and hypercapnia.*

◆ After a tracheotomy, anticipate the patient's needs because they won't be able to cry or call out; provide emotional support. Reassure the patient and their family that the tracheotomy is a short-term intervention (usually from 4 to 7 days). Monitor the patient for rising temperature and pulse rate and hypotension—signs of secondary infection.
◆ The bacterial infection causing epiglottitis is contagious, and airborne or droplet precautions should be followed. Family members should be screened.

::::::: **PREVENTION**
◆ *Perform hand hygiene frequently to prevent infections.*
◆ *Administer the Hib vaccine to children.*

Acute disorders

ACUTE RESPIRATORY DISTRESS SYNDROME

A form of noncardiogenic pulmonary edema that causes acute respiratory failure (ARF), acute respiratory distress syndrome (ARDS), also called *shock lung* or *adult respiratory distress syndrome*, results from increased permeability of the alveolocapillary membrane. Fluid accumulates in the lung interstitium, alveolar spaces, and small airways, causing the lung to stiffen. Effective ventilation is thus impaired, prohibiting adequate oxygenation of pulmonary capillary blood. Severe ARDS can cause intractable and fatal hypoxemia. However, patients who recover may have little or no permanent lung damage. (See *Alveolar changes in ARDS.*)

Causes and incidence

ARDS results from many respiratory and nonrespiratory insults, such as:

♦ aspiration of gastric contents
♦ sepsis (primarily gram-negative), trauma, or oxygen toxicity
♦ shock

PATHOPHYSIOLOGY
Alveolar changes in ARDS

The alveoli undergo major changes in each phase of ARDS.

Phase 1
In *phase 1*, injury reduces normal blood flow to the lungs. Platelets aggregate and release histamine (H), serotonin (S), and bradykinin (B).

Phase 2
In *phase 2*, those substances—especially histamine—inflame and damage the alveolocapillary membrane, increasing capillary permeability. Fluids then shift into the interstitial

Phase 3
In *phase 3*, as capillary permeability increases, proteins and fluids leak out, increasing interstitial osmotic pressure and causing pulmonary edema.

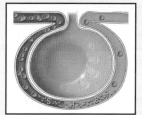
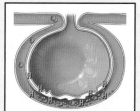
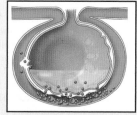

Phase 4
In *phase 4*, decreased blood flow and fluids in the alveoli damage surfactant and impair the cell's ability to produce more. As a result, alveoli collapse, impeding gas exchange and decreasing lung compliance.

Phase 5
In *phase 5*, sufficient oxygen can't cross the alveolocapillary membrane, but carbon dioxide (CO_2) can and is lost with every exhalation. Oxygen (O_2) and CO_2 levels decrease in the blood.

Phase 6
In *phase 6*, pulmonary edema worsens, inflammation leads to fibrosis, and gas exchange is further impeded.

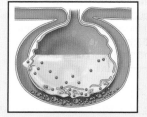
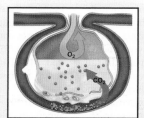
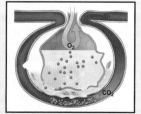

◆ viral, bacterial, or fungal pneumonia or microemboli (fat or air emboli or disseminated intravascular coagulation)
◆ drug overdose (barbiturates, glutethimide, or opioids)
◆ blood transfusion
◆ smoke or chemical inhalation (nitrous oxide, chlorine, or ammonia)
◆ hydrocarbon and paraquat ingestion
◆ pancreatitis, uremia, or miliary tuberculosis (TB; rare)
◆ near drowning
◆ severe traumatic injuries, such as head injury or pulmonary contusions

Altered permeability of the alveolocapillary membrane causes fluid to accumulate in the interstitial space. If the pulmonary lymphatic glands can't remove this fluid, interstitial edema develops. The fluid collects in the peribronchial and peribronchiolar spaces, producing bronchiolar narrowing. Hypoxemia occurs as a result of fluid accumulation in alveoli and subsequent alveolar collapse, causing the shunting of blood through nonventilated lung regions. In addition, alveolar collapse causes a dramatic increase in lung compliance, which makes it more difficult to achieve adequate ventilation.

ARDS affects 10 to 14 people per 100,000, with a mortality rate of 36% to 52%.

Pathophysiology

An acute lung injury can begin the cascade of alveolar damage resulting in an altered permeability of the epithelial barrier and subsequent pulmonary edema. Diffuse alveolar damage progresses and granulation tissue forms in the alveolar spaces creating fibrosis. This fibrotic phase inhibits lung compliance and effective respiration.

Complications

◆ Multisystem failure
◆ Pulmonary fibrosis
◆ Pneumothorax

Signs and symptoms

ARDS initially produces rapid, shallow breathing and dyspnea within hours to days of the initial injury (sometimes after the patient's condition appears to have stabilized). Hypoxemia develops, causing an increased drive for ventilation. Because of the effort required to expand the stiff lung, intercostal and suprasternal retractions result. Fluid accumulation produces crackles and rhonchi; worsening hypoxemia causes restlessness, apprehension, mental sluggishness, motor dysfunction, and tachycardia (possibly with transient increased arterial blood pressure).

 ELDER TIP *The older patient may appear to do well following an initial episode of ARDS. Symptoms commonly appear 2 to 3 days later.*

Severe ARDS causes overwhelming hypoxemia. If uncorrected, this results in hypotension, decreasing urine output, respiratory and metabolic acidosis, and eventually ventricular fibrillation or standstill.

Diagnosis

On room air, ABG analysis initially shows decreased PaO_2 (less than 60 mm Hg) and $PaCO_2$ (less than 35 mm Hg). The resulting pH usually reflects respiratory alkalosis. As ARDS becomes more severe, ABG analysis shows respiratory acidosis (increasing $PaCO_2$ [more than 45 mm Hg]), metabolic acidosis (decreasing bicarbonate [less than 22 mEq/L]), and a decreasing PaO_2 despite oxygen therapy.

Other diagnostic tests include the following:
◆ Pulmonary artery catheterization helps identify the cause of pulmonary edema (cardiac versus noncardiac) by evaluating pulmonary artery wedge pressure (PAWP); allows collection of pulmonary artery blood, which shows decreased oxygen saturation, reflecting tissue hypoxia; measures pulmonary artery pressure (PAP); measures cardiac output by thermodilution techniques; and provides information to allow calculation of the percentage of blood shunted through the lungs.
◆ Serial chest X-rays initially show bilateral infiltrates. In later stages, a ground-glass appearance and eventually (as hypoxemia becomes irreversible), "whiteouts" of both lung fields are apparent. Medical personnel can differentiate ARDS from heart failure by noting the following on serial chest X-rays:
　◆ normal cardiac silhouette
　◆ diffuse bilateral infiltrates that tend to be more peripheral and patchy, as opposed to the usual perihilar "bat wing" appearance of cardiogenic pulmonary edema
　◆ fewer pleural effusions

Differential diagnosis must rule out cardiogenic pulmonary edema, pulmonary vasculitis, and diffuse pulmonary hemorrhage. To establish the etiology, laboratory work should include sputum Gram stain, culture and sensitivity tests, and blood cultures to detect infections; a toxicology screen for drug ingestion; and, when pancreatitis is a consideration, a serum amylase determination.

Treatment

When possible, treatment is designed to correct the underlying cause of ARDS as well as to prevent progression and the potentially fatal complications of hypoxemia and respiratory acidosis. Supportive medical care consists of administering humidified oxygen with CPAP. Hypoxemia that doesn't respond adequately to these measures requires ventilatory support with intubation, volume ventilation, and PEEP. Other supportive measures include fluid restriction, diuretics, and correction of electrolyte and acid–base abnormalities.

When ARDS requires mechanical ventilation, sedatives, opioids, or neuromuscular blocking agents may be ordered to optimize ventilation. Treatment to reverse severe metabolic acidosis with sodium bicarbonate may be necessary, although in severe cases this may worsen the acidosis if CO_2 can't be cleared adequately. Use of fluids and vasopressors may be required to maintain blood pressure. Infections require appropriate anti-infective therapy.

Special considerations

ARDS requires careful monitoring and supportive care.

◆ Frequently assess the patient's respiratory status. Be alert for retractions on inspiration. Note the rate, rhythm, and depth of respirations; watch for dyspnea and the use of accessory muscles of respiration. On auscultation, listen for adventitious or diminished breath sounds. Check for clear, frothy sputum, which may indicate pulmonary edema.

◆ Observe and document the hypoxemic patient's neurologic status (level of consciousness and mental status).

◆ Maintain a patent airway by suctioning, using sterile, nontraumatic technique. Ensure adequate humidification to help liquefy tenacious secretions.

◆ Closely monitor heart rate and blood pressure. Watch for arrhythmias that may result from hypoxemia, acid–base disturbances, or electrolyte imbalance. With pulmonary artery catheterization, know the desired pressure levels. Check readings often and watch for decreasing mixed venous oxygen saturation.

◆ Monitor serum electrolytes and correct imbalances. Measure intake and output; weigh the patient daily.

◆ Check ventilator settings frequently, and empty condensate from tubing promptly to ensure maximum oxygen delivery. Monitor ABG studies and pulse oximetry. The patient with severe hypoxemia may need controlled mechanical ventilation with positive pressure. Give sedatives, as needed, to reduce restlessness.

◆ Because PEEP may decrease cardiac output, check for hypotension, tachycardia, and decreased urine output. Suction only as needed to maintain PEEP or use an in-line suctioning apparatus. Reposition the patient often and record an increase in secretions, temperature, or hypotension that may indicate a deteriorating condition. Monitor peak pressures during ventilation. Because of stiff, noncompliant lungs, the patient is at high risk for barotrauma (pneumothorax), evidenced by increased peak pressures, decreased breath sounds on one side, and restlessness.

◆ Monitor nutrition, maintain joint mobility, and prevent skin breakdown. Accurately record calorie intake. Give tube feedings and parenteral nutrition, as ordered. Perform passive range-of-motion exercises or help the patient perform active exercises, if possible. Provide meticulous skin care. Plan patient care to allow periods of uninterrupted sleep.

◆ Provide emotional support. Warn the family and the patient who's recovering from ARDS that recovery will take some time and that they will feel weak for a while.

◆ Watch for and immediately report all respiratory changes in the patient with injuries that may adversely affect the lungs (especially during the 2- to 3-day period after the injury, when the patient may appear to be improving).

⸭⸭⸭⸭⸭ **PREVENTION** *Prevent VAP through use of the Ventilator Bundle and other best practices, such as continuous removal of subglottic secretions, change of ventilator circuit no more often than every 48 hours, and performance of hand hygiene before and after contact with each patient.*

ACUTE RESPIRATORY FAILURE IN COPD

In patients with essentially normal lung tissue, ARF usually means $PaCO_2$ above 50 mm Hg and PaO_2 below 50 mm Hg. These limits, however, don't apply to patients with COPD, who usually have a consistently high $PaCO_2$ and low PaO_2. In patients with COPD, only acute deterioration in ABG values, with corresponding clinical deterioration, indicates ARF.

Causes and incidence

ARF may develop in patients with COPD as a result of any condition that increases the work of breathing and decreases the respiratory drive. Such conditions include respiratory tract infection (such as bronchitis or pneumonia). The most common precipitating factor is bronchospasm, or accumulating secretions secondary to cough suppression. Other causes of ARF in COPD include the following:

◆ CNS depression—head trauma or injudicious use of sedatives, opioids, tranquilizers, or oxygen (O_2)

- Cardiovascular disorders—myocardial infarction, heart failure, or pulmonary emboli
- Airway irritants—smoke or fumes
- Endocrine and metabolic disorders—myxedema or metabolic alkalosis
- Thoracic abnormalities—chest trauma, pneumothorax, or thoracic or abdominal surgery

The incidence of ARF increases markedly with age and is especially high among people age 65 and older.

Pathophysiology

An acute and progressive exacerbation of COPD is triggered by the cessation of maintenance medications or some type of infection. Damage to the epithelium from ongoing exposure to noxious gases or particles impairs the mucociliary response causing the accumulation of mucus and bacteria and contributing to the obstruction of airways. The permeant enlargement of the airspaces by the terminal bronchioles leads to a decrease in the alveolar surface area for gas exchange and contributes to ineffective ventilation.

Complications

- Respiratory failure
- Pneumonia
- Hypoxemia
- Pneumothorax
- Heart failure

Signs and symptoms

In patients who have COPD with ARF, increased ventilation–perfusion mismatch and reduced alveolar ventilation decrease PaO_2 (hypoxemia) and increase $PaCO_2$ (hypercapnia). This rise in CO_2 lowers the pH. The resulting hypoxemia and acidemia affect all body organs, especially the CNS and the respiratory and cardiovascular systems.

Specific symptoms vary with the underlying cause of ARF but may include these systems:
- Respiratory—Rate may be increased, decreased, or normal depending on the cause; respirations may be shallow, deep, or alternate between the two; and air hunger may occur. Cyanosis may or may not be present, depending on the Hb level and arterial oxygenation. Auscultation of the chest may reveal crackles, rhonchi, wheezing, or diminished breath sounds.
- CNS—When hypoxemia and hypercapnia occur, the patient may show evidence of restlessness, confusion, loss of concentration, irritability, tremulousness, diminished tendon reflexes, and papilledema; the patient may slip into a coma.
- Cardiovascular—Tachycardia, with increased cardiac output and mildly elevated blood pressure secondary to adrenal release of catecholamine, occurs early in response to low PaO_2. With myocardial hypoxia, arrhythmias may develop. Pulmonary hypertension, secondary to pulmonary capillary vasoconstriction, may cause increased pressures on the right side of the heart, jugular vein distention, an enlarged liver, and peripheral edema. Stresses on the heart may precipitate cardiac failure.

Diagnosis

Progressive deterioration in ABG levels and pH, when compared with the patient's "normal" values, strongly suggests ARF in COPD. (In patients with essentially normal lung tissue, pH below 7.35 usually indicates ARF, but patients with COPD display an even greater deviation from this normal value, as they do with $PaCO_2$ and PaO_2.)

Other supporting findings include:
- Bicarbonate—Increased levels indicate metabolic alkalosis or reflect metabolic compensation for chronic respiratory acidosis.
- Hematocrit (HCT) and Hb—Abnormally low levels may be due to blood loss, indicating decreased oxygen-carrying capacity. Elevated levels may occur with chronic hypoxemia.
- Serum electrolytes—Hypokalemia and hypochloremia may result from diuretic and corticosteroid therapies used to treat ARF.
- White blood cell count—Count is elevated if ARF is due to bacterial infection; Gram stain and sputum culture can identify pathogens.
- Chest X-ray—Findings identify pulmonary pathologic conditions, such as emphysema, atelectasis, lesions, pneumothorax, infiltrates, or effusions.
- Electrocardiogram—Arrhythmias commonly suggest cor pulmonale and myocardial hypoxia.

Treatment

ARF in patients with COPD is an emergency that requires cautious O_2 therapy (using nasal prongs or Venturi mask) to raise the PaO_2. In patients with chronic hypercapnia, O_2 therapy can cause hypoventilation by increasing $PaCO_2$ and decreasing the respiratory drive, necessitating mechanical ventilation. The minimum fraction of inspired air (FIO_2) required to maintain ventilation or O_2 saturation greater than 85% to 90% should be used. If significant uncompensated respiratory acidosis or unrefractory hypoxemia exists, mechanical ventilation (through an ET or a tracheostomy tube) or non-invasive ventilation (with a face or nose mask) may be necessary. Treatment routinely includes antibiotics for infection, bronchodilators, and possibly steroids.

Special considerations

◆ Because most patients with ARF are treated in an intensive care unit, orient them to the environment, procedures, and routines to minimize their anxiety.

◆ To reverse hypoxemia, administer O_2 at appropriate concentrations to maintain PaO_2 at a minimum of 50 to 60 mm Hg. Patients with COPD usually require only small amounts of supplemental O_2. Watch for a positive response—such as improvement in the patient's breathing, color, and ABG levels.

◆ Maintain a patent airway. If the patient is retaining CO_2, encourage them to cough and to breathe deeply. Teach them to use pursed-lip and diaphragmatic breathing to control dyspnea. If the patient is alert, have them use an incentive spirometer; if they are intubated and lethargic, turn the patient every 1 to 2 hours. Use postural drainage and chest physiotherapy to help clear secretions.

◆ In an intubated patient, suction the trachea as needed after hyperoxygenation. Observe for a change in quantity, consistency, and color of sputum. Provide humidification to liquefy secretions.

◆ Observe the patient closely for respiratory arrest. Auscultate for chest sounds. Monitor ABG levels and report any changes immediately.

◆ Check the cardiac monitor for arrhythmias.

If the patient requires mechanical ventilation:

◆ Check ventilator settings, cuff pressures, and ABG values often because the FIO_2 setting depends on ABG levels. Draw specimens for ABG analysis 20 to 30 minutes after every FIO_2 change or oximetry check.

◆ Prevent infection by performing hand hygiene and using sterile technique while suctioning.

◆ Stress ulcers are common in the intubated patient. Check gastric secretions for evidence of bleeding if the patient has a nasogastric (NG) tube or if the patient complains of epigastric tenderness, nausea, or vomiting. Monitor Hb level and HCT; check all stools for occult blood. Administer antacids, histamine-2 receptor antagonists, or sucralfate, as ordered.

⁞⁞⁞⁞⁞ PREVENTION
◆ *To prevent VAP, implement Ventilator Bundle.*

◆ *Prevent tracheal erosion, which can result from artificial airway cuff overinflation. Use the minimal leak technique and a cuffed tube with high residual volume (low-pressure cuff), a foam cuff, or a pressure-regulating valve on the cuff.*

◆ *To prevent oral or vocal cord trauma, make sure that the ET tube is positioned midline or moved carefully from side to side every 8 hours.*

◆ To prevent nasal necrosis, keep the nasotracheal tube midline within the patient's nostrils and provide good hygiene. Loosen the tape periodically to prevent skin breakdown. Avoid excessive movement of any tubes; make sure the ventilator tubing is adequately supported.

PULMONARY EDEMA

Pulmonary edema is the accumulation of fluid in the extravascular spaces of the lung. In cardiogenic pulmonary edema, fluid accumulation results from elevations in pulmonary venous and capillary hydrostatic pressures. A common complication of cardiac disorders, pulmonary edema can occur as a chronic condition or it can develop quickly to cause death. (See *How pulmonary edema develops*, page 131.)

Causes and incidence

Pulmonary edema usually results from left-sided heart failure due to arteriosclerotic, hypertensive, cardiomyopathic, or valvular cardiac disease. In such disorders, the compromised left ventricle is unable to maintain adequate cardiac output; increased pressures are transmitted to the left atrium, pulmonary veins, and pulmonary capillary bed. This increased pulmonary capillary hydrostatic force promotes transudation of intravascular fluids into the pulmonary interstitium, decreasing lung compliance and interfering with gas exchange. Other factors that may predispose the patient to pulmonary edema include:

◆ excessive infusion of I.V. fluids

◆ decreased serum colloid osmotic pressure as a result of nephrosis, protein-losing enteropathy, extensive burns, hepatic disease, or nutritional deficiency

◆ impaired lung lymphatic drainage from Hodgkin lymphoma or obliterative lymphangitis after radiation

◆ mitral stenosis, which impairs left atrial emptying

◆ pulmonary veno-occlusive disease

◆ lung damage from a severe infection or exposure to poisonous gas

◆ kidney failure

Pathophysiology

A hemodynamic disturbance or alteration in the permeability of the microvasculature allowing fluid to pass through into the interstitial space. This interstitial edema progresses when the capacity of the lymphatics is exceeded and unable to drain the fluid efficiently and subsequently decreasing lung compliance and shortness of breath.

Complications

◆ respiratory failure

◆ pleural effusion

◆ edema to lower extremities and abdomen
◆ death

Signs and symptoms

The early symptoms of pulmonary edema reflect interstitial fluid accumulation and diminished lung compliance: dyspnea on exertion, paroxysmal nocturnal dyspnea, orthopnea, and coughing. Clinical features include tachycardia, tachypnea, dependent crackles, jugular vein distention, and a diastolic (S_3) gallop. With severe pulmonary edema, the alveoli and bronchioles may fill with fluid and intensify the early symptoms. Respiration becomes labored and rapid, with more diffuse crackles and coughing that produces frothy, bloody sputum. Tachycardia increases, and arrhythmias may occur. Skin becomes cold, clammy, diaphoretic, and cyanotic. Blood pressure falls and the pulse becomes thready as cardiac output falls.

Symptoms of severe heart failure with pulmonary edema may also include signs of hypoxemia, such as anxiety, restlessness, and changes in the patient's level of consciousness.

Diagnosis

Clinical features of pulmonary edema permit a working diagnosis. ABG analysis usually shows hypoxia; the $PaCO_2$ is variable. Profound respiratory alkalosis and acidosis may occur. Chest X-ray shows diffuse haziness of the lung fields and, commonly, cardiomegaly and pleural effusions. Ultrasound (echocardiogram) may show weak heart muscle, leaking or narrow heart valves, and fluid surrounding the heart. Pulmonary artery catheterization helps identify left-sided heart failure by showing elevated PAWPs. This helps to rule out ARDS—in which pulmonary wedge pressure is usually normal.

Treatment

Treatment measures for pulmonary edema are designed to reduce extravascular fluid, improve gas exchange and myocardial function and, if possible, correct any underlying pathologic conditions.

Administration of high concentrations of oxygen by a cannula, a face mask and, if the patient fails to maintain an acceptable PaO_2 level, assisted ventilation improves oxygen delivery to the tissues and usually improves acid–base disturbances. Diuretics—furosemide and bumetanide, for example—promote diuresis, which reduces extravascular fluid.

Treatment of heart failure includes angiotensin-converting enzyme inhibitors, diuretics, inotropic drugs such as digoxin, antiarrhythmic agents, beta-adrenergic blockers, and human B-type natriuretic peptide. Vasodilator drugs, such as nitroprusside, may be used to reduce preload and afterload in acute episodes of pulmonary edema.

Morphine is used to reduce anxiety and dyspnea as well as dilate the systemic venous bed, promoting blood flow from pulmonary circulation to the periphery.

Special considerations

◆ Carefully monitor the vulnerable patient for early signs of pulmonary edema, especially tachypnea, tachycardia, and abnormal breath sounds. Report any abnormalities. Assess for peripheral edema and weight gain, which may also indicate that fluid is accumulating in tissue.
◆ Administer oxygen as ordered.
◆ Monitor the patient's vital signs every 15 to 30 minutes while administering nitroprusside in dextrose 5% in water by I.V. drip. Protect the nitroprusside solution from light by wrapping the bottle or bag with aluminum foil and discard unused solution after 4 hours. Watch for arrhythmias in the patient receiving cardiac glycosides and for marked respiratory depression in the patient receiving morphine.
◆ Assess the patient's condition frequently, and record response to treatment. Monitor ABG levels, oral and I.V. fluid intake, urine output and, in the patient with a pulmonary artery catheter, pulmonary end-diastolic and wedge pressures. Check the cardiac monitor often. Report changes immediately.
◆ Carefully record the time and amount of morphine given.
◆ Reassure the patient, who will be anxious because of hypoxia and respiratory distress. Explain all procedures. Provide emotional support to the family as well.

COR PULMONALE

The World Health Organization defines chronic cor pulmonale as "hypertrophy of the right ventricle resulting from diseases affecting the function or the structure of the lungs, except when these pulmonary alterations are the result of diseases that primarily affect the left side of the heart or of congenital heart disease." Invariably, cor pulmonale follows some disorder of the lungs, pulmonary vessels, chest wall, or respiratory control center. For instance, COPD produces pulmonary hypertension, which leads to right ventricular hypertrophy and right-sided heart failure. Because cor pulmonale generally occurs late during the course of COPD and other irreversible diseases, the prognosis is generally poor.

Causes and incidence

Approximately 85% of patients with cor pulmonale have COPD, and 25% of patients with COPD eventually develop cor pulmonale.

Other respiratory disorders that produce cor pulmonale include:

◆ obstructive lung diseases—for example, bronchiectasis and cystic fibrosis

◆ restrictive lung diseases—for example, pneumoconiosis, interstitial pneumonitis, scleroderma, and sarcoidosis

◆ loss of lung tissue after extensive lung surgery

◆ congenital cardiac shunts—such as a ventricular septal defect

◆ pulmonary vascular diseases—for example, recurrent thromboembolism, primary pulmonary hypertension, schistosomiasis, and pulmonary vasculitis

◆ respiratory insufficiency without pulmonary disease—for example, in chest wall disorders such as kyphoscoliosis, neuromuscular incompetence due to muscular dystrophy and amyotrophic lateral sclerosis, polymyositis, and spinal cord lesions above C6

◆ obesity hypoventilation syndrome (pickwickian syndrome) and upper airway obstruction

◆ living at high altitudes (chronic mountain sickness)

Cor pulmonale accounts for about 25% of all types of heart failure. It's most common in areas of the world where the incidence of cigarette smoking and COPD is high; cor pulmonale affects middle-aged to elderly men more often than women, but the incidence in women is increasing. In children, cor pulmonale may be a complication of cystic fibrosis, hemosiderosis, upper airway obstruction, scleroderma, extensive bronchiectasis, neurologic diseases affecting respiratory muscles, or abnormalities of the respiratory control center.

Pathophysiology

Pulmonary capillary destruction and pulmonary vasoconstriction (usually secondary to hypoxia) reduce the area of the pulmonary vascular bed. Thus, pulmonary vascular resistance is increased, causing pulmonary hypertension. To compensate for the extra work needed to force blood through the lungs, the right ventricle dilates and hypertrophies. In response to low oxygen content, the bone marrow produces more red blood cells (RBCs), causing erythrocytosis. When the HCT exceeds 55%, blood viscosity increases, which further aggravates pulmonary hypertension and increases the hemodynamic load on the right ventricle. Right-sided heart failure is the result.

Complications

◆ Right- and left-sided heart failure
◆ Hepatomegaly
◆ Edema
◆ Ascites
◆ Pleural effusions
◆ Thromboembolism

Signs and symptoms

As long as the heart can compensate for the increased pulmonary vascular resistance, clinical features reflect the underlying disorder and occur mostly in the respiratory system. They include chronic productive cough, exertional dyspnea, wheezing respirations, fatigue, and weakness. Progression of cor pulmonale is associated with dyspnea (even at rest) that worsens on exertion, tachypnea, orthopnea, edema, weakness, and right upper quadrant discomfort. Chest examination reveals findings characteristic of the underlying lung disease.

Signs of cor pulmonale and right-sided heart failure include dependent edema; distended jugular veins; prominent parasternal or epigastric cardiac impulse; hepatojugular reflux; an enlarged, tender liver; ascites; and tachycardia. Decreased cardiac output may cause a weak pulse and hypotension. Chest examination yields various findings, depending on the underlying cause of cor pulmonale.

In COPD, auscultation reveals wheezing, rhonchi, and diminished breath sounds. When the disease is secondary to upper airway obstruction or damage to CNS respiratory centers, chest findings may be normal, except for a right ventricular lift, gallop rhythm, and loud pulmonic component of S_2. Tricuspid insufficiency produces a pansystolic murmur heard at the lower left sternal border; its intensity increases on inspiration, distinguishing it from a murmur due to mitral valve disease. A right ventricular early murmur that increases on inspiration can be heard at the left sternal border or over the epigastrium. A systolic pulmonic ejection click may also be heard. Alterations in the patient's level of consciousness may occur.

Diagnosis

◆ PAP measurements show increased right ventricular and PAPs, stemming from increased pulmonary vascular resistance. Right ventricular systolic and pulmonary artery systolic pressures will exceed 30 mm Hg. Pulmonary artery diastolic pressure will exceed 15 mm Hg.

◆ Echocardiography or angiography indicates right ventricular enlargement; echocardiography can estimate PAP while also ruling out structural and congenital lesions.

◆ Chest X-ray shows large central pulmonary arteries and suggests right ventricular enlargement by rightward enlargement of the heart's silhouette on an anterior chest film.

◆ ABG analysis shows decreased PaO_2 (typically less than 70 mm Hg and usually no more than 90 mm Hg on room air).

◆ Electrocardiogram frequently shows arrhythmias, such as premature atrial and ventricular contractions and atrial fibrillation during severe hypoxia; it may also show right bundle-branch block, right axis deviation, prominent P waves and inverted T wave in right precordial leads, and right ventricular hypertrophy.

◆ PFTs show results consistent with the underlying pulmonary disease.

◆ HCT is typically greater than 50%.

Treatment

Treatment of cor pulmonale is designed to reduce hypoxemia, increase the patient's exercise tolerance and, when possible, correct the underlying condition.

In addition to bed rest, treatment may include administration of:

◆ a cardiac glycoside (digoxin)

◆ antibiotics when respiratory infection is present; culture and sensitivity of a sputum specimen helps select an antibiotic

◆ potent pulmonary artery vasodilators (such as diazoxide, nitroprusside, hydralazine, angiotensin-converting enzyme inhibitors, calcium channel blockers, or prostaglandins) in primary pulmonary hypertension

◆ oxygen by mask or cannula in concentrations ranging from 24% to 40%, depending on PaO_2, as necessary; in acute cases, therapy may also include mechanical ventilation; patients with underlying COPD generally shouldn't receive high concentrations of oxygen because of possible subsequent respiratory depression

◆ a low-sodium diet, restricted fluid intake, and diuretics, such as furosemide, to reduce edema

◆ phlebotomy to reduce the RBC count

◆ anticoagulants to reduce the risk of thromboembolism

Depending on the underlying cause, some variations in treatment may be indicated. For example, a tracheotomy may be necessary if the patient has an upper airway obstruction. Steroids may be used in the patient with a vasculitis autoimmune phenomenon or acute exacerbations of COPD.

Special considerations

◆ Plan diet carefully with the patient and staff dietitian. Because the patient may lack energy and tire easily when eating, provide small, frequent feedings rather than three heavy meals.

◆ Prevent fluid retention by limiting the patient's fluid intake to 1 to 2 qt (1 to 2 L)/day and providing a low-sodium diet.

◆ Monitor serum potassium levels closely if the patient is receiving diuretics. Low serum potassium levels can increase the risk of arrhythmias associated with cardiac glycosides.

◆ Watch the patient for signs of digoxin toxicity, such as complaints of anorexia, nausea, vomiting, and halos around visual images and color perception shifts. Monitor for cardiac arrhythmias. Teach the patient to check their radial pulse before taking digoxin or any cardiac glycoside. They should be instructed to notify the physician if they detect changes in pulse rate.

◆ Reposition bedridden patients often to prevent atelectasis.

◆ Provide meticulous respiratory care, including oxygen therapy and, for the patient with COPD, pursed-lip breathing exercises. Periodically measure ABG levels and watch for signs of respiratory failure: changes in pulse rate, labored respirations, changes in mental status, and increased fatigue after exertion.

Before discharge, maintain the following protocol:

◆ Make sure that the patient understands the importance of maintaining a low-sodium diet, weighing himself daily, and watching for increased edema. Teach patient to detect edema by pressing the skin over a shin with one finger, holding it for a second or two, then checking for a finger impression. Increased weight, increased edema, or respiratory difficulty should be reported to the healthcare provider.

◆ Instruct the patient to plan for frequent rest periods and to do breathing exercises regularly.

◆ If the patient needs supplemental oxygen therapy at home, refer them to an agency that can help obtain the required equipment and, as necessary, arrange for follow-up examinations.

◆ If the patient has been placed on anticoagulant therapy, emphasize the need to watch for bleeding (epistaxis, hematuria, bruising) and to report signs to the physician. Also encourage patient to return for periodic laboratory tests to monitor partial thromboplastin time (PTT), fibrinogen level, platelet count, HCT, Hb level, and prothrombin time.

◆ Because pulmonary infection commonly exacerbates COPD and cor pulmonale, tell the patient to watch for and immediately report early signs of infection, such as increased sputum production, change in sputum color, increased coughing or wheezing, chest pain, fever, and tightness in the chest. Tell the patient to avoid crowds and persons known to have pulmonary infections, especially during the flu season. The patient should receive pneumovax and annual influenza vaccines.

◆ Warn the patient to avoid substances that may depress the ventilatory drive, such as sedatives and alcohol.

LEGIONNAIRES' DISEASE

Legionnaires' disease is an acute bronchopneumonia produced by a gram-negative bacillus, *Legionella pneumophila*. It derives its name and notoriety from the peculiar, highly publicized disease that struck 182 people (29 of whom died) at an American Legion convention in Philadelphia in July 1976. This disease may occur epidemically or sporadically, usually in late summer or early fall. Its severity ranges from a mild illness, with or without pneumonitis, to multilobar pneumonia, with a mortality as high as 15%. A milder, self-limiting form (Pontiac syndrome) subsides within a few days but leaves the patient fatigued for several weeks. This form mimics Legionnaires' disease but produces few or no respiratory symptoms, no pneumonia, and no fatalities.

Causes and incidence

Legionella pneumophila is an aerobic, gram-negative bacillus that's probably transmitted by an airborne route. In past epidemics, it has spread through cooling towers or evaporation condensers in air-conditioning systems. However, *Legionella* bacilli also flourish in soil and excavation sites. The disease doesn't spread from person to person.

Legionnaires' disease is most likely to affect:
♦ middle-aged and elderly people
♦ immunocompromised patients (particularly those receiving corticosteroids, e.g., after a transplant) or those with lymphoma or other disorders associated with delayed hypersensitivity
♦ patients with a chronic underlying disease, such as diabetes, chronic renal failure, or COPD
♦ those with alcoholism
♦ cigarette smokers
♦ those on a ventilator for extended periods

Pathophysiology

When water droplets containing a sufficient amount of the Legionella bacterium enter the atmosphere they can be inhaled into the lungs. There they invade the epithelial cells of the lungs and begin to replicate intracellularly causing a Legionnaires' infection.

Complications

♦ Respiratory failure
♦ Septic shock
♦ Acute kidney failure

Signs and symptoms

The multisystem clinical features of Legionnaires' disease follow a predictable sequence, although the onset of the disease may be gradual or sudden. After a 2- to 10-day incubation period, nonspecific, prodromal signs and symptoms appear, including diarrhea, anorexia, malaise, diffuse myalgias and generalized weakness, headache, and recurrent chills. An unremitting fever develops within 12 to 48 hours with a temperature that may reach 105° F (40.6° C). A cough then develops that's nonproductive initially but eventually may produce grayish, nonpurulent, and occasionally blood-streaked sputum.

Other characteristic features include nausea, vomiting, disorientation, mental sluggishness, confusion, mild temporary amnesia, pleuritic chest pain, tachypnea, dyspnea, and fine crackles. Patients who develop pneumonia may also experience hypoxia. Other complications include hypotension, delirium, heart failure, arrhythmias, ARF, renal failure, and shock (usually fatal).

Diagnosis

The patient history focuses on possible sources of infection and predisposing conditions. Additional tests reveal the following:
♦ Chest X-ray shows patchy, localized infiltration, which progresses to multilobar consolidation (usually involving the lower lobes), pleural effusion and, in fulminant disease, opacification of the entire lung.
♦ Auscultation reveals fine crackles, progressing to coarse crackles as the disease advances.
♦ Abnormal findings include leukocytosis, increased erythrocyte sedimentation rate, an increase in liver enzyme levels (alanine aminotransferase, aspartate aminotransferase, and alkaline phosphatase), hyponatremia, decreased PaO_2 and, initially, decreased $PaCO_2$. Bronchial washings and blood, pleural fluid, and sputum tests rule out other infections.

℞ **CONFIRMING DIAGNOSIS** *Definitive tests include direct immunofluorescence of respiratory tract secretions and tissue, culture of L. pneumophila, and indirect fluorescent antibody testing of serum comparing acute samples with convalescent samples drawn at least 3 weeks later. A convalescent serum showing a fourfold or greater rise in antibody titer for* Legionella *confirms the diagnosis.*

Treatment

Antibiotic treatment begins as soon as Legionnaires' disease is suspected and diagnostic material is collected; it shouldn't await laboratory confirmation. A quinolone (ciprofloxacin, levofloxacin, moxifloxacin, or gatifloxacin) is commonly used, although a macrolide (azithromycin, clarithromycin, or erythromycin) may be prescribed for some patients. Supportive therapy includes administration of antipyretics, fluid replacement, circulatory support with pressor drugs, if necessary, and oxygen administration by mask, cannula, or mechanical ventilation.

Special considerations

◆ Closely monitor the patient's respiratory status. Evaluate chest wall expansion, depth and pattern of respirations, cough, and chest pain. Watch for restlessness as a sign of hypoxemia, which requires suctioning, repositioning, or more aggressive oxygen therapy.

◆ Continually monitor the patient's vital signs, oximetry or ABG values, level of consciousness, and dryness and color of lips and mucous membranes. Watch for signs of shock (decreased blood pressure, thready pulse, diaphoresis, and clammy skin).

◆ Keep the patient comfortable. Provide mouth care frequently. If necessary, apply soothing cream to the nostrils.

◆ Replace fluid and electrolytes, as needed. The patient with renal failure may require dialysis.

◆ Provide mechanical ventilation and other respiratory therapy, as needed. Teach the patient how to cough effectively and encourage deep-breathing exercises. Stress the need to continue these until recovery is complete.

◆ Give antibiotic therapy as indicated and observe carefully for adverse effects.

ATELECTASIS

Atelectasis is incomplete expansion of lobules (clusters of alveoli) or lung segments, which may result in partial or complete lung collapse. Because parts of the lung are unavailable for gas exchange, unoxygenated blood passes through these areas unchanged, resulting in hypoxemia. Atelectasis may be chronic or acute. Many patients undergoing upper abdominal or thoracic surgery experience atelectasis to some degree. The prognosis depends on prompt removal of any airway obstruction, relief of hypoxemia, and re-expansion of the collapsed lung.

Causes

Atelectasis commonly results from bronchial occlusion by mucus plugs. It's a problem in many patients with COPD, bronchiectasis, or cystic fibrosis and in those who smoke heavily. (Smoking increases mucus production and damages cilia.) Atelectasis may also result from occlusion by foreign bodies, bronchogenic carcinoma, and inflammatory lung disease.

Other causes include RDS of the neonate (hyaline membrane disease), oxygen toxicity, and pulmonary edema, in which alveolar surfactant changes increase surface tension and permit complete alveolar deflation.

External compression, which inhibits full lung expansion, or any condition that makes deep breathing painful may also cause atelectasis. Such compression or pain may result from abdominal surgical incisions, rib fractures, pleuritic chest pain, tight dressings around the chest, stab wounds, impalement accidents, car accidents in which the driver slams into the steering column, or obesity (which elevates the diaphragm and reduces tidal volume).

Prolonged immobility may also cause atelectasis by producing preferential ventilation of one area of the lung over another. Mechanical ventilation using constant small tidal volumes without intermittent deep breaths may also result in atelectasis. CNS depression (as in drug overdose) eliminates periodic sighing and is a predisposing factor of progressive atelectasis.

Pathophysiology

Atelectasis results from some type of obstruction or compression of the lungs or bronchus. Retraction of the lung occurs when the blood circulating in the alveolar capillary bed absorbs the gas from the alveolar in the unventilated lung. The alveolar spaces fill with secretions and cells, preventing the complete collapse of the lung. The surrounding tissues distend and displace, shifting the heart and mediastinum toward the ateleactactic area.

Complications

◆ Respiratory failure
◆ Pneumonia
◆ Hypoxemia

Signs and symptoms

Clinical effects vary with the cause of collapse, the degree of hypoxemia, and any underlying disease but generally include some degree of dyspnea. Atelectasis of a small area of the lung may produce only minimal symptoms that subside without specific treatment. However, massive collapse can produce severe dyspnea, anxiety, cyanosis, diaphoresis, peripheral circulatory collapse, tachycardia, and substernal or intercostal retraction. Also, atelectasis may result in compensatory hyperinflation of unaffected areas of the lung, mediastinal shift to the affected side, and elevation of the ipsilateral hemidiaphragm.

Diagnosis

Diagnosis requires an accurate patient history, a physical examination, and a chest X-ray. Auscultation reveals diminished or bronchial breath sounds. When much of the lung is collapsed, percussion reveals dullness. However, extensive areas of "microatelectasis" may exist without abnormalities on the chest X-ray. In widespread atelectasis, the chest X-ray shows characteristic horizontal lines in the lower lung zones. With segmental or lobar collapse, characteristic dense shadows commonly associated with hyperinflation of neighboring lung zones are also apparent. If the cause is unknown, diagnostic procedures may include bronchoscopy to rule out an obstructing neoplasm or a foreign body.

Treatment

Treatment includes incentive spirometry, frequent coughing, and deep-breathing exercises. If atelectasis is secondary to mucus plugging, mucolytics, chest percussion, and postural drainage may be used. If these measures fail, bronchoscopy may be helpful in removing secretions. Humidity and bronchodilators can improve mucociliary clearance and dilate airways.

Atelectasis secondary to an obstructing neoplasm may require surgery or radiation therapy. Postoperative thoracic and abdominal surgery patients require analgesics to facilitate deep breathing, which minimizes the risk of atelectasis.

Special considerations

◆ If mechanical ventilation is used, tidal volume should be maintained at appropriate levels to ensure adequate expansion of the lungs. Use the sigh mechanism on the ventilator, if appropriate, to intermittently increase tidal volume at the rate of 10 to 15 sighs/hour. Implement the Ventilator Bundle to prevent VAP.
◆ Use an incentive spirometer to encourage deep inspiration through positive reinforcement. Teach the patient how to use the spirometer and encourage them to use it every 1 to 2 hours.
◆ Humidify inspired air and encourage adequate fluid intake to mobilize secretions. To promote loosening and clearance of secretions, encourage deep-breathing and coughing exercises and use postural drainage and chest percussion.
◆ If the patient is intubated or uncooperative, provide suctioning, as needed. Use sedatives with discretion because they depress respirations and the cough reflex as well as suppress sighing. However, remember that the patient won't cooperate with treatment if they are in pain.
◆ Assess breath sounds and ventilatory status frequently; report changes at once.
◆ Teach the patient about respiratory care, including postural drainage, coughing, and deep breathing.
◆ Encourage the patient to stop smoking and lose weight, as needed. Refer them to appropriate support groups for help.

◆ Provide reassurance and emotional support; the patient may be anxious because of hypoxia or respiratory distress.

PREVENTION
◆ *In a patient who is bedridden, encourage movement and deep breathing.*
◆ *Administer adequate analgesics.*
◆ *To prevent atelectasis, encourage the postoperative or other high-risk patient to cough and deep-breathe every 1 to 2 hours. To minimize pain during coughing exercises, splint the incision; teach the patient this technique as well. Gently reposition the patient often and encourage ambulation as soon as possible.*
◆ *Teach patients to keep small objects out of reach of children.*

RESPIRATORY ACIDOSIS

An acid–base disturbance characterized by reduced alveolar ventilation and manifested by hypercapnia ($PaCO_2$ greater than 45 mm Hg), respiratory acidosis can be acute (because of a sudden failure in ventilation) or chronic (as in long-term pulmonary disease). The prognosis depends on the severity of the underlying disturbance as well as the patient's general clinical condition.

Causes and incidence

Some predisposing factors in respiratory acidosis include:
◆ Drugs—Opioids, anesthetics, hypnotics, and sedatives, including some of the new designer drugs, such as Ecstasy, decrease the sensitivity of the respiratory center.
◆ CNS trauma—Medullary injury may impair ventilatory drive.
◆ Chronic metabolic alkalosis—Respiratory compensatory mechanisms attempt to normalize pH by decreasing alveolar ventilation.
◆ Ventilation therapy—Use of high-flow oxygen (O_2) in chronic respiratory disorders suppresses the patient's hypoxic drive to breathe.
◆ Neuromuscular diseases (such as myasthenia gravis, Guillain–Barré syndrome, and poliomyelitis)—Failure of the respiratory muscles to respond properly to respiratory drive decreases alveolar ventilation.
◆ In addition, respiratory acidosis can result from airway obstruction or parenchymal lung disease, which interferes with alveolar ventilation; COPD; asthma; severe acute respiratory distress syndrome (SARS); chronic bronchitis; large pneumothorax; extensive pneumonia; and pulmonary edema.

Hypoventilation compromises elimination of CO_2 produced through metabolism. The retained CO_2 then combines with water to form an excess of carbonic acid, decreasing the blood pH. As a result, the concentration of hydrogen ions in body fluids, which directly reflects acidity, increases.

Pathophysiology

Lung diseases or conditions that cause hypoventilation result in CO_2 being produced at a rapid rate. Lack of adequate ventilation quickly increases the partial pressure of arterial CO_2. The increase in $PaCO_2$ also results in the decrease in bicarbonate ration and decreasing the pH to an acidotic state.

Complications

- Shock
- Cardiac arrest

Signs and symptoms

Acute respiratory acidosis produces CNS disturbances that reflect changes in the pH of cerebrospinal fluid rather than increased CO_2 levels in cerebral circulation. Effects range from restlessness, confusion, and apprehension to somnolence, with a fine or flapping tremor (asterixis), or coma. The patient may complain of headaches as well as exhibiting dyspnea and tachypnea with papilledema and depressed reflexes. Unless the patient is receiving O_2, hypoxemia accompanies respiratory acidosis. This disorder may also cause cardiovascular abnormalities, such as tachycardia, hypertension, atrial and ventricular arrhythmias and, in severe acidosis, hypotension with vasodilation (bounding pulses and warm periphery).

Diagnosis

℞ CONFIRMING DIAGNOSIS *ABG analysis confirms the diagnosis: Paco$_2$ exceeds the normal 45 mm Hg; pH is below the normal range of 7.35 to 7.45 unless compensation has occurred; and bicarbonate is normal in the acute stage but elevated in the chronic stage.*

Chest X-ray, CT scan, and PFTs can help determine the cause.

Treatment

Effective treatment of respiratory acidosis requires correction of the underlying source of alveolar hypoventilation.

Significantly reduced alveolar ventilation may require mechanical ventilation until the underlying condition can be treated. In COPD, this includes bronchodilators, O_2, corticosteroids, and antibiotics for infectious conditions; drug therapy for conditions such as myasthenia gravis; removal of foreign bodies from the airway; antibiotics for pneumonia; dialysis or charcoal to remove toxic drugs; and correction of metabolic alkalosis.

Dangerously low blood pH (less than 7.15) can produce profound CNS and cardiovascular deterioration; careful administration of I.V. sodium bicarbonate may be required. In chronic lung disease, elevated CO_2 may persist despite optimal treatment.

Special considerations

- Be alert for critical changes in the patient's respiratory, CNS, and cardiovascular functions. Report such changes as well as any variations in ABG values or electrolyte status immediately. Also, maintain adequate hydration.
- Maintain a patent airway and provide adequate humidification if acidosis requires mechanical ventilation. Perform tracheal suctioning regularly and vigorous chest physiotherapy if ordered. Continuously monitor ventilator settings and respiratory status.
- To prevent respiratory acidosis, closely monitor patients with COPD and chronic CO_2 retention for signs of acidosis. Also, administer O_2 at low flow rates; closely monitor all patients who receive opioids and sedatives. Instruct patients who have received general anesthesia to turn, cough, and perform deep-breathing exercises frequently to prevent the onset of respiratory acidosis.

RESPIRATORY ALKALOSIS

Respiratory alkalosis is an acid–base disturbance characterized by a decrease in the $PaCO_2$ to less than 35 mm Hg, which is due to alveolar hyperventilation. Uncomplicated respiratory alkalosis leads to a decrease in hydrogen ion concentration, which results in elevated blood pH. Hypocapnia occurs when the elimination of CO_2 by the lungs exceeds the production of CO_2 at the cellular level.

Causes

Causes of respiratory alkalosis fall into two categories:

- pulmonary—severe hypoxemia, pneumonia, interstitial lung disease, pulmonary vascular disease, and acute asthma
- nonpulmonary—anxiety, fever, aspirin toxicity, metabolic acidosis, CNS disease (inflammation or tumor), sepsis, hepatic failure, and pregnancy

Pathophysiology

An underlying condition or stimulus that causes hyperventilation, expels an increased amount of CO_2. CO_2 in the circulation is shifted causing hydrogen ions and bicarbonate to change into additional CO_2 via the enzyme carbonic anhydrase which, in turn, decreases the available hydrogen ions and increasing the pH.

Complications
◆ Cardiac arrhythmias
◆ Seizures

Signs and symptoms
The cardinal sign of respiratory alkalosis is deep, rapid breathing, possibly exceeding 40 breaths/minute. This pattern of breathing is similar to Kussmaul's respirations that characterize diabetic acidosis. Such hyperventilation usually leads to CNS and neuromuscular disturbances, such as light-headedness or dizziness (because of below-normal CO_2 levels that decrease cerebral blood flow), agitation, circumoral and peripheral paresthesias, carpopedal spasms, twitching (possibly progressing to tetany), and muscle weakness. Severe respiratory alkalosis may cause cardiac arrhythmias (that may fail to respond to conventional treatment), seizures, or both.

Diagnosis
CONFIRMING DIAGNOSIS *ABG analysis confirms respiratory alkalosis and rules out respiratory compensation for metabolic acidosis: Paco$_2$ less than 35 mm Hg; pH elevated in proportion to the fall in Paco$_2$ in the acute stage but falling toward normal in the chronic stage; and bicarbonate normal in the acute stage, but below normal in the chronic stage.*

Chest X-ray or PFTs may aid in diagnosing possible lung disease.

Treatment
Treatment is designed to eradicate the underlying condition—for example, removal of ingested toxins, treatment of fever or sepsis, providing oxygen for acute hypoxemia, and treatment of CNS disease. When hyperventilation is caused by severe anxiety, the patient may be instructed to breathe into a paper bag, which increases CO_2 levels and helps relieve anxiety.

Prevention of hyperventilation in patients receiving mechanical ventilation requires monitoring ABG levels and adjusting tidal volume and minute ventilation.

Special considerations
◆ Watch for and report any changes in neurologic, neuromuscular, or cardiovascular functions.
◆ Remember that twitching and cardiac arrhythmias may be associated with alkalemia and electrolyte imbalances. Monitor ABG and serum electrolyte levels closely, reporting any variations immediately.
◆ Explain all diagnostic tests and procedures to reduce anxiety.

PNEUMOTHORAX
Pneumothorax is an accumulation of air or gas between the parietal and visceral pleurae. The amount of air or gas trapped in the intrapleural space determines the degree of lung collapse. In tension pneumothorax, the air in the pleural space is under higher pressure than air in adjacent lung and vascular structures. Without prompt treatment, tension or large pneumothorax results in fatal pulmonary and circulatory impairment. (See *Understanding tension pneumothorax*, page 112.)

Causes and incidence
Spontaneous pneumothorax usually occurs in otherwise healthy adults 20 to 40 years old. It may be caused by air leakage from ruptured congenital blebs adjacent to the visceral pleural surface, near the apex of the lung. Secondary spontaneous pneumothorax is a complication of underlying lung disease, such as COPD, asthma, cystic fibrosis, TB, and whooping cough. Spontaneous pneumothorax may also occur in interstitial lung disease, such as eosinophilic granuloma or lymphangiomyomatosis.

Traumatic pneumothorax may result from insertion of a central venous line, thoracic surgery, or a penetrating chest injury, such as a gunshot or knife wound. It may follow a transbronchial biopsy, or it may also occur during thoracentesis or a closed pleural biopsy. When traumatic pneumothorax follows a penetrating chest injury, it frequently coexists with hemothorax (blood in the pleural space).

In *tension pneumothorax*, positive pleural pressure develops as a result of traumatic pneumothorax. When air enters the pleural space through a tear in lung tissue and is unable to leave by the same vent, each inspiration traps air in the pleural space, resulting in positive pleural pressure. This in turn causes collapse of the ipsilateral lung and marked impairment of venous return, which can severely compromise cardiac output and may cause a mediastinal shift. Decreased filling of the great veins of the chest results in diminished cardiac output and lowered blood pressure.

Pathophysiology
Pneumothorax can be classified as open or closed. In *open pneumothorax* (usually the result of trauma), air flows between the pleural space and the outside of the body. In *closed pneumothorax*, air reaches the pleural space directly from the lung.

Complications
◆ Fatal pulmonary and circulatory impairment

Signs and symptoms
The cardinal features of pneumothorax are sudden, sharp, pleuritic pain (exacerbated by movement of the chest, breathing, and

PATHOPHYSIOLOGY
Understanding tension pneumothorax

In tension pneumothorax, air accumulates intrapleurally and can't escape. Intrapleural pressure rises, collapsing the ipsilateral lung.

On inspiration, the mediastinum shifts toward the unaffected lung, impairing ventilation.

On expiration, the mediastinal shift distorts the vena cava and reduces venous return.

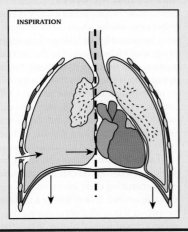

INSPIRATION

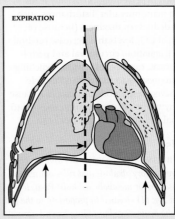

EXPIRATION

coughing); asymmetrical chest wall movement; and shortness of breath. Additional signs of tension pneumothorax are weak and rapid pulse, pallor, jugular vein distention, and anxiety. Tracheal deviations may be present with mediastinal shift. Tension pneumothorax produces the most severe respiratory symptoms; a spontaneous pneumothorax that releases only a small amount of air into the pleural space may cause no symptoms. In a nontension pneumothorax, the severity of symptoms is usually related to the size of the pneumothorax and the degree of preexisting respiratory disease.

Diagnosis

Sudden, sharp chest pain and shortness of breath suggest pneumothorax.

℞ CONFIRMING DIAGNOSIS *Chest X-ray showing air in the pleural space and, possibly, mediastinal shift confirms this diagnosis.*

In the absence of a definitive chest X-ray, the physical examination may reveal:

◆ on inspection—overexpansion and rigidity of the affected chest side; in tension pneumothorax, jugular vein distention with hypotension and tachycardia

◆ on palpation—crackling beneath the skin, indicating subcutaneous emphysema (air in tissue) and decreased vocal fremitus

◆ on percussion—hyperresonance on the affected side

◆ on auscultation—decreased or absent breath sounds over the collapsed lung

If the pneumothorax is significant, ABG findings include pH less than 7.35, PaO_2 less than 80 mm Hg, and $PaCO_2$ above 45 mm Hg.

Treatment

Treatment is conservative for spontaneous pneumothorax in which no signs of increased pleural pressure (indicating tension pneumothorax) appear, lung collapse is less than 30%, and the patient shows no signs of dyspnea or other indications of physiologic compromise. Such treatment consists of bed rest, careful monitoring of blood pressure and pulse and respiratory rates, oxygen administration and, possibly, needle aspiration of air with a large-bore needle attached to a syringe. If more than 30% of the lung is collapsed, treatment to re-expand the lung includes placing a thoracostomy tube in the second or third intercostal space in the midclavicular line (or in the fifth or sixth intercostal space in the midaxillary line), connected to an underwater seal or low suction pressures.

Recurring spontaneous pneumothorax requires thoracotomy and pleurectomy; these procedures prevent recurrence by causing the lung to adhere to the parietal pleura. Traumatic and tension pneumothoraces require chest tube drainage; traumatic pneumothorax may also require surgery.

Special considerations

⚠ **ALERT** *Watch for pallor, gasping respirations, and sudden chest pain. Monitor patient's vital signs at least every hour for signs of shock, increasing respiratory distress, or mediastinal shift. Listen for breath sounds over both lungs. Falling blood pressure and rising pulse and respiratory rates may indicate tension pneumothorax, which can be fatal without prompt treatment.*

◆ Urge the patient to control coughing and gasping during thoracotomy. However, after the chest tube is in place, encourage them to cough and breathe deeply (at least once an hour) to facilitate lung expansion.

◆ If the patient is undergoing chest tube drainage, watch for continuing air leakage (bubbling), indicating the lung defect has failed to close; this may require surgery. Also watch for increasing subcutaneous emphysema by checking around the neck or at the tube insertion site for crackling beneath the skin. If the patient is on a ventilator, watch for difficulty in breathing in time with the ventilator as well as pressure changes on ventilator gauges.

◆ Change dressings around the chest tube insertion site according to your facility's policy. Don't reposition or dislodge the tube. If it dislodges, immediately place a petroleum gauze dressing over the opening to prevent rapid lung collapse.

◆ Secure the chest tube drainage apparatus appropriately. Tape connections securely.

◆ Monitor the patient's vital signs frequently after thoracotomy. Also, for the first 24 hours, assess respiratory status by checking breath sounds hourly. Observe the chest tube site for leakage, noting the amount and color of drainage. Help the patient walk, as ordered (usually on the first postoperative day), to facilitate deep inspiration and lung expansion.

◆ To reassure the patient, explain what pneumothorax is, what causes it, and all diagnostic tests and procedures. Make them as comfortable as possible. (The patient with pneumothorax is usually most comfortable sitting upright.)

PNEUMONIA

Pneumonia is an acute infection of the lung parenchyma that commonly impairs gas exchange. The prognosis is generally good for people who have normal lungs and adequate host defenses before the onset of pneumonia; however, pneumonia is the sixth leading cause of death in the United States. (See *Looking at lobar pneumonia and bronchopneumonia*.)

Looking at lobar pneumonia and bronchopneumonia

Pneumonia can involve the distal airways, alveoli, part of a lobe, or an entire lobe.

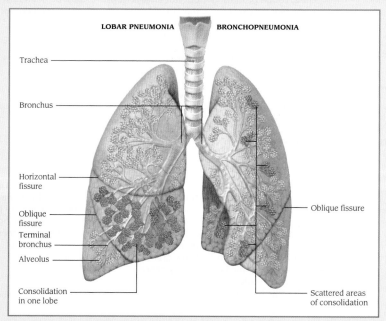

LOBAR PNEUMONIA   BRONCHOPNEUMONIA

Trachea

Bronchus

Horizontal fissure

Oblique fissure

Oblique fissure

Terminal bronchus

Alveolus

Consolidation in one lobe

Scattered areas of consolidation

Causes and incidence

Pneumonia can be classified in several ways:

♦ Microbiologic etiology—Pneumonia can be viral, bacterial, fungal, protozoan, mycobacterial, mycoplasmal, or rickettsial in origin. (See *Diagnosing and treating the types of pneumonia,* pages 114 to 116.)

♦ Location—Bronchopneumonia involves distal airways and alveoli; lobular pneumonia, part of a lobe; and lobar pneumonia, an entire lobe.

♦ Type—Primary pneumonia results from inhalation or aspiration of a pathogen; it includes pneumococcal and viral pneumonia. Secondary pneumonia may follow initial lung damage from a noxious chemical or other insult (superinfection) or may result from hematogenous spread of bacteria from a distant focus.

Predisposing factors for bacterial and viral pneumonia include chronic illness and debilitation, cancer (particularly lung cancer), abdominal and thoracic surgery, atelectasis, common colds or other viral respiratory infections, such as acquired immunodeficiency syndrome, chronic respiratory disease (COPD, asthma,

Diagnosing and treating the types of pneumonia

Type	Signs and symptoms	Diagnosis	Treatment
Aspiration Results from vomiting and aspiration of gastric or oropharyngeal contents into trachea and lungs	♦ Noncardiogenic pulmonary edema that may follow damage to respiratory epithelium from contact with stomach acid ♦ Crackles, dyspnea, cyanosis, hypotension, and tachycardia ♦ May be subacute pneumonia with cavity formation; lung abscess may occur if foreign body is present	♦ *Chest X-ray:* locates areas of infiltrates, which suggest diagnosis	♦ *Antimicrobial therapy:* penicillin G or clindamycin ♦ *Supportive:* oxygen therapy, suctioning, coughing, deep breathing, and adequate hydration
Bacterial Klebsiella	♦ Fever and recurrent chills; cough producing rusty, bloody, viscous sputum (currant jelly); cyanosis of lips and nail beds due to hypoxemia; and shallow, grunting respirations ♦ Common in patients with chronic alcoholism, pulmonary disease, diabetes, or those at risk for aspiration	♦ *Chest X-ray:* typically, but not always, consolidation in the upper lobe that causes bulging of fissures ♦ *White blood cell (WBC) count:* elevated ♦ *Sputum culture and Gram stain:* may show gram-negative *Klebsiella*	♦ *Antimicrobial therapy:* an aminoglycoside and a cephalosporin
Staphylococcus	♦ Temperature of 102° to 104° F (38.9° to 40° C), recurrent shaking chills, bloody sputum, dyspnea, tachypnea, and hypoxemia ♦ Should be suspected with viral illness, such as influenza or measles, and in patients with cystic fibrosis	♦ *Chest X-ray:* multiple abscesses and infiltrates; high incidence of empyema ♦ *WBC count:* elevated ♦ *Sputum culture and Gram stain:* may show gram-positive staphylococci	♦ *Antimicrobial therapy:* nafcillin or oxacillin for 14 days if staphylococci are penicillinase producing ♦ *Supportive:* chest tube drainage of empyema

Diagnosing and treating the types of pneumonia
(continued)

Type	Signs and symptoms	Diagnosis	Treatment
Streptococcus (*Streptococcus pneumoniae*)	Sudden onset of severe, shaking chills and a sustained temperature of 102° to 104° F (38.9° to 40° C); commonly preceded by upper respiratory tract infection	♦ *Chest X-ray:* areas of consolidation, commonly lobar ♦ *WBC count:* elevated ♦ *Sputum culture:* may show gram-positive *S. pneumoniae*; this organism not always recovered	♦ *Antimicrobial therapy:* penicillin G (or erythromycin, if patient is allergic to penicillin) for 7 to 10 days beginning after obtaining culture specimen but without waiting for results. (Resistance to penicillin is becoming much more common and, in the patient with risk factors for resistance [extreme age, day care attendance, or immunosuppression], treatment with vancomycin, imipenem, or levofloxacin should be considered.)
Protozoan *Pneumocystis carinii (jiroveci)*	♦ Occurs in immunocompromised persons ♦ Dyspnea and nonproductive cough ♦ Anorexia, weight loss, and fatigue ♦ Low-grade fever	♦ *Fiber-optic bronchoscopy:* obtains specimens for histologic studies ♦ *Chest X-ray:* nonspecific infiltrates, nodular lesions, or spontaneous pneumothorax	♦ *Antimicrobial therapy:* trimethoprim and sulfamethoxazole or pentamidine by I.V. administration or inhalation. (Prophylactic pentamidine may be used for high-risk patients.) ♦ *Supportive:* oxygen, improved nutrition, and mechanical ventilation
Viral Adenovirus (insidious onset; generally affects young adults)	♦ Sore throat, fever, cough, chills, malaise, small amounts of mucoid sputum, retrosternal chest pain, anorexia, rhinitis, adenopathy, scattered crackles, and rhonchi	♦ *Chest X-ray:* patchy distribution of pneumonia, more severe than indicated by physical examination ♦ *WBC count:* normal to slightly elevated	♦ Treat symptoms only ♦ Mortality low; usually clears with no residual effects
Chicken pox (varicella) (uncommon in children, but present in 30% of adults with varicella)	♦ Cough, dyspnea, cyanosis, tachypnea, pleuritic chest pain, hemoptysis, and rhonchi 1 to 6 days after onset of rash	♦ *Chest X-ray:* shows more extensive pneumonia than indicated by physical examination and bilateral, patchy, diffuse, nodular infiltrates ♦ *Sputum analysis:* predominant mononuclear cells and characteristic intranuclear inclusion bodies, with characteristic skin rash, confirm diagnosis	♦ *Supportive:* adequate hydration, and oxygen therapy in critically ill patients ♦ Therapy with I.V. acyclovir

(continued)

Diagnosing and treating the types of pneumonia
(*continued*)

Type	Signs and symptoms	Diagnosis	Treatment
Viral Cytomegalovirus	♦ Difficult to distinguish from other nonbacterial pneumonias ♦ Fever, cough, shaking chills, dyspnea, cyanosis, weakness, and diffuse crackles ♦ Occurs in neonates as devastating multisystemic infection; in normal adults, resembles mononucleosis; in immunocompromised hosts, varies from clinically inapparent to devastating infection	♦ *Chest X-ray:* in early stages, variable patchy infiltrates; later, bilateral, nodular, and more predominant in lower lobes ♦ *Percutaneous aspiration of lung tissue, transbronchial biopsy, or open lung biopsy:* microscopic examination shows typical intranuclear and cytoplasmic inclusions; the virus can be cultured from lung tissue	♦ Generally, benign and self-limiting in mononucleosis-like form ♦ *Supportive:* adequate hydration and nutrition, oxygen therapy, and bed rest ♦ In immunosuppressed patients, disease is more severe and may be fatal; ganciclovir or foscarnet treatment is warranted
Influenza (prognosis poor even with treatment; 30% mortality)	♦ Cough (initially nonproductive; later, purulent sputum), marked cyanosis, dyspnea, high fever, chills, substernal pain and discomfort, moist crackles, frontal headache, and myalgia ♦ Death results from cardiopulmonary collapse	♦ *Chest X-ray:* diffuse bilateral bronchopneumonia radiating from hilus ♦ *WBC count:* normal to slightly elevated ♦ *Sputum smears:* no specific organisms	♦ *Supportive:* for respiratory failure, endotracheal intubation and ventilator assistance; for fever, hypothermia blanket or antipyretics; and for influenza A, amantadine or rimantadine
Measles (rubeola)	♦ Fever, dyspnea, cough, small amounts of sputum, coryza, rash, and cervical adenopathy	♦ *Chest X-ray:* reticular infiltrates, sometimes with hilar lymph node enlargement ♦ *Lung tissue specimen:* characteristic giant cells	♦ *Supportive:* bed rest, adequate hydration, and antimicrobials; assisted ventilation if necessary
Respiratory syncytial virus (most prevalent in infants and children)	♦ Listlessness, irritability, tachypnea with retraction of intercostal muscles, wheezing, slight sputum production, fine moist crackles, fever, severe malaise, and cough	♦ *Chest X-ray:* patchy bilateral consolidation ♦ *WBC count:* normal to slightly elevated	♦ *Supportive:* humidified air, oxygen, antimicrobials (commonly given until viral etiology confirmed), and aerosolized ribavirin ♦ Usually complete recovery

bronchiectasis, and cystic fibrosis), influenza, smoking, malnutrition, alcoholism, sickle cell disease, tracheostomy, exposure to noxious gases, aspiration, and immunosuppressive therapy.

Predisposing factors for aspiration pneumonia include old age, debilitation, artificial airway use, NG tube feedings, impaired gag reflex, poor oral hygiene, and decreased level of consciousness.

In elderly patients and patients who are debilitated, bacterial pneumonia may follow influenza or a common cold. Respiratory viruses are the most common cause of pneumonia in children 2 to 3 years old. In school-age children, mycoplasma pneumonia is more common.

Pathophysiology
A pathogen or extrinsic agent enters the respiratory tract and invades or insults the alveoli.

When the host defenses are overwhelmed by the inoculum size or virulence of the pathogen, it results in an infection of the lung parenchyma.

Complications
◆ Septic shock
◆ Hypoxemia
◆ Respiratory failure
◆ Empyema
◆ Lung abscess
◆ Bacteremia
◆ Endocarditis
◆ Pericarditis
◆ Meningitis

Signs and symptoms
The main symptoms of pneumonia are coughing, sputum production, pleuritic chest pain, shaking chills, shortness of breath, rapid shallow breathing, and fever. Physical signs vary widely, ranging from diffuse, fine crackles to signs of localized or extensive consolidation and pleural effusion. There may also be associated symptoms of headache, sweating, loss of appetite, excess fatigue, and confusion (in older people).

Complications include hypoxemia, respiratory failure, pleural effusion, empyema, lung abscess, and bacteremia, with spread of infection to other parts of the body, resulting in meningitis, endocarditis, and pericarditis.

Diagnosis
Clinical features, chest X-ray showing infiltrates, and sputum smear demonstrating acute inflammatory cells support the diagnosis. Gram stain and sputum culture may identify the organism. Positive blood cultures in the patient with pulmonary infiltrates strongly suggest pneumonia produced by the organisms isolated from the blood cultures. Pleural effusions, if present, should be tapped and fluid analyzed for evidence of infection in the pleural space. Occasionally, a transtracheal aspirate of tracheobronchial secretions or bronchoscopy with brushings or washings may be done to obtain material for smear and culture. The patient's response to antimicrobial therapy also provides important evidence of the presence of pneumonia.

Treatment
Antimicrobial therapy varies with the causative agent. Therapy should be reevaluated early in the course of treatment. Supportive measures include humidified oxygen therapy for hypoxemia, mechanical ventilation for respiratory failure, a high-calorie diet and adequate fluid intake, bed rest, and an analgesic to relieve pleuritic chest pain. Patients with severe pneumonia on mechanical ventilation may require PEEP to facilitate adequate oxygenation.

Special considerations
Correct supportive care can increase patient comfort, avoid complications, and speed recovery.

The following protocol should be observed throughout the illness:
◆ Maintain a patent airway and adequate oxygenation. Monitor pulse oximetry. Measure ABG levels, especially in hypoxemic patients. Administer supplemental oxygen if the PaO_2 is less than 55 to 60 mm Hg. Patients with underlying chronic lung disease should be given oxygen cautiously.
◆ Teach the patient how to cough and perform deep-breathing exercises to clear secretions; encourage them to do so often. In severe pneumonia that requires ET intubation or tracheostomy (with or without mechanical ventilation), provide thorough respiratory care. Suction often, using sterile technique, to remove secretions.
◆ Obtain sputum specimens as needed, by suction if the patient can't produce specimens independently. Collect specimens in a sterile container and deliver them promptly to the microbiology laboratory.
◆ Administer antibiotics as ordered, sedation, and pain medication as needed; record the patient's response to medications. Fever and dehydration may require I.V. fluids and electrolyte replacement.
◆ Maintain adequate nutrition to offset hypermetabolic state secondary to infection. Ask the dietary department to provide a high-calorie, high-protein diet consisting of soft, easy-to-eat foods. Encourage the patient to eat. As necessary, supplement oral feedings with NG tube feedings or parenteral nutrition. Monitor fluid intake and output. Consider limiting the use of milk products because they may increase sputum production.
◆ Provide a quiet, calm environment for the patient, with frequent rest periods.
◆ Give emotional support by explaining all procedures (especially intubation and suctioning) to the patient and family. Encourage family visits. Provide diversionary activities appropriate to the patient's age.
◆ To control the spread of infection, dispose of secretions properly. Tell the patient to sneeze and cough into a disposable tissue; tape a lined bag to the side of the bed for used tissues.

Pneumonia can be prevented as follows:
◆ Advise the patient to avoid using antibiotics indiscriminately during minor viral infections

because this may result in upper airway colonization with antibiotic-resistant bacteria. If the patient then develops pneumonia, the organisms producing the pneumonia may require treatment with more toxic antibiotics.

◆ Encourage pneumococcal vaccine (pneumovax) and annual influenza vaccination for high-risk patients, such as those with COPD, chronic heart disease, or sickle cell disease.

◆ Urge all bedridden and postoperative patients to perform deep-breathing and coughing exercises frequently. Reposition such patients often to promote full aeration and drainage of secretions. Encourage early ambulation in postoperative patients.

◆ To prevent aspiration during NG tube feedings, elevate the patient's head, check the tube's position, and administer the formula slowly. Don't give large volumes at one time; this could cause vomiting. Keep the patient's head elevated for at least 30 minutes after the feeding. Check for residual formula at 4- to 6-hour intervals.

▓▓▓▓▓ **PREVENTION**
◆ *Perform hand hygiene frequently to prevent infections.*
◆ *Advise patients to avoid taking antibiotics indiscriminately during viral infections.*

IDIOPATHIC BRONCHIOLITIS OBLITERANS WITH ORGANIZING PNEUMONIA

Idiopathic bronchiolitis obliterans with organizing pneumonia (BOOP), also known as *cryptogenic organizing pneumonia*, is one of several types of bronchiolitis obliterans. *Organizing pneumonia* refers to unresolved pneumonia, in which inflammatory alveolar exudate persists and eventually undergoes fibrosis. *Bronchiolitis obliterans* is a generic term used to describe an inflammatory disease of the small airways.

Causes and incidence

BOOP has no known cause. However, other forms of bronchiolitis obliterans and organizing pneumonia may be associated with specific diseases or situations, such as bone marrow, heart, or heart–lung transplantation; collagen vascular diseases, such as rheumatoid arthritis and systemic lupus erythematosus (LE); inflammatory diseases, such as Crohn disease, ulcerative colitis, and polyarteritis nodosa; bacterial, viral, or mycoplasmal respiratory infections; inhalation of toxic gases; and drug therapy with amiodarone, bleomycin, penicillamine, or lomustine.

Much debate still exists about the various pathologies and classifications of bronchiolitis

obliterans. Most patients with BOOP are between 50 and 60 years old. Incidence is equally divided between men and women. A smoking history doesn't seem to increase the risk of developing BOOP.

Pathophysiology

BOOP is the result of an epithelial injury in the lung that progresses to the formation of fibrinoid inflammatory cell clusters and subsequently intra-alveolar fibrosis. Upon biopsy the key characteristic is fibroblastic plugs present in the alveoli, alveolar ducts, and bronchioles.

Complications
◆ Respiratory failure
◆ Interstitial lung disease
◆ Death

Signs and symptoms

The presenting symptoms of BOOP are usually subacute, with a flulike syndrome of fever, persistent and nonproductive cough, dyspnea (especially with exertion), malaise, anorexia, and weight loss lasting for several weeks to several months. Physical assessment findings may reveal dry crackles as the only abnormality. Less common symptoms include a productive cough, hemoptysis, chest pain, generalized aching, and night sweats.

Diagnosis

Diagnosis begins with a thorough patient history meant to exclude any known cause of bronchiolitis obliterans or diseases with a pathophysiology that includes an organizing pneumonia pattern.

◆ Chest X-ray usually shows patchy, diffuse airspace opacities with a ground-glass appearance that may migrate from one location to another. High-resolution CT scans show areas of consolidation. Except for the migrating opacities, these findings are nonspecific and present in many other respiratory disorders.

◆ PFTs may be normal or show reduced capacities. The diffusing capacity for carbon monoxide is generally low.

◆ ABG analysis usually shows mild to moderate hypoxemia at rest, which worsens with exercise.

◆ Blood tests reveal an increased erythrocyte sedimentation rate, an increased C-reactive protein level, and an increased WBC count with a somewhat increased proportion of neutrophils and a minor rise in eosinophils. Immunoglobulin (Ig) G and IgM levels are normal or slightly increased, and the IgE level is normal.

◆ Bronchoscopy reveals normal or slightly inflamed airways. Bronchoalveolar lavage fluid obtained during bronchoscopy shows a moderate elevation in lymphocytes and, sometimes, elevated neutrophil and eosinophil levels. Foamy-looking alveolar macrophages may also be found.

℞ CONFIRMING DIAGNOSIS *Lung biopsy, thoracoscopy, or bronchoscopy is required to confirm the diagnosis of BOOP. Pathologic changes in lung tissue include plugs of connective tissue in the lumen of the bronchioles, alveolar ducts, and alveolar spaces.*

These changes may occur in other types of bronchiolitis and in other diseases that cause organizing pneumonia. They also differentiate BOOP from constrictive bronchiolitis (characterized by inflammation and fibrosis that surrounds and may narrow or completely obliterate the bronchiolar airways). Although the pathologic findings in proliferative and constrictive bronchiolitis are different, the causes and presentations may overlap. Any known cause of bronchiolitis obliterans or organizing pneumonia must be ruled out before the diagnosis of BOOP is made.

Treatment

Corticosteroids are the current treatment for BOOP, although the ideal dosage and duration of treatment remain topics of discussion. Relapse is common when steroids are tapered off or stopped. This usually can be reversed when steroids are increased or resumed. Occasionally, a patient may need to continue corticosteroids indefinitely.

Immunosuppressive-cytotoxic drugs, such as cyclophosphamide, have been used in the few cases of intolerance or unresponsiveness.

Oxygen is used to correct hypoxemia. The patient may need either no oxygen or a small amount of oxygen at rest and a greater amount when they exercise.

Other treatments vary, depending on the patient's symptoms, and may include inhaled bronchodilators, cough suppressants, and bronchial hygiene therapies.

BOOP is very responsive to treatment and usually can be completely reversed with corticosteroid therapy. However, a few deaths have been reported, particularly in patients who had more widespread pathologic changes in the lung or patients who developed opportunistic infections or other complications related to steroid therapy.

Special considerations

◆ Explain all diagnostic tests. The patient may experience anxiety and frustration because of the length of time and number of tests needed to establish the diagnosis.

◆ Explain the diagnosis to the patient and family. This uncommon diagnosis may cause confusion and anxiety.

◆ Monitor the patient for adverse effects of corticosteroid therapy: weight gain, "moon face," glucose intolerance, fluid and electrolyte imbalance, mood swings, cataracts, peptic ulcer disease, opportunistic infections, and osteoporosis leading to bone fractures. In many cases, these effects leave the patient unable to tolerate the treatment. Teach the patient and their family about these adverse effects, emphasizing which reactions should be reported to the physician.

◆ Teach measures that may help prevent complications related to treatment, such as infection control and improved nutrition.

◆ Teach breathing, relaxation, and energy conservation techniques to help the patient manage symptoms.

◆ Monitor oxygenation, both at rest and with exertion. The physician will probably prescribe an oxygen flow rate for use when the patient is at rest and a higher one for exertion. Teach the patient how to increase the oxygen flow rate to the appropriate level for exercise.

◆ If the patient needs oxygen at home, ensure continuity of care by making appropriate referrals to discharge planners, respiratory care practitioners, and home equipment vendors.

PULMONARY EMBOLISM

The most common pulmonary complication in hospitalized patients, pulmonary embolism is an obstruction of the pulmonary arterial bed by a dislodged thrombus, heart valve vegetation, or foreign substance. Although pulmonary infarction that results from embolism may be so mild as to be asymptomatic, massive embolism (more than 50% obstruction of pulmonary arterial circulation) and the accompanying infarction can be rapidly fatal. (See *Looking at pulmonary emboli,* page 120.)

Causes and incidence

Pulmonary embolism generally results from dislodged thrombi originating in the leg veins. More than half of such thrombi arise in the deep veins of the legs. Other less common sources of thrombi are the pelvic veins, renal veins, hepatic vein, right side of the heart, and upper extremities. Such thrombus formation results directly from vascular wall damage, venostasis, or hypercoagulability of the blood. Trauma, clot dissolution, sudden muscle spasm, intravascular pressure changes, or a change in peripheral blood flow can cause the thrombus to loosen or fragment. Then the thrombus— now called an *embolus*—floats to the heart's

Looking at pulmonary emboli

This illustration shows multiple emboli in pulmonary artery branches and a larger embolus that has resulted in an infarcted area in the lung.

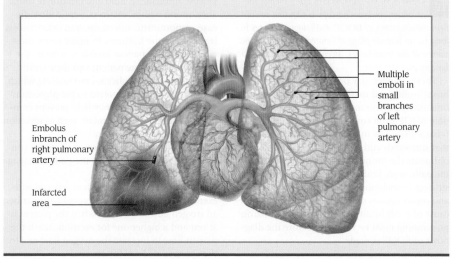

Embolus inbranch of right pulmonary artery

Infarcted area

Multiple emboli in small branches of left pulmonary artery

right side and enters the lung through the pulmonary artery. There, the embolus may dissolve, continue to fragment, or grow.

By occluding the pulmonary artery, the embolus prevents alveoli from producing enough surfactant to maintain alveolar integrity. As a result, alveoli collapse and atelectasis develops. If the embolus enlarges, it may clog most or all of the pulmonary vessels and cause death.

Rarely, the emboli contain air, fat, bacteria, amniotic fluid, talc (from drugs intended for oral administration, which are injected intravenously by addicts), or tumor cells.

Predisposing factors for pulmonary embolism include long-term immobility, chronic pulmonary disease, heart failure or atrial fibrillation, thrombophlebitis, polycythemia vera, thrombocytosis, autoimmune hemolytic anemia, sickle cell disease, varicose veins, recent surgery, advanced age, pregnancy, lower extremity fractures or surgery, burns, obesity, vascular injury, cancer, I.V. drug abuse, or hormonal contraceptives.

Pathophysiology

Once a thrombus dislodges, it travels through to the venous system, through the right side of the heart, and lodges in the pulmonary arteries. The thrombus can completely occlude the vessels or only partially block the flow of blood. Many physiologic factors participate in the potential

outcomes including the ability of the body's thrombolytic system to break down clots, function of the right ventricle, over all condition of lungs, and number and size of emboli.

Complications

◆ Pulmonary infarction
◆ Death

Signs and symptoms

Total occlusion of the main pulmonary artery is rapidly fatal; smaller or fragmented emboli produce symptoms that vary with the size, number, and location of the emboli. Usually, the first symptom of pulmonary embolism is dyspnea, which may be accompanied by anginal or pleuritic chest pain. Other clinical features include tachycardia, productive cough (sputum may be blood-tinged), low-grade fever, and pleural effusion. Less common signs include massive hemoptysis, chest splinting, leg edema and, with a large embolus, cyanosis, syncope, and distended jugular veins.

In addition, pulmonary embolism may cause pleural friction rub and signs of circulatory collapse (weak, rapid pulse, and hypotension) and hypoxia (restlessness and anxiety).

Diagnosis

The patient history should reveal predisposing conditions for pulmonary embolism. A triad of deep vein thrombosis (DVT) formation is stasis, endothelial injury, and hypercoagulability. Risk factors include long car or plane trips, cancer, pregnancy, hypercoagulability, prior DVT, and pulmonary emboli.

◆ Chest X-ray helps to rule out other pulmonary diseases; areas of atelectasis, an elevated diaphragm and pleural effusion, a prominent pulmonary artery and, occasionally, the characteristic wedge-shaped infiltrate suggestive of pulmonary infarction, or focal oligemia of blood vessels, are apparent.

◆ Lung scan shows perfusion defects in areas beyond occluded vessels; however, it doesn't rule out microemboli.

◆ Pulmonary angiography is the most definitive test but requires a skilled angiographer and radiologic equipment; it also poses some risk to the patient. Its use depends on the uncertainty of the diagnosis and the need to avoid unnecessary anticoagulant therapy in a high-risk patient.

◆ Electrocardiography may show right axis deviation; right bundle-branch block; tall, peaked P waves; ST-segment depression and T-wave inversions (indicative of right-sided heart strain); and supraventricular tachyarrhythmias in extensive pulmonary embolism. A pattern sometimes observed is S_1, Q_3, and T_3 (S wave in lead I, Q wave in lead III, and inverted T wave in lead III).

◆ Auscultation occasionally reveals a right ventricular S_3 gallop and increased intensity of the pulmonic component of S_2. Also, crackles and a pleural rub may be heard at the embolism site.

◆ ABG analysis showing a decreased PaO_2 and $PaCO_2$ are characteristic but don't always occur.

If pleural effusion is present, thoracentesis may rule out empyema, which indicates pneumonia.

Treatment

Treatment is designed to maintain adequate cardiovascular and pulmonary function during resolution of the obstruction and to prevent recurrence of embolic episodes. Because most emboli resolve within 10 to 14 days, treatment consists of oxygen therapy as needed and anticoagulation with heparin to inhibit new thrombus formation, followed by oral warfarin. Heparin therapy is monitored by daily coagulation studies (PTT).

Patients with massive pulmonary embolism and shock may need fibrinolytic therapy with thrombolytic therapy (streptokinase, urokinase, or tissue plasminogen activator) to enhance fibrinolysis of the pulmonary

emboli and remaining thrombi. Emboli that cause hypotension may require the use of vasopressors. Treatment of septic emboli requires antibiotics—not anticoagulants—and evaluation for the infection's source, particularly endocarditis.

Surgery is performed on patients who can't take anticoagulants, who have recurrent emboli during anticoagulant therapy, or who have been treated with thrombolytic agents or pulmonary thromboendarterectomy. This procedure (which shouldn't be performed without angiographic evidence of pulmonary embolism) consists of vena cava ligation, plication, or insertion of an inferior vena cava device to filter blood returning to the heart and lungs.

Special considerations

◆ Give oxygen by nasal cannula or mask. Check ABG levels if the patient develops fresh emboli or worsening dyspnea. Be prepared to provide ET intubation with assisted ventilation if breathing is severely compromised.

◆ Administer heparin, as ordered, through I.V. push or continuous drip. Monitor coagulation studies daily. Effective heparin therapy raises the PTT to more than 1½ times normal. Watch closely for nosebleeds, petechiae, and other signs of abnormal bleeding; check stools for occult blood. Patients should be protected from trauma and injury; avoid I.M. injections and maintain pressure over venipuncture sites for 5 minutes, or until bleeding stops, to reduce hematoma.

◆ After the patient is stable, encourage them to move about often, and assist with isometric and range-of-motion exercises. Check pedal pulses, temperature, and color of feet to detect venostasis. *Never* massage the patient's legs. Offer diversional activities to promote rest and relieve restlessness.

◆ Help the patient walk as soon as possible after surgery to prevent venostasis.

◆ Maintain adequate nutrition and fluid balance to promote healing.

◆ Report frequent pleuritic chest pain, so that analgesics can be prescribed. Also, incentive spirometry can assist in deep breathing. Provide tissues and a bag for easy disposal of expectorations.

◆ Warn the patient not to cross their legs; this promotes thrombus formation.

◆ To relieve anxiety, explain procedures and treatments. Encourage the patient's family to participate in their care.

◆ Most patients need treatment with an oral anticoagulant (warfarin) for 3 to 6 months after a pulmonary embolism. Advise these patients to watch for signs of bleeding (bloody stools, blood in urine, and large ecchymoses), to take the prescribed medication exactly as ordered, not to change dosages without consulting their physician, and to avoid taking additional medication (including aspirin and vitamins). Stress the importance of follow-up laboratory tests (international normalized ratio) to monitor anticoagulant therapy.

⁞⁞⁞⁞⁞ PREVENTION
◆ *Encourage early ambulation in patients predisposed to this condition. With close medical supervision, low-dose heparin may be useful prophylactically.*
◆ *In high-risk patients, low–molecular-weight heparin may be given.*

SARCOIDOSIS

Sarcoidosis is a multisystem, granulomatous disorder that characteristically produces lymphadenopathy, pulmonary infiltration, and skeletal, liver, eye, or skin lesions. Acute sarcoidosis usually resolves within 2 years. Chronic, progressive sarcoidosis, which is uncommon, is associated with pulmonary fibrosis and progressive pulmonary disability.

Causes and incidence

The cause of sarcoidosis is unknown, but these factors may play a role:
◆ hypersensitivity response (possibly from T-cell imbalance) to such agents as atypical mycobacteria, fungi, and pine pollen
◆ genetic predisposition (suggested by a slightly higher incidence of sarcoidosis within the same family)
◆ extreme immune response to infection
  Sarcoidosis occurs most commonly in adults 30 to 50 years old. In the United States, sarcoidosis occurs predominantly among blacks, affecting twice as many women as men.

Pathophysiology

In the development of sarcoidosis, T cells play an important role by initiating a significant immune reaction. In sites where there is disease activity, a concentration of CD4 cells exist along with a release of interleukin-2. This results in a disequilibrium of the CD4/CD8 ratio. The exaggerated immune response creates the characteristic noncaseating granulomas, found primarily on the lungs and intrathoracic lymph nodes.

Complications

◆ Pulmonary fibrosis
◆ Pulmonary hypertension
◆ Cor pulmonale

Signs and symptoms

Initial symptoms of sarcoidosis include arthralgia (in the wrists, ankles, and elbows), fatigue, malaise, and weight loss. Other clinical features vary according to the extent and location of the fibrosis:
◆ Respiratory—breathlessness, cough (usually nonproductive), substernal pain; complications in advanced pulmonary disease include pulmonary hypertension and cor pulmonale
◆ Cutaneous—erythema nodosum, subcutaneous skin nodules with maculopapular eruptions, and extensive nasal mucosal lesions
◆ Ophthalmic—anterior uveitis (common), glaucoma, and blindness (rare)
◆ Lymphatic—bilateral hilar and right paratracheal lymphadenopathy and splenomegaly
◆ Musculoskeletal—muscle weakness, polyarthralgia, pain, and punched-out lesions on phalanges
◆ Hepatic—granulomatous hepatitis, usually asymptomatic
◆ Genitourinary—hypercalciuria
◆ Cardiovascular—arrhythmias (premature beats, bundle-branch or complete heart block) and, rarely, cardiomyopathy
◆ CNS—cranial or peripheral nerve palsies, basilar meningitis, seizures, and pituitary and hypothalamic lesions producing diabetes insipidus

Diagnosis

Typical clinical features with appropriate laboratory data and X-ray findings suggest sarcoidosis. A positive skin lesion biopsy supports the diagnosis.
  Other relevant findings include:
◆ Chest X-ray—bilateral hilar and right paratracheal adenopathy with or without diffuse interstitial infiltrates; occasionally large nodular lesions present in lung parenchyma
◆ Lymph node or lung biopsy—noncaseating granulomas with negative cultures for mycobacteria and fungi
◆ Other laboratory data—rarely, increased serum calcium, mild anemia, leukocytosis, and hyperglobulinemia
◆ PFTs—decreased TLC and compliance, and decreased diffusing capacity
◆ ABG analysis—decreased arterial oxygen tension
  Negative tuberculin skin test, fungal serologies, and sputum cultures for mycobacteria and fungi as well as negative biopsy cultures help rule out infection.

Treatment

Sarcoidosis that produces no symptoms requires no treatment. However, those severely affected with sarcoidosis require treatment with corticosteroids. Such therapy is usually continued for 1 to 2 years, but some patients may need lifelong therapy. Immunosuppressive agents, such as methotrexate, azathioprine, and cyclophosphamide, may also be used. If organ failure occurs (although this is rare), transplantation may be required. Other measures include a low-calcium diet and avoidance of direct exposure to sunlight in patients with hypercalcemia.

Special considerations

◆ Watch for and report any complications. Be aware of abnormal laboratory results (e.g., anemia) that could alter patient care.
◆ For the patient with arthralgia, administer analgesics as ordered. Record signs of progressive muscle weakness.
◆ Provide a nutritious, high-calorie diet and plenty of fluids. If the patient has hypercalcemia, suggest a low-calcium diet. Weigh the patient regularly to detect weight loss.
◆ Monitor respiratory function. Check chest X-rays for the extent of lung involvement; note and record any bloody sputum or increase in sputum. If the patient has pulmonary hypertension or end-stage cor pulmonale, check ABG levels, observe for arrhythmias, and administer oxygen, as needed.
◆ Because steroids may induce or worsen diabetes mellitus, perform fingerstick glucose tests at least every 12 hours at the beginning of steroid therapy. Also, watch for other steroid adverse effects, such as fluid retention, electrolyte imbalance (especially hypokalemia), moon face, hypertension, and personality change. During or after steroid withdrawal (particularly in association with infection or other types of stress), watch for and report vomiting, orthostatic hypotension, hypoglycemia, restlessness, anorexia, malaise, and fatigue. Remember that the patient on long-term or high-dose steroid therapy is vulnerable to infection.
◆ When preparing the patient for discharge, stress the need for compliance with prescribed steroid therapy and regular, careful follow-up examinations and treatment. Refer the patient with failing vision to community support and resource groups and the American Foundation for the Blind, if necessary.

SEVERE ACUTE RESPIRATORY SYNDROME

SARS is a viral respiratory infection that can progress to pneumonia and, eventually, death. The disease was first recognized in 2003 with outbreaks in China, Canada, Singapore, Taiwan, and Vietnam, with other countries—including the United States—reporting smaller numbers of cases.

Causes and incidence

SARS is caused by the SARS-associated coronavirus (SARS-CoV). Coronaviruses are a common cause of mild respiratory illnesses in humans, but researchers believe that a virus may have mutated, allowing it to cause this potentially life-threatening disease.

Close contact with a person who's infected with SARS, including contact with infectious aerosolized droplets or body secretions, is the method of transmission. Most people who contracted the disease during the 2003 outbreak contracted it during travel to endemic areas. However, the virus has been found to live on hands, tissues, and other surfaces for up to 6 hours in its droplet form. It has also been found to live in the stool of people with SARS for up to 4 days. The virus may be able to live for months or years in below-freezing temperatures.

Pathophysiology

SARS-CoV is replicated primarily in the lungs but is also found to have the same ability in the gastrointestinal (GI) tract. Once an infection has been established, the virus will cause lysis of cells in the lungs and GI tissues and initiating an immune response. Most tissue damage takes place in the pulmonary tissues and alveoli.

Complications

◆ Respiratory failure
◆ Liver failure
◆ Heart failure
◆ Myelodysplastic syndromes
◆ Death

Signs and symptoms

The incubation period for SARS is typically 3 to 5 days but may last as long as 14 days. Initial signs and symptoms include fever, shortness of breath and other minor respiratory symptoms, general discomfort, headache, rigors, chills, myalgia, sore throat, and dry cough. Some individuals may develop diarrhea or a rash. Later complications include respiratory failure, liver failure, heart failure, myelodysplastic syndromes, and death.

Diagnosis

Diagnosis of severe respiratory illness is made when the patient has a fever greater than 100.4° F (38° C) or upon clinical findings of lower respiratory illness and a chest X-ray demonstrating pneumonia or ARDS. (See *Lungs and alveoli in SARS*, page 124.)

Lungs and alveoli in SARS

Severe acute respiratory syndrome (SARS) is a viral respiratory infection that can progress from minor respiratory symptoms to pneumonia and eventually death.

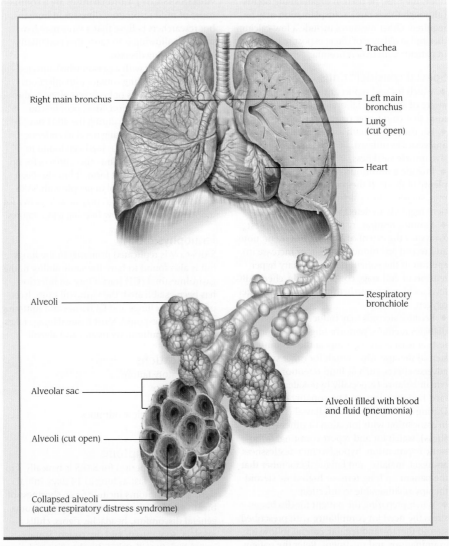

Trachea

Right main bronchus

Left main bronchus

Lung (cut open)

Heart

Alveoli

Respiratory bronchiole

Alveolar sac

Alveoli filled with blood and fluid (pneumonia)

Alveoli (cut open)

Collapsed alveoli (acute respiratory distress syndrome)

Laboratory validation for the virus includes cell culture of SARS-CoV, detection of SARS-CoV ribonucleic acid by the reverse transcription polymerase chain reaction (PCR) test, or detection of serum antibodies to SARS-CoV. Detectable levels of antibodies may not be present until 21 days after the onset of illness, but some individuals develop antibodies within 14 days. A negative PCR, antibody test, or cell culture doesn't rule out the diagnosis.

Treatment

Treatment is symptomatic and supportive and includes maintenance of a patent airway and adequate nutrition. Other treatment measures include supplemental oxygen, chest physiotherapy, or mechanical ventilation. In addition to standard precautions, contact precautions requiring gowns and gloves for all patient contacts and airborne precautions utilizing a negative-pressure isolation room and properly fitted N95 respirators are recommended for patients who are hospitalized. Quarantine may be used to prevent the spread of infection.

Antibiotics may be given to treat bacterial causes of atypical pneumonia. Antiviral medications have also been used. High doses of corticosteroids have been used to reduce lung inflammation. In some serious cases, serum from individuals who have already recovered from SARS (convalescent serum) has been given. The general benefit of these treatments hasn't been determined conclusively.

Special considerations
◆ Report suspected cases of SARS to local and national health organizations.
◆ Frequently monitor the patient's vital signs and respiratory status.
◆ Maintain isolation as recommended. The patient will need emotional support to deal with anxiety and fear related to the diagnosis of SARS and as a result of isolation.
◆ Provide patient and family teaching, including the importance of frequent handwashing, covering the mouth and nose when coughing or sneezing, and avoiding close personal contact while infected or potentially infected. Instruct the patient and family that such items as eating utensils, towels, and bedding shouldn't be shared until they have been washed with soap and hot water and that disposable gloves and household disinfectant should be used to clean any surface that may have been exposed to the patient's body fluids.
◆ Emphasize to the patient the importance of not going to work, school, or other public places, as recommended by the healthcare provider.

LUNG ABSCESS
Lung abscess is a lung infection accompanied by pus accumulation and tissue destruction. The abscess may be putrid (due to anaerobic bacteria) or nonputrid (due to anaerobes or aerobes) and usually has a well-defined border. The availability of effective antibiotics has made lung abscess much less common than it was in the past.

Causes and incidence
Lung abscess is a manifestation of necrotizing pneumonia, generally the result of aspiration of oropharyngeal contents. Poor oral hygiene with dental or gingival (gum) disease is strongly associated with putrid lung abscess. Septic pulmonary emboli commonly produce cavitary lesions. Infected cystic lung lesions and cavitating bronchial carcinoma must be distinguished from lung abscesses.

Pathophysiology
The development of a lung abscess is a response to the introduction of a pathogen, likely from the mouth, into the lower airways. These anaerobes are not cleared away with the body's initial immune response and create a thick-walled cavity filled with purulent material in response to the infection. They can lead to tissue necrosis or possibly the destruction of the involved lung parenchyma.

Complications
◆ Rupture into pleural space, resulting in empyema
◆ Massive hemorrhage

Signs and symptoms
The clinical effects of lung abscess include a cough that may produce bloody, purulent, or foul-smelling sputum, pleuritic chest pain, dyspnea, excessive sweating, chills, fever, headache, malaise, diaphoresis, and weight loss. Chronic lung abscess may cause localized bronchiectasis. Failure of an abscess to improve with antibiotic treatment suggests possible underlying neoplasm or other causes of obstruction.

Diagnosis
◆ Auscultation of the chest may reveal crackles and decreased breath sounds.
◆ Chest X-ray shows a localized infiltrate with one or more clear spaces, usually containing air–fluid levels.
◆ Percutaneous aspiration or bronchoscopy may be used to obtain cultures to identify the causative organism. Bronchoscopy is only used if abscess resolution is eventful and the patient's condition permits it.
◆ Blood cultures, Gram stain, and sputum culture are also used to detect the causative organism; leukocytosis (WBC count greater than 10,000/µL) is commonly present.

Treatment
Treatment consists of prolonged antibiotic therapy, commonly lasting for months, until radiographic resolution or definite stability occurs. Symptoms usually disappear in a few weeks. Postural drainage may facilitate discharge of necrotic material into the upper airways where expectoration is possible; oxygen therapy may relieve hypoxemia. Poor response to therapy requires resection of the lesion or removal of the diseased section of the lung. All patients need rigorous follow-up and serial chest X-rays.

Special considerations

◆ Help the patient with chest physiotherapy (including coughing and deep breathing), increase fluid intake to loosen secretions, and provide a quiet, restful atmosphere.

◆ To prevent lung abscess in the unconscious patient and the patient with seizures, first prevent aspiration of secretions. Do this by suctioning the patient and by positioning in such a way to promote drainage of secretions.

HEMOTHORAX

In hemothorax, blood from damaged intercostal, pleural, mediastinal, and (infrequently) lung parenchymal vessels enters the pleural cavity. Depending on the amount of bleeding and the underlying cause, hemothorax may be associated with varying degrees of lung collapse and mediastinal shift. Pneumothorax—air in the pleural cavity—commonly accompanies hemothorax.

Causes and incidence

Hemothorax usually results from blunt or penetrating chest trauma; in fact, about 25% of patients with such trauma have hemothorax. In some cases, it results from thoracic surgery, pulmonary infarction, neoplasm, dissecting thoracic aneurysm, or as a complication of TB or anticoagulant therapy.

Pathophysiology

A hemothorax occurs when a disruption of the chest wall tissues or intrathoracic structures allows blood to enter the pleural space. Depending on the speed and volume of the circulating blood, there can be a significant hemodynamic shift including the early stages of shock.

Complications

◆ Mediastinal shift
◆ Ventilatory compromise
◆ Lung collapse
◆ Cardiopulmonary arrest

Signs and symptoms

The patient with hemothorax may experience chest pain, tachypnea, and mild to severe dyspnea, depending on the amount of blood in the pleural cavity and associated pathologic conditions. If respiratory failure results, the patient may appear anxious, restless, possibly stuporous, and cyanotic; marked blood loss produces hypotension and shock. The affected side of the chest expands and stiffens, whereas the unaffected side rises and falls with the patient's breaths.

Diagnosis

Characteristic clinical signs and a history of trauma strongly suggest hemothorax. Percussion and auscultation reveal dullness and decreased to absent breath sounds over the affected side. Thoracentesis yields blood or serosanguineous fluid; chest X-rays show pleural fluid with or without mediastinal shift. ABG analysis may reveal respiratory failure; Hb may be decreased, depending on the amount of blood lost.

Treatment

Treatment is designed to stabilize the patient's condition, stop the bleeding, evacuate blood from the pleural space, and re-expand the underlying lung. Mild hemothorax usually clears in 10 to 14 days, requiring only observation for further bleeding. In severe hemothorax, thoracentesis not only serves as a diagnostic tool, but also removes fluid from the pleural space.

After the diagnosis is confirmed, a chest tube is inserted into the sixth intercostal space at the posterior axillary line. Suction may be used; a large-bore tube is used to prevent clot blockage. If the chest tube doesn't improve the patient's condition, they may need a thoracotomy to evacuate blood and clots and to control bleeding.

Special considerations

◆ Give oxygen by face mask or nasal cannula.

◆ Give I.V. fluids and blood transfusions, as ordered, to treat shock. Monitor pulse oximetry and ABG levels often.

◆ Explain all procedures to the patient to allay their fears. Assist with thoracentesis. Warn the patient not to cough during this procedure.

◆ Carefully observe chest tube drainage and record the volume drained (at least every hour). Milk the chest tube (only if necessary and according to facility and physician protocols) to keep it open and free from clots. If the tube is warm and full of blood and the bloody fluid level in the water-seal bottle is rising rapidly, report this at once. The patient may need immediate surgery.

◆ Watch the patient closely for pallor and gasping respirations. Monitor vital signs diligently. Falling blood pressure, rising pulse rate, and rising respiratory rate may indicate shock or massive bleeding.

PULMONARY HYPERTENSION

Pulmonary hypertension occurs when PAP rises above normal for reasons other than aging or altitude. No definitive set of values is used to diagnose pulmonary hypertension, but the

National Institutes of Health requires a mean PAP of 25 mm Hg or more. The prognosis depends on the cause of the underlying disorder, but the long-term prognosis is poor. Within 5 years of diagnosis, only 25% of patients are still alive.

Causes and incidence

Pulmonary hypertension begins as hypertrophy of the small pulmonary arteries. The medial and intimal muscle layers of these vessels thicken, decreasing distensibility and increasing resistance. This disorder then progresses to vascular sclerosis and obliteration of small vessels.

In most cases, pulmonary hypertension occurs secondary to an underlying disease process, including:

◆ *alveolar hypoventilation* from COPD (most common cause in the United States), sarcoidosis, diffuse interstitial disease, pulmonary metastasis, and certain diseases such as scleroderma. (In these disorders, pulmonary vascular resistance occurs secondary to hypoxemia and destruction of the alveolocapillary bed. Other disorders that cause alveolar hypoventilation without lung tissue damage include obesity, kyphoscoliosis, and obstructive sleep apnea.)

◆ *vascular obstruction* from pulmonary embolism, vasculitis, and disorders that cause obstruction of small or large pulmonary veins, such as left atrial myxoma, idiopathic venoocclusive disease, fibrosing mediastinitis, and mediastinal neoplasm

◆ *primary cardiac disease*, which may be congenital or acquired. Congenital defects that cause left-to-right shunting of blood—such as patent ductus arteriosus or atrial or ventricular septal defect—increase blood flow into the lungs and, consequently, raise pulmonary vascular pressure. Acquired cardiac diseases, such as rheumatic valvular disease and mitral stenosis, increase pulmonary venous pressure by restricting blood flow returning to the heart

Primary (or idiopathic) pulmonary hypertension is rare, occurring most commonly—and with no known cause—in women between 20 and 40 years old. Secondary pulmonary hypertension results from existing cardiac, pulmonary, thromboembolic, or collagen vascular diseases or from the use of certain drugs.

Pathophysiology

The primary pathogenic mechanism involved in pulmonary hypertension is vascular resistance. This resistance typically results from vasoconstriction, remodeling, or a formation of a microthrombus in the pulmonary arteries or arterioles.

Complications
◆ Cor pulmonale
◆ Cardiac failure
◆ Cardiac arrest

Signs and symptoms

Most patients complain of increasing dyspnea on exertion, weakness, syncope, and fatigability. Many also show signs of right-sided heart failure, including peripheral edema, ascites, jugular vein distention, and hepatomegaly. Other clinical effects vary with the underlying disorder.

Diagnosis

Characteristic diagnostic findings include:

◆ Auscultation reveals abnormalities associated with the underlying disorder.

◆ ABG analysis indicates hypoxemia (decreased PaO_2).

◆ Electrocardiography shows right axis deviation and tall or peaked P waves in inferior leads in the patient with right ventricular hypertrophy.

◆ Cardiac catheterization reveals pulmonary systolic pressure above 30 mm Hg as well as increased PAWP if the underlying cause is left atrial myxoma, mitral stenosis, or left-sided heart failure (otherwise normal).

◆ Pulmonary angiography detects filling defects in pulmonary vasculature such as those that develop in patients with pulmonary emboli.

◆ PFTs may show decreased flow rates and increased residual volume in underlying obstructive disease and decreased TLC in underlying restrictive disease.

Treatment

Treatment usually includes oxygen therapy to decrease hypoxemia and resulting pulmonary vascular resistance. It may also include vasodilator therapy (nifedipine [Procardia], diltiazem [Cardizem], or prostaglandin E). For patients with right-sided heart failure, treatment also includes fluid restriction, cardiac glycosides to increase cardiac output, and diuretics to decrease intravascular volume and extravascular fluid accumulation. Treatment also aims to correct the underlying cause.

Some patients with pulmonary hypertension may be candidates for heart–lung transplantation to improve their chances of survival.

Special considerations

Pulmonary hypertension requires keen observation and careful monitoring as well as skilled supportive care.

◆ Administer oxygen therapy as ordered and observe the patient's response. Report any signs of increasing dyspnea to the physician so they can adjust treatment accordingly.

◆ Monitor ABG levels for acidosis and hypoxemia. Report any change in the patient's level of consciousness at once.

◆ When caring for a patient with right-sided heart failure, especially one receiving diuretics, record their weight daily, carefully measure intake and output, and explain all medications and diet restrictions. Check for worsening jugular vein distention, which may indicate fluid overload.

◆ Monitor the patient's vital signs, especially blood pressure and heart rate. Watch for hypotension and tachycardia. If they have a pulmonary artery catheter, check PAP and PAWP, as indicated. Report any changes.

◆ Before discharge, help the patient adjust to the limitations imposed by this disorder. Advise against overexertion and suggest frequent rest periods between activities. Refer the patient to the social services department if they will need special equipment, such as oxygen equipment, for home use. Make sure that they understand the prescribed medications and diet and the need to weigh themselves daily.

PLEURAL EFFUSION AND EMPYEMA

Pleural effusion is an excess of fluid in the pleural space. Normally, this space contains a small amount of extracellular fluid that lubricates the pleural surfaces. Increased production or inadequate removal of this fluid results in pleural effusion. Empyema is the accumulation of pus and necrotic tissue in the pleural space. Blood (hemothorax) and chyle (chylothorax) may also collect in this space.

Causes and incidence

The balance of osmotic and hydrostatic pressures in parietal pleural capillaries normally results in fluid movement into the pleural space. Balanced pressures in visceral pleural capillaries promote reabsorption of this fluid. Effusions frequently result from heart failure, hepatic disease with ascites, peritoneal dialysis, hypoalbuminemia, and disorders resulting in overexpanded intravascular volume.

Exudative pleural effusions occur with TB, subphrenic abscess, pancreatitis, bacterial or fungal pneumonitis or empyema, malignancy, pulmonary embolism with or without infarction, collagen disease (LE and rheumatoid arthritis), myxedema, and chest trauma.

Empyema is usually associated with infection in the pleural space. Such infection may be idiopathic or may be related to pneumonitis, carcinoma, perforation, or esophageal rupture.

Pathophysiology

Pleural effusions result from excessive hydrostatic pressure or decreased osmotic pressure causing excessive amounts of fluid to pass across intact capillaries. The result is a transudative pleural effusion, an ultrafiltrate of plasma containing low concentrations of protein. Exudative pleural effusions result when capillaries exhibit increased permeability with or without changes in hydrostatic and colloid osmotic pressures, allowing protein-rich fluid to leak into the pleural space. An empyema results from an infection in the pleural space or accumulated fluid.

Complications
◆ Atelectasis
◆ Infection
◆ Hypoxemia

Signs and symptoms

Patients with pleural effusion characteristically display symptoms relating to the underlying pathologic condition. Most patients with large effusions, particularly those with underlying pulmonary disease, complain of dyspnea. Those with effusions associated with pleurisy complain of pleuritic chest pain. Other clinical features depend on the cause of the effusion. Patients with empyema also develop fever and malaise.

Diagnosis

Auscultation of the chest reveals decreased breath sounds; percussion detects dullness over the effused area, which doesn't change with breathing. Chest X-ray shows fluid in dependent regions. However, diagnosis also requires other tests to distinguish transudative from exudative effusions and to help pinpoint the underlying disorder.

The most useful test is thoracentesis, in which pleural fluid is analyzed in the laboratory to show components. Acute inflammatory WBCs and microorganisms may be evident in empyema.

In addition, if a pleural effusion results from esophageal rupture or pancreatitis, fluid amylase levels are usually higher than serum levels. Aspirated fluid may be tested for LE cells, antinuclear antibodies, and neoplastic cells. It may also be analyzed for color and consistency; acid-fast bacillus (AFB), fungal, and bacterial cultures; and triglycerides (in chylothorax). Cell analysis shows leukocytosis in empyema. A negative tuberculin skin test strongly rules against TB as the cause. In exudative pleural effusions in which thoracentesis isn't definitive, pleural biopsy may be done. This is particularly useful for confirming TB or malignancy.

Treatment

Depending on the amount of fluid present, symptomatic effusion may require thoracentesis to remove fluid or careful monitoring of the patient's own reabsorption of the fluid. Hemothorax requires drainage to prevent fibrothorax formation. Pleural effusions associated with lung cancer commonly reaccumulate quickly. If a chest tube is inserted to drain the fluid, a sclerosing agent, such as talc, may be injected through the tube to cause adhesions between the parietal and visceral pleura, thereby obliterating the potential space for fluid to recollect.

Treatment of empyema requires insertion of one or more chest tubes after thoracentesis, to allow drainage of purulent material, and possibly decortication (surgical removal of the thick coating over the lung) or rib resection to allow open drainage and lung expansion. Empyema also requires parenteral antibiotics. Associated hypoxia requires oxygen administration.

Special considerations

◆ Explain thoracentesis to the patient. Before the procedure, tell the patient to expect a stinging sensation from the local anesthetic and a feeling of pressure when the needle is inserted. Instruct them to tell you immediately if they feel uncomfortable or has difficulty breathing during the procedure.

◆ Reassure the patient during thoracentesis. Remind them to breathe normally and avoid sudden movements, such as coughing or sighing. Monitor vital signs and watch for syncope. If fluid is removed too quickly, the patient may suffer bradycardia, hypotension, pain, pulmonary edema, or even cardiac arrest. Watch for respiratory distress or pneumothorax (sudden onset of dyspnea and cyanosis) after thoracentesis.

◆ Administer oxygen and, in empyema, antibiotics, as ordered.

◆ Encourage the patient to perform deep-breathing exercises to promote lung expansion. Use an incentive spirometer to promote deep breathing.

◆ Provide meticulous chest tube care, and use sterile technique for changing dressings around the tube insertion site in empyema. Ensure tube patency by watching for fluctuations of fluid or air bubbling in the underwater seal chamber. Continuous bubbling may indicate an air leak. Record the amount, color, and consistency of any tube drainage.

◆ If the patient has open drainage through a rib resection or intercostal tube, use hand and dressing precautions. Because weeks of such drainage are usually necessary to obliterate the space, make visiting nurse referrals for the patient who will be discharged with the tube in place.

◆ If pleural effusion was a complication of pneumonia or influenza, advise prompt medical attention for upper respiratory infections.

PLEURISY

Pleurisy, also known as *pleuritis*, is an inflammation of the visceral and parietal pleurae that line the inside of the thoracic cage and envelop the lungs.

Causes and incidence

Pleurisy develops as a complication of pneumonia, TB, viruses, systemic LE, rheumatoid arthritis, uremia, Dressler syndrome, certain cancers, pulmonary infarction, and chest trauma. Pleuritic pain is caused by the inflammation or irritation of sensory nerve endings in the parietal pleura. As the lungs inflate and deflate, the visceral pleura covering the lungs moves against the fixed parietal pleura lining the pleural space, causing pain. This disorder usually begins suddenly.

In the United States, pleural effusions develop in 36% to 66% of hospitalized patients with bacterial pneumonia.

Pathophysiology

There are pain fibers located in the two layers of the pleura; the visceral pleural covers the lung and the parietal pleural line the inner chest wall. Pleurisy or pleuritis is the result of the inflammation of these pleuritic layers, usually from an infectious source.

Complications

◆ Pneumonia
◆ Pleural effusion
◆ Lung collapse

Signs and symptoms

Sharp, stabbing pain that increases with deep breathing may be so severe that it limits movement on the affected side. Dyspnea also occurs. Other symptoms vary according to the underlying pathologic process.

Diagnosis

Auscultation of the chest reveals a characteristic pleural friction rub—a coarse, creaky sound heard during late inspiration and early expiration, directly over the area of pleural inflammation. Palpation over the affected area may reveal coarse vibration. Chest X-ray, ultrasound of the chest, and thoracentesis may aid in diagnosis.

Treatment
Treatment is directed at the underlying cause; bacterial infections are treated with appropriate antibiotics, TB requires special treatment, and viral infections may be permitted to run their course. Treatment also includes measures to relieve symptoms, such as anti-inflammatory agents, analgesics, and bed rest. Severe pain may require an intercostal nerve block of two or three intercostal nerves. Pleurisy with pleural effusion calls for thoracentesis as a therapeutic and diagnostic measure.

Special considerations
◆ Stress the importance of bed rest and plan your care to allow the patient as much uninterrupted rest as possible.
◆ Administer antitussives and pain medication, as ordered, but be careful not to overmedicate. If the pain requires an opioid analgesic, warn the patient who's about to be discharged to avoid overuse because such medication depresses coughing and respiration.
◆ Encourage the patient to cough. Tell them to apply firm pressure at the site of the pain during coughing exercises to minimize pain.

Chronic disorders
CHRONIC OBSTRUCTIVE PULMONARY DISEASE
COPD is chronic airway obstruction that results from emphysema, chronic bronchitis, asthma, or any combination of these disorders. (See *How pulmonary edema develops,* page 131. Also see *Lung changes in emphysema,* page 132.) Usually, more than one of these underlying conditions coexist; in most cases, bronchitis and emphysema occur together. It doesn't always produce symptoms and causes only minimal disability in many patients. However, COPD tends to worsen with time.

Causes and incidence
Predisposing factors include cigarette smoking, recurrent or chronic respiratory infections, air pollution, occupational exposure to chemicals, and allergies. Early inflammatory changes may reverse if the patient stops smoking before lung destruction is extensive. Familial and hereditary factors (such as deficiency of alpha$_1$-antitrypsin) may also predispose a person to COPD.

The most common chronic lung disease, COPD (also known as *chronic obstructive lung disease*) affects an estimated 17 million Americans, and its incidence is rising. It affects more males than females, probably because until recently men were more likely to smoke heavily. COPD occurs mostly in people older than age 40.

Pathophysiology
Repeated exposure to carcinogens, such as smoking, is by far the most important causative action—it impairs ciliary action and macrophage function, inflames airways, increases mucus production, destroys alveolar septae, and causes peribronchiolar fibrosis.

Complications
◆ Overwhelming disability
◆ Cor pulmonale
◆ Severe respiratory failure
◆ Death

Signs and symptoms
The typical patient, a long-term cigarette smoker, has no symptoms until middle age. The ability to exercise or do strenuous work gradually starts to decline, and the patient begins to develop a productive cough. These signs are subtle at first but become more pronounced as the patient gets older and the disease progresses. Eventually the patient may develop dyspnea on minimal exertion, frequent respiratory infections, intermittent or continuous hypoxemia, and grossly abnormal pulmonary function studies. Advanced COPD may cause severe dyspnea, overwhelming disability, cor pulmonale, severe respiratory failure, and death.

Diagnosis
For specific diagnostic tests used to determine COPD, see *Types of chronic obstructive pulmonary disease.*

Treatment
Treatment is designed to relieve symptoms and prevent complications. Because most patients with COPD receive outpatient treatment, they need comprehensive teaching to help them comply with therapy and understand the nature of this chronic, progressive disease. If programs in pulmonary rehabilitation are available, encourage patient to enroll.

Urge the patient to stop smoking. Provide smoking cessation counseling or refer them to a program. Avoid other respiratory irritants, such as secondhand smoke, aerosol spray products, and outdoor air pollution. An air conditioner with an air filter in the home may be helpful.

PATHOPHYSIOLOGY
How pulmonary edema develops

In pulmonary edema, diminished function of the left ventricle causes blood to pool there and in the left atrium. Eventually, blood backs up into the pulmonary veins and capillaries.

Increasing capillary hydrostatic pressure pushes fluid into the interstitial spaces and alveoli. The illustrations below show a normal alveolus and the effects of pulmonary edema.

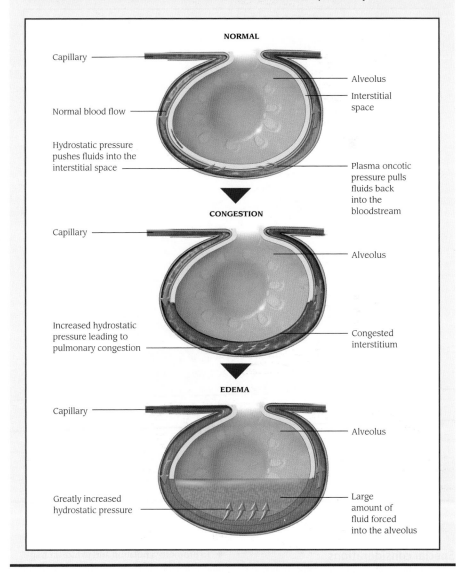

NORMAL

Capillary

Alveolus

Interstitial space

Normal blood flow

Hydrostatic pressure pushes fluids into the interstitial space

Plasma oncotic pressure pulls fluids back into the bloodstream

CONGESTION

Capillary

Alveolus

Increased hydrostatic pressure leading to pulmonary congestion

Congested interstitium

EDEMA

Capillary

Alveolus

Greatly increased hydrostatic pressure

Large amount of fluid forced into the alveolus

The patient is usually treated with beta-agonist bronchodilators (albuterol or salmeterol), anticholinergic bronchodilators (ipratropium), and corticosteroids (beclomethasone or triamcinolone). These are usually given by metered-dose inhaler, requiring that the patient be taught the correct administration technique.

Antibiotics are used to treat respiratory infections. Stress the need to complete the prescribed course of antibiotic therapy.

Lung changes in emphysema

A form of chronic obstructive pulmonary disease, emphysema is the abnormal, permanent enlargement of the acini accompanied by the destruction of the alveolar walls. Obstruction results from tissue changes, rather than mucus production, as occurs in asthma and chronic bronchitis. The distinguishing characteristic of emphysema is airflow limitation caused by a lack of elastic recoil in the lungs.

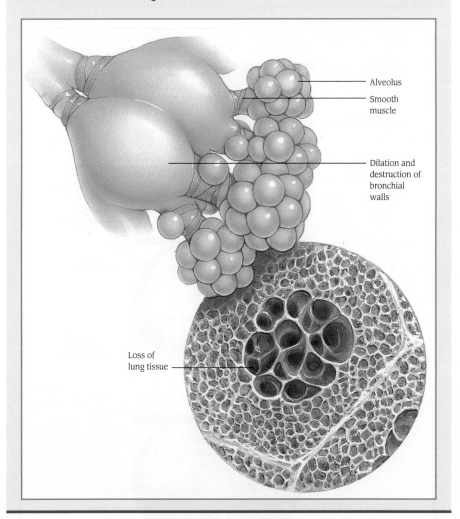

Alveolus

Smooth muscle

Dilation and destruction of bronchial walls

Loss of lung tissue

Special considerations

◆ Teach the patient and family how to recognize early signs of infection; warn the patient to avoid contact with people with respiratory infections. Encourage good oral hygiene to help prevent infection. Pneumococcal vaccination and annual influenza vaccinations are important preventive measures.

◆ To promote ventilation and reduce air trapping, teach the patient to breathe slowly, prolong expirations to two to three times the duration of inspiration, and to exhale through pursed lips.

◆ To help mobilize secretions, teach the patient how to cough effectively. If the patient with copious secretions has difficulty mobilizing secretions, teach his or her family how to perform postural drainage and chest physiotherapy. If secretions are thick, urge the patient to drink 12 to 15 glasses of fluid per day. A home humidifier may be beneficial, particularly in the winter.

◆ Administer low concentrations of oxygen as ordered. Perform blood gas analysis to determine the patient's oxygen needs and to avoid CO_2 narcosis. If the patient is to continue oxygen therapy at home, teach them how to use the equipment correctly. The patient with COPD rarely requires more than 2 to 3 L/minute to maintain adequate oxygenation. Higher flow rates will further increase the PaO_2, but the patient whose ventilatory drive is largely based on hypoxemia commonly develops markedly increased $PaCO_2$. In these cases, chemoreceptors in the brain are relatively insensitive to the increase in CO_2. Teach the patient and family that excessive oxygen therapy may eliminate the hypoxic respiratory drive, causing confusion and drowsiness, signs of CO_2 narcosis.

◆ Emphasize the importance of a balanced diet. Because the patient may tire easily when eating, suggest that they eat frequent, small meals and consider using oxygen, administered by nasal cannula, during meals.

◆ Help the patient and family adjust their lifestyles to accommodate the limitations imposed by this debilitating chronic disease. Instruct the patient to allow for daily rest periods and to exercise daily as the provider directs.

◆ As COPD progresses, encourage the patient to discuss their fears.

◆ To help prevent COPD, advise all patients, especially those with a family history of COPD or those in its early stages, not to smoke.

◆ Assist in the early detection of COPD by urging persons to have periodic physical examinations, including spirometry and medical evaluation of a chronic cough, and to seek treatment for recurring respiratory infections promptly.

◆ Lung volume reduction surgery is a new procedure for carefully selected patients with primarily emphysema. Nonfunctional parts of the lung (tissue filled with disease and providing little ventilation or perfusion) are surgically removed. Removal allows more functional lung tissue to expand and the diaphragm to return to its normally elevated position.

BRONCHIECTASIS

A condition marked by chronic abnormal dilation of bronchi and destruction of bronchial walls, bronchiectasis can occur throughout the tracheobronchial tree or can be confined to one segment or lobe. However, it's usually bilateral and involves the basilar segments of the lower lobes. This disease has three forms: cylindrical (fusiform), varicose, and saccular (cystic). Bronchiectasis is irreversible once established.

Causes and incidence

Because of the availability of antibiotics to treat acute respiratory tract infections, the incidence of bronchiectasis has dramatically decreased in the past 20 years. Incidence is highest among Eskimos and the Maoris of New Zealand. It affects people of both sexes and all ages.

The different forms of bronchiectasis may occur separately or simultaneously. In *cylindrical bronchiectasis*, the bronchi expand unevenly, with little change in diameter, and end suddenly in a squared-off fashion. In *varicose bronchiectasis*, abnormal, irregular dilation and narrowing of the bronchi give the appearance of varicose veins. In *saccular bronchiectasis*, many large dilations end in sacs. These sacs balloon into pus-filled cavities as they approach the periphery and are then called saccules. (See *Forms of bronchial dilatation*, page 134.)

This disease results from conditions associated with repeated damage to bronchial walls and abnormal mucociliary clearance, which cause a breakdown of supporting tissue adjacent to airways. Such conditions include:

◆ cystic fibrosis

◆ immunologic disorders (e.g., agammaglobulinemia)

◆ recurrent, inadequately treated bacterial respiratory tract infections, such as TB, and complications of measles, pneumonia, pertussis, or influenza

◆ obstruction (by a foreign body [most common in children], tumor, or stenosis) in association with recurrent infection

◆ inhalation of corrosive gas or repeated aspiration of gastric juices into the lungs

◆ congenital anomalies (uncommon), such as bronchomalacia, congenital bronchiectasis, immotile cilia syndrome, and Kartagener syndrome, a variant of immotile cilia syndrome characterized by situs inversus, bronchiectasis, and either nasal polyps or sinusitis

Pathophysiology

In bronchiectasis, hyperplastic squamous epithelium denuded of cilia replaces ulcerated columnar epithelium. Abscess formation involving all layers of the bronchial wall produces inflammatory cells and fibrous tissue, resulting in dilation and narrowing of the airways. Mucus plugs or fibrous tissue obliterates smaller bronchioles, whereas peribronchial lymphoid tissue becomes hyperplastic. Extensive vascular proliferation of bronchial circulation occurs and produces frequent hemoptysis.

Forms of bronchial dilatation

Dilatations of the air sacs occur because of bronchiectasis, as depicted below.

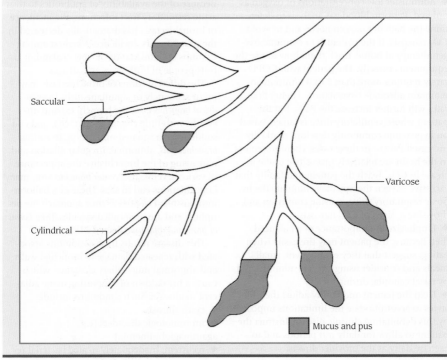

Complications
◆ Chronic malnutrition
◆ Amyloidosis
◆ Right ventricular failure
◆ Cor pulmonale

Signs and symptoms
Initially, bronchiectasis may be asymptomatic. When symptoms do arise, they're commonly attributed to other illnesses. The patient usually complains of frequent bouts of pneumonia or hemoptysis. The classic symptom, however, is a chronic cough that produces foul-smelling, mucopurulent secretions in amounts ranging from less than 10 mL/day to more than 150 mL/day.

Cough and sputum production are observed in greater than 90% of bronchiectasis patients. Characteristic findings include coarse crackles during inspiration over involved lobes or segments, occasional wheezing, dyspnea, sinusitis, weight loss, anemia, malaise, clubbing, recurrent fever, chills, and other signs of infection.

Advanced bronchiectasis may produce chronic malnutrition as well as right-sided heart failure and cor pulmonale because of hypoxic pulmonary vasoconstriction.

Diagnosis
A history of recurrent bronchial infections, pneumonia, and hemoptysis in a patient whose chest X-rays show peribronchial thickening, areas of atelectasis, and scattered cystic changes suggest bronchiectasis.

In recent years, CT scanning has supplanted bronchography as the most useful diagnostic test for bronchiectasis. It's sometimes used with high-resolution techniques to better determine anatomic changes. Bronchoscopy doesn't establish the diagnosis of bronchiectasis, but it does help to identify the source of secretions. Bronchoscopy can also be instrumental in pinpointing the site of bleeding in hemoptysis.

Other helpful laboratory tests include:
♦ sputum culture and Gram stain to identify predominant organisms
♦ complete blood count to detect anemia and leukocytosis
♦ PFTs to detect decreased vital capacity, expiratory flow rate, and hypoxemia. These tests also help determine the physiologic severity of the disease and the effects of therapy and help evaluate patients for surgery

When cystic fibrosis is suspected as the underlying cause of bronchiectasis, a sweat electrolyte test is useful.

Treatment

Treatment includes antibiotics, given orally or I.V., for 7 to 10 days or until sputum production decreases. Bronchodilators, combined with postural drainage and chest percussion, help remove secretions if the patient has bronchospasm and thick, tenacious sputum. Bronchoscopy may be used to remove obstruction and secretions. Hypoxia requires oxygen therapy; severe hemoptysis commonly requires lobectomy, segmental resection, or bronchial artery embolization if pulmonary function is poor. Long-term antibiotic therapy isn't appropriate because it may predispose the patient to serious gram-negative infections and resistant organisms.

Special considerations

♦ Provide supportive care and help the patient adjust to the permanent changes in lifestyle that irreversible lung damage necessitates. Thorough teaching is vital.
♦ Administer antibiotics as ordered and explain all diagnostic tests. Perform chest physiotherapy, including postural drainage and chest percussion designed for involved lobes, several times a day. The best times to do this are early morning and just before bedtime. Instruct the patient to maintain each position for 10 minutes, and then perform percussion and tell them to cough. Show family members how to perform postural drainage and percussion. Also teach the patient coughing and deep-breathing techniques to promote good ventilation and the removal of secretions.
♦ Advise the patient to stop smoking, if appropriate, to avoid stimulating secretions and irritating the airways. Refer them to a local self-help group.
♦ Provide a warm, quiet, comfortable environment, and urge the patient to rest as much as possible. Encourage balanced, high-protein meals to promote good health and tissue

healing and plenty of fluids (2 to 3 qt [2 to 3 L])/day to hydrate and thin bronchial secretions. Give frequent mouth care to remove foul-smelling sputum. Teach the patient to dispose of all secretions properly. Instruct them to seek prompt attention for respiratory infections.
♦ Tell the patient to avoid air pollutants and people with upper respiratory tract infections. Instruct them to take medications (especially antibiotics) exactly as prescribed.

▓▓▓▓▓ **PREVENTION**
♦ *Treat bacterial pneumonia vigorously.*
♦ *Stress the need for immunization to prevent childhood diseases.*

IDIOPATHIC PULMONARY FIBROSIS

Idiopathic pulmonary fibrosis (IPF) is a chronic and usually fatal interstitial pulmonary disease. About 50% of patients with IPF die within 5 years of diagnosis. Once thought to be a rare condition, it's now diagnosed with much greater frequency. IPF has been known by several other names over the years, including cryptogenic fibrosing alveolitis, diffuse interstitial fibrosis, idiopathic interstitial pneumonitis, and Hamman–Rich syndrome.

Causes and incidence

IPF is the result of a cascade of events that involve inflammatory, immune, and fibrotic processes in the lung. However, despite many studies and hypotheses, the stimulus that begins the progression remains unknown. Speculation has revolved around viral and genetic causes, but no good evidence has been found to support either theory. However, it's clear that chronic inflammation plays an important role. Inflammation develops the injury and the fibrosis that ultimately distorts and impairs the structure and function of the alveolocapillary gas exchange surface.

IPF is slightly more common in men than in women and is more common in smokers than in nonsmokers. It usually affects people 50 to 70 years old.

Pathophysiology

IPF pathophysiology is thought to be initiated when alveolar epithelial cells signal an injury and then activates the excessive formation of fibroblast migration and differentiation. Scarring to the lung structures occurs when the fibroblasts and myofibroblasts secrete large amounts of extracellular matrix proteins, such as collagens, decreasing the overall lung volume.

Complications
◆ Respiratory failure
◆ Pneumonia
◆ Hypoxemia
◆ Pneumothorax
◆ Pulmonary hypertension

Signs and symptoms
The usual presenting symptoms of IPF are dyspnea and a dry, hacking, and typically paroxysmal cough. Most patients have had these symptoms for several months to 2 years before seeking medical help. Expiratory crackles, especially in the bases of the lungs, are usually heard early in the disease. Bronchial breath sounds appear later, when airway consolidation develops. Rapid, shallow breathing occurs, especially with exertion, and clubbing has been noted in more than 40% of patients. Late in the disease, cyanosis and evidence of pulmonary hypertension (augmented S_2 and S_3 gallop) commonly occur. As the disease progresses, profound hypoxemia and severe, debilitating dyspnea are the hallmark signs.

Diagnosis
Diagnosis begins with a thorough patient history to exclude a more common cause of interstitial lung disease.

℞ CONFIRMING DIAGNOSIS *Lung biopsy is helpful in the diagnosis of IPF. In the past, an open lung biopsy was the only acceptable procedure, but now biopsies may be done through a thoracoscope or bronchoscope.*

Histologic features of the biopsy tissue vary, depending on the stage of the disease and other factors that aren't yet completely understood. The alveolar walls are swollen with chronic inflammatory cellular infiltrate composed of mononuclear cells and polymorphonuclear leukocytes. Intra-alveolar inflammatory cells may be found in early stages. As the disease progresses, excessive collagen and fibroblasts fill the interstitium. In advanced stages, alveolar walls are destroyed and are replaced by honeycombing cysts.

Chest X-rays may show one of four distinct patterns: interstitial, reticulonodular, ground-glass, or honeycomb. Although chest X-rays are helpful in identifying the presence of an abnormality, they don't correlate well with histologic findings or PFTs in determining the severity of the disease. They also don't help distinguish inflammation from fibrosis. However, serial X-rays may help track the progression of the disease.

High-resolution CT scans provide superior views of the four patterns seen on routine X-ray film and are used routinely to help establish the diagnosis of IPF. Research is currently underway to determine whether the four patterns of abnormality seen on these scans correlate with responsiveness to treatment.

PFTs show reductions in vital capacity and TLC and impaired diffusing capacity for carbon monoxide. ABG analysis and pulse oximetry reveal hypoxemia, which may be mild when the patient is at rest early in the disease but may become severe later in the disease. Oxygenation will always deteriorate, usually to a severe level, with exertion. Serial PFTs (especially carbon monoxide diffusing capacity) and ABG values may help track the course of the disease and the patient's response to treatment.

Treatment
Although it can't change the pathophysiology of IPF, oxygen therapy can prevent the problems related to dyspnea and tissue hypoxia in the early stages of the disease process. The patient may require little or no supplemental oxygen while at rest initially, but he or she will need more as the disease progresses and during exertion.

No known cure exists. Corticosteroids and cytotoxic drugs may be given to suppress inflammation but are usually unsuccessful. Recently, interferon gamma-1b has shown some promise in treating the disease.

Lung transplantation may be successful for younger, otherwise healthy individuals.

Special considerations
◆ Explain all diagnostic tests to the patient, who may experience anxiety and frustration about the many tests required to establish the diagnosis.
◆ Monitor oxygenation at rest and with exertion. The physician may prescribe one oxygen flow rate for use when the patient is at rest and a higher one for use during exertion to maintain adequate oxygenation. Instruct the patient to increase oxygen flow rate to the appropriate level for exercise.
◆ As IPF progresses, the patient's oxygen requirements will increase. They may need a nonrebreathing mask to supply high oxygen percentages. Eventually, maintaining adequate oxygenation may become impossible despite maximum oxygen flow.
◆ Most patients will need oxygen at home. Make appropriate referrals to discharge planners, respiratory care practitioners, and

home equipment vendors to ensure continuity of care.

◆ Teach breathing, relaxation, and energy conservation techniques to help the patient manage severe dyspnea.

◆ Encourage the patient to be as active as possible. Refer them to a pulmonary rehabilitation program.

◆ Monitor the patient for adverse reactions to drug therapy.

◆ Teach the patient about prescribed medications, especially adverse effects. Teach the patient and their family members infection prevention techniques.

◆ Encourage good nutritional habits. Small, frequent meals with high nutritional value may be necessary if dyspnea interferes with eating.

◆ Provide emotional support for the patient and their family as they deal with the patient's increasing disability, dyspnea, and probable death. Consult hospice as appropriate.

TUBERCULOSIS

An acute or chronic infection caused by *Mycobacterium tuberculosis*, TB is characterized by pulmonary infiltrates, formation of granulomas with caseation, fibrosis, and cavitation. (See *Understanding tuberculosis invasion*.) People who live in crowded, poorly ventilated conditions and those who are immunocompromised are most likely to become infected. In patients with strains that are sensitive to the usual antitubercular agents, the prognosis is excellent with correct treatment. However, in those with strains that are resistant to two or more of the major antitubercular agents, mortality is 50%.

Causes and incidence

After exposure to *M. tuberculosis*, roughly 5% of infected people develop active TB within 1 year; in the remainder, microorganisms cause a latent infection. The host's immune system usually

---

PATHOPHYSIOLOGY
Understanding tuberculosis invasion

After infected droplets are inhaled, they enter the lungs and are deposited either in the lower part of the upper lobe or in the upper part of the lower lobe. Leukocytes surround the droplets, which leads to inflammation. As part of the inflammatory response, some mycobacteria are carried off in the lymphatic circulation by the lymph nodes.

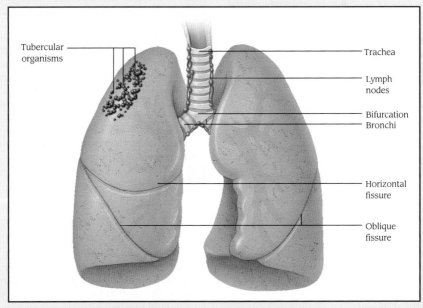

controls the tubercle bacillus by enclosing it in a tiny nodule (tubercle). The bacillus may lie dormant within the tubercle for years and later reactivate and spread.

Although the primary infection site is the lungs, mycobacteria commonly exist in other parts of the body. Several factors increase the risk of infection reactivation: gastrectomy, uncontrolled diabetes mellitus, Hodgkin lymphoma, leukemia, silicosis, acquired immunodeficiency syndrome, treatment with corticosteroids or immunosuppressants, and advanced age.

Cell-mediated immunity to the mycobacteria, which develops 3 to 6 weeks later, usually contains the infection and arrests the disease. If the infection reactivates, the body's response characteristically leads to caseation—the conversion of necrotic tissue to a cheese-like material. The caseum may localize, undergo fibrosis, or excavate and form cavities, the walls of which are studded with multiplying tubercle bacilli. If this happens, infected caseous debris may spread throughout the lungs by the tracheobronchial tree. Sites of extrapulmonary TB include the pleurae, meninges, joints, lymph nodes, peritoneum, genitourinary tract, and bowel.

The incidence of TB has been increasing in the United States secondary to homelessness, drug abuse, and human immunodeficiency virus infection. Globally, TB is the leading infectious cause of morbidity and mortality, generating 8 to 10 million new cases each year.

Pathophysiology

Transmission is by droplet nuclei produced when infected persons cough or sneeze. Persons with a cavitary lesion are particularly infectious because their sputum usually contains 1 to 100 million bacilli per milliliter. If an inhaled tubercle bacillus settles in an alveolus, infection occurs, with alveolocapillary dilation and endothelial cell swelling. Alveolitis results, with replication of tubercle bacilli and influx of polymorphonuclear leukocytes. These organisms spread through the lymph system to the circulatory system and then through the body.

Complications

◆ Respiratory failure
◆ Bronchopleural fistulas
◆ Pneumothorax
◆ Hemorrhage
◆ Pleural effusion
◆ Pneumonia

Signs and symptoms

After an incubation period of 4 to 8 weeks, TB is usually asymptomatic in primary infection but may produce nonspecific symptoms, such as fatigue, weakness, anorexia, weight loss, night sweats, and low-grade fever.

ELDER TIP *Fever and night sweats, the typical hallmarks of TB, may not be present in elderly patients, who instead may exhibit a change in activity or weight. Assess older patients carefully.*

In reactivation, symptoms may include a cough that produces mucopurulent sputum, occasional hemoptysis, and chest pains.

Diagnosis

CONFIRMING DIAGNOSIS *Diagnostic tests include chest X-rays, a tuberculin skin test, and sputum smears and cultures to identify M. tuberculosis. The diagnosis must be precise because several other diseases (such as lung cancer, lung abscess, pneumoconiosis, and bronchiectasis) may mimic TB.*

These procedures aid in diagnosis:
◆ Auscultation detects crepitant crackles, bronchial breath sounds, wheezing, and whispered pectoriloquy.
◆ Chest percussion detects dullness over the affected area, indicating consolidation or pleural fluid.
◆ Chest X-ray shows nodular lesions, patchy infiltrates (mainly in upper lobes), cavity formation, scar tissue, and calcium deposits; however, it may not be able to distinguish active from inactive TB.
◆ Tuberculin skin test detects TB infection. Intermediate-strength purified protein derivative or 5 tuberculin units (0.1 mL) are injected intracutaneously on the forearm. The test results are read in 48 to 72 hours; a positive reaction (induration of 5 to 15 mm or more, depending on risk factors) develops 2 to 10 weeks after infection in active and inactive TB. However, severely immunosuppressed patients may never develop a positive reaction.

CONFIRMING DIAGNOSIS *Stains and cultures (of sputum, cerebrospinal fluid, urine, drainage from abscess, or pleural fluid) show heat-sensitive, nonmotile, aerobic, acid-fast bacilli.*

Treatment

First-line agents for the treatment of TB are isoniazid (INH), rifampin (RIF), ethambutol (EMB), and pyrazinamide. Latent TB is usually treated with daily INH for 9 months. RIF daily for 4 months may be used for people with latent TB whose contacts are INH resistant. For most adults with active TB, the recommended dosing includes the administration of all four drugs daily for 2 months, followed by 4 months of INH and RIF. Drug therapy must be selected according to patient condition and organism susceptibility. Another first-line drug used for TB is rifapentine. Second-line agents, such as cycloserine, ethionamide, p-aminosalicylic acid, streptomycin, and capreomycin, are reserved for special circumstances or drug-resistant strains. Interruption of drug therapy may require initiation of therapy from the beginning of the regimen or additional treatment.

Directly observed therapy (DOT) may be selected or required. In this therapy, an assigned caregiver directly observes the administration of the drug. The goal of DOT is to monitor the treatment regimen and reduce the development of resistant organisms.

Special considerations

◆ Initiate AFB isolation precautions immediately for all patients suspected or confirmed to have TB. AFB isolation precautions include the use of a private room with negative pressure in relation to surrounding areas and a minimum of six air exchanges per hour (air should be exhausted directly to the outside).
◆ Continue AFB isolation until there's clinical evidence of reduced infectiousness

(substantially decreased cough, fewer organisms on sequential sputum smears).
◆ Teach the infectious patient to cough and sneeze into tissues and to dispose of all secretions properly. Place a covered trash can nearby or tape a lined bag to the side of the bed to dispose of used tissues.
◆ Instruct the patient to wear a mask when outside his or her room.
◆ Visitors and staff members should wear particulate respirators that fit closely around the face when they're in the patient's room.
◆ Remind the patient to get plenty of rest. Stress the importance of eating balanced meals to promote recovery. If the patient is anorexic, urge him or her to eat small meals frequently. Record weight weekly.
◆ Be alert for adverse effects of medications. Because INH sometimes leads to hepatitis or peripheral neuritis, monitor aspartate aminotransferase and alanine aminotransferase levels. To prevent or treat peripheral neuritis, give pyridoxine (vitamin B_6), as ordered. If the patient receives EMB, watch for optic neuritis; if it develops, discontinue the drug. If the patient receives RIF, watch for hepatitis and purpura. Observe the patient for other complications, such as hemoptysis.
◆ Before discharge, advise the patient to watch for adverse effects from the medication and

PREVENTION

Preventing tuberculosis

The best way to prevent tuberculosis (TB) is early detection to prevent it from becoming active. Hospitalized patients with TB should be isolated from other patients using airborne precautions. Staff members should also use disposable high-efficiency particulate air filter masks, which serve as adequate respiratory protection when caring for patients who are in airborne isolation.

Other ways to prevent the spread of TB include:
◆ If a patient has a weakened immune system or has human immunodeficiency virus, it is recommended that they receive annual TB testing. Annual testing is also recommended for healthcare workers, those who work in a prison or a long-term care facility, and those with a substantially increased risk of exposure to the disease.
◆ If a patient tests positive for latent TB infection but has no evidence of active TB, he or she may be able to reduce the risk of developing active TB by taking a course of therapy with isoniazid.

To prevent the spread of disease from those with active TB or from those who are receiving treatment, the following recommendations should be followed:
◆ Stress the need to maintain the treatment regimen and to not stop or skip doses. When the treatment regimen is stopped, the TB bacteria can mutate and become drug resistant.
◆ The patient who is on a treatment regimen is still contagious until he or she has been taking the medications for 2 to 3 weeks. Encouraging the patient to stay indoors and home from school or work is recommended. If the patient must leave home, a mask is recommended during this initial treatment time to lessen the risk of transmission.

report them immediately. Emphasize the importance of regular follow-up examinations. Instruct the patient and family concerning the signs and symptoms of recurring TB. Stress the need to follow long-term treatment faithfully.

◆ Emphasize to the patient the importance of taking the medications daily as prescribed. The patient may enroll in a supervised administration program to avoid the development of drug-resistant organisms. (See *Preventing tuberculosis*, page 139.)

Pneumoconioses

SILICOSIS

Silicosis is a progressive disease characterized by nodular lesions that commonly progress to fibrosis. The most common form of pneumoconiosis, silicosis can be classified according to the severity of pulmonary disease and the rapidity of its onset and progression. It usually occurs as a simple asymptomatic illness.

Acute silicosis develops after 1 to 3 years in workers exposed to very high concentrations of respirable silica (sand blasters and tunnel workers). *Accelerated silicosis* appears after an average of 10 years of exposure to lower concentrations of free silica. *Chronic silicosis* develops after 20 or more years of exposure to lower concentrations of free silica. (Chronic silicosis is further subdivided into simple and complicated forms.)

The prognosis is good unless the disease progresses into the complicated fibrotic form, which causes respiratory insufficiency and cor pulmonale. It's also associated with pulmonary TB.

Causes and incidence

Silicosis results from the inhalation and pulmonary deposition of respirable crystalline silica dust, mostly from quartz. The danger to the worker depends on the concentration of dust in the atmosphere, the percentage of respirable free silica particles in the dust, and the duration of exposure. Respirable particles are less than 10 μm in diameter, but the disease-causing particles deposited in the alveolar space are usually 1 to 3 μm in diameter.

Industrial sources of silica in its pure form include the manufacture of ceramics (flint) and building materials (sandstone). It occurs in mixed form in the production of construction materials (cement). It's found in powder form (silica flour) in paints, porcelain, scouring soaps, and wood fillers as well as in the mining of gold, coal, lead, zinc, and iron. Foundry workers, boiler scalers, and stonecutters are all exposed to silica dust and, therefore, are at high risk for developing silicosis.

The incidence of silicosis has decreased since the Occupational Safety and Health Administration instituted regulations requiring the use of protective equipment that limits the amount of silica dust inhaled.

Pathophysiology

Nodules result when alveolar macrophages ingest silica particles, which they're unable to process. As a result, the macrophages die and release proteolytic enzymes into the surrounding tissue. The subsequent inflammation attracts other macrophages and fibroblasts into the region to produce fibrous tissue and wall off the reaction. The resulting nodule has an onionskin appearance when viewed under a microscope. Nodules develop adjacent to terminal and respiratory bronchioles, concentrate in the upper lobes, and are commonly accompanied by bullous changes in both lobes. If the disease process doesn't progress, minimal physiologic disturbances and no disability occur. Occasionally, however, the fibrotic response accelerates, engulfing and destroying large areas of the lung (progressive massive fibrosis or conglomerate lesions). Fibrosis may continue even after exposure to dust has ended.

Complications

◆ Pulmonary fibrosis
◆ Cor pulmonale
◆ Ventricular or respiratory failure
◆ Pulmonary TB

Signs and symptoms

Initially, silicosis may be asymptomatic or may produce dyspnea on exertion, usually attributed to being "out of shape" or "slowing down." If the disease progresses to the chronic and complicated stage, dyspnea on exertion worsens, and other symptoms—usually tachypnea and an insidious dry cough that's most pronounced in the morning—appear.

Progression to the advanced stage causes dyspnea on minimal exertion, worsening cough, and pulmonary hypertension, which in turn leads to right-sided heart failure and cor pulmonale. Patients with silicosis have a high incidence of active TB, which should be considered when evaluating patients with this disease. CNS changes—confusion, lethargy, and a decrease in the rate and depth of respiration as the $PaCO_2$ increases—also occur in advanced silicosis.

Other clinical features include malaise, disturbed sleep, and hoarseness. The severity of these symptoms may not correlate with chest X-ray findings or the results of PFTs.

Diagnosis

The patient history reveals occupational exposure to silica dust. The physical examination is normal in simple silicosis; in chronic silicosis with conglomerate lesions, it may reveal decreased chest expansion, diminished intensity of breath sounds, areas of hyporesonance and hyperresonance, fine to medium crackles, and tachypnea.

In simple silicosis, chest X-rays show small, discrete, nodular lesions distributed throughout both lung fields but typically concentrated in the upper lung zones; the hilar lung nodes may be enlarged and exhibit "eggshell" calcification. In complicated silicosis, X-rays show one or more conglomerate masses of dense tissue.

PFTs show:

◆ FVC—reduced in complicated silicosis

◆ FEV_1—reduced in obstructive disease (emphysematous areas of silicosis); reduced in complicated silicosis, but ratio of FEV_1 to FVC is normal or high

◆ Maximal voluntary ventilation—reduced in restrictive and obstructive diseases

◆ CO_2 diffusing capacity—reduced when fibrosis destroys alveolar walls and obliterates pulmonary capillaries or when fibrosis thickens the alveolocapillary membrane

Treatment

The goal of treatment is to relieve respiratory symptoms, to manage hypoxemia and cor pulmonale, and to prevent respiratory tract irritation and infections. Treatment also includes careful observation for the development of TB. Respiratory symptoms may be relieved through daily use of inhaled bronchodilators and increased fluid intake (at least 3 qt [3 L] daily). Steam inhalation and chest physiotherapy techniques, such as controlled coughing and segmental bronchial drainage with chest percussion and vibration, help clear secretions. In severe cases, it may be necessary to administer oxygen by cannula or mask (1 to 2 L/minute) for the patient with chronic hypoxemia or by mechanical ventilation if arterial oxygen can't be maintained above 40 mm Hg. Respiratory infections require prompt administration of antibiotics.

Special considerations

◆ Teach the patient to prevent infections by avoiding crowds and persons with respiratory infections and by receiving influenza and pneumococcal vaccines.

◆ Increase exercise tolerance by encouraging regular activity. Advise the patient to plan his or her daily activities to decrease the work of breathing. The patient should be instructed to pace himself or herself, rest often, and generally move slowly through his or her daily routine.

ASBESTOSIS

Asbestosis is a form of pneumoconiosis characterized by diffuse interstitial fibrosis. It can develop as long as 15 to 20 years after regular exposure to asbestos has ended. Asbestos also causes pleural plaques and mesotheliomas of pleura and the peritoneum. A potent co-carcinogen, asbestos increases the risk of lung cancer in cigarette smokers.

Causes and incidence

Asbestosis results from the inhalation of respirable asbestos fibers (50 μm or more in length and 0.5 μm or less in diameter), which assume a longitudinal orientation in the airway and move in the direction of airflow. The fibers penetrate respiratory bronchioles and alveolar walls. Sources include the mining and milling of asbestos, the construction industry, and the fireproofing and textile industries. Asbestos was also used in the production of paints, plastics, and brake and clutch linings.

Asbestos-related diseases develop in families of asbestos workers as a result of exposure to fibrous dust shaken off workers' clothing at home. Such diseases develop in the general public as a result of exposure to fibrous dust or waste piles from nearby asbestos plants, but exposures for occupants of typical buildings are quite low and not in a range associated with asbestosis.

Inhaled fibers become encased in a brown, protein-like sheath rich in iron (ferruginous bodies or asbestos bodies), found in sputum and lung tissue. Interstitial fibrosis develops in lower lung zones, causing obliterative changes in lung parenchyma and pleurae. Raised hyaline plaques may form in parietal pleura, diaphragm, and pleura contiguous with the pericardium.

Asbestosis occurs in 4 of every 10,000 people.

Pathophysiology

Asbestos fibers penetrate the pleura tissues and are phagocytosed permanently within the lungs. This sets up cycles of cellular events and the release of cytokines. The initial irritation occurs in the alveoli and initiates a surge of asbestos-activated macrophages. These specified macrophages then produce multiple varieties of growth factors that interact to produce fibroblast proliferation.

Complications

◆ Pulmonary fibrosis
◆ Respiratory failure
◆ Pulmonary hypertension
◆ Cor pulmonale

A close look at asbestosis

After years of exposure to asbestos, healthy lung tissue progresses from simple asbestosis to massive pulmonary fibrosis, as shown below.

Simple asbestosis

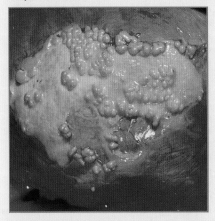

Progressive massive pulmonary fibrosis

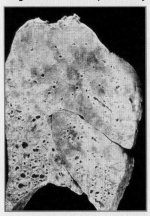

Signs and symptoms

Clinical features may appear before chest X-ray changes. The first symptom is usually dyspnea on exertion, typically after 10 years' exposure. As fibrosis extends, dyspnea on exertion increases until, eventually, dyspnea occurs even at rest. Advanced disease also causes a dry cough (may be productive in smokers), chest pain (commonly pleuritic), recurrent respiratory infections, and tachypnea. (See *A close look at asbestosis*.)

Cardiovascular complications include pulmonary hypertension, right ventricular hypertrophy, and cor pulmonale. Finger clubbing commonly occurs.

Diagnosis

The patient history reveals occupational, family, or neighborhood exposure to asbestos fibers. Physical examination reveals characteristic dry crackles at lung bases. Chest X-rays show fine, irregular, and linear diffuse infiltrates; extensive fibrosis results in a "honeycomb" or "ground-glass" appearance. X-rays may also show pleural thickening and calcification, with bilateral obliteration of costophrenic angles. In later stages, an enlarged heart with a classic "shaggy" heart border may be evident. CT scan of the lungs also aids in diagnosis.

PFTs show:
◆ Vital capacity, FVC, and TLC—decreased
◆ FEV_1—decreased or normal

◆ Carbon monoxide diffusing capacity—reduced when fibrosis destroys alveolar walls and thickens alveolocapillary membranes
ABG analysis reveals:
◆ PaO_2—decreased
◆ $PaCO_2$—low due to hyperventilation

Treatment

The goal of treatment is to relieve respiratory symptoms and, in advanced disease, manage hypoxemia and cor pulmonale. Respiratory symptoms may be relieved by chest physiotherapy techniques, such as controlled coughing and segmental bronchial drainage, chest percussion, and vibration. Aerosol therapy, inhaled mucolytics, and increased fluid intake (at least 3 qt [3 L] daily) may also relieve symptoms.

Diuretics, cardiac glycosides, and salt restriction may be indicated for patients with cor pulmonale. Hypoxemia requires oxygen administration by cannula or mask (1 to 2 L/minute) or by mechanical ventilation if arterial oxygen can't be maintained above 40 mm Hg. Respiratory infections require prompt administration of antibiotics.

Special considerations

◆ Teach the patient to prevent infections by avoiding crowds and persons with infections and by receiving influenza and pneumococcal vaccines.
◆ Improve the patient's ventilatory efficiency by encouraging physical reconditioning, energy conservation in daily activities, and relaxation techniques.

COAL WORKER'S PNEUMOCONIOSIS

A progressive nodular pulmonary disease, coal worker's pneumoconiosis (CWP) occurs in two forms. Simple CWP is characterized by small lung opacities; in complicated CWP, also known as *progressive massive fibrosis*, masses of fibrous tissue occasionally develop in the patient's lungs. The risk of developing CWP (also known as *black lung disease, coal miner's disease, miner's asthma, anthracosis*, and *anthracosilicosis*) depends on the duration of exposure to coal dust (usually 15 years or longer), intensity of exposure (dust count and particle size), location of the mine, silica content of the coal (anthracite coal has the highest silica content), and the worker's susceptibility.

The prognosis varies. Simple asymptomatic disease is self-limiting, although progression to complicated CWP is more likely if CWP begins after a relatively short period of exposure. Complicated CWP may be disabling, resulting in severe ventilatory failure and cor pulmonale.

Causes and incidence

CWP is caused by the inhalation and prolonged retention of respirable coal dust particles (less than 5 μm in diameter). Simple CWP results in the formation of macules (accumulations of macrophages laden with coal dust) around the terminal and respiratory bronchioles, surrounded by a halo of dilated alveoli. Macule formation leads to atrophy of supporting tissue, causing permanent dilation of small airways (focal emphysema).

Simple disease may progress to complicated CWP, involving one or both lungs. In this form of the disease, fibrous tissue masses enlarge and coalesce, causing gross distortion of pulmonary structures (destruction of vasculature alveoli and airways).

The incidence of CWP is highest among anthracite coal miners in the eastern United States.

Pathophysiology

When coal dust particles are inhaled into the lung bronchioles, the carbon is phagocytosed and transported by macrophages and microciliary into the mucus. An immune response is triggered as the coal-filled macrophages accumulate in the alveoli. Reticulin is secreted from the fibroblasts which then entrap the macrophages and become strangulated from the resultant interstitial fibrosis.

Complications

◆ Pulmonary hypertension
◆ Pulmonary TB
◆ Cor pulmonale

Signs and symptoms

Simple CWP produces no symptoms, especially in nonsmokers. Symptoms of complicated CWP include exertional dyspnea and a cough that occasionally produces inky-black sputum (when fibrotic changes undergo avascular necrosis and their centers cavitate). Other clinical features of CWP include increasing dyspnea and a cough that produces milky, gray, clear, or coal-flecked sputum. Recurrent bronchial and pulmonary infections produce yellow, green, or thick sputum.

Complications include pulmonary hypertension, right ventricular hypertrophy, cor pulmonale, and pulmonary TB. In cigarette smokers, chronic bronchitis and emphysema may also complicate the disease.

Diagnosis

The patient history reveals exposure to coal dust. Physical examination shows barrel chest, hyperresonant lungs with areas of dullness, diminished breath sounds, crackles, rhonchi, and wheezes. In *simple CWP*, chest X-rays show small opacities (less than 10 mm in diameter). These may be present in all lung zones but are more prominent in the upper lung zones. In *complicated CWP*, one or more large opacities (1 to 5 cm in diameter), possibly exhibiting cavitation, are seen.

PFTs show:
◆ Vital capacity—normal in simple CWP but decreased with complicated CWP
◆ FEV_1—decreased in complicated disease
◆ Residual volume and TLC—normal in simple CWP; decreased in complicated CWP
◆ Carbon monoxide diffusing capacity—significantly decreased in complicated CWP as alveolar septae are destroyed and pulmonary capillaries obliterated
◆ $PaCO_2$—may be increased with concomitant COPD

Treatment

There's no specific treatment. The goal of treatment is to relieve respiratory symptoms, manage hypoxia and cor pulmonale, and avoid respiratory tract irritants and infections. Treatment also includes careful observation for the development of TB. Chest physiotherapy techniques, such as controlled coughing and segmental bronchial drainage combined with chest percussion and vibration, help remove secretions.

Other measures include increased fluid intake (at least 3 qt [3 L] daily) and respiratory therapy techniques, such as aerosol therapy, inhaled mucolytics, and intermittent positive-pressure breathing. Diuretics, cardiac glycosides, and salt restriction may be indicated in cor pulmonale. In severe cases, it may be necessary to administer oxygen for hypoxemia by cannula or mask (1 to 2 L/minute) if the patient has chronic hypoxia; mechanical ventilation is utilized if PaO_2 can't be maintained above 40 mm Hg. Respiratory infections require prompt administration of antibiotics.

Special considerations

◆ Teach the patient to prevent infections by avoiding crowds and persons with respiratory infections and by receiving pneumococcal vaccine polyvalent and annual influenza vaccines.
◆ Encourage the patient to stay active to avoid a deterioration in his or her physical condition but to pace activities and practice relaxation techniques.

SELECTED REFERENCES

Al-Dabbagh, M., et al. (2011). Drug-resistant tuberculosis: Pediatric guidelines. *Pediatric Infectious Disease Journal*, 30(6), 501–505.

Arakawa, H., et al. (2016). Asbestosis and other pulmonary fibrosis in asbestos-exposed workers: High-resolution CT features with pathological correlations. *European Radiology*, 26, 1485–1492. doi:10.1007/s00330-015-3973-z

Bhattacharya, S., et al. (2016, May–August). Silicosis in the form of progressive massive fibrosis: A diagnostic challenge. *Indian Journal of Occupational and Environmental Medicine*, 20(2), 114–117. doi:10.4103/0019-5278.197548

Butt, Y., et al. (2016, April). Acute lung injury a clinical and molecular review. *Archives of Pathophysiology and Laboratory Medicine*, 140, 345–350.

Criner, R. N., & Han, M. K. (2018, May). COPD care in the 21st century: A public health priority. *Respiratory Care*, 63(5), 591–600. doi:10.4187/respcare.06276

Cruz, A. T., & Stark, J. R. (2018, February). Completion rate and safety of Tuberculosis infection treatment with shorter regimens. *Pediatrics*, 141(2), 1–9. doi:10.1542/peds.2017-2838

Dodia, B. K., et al. (2015, April–June). Role of chest physiotherapy in resolving post operative massive atelectasis. *Indian Journal of Physiotherapy and Occupational Therapy*, 9(2), 40–42. doi:10.5958/0973-5674.2015.00050.7

Faisy, C., et al. (2016). Effect of acetazolamide vs placebo on duration of invasive mechanical ventilation among patients with chronic obstructive pulmonary disease. *Journal of the American Medical Association*, 315(5), 480–488. doi:10.1001/jama.2016.0019

Garrison, L. E., et al. (2016). Vital signs: Deficiencies in environmental control identified in outbreaks of Legionnaires' Disease—North America, 2000–2014. *MMWR: Morbidity and Mortality Weekly Report*, 65(22), 576–584. doi:10.15585/mmwr.mm6522e1

Grazel, R., et al. (2010). Implementation of the American Academy of Pediatrics Recommendations to reduce sudden infant death syndrome risk in neonatal intensive care units: An evaluation of nursing knowledge and practice. *Advances in Neonatal Care*, 10(6), 332–342.

Guerin, C., & Matthay, M. A. (2016). Acute cor pulmonale and the acute respiratory distress syndrome. *Intensive Care Medicine*, 42, 934–936. doi:10.1007/s00134-015-4197-z

Hauk, L. (2017). SIDS and safe sleeping environments for infants: AAP updates recommendations. *American Family Physician*, 95(12), 806–807.

Havermans, T., et al. (2011). Siblings of children with cystic fibrosis: Quality of life and the impact of illness. *Child: Care, Health and Development*, 37(2), 252–260.

Herchline, T. E. (2017). *Tuberculosis*. Retrieved from https://emedicine.medscape.com/article/230802-overview#a4

Janda, S., et al. (2011). Diagnostic accuracy of echocardiography for pulmonary hypertension: A systematic review and meta-analysis. *Heart*, 97(8), 612–622.

Jeffries, M., et al. (2017, May–June). Evidence to support the use of occlusive dry sterile dressings for chest tubes. *MEDSURG Nursing*, 26(3), 171–174.

Johnson, D. W. (2016, September 16). Croup. *American Family Physician*, 94(6), 476–478.

Jung, I. Y., et al. (2015). A case of bronchiolitis obliterans organizing pneumonia in an HIV-infected Korean patient successfully treated with clarithromycin. *BMC Infectious Disease*, 15(280), 1–4. doi:10.1186/s12879-015-1025-6

Kak, C. C., et al. (2016). Safety of indwelling pleural catheter use in patients undergoing chemotherapy: A five-year retrospective evaluation. *BMC Pulmonary Medicine*, 16(41), 1–7. doi:10.1186/s12890-016-0203-7

Kamanger, N. (2018). *Lung abscess*. Retrieved from https://emedicine.medscape.com/article/299425-overview#a5

Kaufman, J. S. (2017, June). Acute exacerbation of COPD: Diagnosis and management. *The Nurse Practitioner*, 42(6), 1–7. doi:10.1097/01.NPR.0000515997.35046.b8

Khan, F. J. (2015). *Coal worker's pneumoconiosis*. Retrieved from https://emedicine.medscape.com/article/297887-overview

Kim, J. J., et al. (2015). Life-threatening hemothorax due to the inferior pulmonary ligament injury without obvious organ injuries: A case report. *Journal of Cardiothoracic Surgery*, 10(35), 1–3. doi:10.1186/s13019-015-0243-8

Kjaerulff, A. M., et al. (2018). Clinical evaluation of intravenous ampicillin as empirical antimicrobial treatment of acute epiglottitis. *Acta Oto-Laryngologica*, 138(1), 60–65. doi:10.1080/00016489.2017.1363912

Kong, V. Y., et al. (2015). Open pneumothorax: The spectrum and outcome of management based on advanced trauma life support recommendations. *European Journal of Trauma and Emergency Surgery*, 41(4), 401–404. doi:10.1007/s00068-014-0469-5

Li, H., et al. (2018). A simplified ultrasound comet tail grading scoring to assess pulmonary congestion in patients with heart failure. *BioMed Research International*, 1–10. doi:10.1155/2018/8474839

Locci, G., et al. (2014). Hyaline membrane disease (HMD): The role of the perinatal pathologist. *The Journal of Pediatric of Neonatal Individualized Medicine*, 3(2), 1–9. doi:10.7363/030255

Madappa, T. (2017). *Atelectasis*. Retrieved from https://emedicine.medscape.com/article/296468-overview

Madhani, K., et al. (2016, July–September). A 10-year retrospective review of pediatric lung abscesses from a single center. *Annals of Thoracic Medicine*, 11(3), 191–196. doi:10.4103/1817-1737.185763

Mancini, M. C. (2017). *Hemothorax*. Retrieved from https://emedicine.medscape.com/article/2047916-overview

Masa, J. F., et al. (2016). Noninvasive ventilation for severely acidotic patients in respiratory intermediate care units. *BMC Pulmonary Medicine*, 16(97), 1–13. doi:10.1186/s12890-016-0262-9

Mazurek, J. M., et al. (2017, July 21). Surveillance for silicosis deaths among persons aged 15–44 years—United States, 1999–2015. *Morbidity and Mortality Weekly Report*, 66(28), 747–752.

Mennella, H., & Schub, T. (2017, November 17). Severe acute respiratory syndrome (SARS). *CINAHL Nursing Guide*.

Mosenifar, Z. (2017). *Chronic obstructive pulmonary disease (COPD)*. Retrieved from https://emedicine.medscape.com/article/297664-overview

National Heart, Lung, and Blood Institute. *Guidelines for diagnosis and treatment of asthma (EPR-3)*. Retrieved from http://www.nhlbi.nih.gov/guidelines/asthma/index.htm

Ozdemir, L., & Ozdemir, B. (2018). A prospective review of the results of patients treated and followed up for a diagnosis of sarcoidosis. *Turkish Thoracic Journal, 19*, 1–6. doi:10.5152/TurkThoracJ.2017.17028

Pleural effusion. (2017). *Mayo Clinic Health Letter, 35*(1), 1–5.

Rajpurohit, V., et al. (2017). Metatarsal fracture leading to massive pulmonary embolism. *Indian Journal of Critical Care Medicine, 21*(6), 67–69. doi:10.4103/ijccm. IJCCM_125_17

Ramsey, C., et al. (2011). H1N1: Viral pneumonia as a cause of acute respiratory distress syndrome. *Current Opinion in Critical Care, 17*(1), 64–71.

Singh, I., et al. (2016, April). Pathophysiology of pulmonary hypertension in chronic parenchymal lung disease. *American Journal of Medicine, 129*(4), 366–371. doi:10.1016/j.amjmed.2015.11.026

Subira, C., et al. (2018, April). Minimizing asynchronies in mechanical ventilation: Current and future trends. *Respiratory Care, 63*(4), 464–478. doi:10.4187/respcare.05949

Tambascio, J., et al. (2017, August). Effects of an airway clearance device on inflammation, bacteriology, and mucus transport in bronchiectasis. *Respiratory Care, 62*(8), 1067–1074. doi:10.4187/respcare.05214

Tolentino-Delos Reyes, A., et al. (2007). Evidence-based practice: Use of the ventilator bundle to prevent ventilator-associated pneumonia. *American Journal of Critical Care, 16*(1), 20–27.

Udeani, J. (2016). *Pediatric epiglottitis*. Retrieved from https://emedicine.medscape.com/article/963773-overview

Varkey, B. (2015). *Asbestosis*. Retrieved from https://emedicine.medscape.com/article/295966-overview

Vega-Olivo, M., & Criner, G. J. (2018, May). Idiopathic pulmonary fibrosis: A guide for nurse practitioners. *The Nurse Practitioner, 43*(5), 48–54. doi:10.1097/01 .NPR.0000531121.07294.36

Zheng, Y., et al. (2017). Cross-section analysis of coal workers' pneumoconiosis and higher brachial-ankle pulse wave velocity within Kailuan study. *BMC Public Health, 17*(148), 1–8. doi:10.1186/s12889-017-4048-7

3

NEUROLOGIC DISORDERS

Introduction

The neurologic system, the body's communications network, coordinates and organizes the functions of all body systems. This intricate network has three main divisions:

◆ *central nervous system (CNS):* the control center, made up of the brain, the brainstem, and the spinal cord

◆ *peripheral nervous system:* motor and sensory nerves that connect the CNS to remote body parts and relay and receive messages from them

◆ *autonomic nervous system (part of the peripheral nervous system):* regulates involuntary functioning of the internal organs and vascular system.

FUNDAMENTAL UNIT

The fundamental unit of the nervous system is the neuron, a highly specialized conductor cell that receives and transmits electrochemical nerve impulses. Its structure contains delicate, thread-like nerve fibers that extend from the central cell body and transmit signals: *axons,* which carry impulses *away* from the cell body, and *dendrites,* which carry impulses *to* it. Most neurons have multiple dendrites but only one axon. *Sensory (afferent) neurons* transmit impulses from special receptors to the spinal cord or the brain, *motor (efferent) neurons* transmit impulses from the CNS to regulate activity of muscles or glands, and *interneurons (connecting or association neurons)* shuttle signals through complex pathways between sensory and motor neurons. Interneurons account for 99% of all the neurons in the nervous system and include most of the neurons in the brain. (See *Parts of a neuron,* page 147.)

INTRICATE CONTROL SYSTEM

This intricate network of interlocking receptors and transmitters forms, together with the brain and spinal cord, a dynamic control system—a living computer—that controls and regulates every mental and physical function. From birth to death, this astonishing system efficiently organizes the body's affairs—controlling the smallest action, thought, or feeling; monitoring communication and instinct for survival; and allowing introspection, wonder, abstract thought, and awareness of one's own intelligence. The brain, the primary center of the CNS, is the large soft mass of nervous tissue housed in the cranium and protected and supported by the meninges and skull bones.

The fragile brain, brainstem, and spinal cord are protected by bone (the skull and vertebrae), cushioning *cerebrospinal fluid (CSF),* and three protective membranes, called *meninges:*

◆ The *dura mater,* or outer sheath, is made of tough white fibrous tissue.

◆ The *arachnoid membrane,* the middle layer, is delicate and lacelike.

◆ The *pia mater,* the inner meningeal layer, is made of fine blood vessels held together by connective tissue. It's thin and transparent and clings to the brain and spinal cord surfaces, carrying branches of the cerebral arteries deep into the brain's fissures and sulci.

Between the dura mater and the arachnoid membrane is the *subdural space;* between the pia mater and the arachnoid membrane is the *subarachnoid space.* The subarachnoid space and the brain's four ventricles contain *CSF,* a clear

Parts of a neuron

A typical neuron, like the one shown here, has one axon and many dendrites. A myelin sheath encloses the axon.

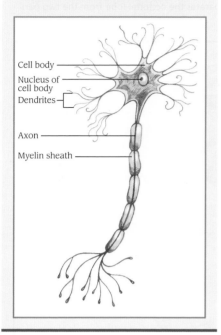

Cell body

Nucleus of cell body

Dendrites

Axon

Myelin sheath

---

the brain through the pyramidal tract cross in the medulla, the right hemisphere controls the left side of the body and the left hemisphere, the right side of the body. Several fissures divide the cerebrum into lobes, each of which is associated with specific functions. (See *A look at the lobes*, page 148.)

The *thalamus*, a relay center below the corpus callosum, further organizes cerebral function by transmitting impulses to and from appropriate areas of the cerebrum. In addition to its primary relay function, it's responsible for primitive emotional responses, such as fear, and for distinguishing pleasant stimuli from unpleasant ones.

The *hypothalamus*, which lies beneath the thalamus, is an autonomic center that has connections with the brain, spinal cord, autonomic nervous system, and pituitary gland. It regulates temperature control, appetite, blood pressure, breathing, sleep patterns, and peripheral nerve discharges that occur with behavioral and emotional expression. It also has partial control of pituitary gland secretion and stress reaction.

THE BASE OF THE BRAIN

Beneath the cerebrum, at the base of the brain, is the *cerebellum*. It's responsible for smooth muscle movements, coordinating sensory impulses with muscle activity, and maintaining muscle tone and equilibrium.

The brainstem houses cell bodies for most of the cranial nerves and includes the *midbrain*, the *pons*, and the *medulla oblongata*. With the thalamus and the hypothalamus, it makes up a nerve network called the *reticular formation*, which acts as an arousal mechanism and controls wakefulness. It also relays nerve impulses between the spinal cord and other parts of the brain. The midbrain is the reflex center for the third and fourth cranial nerves and mediates pupillary reflexes and eye movements. The pons helps regulate respirations; it's also the reflex center for the fifth through eighth cranial nerves and mediates chewing, taste, saliva secretion, hearing, and equilibrium. The medulla oblongata affects cardiac, respiratory, and vasomotor functions.

BLOODLINE TO THE BRAIN

Four major arteries—two vertebral and two carotid—supply the brain with oxygenated blood. These arteries originate in or near the aortic arch. The two vertebral arteries (branches of the subclavian) converge to become the basilar artery, which supplies the posterior brain. The common carotids branch into the two internal

---

liquid containing water and traces of organic materials (especially protein), glucose, and minerals.

CSF is formed from blood in capillary networks called *choroid plexus*, which are located primarily in the brain's lateral ventricles. This fluid is eventually reabsorbed into the venous blood through the *arachnoid villi*, in dural sinuses on the brain's surface.

The *cerebrum*, the largest portion of the brain, is the nerve center that controls sensory and motor activities and intelligence. The outer layer of the cerebrum, the *cerebral cortex*, consists of neuron cell bodies (*gray matter*); the inner layers consist of axons (*white matter*) and basal ganglia, which control motor coordination and steadiness. The cerebral surface is deeply convoluted, furrowed with elevations (*gyri*) and depressions (*sulci*). A *longitudinal fissure* divides the cerebrum into two hemispheres connected by a wide band of nerve fibers called the *corpus callosum*, through which the hemispheres share information. The hemispheres don't share equally; one always dominates, giving one side control over the other. Because motor impulses descending from

A look at the lobes

Several fissures divide the cerebrum into hemispheres and lobes; each lobe has a specific function. The *fissure of Sylvius* (lateral sulcus) separates the temporal lobe from the frontal and parietal lobes. The *fissure of Rolando* (central sulcus) separates the frontal lobes from the parietal lobe. The *parieto-occipital fissure* separates the occipital lobe from the two parietal lobes.

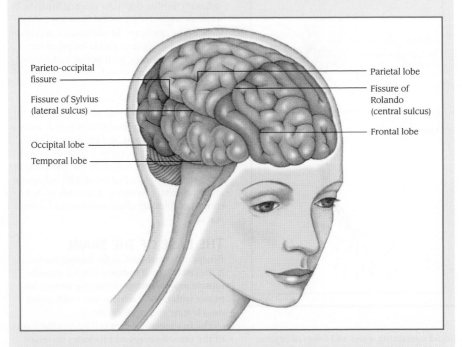

♦ The *frontal lobe* controls voluntary muscle movements and contains motor areas (including the motor area for speech, or Broca area). It's the center for personality, behavioral, and intellectual functions, such as judgment, memory, and problem solving; for autonomic functions; and for cardiac and emotional responses.
♦ The *temporal lobe* is the center for taste, hearing, and smell; in the brain's dominant hemisphere, it interprets spoken language.
♦ The *parietal lobe* coordinates and interprets sensory information from the opposite side of the body.
♦ The *occipital lobe* interprets visual stimuli.

carotids, which divide further to supply the anterior brain and the middle brain. These arteries interconnect through the *circle of Willis*, at the base of the brain. This anastomosis usually ensures continual circulation to the brain.

THE SPINAL CORD: CONDUCTOR PATHWAY

Extending downward from the brain through the vertebrae, to the level of approximately the second lumbar vertebra, is the spinal cord, a two-way conductor pathway between the brainstem and the peripheral nervous system. The spinal cord is also the reflex center for activities that don't require brain control, such as deep tendon reflexes, the jerking reaction elicited by tapping with a reflex hammer.

A cross section of the spinal cord shows an internal H-shaped mass of gray matter divided into horns, which consist primarily of neuron cell bodies. (See *Cross section of the spinal cord,* page 149.) Cell bodies in the posterior, or dorsal, horn primarily relay sensations; those in the anterior, or ventral, horn are needed for voluntary or reflex motor activity. The white matter surrounding the outer part of these horns consists of myelinated nerve fibers grouped functionally in vertical columns, called *tracts*. The sensory, or ascending, tracts carry sensory impulses up the spinal cord to the brain; the motor, or descending, tracts carry motor impulses down the spinal cord. The brain's motor impulses reach a descending tract and continue through the peripheral nervous system via upper motor neurons. These neurons originate in the brain and form two major systems:

◆ The *pyramidal system* (corticospinal tract) is responsible for fine, skilled movements of skeletal muscle. An impulse in this system originates in the frontal lobe's motor cortex and travels downward to the pyramids of the medulla, where it crosses to the opposite side of the spinal cord.

◆ The *extrapyramidal system* (extracorticospinal tract) controls gross motor movements. An impulse traveling in this system originates in the frontal lobe's motor cortex and is mediated by basal ganglia, the thalamus, cerebellum, and reticular formation before descending to the spinal cord.

OUTLYING AREAS

Messages transmitted through the spinal cord reach outlying areas through the peripheral nervous system, which originates in 31 pairs of segmentally arranged spinal nerves attached to the spinal cord. Spinal nerves are numbered according to their point of origin in the cord:

◆ 8 cervical: C1 to C8
◆ 12 thoracic: T1 to T12
◆ 5 lumbar: L1 to L5
◆ 5 sacral: S1 to S5
◆ 1 coccygeal.

On the cross section of the spinal cord, you'll see that these spinal nerves are attached to the spinal cord by two roots:

◆ The *anterior*, or *ventral*, root consists of motor fibers that relay impulses from the cord to glands and muscles.

◆ The *posterior*, or *dorsal*, root consists of sensory fibers that relay sensory information from receptors to the cord. The posterior root has an enlarged area—the posterior root ganglion—which is made up of sensory neuron cell bodies.

After leaving the vertebral column, each spinal nerve separates into *rami* (branches),

Cross section of the spinal cord

The cross section of the spinal cord below shows the anterior and posterior segments.

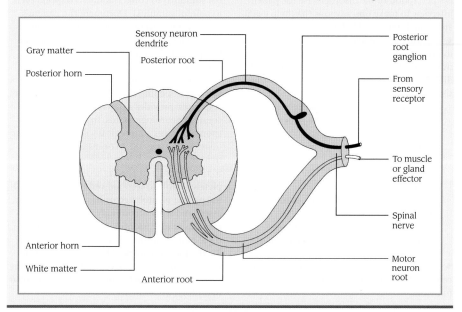

Sensory neuron dendrite
Gray matter
Posterior root
Posterior horn
Posterior root ganglion
From sensory receptor
To muscle or gland effector
Spinal nerve
Motor neuron root
Anterior horn
White matter
Anterior root

distributed peripherally, with extensive but organized overlapping. This overlapping reduces the chance of lost sensory or motor function from interruption of a single spinal nerve.

TWO FUNCTIONAL SYSTEMS

◆ The *somatic (voluntary) nervous system* is activated by will but can also function independently. It's responsible for all conscious and higher mental processes and for subconscious and reflex actions such as shivering.

◆ The *autonomic (involuntary) nervous system* regulates unconscious processes to control involuntary body functions, such as digestion, respiration, and cardiovascular function. It's usually divided into two competing systems: The sympathetic nervous system controls energy expenditure, especially in stressful situations, by releasing adrenergic catecholamines. The parasympathetic nervous system helps conserve energy by releasing the cholinergic neurohormone acetylcholine. These systems balance each other to support homeostasis under normal conditions.

ASSESSING NEUROLOGIC FUNCTION

A complete neurologic assessment helps confirm the diagnosis when a neurologic disorder is suspected. It establishes a clinical baseline and can offer lifesaving clues to rapid deterioration. Neurologic assessment includes:

◆ *Patient history:* In addition to the usual information, try to elicit the patient's and the family's perception of the disorder. Use the patient interview to make observations that help evaluate mental status and behavior.

◆ *Physical examination:* Pay particular attention to obvious abnormalities that may signal serious neurologic problems; for example, fluid draining from the nose or ears. Check for these significant symptoms:

  ◆ headaches, especially if they're more severe in the morning, wake the patient, or the pain is unusually intense

  ◆ change in visual acuity, especially sudden change

  ◆ numbness or tingling in one or more extremities

  ◆ clumsiness or complete loss of function in an extremity

  ◆ mood swings or personality changes

  ◆ any new onset of seizures or change in seizure activity.

◆ *Neurologic examination:* Determine cerebral, cerebellar, motor, sensory, and cranial nerve function.

Obviously, there isn't always time for a complete neurologic examination during bedside assessment. It's therefore necessary to select priorities; for example, typical bedside assessment focuses on level of consciousness (LOC), pupillary response, motor function, reflexes, sensory functions, and vital signs. However, when time permits, a complete neurologic examination can provide valuable information regarding total neurologic function.

ASSESSING MENTAL STATUS, INTELLECT, AND BEHAVIOR

Mental status and behavior are good indicators of cerebral function, and they're easy to assess. Note the patient's appearance, mannerisms, posture, facial expression, grooming, and tone of voice. Check for orientation to time, place, and person and for memory of recent and past events. To test intellect, ask the patient to count backward from 100 by 7s, to read aloud, or to interpret a common proverb, and see how well they understand and follow commands. To assess executive function, ask the patient to follow a series of commands. If you make such checks frequently, vary the questions to avoid a programmed response.

ASSESSING LEVEL OF CONSCIOUSNESS

LOC is a valuable indicator of neurologic function. It can vary from alertness (response to verbal stimulus) to coma (failure to respond even to painful stimulus). Document the patient's exact response to the stimulus; for example, write, "Patient pulled away in response to nail bed pressure," rather than a simple adjective like "stuporous."

The Glasgow Coma Scale (GCS), which assesses eye opening as well as verbal and motor responses, provides a quick, standardized account of neurologic status. In this test, each response receives a numerical value. (See *Glasgow Coma Scale*, page 151.) For instance, if the patient readily responds verbally and is oriented to time, place, and person, scores a 5; if completely unable to respond verbally, scores a 1. If the patient is intubated or has a tracheostomy, assess and score accordingly, such as 5/T ("T" meaning tracheostomy). A score of 15 for all three parts is normal; 7 or less indicates coma; 3—the lowest score possible—generally (but not always) indicates brain death. Although the GCS is useful, it isn't a substitute for a complete neurologic assessment.

ASSESSING MOTOR FUNCTION

The inability to perform the following simple tests, or the presence of tics, tremors, or other abnormalities during such testing, suggests cerebellar dysfunction.

◆ Ask the patient to touch the nose with each index finger, alternating hands. Repeat this test with the eyes closed.

◆ Instruct the patient to tap the index finger and thumb of each hand together rapidly.

◆ Have the patient draw a figure eight in the air with one foot.

◆ To test tandem walk, ask the patient to walk heel to toe in a straight line.

◆ To test balance, perform the Romberg test: Ask the patient to stand with feet together, eyes closed, and arms outstretched without losing balance.

Motor function is a good indicator of LOC and can also point to central or peripheral nervous system damage. During all tests of motor function, watch for differences between right and left side functions.

◆ To check gait, ask the patient to walk while you observe posture, balance, and coordination of leg movement and arm swing.

◆ To check muscle tone, palpate muscles at rest and in response to passive flexion. Look for flaccidity, spasticity, and rigidity. Measure muscle size, and look for involuntary movements, such as rapid jerks, tremors, or contractions.

◆ To evaluate muscle strength, have the patient grip your hands and squeeze. Then ask the patient to push against your palm with a foot. Compare muscle strength on each side, using a 5-point scale (5 is normal strength, 0 is complete paralysis). Insert table of motor strength; also test the patient's ability to extend and flex the neck, elbows, wrists, fingers, toes, hips, and knees; to extend the spine; to contract and relax the abdominal muscles; and to rotate the shoulders.

◆ Rate reflexes on a 4-point scale (4 is clonus, 2 is normal, 0 is absent reflex). Before testing reflexes, make sure that the patient is comfortable and relaxed. To test deep reflexes, use a reflex hammer to briskly tap the biceps, the triceps, and the brachioradialis, patellar, and Achilles tendon regions. A normal response is rapid extension and contraction. Then, to test superficial reflexes, stroke the skin of the abdominal, gluteal, plantar, and scrotal regions with a moderately sharp object that won't puncture the skin. For the superficial reflexes, abdominal gluteal and scrotal contraction should move toward the stimulus. The plantar reflex toes should curl down.

Glasgow Coma Scale

To quickly assess a patient's level of consciousness and to uncover baseline changes, use the Glasgow Coma Scale. This assessment tool grades consciousness in relation to eye opening and motor and verbal responses. A decreased reaction score in one or more categories warns of an impending neurologic crisis. A patient scoring 7 or less is comatose and probably has severe neurologic damage.

Test	Patient's reaction	Score
Best eye opening response	Open spontaneously	4
	Open to verbal command	3
	Open to pain	2
	No response	1
Best motor response	Obeys verbal command	6
	Localizes painful stimuli	5
	Flexion-withdrawal	4
	Flexion-abnormal (decorticate rigidity)	3
	Extension (decerebrate rigidity)	2
	No response	1
Best verbal response	Oriented and converses	5
	Disoriented and converses	4
	Inappropriate words	3
	Incomprehensible sounds	2
	No response	1
Total		3 to 15

ASSESSING SENSORY FUNCTION

Impaired or absent sensation in the trunk or extremities can point to brain, spinal cord, or peripheral nerve damage. Determining the extent of sensory dysfunction is important because it helps locate neurologic damage. For instance, localized dysfunction indicates local peripheral nerve damage, dysfunction over a single dermatome (an area served by 1 of the 31 pairs of spinal nerves) indicates damage to the nerve's dorsal root, and dysfunction extending over more than one dermatome suggests brain or spinal cord damage.

In assessing sensory function, always test both sides of symmetrical areas—for instance, both arms, not just one. Reassure the patient that the test won't be painful.

◆ *Superficial pain perception:* Lightly press the point of an open safety pin against the patient's skin. Don't press hard enough to scratch the skin. Discard pin after use.

◆ *Thermal sensitivity:* The patient tells what it feels like when you place a test tube filled with hot water and one filled with cold water against the skin.

◆ *Tactile sensitivity:* Ask the patient to close the eyes and tell you what is felt when touched lightly on hands, wrists, arms, thighs, lower legs, feet, and trunk with a wisp of cotton.

◆ *Sensitivity to vibration:* Place the base of a vibrating tuning fork against the patient's wrists, elbows, knees, or other bony prominences. Hold it in place, and ask the patient to tell you when it stops vibrating.

◆ *Position sense:* Hold the lateral medial portion of the patient's fingers and toes and move them up, down, and to the side. Ask the patient to tell you the direction of movement.

◆ *Discriminatory sensation:* Ask the patient to close the eyes and identify familiar textures (velvet or burlap) or objects placed in the hand or numbers and letters traced on the palm.

◆ *Two-point discrimination:* Using calipers or other sharp objects, touch the patient in two different places simultaneously. Ask if the patient can feel one or two points. Record how many millimeters of separation are required for the patient to feel two points.

ASSESSING CRANIAL NERVE FUNCTION

By using the simple tests that follow, you can reliably localize cranial nerve dysfunction.

◆ *Olfactory nerve (I):* Have the patient close both eyes and, using each nostril separately, try to identify common nonirritating smells, such as cinnamon, coffee, or peppermint.

◆ *Optic nerve (II):* Examine the patient's eyes with an ophthalmoscope, and have them read a Snellen eye chart or a newspaper. To test peripheral vision, ask the patient to cover one eye and fix the other eye on a point directly in front of him. Then, ask if the patient can see you wiggle your finger in the four quadrants; you'd expect them to see your finger in all four.

◆ *Oculomotor nerve (III):* Compare the size and shape of the patient's pupils and the equality of pupillary response to a small light in a darkened room. Shine the light from a lateral position, not directly in front of the patient's eyes.

◆ *Trochlear nerve (IV) and abducens nerve (VI):* To assess for conjugate and lateral eye movement, ask the patient to follow your finger with both eyes as you slowly move it from the far left to the far right.

◆ *Trigeminal nerve (V):* To test all three portions of this cranial nerve, test facial sensation by stroking the patient's jaws, cheeks, and forehead with a cotton swab, the point of a pin, or test tubes filled with hot or cold water. Because testing for a blink reflex is irritating to the patient, it's not commonly done. If you must test for this response (it may be decreased in patients who wear contact lenses), touch the cornea lightly with a wisp of cotton or tissue, and avoid repeating the test, if possible. To test for jaw jerk, ask the patient to hold their mouth slightly open; then tap the middle of their chin lightly with a reflex hammer. The jaw should jerk closed.

◆ *Facial nerve (VII):* To test upper and lower facial motor function, ask the patient to raise the eyebrows, close the eyes, wrinkle the forehead, and show the teeth. To test sense of taste, ask the patient to identify the taste of salty, sour, sweet, and bitter substances, which you have placed on their tongue.

◆ *Acoustic nerve (VIII):* Ask the patient to identify common sounds such as a ticking clock. With a tuning fork, test for air and bone conduction.

◆ *Glossopharyngeal nerve (IX):* To test gag reflex, touch a tongue blade to each side of the patient's pharynx.

◆ *Vagus nerve (X):* Observe ability to swallow, and watch for symmetrical movements of soft palate when the patient says, "Ah."

◆ *Spinal accessory nerve (XI):* To test shoulder muscle strength, palpate the patient's shoulders, and ask the patient to shrug against a resistance.

◆ *Hypoglossal nerve (XII):* To test tongue movement, ask the patient to stick out his or her tongue. Inspect it for tremor, atrophy, or lateral deviation. To test for strength, ask the patient to move his or her tongue from side to side while you hold a tongue blade against it.

TESTING FOR A FIRM DIAGNOSIS

A firm diagnosis of many neurologic disorders usually requires a wide range of diagnostic tests—both noninvasive and invasive. Noninvasive tests are done first and may include the following:

◆ Skull X-ray identifies skull malformations, fractures, erosion, or thickening. Changes in landmarks may indicate a space-occupying lesion.

◆ Computed tomography (CT) scan produces three-dimensional images that can identify hemorrhage, intracranial tumors, malformation, and cerebral atrophy, edema, calcification, and infarction. If a contrast medium is used, the procedure is invasive. CT angiography uses CT technology with contrast media to produce images of the intracranial vessels to identify aneurysms and arteriovenous malformations (AVMs).

◆ Magnetic resonance imaging (MRI) views the CNS in greater detail than a CT scan and is the procedure of choice for detecting multiple sclerosis (MS); intraluminal clots, brainstem, posterior fossa, and spinal cord lesions; early cerebral infarction; and brain tumors. A noniodinated contrast medium may be used to enhance lesions. MR angiography uses MR technique with contrast media to evaluate the cerebral vessels. MR spectroscopy provides a measure of brain chemistry. It can be used to monitor biochemical changes in tumors, epilepsy, metabolic disorders, infection, and neurodegenerative diseases.

◆ EEG detects abnormal electrical activity in the brain (e.g., from a seizure, metabolic disorder, or drug overdose).

◆ Ultrasonography detects carotid lesions or changes in carotid blood flow and velocity. High frequency sound waves reflect back the velocity of blood flow, which is then reported as a graphic recording of a waveform.

◆ Transcranial Doppler sonography uses ultrasound high frequency sound waves to measure the rate and direction of blood flow in the intracranial vessels.

◆ Evoked potentials evaluate the visual, auditory, and somatosensory nerve pathways by measuring the brain's electrical response to stimulation of the sensory organs or peripheral nerves.

Invasive tests may include the following:

◆ In lumbar puncture, a needle is inserted into the subarachnoid space of the spinal cord, usually between L3 and L4 (or L4 and L5). This allows aspiration of CSF for analysis to detect infection or hemorrhage; to determine cell count and glucose, protein, and globulin levels; and to measure CSF pressure. Lumbar puncture is usually contraindicated in hydrocephalus and in increased intracranial pressure (ICP) because a quick pressure reduction may cause brain herniation. (See *What happens in increased ICP*, page 154.)

◆ Myelography follows a lumbar puncture and CSF removal. In this procedure, a radiologic dye is instilled and X-rays show spinal abnormalities and determine spinal cord and or nerve root compression related to back pain or extremity weakness.

◆ In cerebral arteriography, also known as *angiography*, a catheter is inserted into an artery—usually the femoral artery—and is threaded up to the carotid artery. Then a radiopaque dye is injected, allowing X-ray visualization of the cerebral vasculature. Sometimes the catheter is threaded directly into the brachial or carotid artery. This test can show cerebrovascular abnormalities and spasms plus arterial changes due to a tumor, arteriosclerosis, hemorrhage, an aneurysm, or blockage. A patient undergoing this procedure is at risk for a stroke and for increased ICP.

◆ Brain scan measures gamma rays produced by a radioisotope injected I.V. Uptake and distribution of the isotope in the brain highlights intracranial masses, vascular lesions, and other problems.

◆ ICP monitoring can be a direct, invasive method of identifying trends in ICP. A subarachnoid screw or an intraventricular catheter converts CSF pressure readings into waveforms that are displayed digitally on an oscilloscope monitor. Another method uses a fiber-optic catheter inserted in the subdural space or the brain parenchyma; with this indirect method, pressure changes are reported digitally or in waveform.

◆ Electromyography detects lower motor neuron disorders, neuromuscular disorders, and nerve damage. A needle inserted into selected muscles at rest and during voluntary contraction picks up nerve impulses and measures nerve conduction time.

PATHOPHYSIOLOGY
What happens in increased ICP

Intracranial pressure (ICP) is the pressure exerted within the intact skull by the intracranial volume—about 10% blood, 10% cerebrospinal fluid (CSF), and 80% brain tissue water. The rigid skull allows very little space for expansion of these substances. When ICP increases to pathologic levels, brain damage can result.

The brain compensates for increases in ICP by regulating the volumes of the three substances in the following ways:
♦ limiting blood flow to the head
♦ displacing CSF into the spinal canal
♦ increasing absorption or decreasing production of CSF—withdrawing water from brain tissue into the blood and excreting it through the kidneys. When compensatory mechanisms become overworked, small changes in volume lead to large changes in pressure.

The chart at right will help you understand the pathophysiology of increased ICP.

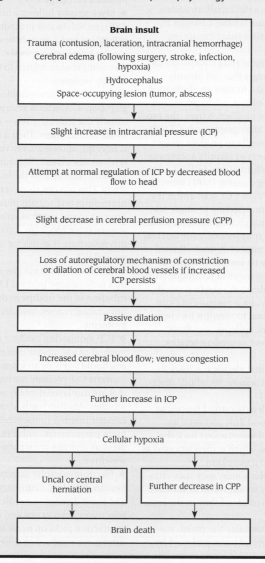

Congenital anomalies

CEREBRAL PALSY

The most common cause of crippling in children, cerebral palsy (CP) is a group of neuromuscular disorders resulting from prenatal, perinatal, or postnatal CNS damage. Although nonprogressive, these disorders may become more obvious as an affected infant grows older. Three major types of CP occur—spastic, athetoid, and ataxic—sometimes in mixed forms. Motor impairment may be minimal (sometimes apparent only during physical activities such as running) or severely disabling. Associated defects, such as seizures, speech disorders, and mental retardation, are common. The prognosis varies; in cases of mild impairment, proper treatment may make a near-normal life possible.

Causes and incidence

See *Causes of cerebral palsy* for a more detailed description of the causes of CP. Incidence is slightly higher in premature neonates (anoxia plays the greatest role in contributing to CP) and in neonates who are small for their gestational age. CP is slightly more common in males than in females. For every 1,000 births, 2 to 4 neonates are affected.

Spastic CP is the most common type of CP, affecting about 50% of CP patients. Athetoid CP affects about 20% of CP patients, ataxic CP accounts for another 10% of these patients, and the remaining 20% of patients are mixed, with a combination of symptoms.

Pathophysiology

During the early stages of brain development, a structural abnormality occurs which results in impaired motor function or a cognitive deficit.

The defects are present at birth but because of relative immaturity of the CNS at birth the neurologic deficits become apparent later on.

Complications

◆ Seizure disorder
◆ Injuries from falls
◆ Speech, vision, and hearing problems
◆ Language and perception deficits
◆ Respiratory problems (poor swallowing and gag reflexes)
◆ Dental problems
◆ Mental retardation

Signs and symptoms

Spastic CP is characterized by hyperactive deep tendon reflexes, increased stretch reflexes, rapid alternating muscle contraction and relaxation, muscle weakness, underdevelopment of affected limbs, muscle contraction in response to manipulation, and a tendency to contractures. Typically, a child with spastic CP walks on his or her toes with a scissors gait, crossing one foot in front of the other.

In athetoid CP, involuntary movements—grimacing, wormlike writhing, dystonia, and sharp jerks—impair voluntary movement. Usually, these involuntary movements affect the arms more severely than the legs; involuntary facial movements may make speech difficult. These athetoid movements become more severe during stress, decrease with relaxation, and disappear entirely during sleep.

Ataxic CP is characterized by disturbed balance, incoordination (especially of the arms), hypoactive reflexes, nystagmus, muscle weakness, tremor, lack of leg movement during infancy, and a wide-based gait as the child begins to walk. Ataxia makes sudden or fine movements almost impossible.

Causes of cerebral palsy

Cerebral palsy (CP) is caused by a developmental brain malformation or neurologic damage.
◆ Prenatal conditions that may increase risk of CP: maternal infection (especially rubella), maternal drug ingestion, radiation, anoxia, toxemia, maternal diabetes, abnormal placental attachment, malnutrition, and isoimmunization
◆ Perinatal and birth difficulties that increase the risk of CP: forceps delivery, breech presentation, placenta previa, abruptio placentae, metabolic or electrolyte disturbances, abnormal maternal vital signs from general or spinal anesthetic, prolapsed cord with delay in delivery of head, premature birth, prolonged or unusually rapid labor, and multiple birth (especially infants born last in a multiple birth)
◆ Infection or trauma during infancy: poisoning, severe kernicterus resulting from erythroblastosis fetalis, brain infection, head trauma, prolonged anoxia, brain tumor, cerebral circulatory anomalies causing blood vessel rupture, and systemic disease resulting in cerebral thrombosis or embolus

Some children with CP display a combination of these clinical features. In most, impaired motor function makes eating (especially swallowing) difficult and retards growth and development. Up to 40% of these children are mentally retarded, about 25% have seizure disorders, and about 80% have impaired speech. Many also have dental abnormalities, vision and hearing defects, and reading disabilities.

Diagnosis

Early diagnosis is essential for effective treatment and requires precise neurologic assessment and careful clinical observation during infancy. CT scan and MRI can reveal structural or congenital abnormalities. Suspect CP whenever an infant:

◆ has difficulty sucking or keeping the nipple or food in his or her mouth
◆ seldom moves voluntarily or has arm or leg tremors with voluntary movement
◆ crosses legs when lifted from behind rather than pulling them up or "bicycling" like a normal infant
◆ has legs that are difficult to separate, making diaper changing difficult
◆ persistently uses only one hand or, as they get older, uses hands well but not legs.

Infants at particular risk include those with low birth weight, low Apgar scores at 5 minutes, seizures, and metabolic disturbances. However, all infants should have a screening test for CP as a regular part of their 6-month checkup.

Treatment

CP can't be cured, but proper treatment can help affected children reach their full potential within the limitations set by this disorder. Such treatment requires a comprehensive and cooperative effort involving physicians, nurses, teachers, psychologists, the child's family, and occupational, physical, and speech therapists. Home care is usually possible. Treatment usually includes interventions that encourage optimum development:

◆ Braces or splints and special appliances, such as adapted eating utensils and a low toilet seat with arms, help these children perform activities independently.
◆ An artificial urinary sphincter may be indicated for the incontinent child who can use the hand controls.
◆ Range-of-motion stretches minimize contractures.
◆ Orthopedic surgery may be indicated to correct contractures. Botulinum toxin has been shown to reduce or delay the need for surgery.

◆ Phenytoin, phenobarbital, or another anticonvulsant may be used to control seizures.
◆ Muscle relaxants or neurosurgery may be required to decrease spasticity.

Children with milder forms of CP should attend a regular school; severely afflicted children may need special education.

Special considerations

◆ A child with CP may be hospitalized for orthopedic surgery or for treatment of other complications.
◆ Speak slowly and distinctly. Encourage the child to ask for things he or she wants. Listen patiently and don't rush.
◆ Plan a high-calorie diet that's adequate to meet the child's high-energy needs.
◆ During meals, maintain a quiet, unhurried atmosphere with as few distractions as possible. The child should be encouraged to feed himself and may need special utensils and a chair with a solid footrest. Teach the patient to place food far back in his or her mouth to facilitate swallowing.
◆ Encourage the child to chew food thoroughly, drink through a straw, and suck on lollipops to develop the muscle control needed to minimize drooling.
◆ Allow the child to wash and dress independently, assisting only as needed. The child may need clothing modifications.
◆ Give all care in an unhurried manner; otherwise, muscle spasticity may increase.
◆ Encourage the child and their family to participate in the plan of care so they can continue it at home.
◆ Care for associated hearing or visual disturbances, as necessary.
◆ Give frequent mouth care and dental care, as necessary.
◆ Reduce muscle spasms that increase postoperative pain by moving and turning the child carefully after surgery; provide analgesics as needed.
◆ After orthopedic surgery, provide cast care. Reposition the child often, check for foul odor, and ventilate under the cast with a cool air blow-dryer. Use a flashlight to check for skin breakdown beneath the cast. Help the child relax, perhaps by giving a warm bath, before reapplying a bivalved cast.

To help the parents:
◆ Encourage them to set realistic individual goals.
◆ Assist in planning crafts and other activities.
◆ Stress the child's need to develop peer relationships; warn the parents against being overprotective.

◆ Identify and deal with family stress. The parents may feel unreasonable guilt about their child's handicap and may need psychological counseling.

◆ Refer the parents to supportive community organizations. For more information, tell them to contact the United Cerebral Palsy Association or their local chapter.

HYDROCEPHALUS

Hydrocephalus is an excessive accumulation of CSF within the ventricular spaces of the brain. The resulting compression can damage brain tissue. With early detection and surgical intervention, the prognosis improves but remains guarded. Even after surgery, such complications as mental retardation, impaired motor function, and vision loss can persist. Without surgery, the prognosis is poor: Mortality may result from increased ICP; infants may also die prematurely of infection and malnutrition.

Causes and incidence

Hydrocephalus may result from an obstruction in CSF flow (noncommunicating hydrocephalus) or from faulty absorption of CSF (communicating hydrocephalus). (See *Normal circulation of CSF*.)

Hydrocephalus occurs most commonly in neonates but can also occur in adults as a result of injury or disease. It affects 1 of every 1,000 people.

Complications

◆ Mental retardation
◆ Impaired motor function
◆ Vision loss
◆ Death

Normal circulation of CSF

Cerebrospinal fluid (CSF) is produced from blood in a capillary network (choroid plexus) in the brain's lateral ventricles. From the lateral ventricles, CSF flows through the interventricular foramen (foramen of Monro) to the third ventricle. From there, it flows through the aqueduct of Sylvius to the fourth ventricle and through the foramina of Luschka and Magendie to the cisterna of the subarachnoid space.

Then, the fluid passes under the base of the brain, upward over the brain's upper surfaces, and down around the spinal cord. Eventually, CSF reaches the arachnoid villi, where it's reabsorbed into venous blood at the venous sinuses.

Normally, the amount of fluid produced (about 500 mL/day) equals the amount absorbed. The average amount circulated at one time is 150 to 175 mL.

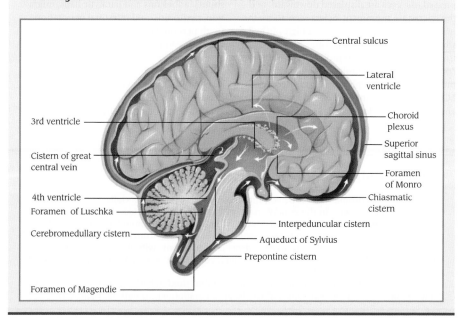

Pathophysiology

In noncommunicating hydrocephalus, the obstruction occurs most frequently between the third and fourth ventricles, at the aqueduct of Sylvius, but it can also occur at the outlets of the fourth ventricle (foramina of Luschka and Magendie) or, rarely, at the foramen of Monro. This obstruction may result from faulty fetal development, infection (syphilis, granulomatous diseases, meningitis), a tumor, cerebral aneurysm, or a blood clot (after intracranial hemorrhage). In communicating hydrocephalus, faulty absorption of CSF may result from surgery to repair a myelomeningocele, adhesions between meninges at the base of the brain, or meningeal hemorrhage. Rarely, a tumor in the choroid plexus causes overproduction of CSF, producing hydrocephalus.

Complications

◆ Mental retardation
◆ Impaired motor function
◆ Vision loss
◆ Death

Signs and symptoms

In infants, the unmistakable sign of hydrocephalus is rapidly increasing head circumference, clearly disproportionate to the infant's growth. Other characteristic changes include widening and bulging of the fontanels; distended scalp veins; thin, shiny, and fragile-looking scalp skin; and underdeveloped neck muscles. In severe hydrocephalus, the roof of the orbit is depressed, the eyes are displaced downward, and the sclerae are prominent. Sclera seen above the iris is called the *setting-sun sign*. A high-pitched, shrill cry; abnormal muscle tone of the legs; irritability; anorexia; and projectile vomiting commonly occur. In adults and older children, indicators of hydrocephalus include decreased LOC, ataxia, incontinence, loss of coordination, and impaired intellect.

Diagnosis

In infants, abnormally large head size for the patient's age strongly suggests hydrocephalus. Measurement of head circumference is a most important diagnostic technique. Skull X-rays show thinning of the skull with separation of sutures and widening of fontanels.

Other diagnostic tests for hydrocephalus, including arteriography, CT scan, and MRI, can differentiate between hydrocephalus and intracranial lesions and can also demonstrate the Arnold–Chiari deformity, which may occur in an infant with hydrocephalus. (See *Arnold–Chiari syndrome*, page 158.)

Treatment

Surgical correction is the only treatment for hydrocephalus. Surgery typically consists of insertion of a ventriculoperitoneal shunt, which transports excess fluid from the lateral ventricle into the peritoneal cavity. A less common procedure is insertion of a ventriculoatrial shunt, which drains fluid from the brain's lateral ventricle into the right atrium of the heart, where the fluid makes its way into the venous circulation.

Another procedure that can be done for noncommunicating hydrocephalus is an endoscopic third ventriculostomy. This involves inserting an endoscope into the third ventricle and fenestrating the floor of the ventricle to allow CSF to flow out.

Complications of surgery include shunt infection, septicemia (after ventriculoatrial shunt), adhesions and paralytic ileus, migration, peritonitis, and intestinal perforation (with peritoneal shunt) or failure of the third ventriculostomy and return of hydrocephalus.

Special considerations

◆ On initial assessment, obtain a complete history from the patient or their family. Note general behavior, especially irritability, apathy,

Arnold–Chiari syndrome

Arnold–Chiari syndrome frequently accompanies hydrocephalus, especially when a myelomeningocele is also present. In this condition, an elongation or tonguelike downward projection of the cerebellum and medulla extends through the foramen magnum into the cervical portion of the spinal canal, impairing cerebrospinal fluid drainage from the fourth ventricle.

In addition to signs and symptoms of hydrocephalus, infants with Arnold–Chiari syndrome have nuchal rigidity, noisy respirations, irritability, vomiting, weak sucking reflex, and a preference for hyperextension of the neck.

Treatment requires surgery to insert a shunt like that used in hydrocephalus. Surgical decompression of the cerebellar tonsils at the foramen magnum is sometimes indicated.

or decreased LOC. Perform a neurologic assessment. Examine the eyes: pupils should be equal and reactive to light. In adults and older children, evaluate movements and motor strength in extremities. Watch especially for ataxia, confusion, and incontinence. Ask if the patient has headaches, and watch for projectile vomiting; both are signs of increased ICP. Also watch for seizures. Note changes in vital signs.

Before surgery to insert a shunt:
◆ Encourage maternal–infant bonding when possible. When caring for the infant yourself, hold on your lap for feeding; stroke and cuddle him, and speak soothingly.
◆ Check fontanels for tension or fullness, and measure and record head circumference. On the patient's chart, draw a picture showing where to measure the head so that other staff members measure it in the same place, or mark the forehead with ink.
◆ To prevent post feeding aspiration and hypostatic pneumonia, place the infant on his or her side and reposition every 2 hours, or prop up in an infant seat.
◆ To prevent skin breakdown, make sure the infant's earlobe is flat, and place a sheepskin or rubber foam under the infant's head.
◆ When turning the infant, move the head, neck, and shoulders with the body to reduce strain on the neck.
◆ Feed the infant slowly. To lessen strain from the weight of the infant's head on your arm while holding during feeding, place head, neck, and shoulders on a pillow.

After surgery:
◆ Place the infant on the side opposite the operative site with the head level with the body unless the physician's orders specify otherwise.
◆ Check temperature, pulse rate, blood pressure, and LOC. Also check fontanels for fullness daily. Watch for vomiting, which may be an early sign of increased ICP and shunt malfunction.
◆ Watch for signs of infection, especially meningitis: fever, stiff neck, irritability, or tense fontanels. Also watch for redness, swelling, or other signs of local infection over the shunt tract. Check dressing often for drainage.
◆ Listen for bowel sounds after ventriculoperitoneal shunt.
◆ Check the infant's growth and development periodically, and help the parents set goals consistent with ability and potential. Help parents focus on their child's strengths, not their weaknesses. Discuss special education programs, and emphasize the infant's need for sensory stimulation appropriate for age. Teach parents to watch for signs of shunt malfunction, infection, and paralytic ileus. Tell them that surgery for lengthening the shunt will be required periodically as the child grows older. Surgery may also be required to correct shunt malfunctioning or to treat infection. Emphasize that hydrocephalus is a lifelong problem and that the child will require regular, continuing evaluation.

CEREBRAL ANEURYSM

Cerebral aneurysm is a localized dilation of a cerebral artery that typically results from a congenital weakness in the arterial wall. Its most common form is the berry aneurysm, a saclike outpouching in a cerebral artery. Cerebral aneurysms may arise at an arterial junction in the circle of Willis, the circular anastomosis forming the major cerebral arteries at the base of the brain. Cerebral aneurysms can rupture and cause subarachnoid hemorrhage. (See *How a cerebral aneurysm forms,* page 160.)

The prognosis is guarded. About 40% of the patients with subarachnoid hemorrhages die immediately; of those who survive untreated, 35% die from the effects of hemorrhage; another 15% die later from recurring hemorrhage. Sixty percent of patients who recover are left with neurologic deficit. Advances in imaging and interventional procedures are improving the outcome overall.

Causes and incidence

Cerebral aneurysm may result from a congenital defect, a degenerative process, or a combination. For example, hypertension and atherosclerosis may disrupt blood flow and exert pressure against a congenitally weak arterial wall, stretching it like an overblown balloon and making it likely to rupture. After such rupture, blood spills into the space normally occupied by CSF, resulting in subarachnoid hemorrhage. Blood may also spill into the brain tissue and form a clot, which can result in potentially fatal increased ICP and brain tissue damage.

Incidence is slightly higher in women than in men, especially those in their late 40s or early to mid-50s, but cerebral aneurysm may occur at any age, in both women and men.

Pathophysiology

The pressure of arterial blood flow against a weak congenital vessel abnormality stretches the vessel walls—the walls also become thin from the pressure making rupture likely. When the aneurysm ruptures, it spills blood into the subarachnoid space, which is normally occupied by the cerebral spinal fluid. Depending on the location of the aneurysm in the cerebral circulation, blood can also be forced into the ventricular system and/or the brain parenchyma.

How a cerebral aneurysm forms

In an intracranial or cerebral aneurysm, a weakness in the wall of the cerebral artery causes localized dilation. Cerebral aneurysms usually arise at an arterial junction in the circle of Willis, the circular anastomosis connecting the major cerebral arteries at the base of the brain. Many cerebral aneurysms rupture, causing a subarachnoid hemorrhage.

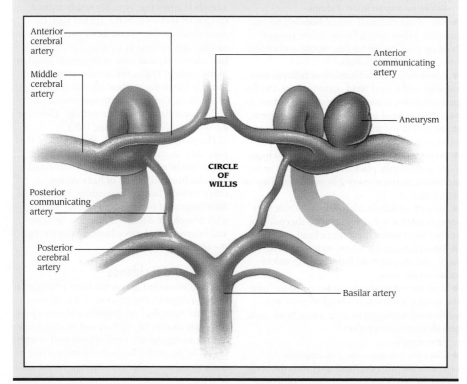

Complications
(Most common after a rupture)
- Subarachnoid hemorrhage
- Brain tissue infarction
- Rebleeding
- Meningeal irritation
- Hydrocephalus

Signs and symptoms
Occasionally, rupture of a cerebral aneurysm causes premonitory symptoms that last several days, such as headache, nuchal rigidity, stiff back and legs, and intermittent nausea. Usually, however, onset is abrupt and without warning, causing a sudden severe headache, nausea, vomiting and, depending on the severity and location of bleeding, altered consciousness (including deep coma).

Bleeding causes meningeal irritation, resulting in nuchal rigidity, back and leg pain, fever, restlessness, irritability, occasional seizures, and blurred vision. Bleeding into the brain tissues causes hemiparesis, hemisensory defects, dysphagia, and visual defects. If the aneurysm is near the internal carotid artery, it compresses the oculomotor nerve and causes diplopia, ptosis, dilated pupil, and inability to rotate the eye.

The severity of symptoms varies considerably from patient to patient, depending on the site and amount of bleeding. To better describe their conditions, patients with ruptured cerebral aneurysms are grouped as follows:
- *Grade I (minimal bleed):* Patient is alert with no neurologic deficit; he or she may have a slight headache and nuchal rigidity.
- *Grade II (mild bleed):* Patient is alert, with a mild to severe headache, nuchal rigidity and, possibly, third-nerve palsy.

◆ *Grade III (moderate bleed):* Patient is confused or drowsy, with nuchal rigidity and, possibly, a mild focal deficit.

◆ *Grade IV (severe bleed):* Patient is stuporous, with nuchal rigidity and, possibly, mild to severe hemiparesis.

◆ *Grade V (moribund; commonly fatal):* If nonfatal, patient is in deep coma or decerebrate.

Generally, cerebral aneurysm poses three major threats:

◆ *Death from increased ICP:* Increased ICP may push the brain downward, impair brainstem function, and cut off blood supply to the part of the brain that supports vital functions.

◆ *Rebleed:* Generally, after the initial bleeding episode, a clot forms and seals the rupture, which reinforces the wall of the aneurysm for 7 to 10 days. However, after the seventh day, fibrinolysis begins to dissolve the clot and increases the risk of rebleeding. Signs and symptoms are similar to those accompanying the initial hemorrhage. Rebleeds during the first 24 hours after initial hemorrhage aren't uncommon, and they contribute to cerebral aneurysm's high mortality.

◆ *Vasospasm:* Why this occurs isn't clearly understood. Usually, vasospasm occurs in blood vessels adjacent to the cerebral aneurysm, but it may extend to major vessels of the brain, causing ischemia and altered brain function.

◆ *Risk of vasospasm can be predicted by use of the Fisher Grading scale.*

Fisher grade	Blood on CT	Risk of vasospasm
II	Diffuse or vertical layer of subarachnoid blood < 1 mm thick	Low (range 0% to 25%)
III	Localized clot and/or vertical layer within the subarachnoid space > 1 mm thick	Low to high (range 23% to 96%)
IV	ICH or IVH with diffuse or no SAH	Low to moderate (range 0% to 35%)

ICH, intracranial hemorrhage; IVH, intraventricular hemorrhage; SAH, subarachnoid hemorrhage

Other complications of cerebral aneurysm include pulmonary embolism (a possible adverse effect of deep vein thrombosis or aneurysm treatment) and acute hydrocephalus, occurring as CSF accumulates in the cranial cavity because of blockage by blood or adhesions.

Diagnosis

Diagnosis of cerebral aneurysm is based on the patient history and a neurologic examination; CT scan, which reveals subarachnoid or ventricular blood; or MRI, which can identify a cerebral aneurysm as a flow void.

Cerebral angiography remains the procedure of choice for diagnosing cerebral aneurysm. A CT angiography is less invasive. Lumbar puncture may be used to identify blood in CSF if other studies are negative and the patient has no signs of increased ICP. Lumbar puncture should be performed if no contraindication is present and you strongly suspect a bleed, because imaging studies may miss a bleed.

Other baseline laboratory studies include complete blood count (CBC), urinalysis, arterial blood gas (ABG) analysis, coagulation studies, serum osmolality, and electrolyte and glucose levels.

Treatment

Coil embolization or clipping of the aneurysm aims to reduce the risk of bleeding, rebleeding after subarachnoid hemorrhage, and cerebral infarction. (See *Repair of cerebral aneurysm,* page 162.) Both methods have advantages and disadvantages. Reinforcing the aneurysm with wrapping when the vessel is easily accessible is an alternative in specific situations. Vasospasm, which previously had been the source of morbidity and mortality associated with successful surgical intervention, has shown therapeutic promise with transluminal balloon intraarterial nimodipine, nicardipine, verapamil, and milrinone. Newer drugs in clinical trials (fasudil hydrochloride and colforsin daropate) are still under investigation.

When surgical correction is delayed or hazardous because of aneurysmal location or fitness of the patient, treatment includes:

◆ careful control of blood pressure (Calcium antagonists are preferred.)

◆ bed rest and avoidance of head-down position

◆ avoidance of stimulants, including caffeine and catecholamines

◆ avoidance of platelet inhibitors such as aspirin

◆ corticosteroids (sometimes used to decrease headache that results from meningeal irritation from the blood products but studies are not conclusive)

◆ anticonvulsants

◆ sedatives.

After surgical repair, the patient's condition depends on the extent of damage from the initial bleed and the success of treatment for any

Repair of cerebral aneurysm

Clipping a cerebral aneurysm
The clip, which is made of materials that won't affect metal detectors and will not rust, is placed at the base of the aneurysm to stop the blood supply. The clip remains in place permanently.

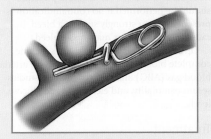

Coil embolization
In coil embolization, soft platinum coils are inserted into the aneurysm through the femoral artery. Usually five to six coils are needed to fill the aneurysm. The goal is to prevent blood flow into the aneurysm sac by filling the aneurysm with coils and thrombus.

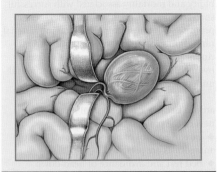

resulting complications. Surgery can't improve the patient's neurologic condition unless it removes a hematoma or reduces the compression effect.

Special considerations
◆ An accurate neurologic assessment, good patient care, patient and family teaching, and psychological support can speed recovery and reduce complications.

◆ During initial treatment after hemorrhage, establish and maintain a patent airway if the patient needs supplementary oxygen. Position the patient to promote pulmonary drainage and prevent upper airway obstruction. If he or she is intubated, administering 100% oxygen before suctioning to remove secretions will prevent hypoxia and vasodilation from carbon dioxide accumulation. Suction no longer than 20 seconds to avoid increased ICP. Give frequent nose and mouth care.

◆ Impose aneurysm precautions to minimize the risk of rebleed and to avoid increased ICP. Such precautions include bed rest in a quiet, darkened room (keep the head of the bed flat or under 30 degrees, as ordered); limited visitors; avoiding strenuous physical activity and straining with bowel movements; and restricted fluid intake. Be sure to explain why these restrictive measures are necessary.

Preventive measures and good patient care can minimize other complications:

◆ Turn the patient often. Encourage occasional deep breathing and leg movement. Warn the patient to avoid all unnecessary physical activity. Assist with active range-of-motion exercises; if the patient is paralyzed, perform regular passive range-of-motion exercises.

◆ Monitor ABG levels, LOC, and vital signs often, and accurately measure intake and output. Avoid taking temperature rectally because vagus nerve stimulation may cause cardiac arrest.

◆ Watch for these danger signals, which may indicate an enlarging aneurysm, rebleeding, intracranial clot, vasospasm, or other complication: decreased LOC, unilateral enlarged pupil, onset or worsening of hemiparesis or motor deficit, increased blood pressure, slowed pulse, worsening of headache or sudden onset of a headache, renewed or worsened nuchal rigidity, and renewed or persistent vomiting. Intermittent signs such as restlessness, extremity weakness, and speech alterations can also indicate increasing ICP.

◆ Give fluids as ordered, and monitor I.V. infusions to avoid increased ICP.

◆ If the patient has facial weakness, assess the gag reflex and assist during meals, placing food in the unaffected side of the mouth. If the patient can't swallow, insert a nasogastric tube as ordered, and give all tube feedings slowly. Prevent skin breakdown by taping the tube so it doesn't press against the nostril. If the patient can eat, provide a high-fiber diet to prevent straining at stool, which can increase ICP. Obtain an order for a stool softener, such as dioctyl sodium sulfosuccinate, or a mild laxative, and administer as ordered. Don't force fluids. Implement a bowel program on the basis of previous habits. If the patient is receiving steroids, check the stool for blood.

◆ With third or facial nerve palsy, administer artificial tears or ointment to the affected eye, and tape the eye shut at night to prevent corneal damage.

◆ To minimize stress, encourage relaxation techniques. If possible, avoid using restraints because these can cause agitation and raise ICP.

◆ Administer antihypertensives as indicated. Carefully monitor blood pressure and immediately report *any* significant change, but especially a rise in systolic pressure.

◆ Prevent deep vein thrombosis by applying antiembolism stockings or sequential compression sleeves.

◆ If the patient can't speak, establish a simple means of communication, or use cards or a notepad. Try to limit conversation to topics that won't frustrate the patient. Encourage the family to speak in a normal tone, even if the patient doesn't seem to respond.

◆ Provide emotional support, and include the patient's family in the care as much as possible. Encourage family members to adopt a realistic attitude, but don't discourage hope.

◆ Before discharge, make a referral to a visiting nurse or a rehabilitation center when necessary.

ARTERIOVENOUS MALFORMATIONS

Cerebral AVM is a disorder of the blood vessels consisting of an abnormal connection between the arteries and the veins in the brain. It's a congenital disorder commonly resulting in tangled masses of thin-walled, dilated blood vessels between arteries and veins that aren't connected by capillaries. AVM primarily occurs in the posterior portion of the cerebral hemispheres. (See *Where a cerebral AVM commonly occurs*, page 164.) Adequate perfusion of brain tissue is prevented because of abnormal channels between the arterial and venous systems that allow mixing of oxygenated and unoxygenated blood. AVMs range in size from a few millimeters to large malformations that extend from the cerebral cortex to the ventricles. Patients typically present with multiple AVMs.

Complications of AVM include development of aneurysm and subsequent rupture, hemorrhage (intracerebral, subarachnoid, or subdural, depending on the location of the AVM), and hydrocephalus.

Causes and incidence

Although some AVMs occur as a result of penetrating injuries such as trauma, most are present at birth. However, symptoms typically don't occur until between ages 10 and 20. Very large AVMs may short-circuit blood flow enough to cause cardiac decompensation, in which the heart can't pump enough blood to compensate for arteriovenous shunting in the brain. This typically occurs in infants and young children.

The vessels of an AVM are very thin and one or more arteries feed into it, causing it to appear dilated and tortuous. Typically, high-pressured arterial flow moves into the venous system through the connecting channels to increase venous pressure, engorging and dilating the venous structures. If the AVM is large enough, the shunting can deprive the surrounding tissue of adequate blood flow. Thin-walled vessels may ooze small amounts of blood—they may even rupture—causing hemorrhage into the brain or subarachnoid space.

Cerebral AVMs occur in approximately 3 of 10,000 people. Although the lesion is present at birth, symptoms may occur at any time. Two thirds of cases occur before age 40. Evidence suggests that AVMs run in families. Males and females are affected equally.

Pathophysiology

AVMs lack the typical structural characteristics of blood vessels. The vessel walls are thin, can have several arteries that feed into it causing it to dilate. The arterial flow moves directly into the venous channel without the normal channel that allows for the dissipation of pressure. This causes the venous side to dilate and it can act like a mass lesion causing pressure on the brain structures.

Complications

◆ Aneurysm and subsequent rupture
◆ Intracerebral, subarachnoid, or subdural hemorrhage
◆ Hydrocephalus

Signs and symptoms

An AVM may be asymptomatic until complications occur; these may include rupture and a resulting sudden bleed in the brain, known as a hemorrhagic stroke. AVMs vary in size and location within the brain. Systolic bruit may be auscultated over the carotid artery, mastoid process, or orbit on examination.

Symptoms that occur before an AVM rupture are related to smaller and slower bleeding from the abnormal vessels, which are usually fragile

Where a cerebral AVM commonly occurs

A cerebral arteriovenous malformation (AVM) is a disorder of blood vessels in which there is an abnormal connection between the arteries and the veins. It is a congenital disorder. Cerebral AVMs commonly occur in the posterior portion of the cerebral hemisphere.

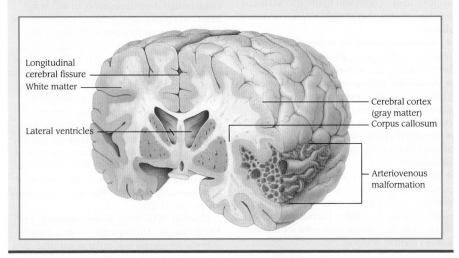

Longitudinal cerebral fissure
White matter
Lateral ventricles
Cerebral cortex (gray matter)
Corpus callosum
Arteriovenous malformation

because their structure is abnormal or if the AVM is larger symptoms are associated with mass effect on the surrounding brain.

In more than half of patients with AVM, hemorrhage from the malformation is the first symptom. Depending on the location and the severity of the bleed, the hemorrhage can be profoundly disabling or fatal. The risk of bleeding from an AVM is approximately 2% to 4% per year.

The first symptoms often include headache, seizure, or other sudden neurologic problems, such as vision problems, weakness, inability to move a limb or a side of the body, lack of sensation in part of the body, or abnormal sensations, such as ringing and numbness. Symptoms are the same as for stroke. The individual with an AVM may complain of chronic mild headache, a sudden and severe headache, or a localized or general headache. The headache may resemble migraine and vomiting may occur. Seizures may result from focal neurologic deficits (depending on the location of the AVM) resulting from compression and diminished perfusion. Symptoms of intracranial (intracerebral, subarachnoid, or subdural) hemorrhage result. Muscle weakness and decreased sensation can occur in any part of the body. Mental

status change can occur where the individual appears sleepy, stuporous, lethargic, confused, disoriented, or irritable. Additional symptoms may include stiff neck, speech or sense of smell impairment, dysfunctional movement, fainting, facial paralysis, eyelid drooping, tinnitus, dizziness, and decreased LOC.

Intracerebral or subarachnoid hemorrhages are the most common first symptoms of cerebral AVM. In some cases, symptoms may also occur because of lack of blood flow to an area of the brain (ischemia), compression or distortion of brain tissue by large AVMs, or abnormal brain development in the area of the malformation. Progressive loss of nerve cells in the brain may occur, caused by mechanical (pressure) and ischemic (lack of blood supply) factors.

Diagnosis

Tests used to diagnose AVM include head CT scan, cranial MRI, and MR angiography. An EEG may be performed if symptoms include seizures, but this test isn't diagnostic of the specific area of the lesion.

Cerebral arteriogram confirms the presence of AVMs and evaluates blood flow. Doppler ultrasonography of cerebrovascular system indicates abnormal, turbulent blood flow.

Treatment

General support measures include aneurysm precautions to prevent possible rupture. This involves placing the patient on bed rest or with limited activity and maintaining a quiet atmosphere. Analgesics may be given for headache, and sedatives may be given to help calm the patient and prevent rupture. Stool softeners may be given to prevent straining at stool, which increases ICP.

Hemorrhage from an AVM is a medical emergency requiring immediate hospitalization. The goal of treatment is to prevent further complications by limiting bleeding, controlling seizures, and controlling ICP. Surgery for correction may include block dissection, laser, or ligation to repair the communicating channels and remove the feeding vessels. In most cases this is performed in a delayed fashion to give the patient the opportunity to recover from the hemorrhage. Embolization or radiation therapy may be done before surgery to close the communicating channels and feeder vessels, thereby reducing blood flow to the AVM or may be done as the treatment of choice in difficult to reach malformations. Open brain surgery, endovascular treatment, and radiosurgery may be used separately or in any combination, depending on the physician and the patient's individual situation. Surgery is dependent on the accessibility and size of the lesion and the patient's status. Open brain surgery involves the actual removal of the malformation in the brain through an opening made in the skull. This surgery is particularly risky because the surgery itself may cause the AVM to bleed uncontrollably.

Embolization (injecting a glue-like substance into the abnormal vessels to stop aberrant blood flow into the AVM) may be an alternative if surgery isn't feasible because of the size or location of the lesion. Stereotactic radiosurgery may also be an alternative for patients with inoperable AVMs. It's particularly useful for small, deep lesions, which are difficult to remove by surgery.

Anticonvulsant medications such as phenytoin are usually prescribed if seizures occur.

Special considerations

◆ Monitor vital signs and adjust medications to control hypertension.
◆ Monitor neurologic status.
◆ Monitor for seizure activity and institute seizure precautions.
◆ Maintain a quiet atmosphere and provide relaxation techniques.
◆ Discuss the importance of reporting any signs of intracranial bleeding immediately (sudden severe headache, vision changes, decreased movement in extremities, and change in LOC).
◆ Refer to social service for support services if neurologic deficits have occurred from a ruptured AVM.

Paroxysmal disorders

HEADACHE

The most common patient complaint, headache usually occurs as a symptom of an underlying disorder. Ninety percent of all headaches are vascular, muscle contraction, or a combination; 10% are due to underlying intracranial, systemic, or psychological disorders. Migraine headaches, probably the most intensively studied, are throbbing, vascular headaches that usually begin to appear in childhood or adolescence and recur throughout adulthood.

Causes and incidence

Most chronic headaches result from tension (muscle contraction), which may be caused by emotional stress, fatigue, menstruation, or environmental stimuli (noise, crowds, or bright lights). Other possible causes include glaucoma; inflammation of the eyes or mucosa of the nasal or paranasal sinuses; diseases of the scalp, teeth, extracranial arteries, or external or middle ear; muscle spasms of the face, neck, or shoulders; and cervical arthritis. In addition, headaches may be caused by vasodilators (nitrates, alcohol, and histamine), systemic disease, hypoxia, hypertension, head trauma and tumor, intracranial bleeding, abscess, or aneurysm.

The cause of migraine headache is unknown, but it's associated with constriction and dilation of intracranial and extracranial arteries. Certain biochemical abnormalities are thought to occur during a migraine attack. These include local leakage of a vasodilator polypeptide called *neurokinin* through the dilated arteries and a decrease in the plasma level of serotonin.

Headache pain may emanate from the pain-sensitive structures of the skin, scalp, muscles, arteries, and veins; cranial nerves V, VII, IX, and X; or cervical nerves 1, 2, and 3. Intracranial mechanisms of headaches include traction or displacement of arteries, venous sinuses, or venous tributaries and inflammation or direct pressure on the cranial nerves with afferent pain fibers.

Affecting up to 10% of Americans, headaches are more common in females and have a strong familial incidence. Drops in estrogen level may precipitate migraine headaches.

Pathophysiology

The pathophysiology of headache varies with the type of headache—migraine is thought to be the result of vascular alterations, dilation of the intracranial blood vessels which allow the leakage of neurokinin. In tension headaches, there is a central stimulus of the trigeminal nerve that involves a hypersensitivity of pain fibers. There is also a peripheral sensitization of the myofascial sensory nerves that contribute to the pain. Headaches associated with intracranial lesions such as hematomas or tumors are the result of increased ICP.

Complications

◆ Worsening of preexisting hypertension
◆ Photophobia
◆ Emotional lability
◆ Motor weakness

Signs and symptoms

Initially, migraine headaches usually produce unilateral, pulsating pain, which later becomes more generalized. They're commonly preceded by a scintillating scotoma, hemianopsia, unilateral paresthesia, or speech disorders. The patient may experience irritability, anorexia, nausea, vomiting, and photophobia. (See *Clinical features of migraine headaches*, pages 166 and 167.)

Both muscle contraction and traction-inflammatory vascular headaches produce a dull, persistent ache; tender spots on the head and neck; and a feeling of tightness around the head, with a characteristic "hatband" distribution. The pain is usually severe and unrelenting. If caused by intracranial bleeding, these headaches may result in mental changes and neurologic deficits, such as paresthesia and muscle weakness; narcotics may fail to relieve pain in these cases. If caused by a tumor, pain is most severe when the patient awakens.

Clinical features of migraine headaches

Type	Signs and symptoms
Common migraine (most prevalent) Usually occurs on weekends and holidays	◆ Prodromal symptoms (fatigue, nausea, vomiting, and fluid imbalance) precede headache by about 1 day. ◆ Sensitivity to light and noise (most prominent feature) ◆ Headache pain (unilateral or bilateral, aching or throbbing)
Classic migraine Usually occurs in compulsive personalities and within families	◆ Prodromal symptoms include visual disturbances, such as zigzag lines and bright lights (most common), sensory disturbances (tingling of face, lips, and hands), or motor disturbances (staggering gait). ◆ Recurrent and periodic headaches
Hemiplegic and ophthalmoplegic migraine (rare) Usually occurs in young adults	◆ Severe, unilateral pain ◆ Extraocular muscle palsies (involving third cranial nerve) and ptosis ◆ With repeated headaches, possible permanent third cranial nerve injury ◆ In hemiplegic migraine, neurologic deficits (hemiparesis, hemiplegia) may persist after the headache subsides.
Basilar artery migraine Occurs in young women before their menstrual periods	◆ Prodromal symptoms usually include partial vision loss followed by vertigo, ataxia, dysarthria, tinnitus and, sometimes, tingling of the fingers and toes, lasting from several minutes to almost an hour. ◆ Headache pain, severe occipital throbbing, vomiting

Clinical features of migraine headaches (*continued*)

Type	Signs and symptoms
Cluster headaches Occur in men more commonly than in women and occur at all ages, but more commonly in adolescents and middle-aged people	♦ Episodic type (more common) and involves one to three short-lived attacks of periorbital pain per day over a 4- to 8-week period followed by a pain-free interval averaging 1 year. Chronic type occurs after an episodic pattern is established. ♦ Unilateral pain occurs without warning, reaching a crescendo within 5 minutes, and is described as excruciating and deep, with attacks lasting from 30 minutes to 2 hours. ♦ Associated symptoms may include tearing, reddening of the eye, nasal stuffiness, lid ptosis, and nausea.

Diagnosis

Diagnosis requires a history of recurrent headaches and physical examination of the head and neck. Such examination includes percussion, auscultation for bruits, inspection for signs of infection, and palpation for defects, crepitus, or tender spots (especially after trauma). Firm diagnosis also requires a complete neurologic examination, assessment for other systemic diseases—such as hypertension—and a psychosocial evaluation, when such factors are suspected.

Diagnostic tests include cervical spine and sinus X-rays, CT scan—performed before lumbar puncture to rule out increased ICP—or MRI. A lumbar puncture isn't done if there's evidence of increased ICP or if a brain tumor is suspected because rapidly reducing pressure by removing spinal fluid can cause brain herniation.

Treatment

Depending on the type of headache, analgesics—ranging from aspirin to codeine or ketorolac—may provide symptomatic relief. Other measures include identification and elimination of causative factors and, possibly, psychotherapy for headaches caused by emotional stress. Chronic tension headaches may also respond to muscle relaxants. A new preventive treatment for migraine has just been released. Erenumab (Aimovig) is a human monoclonal antibody that blocks a protein fragment CGRP that instigates and perpetuates migraine. It is the first drug of its kind to specifically target migraine prevention.

For migraine headaches, ergotamine alone or with caffeine may be an effective treatment. The Food and Drug Administration allows labeling of various analgesic preparations that include caffeine to state that they're for the treatment of migraine headaches. Remember that these medications can't be taken by pregnant women because they stimulate uterine contractions. These drugs and others, such as metoclopramide or nonsteroidal anti-inflammatory drugs, work best when taken early in the course of an attack. If nausea and vomiting make oral administration impossible, drugs may be given as rectal suppositories.

Drugs in the class of sumatriptan are considered by many clinicians to be the drug of choice for acute migraine attacks or cluster headaches. Drugs that can help prevent migraine headaches include antidepressants (such as nortriptyline or fluoxetine), beta-adrenergic blockers (propranolol), and calcium channel blockers (verapamil). Corticosteroids provide short-term relief for some patients with cluster headaches.

Special considerations

♦ Headaches seldom require hospitalization unless caused by a serious disorder. If that's the case, direct your care to the underlying problem.
♦ Obtain a complete patient history: duration and location of the headache; time of day it usually begins; nature of the pain; concurrence with other symptoms such as blurred vision; precipitating factors, such as tension, menstruation, loud noises, menopause, or alcohol; medications taken such as oral contraceptives; or prolonged fasting. Exacerbating factors can also be assessed through ongoing observation of the patient's personality, habits, activities of daily living, family relationships, coping mechanisms, and relaxation activities.

◆ Using the history as a guide, help the patient avoid exacerbating factors. Advise the patient to lie down in a dark, quiet room during an attack and to place ice packs on the forehead or a cold cloth over the eyes.

◆ Instruct the patient to take the prescribed medication at the onset of migraine symptoms, to prevent dehydration by drinking plenty of fluids after nausea and vomiting subside, and to use other headache relief measures.

◆ The patient with a migraine headache usually needs to be hospitalized only if nausea and vomiting are severe enough to induce dehydration and possible shock.

◆ Avoid repeated use of narcotics—overuse of pain medication, especially narcotics, can produce rebound headache.

:::::: **PREVENTION** *Advise patient to:*
◆ *get adequate sleep*
◆ *eat a well-balanced diet and drink plenty of water*
◆ *do upper-body stretching exercises*
◆ *quit smoking*
◆ *learn relaxation techniques such as yoga, medication, and deep breathing*
◆ *avoid known causative triggers.*

SEIZURE DISORDER

Seizure disorder, also called *epilepsy*, is a condition of the brain marked by a susceptibility to recurrent seizures—paroxysmal events associated with abnormal electrical discharges of neurons in the brain.

Causes and incidence

In about half the cases of seizure disorder, the cause is unknown. However, some possible causes of seizure disorder include:

◆ birth trauma (inadequate oxygen supply to the brain, blood incompatibility, or hemorrhage)
◆ perinatal infection
◆ anoxia (after respiratory or cardiac arrest)
◆ infectious diseases (meningitis, encephalitis, or brain abscess)
◆ ingestion of toxins (mercury, lead, or carbon monoxide)
◆ tumors of the brain
◆ inherited disorders or degenerative disease, such as phenylketonuria or tuberous sclerosis
◆ head injury or trauma
◆ metabolic disorders, such as hypoglycemia or hypoparathyroidism
◆ stroke (hemorrhage, thrombosis, or embolism).

Alcohol withdrawal can cause nonepileptic seizures.

Seizure disorder affects 1% to 2% of the population. However, 80% of patients have good seizure control if they strictly adhere to the prescribed treatment regimen.

Pathophysiology

Seizures are the result of abnormal synaptic transmission, an imbalance in the brain neurotransmitters or the development of abnormal nerve connections after an injury. The result is a group of hypersensitive neurons that exhibit paroxysmal depolarization. In the tonic phase of a seizure, there is excitation of subcortical, thalamic, and brainstem areas, which results in loss of consciousness. The clonic phase of the seizure is the result of inhibitory neurons in the cortex, subthalamus, and basal ganglia reacting to the cortical excitation.

During the seizure oxygen is consumed at a high rate as is glucose, cerebral blood flow increases, and lactate increases in the cerebral tissues.

Complications

◆ Anoxia (during a seizure)
◆ Fall injuries

Signs and symptoms

The hallmarks of seizure disorder are recurring seizures, which can be classified as partial or generalized (some patients may be affected by more than one type).

Partial seizures arise from a localized area of the brain, causing specific symptoms. In some patients, partial seizure activity may spread to the entire brain, causing a generalized seizure. Partial seizures include simple partial (jacksonian) and complex partial seizures (psychomotor or temporal lobe).

A simple partial motor-type seizure begins as a localized motor seizure characterized by a spread of abnormal activity to adjacent areas of the brain. It typically produces stiffening or jerking in one extremity, accompanied by a tingling sensation in the same area. For example, it may start in the thumb and spread to the entire hand and arm. The patient seldom loses consciousness, although the seizure may progress to a generalized seizure.

A simple partial sensory-type seizure involves perceptual distortion, which can include hallucinations.

The symptoms of a complex partial seizure vary but usually include purposeless behavior. The patient experiences an aura immediately before the seizure. An aura represents the beginning of abnormal electrical discharges within a focal area of the brain and may include a pungent smell, gastrointestinal (GI) distress (nausea or indigestion), a rising or sinking feeling in the stomach, a dreamy feeling, an unusual taste, or a visual disturbance. Overt signs of a complex partial seizure include a glassy stare, picking at one's clothes, aimless wandering, lip-smacking or chewing motions, and unintelligible speech; these signs may last for just a few seconds or as long as 20 minutes. Mental confusion may last several minutes after the seizure; as a result, an observer may mistakenly suspect intoxication with alcohol or drugs or psychosis.

Generalized seizures, as the term suggests, cause a generalized electrical abnormality within the brain and include several distinct types:

◆ Absence (*petit mal*) seizures occur most commonly in children, although they may affect adults as well. They usually begin with a brief change in LOC, indicated by blinking or rolling of the eyes, a blank stare, and slight mouth movements. There's little or no tonic–clonic movement. The patient retains posture and continues preseizure activity without difficulty. Typically, each seizure lasts from 1 to 10 seconds. If not properly treated, seizures can recur as often as 100 times/day. An absence seizure may progress to generalized tonic–clonic seizures.

◆ A myoclonic (*bilateral massive epileptic myoclonus*) seizure is characterized by brief, involuntary muscular jerks of the body or extremities, which may occur in a rhythmic fashion and may precede generalized tonic–clonic seizures by months or years.

◆ A generalized tonic–clonic (*grand mal*) seizure typically begins with a loud cry, precipitated by air rushing from the lungs through the vocal cords. The patient then falls to the ground, losing consciousness. The body stiffens (tonic phase) and then alternates between episodes of muscular spasm and relaxation (clonic phase). Tongue-biting, incontinence, labored breathing, apnea, and subsequent cyanosis may also occur. The seizure stops in 2 to 5 minutes, when abnormal electrical conduction of the neurons is completed. The patient then regains consciousness but is somewhat confused and may have difficulty talking. If the patient can talk, they may complain of drowsiness, fatigue, headache, muscle soreness, and arm or leg weakness. The patient may fall into deep sleep after the seizure. These seizures may start as facial seizures and spread to become generalized.

An akinetic seizure is characterized by a general loss of postural tone (the patient falls in a flaccid state) and a temporary loss of consciousness. It occurs in young children and is sometimes called a *drop attack* because it causes the child to fall.

Status epilepticus is a continuous seizure state that can occur in all seizure types. The most life-threatening example is generalized tonic–clonic status epilepticus, a continuous generalized tonic–clonic seizure without intervening return of consciousness. Status epilepticus is accompanied by respiratory distress. It can result from abrupt withdrawal of anticonvulsant medications, hypoxic encephalopathy, acute head trauma, metabolic encephalopathy, or septicemia secondary to encephalitis or meningitis.

Diagnosis

Clinically, the diagnosis of seizure disorder is based on the occurrence of one or more seizures and proof or the assumption that the condition that led to them is still present.

Diagnostic information is obtained from the patient's history and description of seizure activity and from family history, physical and neurologic examinations, and CT scan or MRI. These scans offer density readings of the brain and may indicate abnormalities in internal structures. Paroxysmal abnormalities on the EEG confirm the diagnosis by providing evidence of the continuing tendency to have seizures. A negative EEG doesn't rule out seizure disorder because the paroxysmal abnormalities occur intermittently. Other tests may include serum glucose and calcium studies, skull X-rays, lumbar puncture, brain scan, and cerebral angiography.

Treatment

Generally, treatment of seizure disorder consists of anticonvulsant therapy to reduce the number of future seizures. The most commonly prescribed drugs include phenytoin, carbamazepine, phenobarbital, gabapentin, primidone, levetiracetam administered individually for generalized tonic–clonic seizures and complex partial seizures. Valproic acid, clonazepam, and ethosuximide are commonly prescribed for absence seizures. Gabapentin and felbamate are also anticonvulsant drugs.

A patient taking anticonvulsant medications requires monitoring for toxic signs: nystagmus, ataxia, lethargy, dizziness, drowsiness, slurred speech, irritability, nausea, and vomiting.

If drug therapy fails, treatment may include surgical removal of a demonstrated focal lesion to attempt to stop seizures. Emergency treatment of status epilepticus usually consists of diazepam (Valium) or lorazepam (Ativan), phenytoin or phenobarbital (Solfoton); dextrose 50% I.V. (when seizures are secondary to hypoglycemia); and thiamine I.V. (in chronic alcoholism or withdrawal).

Special considerations

A key to support is a true understanding of the nature of seizure disorder and of the misconceptions that surround it.

◆ Encourage the patient and family to express their feelings about the patient's condition. Answer their questions, and help them cope by dispelling some of the myths about seizure disorder, for example, the myth that seizure disorder is contagious. Assure them that seizure disorder is controllable for most patients who follow a prescribed regimen of medication and that most patients maintain a normal lifestyle.

◆ Because drug therapy is the treatment of choice for most people with seizure disorder, information about medications is invaluable.

◆ Stress the need for compliance with the prescribed drug schedule. Reinforce dosage instructions and stress the importance of taking medication regularly, at scheduled times. Caution the patient to monitor the quantity of medication so it does not run out.

◆ Warn against possible adverse effects—drowsiness, lethargy, hyperactivity, confusion, and visual and sleep disturbances—all of which indicate the need for dosage adjustment. Phenytoin therapy may lead to hyperplasia of the gums, which may be relieved by conscientious oral hygiene. Instruct the patient to report adverse effects immediately.

◆ When administering phenytoin I.V., use a large vein and monitor vital signs frequently or administer fosphenytoin (Cerebyx), which has fewer vascular side effects. Avoid I.M. administration and mixing with dextrose solutions. Another I.V. alternative is levetiracetam.

◆ Emphasize the importance of having anticonvulsant blood levels checked at regular intervals, even if the seizures are under control.

◆ Warn the patient against drinking alcoholic beverages.

◆ Know which social agencies in your community can help epileptic patients. Refer the patient to the Epilepsy Foundation of America for general information and to the state motor vehicle department for information about a driver's license.

The primary goals of the healthcare professional and family members caring for a patient having a seizure are protection from injury, protection from aspiration, and observation of the seizure activity. Generalized tonic–clonic seizures may necessitate first aid. Show the patient's family members how to administer first aid correctly:

◆ Avoid restraining the patient during a seizure. Help the patient to a lying position, loosen any tight clothing, and place something flat and soft, such as a pillow, jacket, or hand, under head. Clear the area of hard objects. *Don't* force anything into the patient's mouth if the teeth are clenched—a tongue blade or spoon could lacerate a mouth and lips or displace teeth, precipitating respiratory distress. However, if the patient's mouth is open, protect the tongue by placing a soft object (such as a folded cloth) between the teeth. Turn the head to provide an open airway. After the seizure subsides, reassure the patient that he or she is all right, orient to time and place, and inform that he or she has had a seizure.

◆ *Don't* restrain the patient during a complex partial seizure. Clear the area of any hard objects. Protect the patient from injury by gently calling his or her name and directing away from the source of danger. After the seizure passes, reassure and tell the patient that he or she has just had a seizure.

Brain and spinal cord disorders

STROKE

A stroke, also called *cerebrovascular accident* or *brain attack,* is a sudden impairment of cerebral circulation in one or more of the blood vessels supplying the brain. A stroke interrupts or diminishes oxygen supply and commonly causes serious damage or necrosis in brain tissues. The sooner circulation returns to normal after a stroke, the better chances are for complete recovery. However, about half of those who survive a stroke remain permanently disabled and experience a recurrence within weeks, months, or years.

Causes and incidence

A stroke results from obstruction of a blood vessel, typically in extracerebral vessels, but occasionally in intracerebral vessels. Factors that increase the risk of stroke include history of transient ischemic attacks (TIAs), atherosclerosis, hypertension, kidney disease, arrhythmias (specifically atrial fibrillation), electrocardiogram changes, rheumatic heart disease, diabetes mellitus, postural hypotension, cardiac or myocardial enlargement, high serum triglyceride levels, lack of exercise, use of oral contraceptives, cigarette smoking, and a family history of stroke. (See *Transient ischemic attack,* page 171.)

Transient ischemic attack

A transient ischemic attack (TIA) is a transient episode of neurologic dysfunction caused by a brain ischemia without acute infarct. It's usually considered a warning sign of an impending thrombotic stroke. In fact, TIAs have been reported in 50% to 80% of patients who have had a cerebral infarction from such thrombosis. The age of onset varies. Incidence rises dramatically after age 50 and is highest among blacks and men.

Causes
In TIA, microemboli released from a thrombus probably temporarily interrupt blood flow, especially in the small distal branches of the arterial tree in the brain. Small spasms in those arterioles may impair blood flow and also precede TIA. Predisposing factors are the same as for thrombotic strokes. The most distinctive characteristics of TIAs are the transient duration of neurologic deficits and complete return of normal function. The symptoms of TIA easily correlate with the location of the affected artery. These symptoms include double vision, speech deficits (slurring or thickness), unilateral blindness, staggering or uncoordinated gait, unilateral weakness or numbness, falling because of weakness in the legs, and dizziness.

Treatment
During an active TIA, treatment aims to prevent a completed stroke and consists of aspirin or anticoagulants to minimize the risk of thrombosis. After or between attacks, preventive treatment includes carotid endarterectomy or cerebral microvascular bypass.

The major causes of stroke are thrombosis, embolism, and hemorrhage. Thrombosis is the most common cause in middle-aged and elderly people, who have a higher incidence of atherosclerosis, diabetes, and hypertension. Thrombosis causes ischemia in brain tissue supplied by the affected vessel as well as congestion and edema; the latter may produce more clinical effects than thrombosis itself, but these symptoms subside with the edema. Thrombosis may develop while the patient sleeps or shortly after the patient awakens; it can also occur during surgery or after a myocardial infarction. The risk increases with obesity, smoking, or the use of oral contraceptives. Cocaine-induced ischemic stroke is now being seen in younger patients.

Embolism, the second most common cause of stroke, is an occlusion of a blood vessel caused by a fragmented clot, a tumor, fat, bacteria, or air. It can occur at any age, especially among patients with a history of rheumatic heart disease, endocarditis, posttraumatic valvular disease, myocardial fibrillation and other cardiac arrhythmias, or after open heart surgery. It usually develops rapidly—in 10 to 20 seconds—and without warning. When an embolus reaches the cerebral vasculature, it cuts off circulation by lodging in a narrow portion of an artery, most commonly the middle cerebral artery, causing necrosis and edema. (See *Ischemic stroke*, page 172.) If the embolus is septic and infection extends beyond the vessel wall, encephalitis or an abscess may develop.

Hemorrhage, the third most common cause of stroke, may, like embolism, occur suddenly, at any age, and affects more women than men. Hemorrhage results from chronic hypertension or aneurysms, which cause sudden rupture of a cerebral artery, thereby diminishing blood supply to the area served by the artery. In addition, blood accumulates deep within the brain, further compressing neural tissue and causing even greater damage.

Strokes are classified according to their course of progression. A progressive stroke, or stroke-in-evolution (thrombus-in-evolution), begins with a slight neurologic deficit and worsens in a day or two. In a completed stroke, usually embolic in nature, neurologic deficits are maximal at onset.

Stroke is the third most common cause of death in most developed countries today and the most common cause of neurologic disability. It occurs in 1 of 15 deaths in the United States each year.

Pathophysiology
Cerebral infarction occurs when an area of the brain has lost its blood supply. This results in a core of irreversible ischemia and necrosis. The central core is surrounded by a border of ischemic tissue which is still salvageable tissue. The best window of time to preserve the tissue in the penumbra is within the first 3 hours.

Within 6 to 12 hours the affected areas pale and soften; necrosis, swelling, and mushy disintegration of the infarcted area appears within 48 to 72 hours.

Ischemic stroke

The illustrations below show common sites of cardiac thrombosis and the resulting sites of embolism and infarction.

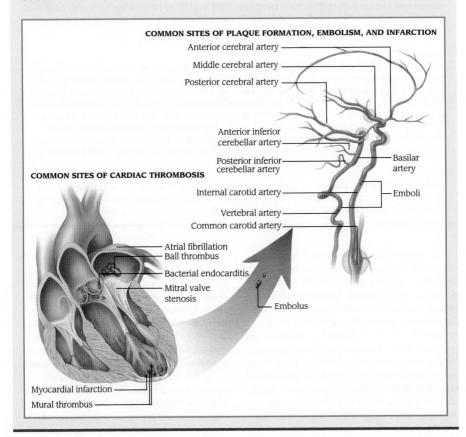

COMMON SITES OF PLAQUE FORMATION, EMBOLISM, AND INFARCTION

Anterior cerebral artery

Middle cerebral artery

Posterior cerebral artery

Anterior inferior cerebellar artery

Posterior inferior cerebellar artery

Basilar artery

COMMON SITES OF CARDIAC THROMBOSIS

Internal carotid artery

Emboli

Vertebral artery

Common carotid artery

Atrial fibrillation

Ball thrombus

Bacterial endocarditis

Mitral valve stenosis

Embolus

Myocardial infarction

Mural thrombus

Complications
◆ Unstable blood pressure
◆ Fluid imbalances
◆ Infection
◆ Sensory impairment
◆ Altered LOC
◆ Aspiration
◆ Pulmonary emboli

Signs and symptoms
Clinical features of stroke vary with the artery affected (and, consequently, the portion of the brain it supplies), the severity of damage, and the extent of collateral circulation that develops to help the brain compensate for decreased blood supply. If the stroke occurs in the left hemisphere, it produces symptoms on the right side; if in the right hemisphere, symptoms are on the left side. However, a stroke that causes cranial nerve damage produces signs of cranial nerve dysfunction on the same side as the hemorrhage.

Symptoms are usually classified according to the artery affected:
◆ *Middle cerebral artery:* aphasia, dysphasia, visual field cuts, and hemiparesis on affected side (more severe in the face and arm than in the leg)
◆ *Carotid artery:* weakness, paralysis, numbness, sensory changes, and visual disturbances on affected side; altered LOC, bruits, headaches, aphasia, and ptosis
◆ *Vertebrobasilar artery:* weakness on affected side, numbness around lips and mouth, visual field cuts, diplopia, poor coordination, dysphagia, slurred speech, dizziness, amnesia, and ataxia

◆ *Anterior cerebral artery:* confusion, weakness, and numbness (especially in the leg) on affected side, incontinence, loss of coordination, impaired motor and sensory functions, and personality changes

◆ *Posterior cerebral arteries:* visual field cuts, sensory impairment, dyslexia, coma, and cortical blindness; typically, paralysis is absent.

Symptoms can also be classified as premonitory, generalized, and focal. Premonitory symptoms, such as drowsiness, dizziness, headache, and mental confusion, are rare. Generalized symptoms, such as headache, vomiting, mental impairment, seizures, coma, nuchal rigidity, fever, and disorientation, are typical. Focal symptoms, such as sensory and reflex changes, reflect the site of hemorrhage or infarct and may worsen.

Diagnosis

Diagnosis of stroke is based on the observation of clinical features, a history of risk factors, and the results of diagnostic tests:

◆ CT scan shows evidence of hemorrhagic stroke immediately but may not show evidence of thrombotic infarction for 48 to 72 hours.

◆ MRI may help identify ischemic or infarcted areas and cerebral swelling.

◆ Electrocardiogram can help diagnose underlying heart disorders.

◆ Carotid duplex may detect carotid artery stenosis.

Angiography outlines blood vessels and pinpoints occlusion or rupture site.

Other baseline laboratory studies may be done to exclude immune conditions or abnormal clotting that can lead to clot formation.

Treatment

Surgery performed to improve cerebral circulation for patients with thrombotic or embolic stroke includes endarterectomy (removal of atherosclerotic plaques from the inner arterial wall) and microvascular bypass (surgical anastomosis of an extracranial vessel to an intracranial vessel). Angioplasty and stenting can improve arterial circulation to the brain. Mechanical embolectomy/clot removal can be done within 8 hours of onset of symptoms.

Medications useful in stroke include the following:

◆ Tissue plasminogen activator has been used successfully in clot dissolution when administered within 3 hours of the onset of symptoms. In other circumstances, heparin and warfarin (Coumadin) may be used, as well as aspirin and other antiplatelet drugs.

◆ Clopidogrel, an antiplatelet drug, may be more effective than aspirin in preventing stroke

and reducing the risk of recurrent stroke after therapy has begun.

◆ Anticonvulsants may be used to treat or prevent seizures.

◆ Stool softeners may be used to prevent straining, which increases ICP.

◆ Analgesics may be used to relieve the headache that typically follows hemorrhagic stroke.

Special considerations

During the acute phase, efforts focus on survival needs and prevention of further complications. Effective care emphasizes continuing neurologic assessment, support of respiration, continuous monitoring of vital signs, careful positioning to prevent aspiration and contractures, management of GI problems, and careful monitoring of fluid, electrolyte, and nutritional status. Patient care must also include measures to prevent complications such as infection.

◆ Maintain a patent airway and oxygenation. Loosen constricting clothes. Watch for ballooning of the cheek with respiration. The side that balloons is the side affected by the stroke. If the patient is unconscious, it is possible that he or she could aspirate saliva, so keep the patient in a lateral position to allow secretions to drain naturally or suction secretions, as needed. Insert an artificial airway, and start mechanical ventilation or supplemental oxygen, if necessary.

◆ Check vital signs and neurologic status, record observations, and report any significant changes to the physician. Monitor blood pressure, LOC, pupillary changes, motor function (voluntary and involuntary movements), sensory function, speech, skin color, temperature, signs of increased ICP, and nuchal rigidity or flaccidity. Remember, if stroke is impending, blood pressure rises suddenly, pulse is rapid and bounding, and the patient may complain of a headache. Also, watch for signs of pulmonary emboli, such as chest pains, shortness of breath, dusky color, tachycardia, fever, and changed sensorium. If the patient is unresponsive, monitor the blood gases often and alert the physician to increased partial pressure of carbon dioxide or decreased partial pressure of oxygen.

◆ Maintain fluid and electrolyte balance. If the patient can take liquids orally, offer them as often as fluid limitations permit. Administer I.V. fluids as ordered; never give too much too fast because this can increase ICP. Offer the urinal or bedpan every 2 hours. If the patient is incontinent, he or she may need an indwelling urinary catheter, but this should be avoided, if possible, because of the risk of infection.

◆ Ensure adequate nutrition. Check for gag reflex before offering small oral feedings of semisolid foods. Place the food tray within the patient's visual field because loss of peripheral vision is common. If oral feedings aren't possible, insert a nasogastric tube.

◆ Manage GI problems. Be alert to signs that the patient is straining at elimination because this increases ICP. Modify diet, administer stool softeners, as indicated, and give laxatives, if necessary. If the patient vomits (usually during the first few days), keep positioned on the side to prevent aspiration.

◆ Provide careful mouth care. Clean and irrigate the patient's mouth to remove food particles. Care for the dentures as needed.

◆ Provide meticulous eye care. Remove secretions with a cotton ball and sterile normal saline solution. Instill eye drops as ordered. Patch the patient's affected eye if the patient can't close the lid.

◆ Position the patient and align the extremities correctly. Use splints to prevent foot drop and contracture, use convoluted foam, flotation, or pulsating mattresses, or sheepskin, to prevent pressure ulcers. To prevent pneumonia, turn the patient at least every 2 hours. Elevate the affected hand to control dependent edema, and place it in a functional position. Mobilize the patient as soon as hemodynamic stability is achieved.

◆ Assist the patient with exercise. Perform range-of-motion exercises for both the affected and unaffected sides. Teach and encourage the patient to use the unaffected side to exercise the affected side.

◆ Give medications as ordered, and watch for and report adverse effects.

◆ Establish and maintain communication with the patient. If the patient is aphasic, set up a simple method of communicating basic needs. Then, remember to phrase your questions so the patient will be able to answer using this system. Repeat yourself quietly and calmly, and use gestures if necessary to help the patient understand. Even an unresponsive patient may be able to hear, so don't say anything in their presence you wouldn't want the patient to hear and remember.

◆ Provide psychological support. Set realistic short-term goals. Involve the patient's family in care when possible, and explain the deficits and strengths.

◆ If the patient has a visual field deficit, make sure caregivers and family members approach the patient from his visually intact side.

◆ For a patient who has had a stroke, start rehabilitation at admission. The amount of teaching you'll have to do depends on the extent of neurologic deficit.

◆ If necessary, teach the patient to comb hair, dress, and wash. With the aid of a physical therapist and an occupational therapist, obtain appliances, such as walking frames, hand bars by the toilet, and ramps, as needed. The patient may fail to recognize that they have a paralyzed side (called *unilateral neglect*) and must be taught to inspect that side of the body for injury and to protect it from harm. If speech therapy is indicated, encourage the patient to begin as soon as possible and to follow through with the speech pathologist's suggestions. To reinforce teaching, involve the patient's family in all aspects of rehabilitation. With their cooperation and support, devise a realistic discharge plan, and let them help decide when the patient can return home.

◆ Before discharge, warn the patient or family to report any premonitory signs of a stroke, such as severe headache, drowsiness, confusion, and dizziness. Emphasize the importance of regular follow-up visits.

◆ If aspirin has been prescribed to minimize the risk of embolic stroke, tell the patient to watch for possible GI bleeding. Make sure the patient and family realize that acetaminophen isn't a substitute for aspirin.

To help prevent stroke:

◆ Stress the need to control diseases, such as diabetes or hypertension.

◆ Teach all patients (especially those at high risk) the importance of following a low-cholesterol, low-salt diet; watching their weight; increasing activity; avoiding smoking and prolonged bed rest; and minimizing stress. (See *Preventing stroke*, page 175.)

◆ Ensure that the patient understands that if symptoms develop, he or she should go to the emergency department immediately.

MENINGITIS

In meningitis, the brain and the spinal cord meninges become inflamed, usually as a result of a viral or, less commonly, a bacterial infection. Such inflammation may involve all three meningeal membranes—the dura mater, the arachnoid, and the pia mater. (See *Meningeal inflammation in meningitis*, page 175.) Viral meningitis is usually mild and often clears on its own in 10 days or less. Bacterial meningitis requires prompt treatment with I.V. antibiotics.

Causes and incidence

Bacterial meningitis is almost always a complication of another bacterial infection—bacteremia (especially from pneumonia, empyema, osteomyelitis, or endocarditis), sinusitis, otitis media, encephalitis, myelitis, or brain abscess—usually caused by *Neisseria meningitidis, Haemophilus*

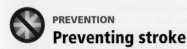

Preventing stroke

Lifestyle modifications can help prevent heart attack and stroke. The American Heart Association recommends the following:

Healthy diet
Give patients the following advice:
♦ Eat five or more servings of fruit and vegetables daily.
♦ Eat six or more servings a day of grain products including whole grains.
♦ Eat fish at least twice a week, especially mackerel, lake trout, herring, sardines, albacore tuna, and salmon.
♦ Include fat-free and low-fat milk products, beans, lean meats, and skinless poultry.
♦ Choose fats and oils with 2 g or less of saturated fat per serving (1 tablespoon).
♦ Limit your intake of foods high in calories or low in protein, such as carbonated beverages, high-sugar foods, and candy.
♦ Eat less than 6 g of salt per day (1 teaspoon).
♦ Limit foods high in saturated fat, trans fat, or cholesterol, such as whole milk, fatty meats, tropical oils, and partially hydrogenated vegetable oils.

Exercise
Regular physical activity is defined by the American Heart Association as moderate to vigorous exercise 30 minutes a day on most or all days of the week. A lack of physical activity can lead to obesity and increase the risk of hypertension, heart attack, and stroke.

Smoking cessation
Even smoking filtered and light or ultralight cigarettes can lead to atherosclerosis. Quitting or not starting is the only thing that can prevent this major risk factor for heart attack and stroke.

Blood pressure awareness
Individuals should know what their blood pressure is by having it checked by a practitioner. If it's high, it may be able to be lowered by following a healthy diet and including exercise in their daily routine. If diet and exercise don't lower blood pressure, medication may be needed. Adherence to the medication regimen is foremost in reducing blood pressure and preventing stroke.

Meningeal inflammation in meningitis

The illustration below shows normal meninges and how the meninges become inflamed in meningitis.

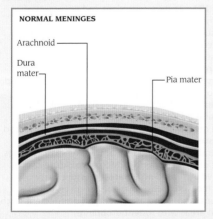

NORMAL MENINGES

Arachnoid
Dura mater
Pia mater

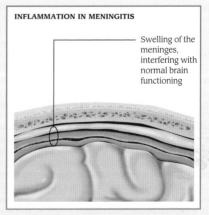

INFLAMMATION IN MENINGITIS

Swelling of the meninges, interfering with normal brain functioning

influenzae (in children and young adults), or *Streptococcus pneumoniae* (in adults). In some cases, a virus is suspected. (See *Lymphocytic choriomeningitis*.) Meningitis may also follow skull fracture, a penetrating head wound, lumbar puncture, or a ventricular shunting procedure. Aseptic meningitis may result from a virus or other organism. Sometimes, no causative organism can be found. Meningitis commonly begins as an inflammation of the pia-arachnoid, which may progress to congestion of adjacent tissues and destruction of some nerve cells.

The incidence of meningitis is high among Blacks and Native Americans. Male infants have a high incidence of gram-negative neonatal meningitis.

Pathophysiology

Microorganisms invade the CNS through the nose or mouth, along a cranial or peripheral nerve, through a direct opening such as trauma or through the bloodstream. This sets off an inflammatory response in the meninges, exudate forms in the subarachnoid space causing the CSF to thicken. The exudate also irritates the cerebral cortex. This results in increased ICP.

Complications
◆ Visual impairment
◆ Optic neuritis
◆ Cranial nerve palsies
◆ Personality changes
◆ Headache
◆ Paresis or paralysis
◆ Vasculitis
◆ Endocarditis

Signs and symptoms

The cardinal signs of meningitis are infection (fever, chills, and malaise) and increased ICP (headache, vomiting, and, rarely, papilledema). Signs of meningeal irritation include nuchal rigidity, positive Brudzinski and Kernig signs, exaggerated and symmetrical deep tendon reflexes, and opisthotonos (a spasm in which the back and extremities arch backward so that the body rests on the head and heels). (See *Two signs of meningitis*, page 177.) Other manifestations of meningitis are irritability; sinus arrhythmias; photophobia, diplopia, and other visual problems; and delirium, deep stupor, and coma.

Lymphocytic choriomeningitis

Lymphocytic choriomeningitis (LCM) is a mild, biphasic, febrile illness lasting about 2 weeks. Infection occurs through inhalation of the LCM virus or arenavirus from infectious aerosolized particles of the host (rodents such as mice or hamsters) or its excreta (urine, feces, or saliva) 1 to 3 weeks before the onset of symptoms. It can also result from contact with food contaminated with the virus or by contamination of mucous membranes, skin lesions, or cuts with infected body fluids. Handlers of infected animals or their excreta are at risk for this disease. Most cases occur in the northeast and eastern seaboard areas of the United States. LCM is more common during fall and winter.

The incubation period is 8 to 13 days after exposure. Early characteristics include fever, malaise, anorexia, weakness, muscle aches, retro-orbital headache, nausea, and vomiting. Sore throat, nonproductive cough, joint pain, chest pain, testicular pain, and parotid (salivary gland) pain may occur. Meningeal symptoms appear in 15 to 21 days, with signs and symptoms of meningitis (fever, increased headache, and stiff neck) or encephalitis (drowsiness, confusion, sensory disturbances, and motor abnormalities such as paralysis). Alopecia may also occur.

Complications include temporary or permanent neurologic damage, possible maternal transmission (pregnancy-related infection is associated with spontaneous abortion, congenital hydrocephalus, chorioretinitis, and mental retardation), myelitis, Guillain–Barré-type syndrome, orchitis or parotitis, myocarditis, psychosis, joint pain and arthritis, and prolonged convalescence with continuing dizziness, somnolence, and fatigue.

Diagnosis is made by detection of immunoglobulin M antibodies by enzyme-linked immunosorbent assay from serum or cerebrospinal fluid (CSF) (the preferred diagnostic test). Lumbar puncture CSF is typically abnormal and reveals increased opening pressure, increased protein levels, and a lymphocytic pleocytosis, usually in the range of several hundred white blood cells. Treatment is generally supportive and includes bed rest, anti-inflammatory drugs, and analgesics. Ribavirin has been shown to be effective against LCM in vitro. Acute hydrocephalus may require surgical shunting to relieve increased intracranial pressure.

Prevention involves teaching rodent control measures, basic hygiene practices, use of a personal respirator, importance of adequate ventilation, and use of a liquid disinfectant, such as a diluted household bleach solution, to clean areas with rodent droppings.

Two signs of meningitis

Brudzinski sign: Place the patient in a dorsal recumbent position, put your hands behind the patient's neck, and bend it forward. Pain and resistance may indicate meningeal inflammation, neck injury, or arthritis. If the patient also flexes hips and knees in response to this manipulation, chances are the patient has meningitis.

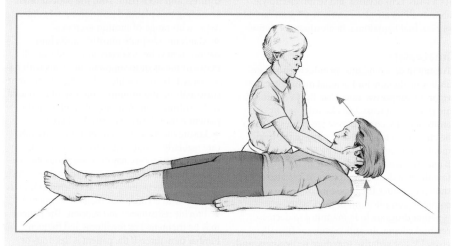

Kernig sign: Place the patient in a supine position. Flex the leg at the hip and knee and then straighten the knee. Pain or resistance points to meningitis.

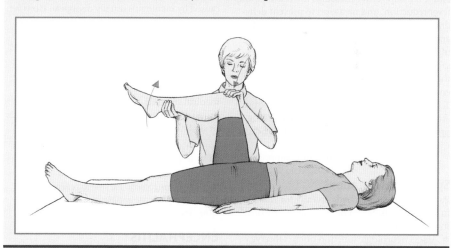

An infant may not show clinical signs of infection but may be fretful and refuse to eat. Such an infant may vomit often, leading to dehydration; this prevents a bulging fontanel and thus masks this important sign of increased ICP. As the illness progresses, twitching, seizures (in 30% of infants), or coma may develop. Most older children have the same symptoms as adults. In subacute meningitis, the onset may be insidious.

Diagnosis

A lumbar puncture showing typical CSF findings, when accompanied by positive Brudzinski and Kernig signs, usually establishes a diagnosis. The following tests can uncover the primary sites of infection: cultures of blood, urine, and nose and throat secretions; chest X-ray; electrocardiogram; and a physical examination, with special attention to skin, ears, and sinuses. Lumbar puncture usually indicates elevated CSF pressure, from obstructed outflow at the arachnoid villi. The fluid may appear cloudy or milky white, depending on the number of white blood cells present. CSF protein levels tend to be high; glucose levels may be low. (In subacute meningitis, CSF findings may vary.) CSF culture and sensitivity tests usually identify the infecting organism, unless it's a virus. Leukocytosis and serum electrolyte abnormalities are also common. CT scan can rule out cerebral hematoma, hemorrhage, or tumor.

Treatment

Treatment of meningitis includes appropriate antibiotic therapy for bacterial meningitis and vigorous supportive care. Usually, I.V. antibiotics are given for at least 2 weeks, followed by oral antibiotics. Dexamethasone has been shown to be effective as adjunctive therapy in the treatment of meningitis caused by *H. influenzae* type B and in pneumococcal meningitis if given before the first dose of antibiotic. It has also been shown to reduce the incidence of deafness, a common complication of meningitis.

Other drugs include mannitol to decrease cerebral edema, an anticonvulsant (usually given I.V.) or sedative to reduce restlessness, and aspirin or acetaminophen to relieve headache and fever. Supportive measures include bed rest, fever reduction, and measures to prevent dehydration. The patient's room is kept darkened and quiet because any increase in sensory stimulation may cause a seizure. Isolation is necessary if nasal cultures are positive. Appropriate therapy for any coexisting conditions, such as endocarditis or pneumonia, is included as well. To prevent meningitis, prophylactic antibiotics are sometimes used after ventricular shunting procedures, skull fracture, or penetrating head wounds, but this use is controversial.

For viral meningitis, treatment is supportive.

Special considerations

Patients must be watched carefully for changes in neurologic function or other signs of worsening condition.

◆ Assess neurologic function often. Observe LOC and signs of increased ICP (plucking at the bedcovers, vomiting, seizures, and a change in motor function and vital signs). Watch for signs of cranial nerve involvement (ptosis, strabismus, and diplopia).

⚠ **ALERT** *Be especially alert for a temperature increase up to 102° F (38.9° C), deteriorating LOC, onset of seizures, and altered respirations, all of which may signal an impending crisis.*

◆ Monitor fluid balance. Maintain adequate fluid intake to avoid dehydration, but avoid fluid overload because of the danger of cerebral edema. Measure central venous pressure and intake and output accurately.

◆ Watch for adverse effects of I.V. antibiotics and other drugs. To avoid infiltration and phlebitis, check I.V. site often, and change the site according to hospital policy.

◆ Position the patient carefully to prevent joint stiffness and neck pain. Turn the patient often, according to a planned positioning schedule. Assist with range-of-motion exercises.

◆ Maintain adequate nutrition and elimination. It may be necessary to provide small, frequent meals or to supplement meals with nasogastric tube or parenteral feedings. To prevent constipation and minimize the risk of increased ICP resulting from straining at stool, give the patient a mild laxative or stool softener.

◆ Ensure the patient's comfort. Provide mouth care regularly. Maintain a quiet environment. Darkening the room may decrease photophobia. Relieve headache with a nonopioid analgesic, such as aspirin or acetaminophen, as ordered. (Opioids interfere with accurate neurologic assessment.)

◆ Provide reassurance and support. The patient may be frightened by the illness and frequent lumbar punctures. If the patient is delirious or confused, attempt to reorient often. Reassure the family that the delirium and behavior changes caused by meningitis usually disappear. However, if a severe neurologic deficit appears permanent, refer the patient to a rehabilitation program as soon as the acute phase of this illness has passed.

◆ To help prevent development of meningitis, teach patients with chronic sinusitis or other chronic infections the importance of proper medical treatment. Follow strict sterile technique when treating patients with head wounds or skull fractures.

▦▦ **PREVENTION**
◆ *Give* Haemophilus influenzae *Type B and pneumococcal vaccines to children.*
◆ *Give meningococcal vaccine to college students.*
◆ *Give prophylactic antibiotics to those who have been exposed to a patient with meningitis.*

ENCEPHALITIS

Encephalitis is a severe inflammation of the brain, commonly caused by a mosquito-borne or, in some areas, a tick-borne virus. However, transmission by means other than arthropod bites may occur through ingestion of infected goat's milk and accidental injection or inhalation of the virus. Person-to-person, airborne transmission of viruses (such as measles or mumps) may also lead to encephalitis in nonimmunized populations. Eastern equine encephalitis may produce permanent neurologic damage and is commonly fatal. (See *Types of encephalitis*, pages 179 to 181.)

Types of encephalitis

Four main viral agents cause most cases of encephalitis in the United States: eastern equine encephalitis (EEE), western equine encephalitis (WEE), St. Louis encephalitis, and La Crosse (LAC) encephalitis, all of which are transmitted by mosquitoes. Another virus, Powassan (POW) virus, is a minor cause of encephalitis in the northern United States; this virus is transmitted by ticks. Most cases of arboviral encephalitis occur from June through September, when arthropods are most active. In milder parts of the country, where arthropods are active late into the year, cases can occur into the winter months.

No vaccines are available for these U.S.-based diseases. However, a Japanese encephalitis (JE) vaccine is available for those who will be traveling to Japan, a tick-borne encephalitis vaccine is available for those who will be traveling to Europe, and an equine vaccine is available for EEE, WEE, and Venezuelan equine encephalitis (VEE). Public health measures often require spraying of insecticides to kill larvae and adult mosquitoes as well as controlling standing water that can provide mosquito breeding sites.

Eastern equine encephalitis
♦ EEE is caused by an alphavirus transmitted to humans and horses by the bite of an infected mosquito.
♦ Incubation is 4 to 10 days.
♦ Symptoms begin with a sudden onset of fever, general muscle pains, and a headache of increasing severity; can progress to seizures and coma.
♦ One third of those afflicted will die from the disease and of those who recover, many will suffer irreversible brain damage requiring care.
♦ Human cases are usually preceded by outbreaks in horses.
♦ The virus occurs in natural cycles involving birds in swampy areas nearly every year during the warm months. The virus doesn't escape from these areas, however, and this mosquito doesn't usually bite humans or other mammals.

Western equine encephalitis
♦ The alphavirus WEE is the causative agent. The virus is closely related to the EEE and VEE viruses.
♦ The enzootic cycle of WEE involves passerine birds, in which the infection is inapparent, and culicine mosquitoes, principally *Culex tarsalis*, a species associated with irrigated agriculture and stream drainages.
♦ Human WEE cases are usually first seen in June or July.
♦ Most WEE infections are asymptomatic or present as mild, nonspecific illness. Patients with clinically apparent illness usually have a sudden onset with fever, headache, nausea, vomiting, anorexia, and malaise, followed by altered mental status, weakness, and signs of meningeal irritation.
♦ Children, especially those younger than age 1, are affected more severely than adults and may be left with permanent sequelae, which are seen in 5% to 30% of young patients.
♦ Mortality is about 3%.

St. Louis encephalitis
♦ The leading cause of St. Louis encephalitis is a flavivirus. St. Louis encephalitis is the most common mosquito-transmitted human pathogen in the United States.
♦ Mosquitoes become infected by feeding on birds infected with the St. Louis encephalitis virus. Infected mosquitoes then transmit virus to humans and animals during the feeding process. The virus grows both in the infected mosquito and the infected bird, but doesn't make either one sick.
♦ Less than 1% of St. Louis encephalitis viral infections are clinically apparent; the majority are undiagnosed.
♦ Illness ranges in severity from a simple febrile headache to meningoencephalitis, with an overall case–fatality ratio of 30%.
♦ The incubation period is 5 to 15 days.
♦ Mild infections present with fever and headache. More severe infection is marked by headache, high fever, neck stiffness, stupor, disorientation, coma, tremors, occasional convulsions (especially in infants), and spastic (but rarely flaccid) paralysis.
♦ The disease is generally milder in children than in adults, but in those children who do have disease, there's a high rate of encephalitis.
♦ Elderly people are at highest risk for severe disease and death.
♦ During the summer season, St. Louis encephalitis virus is maintained in a mosquito–bird–mosquito cycle, with periodic amplification by peridomestic birds and *Culex* mosquitoes.

(continued)

Types of encephalitis (*continued*)

La Crosse encephalitis
♦ The LAC virus, a bunyavirus, is a zoonotic pathogen cycled between the daytime-biting tree hole mosquito, *Aedes triseriatus*, and vertebrate amplifier hosts (chipmunks, tree squirrels) in deciduous forest habitats. The virus is maintained over the winter by transmission in mosquito eggs. If the female mosquito is infected, she may lay eggs that carry the virus. The vector uses artificial containers (tires, buckets, and so forth) in addition to tree holes.
♦ LAC encephalitis initially presents as a nonspecific summertime illness with fever, headache, nausea, vomiting, and lethargy.
♦ Severe disease occurs most commonly in children younger than 16 and is characterized by seizures, coma, paralysis, and a variety of neurologic sequelae after recovery.
♦ Death occurs in less than 1% of clinical cases.
♦ Cases are often reported as aseptic meningitis or viral encephalitis of unknown etiology.
♦ During an average year, about 75 cases of LAC encephalitis are reported to the Centers for Disease Control and Prevention.

Powassan encephalitis
♦ The POW virus is a flavivirus.
♦ Recently a Powassan-like virus was isolated from the deer tick, *Ixodes scapularis*. The virus has been recovered from ticks (*Ixodes marxi* and *Dermacentor andersoni*) and from the tissues of an eastern spotted skunk.
♦ It's a rare cause of acute viral encephalitis.
♦ Patients who recover may have residual neurologic problems.

Venezuelan equine encephalitis
♦ Like EEE and WEE viruses, VEE is an alphavirus that causes encephalitis in horses and humans. VEE is a significant veterinary and public health problem in Central and South America.
♦ Infection of humans with the VEE virus is less severe than with EEE and WEE viruses, and fatalities are rare.
♦ Adults usually develop only an influenza-like illness; overt encephalitis is usually confined to children.
♦ Effective VEE virus vaccines are available for equines.

Japanese encephalitis
♦ JE virus, which is related to St. Louis encephalitis, is a flavivirus. It's widespread throughout Asia.
♦ Epidemics occur in late summer in temperate regions, but the infection is enzootic and occurs throughout the year in many tropical areas of Asia.
♦ The virus is maintained in a cycle involving culicine mosquitoes and waterbirds. It's transmitted to humans by *Culex* mosquitoes, primarily *Culex tritaeniorhynchus*, which breed in rice fields.
♦ Mosquitoes become infected by feeding on domestic pigs and wild birds infected with the JE virus. Infected mosquitoes then transmit the virus to humans and animals during the feeding process. The virus is amplified in domestic pigs and wild birds.
♦ The incubation period is 5 to 14 days.
♦ Mild infections occur without apparent symptoms other than fever with headache. More severe infection is marked by quick onset, headache, high fever, neck stiffness, stupor, disorientation, coma, tremors, occasional seizures (especially in infants), and spastic (but rarely flaccid) paralysis.
♦ The illness resolves in 5 to 7 days if there's no central nervous system involvement.
♦ The mortality is less than 10%, but is higher in children and can exceed 30%. Neurologic sequelae in patients who recover are reported in up to 30% of cases.
♦ A vaccine is currently available for human use in the United States for individuals who might be traveling to endemic countries.

Tick-borne encephalitis
♦ Tick-borne encephalitis (TBE) is caused by two closely related flaviviruses. The eastern subtype causes Russian spring-summer encephalitis (RSSE) and is transmitted by *Ixodes persulcatus*, whereas the western subtype is transmitted by *Ixodes ricinus* and causes Central European encephalitis (CEE).
♦ RSSE is the more severe infection, having a mortality of up to 25% in some outbreaks, whereas mortality in CEE seldom exceeds 5%.
♦ The incubation period is 7 to 14 days.

Types of encephalitis (*continued*)

♦ Infection usually presents as a mild, influenza-type illness or as benign, aseptic meningitis, but may result in fatal meningoencephalitis.
♦ Fever is often biphasic, and there may be severe headache and neck rigidity, with transient paralysis of the limbs, shoulders or, less commonly, the respiratory musculature. A few patients are left with residual paralysis.
♦ Although the great majority of TBE infections follow exposure to ticks, infection has occurred through the ingestion of infected cows' or goats' milk.
♦ An inactivated TBE vaccine is currently available in Europe and Russia.

West Nile encephalitis
♦ West Nile virus (WNV) is a flavivirus belonging to the Japanese encephalitis serocomplex that includes the closely related St. Louis encephalitis virus, Kunjin, and Murray Valley encephalitis (MVE) viruses, as well as others.
♦ WNV can infect a wide range of vertebrates; in humans it usually produces either asymptomatic infection or mild febrile disease, but can cause severe and fatal infection in a small percentage of patients.
♦ The incubation period is thought to range from 3 to 14 days.
♦ Symptoms generally last 3 to 6 days.
♦ Like St. Louis encephalitis virus, WNV is transmitted principally by *Culex* species mosquitoes, but also can be transmitted by *Aedes*, *Anopheles*, and other species.
♦ The mild form of WNV infection has presented as a febrile illness of sudden onset often accompanied by malaise, anorexia, nausea, vomiting, eye pain, headache, myalgia, rash, and lymphadenopathy.
♦ A minority of patients with severe disease develop a maculopapular or morbilliform rash involving the neck, trunk, arms, or legs. Some patients experience severe muscle weakness and flaccid paralysis. Neurologic presentations include ataxia, cranial nerve abnormalities, myelitis, optic neuritis, polyradiculitis, and seizures. Although not observed in recent outbreaks, myocarditis, pancreatitis, and fulminant hepatitis have been described.

Murray Valley encephalitis
♦ MVE is endemic in New Guinea and in parts of Australia.
♦ It's related to the St. Louis encephalitis, WNV, and JE viruses.
♦ Infections are common, and the small number of fatalities has mostly been in children.

In encephalitis, intense lymphocytic infiltration of brain tissues and the leptomeninges causes cerebral edema, degeneration of the brain's ganglion cells, and diffuse nerve cell destruction.

Causes and incidence
Encephalitis typically results from infection with arboviruses specific to rural areas. However, in urban areas, it's most frequently caused by enteroviruses (coxsackievirus, poliovirus, and echovirus) and flaviviruses (WNV). Other causes include herpesvirus, mumps virus, human immunodeficiency virus, adenoviruses, rabies, and demyelinating diseases after measles, varicella, rubella, or vaccination.

Pathophysiology
Infectious organisms from a mosquito or tick causes a lymphocytic infiltration of brain tissues and the leptomeninges which causes cerebral edema, degeneration of the ganglion cells of the brain with diffuse nerve cell destruction.

Complications
♦ Bronchial pneumonia
♦ Urine retention
♦ Urinary tract infection
♦ Pressure ulcers
♦ Seizure disorder
♦ Parkinsonism
♦ Mental deterioration
♦ Coma

Signs and symptoms
All viral forms of encephalitis have similar clinical features, although certain differences do occur. Usually, the acute illness begins with sudden onset of fever, headache, and vomiting and progresses to include signs and symptoms of meningeal irritation (stiff neck and back) and neuronal damage (drowsiness, coma, paralysis,

seizures, ataxia, tremors, nausea, vomiting, and organic psychoses). After the acute phase of the illness, coma may persist for days or weeks.

The severity of arbovirus encephalitis may range from subclinical to rapidly fatal necrotizing disease. Herpes encephalitis also produces signs and symptoms that vary from subclinical to acute and commonly fatal fulminating disease. Associated effects include disturbances of taste or smell.

Diagnosis

During an encephalitis epidemic, diagnosis is readily made on clinical findings and patient history. However, sporadic cases are difficult to distinguish from other febrile illnesses, such as gastroenteritis or meningitis. Diagnosis may be assisted by serologic assays, such as immunoglobulin (Ig) M-capture ELISA (MAC-ELISA) and Ig ELISA. Early in infection, IgM antibody is more specific, whereas later, IgG is more reactive. Monoclonal antibody studies show promise in diagnosis. Polymerase chain reaction is also being investigated.

When possible, identification of the virus in CSF or blood confirms this diagnosis. The common viruses that also cause herpes, measles, and mumps are easier to identify than arboviruses. Both herpesviruses and arboviruses can be isolated by inoculating young mice with a specimen taken from the patient. In herpes encephalitis, serologic studies may show rising titers of complement-fixing antibodies.

In all forms of encephalitis, CSF pressure is elevated and despite inflammation, the fluid is usually clear. White blood cell and protein levels in CSF are slightly elevated, but the glucose level remains normal. An EEG reveals abnormalities. Occasionally, a CT scan or MRI may be ordered to rule out cerebral hematoma.

Treatment

The antiviral acyclovir must be prescribed for herpes encephalitis. Antibiotics may be prescribed if the infection is thought to be caused by bacteria. Treatment of all other forms of encephalitis is entirely supportive. Drug therapy includes phenytoin or another anticonvulsant, usually given I.V.; steroids such as dexamethasone to reduce cerebral inflammation and edema; corticosteroids; mannitol to reduce cerebral swelling (although the evidence for benefit is weak); sedatives for restlessness; and aspirin or acetaminophen to relieve headache and reduce fever. Ribavirin and interferon alpha-2b were found to have some effect on West Nile encephalitis. Other supportive measures include adequate fluid and electrolyte intake to prevent dehydration and antibiotics for an associated infection such as pneumonia. Isolation is unnecessary. (See *Preventing mosquito-borne encephalitis*.)

Special considerations

During the acute phase of the illness:
◆ Assess neurologic function often. Observe LOC and signs of increased ICP (increasing restlessness, plucking at the bedcovers, vomiting, seizures, and changes in pupil size, motor function, and vital signs—such as rising blood pressure, widening pulse pressure, and slowly falling pulse). Watch for cranial nerve involvement (ptosis, strabismus, and diplopia), abnormal sleep patterns, and behavior changes.
◆ Maintain adequate fluid intake to prevent dehydration, but avoid fluid overload, which may increase cerebral edema. Measure and record intake and output accurately, and assess daily weights.
◆ Carefully position the patient to prevent joint stiffness and neck pain, and turn the patient often. Assist with range-of-motion exercises.

PREVENTION

Preventing mosquito-borne encephalitis

Help patients prevent mosquito-borne encephalitis by urging them to follow these steps:
♦ Wear long-sleeved shirts and long pants if going outside between dusk and dawn.
♦ A mosquito repellent with a 10% to 30% concentration of *N,N*-diethyl-meta-toluamide (DEET) is recommended and should be applied to skin and clothing. Don't use DEET on the hands of young children or on infants under 2 months of age. Cover an infant's stroller or playpen with mosquito netting when outside.
♦ Refrain from unnecessary activity in places where mosquitoes are most prevalent.
♦ Repair holes in screens on doors and windows to prevent mosquitoes from entering the home.
♦ Eliminate areas that attract mosquitoes, such as standing water in birdbaths, wheelbarrows, flower pots, old tires, and unused containers. These items are excellent breeding areas for mosquitoes.

◆ Maintain adequate nutrition. It may be necessary to give the patient small, frequent meals or to supplement meals with nasogastric tube or parenteral feedings.

◆ To prevent constipation and minimize the risk of increased ICP resulting from straining at stool, give a mild laxative or stool softener.

◆ Provide mouth care.

◆ Maintain a quiet environment. Darkening the room may decrease photophobia and headache. If the patient naps during the day and is restless at night, plan daytime activities to minimize napping and promote sleep at night.

◆ Provide emotional support and reassurance because the patient is apt to be frightened by the illness and frequent diagnostic tests.

◆ If the patient is delirious or confused, attempt to reorient often. Providing a calendar or a clock in the patient's room may be helpful.

◆ Reassure the patient and family that behavior changes caused by encephalitis usually disappear. If a neurologic deficit is severe and appears permanent, refer the patient to a rehabilitation program as soon as the acute phase has passed.

BRAIN ABSCESS

Brain abscess, also known as an *intracranial abscess*, is a free or encapsulated collection of pus usually in the temporal lobe, cerebellum, or frontal lobes. It can vary in size and may occur singly or in more than one location.

Untreated brain abscess is usually fatal; even with treatment, the prognosis is only fair, and about 30% of patients develop focal seizures. Multiple metastatic abscesses secondary to systemic or other infections have the poorest prognosis.

Causes and incidence

Brain abscess is usually secondary to some other infection, especially otitis media, sinusitis, dental abscess, and mastoiditis. Other causes include subdural empyema; bacterial endocarditis; human immunodeficiency virus infection; bacteremia; pulmonary or pleural infection; pelvic, abdominal, and skin infections; and cranial trauma, such as a penetrating head wound or compound skull fracture. Brain abscess also occurs in those with congenital heart disease and congenital blood vessel abnormalities of the lungs such as Osler–Weber–Rendu disease. These disorders carry a high risk of infection of the heart or lungs, which can then spread to the brain. Penetrating head trauma or bacteremia usually leads to staphylococcal infection; pulmonary disease, to streptococcal infection.

Brain abscess has a relatively low incidence. It has a 10% mortality rate.

Pathophysiology

Brain abscess usually begins with localized inflammatory necrosis and edema, septic thrombosis of vessels, and suppurative encephalitis. This is followed by thick encapsulation of accumulated pus and adjacent meningeal infiltration by neutrophils, lymphocytes, and plasma cells. The abscess acts like a space-occupying lesion. If the capsule of the abscess ruptures, it creates a more diffuse inflammation with more global increased ICP.

Complications

◆ Seizures
◆ Permanent weakness or paralysis
◆ Meningitis
◆ Memory difficulty
◆ Speech difficulty

Signs and symptoms

Onset varies according to cause, but generally brain abscess produces clinical effects similar to those of a brain tumor. Early symptoms result from increased ICP and include constant intractable headache, worsened by straining; nausea; vomiting; and focal or generalized seizures. Typical later symptoms include ocular disturbances, such as nystagmus, decreased vision, and unequal pupil size.

Other features differ with the site of the abscess:

◆ *temporal lobe abscess:* auditory-receptive dysphasia, central facial weakness, and hemiparesis

◆ *cerebellar abscess:* dizziness, coarse nystagmus, gaze weakness on lesion side, tremor, and ataxia

◆ *frontal lobe abscess:* expressive dysphasia, hemiparesis with unilateral motor seizure, drowsiness, inattention, and mental function impairment.

Signs of infection, such as fever, pallor, and bradycardia, are absent until late stages unless they result from the predisposing condition. If the abscess is encapsulated, they may never appear. Depending on abscess size and location, LOC varies from drowsiness to deep stupor.

Diagnosis

A history of infection—especially of the middle ear, mastoid, nasal sinuses, heart, or lungs—or a history of congenital heart disease, along with a physical examination showing such characteristic clinical features as increased ICP, points to brain abscess. A CT scan or MRI and, occasionally, arteriography (which highlights brain abscess by a halo) help locate the site. Blood culture will reveal any bacteria in the bloodstream. Chest X-ray may reveal lung infection.

Examination of CSF can help confirm infection, but lumbar puncture is risky because it can release the increased ICP and provoke cerebral herniation. A CT-guided stereotactic biopsy may be performed to drain and culture the abscess. Other tests include culture and sensitivity of drainage to identify the causative organism, skull X-rays, and a radioisotope scan.

Treatment

Management of patients with brain abscess has become increasingly challenging because of the proliferation of unusual bacterial, fungal, and parasitic infections, particularly in immunocompromised patients. Therapy consists of antibiotics to combat the underlying infection and surgical aspiration or drainage of the abscess. Surgical drainage or excision may be performed (CT scan or MRI can help determine the need for these procedures). Antimicrobials may be injected directly into the mass. Administration of antibiotics for at least 2 weeks before surgery can reduce the risk of spreading infection.

Other treatments during the acute phase are palliative and supportive and include mechanical ventilation, administration of I.V. fluids with diuretics (urea, mannitol, or hypertonic saline), to combat increased ICP and cerebral edema. Anticonvulsants, such as phenytoin, levetiracetam, or phenobarbital, help prevent seizures.

Special considerations

The patient with an acute brain abscess requires intensive monitoring.

◆ Frequently assess neurologic status, especially LOC, speech, and sensorimotor and cranial nerve functions. Watch for signs of increased ICP (decreased LOC, vomiting, abnormal pupil response, and depressed respirations), which may lead to cerebral herniation with such signs as fixed and dilated pupils, widened pulse pressure, bradycardia or tachycardia, and absent respirations.

◆ Assess and record vital signs at least every hour.

◆ Monitor fluid intake and output carefully because fluid overload can contribute to cerebral edema.

If surgery is necessary, explain the procedure to the patient and answer any questions. After surgery:

◆ Continue frequent neurologic assessment. Monitor vital signs and intake and output.

◆ Watch for signs of meningitis (nuchal rigidity, headaches, chills, and sweats), an ever present threat.

◆ Be sure to change a damp dressing often, using sterile technique and noting the amount of drainage. Never allow bandages to remain damp. To promote drainage and prevent reaccumulation of purulent material in the abscess, position the patient on the operative side.

◆ If the patient remains stuporous or comatose for an extended period, give meticulous skin care to prevent pressure ulcers, and position to preserve function and prevent contractures.

◆ Encourage the patient to ambulate as soon as possible to prevent immobility and encourage independence.

⠿⠿⠿⠿ **PREVENTION**
◆ *Stress the need for treatment of otitis media, mastoiditis, dental abscess, and other infections.*
◆ *Give prophylactic antibiotics after compound skull fracture or penetrating head wound.*

HUNTINGTON DISEASE

Also called *Huntington chorea*, hereditary chorea, chronic progressive chorea, or adult chorea, Huntington disease is a hereditary disease in which degeneration in the cerebral cortex and basal ganglia causes chronic progressive chorea and mental deterioration, ending in dementia.

Causes and incidence

Huntington disease is inherited as a single faulty gene on chromosome 4 whereby part of the gene is repeated in multiple copies. It's transmitted as an autosomal dominant trait; either sex can transmit and inherit it. Each child of a parent with this disease has a 50% chance of inheriting it.

The disease usually strikes people between ages 35 and 55; however, 2% of cases occur in children, and 5% of cases occur as late as age 60. Death usually results 10 to 15 years after onset, from suicide, heart failure, or pneumonia. Genetic testing is available for persons with a family history of the disease.

Pathophysiology

Huntington disease involves a disturbance in neurotransmitters—primarily gamma-aminobutyric acid (GABA) and dopamine. GABA neurons in the basal ganglia, frontal cortex, and cerebellum are destroyed and replaced by glial cells which create a deficiency of GABA and an excess of dopamine. This imbalance alters neural transmission along the affected pathway.

Complications

◆ Aspiration
◆ Pneumonia
◆ Heart failure
◆ Infections
◆ Suicidal ideation

Signs and symptoms

Onset is insidious. The patient eventually becomes totally dependent—emotionally and physically—through loss of musculoskeletal control, and develops progressively severe choreic movements. Such movements are rapid, usually violent, and purposeless. Initially, they're unilateral and more prominent in the face and arms than in the legs, progressing from mild fidgeting to grimacing, tongue smacking, dysarthria (indistinct speech), athetoid movements (especially of the hands) related to emotional state, and torticollis.

Ultimately, the patient with Huntington disease develops progressive dementia, although the dementia doesn't always progress at the same rate as the chorea. Dementia can be mild at first, but eventually causes severe disruption of the personality. Personality changes include obstinacy, carelessness, untidiness, moodiness, apathy, inappropriate behavior, loss of memory and concentration and, occasionally, paranoia.

Diagnosis

Huntington disease can be detected by positron emission tomography and deoxyribonucleic acid analysis. Diagnosis is based on a characteristic clinical history: progressive chorea and dementia, onset in early middle age (35 to 40 years old), and confirmation of a genetic link. CT scan and MRI demonstrate brain atrophy. Molecular genetics may detect the gene for Huntington disease in people at risk while they're still asymptomatic.

Treatment

Because Huntington disease has no known cure, treatment is supportive, protective, and symptomatic. Dopamine blockers, such as phenothiazine or haloperidol, help control choreic movements and reduce abnormal behaviors. Reserpine and other drugs have been used with varying success to control choreic movements and reduce abnormal behavior. Drugs such as tetrabenazine and amantadine are used to control extra movements. Some evidence suggests that co-enzyme Q10 may minimally decrease progression of the disease. Institutionalization may be necessary because of mental deterioration, which can't be halted or managed by drugs.

Special considerations

Patient comfort and support are the primary considerations.

◆ Provide physical support by attending to the patient's basic needs, such as hygiene, skin care, bowel and bladder care, and nutrition. Increase this support as mental and physical deterioration make the patient increasingly immobile.

◆ Offer emotional support to the patient and family. Teach them about the disease, and listen to their concerns and special problems. Keep in mind the patient's dysarthria, and allow extra time to express himself, thereby decreasing frustration. Teach the family to participate in the patient's care.

◆ Stay alert for possible suicide attempts. Control the patient's environment to protect from suicide or other self-inflicted injury. Pad the side rails of the bed, but avoid restraints, which may cause the patient to injure himself with violent, uncontrolled movements.

◆ If the patient has difficulty walking, provide a walker to help maintain balance.

◆ Make sure affected families receive genetic counseling. All affected family members should realize that each of their offspring has a 50% chance of inheriting this disease.

◆ Refer people at risk who desire genetic testing to centers specializing in Huntington's care, where psychosocial support is available.

◆ Refer the patient and family to the appropriate community organizations.

◆ For more information about this degenerative disease, refer the patient and family to the Huntington's Disease Society of America.

PARKINSON DISEASE

Named for James Parkinson, the English physician who wrote the first accurate description of the disease in 1817, Parkinson disease characteristically produces progressive muscle rigidity, akinesia, involuntary tremor, and dementia. Death may result from aspiration pneumonia or an infection.

Causes and incidence

Although the cause of Parkinson disease is unknown, study of the extrapyramidal brain nuclei (corpus striatum, globus pallidus, and substantia nigra) has established that a dopamine deficiency prevents affected brain cells from performing their normal inhibitory function within the CNS. Parkinson disease occurs in families in some cases.

Parkinson disease, also called *parkinsonism*, paralysis agitans, and shaking palsy, is one of the most common crippling diseases in the United States. Parkinson disease strikes 2 in every 1,000 people, most often developing in those older than 50; however, it also occurs in children and young adults. Because of increased longevity, this amounts to roughly 60,000 new cases diagnosed annually in the United States alone. Incidence increases in persons with repeated brain injury, including professional athletes, and persons using psychoactive substances, whether prescribed or illicit.

Pathophysiology

Parkinson is a degenerative process involving the dopaminergic neurons in the substantia nigra. Stimulation of the basal ganglia usually results in refined motor response because acetylcholine (excitatory) and dopamine (inhibitory) are balanced. The degeneration of the dopaminergic neurons results in an imbalance leading to excess acetylcholine at the synapse. The result is rigidity, tremors, and bradykinesia.

Complications

◆ Injury from falls
◆ Aspiration
◆ Urinary tract infections
◆ Skin breakdown

Signs and symptoms

The cardinal symptoms of Parkinson disease are muscle rigidity and akinesia and an insidious resting tremor that begins in the fingers (unilateral pill-roll tremor), increases during stress or anxiety, and decreases with purposeful movement and sleep. Muscle rigidity results in resistance to passive muscle stretching, which may be uniform (lead-pipe rigidity) or jerky (cogwheel rigidity). Akinesia causes the patient to walk with difficulty (gait lacks normal parallel motion and may be retropulsive or propulsive) and produces a high-pitched, monotone voice; drooling; a masklike facial expression; loss of posture control (the patient walks with body bent forward); and dysarthria, dysphagia, or both. Occasionally, akinesia may also cause oculogyric crises (eyes are fixed upward, with involuntary tonic movements) or blepharospasm (eyelids are completely closed). Parkinson disease itself doesn't impair the intellect, but a coexisting disorder, such as arteriosclerosis, may do so.

Diagnosis

Generally, laboratory data are of little value in identifying Parkinson disease; consequently, diagnosis is based on the patient's age, history, and characteristic clinical picture.

Conclusive diagnosis is possible only after ruling out other causes of tremor, involutional depression, cerebral arteriosclerosis and, in patients younger than 30, intracranial tumors, Wilson disease, or phenothiazine or other drug toxicity.

Treatment

Because Parkinson disease has no cure, the primary aim of treatment is to relieve symptoms and keep the patient functional as long as possible. Treatment consists of drugs, physical therapy and, in severe disease states unresponsive to drugs, stereotactic neurosurgery or the controversial treatment called fetal cell transplantation. In this treatment, fetal brain tissue is injected into the patient's brain. If the injected cells grow within the recipient's brain, they will allow the brain to process dopamine, thereby either halting or reversing disease progression. Neurotransplantation techniques, including the use of nerve cells from other parts of the patient's body, have been attempted with varying results.

Drug therapy usually includes levodopa, a dopamine replacement that's most effective during early stages. It's given in increasing doses until symptoms are relieved or adverse effects appear. Because adverse effects can be serious, levodopa is usually given in combination with carbidopa to halt peripheral dopamine synthesis. Occasionally, levodopa proves ineffective, producing dangerous adverse effects that include postural hypotension, hallucinations, and increased libido leading to inappropriate sexual behavior. In that case, alternative drug therapy includes anticholinergics such as trihexyphenidyl, antihistamines such as diphenhydramine, and amantadine, an antiviral agent.

Research into the oxidative stress theory has caused a controversy in drug therapy for Parkinson disease. Traditionally, levodopa–carbidopa has been a first-line drug in management; however, it has also been associated with an acceleration of disease process. Inclusion of entacapone potentiates the effects of levodopa–carbidopa treatment so that less frequent doses are required.

Selegiline, an enzyme-inhibiting agent, allows conservation of dopamine and enhances the therapeutic effect of levodopa. Selegiline used with tocopherols delays the time when the patient with Parkinson disease becomes disabled.

ELDER TIP *Elderly patients may need smaller doses of antiparkinsonian drugs because of reduced tolerance. Be alert for and report orthostatic hypotension, irregular pulse, blepharospasm, and anxiety or confusion.*

When drug therapy fails, stereotactic neurosurgery, such as subthalamotomy and pallidotomy, may be an alternative. In these procedures, electrical coagulation, freezing, radioactivity, or ultrasound destroys the ventrolateral nucleus of the thalamus to prevent involuntary movement. This is most effective in young, otherwise healthy people with unilateral tremor or muscle rigidity. Neurosurgery can only relieve symptoms. Brain stimulator implantation alters the activity of the area where Parkinson disease symptoms originate. A pacemaker is implanted into the chest wall, and the electrode is threaded (using MRI for guidance) to the thalamus, pallidum, or subthalamic nucleus. A successful procedure reduces the need for medication, thus reducing the medication-related adverse effects experienced by the patient.

Individually planned physical therapy complements drug treatment and neurosurgery to maintain normal muscle tone and function. Appropriate physical therapy includes both active and passive range-of-motion exercises, routine daily activities, walking, and baths and massage to help relax muscles.

Special considerations

Effectively caring for the patient with Parkinson disease requires careful monitoring of drug treatment, emphasis on teaching self-reliance, and generous psychological support.

◆ Monitor drug treatment and adjust dosage, if necessary, to minimize adverse effects.

◆ If the patient has surgery, watch for signs of hemorrhage and increased ICP by frequently checking LOC and vital signs.

◆ Encourage independence. The patient with excessive tremor may achieve partial control of his or her body by sitting on a chair and using its arms to steady themselves. Advise the patient to change position slowly and dangle the legs before getting out of bed. Remember that fatigue may cause the patient to depend more on others.

◆ Help the patient overcome problems related to eating and elimination. For example, if the patient has difficulty eating, offer supplementary or small, frequent meals to increase caloric intake. Help establish a regular bowel routine by encouraging the patient to drink at least 2 qt (about 2 L) of liquids daily and eat high-fiber foods. The patient may need an elevated toilet seat to assist from a standing to a sitting position.

◆ Give the patient and family emotional support. Teach them about the disease, its progressive stages, and drug adverse effects. Show the family how to prevent pressure ulcers and contractures by proper positioning. Inform them of the dietary restrictions levodopa imposes, and explain household safety measures to prevent accidents. Help the patient and family express their feelings and frustrations about the progressively debilitating effects of the disease. Establish long- and short-term treatment goals, and be aware of the patient's need for intellectual stimulation and diversion. Refer the patient and family to the National Parkinson Foundation or the United Parkinson Foundation for more information.

MYELITIS AND ACUTE TRANSVERSE MYELITIS

Myelitis, or inflammation of the spinal cord, can result from several diseases. Poliomyelitis affects the cord's gray matter and produces motor dysfunction; leukomyelitis affects only the white matter and produces sensory dysfunction. These types of myelitis can attack any level of the spinal cord, causing partial destruction or scattered lesions. Acute transverse myelitis, which affects the entire thickness of the spinal cord, produces both motor and sensory dysfunctions. It has a rapid onset and is the most devastating form of myelitis.

The prognosis depends on the severity of cord damage and prevention of complications. If spinal cord necrosis occurs, prognosis for complete recovery is poor. Even without necrosis, residual neurologic deficits usually persist after recovery. Patients who develop spastic reflexes early in the course of the illness are more likely to recover than those who don't.

Causes and incidence

Acute transverse myelitis has a variety of causes. It commonly follows acute infectious diseases, such as measles or pneumonia (the inflammation occurs after the infection has subsided), and primary infections of the spinal cord itself, such as syphilis or acute disseminated encephalomyelitis. Acute transverse myelitis can accompany demyelinating diseases, such as an acute exacerbation of MS, and inflammatory and necrotizing disorders of the spinal cord such as hematomyelia.

Certain toxic agents (carbon monoxide, lead, and arsenic) can cause a type of myelitis in which acute inflammation (followed by hemorrhage and possible necrosis) destroys the entire circumference (myelin, axis cylinders, and neurons) of the spinal cord. Other forms of myelitis may result from poliovirus, herpes zoster, herpesvirus B, or rabies virus; disorders that cause meningeal inflammation, such as syphilis, abscesses and other suppurative conditions, and tuberculosis; smallpox or polio vaccination; parasitic and fungal infections; and chronic adhesive arachnoiditis.

Peak incidence occurs between 10 and 19 years old, then again between 30 and 39.

Approximately 1,400 new cases are diagnosed each year in the United States. About 33,000 Americans have some type of disability from this disorder.

Pathophysiology

Caused by an acute infection, myelitis is an inflammation of the spinal cord. It can affect only the gray matter—which leads to motor dysfunction, or it can affect the white matter which leads to sensory dysfunction. In acute transvers myelitis the entire cord is affected leading to both motor and sensory deficits.

Complications

◆ Hypertension
◆ Urinary tract infection
◆ Urolithiasis
◆ Pneumonia
◆ Skeletal and smooth muscle deformities
◆ Myocarditis
◆ Paralytic ileus

Signs and symptoms

In acute transverse myelitis, onset is rapid, with motor and sensory dysfunctions below the level of spinal cord damage appearing in 1 to 2 days.

Patients with acute transverse myelitis develop flaccid paralysis of the legs (sometimes beginning in just one leg) with loss of sensory and sphincter functions. Such sensory loss may follow pain in the legs or trunk. Reflexes disappear in the early stages but may reappear later. The extent of damage depends on the level of the spinal cord affected; transverse myelitis seldom involves the arms. If spinal cord damage is severe, it may cause shock (hypotension and hypothermia).

Diagnosis

Paraplegia of rapid onset usually points to acute transverse myelitis. In such patients, neurologic examination confirms paraplegia or neurologic deficit below the level of the spinal cord lesion and absent (or, in later stages) hyperactive reflexes. CSF may be normal or show increased lymphocytes or elevated protein levels. Diagnostic evaluation must rule out spinal cord tumor and identify the cause of any underlying infection.

Treatment

No effective treatment exists for acute transverse myelitis. However, this condition requires appropriate treatment of any underlying infection. Some patients with postinfectious or MS-induced myelitis have received steroid therapy, but its benefits aren't clear.

Special considerations

Managing symptoms and treating the underlying infection are the primary considerations.
◆ Frequently assess vital signs. Watch carefully for signs of spinal shock (hypotension and excessive sweating).
◆ Prevent contractures with range-of-motion exercises and proper alignment.
◆ Watch for signs of urinary tract infections from indwelling urinary catheters.
◆ Prevent skin infections and pressure ulcers with meticulous skin care. Check pressure points often and keep skin clean and dry; use a low-pressure specialty or rotational bed or other pressure-relieving device.
◆ Initiate rehabilitation immediately. Assist the patient with physical therapy, bowel and bladder training, and the lifestyle changes the condition requires.

ALZHEIMER DISEASE

Alzheimer disease, also called *primary degenerative dementia*, accounts for more than half of all dementias. It results in memory loss, confusion, impaired judgment, personality changes, disorientation, and loss of language skills. Because this is a primary progressive dementia, the prognosis for a patient with this disease is poor.

Causes and incidence

The cause of Alzheimer disease is unknown; however, several factors are thought to be implicated in this disease. These include *neurochemical factors*, such as deficiencies in the neurotransmitter acetylcholine, somatostatin, substance P, and norepinephrine; *environmental factors*; and *genetic immunologic factors*. Genetic studies show that an autosomal dominant form of Alzheimer disease is associated with early onset and early death, accounting for about 100,000 deaths a year. A family history of Alzheimer disease and the presence of Down syndrome are two established risk factors. Alzheimer disease isn't exclusive to the elder population; its onset begins in middle age in 1% to 10% of cases.

The brain tissue of patients with Alzheimer disease has three hallmark features: neurofibrillary tangles, neuritic plaques, and granulovascular degeneration. Examination of the brain after death also finds that it's atrophic, commonly weighing less than 1,000 g, compared with a normal brain weight of about 1,380 g. (See *Tissue changes in Alzheimer disease*, page 189.)

Tissue changes in Alzheimer disease

The illustrations below show the progressive tissue changes that occur in Alzheimer disease.

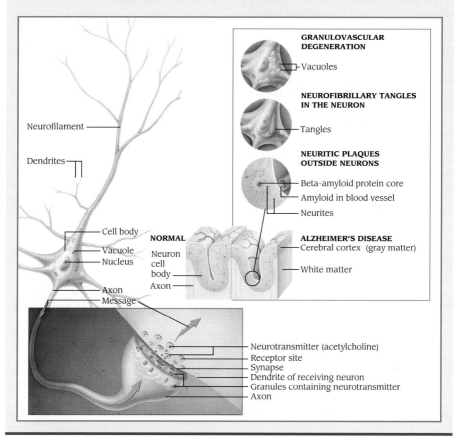

About 360,000 new cases of Alzheimer disease are diagnosed each year.

Pathophysiology

Structural changes in the brain that occur in Alzheimer disease are neurofibrillary tangle (which are fibrous proteins), neuritic plaques (which are degenerative axons and dendrites), and granulovascular changes. There is significant brain tissue loss and loss of cholinergic pathways in the frontal lobe and hippocampus which are responsible for memory and cognitive function.

Complications

◆ Injury
◆ Pneumonia
◆ Infection
◆ Malnutrition
◆ Dehydration

Signs and symptoms

Onset is insidious. Initially, the patient undergoes almost imperceptible changes, such as forgetfulness, recent memory loss, difficulty learning and remembering new information, deterioration in personal hygiene and appearance, and an inability to concentrate. Gradually, tasks that require abstract thinking and activities that require judgment become more difficult. Progressive difficulty in communication and severe deterioration in memory, language, and motor function result in a loss of coordination and an inability to write or speak. Personality changes (restlessness, irritability) and nocturnal awakenings are common.

Patients also exhibit loss of eye contact, a fearful look, wringing of the hands, and other signs of anxiety. When someone with Alzheimer disease is overwhelmed with anxiety, he or she becomes dysfunctional, acutely confused, agitated, compulsive, or fearful.

Eventually, the patient becomes disoriented, and emotional lability and physical and intellectual disability progress. The patient becomes susceptible to infection and accidents. Usually, death results from infection.

Diagnosis

Early diagnosis of Alzheimer disease is difficult because the patient's signs and symptoms are subtle. (See *Organic brain syndrome*.) Diagnosis relies on an accurate history from a reliable family member, mental status and neurologic examinations, and psychometric testing. A positron emission tomography scan measures the metabolic activity of the cerebral cortex and may help in early diagnosis. An EEG and a CT scan may help in later diagnosis. Currently, the disease is diagnosed by exclusion; that is, tests are performed to rule out other disorders. The presence of Alzheimer disease can't be confirmed until death, when pathologic findings are revealed at autopsy.

Treatment

Therapy consists of attempts to slow disease progression, manage behavioral problems, modify the home environment, and elicit family support. Some medications have proven helpful. Tacrine, a centrally acting anticholinesterase agent, is given to treat memory deficits. It has slowed progression of the disease and improved cognitive function in some patients. Other agents include donepezil and rivastigmine. Memantine

hydrochloride reduces chemical actions in the brain that contribute to the symptoms of Alzheimer disease. Underlying disorders that contribute to the patient's confusion, such as hypoxia, are also identified and treated.

Special considerations

Overall care is focused on supporting the patient's remaining abilities and compensating for those lost.

◆ Establish an effective communication system with the patient and family to help them adjust to the patient's altered cognitive abilities.

◆ Offer emotional support to the patient and family members. Behavior problems may be worsened by excess stimulation or change in established routine. Teach them about the disease, and refer them to social service and community resources for legal and financial advice and support.

◆ Anxiety may cause the patient to become agitated or fearful. Intervene by helping the patient focus on another activity.

◆ Provide the patient with a safe environment. Encourage the patient to exercise, as ordered, to help maintain mobility.

CREUTZFELDT–JAKOB DISEASE

Creutzfeldt–Jakob disease (CJD) is a rare, rapidly progressive viral disease that attacks the CNS, causing dementia and neurologic signs and symptoms, such as myoclonic jerking, ataxia, aphasia, visual disturbances, and paralysis. CJD is always fatal. A new variant of CJD (vCJD) emerged in Europe in 1996. (See *Understanding vCJD*, page 191.)

Organic brain syndrome

Although many behavioral disturbances are clearly linked to organic brain dysfunction, the clinical syndromes associated with this type of impairment are sometimes hard to detect because they aren't always determined by the affected area of the brain or even by the extent of tissue damage. Instead, the way the patient's personality interacts with the brain injury determines the specific clinical effects. General symptoms often include impairment of orientation, memory, and intellectual and emotional function. These primary cognitive deficits help to distinguish organic brain syndromes from neurosis and depression.

Diagnosis

Diagnosis of an organic brain syndrome depends on a detailed history of the onset of cognitive and behavioral disturbances; a complete neurologic assessment; and such tests as EEG, computed tomography scans, brain X-rays, cerebrospinal fluid analysis, and psychological studies. Organic brain syndromes are classified by etiology and specific clinical effects. Causes include infection, brain trauma, nutritional deficiency, cerebrovascular disease, degenerative disease, tumor, toxins, and metabolic or endocrine disorders.

Treatment

Effective treatment requires correction of the underlying cause. Special considerations may include reality orientation, emotional support for the patient and the family, a safe environment, mat therapy for an agitated or aggressive patient, and referral for psychological counseling.

Understanding vCJD

Like conventional Creutzfeldt–Jakob disease (CJD), the variant of the disease (vCJD) is a rare, fatal neurodegenerative disease. Most cases have been reported in the United Kingdom. vCJD is most likely caused by exposure to bovine spongiform encephalopathy (BSE)—a fatal brain disease in cattle also known as *mad cow disease*—via ingestion of beef products from cattle with BSE.

vCJD affects patients at a much younger age (younger than 55) than CJD, and the duration of the illness is much longer (14 months).

Regulations have been established in Europe to control outbreaks of BSE in cattle and to prevent contaminated meat from entering the food supply.

Causes and incidence

The causative organism is difficult to identify because no foreign ribonucleic acid or deoxyribonucleic acid has been linked to the disease. CJD is believed to be caused by a specific protein called a *prion*, which lacks nucleic acids, resists proteolytic digestion, and spontaneously aggregates in the brain. Most cases are sporadic; 5% to 15% are familial, with an autosomal dominant pattern of inheritance. Although CJD isn't transmitted by normal casual contact, human-to-human transmission can occur as a result of certain medical procedures, such as corneal and cadaveric dura mater grafts. Isolated cases have resulted from childhood treatment with harvested human growth hormone and from improperly decontaminated neurosurgical instruments and brain electrodes.

CJD typically affects adults 40 to 65 years old and occurs in more than 50 countries. Males and females are affected equally. In people younger than 30, the incidence is 5 in 1 billion; in all other age groups, the incidence is 1 in 1 million.

Pathophysiology

Caused by prions which are deviant forms of harmless proteins found in the brains of mammals and birds. As the prions replicate, they convert normal forms of the protein into their abnormal shape. As the prions accumulate into the nerve cell, they cause neurodegeneration.

Complications

◆ Impaired gait
◆ Incontinence
◆ Akinetic mute state
◆ Bronchopneumonia
◆ Death

Signs and symptoms

Early signs and symptoms of mental impairment may include slowness in thinking, difficulty concentrating, impaired judgment, and memory loss. Dementia is progressive and occurs early. Involuntary movements, such as muscle twitching, trembling, and peculiar body movements, and visual disturbances appear with disease progression and advancing mental deterioration. Hallucinations are also common. The duration of the typical illness is 4 months.

Diagnosis

CJD must be considered for anyone with signs of progressive dementia. Neurologic examination is the most effective tool in diagnosing CJD. Difficulty with rapid alternating movements and point-to-point movements are typically evident early in the disease.

An EEG may be performed to assess the patient for typical changes in brain wave activity. CT scan, MRI of the brain, and lumbar puncture may be useful in ruling out other disorders that cause dementia. Though not diagnostic, the presence of the 14-3-3 protein in the spinal fluid is highly suggestive of the disease when it's accompanied by other characteristic symptoms. Definitive diagnosis usually isn't obtained until an autopsy is done and brain tissue is examined.

Treatment

There's no cure for CJD, and its progress can't be slowed. Palliative care is provided to make the patient comfortable and to ease symptoms. Medications may be needed to control aggressive behaviors. These include sedatives and antipsychotics.

The need to provide a safe environment, control aggressive or agitated behavior, and meet physiologic needs may require monitoring and assistance in the home or in an institutionalized setting. Family counseling may help in coping with the changes required for home care.

Behavior modification may be helpful, in some cases, for controlling unacceptable or dangerous behaviors. Reality orientation, with repeated reinforcement of environmental and other cues, may help reduce disorientation.

Legal advice may be appropriate early in the course of the disorder regarding advance directives, power of attorney, and other legal actions that may make it easier to make ethical decisions regarding the care of an individual with CJD.

Special considerations

◆ Offer emotional support to the patient and family. Teach them about the disease, and assist them through the grieving process. Refer the patient and family to CJD support groups, and encourage participation.

◆ Contact social services and hospice, as appropriate, to assist the family with their needs.

◆ Encourage the patient and family to discuss and complete advance directives.

◆ To prevent disease transmission, use caution when handling body fluids and other materials from patients suspected of having CJD.

REYE SYNDROME

Reye syndrome is an acute illness affecting children and, less commonly, adults. It causes fatty infiltration of the liver with concurrent hyperammonemia, encephalopathy, and increased ICP. In addition, fatty infiltration of the kidneys, brain, and myocardium may occur.

Prognosis depends on the severity of CNS depression. Until recently, mortality was as high as 90%. Today, ICP monitoring and, consequently, early treatment of increased ICP, along with other treatment measures, have cut mortality to about 20%. Death is usually a result of cerebral edema or respiratory arrest. Comatose patients who survive may have residual brain damage.

Causes and incidence

Reye syndrome typically begins within 1 to 3 days of an acute viral infection, such as an upper respiratory tract infection, type B influenza, or varicella (chickenpox). Incidence commonly rises during influenza outbreaks and may be linked to salicylate use. For this reason, use of aspirin for children younger than 15 isn't recommended. The Reye's Syndrome Foundation warns against the use of salicylates, even in topical preparations, when a viral illness is suspected.

In Reye syndrome, damaged hepatic mitochondria disrupt the urea cycle, which normally changes ammonia to urea for its excretion from the body. This results in hyperammonemia, hypoglycemia, and an increase in serum short-chain fatty acids, leading to encephalopathy. Simultaneously, fatty infiltration occurs in renal tubular cells, neuronal tissue, and muscle tissue, including the heart.

Reye syndrome affects children from infancy to adolescence and occurs equally in boys and girls. Peak incidence is at 6 years old.

Pathophysiology

Reye syndrome is the result of damaged hepatic mitochondria which disrupts the urea cycle. The result is hyperammonemia, hypoglycemia, and an increase in serum short-chain fatty acids which leads to encephalopathy.

Complication

◆ Increased ICP

Signs and symptoms

The severity of the child's signs and symptoms varies with the degree of encephalopathy and cerebral edema. In any case, Reye syndrome develops in five stages. After the initial viral infection, a brief recovery period follows when the child doesn't seem seriously ill. A few days later, the patient develops intractable vomiting; lethargy; rapidly changing mental status (mild to severe agitation, confusion, irritability, and delirium); rising blood pressure, respiratory rate, and pulse rate; and hyperactive reflexes.

Reye syndrome commonly progresses to coma. As coma deepens, seizures develop, followed by decreased tendon reflexes and, usually, respiratory failure.

Increased ICP, a serious complication, is now considered the result of an increased cerebral blood volume causing intracranial hypertension. Such swelling may develop as a result of acidosis, increased cerebral metabolic rate, and an impaired autoregulatory mechanism.

Diagnosis

A history of a recent viral disorder with typical clinical features strongly suggests Reye syndrome. An increased serum ammonia level, abnormal clotting studies, and hepatic dysfunction confirm it. Testing serum salicylate level rules out aspirin use. Absence of jaundice despite increased liver aminotransferase levels rules out acute hepatic failure and hepatic encephalopathy.

Abnormal test results may include:

◆ Liver function studies—aspartate aminotransferase and alanine aminotransferase elevated to twice normal levels; bilirubin level usually normal.

◆ Liver biopsy—fatty droplets uniformly distributed throughout cells.

◆ CSF analysis—white blood cell count less than 10/µL; with coma, increased CSF pressure.

◆ Coagulation studies—prothrombin time and partial thromboplastin time prolonged.

◆ Blood values—serum ammonia levels elevated; serum glucose levels normal or, in 15% of cases, low; serum fatty acid and lactate levels increased.

Treatment

For treatment guidelines, see *Stages of treatment for Reye syndrome.*

Stages of treatment for Reye syndrome

Signs and symptoms	Baseline treatment	Baseline intervention
Stage I: vomiting, lethargy, hepatic dysfunction	◆ To decrease intracranial pressure (ICP) and brain edema, give I.V. fluids at $^2/_3$ maintenance. Also give an osmotic diuretic or furosemide. ◆ To treat hypoprothrombinemia, give vitamin K; if vitamin K is unsuccessful, give fresh frozen plasma. ◆ Monitor serum ammonia and blood glucose levels and plasma osmolality every 4 to 8 hours to check progress.	◆ Monitor the patient's vital signs and check the level of consciousness for increasing lethargy. Take vital signs more often as the patient's condition deteriorates. ◆ Monitor fluid intake and output to prevent fluid overload. Maintain urine output at 1.0 mL/kg/hour; plasma osmolality, 290 mOsm; and blood glucose, 150 mg/mL. (*Goal:* Keep glucose level high, osmolality normal to high, and ammonia level low.) Also, restrict protein.
Stage II: hyperventilation, delirium, hepatic dysfunction, hyperactive reflexes	◆ Continue baseline treatment.	◆ Maintain seizure precautions. ◆ Immediately report any signs of coma that require invasive, supportive therapy, such as intubation. ◆ Keep the head of the bed at a 30-degree angle.
Stage III: coma, hyperventilation, decorticate rigidity, hepatic dysfunction	◆ Continue baseline and seizure treatment. ◆ Monitor ICP with a subarachnoid screw or other invasive device. ◆ Provide endotracheal intubation and mechanical ventilation to control the partial pressure of arterial carbon dioxide ($PaCO_2$) levels. A paralyzing agent, such as atracurium or pancuronium I.V., may help maintain ventilation. ◆ Give mannitol I.V. or glycerol by nasogastric tube.	◆ Monitor ICP (should be less than 20 mm Hg before suctioning) or give a barbiturate I.V., as ordered; hyperventilate the patient as necessary. ◆ When ventilating the patient, maintain $PaCO_2$ between 25 and 30 mm Hg and the partial pressure of arterial oxygen between 80 and 100 mm Hg. ◆ Closely monitor cardiovascular status with a pulmonary artery catheter or central venous pressure line. ◆ Give skin and mouth care and perform range-of-motion exercises.
Stage IV: deepening coma; decerebrate rigidity; large, fixed pupils; minimal hepatic dysfunction	◆ Continue baseline and supportive care. ◆ If all previous measures fail, some pediatric centers use barbiturate coma, decompressive craniotomy, hypothermia, or exchange transfusion.	◆ Check the patient for loss of reflexes and signs of flaccidity. ◆ Give the patient's family the extra support they need, considering their child's poor prognosis.
Stage V: seizures, loss of deep tendon reflexes, flaccidity, respiratory arrest, ammonia level above 300 mg/dL	◆ Continue baseline and supportive care.	◆ Help the patient's family to face impending death.

!!!!!! **PREVENTION** *Advise parents to give nonsalic-ylate analgesics and antipyretics such as acet-aminophen. For more information, refer parents to the National Reye's Syndrome Foundation.*

GUILLAIN–BARRÉ SYNDROME

Guillain–Barré syndrome is an acute, rapidly progressive, and potentially fatal form of poly-neuritis that causes muscle weakness and mild distal sensory loss. Recovery is spontaneous and complete in about 95% of patients, although mild motor or reflex deficits in the feet and legs may persist. The prognosis is best when symp-toms clear between 15 and 20 days after onset.

Causes and incidence

Precisely what causes Guillain–Barré syndrome is unknown, but it may be a cell-mediated immunologic attack on peripheral nerves in response to a virus. The major pathologic effect is segmental demyelination of the peripheral nerves. Because this syndrome causes inflam-mation and degenerative changes in both the posterior (sensory) and anterior (motor) nerve roots, signs of sensory and motor losses occur simultaneously.

This syndrome (also called infectious poly-neuritis, Landry–Guillain–Barré syndrome, and acute idiopathic polyneuritis) can occur at any age but is most common between 30 and 50 years old; it affects both sexes equally. In the United States, it has an incidence of 0.6 to 2.4 cases per 100,000 people.

Pathophysiology

Guillain–Barré is the result of segmental de-myelination of the peripheral nerves resulting in inflammation and swelling. The result is impairment of impulse transmission along the dorsal and anterior nerve roots—motor and sensory loss occurs simultaneously.

Complications

- Thrombophlebitis
- Pressure ulcers
- Contractures
- Muscle wasting
- Aspiration
- Respiratory tract infections
- Respiratory and cardiac compromise

Signs and symptoms

About 50% of patients with Guillain–Barré syndrome have a history of minor febrile illness (10 to 14 days before onset), usually an upper respiratory tract infection or, less commonly, gastroenteritis with *Campylobacter jejuni*. When infection precedes onset of Guillain–Barré syndrome, signs of infection subside before neurologic features appear. Other possible precipitating factors include surgery; rabies or swine influenza vaccination, viral illness such as Epstein–Barr virus, cytomegalovirus, hepatitis, and HIV; Hodgkin or other malignant disease; and lupus erythematosus.

Symmetrical muscle weakness, the major neurologic sign, usually appears in the legs first (ascending type) and then extends to the arms and facial nerves in 24 to 72 hours. Some-times, muscle weakness develops in the arms first (descending type) or in the arms and legs simultaneously. (See *Testing for thoracic sensa-tion*, page 195.) In milder forms of this disease, muscle weakness may affect only the cranial nerves or may not occur at all.

Another common neurologic sign is par-esthesia, which sometimes precedes muscle weakness but tends to vanish quickly. However, some patients with this disorder never develop this symptom. Other clinical features may include facial diplegia (possibly with ophthal-moplegia), dysphagia or dysarthria and, less commonly, weakness of the muscles supplied by cranial nerve XI. Muscle weakness develops so quickly that muscle atrophy doesn't occur, but hypotonia and areflexia do. Stiffness and pain in the form of a severe "charley horse" commonly occur.

The clinical course of Guillain–Barré syn-drome is divided into three phases. The initial phase begins when the first definitive symptom appears and ends 1 to 3 weeks later, when no further deterioration manifests. The plateau phase lasts several days to 2 weeks and is fol-lowed by the recovery phase, which is believed to coincide with remyelination and axonal pro-cess regrowth. The recovery phase extends over a period of 4 to 6 months; patients with severe disease may take up to 2 years to recover, and recovery may not be complete.

Diagnosis

A history of febrile illness (usually a respiratory tract infection) and typical clinical features sug-gest Guillain–Barré syndrome.

Several days after onset of signs and symptoms, CSF protein levels begin to rise, peaking in 4 to 6 weeks, probably as a result of widespread inflammatory disease of the nerve roots. CSF white blood cell count remains normal, but in severe disease, CSF pressure may rise above normal. Probably because of predisposing infection, CBC shows leukocy-tosis and a shift to immature forms early in

Testing for thoracic sensation

When Guillain–Barré syndrome progresses rapidly, test for ascending sensory loss by touching the patient or pressing the skin lightly with a pin every hour. Move systematically from the iliac crest (T12) to the scapula, occasionally substituting the blunt end of the pin to test the patient's ability to discriminate between sharp and dull.

Mark the level of diminished sensation to measure any change. If diminished sensation ascends to T8 or higher, the patient's intercostal muscle function (and consequently respiratory function) will probably be impaired. As Guillain–Barré syndrome subsides, sensory and motor weakness descends to the lower thoracic segments, heralding a return of intercostal and extremity muscle function.

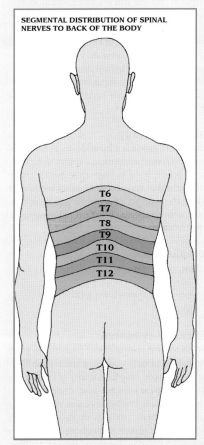

SEGMENTAL DISTRIBUTION OF SPINAL NERVES TO BACK OF THE BODY

T6
T7
T8
T9
T10
T11
T12

Key: T, thoracic segments.

the illness, but blood studies soon return to normal. Electromyography may show repeated firing of the same motor unit instead of widespread sectional stimulation. Nerve conduction velocities are slowed soon after paralysis develops and show demyelination. Diagnosis must rule out similar diseases such as acute poliomyelitis.

Treatment
Treatment is primarily supportive, including such measures as endotracheal (ET) intubation or tracheotomy if the patient has difficulty clearing secretions. Preventing complications is another goal of treatment.

Plasmapheresis is useful in decreasing severity of symptoms, thereby facilitating a more rapid recovery. I.V. immune globulin is equally effective in reducing the severity and duration of symptoms.

Special considerations
Monitoring the patient for escalation of symptoms is of special concern.
◆ Watch for ascending sensory loss, which precedes motor loss. Also, monitor vital signs and LOC.
◆ Assess and treat respiratory dysfunction. If respiratory muscles are weak, take serial vital capacity recordings. Use a respirometer with a mouthpiece or a face mask for bedside testing.
◆ Obtain ABG measurements. Because neuromuscular disease results in primary hypoventilation with hypoxemia and hypercapnia, watch for respiratory failure. Be alert to signs of rising partial pressure of carbon dioxide (such as confusion and tachypnea).
◆ Auscultate breath sounds, turn and position the patient, and encourage coughing and deep breathing. Begin respiratory support at the first sign of dyspnea or with decreasing partial pressure of arterial oxygen.
◆ If respiratory failure becomes imminent, establish an emergency airway with an ET tube.
◆ Give meticulous skin care to prevent skin breakdown and contractures. Establish a strict turning schedule; inspect the skin (especially sacrum, heels, and ankles) for breakdown, and reposition the patient every 2 hours. After each position change, stimulate circulation by carefully massaging pressure points. Also, use foam, gel, or alternating pressure pads at points of contact.
◆ Perform passive range-of-motion exercises within the patient's pain limits. When the patient's condition stabilizes, change to gentle stretching and active assistance exercises.

◆ To prevent aspiration, test the gag reflex, and elevate the head of the bed before giving the patient anything to eat. If the gag reflex is absent, give nasogastric feedings until this reflex returns. If the patient has severe paralysis and is expected to have a long recovery period, a gastrostomy tube may be necessary to provide adequate nourishment.

◆ As the patient regains strength and can tolerate a vertical position, be alert to postural hypotension. Monitor blood pressure and pulse during tilting periods and, if necessary, apply toe-to-groin elastic bandages to prevent postural hypotension.

◆ Inspect the patient's legs regularly for signs of thrombophlebitis (localized pain, tenderness, erythema, edema, and positive Homans sign), a common complication of Guillain–Barré syndrome. To prevent thrombophlebitis, apply antiembolism stockings and give prophylactic anticoagulants, as ordered.

◆ If the patient has facial paralysis, give eye and mouth care every 4 hours.

◆ Watch for urine retention. Measure and record intake and output every 8 hours, and offer the bedpan every 3 to 4 hours. Encourage adequate fluid intake of 2 qt (about 2 L) per day, unless contraindicated. If urine retention develops, begin intermittent catheterization as ordered. Because the abdominal muscles are weak, the patient may need manual pressure on the bladder (Credé method) before they can urinate.

◆ To prevent or relieve constipation, offer the patient plenty of water, prune juice, and a high-bulk diet. If necessary, give daily or alternate-day suppositories (glycerin or bisacodyl) or enemas, as ordered.

◆ Before discharge, prepare a home care plan. Teach the patient how to transfer from bed to wheelchair, from wheelchair to toilet or tub, and how to walk short distances with a walker or a cane. Teach the family how to help the patient eat, compensating for facial weakness, and how to help avoid skin breakdown. Stress the need for a regular bowel and bladder routine. Refer the patient for physical therapy as needed.

◆ Refer the patient's family to the Guillain–Barré Syndrome Foundation International.

Neuromuscular disorders

MYASTHENIA GRAVIS

Myasthenia gravis produces sporadic but progressive weakness and abnormal fatigability of striated (skeletal) muscles, exacerbated by exercise and repeated movement, but improved by anticholinesterase drugs. Usually, this disorder affects muscles innervated by the cranial nerves (face, lips, tongue, neck, and throat), but it can affect any muscle group. Myasthenia gravis follows an unpredictable course of recurring exacerbations and periodic remissions. There's no known cure. Drug treatment has improved prognosis and allows patients to lead relatively normal lives except during exacerbations. When the disease involves the respiratory system, it may be life threatening.

Causes and incidence

Myasthenia gravis causes a failure in transmission of nerve impulses at the neuromuscular junction. Theoretically, such impairment may result from an autoimmune response, ineffective acetylcholine release, or inadequate muscle fiber response to acetylcholine. (See *What happens in myasthenia gravis*, page 197.)

Myasthenia gravis affects 3 of every 10,000 people at any age, but it's more common in young women and older men. About 20% of neonates born to mothers with myasthenia gravis have transient (or occasionally persistent) myasthenia. This disease may coexist with immunologic and thyroid disorders; about 15% of patients with myasthenia gravis have thymomas. Remissions occur in about 25% of patients.

Pathophysiology

Myasthenia gravis is a breakdown of transmission across the neuromuscular junction. The site of action is the postsynaptic membrane. It is thought that receptor antibodies weaken or reduce the number of acetylcholine receptors at the neuromuscular junction reducing muscle depolarization.

Complications

◆ Respiratory distress
◆ Pneumonia
◆ Chewing and swallowing difficulties
◆ Aspiration

Signs and symptoms

The dominant symptoms of myasthenia gravis are skeletal muscle weakness and fatigability. In the early stages, easy fatigability of certain muscles may appear with no other findings. Later, it may be severe enough to cause paralysis. Typically, myasthenic muscles are strongest in the morning but weaken throughout the day, especially after exercise. Short rest periods temporarily restore muscle function. Muscle weakness is progressive; more and more muscles become

What happens in myasthenia gravis

During normal neuromuscular transmission, a motor nerve impulse travels to a motor nerve terminal, stimulating the release of a chemical neurotransmitter called *acetylcholine*. When acetylcholine diffuses across the synapse, receptor sites in the motor end plate react and depolarize the muscle fiber. The depolarization spreads through the muscle fiber, causing muscle contraction.

In myasthenia gravis, antibodies attach to the acetylcholine receptor sites. They block, destroy, and weaken these sites, leaving them insensitive to acetylcholine, thereby blocking neuromuscular transmission.

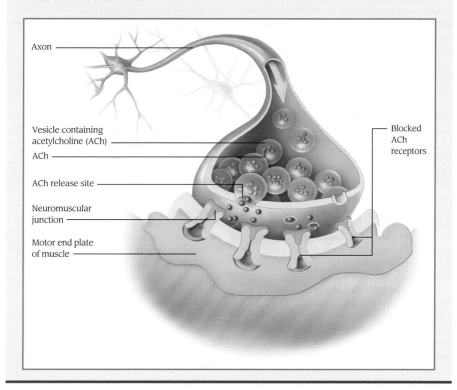

weak, and eventually some muscles may lose function entirely. Resulting symptoms depend on the muscle group affected; they become more intense during menses and after emotional stress, prolonged exposure to sunlight or cold, or infections.

Onset may be sudden or insidious. In many patients, weak eye closure, ptosis, and diplopia are the first signs that something is wrong. Patients with myasthenia gravis usually have blank, expressionless faces and nasal vocal tones. They experience frequent nasal regurgitation of fluids and have difficulty chewing and swallowing. Because of this, they usually worry about choking. Their eyelids droop (ptosis),

and they may have to tilt their heads back to see. Their neck muscles may become too weak to support their heads without bobbing.

In patients with weakened respiratory muscles, decreased tidal volume and vital capacity make breathing difficult and predispose to pneumonia and other respiratory tract infections. Respiratory muscle weakness (myasthenic crisis) may be severe enough to require an emergency airway and mechanical ventilation.

Diagnosis

Repeated muscle use over a very short time that fatigues and then improves with rest suggests a diagnosis of myasthenia gravis. Tests for this neurologic condition record the effect of exercise and subsequent rest on muscle weakness. Electromyography, with repeated neural stimulation, may help confirm this diagnosis. Acetylcholine receptor antibodies may be present in the blood.

℞ CONFIRMING DIAGNOSIS *The classic proof of myasthenia gravis is improved muscle function after an I.V. injection of edrophonium or neostigmine (anticholinesterase drugs).*

In patients with myasthenia gravis, muscle function improves within 30 to 60 seconds and lasts up to 30 minutes. Long-standing ocular muscle dysfunction may fail to respond to such testing. This test can differentiate a myasthenic crisis from a cholinergic crisis (caused by acetylcholine overactivity at the neuromuscular junction). The acetylcholine receptor antibody titer may be elevated in generalized myasthenia. Evaluation should rule out thyroid disease and thymoma.

Treatment

Treatment is symptomatic. Anticholinesterase drugs, such as neostigmine and pyridostigmine, counteract fatigue and muscle weakness and allow about 80% of normal muscle function. However, these drugs become less effective as the disease worsens. Corticosteroids may relieve symptoms. Immunosuppressants are also used. Plasmapheresis is used in severe myasthenic exacerbation.

Patients with thymomas require thymectomy, which may cause remission in some cases of adult-onset myasthenia. Acute exacerbations that cause severe respiratory distress necessitate emergency treatment. Tracheotomy, positive-pressure ventilation, and vigorous suctioning to remove secretions usually produce improvement in a few days. Because anticholinesterase drugs aren't effective in myasthenic crisis, they're stopped until respiratory function improves. Myasthenic crisis requires immediate hospitalization and vigorous respiratory support.

Special considerations

Careful baseline assessment, early recognition and treatment of potential crises, supportive measures, and thorough patient teaching can minimize exacerbations and complications. Continuity of care is essential.

◆ Establish an accurate neurologic and respiratory baseline. Thereafter, monitor tidal volume and vital capacity regularly. The patient may need a ventilator and frequent suctioning to remove accumulating secretions.

◆ Be alert to signs of an impending crisis (increased muscle weakness, respiratory distress, and difficulty in talking or chewing).

◆ To prevent relapses, adhere closely to the ordered drug administration schedule. Be prepared to give atropine for anticholinesterase overdose or toxicity.

◆ Plan exercise, meals, patient care, and activities to make the most of energy peaks. For example, give medication 20 to 30 minutes before meals to facilitate chewing or swallowing. Allow the patient to participate in care.

◆ When swallowing is difficult, give soft, solid foods instead of liquids to lessen the risk of choking.

◆ Patient teaching is essential because myasthenia gravis is usually a lifelong condition. Help the patient plan daily activities to coincide with energy peaks. Stress the need for frequent rest periods throughout the day. Emphasize that periodic remissions, exacerbations, and day-to-day fluctuations are common.

◆ Teach the patient how to recognize adverse effects and signs of toxicity of anticholinesterase drugs (headaches, weakness, sweating, abdominal cramps, nausea, vomiting, diarrhea, excessive salivation, and bronchospasm) and corticosteroids (euphoria, insomnia, edema, and increased appetite).

◆ Warn the patient to avoid strenuous exercise, stress, infection, and needless exposure to the sun or cold. All of these things may worsen signs and symptoms.

◆ For more information and an opportunity to meet other myasthenia gravis patients who lead full, productive lives, refer the patient to the Myasthenia Gravis Foundation.

AMYOTROPHIC LATERAL SCLEROSIS

Amyotrophic lateral sclerosis (ALS), also called *Lou Gehrig disease*, is the most common of the motor neuron diseases that cause muscle atrophy. (See *Motor neuron disease*, page 199.) Other motor neuron diseases include progressive muscular atrophy and progressive bulbar palsy. A chronic, progressively debilitating disease, ALS may be fatal in less than 1 year or may continue for 10 years or more, depending on the muscles it affects.

Causes and incidence

ALS affects about 1 of 100,000 people. The exact cause of ALS is unknown, but about 10% of cases have a genetic component. In these patients, it's an autosomal dominant trait and affects men and women equally.

Other than a family member affected with the hereditary form, there are no known risk factors.

Pathophysiology

The principle feature in ALS is the loss of both upper and lower motor neurons. Loss of the motor neurons results in axonal degeneration and secondary demyelination with glial proliferation and sclerosis.

Complications

- Pneumonia
- Aspiration
- Pressure ulcers
- Contractures

Signs and symptoms

Progressive loss of muscle strength and coordination eventually interfere with everyday activities. Patients with ALS develop fasciculations, accompanied by atrophy and weakness, especially in the muscles of the feet and the hands. Other signs include impaired speech; difficulty chewing, swallowing, and breathing; and, occasionally, choking and excessive drooling. Mental deterioration doesn't occur, but patients may become depressed as a reaction to the disease.

Diagnosis

Characteristic clinical features indicate a combination of upper and lower motor neuron involvement without sensory impairment. Electromyography and muscle biopsy indicate that the motor nerves aren't functioning, yet sensory nerves are normal. CT scan and MRI may help rule out other conditions, such as MS, spinal cord neoplasm, CNS syphilis, polyarteritis, syringomyelia, myasthenia gravis, progressive muscular dystrophy, and progressive strokes.

Treatment

Management aims to control symptoms and provide emotional, psychological, and physical support. Riluzole may increase quality of life and survival but doesn't reverse or stop disease progression.

Baclofen or diazepam helps control spasticity that interferes with activities of daily living. Trihexyphenidyl or amitriptyline may be used for impaired ability to swallow saliva. Gastrostomy may be needed early to prevent choking; referral to an otolaryngologist is advised. Physical therapy, rehabilitation, and use of appliances or orthopedic intervention may be required to maximize function. Devices to assist in breathing at night or mechanical ventilation should be discussed, but the patient's wishes should be respected.

Special considerations

Because mental status remains intact while progressive physical degeneration takes place, the patient acutely perceives every change. This threatens the patient's relationships, career, income, muscle coordination, sexuality, and energy.

- Implement a rehabilitation program designed to maintain independence for as long as possible.
- Help the patient obtain assistive equipment, such as a walker and a wheelchair. Arrange for a visiting nurse to oversee the patient's status, to provide support, and to teach the family about the illness.
- Depending on the patient's muscular capacity, assist with bathing, personal hygiene, and transfers from wheelchair to bed. Help establish a regular bowel and bladder routine.
- To help the patient handle increased accumulation of secretions and dysphagia, teach them how to perform self-suction. He should have a suction machine handy at home to reduce the fear of choking.
- To prevent skin breakdown, provide good skin care when the patient is bedridden. Turn the patient often, keep skin clean and dry, and use pressure-reducing devices such as alternating air mattress.

Motor neuron disease

In its final stages, motor neuron disease affects both upper and lower motor neuron cells. However, the site of initial cell damage varies according to the specific disease:

- *progressive bulbar palsy:* degeneration of upper motor neurons in the medulla oblongata
- *progressive muscular atrophy:* degeneration of lower motor neurons in the spinal cord
- *amyotrophic lateral sclerosis:* degeneration of upper motor neurons in the medulla oblongata and lower motor neurons in the spinal cord.

◆ If the patient has trouble swallowing, give soft, solid foods and position upright during meals. Gastrostomy and nasogastric tube feedings may be necessary if the patient can no longer swallow. Teach the patient (if still able to feed self) or family how to administer gastrostomy feedings.

◆ Provide emotional support. A discussion of directives regarding healthcare decisions should be instituted before the patient becomes unable to communicate his or her wishes. Prepare the patient and family members for eventual death, and encourage the start of the grieving process. Patients with ALS may benefit from a hospice program or the local ALS support group chapter.

MULTIPLE SCLEROSIS

MS is a progressive disease caused by demyelination of the white matter of the brain and spinal cord. (See *Understanding myelin breakdown*, page 201.) In this disease, sporadic patches of demyelination throughout the CNS induce widely disseminated and varied neurologic dysfunction. Characterized by exacerbations and remissions, MS is a major cause of chronic disability in young adults.

The prognosis varies; MS may progress rapidly, disabling some patients by early adulthood or causing death within months of onset. However, 70% of patients lead active, productive lives with prolonged remissions.

Causes and incidence

The exact cause of MS is unknown, but current theories suggest a slow-acting or latent viral infection and an autoimmune response. Other theories suggest that environmental and genetic factors may also be linked to MS. Emotional stress, overwork, fatigue, pregnancy, and acute respiratory tract infections have been known to precede the onset of this illness.

MS usually begins between 20 and 40 years old. It affects more women than men. A family history of MS and living in a geographical area with a higher incidence of MS (northern Europe, northern United States, southern Australia, and New Zealand) increase the risk.

Pathophysiology

There is sporadic patchy axon demyelination and nerve fiber loss throughout the CNS. Loss of the myelin sheath disrupts nerve conduction with subsequent neuronal death and atrophy.

Complications

◆ Injuries from falls
◆ Urinary tract infections
◆ Constipation
◆ Joint contractures
◆ Pressure ulcers
◆ Rectal distention
◆ Pneumonia

Signs and symptoms

Clinical findings in MS depend on the extent and site of myelin destruction, the extent of remyelination, and the adequacy of subsequent restored synaptic transmission.

Signs and symptoms in MS may be transient, or they may last for hours or weeks. They may wax and wane with no predictable pattern, vary from day to day, and be bizarre and difficult for the patient to describe.

In most patients, visual problems and sensory impairment, such as numbness and tingling sensations (paresthesia), are the first signs that something may be wrong.

Other characteristic changes include:
◆ *ocular disturbances*—optic neuritis, diplopia, ophthalmoplegia, blurred vision, and nystagmus
◆ *muscle dysfunction*—weakness, paralysis ranging from monoplegia to quadriplegia, spasticity, hyperreflexia, intention tremor, and gait ataxia
◆ *urinary disturbances*—incontinence, frequency, urgency, and frequent infections
◆ *emotional lability*—characteristic mood swings, irritability, euphoria, and depression.

Associated signs and symptoms include poorly articulated or scanning speech and dysphagia. Clinical effects may be so mild that the patient is unaware of them or so bizarre that they appear hysterical.

Diagnosis

A misdiagnosis of psychiatric problems is common. Because early symptoms may be mild, years may elapse between onset of the first signs and the diagnosis, which typically requires evidence of multiple neurologic attacks and characteristic remissions and exacerbations. MRI may detect MS lesions; however, diagnosis still remains difficult. Periodic testing and close observation of the patient are necessary, perhaps for years, depending on the course of the disease.

Abnormal EEG findings occur in one third of patients. Lumbar puncture shows elevated gamma globulin fraction of immunoglobulin G but normal total CSF protein levels. Elevated CSF gamma globulin is significant only when serum gamma globulin levels are normal because it reflects hyperactivity of the immune system due to chronic demyelination. Oligoclonal bands of immunoglobulin can be detected

Understanding myelin breakdown

Myelin plays a key role in speeding electrical impulses to the brain for interpretation. The myelin sheath is a lipoprotein complex formed of glial cells. It protects the neuron's long nerve fiber (axon) much like the insulation on an electrical wire. Because of its high electrical resistance and weak ability to store an electrical charge, the myelin sheath permits conduction of nerve impulses from one node of Ranvier to the next.

Effects of injury

Myelin can be injured by hypoxemia, toxic chemicals, vascular insufficiency, or autoimmune responses. When this occurs, the myelin sheath becomes inflamed and the membrane layers break down into smaller components. These components become well-circumscribed plaques filled with microglial elements, macroglia, and lymphocytes. This process is called *demyelination*.

The damaged myelin sheath impairs normal conduction, causing partial loss or dispersion of the action potential and consequent neurologic dysfunction.

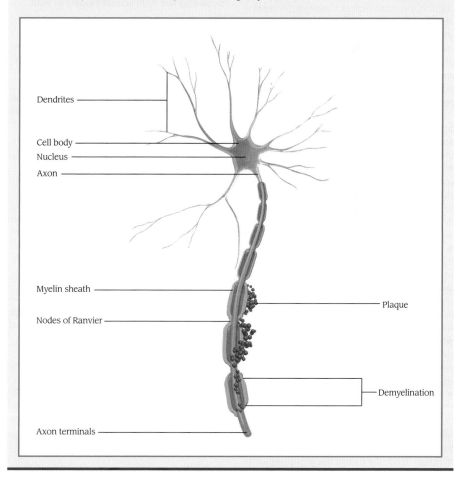

when gamma globulin in CSF is examined by electrophoresis, and these bands are present in most patients, even when the percentage of gamma globulin in CSF is normal. In addition, the white blood cell count in CSF may rise.

Differential diagnosis must rule out spinal cord compression, foramen magnum tumor (may mimic the exacerbations and remissions of MS), multiple small strokes, syphilis or other infection, and psychological disturbances.

Treatment

The aim of treatment is to shorten exacerbations and relieve neurologic deficits so that the patient can resume a normal lifestyle. Those with relapsing–remitting courses are placed on immune modulating therapy, with interferon or glatiramer acetate. Steroids are used to reduce the associated edema of the myelin sheath during exacerbations.

Other drugs include baclofen, tizanidine, or diazepam to relieve spasticity; cholinergic agents to relieve urine retention and minimize frequency and urgency; amantadine to relieve fatigue; and antidepressants to help with mood or behavioral symptoms. During acute exacerbations, supportive measures include bed rest, comfort measures such as massages, prevention of fatigue, prevention of pressure ulcers, bowel and bladder training (if necessary), administration of antibiotics for bladder infections, physical therapy, and counseling. Physical therapy, speech therapy, occupational therapy, and support groups are also useful. Planned exercise programs help with maintaining muscle tone.

Special considerations

Management considerations focus on educating the patient and family.
◆ Assist with physical therapy. Increase patient comfort with massages and relaxing baths. Assist with active, resistive, and stretching exercises to maintain muscle tone and joint mobility, decrease spasticity, improve coordination, and boost morale.
◆ Educate the patient and family concerning the chronic course of MS. Emphasize the need to avoid temperature extremes, stress, fatigue, and infections and other illnesses, all of which can trigger an MS attack. Advise the patient to maintain independence by developing new ways of performing daily activities.
◆ Stress the importance of eating a nutritious, well-balanced diet that contains sufficient roughage and adequate fluids to prevent constipation.
◆ Evaluate the need for bowel and bladder training during hospitalization. Encourage adequate fluid intake and regular urination. Eventually, the patient may require urinary drainage by self-catheterization or, in men, condom drainage. Teach the correct use of suppositories to help establish a regular bowel schedule.
◆ Promote emotional stability. Help the patient establish a daily routine to maintain optimal functioning. Activity level is regulated by tolerance level. Encourage regular rest periods to prevent fatigue and daily physical exercise.
◆ Inform the patient that exacerbations are unpredictable, necessitating physical and emotional adjustments in lifestyle.
◆ For more information, refer the patient to the National Multiple Sclerosis Society.

Cranial nerve disorders

TRIGEMINAL NEURALGIA

Trigeminal neuralgia, also called *tic douloureux*, is a painful disorder of one or more branches of the fifth cranial (trigeminal) nerve that produces paroxysmal attacks of excruciating facial pain precipitated by stimulation of a trigger zone. It can subside spontaneously, and remissions may last from several months to years.

Causes and incidence

Although the cause remains undetermined, trigeminal neuralgia may reflect an afferent reflex in the brainstem or in the sensory root of the trigeminal nerve. Such neuralgia may also be related to compression of the nerve root by posterior fossa tumors, middle fossa tumors, or vascular lesions (subclinical aneurysm), although such lesions usually produce simultaneous loss of sensation. Occasionally, trigeminal neuralgia is a manifestation of MS or herpes zoster. Regardless of the cause, the pain of trigeminal neuralgia is probably produced by an interaction or short-circuiting of touch and pain fibers.

Trigeminal neuralgia occurs mostly in people older than 40, in women more commonly than in men, and on the right side of the face more commonly than on the left. The incidence is 4 to 5 cases per 100,000 people.

Pathophysiology

The exact pathophysiology of trigeminal neuralgia is controversial. It can be either centrally mediated or peripherally mediated. The trigeminal nerve itself can cause the pain as its major function is sensory. There is also a belief that the pain is mediated by vascular compression of the nerve but in 85% of people there is no structural lesion. Microanatomic small and large fiber demyelination is often seen at the root entry zone. There is a lack of inhibitory inputs and a re-entry mechanism causes an amplification of sensory inputs.

Complications

◆ Double vision
◆ Jaw weakness
◆ Loss of corneal reflex
◆ Malnutrition
◆ Numbness of face

Signs and symptoms

Typically, the patient reports a searing or burning pain that occurs in lightning like jabs and lasts from 1 to 15 minutes (usually 1 to 2 minutes) in an area innervated by one of the divisions of the trigeminal nerve, primarily the superior mandibular or maxillary division. The pain rarely affects more than one division and seldom the first division (ophthalmic) or both sides of the face. It affects the second (maxillary) and third (mandibular) divisions of the trigeminal nerve equally. (See *Trigeminal nerve function and distribution.*)

These attacks characteristically follow stimulation of a trigger zone, usually by a light touch to a hypersensitive area, such as the tip of the nose, the cheeks, or the gums. Although attacks can occur at any time, they may follow a draft of air, exposure to heat or cold, eating, smiling, talking, or drinking hot or cold beverages. The frequency of attacks varies greatly, from many times a day to several times a month or year.

Between attacks, most patients are free from pain, although some have a constant, dull ache. No patient is ever free from the fear of the next attack.

Diagnosis

The patient's pain history is the basis for diagnosis because trigeminal neuralgia produces no objective clinical or pathologic changes. Physical examination shows no impairment of sensory or motor function; indeed, sensory impairment implies a space-occupying lesion as the cause of pain.

Observation during the examination shows the patient favoring (splinting) the affected area. To ward off a painful attack, the patient commonly holds the face immobile when talking. The patient may also leave the affected side of the face unwashed and unshaven or protect it with a coat or shawl. When asked where the pain occurs, the patient points to—but never touches—the affected area. Witnessing a typical attack helps to confirm diagnosis. Rarely, a tumor in the posterior fossa can produce pain that's clinically indistinguishable from trigeminal neuralgia. Skull X-rays, CT scan, and MRI rule out sinus or tooth infections and tumors. If the patient has trigeminal neuralgia, these test results are normal.

Treatment

Oral administration of carbamazepine (Tegretol), gabapentin (Neurontin), or phenytoin may temporarily relieve or prevent pain. Opioids are of little help during the pain episode. Caution should be used when treating a chronic problem with opioids.

When these medical measures fail or attacks become increasingly frequent or severe, neurosurgical procedures may provide permanent relief. The preferred procedure is percutaneous electrocoagulation of nerve rootlets under a local anesthetic. Other treatments include a percutaneous radio frequency procedure, which causes partial root destruction and relieves pain, and microsurgery for vascular decompression of the trigeminal nerve. Gamma knife radiosurgery, the least invasive procedure, can be done for patients refractory to medications or patients who have multiple medical comorbidities.

Special considerations

The focus here is management of pain.

◆ Observe and record the characteristics of each attack, including the patient's protective mechanisms.

Trigeminal nerve function and distribution

Function

◆ Motor: chewing movements
◆ Sensory: sensations of face, scalp, and teeth (mouth and nasal chamber)

Distribution

I. Ophthalmic
II. Maxillary
III. Mandibular

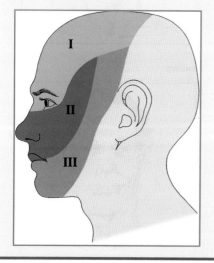

◆ Provide adequate nutrition in small, frequent meals served at room temperature.

◆ Avoid jarring the bed and causing increased discomfort.

◆ If the patient is receiving neuroleptics, watch for cutaneous and hematologic reactions (erythematous and pruritic rashes, urticaria, photosensitivity, exfoliative dermatitis, leukopenia, agranulocytosis, eosinophilia, aplastic anemia, and thrombocytopenia) and, possibly, urine retention and transient drowsiness. For the first 3 months of therapy, monitor CBC and liver function weekly, then monthly thereafter. Warn the patient to immediately report fever, sore throat, mouth ulcers, easy bruising, or petechial or purpuric hemorrhage because these may signal thrombocytopenia or aplastic anemia and may require discontinuation of drug therapy.

◆ If the patient is receiving phenytoin, also watch for adverse effects, including ataxia, skin eruptions, gingival hyperplasia, and nystagmus.

◆ After resection of the first branch of the trigeminal nerve, tell the patient to avoid rubbing their eyes and using aerosol spray. Advise the patient to wear glasses or goggles outdoors and to blink often.

◆ After surgery to sever the second or third branch, tell the patient to avoid hot foods and drinks, which could burn the mouth, and to chew carefully to avoid biting the mouth. The patient may need to eat pureed food, possibly through a straw. Advise the patient to place food in the unaffected side of the mouth when chewing, to brush teeth and rinse the mouth often, and to see the dentist twice a year to detect cavities because they won't experience pain from cavities in the area of the severed nerve.

◆ After surgical decompression of the root or partial nerve dissection, check neurologic and vital signs often.

◆ Provide emotional support, and encourage the patient to express their feelings. Promote independence through self-care and maximum physical activity. Reinforce natural avoidance of stimulation (air, heat, and cold) of trigger zones (lips, cheeks, and gums).

BELL PALSY

Bell palsy is a disease of the seventh cranial nerve (facial) that produces unilateral or bilateral facial weakness or paralysis. (See *Recognizing unilateral Bell palsy*.) Onset is rapid. In 80% to 90% of patients, Bell palsy subsides spontaneously, with complete recovery in 1 to 8 weeks; however, recovery may be delayed in the elderly. If recovery is partial, contractures may develop on the paralyzed side of the face. Bell palsy may recur on the same or opposite side of the face.

Recognizing unilateral Bell palsy

Bell palsy usually causes a unilateral facial paralysis. This produces a distorted appearance with an inability to wrinkle the forehead, close the eyelid, smile, show the teeth, or puff out the cheek.

Distorted appearance

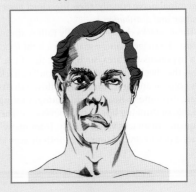

Wrinkling the forehead

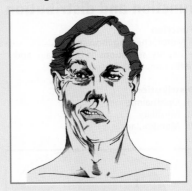

Smiling

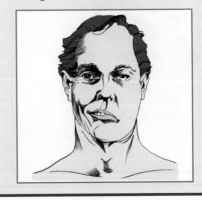

Causes and incidence

Bell palsy blocks the seventh cranial nerve, which is responsible for motor innervation of the muscles of the face. The conduction block is from an inflammatory reaction around the nerve (usually at the internal auditory meatus), which may result from infection, hemorrhage, tumor, meningitis, local trauma, hypertension, sarcoidosis, Lyme disease, or infarction of the nerve.

Bell palsy affects all age groups and males and females nearly equally, although females are slightly more likely to develop it during their late teens and early 20s. In the United States, the incidence is 23 cases per 100,000 people.

Pathophysiology

Bell palsy is thought to occur related to inflammation of the seventh cranial nerve; pressure is produced where the nerve exits the skull through a bony foramen blocking the transmission of the nerve impulse.

Complications

- ◆ Corneal ulcers
- ◆ Blindness
- ◆ Impaired nutrition

Signs and symptoms

Bell palsy usually produces unilateral facial weakness, occasionally with aching pain around the angle of the jaw or behind the ear. On the weak side, the mouth droops (causing the patient to drool saliva from the corner of the mouth), and taste perception is distorted over the affected anterior portion of the tongue. The forehead appears smooth, and the patient's ability to close his eye on the weak side is markedly impaired. When the patient tries to close this eye, it rolls upward (Bell phenomenon) and shows excessive tearing. Although Bell phenomenon occurs in normal people, it isn't apparent because the eyelids close completely and cover this eye motion. In Bell palsy, incomplete eye closure makes this upward motion obvious. Other symptoms may include loss of taste and ringing in the ear.

Diagnosis

Diagnosis is based on clinical presentation: distorted facial appearance and the inability to raise the eyebrow, close the eyelid, smile, show the teeth, or puff out the cheek. Electromyography helps determine the severity of nerve damage. Blood tests may be done to rule out acute causes (sarcoidosis or Lyme disease). If no improvement is evident within several weeks of onset, MRI will rule out other causes of dysfunction.

Treatment

Treatment consists of corticosteroids to reduce facial nerve edema and improve nerve conduction and blood flow. They must be given early—within 24 hours of onset of paralysis—to be most effective. Lubricants or an eye ointment may be needed to protect the eye, as well as patching during sleep.

Special considerations

Patient care includes observation for adverse drug effects, pain relief, and emotional support.
- ◆ During treatment with corticosteroids, watch for adverse effects, such as GI distress and fluid retention. If GI distress is troublesome, a concomitant antacid usually provides relief. If the patient has diabetes, frequent monitoring of serum glucose levels is necessary.
- ◆ To reduce pain, apply moist heat to the affected side of the face, taking care not to burn the skin.
- ◆ To help maintain muscle tone, massage the patient's face with a gentle upward motion two to three times daily for 5 to 10 minutes, or have the patient massage the face himself. When the patient is ready for active exercises, teach how to exercise by grimacing in front of a mirror.
- ◆ Advise the patient to protect the eye by covering it with an eye patch, especially when outdoors. Tell the patient to keep warm and avoid exposure to dust and wind. When exposure is unavoidable, instruct the patient to cover the face.
- ◆ Instruct the patient to chew on the unaffected side of the mouth. Provide a soft, nutritionally balanced diet, eliminating hot foods and fluids. Give the patient frequent mouth care, being particularly careful to remove residual food that collects between the cheeks and gums.
- ◆ Offer psychological support.

PERIPHERAL NEURITIS

Peripheral neuritis (also called *multiple neuritis, peripheral neuropathy,* and *polyneuritis*) is the degeneration of peripheral nerves supplying mainly the distal muscles of the extremities. It results in muscle weakness with sensory loss and atrophy and decreased or absent deep tendon reflexes. This syndrome is associated with a noninflammatory degeneration of the axon and myelin sheaths, chiefly affecting the distal muscles of the extremities. Because onset is usually insidious, patients may compensate by overusing unaffected muscles. If the cause can be identified and eliminated, the prognosis is good.

Causes and incidence

Causes of peripheral neuritis include:
◆ hereditary disorders (Charcot–Marie–Tooth disease or Friedreich ataxia)
◆ exposure to toxic compounds (sniffing glue or toxic compounds, nitrous oxide, industrial agents—especially solvents, and heavy metals, such as lead, arsenic, or mercury)
◆ infectious or inflammatory diseases (acquired immunodeficiency syndrome, botulism, Colorado tick fever, hepatitis, human immunodeficiency virus infection, leprosy, rheumatoid arthritis, sarcoidosis, systemic lupus erythematosus, diphtheria, syphilis, and Guillain–Barré syndrome)
◆ systemic or metabolic disorders (diabetes mellitus, dietary deficiencies [especially B_{12}], excessive use of alcohol, uremia, and cancer)
◆ neuropathy secondary to drugs
◆ miscellaneous causes (ischemia and prolonged exposure to cold temperature).

Peripheral neuropathy is common. Risk factors include diabetes, heavy alcohol use, and exposure to certain drugs and chemicals. Prolonged pressure on a nerve (such as with a cast, splint, or other device) is also a risk factor for developing nerve injury. Although it can occur at any age, incidence is highest in men between 30 and 50 years old.

Pathophysiology

The pathophysiology of peripheral neuritis is unclear. However, evidence suggests that the manifestation is related to an increased number of sodium channels or an abnormal sodium channel subtype in the injured nerve—creating abnormal nerve activity.

Complications

◆ Impotence
◆ Difficulty breathing
◆ Dysphagia

Signs and symptoms

The clinical effects of peripheral neuritis develop slowly, and the disease usually affects the motor and sensory nerve fibers. Symptoms vary according to which type of nerve is affected (sensory, motor, or autonomic). Neuropathy can affect any one or be a combination of all three types.
◆ *Sensory changes:* Damage to sensory fibers results in changes in sensation, ranging from abnormal sensations, such as burning, nerve pain, or tingling, to numbness or an inability to determine joint position in the area. Sensation changes often begin in the feet and progress toward the center of the body with involvement of other areas as the condition worsens.
◆ *Motor changes:* Damage to the motor fibers interferes with muscle control and can cause weakness, loss of muscle bulk, and loss of dexterity. Muscle cramping may be a sign of motor nerve involvement. Other muscle-related symptoms include lack of muscle control, difficulty or inability to move a part of the body (paralysis), muscle atrophy, muscle twitching (fasciculation) or cramping, difficulty breathing or swallowing, falling (from legs buckling or tripping over toes), or lack of dexterity (such as the inability to button a shirt).
◆ *Autonomic changes:* The autonomic nerves control involuntary or semi-voluntary functions, such as control of internal organs and blood pressure. Damage to autonomic nerves can cause blurred vision, decreased ability to sweat (anhidrosis), dizziness that occurs when standing up or fainting associated with a fall in blood pressure, heat intolerance with exertion (decreased ability to regulate body temperature), nausea or vomiting after meals, abdominal bloating (swelling), feeling full after eating a small amount (early satiety), diarrhea, constipation, unintentional weight loss (more than 5% of body weight), urinary incontinence, feeling of incomplete bladder emptying, difficulty beginning to urinate (urinary hesitancy), and male impotence.

Diagnosis

Patient history and physical examination delineate characteristic distribution of motor and sensory deficits. Electromyography may show a delayed action potential if this condition impairs motor nerve function. Nerve biopsy and nerve conduction tests can facilitate diagnosis.

Treatment

Effective treatment of peripheral neuritis consists of supportive measures to relieve pain, adequate bed rest, and physical therapy, vocational therapy, occupational therapy, and orthopedic interventions to promote independence, as needed. Most importantly, however, the underlying cause must be identified and corrected. For instance, it's essential to identify and remove the toxic agent, correct nutritional and vitamin deficiencies (the patient needs a high-calorie diet rich in vitamins, especially B-complex), and counsel the patient to avoid alcohol.

Over-the-counter analgesics or prescription pain medications may be needed to control nerve pain. Anticonvulsants (phenytoin, carbamazepine, and gabapentin) or tricyclic antidepressants may be used to reduce the stabbing pains that some patients experience. Whenever possible, medication use should be minimized to avoid adverse effects.

Fludrocortisone or similar medications may be beneficial in reducing postural hypotension for some patients. Medications that increase gastric motility, such as metoclopramide, are helpful for patients with reduced gastric motility.

For patients with bladder dysfunction, manual expression of urine (pressing over the bladder with the hands), intermittent catheterization, or medications such as bethanechol may be necessary.

Special considerations
Patient care includes promoting maximal independence and control of symptoms.
◆ Exercises and retraining may be used to increase muscle strength and control. Appliances, such as wheelchairs, braces, and splints, may improve mobility or the ability to use an affected extremity.
◆ The patient with decreased sensation should be taught to check feet or other affected areas frequently for bruises, open skin areas, or other injuries. A podiatrist can usually determine whether special orthotic devices are needed.
◆ Discuss safety measures in the home. Safety measures for the patient experiencing difficulty with movement may include railings, specialized appliances, removal of obstacles (such as loose rugs that may slip on the floor), and other measures, as appropriate. Safety measures for the patient with diminished sensation include adequate lighting (including lights left on at night), testing water temperature before bathing or immersing the body in water, and the use of protective shoes (no open toes and no high heels). Shoes should be checked often for grit or rough spots that may cause injury to the feet.
◆ The patient with neuropathy (especially the patient with polyneuropathy or mononeuropathy multiplex) is prone to new nerve injury at pressure points, such as the knees and elbows. Caution the patient to avoid prolonged pressure on these areas from leaning on the elbows, crossing the knees, or similar positions.
◆ Advise the patient with orthostatic hypotension to use elastic stockings and sleep with the head elevated.

◆ Instruct the patient with reduced gastric motility to eat small, frequent meals and sleep with the head elevated.
◆ Assist the patient with bladder dysfunction with manual expression of urine and intermittent catheterization, as necessary.
◆ To prevent pressure ulcers, assist in turning and repositioning every 2 hours and apply a food cradle. To prevent contractures, provide range-of-motion exercises as well as arrange for the patient to obtain splints, boards, braces, or other orthopedic appliances.
◆ Suggest that the patient's family contact the Neuropathy Association for additional information.

Pain disorders
COMPLEX REGIONAL PAIN SYNDROME
Complex regional pain syndrome (CRPS), also known as *reflex sympathetic dystrophy* (CRPS1) or *causalgia* (CRPS2), is a chronic pain disorder that results from abnormal healing after an injury—either minor or major—to a bone, muscle, or nerve. The development of symptoms is commonly disproportionate to the severity of the injury and seems to result from abnormal functioning of the sympathetic nervous system, the part of the nervous system that controls the diameter of blood vessels. One or more limbs and other parts of the body may be affected.

Causes and incidence
The exact cause of CRPS is unknown. Impaired communication between the damaged nerves of the sympathetic nervous system and the brain may cause interference with normal signals for sensations, temperature, and blood flow. This leads to problems in the nerves, blood vessels, skin, bones, and muscles. Infection or injury to an arm or leg may initiate CRPS. It can also occur after heart attacks and strokes. However, the condition can sometimes appear without obvious injury to the affected limb. This condition is more common in people between 40 and 60 years old but has been seen in younger people too. CRPS may also be seen in postoperative patients and in patients with diseases that can cause chronic pain, such as cancer and arthritis. The annual incidence is unknown because CRPS is often misdiagnosed. However, it has been reported in 1% to 2% of patients with various fractures and in 2% to 5% of patients with peripheral nerve injury.

Pathophysiology

The exact mechanism of CRPS is not well understood. Research suggests that it is multifactorial involving both sympathetic and central fibers, resulting in peripheral and central sensitization, inflammation and altered sympathetic and catecholinergic function and psychophysiologic functions.

Complications

◆ Depression
◆ Drug dependence

Signs and symptoms

Patients usually report severe and constant pain; severe pain is common with CRPS2 in particular. The affected area may have altered blood flow, feeling either warm or cool to the touch, with discoloration, sweating, or swelling. In time, skin, hair, and nail changes may occur along with impaired mobility and muscle wasting, especially if adequate treatment is delayed.

Diagnosis

There's no laboratory test for CRPS, so the diagnosis is based on the patient's history and clinical findings. A history of injury to an extremity may point to CRPS. Bone X-rays may aid in ruling out other conditions, such as osteomyelitis and stress fractures, which cause similar signs and symptoms. Additional tests may include bone scans, nerve conduction studies, and thermography (a test to show temperature changes and lack of blood supply in the painful area of the affected limb). With early diagnosis, prognosis improves.

Treatment

Treatment typically includes a combination of therapies such as drug therapy, with an anti-inflammatory, antidepressant, vasodilator, and analgesic used singly or in varying combinations, depending on the patient and the severity of symptoms. Steroids may be given in some patients; others may be given bone loss medications such as Actonel. Physical therapy to the injured area, application of heat and cold, the use of a transcutaneous electrical nerve stimulator unit, biofeedback, and psychological support are helpful for some patients.

Treatment may also include techniques for interrupting the hyperactivity of the sympathetic nervous system, such as nerve or regional blocks. Surgical sympathectomy—radical surgery that involves cutting the nerves to destroy the pain—may be done in severe cases; however, this method is rarely used because other sensation may be destroyed in the process.

Special considerations

◆ Offer emotional support to the patient and the family. Teach them about the disease.
◆ Monitor effects of prescribed medications.
◆ In addition to attending physical therapy sessions, the patient may need a home therapy regimen that includes stretching, active and passive exercises, strengthening exercises, compressive stockings or gloves to control edema, and heat or cold pack applications.
◆ Consult a pain care specialist to provide additional options for the patient, and help manage discomfort.
◆ Because chronic pain can be an emotional burden to the patient and the family, provide information on resources, such as counseling, support groups, stress reduction methods, meditation, relaxation training, and hypnosis.

SELECTED REFERENCES

Balami, J. S., et al. (2018). Complications of endovascular treatment for acute ischemic stroke: Prevention and management. *International Journal of Stroke, 13*(4), 348–361.

Borchers, A. T., & Gershwin, M. E. (2014). Complex regional pain syndrome: A comprehensive and critical review. *Autoimmunity Reviews, 13*(3), 242–265.

Diringer, M. N., & Zazulia, A. R. (2017, December). Aneurysmal subarachnoid hemorrhage: Strategies for preventing vasospasm in the intensive care unit. In *Seminars in respiratory and critical care medicine* (Vol. 38, No. 06, pp. 760–767). New York: Thieme Medical Publishers.

Hirsch, L., et al. (2016). The incidence of Parkinson's disease: A systematic review and meta-analysis. *Neuroepidemiology, 46*(4), 292–300.

Kumar, A., & Singh, A. (2015). A review on Alzheimer's disease pathophysiology and its management: An update. *Pharmacological Reports, 67*(2), 195–203.

Massimi, L., et al. (2011). Endoscopic third ventriculostomy for the management of Chiari I and related hydrocephalus: Outcome and pathogenetic implications. *Neurosurgery, 68*(4), 950–956.

Rubio-Ochoa, J., et al. (2016). Physical examination tests for screening and diagnosis of cervicogenic headache: A systematic review. *Manual Therapy, 21*, 35–40.

Zarei, S., et al. (2015). A comprehensive review of amyotrophic lateral sclerosis. *Surgical Neurology International, 6*, 171.

4

GASTROINTESTINAL DISORDERS

Introduction

The gastrointestinal (GI) tract, also known as the *alimentary canal*, is a long, hollow, musculomembranous tube consisting of glands and accessory organs (salivary glands, liver, gallbladder, and pancreas). (See *Reviewing GI anatomy and physiology*, page 210. See also *Histology of the GI tract*, page 211.) The GI tract breaks down food—carbohydrates, fats, and proteins—into molecules small enough to permeate cell membranes, thus providing cells with the necessary energy to function properly; it prepares food for cellular absorption by altering its physical and chemical composition. (See *Primary source of digestive hormones*, page 211.) Consequently, a malfunction along the GI tract can produce far-reaching metabolic effects, eventually threatening life itself. The GI tract is an unsterile system filled with bacteria and other flora; these organisms can cause superinfection from antibiotic therapy or they can infect other systems when a GI organ ruptures. A common indication of GI problems is referred pain, which makes diagnosis especially difficult.

ACCURATE ASSESSMENT VITAL

Your assessment of the patient with suspected GI disease must begin with a careful history that includes occupation, family history, and recent travel. The medical history should include previous hospital admissions; surgical procedures (including recent tooth extraction); family history of ulcers, colitis, liver disease, or cancer; and current medications, whether prescribed, over-the-counter, or herbal remedies, with particular attention to aspirin, steroids, and anticoagulants. In addition, assess for food or drug allergies.

Have the patient describe the chief concern in subjective words. Does he or she have abdominal pain, indigestion, heartburn, or rectal bleeding? How long has this been present? What relieves these symptoms or makes them worse? Has the patient experienced nosebleeds or difficulty in swallowing recently? Has there been recent unintentional weight loss or gain? Is the patient on a special diet? Does the patient drink alcoholic beverages or smoke? If yes to either, how much and how often? Ask about bowel habits. Is there regular use of laxatives or enemas? If the patient experiences nausea and vomiting, what does the vomitus look like? Does changing position relieve nausea?

Next, try to define and locate any pain. Ask the patient to describe the pain. Is it dull, sharp, burning, aching, spasmodic, or intermittent? Where is it located? Does it radiate? How long does it last? When does it occur? What triggers it? What relieves it?

VISUAL ASSESSMENT

Observe how the patient looks, and note appropriateness of behavior. Changes in fluid and electrolyte balance, severe infection, drug toxicity, and hepatic disease may cause abnormal behavior. Your visual examination should check:
◆ *Skin*—loss of turgor, jaundice, cyanosis, pallor, diaphoresis, petechiae, bruises, edema, and texture (dry or oily)

Reviewing GI anatomy and physiology

The GI tract includes the mouth, pharynx, esophagus, stomach (fundus, body, and antrum), small intestine (duodenum, jejunum, and ileum), and large intestine (cecum, colon, rectum, and anal canal).

Digestion begins in the mouth through chewing and through the action of an enzyme secreted in saliva—ptyalin (amylase)—which breaks down starch. Digestion continues in the stomach, where the lining secretes gastric juice that contains hydrochloric acid and the enzymes pepsin (begins protein digestion), lipase (speeds hydrolysis of emulsified fats) and, in infants, rennin (curdles milk).

Through a churning motion, the stomach breaks food into tiny particles, mixes them with gastric juice, and pushes the mass toward the pylorus. The liquid portion (chyme) enters the duodenum in small amounts; any solid material remains in the stomach until it liquefies (usually from 1 to 6 hours). The stomach also produces an intrinsic factor necessary for the absorption of vitamin B_{12}. Although limited amounts of water, alcohol, and some drugs are absorbed in the stomach, chyme passes unabsorbed into the duodenum.

Small intestine's role

Most digestion and absorption occur in the small intestine, where the surface area is increased by millions of villi in the mucous membrane lining. For digestion, the small intestine relies on a vast array of enzymes produced by the pancreas or by the intestinal lining itself. Pancreatic enzymes include trypsin, which digests protein to amino acids; lipase, which digests fat to fatty acids and glycerol; and amylase, which digests starches to sugars. Intestinal enzymes include erepsin, which digests protein to amino acids; lactase, maltase, and sucrase, which digest complex sugars such as glucose, fructose, and galactose; and enterokinase, which activates trypsin.

In addition, bile, secreted by the liver and stored in the gallbladder, helps neutralize stomach acid and aids the small intestine to emulsify and absorb fats and fat-soluble vitamins.

Final stages

By the time the ingested material reaches the ileocecal valve (where the small intestine joins the large intestine), all nutritional value has been absorbed through the villi of the small intestine into the bloodstream.

The large intestine, so named because it's larger in diameter than the small intestine, absorbs water from the digestive material before passing it on for elimination. Rectal distention by feces stimulates the defecation reflex, which, when assisted by voluntary sphincter relaxation, permits defecation.

Throughout the GI tract, peristalsis (a coordinated, rhythmic contraction of smooth muscle) propels ingested material along; sphincters prevent its reflux.

♦ *Head*—color of sclerae, sunken eyes, dentures, caries, lesions, tongue (color, swelling, dryness), and breath odor
♦ *Chest*—shape (asymmetrical, barrel, or sunken)
♦ *Lungs*—rate, rhythm, and quality of respirations
♦ *Abdomen*—size and shape (distention, contour, visible masses, and protrusions), abdominal scars or fistulae, excessive skin folds (may indicate wasting), and abnormal respiratory movements (inflammation of diaphragm)

AUSCULTATION, PALPATION, AND PERCUSSION

Auscultation provides helpful clues to GI abnormalities and should always be performed before palpation and percussion to avoid altering the assessment. For example, the absence of bowel sounds over the area to the lower right of the umbilicus may indicate peritonitis. High-pitched sounds that coincide with colicky pain may indicate small bowel obstruction. Less intense, low-pitched rumbling noises may accompany minor irritation.

Palpating the abdomen after auscultation helps detect tenderness, muscle guarding, and abdominal masses. Watch for muscle tone (boardlike rigidity points to peritonitis or hemorrhage; transient rigidity suggests severe pain) and tenderness (rebound tenderness may indicate peritoneal inflammation).

Percussion helps detect air, fluid, and solid matter in the abdominal region.

Histology of the GI tract

The GI tract consists of four tissue layers, the structure of which varies in different organs:
♦ *Mucous membrane*—innermost layer; secretes gastric juice, protects the tract, and absorbs nutrients
♦ *Submucosa*—connective tissue that contains the major blood vessels and nerves
♦ *External muscle coat (muscularis externa)*—double layer of smooth muscle fibers; inner circular and outer longitudinal layers propel gastric contents downward by peristalsis
♦ *Fibroserous coat (serosa)*—outermost protective layer of connective tissue; forms the peritoneum, which is the largest serous membrane of the body. The peritoneum's parietal layer covers the walls of the abdominal cavity. An extension of the parietal peritoneum, called the *mesentery*, anchors the small intestine to the abdominal wall. The visceral layer drapes most of the abdominal organs, covering the upper surface of the pelvic organs.

DIAGNOSTIC TESTS

After physical assessment, several tests can identify GI malfunction.
♦ A barium or Gastrografin swallow is used primarily to examine the esophagus. Gastrografin may be used instead of barium. Like barium, Gastrografin facilitates X-ray imaging. However, if Gastrografin escapes from the GI tract, it's absorbed by the surrounding tissue, whereas escaped barium isn't absorbed and can cause complications.
♦ In an upper GI series, swallowed barium sulfate travels through the esophagus, stomach, and duodenum to reveal abnormalities. The barium outlines stomach walls and delineates ulcer craters and defects.
♦ A small bowel series, an extension of the upper GI series, visualizes barium flowing through the small intestine to the ileocecal valve.
♦ A barium enema (lower GI series) allows X-ray visualization of the colon.
♦ A stool specimen is useful to detect suspected GI bleeding, infection, or malabsorption as well as the presence of parasites. Guaiac test for occult blood, microscopic stool examination for ova and parasites, and tests for fat require several specimens.

Primary source of digestive hormones

This cross section of the stomach shows the G-cells (which secrete gastrin) in the pyloric glands. The cross sections of the duodenum and jejunum show the S-cells (which secrete secretin) in the duodenal and jejunal glands.

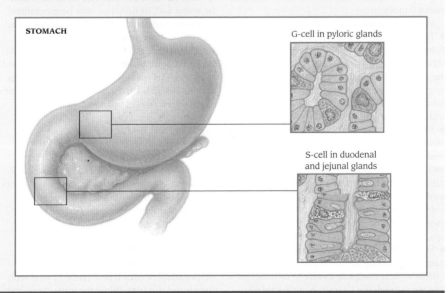

STOMACH

G-cell in pyloric glands

S-cell in duodenal and jejunal glands

◆ In esophagogastroduodenoscopy, insertion of a fiberoptic scope allows direct visual inspection of the esophagus, stomach, and duodenum. These structures are examined for varices, tumors, inflammation, hernias, polyps, ulcers, and obstruction.

◆ Proctosigmoidoscopy permits inspection of the rectum and distal sigmoid colon; colonoscopy is used for inspection of the descending, transverse, and ascending colon. These tests help visualize tumors, polyps, hemorrhoids, or ulcers.

◆ Gastric analysis examines gastric secretions for the presence of high levels of gastrin and the amount of acid produced.

◆ Endoscopic retrograde cholangiopancreatography (ERCP) directly visualizes the esophagus, stomach, proximal duodenum, and fluoroscopically visualizes the pancreatic, hepatic, and biliary ducts. This test can help visualize duct obstruction, benign structures, cysts, anatomic variations, and malignant tumors. ERCP can be used to relieve or remove obstructions of the biliary tree.

INTUBATION

Certain GI disorders require nasogastric (NG) intubation to empty the stomach and intestine, to aid diagnosis and treatment, to decompress obstructed areas, to detect and treat GI bleeding, and to administer medications or feedings. Tubes generally inserted through the nose are the short NG tubes (the Levin, the Salem Sump, and the specialized Sengstaken–Blakemore) and the long intestinal tubes (Cantor and Miller–Abbott). The larger Ewald tube is usually inserted orally.

When caring for the patient with a tube:

◆ Explain the procedure before intubation.

◆ Maintain accurate intake and output records. Measure gastric drainage every 8 hours; record the amount, color, odor, and consistency. When irrigating the tube, note the amount of saline solution instilled and aspirated. Check for fluid and electrolyte imbalances.

◆ Provide good oral and nasal care. Brush the patient's teeth frequently and provide mouthwash. Make sure that the tube is secure, but isn't causing pressure on the nostrils. Change the tape to the nose every 24 hours. Gently wash the area around the tube, and apply a water-soluble lubricant to soften crusts. These measures help prevent sore throat and nose, dry lips, nasal excoriation, and parotitis.

◆ Ensure maximum patient comfort. After insertion of a long intestinal tube, instruct the patient to turn from side to side to facilitate its passage through the GI tract. Note the tube's progress. Never attach an intestinal tube to a patient's gown, bed linens, side rails of the bed, and so forth.

◆ With both types of tubes, tell the patient to expect a feeling of dryness or a lump in the throat; if allowed, suggest that the patient chew gum or eat hard candy to relieve discomfort.

◆ Always keep scissors taped to the wall near the bed when the patient has a Sengstaken–Blakemore tube in place. If the tube should dislodge and obstruct the bronchus, cut the lumen to the balloons immediately. Sometimes the tube is taped to the face piece of a football helmet worn by the patient to prevent the tube from dislodging and to put traction on the tube.

◆ After removing the tube from a patient with GI bleeding, watch for signs and symptoms of recurrent bleeding, such as hematemesis, decreased hemoglobin level, pallor, chills, diaphoresis, hypotension, and rapid pulse.

◆ Provide emotional support because the patient may panic at the sight of a tube. A calm, reassuring manner can help minimize fear.

Mouth and esophagus

STOMATITIS AND OTHER ORAL INFECTIONS

Stomatitis is an inflammation of the oral mucosa that may extend to the buccal mucosa, lips, and palate. It's a common infection that may occur alone or as part of a systemic disease. There are two main types: acute herpetic stomatitis and aphthous stomatitis. Acute herpetic stomatitis is usually self-limiting; however, it may be severe and, in neonates, may be generalized and potentially fatal. Aphthous stomatitis, also known as *canker sores*, usually heals spontaneously, without a scar, in 10 to 14 days. It may be an extraintestinal symptom of irritable bowel disease. Other oral infections include gingivitis, candidiasis, glossitis, periodontitis, and Vincent's angina. (See *Types of oral infections*, page 213.)

Causes and incidence

Acute herpetic stomatitis results from the herpes simplex virus. It's common in children 6 months to 5 years old. The cause of aphthous stomatitis is unknown, but predisposing factors include stress, fatigue, anxiety, febrile states, trauma, and solar overexposure. This type is common in young and teenage girls.

Pathophysiology

Tissue destruction takes place as a result of herpes simplex virus type 1 (HSV-1) viral replication and cell lysis. When the virus enters into

Types of oral infections

Disease and causes	Signs and symptoms	Treatment
Candidiasis *(infection of the oropharyngeal mucosa)*		
♦ Fungal infection caused by *Candida albicans* or related species ♦ High-risk patients include premature neonates, older adults, the immunosuppressed, and those taking antibiotics or long-term steroids	♦ Cream-colored or bluish white patches of exudate on the tongue, mouth, or pharynx ♦ Painful fissures at the corners of the mouth	♦ Antifungals for infection ♦ May benefit from eating active-culture yogurt or other live lactobacillus ♦ Topical anesthetic to relieve discomfort ♦ Nonirritating mouthwash to loosen tenacious secretions
Gingivitis *(inflammation of the gingiva)*		
♦ Early sign of hypovitaminosis, diabetes, blood dyscrasias ♦ Occasionally related to use of hormonal contraceptives	♦ Inflammation with painless swelling, redness, change in normal contours, bleeding, and periodontal pocket (gum detachment from teeth)	♦ Removal of irritating factors (calculus, faulty dentures) ♦ Good oral hygiene, regular dental checkups, vigorous chewing ♦ Oral or topical corticosteroids
Glossitis *(inflammation of the tongue)*		
♦ Streptococcal infection ♦ Irritation or injury; jagged teeth; ill-fitting dentures; biting during seizures; alcohol; spicy foods; smoking; sensitivity to toothpaste or mouthwash ♦ Vitamin B deficiency; anemia ♦ Skin conditions: lichen planus, erythema multiforme, pemphigus vulgaris	♦ Reddened, ulcerated, or swollen tongue (may obstruct airway) ♦ Painful chewing and swallowing ♦ Speech difficulty ♦ Painful tongue without inflammation	♦ Treatment of underlying cause ♦ Topical anesthetic mouthwash or systemic analgesics (acetaminophen) for painful lesions ♦ Good oral hygiene, regular dental checkups, vigorous chewing ♦ Avoidance of hot, cold, or spicy foods and alcohol
Periodontitis *(gingival infection and recession, loosening of teeth)*		
♦ Early sign of hypovitaminosis, diabetes, blood dyscrasias ♦ Occasionally related to use of hormonal contraceptives ♦ Dental factors: calculus, poor oral hygiene, malocclusion; major cause of tooth loss after middle age	♦ Acute onset of bright red gum inflammation, painless swelling of interdental papillae, easy bleeding ♦ Loosening of teeth, typically without inflammatory symptoms, progressing to loss of teeth and alveolar bone ♦ Acute systemic infection (fever, chills)	♦ Scaling, root planing, and curettage for infection control ♦ Periodontal surgery to prevent recurrence ♦ Good oral hygiene, regular dental checkups, vigorous chewing
Vincent's angina *("trench mouth," necrotizing ulcerative gingivitis)*		
♦ Fusiform bacillus or spirochete infection ♦ Predisposing factors: stress, poor oral hygiene, insufficient rest, nutritional deficiency, smoking	♦ Sudden onset: painful, superficial bleeding; gingival ulcers (rarely, on buccal mucosa) covered with a gray-white membrane ♦ Ulcers become punched-out lesions after slight pressure or irritation ♦ Malaise, mild fever, excessive salivation, bad breath, pain on swallowing or talking, enlarged submaxillary lymph nodes	♦ Removal of devitalized tissue with ultrasonic cavitron ♦ Antibiotics for infection ♦ Analgesics, as needed ♦ Hourly mouth rinses (with equal amounts of hydrogen peroxide and warm water) ♦ Soft, nonirritating diet; rest; no smoking ♦ With treatment, improvement common within 24 hours

the sensory and autonomic nerve endings, it is transported to the cell nuclei and can remain latent until reactivation.

Complications
◆ Nutritional deficiencies
◆ Esophagitis
◆ Sepsis

Signs and symptoms
Acute herpetic stomatitis begins suddenly with mouth pain, malaise, lethargy, anorexia, irritability, and fever, which may persist for 1 to 2 weeks. Gums are swollen and bleed easily, and the mucous membrane is extremely tender.

Papulovesicular ulcers appear in the mouth and throat and eventually become punched-out lesions with reddened areolae. Submaxillary lymphadenitis is common. Pain usually disappears 2 to 4 days before healing of ulcers is complete. If the child with stomatitis sucks his or her thumb, these lesions spread to the hand.

A patient with aphthous stomatitis typically reports burning, tingling, and slight swelling of the mucous membrane. Single or multiple shallow ulcers with whitish centers and red borders appear and heal at one site and then reappear at another. (See *Looking at aphthous stomatitis*.)

Looking at aphthous stomatitis

In aphthous stomatitis, numerous small, round vesicles appear. They soon break and leave shallow ulcers with red areolae.

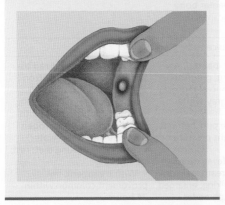

Diagnosis
Diagnosis is based on the physical examination; in Vincent's angina, a smear of ulcer exudate allows for identification of the causative organism.

Treatment
For acute herpetic stomatitis, treatment is conservative. For local symptoms, supportive measures include warm saltwater mouth rinses (antiseptic mouthwashes are contraindicated because they are irritating) and a topical anesthetic to relieve mouth ulcer pain. Topical antihistamines, antacids, or corticosteroids may also be recommended. Supplementary treatment includes a bland or liquid diet and, in severe cases, I.V. fluids and bed rest.

For aphthous stomatitis, primary treatment is application of a topical anesthetic. Effective long-term treatment requires alleviation or prevention of precipitating factors.

GASTROESOPHAGEAL REFLUX DISEASE
Gastroesophageal reflux disease (GERD) is a disease process that results from continued backflow of gastric or duodenal contents, or both, into the esophagus and past the lower esophageal sphincter (LES) without associated belching or vomiting. Reflux may cause symptoms or pathologic changes. Persistent reflux may cause reflux esophagitis (inflammation of the esophageal mucosa). Prognosis varies with the underlying cause.

Causes and incidence
The function of the LES—a high-pressure area in the lower esophagus, just above the stomach—is to prevent gastric contents from backing up into the esophagus. Normally, the LES creates pressure, closing the lower end of the esophagus, but relaxes after each swallow to allow food into the stomach. Reflux occurs when LES pressure is deficient or when pressure within the stomach exceeds LES pressure. (See *Influences on LES pressure*, page 215.)

In 2015, there were 7 million diagnoses of gastroesophageal reflux. True figures may be even higher because many people with GERD take over-the-counter remedies without reporting their symptoms. Studies show that GERD is common and may be overlooked in infants and children. It can cause repeated vomiting, coughing, and other respiratory problems. An immature digestive system is usually responsible, and most infants grow out of GERD by the time they are age 1.

Influences on lower esophageal sphincter (LES) pressure

Several factors can influence LES pressure, thereby affecting reflux, as noted here.

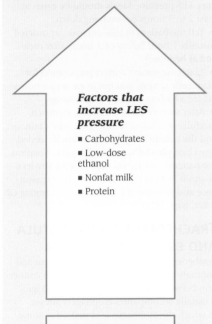

Factors that increase LES pressure

- Carbohydrates
- Low-dose ethanol
- Nonfat milk
- Protein

Factors that decrease LES pressure

- Antiflatulents (simethicone)
- Chocolate
- Cigarette smoking
- Fat
- High-dose ethanol
- Lying on right or left side
- Orange juice
- Peppermint
- Sitting
- Tomatoes
- Whole milk

Patients with symptom-producing reflux can't swallow often enough to create sufficient peristaltic amplitude to clear gastric acid from the lower esophagus. This results in prolonged periods of acidity in the esophagus when reflux occurs.

Predisposing factors include:

◆ pyloric surgery (alteration or removal of the pylorus), which allows reflux of bile or pancreatic juice

◆ long-term NG intubation (>4 days)

◆ any agent that lowers LES pressure, such as food, alcohol, cigarettes, anticholinergics (atropine, belladonna, and propantheline), or other drugs (morphine, diazepam, calcium channel blockers, and meperidine)

◆ hiatal hernia with an incompetent sphincter

◆ any condition or position that increases intra-abdominal pressure, such as straining, bending, coughing, pregnancy, obesity, and recurrent or persistent vomiting

Pathophysiology

Most commonly, the excessive relaxation of the LES is the cause of GERD; this allows reflux contents into the esophagus, and the esophageal mucosa is then exposed to acidic contents.

Signs and symptoms

GERD doesn't always cause symptoms, and in patients showing clinical effects, it isn't always possible to confirm physiologic reflux. The most common feature of GERD is heartburn, which may become more severe with vigorous exercise, bending, or lying down, and may be relieved by antacids or sitting upright. The pain of esophageal spasm resulting from reflux esophagitis tends to be chronic and may mimic angina pectoris, radiating to the neck, jaws, and arms.

Other symptoms include odynophagia, which may be followed by a dull substernal ache from severe, long-term reflux; dysphagia from esophageal spasm, stricture, or esophagitis; and bleeding (bright red or dark brown). Nocturnal regurgitation can awaken the patient with coughing, choking, and a mouthful of saliva. Reflux may be associated with hiatal hernia. Direct hiatal hernia becomes clinically significant only when reflux is confirmed.

Pulmonary symptoms result from reflux of gastric contents into the throat and subsequent aspiration; they include chronic pulmonary disease or nocturnal wheezing, bronchitis, asthma, morning hoarseness, and cough. In children, other signs consist of failure to thrive and forceful vomiting from esophageal irritation. Such vomiting sometimes causes aspiration pneumonia.

Complications

- Esophageal ulcer
- Esophageal stricture
- Barrett's esophagus
- Hoarseness
- Reflux esophagitis

Diagnosis

CONFIRMING DIAGNOSIS *After a careful history and physical examination, tests to confirm GERD include barium swallow fluoroscopy, esophageal pH probe, esophageal manometry, and esophagoscopy. In children, barium esophagography under fluoroscopic control can show reflux.*

Recurrent reflux after age 6 weeks is abnormal. An acid perfusion (Bernstein) test can show that reflux is the cause of symptoms. Finally, endoscopy and biopsy allow visualization and confirmation of any pathologic changes in the mucosa.

Treatment

Promotility agents help increase LES sphincter tone and stimulate upper GI motility. Proton pump inhibitors and histamine-2 (H_2) receptor antagonists help reduce gastric acidity. If possible, NG intubation shouldn't be continued for more than 5 days because the tube interferes with sphincter integrity and allows reflux, especially when the patient lies flat.

PEDIATRIC TIP *Positional therapy is especially useful in infants and children who experience GERD without complications. Strategies, such as burping the infant several times during feeding, keeping the infant in an upright position for 30 minutes after feeding, and avoiding feeding 2 to 3 hours before bedtime, may help.*

Surgery may be necessary to control severe and refractory symptoms, such as pulmonary aspiration, hemorrhage, obstruction, severe pain, perforation, an incompetent LES, or associated hiatal hernia. Surgical procedures that create an artificial closure at the gastroesophageal junction may be needed in some patients. These include a procedure that invaginates the esophagus into the stomach and procedures that create a gastric wraparound with or without fixation. The fundoplication procedure can be performed endoscopically.

Special considerations

Teach the patient what causes reflux, how to avoid reflux with an antireflux regimen (medication, diet, and positional therapy), and what symptoms to watch for and report.

- Instruct the patient to avoid circumstances that increase intra-abdominal pressure (such as bending, coughing, vigorous exercise, tight clothing, constipation, and obesity) as well as substances that reduce sphincter control (cigarettes, alcohol, fatty foods, and caffeine).
- Advise the patient to sit upright, particularly after meals, and to eat small, frequent meals. Tell him to avoid highly seasoned food, acidic juices, alcoholic drinks, bedtime snacks, and foods high in fat or carbohydrates, which reduce LES pressure. Meals should be eaten at least 2 to 3 hours before lying down.
- Tell the patient to take antacids, as ordered (usually 1 hour before or 3 hours after meals and at bedtime).
- Teach the patient correct preparation for diagnostic testing, and not to eat 6 to 8 hours before a barium swallow or endoscopy.
- After surgery using a thoracic approach, carefully watch and record chest tube drainage and the patient's respiratory status. If needed, give chest physiotherapy and oxygen. Position the patient with an NG tube in semi-Fowler's position to help prevent reflux. Offer reassurance and emotional support. (See *Preventing GI reflux*, page 217.)

TRACHEOESOPHAGEAL FISTULA AND ESOPHAGEAL ATRESIA

Tracheoesophageal fistula is a developmental anomaly characterized by an abnormal connection between the trachea and the esophagus. It usually accompanies esophageal atresia, in which the esophagus is closed off at some point. Although these malformations have numerous anatomic variations, the most common, by far, is esophageal atresia with fistula to the distal segment. (See *Types of tracheoesophageal anomalies*, page 218.)

These disorders, two of the most serious surgical emergencies in neonates, require immediate diagnosis and correction. They may coexist with other serious anomalies, such as congenital heart disease, imperforate anus, genitourinary abnormalities, and intestinal atresia.

Causes and incidence

Tracheoesophageal fistula and esophageal atresia result from failure of the embryonic esophagus and trachea to develop and separate correctly. Respiratory system development begins at about day 26 of gestation. Abnormal development of the septum during this time can lead to tracheoesophageal fistula. The most common abnormality is type C tracheoesophageal fistula with esophageal atresia, in which the upper section of the esophagus terminates in a blind pouch, and the lower section ascends

PREVENTION

Preventing GI reflux

Changing lifestyle will help the patient to prevent GI reflux.

Diet and eating habits
Foods, such as caffeine, chocolate, spicy food, carbonated beverages, orange juice, liquor, wine, and tomato sauce, stimulate the production of acid. Large meals expand the stomach and put pressure on the lower esophageal sphincter (LES). Gravity helps keep the stomach juices from backing up into the esophagus: Don't allow the patient to lie down for 2 hours after eating. If nighttime heartburn is a concern, raise the head of the bed 6" to 8" because a flat position places pressure on the LES.

Weight
Being overweight increases abdominal pressure, which can then push stomach contents up into the esophagus.

Smoking
Nicotine relaxes the esophageal sphincter and stimulates the production of stomach acid. Smoking also may injure the esophagus by causing irritation making it more susceptible to damage from acid reflux. Smoking can decrease gastric motility and reduce the effectiveness of digestion because the stomach takes longer to empty.

Stress
Although stress itself doesn't cause heartburn, the anxiety that comes along with stress can lead to behaviors that increase the risk of heartburn, such as overeating, drinking, and smoking.

Alcohol
Alcohol can increase the production of stomach acid and can also lower the esophageal sphincter, which allows stomach acids to move up into the esophagus. Alcohol also makes the esophagus more sensitive to stomach acid.

---

from the stomach and connects with the trachea by a short fistulous tract. Esophageal atresia occurs in about 1 of every 2,500 to 4,000 live births.

Pathophysiology

In type A atresia, both esophageal segments are blind pouches, and neither is connected to the airway. In type E (or H-type), tracheoesophageal fistula without atresia, the fistula may occur anywhere between the level of the cricoid cartilage and the midesophagus, but is usually higher in the trachea than in the esophagus. Such a fistula may be as small as a pinpoint. In types B and D, the upper portion of the esophagus opens into the trachea; neonates with this anomaly may experience life-threatening aspiration of saliva or food.

Complications

♦ Recurrent fistulas
♦ Abnormal esophageal motility
♦ Pneumothorax
♦ Esophageal stricture

Signs and symptoms

A neonate with type C tracheoesophageal fistula with esophageal atresia appears to swallow normally but soon after swallowing coughs, struggles, becomes cyanotic, and stops breathing as he aspirates fluids returning from the blind pouch of the esophagus through his nose and mouth. Stomach distention may cause respiratory distress; air and gastric contents (bile and gastric secretions) may reflux through the fistula into the trachea, resulting in chemical pneumonitis.

An infant with type A esophageal atresia appears normal at birth. The infant swallows normally, but as secretions fill the esophageal sac and overflow into the oropharynx, they develop mucus in the oropharynx and drools excessively. When the infant is fed, regurgitation and respiratory distress follow aspiration. Suctioning the mucus and secretions temporarily relieves these symptoms. Excessive secretions and drooling in the neonate strongly suggest esophageal atresia.

Types of tracheoesophageal anomalies

Congenital malformations of the esophagus occur in about 1 in 3,500 live births. Anatomic variations of tracheoesophageal anomalies are classified as follows.

- Type A: esophageal atresia without fistula
- Type B: esophageal atresia with tracheoesophageal fistula to the proximal segment
- Type C (the most common): esophageal atresia with fistula to the distal segment
- Type D: esophageal atresia with fistula to both segments
- Type E (or H-Type): tracheoesophageal fistula without atresia

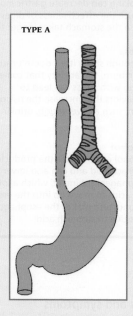

TYPE A

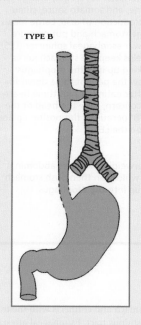

TYPE B

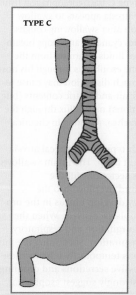

TYPE C

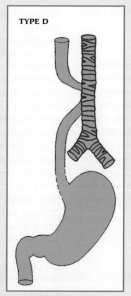

TYPE D

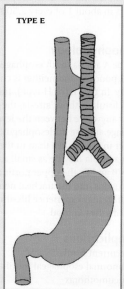

TYPE E

Repeated episodes of pneumonitis, pulmonary infection, and abdominal distention may signal type E (or H-type) tracheoesophageal fistula. When a child with this disorder drinks, he or she coughs, chokes, and becomes cyanotic. Excessive mucus builds up in the oropharynx. Crying forces air from the trachea into the esophagus, producing abdominal distention. Because such a child may appear normal at birth, this type of tracheoesophageal fistula may be overlooked, and diagnosis may be delayed as long as 1 year.

Type B (proximal fistula) and type D (fistula to both segments) cause immediate aspiration of saliva into the airway and bacterial pneumonitis.

Diagnosis
Respiratory distress and drooling in a neonate suggest tracheoesophageal fistula and esophageal atresia. The following procedures confirm the diagnosis:

◆ A size 10 or 12 French catheter passed through the nose meets an obstruction (esophageal atresia) approximately 4″ to 5″ (10 to 12.5 cm) distal from the nostrils. Aspirate of gastric contents is less acidic than normal.

◆ Chest X-ray demonstrates the position of the catheter and can also show a dilated, air-filled upper esophageal pouch, pneumonia in the right upper lobe, or bilateral pneumonitis. Both pneumonia and pneumonitis suggest aspiration.

◆ Abdominal X-ray shows gas in the bowel in a distal fistula (type C) but none in a proximal fistula (type B) or in atresia without fistula (type A).

◆ Cinefluorography allows visualization on a fluoroscopic screen. After a size 10 or 12 French catheter is passed through the patient's nostril into the esophagus, a small amount of contrast medium is instilled to define the tip of the upper pouch and to differentiate between overflow aspiration from a blind end (atresia) and aspiration due to passage of liquid through a tracheoesophageal fistula.

Treatment
Tracheoesophageal fistula and esophageal atresia require surgical correction and are usually surgical emergencies. The type and timing of surgical procedure depend on the nature of the anomaly, the patient's general condition, and the presence of coexisting congenital defects. In premature neonates who are poor surgical risks, correction of combined tracheoesophageal fistula and esophageal atresia is done in two stages: first, gastrostomy (for gastric

decompression, prevention of reflux, and feeding) and closure of the fistula; then, 1 to 2 months later, anastomosis of the esophagus.

Before and after surgery, positioning varies with the physician's philosophy and the infant's anatomy: the infant may be placed supine, with the head positioned low to facilitate drainage, or with the head elevated to prevent aspiration.

The infant should receive I.V. fluids, as necessary, and appropriate antibiotics for superimposed infection.

Postoperative complications after correction of tracheoesophageal fistula include recurrent fistulas, esophageal motility dysfunction, esophageal stricture, recurrent bronchitis, pneumothorax, and failure to thrive. Esophageal motility dysfunction or hiatal hernia may develop after surgery to correct esophageal atresia.

Correction of esophageal atresia alone requires anastomosis of the proximal and distal esophageal segments in one or two stages. End-to-end anastomosis commonly produces postoperative stricture; end-to-side anastomosis is less likely to do so. If the esophageal ends are widely separated, treatment may include a colonic interposition (grafting a piece of the colon) or elongation of the proximal segment of the esophagus by bougienage. About 10 days after surgery, and again 1 and 3 months later, X-rays are required to evaluate the effectiveness of surgical repair.

Postoperative treatment includes placement of a suction catheter in the upper esophageal pouch to control secretions and prevent aspiration, maintaining the infant in an upright position to avoid reflux of gastric juices into the trachea, I.V. fluids (nothing by mouth), gastrostomy to prevent reflux and allow feeding, and appropriate antibiotics for pneumonia.

Postoperative complications may include impaired esophageal motility (in one third of patients), hiatal hernia, and reflux esophagitis.

Special considerations
Postoperative care should include the following:

◆ Monitor the infant's respiratory status. Administer oxygen and perform pulmonary physiotherapy and suctioning, as needed. Provide a humid environment.

◆ Administer antibiotics and parenteral fluids, as ordered. Keep accurate intake and output records.

◆ If the infant has chest tubes postoperatively, check them frequently for patency. Maintain proper suction; measure and mark drainage periodically.

◆ Observe carefully for signs of complications.

◆ Maintain gastrostomy tube feedings, as ordered. Such feedings initially consist of dextrose and water (not >5% solution); later, add a proprietary formula (first diluted and then full strength). If the infant develops gastric atony, use an iso-osmolar formula. Oral feedings can usually resume 8 to 10 days postoperatively. If gastrostomy feedings and oral feedings are impossible because of intolerance to them or decreased intestinal motility, the infant requires total parenteral nutrition (TPN).

◆ If the infant can safely handle secretions, give a pacifier to satisfy sucking needs; however, this is done *only* when the child can safely handle secretions because sucking stimulates saliva secretion.

◆ Offer the parents support and guidance in dealing with their infant's acute illness. Encourage them to participate in the infant's care and to hold and touch as much as possible to facilitate bonding.

CORROSIVE ESOPHAGITIS AND STRICTURE

Corrosive esophagitis is inflammation and damage to the esophagus after ingestion of a caustic chemical. Severe injury can quickly lead to esophageal perforation, mediastinitis, and death from infection, shock, and massive hemorrhage (due to aortic perforation).

Causes and incidence

The most common chemical injury to the esophagus follows the ingestion of lye or other strong alkali; ingestion of strong acids is less common. The type and amount of chemical ingested determine the severity and location of the damage. In children, household chemical ingestion is accidental; in adults, it's usually a suicide attempt or gesture.

Esophageal tissue damage occurs in three phases: the acute phase, consisting of edema and inflammation; the latent phase, with ulceration, exudation, and tissue sloughing; and the chronic phase, in which there is diffuse scarring.

Corrosive strictures account for less than 5% of all stricture cases.

Pathophysiology

In corrosive esophagitis, the chemical may damage only the mucosa or submucosa or it may damage all layers of the esophagus. Similar to a burn, this injury may be temporary or may lead to permanent stricture (narrowing or stenosis) of the esophagus that's correctable only through surgery.

Complications

◆ Esophageal perforation
◆ Mediastinitis
◆ Infection, massive hemorrhage, shock

Signs and symptoms

Effects vary from none at all to intense pain and edema in the mouth, anterior chest pain, marked salivation, inability to swallow, and tachypnea. Bloody vomitus containing pieces of esophageal tissue signals severe damage. Signs of esophageal perforation and mediastinitis, especially crepitation, indicate destruction of the entire esophagus. Inability to speak implies laryngeal damage.

The acute phase subsides in 3 to 4 days, enabling the patient to eat again. Fever suggests secondary infection. Symptoms of dysphagia return if stricture develops, usually within weeks; rarely, stricture is delayed and develops several years after the injury.

Diagnosis

℞ **CONFIRMING DIAGNOSIS** *A history of chemical ingestion and physical examination revealing oropharyngeal burns (including white membranes and edema of the soft palate and uvula) usually confirm the diagnosis.*

The type and amount of the chemical ingested must be identified; this may be done by examining the container of the ingested material or by calling the poison control center.

Two procedures are helpful in evaluating the severity of the injury:

◆ Endoscopy (in the first 24 hours after ingestion) delineates the extent and location of the esophageal injury and assesses the depth of the burn. This procedure may also be performed a week after ingestion to assess stricture development.

◆ Barium swallow (1 week after ingestion and every 3 weeks thereafter) may identify segmental spasm or fistula, but doesn't always show mucosal injury.

Treatment

Conservative treatment of corrosive esophagitis and stricture includes monitoring the patient's condition; early endoscopy; administering corticosteroids, such as prednisone and hydrocortisone, to control inflammation and inhibit fibrosis; and using a broad-spectrum antibiotic, such as ampicillin, to protect the corticosteroid-immunosuppressed patient against infection by his own mouth flora.

Treatment may also include bougienage, a procedure in which a slender, flexible, cylindrical instrument called a *bougie* is passed into the esophagus to dilate it and minimize stricture. Some physicians begin bougienage immediately and continue it regularly to maintain a patent lumen and prevent stricture; others delay it for a week to avoid the risk of esophageal perforation.

Surgery is needed immediately for esophageal perforation or later to correct stricture untreatable with bougienage. Corrective surgery may involve transplanting a piece of the colon to the damaged esophagus. However, even after surgery, stricture may recur at the site of the anastomosis.

Supportive treatment includes I.V. therapy to replace fluids or TPN while the patient can't swallow, gradually progressing to clear liquids and a soft diet.

Special considerations

If you're the first healthcare professional to see the patient who has ingested a corrosive chemical, the quality of your emergency care will be critical. Carefully follow these important guidelines:

◆ *Don't* induce vomiting or lavage because this will expose the esophagus and oropharynx to additional injury.

◆ *Don't* perform gastric lavage because the corrosive chemical may cause further damage to the mucous membrane of the GI lining.

◆ Provide vigorous support of vital functions, as needed, such as oxygen, mechanical ventilation, administration of I.V. fluids, and treatment for shock, depending on the severity of the injury.

◆ Carefully observe and record intake and output.

◆ Before X-rays and endoscopy, explain the procedure to the patient to lessen anxiety during the tests and to obtain consent.

◆ Because the adult who has ingested a corrosive agent may have done so with suicidal intent, assist the patient and family in seeking psychological counseling. Monitor the patient according to facility protocol if the attempt was a suicide.

◆ Provide emotional support for parents whose child has ingested a chemical. They'll be distraught and may feel guilty about the accident. Also be alert in case there is any suspicion of child abuse that may have accompanied the ingestion. Report according to facility and demographic protocol.

◆ Encourage long-term follow-up because of the increased risk of squamous cell carcinoma.

▦ PREVENTION *Tell parents to lock accessible cabinets and keep all corrosive agents out of a child's reach.*

MALLORY–WEISS SYNDROME

Mallory–Weiss syndrome is mild to massive, usually painless bleeding due to a tear in the mucosa or submucosa of the cardia or lower esophagus. Such a tear, usually singular and longitudinal, results from prolonged or forceful vomiting.

Causes and incidence

Forceful or prolonged vomiting can cause esophageal tearing when the upper esophageal sphincter fails to relax during vomiting; this lack of sphincter coordination seems more common after excessive alcohol intake. Other factors that can increase intra-abdominal pressure and predispose a person to this type of tear include coughing, straining during bowel movements, traumatic injury, seizures, childbirth, hiatal hernia, esophagitis, gastritis, and atrophic gastric mucosa. The incidence of Mallory–Weiss syndrome among patients with upper GI bleeding ranges from 8% to 15%. The condition most commonly occurs in patients under 40.

Pathophysiology

The pathophysiology of Mallory–Weiss syndrome is not completely understood, but it is thought that mucosal lacerations develop after a sudden increase in intra-abdominal pressure.

Complications

◆ Hypovolemia (if bleeding is excessive)
◆ Fatal shock

Signs and symptoms

Mallory–Weiss syndrome typically begins with vomiting of blood or passing large amounts of blood rectally a few hours to several days after forceful vomiting. The bleeding, which may be accompanied by epigastric or back pain, may range from mild to massive, but is usually more profuse than in esophageal rupture. In Mallory–Weiss syndrome, the blood vessels are only partially severed, preventing retraction and closure of the lumen.

▼ ALERT *Massive bleeding—most likely when the tear is on the gastric side, near the cardia—may quickly lead to fatal shock.*

Diagnosis

℞ CONFIRMING DIAGNOSIS *Fiberoptic endoscopy (esophagogastroduodenoscopy) confirms Mallory–Weiss syndrome by identifying esophageal tears. Recent tears appear as erythematous longitudinal cracks in the mucosa; older tears appear as raised white streaks surrounded by erythema.*

Treatment

Treatment varies with the severity of bleeding. GI bleeding usually stops spontaneously, thereafter requiring supportive measures and careful observation but no definitive treatment. However, if bleeding continues, treatment may include:
◆ proton pump inhibitors or H_2 receptor antagonists to help decrease acidity
◆ blood transfusions if blood loss is great
◆ endoscopy with electrocoagulation or heater probe for hemostasis
◆ transcatheter embolization or thrombus formation with an autologous blood clot or other hemostatic material (such as a shredded adsorbent gelatin sponge)
◆ surgery to suture each esophageal laceration

Special considerations

Observation is necessary to determine whether bleeding is transitory or ongoing.
◆ Evaluate the patient's respiratory status, monitor arterial blood gas values, and administer oxygen as necessary.
◆ Assess the amount of blood lost and record the color, amount, consistency, and frequency of hematemesis and melena.
◆ Draw blood for coagulation studies (prothrombin time, partial thromboplastin time, and platelet count), and type and crossmatch.
◆ Keep 3 units of blood available at all times. Insert a 14G to 18G I.V. line, and start an infusion of I.V. solution, as ordered. (If the I.V. infusion is for blood transfusion, use normal saline solution; if the infusion is for fluid replacement, use lactated Ringer's solution or another appropriate solution, depending on the results of laboratory tests.)
◆ Monitor the patient's vital signs, central venous pressure, urine output, neurologic status, and overall clinical status.
◆ Explain diagnostic tests to the patient.
◆ Keep the patient warm and maintain a safe environment.
◆ Obtain a detailed history of recent medications taken, dietary habits, and alcohol ingestion.
◆ Administer antiemetics, as ordered, to prevent postoperative retching and vomiting.
◆ Advise the patient to avoid aspirin, alcohol, and other irritating substances.

ESOPHAGEAL DIVERTICULA

Esophageal diverticula are hollow outpouchings of one or more layers of the esophageal wall. They occur in three main areas: immediately above the upper esophageal sphincter (Zenker's, or pulsion, diverticulum, the most common type); near the

midpoint of the esophagus (traction diverticulum); and immediately above the LES (epiphrenic diverticulum). Generally, esophageal diverticula occur later in life—although they can affect infants and children—and are three times more common in men than in women. Epiphrenic diverticula usually occur in middle-aged men, whereas Zenker's diverticula typically affect men older than 60 (and often older than 75).

Causes and incidence

Some esophageal diverticula arise from primary muscular abnormalities. Most diverticula occur in middle-aged and elderly patients. Zenker's diverticula occur most commonly in patients older than 50 and are especially prevalent in patients in their 70s and 80s.

Pathophysiology

Zenker's diverticulum occurs when the pouch results from increased intraesophageal pressure; traction diverticulum occurs when the pouch is pulled out by adjacent inflamed tissue or lymph nodes. Zenker's diverticulum results from developmental muscular weakness of the posterior pharynx above the border of the cricopharyngeal muscle. The pressure of swallowing aggravates this weakness, as does contraction of the pharynx before relaxation of the sphincter.

Esophageal diverticula are due to primary muscular abnormalities that may be congenital or to inflammatory processes adjacent to the esophagus. Some authorities classify all diverticula as traction diverticula. A midesophageal (traction) diverticulum is a response to scarring and pulling on esophageal walls by an external inflammatory process such as tuberculosis. An epiphrenic diverticulum (rare) is generally right-sided and usually accompanies an esophageal motor disturbance, such as esophageal spasm or achalasia. It's thought to be caused by traction and pulsation.

Complications
◆ Malnutrition
◆ Dehydration

Signs and symptoms

Midesophageal and epiphrenic diverticula with an associated motor disturbance (achalasia or spasm) seldom produce symptoms, although the patient may experience dysphagia and heartburn. Zenker's diverticulum, however, produces distinctly staged symptoms, beginning with initial throat irritation followed by dysphagia and near-complete obstruction. In early stages, regurgitation occurs soon after eating; in later stages, regurgitation after eating is delayed and may even occur during sleep, leading to food aspiration and pulmonary infection.

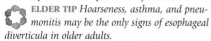 **ELDER TIP** *Hoarseness, asthma, and pneumonitis may be the only signs of esophageal diverticula in older adults.*

Other signs and symptoms include noise when liquids are swallowed, chronic cough, hoarseness, a bad taste in the mouth or foul breath and, rarely, bleeding.

Diagnosis

CONFIRMING DIAGNOSIS *X-rays taken following a barium swallow usually confirm the diagnosis by showing characteristic outpouching.*

Esophagoscopy can rule out another lesion; however, the procedure risks rupturing the diverticulum by passing the scope into it rather than into the lumen of the esophagus, a special danger with Zenker's diverticulum.

Treatment

Treatment of Zenker's diverticulum is usually palliative and includes a bland diet, thorough chewing, and drinking water after eating to flush out the sac. However, severe symptoms or a large diverticulum necessitates surgery to remove the sac or facilitate drainage. An esophagomyotomy may be necessary to prevent recurrence. Endoscopic stapling or laser surgery using CO_2 microscopy is commonly performed in patients who can't tolerate traditional surgeries.

A midesophageal diverticulum seldom requires therapy except when esophagitis aggravates the risk of rupture, in which case treatment includes antacids and an antireflux regimen: keeping the head elevated, maintaining an upright position for 2 hours after eating, eating small meals, controlling chronic coughing, and avoiding constrictive clothing.

Epiphrenic diverticulum requires treatment of accompanying motor disorders. Achalasia is treated by repeated dilations of the esophagus; acute spasm is controlled by anticholinergic administration and diverticulum excision; and dysphagia or severe pain is relieved by surgical excision or suspending the diverticulum to promote drainage. Treatment may also include parenteral feeding to improve the patient's nutritional status.

Special considerations

Care includes documenting the patient's symptoms and nutritional status and providing education about the disorder.

◆ Regularly assess the patient's nutritional status (weight, calorie intake, and appearance).

◆ If the patient regurgitates food and mucus, protect against aspiration by careful positioning (head elevated or turned to one side). To prevent aspiration, tell the patient to empty any visible outpouching in the neck by massage or postural drainage before retiring.

◆ If the patient has dysphagia, record well-tolerated foods and what circumstances ease swallowing. Provide a pureed diet, with vitamin or protein supplements, and encourage thorough chewing.

◆ Teach the patient about this disorder. Explain treatment instructions and diagnostic procedures.

HIATAL HERNIA

Hiatal hernia, also called *hiatus hernia*, is a defect in the diaphragm that permits a portion of the stomach to pass through the diaphragmatic opening into the chest. Hiatal hernia is the most common problem of the diaphragm affecting the alimentary canal. Four types of hiatal hernia can occur: sliding hiatal hernia (Type I), paraesophageal hiatal hernia (Type II), mixed hiatal hernia (Type III), or a Type IV, which is an aggravated form of Type II that includes other abdominal visceral herniation. (See *Types of hiatal hernia*, page 224.)

Causes and incidence

Hiatal hernia typically results from muscle weakening that's common with aging and may be secondary to esophageal carcinoma, kyphoscoliosis, trauma, or certain surgical procedures. It may also result from certain diaphragmatic malformations that may cause congenital weakness. Obesity and smoking are common risk factors.

In hiatal hernia, the muscular collar around the esophageal and diaphragmatic junction loosens, permitting the lower portion of the esophagus and the stomach to rise into the chest when intra-abdominal pressure increases (possibly causing gastroesophageal reflux). Such increased intra-abdominal pressure may result from ascites, pregnancy, obesity, constrictive clothing, bending, straining, coughing, Valsalva's maneuver, or extreme physical exertion.

Sliding hernias are more common than paraesophageal hernias. The incidence of hiatal hernia increases with age (most occur in people older than 40), and prevalence is higher in women than in men (especially the paraesophageal type). Contributing factors include obesity and trauma.

Types of hiatal hernia

A hiatal hernia is a displacement of the normal anatomy, as shown in the illustrations below.

Normal stomach

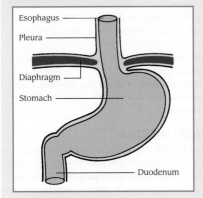

Esophagus
Pleura
Diaphragm
Stomach
Duodenum

Mixed hiatal hernia

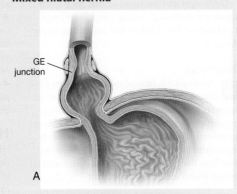

GE junction

A

Sliding hiatal hernia

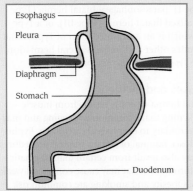

Esophagus
Pleura
Diaphragm
Stomach
Duodenum

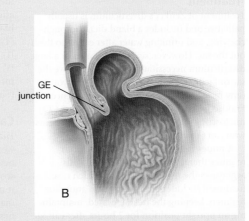

GE junction

B

Paraesophageal hernia

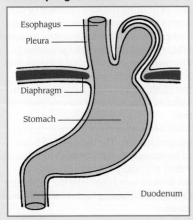

Esophagus
Pleura
Diaphragm
Stomach
Duodenum

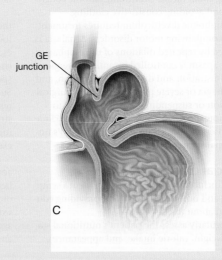

GE junction

C

Pathophysiology

In a sliding hiatal hernia, the stomach and the gastroesophageal junction slip up into the chest, so the gastroesophageal junction is above the diaphragmatic hiatus. In paraesophageal hiatal hernia, a part of the greater curvature of the stomach rolls through the diaphragmatic defect. A mixed hiatal hernia is a combination of Type I and Type II hernias, and often occurs with other diseases such as GERD, peptic ulcer disease (PUD), cholecystitis, cholelithiasis, chronic pancreatitis, and diverticulosis. In Type IV hiatal hernias, the entire stomach and other abdominal organs slide into the thorax.

Complications

- ◆ Dysphagia
- ◆ Gastroesophageal reflux
- ◆ Barrett's esophagus
- ◆ Esophageal adenocarcinoma

Signs and symptoms

Typically, a paraesophageal hernia produces no symptoms; it's usually an incidental finding during a barium swallow or when testing for occult blood. Because this type of hernia leaves the closing mechanism of the cardiac sphincter unchanged, it rarely causes acid reflux or reflux esophagitis. Symptoms result from displacement or stretching of the stomach and may include a feeling of fullness in the chest or pain resembling angina pectoris. Even if it produces no symptoms, this type of hernia needs surgical treatment because of the high risk of strangulation that can occur when a large portion of the stomach becomes caught above the diaphragm.

A sliding hernia without an incompetent sphincter produces no reflux or symptoms and, consequently, doesn't require treatment. When a sliding hernia causes symptoms, they are typical of gastric reflux, resulting from the incompetent LES, and may include the following:

- ◆ Pyrosis (heartburn) occurs 1 to 4 hours after eating (especially overeating) and is aggravated by reclining, belching, and increased intra-abdominal pressure. It may be accompanied by regurgitation or vomiting.
- ◆ Retrosternal or substernal chest pain results from reflux of gastric contents, stomach distention, and spasm or altered motor activity. Chest pain usually occurs after meals or at bedtime and is aggravated by reclining, belching, and increased intra-abdominal pressure.

Other common symptoms reflect possible complications:

- ◆ Dysphagia occurs when the hernia produces esophagitis, esophageal ulceration, or stricture,

especially with ingestion of very hot or cold foods, alcoholic beverages, or a large amount of food.

- ◆ Bleeding may be mild or massive, frank or occult; the source may be esophagitis or erosions of the gastric pouch.
- ◆ Severe pain and shock result from incarceration, in which a large portion of the stomach is caught above the diaphragm (usually occurs with paraesophageal hernia). Incarceration may lead to perforation of the gastric ulcer and strangulation and gangrene of the herniated portion of the stomach. It requires immediate surgery.

Diagnosis

Diagnosis of hiatal hernia is based on typical clinical features and on the results of these laboratory studies and procedures:

- ◆ In barium study, hernia may appear as an outpouching containing barium at the lower end of the esophagus. Small hernias, however, are difficult to recognize. This study also shows diaphragmatic abnormalities.
- ◆ Endoscopy (esophagogastroduodenoscopy) and biopsy differentiate among hiatal hernia, varices, and other small gastroesophageal lesions; identify the mucosal junction and the edge of the diaphragm indenting the esophagus; and can rule out malignancy that otherwise may be difficult to detect.
- ◆ Esophageal motility studies assess the presence of esophageal motor abnormalities before surgical repair of the hernia.
- ◆ pH studies assess for reflux of gastric contents.

Treatment

The primary goals of treatment are to relieve symptoms by minimizing or correcting the incompetent cardia and to manage and prevent complications. Medical intervention is used first because symptoms usually respond to it and because hiatal hernia tends to recur after surgery. Such treatment attempts to modify or reduce reflux by changing the quantity or quality of refluxed gastric contents, by strengthening the LES muscle pharmacologically, or by decreasing the amount of reflux through gravity. These measures include restricting any activity that raises intra-abdominal pressure (coughing, straining, or bending), giving antiemetics, avoiding constrictive clothing, modifying diet, giving stool softeners or laxatives to prevent straining at stool, and discouraging smoking because it stimulates gastric acid production.

Modifying the diet means eating small, frequent, bland meals at least 2 hours before lying down, avoidance of bedtime snacking, eating slowly, and avoiding spicy foods, fruit juices, alcoholic beverages, and coffee. Antacids also modify the fluid refluxed into the esophagus and are effective treatment for intermittent reflux.

To reduce the amount of reflux, the patient who is overweight should lose weight to decrease intra-abdominal pressure. Elevating the head of the bed 6" (15 cm) reduces gastric reflux by gravity.

Drug therapy includes antacids to neutralize stomach acid, medications to reduce acid production, and medications to block acid production and to heal the esophagus.

Surgical repair is necessary when symptoms can't be controlled medically or with the onset of complications, such as stricture, bleeding, pulmonary aspiration, strangulation, or incarceration. Surgery typically involves creating an artificial closing mechanism at the gastroesophageal junction to strengthen the LES's barrier function. The surgeon may use an abdominal or a thoracic approach, or may repair the hernia by laparoscopic surgery, which allows for less dependence on an NG tube and a shorter hospital stay.

Special considerations

To enhance compliance with treatment, teach the patient about this disorder. Explain treatments, diagnostic tests, and significant symptoms.

◆ Prepare the patient for diagnostic tests as needed. After endoscopy, watch for signs of perforation (falling blood pressure, rapid pulse, shock, and sudden pain).

◆ If surgery is scheduled, review preoperative and postoperative considerations with the patient.

◆ After surgery, carefully record intake and output, including NG tube and wound drainage.

◆ While the NG tube is in place, provide meticulous mouth and nose care, but don't manipulate the tube. Give ice chips, if permitted, to moisten oral mucous membranes.

◆ If the surgeon used a thoracic approach, the patient may have chest tubes in place. Carefully observe chest tube drainage and the patient's respiratory status, and perform pulmonary physiotherapy.

◆ Before discharge, tell the patient what foods he or she can eat, and recommend small, frequent meals. Teach about avoidance of activities that cause increased intra-abdominal pressure, and recommend a slow return to normal functions (within 6 to 8 weeks).

Stomach, intestine, and pancreas

GASTRITIS

Gastritis, an inflammation of the gastric mucosa, may be acute or chronic. Acute gastritis produces mucosal reddening, edema, hemorrhage, and erosion. Chronic gastritis is common among elderly people and people with pernicious anemia. It typically occurs as chronic atrophic gastritis, in which all stomach mucosal layers are inflamed, with reduced numbers of chief and parietal cells. Acute or chronic gastritis can occur at any age.

Causes and incidence

Acute gastritis has numerous causes, including:
◆ chronic ingestion of (or an allergic reaction to) irritating foods or beverages, such as hot peppers or alcohol
◆ drugs, such as aspirin and other nonsteroidal anti-inflammatory drugs (NSAIDs; in large doses), cytotoxic agents, corticosteroids, antimetabolites, phenylbutazone, and indomethacin
◆ ingestion of poisons, especially DDT, ammonia, mercury, carbon tetrachloride, and corrosive substances
◆ endotoxins released from infecting bacteria, such as staphylococci, *Escherichia coli*, or salmonella

Acute gastritis leading to stress ulcers also may develop in acute illnesses, especially when the patient has had major traumatic injuries; burns; severe infection; hepatic, renal, or respiratory failure; or major surgery.

Chronic gastritis can occur at any age, and may be associated with PUD or gastrostomy, both of which cause chronic reflux of pancreatic secretions, bile, and bile acids from the duodenum into the stomach. Recurring exposure to irritating substances, such as drugs, alcohol, cigarette smoke, or environmental agents, may also lead to chronic gastritis. Chronic gastritis may occur with pernicious anemia, renal disease, or diabetes mellitus. Pernicious anemia is commonly associated with atrophic gastritis, a chronic inflammation of the stomach resulting from degeneration of the gastric mucosa. In pernicious anemia, the stomach can no longer secrete intrinsic factor, which is needed for vitamin B_{12} absorption.

Bacterial infection with *Helicobacter pylori* is a common cause of nonerosive chronic gastritis. About 50% of adults are infected with *H. pylori*, with a higher prevalence in developing nations.

Pathophysiology

Acute gastritis is caused by injury of the protective mucosal barrier; mechanisms of injury include drugs, chemicals, or *H. pylori* infection. NSAIDs inhibit the action of cyclooxygenase-1 (COX-1) and cause gastritis because of the inhibited prostaglandin synthesis which normally stimulates mucus secretion and suppresses inflammation.

Chronic gastritis is classified as type A (immune, or fundal), type B (nonimmune, or antral) associated with *H. pylori*, type AB (when types A and B occur at the same time), or type C (which is associated with bile reflux and pancreatic secretions into the stomach).

Complications

◆ Hemorrhage
◆ Shock
◆ Obstruction
◆ Perforation
◆ Peritonitis
◆ Gastric cancer

Signs and symptoms

After exposure to the offending substance, the patient with acute gastritis typically reports a rapid onset of symptoms, such as epigastric discomfort, indigestion, cramping, anorexia, nausea, vomiting, and hematemesis. The symptoms last from a few hours to a few days.

The patient with chronic gastritis may describe similar symptoms or may have only mild epigastric discomfort. Concerns may be vague, such as intolerance for spicy or fatty foods or slight pain relieved by eating.

Diagnosis

℞ **CONFIRMING DIAGNOSIS** *Esophagogastroduodenoscopy or gastroscopy (with biopsy) confirms gastritis when done before lesions heal (usually within 24 hours). This test is contraindicated after ingestion of a corrosive agent.*

Laboratory analyses can detect occult blood in vomitus or stool (or both) if the patient has gastric bleeding. Hemoglobin level and hematocrit are decreased if the patient has developed anemia from bleeding.

Treatment

Treatment for gastritis focuses on eliminating the cause; for example, bacterial gastritis is treated with antibiotics, whereas gastritis caused by ingested poison is treated by neutralizing the poison with the appropriate antidote. Proton pump inhibitors or H_2 receptor antagonists may reduce gastric acid production. Many over-the-counter preparations are available. Antacids may be used as buffers.

For critically ill patients, antacids administered hourly, with or without H_2-receptor antagonists, may reduce the frequency of gastritis attacks. Some patients also require analgesics. Until healing occurs, patients' oxygen needs, blood volume, and fluid and electrolyte balance must be monitored.

When gastritis causes massive bleeding, treatment includes blood replacement; iced saline lavage, possibly with norepinephrine; angiography with vasopressin infused in normal saline solution; and, sometimes, surgery.

Vagotomy and pyloroplasty achieve limited success when conservative treatments fail. Rarely, partial or total gastrectomy may be required.

Simply avoiding aspirin and spicy foods may prevent exacerbations of chronic gastritis. If symptoms develop or persist, antacids may be taken. If pernicious anemia is the cause, vitamin B_{12} may be administered parenterally. A combination of two antibiotics, such as clarithromycin and amoxicillin, is typically given for 14 days to treat *H. pylori*. Acid-reducing medications may help to enhance the effectiveness of the antibiotics.

Special considerations

Patient care includes education and attention to various aspects of nutritional status to control symptoms and prevent their recurrence.

◆ For vomiting, give antiemetics and I.V. fluids, as ordered. Monitor fluid intake and output and electrolyte levels.
◆ Monitor the patient for recurrent symptoms as food is reintroduced; provide a bland diet.
◆ Offer smaller, more frequent meals to reduce irritating gastric secretions. Eliminate foods that cause gastric upset.
◆ Administer proton pump inhibitors, H_2-receptor antagonists, and antacids, as ordered.
◆ If pain or nausea interferes with the patient's appetite, give analgesics or antiemetics 1 hour before meals.
◆ Teach the patient to avoid alcohol, caffeine, and irritating foods such as spicy or highly seasoned foods.
◆ If the patient smokes, provide referral to a smoking-cessation program.
◆ Urge the patient to seek immediate attention for recurring symptoms, such as hematemesis, nausea, or vomiting.
◆ To prevent exacerbation, urge the patient to take prophylactic medications, as ordered.

░ **PREVENTION** *Advise the patient to take steroids with milk, food, or antacids. Instruct to take antacids between meals and at bedtime and to avoid aspirin-containing compounds.*

GASTROENTERITIS

A self-limiting disorder, gastroenteritis is characterized by diarrhea, nausea, vomiting, and acute or chronic abdominal cramping. Also called *intestinal flu, traveler's diarrhea, viral enteritis,* or *food poisoning,* it occurs in persons of all ages and is a major cause of morbidity and mortality in underdeveloped nations. It also can be life-threatening in elderly or debilitated people.

Causes and incidence

Gastroenteritis has many possible causes, including:
◆ bacteria (responsible for acute food poisoning), such as *Staphylococcus aureus, Salmonella, Shigella, Clostridium botulinum, C. perfringens,* and *E. coli*
◆ amebae, especially *Entamoeba histolytica*
◆ parasites, such as *Ascaris, Enterobius,* and *Trichinella spiralis*
◆ viruses (may be responsible for traveler's diarrhea) such as adenoviruses, echoviruses, or coxsackieviruses
◆ ingestion of toxins, including plants or toadstools
◆ drug reactions; for example, to antibiotics
◆ enzyme deficiencies
◆ food allergens

The bowel reacts to any of these enterotoxins with hypermotility, producing severe diarrhea and secondary depletion of intracellular fluid. Chronic gastroenteritis is usually the result of another GI disorder such as ulcerative colitis. The incidence of gastroenteritis is relevant to the causative agent. The prevalence of norovirus is approximately 18%, and higher in low-mortality developing and developed countries versus high-mortality developing and developed countries.

Pathophysiology

Pathophysiology of gastroenteritis is related to the causative agent.

Complications

◆ Severe dehydration
◆ Electrolyte loss
◆ Shock
◆ Vascular collapse
◆ Renal failure

Signs and symptoms

Signs and symptoms vary depending on the pathologic organism and on the level of the GI tract involved. However, gastroenteritis in adults is usually an acute, self-limiting, nonfatal disease producing diarrhea, abdominal discomfort (ranging from cramping to pain), nausea, and vomiting. Other possible signs and symptoms include fever, malaise, and borborygmi. In children, older adults, and the immunocompromised, gastroenteritis produces the same symptoms, but these patients' intolerance to electrolyte and fluid losses leads to a higher mortality.

Diagnosis

Patient history can aid in the diagnosis of gastroenteritis. Stool culture (by direct rectal swab) or blood culture identifies the causative bacteria or parasites.

Treatment

Treatment is usually supportive and consists of rest, nutritional support, and increased fluid intake. When gastroenteritis is severe or affects a young child or an elderly or debilitated person, treatment may necessitate hospitalization, specific antimicrobials, I.V. fluid and electrolyte replacement and, possibly, antiemetics (given orally, I.M., or by rectal suppository).

Special considerations

Patient care includes education, administering medications, and assessing symptoms for signs of improvement or worsening.
◆ Administer medications as ordered; correlate dosages, routes, and times appropriately with the patient's meals and activities (e.g., give antiemetics 30 to 60 minutes before meals).
◆ If the patient can eat and is not dehydrated, replace lost fluids and electrolytes with foods and diluted fruit juice, sports drinks. No specific diet is required, yet a bland diet may be better tolerated. Saltine crackers, broths, soups, broiled starches or cereals, bananas, and vegetables can help to meet fluid and sodium needs. Vary the diet to make it more enjoyable, and allow some choice of foods. Teach the patient to avoid milk and milk products, which may provoke recurrence.
◆ Record intake and output carefully and obtain serial weight measurements. Watch for signs of dehydration, such as dry skin and mucous membranes, fever, and sunken eyes.
◆ Wash hands thoroughly after giving care to avoid spreading infection.
◆ To ease anal irritation, provide warm sitz baths or apply witch hazel compresses.
◆ If food poisoning is the likely cause of gastroenteritis, contact public health authorities so they can interview patients and food handlers, and take samples of the suspected contaminated food.

PREVENTION *Teach good hygiene to prevent recurrence. Instruct patients to cook foods—especially pork—thoroughly; to refrigerate perishable foods, such as milk, mayonnaise, potato salad, and cream-filled pastries; to always wash hands thoroughly with warm water and soap before handling food, and especially after using the bathroom; to clean utensils thoroughly; to avoid drinking water or eating raw fruit or vegetables when visiting a foreign country; and to eliminate flies and roaches in the home.*

PEPTIC ULCERS

Peptic ulcers—circumscribed lesions in the mucosal membrane—can develop in the lower esophagus, stomach, pylorus, duodenum, or jejunum. Most peptic ulcers are duodenal ulcers, which affect the proximal part of the small intestine.

Gastric ulcers, which affect the stomach mucosa, are commonly seen in chronic users of NSAIDs, alcohol, or tobacco. Duodenal ulcers usually follow a chronic course, with remissions and exacerbations; a small percentage of patients develop complications that necessitate surgery.

Causes and incidence

Researchers recognize two primary major causes of PUD: infection with *H. pylori* (formerly known as *Campylobacter pylori*), and use of NSAIDs, and pathologic hypersecretory disorders such as Zollinger–Ellison syndrome.

Pathophysiology

In the United States, about 1.6 million people develop peptic ulcers yearly. Men and women

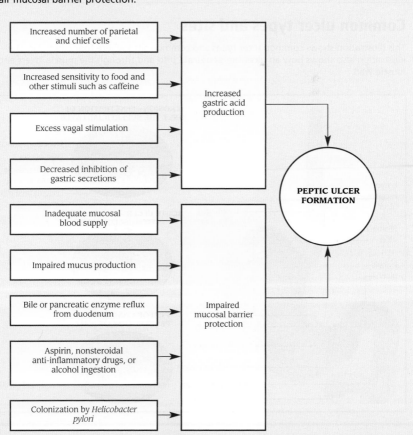

PATHOPHYSIOLOGY
How peptic ulcers develop

Peptic ulcers can result from factors that increase gastric acid production or from factors that impair mucosal barrier protection.

Increased number of parietal and chief cells →

Increased sensitivity to food and other stimuli such as caffeine →

Excess vagal stimulation →

Decreased inhibition of gastric secretions →

→ Increased gastric acid production

Inadequate mucosal blood supply →

Impaired mucus production →

Bile or pancreatic enzyme reflux from duodenum →

Aspirin, nonsteroidal anti-inflammatory drugs, or alcohol ingestion →

Colonization by *Helicobacter pylori* →

→ Impaired mucosal barrier protection

PEPTIC ULCER FORMATION

are affected equally, and incidence increases with age. A higher percentage of *H. pylori* infection occurs in people older than age 50. See box *how peptic ulcers develop* for pathophysiology.

Helicobacter pylori produces an ulcer by damaging the mucous coating that protects the stomach and duodenum.

Salicylates and other NSAIDs encourage ulcer formation by inhibiting the secretion of prostaglandins (the substances that suppress ulceration). Certain illnesses, such as pancreatitis, hepatic disease, Crohn disease, preexisting gastritis, and Zollinger–Ellison syndrome, are also known causes.

Besides peptic ulcer's main causes, several predisposing factors are acknowledged. They include blood type (gastric ulcers tend to strike people with type A blood; duodenal ulcers tend to afflict people with type O blood) and other genetic factors. Exposure to irritants, such as alcohol, coffee, and tobacco, may contribute by accelerating gastric acid emptying and promoting mucosal breakdown. Ulceration occurs when the acid secretion exceeds the buffering factors. Physical trauma, emotional stress, and normal aging are additional predisposing conditions. (See *Common ulcer types and sites.*)

Complications
- GI hemorrhage
- Hypovolemic shock
- Perforation
- Obstruction
- Extension of ulcer into adjacent structures
- Dumping syndrome
- Vitamin deficiency

Signs and symptoms
Heartburn and indigestion usually signal the beginning of a gastric ulcer attack. Eating stretches the gastric wall and may cause or, in some cases, relieve pain and feelings of fullness and distention. Other typical effects include weight loss and repeated episodes of massive GI bleeding.

Duodenal ulcers produce heartburn, well-localized midepigastric pain (relieved by food),

Common ulcer types and sites

This illustration shows common ulcer types and common sites where they can occur. The illustration also shows how an ulcer can penetrate into and through the muscle layers and muscle wall.

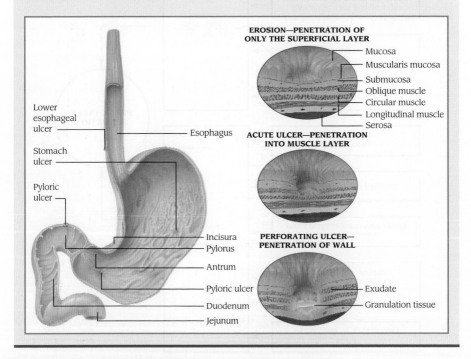

weight gain (because the patient eats to relieve discomfort), and a peculiar sensation of hot water bubbling in the back of the throat. Attacks usually occur about 2 hours after meals, whenever the stomach is empty, or after consumption of orange juice, coffee, aspirin, or alcohol. Exacerbations tend to recur several times per year and then fade into remission. Vomiting and other digestive disturbances are rare.

Ulcers may penetrate the pancreas and cause severe back pain. Other complications of peptic ulcers include perforation, hemorrhage, and pyloric obstruction. Ulcers may, on occasion, produce no symptoms.

Diagnosis

℞ CONFIRMING DIAGNOSIS *Esophagogastroduodenoscopy confirms the presence of an ulcer and permits cytologic studies and biopsy to rule out H. pylori or cancer.*

Diagnosis may be confirmed by the following tests:

◆ Barium swallow or upper GI and small bowel series may reveal the presence of the ulcer. This is the initial test performed on a patient whose symptoms aren't severe.
◆ Laboratory analysis may detect occult blood in stools.
◆ Serologic testing may disclose clinical signs of infection such as an elevated white blood cell count.
◆ Carbon 13 (^{13}C) urea breath test results reflect activity of *H. pylori.*

Treatment

Experts recommend treating the patient with two antibiotics and a proton pump inhibitor or H$_2$ receptor antagonists to eradicate *H. pylori.* The patient taking NSAIDs may take a prostaglandin analog (misoprostol) to suppress ulceration (or the patient may take the analog with NSAIDs to prevent ulceration). H$_2$ receptor antagonists or proton pump inhibitors may reduce acid secretion. A coating agent or bismuth may be administered to the patient with a duodenal ulcer to protect the lining.

If GI bleeding occurs, emergency treatment begins with passage of an NG tube to allow for iced saline lavage, possibly containing norepinephrine. Gastroscopy allows visualization of the bleeding site and coagulation by laser or cautery to control bleeding. This type of therapy allows postponement of surgery until the patient's condition stabilizes. Surgery is indicated for perforation, unresponsiveness to conservative treatment, and suspected malignancy. Surgery for peptic ulcers may include:

◆ Vagotomy and pyloroplasty—severing one or more branches of the vagus nerve to reduce hydrochloric acid secretion and refashioning the pylorus to create a larger lumen and facilitate gastric emptying
◆ Distal subtotal gastrectomy (with or without vagotomy)—excising the antrum of the stomach, thereby removing the hormonal stimulus of the parietal cells, followed by anastomosis of the rest of the stomach to the duodenum or the jejunum
◆ Pyloroplasty—surgical enlargement of the pylorus to provide drainage of gastric secretions.

Special considerations

Management of peptic ulcers requires careful administration of medications, thorough patient teaching, and skillful postoperative care.
◆ Watch for adverse reactions to H$_2$-receptor antagonists and proton pump inhibitors (dizziness, fatigue, rash, and mild diarrhea).
◆ Advise any patient who uses antacids, who has a history of cardiac disease, or who follows a sodium-restricted diet to take only those antacids that contain low amounts of sodium.
◆ Warn the patient to avoid NSAIDs because they irritate the gastric mucosa. For the same reason, advise the patient to stop smoking and to avoid stressful situations, excessive intake of coffee, and drinking alcoholic beverages during exacerbations of PUD.

After gastric surgery:
◆ Keep the NG tube patent. If the tube isn't functioning, don't reposition it; you might damage the suture line or anastomosis. Notify the surgeon promptly.
◆ Monitor intake and output, including NG tube drainage. Check for bowel sounds, and allow the patient nothing by mouth until peristalsis resumes and the NG tube is removed or clamped.
◆ Replace fluids and electrolytes. Assess the patient for signs of dehydration, sodium deficiency, and metabolic alkalosis, which may occur secondary to gastric suction.
◆ Monitor the patient for possible dumping syndrome (a rapid gastric emptying, causing distention of the duodenum or jejunum produced by a bolus of food). Signs and symptoms of dumping syndrome include diaphoresis, weakness, nausea, flatulence, explosive diarrhea, distention, and palpitations within 30 minutes after a meal.
◆ To avoid dumping syndrome, advise the patient to lie down after meals, to drink fluids *between* meals rather than with meals, to avoid eating large amounts of carbohydrates, and to eat four to six small, high-protein, low-carbohydrate meals during the day.

PATHOPHYSIOLOGY
Mucosal changes in ulcerative colitis

In ulcerative colitis, the colon goes through inflammation and ulceration.

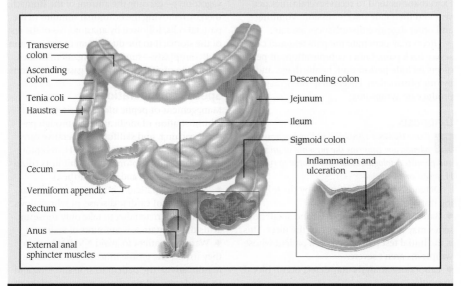

ULCERATIVE COLITIS

Ulcerative colitis is an inflammatory, usually chronic disease that affects the mucosa of the colon. It invariably begins in the rectum and sigmoid colon and commonly extends upward into the entire colon; it rarely affects the small intestine, except for the terminal ileum. Ulcerative colitis produces edema (leading to mucosal friability) and ulcerations. Severity is categorized as mild, moderate, or severe. (See *Mucosal changes in ulcerative colitis*.)

Causes and incidence

Although the etiology of ulcerative colitis is unknown, it's thought to be related to abnormal immune response in the GI tract, possibly associated with food or bacteria such as *E. coli*. Stress was once thought to be a cause of ulcerative colitis, but studies show that it isn't a cause, although it does increase the severity of the attack.

Ulcerative colitis occurs primarily in young adults. It's also more prevalent among those of Jewish ancestry, indicating a possible familial tendency. In North America, the incidence of the disease has risen in the past decade, with approximately 286 of every 100,000 persons affected. The onset of symptoms is generally noted between 15 and 40 years old, with a second peak between 50 and 80.

Pathophysiology
Complications
◆ Nutritional deficiency
◆ Perineal sepsis
◆ Anal fissure or fistula
◆ Perirectal abscess
◆ Hemorrhage
◆ Toxic megacolon
◆ Coagulation deficit

Signs and symptoms

The hallmark of ulcerative colitis is recurrent attacks of bloody diarrhea, in many cases containing pus and mucus, interspersed with asymptomatic remissions. The intensity of these attacks varies with the extent of inflammation. It isn't uncommon for a patient with ulcerative colitis to have as many as 15 to 20 liquid, bloody stools daily. Other symptoms include spastic rectum and anus, abdominal pain, irritability, weight loss, weakness, anorexia, nausea, and vomiting.

Ulcerative colitis may lead to complications, such as hemorrhage, stricture, or perforation of the colon. Other complications include joint inflammation, ankylosing spondylitis, eye lesions, mouth ulcers, liver disease, and pyoderma gangrenosum. Researchers anticipate that these complications occur when the immune system triggers inflammation in other parts of the body. These disorders are usually mild and disappear when the colitis is treated.

Patients with ulcerative colitis have an increased risk of developing colorectal cancer; children with ulcerative colitis may experience impaired growth and sexual development.

Diagnosis

℞ **CONFIRMING DIAGNOSIS** *Sigmoidoscopy showing increased mucosal friability, decreased mucosal detail, pinpoint hemorrhages, and thick inflammatory exudate suggests this diagnosis. Biopsy can help confirm it.*

Colonoscopy may be required to determine the extent of the disease and to evaluate stricture areas and pseudopolyps for which a biopsy would then be done during the colonoscopy. Barium enema can assess the extent of the disease and detect complications, such as strictures and carcinoma.

A stool sample should be cultured and analyzed for leukocytes, ova, and parasites. Other supportive laboratory values include decreased serum levels of potassium, magnesium, hemoglobin, and albumin as well as leukocytosis and increased prothrombin time. An elevated erythrocyte sedimentation rate correlates with the severity of the attack.

Treatment

The goals of treatment are to control inflammation, replace nutritional losses and blood volume, and prevent complications. Supportive treatment includes bed rest, I.V. fluid replacement, and a clear-liquid diet. For patients awaiting surgery or showing signs of dehydration and debilitation from excessive diarrhea, TPN rests the intestinal tract, decreases stool volume, and restores positive nitrogen balance. Blood transfusions or iron supplements may be needed to correct anemia.

Sulfasalazine and mesalamine are used for their anti-inflammatory action. Immune system suppressors may be used to decrease the frequency of attacks. Drug therapy to control inflammation may include steroids. Antispasmodics and antidiarrheals are used only in patients whose ulcerative colitis is under control but who have frequent, loose stools.

⚠ **ALERT** *Antispasmodics and antidiarrheals may lead to massive dilation of the colon (toxic megacolon) and are generally contraindicated.*

Surgery is the last resort if the patient has toxic megacolon, fails to respond to drugs and supportive measures, or finds symptoms unbearable. A common surgical technique is proctocolectomy with ileostomy. Another procedure, the ileoanal pull-through, is being performed in more cases. This procedure entails performing a total proctocolectomy and mucosal stripping, creating a pouch from the terminal ileum, and anastomosing the pouch to the anal canal. A temporary ileostomy is created to divert stool and allow the rectal anastomosis to heal. The ileostomy is closed in 2 to 3 months, and the patient can then evacuate stool rectally. This procedure removes all the potentially malignant epithelia of the rectum and colon. Total colectomy and ileorectal anastomosis isn't as common because of its mortality rate. This procedure removes the entire colon and anastomoses the terminal ileum to the rectum; it requires observation of the remaining rectal stump for any signs of cancer or colitis.

Pouch ileostomy (Kock pouch or continent ileostomy), in which the surgeon creates a pouch from a small loop of the terminal ileum and a nipple valve from the distal ileum, may be an option. The resulting stoma opens just above the pubic hairline, and the pouch is emptied periodically through a catheter inserted in the stoma. In ulcerative colitis, a colectomy may have to be performed after colonic perforation (although this is rare) or after years of active disease because of the increased incidence of colon cancer in these cases. Performing a partial colectomy to prevent colon cancer is controversial.

Special considerations

Patient care includes close monitoring for changes in status.

◆ Accurately record intake and output, particularly the frequency and volume of stools. Watch for signs of dehydration and electrolyte imbalances, especially signs and symptoms of hypokalemia (muscle weakness and paresthesia) and hypernatremia (tachycardia, flushed skin, fever, and dry tongue). Monitor hemoglobin level and hematocrit, and give blood transfusions as ordered. Provide good mouth care for the patient who's allowed nothing by mouth.

◆ After each bowel movement, thoroughly clean the skin around the rectum. Provide an air mattress or sheepskin to help prevent skin shear and breakdown.

◆ Administer medications, as ordered. Monitor for adverse effects of prolonged corticosteroid therapy (moon face, hirsutism, edema, and gastric irritation). Be aware that corticosteroid therapy may mask infection.

◆ If the patient needs TPN, change dressings as ordered, assess for inflammation at the insertion site, and check capillary blood glucose levels every 4 to 6 hours.

◆ Take precautionary measures if the patient is prone to bleeding. Watch closely for signs of complications, such as a perforated colon and peritonitis (fever, severe abdominal pain, abdominal rigidity and tenderness, and cool, clammy skin) and toxic megacolon (abdominal distention and decreased bowel sounds).

For the patient requiring surgery:

◆ Carefully prepare the patient for surgery, and teach about ileostomy.

◆ Perform bowel preparation, as ordered.

◆ After surgery, provide meticulous supportive care and continue teaching correct stoma care.

◆ Keep the NG tube patent. After removal of the tube, provide a clear-liquid diet and gradually advance to a low-residue diet, as tolerated.

◆ After a proctocolectomy and ileostomy, teach good stoma care. Wash the skin around the stoma with soapy water and dry it thoroughly. Apply karaya gum around the stoma's base to avoid irritation, and make a watertight seal. Attach the pouch over the karaya ring. Cut an opening in the ring to fit over the stoma, and secure the pouch to the skin. Empty the pouch when it's one third full. Encourage the patient to report stoma color changes or purulent drainage to the healthcare provider.

◆ After a pouch ileostomy, uncork the catheter every hour to allow contents to drain. After 10 to 14 days, gradually increase the length of time the catheter is left corked until it can be opened every 3 hours. Then remove the catheter and reinsert it every 3 to 4 hours for drainage. Teach the patient how to insert the catheter and how to take care of the stoma.

◆ Encourage the patient to have regular physical examinations.

NECROTIZING ENTEROCOLITIS

Necrotizing enterocolitis (NEC) is characterized by diffuse or patchy intestinal necrosis, accompanied by fatal sepsis in about one third of cases. Sepsis usually involves *E. coli*, *Clostridia*, *Salmonella*, *Pseudomonas*, or *Klebsiella*. Initially, necrosis is localized, occurring anywhere along the intestine, but usually in the ileum, ascending colon, or rectosigmoid. If diffuse bleeding occurs, NEC usually results in disseminated intravascular coagulation (DIC).

Causes and incidence

The exact cause of NEC is not fully understood, although it is thought to be related to mucosal injury by cytotoxic drugs, profound neutropenia, and/or impaired host defense when invaded by microorganisms.

NEC usually occurs in premature infants (<32 weeks of gestation) and those of very low birth weight (<1,500 g). NEC is more common in some geographic areas, thought to be due to the higher incidence of premature neonates and neonates who have low birth weights in these areas. In the United States, it is estimated that this condition occurs in 1 to 3 per 1,000 live births.

Pathophysiology

The etiology of NEC is not fully known, although it is thought to be related to mucosal injury as noted above. Other predisposing factors are thought to include birth asphyxia, postnatal hypotension, respiratory distress, hypothermia, umbilical vessel catheterization, exchange transfusion, or patent ductus arteriosus. NEC may also be a response to significant prenatal stress, such as premature rupture of membranes, placenta previa, maternal sepsis, toxemia of pregnancy, or breech or cesarean birth.

NEC may develop when the infant suffers perinatal hypoxemia due to shunting of blood from the gut to more vital organs. Subsequent mucosal ischemia provides an ideal medium for bacterial growth. Accumulation of gas in the intestine can cause pressure that impedes blood flow; vasoconstriction may play a role in contribution to this condition. Hypertonic formula may increase bacterial activity because—unlike maternal breast milk—it doesn't provide protective immunologic activity and it contributes to the production of hydrogen gas. As the bowel swells and breaks down, gas-forming bacteria invade damaged areas, producing free air in the intestinal wall. This may result in fatal perforation and peritonitis.

Complications

◆ Perforation

◆ Mechanical and functional abnormalities of the intestine

Signs and symptoms

Neonates who have suffered from perinatal hypoxemia have the potential for developing NEC. A distended (especially tense or rigid) abdomen with gastric retention is the earliest and most common sign of oncoming NEC, which usually appears 1 to 10 days after birth. Other clinical features are increasing residual gastric contents (which may contain bile), bile-stained vomitus, and occult blood in the stool. A portion of patients may have bloody diarrhea. A red or shiny, taut abdomen may indicate peritonitis.

Nonspecific signs and symptoms include thermal instability, lethargy, metabolic acidosis, jaundice, and DIC. The major complication is perforation, which requires surgery. Recurrence of NEC and mechanical and functional abnormalities of the intestine, especially stricture, are the usual cause of residual intestinal malfunction in any infant who survives acute NEC; this complication may develop as late as several months postoperatively.

Diagnosis

Successful treatment of NEC is reliant upon early recognition.

CONFIRMING DIAGNOSIS *Abdominal X-rays confirm the diagnosis, showing nonspecific intestinal dilation and, in later stages of NEC, pneumatosis cystoides intestinalis (gas or air in the intestinal wall).*

Blood studies show several abnormalities. Platelet count may fall below 50,000/µL. Serum sodium levels are decreased, and arterial blood gas levels indicate metabolic acidosis (a result of sepsis). Infection-induced red blood cell breakdown elevates bilirubin levels. Blood and stool cultures identify the infecting organism, clotting studies and the hemoglobin level reveal associated DIC, and the guaiac test detects occult blood in the stool.

Treatment

The first signs of NEC necessitate removal of the umbilical catheter (arterial or venous) and discontinuation of oral intake for 7 to 10 days to rest the injured bowel. I.V. fluids, including TPN, maintain fluid and electrolyte balance and nutrition during this time; passage of an NG tube aids bowel decompression. If coagulation studies indicate a need for transfusion, the infant usually receives dextran to promote hemodilution, increase mesenteric blood flow, and reduce platelet aggregation. Antibiotic therapy consists of parenteral agents—administered through an NG tube, if necessary—to suppress bacterial flora and prevent bowel perforation. Anteroposterior and lateral X-rays are repeated to monitor disease progression.

Surgery is indicated if the patient shows any of these signs or symptoms: signs of perforation (free intraperitoneal air on X-ray or symptoms of peritonitis), respiratory insufficiency (caused by severe abdominal distention), progressive and intractable acidosis, or DIC. Surgery removes all necrotic and acutely inflamed bowel and creates a temporary colostomy or ileostomy. At least 12″ (30.5 cm) of bowel must remain or the infant may suffer from malabsorption or chronic vitamin B_{12} deficiency.

Special considerations

ALERT *Be alert for signs or symptoms of gastric distention and perforation: apnea, cardiovascular shock, sudden drop in temperature, bradycardia, sudden listlessness, rag-doll limpness, increasing abdominal tenderness, edema, erythema, or involuntary abdominal rigidity.*

◆ To avoid perforating the bowel, *don't* take rectal temperatures.

◆ Prevent cross-contamination by disposing of soiled diapers properly and washing hands immediately after diaper changes.

◆ After surgery, the infant needs mechanical ventilation. Gently suction secretions, and assess breathing often.

◆ Replace fluids lost through NG tube and stoma drainage. Include drainage losses in output records. Weigh the infant daily. A daily weight gain of 10 to 20 g indicates a favorable response to therapy.

◆ An infant with a temporary colostomy or ileostomy needs special care. Explain to the parents what a colostomy or ileostomy is and why it's necessary. Encourage them to participate in their infant's physical care after the condition is no longer critical.

◆ Because of the infant's small abdomen, the suture line is near the stoma; as a result, keeping the suture line clean can be a problem. Good skin care is essential because the immature infant's skin is fragile and vulnerable to excoriation and the active enzymes in bowel secretions are corrosive. Improvise premature-sized colostomy bags from urine collection bags, medicine cups, or condoms. Karaya gum is helpful in making a seal. Watch for wound disruption, infection, and excoriation—potential dangers because of severe catabolism.

◆ Watch for intestinal malfunction from stricture or short-gut syndrome. Such complications usually develop a month after the infant resumes normal feedings.

PREVENTION *Encourage mothers to breast-feed because breast milk contains live macrophages that fight infection and has a low pH that inhibits the growth of many organisms. Also, colostrum—fluid secreted from the breast before the milk—contains high concentrations of immunoglobulin A, which directly protects the gut from infection and which the neonate lacks for several days postpartum. Tell mothers that they may refrigerate their milk for 48 hours but shouldn't freeze or heat it because this destroys antibodies.*

CROHN DISEASE

Crohn disease, also known as *regional enteritis* and *granulomatous colitis*, is an idiopathic inflammation of any part of the GI tract from mouth to anus (usually the ileum or proximal portion of the colon).

Causes and incidence

In Crohn disease, lacteal blockage in the intestinal wall leads to edema and, eventually, inflammation, ulceration, and stenosis. Abscesses and fistulas may also occur.

Although the exact cause of Crohn disease is unknown, risk factors include family history, smoking cigarettes, Jewish ethnicity, urban residency, age of less than 40, and an altered gut microbiome. It is most prevalent in adults 15 to 30 years old. It's two to three times more common in those of Jewish ancestry.

The incidence of Crohn disease has risen steadily over the past 50 years; it now affects 20.2 of every 100,000 people.

Pathophysiology

Crohn disease involves "skip lesions" (granulomas surrounded by normal mucosa) with mixed areas of transmural inflammation (versus areas that are noninflamed) noncaseating granulomas, fistulas, and deep ulcers. The surface of the inflamed GI tract usually has a cobblestone appearance, which is different from alternating areas of inflammation and fissure crevices. The progression of Crohn disease involves neutrophil infiltration of the crypts, which leads to the formation of abscesses and crypt destruction.

Complications

+ Anal fistula
+ Perineal abscess
+ Intestinal obstruction
+ Nutritional deficiency
+ Peritonitis (rare)

Signs and symptoms

Clinical effects may be mild and nonspecific initially; they vary according to the location and extent of the lesion. Acute inflammatory signs and symptoms mimic appendicitis and include steady, colicky pain in the right lower quadrant, cramping, tenderness, flatulence, nausea, fever, and diarrhea. Bleeding may occur and, although usually mild, may be massive. Bloody stools may also occur.

Chronic symptoms, which are more typical of the disease, are more persistent and less severe; they include diarrhea (four to six stools per day) with pain in the right lower abdominal quadrant, steatorrhea (excess fat in feces), marked weight loss and, rarely, clubbing of fingers. The patient may complain of weakness and fatigue. Complications include intestinal

The "String Sign"

The characteristic "string sign" (marked narrowing of the bowel), resulting from inflammatory disease and scarring, strengthens the diagnosis of Crohn disease.

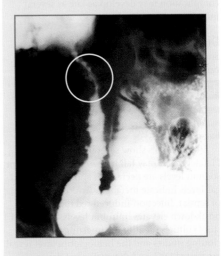

obstruction, fistula formation between the small bowel and the bladder, perianal and perirectal abscesses and fistulas, intra-abdominal abscesses, and perforation.

Diagnosis

℞ **CONFIRMING DIAGNOSIS** *Barium enema showing the string sign (segments of stricture separated by normal bowel) supports a diagnosis of Crohn disease. (See The "String Sign.")*

Sigmoidoscopy and colonoscopy may show patchy areas of inflammation, thus helping to rule out ulcerative colitis. However, biopsy is required for a definitive diagnosis.

Laboratory findings commonly indicate increased white blood cell count and erythrocyte sedimentation rate, hypokalemia, hypocalcemia, hypomagnesemia, and a decreased hemoglobin level.

Treatment

To control the inflammatory process, medications, such as mesalamine and sulfasalazine, may be prescribed. Corticosteroids and immune system suppressors, such as azathioprine (Imuran) and mercaptopurine (Purinethol), may be prescribed if mesalamine isn't effective or in patients with severe Crohn disease. In debilitated patients, therapy includes TPN to maintain nutritional status while resting the bowel. If abscesses or fistulas occur, antibiotics may be prescribed. Infliximab (Remicade), an antibody to tumor necrosis factor-alpha (an immune chemical that promotes inflammation), may also be prescribed. Other medications prescribed for refractory Crohn disease include certolizumab (Cimzia), adalimumab (Humira), and natalizumab (Tysabri). Some clinicians start with these medications in patients with severe Crohn disease, where others step up to these medications when the patient fails traditional treatment.

Effective treatment requires important changes in lifestyle: physical rest, restricted diet (specific foods vary from person to person), vitamin B_{12} injections and supplements, and elimination of dairy products for lactose intolerance.

Surgery may be necessary to correct bowel perforation, massive hemorrhage, fistulas, or acute intestinal obstruction. Colectomy with ileostomy is necessary in many patients with extensive disease of the large intestine and rectum.

Special considerations

Although treatment is based largely on symptoms, monitor the patient's status carefully for signs of worsening.

◆ Record fluid intake and output (including the amount of stool), and weigh the patient daily. Watch for dehydration, and maintain fluid and electrolyte balance. Be alert for signs of intestinal bleeding (bloody stools); check stools daily for occult blood.

◆ Check hemoglobin level and hematocrit regularly. Give iron supplements and blood transfusions, as ordered.

◆ Provide hygiene and mouth care if the patient is restricted to having nothing by mouth. After each bowel movement, provide thorough skin care. Always keep a clean, covered bedpan within the patient's reach. Ventilate the room to eliminate odors.

◆ Observe the patient for fever and pain or pneumaturia, which may signal bladder fistula. Abdominal pain and distention and fever may indicate intestinal obstruction. Watch for stools from the vagina and an enterovaginal fistula.

◆ Before ileostomy, arrange for a visit by an enterostomal therapist.

◆ After surgery, frequently check the patient's I.V. line and NG tube for proper functioning. Monitor vital signs and fluid intake and output. Watch for wound infection. Provide meticulous stoma care and teach proper care to the patient

and family. Realize that ileostomy changes the patient's body image; provide reassurance and emotional support.

◆ Stress the need for a severely restricted diet and bed rest, which may be challenging, particularly for a young patient. Encourage reduction in tension. If stress is clearly an aggravating factor, refer the patient for counseling.

◆ Refer the patient to a support group such as the Crohn's and Colitis Foundation of America.

PSEUDOMEMBRANOUS ENTEROCOLITIS

Pseudomembranous enterocolitis is an acute inflammation and necrosis of the small and large intestines, which usually affects the mucosa but may extend into the submucosa and, rarely, other layers. Marked by severe diarrhea, this rare condition is generally fatal in 1 to 7 days due to severe dehydration and toxicity, peritonitis, or perforation.

Causes and incidence

The exact cause of pseudomembranous enterocolitis is unknown. The incidence of antibiotic-related diarrhea varies from 5% to 39%, depending on the antibiotic. Pseudomembranous enterocolitis complicates 10% of these cases.

PEDIATRIC TIP *Ampicillin is the most common antibiotic associated with pseudomembranous enterocolitis in children.*

Pathophysiology

Although the pathophysiology of pseudomembranous enterocolitis is not fully understood, *Clostridium difficile* is thought to produce a toxin that may play a role in its development. Pseudomembranous enterocolitis has occurred postoperatively in debilitated patients who undergo abdominal surgery and in patients treated with broad-spectrum antibiotics. Irrespective of the cause, necrotic mucosa is replaced by a pseudomembrane filled with staphylococci, leukocytes, mucus, fibrin, and inflammatory cells.

Complications

◆ Severe dehydration
◆ Electrolyte imbalance
◆ Hypotension
◆ Shock
◆ Colonic perforation
◆ Peritonitis

Signs and symptoms

Pseudomembranous enterocolitis begins suddenly with copious watery or bloody diarrhea that may contain pus or mucus, abdominal pain, and fever. Serious complications, including severe dehydration, electrolyte imbalance, hypotension, shock, and colonic perforation, may occur in this disorder.

Diagnosis

Diagnosis is difficult in many cases because of the abrupt onset of enterocolitis and the emergency situation it creates, so consideration of patient history is essential. A rectal biopsy through sigmoidoscopy confirms pseudomembranous enterocolitis. Stool cultures can identify *C. difficile*.

Treatment

A patient receiving broad-spectrum antibiotic therapy must discontinue antibiotics at once. Effective treatment usually includes metronidazole. Oral vancomycin is superior to metronidazole for all cases. A patient with mild pseudomembranous enterocolitis may receive anion exchange resins, such as cholestyramine, to bind the toxin produced by *C. difficile*. Supportive treatment must maintain fluid and electrolyte balance, and combat hypotension and shock with a pressor, such as dopamine.

Special considerations

Careful observation for signs of worsening is essential.
◆ Monitor the patient's vital signs, skin color, and level of consciousness. Immediately report signs of shock.
◆ Record fluid intake and output, including fluid lost in stools. Watch for symptoms that indicate dehydration (poor skin turgor, sunken eyes, and decreased urine output).
◆ Check serum electrolyte levels daily, and watch for clinical signs of hypokalemia, especially malaise, and a weak, rapid, irregular pulse.
⫶⫶⫶⫶⫶ **PREVENTION** *Antibiotics should be used only as prescribed by healthcare providers. Research indicates that the use of probiotics along with antibiotics may help address a variety of GI problems.*

IRRITABLE BOWEL SYNDROME

Irritable bowel syndrome (IBS) is a condition marked by abdominal pain and altered bowel habits. Some patients experience chronic or periodic diarrhea, alternating with constipation, while others experience only one or the other (IBS-D, for diarrhea, or IBS-C, for constipation). Supportive treatment or avoidance of a known irritant often relieves symptoms.

Causes and incidence

This brain-gut disorder has been associated with psychological stress, yet it is important to recognize that continuing research shows that it is a multisystem interaction that causes the symptoms. Physical factors such as diverticular disease, hormonal changes during the menstrual cycle, ingestion of irritants (coffee, raw fruits, or vegetables), lactose intolerance, laxative abuse, food poisoning, or colon cancer may contribute to symptoms. Some patients may experience a disturbance in the movement of the intestine or a lower tolerance for stretching and movement of the intestine.

IBS affects approximately 12% of North American individuals, is more common in women than in men, and has a higher prevalence in youth and middle-aged people.

Pathophysiology

The pathophysiology of IBS is not fully understood. A multisystem interaction is anticipated, including visceral hypersensitivity; abnormal GI permeability, motility, secretion, and sensitivity; alteration in gut microbes; food allergy or intolerance; and psychological factors.

Complications

◆ Hemorrhoid aggravation
◆ Malnourishment

Signs and symptoms

IBS characteristically produces lower abdominal pain (usually relieved by defecation or passage of gas) and diarrhea or constipation that typically occurs during the day. Stools are commonly small and contain visible mucus. Dyspepsia and abdominal distention may occur. (See *Effects of irritable bowel syndrome*, page 239.)

Symptoms of IBS are two to three times more common in women than in men, and are often noted in patients who have anxiety, depression, or reduced quality of life.

Diagnosis

The diagnosis of IBS requires a careful history to determine contributing factors. Psychological factors should be assessed in addition to physiological contributors. Diagnosis must also rule out other disorders, such as amebiasis, diverticulitis, colon cancer, and lactose intolerance. Appropriate diagnostic procedures include sigmoidoscopy, colonoscopy, barium enema, rectal biopsy, and stool examination for blood, parasites, and bacteria.

Treatment

Therapy aims to relieve symptoms. Strict dietary restrictions aren't beneficial, but food irritants should be investigated, and the patient should

Effects of irritable bowel syndrome

The illustration below shows partial obstructing in the bowel caused by irritable bowel syndrome.

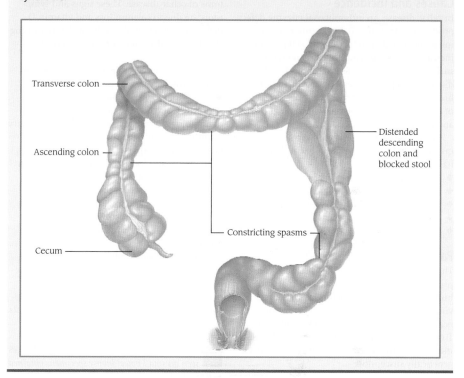

Transverse colon

Ascending colon

Cecum

Distended descending colon and blocked stool

Constricting spasms

be instructed to avoid them. Rest and heat applied to the abdomen may be helpful, as is extremely judicious use of sedatives and antispasmodics. However, with chronic use, the patient may become dependent on these drugs. If the cause of IBS involves chronic laxative abuse, bowel training may help correct the condition. If psychological factors appear to contribute to the syndrome, counseling to help the patient understand the relationship between stress and illness can be helpful. Current strategies of treating patients with IBS may include antidepressants such as amitriptyline to decrease sensitivity to pain and probiotics to correct the underlying problematic bowel pattern. Lubiprostone (Amitiza) and rifaximin (Xifaxan) are helpful treatments for patients with IBS.

Special considerations

Because the patient with IBS usually isn't hospitalized, focus care on patient teaching.

◆ Tell the patient to avoid irritating foods, and encourage development of regular bowel habits.
◆ Help the patient identify concerns associated with stress.
◆ Teach about dependence on sedatives or antispasmodics.
◆ Encourage regular checkups because IBS is associated with a higher-than-normal incidence of diverticulitis and colon cancer. For patients older than 40, emphasize the need for consideration of an annual sigmoidoscopy and rectal examination.

CELIAC DISEASE

Celiac disease (also known as *celiac sprue* and *gluten-sensitive enteropathy*) is characterized by poor food absorption and intolerance of gluten, a protein in wheat and wheat products. Malabsorption in the small bowel results from atrophy of the villi and a decrease in the activity and amount of enzymes in the surface epithelium. The prognosis is good with treatment (eliminating gluten from the patient's diet), but residual bowel changes may persist in adults.

Causes and incidence

In celiac disease, an intramucosal enzyme defect produces an inability to digest gluten. Resulting tissue toxicity produces rapid cell turnover, increases epithelial lymphocytes, and damages surface epithelium of the small bowel. Celiac disease has a prevalence of approximately 1%; however, evidence indicates that only a fraction of those affected have actually been diagnosed and treated.

Celiac disease is present with greater frequency in individuals (especially children) who have:
◆ Type I diabetes
◆ Autoimmune thyroid or liver disease
◆ Down, Turner, or Williams syndrome
◆ Selective IgA deficiency
◆ Addison disease

Pathophysiology

The pathophysiology of celiac disease is complicated, involving genetic, and cellular and humoral immunologic factors, as well as environmental factors. The major characteristic is an HLA-DQ2- or HLA-DQ8-induced $CD4^+$ T-cell-mediated autoimmune injury to the small intestinal epithelial cells of individuals who are genetically susceptible.

Complications

◆ Anemia from malabsorption
◆ Syncope, heart failure, and angina from anemia
◆ Bleeding disorders from vitamin K deficiency
◆ Intestinal lymphoma (higher incidence)

Signs and symptoms

Celiac disease produces clinical effects on many body systems:
◆ GI symptoms include recurrent attacks of diarrhea, steatorrhea, abdominal distention due to flatulence, stomach cramps, weakness, anorexia and, occasionally, increased appetite without weight gain. Atrophy of intestinal villi leads to malabsorption of fat, carbohydrates, and protein as well as loss of calories, fat-soluble vitamins (A, D, and K), calcium, and essential minerals and electrolytes. In adults, celiac disease produces multiple nonspecific ulcers in the small bowel, which may perforate or bleed.
◆ Hematologic effects include normochromic, hypochromic, or macrocytic anemia due to poor absorption of folate, iron, and vitamin B_{12}

and to hypoprothrombinemia from jejunal loss of vitamin K.
◆ Osteomalacia, osteoporosis, tetany, and bone pain (especially in the lower back, rib cage, and pelvis) are some of the musculoskeletal symptoms of celiac disease. These signs and symptoms are due to calcium loss and vitamin D deficiency, which weakens the skeleton, causing rickets in children and compression fractures in adults.
◆ Neurologic effects may include peripheral neuropathy, seizures, or paresthesia.
◆ Dry skin, eczema, psoriasis, dermatitis herpetiformis, and acne rosacea are some of the dermatologic effects of celiac disease. Deficiency of sulfur-containing amino acids may cause generalized fine, sparse, prematurely gray hair; brittle nails; and localized hyperpigmentation on the face, lips, or mucosa.
◆ Endocrine symptoms include amenorrhea, hypometabolism and, possibly, with severe malabsorption, adrenocortical insufficiency.
◆ Psychosocial effects include mood changes and irritability.

Symptoms may develop as early as the first year of life, when gluten is introduced into the child's diet; in half of affected children, onset occurs by 18 months old. The severity of symptoms varies greatly between affected individuals.

Diagnosis

℞ **CONFIRMING DIAGNOSIS** *Histologic changes seen on small bowel biopsy specimens obtained with an esophagogastroduodenoscopy confirm the diagnosis: a mosaic pattern of alternating flat and bumpy areas on the bowel surface due to an almost total absence of villi and an irregular, blunt, and disorganized network of blood vessels. These changes appear most prominently in the jejunum.*

An elevated alkaline phosphatase level may indicate bone loss, which is commonly experienced before diagnosis. Low cholesterol and albumin levels may reflect malabsorption and malnutrition. Mildly elevated liver enzymes and abnormal blood clotting may also be noted as well as anemia.

Antibody blood tests useful in screening for celiac disease include IgA antiendomysial antibody, anti-tissue transglutaminase, antigliadin (IgA and IgG), and total serum IgA. Combined, these antibodies provide a sensitive and specific indicator for the presence of celiac disease.

Treatment

Treatment requires elimination of gluten from the patient's diet for life—educate the patient to follow this gluten-free diet (GFD). Even with this exclusion, a full return to normal absorption and bowel histology may not occur for months or may never occur.

Supportive treatment may include supplemental iron, vitamin B_{12}, and folic acid; reversal of electrolyte imbalance (by I.V. infusion, if necessary); I.V. fluid replacement for dehydration; corticosteroids to treat accompanying adrenal insufficiency; and vitamin K for hypoprothrombinemia.

Special considerations

Explain the necessity of the GFD to the patient (and to the parents or caregivers, if the patient is a child). Advise eliminating wheat, barley, rye, and oats as well as foods made from these grains, such as breads and baked goods; suggest substituting corn or rice. Consult a dietitian for nutritional instruction on the GFD. Depending on individual tolerance, the diet initially consists of proteins and gradually expands to include other foods. Assess the patient's acceptance and understanding of the disease, and encourage regular reevaluation.

⚠ ALERT *Because many foods contain hidden sources of gluten, teach the patient to read food labels carefully and thoroughly.*

◆ Observe the patient's nutritional status and progress by daily calorie counts and weight checks. Evaluate tolerance to new foods. In the early stages, offer small, frequent meals to counteract anorexia.

◆ Assess the patient's fluid status: record intake, urine output, and number of stools (which may exceed 10 per day). Watch for signs of dehydration, such as dry skin and mucous membranes, and poor skin turgor.

◆ Check serum electrolyte levels. Watch for signs of hypokalemia (weakness, lethargy, rapid pulse, nausea, and diarrhea) and low calcium levels (impaired blood clotting, muscle twitching, and tetany).

◆ Monitor prothrombin time, hemoglobin level, and hematocrit. Protect the patient from bleeding and bruising. The patient may need iron replenishment. If the patient can tolerate oral iron, give it between meals, when absorption is best. Dilute oral iron preparations, and give them through a straw to prevent staining teeth.

◆ Protect the patient with osteomalacia from injury by keeping the bed side rails up and assisting with ambulation, as necessary.

◆ Advise the patient to contact the Gluten Intolerance Group of North America or the Celiac Disease Foundation for information and support.

DIVERTICULAR DISEASE

In diverticular disease, bulging pouches (diverticula) in the GI wall push the mucosal lining through the surrounding muscle. The most common site for diverticula is in the sigmoid colon, but they may develop anywhere, from the proximal end of the pharynx to the anus. Other typical sites are the duodenum, near the pancreatic border or the ampulla of Vater, and the jejunum. Diverticular disease of the stomach is rare and is usually a precursor of peptic or neoplastic disease. Diverticular disease of the ileum (Meckel's diverticulum) is the most common congenital anomaly of the GI tract. (See *Meckel's diverticulum.*)

Meckel's diverticulum

In Meckel's diverticulum, a congenital abnormality—a blind tube, like the appendix—opens into the distal ileum near the ileocecal valve. This disorder results from failure of the intra-abdominal portion of the yolk sac to close completely during fetal development. It occurs in approximately 1.2% to 2% of the population, mostly in males.

Uncomplicated Meckel's diverticulum produces no symptoms, but complications cause abdominal pain, especially around the umbilicus, and dark red melena or hematochezia. The lining of the diverticulum is gastric mucosa. This disorder may lead to peptic ulceration, perforation, and peritonitis and may resemble acute appendicitis.

Meckel's diverticulum also may cause bowel obstruction when a fibrous band that connects the diverticulum to the abdominal wall, the mesentery, or other structures snares a loop of the intestine. This may cause intussusception into the diverticulum or volvulus near the diverticular attachment to the back of the umbilicus or another intra-abdominal structure. Meckel's diverticulum should be considered in cases of GI obstruction or hemorrhage, especially when routine GI X-rays are negative.

Treatment consists of surgical resection of the inflamed bowel and antibiotic therapy if infection is present.

Diverticular disease has two clinical forms. In *diverticulosis*, asymptomatic diverticula are present. In *diverticulitis*, diverticula are inflamed and may cause potentially fatal obstruction, infection, or hemorrhage.

Causes and incidence

Diet may be a contributing factor to diverticular disease because insufficient fiber reduces fecal residue, narrows the bowel lumen, and leads to higher intra-abdominal pressure during defecation. Diverticulosis is age-dependent; less than 20% of patients develop this before age 40, yet 60% have been diagnosed by age 60; between 4% and 15% of those with diverticulosis develop diverticulitis, with a mean age at admission of 63. Left-sided diverticulitis is more common in North America; right-sided diverticulitis is most commonly seen in Asian countries.

ELDER TIP *Many older adults develop diverticulosis. In older adults, a rare complication of diverticulosis (without diverticulitis) is hemorrhage from colonic diverticula. Such hemorrhage is usually mild to moderate and easily controlled, yet may occasionally be massive and life-threatening.*

Pathophysiology

In diverticulitis, retained undigested food mixed with bacteria accumulates in the diverticular sac, forming a hard mass (fecalith). This substance cuts off the blood supply to the thin walls of the sac, making them more susceptible to attack by colonic bacteria. Inflammation follows, possibly leading to perforation, abscess, peritonitis, obstruction, or hemorrhage. Occasionally, the inflamed colon segment may produce a fistula by adhering to the bladder or other organs.

Diverticula probably result from high intraluminal pressure on areas of weakness in the GI wall, where blood vessels enter.

Complications

◆ Rectal hemorrhage
◆ Portal pyemia
◆ Fistula

Signs and symptoms

Diverticulosis usually produces no symptoms but may cause recurrent left lower quadrant pain, which is commonly accompanied by alternating constipation and diarrhea and is relieved by defecation or the passage of flatus. Symptoms resemble IBS and suggest that the disorders may coexist.

Mild diverticulitis produces moderate left lower abdominal pain, mild nausea, gas,

irregular bowel habits, low-grade fever, and leukocytosis. In severe diverticulitis, the diverticula can rupture and produce abscesses or peritonitis, which occurs in approximately one in five of patients. Symptoms of rupture include abdominal rigidity and left lower quadrant pain. Peritonitis follows release of fecal material from the rupture site and causes signs of sepsis and shock (high fever, chills, and hypotension). Rupture of the diverticulum near a vessel may cause microscopic or massive hemorrhage, depending on the vessel's size.

Chronic diverticulitis may cause fibrosis and adhesions that narrow the bowel's lumen and lead to bowel obstruction. Symptoms of incomplete obstruction are constipation, ribbonlike stools, intermittent diarrhea, and abdominal distention. Increasing obstruction causes abdominal rigidity and pain, diminishing or absent bowel sounds, nausea, and vomiting.

Diagnosis

In many cases, diverticular disease produces no symptoms and is found during an upper GI series performed as part of a differential diagnosis.

Tests showing diverticular disease include computed tomography (CT; reveals areas of inflammation), colonoscopy, sigmoidoscopy, and barium enema.

CONFIRMING DIAGNOSIS *A barium study confirms the diagnosis. An upper GI series confirms or rules out diverticulosis of the esophagus and upper bowel; a barium enema confirms or rules out diverticulosis of the lower bowel.*

Barium-filled diverticula can be single, multiple, or clustered and may have a wide or narrow mouth. Barium outlines—but doesn't fill—diverticula blocked by impacted feces. In patients with acute diverticulitis, a barium enema may rupture the bowel, so this procedure requires caution. If IBS accompanies diverticular disease, X-rays may reveal colonic spasm.

Biopsy rules out cancer; however, a colonoscopic biopsy isn't recommended during acute diverticular disease because of the strenuous bowel preparation it requires. Blood studies may show an elevated erythrocyte sedimentation rate in diverticulitis, especially if the diverticula are infected.

Treatment

Asymptomatic diverticulosis doesn't necessitate treatment. Intestinal diverticulosis with pain, mild GI distress, constipation, or difficult defecation may respond to a liquid or bland diet, stool softeners, and occasional doses of mineral oil. These measures relieve symptoms, minimize irritation, and lessen the risk of progression to diverticulitis. After pain subsides, patients also benefit from a high-residue diet and bulk medication such as psyllium.

Treatment of mild diverticulitis without signs of perforation must prevent constipation and combat infection. It may include bed rest, a liquid diet, stool softeners, and a broad-spectrum antibiotic.

If diverticulitis is refractory to medical treatment, a colon resection is necessary to remove the involved segment. Perforation, peritonitis, obstruction, or fistula that accompanies diverticulitis may require a temporary colostomy to drain abscesses and rest the colon, followed by later reanastomosis 6 weeks to 3 months after initial surgery.

Special considerations

Management of uncomplicated diverticulosis chiefly involves thorough patient education about fiber and dietary habits.

◆ Make sure that the patient understands the importance of dietary fiber and the harmful effects of constipation and straining during defecation. Encourage increased intake of foods high in indigestible fiber, including fresh fruits and vegetables, whole grain bread, and wheat or bran cereals. Warn that a high-fiber diet may temporarily cause flatulence and discomfort. Teach the patient to relieve constipation with stool softeners or bulk-forming cathartics. However, caution the patient against taking bulk-forming cathartics without plenty of water; if swallowed dry, they may absorb enough moisture in the mouth and throat to swell and obstruct the esophagus or trachea.

◆ If the patient with diverticular disease is hospitalized, observe stools carefully for frequency, color, and consistency, and keep accurate pulse and temperature charts because changes may signal developing inflammation or complications.

After surgery to resect the colon:

◆ Monitor for signs of infection.

◆ Provide meticulous wound care because perforation may already have infected the area.

◆ Check drain sites frequently for signs of infection (purulent drainage or foul odor) or fecal drainage.

◆ Change dressings as necessary.

◆ Encourage coughing and deep breathing to prevent atelectasis.

◆ Watch for signs of postoperative bleeding (hypotension and decreased hemoglobin level and hematocrit).

◆ Record intake and output accurately.

◆ Keep the NG tube patent.

◆ Teach ostomy care as needed.

◆ Arrange for a visit by an enterostomal therapist.

APPENDICITIS

Appendicitis is inflammation of the vermiform appendix.

Causes and incidence

Appendicitis, the most common surgical emergency of the abdomen, is thought to result from an obstruction of the appendiceal lumen caused by a fecal mass, stricture, barium ingestion, or viral infection. This obstruction sets off an inflammatory process that can lead to infection, thrombosis, necrosis, and perforation. If the appendix ruptures or perforates, the infected contents spill into the abdominal cavity, causing peritonitis, the most common and most perilous complication of appendicitis.

Appendicitis occurs more commonly in men than in women, in the second or third decades of life.

Pathophysiology

Although the pathophysiology of appendicitis is not fully understood, causes are postulated to be obstruction of the lumen with stool, tumors, or foreign bodies which cause increased intraluminal pressure, ischemia, bacterial infection, and inflammation.

Complications

◆ Perforation

◆ Peritonitis

◆ Appendiceal abscess

◆ Pyelophlebitis

Signs and symptoms

Typically, appendicitis begins with generalized or localized abdominal pain in the right upper abdomen, followed by anorexia, nausea, and vomiting (rarely profuse). Pain eventually localizes in the right lower abdomen (McBurney's point) with abdominal "boardlike" rigidity, retractive respirations, increasing tenderness, increasingly severe abdominal spasms and, almost invariably, rebound tenderness. (Rebound tenderness on the opposite side of the abdomen suggests peritoneal inflammation.)

Later signs and symptoms include constipation or diarrhea, slight fever, and tachycardia. The patient may walk bent over or lie with his right knee flexed to reduce pain.

ALERT *Sudden cessation of abdominal pain indicates perforation or infarction of the appendix; this is considered an emergent condition.*

Diagnosis

Diagnosis of appendicitis is based on physical findings and characteristic clinical symptoms. Supportive findings include a low-grade temperature up to approximately 101° F (38.33° C) and a moderately elevated white blood cell count (>10,000/μL), with increased immature neutrophil cells.

Diagnosis must rule out illnesses with similar symptoms: gastritis, gastroenteritis, ileitis, colitis, diverticulitis, pancreatitis, renal colic, bladder infection, ovarian cyst, and uterine disease. It may be strongly suspected based on abdominal sonography or CT scan. Appendicitis can be confirmed by exploratory laparoscopy.

Treatment

Appendectomy is the only effective treatment. Laparoscopic appendectomies decrease the recovery time and thus the hospital stay. If peritonitis develops, treatment involves GI intubation, parenteral replacement of fluids and electrolytes, and administration of antibiotics.

Special considerations

If appendicitis is suspected, or during preparation for appendectomy:

◆ Administer I.V. fluids to prevent dehydration. *Never* administer cathartics or enemas, which may rupture the appendix. Give the patient nothing by mouth, and administer analgesics judiciously because they may mask symptoms.

◆ To lessen pain, place the patient in Fowler's position.

! ALERT *Never apply heat to the right lower abdomen; this may cause the appendix to rupture.*

An ice bag may be used for pain relief.

After appendectomy:

◆ Monitor the patient's vital signs and intake and output. Give analgesics, as ordered.

◆ Encourage the patient to cough, breathe deeply, and turn frequently to prevent pulmonary complications.

◆ Document bowel sounds, passing of flatus, and bowel movements. In a patient whose nausea and abdominal rigidity have subsided, these signs indicate readiness to resume oral fluids.

◆ Watch closely for possible surgical complications. Continuing pain and fever may signal an abscess. The complaint that "something gave way" or "popped" may indicate wound dehiscence. If an abscess or peritonitis develops, incision and drainage may be necessary. Frequently assess the dressing for wound drainage.

◆ Help the patient ambulate as soon as possible after surgery.

◆ In appendicitis complicated by peritonitis, an NG tube may be needed to decompress the stomach and reduce nausea and vomiting. If so, record drainage and provide mouth and nose care.

PERITONITIS

Peritonitis is an acute or chronic inflammation of the peritoneum, the membrane that lines the abdominal cavity and covers the visceral organs. Inflammation may extend throughout the peritoneum or may be localized as an abscess. Peritonitis commonly decreases intestinal motility and causes intestinal distention with gas. Death can occur as a result of bowel obstruction.

Causes and incidence

Although the GI tract normally contains bacteria, the peritoneum is sterile. When bacteria invade the peritoneum due to inflammation and perforation of the GI tract, peritonitis results. Because there are varying conditions that contribute to peritonitis, incidence is difficult to determine.

Pathophysiology

Bacterial invasion of the peritoneum typically results from appendicitis, diverticulitis, peptic ulcer, ulcerative colitis, volvulus, strangulated obstruction, abdominal neoplasm, or a stab wound. Peritonitis may also occur following chemical inflammation, as in the rupture of a fallopian or ovarian tube or the bladder, perforation of a gastric ulcer, or released pancreatic enzymes. It may also be associated with peritoneal dialysis.

In chemical and bacterial inflammation, accumulated fluids containing protein and electrolytes make the transparent peritoneum opaque, red, inflamed, and edematous. Because the peritoneal cavity is so resistant to contamination, infection is commonly localized as an abscess instead of disseminated as a generalized infection.

Complications

◆ Abscess
◆ Septicemia
◆ Respiratory compromise
◆ Bowel obstruction
◆ Shock

Signs and symptoms

The key symptom of peritonitis is sudden, severe, and diffuse abdominal pain that tends to intensify and localize in the area of the underlying disorder. For instance, if appendicitis causes the rupture, pain eventually localizes in the right lower quadrant. Many patients display weakness, pallor, excessive sweating, and cold skin as a result of excessive loss of fluid, electrolytes, and protein into the abdominal cavity. Decreased intestinal motility and paralytic ileus result from the effect of bacterial toxins on the intestinal muscles. Intestinal obstruction causes nausea, vomiting, and abdominal rigidity.

Other clinical characteristics include hypotension, tachycardia, signs and symptoms of dehydration (oliguria, thirst, dry swollen tongue, and pinched skin), an acutely tender abdomen associated with rebound tenderness, temperature of 103° F (39.4° C) or higher, and hypokalemia. Inflammation of the diaphragmatic peritoneum may cause shoulder pain and hiccups. Abdominal distention and resulting upward displacement of the diaphragm may decrease respiratory capacity. Typically, the patient with peritonitis tends to breathe shallowly and move as little as possible to minimize pain. The patient may prefer to lie on his or her back, with knees flexed, to relax abdominal muscles.

Diagnosis

Severe abdominal pain in a person with direct or rebound tenderness suggests peritonitis. Abdominal X-rays or CT scan showing edematous and gaseous distention of the small and large bowel support the diagnosis. In the case of perforation of a visceral organ, the X-ray shows air lying under the diaphragm in the abdominal cavity. Other appropriate tests include the following:

◆ Chest X-ray may show elevation of the diaphragm.
◆ Blood studies show leukocytosis (>20,000/µL).
◆ Paracentesis reveals bacteria, exudate, blood, pus, or urine.
◆ Laparotomy may be necessary to identify the underlying cause.

Treatment

Early treatment of GI inflammatory conditions and preoperative and postoperative antibiotic therapy help prevent peritonitis. After peritonitis develops, emergency treatment must combat infection, restore intestinal motility, and replace fluids and electrolytes.

Antibiotic therapy depends on the infecting organisms. If peritonitis is associated with peritoneal dialysis, antibiotics may be infused through the dialysis catheter; however, if the infection is severe, the catheter must be removed. To decrease peristalsis and prevent perforation, the patient should receive nothing by mouth;

supportive fluids and electrolytes should be given parenterally.

Other supplementary treatment measures include preoperative and postoperative administration of an analgesic, NG intubation to decompress the bowel and, possibly, using a rectal tube to facilitate passage of flatus. When peritonitis results from perforation, surgery is necessary as soon as possible. Surgery aims to eliminate the source of infection by evacuating the spilled contents and inserting drains.

Special considerations

Patient care includes monitoring and measures to prevent complications and the spread of infection.

◆ Monitor the patient's vital signs, fluid intake and output, and amount of NG drainage or vomitus.
◆ Place the patient in semi-Fowler's position to facilitate deep breathing with less pain; this helps to prevent pulmonary complications and localize purulent exudate in the lower abdomen or pelvis.

After surgery to evacuate the peritoneum:
◆ Maintain parenteral fluid and electrolyte administration, as ordered. Accurately record fluid intake and output, including NG tube and any drain output.
◆ Place in semi-Fowler's position to promote drainage (through drainage tube) by gravity. Move the patient carefully because the slightest movement will intensify the pain.
◆ Implement other safety measures if fever and pain disorient the patient.
◆ Encourage and assist ambulation, as ordered, usually on the first postoperative day.
◆ Watch for signs of dehiscence (the patient may complain that "something gave way" or "popped") and abscess formation (continued abdominal tenderness and fever).
◆ Frequently assess for peristaltic activity by listening for bowel sounds and checking for gas, bowel movements, and a soft abdomen.
◆ Gradually decrease parenteral fluids and increase oral fluids.

INTESTINAL OBSTRUCTION

Intestinal obstruction is the partial or complete blockage of the lumen in the small or large bowel. Small bowel obstruction, far more common, is usually more serious. Complete obstruction in any part of the bowel, if untreated, can cause death within hours from shock and vascular collapse. Intestinal obstruction usually occurs after abdominal surgery or in persons with congenital bowel deformities.

Causes and incidence

Adhesions and strangulated hernias usually cause small bowel obstruction; large-bowel obstruction is typically due to carcinomas. Mechanical intestinal obstruction results from foreign bodies (fruit pits, gallstones, or worms) or compression of the bowel wall due to stenosis, intussusception, volvulus of the sigmoid or cecum, tumors, or atresia. Nonmechanical obstruction results from physiologic disturbances, such as paralytic ileus, electrolyte imbalances, toxicity (uremia or generalized infection), neurogenic abnormalities (spinal cord lesions), and thrombosis or embolism of mesenteric vessels. (See *Paralytic ileus*.)

Intestinal obstruction develops in three forms:

◆ *Simple:* Blockage prevents intestinal contents from passing, with no other complications or with a change in blood flow.

◆ *Strangulated:* The blood supply to part or all of the obstructed section is cut off, in addition to blockage of the lumen.

◆ *Close-looped:* Both ends of a bowel section are occluded, isolating it from the rest of the intestine. (See *Causes of intestinal obstruction*, page 247.)

Pathophysiology

See box for *pathophysiology of intestinal obstruction*.

The physiologic effects are similar in all three forms of obstruction: When intestinal obstruction occurs, fluid, air, and gas collect near the site. Peristalsis increases temporarily as the bowel tries to force its contents through the obstruction, injuring intestinal mucosa and causing distention at and above the site of the obstruction. Distention blocks the flow of venous blood and halts normal absorptive processes; as a result, the bowel begins to secrete water, sodium, and potassium into the fluid pooled in the lumen.

Obstruction in the small intestine results in metabolic alkalosis from dehydration and loss of gastric hydrochloric acid; lower bowel obstruction causes slower dehydration and loss of intestinal alkaline fluids, resulting in metabolic acidosis. Ultimately, intestinal obstruction may lead to ischemia, necrosis, and death. (See *Symptom progression in intestinal obstruction*, page 248.)

⬡ **ELDER TIP** *Watch for air-fluid lock syndrome in older adults who remain recumbent for extended periods. In this syndrome, fluid first collects in the dependent bowel loops. Then peristalsis is too weak to push fluid "uphill." The resulting obstruction primarily occurs in the large bowel.*

Paralytic ileus

Paralytic ileus is a physiologic form of intestinal obstruction that usually develops in the small bowel after abdominal surgery. It causes decreased or absent intestinal motility that usually recovers spontaneously after 2 to 3 days. The clinical effects of paralytic ileus include severe abdominal distention, extreme distress, and, possibly, vomiting. The patient may be severely constipated or may pass flatus and small, liquid stools.

Causes

This condition can develop as a response to trauma, toxemia, or peritonitis or as a result of electrolyte deficiencies (especially hypokalemia) and the use of certain drugs, such as ganglionic blocking agents and anticholinergics. It can also result from vascular causes, such as thrombosis or embolism. Excessive air swallowing may contribute to it, but paralytic ileus brought on by this factor alone seldom lasts more than 24 hours.

Treatment

Paralytic ileus lasting longer than 48 hours requires intubation for decompression and nasogastric suctioning. Because of the absence of peristaltic activity, a long, weighted intestinal tube—called a *Miller–Abbott tube*—may be necessary in the patient with extraordinary abdominal distention. However, such procedures must be used with extreme caution because additional trauma to the bowel can aggravate ileus. When paralytic ileus results from surgical manipulation of the bowel, treatment may also include cholinergic agents, such as neostigmine (Bloxiverz) or bethanechol (Urecholine).

When caring for patients with paralytic ileus, warn those receiving cholinergic agents to expect certain paradoxical adverse effects, such as intestinal cramps and diarrhea. Remember that neostigmine produces cardiovascular adverse effects, usually bradycardia and hypotension. Check frequently for returning bowel sounds.

Causes of intestinal obstruction

Intestinal obstruction is a partial or complete blockage of the lumen in the small or large bowel. Adhesions and strangulated hernias usually cause small bowel obstruction; large-bowel obstruction is typically due to carcinomas. Other causes include intussusception, volvulus, and inguinal hernia.

Intussusception with invagination
The bowel is shortened by the involution of one segment of the bowel into another.

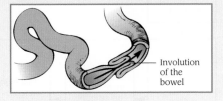

Involution of the bowel

Volvulus
In most cases, the bowel twists counterclockwise.

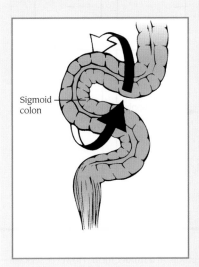

Sigmoid colon

Inguinal hernia
Intestine, omentum, and the other abdominal contents pass through the hernia opening.

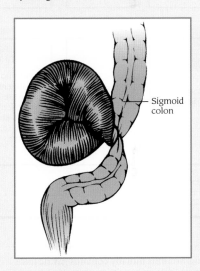

Sigmoid colon

Complications
◆ Perforation
◆ Peritonitis
◆ Septicemia
◆ Secondary infection
◆ Metabolic acidosis or alkalosis
◆ Hypovolemic or septic shock

Signs and symptoms
Colicky pain, nausea, vomiting, constipation, and abdominal distention characterize small bowel obstruction. It may also cause drowsiness, intense thirst, malaise, and aching and may dry up oral mucous membranes and the tongue. Auscultation reveals bowel sounds, borborygmi, and rushes; occasionally, these are loud enough to be heard without a stethoscope. Palpation elicits abdominal tenderness, with moderate distention; rebound tenderness occurs when obstruction has caused strangulation with ischemia. In late stages, signs of hypovolemic shock result from progressive dehydration and plasma loss.

In complete small bowel obstruction, vigorous peristaltic waves propel bowel contents toward the mouth instead of the rectum. Spasms may occur every 3 to 5 minutes and last about 1 minute each, with persistent epigastric or periumbilical pain. Passage of small amounts of mucus and blood may occur. The higher the

PATHOPHYSIOLOGY
Symptom progression in intestinal obstruction

A partial or complete blockage of the small or large intestine creates an obstruction with resultant symptoms.

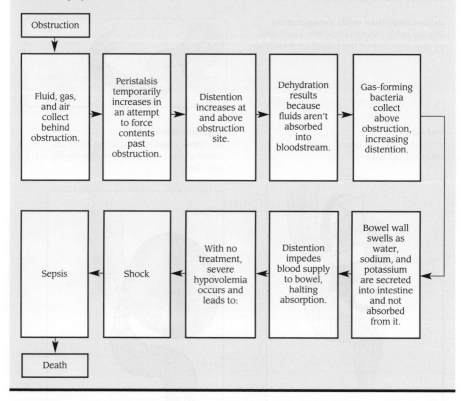

obstruction, the earlier and more severe the vomiting. Vomitus initially contains gastric juice, then bile, and finally contents of the ileum.

Symptoms of large-bowel obstruction develop more slowly because the colon can absorb fluid from its contents and distend well beyond its normal size. Constipation may be the only clinical effect for days. Colicky abdominal pain may then appear suddenly, producing spasms that last less than 1 minute each and recur every few minutes. Continuous hypogastric pain and nausea may develop, but vomiting is usually absent at first. Large-bowel obstruction can cause dramatic abdominal distention; loops of the large bowel may become visible on the abdomen. Eventually, complete large-bowel obstruction may cause fecal vomiting, continuous pain, or localized peritonitis.

Patients with partial obstruction may display any of the previously discussed signs and symptoms in a milder form. However, leakage of liquid stool around the obstruction is common in partial obstruction.

Diagnosis
Progressive, colicky, abdominal pain and distention, with or without nausea and vomiting, suggest bowel obstruction.

CONFIRMING DIAGNOSIS *Tests that show obstruction include barium enema, abdominal CT, upper GI and small bowel series, and abdominal films. Abdominal films show the presence and location of intestinal gas or fluid. In small bowel obstruction, a typical "stepladder" pattern emerges, with alternating fluid and gas levels apparent in 3 to 4 hours. In large-bowel obstruction, barium enema reveals a distended, air-filled colon or a closed loop of sigmoid with extreme distention (in sigmoid volvulus).*

Laboratory results supporting this diagnosis include:
◆ decreased sodium, chloride, and potassium levels (due to vomiting)
◆ a slightly elevated white blood cell count (with necrosis, peritonitis, or strangulation)
◆ an increased serum amylase level (possibly from irritation of the pancreas by bowel loop).

Treatment

Preoperative therapy consists of correction of fluid and electrolyte imbalances, decompression of the bowel to relieve vomiting and distention, and treatment of shock and peritonitis. Strangulated obstruction usually necessitates blood replacement as well as I.V. fluid administration. Decompression of the intestine may be accomplished with the use of an NG tube inserted into the stomach or intestine to relieve distention and vomiting.

Close monitoring of the patient's condition determines the duration of treatment; if the patient fails to improve or if the condition deteriorates, surgery is necessary. In large-bowel obstruction, surgical resection with anastomosis, colostomy, or ileostomy commonly follows decompression with an NG tube.

TPN may be appropriate if the patient suffers a protein deficit from chronic obstruction, postoperative or paralytic ileus, or infection. Drug therapy includes analgesics, sedatives, and antibiotics for peritonitis due to bowel strangulation or infarction.

Special considerations

Effective management of intestinal obstruction, a life-threatening condition that commonly causes overwhelming pain and distress, requires skillful supportive care and close observation.

◆ **ALERT** *Monitor the patient's vital signs frequently. A drop in blood pressure may indicate reduced circulating blood volume due to blood loss from a strangulated hernia. Observe the patient closely for signs of shock (pallor, rapid pulse, and hypotension).*

◆ Stay alert for signs and symptoms of metabolic alkalosis (changes in sensorium; slow, shallow respirations; hypertonic muscles; and tetany) or acidosis (shortness of breath on exertion, disorientation and, later, deep, rapid breathing, weakness, and malaise).
◆ Watch for signs and symptoms of secondary infection, such as fever and chills.
◆ Monitor the patient's urine output carefully to assess renal function, circulating blood volume, and possible urine retention caused by bladder compression by the distended intestine. If bladder compression is suspected, catheterize

the patient for residual urine immediately after voiding. Also, measure abdominal girth frequently to detect progressive distention.
◆ Provide mouth and nose care if the patient has vomited or undergone decompression by intubation. Assess for signs of dehydration (thick, swollen tongue; dry, cracked lips; and dry oral mucous membranes).
◆ Record the amount and color of drainage from the decompression tube. Irrigate the tube with normal saline solution to maintain patency. If a weighted tube has been inserted, check periodically to make sure it's advancing. Help the patient turn from side to side (or walk around, if able) to facilitate passage of the tube.
◆ Keep the patient in Fowler's position as much as possible to promote pulmonary ventilation and ease respiratory distress from abdominal distention. Listen for bowel sounds, and watch for signs of returning peristalsis (passage of flatus and mucus through the rectum).
◆ Explain all diagnostic and therapeutic procedures to the patient, and answer any questions. Make sure the patient understands that these procedures are necessary to relieve the obstruction and reduce pain. Teach to lie on the left side for about a half hour before X-rays are taken.
◆ Prepare the patient and family for the possibility of surgery, and provide emotional support and positive reinforcement afterward. Arrange for an enterostomal therapist to visit the patient who has had an ostomy.

INGUINAL HERNIA

A hernia occurs when part of an internal organ protrudes through an abnormal opening in the containing wall of its cavity. Hernias typically occur in the abdominal cavity. Although many kinds of abdominal hernias are possible, inguinal hernias are most common. (See *Common sites of hernia*, page 250.) In an inguinal hernia, the large or small intestine, omentum, or bladder protrudes into the inguinal canal. Hernias can be reduced (if the hernia can be manipulated back into place with relative ease), incarcerated (if the hernia can't be reduced because adhesions have formed, obstructing the intestinal flow), or strangulated (part of the herniated intestine becomes twisted or edematous, seriously interfering with normal blood flow and peristalsis, and possibly leading to intestinal obstruction and necrosis).

Causes and incidence

An inguinal hernia may be indirect or direct. An indirect inguinal hernia may develop at any age, is more common in males, occurs more often

Common sites of hernia

Femoral hernia occurs where the femoral artery passes into the femoral canal. Typically, a fatty deposit within the femoral canal enlarges and eventually creates a hole big enough to accommodate part of the peritoneum and bladder. A femoral hernia appears as a swelling or bulge at the pulse point of the large femoral artery. It's usually a soft, pliable, reducible, nontender mass, but commonly becomes incarcerated or strangulated.

Umbilical hernia results from abnormal muscular structures around the umbilical cord. This hernia is quite common in neonates, but also occurs in women who are obese or who have had several pregnancies. Because most umbilical hernias in infants close spontaneously, surgery is warranted only if the hernia persists for more than 4 or 5 years. Taping or binding the affected area or supporting it with a truss may relieve symptoms until the hernia closes. Severe congenital umbilical hernia allows the abdominal viscera to protrude outside the body. This condition necessitates immediate repair.

Incisional (ventral) hernia develops at the site of previous surgery, usually along vertical incisions. This hernia may result from a weakness in the abdominal wall, perhaps as a result of an infection or impaired wound healing. Inadequate nutrition, extreme abdominal distention, or obesity also predispose the patient to incisional hernia. Palpation of an incisional hernia may reveal several defects in the surgical scar. Effective repair requires pulling the layers of the abdominal wall together without creating tension. If this isn't possible, surgical reconstruction uses Teflon, Marlex mesh, or tantalum mesh to close the opening.

Inguinal hernia can be direct or indirect. Indirect inguinal hernia causes the abdominal viscera to protrude through the inguinal ring and follow the spermatic cord (in males) or round ligament (in females). Direct inguinal hernia results from a weakness in the fascial floor of the inguinal canal.

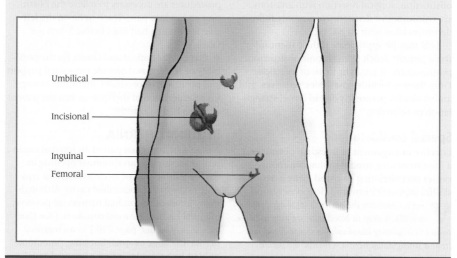

Umbilical

Incisional

Inguinal

Femoral

in those of Caucasian ethnicity, and can occur in infants younger than 1. The lifetime risk of developing a groin hernia is approximately 25% in men, and less than 5% in women.

Pathophysiology

An indirect inguinal hernia, the more common form, results from weakness in the fascial margin of the internal inguinal ring. In an indirect hernia, abdominal viscera leave the abdomen through the inguinal ring and follow the spermatic cord (in males) or round ligament (in females); they emerge at the external ring and extend down the inguinal canal, commonly into the scrotum or labia. A direct inguinal hernia results from a weakness in the fascial floor of the inguinal canal. Instead of entering the canal through the internal ring, the hernia passes through the posterior inguinal wall, protrudes directly through the transverse fascia of the canal (in an area known as *Hesselbach's triangle*), and comes out at the external ring.

In males, during the seventh month of gestation, the testicle normally descends into the scrotum, preceded by the peritoneal sac. If the sac closes improperly, it leaves an opening through which the intestine can slip. In either sex, a hernia can result from weak abdominal muscles (caused by congenital malformation, trauma, or aging) or increased intra-abdominal pressure (due to heavy lifting, pregnancy, obesity, or straining).

Complications
◆ Incarceration or strangulation of the bowel
◆ Intestinal obstruction
◆ Intestinal necrosis

Signs and symptoms
Inguinal hernia usually causes a lump to appear over the herniated area when the patient stands or strains. The lump disappears when the patient is supine. Tension on the herniated contents may cause a sharp, steady pain in the groin, which fades when the hernia is reduced. Strangulation produces severe pain and may lead to partial or complete bowel obstruction and even intestinal necrosis. Partial bowel obstruction may cause anorexia, vomiting, pain and tenderness in the groin, an irreducible mass, and diminished bowel sounds. Complete obstruction may cause shock, high fever, absent bowel sounds, and bloody stools.

PEDIATRIC TIP *In an infant, an inguinal hernia commonly coexists with an undescended testicle or a hydrocele.*

Diagnosis
In a patient with a large hernia, physical examination reveals an obvious swelling or lump in the inguinal area. In the patient with a small hernia, the affected area may simply appear full. Palpation of the inguinal area while the patient is performing Valsalva's maneuver confirms the diagnosis. To detect a hernia in a male patient, the patient is asked to stand with his ipsilateral leg slightly flexed and his weight resting on the other leg. The examiner inserts an index finger into the lower part of the scrotum and invaginates the scrotal skin so the finger advances through the external inguinal ring to the internal ring (about 1½" to 2" [4 to 5 cm] through the inguinal canal). The patient is then told to cough. If the examiner feels pressure against the fingertip, an indirect hernia exists; if pressure is felt against the side of the finger, a direct hernia exists.

A patient history of sharp or "catching" pain when lifting or straining may help confirm the diagnosis. Suspected bowel obstruction requires X-rays and a white blood cell count (may be elevated).

Treatment
If the hernia is reducible, the pain may be temporarily relieved by pushing the hernia back into place. A truss may keep the abdominal contents from protruding into the hernial sac; however, this won't cure the hernia. This device is especially beneficial for an older adult or debilitated patient for whom surgery might be hazardous.

For infants, adults, and otherwise healthy older adult patients, herniorrhaphy is the treatment of choice. Herniorrhaphy replaces the contents of the hernial sac into the abdominal cavity and closes the opening. In many cases, this procedure is performed under local anesthesia in a short-term unit or as a single-day admission. Another effective surgical procedure for repairing hernia is hernioplasty, which reinforces the weakened area with steel mesh, fascia, or wire.

A strangulated or necrotic hernia necessitates bowel resection. Rarely, an extensive resection may require temporary colostomy. In either case, bowel resection lengthens postoperative recovery and requires antibiotics, parenteral fluids, and electrolyte replacement.

Special considerations
Care includes managing symptoms to increase patient comfort and prevent worsening.
◆ Apply a truss only after a hernia has been reduced. For best results, apply it in the morning, before the patient gets out of bed.
◆ To prevent skin irritation, tell the patient to bathe daily and apply cornstarch. Teach against applying the truss over clothing because this reduces the effectiveness of the device and may make it slip.

ALERT *If incarceration and strangulation occur, don't try to reduce the hernia because this may perforate the bowel. If severe intestinal obstruction develops because of hernial strangulation, inform the healthcare provider immediately. An NG tube may be inserted promptly to empty the stomach and relieve pressure on the hernial sac.*
◆ Before surgery for an incarcerated hernia, closely monitor the patient's vital signs. Administer I.V. fluids and analgesics, as ordered. Place the patient in Trendelenburg's position to reduce pressure on the hernia site.
◆ Give special reassurance and emotional support to a child and parents or caregivers when hernia repair is scheduled. Encourage questions, and answer them as thoroughly as possible.

◆ After outpatient surgery, make sure that the patient voids before leaving the hospital. Teach the patient to check the incision and dressing for drainage, inflammation, or swelling and to watch for fever. If any of these occur, notify the healthcare provider.

◆ To reduce scrotal swelling, have the patient support the scrotum with a rolled towel and apply an ice bag.

◆ Instruct the patient to drink plenty of fluids to maintain hydration and prevent constipation.

◆ Before discharge, teach the patient to avoid lifting heavy objects or straining during bowel movements. Additionally, instruct to watch for signs and symptoms of infection (oozing, tenderness, warmth, and redness) at the incision site and to keep the incision clean and covered until the sutures are removed.

◆ Advise the patient not to resume normal activity or return to work without the surgeon's permission.

INTUSSUSCEPTION

Intussusception is a telescoping (invagination) of a proximal segment into a distal segment of the intestine, which causes an obstruction. Intussusception may be fatal, especially if treatment is delayed for more than 24 hours.

Causes and incidence

The cause of intussusception is idiopathic; however, it has been associated with lead points (polyps or tumors, Meckel's diverticulum, intestinal adhesions), cystic fibrosis, and as occurring immediately after abdominal surgery. Although it can affect adults, intussusception is most common in infants between 5 and 7

months of age. It occurs more often in males than in females, with 4 to 5.5 per 10,000 children hospitalized in the United States annually for this condition.

Seasonal peaks—between fall and winter—coinciding with the peak incidence of respiratory tract infections—have been noted in the incidence of intussusception, suggesting a connection to viral infections. Other potential causes include a mass, such as a lymph node, polyp, or tumor that telescopes the gut and leads to intussusception.

Pathophysiology

When a bowel segment (the intussusceptum) invaginates, peristalsis propels it along the bowel, pulling more bowel along with it; the receiving segment is the intussuscipiens. This invagination produces edema, hemorrhage from venous engorgement, incarceration, and obstruction. If treatment is delayed for longer than 24 hours, strangulation of the intestine usually occurs, with gangrene, shock, and perforation. (See *Understanding intussusception*.)

Complications

◆ Strangulation of intestine
◆ Gangrene
◆ Shock
◆ Perforation
◆ Peritonitis

Signs and symptoms

PEDIATRIC TIP *In an infant or child, intussusception produces four cardinal clinical effects:*
◆ *Intermittent attacks of colicky pain cause the child to scream, draw the legs up to the abdomen, turn pale and diaphoretic and, possibly, display grunting respirations.*
◆ *Vomiting of stomach contents may occur initially, followed by further vomiting of bile-stained or fecal material.*
◆ *"Currant-jelly" stools, containing a mixture of blood and mucus, may be observed.*
◆ *The patient will have a tender, distended abdomen, with a palpable, sausage-shaped abdominal mass; the viscera are usually absent from the right lower quadrant.*

In adults, intussusception produces nonspecific, chronic, and intermittent symptoms, including colicky abdominal pain and tenderness, vomiting, diarrhea (occasionally constipation), bloody stools, and weight loss. Abdominal pain usually localizes in the right lower quadrant, radiates to the back, and increases with eating. Adults with severe intussusception may develop strangulation with excruciating pain, abdominal distention, and tachycardia.

Understanding intussusception

In intussusception, a bowel section invaginates and is propelled along by peristalsis, pulling in more bowel. Intussusception typically produces edema, hemorrhage from venous engorgement, incarceration, and obstruction.

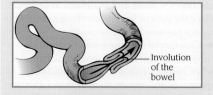

Involution of the bowel

Diagnosis

℞ CONFIRMING DIAGNOSIS *Abdominal ultrasound and radiographic imaging studies can confirm the presence of intussusception.*

Upright abdominal X-rays may show a soft-tissue mass and signs of complete or partial obstruction, with dilated loops of bowel. Signs of dehydration or shock support the diagnosis, as does the presence of a palpable mass in the abdomen.

Treatment

In children, spontaneous reduction may occur; in the absence of spontaneous reduction, therapy may include hydrostatic reduction or surgery. Surgery is indicated for children with recurrent intussusception, for those who show signs of shock or peritonitis, and for those in whom symptoms have been present longer than 24 hours. In adults, surgery is always the treatment of choice.

During hydrostatic reduction, the radiologist drips a barium solution into the rectum from a height of no more than 3′ (1 m); fluoroscopy traces the progress of the barium. If the procedure is successful, the barium backwashes into the ileum, and the mass disappears. If not, the procedure is stopped, and the patient is prepared for surgery.

During surgery, manual reduction is attempted first. After compressing the bowel above the intussusception, the physician attempts to milk the intussusception back through the bowel. However, if manual reduction fails or if the bowel is gangrenous or strangulated, the physician will perform a resection of the affected bowel segment.

Special considerations

Care focuses on changes in the patient's condition that might indicate worsening of the condition.

⚠ ALERT *Monitor the patient's vital signs before and after surgery. A change in temperature may indicate sepsis; infants may become hypothermic at the onset of infection. Rising pulse rate and falling blood pressure may be signs of peritonitis.*

◆ Check the patient's intake and output. Watch for signs of dehydration and bleeding.

◆ An NG tube is inserted to decompress the intestine and minimize vomiting. Monitor tube drainage and replace volume lost, as ordered.

◆ Monitor the patient who has undergone hydrostatic reduction for passage of stools and barium, a sign that the reduction was successful. Keep in mind that the patient may have a recurrence of intussusception, usually within the first 24 to 36 hours after the reduction.

◆ After surgery, administer antibiotics, as ordered. Closely check the incision for inflammation, drainage, or suture separation.

◆ Encourage deep breathing and productive coughing. Teach the patient to splint the incision when coughing.

◆ The NG tube may be removed when bowel sounds and peristalsis resume. The patient's diet can be advanced as tolerated.

◆ Check for abdominal distention after the patient resumes a normal diet, and monitor general condition.

◆ Offer special reassurance and emotional support to the child and parents or caregivers. This condition is considered a pediatric emergency, and parents or caregivers are generally unprepared for their child's hospitalization and possible surgery. They may feel guilty for not seeking medical aid sooner. Similarly, the child is unprepared for a separation from parents and home.

To minimize the stress of hospitalization, encourage parents or caregivers to participate in their child's care as much as possible.

VOLVULUS (TORSION)

Volvulus (torsion) is a twisting of the intestine at least 180 degrees on its mesenteric pedicle, which results in blood vessel compression and ischemia.

Causes and incidence

Twisting in volvulus may result from an anomaly of rotation, an ingested foreign body, or an adhesion; in some cases, however, the cause is unknown. Volvulus usually occurs in a bowel segment with a mesentery long enough to twist. The most common area, particularly in adults, is the sigmoid; the small bowel is a common site in children. Other common sites include the stomach and cecum. Volvulus secondary to meconium ileus may occur in patients with cystic fibrosis.

◆ Acute gastric volvulus has a high-mortality rate. There's no racial predilection, and it affects males and females equally. Peak incidence occurs in people over the age of 50.

Pathophysiology

Volvulus is a twisting of the intestine on its mesenteric pedicle, with blood supply occlusion; it is often associated with fibrous adhesions in the small intestine, although it occurs more frequently in the large intestine in older adults.

Complications

◆ Strangulation of the twisted intestinal loop
◆ Ischemia

♦ Infarction
♦ Perforation
♦ Fatal peritonitis

Signs and symptoms

Vomiting and rapid, marked abdominal distention follow sudden onset of severe abdominal pain. Nausea, vomiting, bloody stools, constipation, and shock may occur. Without immediate treatment, volvulus can lead to strangulation of the twisted bowel loop, ischemia, infarction, perforation, and fatal peritonitis.

Diagnosis

The sudden onset of severe abdominal pain and physical examination that may reveal a palpable mass suggest volvulus. Appropriate tests include the following:

♦ X-rays—Abdominal X-rays may show obstruction and abnormal air-fluid levels in the sigmoid and cecum; in midgut volvulus, abdominal X-rays may be normal.

♦ CT scan—may show evidence of intestinal obstruction.

♦ Barium enema—In cecal volvulus, barium fills the colon distal to the section of cecum; in sigmoid volvulus in children, barium may twist to a point and, in adults, it may take on an "ace of spades" configuration.

♦ Upper GI series (with small bowel follow-through)—In midgut volvulus, obstruction and possibly a twisted contour show in a narrow area near the duodenojejunal junction, where barium won't pass.

♦ White blood cell count—In strangulation, the count is greater than 15,000/μL; in bowel infarction, greater than 20,000/μL.

Treatment

Treatment varies according to the severity and location of the volvulus. For children with midgut volvulus, treatment is surgical. For adults with sigmoid volvulus, a proctoscopic examination is performed to check for infarction, and nonsurgical treatment includes reduction by careful insertion of a sigmoidoscope or a long rectal tube to deflate the bowel.

The success of nonsurgical reduction is indicated by expulsion of gas and immediate relief from abdominal pain. If the bowel is distended but viable, surgery consists of detorsion (untwisting); if the bowel is necrotic, surgery includes resection and anastomosis.

Special considerations

After surgical correction of volvulus:

♦ Monitor the patient's vital signs, watching for temperature changes (a sign of sepsis) and a rapid pulse rate and falling blood pressure (signs of shock and peritonitis). Carefully monitor fluid intake and output (including stools), electrolyte values, and complete blood count. Be sure to measure and record drainage from the NG tube and drains.

♦ Encourage frequent coughing and deep breathing with splinting of the incision.

♦ Reposition the patient often and perform suction as needed.

♦ Record excessive or unusual drainage.

♦ Check for incisional inflammation and separation of sutures.

♦ When bowel sounds and peristalsis return, remove the NG tube and begin oral feedings with clear liquids, as ordered. When solid food can be tolerated, gradually expand the diet. Reassure the patient and family or caregivers appropriately, and explain all diagnostic procedures. If the patient is a child, encourage parents or caregivers to participate in their child's care to minimize the stress of hospitalization.

PANCREATITIS

Pancreatitis, inflammation of the pancreas, occurs in acute and chronic forms and may be due to edema, necrosis, or hemorrhage. Alcohol use is associated with approximately 30% of cases of acute pancreatitis in the United States. The prognosis is better when pancreatitis follows biliary tract disease, but poor when it follows alcoholism. Mortality rises are high when pancreatitis is associated with necrosis and hemorrhage. (See *Chronic pancreatitis*.)

Chronic pancreatitis

Chronic pancreatitis is associated with alcoholism in more than 45% of patients, but it also may follow hyperparathyroidism (causing hypercalcemia), hyperlipidemia or, infrequently, gallstones, trauma, or peptic ulcer. Inflammation and fibrosis cause progressive pancreatic insufficiency and eventually destroy the pancreas.

Symptoms of chronic pancreatitis include constant dull pain with occasional exacerbations, malabsorption, severe weight loss, and hyperglycemia (leading to diabetic symptoms). Diagnosis is based on the patient history, X-rays showing pancreatic calcification, an elevated erythrocyte sedimentation rate, and examination of stool for steatorrhea.

Chronic pancreatitis
(*continued*)

In many cases, the severe pain of chronic pancreatitis requires large doses of analgesics or opioids, making addiction a serious problem. Treatment also includes a low-fat diet and oral administration of pancreatic enzymes, such as pancreatin or pancrelipase, to control steatorrhea; insulin or oral hypoglycemics to curb hyperglycemia; and, occasionally, surgical repair of biliary or pancreatic ducts or the sphincter of Oddi to reduce pressure and promote the flow of pancreatic juice. The prognosis is favorable if the patient can avoid alcohol, but poor if not avoided.

Causes and incidence

The most common causes of pancreatitis are biliary tract disease and alcoholism, but it can also result from pancreatic cancer, trauma, or use of certain drugs, such as glucocorticoids, sulfonamides, chlorothiazide, and azathioprine. This disease also may develop as a complication of peptic ulcer, mumps, or hypothermia.

Rarer causes are stenosis or obstruction of the sphincter of Oddi, hyperlipidemia, metabolic endocrine disorders (hyperparathyroidism and hemochromatosis), vasculitis or vascular disease, viral infections, mycoplasmal pneumonia, and pregnancy.

Diabetes, pancreatic insufficiency, and calcification occur in young people, probably from malnutrition and alcoholism, and lead to pancreatic atrophy. (See *Necrotizing pancreatitis*.)

The incidence of acute pancreatitis varies; its incidence ranges from 4.9 to 35 per 100,000 affected. Alcohol is estimated to account for 45% of cases of chronic pancreatitis in the United States.

Pathophysiology

Regardless of the cause, pancreatitis involves autodigestion: The enzymes normally excreted by the pancreas digest pancreatic tissue. Autodigestion causes vascular damage, coagulative and fat necrosis, and pseudocyst formation.

Complications

◆ Diabetes mellitus (if islets of Langerhans are damaged)
◆ Massive hemorrhage
◆ Destruction of pancreas

PATHOPHYSIOLOGY
Necrotizing pancreatitis

Acute pancreatitis can occur as necrotizing pancreatitis when there is cell death and tissue damage.

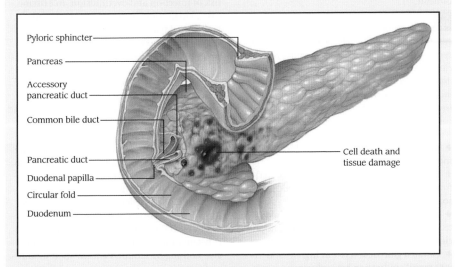

Pyloric sphincter
Pancreas
Accessory pancreatic duct
Common bile duct
Pancreatic duct
Duodenal papilla
Circular fold
Duodenum
Cell death and tissue damage

◆ Diabetes acidosis
◆ Shock
◆ Coma
◆ Adult respiratory distress syndrome
◆ Atelectasis
◆ Pulmonary effusion
◆ Pneumonia
◆ GI bleeding
◆ Pancreatic abscess

Signs and symptoms

In many patients, the first and only symptom of mild pancreatitis is steady epigastric pain centered close to the umbilicus, radiating between the tenth thoracic and sixth lumbar vertebrae, and unrelieved by vomiting. However, a severe attack causes extreme pain, persistent vomiting, abdominal rigidity, diminished bowel activity (suggesting peritonitis), crackles at lung bases, and left pleural effusion. Progression produces extreme malaise and restlessness, with mottled skin, tachycardia, low-grade fever (100° to 102° F [37.7° to 38.8° C]), and cold, sweaty extremities. The proximity of the inflamed pancreas to the bowel may cause ileus.

If pancreatitis damages the islets of Langerhans, complications may include diabetes mellitus. Fulminant pancreatitis causes massive hemorrhage and total destruction of the pancreas, resulting in diabetic acidosis, shock, or coma.

Diagnosis

A thorough patient history (especially for alcoholism) and physical examination are the first steps in diagnosis, but the retroperitoneal position of the pancreas makes physical assessment difficult.

℞ CONFIRMING DIAGNOSIS *Dramatically elevated serum amylase levels—in many cases over 500 U/L—confirm pancreatitis and rule out perforated peptic ulcer, acute cholecystitis, appendicitis, and bowel infarction or obstruction. Similarly, dramatic elevations of amylase also occur in urine, ascites, or pleural fluid. Characteristically, amylase levels return to normal 48 hours after the onset of pancreatitis, despite continuing symptoms.*

Supportive laboratory values include:
◆ increased serum lipase levels, which rise more slowly than serum amylase
◆ low serum calcium levels (hypocalcemia) from fat necrosis and formation of calcium soaps
◆ white blood cell counts ranging from 8,000 to 20,000/µL, with increased polymorphonuclear leukocytes
◆ elevated glucose levels—as high as 500 to 900 mg/dL, indicating hyperglycemia

Tests used to diagnose pancreatitis may include the following:
◆ Abdominal X-rays or CT scans show dilation of the small or large bowel or calcification of the pancreas.
◆ Ultrasound or CT scan reveals an increased pancreatic diameter and helps distinguish acute cholecystitis from acute pancreatitis.

Treatment

The goal of therapy is to maintain circulation and fluid volume. Treatment measures must also relieve pain and decrease pancreatic secretions.

Emergency treatment of shock (which is the most common cause of death in early-stage pancreatitis) consists of vigorous I.V. replacement of electrolytes and proteins. Metabolic acidosis that develops secondary to hypovolemia and impaired cellular perfusion requires vigorous fluid volume replacement.

Drug treatment may include meperidine for pain, diazepam for restlessness and agitation, and antibiotics for bacterial infections. Morphine and codeine are usually avoided as pain medications because of their effect on the sphincter of Oddi. If the patient has hypocalcemia, they may need an infusion of 10% calcium gluconate. Elevated serum glucose levels may require insulin therapy.

After the emergency phase, continuing I.V. therapy should provide adequate electrolytes and protein solutions that don't stimulate the pancreas for 5 to 7 days. If the patient isn't ready to resume oral feedings by then, TPN may be necessary. Nonstimulating elemental gavage feedings may be safer because of the decreased risk of infection and overinfusion. In extreme cases, laparotomy to debride the pancreatic bed, partial pancreatectomy, or a combination of both and feeding jejunostomy may be necessary.

Special considerations

Acute pancreatitis is a life-threatening emergency, requiring meticulous supportive care and continuous monitoring of vital systems.
◆ Monitor the patient's vital signs and pulmonary artery pressure or central venous pressure closely. Give plasma or albumin, if ordered, to maintain blood pressure. Record fluid intake and output, check urine output hourly, and monitor electrolyte levels. Assess for crackles, rhonchi, or decreased breath sounds.
◆ For bowel decompression, maintain constant or intermittent NG suctioning, and give nothing by mouth. Perform good mouth and nose care.

◆ Watch for signs and symptoms of calcium deficiency—tetany, cramps, carpopedal spasm, and seizures. If hypocalcemia is suspected, keep airway and suction apparatus handy and pad side rails.

◆ Administer analgesics as needed to relieve the patient's pain and anxiety. Remember that anticholinergics reduce salivary and sweat gland secretions. Teach the patient that dry mouth and facial flushing may be experienced. *Caution:* Narrow-angle glaucoma contraindicates the use of atropine or its derivatives.

◆ Monitor glucose levels.

◆ Watch for complications due to TPN, such as sepsis, hypokalemia, overhydration, and metabolic acidosis. Watch for fever, cardiac irregularities, changes in arterial blood gas measurements, and deep respirations. Use strict aseptic technique when caring for the catheter insertion site.

Anorectum

HEMORRHOIDS

Hemorrhoids are varicosities in the superior or inferior hemorrhoidal venous plexus. Dilation and enlargement of the superior plexus produce internal hemorrhoids; dilation and enlargement of the inferior plexus produce external hemorrhoids that may protrude from the rectum. (See *Types of hemorrhoids.*) Hemorrhoids occur in both sexes; incidence is self-reported to be at the highest between 45 and 65 years old.

Causes and incidence

Predisposing factors include occupations that require prolonged standing or sitting; straining due to constipation, diarrhea, coughing, sneezing, or vomiting; heart failure; hepatic disease, such as cirrhosis, amebic abscesses, or hepatitis; alcoholism; anorectal infections; loss of muscle tone due to old age, rectal surgery, or episiotomy; anal intercourse; and pregnancy.

Pathophysiology

Hemorrhoids are thought to result from increased venous pressure in the hemorrhoidal plexus.

Complications

◆ Local infection
◆ Thrombosis

Signs and symptoms

Although hemorrhoids may be asymptomatic, they characteristically cause painless, intermittent bleeding, which occurs on defecation. Bright red blood appears streaked on stool or on toilet paper due to injury of the fragile mucosa covering the hemorrhoid. These first-degree hemorrhoids may itch because of poor anal hygiene. When second-degree hemorrhoids prolapse, they're usually painless and spontaneously return to the anal canal following defecation. Third-degree hemorrhoids cause constant discomfort and prolapse in response to any increase in intra-abdominal pressure. They must be manually reduced. Thrombosis of external hemorrhoids produces sudden rectal pain and a subcutaneous, large, firm lump that the patient can feel. If hemorrhoids cause severe or recurrent bleeding, they may lead to secondary anemia with significant pallor, fatigue, and weakness; however, such systemic complications are rare.

Diagnosis

Physical examination confirms external hemorrhoids. Proctoscopy confirms internal hemorrhoids and rules out rectal polyps.

Treatment

Treatment depends on the type and severity of the hemorrhoid and on the patient's overall condition. Generally, treatment includes measures to ease pain, combat swelling, and

---

Types of hemorrhoids

Covered by mucosa, *internal hemorrhoids* bulge into the rectal lumen and may prolapse during defecation. Covered by skin, *external hemorrhoids* protrude from the rectum and are more likely to thrombose than internal hemorrhoids.

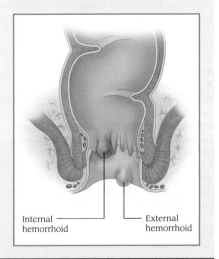

Internal hemorrhoid

External hemorrhoid

regulate bowel habits. The patient can relieve constipation by increasing the amount of raw vegetables, fruit, and whole grains consumed in the diet or by occasionally using stool softeners. Venous congestion can be prevented by avoiding prolonged sitting; local swelling and pain can be decreased with local anesthetic agents (lotions, creams, or suppositories), astringents, or cold compresses, followed by warm sitz baths or thermal packs. Rarely, the patient with chronic, profuse bleeding may require a blood transfusion. Other nonsurgical treatments include injection of a sclerosing solution to produce scar tissue that decreases prolapse, manual reduction, and hemorrhoid band ligation or laser ablation.

Hemorrhoidectomy, the most effective treatment, is necessary for patients with severe bleeding, intolerable pain and pruritus, and large prolapse. This procedure is contraindicated in patients with blood dyscrasias (acute leukemia, aplastic anemia, or hemophilia) or GI carcinoma and during the first trimester of pregnancy.

Special considerations

Patient care includes preoperative and postoperative support.

◆ To prepare the patient for hemorrhoidectomy, administer an enema as appropriate (usually 2 to 4 hours before surgery), and record results. Prepare the area as ordered.

◆ Postoperatively, check for signs of prolonged rectal bleeding, administer adequate analgesics, and provide sitz baths as ordered.

◆ As soon as the patient can resume oral intake, administer a bulk medication, such as psyllium, about 1 hour after the evening meal, to ensure a daily stool. Teach to refrain from using stool-softening medications soon after hemorrhoidectomy because a firm stool acts as a natural dilator to prevent anal stricture from the scar tissue. (The patient may need repeated digital dilation to prevent such narrowing.)

◆ Keep the wound site clean to prevent infection and irritation.

◆ Before discharge, stress the importance of regular bowel habits and good anal hygiene. Discourage too vigorous wiping with washcloths and using harsh soaps. Encourage the use of medicated astringent pads and white toilet paper (the fixative in colored paper can irritate the skin).

ANORECTAL ABSCESS AND FISTULA

Anorectal abscess is a localized collection of pus due to inflammation of the soft tissue near the rectum or anus. Inflammation may produce an anal fistula—an abnormal opening in the anal skin—that may communicate with the rectum.

Causes and incidence

Causes of anorectal abscess and fistula are many (see *Pathophysiology* below). The peak incidence of anorectal abscess occurs in people in their 30s and 40s, but there's also a high occurrence in infants. Men are affected two to three times more often than women. About 30% of patients have a previous history of abscess.

Pathophysiology

The inflammatory process that leads to abscess may begin with an abrasion or tear in the lining of the anal canal, rectum, or perianal skin and subsequent infection by *E. coli*, staphylococci, or streptococci. Trauma may result from injections for treatment of internal hemorrhoids, enema-tip abrasions, puncture wounds from ingested eggshells or fish bones, or insertion of foreign objects. Other preexisting lesions include infected anal fissure, infections from the anal crypt through the anal gland, ruptured anal hematoma, prolapsed thrombosed internal hemorrhoids, and septic lesions in the pelvis, such as acute appendicitis, acute salpingitis, and diverticulitis. Systemic illnesses that may cause abscesses include ulcerative colitis and Crohn disease. However, many abscesses develop without preexisting lesions.

As the abscess (particularly from an infected anal crypt gland) produces more pus, a fistula may form in the soft tissue beneath the muscle fibers of the sphincters (especially the external sphincter), usually extending into the perianal skin. The internal (primary) opening of the abscess or fistula is usually near the anal glands and crypts; the external (secondary) opening, in the perianal skin.

Complications

◆ Anorectal fistula
◆ Perineal cellulitis
◆ Scar tissue formation
◆ Anal stricture

Signs and symptoms

Characteristics are throbbing pain and tenderness at the site of the abscess. A hard, painful lump develops on one side, preventing comfortable sitting. Discharge of pus may occur from the rectum, and there may be constipation or pain associated with bowel movements.

Diagnosis

Anorectal abscess is detectable on physical examination. If the abscess drains by forming a fistula, the pain usually subsides and the major signs become pruritic drainage and subsequent perianal irritation. The external opening of a fistula generally appears as a pink or red, elevated, discharging sinus or ulcer on the skin near the anus. Depending on the severity of the infection, the patient may have chills, fever, nausea, vomiting, and malaise. Digital examination may reveal a palpable indurated tract and a drop or two of pus on palpation. The internal opening may be palpated as a depression or ulcer in the midline anteriorly or at the dentate line posteriorly. Examination with a probe may require an anesthetic. A proctosigmoidoscopy may be performed to exclude associated diseases.

Treatment

Anorectal abscesses require surgical incision under caudal anesthesia to promote drainage. Fistulas require a fistulotomy—removal of the fistula and associated granulation tissue—under caudal anesthesia. If the fistula tract is epithelialized, treatment requires fistulectomy—removal of the fistulous tract—followed by insertion of drains, which remain in place for 48 hours. Warm sitz baths are useful to relieve inflammation; however, pain medication and antibiotics may be needed.

Special considerations

After incision to drain anorectal abscess, follow these guidelines:
◆ Provide adequate medication for pain relief, as ordered.
◆ Examine the wound frequently to assess proper healing, which should progress from the inside out. Healing should be complete in 4 to 5 weeks for perianal fistulas; in 12 to 16 weeks for deeper wounds.
◆ Inform the patient that complete recovery takes time, and offer encouragement.
◆ Stress the importance of perianal cleanliness.
◆ Be alert for the first postoperative bowel movement. The patient may suppress the urge to defecate because of anticipated pain; the resulting constipation increases pressure at the wound site. Such a patient may benefit from a stool-softening laxative.

RECTAL POLYPS

Rectal polyps are masses of tissue that rise above the mucosal membrane and protrude into the GI tract. Types of polyps include common polypoid adenomas, villous adenomas, hereditary polyposis, focal polypoid hyperplasia, and juvenile polyps (hamartomas). Most rectal polyps are benign; however, villous and hereditary polyps show a marked inclination to

become malignant. Indeed, a striking feature of familial polyposis is that it's commonly associated with rectosigmoid adenocarcinoma.

Causes and incidence

Polyps form as a result of unrestrained cell growth in the upper epithelium. Predisposing factors include heredity, age, infection, and diet.

Villous adenomas are most prevalent in men over 50 years old, and are more common in African American men than those of other ethnicity. Incidence in both sexes rises after 70 years old.

Pathophysiology

Polyps are masses or finger-like projections that arise from the intestinal mucosal epithelium. Adenomatous polyps form in an area where there is hyperproliferation of epithelial cells and crypt dysplasia; after traversing the muscularis mucosae, the polyp can become invasive and malignant.

Complications

◆ Anemia from slow bleeding
◆ Bowel obstruction
◆ Colorectal cancer

Signs and symptoms

Because rectal polyps don't generally cause symptoms, they're usually discovered incidentally during a digital examination or rectosigmoidoscopy. Rectal bleeding is a common sign; high rectal polyps leave a streak of blood on the stool, whereas low rectal polyps bleed freely.

Rectal polyps vary in appearance. Common polypoid adenomas are small, multiple lesions that are redder than normal mucosa. They're commonly pedunculated (attached to rectal mucosa by a long, thin stalk) and granular, with a red, lobular, or eroded surface.

Villous adenomas are usually sessile (attached to the mucosa by a wide base) and vary in size from 0.5 to 12 cm. They are soft, friable, and finely lobulated. They may grow large and cause painful defecation; however, because adenomas are soft, they rarely cause bowel obstruction. Sometimes adenomas prolapse outside the anus, expelling parts of the adenoma with feces. These polyps may cause diarrhea, bloody stools, and subsequent fluid and electrolyte depletion, with hypotension and oliguria.

In hereditary polyposis, rectal polyps resemble benign adenomas but occur as hundreds of small (0.5 cm) lesions carpeting the entire mucosal surface. Associated signs include diarrhea, bloody stools, and secondary anemia. In patients with hereditary polyposis, changes in bowel habits with abdominal pain usually signal rectosigmoid cancer.

Juvenile polyps are large, inflammatory lesions, commonly without an epithelial covering. Mucus-filled cysts cover their usually smooth surface.

Focal polypoid hyperplasia produces small (<3 mm), granular, sessile lesions, similar to the colon in color, or gray or translucent. They usually occur at the rectosigmoid junction.

Diagnosis

CONFIRMING DIAGNOSIS *Firm diagnosis of rectal polyps requires identification of the polyps through proctosigmoidoscopy or colonoscopy and rectal biopsy.*

Barium enema can help identify polyps that are located high in the colon. Supportive laboratory findings include occult blood in the stools, low hemoglobin level and hematocrit (with anemia) and, possibly, serum electrolyte imbalances in patients with villous adenomas.

Treatment

Treatment varies according to the type and size of the polyps and their location in the colon. Common polypoid adenomas less than 1 cm require polypectomy, usually by fulguration (destruction by high-frequency electricity) during endoscopy. For common polypoid adenomas larger than 4 cm and all invasive villous adenomas, treatment usually consists of abdominoperineal resection or low anterior resection.

Focal polypoid hyperplasia can be obliterated by biopsy. Depending on GI involvement, hereditary polyps necessitate total abdominoperineal resection with a permanent ileostomy, subtotal colectomy with ileoproctostomy, or ileoanal anastomosis. Juvenile polyps are prone to autoamputation; if this doesn't occur, snare removal during colonoscopy is the treatment of choice.

Special considerations

During diagnostic evaluation:
◆ Check sodium, potassium, and chloride levels daily in the patient with fluid imbalances; adjust fluid and electrolytes, as necessary. Administer normal saline solution with potassium I.V., as ordered. Weigh the patient daily, and record the amount of diarrhea. Watch for signs of dehydration (decreased urine output and increased blood urea nitrogen levels).
◆ Tell the patient to watch for and report evidence of rectal bleeding.

After biopsy and fulguration:
◆ Check for signs of perforation and hemorrhage, such as sudden hypotension, a decrease

in hemoglobin level or hematocrit, shock, abdominal pain, and passage of red blood through the rectum.
◆ Have the patient walk as soon as possible after the procedure.
◆ Watch for and record the first bowel movement, which may not occur for 2 to 3 days.
◆ Provide sitz baths for 3 days.
◆ If the patient has benign polyps, stress the need for routine follow-up studies to check the polypoid growth rate.
◆ Prepare the patient with precancerous or familial lesions for abdominoperineal resection. Provide emotional support and preoperative instruction.

After ileostomy or subtotal colectomy with ileoproctostomy:
◆ Properly care for abdominal dressings, I.V. lines, and indwelling urinary catheters. Record intake and output, and check the patient's vital signs for hypotension and surgical complications. Administer pain medication, as ordered.
◆ To prevent embolism, have the patient walk as soon as possible, and apply antiembolism stockings; encourage range-of-motion exercises.
◆ Provide enterostomal therapy and teach the patient proper stoma care.

PILONIDAL DISEASE

In pilonidal disease, a coccygeal cyst forms in the intergluteal cleft on the posterior surface of the lower sacrum. It usually contains hair and becomes infected, producing an abscess, a draining sinus, or a fistula. Incidence is highest among hirsute white men around age 19.

Causes and incidence

Pilonidal disease may develop congenitally from a tendency to hirsutism, or it may be acquired from stretching or irritation of the sacrococcygeal area (intergluteal fold) from prolonged rough exercise (such as horseback riding), heat, excessive perspiration, or constrictive clothing.

The incidence rate of pilonidal disease is 0.7%. It affects men two to four times more often than women, but the onset is earlier in females, possibly because they begin puberty at an earlier age.

Pathophysiology

The pathophysiology of pilonidal disease is not fully understood; however, hair and inflammation present in the natal cleft are recognized as contributing factors. As the patient sits or bends, the natal cleft stretches, hair follicles are damaged or broken, and a pore is opened. This pore collects debris and serves as a receptacle for shed hairs from others parts of the body to become embedded. Negative pressure is created in the subcutaneous space as the skin becomes taut over the natal cleft; this draws the hairs deeper into the pore, and friction then causes the hairs to form a sinus.

Complications
◆ Impaired social interaction due to pain and discomfort
◆ Difficulty performing work-related activities

Signs and symptoms
Generally, a pilonidal cyst produces no symptoms until it becomes infected, causing local pain, tenderness, swelling, or heat. Other clinical features include continuous or intermittent purulent drainage, followed by development of an abscess, chills, fever, headache, and malaise.

Diagnosis
℞ **CONFIRMING DIAGNOSIS** *Physical examination confirms the diagnosis and may reveal a series of openings along the midline, with thin, brown, foul-smelling drainage or a protruding tuft of hair.*

Pressure on the sinus tract may produce purulent drainage. Passing a probe back through the sinus tract toward the sacrum shouldn't reveal a perforation between the anterior sinus and the anal canal. Cultures of discharge from the infected sinus may show staphylococci or skin bacteria, but don't usually contain bowel bacteria.

Treatment
Conservative treatment of pilonidal disease consists of incision and drainage of abscesses, regular extraction of protruding hairs, and sitz baths (four to six times daily). However, persistent infections may necessitate surgical excision of the entire affected area.

After excision of a pilonidal abscess, the patient requires regular follow-up care to monitor wound healing. The surgeon may periodically palpate the wound during healing with a cotton-tipped applicator, curette excess granulation tissue, and extract loose hairs to promote wound healing from the inside out and to prevent dead cells from collecting in the wound. Complete healing may take several months.

Special considerations
Care includes preoperative and postoperative support and patient education.
◆ Before incision and drainage of a pilonidal abscess, assure the patient adequate pain medication will first be administered.

◆ After surgery, check the compression dressing for signs of excessive bleeding, and change the dressing as directed.
◆ Encourage the patient to walk as soon as possible after the procedure.
◆ Tell the patient to place a gauze pad over the wound site after the dressing is removed to allow ventilation and prevent friction from clothing. Teach the patient to take sitz baths and to let the area air-dry instead of rubbing or patting it dry with a towel.
◆ After healing, the patient should briskly wash the area daily with a washcloth to remove loose hairs. Encourage the patient with obesity to establish a weight loss plan.

RECTAL PROLAPSE
Rectal prolapse is the circumferential protrusion of one or more layers of the mucous membrane through the anus. Prolapse may be complete (with displacement of the anal sphincter or bowel herniation) or partial (mucosal layer). (See *Types of rectal prolapse,* page 262.)

Causes and incidence
Rectal prolapse usually occurs in older multiparous females who have given birth vaginally. It's commonly associated with other conditions, such as prior pelvic surgery, history of chronic straining, chronic constipation or diarrhea, cystic fibrosis, dementia, stroke, pelvic floor dysfunction, and pelvic floor anatomic defects.

True incidence figures are unavailable because many cases go unreported.

Pathophysiology
See *Types of rectal prolapse* box for pathophysiology.

Complications
◆ Rectal ulceration
◆ Bleeding
◆ Incontinence

Signs and symptoms
In rectal prolapse, protrusion of tissue from the rectum may occur during defecation or walking. Other symptoms include a persistent sensation of rectal fullness, bloody diarrhea, pain in the lower abdomen due to ulceration, a feeling of incomplete evacuation, and rectal incontinence. Hemorrhoids or rectal polyps may coexist with a prolapse.

Diagnosis
Typical clinical features and visual examination confirm the diagnosis. In complete prolapse, examination reveals the full thickness of the

Types of rectal prolapse

Partial rectal prolapse involves only the rectal mucosa and a small mass of radial mucosal folds. However, in complete rectal prolapse (also known as procidentia), the full rectal wall, sphincter muscle, and a large mass of concentric mucosal folds protrude. Ulceration is possible after complete prolapse.

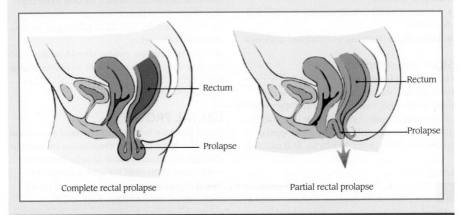

Complete rectal prolapse   Partial rectal prolapse

bowel wall and, possibly, the sphincter muscle protruding and mucosa falling into bulky, concentric folds. In partial prolapse, examination reveals only partially protruding mucosa and a smaller mass of radial mucosal folds. Straining during examination may disclose the full extent of prolapse.

Treatment

In some cases, eliminating the underlying cause is the only treatment necessary. The rectal mucosa can be returned to the rectum manually. While the patient is in a knee-chest position, a soft, warm, wet cloth may be used to apply gentle pressure to the mass to push it back through the anal opening, thereby allowing gravity to help return the prolapse into place. In an older adult, injection of a sclerosing agent to cause a fibrotic reaction fixes the rectum in place. Severe or chronic prolapse requires surgical repair by strengthening or tightening the sphincters with wire or by anterior or rectal resection of prolapsed tissue.

Special considerations

Provide the patient with education regarding underlying causes and preoperative and postoperative support.

▦ PREVENTION *Help the patient prevent consti-*
pation by teaching the correct diet and
stool-softening regimen.

◆ Advise the patient with severe prolapse and incontinence to wear a perineal pad.
◆ Before surgery, explain possible complications, including permanent rectal incontinence.
◆ After surgery, monitor for immediate complications (hemorrhage) and later ones (pelvic abscess, fever, pus drainage, pain, rectal stenosis, constipation, or pain on defecation). Teach perineal strengthening exercises: Have the patient lie down, with the back flat on the mattress; then ask the patient to pull in the abdomen and squeeze while taking a deep breath. Also have the patient repeatedly squeeze and relax the buttocks while sitting on a chair.

ANAL FISSURE

Anal fissure is a laceration or crack in the lining of the anus that extends to the circular muscle. Most fissures heal on their own and don't require treatment, aside from good diaper hygiene. However, some fissures may require medical treatment. The prognosis is very good, especially with fissurectomy and good anal hygiene.

Causes and incidence

Anal fissure results from passage of large, hard stools that stretch the lining beyond its limits. It may also be due to prolonged diarrhea, strain on the perineum during childbirth and, rarely, from scar stenosis. Occasionally, anal fissure is secondary to proctitis, anal tuberculosis, cancer, or Crohn disease.

Anal fissures are common in young infants and most often affect those who are middle-aged. Actual incidence is unknown since many cases are attributed to hemorrhoids.

Pathophysiology

A tear to the anoderm within the distal half of the anal canal usually begins an anal fissure; a cycle of anal pain and bleeding may result. Spasms may result from the exposed internal sphincter muscle, which can also restrict blood flow to the area, preventing healing.

Complications

◆ Abscess, fistula, and septicemia (rare)
◆ Scar tissue
◆ Hampered bowel elimination

Signs and symptoms

The onset of an acute anal fissure is characterized by tearing, cutting, or burning pain during or immediately after a bowel movement. A few drops of blood may streak toilet paper or underclothes. Painful anal sphincter spasms result from ulceration of a "sentinel pile" (swelling at the lower end of the fissure). A fissure may heal spontaneously and completely, or it may partially heal and break open again. Chronic fissure produces scar tissue that hampers normal bowel evacuation.

Diagnosis

Anoscopy showing a longitudinal tear and typical clinical features help establish the diagnosis. Digital examination that elicits pain and bleeding supports the diagnosis. Gentle traction on perianal skin can create sufficient eversion to visualize the fistula directly.

Treatment

Treatment varies according to the severity of the tear. Conservative treatment measures include stool softeners, dietary adjustment (addition of bulk to absorb water while in the intestinal tract), use of petroleum jelly and sitz baths, and cleaning more gently. Anesthetic ointment may be useful if pain interferes with normal bowel movements. Topical muscle relaxants may also be soothing. These measures generally heal most anal fissures. For fissures that don't heal with these treatments, a minor surgical procedure to relax the sphincter may be necessary.

For superficial fissures without hemorrhoids, forcible digital dilatation of the anal sphincter under local anesthesia stretches the lower portion of the sphincter. For complicated fissures, treatment includes surgical excision of tissue, adjacent skin, and mucosal tags and division of hypertrophied internal sphincter muscle to release tension.

Special considerations

Care consists of patient education and support.
◆ Prepare the patient for rectal examination; explain the necessity for the procedure.
◆ Provide warm sitz baths, warm soaks, and local anesthetic ointment to relieve pain. A low-residue diet, adequate fluid intake, and stool softeners prevent straining during defecation.
◆ Give diphenoxylate (Lomotil) or other antidiarrheals to control diarrhea.

ANAL PRURITUS

Anal pruritus is perianal itching, irritation, or superficial burning.

Causes and incidence

Factors that contribute to pruritus ani include overcleaning of the perianal area (harsh soap, vigorous rubbing with a washcloth or toilet paper); minor trauma caused by straining to defecate; poor hygiene; sensitivity to spicy foods, coffee, alcohol, food preservatives, perfumed or colored toilet paper, detergents, or certain fabrics; specific medications (antibiotics, antihypertensives, or antacids that cause diarrhea); excessive sweating (in occupations associated with physical labor or high stress levels); anal skin tags; systemic disease, especially diabetes; skin disorders, such as psoriasis or eczema; certain skin lesions, such as those associated with squamous cell carcinoma, basal cell carcinoma, Bowen disease, Paget disease, melanoma, syphilis, and tuberculosis; fungal or parasitic infection; and local anorectal disease (fissure, hemorrhoids, and fistula). This disorder is more common in males than in females, and often occurs between 40 and 60 years old.

Pathophysiology

Pathophysiology is associated with the root cause of the pruritus. Idiopathic anal pruritus is thought to be associated with perianal fecal contamination, and subsequent traumatic wiping or scratching.

Signs and symptoms

The key symptom of anal pruritus is perianal itching or burning after a bowel movement, during stress, or at night. In acute anal pruritus, scratching produces reddened skin, with weeping excoriations; in chronic anal pruritus, skin becomes thick and leathery, with excessive pigmentation.

Diagnosis
A detailed patient history is essential. Rectal examination rules out fissures and fistulas; biopsy rules out cancer. Allergy testing may also be helpful.

Treatment
After elimination of the underlying cause, treatment is symptomatic, such as advising the patient to avoid scratching or rubbing the itchy areas. Lukewarm baths and a skin-soothing oatmeal or cornstarch bath may be comforting. Temporary relief may be obtained with cold compresses. Topical over-the-counter ointments or creams containing hydrocortisone or zinc oxide are also useful.

Special considerations
◆ Make sure that the patient understands the condition and its causes.
◆ Recommend keeping fingernails short to avoid skin damage from inadvertent scratching. Suggest using cool, light, loose bedclothes and avoiding wearing rough clothing, particularly wool, over the irritated area.
◆ Advise the patient to avoid prolonged exposure to excessive heat and humidity.
◆ Advise the patient to avoid self-prescribed creams or powders, perfumed soaps, colored toilet paper, and moistened wipes because they may be irritating.
◆ Teach the patient to keep the perianal area clean and dry. Suggest witch hazel pads for wiping and cotton balls tucked between the buttocks to absorb moisture.

PROCTITIS
Proctitis is an acute or chronic inflammation of the rectal mucosa. It can result in discomfort, bleeding, and possibly a discharge of mucus or pus.

Causes and incidence
Proctitis caused by sexually transmitted disease (STD) occurs with high frequency among individuals who engage in anal intercourse. STDs that can cause proctitis include gonorrhea, herpes, chlamydia, and lymphogranuloma venereum.

In children, beta-hemolytic streptococcus may cause proctitis. Autoimmune proctitis is associated with such diseases as ulcerative colitis or Crohn disease. Proctitis may also be caused by medications, radiation, or noxious agents such as chemicals inserted into the rectum.

Other contributing factors include chronic constipation, habitual laxative use, emotional upset, radiation (especially for cancer of the cervix or uterus), endocrine dysfunction, rectal injury, rectal medications, bacterial infections, allergies (especially to milk), vasomotor disturbance that interferes with normal muscle control, and food poisoning.

Pathophysiology
Pathophysiology is associated with the root cause mechanism.

Complications
Complications are congruent with root cause mechanism.

Signs and symptoms
Key symptoms include tenesmus, constipation, a feeling of rectal fullness, and abdominal cramps on the left side. The patient feels an intense urge to defecate, which produces a small amount of stool that may contain blood and mucus.

Diagnosis
A detailed patient history is essential. In acute proctitis, sigmoidoscopy or proctoscopy reveals edematous, bright red or pink rectal mucosa that's thick, shiny, friable and, possibly, ulcerated. In chronic proctitis, sigmoidoscopy shows thickened mucosa, loss of vascular pattern, and stricture of the rectal lumen. Other supportive tests include biopsy to rule out cancer as well as rectal culture and examination of a stool sample.

Treatment
Primary treatment eliminates the underlying cause (fecal impaction, laxatives, or other medications). Proctitis caused by infection is treated with antibiotics specific for the causative organism. Corticosteroids or mesalamine suppositories may relieve symptoms in Crohn disease or ulcerative colitis. Soothing enemas or steroid (hydrocortisone) suppositories or enemas may be helpful if proctitis is due to radiation.

Special considerations
◆ Tell the patient to watch for and report bleeding and other persistent symptoms.
◆ Fully explain proctitis and its treatment to the patient to foster understanding of the disorder and prevent its recurrence.
◆ Offer explanations, emotional support, and reassurance during rectal examinations and treatment.

SELECTED REFERENCES

Ahmed, S., et al. (2014). Global prevalence of norovirus in cases of gastroenteritis: A systematic review and meta-analysis. *Lancet Infectious Disease, 14*(8), 725–730.

Aziz, Q., et al. (2016). Functional esophageal disorders. *Gastroenterology, 150*(6), 1368–1379.

Bagdasarian, N., et al. (2015). Diagnosis and treatment of *Clostridium difficile* in adults: A systematic review. *JAMA, 313*(4), 398–408.

Bergsland, E. (2017). *Zollinger-Ellison syndrome (gastrinoma): Clinical manifestations and diagnosis.* Retrieved from https://www.uptodate.com/contents/zollinger-ellison-syndrome-gastrinoma-clinical-manifestations-and-diagnosis

Bleday, R., & Breen, E. (2017). *Hemorrhoids: Clinical manifestations and diagnosis.* Retrieved from https://www.uptodate.com/contents/hemorrhoids-clinical-manifestations-and-diagnosis

Breen, E., & Bleday, R. (2016). *Approach to the patient with anal pruritus.* Retrieved from https://www.uptodate.com/contents/approach-to-the-patient-with-anal-pruritus

Centers for Disease Control and Prevention. (2018). *Birth defects homepage: Data and statistics.* Retrieved from www.cdc.gov/ncbddd/birthdefects/data.html

Crowe, S. (2016). *Bacteriology and epidemiology of Helicobacter pylori infection.* Retrieved from https://www.uptodate.com/contents/bacteriology-and-epidemiology-of-helicobacter-pylori-infection

Fishman, D. (2018). *Caustic esophageal injury in children.* Retrieved from https://www.uptodate.com/contents/caustic-esophageal-injury-in-children

Fleshner, P. (2018). *Surgical management of ulcerative colitis.* Retrieved from https://www.uptodate.com/contents/surgical-management-of-ulcerative-colitis

Freedman, S., & Lewis, M. (2016). *Etiology and pathogenesis of chronic pancreatitis in adults.* Retrieved from https://www.uptodate.com/contents/etiology-and-pathogenesis-of-chronic-pancreatitis-in-adults

Guelrud, M. (2017). *Mallory-Weiss syndrome.* Retrieved from https://www.uptodate.com/contents/mallory-weiss-syndrome

Ignatavicius, D., et al. (2018). *Medical-surgical nursing: Concepts for interprofessional collaborative care* (9th ed.). St. Louis: Elsevier.

Javid, P., & Pauly, E. (2018). *Meckel's diverticulum.* Retrieved from https://www.uptodate.com/contents/meckels-diverticulum

Johnson, E. (2018). *Pilonidal disease.* Retrieved from https://www.uptodate.com/contents/pilonidal-disease

Keels, M., & Clements, D. (2018). *Herpetic gingivostomatitis in young children.* Retrieved from https://www.uptodate.com/contents/herpetic-gingivostomatitis-in-young-children

Klein, R. (2016). *Clinical manifestations and diagnosis of herpes simplex virus type 1 infection.* Retrieved from https://www.uptodate.com/contents/clinical-manifestations-and-diagnosis-of-herpes-simplex-virus-type-1-infection

Kohn, G. P., et al. (2013). Guidelines for the management of hiatal hernia. *Surgical Endoscopy, 27*(12), 4409–4428.

Law, R., et al. (2014). Zenker's diverticulum. *Clinical Gastroenterology and Hepatology, 12*(11), 1773–1782.

Malfertheiner, P., et al. (2017). Management of Helicobacter pylori infection-the Maastricht V/Florence Consensus Report. *Gut, 66*(1), 6–30.

Martin, R. (2018). *Acute appendicitis in adults: Clinical manifestations and differential diagnosis.* Retrieved from https://www.uptodate.com/contents/acute-appendicitis-in-adults-clinical-manifestations-and-differential-diagnosis

McCance, K., & Huether, S. (2019). *Pathophysiology: The biological basis for disease in adults and children* (8th ed.) St. Louis: Elsevier.

McDonald, L. C., et al. (2018). Clinical practice guidelines for *Clostridium difficile* infection in adults and children: 2017 Update by the Infectious Diseases Society of America (IDSA) and Society for Healthcare Epidemiology of America (SHEA). *Clinical Infectious Diseases, 66*(7), e1–e48.

Menees, S. B., et al. (2015). A meta-analysis of the utility of C-reactive protein, erythrocyte sedimentation rate, fecal calprotectin, and fecal lactoferrin to exclude inflammatory bowel disease in adults with IBS. *American Journal of Gastroenterology, 110*(3), 444–454.

Mulder, C., & van Delft, F. (2017). *Zenker's diverticulum.* Retrieved from https://www.uptodate.com/contents/zenkers-diverticulum

Peery, A. F., et al. (2015). Burden of gastrointestinal, liver, and pancreatic diseases in the United States. *Gastroenterology, 149*(7), 1731–1741.

Pemberton, J. (2017). *Colonic diverticulosis and diverticular disease: Epidemiology, risk factors, and pathogenesis.* Retrieved from https://www.uptodate.com/contents/colonic-diverticulosis-and-diverticular-disease-epidemiology-risk-factors-and-pathogenesis

Peppercorn, M., & Cheifetz, A. (2018). *Definition, epidemiology, and risk factors in inflammatory bowel disease.* Retrieved from https://www.uptodate.com/contents/definition-epidemiology-and-risk-factors-in-inflammatory-bowel-disease

Peppercorn, M., & Kane, S. (2017). *Clinical manifestations, diagnosis, and prognosis of ulcerative colitis in adults.* Retrieved from https://www.uptodate.com/contents/clinical-manifestations-diagnosis-and-prognosis-of-ulcerative-colitis-in-adults

Sartor, R. (2015). *Probiotics for gastrointestinal diseases.* Retrieved from https://www.uptodate.com/contents/probiotics-for-gastrointestinal-diseases

Sfeir, R., et al. (2013). Epidemiology of esophageal atresia. *Diseases of the Esophagus, 26*(4), 354–355.

Stewart, D. (2017). *Anal fissure: Clinical manifestations, diagnosis, prevention.* Retrieved from https://www.uptodate.com/contents/anal-fissure-clinical-manifestations-diagnosis-prevention

Taylor, M. R., & Lalani, N. (2013). Adult small bowel obstruction. *Academic Emergency Medicine, 20*(6), 528–544.

Thangarajah, T., et al. (2018). A review article on gastric volvulus: A challenge to diagnosis and management. *International Journal of Surgery, 8*(1), 18.

University of Chicago. (2013). *Tracheoesophageal fistula.* Retrieved from https://pedclerk.bsd.uchicago.edu/page/tracheoesophageal-fistula

Varma, M., & Steele, S. (2017). *Overview of rectal procidentia (rectal prolapse).* Retrieved from https://www.uptodate.com/contents/overview-of-rectal-procidentia-rectal-prolapse

Vega, S. (2018). *Etiology of acute pancreatitis.* Retrieved from https://www.uptodate.com/contents/etiology-of-acute-pancreatitis

Wee, J. (2018). *Gastric volvulus in adults.* Retrieved from https://www.uptodate.com/contents/gastric-volvulus-in-adults

Wong Kee Song, L., & Marcon, N. (2018). *Neutropenic enterocolitis (typhlitis).* Retrieved from https://www.uptodate.com/contents/neutropenic-enterocolitis-typhlitis

5

HEPATOBILIARY DISORDERS

Introduction

The liver is the largest internal organ in the body, weighing slightly more than 3 lb (1,200 to 1,600 g) in the average adult. It is also one of the busiest, performing well over 100 separate functions. The most important of these are the formation and secretion of bile; detoxification of harmful substances; storage of vitamins; metabolism of carbohydrates, fats, and proteins; and production of plasma proteins. This remarkably resilient organ serves as the body's warehouse and is essential to life.

LOBULAR STRUCTURE

Located above the right kidney, stomach, pancreas, and intestines and immediately below the diaphragm, the liver divides into a left and a right lobe separated by the falciform ligament. The right lobe is six times larger than the left. Glisson's capsule, a network of connective tissue, covers the entire organ and extends into the parenchyma along blood vessels and bile ducts. Within the parenchyma, cylindrical lobules comprise the basic functional units of the liver, consisting of cellular plates that radiate from a central vein, somewhat like spokes in a wheel. Small bile canaliculi fit between the cells in the plates and empty into terminal bile ducts, which join two larger ones that merge into a single hepatic duct upon leaving the liver. The hepatic duct then joins the cystic duct to form the common bile duct.

The liver receives blood from two major sources: the hepatic artery and the portal vein.

The two vessels carry approximately 1,500 mL of blood to the liver per minute, nearly 75% of which is supplied by the portal vein. Sinusoids—offshoots of the hepatic artery and portal vein—run between each row of the hepatic cells. Phagocytic Kupffer's cells, part of the reticuloendothelial system, line the sinusoids, destroying old or defective red blood cells and detoxifying harmful substances. The liver has a large lymphatic supply; consequently, cancer frequently metastasizes there.

LIVER FUNCTION

One of the liver's most important functions is the conversion of bilirubin, a breakdown product of hemoglobin, into bile. Liberated by the spleen into plasma and bound loosely to albumin, bilirubin reaches the liver in an unconjugated (water-insoluble) state. The liver then conjugates or dissociates it, converting it to a water-soluble derivative before excreting it as bile. All hepatic cells continually form bile.

The liver also detoxifies many substances through inactivation or through conjugation. Inactivation involves reduction, oxidation, and hydroxylation. An important liver function is the inactivation of many drugs that are metabolized primarily in the liver. Such drugs must be used with caution in hepatic disease because their effects may be markedly prolonged.

ELDER TIP *In elderly people, the blood supply to the liver decreases, and certain liver enzymes become less active. As a result, the liver loses some of its ability to metabolize drugs, and higher levels of drugs remain in the circulation, causing more intense drug effects. This increases the risk of drug toxicity.*

As still another example of its amazing versatility, the liver forms vitamin A from certain vegetables and stores vitamins K, D, and B$_{12}$. It also stores iron in the form of ferritin.

METABOLIC FUNCTIONS

The liver figures indispensably in the metabolism of the three major food groups: carbohydrates, fats, and proteins. In carbohydrate metabolism, the liver plays one of its most vital roles by extracting excess glucose from the blood and reserving it for times when blood glucose levels fall below normal, when it releases glucose into the circulation, and then replenishes the supply by a process called *glyconeogenesis*. To prevent dangerously low blood glucose levels, the liver can also convert galactose or amino acids into glucose (gluconeogenesis). The liver also forms many critical chemical compounds from the intermediate products of carbohydrate metabolism.

The liver performs more than half the body's preliminary breakdown of fats because liver cells metabolize fats more quickly and efficiently than do other body cells. Liver cells break fats down into glycerol and fatty acids and convert the fatty acids into small molecules that can be oxidized. The liver also produces substantial quantities of cholesterol and phospholipids, manufactures lipoproteins, and synthesizes fat from carbohydrates and proteins to be transported in lipoproteins for eventual storage in adipose tissue.

Like so many of its functions, the liver's role in protein metabolism is essential to life. The liver deaminates amino acids so they can be used for energy or converted into fats or carbohydrates. It forms urea to remove ammonia from body fluids and forms all plasma proteins (as much as 50 to 100 g/day) except gamma globulin. The liver is such an effective synthesizer of protein that it can replenish as much as half its plasma proteins in 4 to 7 days. The liver also synthesizes nonessential amino acids and forms other important chemical compounds from amino acids.

PRODUCTION OF PLASMA PROTEINS

The liver synthesizes most of the body's large molecules of plasma proteins, including all of the albumin, which binds many substances in plasma and maintains colloid osmotic pressure.

Normally, plasma proteins and amino acid levels maintain equilibrium in the blood. When amino acid levels decrease, plasma proteins split into amino acids to restore this equilibrium. Reacting to decreased levels of amino acids, the liver steps up the production of plasma proteins. The liver may synthesize approximately 400 g of protein daily; for this reason, significant liver damage leads to hyperproteinemia, which in turn disrupts the colloid osmotic pressure and amino acid levels.

The liver also produces most of the plasma proteins necessary for blood coagulation, including prothrombin and fibrinogen, which are the most abundant. The liver forms prothrombin in a process dependent on vitamin K and the production of bile. Fibrinogen, a large-molecule protein formed entirely by the liver, is an essential factor in the coagulation cascade.

Together, the plasma proteins maintain colloid osmotic pressure throughout the capillaries. Because the plasma protein molecules are too large to cross the capillary membrane, they concentrate at the capillary line and produce an osmotic pressure of pull. This constant colloid osmotic pressure at the arteriolar and venular sections of the capillary provides the major osmotic force regulating the return of fluid to the intravascular compartment.

Because of their large molecular size, plasma proteins don't easily cross into the interstitial spaces. Their only route for return to the bloodstream is through lymphatic drainage. The lymphatic vessels drain into the lymphatic and thoracic ducts, which drain directly into the superior vena cava.

ASSESSING FOR LIVER DISEASE

In many cases, a careful physical examination and patient history can detect hepatic disease. Watch especially for its cardinal signs: jaundice (a result of increased serum bilirubin levels), ascites (commonly with hemoconcentration, edema, and oliguria), and hepatomegaly. Other signs and symptoms may include right upper quadrant abdominal pain, lassitude, anorexia, nausea, and vomiting. The presence of a palpable left lobe is always pathologic and usually suggestive of chronic liver disease. Another primary sign is portal hypertension (portal vein pressure >6 cm H$_2$O) revealed by the presence of caput medusae (dilated veins seen on the abdomen). Surgical insertion of a catheter into the portal vein allows measurement of portal vein pressure.

ALERT *Carefully assess the patient's neurologic status because neurologic symptoms, such as those associated with hepatic encephalopathy (confusion, muscle tremors, and asterixis), may signal the onset of life-threatening hepatic failure.*

Other common signs of hepatic disease include pallor (commonly linked to cirrhosis or carcinoma), parotid gland enlargement (in alcohol-induced liver damage), Dupuytren's contracture, gynecomastia, testicular atrophy, decreased axillary or pubic hair, bleeding disorders (ecchymosis and purpura), spider angiomas, and palmar erythema.

Careful abdominal palpation and auscultation can also detect hepatocellular carcinoma or metastasis, which turns the liver rock-hard and causes abdominal bruits. In hepatitis, the liver is usually enlarged; palpation may elicit tenderness at the liver's edge. In cirrhosis, the atrophic liver is difficult to palpate. In neoplastic disease or hepatic abscess, auscultation may detect a pleural friction rub.

COMPREHENSIVE HISTORY

ESSENTIAL

Ask if the patient has ever had jaundice, anemia, or a splenectomy. Ask about occupational or other exposure to toxins (carbon tetrachloride, beryllium, or vinyl chloride), which may predispose the patient to hepatic disease. Consider recent travel or contact with persons who have traveled to areas where hepatic disease is endemic.

Make sure to ask about alcohol consumption, a significant factor in suspected hepatic disease. Remember, an alcoholic may deliberately underestimate their alcohol intake, so interview the patient's family as well. Ask about recent contact with a jaundiced person and about any recent blood or plasma transfusions, blood tests, body piercings, tattoos, or dental work. Find out if the patient takes any drugs that may cause liver damage, such as sedatives, tranquilizers, analgesics, and diuretics that cause potassium loss. Ask if the onset of symptoms was abrupt or insidious or if it followed abdominal injury that could have damaged the liver. Ask if the patient bruises or bleeds easily. Check for light or clay-colored stools and dark urine, and ask about any change in bowel habits. Also ask if the patient's weight has fluctuated recently.

LIVER FUNCTION STUDIES

Numerous tests are available to detect hepatic disease. Perhaps the most useful tests are liver function studies, which measure serum enzymes and other substances. Typical findings in hepatic disease include the following:
- Increased bilirubin levels
- Increased alkaline phosphatase and 5′-nucleotidase levels
- Elevated levels of aspartate aminotransferase (AST) and alanine aminotransferase (ALT):

possible hepatocellular damage, viral hepatitis, or acute hepatic necrosis
- Elevated gamma-glutamyltransferase levels: sensitive for alcoholic liver disease
- Hypoalbuminemia: subacute or massive hepatic necrosis or cirrhosis
- Hyperglobulinemia: chronic inflammatory disorders
- Prolonged prothrombin time or partial thromboplastin time: hepatitis or cirrhosis
- Elevated serum ammonia levels: hepatic encephalopathy
- Decreased serum total cholesterol levels: liver disease
- Positive antinuclear antibodies (ANA) test (in chronic active hepatitis and the presence of hepatitis B antigen)

Liver function studies are less reliable after liver trauma. For instance, tests done long after the injury might miss an initial rise in serum AST and ALT levels. Several less specific blood tests for detecting hepatic disease are urine urobilinogen, lactate dehydrogenase, and ornithine carbamoyltransferase.

Other useful diagnostic tests include the following:
- Plain abdominal X-rays may indicate gross hepatomegaly and hepatic masses by elevation or distortion of the diaphragm and may show calcification in the gallbladder, biliary tree, pancreas, and liver.
- Abdominal ultrasounds show fatty infiltration, hepatomegaly, gallbladder inflammation or obstruction, ascites, and cirrhosis. Doppler ultrasound demonstrates blood flow.
- Magnetic resonance imaging shows masses, fatty infiltration, and cirrhosis and its complications.
- Percutaneous transhepatic cholangiography distinguishes mechanical biliary obstruction from intrahepatic cholestasis.
- Angiography demonstrates hepatic arterial circulation (altered in cirrhosis) and helps diagnose primary or secondary hepatic tumor masses.
- Radioisotope liver scans (scintiscans) may show an area of decreased uptake (a "hole") using a colloidal or bengal scan or an area of increased uptake (a "hot spot") using a gallium scan in hepatoma or hepatic abscess.
- Computed tomography (CT) scan produces in-depth, three-dimensional images of the biliary tract (the liver as well as the pancreas) that help distinguish between obstructive and nonobstructive jaundice and also helps identify space-occupying hepatic lesions.
- Portal and hepatic vein manometry localizes obstructions in the extrahepatic portion of

the portal vein and portal inflow system or increased pressure in the presinusoidal vessels.
◆ Percutaneous or transvenous liver biopsy can determine the cause of unexplained hepatomegaly, hepatosplenomegaly, cholestasis, or persistently abnormal liver function tests; it's also useful when systemic infiltrative disease (such as sarcoidosis) or primary or metastatic hepatic tumors are suspected.
◆ Laparoscopy visualizes the serosal lining, liver, gallbladder, spleen, and other organs and is useful in unexplained hepatomegaly, ascites, or an abdominal mass.

GALLBLADDER ANATOMY

The gallbladder is a pear-shaped organ that lies in the fossa on the underside of the liver and is capable of holding 50 mL of bile. Attached to the large organ above by connective tissue, the peritoneum, and blood vessels, the gallbladder is divided into four parts: the fundus, or broad inferior end; the body, which is funnel-shaped and bound to the duodenum; the neck, which empties into the cystic duct; and the infundibulum, which lies between the body and the neck and sags to form Hartmann's pouch. The hepatic artery supplies the cystic and hepatic ducts with blood, which drains out of the gallbladder through the cystic vein. Rich lymph vessels in the submucosal layer also drain the gallbladder as well as the head of the pancreas.

The biliary duct system provides a passage for bile from the liver to the intestine and regulates bile flow. The gallbladder itself collects, concentrates, and stores bile. The normally functioning gallbladder also removes water and electrolytes from hepatic bile, increases the concentration of the larger solutes, and reduces its pH to less than 7. In gallbladder disease, bile becomes more alkaline, altering bile salts and cholesterol and predisposing the organ to stone formation.

MECHANISMS OF CONTRACTION

The gallbladder responds to sympathetic and parasympathetic innervation. Sympathetic stimulation inhibits muscle contraction, mild vagal stimulation causes the gallbladder to contract and the sphincter of Oddi to relax, and stronger stimulation causes the sphincter to contract. The gallbladder also responds to substances released by the intestine. For instance, after chyme (semiliquid, partially digested food) enters the duodenum from the stomach, the duodenum releases cholecystokinin (CCK) and pancreozymin (PCZ) into the bloodstream and stimulates the gallbladder to contract. The gallbladder also produces secretin, which stimulates the liver to secrete bile and CCK-PCZ.

The gallbladder may also respond to some type of hormonal control, a theory based in part on the fact that the gallbladder empties more slowly during pregnancy.

ASSESSING FOR GALLBLADDER DISEASE

During your physical examination of a patient with suspected gallbladder disease, look for its telltale signs and symptoms: pain, jaundice (a result of blockage of the common bile duct), fever, chills, indigestion, nausea, and intolerance of fatty foods. Pain may range from vague discomfort (as when pressure within the common bile duct gradually increases) to deep visceral pain (as when the gallbladder suddenly distends). Abrupt onset of pain with epigastric distress indicates gallbladder inflammation or obstruction of bile outflow by a stone or spasm.

The onset of jaundice also varies. If the gallbladder is healthy, jaundice may be delayed several days after bile duct blockage; if the gallbladder is absent or diseased, jaundice may appear within 24 hours after the blockage. Other effects of obstruction—pruritus, steatorrhea, and bleeding tendencies—may accompany jaundice. Gallbladder disorders rarely cause internal bleeding, but when they do—as in cholecystitis or obstructive clots in the biliary tree from gastrointestinal (GI) bleeding—they can be fatal.

DIAGNOSTIC TESTS

After taking a thorough patient history and carefully assessing the clinical features, the next step in accurate diagnosis of gallbladder disease is to perform diagnostic testing.

Diagnostic tests for gallbladder disease include the following:
◆ Magnetic resonance cholangiopancreatography (MRCP), CT, or ultrasound are used to diagnose gallbladder disease. An MRCP uses magnetic resonance imaging that creates images of the bile and pancreatic ducts. The CT identifies gallstones and pancreatic cancer and is the preferred method for assessing pancreatitis. The ultrasound visualizes the bile ducts, liver, and pancreas. It is less effective in obese patients.
◆ Percutaneous transhepatic cholangiography differentiates extrahepatic from intrahepatic obstructive jaundice and helps detect biliary masses and calculi. Needle insertion in a bile duct permits withdrawal of bile and injection of dye. Fluoroscopic tests evaluate the filling of the hepatic and biliary trees. The test also permits palliative internal or external placement of biliary catheters for free flow of bile.

◆ Endoscopic ultrasound is used to diagnose and stage gallbladder cancer. An endoscope with an ultrasound transducer on the end is passed down into the intestines, where it can visualize the bile ducts, gallbladder, and pancreatic ducts.

◆ In endoscopic retrograde cholangiopancreatography (ERCP), duodenal endoscopy with dye injection and fluoroscopy are used to cannulate and visualize bile ducts and pancreatic ducts. This test is useful in locating obstruction, calculi, carcinoma, or stricture and for obtaining bile or pancreatic juice for analysis. Internal stents can be inserted to allow free flow of bile or pancreatic juice.

◆ A hepatobiliary iminodiacetic acid scan (HIDA) creates pictures of liver, gallbladder, bile duct, and small intestine. It is a nuclear scan, which requires that the patient take nothing by mouth after midnight, the night before the test. A radioactive tracer is administered intravenously and then filmed by the HIDA camera. The test takes approximately 2 hours.

◆ In gallbladder ultrasound, sound waves are used to visualize the gallbladder and locate obstruction, stones, and tumors. This test is 95% accurate in detecting stones.

Other appropriate tests for biliary disease are the same as those for hepatic disease.

Liver disorders

VIRAL HEPATITIS

Viral hepatitis is a fairly common systemic disease, marked by hepatic cell destruction, necrosis, and autolysis, leading to anorexia, jaundice, and hepatomegaly. In most patients, hepatic cells eventually regenerate with little or no residual damage. However, old age and serious underlying disorders make complications more likely. The prognosis is poor if edema and hepatic encephalopathy develop.

Pathophysiology

Hepatitis occurs in these forms:

◆ Type A (infectious or short-incubation hepatitis—15 to 45 days) is an acute-onset infection and most often affects children and young adults. Hepatitis A does not persist and, thus, does not lead to chronic hepatitis.

◆ Type B (serum or long-incubation hepatitis—40 to 150 days) is an insidious-onset infection and affects all age groups. It may be directly cytopathic to hepatocytes. The immune system–mediated cytotoxicity plays a predominant role in causing liver damage. This is driven by human leukocyte antigen class I–restricted CD8 cytotoxic T lymphocytes that recognize

hepatitis B core antigen (HBcAg) and hepatitis B e antigen (HBeAg) on the cell membranes of infected hepatocytes. Routine screening of donor blood for the hepatitis B surface antigen (HBsAg) has decreased the incidence of posttransfusion cases, but transmission by needles shared by drug abusers and sexual transmission remain major problems.

◆ Type C accounts for about 20% of all viral hepatitis cases. Incubation period is generally around 8 weeks. It tends to follow a mild course. With aminotransferase levels rarely higher than 1,000 U/L, approximately 15% to 45% of patients acutely infected with hepatitis C virus lose virologic markers. As much as 55% to 85% of patients remain viremic and could develop chronic liver disease. Most cases are related to injectable drug use.

◆ Type D (delta hepatitis) is responsible for about 50% of all cases of fulminant hepatitis, which has a high mortality. Developing in 1% of patients, fulminant hepatitis causes unremitting liver failure with encephalopathy. It progresses to coma and commonly leads to death within 2 weeks. Type D is uncommon in the United States.

◆ Type E (formerly grouped with type C under the name non-A, non-B hepatitis) has an incubation period of 2 to 10 weeks. This is characterized by fluctuating aminotransferase levels. It occurs primarily among patients who have recently returned from an endemic area (such as India, Africa, Asia, or Central America); it is more common in young adults and more severe in pregnant women.

Causes and incidence

The major forms of viral hepatitis result from infection with the causative viruses: A, B, C, D, or E. (See *Viral hepatitis from A to E,* page 271.)

Type A hepatitis is highly contagious and is usually transmitted by the fecal-oral route. However, it may also be transmitted parenterally, sexually (especially with oral or anal contact), and perinatally. Hepatitis A usually results from ingestion of contaminated food, milk, or water. Many outbreaks of this type are traced to ingestion of seafood from polluted water. In 2008, there were more than 25,000 acute cases of hepatitis A infection reported in the United States.

Type B hepatitis, once thought to be transmitted only by the direct exchange of contaminated blood, is now known to be transmitted also by contact with bodily fluids. As a result, nurses, physicians, laboratory technicians, and dentists are frequently exposed to type B hepatitis, in many cases as a result of wearing defective

Viral hepatitis from A to E

The following chart compares the features of each type of viral hepatitis.

Feature	Hepatitis A	Hepatitis B	Hepatitis C	Hepatitis D	Hepatitis E
Incubation	15 to 45 days	30 to 180 days	15 to 160 days	14 to 64 days	14 to 60 days
Onset	Acute	Insidious	Insidious	Acute	Acute
Age group most affected	Children, young adults	Any age	More common in adults	Any age	Ages 20 to 40
Transmission	Fecal-oral, sexual (especially oral-anal contact), nonpercutaneous (sexual, maternal-neonatal), percutaneous (rare)	Blood-borne; parenteral route, sexual, maternal-neonatal; virus is shed in all body fluids	Blood-borne; parenteral route	Parenteral route; most people infected with hepatitis D are also infected with hepatitis B	Primarily fecal-oral
Severity	Mild	Usually severe	Moderate	Can be severe and lead to fulminant hepatitis	Highly virulent with common progression to fulminant hepatitis and hepatic failure, especially in pregnant patients
Prognosis	Generally good	Worsens with age and debility	Moderate	Fair; worsens in chronic cases; can lead to chronic hepatitis D and chronic liver disease	Good unless pregnant
Progression to chronicity	None	Occasional	10% to 50% of cases	Occasional	None

gloves. Transmission also occurs during intimate sexual contact as well as through perinatal transmission. Hepatitis B may also be transmitted by the parenteral route through equipment that has been contaminated. An estimated 38,000 new cases of hepatitis B virus (HBV) and 3,000 deaths from HBV occurred in the United States in 2008.

Historically, hepatitis C is transmitted through transfused blood from asymptomatic donors. Hepatitis C may be transmitted parenterally through the use of contaminated equipment. Hepatitis C accounted for 18,000 new infections and 12,000 deaths in the United

States in 2008. Most exposures (60%) occur through the use of illicit I.V. drugs. However, sexual transmission is responsible for a small number of cases. Approximately, 3.2 million people in the United States have chronic hepatitis C infection.

Type D hepatitis is found only in patients with an acute or chronic episode of hepatitis B and requires the presence of HBsAg. The type D virus depends on the double-shelled type B virus to replicate. For this reason, type D infection can't outlast a type B infection. About 15 million people are infected with hepatitis D worldwide. It's more common in adults than in children. People with a history of illicit I.V. drug use and people who live in the Mediterranean basin have a higher incidence.

Type E hepatitis is transmitted enterically, much like type A. Because this virus is inconsistently shed in feces, detection is difficult. In the United States, the prevalence of hepatitis E is less than 2%. It is typically found in developing countries that lie near the Equator. Incidence is highest among people in the age group of 15 to 40 years.

Other proposed causative factors, such as non-ABCDE viral hepatitis and type F, are under investigation.

Complications
◆ Chronic active hepatitis (with late hepatitis B or C)
◆ Primary liver cancer (hepatitis B or C)
◆ Pancreatitis
◆ Cirrhosis
◆ Lymphoma
◆ Aplastic anemia
◆ Peripheral neuropathy

Signs and symptoms
Assessment findings are similar for the different types of hepatitis. Typically, signs and symptoms progress in several stages.

In the prodromal (preicteric) stage, the patient typically complains of easy fatigue and anorexia (possibly with mild weight loss), generalized malaise, depression, headache, weakness, arthralgia, myalgia, photophobia, and nausea with vomiting. The patient also may describe changes in senses of taste and smell.

Assessment of the patient's vital signs may reveal a fever of 100° to 102° F (37.8° to 38.9° C). As the prodromal stage ends, usually 1 to 5 days before the onset of the clinical jaundice stage, inspection of urine and stool specimens may reveal dark-colored urine and clay-colored stools.

If the patient has progressed to the clinical jaundice stage, they may report pruritus, abdominal pain or tenderness, and indigestion. Early in this stage, the patient may complain of anorexia; later, the appetite may return. Inspection of the sclerae, mucous membranes, and skin may reveal jaundice, which can last for 1 to 2 weeks. Jaundice indicates that the damaged liver is unable to remove bilirubin from the blood; however, its presence doesn't indicate the severity of the disease. Occasionally, hepatitis occurs without jaundice (anicteric hepatitis).

During the clinical jaundice stage, inspection of the skin may detect rashes, erythematous patches, or urticaria, especially if the patient has hepatitis B or C. Palpation may disclose abdominal tenderness in the right upper quadrant, an enlarged and tender liver, and, in some cases, splenomegaly and cervical adenopathy.

During the recovery (posticteric) stage, most of the patient's symptoms decrease or subside. On palpation, a decrease in liver enlargement may be noted. The recovery phase commonly lasts from 2 to 12 weeks, although sometimes this phase lasts longer in the patient with hepatitis B, C, or E.

Diagnosis
A hepatitis profile, which identifies antibodies specific to the causative virus and establishes the type of hepatitis, is routine in suspected viral hepatitis.
◆ Type A: Detection of an antibody to hepatitis A confirms the diagnosis.
◆ Type B: The presence of HBsAg or hepatitis B IgM antibodies confirms the diagnosis.
◆ Type C: Hepatitis C antibody positively confirms exposure (usually 4 to 10 weeks after exposure). Hepatitis C serum RNA is detectable 2 to 3 weeks after exposure.
◆ Type D: Detection of intrahepatic delta antigens or immunoglobulin antidelta antigens in acute disease (or IgM and IgG in chronic disease) establishes the diagnosis.
◆ Type E: Detection of hepatitis E antigens confirms the diagnosis.

Additional findings from liver function studies support the diagnosis:
◆ Serum aspartate aminotransferase and serum alanine aminotransferase levels are increased in the prodromal stage of acute viral hepatitis.
◆ Serum alkaline phosphatase levels are slightly increased.
◆ Serum bilirubin levels are elevated. Levels may continue to be high late in the disease, especially in severe cases.
◆ Prothrombin time can be prolonged (>3 seconds longer than normal indicates severe liver damage).
◆ White blood cell (WBC) counts commonly reveal transient neutropenia and lymphopenia followed by lymphocytosis.
◆ Liver biopsy is performed if chronic hepatitis is suspected; however, it is performed for acute hepatitis only if the diagnosis is questionable.

Treatment
No specific drug therapy has been developed for hepatitis, with the exception of hepatitis B and hepatitis C. Chronic hepatitis B can be treated with interferon alfa, pegylated interferon, lamivudine, adefovir dipivoxil, telbivudine, and tenofovir. Hepatitis C is treated with pegylated

interferon, ribavirin, Victrelis (boceprevir), Olysio (simeprevir), Sovaldi (sofosbuvir), Harvoni (ledipasvir/sofosbuvir), Zepatier (elbasvir/grazoprevir), and Epclusa (sofosbuvir/velpatasvir). Patients are advised to rest in the early stages of the illness and to combat anorexia by eating small, high-calorie, high-protein meals. (Protein intake should be reduced if signs or symptoms of precoma—lethargy, confusion, and mental changes—develop.) Large meals are usually better tolerated in the morning because many patients experience nausea late in the day.

In acute viral hepatitis, hospitalization usually is required only for the patient with severe symptoms or complications. Parenteral nutrition may be required if the patient experiences persistent vomiting and is unable to maintain oral intake.

Antiemetics may be given 30 minutes before meals to relieve nausea and prevent vomiting; phenothiazines have a cholestatic effect and should be avoided. For severe pruritus, the resin cholestyramine may be given.

Special considerations

Use enteric precautions when caring for patients with type A or E hepatitis. Practice standard precautions for all patients.

◆ Inform visitors about isolation precautions.
◆ Provide rest periods throughout the day. Schedule treatments and tests so that the patient can rest between bouts of activity.
◆ Because inactivity may make the patient anxious, include diversionary activities as part of the daily care regimen. Gradually add activities to the patient's schedule as the patient begins to recover.
◆ Encourage the patient to eat. Don't overload the meal tray or overmedicate the patient because this will diminish the patient's appetite.
◆ Encourage fluids (at least 4 qt [4 L]/day). Encourage the anorectic patient to drink fruit juice. Also offer chipped ice and effervescent soft drinks to maintain hydration without inducing vomiting.
◆ Administer supplemental vitamins and commercial feedings, as ordered. If symptoms are severe and the patient can't tolerate oral intake, provide I.V. therapy and parenteral nutrition, as ordered by the physician.
◆ Record the patient's weight daily, and keep intake and output records. Observe stools for color, consistency, and amount and record the frequency of bowel movements.
◆ Watch for signs of fluid shift, such as weight gain and orthostasis.
◆ Watch for signs of hepatic coma, dehydration, pneumonia, vascular problems, and pressure ulcers.

◆ In fulminant hepatitis, maintain electrolyte balance and a patent airway, prevent infections, and control bleeding. Correct hypoglycemia and other complications while awaiting liver regeneration and repair.
◆ Before discharge, emphasize the importance of having regular medical checkups for at least 1 year. The patient will have an increased risk of developing hepatoma. Warn the patient against using alcohol or over-the-counter drugs during this period. Teach the patient to recognize the signs of a recurrence.
◆ Inform the patient about the availability of support groups for people with all types of hepatitis and provide contact information if he's interested.

⦙⦙⦙⦙⦙ **PREVENTION** *Review the following with your patient to prevent the spread of hepatitis:*
◆ *Stress the importance of thorough and frequent hand washing.*
◆ *Tell the patient not to share food, eating utensils, or toothbrushes.*
◆ *If the patient has hepatitis A or E, warn them not to contaminate food or water with fecal matter, because the disease is transmitted by the fecal-oral route.*
◆ *If the patient has hepatitis B, C, or D explain that transmission occurs through exchange of blood or body fluids that contain blood. While infected, the patient shouldn't donate blood or have sexual contact.*
◆ *Advise the patient to take extra care to avoid cutting himself.*

NONVIRAL HEPATITIS

Nonviral inflammation of the liver is a form of hepatitis that is classified as toxic, drug-induced (idiosyncratic), or autoimmune. Most patients recover from drug-induced hepatitis, although a few develop fulminating hepatitis or cirrhosis.

Causes, incidence, and pathophysiology

Various hepatotoxins—carbon tetrachloride, acetaminophen, trichloroethylene, poisonous mushrooms, and vinyl chloride—can cause the toxic form of this disease. Liver damage usually occurs within 24 to 48 hours after exposure to these agents, depending on the size of the dose or degree of exposure. Alcohol, anoxia, and preexisting liver disease exacerbate the toxic effects of some of these agents.

Drug-induced (idiosyncratic) hepatitis may stem from a hypersensitivity reaction unique to the affected individual, unlike toxic hepatitis, which appears to affect all people indiscriminately. Among the drugs that may cause this type of hepatitis are niacin, halothane, sulfonamides, isoniazid, methyldopa, and phenothiazines (cholestasis-induced hepatitis). Other drugs that have been associated with this form of hepatitis include amoxicillin and clavulanic acid, stains, methotrexate, amiodarone, nonsteroidal anti-inflammatory drugs, and vitamin A. In hypersensitive people, symptoms of hepatic dysfunction may appear at any time during or after exposure to these drugs but usually emerge after 2 to 5 weeks of therapy. Not all adverse drug reactions are toxic. Hormonal contraceptives, for example, may impair liver function and produce jaundice without causing necrosis, fatty infiltration of liver cells, or hypersensitivity.

Autoimmune hepatitis, also known as *lupoid hepatitis*, is a disease in which the body's immune system attacks liver cells, causing them to become inflamed. Researchers think a genetic factor may predispose some people to autoimmune diseases. An environmental agent may trigger the autoimmune response against liver antigens, causing inflammatory liver damage. About 70% of those with autoimmune hepatitis are women, most in the age range of 15 to 40 years. It is usually chronic and can lead to cirrhosis.

Complications
◆ Cirrhosis
◆ Chronic hepatitis
◆ Liver failure

Signs and symptoms
Clinical features of toxic and drug-induced hepatitis vary with the severity of the liver damage and the causative agent. In most patients, signs and symptoms resemble those of viral hepatitis: anorexia, nausea, vomiting, jaundice, dark urine, hepatomegaly, possible abdominal pain (with acute onset and massive necrosis), and clay-colored stools or pruritus with the cholestatic form of hepatitis. Carbon tetrachloride poisoning also produces headache, dizziness, drowsiness, and vasomotor collapse; halothane-related hepatitis produces fever, moderate leukocytosis, and eosinophilia; chlorpromazine toxicity produces abrupt fever, rash, arthralgia, lymphadenopathy, and epigastric or right upper quadrant pain.

Diagnosis
Diagnostic findings include elevations in serum aspartate aminotransferase and alanine aminotransferase, total and direct bilirubin (with cholestasis), alkaline phosphatase, WBC count, and eosinophil count (possible in drug-induced type). To diagnose autoimmune hepatitis, antibodies, including antinuclear antibodies (ANA), anti-smooth muscle antibodies (ASMA/anti-liver-kidney), or liver and kidney microsome antibodies (anti-LKM), will be elevated. Liver biopsy may help identify the underlying pathology, especially infiltration with WBCs and eosinophils. Liver function tests have limited value in distinguishing between nonviral and viral hepatitis.

Treatment
Effective treatment must remove the causative agent by lavage, catharsis, or hyperventilation, depending on the route of exposure. Acetylcysteine (Acetadote) serves as an antidote for toxic hepatitis caused by acetaminophen poisoning but doesn't prevent drug-induced hepatitis caused by other substances. Corticosteroids may be ordered for patients with drug-induced and autoimmune hepatitis. Azathioprine (Imuran), an immunosuppressant, may also be used in conjunction with corticosteroids to treat autoimmune hepatitis.

Special considerations
◆ Monitor laboratory studies and note trends.
◆ Monitor the patient's vital signs and provide support to maintain vital functioning, depending on the severity of symptoms.
◆ Preventive measures should include instructing the patient about the proper use of drugs and the proper handling of cleaning agents and solvents.

CIRRHOSIS AND FIBROSIS
Cirrhosis is a chronic hepatic disease characterized by diffuse destruction and fibrotic regeneration of hepatic cells. As necrotic tissue yields to fibrosis, this disease alters liver structure and normal vasculature, impairs blood and lymph flow, and ultimately causes hepatic insufficiency. The prognosis is better in noncirrhotic forms of hepatic fibrosis, which cause minimal hepatic dysfunction and don't destroy liver cells. (See *Cirrhotic changes in the liver*, page 275.)

Causes and incidence
These clinical types of cirrhosis reflect its diverse etiology:
◆ Portal, nutritional, or alcoholic (Laennec) cirrhosis, the most common type, occurs in 30% to 50% of cirrhotic patients, up to 90% of whom have a history of alcoholism. Liver damage has been associated with malnutrition, especially of dietary protein, and chronic alcohol ingestion. Fibrous tissue forms in portal areas and around central veins.

PATHOPHYSIOLOGY
Cirrhotic changes in the liver

The following illustration shows the nodular changes that occur in cirrhosis.

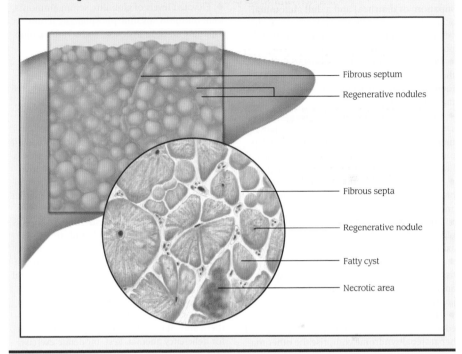

Fibrous septum

Regenerative nodules

Fibrous septa

Regenerative nodule

Fatty cyst

Necrotic area

◆ Biliary cirrhosis (15% to 20% of patients) results from injury or prolonged obstruction.
◆ Postnecrotic (posthepatic) cirrhosis (10% to 30% of patients) stems from various types of hepatitis.
◆ Pigment cirrhosis (5% to 10% of patients) may result from disorders such as hemochromatosis.
◆ Cardiac cirrhosis (rare) refers to cirrhosis caused by right-sided heart failure.
◆ Idiopathic cirrhosis (about 10% of patients) has no known cause.

Noncirrhotic fibrosis may result from schistosomiasis or congenital hepatic fibrosis or may be idiopathic.

Pathophysiology

Growth regulators induce hepatocellular hyperplasia (producing regenerating nodules) and arterial growth (angiogenesis). Among the growth regulators are cytokines and hepatic growth factors (e.g., epithelial growth factor, hepatocyte growth factor, transforming growth factor-alpha, tumor necrosis factor). Insulin, glucagon, and patterns of intrahepatic blood flow determine how and where nodules develop.

Angiogenesis produces new vessels within the fibrous sheath that surrounds nodules. These vessels connect the hepatic artery and portal vein to hepatic venules, restoring the intrahepatic circulatory pathways. Such interconnecting vessels provide relatively low-volume, high-pressure venous drainage that cannot accommodate as much blood volume as normal. As a result, portal vein pressure increases. Such distortions in blood flow contribute to portal hypertension, which increases because the regenerating nodules compress hepatic venules.

Complications

◆ Portal hypertension
◆ Esophageal varices
◆ Hepatic encephalopathy
◆ Hepatorenal syndrome
◆ Ascites
◆ Liver cancer

Signs and symptoms

Clinical manifestations of cirrhosis and fibrosis are similar for all types, regardless of the cause. Early indications are vague, but usually include GI signs and symptoms (anorexia, indigestion, nausea, vomiting, cachexia, constipation, or diarrhea) and a dull abdominal ache. Major and late signs and symptoms develop as a result of hepatic insufficiency and portal hypertension:

♦ Respiratory—pleural effusion and limited thoracic expansion due to abdominal ascites, interfering with efficient gas exchange and leading to hypoxia

♦ Central nervous system—progressive signs or symptoms of hepatic encephalopathy—lethargy, mental changes, slurred speech, asterixis (flapping tremor), peripheral neuritis, paranoia, hallucinations, extreme obtundation, and coma

♦ Hematologic—bleeding tendencies (nosebleeds, easy bruising, and bleeding gums) and anemia

♦ Endocrine—testicular atrophy, menstrual irregularities, gynecomastia, and loss of chest and axillary hair

♦ Skin—severe pruritus, extreme dryness, poor tissue turgor, abnormal pigmentation, spider angiomas, palmar erythema, and possibly jaundice

♦ Hepatic—jaundice, hepatomegaly, ascites, edema of the legs, hepatic encephalopathy, and hepatorenal syndrome comprise the other major effects of full-fledged cirrhosis

♦ Miscellaneous—musty breath, enlarged superficial abdominal veins, muscle atrophy, pain in the right upper abdominal quadrant that worsens when the patient sits up or leans forward, palpable liver or spleen, and temperature of 101° to 103° F (38.3° to 39.4° C). Bleeding from esophageal varices results from portal hypertension.

Diagnosis

℞ CONFIRMING DIAGNOSIS *Liver biopsy, the definitive test for cirrhosis, detects destruction and fibrosis of hepatic tissue.*

Liver imaging, including CT scan, ultrasound, and magnetic resonance imaging, may confirm the diagnosis of cirrhosis through visualization of masses, abnormal growths, metastases, and venous malformations. Liver scan shows abnormal thickening and a liver mass. Cholecystography and cholangiography visualize the gallbladder and the biliary duct system, respectively; splenoportal venography visualizes the portal venous system. Percutaneous transhepatic cholangiography differentiates extrahepatic from intrahepatic obstructive jaundice and discloses hepatic pathology and the presence of gallstones.

Laboratory findings that are characteristic of cirrhosis include the following:

♦ Decreased WBC count, hemoglobin level and hematocrit, albumin, or platelets

♦ Elevated levels of globulin, serum ammonia, total bilirubin, alkaline phosphatase, serum aspartate aminotransferase, and serum alanine aminotransferase

♦ Prolonged prothrombin and partial thromboplastin times

♦ Deficiencies of folic acid, iron, and vitamins A, B_{12}, C, and K are common.

Treatment

Treatment is designed to remove or alleviate the underlying cause of cirrhosis or fibrosis, prevent further liver damage, and prevent or treat complications. The patient may benefit from a high-calorie and moderate- to high-protein diet. Developing hepatic encephalopathy mandates restricted protein intake. In addition, sodium is usually restricted 2 g/day and fluids to 1 to 1½ qt (about 1 to 1.5 L)/day.

If the patient's condition deteriorates, the patient may need tube feedings or total parenteral nutrition. the patient also may need supplemental vitamins—A, B complex, D, and K—to compensate for the liver's inability to store them and vitamin B_{12}, folic acid, and thiamine for deficiency anemia. Rest, moderate exercise, and avoidance of infections and toxic agents are essential.

Drug therapy requires special caution because the cirrhotic liver can't detoxify harmful substances efficiently. If required, octreotide may be prescribed for esophageal varices, and diuretics may be given for edema. However, diuretics require careful monitoring because fluid and electrolyte imbalance may precipitate hepatic encephalopathy. Encephalopathy is treated with lactulose. Antibiotics are used to decrease intestinal bacteria and reduce ammonia production, which is one of the causes of encephalopathy. Coagulopathy may be treated with blood products or vitamin K.

Paracentesis and infusions of salt-poor albumin, in addition to fluid and salt restriction, may alleviate ascites. Surgical procedures include treatment of varices by upper endoscopy with banding or the TIPS (transjugular intrahepatic portosystemic shunt) procedure to relieve portal hypertension. (See *Understanding portal hypertension and esophageal varices*, page 277, and *Circulation in portal hypertension*, page 278.)

Low-protein diets are controversial. They aid in managing acute hepatic encephalopathy

Understanding portal hypertension and esophageal varices

Portal hypertension—elevated pressure in the portal vein—occurs when blood flow meets increased resistance. The disorder is a common result of cirrhosis, but may also stem from mechanical obstruction and occlusion of the hepatic veins (Budd–Chiari syndrome) or portal vein. As portal pressure rises, blood backs up into the spleen and flows through collateral channels to the venous system, bypassing the liver. Consequently, portal hypertension produces splenomegaly with thrombocytopenia, dilated collateral veins (esophageal varices, hemorrhoids, or prominent abdominal veins), and ascites. In many patients, the first sign of portal hypertension is bleeding from esophageal varices—dilated tortuous veins in the submucosa of the lower esophagus. Bleeding esophageal varices commonly cause massive hematemesis, requiring emergency treatment to control hemorrhage and prevent hypovolemic shock.

Diagnosis and treatment

These procedures help diagnose and correct esophageal varices.

♦ Endoscopy identifies the ruptured varix as the bleeding site, excludes other potential sources in the upper gastrointestinal (GI) tract, and allows for banding ligation of actively bleeding varices.

♦ Angiography may aid diagnosis, but is less precise than endoscopy.

♦ Vasopressin infused into the superior mesenteric artery may temporarily stop bleeding. When angiography is unavailable, vasopressin may be infused by I.V. drip or diluted with 5% dextrose in water (except in patients with coronary vascular disease), but this route is usually less effective.

♦ Octreotide is administered intravenously to slow the blood flow into the portal vein and decreases portal hypertension. It is used in combination with endoscopic therapy to treat bleeding esophageal varices. Octreotide is currently used more frequently than vasopressin.

♦ A Sengstaken–Blakemore or Minnesota tube may also help control hemorrhage by applying pressure on the bleeding site. Iced saline lavage through the tube may help control bleeding.

The use of vasopressin or octreotide or a Minnesota or Sengstaken–Blakemore tube is a temporary measure, especially in the patient with a severely deteriorated liver. Fresh blood and fresh frozen plasma, if available, are preferred for blood transfusions to replace clotting factors. Treatment with lactulose promotes elimination of old blood from the GI tract, which combats excessive ammonia production and accumulation.

An appropriate bypass procedure is the transjugular intrahepatic portosystemic shunt (TIPS), which creates an artificial path for the blood traveling from the intestines, through the liver, and back to the heart. The procedure is done in the interventional radiology department. A tube is placed between the portal vein and the hepatic vein, causing the blood to bypass a portion of the liver and to be shunted to the heart. This reduces portal vein pressure and the hypertension complications of recurrent variceal bleeding and ascites. TIPS is an effective therapeutic measure to reduce portal hypertension. The TIPS procedure provides a salvage therapy for those patients who have failed medical treatment and may be used as a bridge for patients awaiting transplant. A complication of the TIPS procedure is encephalopathy, which may occur as a result of the shunted blood bypassing the liver and being sent into the systemic circulation without being detoxified by the liver.

Patient care

Care for the patient who has portal hypertension with esophageal varices focuses on careful monitoring for signs and symptoms of hemorrhage and subsequent hypotension, compromised oxygen supply, and altered level of consciousness (LOC).

♦ Monitor the patient's vital signs, urine output, and central venous pressure to determine fluid volume status.

♦ Assess the patient's LOC often.

♦ Provide emotional support and reassurance after massive GI bleeding, which is always frightening.

♦ Keep the patient as quiet and comfortable as possible, but remember that tolerance of sedatives and tranquilizers may be decreased because of liver damage.

♦ Clean the patient's mouth, which may be dry and flecked with dried blood.

♦ Carefully monitor the patient with a Minnesota or Sengstaken–Blakemore tube in place for persistent bleeding in gastric drainage, signs of asphyxiation from tube displacement, proper inflation of balloons, and correct traction to maintain tube placement.

PATHOPHYSIOLOGY
Circulation in portal hypertension

As portal vein pressure rises, blood backs up into the spleen and flows through collateral channels to the venous system, bypassing the liver and resulting in esophageal varices.

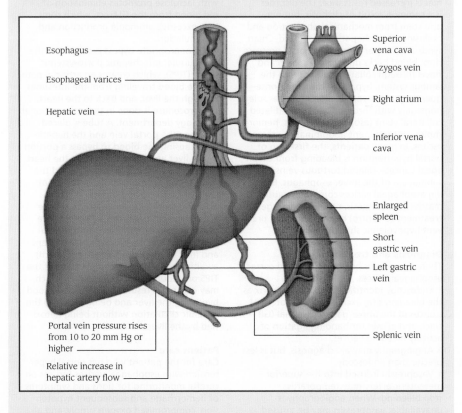

Esophagus

Esophageal varices

Hepatic vein

Superior vena cava

Azygos vein

Right atrium

Inferior vena cava

Enlarged spleen

Short gastric vein

Left gastric vein

Portal vein pressure rises from 10 to 20 mm Hg or higher

Relative increase in hepatic artery flow

Splenic vein

---

but are rarely necessary in chronic conditions because of the underlying protein-calorie malnutrition.

> **ALERT** *If cirrhosis progresses and becomes life-threatening, a liver transplant should be considered.*

Special considerations

The patient with cirrhosis needs close observation, first-rate supportive care, and sound nutritional counseling.

◆ Check the patient's skin, gums, stools, and vomitus regularly for bleeding. Apply pressure to injection sites to prevent bleeding. Warn the patient against taking nonsteroidal anti-inflammatory drugs, straining at stool, and blowing the nose or sneezing too vigorously. Suggest using an electric razor and soft toothbrush.

> **ALERT** *Observe the patient closely for changes in behavior or personality. Report increasing stupor, lethargy, hallucinations, or neuromuscular dysfunction. Awaken the patient periodically to determine their level of consciousness. Watch for asterixis, a sign of developing hepatic encephalopathy.*

◆ To assess fluid retention, weigh the patient and measure abdominal girth at least daily, inspect ankles and sacrum for dependent edema, and accurately record intake and output. Carefully evaluate the patient before, during, and after paracentesis.

◆ To prevent skin breakdown associated with edema and pruritus, avoid using soap when you bathe the patient; instead, use lubricating lotion or moisturizing agents. Handle the patient gently, and turn and reposition often to keep skin intact.

◆ Tell the patient that rest and good nutrition will conserve energy and decrease metabolic demands on the liver. Urge the patient to eat frequent, small meals. Stress the need to avoid infections and abstain from alcohol. Refer the patient to Alcoholics Anonymous, if necessary.

LIVER ABSCESS

A liver abscess occurs when bacteria or protozoa destroy hepatic tissue, producing a cavity, which fills with infectious organisms, liquefied liver cells, and leukocytes. Necrotic tissue then walls off the cavity from the rest of the liver.

Although liver abscess is relatively uncommon, it carries a mortality of 10% to 30%. Complications include rupture into the peritoneum, pleura, or pericardium, as well as sepsis and multi-organ failure, significantly increasing mortality.

Causes and incidence

In pyogenic liver abscesses, the common infecting organisms are *Escherichia coli*, *Klebsiella*, *Staphylococcus*, *Streptococcus*, *Bacteroides*, and enterococcus.

An amebic abscess results from infection with a protozoa.

There are 8 to 16 cases of liver abscess for every 100,000 people hospitalized, and the mortality rate is 5% to 30%. Most cases occur in people in their 60s and 70s.

Pathophysiology

In pyogenic liver abscess, the infecting organisms may invade the liver directly after a liver wound, or they may spread from the lungs, skin, or other organs by the hepatic artery, portal vein, or biliary tract. Biliary tract disease is the most common form. Obstruction of bile allows for bacterial growth. Pyogenic abscesses are generally multiple and can follow cholecystitis, peritonitis, pneumonia, appendicitis, and bacterial endocarditis.

An amebic abscess results from infection with the protozoa *Entamoeba histolytica*, the organism that causes amebic dysentery. Amebic liver abscesses usually occur singly, in the right lobe.

Complication

◆ Abscess rupture into pleura, peritoneum, or pericardium

Signs and symptoms

The clinical manifestations of a liver abscess depend on the degree of involvement. Some patients are acutely ill; in others, the abscess is

recognized only at autopsy, after death from another illness. The onset of symptoms of a pyogenic abscess is usually sudden; in an amebic abscess, the onset is more insidious. Common signs and symptoms include right abdominal and shoulder pain, weight loss, fever, chills, diaphoresis, nausea, vomiting, and anemia. Signs of right pleural effusion, such as dyspnea and pleural pain, develop if the abscess extends through the diaphragm. Liver damage may cause jaundice.

Diagnosis

℞ CONFIRMING DIAGNOSIS *Ultrasound and computed tomography (CT) scan with contrast medium can accurately define intrahepatic lesions and assess intra-abdominal pathology. Percutaneous needle aspiration and drainage of the abscess can be performed using ultrasound or CT guidance to identify the causative organism.*

Relevant laboratory values include elevated serum aspartate aminotransferase, alanine aminotransferase, alkaline phosphatase, and bilirubin levels; increased WBC count; and decreased serum albumin levels. A blood culture can identify the bacterial agent; in amebic abscess, a stool culture and serologic and hemagglutination tests can assist in diagnosis.

Treatment

If the organism causing the liver abscess is unknown, long-term antibiotic therapy begins immediately. When culture results are obtained, antibiotics are prescribed specific to treat the organism. I.V. antibiotic therapy usually continues for 14 days and then is replaced with an oral preparation to complete a 6-week course. Surgery is usually avoided, but it may be done for a single pyogenic abscess or for an amebic abscess that fails to respond to antibiotics. Placement of drains (using CT or ultrasound guidance), particularly in large abscesses, reduces the need for abdominal surgery. In acutely toxic patients, percutaneous needle aspiration and decompression may be needed to remove the abscess.

Special considerations

◆ Provide supportive care, monitor the patient's vital signs (especially temperature), and maintain fluid and nutritional intake.
◆ Administer anti-infectives and antibiotics as ordered, and watch for possible adverse effects. Stress the importance of compliance with therapy.
◆ Explain diagnostic and surgical procedures.
◆ Watch carefully for complications of abdominal surgery, such as hemorrhage or sepsis.

FATTY LIVER

Fatty liver, also known as *steatosis* or *nonalcoholic steatohepatitis (NAFLD)*, is a common clinical finding consisting of accumulated triglycerides and other fats in liver cells. In severe fatty liver, fat comprises as much as 40% of the liver's weight (as opposed to 5% in a normal liver), and the weight of the liver may increase from 3.31 lb (1.5 kg) to as much as 11 lb (4.9 kg). Minimal fatty changes are temporary and as-ymptomatic; severe or persistent changes may cause liver dysfunction. Fatty liver is reversible by simply eliminating the cause.

Causes and incidence

Chronic alcoholism is the most common cause of fatty liver in the United States and in Europe, with the severity of hepatic disease directly related to the amount of alcohol consumed. (Fatty liver can occur in people who consume as little as 10 oz of alcohol per week.)

Other causes of nonalcoholic steatohepatitis include malnutrition (especially protein deficiency), obesity, diabetes mellitus, jejunoileal bypass surgery, Cushing syndrome, Reye syndrome, pregnancy, large doses of hepatotoxins such as I.V. tetracycline, carbon tetrachloride intoxication, prolonged parenteral nutrition, and DDT poisoning. Whatever the cause, fatty infiltration of the liver probably results from mobilization of fatty acids from adipose tissues or altered fat metabolism.

Pathophysiology

Steatosis, the earliest response of the liver to alcohol abuse, is characterized by the accumulation of fat (mainly triglycerides, phospholipids, and cholesterol esters) in hepatocytes. Early studies indicated that alcohol consumption increases the ratio of reduced nicotinamide adenine dinucleotide/oxidized nicotinamide adenine dinucleotide in hepatocytes, which disrupts mitochondrial beta-oxidation of fatty acids and results in steatosis. Alcohol intake has also been shown to augment the supply of lipids to the liver from the small intestine, increasing mobilization of fatty acids from adipose tissue and uptake of fatty acids by the liver.

Nonalcoholic steatohepatitis mechanism is complex and incompletely understood; a two-hit hypothesis has been proposed, in which the first hit involves an imbalance of fatty acid metabolism that leads to hepatic triglyceride accumulation (steatosis). The second hit may be oxidative or metabolic stress and dysregulated cytokine production resulting from efforts to compensate for altered lipid homeostasis, leading to

subsequent inflammation and fibrosis. Data show that hepatic mitochondrial dysfunction is crucial to the pathogenesis of NAFLD.

Complications
◆ Cirrhosis
◆ Portal hypertension
◆ Metabolic disturbances and insulin assistance
◆ Renal failure
◆ Coma

Signs and symptoms

Clinical features of fatty liver vary with the degree of lipid infiltration, and many patients are asymptomatic. The most typical sign is a large, tender liver (hepatomegaly). Common signs and symptoms include right upper quadrant pain (with massive or rapid infiltration), ascites, edema, jaundice, and fever (all with hepatic necrosis or biliary stasis). (See *Signs of liver failure*, page 281.) Nausea, vomiting, and anorexia are less common. Splenomegaly frequently accompanies cirrhosis. Rarer changes are spider angiomas, varices, transient gynecomastia, and menstrual disorders.

Diagnosis

Typical clinical features—especially in patients with chronic alcoholism, malnutrition, poorly controlled diabetes mellitus, or obesity—suggest fatty liver.

 CONFIRMING DIAGNOSIS *A liver biopsy confirms excessive fat in the liver. These liver function tests support this diagnosis:*
◆ *Albumin—somewhat low*
◆ *Globulin—usually elevated*
◆ *Cholesterol—usually elevated*
◆ *Total bilirubin—elevated*
◆ *Alkaline phosphatase—elevated*
◆ *Transaminase—elevated*
◆ *Prothrombin time—possibly prolonged.*

Other findings may include anemia, leukocytosis, elevated WBC count, albuminuria, hyperglycemia or hypoglycemia, and iron, folic acid, and vitamin B_{12} deficiencies.

Treatment

Treatment of fatty liver is essentially supportive and consists of correcting the underlying condition or eliminating its cause. For instance, when fatty liver results from parenteral nutrition, decreasing the rate of carbohydrate infusion may correct the disease. In alcoholic fatty liver, abstinence from alcohol and a proper diet can begin to correct liver changes within 4 to 8 weeks. In nonalcoholic fatty liver disease, gradual weight loss is the standard treatment.

Signs of liver failure

Liver failure may be a complication of hepatitis, cirrhosis, and fatty liver. The signs of liver failure may be visible in many areas of the body.

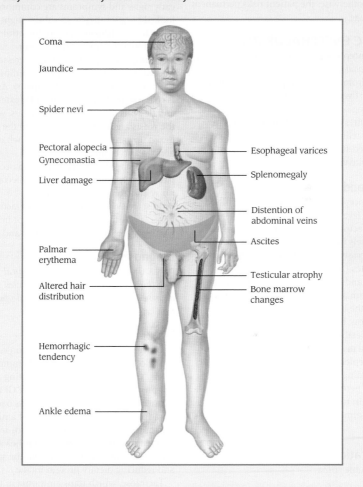

Coma

Jaundice

Spider nevi

Pectoral alopecia
Gynecomastia

Liver damage

Palmar erythema

Altered hair distribution

Hemorrhagic tendency

Ankle edema

Esophageal varices

Splenomegaly

Distention of abdominal veins

Ascites

Testicular atrophy

Bone marrow changes

Special considerations

Providing support to the patient and family is an important element in the care of the patient with steatosis.

◆ Suggest counseling for the alcoholic patient and provide emotional support for the family.

◆ Teach the patient with diabetes—and family—about proper care, such as the purpose of insulin injections, diet, and exercise. Refer the patient to home health nurses or to group classes, as necessary, to promote compliance with treatment. Emphasize the need for long-term medical supervision and urge the patient to report any changes in health immediately.

◆ Instruct an obese patient and their family about proper diet. Warn against fad diets, which are usually nutritionally inadequate. Recommend medical supervision for a patient who's more than 20% overweight. Encourage attendance at group diet and exercise programs and, if necessary, suggest behavior modification programs to correct eating habits. Be sure to follow up on the patient's progress and provide positive reinforcement for any weight loss.

◆ Assess for malnutrition, especially protein deficiency, in the patient with chronic illness. Suggest dietary changes and refer the patient to a dietitian.

♦ Advise patients receiving hepatotoxins and those at risk for occupational exposure to watch for and immediately report signs of toxicity.
♦ Inform the patient that fatty liver is reversible *only* if they strictly follow the therapeutic program; otherwise, the patient risks permanent liver damage.

HEPATIC ENCEPHALOPATHY

Hepatic encephalopathy, also known as *portosystemic encephalopathy* or *hepatic coma*, is a neurologic syndrome that develops as a complication of chronic liver disease. It may be acute and self-limiting or chronic and progressive. Treatment requires correction of the precipitating cause and reduction of blood ammonia levels. In advanced stages, the prognosis is extremely poor despite vigorous treatment.

Causes and incidence

Hepatic encephalopathy follows rising blood ammonia levels.

Other factors that predispose to rising ammonia levels include excessive protein intake, sepsis, excessive accumulation of nitrogenous body wastes (from constipation or GI hemorrhage), and bacterial action on protein and urea to form ammonia. Certain other factors heighten the brain's sensitivity to ammonia intoxication: hypoxia, azotemia, impaired glucose metabolism, infection, and administration of sedatives, narcotics, and general anesthetics. Depletion of the intravascular volume, from bleeding or diuresis, reduces hepatic and renal perfusion and leads to contraction alkalosis. In turn, hypokalemia and alkalosis increase ammonia production and impair its excretion.

Complication

♦ Irreversible coma
♦ Death

Pathophysiology

Most common in patients with cirrhosis, this syndrome is due primarily to ammonia intoxication of the brain. Normally, the ammonia produced by protein breakdown in the bowel is metabolized to urea in the liver. When portal blood shunts past the liver, ammonia directly enters the systemic circulation and is carried to the brain. Such shunting may result from the collateral venous circulation that develops in portal hypertension or from surgically created portosystemic shunts (such as a TIPS). Cirrhosis further compounds this problem because impaired hepatocellular function prevents conversion of ammonia that reaches the liver.

Signs and symptoms

Clinical manifestations of hepatic encephalopathy vary (depending on the severity of neurologic involvement) and develop in four stages:
♦ In stage I (minimal hepatic encephalopathy), early signs and symptoms are commonly overlooked because they're so subtle: slight personality changes (disorientation, forgetfulness, and slurred speech) and a slight tremor.
♦ During the stage II, tremor progresses into asterixis (liver flap and flapping tremor), the hallmark of hepatic encephalopathy. Asterixis is characterized by quick, irregular extensions and flexions of the wrists and fingers, when the wrists are held out straight and the hands flexed upward. Lethargy, aberrant behavior, and apraxia also occur.
♦ At the stage III, hyperventilation occurs; the patient is typically stuporous, but becomes noisy and abusive when aroused.
♦ In stage IV, the patient has hyperactive reflexes, a positive Babinski sign, fetor hepaticus (musty, sweet odor to the breath), and coma.

Diagnosis

℞ **CONFIRMING DIAGNOSIS** *Clinical features, a history of liver disease, and elevated serum ammonia levels in venous and arterial samples confirm hepatic encephalopathy.*

Treatment

Effective treatment stops progression of encephalopathy by reducing blood ammonia levels. Treatment includes eliminating ammonia-producing substances from the GI tract by administering rifaximin to suppress bacterial flora (preventing the conversion of amino acids into ammonia), performing sorbitol-induced catharsis to produce osmotic diarrhea and continuous aspiration of blood from the stomach, and reducing dietary protein intake.

Lactulose, which traps ammonia in the bowel and promotes its excretion, is administered to reduce blood ammonia levels. Bacterial enzymes change lactulose to lactic acid, thereby rendering the colon too acidic for bacterial growth. At the same time, the resulting increase in free hydrogen ions prevents diffusion of ammonia through the mucosa; lactulose promotes conversion of systemically absorbable ammonia to ammonium, which is poorly absorbed and can be excreted. It is usually given orally. However, if the patient is in a coma, it may be administered by retention enema.

Treatment may also include potassium supplements to correct alkalosis due to increased ammonia levels, especially if the patient is taking diuretics. Hemodialysis may sometimes be used to clear toxic blood temporarily. Salt-poor albumin may be used to maintain fluid and electrolyte balance, replace depleted albumin levels, and restore plasma. Sedatives, tranquilizers, and other medications metabolized or excreted by the liver should be avoided if possible. Medications containing ammonium (including certain antacids) should also be avoided.

Special considerations
Patient care includes monitoring symptoms and support.
◆ Assess and record the patient's level of consciousness frequently. Continually orient the patient to place and time. Keep a daily record of the patient's handwriting to monitor the progression of neurologic involvement.
◆ Monitor the patient's intake, output, and fluid and electrolyte balance. Check daily weight and measure abdominal girth. Watch for, and immediately report, signs of anemia (decreased hemoglobin level), infection, alkalosis (increased serum bicarbonate), and GI bleeding (melena and hematemesis).
◆ If the encephalopathy is acute, ask the dietary department to provide the specified low-protein diet, with carbohydrates supplying most of the calories.
◆ Promote rest, comfort, and a quiet atmosphere. Prevent falls.
◆ Use restraints, if necessary, but avoid sedatives. Protect the comatose patient's eyes from corneal injury by using artificial tears or eye patches.
◆ Provide emotional support for the patient's family in the terminal stage of encephalopathy.

Gallbladder and duct disorders

CHOLELITHIASIS AND RELATED DISORDERS
Diseases of the gallbladder and biliary tract are common and, in many cases, painful conditions that frequently require surgery and may be life-threatening. They are generally associated with deposition of calculi and inflammation. (See *Understanding gallstone formation*, page 284.)

Causes and incidence
Cholelithiasis, stones or calculi (gallstones) in the gallbladder, results from changes in bile components. Gallstones are made of cholesterol, calcium bilirubinate, or a mixture of cholesterol and bilirubin pigment. They arise during periods of sluggishness in the gallbladder due to pregnancy, hormonal contraceptives,

diabetes mellitus, celiac disease, cirrhosis of the liver, and pancreatitis. Cholelithiasis is a common health problem, affecting about 50% of white women and 30% of white men. The prognosis is usually good with treatment unless infection occurs, in which case the prognosis depends on its severity and response to antibiotics.

One out of every 10 patients with gallstones develops *choledocholithiasis*, or gallstones in the common bile duct (sometimes called *common duct stones*). This occurs when stones passed out of the gallbladder lodge in the hepatic and common bile ducts and obstruct the flow of bile into the duodenum. Prognosis is good unless infection occurs.

Cholangitis, infection of the bile duct, is commonly associated with choledocholithiasis and may follow percutaneous transhepatic cholangiography or occlusion of endoscopic stents. Predisposing factors may include bacterial or metabolic alteration of bile acids. Widespread inflammation may cause fibrosis and stenosis of the common bile duct. The prognosis for this condition is poor without stenting or surgery.

Cholecystitis, acute or chronic inflammation of the gallbladder, is usually associated with a gallstone impacted in the cystic duct, causing painful distention of the gallbladder. Cholecystitis accounts for most patients requiring gallbladder surgery. The acute form is most common during middle age; the chronic form usually occurs among elderly patients. The prognosis is good with treatment.

Biliary cirrhosis is a disorder whose primary cause is unknown. This condition usually leads to obstructive jaundice and involves the portal and periportal spaces of the liver. It is nine times more common among women 40 to 60 years old than among men. The prognosis is poor without liver transplantation.

Gallstone ileus results from a gallstone lodging at the terminal ileum; it's more common in the elderly. The prognosis is good with surgery.

Postcholecystectomy syndrome is the presence of GI symptoms after cholecystectomy. It occurs in 10% to 15% of all patients whose gallbladders have been surgically removed and may produce right upper quadrant abdominal pain, biliary colic, fatty food intolerance, dyspepsia, and indigestion. The prognosis is good with selected radiologic procedures, endoscopic procedures, or surgery.

Acalculous cholecystitis is more common in critically ill patients, accounting for about 5% of cholecystitis cases. It may result from primary infection with such organisms as *Salmonella typhi*, *E. coli*, or *Clostridium* or from obstruction

PATHOPHYSIOLOGY
Understanding gallstone formation

Abnormal metabolism of cholesterol and bile salts plays an important role in gallstone formation. Bile is made continuously by the liver and is concentrated and stored in the gallbladder until the duodenum needs it to help digest fat. Changes in the composition of bile may allow gallstones to form. Changes to the absorptive ability of the gallbladder lining may also contribute to gallstone formation.

Too much cholesterol

Certain conditions, such as age, obesity, and estrogen imbalance, cause the liver to secrete bile that's abnormally high in cholesterol or lacking the proper concentration of bile salts.

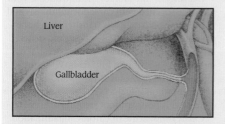

Jaundice, irritation, inflammation

If a stone lodges in the common bile duct, the bile flow into the duodenum becomes obstructed. Bilirubin is absorbed into the blood, causing jaundice.

Biliary narrowing and swelling of the tissue around the stone can also cause irritation and inflammation of the common bile duct.

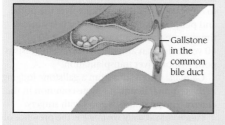

Inside the gallbladder

When the gallbladder concentrates this bile, inflammation may occur. Excessive water and bile salts are reabsorbed, making the bile less soluble. Cholesterol, calcium, and bilirubin precipitate into gallstones.

Fat entering the duodenum causes the intestinal mucosa to secrete the hormone cholecystokinin, which stimulates the gallbladder to contract and empty. If a stone lodges in the cystic duct, the gallbladder contracts but can't empty.

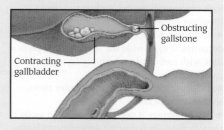

Up the biliary tree

Inflammation can progress up the biliary tree and cause infection of any of the bile ducts. This causes scar tissue, fluid accumulation, cirrhosis, portal hypertension, and bleeding.

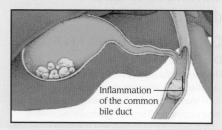

---

of the cystic duct due to lymphadenopathy or a tumor. It appears that ischemia, usually related to a low cardiac output, also has a role in the pathophysiology of this disease. Signs and symptoms of acalculous cholecystitis include unexplained sepsis, right upper quadrant pain, fever, leukocytosis, and a palpable gallbladder.

Each of these disorders produces its own set of complications. Cholelithiasis may lead to any of the disorders associated with gallstone formation: cholangitis, cholecystitis, choledocholithiasis, and gallstone ileus. Cholecystitis can progress to gallbladder complications, such as empyema, hydrops or mucocele, or gangrene.

Gangrene may lead to perforation, resulting in peritonitis, fistula formation, pancreatitis, limy bile, and porcelain gallbladder. Other complications include chronic cholecystitis and cholangitis.

Choledocholithiasis may lead to cholangitis, obstructive jaundice, pancreatitis, and secondary biliary cirrhosis. Cholangitis, especially in the suppurative form, may progress to septic shock and death. Gallstone ileus may cause bowel obstruction, which can lead to intestinal perforation, peritonitis, septicemia, secondary infection, and septic shock.

In most cases, gallbladder and bile duct diseases occur in people who are older than 40 years; they are more prevalent in women and Native Americans.

Complications

Each of these disorders produces a set of complications.

◆ Cholelithiasis may lead to any of the disorders associated with gallstone formation: cholangitis, cholecystitis, choledocholithiasis, and gallstone ileus.

◆ Cholecystitis can progress to gallbladder complications, such as empyema, hydrops or mucocele, and gangrene. Gangrene may lead to perforation, resulting in peritonitis, fistula formation, pancreatitis, limy bile syndrome, and porcelain gallbladder. Other complications include chronic cholecystitis and cholangitis.

◆ Cholecholithiasis may lead to cholangitis, obstructive jaundice, pancreatitis, and secondary biliary cirrhosis.

◆ Cholangitis may progress to septic shock and death, especially in the suppurative form.

◆ Gallstone ileus may cause bowel obstruction, which can lead to intestinal perforation, peritonitis, septicemia, secondary infection, and septic shock.

Signs and symptoms

Although gallbladder disease may produce no symptoms, acute cholelithiasis, acute cholecystitis, and choledocholithiasis produce the symptoms of a classic gallbladder attack. Attacks usually follow meals rich in fats or may occur at night, suddenly awakening the patient. They begin with acute abdominal pain in the right upper quadrant that may radiate to the back, between the shoulders, or to the front of the chest; the pain may be so severe that the patient seeks emergency department care. Other features may include recurring fat intolerance, biliary colic, belching, flatulence, indigestion, diaphoresis, nausea, vomiting, chills, low-grade fever, jaundice (if a stone obstructs the common

bile duct), and clay-colored stools (with choledocholithiasis).

Clinical features of cholangitis include a rise in neutrophils, jaundice, right upper quadrant abdominal pain, high fever, and chills; biliary cirrhosis may produce jaundice, related itching, weakness, fatigue, slight weight loss, and abdominal pain. Gallstone ileus produces signs and symptoms of small-bowel obstruction—nausea, vomiting, abdominal distention, and absent bowel sounds if the bowel is completely obstructed. Its most telling symptom is intermittent recurrence of colicky pain over several days.

Diagnosis

Ultrasonography detects gallstones. Other tests may include the following:

◆ Abdominal CT scan may detect stones in the gallbladder.

◆ Percutaneous transhepatic cholangiography, done under fluoroscopic control, distinguishes between gallbladder or bile duct disease and cancer of the pancreatic head in patients with jaundice.

◆ ERCP visualizes the biliary tree after insertion of an endoscope down the esophagus into the duodenum, cannulation of the common bile and pancreatic ducts, and injection of contrast medium.

◆ HIDA scan detects obstruction of the cystic duct.

◆ Magnetic resonance cholangiopancreatography can detect gallstones, choledocholithiasis, masses, biliary strictures, and dilation.

Elevated total bilirubin, urine bilirubin, and alkaline phosphatase levels support the diagnosis. The WBC count is slightly elevated during a cholecystitis attack. Differential diagnosis is essential because gallbladder disease can mimic other diseases (myocardial infarction, angina, pancreatitis, pancreatic head cancer, pneumonia, peptic ulcer, hiatal hernia, esophagitis, and gastritis). Serum amylase levels distinguish gallbladder disease from pancreatitis. With suspected heart disease, serial cardiac enzyme tests and electrocardiography should precede gallbladder and upper GI diagnostic tests.

Treatment

Surgery, usually elective, is the treatment of choice for gallbladder and bile duct diseases. Laparoscopic cholecystectomy and cholecystectomy with operative cholangiography are the most frequently performed surgeries. Open cholecystectomy is reserved from complicated cases. Other treatments include a low-fat diet to prevent attacks and vitamin K for itching, jaundice, and bleeding tendencies due to vitamin K deficiency. Treatment during an acute attack may include insertion of a nasogastric tube and an I.V. line and, possibly, antibiotic administration.

ERCP with sphincterotomy is the treatment of choice for choledocholithiasis with obstruction or cholangitis due to obstruction.

Ursodeoxycholic acid, which dissolves radiolucent stones, provides an alternative for patients who are poor surgical risks or who refuse surgery.

Special considerations

Patient care for gallbladder and bile duct diseases focuses on supportive care and close postoperative observation.

◆ Before surgery, teach the patient to deep-breathe, cough, expectorate, and perform leg exercises that are necessary after surgery. Also teach splinting, repositioning, and ambulation techniques. Explain the procedures that will be performed before, during, and after surgery to help ease the patient's anxiety and to help ensure cooperation.

◆ After surgery, monitor the patient's vital signs for signs of bleeding, infection, or atelectasis.

◆ Evaluate the incision site for bleeding. Serosanguineous drainage is common during the first 24 to 48 hours if the patient has a wound drain. If, after a choledochostomy, a T-tube drain is placed in the duct and attached to a drainage bag, make sure that the drainage tube has no kinks. Also check that the connecting tubing from the T-tube is well secured to the patient to prevent dislodgment.

◆ Measure and record T-tube drainage daily (200 to 300 mL is normal).

◆ Teach patients who will be discharged with a T-tube how to perform dressing changes and routine skin care.

◆ Monitor the patient's intake and output. Allow the patient nothing by mouth for 24 to 48 hours or until bowel sounds return and nausea and vomiting cease (postoperative nausea may indicate a full bladder).

◆ If the patient doesn't void within 8 hours (or if the amount voided is inadequate based on I.V. fluid intake), percuss over the symphysis pubis for bladder distention (especially in the patient receiving anticholinergics). The patient who has had a laparoscopic cholecystectomy may be discharged the same day or within

24 hours after surgery. The patient should have minimal pain, be able to tolerate a regular diet within 24 hours after surgery, and be able to return to normal activity within a few days to a week.

◆ Encourage deep-breathing and leg exercises every hour. The patient should ambulate after surgery. Provide elastic stockings to support the leg muscles and promote venous blood flow, thus preventing stasis and clot formation.

◆ Evaluate the location, duration, and character of any pain. Administer adequate medication to relieve pain, especially before such activities as deep breathing and ambulation, which increase pain.

◆ At discharge, advise the patient against heavy lifting or straining for 6 weeks. Urge the patient to walk daily. Tell them that food restrictions are unnecessary unless they have intolerance to a specific food or some underlying condition (such as diabetes, atherosclerosis, celiac disease or allergy, or obesity) that requires such restriction.

◆ Instruct the patient to notify the surgeon if they have pain for more than 24 hours or notices any jaundice, anorexia, nausea or vomiting, fever, or tenderness in the abdominal area because these may indicate a biliary tract injury from cholecystectomy, requiring immediate attention.

SELECTED REFERENCES

American Liver Foundation. (2018). *Advances in medicine to treat hepatitis C*. Retrieved from https://liverfoundation.org/for-patients/about-the-liver/diseases-of-the-liver/hepatitis-c/treating-hepatitis-c/

Civan, J. (2018). *Cirrhosis*. Retrieved from https://www.merckmanuals.com/professional/hepatic-and-biliary-disorders/fibrosis-and-cirrhosis/cirrhosis

Gao, B., & Baraller, R. (2011). Alcoholic liver disease: Pathogenesis and new therapeutic targets. *Gastroenterology, 141*(5), 1572–1585. doi:10.1053/j.gastro.2011.09.002

Peralta, R. (2017). *Liver abscess*. Retrieved from https://emedicine.medscape.com/article/188802-overview?pa=maup44Yk3I-aygCmJtrhQE5v9dMiuGzCpUCayfYh6JNLjvUx60Lt-2ViVgLNN9zZHMDhpXzs5obC2teoj0OoLcChiNxS-J9G4l%2BTQuhj9GxWnk%3D#a5

Samji, N. (2017). *Viral hepatitis*. Retrieved from https://emedicine.medscape.com/article/775507-overview#a3

Wolf, D. (2017). *Autoimmune hepatitis*. Retrieved from https://emedicine.medscape.com/article/172356-overview#a4

Yeg, M. (2017). *Pathology of nonalcoholic steatohepatitis*. Retrieved from https://emedicine.medscape.com/article/2038493-overview#a2

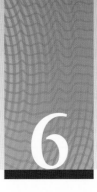

MUSCULOSKELETAL DISORDERS

Introduction

A complex system of bones, muscles, ligaments, tendons, and other connective tissue, the musculoskeletal system gives the body its form and shape. It also protects vital organs, makes movement possible, stores calcium and other minerals, and provides sites for hematopoiesis. A fibrous layer called the *periosteum* covers all bones, except at joints, where they're covered by articular cartilage.

The human skeleton contains 206 bones, which are composed of inorganic salts, such as calcium and phosphate, embedded in a framework of collagen fibers. Bones are classified by shape as long, short, flat, or irregular.

LONG BONES

Long bones, which are found in the limbs, include the humerus, radius, and ulna of the arm; the femur, tibia, and fibula of the leg; and the phalanges, metacarpals, and metatarsals in the hands and feet. These bones have a long shaft, or *diaphysis*, and widened, bulbous ends, called *epiphyses*. A long bone is made up mainly of compact bone, which surrounds the medullary cavity (also called the *yellow marrow*), a storage site for fat. The lining of the medullary cavity (the *endosteum*) is a thin layer of connective tissue. The outer layer is the periosteum. (See *Long-bone structure*, page 288.)

In children and young adults, lengthwise growth occurs at the epiphyseal cartilage between the diaphysis and epiphysis. In adults, in whom bone growth is complete, this cartilage is ossified and forms the epiphyseal line. The epiphysis also has a surface layer made up of compact bone, but its center is made of spongy or cancellous bone. Cancellous bone contains open spaces between thin threads of bone, called *trabeculae*, which are arranged in various directions to correspond with the lines of maximum stress or pressure. This configuration gives the bone added structural strength.

Unlike cancellous bone, adult compact bone consists of numerous orderly networks of interconnecting canals that run parallel to the bone's long axis. Each of these networks, called a *haversian system*, consists of a central haversian canal surrounded by layers (*lamellae*) of bone. Between adjacent lamellae are small openings (*lacunae*), which contain bone cells (*osteocytes*). All lacunae are joined by an interconnecting network of tiny canals (*canaliculi*), each of which contains one or more capillaries and provides a route for movement of tissue fluids. The haversian system carries blood to the bone through blood vessels that enter the system through channels called *Volkmann's canals*.

SHORT, FLAT, OR IRREGULAR BONES

Short bones include the tarsal and carpal bones; flat bones, the frontal and parietal bones of the cranium, ribs, sternum, scapulae, ilium, and pubis; and irregular bones, the bones of the spine (vertebrae, sacrum, and coccyx) and certain bones of the skull (sphenoid, ethmoid, and mandible).

Short, flat, and irregular bones have an outer layer of compact bone and an inner portion of spongy bone. In the sternum and certain areas in the flat bones of the skull, the spongy bone contains red marrow.

Long-bone structure

Long-bone composition is depicted below, with an illustrated cross section.

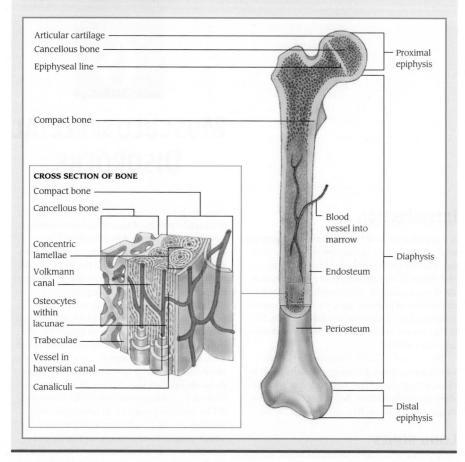

Articular cartilage
Cancellous bone
Epiphyseal line
Compact bone
Proximal epiphysis

CROSS SECTION OF BONE
Compact bone
Cancellous bone
Concentric lamellae
Volkmann canal
Osteocytes within lacunae
Trabeculae
Vessel in haversian canal
Canaliculi

Blood vessel into marrow
Endosteum
Periosteum
Diaphysis
Distal epiphysis

JOINTS

The tissues connecting two bones make up a joint, which permits motion between the bones and provides stability. Joints, like bones, have varying forms.

◆ Fibrous joints (*synarthroses*) have only minute motion and provide stability when tight union is necessary, as in the seams, called *sutures*, that join the cranial bones.

◆ Cartilaginous joints (*amphiarthroses*) have limited motion, as between vertebrae and symphysis pubis.

◆ Synovial joints (*diarthroses*) are the most common and have the greatest degree of movement. Such joints include the elbows, shoulders, and knees. Synovial joints have special characteristics: the articulating surfaces of each bone have a smooth hyaline covering (articular cartilage), which is resilient to pressure; their opposing surfaces are congruous and glide smoothly on each other without touching each other; a fibrous (articular) capsule holds them together. Beneath the capsule and lining the joint cavity, the synovial membrane secretes the clear, viscous synovial fluid. This fluid lubricates the two opposing surfaces during motion and also nourishes the articular cartilage. Surrounding a synovial joint are ligaments, muscles, and tendons, which strengthen and stabilize the joint but allow free movement.

In some synovial joints, the synovial membrane forms two additional structures—bursae and tendon sheaths—which reduce friction that normally accompanies movement. Bursae are small, cushionlike sacs lined with synovial membranes and filled with synovial fluid; most are located between tendons and bones. Tendon sheaths wrap around the tendon and cushion it as it crosses the joint.

The synovial joints permit angular and circular movements. Angular movements include *flexion* (decrease in joint angle), *extension* (increase in joint angle), and *hyperextension* (increase in the angle of extension beyond the usual arc). Joints of the knees, elbows, and phalanges permit such movement. Other angular movements are *abduction* (movement away from the body's midline) and *adduction* (movement toward the body's midline).

Circular movements include *rotation* (motion around a central axis), as in the ball-and-socket joints of the hips and shoulders; *pronation* (wrist motion to place palmar surface of the hand down, with the thumb toward the body); *supination* (begging position, with palm up). Other kinds of movement are *inversion* (movement facing inward), *eversion* (movement facing outward), *protraction* (as in forward motion of the mandible), and *retraction* (returning protracted part into place).

MUSCLES

Muscle tissues' most specialized feature—*contractility*—makes movement of bones and joints possible. Muscles also pump blood through the body, move food through the intestines, and make breathing possible. Muscular activity produces heat, so it's an important component in temperature regulation. Muscles maintain body positions, such as sitting and standing. Muscle mass accounts for about 40% of the body weight of a person of average size.

Muscles are classified in many ways. *Skeletal* muscles are attached to bone, *visceral* muscles permit function of internal organs, and *cardiac* muscles make up the heart wall. Also, muscles may be striated or nonstriated (smooth), depending on their cellular configuration.

Muscles classified according to activity are called *voluntary* or *involuntary*. Voluntary muscles can be controlled at will and are under the influence of the somatic nervous system; these are the skeletal muscles. Involuntary muscles, controlled by the autonomic nervous system, include the cardiac and visceral muscles.

Each skeletal muscle consists of many elongated muscle cells, called *muscle fibers*, through which run slender threads of protein, called *myofibrils*. Muscle fibers are held together in bundles by sheaths of fibrous tissue, called *fascia*. Blood vessels and nerves pass through the fascia to reach the individual muscle fibers.

Skeletal muscles are attached to bone directly or indirectly by fibrous cords called *tendons*. The least movable end of the muscle attachment is called *the point of origin*; the most movable end is *the point of insertion*.

MECHANISM OF CONTRACTION

To stimulate muscle contraction and movement, the brain sends motor impulses through the peripheral motor nerves to motor nerve fibers in the voluntary muscle. These nerve fibers reach membranes of skeletal muscle cells at neuromuscular (*myoneural*) junctions. When an impulse reaches the myoneural junction, it triggers the following sequence: release of the neurochemical acetylcholine, transient release of calcium from the sarcoplasmic reticulum (a membranous network in the muscle fiber), and muscle contraction. The arriving impulse at the myoneural junction also triggers release of adenosine triphosphate, the energy source for muscle contraction. Muscle relaxation is believed to take place by reversal of the above mechanisms.

MUSCULOSKELETAL ASSESSMENT

Most patients with musculoskeletal disorders are elderly, have concurrent medical conditions, or have experienced trauma. Younger patients tend to experience more benign, self-limited conditions. Generally, they face prolonged immobilization. These factors make thorough assessment essential. Your assessment should include a complete history and a careful physical examination to determine a possible cause of the symptoms.

Interview the patient carefully to obtain a complete medical, social, and personal history. Ask about general activity, for example jogging daily or sedentary life which may be significantly altered by musculoskeletal disease or trauma. Does the patient have any systemic symptoms, such as fever, chills, weight loss, or skin rashes? Obtain information about occupation, diet, sexual activity, and elimination habits, drugs taken, and use of safety devices, and try to assess how the problem will affect body image. Also, ask how the patient functions at home. Is the patient independent with activities of daily living, are there stairs to the bedroom or bathroom, any prosthetic devices, any family members who help with personal care?

Get an accurate account of the musculoskeletal problem. Ask if it has caused any changes to everyday routines. When did symptoms begin and how did they progress? Has the patient received treatment for this problem? Has there been any trauma? If so, find out the details.

Assess the level of pain. Is the patient in pain now? Ask what makes the discomfort worse or better (movement, position, and so forth). Evaluate past and present responses to treatment. For instance, if the patient has arthritis and uses corticosteroids, ask about their effectiveness. Is more of less medication needed than before? Are there any issues with adherence to the prescribed treatment?

Physical examination helps to determine the diagnosis and reveals any existing disabilities. (These baseline data will help when the effects of treatment are evaluated.) Observe the patient's appearance. Look for localized edema, pigmentation, redness and tenderness at pressure points, and other deformities such as atrophy. Note mobility, strength, and gait. To check range of motion (ROM), ask the patient to abduct, adduct, or flex the muscles in question. Obtain height, weight, and vital signs. Check neurovascular status, including motion sensation and circulation. Measure and record discrepancies in muscle circumference or leg length. Compare one side or limb to the other. If a neck injury is suspected, don't force ROM.

DIAGNOSTIC TOOLS

◆ X-rays are a useful diagnostic tool to evaluate musculoskeletal diseases. They can help to identify joint disruption, bone deformities, calcifications, and bone destruction and fractures. X-rays also measure bone density.
◆ Myelography is an invasive procedure used to evaluate abnormalities of the spinal canal and cord. It entails injection of a radiopaque contrast medium into the subarachnoid space of the spine. Serial X-rays visualize the progress of the contrast medium as it passes through the subarachnoid space. Displacement of the medium indicates a space-occupying lesion, such as a herniated disk or a tumor.
◆ Magnetic resonance imaging (MRI) is useful in evaluating soft-tissue injuries or ligament tears, such as rotator cuff tears or meniscal tears.
◆ Computed tomography (CT) scan can be used to identify injuries to bones, soft tissue, ligaments, tendons, and muscles.
◆ Arthroscopy is the visual examination of the interior of a joint with a fiberoptic endoscope.

Other useful tests include bone and muscle biopsies, electromyography, microscopic examination of synovial fluid, and multiple laboratory studies of urine and blood to identify systemic abnormalities.

PATIENT CARE

Each patient with musculoskeletal disease needs an individual care plan formulated early in the hospital stay by the entire clinical team, including the physician, physical therapist, and occupational therapist. Develop this plan with short- and long-term goals, during and after hospitalization.

Caring for the patient with a musculoskeletal disease usually includes at least one of the following: traction, casts, braces, splints, crutches, intermittent ROM devices, prolonged immobilization, physical therapy, occupational therapy, and self-care measures; adequate vitamin D intake, weight loss, dietary modifications, and drugs.

Traction is the manual or mechanical application of a steady pulling force to reduce a fracture, minimize muscle spasms, or immobilize or align a joint.
◆ Skin traction is the indirect application of traction to the skeletal system through skin and soft tissues.
◆ Skeletal traction is the direct application of traction to bones by means of a pin (Steinmann pin) or wire (Kirschner wire) through the affected bone or by calipers or a tonglike device (Gardner-Wells tongs) that grips the bone.
◆ Manual traction, for emergency use, is the direct application of traction to a body part by hand.

During the use of all types of traction:
◆ Explain to the patient how traction works and advise the patient about permissible amounts of activity and elevation of the head of the bed. Inform the patient of the anticipated duration of traction and whether the traction is removable. Teach active ROM exercises.
◆ Check neurovascular status to prevent nerve damage. Also, make sure the mattress is firm, that the traction ropes aren't frayed, that they're on the center track of the pulley, and that traction weights are hanging free. Thoroughly investigate any complaint the patient makes.
◆ Check for signs of infection (odor, local inflammation and drainage, or fever) at pin sites if the patient is in skeletal traction. Also, check with the physician's or the facility's procedure regarding pin-site care, such as use of peroxide or povidone–iodine.

Ideally, a cast immobilizes without adding too much weight. It's snug-fitting but doesn't constrict and has a smooth inner surface and smooth edges to prevent pressure or skin irritation. Casts require comprehensive patient education.
◆ A plaster cast takes 24 to 48 hours to dry. To prevent indentations, tell the patient not to

squeeze the cast, not to cover or walk on the cast until it has dried, and not to bump a damp cast on hard surfaces because dents can cause pressure areas. Warn the patient that while the cast is drying, there may be a temporary sensation of heat under the cast.

◆ If fiberglass is used, the cast may feel dry and the patient may be able to bear weight immediately. Advise the patient, however, not to get the cast wet. Although the fiberglass won't disintegrate as plaster would, the padding will become wet and potentially cause maceration of the skin.

◆ Emphasize the need to keep the cast above heart level for *24 hours* after its application to reduce swelling in the limb.

◆ While the cast is drying and after drying is complete, the patient should watch for and immediately report persistent pain in the limb inside or distal to the cast as well as edema, changes in skin color, coldness, or tingling or numbness in this area. If any of these signs occur, tell the patient to position the casted body part above heart level and notify the physician.

◆ The patient should also report drainage through the cast or an odor that may indicate infection. Warn against inserting foreign objects under the cast, getting it wet, pulling out its padding, or scratching inside it. Tell the patient to seek immediate attention for a broken cast.

◆ Instruct the patient to exercise the joints above and below the cast to prevent stiffness and contracture.

Braces, splints, and slings also provide alignment, immobilization, and pain relief for musculoskeletal diseases. Slings and splints are usually used for short-term immobilization. Explain to the patient and the family why these appliances are necessary and show them the proper way to apply the sling, splint, or brace for optimal benefit. Tell the patient how long the appliance will have to be worn and advise the patient of any activity limitations that must be observed. If the patient has a brace, check with the orthotist (orthopedic appliance specialist) about proper care. Encourage the patient to refer additional questions to the physician. Teach proper crutch walking.

COPING WITH IMMOBILITY

Immobilized patients require meticulous care to prevent complications. Without constant care, the bedridden patient becomes susceptible to pressure ulcers, caused by the increased pressure on tissue over bony prominences, and is especially vulnerable to cardiopulmonary complications.

◆ To prevent pressure ulcers, turn the patient every 2 hours and, if possible, reposition in a 30-degree side-lying position for short periods. In addition, place a flotation pad or sheepskin pad under bony prominences, or use an alternating-air-current, convoluted foam, or foam mattress. Show the patient how to use a Balkan frame with a trapeze to move about in bed.

◆ Keep the patient's skin dry and clean.

◆ Keep the sheets wrinkle-free.

◆ Increase fluid intake to minimize risk of renal calculi.

◆ Provide adequate nutrition; a high-protein diet is preferred, if tolerated.

◆ Perform passive ROM exercises on the affected side, as ordered, to prevent contractures, and instruct the patient in active ROM exercises on the unaffected side. Apply footboards or high-topped sneakers to prevent footdrop. Keep the patient's heels off the bed to prevent heel breakdown. Also, watch for reddened elbows.

◆ Because most bedridden patients involuntarily perform a Valsalva's maneuver when using the upper arms and trunk to move, instruct the patient to exhale (instead of holding their breath) while turning. This will prevent possible cardiac complications that result from increased intrathoracic pressure.

◆ Emphasize the importance of coughing and deep breathing and teach the patient how to use the incentive spirometer if ordered.

◆ Because constipation is a common problem in bedridden patients, establish a bowel program (fluids, fiber, laxatives, stool softeners), as needed.

REHABILITATION

Restoring the patient to a former state of health isn't always possible. When it isn't, help the patient adjust to a modified lifestyle. During hospitalization, promote independence by letting patients finish difficult tasks independently. If necessary, refer the patient to a community facility for continued rehabilitation.

Congenital disorders

CLUBFOOT

Clubfoot, or *talipes*, is the most common congenital disorder of the lower limbs. It's marked primarily by a deformed talus and shortened Achilles tendon, which give the foot a characteristic clublike appearance. In talipes equinovarus, the foot points downward (equinus) and turns inward (varus), whereas the front of the foot curls toward the heel (forefoot adduction).

Causes and incidence

It is no longer believed that clubfoot is caused by fetal position in utero. Heredity is a definite factor in some cases, although the mechanism of transmission is undetermined. In children without a family history of clubfoot, this anomaly seems linked to arrested development during the 9th and 10th weeks of embryonic life, when the feet are formed. Researchers also suspect muscle abnormalities, leading to variations in length and tendon insertions, as possible causes of clubfoot. Environmental factors play a role. Studies strongly link clubfoot to cigarette smoking during pregnancy, especially if there is a family history of clubfoot.

Clubfoot, which has an incidence of about 1 per 1,000 live births, usually occurs bilaterally and is twice as common in boys. It may be associated with other birth defects, such as myelomeningocele, spina bifida, and arthrogryposis. However, most cases are sporadic occurrences.

Pathophysiology

Abnormal development of the foot during fetal growth leads to abnormal muscles and joints and contracture of soft tissue. Clubfoot can also occur because of paralysis, poliomyelitis, or cerebral palsy. The condition called *apparent clubfoot* results when a fetus maintains a position in utero that gives feet a clubfoot appearance at birth; it can usually be corrected manually. Another form of apparent clubfoot is inversion of the feet, resulting from the denervation type of progressive muscular atrophy and progressive muscular dystrophy.

Complication

◆ Retention deformity

Signs and symptoms

Talipes equinovarus varies greatly in severity. Deformity may be so extreme that the toes touch the inside of the ankle, or it may be only vaguely apparent. In every case, the talus is deformed, the Achilles tendon shortened, and the calcaneus somewhat shortened and flattened. Depending on the degree of the varus deformity, the calf muscles are shortened and underdeveloped, and soft-tissue contractures form at the site of the deformity. The foot is tight in its deformed position and resists manual efforts to push it into normal position. Clubfoot is painless, except in elderly, arthritic patients. In older children, clubfoot may be secondary to paralysis, poliomyelitis, or cerebral palsy, in which case treatment must include management of the underlying disease.

Diagnosis

Early diagnosis of clubfoot is usually possible because the deformity is obvious. In subtle deformity, however, true clubfoot must be distinguished from apparent clubfoot (metatarsus varus or pigeon toe). Apparent clubfoot is inversion of the feet, resulting from the peroneal type of progressive muscular atrophy and progressive muscular dystrophy. In true clubfoot, X-rays show superimposition of the talus and the calcaneus and a ladderlike appearance of the metatarsals. (See *Recognizing clubfoot.*)

Treatment

Clubfoot is correctable with prompt treatment, which is performed in three stages: correcting the deformity, maintaining the correction until the foot regains normal muscle balance, and observing the foot closely for several years to prevent the deformity from recurring. In neonates with true clubfoot, corrective treatment should begin at once. An infant's foot contains large amounts of cartilage; the muscles, ligaments, and tendons are supple. The ideal time to begin treatment is during the first few days and weeks of life, when the foot is most malleable.

Clubfoot deformities are usually corrected in sequential order. Several therapeutic methods have been found effective in correcting clubfoot. In all patients, the first procedure should be simple manipulation and casting, whereby the foot is gently manipulated into a partially corrected position and held in place by a cast for several days or weeks. (The skin should be painted with a nonirritating adhesive liquid beforehand to prevent the cast from slipping.) After the cast is

Recognizing clubfoot

Congenital skeletal anomalies frequently involve the foot and the ankle and are referred to as "clubfoot."

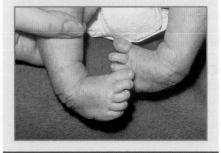

removed, the foot is manipulated into an even better position and casted again. This procedure is repeated as many times as necessary. In some cases, the shape of the cast can be transformed through a series of wedging maneuvers instead of changing the cast each time.

After correction of clubfoot, proper foot alignment should be maintained through exercise, night splints, and orthopedic shoes. With manipulating and casting, correction usually takes about 3 months. The Denis Browne splint, a device that consists of two padded, metal footplates connected by a flat, horizontal bar, is sometimes used as a follow-up measure to help promote bilateral correction and strengthen the foot muscles.

Resistant clubfoot may require surgery. Older children, for example, with recurrent or neglected clubfoot usually need surgery. Tenotomy, tendon transfer, stripping of the plantar fascia, and capsulotomy are some of the surgical procedures that may be used. In severe cases, bone surgery (wedge resections, osteotomy, or astragalectomy) may be appropriate. After surgery, a cast is applied to preserve the correction. Clubfoot severe enough to require surgery is rarely totally correctable; however, surgery can usually ameliorate the deformity.

Special considerations

The primary concern is recognition of clubfoot as early as possible, preferably in neonates.

♦ Look for any exaggerated attitudes in an infant's feet. Make sure you recognize the difference between true clubfoot and apparent clubfoot. Don't use excessive force in trying to manipulate a clubfoot. The foot with apparent clubfoot moves easily.

♦ Stress to parents the importance of prompt treatment. Make sure they understand that clubfoot demands immediate therapy and orthopedic supervision until growth is completed.

♦ After casting, elevate the child's feet with pillows. Check the toes every 1 to 2 hours for temperature, color, sensation, motion, and capillary refill time; watch for edema. Before a child in a clubfoot cast is discharged, teach parents to recognize circulatory impairment.

♦ Insert plastic petals over the top edges of a new cast while it's still wet to keep urine from soaking and softening the cast. This is done as follows: Cut a plastic sheet into strips long enough to cover the outside of the cast and tuck them about a finger length beneath the cast edges. Using overlapping strips of tape, tack the corner of each petal to the outside of the cast. When the cast is dry, petal the edges with

adhesive tape to keep out plaster crumbs and prevent skin irritation. Perform good skin care under the cast edges every 4 hours, washing and carefully drying the skin. (Don't rub the skin with alcohol, and don't use oils or powders, which tend to macerate the skin.)

♦ If the child is old enough to walk, caution parents not to let the foot part of the cast get soft and thin from wear. If it does, much of the correction may be lost.

♦ When the wedging method of shaping the cast is being used, check circulatory status frequently; it may be impaired by increased pressure on tissues and blood vessels. The equinus (posterior release) correction especially places considerable strain on ligaments, blood vessels, and tendons.

♦ After surgery, elevate the child's feet with pillows to decrease swelling and pain. Report signs of discomfort or pain right away. Try to locate the source of pain; it may result from cast pressure rather than from the incision. If bleeding occurs under the cast, circle the location and mark the time on the cast. If bleeding spreads, report it.

♦ Explain to the older child and the parents that surgery can improve clubfoot with good function but can't totally correct it; the affected calf muscle will remain slightly underdeveloped.

♦ Emphasize the need for long-term orthopedic care to maintain correction. Teach parents the prescribed exercises that the child can do at home. Urge them to make the child wear the corrective shoes ordered and the splints during naps and at night. Make sure they understand that treatment for clubfoot continues during the entire growth period. Correcting this defect permanently takes time and patience.

DEVELOPMENTAL DYSPLASIA OF THE HIP

Developmental dysplasia of the hip (DDH), an abnormality of the hip joint present from birth, is the most common disorder affecting hip joints of children younger than 3 years old. DDH can be unilateral or bilateral. (See *Characteristics of developmental hip dysplasia*, page 294.) This abnormality occurs in three forms of varying severity: *unstable hip dysplasia*, in which the hip is positioned normally but can be dislocated by manipulation; *subluxation or incomplete dislocation*, in which the femoral head rides on the edge of the acetabulum; and *complete or true congenital dislocation*, in which the femoral head is totally outside the acetabulum.

Characteristics of developmental hip dysplasia

The classic characteristics of developmental hip dysplasia are illustrated below.

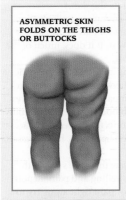

ASYMMETRIC SKIN FOLDS ON THE THIGHS OR BUTTOCKS

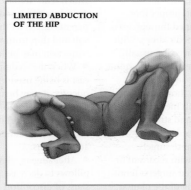

LIMITED ABDUCTION OF THE HIP

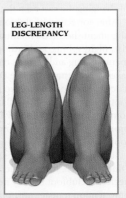

LEG-LENGTH DISCREPANCY

Developmental hip subluxation or dislocation can cause abnormal acetabular development and permanent disability.

Causes and incidence

Experts are uncertain about the causes of DDH. Dislocation is 10 times more common after breech delivery (malpositioning in utero) than after cephalic delivery, and it's also more common among large neonates and twins. It's a lot more common in firstborn children. Girls are affected more often than boys and white children more than black children. Genetic factors may also play a role.

Although DDH is found throughout the world, incidence is particularly high among Native Americans.

Pathophysiology

The precise cause of congenital dislocation is unknown. Excessive or abnormal movement of the joint during a traumatic birth may cause dislocation. Displacement of bones within the joint may damage joint structures, including articulating surfaces, blood vessels, tendons, ligaments, and nerves. This may lead to ischemic necrosis because of the disruption of blood flow to the joint.

Complications

◆ Degenerative hip changes (if treatment is delayed)
◆ Lordosis
◆ Joint malformation
◆ Crippling osteoarthritis

Signs and symptoms

Clinical effects of hip dysplasia vary with age. In neonates, dysplasia doesn't cause gross deformity or pain. However, in complete dysplasia, the hip rides above the acetabulum, causing the level of the knees to be uneven. As the child grows older and begins to walk, the abduction on the dislocated side is limited. Uncorrected bilateral dysplasia may cause the child to sway from side to side, a condition known as "duck waddle"; unilateral dysplasia may produce a limp. If corrective treatment isn't begun until after age 2, DDH may cause degenerative hip changes, lordosis, joint malformation, and soft-tissue damage.

Diagnosis

Several observations during physical examination of the relaxed child strongly suggest DDH. First, place the child on the back, and inspect the folds of skin over the thighs. Usually, a child in this position has an equal number of thigh folds on each side, but a child with subluxation or dislocation may have an extra fold on the affected side (this extra fold is also apparent when the child lies prone). Next, with the child lying prone, check for alignment of the buttock fold. In a child with dysplasia, the buttock fold on the affected side is higher. In addition, abduction of the affected hip is restricted.

℞ **CONFIRMING DIAGNOSIS** *A positive Ortolani or Trendelenburg sign confirms DDH. To elicit Ortolani sign, place the infant on back, with hip flexed and abducted. Adducting the hip while pressing the femur downward will dislocate the hip.*

Then, abducting the hip while moving the femur upward will move the femoral head over the acetabular rim. If you hear a click or feel a jerk as the femoral head moves, the test is positive. This sign indicates subluxation in a neonate younger than 1 month and subluxation or complete dislocation in an older infant.

To elicit Trendelenburg sign, have the child put weight on the side of the dislocation and lift the other knee. The pelvis drops on the normal side because of weak abductor muscles in the affected hip. However, when the child stands with weight on the normal side and lifts the other knee, the pelvis remains horizontal.

Ultrasound of the hip reveals hip deformity. X-rays show the location of the femur head and a shallow acetabulum. X-rays may also show acetabular dysplasia or a teratologica dislocation. MRI may also be used to assess reduction.

Treatment

The earlier the infant receives treatment, the better the chances are for normal development. Treatment varies with the patient's age and is tailored to the specific pathological condition. In infants younger than 6 months, treatment includes *gentle* manipulation to reduce the dislocation, followed by holding the hips in a flexed and abducted position with a splint-brace or harness to maintain the reduction. The infant must wear this apparatus continuously for 2 to 3 months and then use a night splint for another month, so the joint capsule can tighten and stabilize in correct alignment.

If treatment doesn't begin until after age 3 months, it may include bilateral skin traction (in infants) or skeletal traction (in children who have started walking) to reduce the dislocation by gradually abducting the hips. In Bryant's traction, or divarication traction, both legs are placed in traction, even if only one is affected, to help maintain immobilization. This type of traction is used in children who are younger than 3 years and weigh less than 35 lb (16 kg). The length of treatment is 2 to 3 weeks.

If traction fails, gentle closed reduction under general anesthetic can further abduct the hips; the child is then placed in a spica cast for 4 to 6 months. If closed treatment fails, open reduction, followed by immobilization in a spica cast for an average of 6 months, or osteotomy may be considered.

In the child 2 to 5 years old, treatment is difficult and includes skeletal traction and subcutaneous adductor tenotomy. Treatment begun after age 5 rarely restores satisfactory hip function.

Special considerations

The child who must wear a splint, brace, or body cast needs special personal care that requires parent education.

◆ Teach parents how to correctly splint or brace the hips, as ordered. Stress the need for frequent checkups.

◆ Listen sympathetically to the parents' expressions of anxiety and fear. Explain possible causes of DDH, and give reassurance that early, prompt treatment will probably result in complete correction.

◆ During the child's first few days in a cast or splint-brace, expect some irritability due to the unaccustomed restricted movement. Encourage the parents to stay with the child as much as possible and to calm to provide reassurance.

◆ Assure parents that the child will adjust to this restriction and return to normal sleeping, eating, and playing behavior in a few days.

◆ Instruct parents to remove braces and splints while bathing the infant but to replace them immediately afterward. Stress good hygiene; parents should bathe and change the child frequently and wash perineum with warm water and soap at each diaper change.

If treatment requires a spica cast:

◆ When transferring the child immediately after casting, use your palms to avoid making dents in the cast. Such dents predispose the patient to pressure sores. Remember that the plaster cast needs 24 to 48 hours to dry naturally. Don't use heat to make it dry faster because heat also makes it more fragile.

◆ Immediately after the cast is applied, use a plastic sheet to protect it from moisture around the perineum and buttocks. Cut the sheet into strips long enough to cover the outside of the cast and tuck them about a finger length beneath the cast edges. Using overlapping strips of tape, tack the corner of each petal to the outside of the cast. Remove the plastic under the cast every 4 hours; then wash, dry, and retuck it. Disposable diapers folded lengthwise over the perineum may also be used.

◆ Position the child either on a Bradford frame elevated on blocks, with a bedpan under the frame, or on pillows to support the child's legs. Be sure to keep the cast dry and change the child's diapers often.

◆ Turn the child every 2 hours during the day and every 4 hours at night. Check color, sensation, and motion of the infant's legs and feet. Be sure to examine all toes. Notify the physician of dusky, cool, or numb toes.

◆ Check the cast daily for odors, which may herald infection.

◆ If the child complains of itching, he may benefit from diphenhydramine, or you may aim a hair dryer set on cool at the cast edges to relieve itching. Don't scratch or probe under the cast. Investigate any persistent itching.

◆ Provide adequate nutrition and maintain adequate fluid intake to avoid renal calculi and constipation, both complications of inactivity.

◆ Provide adequate stimuli to promote growth and development.

◆ Tell parents to watch for signs that the child is outgrowing the cast (cyanosis, cool limbs, or pain).

◆ Tell parents that treatment may be prolonged and requires patience.

◆ The patient in Bryant's traction may be cared for at home if the parents are taught traction application and maintenance.

◆ Encourage the parents to cuddle and hold the child and encourage interactions with siblings and friends.

◆ Maintain skin integrity and check circulation at least every 2 hours.

◆ Feed the child carefully to avoid aspiration and choking.

◆ Refer the child and parents to a child life specialist to ensure continued developmental progress.

MUSCULAR DYSTROPHY

Muscular dystrophy is a group of congenital disorders characterized by progressive symmetrical wasting of skeletal muscles without neural or sensory defects. Paradoxically, these wasted muscles tend to enlarge because of connective tissue and fat deposits, giving an erroneous impression of muscle strength. The main types of muscular dystrophy are Duchenne (pseudohypertrophic), Becker (benign pseudohypertrophic), facioscapulohumeral (Landouzy–Dejerine), limb-girdle dystrophy, Emery–Dreifuss muscular dystrophy, and myotonia congenita.

The prognosis varies. Duchenne muscular dystrophy generally strikes during early childhood and usually results in death in the 20s or early 30s. Patients with Becker muscular dystrophy typically live into their 40s. Facioscapulohumeral and limb-girdle dystrophies usually don't shorten life.

Causes and incidence

Muscular dystrophy is caused by various genetic mechanisms. Duchenne and Becker muscular dystrophies are X-linked recessive disorders. Both result from defects in the gene coding for the muscle protein dystrophin; the gene has been mapped to the Xp21 locus.

The incidence of muscular dystrophy is about 1 in 651,450 persons in the United States. Duchenne and Becker muscular dystrophies affect males almost exclusively.

Facioscapulohumeral dystrophy is an autosomal dominant disorder. Limb-girdle dystrophy is usually autosomal recessive. These two types affect both sexes about equally.

Pathophysiology

Abnormally permeable cell membranes allow leakage of various muscle enzymes, particularly creatine kinase. This metabolic defect that causes the muscle cells to die is present from fetal life onward. The absence of progressive muscle wasting at birth suggests that other factors compound the effect of dystrophin deficiency. The specific trigger is unknown, but phagocytosis of the muscle cells by inflammatory cells causes scarring and loss of muscle function.

As the disease progresses, skeletal muscle becomes almost totally replaced by fat and connective tissue. The skeleton eventually becomes deformed, causing progressive immobility. Cardiac and smooth muscle of the gastrointestinal (GI) tract typically become fibrotic. No consistent structural abnormalities are seen in the brain.

Complications

◆ Inhibited pulmonary function due to deformities

◆ Greater risk for pneumonia

◆ Respiratory problems lead to arrhythmias and hypertrophy

Signs and symptoms

Although all four types of muscular dystrophy cause progressive muscular deterioration, the degree of severity and age of onset vary.

Duchenne muscular dystrophy begins insidiously, between ages 2 and 3. Initially, it affects leg and pelvic muscles but eventually spreads to the involuntary muscles. Muscle weakness produces a waddling gait, toe walking, and lordosis. Children with this disorder have difficulty climbing stairs, fall often, can't run properly, and their scapulae flare out (or "wing") when they raise their arms. Calf muscles especially become enlarged and firm. Muscle deterioration progresses rapidly, and contractures develop. Some have abrupt intermittent oscillations of the irises in response to light (Gower sign). Usually, these children are confined to wheelchairs by ages 9 to 12. Late in the disease, progressive weakening of cardiac muscle causes tachycardia, electrocardiogram abnormalities, and pulmonary complications. Death commonly results from sudden heart failure, respiratory failure, or infection.

Signs and symptoms of Becker muscular dystrophy resemble those of Duchenne muscular dystrophy, but they progress more slowly. It generally affects older boys and young men. Children affected usually walk through their teens and into adulthood—sometimes into their 40s. Cardiac involvement is much less frequent.

Facioscapulohumeral dystrophy is a slowly progressive and relatively benign form of muscular dystrophy that commonly occurs before age 10 but may develop during early adolescence. The earlier the disease occurs, the more rapid and progressive it is. Initially, it weakens the muscles of the face, shoulders, and upper arms but eventually spreads to all voluntary muscles, producing a pendulous lower lip and absence of the nasolabial fold. Early symptoms include the inability to pucker the mouth or whistle, abnormal facial movements, and the absence of facial movements when laughing or crying. Other signs consist of diffuse facial flattening that leads to a mask-like expression, winging of the scapulae, the inability to raise the arms above the head and, in infants, the inability to suckle.

Limb-girdle dystrophy follows a similarly slow course and commonly causes only slight disability. Usually, it begins between ages 6 and 10; less commonly, in early adulthood. The later the onset, the more rapid the progression. Muscle weakness first appears in the upper arm and pelvic muscles. Other symptoms include winging of the scapulae, lordosis with abdominal protrusion, waddling gait, poor balance, and the inability to raise the arms.

Diagnosis

Diagnosis depends on typical clinical findings, family history, and diagnostic test findings. If another family member has muscular dystrophy, its clinical characteristics can indicate the type of dystrophy the patient has and how he may be affected.

Electromyography typically demonstrates short, weak bursts of electrical activity or high-frequency, repetitive waxing and waning discharges in affected muscles. Muscle biopsy shows variations in the size of muscle fibers and, in later stages, shows fat and connective tissue deposits; dystrophin is absent in Duchenne dystrophy and diminished in Becker dystrophy. Serum creatine kinase level is markedly elevated in Duchenne, but only moderately elevated in Becker and facioscapulohumeral dystrophies.

Immunologic and molecular biologic assays available in specialized medical centers facilitate accurate prenatal and postnatal diagnosis of Duchenne and Becker muscular dystrophies and are replacing muscle biopsy and elevated serum creatine kinase levels in diagnosing these dystrophies. These assays can also help to identify carriers.

Treatment

No treatment stops the progressive muscle impairment of muscular dystrophy. However, orthopedic appliances, exercise, physical therapy, and surgery to correct contractures can help preserve the patient's mobility and independence. Prednisone improves muscle strength in patients with Duchenne.

Special considerations

Comprehensive long-term care and follow-up, patient and family teaching, and psychological support can help the patient and the family deal with this disorder.

♦ When respiratory involvement occurs in Duchenne muscular dystrophy, encourage coughing, deep-breathing exercises, and diaphragmatic breathing. Teach parents how to recognize early signs of respiratory complications.

♦ Encourage and assist with active and passive ROM exercises to preserve joint mobility and prevent muscle atrophy.

♦ Advise the patient to avoid long periods of bed rest and inactivity; if necessary, limit TV viewing and other sedentary activities.

♦ Refer the patient for physical therapy. Splints, braces, trapeze bars, overhead slings, and a wheelchair can help preserve mobility. A footboard or high-topped sneakers and a foot cradle increase comfort and prevent footdrop.

♦ Refer the patient to surgery to correct contractures.

♦ Because inactivity may cause constipation, encourage adequate fluid intake, increase dietary bulk, and obtain an order for a stool softener. The patient is prone to obesity due to reduced physical activity; assist with planning a low-calorie, high-protein, high-fiber diet if needed.

♦ Always allow the patient plenty of time to perform even simple physical tasks because if feeling slow and awkward.

♦ Encourage communication between the patient's family members to help them deal with the emotional strain this disorder produces. Provide emotional support to help the patient cope with continual changes in body image.

PEDIATRIC TIP *Help the child with Duchenne muscular dystrophy to maintain* *peer relationships and to realize the intellectual potential by encouraging the parents to keep the child in a regular school if possible.*

◆ If necessary, refer adult patients for counseling. Refer those who must acquire new job skills for vocational rehabilitation. (Contact the Department of Labor and Industry in your state for more information.) For information on social services and financial assistance, refer these patients and their families to the Muscular Dystrophy Association.

◆ Refer the patient's family members for genetic counseling.

Joints

SEPTIC ARTHRITIS

Septic, or infectious, arthritis is a medical emergency that occurs when bacterial invasion of a joint causes inflammation of the synovial lining, effusion and pyogenesis, and destruction of bone and cartilage. Septic arthritis can lead to ankylosis and even fatal septicemia. However, prompt antibiotic therapy and joint aspiration or drainage cures most patients.

Causes and incidence

In most cases of septic arthritis, bacteria spread from a primary site of infection—usually in adjacent bone or soft tissue—through the bloodstream to the joint. Common infecting organisms in children are group B *Streptococcus* and *Haemophilus influenzae*. Adults are usually infected by *Staphylococcus, Streptococcus, Neisseria gonorrhoeae* (pneumonia), and group B *Streptococcus*, whereas chronic septic arthritis is caused by *Mycobacterium tuberculosis* and *Candida albicans.*

Various factors can predispose a person to septic arthritis. Any concurrent bacterial infection (of the genitourinary or the upper respiratory tract, for example) or serious chronic illness (such as malignancy, renal failure, rheumatoid arthritis, systemic lupus erythematosus, diabetes, or cirrhosis) heightens susceptibility. Consequently, elderly people and those who abuse I.V. drugs run a higher risk of developing septic arthritis. Of course, diseases that depress the immune system and immunosuppressant therapy increase susceptibility. Other predisposing factors include recent articular trauma, joint arthroscopy or other surgery, intra-articular injections, local joint abnormalities, animal or human bites, and nail puncture wounds.

Septic arthritis may be seen at any age in children, but it occurs most often in children younger than 3 years old. It's uncommon from age 3 until adolescence, at which time the incidence increases again.

Pathophysiology

Previously damaged joints, especially those damaged by rheumatoid arthritis, are the most susceptible to infection. The synovial membranes of these joints exhibit neovascularization and increased adhesion factors; both conditions increase the chance of bacteremia, resulting in a joint infection. Some microorganisms have properties that promote their tropism to the synovium. *Staphylococcus aureus* readily binds to articular sialoprotein, fibronectin collage, elastin, hyaluronic acid, and prosthetic material via specific tissue adhesion factors (microbial surface components recognizing adhesive matrix molecules). In adults, the arteriolar anastomosis between the epiphysis and the synovium permits the spread of osteomyelitis into the joint space.

Complications

◆ Joint degeneration
◆ Osteomyelitis

Signs and symptoms

Acute septic arthritis begins abruptly, causing intense pain, inflammation, and swelling of the affected joint and low-grade fever. It usually affects a single joint. It most commonly develops in the large joints but can strike any joint, including the spine and small peripheral joints. The hip is a frequent site in infants. Systemic signs of inflammation may not appear in some patients. Migratory polyarthritis sometimes precedes localization of the infection. If the bacteria invade the hip, pain may occur in the groin, upper thigh, or buttock or may be referred to the knee.

Diagnosis

℞ **CONFIRMING DIAGNOSIS** *Identifying the causative organism in a Gram stain or culture of synovial fluid or a biopsy of synovial membrane confirms septic arthritis. When synovial fluid culture is negative, positive blood culture may confirm the diagnosis. Ultrasound of the hip is the modality of choice to detect fluid collections in the hip joint and can serve as a guide during aspiration procedures.*

Joint fluid analysis shows gross pus or watery, cloudy fluid of decreased viscosity, usually with 50,000/µL or more white cells, primarily neutrophils. Synovial fluid glucose concentration is usually greater than 40 mg/dL. (See *Other types of arthritis,* page 299.)

Other diagnostic measures include the following:

◆ X-rays can show typical changes as early as 1 week after initial infection—distention of joint capsules, for example, followed by narrowing of joint space (indicating cartilage damage) and erosions of bone (joint destruction).

Other types of arthritis

Hemophilic arthrosis
Hemophilic arthrosis produces transient or permanent joint changes. Often precipitated by trauma, hemophilic arthrosis usually arises between ages 1 and 5 and tends to recur until about age 10. It usually affects only one joint at a time—most commonly the knee, elbow, or ankle—and tends to recur in the same joint. Initially, the patient may feel only mild discomfort; later, he may experience warmth, swelling, tenderness, and severe pain with adjacent muscle spasm that leads to flexion of the extremity.

Mild hemophilic arthrosis may cause only limited stiffness that subsides within a few days. In prolonged bleeding, however, symptoms may subside after weeks or months or not at all. Severe hemophilic arthrosis may be accompanied by fever and leukocytosis; severe, prolonged, or repeated bleeding may lead to chronic hemophilic joint disease.

Effective treatment includes I.V. infusion of the deficient clotting factor, bed rest with the affected extremity elevated, application of ice packs, analgesics, and joint aspiration. Physical therapy includes progressive range-of-motion and muscle-strengthening exercises to restore motion and to prevent contractures and muscle atrophy.

Intermittent hydrarthrosis
Intermittent hydrarthrosis is a rare, benign condition characterized by regular, recurrent joint effusions. It most commonly affects the knee. The patient may have difficulty moving the affected joint but have no other arthritic symptoms. The cause of intermittent hydrarthrosis is unknown; onset is usually at or soon after puberty and may be linked to familial tendencies, allergies, or menstruation. No effective treatment exists.

Henoch–Schönlein purpura
Henoch–Schönlein purpura—a vasculitic syndrome—is marked by palpable purpura, abdominal pain, and arthralgia that most commonly affects the knees and ankles, producing swollen, warm, and tender joints without joint erosion or deformity. Renal involvement is also common. Most patients have microscopic hematuria and proteinuria 4 to 8 weeks after onset. Incidence is highest in children and young adults, occurring most often in the spring after a respiratory infection. Treatment may include corticosteroids.

Traumatic arthritis
Traumatic arthritis results from blunt, penetrating, or repeated trauma or from forced inappropriate motion of a joint or ligament. Clinical effects may include swelling, pain, tenderness, joint instability, and internal bleeding. Treatment includes analgesics, nonsteroidal anti-inflammatory drugs, application of cold followed by heat and, if needed, compression dressings, splinting, joint aspiration, casting, or possibly surgery.

◆ White blood cell (WBC) count may be elevated, with many polymorphonuclear cells; erythrocyte sedimentation rate is increased.
◆ Triple-phase bone scan is often used in children. A whole body scan is preferred in very young children.
◆ CT and MRI can provide useful images to delineate the extent of the infection.

Treatment
Antibiotic therapy should begin as soon as a Gram stain has been done; it may be modified when drug sensitivity of the infecting organism is known. Bioassays or bactericidal assays of synovial fluid and bioassays of blood may confirm clearing of the infection.

Rest, immobilization, elevation, and warm compresses help with pain relief. Analgesics are given for pain, if needed. The affected joint can be immobilized with a splint or put into traction until the patient can tolerate movement.

In severe cases, needle aspiration (arthrocentesis) or surgery may be done under sterile conditions to remove grossly purulent or infected joint fluid. Late reconstructive surgery is warranted only for severe joint damage and only after all signs of active infection have disappeared, which usually takes several months. Recommended procedures include arthroplasty and joint fusion. Prosthetic replacement remains controversial because it may exacerbate the infection, but it has helped patients with damaged femoral heads or acetabula.

Special considerations
Management of septic arthritis demands meticulous supportive care, close observation, and control of infection.

◆ Practice strict sterile technique for all procedures. Wash hands carefully before and after giving care. Dispose of soiled linens and dressings properly. Prevent contact between immunosuppressed patients and infected patients.

◆ Watch for signs of joint inflammation: heat, redness, swelling, pain, or drainage. Monitor vital signs and fever pattern. Remember that corticosteroids mask signs of infection.

◆ Check splints or traction regularly. Keep the joint in proper alignment but avoid prolonged immobilization. Start passive ROM exercises immediately, and progress to active exercises as soon as the patient can move the affected joint and put weight on it.

◆ Monitor pain levels and medicate accordingly, especially before exercise, remembering that the pain of septic arthritis is easy to underestimate. Administer analgesics and opioids for acute pain and heat or ice packs for moderate pain.

ELDER TIP *Monitor older adults who are on long-term opioid therapy because these drugs can impair mental status and may contribute to falls and other accidents.*

◆ Warn the patient before the first aspiration that it will be *extremely* painful. Carefully evaluate the patient's condition after joint aspiration.

GOUT

Gout, also called *gouty arthritis*, is a metabolic disease marked by urate deposits, which cause painfully arthritic joints. (See *Gouty deposits*.) It can strike any joint but favors those in the feet and legs. Gout follows an intermittent course and typically leaves patients totally free from symptoms for years between attacks. It can cause chronic disability or incapacitation and, rarely, severe hypertension and progressive renal disease. The prognosis is good with treatment.

Causes and incidence

Although the exact cause of primary gout remains unknown, it appears to be linked to a genetic defect in purine metabolism, which causes elevated blood levels of uric acid (hyperuricemia) due to overproduction of uric acid, retention of uric acid, or both. In secondary gout, which develops during the course of another disease (such as obesity, diabetes mellitus, hypertension, sickle cell anemia, and renal disease), hyperuricemia results from the breakdown of nucleic acids. Myeloproliferative and lymphoproliferative diseases, psoriasis, and hemolytic anemia are the most common causes. Primary gout usually occurs in men and in postmenopausal women; secondary gout occurs in elderly people.

Gouty deposits

The final stage of gout is marked by painful polyarthritis, with large, subcutaneous, tophaceous deposits in cartilage, synovial membranes, tendons, and soft tissue. The skin over the tophus is shiny, thin, and taut.

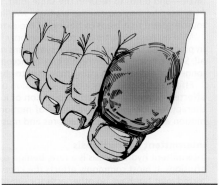

Secondary gout can also follow drug therapy that interferes with uric acid excretion. Increased concentration of uric acid leads to urate deposits (*tophi*) in joints or tissues and consequent local necrosis or fibrosis. The risk is greater in men, postmenopausal women, and those who use alcohol.

Pathophysiology

When uric acid becomes supersaturated in blood and other body fluids, it crystallizes and forms a precipitate of urate salts that accumulate in connective tissue throughout the body; these deposits are called *tophi*. The presence of the crystals triggers an acute inflammatory response when neutrophils begin to ingest the crystals. Tissue damage begins when the neutrophils release their lysosomes (see Chapter 8). The lysosomes not only damage the tissues but also perpetuate the inflammation.

In asymptomatic gout, the serum urate level increases, but the urate doesn't crystallize or produce symptoms. As the disease progresses, it may cause hypertension or urate kidney stones may form.

Complications
◆ Renal calculi
◆ Atherosclerotic disease
◆ Cardiovascular disease
◆ Stroke
◆ Coronary thrombosis
◆ Hypertension
◆ Infection when tophi rupture

Signs and symptoms

Gout develops in four stages: asymptomatic, acute, intercritical, and chronic. In asymptomatic gout, serum urate levels rise but produce no symptoms. As the disease progresses, it may cause hypertension or nephrolithiasis, with severe back pain. The first acute attack strikes suddenly and peaks quickly. Although it generally involves only one or a few joints, this initial attack is extremely painful. Affected joints are hot, tender, inflamed, and appear dusky-red or cyanotic. The metatarsophalangeal joint of the great toe usually becomes inflamed first (*podagra*), followed by the instep, ankle, heel, knee, or wrist joints. Sometimes a low-grade fever is present. Mild acute attacks usually subside quickly but tend to recur at irregular intervals. Severe attacks may persist for days or weeks.

Intercritical periods are the symptom-free intervals between gout attacks. Most patients have a second attack within 6 months to 2 years, but in some the second attack doesn't occur for 5 to 10 years. Delayed attacks are more common in untreated patients and tend to be longer and more severe than initial attacks. Such attacks are also polyarticular, invariably affecting joints in the feet and legs, and are sometimes accompanied by fever. A migratory attack sequentially strikes various joints and the Achilles tendon and is associated with either subdeltoid or olecranon bursitis.

Eventually, chronic polyarticular gout sets in. This final, unremitting stage of the disease is marked by persistent painful polyarthritis, with large, subcutaneous tophi in cartilage, synovial membranes, tendons, and soft tissue. Tophi form in fingers, hands, knees, feet, ulnar sides of the forearms, helix of the ear, Achilles tendons and, rarely, internal organs, such as the kidneys and myocardium. The skin over the tophus may ulcerate and release a chalky, white exudate or pus. Chronic inflammation and tophaceous deposits precipitate secondary joint degeneration, with eventual erosions, deformity, and disability. Kidney involvement, with associated tubular damage, leads to chronic renal dysfunction. Hypertension and albuminuria occur in some patients; urolithiasis is common.

Diagnosis

CONFIRMING DIAGNOSIS *The presence of monosodium urate monohydrate crystals in synovial fluid taken from an inflamed joint or tophus establishes the diagnosis.*

Aspiration of synovial fluid (arthrocentesis) or of tophaceous material reveals needlelike intracellular crystals of sodium urate. Although hyperuricemia isn't specifically diagnostic of gout, serum uric acid is above normal. Urinary uric acid is usually higher in secondary gout than in primary gout. In acute attacks, erythrocyte sedimentation rate and WBC count may be elevated, and WBC count shifts to the left.

Initially, X-rays are normal. However, in chronic gout, X-rays show "punched out" erosions, sometimes with periosteal overgrowth. Outward displacement of the overhanging margin from the bone contour characterizes gout. X-rays rarely show tophi. (See *Understanding pseudogout.*)

Understanding pseudogout

Also known as *calcium pyrophosphate disease*, pseudogout results when calcium pyrophosphate crystals collect in periarticular joint structures.

Signs and symptoms
Like true gout, pseudogout causes sudden joint pain and swelling, most commonly of the knee, wrist, and ankle or other peripheral joints.

Pseudogout attacks are self-limiting and triggered by stress, trauma, surgery, severe dieting, thiazide therapy, or alcohol abuse. Associated symptoms resemble those of rheumatoid arthritis and osteoarthritis. Many patients may be asymptomatic.

Establishing a diagnosis
Diagnosis of pseudogout hinges on joint aspiration and synovial biopsy to detect calcium pyrophosphate crystals. X-rays show calcium deposits in the fibrocartilage and linear markings along the bone ends. Blood tests may detect an underlying endocrine or metabolic disorder.

Relief for pressure and inflammation
Management of pseudogout may include aspirating the joint to relieve pressure; instilling corticosteroids and administering analgesics, salicylates, phenylbutazone, or other nonsteroidal anti-inflammatory drugs to treat inflammation and, if appropriate, treating the underlying disorder. Without treatment, pseudogout leads to permanent joint damage in about half of those it affects, most of whom are older adults.

Treatment

Correct management seeks to terminate an acute attack, reduce hyperuricemia, and prevent recurrence, complications, and the formation of renal calculi. (See *Preventing gout*.) Colchicine is effective in reducing pain, swelling, and inflammation; pain often subsides within 12 hours of treatment and is completely relieved in 48 hours. Treatment for the patient with acute gout consists of bed rest; immobilization and protection of the inflamed, painful joints; and local application of heat or cold, whichever works for the patient. Maximal doses of non-steroidal anti-inflammatory drugs (NSAIDs) usually provide excellent relief for patients who can tolerate them; doses should be gradually reduced after several days.

ELDER TIP *Older patients are at risk for GI bleeding associated with NSAID use. Encourage the elderly patient to take these drugs with meals and monitor the patient's stools for occult blood.*

Resistant inflammation may require oral corticosteroids or intra-articular corticosteroid injection to relieve pain. Treatment for chronic gout aims to decrease serum uric acid level. Continuing maintenance dosage of allopurinol may be given to suppress uric acid formation or control uric acid levels, preventing further attacks. However, this powerful drug should be used cautiously in patients with renal failure. Uricosuric agents promote uric acid excretion and inhibit accumulation of uric acid, but their value is limited in patients with renal impairment. These medications shouldn't be given to patients with renal calculi.

Adjunctive therapy emphasizes a few dietary restrictions, primarily the avoidance of alcohol and purine-rich foods (organ meats, beer, wine, and certain types of fish are high in purines). Obese patients should try to lose weight because obesity puts additional stress on painful joints.

In some cases, surgery may be necessary to improve joint function or correct deformities. Tophi must be excised and drained if they become infected or ulcerated. They can also be excised to prevent ulceration, improve the patient's appearance, or make it easier for the patient to wear shoes or gloves.

Special considerations

Patient care for gout includes these interventions:

◆ Encourage bed rest but use a bed cradle to keep bedcovers off extremely sensitive, inflamed joints.

◆ Give pain medication, as needed, especially during acute attacks. Apply hot or cold packs to inflamed joints according to what the patient finds effective. Administer anti-inflammatory medication and other drugs, as ordered. Watch for adverse effects. Be alert for GI disturbances with colchicine.

◆ Watch for acute gout attacks 24 to 96 hours after surgery. Even minor surgery can precipitate an attack. Before and after surgery, administer colchicine as ordered, to help prevent gout attacks.

◆ Tell the patient to avoid high-purine foods, such as anchovies, liver, sardines, kidneys, sweetbreads, lentils, and alcoholic

---

PREVENTION

Preventing gout

Because the cause of gout is unknown, the disease can't be prevented. However, it's important to teach your patients how to prevent acute gout attacks to reduce the risk of joint damage. Acute gout attacks can be prevented by dietary changes, weight reduction, adequate fluid intake, and drugs.

Dietary restrictions
Dietary changes include avoidance of foods high in purine, such as alcohol (especially beer and wine), organ meats, sardines, sweetbreads, peas, and lentils.

Weight reduction
Obese patients need to lose weight at a slow rate. Losing weight rapidly may temporarily increase uric acid levels.

Fluid intake
It's also important to drink adequate amounts of fluids to dilute the amount of uric acid in the blood. This will help decrease the risk of kidney stone formation. Taking the prescribed drug slows the production of uric acid and speeds its elimination from the body.

beverages—especially beer and wine—which raise the urate level. Explain the principles of a gradual weight-reduction diet to obese patients.

◆ Advise the patient to report any adverse effects of allopurinol, such as drowsiness, dizziness, nausea, vomiting, urinary frequency, or dermatitis.

NEUROGENIC ARTHROPATHY

Neurogenic arthropathy, also called *Charcot arthropathy*, is a progressively degenerative disease of peripheral and axial joints, resulting from impaired sensory innervation. The loss of sensation in the joints causes progressive deterioration, resulting from trauma or primary disease, which leads to laxity of supporting ligaments and eventual disintegration of the affected joints.

Causes and incidence

Neurogenic arthropathy is most common in men older than 40 years. In adults, the most common cause of neurogenic arthropathy is diabetes mellitus. Other causes include tabes dorsalis (especially among patients 40 to 60 years old), syringomyelia (progresses to neurogenic arthropathy in about 25% of patients), myelopathy of pernicious anemia, spinal cord trauma, paraplegia, hereditary sensory neuropathy, and Charcot–Marie–Tooth disease. Amyloidosis, peripheral nerve injury, myelomeningocele (in children), leprosy, and alcoholism may cause neurogenic arthropathy, but only in rare occurrences.

Frequent intra-articular injection of corticosteroids has also been linked to neurogenic arthropathy. The analgesic effect of the corticosteroids may mask symptoms and allow continuous stress to accelerate joint destruction.

Pathophysiology

Many conditions predispose to neurogenic arthropathy. Impaired deep pain sensation or proprioception affects the joint's normal protective reflexes, often allowing trauma (especially repeated minor episodes) and small periarticular fractures to go unrecognized. Increased blood flow to bone from reflex vasodilation, resulting in active bone resorption, contributes to bone and joint damage.

Each new injury sustained by the joint causes more distortion as it heals. Hemorrhagic joint effusions and multiple small fractures can occur, accelerating disease progression. Ligamentous laxity, muscular hypotonia, and rapid destruction of joint cartilage are common, predisposing to joint dislocations, which also accelerate disease progression. Advanced neurogenic arthropathy can cause hypertrophic changes, destructive changes, or both.

Complications

◆ Joint subluxation or dislocation
◆ Pathologic fractures
◆ Infection
◆ Pseudogout
◆ Neurovascular compression

Signs and symptoms

Neurogenic arthropathy begins insidiously with swelling, warmth, decreased mobility, and instability in a single joint or in many joints. It can progress to deformity. The first clue to vertebral neuroarthropathy, which progresses to gross spinal deformity, may be nothing more than a mild, persistent backache. Characteristically, pain is minimal despite obvious deformity.

The specific joint affected varies according to the underlying cause. Diabetes usually attacks the joints and bones of the feet; tabes dorsalis attacks the large weight-bearing joints, such as the knee, hip, ankle, or lumbar and dorsal vertebrae (Charcot spine); syringomyelia causes occurrence in the shoulder, elbow, or cervical intervertebral joint. Neurogenic arthropathy caused by intra-articular injection of corticosteroids usually develops in the hip or knee joint.

Diagnosis

Patient history of painless joint deformity and underlying primary disease suggests neurogenic arthropathy. Physical examination may reveal bone fragmentation in advanced disease. X-rays confirm diagnosis and assess severity of joint damage. In the early stage of the disease, soft-tissue swelling or effusion may be the only overt effect; in the advanced stage, articular fracture, subluxation, erosion of articular cartilage, periosteal new bone formation, and excessive growth of marginal loose bodies (osteophytosis) or resorption may be seen. CT scan helps define the extent of disease.

Other diagnostic measures include:
◆ vertebral examination: narrowing of disk spaces, deterioration of vertebrae, and osteophyte formation, leading to ankylosis and deforming kyphoscoliosis
◆ synovial biopsy: bony fragments and bits of calcified cartilage.

Treatment

Effective management relieves pain with analgesics and immobilization using crutches, splints, braces, and restriction of weight bearing to the affected joint.

In severe disease, surgery may include arthrodesis or, in severe diabetic neuropathy, amputation. However, surgery risks further damage through nonunion and infection.

Special considerations

Assess the pattern of pain and give analgesics, as needed. Check sensory perception, ROM, alignment, joint swelling, and the status of underlying disease.

◆ Teach the patient to use joint protection techniques, to avoid physically stressful actions that may cause pathologic fractures, and to take safety precautions, such as removing throw rugs and other objects over which the patient may trip.

◆ Advise the patient to report severe joint pain, swelling, or instability. Warm compresses may be applied to relieve local pain and tenderness.

◆ Instruct the patient in the proper technique for crutches or other orthopedic devices. Stress the importance of proper fitting and regular professional readjustment of such devices. Warn the patient that impaired sensation might allow damage from these aids to occur and progress without discomfort.

◆ Emphasize the need to continue regular treatment of the underlying disease.

OSTEOARTHRITIS

Osteoarthritis, the most common form of arthritis, is a chronic disease that causes deterioration of the joint cartilage and formation of reactive new bone at the margins and subchondral areas of the joints. This degeneration results from a breakdown of chondrocytes, most commonly in the distal interphalangeal and proximal interphalangeal joints, but also in the hip and knee joints.

Osteoarthritis is widespread, occurring equally in both sexes. Its earliest symptoms typically begin after age 40 and may progress with advancing age.

Disability depends on the site and severity of involvement and can range from minor limitation of the dexterity of the fingers to severe disability in persons with hip or knee involvement. The rate of progression varies, and joints may remain stable for years in an early stage of deterioration.

Causes and incidence

Studies indicate that osteoarthritis is acquired and probably results from a combination of metabolic, genetic, chemical, and mechanical factors. Secondary osteoarthritis usually follows an identifiable predisposing event—most commonly trauma, metabolic conditions, congenital deformity, or obesity—and leads to degenerative changes.

Osteoarthritis may first appear between ages 30 and 40 and is present in almost everyone by age 70. Before age 55, it affects men and women equally, but after age 55 the incidence is higher in women.

> **ELDER TIP** *Primary osteoarthritis is strongly associated with aging, and indeed aging may predispose to the cartilage degeneration common in persons with osteoarthritis.*

Pathophysiology

The major defect in primary and secondary osteoarthritis is loss of articular cartilage. Articular cartilage is probably lost through enzymatic breakdown of the cartilage matrix—the proteoglycans, glycosaminoglycans, and collagen. Other studies indicate that interleukin-1 may play a part in cartilage destruction.

Osteoarthritis occurs in synovial joints. The joint cartilage deteriorates, and reactive new bone forms at the margins and subchondral areas of the joints. The degeneration results from damage to the chondrocytes. Cartilage softens with age, narrowing the joint space. Mechanical injury erodes articular cartilage, leaving the underlying bone unprotected. This causes sclerosis or thickening and hardening of the bone underneath the cartilage.

Articular cartilage particles within the joint irritate the synovial lining, which becomes fibrotic and limits joint movement. Synovial fluid may be forced into defects in the bone, causing cysts. New bone, called *osteophyte* (bone spur), forms at joint margins as the articular cartilage erodes, causing gross alteration of the bony contours and enlargement of the joint. The spurlike bony projections enlarge until small pieces called joint mice break off into the synovial cavity.

Complications

◆ Flexion contractures
◆ Subluxation and deformity
◆ Ankylosis
◆ Bony cysts
◆ Gross bone overgrowth
◆ Central cord syndrome
◆ Nerve root compression
◆ Cauda equina syndrome

Signs and symptoms

The most common symptom of osteoarthritis is a deep, aching joint pain, particularly after exercise or weight bearing, usually relieved by rest. Other symptoms include stiffness in the morning and after inactivity (improves with activity), aching during changes in weather, "grating" of the joint during motion, altered gait contractures, joint instability, and limited movement. These symptoms increase with poor posture, obesity, and stress to the affected joint.

Osteoarthritis of the interphalangeal joints produces irreversible joint changes and node formation. The nodes eventually become red, swollen, and tender, causing numbness and loss of dexterity. (See *What happens in osteoarthritis*.)

What happens in osteoarthritis

The characteristic breakdown of articular cartilage is a gradual response to aging or to predisposing factors, such as joint abnormalities or traumatic injury.

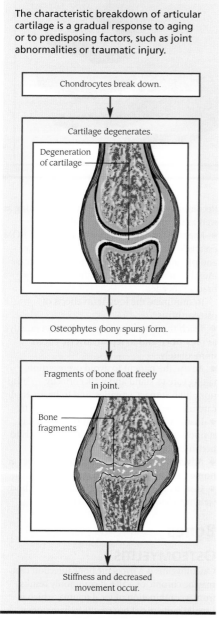

Chondrocytes break down.

↓

Cartilage degenerates.

Degeneration of cartilage —

↓

Osteophytes (bony spurs) form.

↓

Fragments of bone float freely in joint.

Bone fragments —

↓

Stiffness and decreased movement occur.

Diagnosis

A thorough physical examination confirms typical symptoms, and absence of systemic symptoms rules out an inflammatory joint disorder. X-rays of the affected joint help confirm diagnosis of osteoarthritis but may be normal in the early stages. X-rays may require many views and typically show:
◆ narrowing of joint space or margin
◆ cystlike bony deposits in joint space and margins and sclerosis of the subchondral space
◆ joint deformity due to degeneration or articular damage
◆ bony growths at weight-bearing areas
◆ fusion of joints. (See *A close look at the effects of osteoarthritis*, page 306.)

MRI and CT scans may be used to show cartilage breakdown and bone abnormalities. Importantly, MRI can detect signs of inflammation of the bone or the synovial membrane.

Treatment

Treatment is aimed at relieving pain, maintaining or improving mobility, and minimizing disability. Medications include NSAIDs, cyclo-oxygenase-2 inhibitors and, in some cases, intra-articular injections of corticosteroids. Studies indicate that glucosamine and chondroitin may be useful in controlling symptoms and reducing functional impairment. Injecting artificial joint fluid into the knee can provide relief of pain for up to 6 months.

Effective treatment also reduces stress by weight loss and supporting or stabilizing the joint with crutches, braces, cane, walker, cervical collar, or traction. Exercise, such as through physical therapy, is integral to maintaining or improving joint mobility. Other supportive measures include massage, moist heat, paraffin dips for hands, protective techniques to prevent undue stress on the joints, and adequate rest (particularly after activity).

Surgical treatment, such as one of the following, is reserved for patients who have severe disability or uncontrollable pain:
◆ Arthroplasty (partial or total): replacement of deteriorated part of joint with prosthetic appliance
◆ Arthrodesis: surgical fusion of bones, used primarily in spinal surgery (laminectomy)
◆ Osteoplasty: scraping and lavage of deteriorated bone from joint
◆ Osteotomy: change in alignment of bone to relieve stress by excision of wedge of bone or cutting of bone

A close look at the effects of osteoarthritis

Involvement of the interphalangeal (finger bone) joints produces irreversible changes in the distal joints (Heberden nodes) and the proximal joints (Bouchard nodes), as shown below. These nodes can be painless initially, with gradual progression to or sudden flare-ups of redness, swelling, tenderness, and impaired sensation and dexterity.

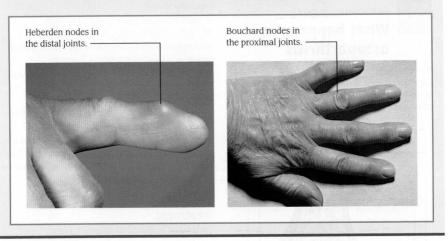

Heberden nodes in the distal joints.

Bouchard nodes in the proximal joints.

Special considerations

Patient care for osteoarthritis includes the following:

◆ Promote adequate rest, particularly after activity. Plan rest periods during the day and provide for adequate sleep at night. Moderation is the key—teach the patient to pace daily activities.

◆ Assist with physical therapy, and encourage the patient to perform gentle, isometric ROM exercises.

◆ Provide emotional support and reassurance to help the patient cope with limited mobility. Explain that osteoarthritis *isn't* a systemic disease.

Specific patient care depends on the affected joint:

◆ *Hand:* Apply hot soaks and paraffin dips to relieve pain, as ordered.

◆ *Spine (lumbar and sacral):* Recommend a firm mattress (or bed board) to decrease morning pain.

◆ *Spine (cervical):* Check cervical collar for constriction; watch for redness with prolonged use.

◆ *Hip:* Use moist heat pads to relieve pain and administer antispasmodic drugs, as ordered. Assist with ROM and strengthening exercises, always making sure the patient gets the proper rest afterward. Check crutches, cane, braces, and walker for proper fit, and teach the patient to use them correctly. For example, the patient with unilateral joint involvement should use an orthopedic appliance such as a walker or a cane.

Recommend the use of cushions when sitting as well as the use of an elevated toilet seat.

◆ *Knee:* Twice daily, assist with prescribed ROM exercises, exercises to maintain muscle tone, and progressive resistance exercises to increase muscle strength. Provide elastic supports or braces if needed.

To minimize the long-term effects of osteoarthritis:

◆ Teach the patient to take medication exactly as prescribed and to report adverse effects immediately.

◆ Advise the patient to avoid overexertion, taking care to stand and walk correctly, to minimize high-impact activities, and to be especially careful when stooping or picking up objects.

◆ Instruct the patient to wear proper-fitting, supportive shoes and not to allow the heels to become worn down.

◆ Advise the patient to install safety devices at home such as guard rails in the bathroom.

◆ Instruct the patient to maintain proper body weight to lessen strain on joints.

Bones

OSTEOMYELITIS

Osteomyelitis is a pyogenic bone infection that may be chronic or acute. It commonly results from a combination of local trauma, which is usually quite trivial but results in hematoma formation, and an acute infection originating elsewhere in the body. Although osteomyelitis usually remains localized, it can spread through the bone to the marrow, cortex, and periosteum. Acute osteomyelitis is usually a blood-borne disease, which most commonly affects rapidly growing children. Chronic osteomyelitis, which is rare, is characterized by multiple draining sinus tracts and metastatic lesions. (See *Stages of osteomyelitis*.)

Causes and incidence

Virtually any pathogenic bacteria can cause osteomyelitis under the right circumstances. Typically, these organisms find a culture site in a hematoma from recent trauma or in a weakened area, such as the site of surgery or local infection (for example, furunculosis), and spread directly to bone. As the organisms grow and form pus within the bone, tension builds within the rigid medullary cavity, forcing pus through the haversian canals. This forms a subperiosteal abscess that deprives the bone of its blood supply and may eventually cause necrosis. In turn, necrosis stimulates the periosteum to create new bone (*involucrum*); the old bone (*sequestrum*) detaches and works its way out through an abscess or the sinuses. By the time sequestrum forms, osteomyelitis is chronic.

Osteomyelitis occurs more commonly in children (especially boys) than in adults—usually as a complication of an acute localized infection. The most common sites in children are the lower end of the femur and the upper end of the tibia, humerus, and radius. The most common sites in adults are the pelvis and vertebrae, generally because of contamination associated with surgery or trauma. Other common sites are sternoclavicular,

sacroiliac, and symphysis pubis. The incidence of both chronic and acute osteomyelitis is declining, except in drug abusers. With prompt treatment, the prognosis for acute osteomyelitis is very good; for chronic osteomyelitis, which is more prevalent in adults, the prognosis is still poor.

Pathophysiology

Typically, bacteria find a culture site in a hematoma from recent trauma or in a weakened area, such as the site of local infection (e.g., furunculosis), and travel through the bloodstream to the metaphysis, the section of a long bone that's continuous with the epiphysis plates, where the blood flows into sinusoids. Predisposing factors include diabetes mellitus, sickle cell disease, and being immunocompromised.

Complications
◆ Chronic osteomyelitis
◆ Poor joint function
◆ Amputation of limb

Signs and symptoms

The onset of acute osteomyelitis is usually rapid, with sudden pain accompanied by tenderness, heat, swelling, and restricted movement of the affected area. Associated systemic symptoms may include tachycardia, sudden fever, nausea, and malaise. Generally, the clinical features of both chronic and acute osteomyelitis are the same, except that chronic infection can persist intermittently for years, flaring up spontaneously after minor trauma. Sometimes, however, the only symptom of chronic infection is the persistent drainage of pus from an old pocket in a sinus tract.

PATHOPHYSIOLOGY
Stages of osteomyelitis

The illustrations show the progression of osteomyelitis.

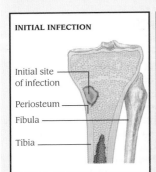

INITIAL INFECTION

Initial site of infection
Periosteum
Fibula
Tibia

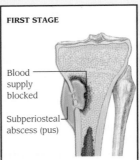

FIRST STAGE

Blood supply blocked
Subperiosteal abscess (pus)

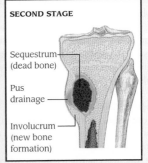

SECOND STAGE

Sequestrum (dead bone)
Pus drainage
Involucrum (new bone formation)

Diagnosis

Patient history, physical examination, and blood tests help to confirm osteomyelitis:

♦ WBC count shows leukocytosis.

♦ Erythrocyte sedimentation rate or C-reactive protein is usually elevated but nonspecific in acute cases.

♦ Cultures of the lesion indicate the source of the organism. Blood cultures help identify causative organism.

♦ MRI is best for detecting spinal infection.

♦ CT is best for visualizing islands of dead bone.

X-rays may not show bone involvement until the disease has been active for some time, usually 2 to 3 weeks. Bone scans can detect early infection. Diagnosis must rule out poliomyelitis, rheumatic fever, myositis, and bone fractures.

℞ CONFIRMING DIAGNOSIS *The gold standard for diagnosing osteomyelitis is histopathologic and microscopic examination of bone.*

Treatment

Treatment for acute osteomyelitis should begin before definitive diagnosis. Treatment includes administration of antibiotics after blood cultures are taken; early surgical drainage to relieve pressure buildup and sequestrum formation; immobilization of the affected bone by a cast, traction, or bed rest; and supportive measures, such as analgesics and I.V. fluids.

If an abscess forms, treatment includes incision and drainage, followed by a culture of the drained fluid. Intracavitary instillation of antibiotics may be done through closed-system continuous irrigation with low intermittent suction; limited irrigation with blood drainage system with suction; or local application of packed, wet, antibiotic-soaked dressings.

In addition to these therapies, chronic osteomyelitis usually requires surgery to remove dead bone (*sequestrectomy*) and to promote drainage (*saucerization*). The area may be filled with bone graft or packing material to promote new bone tissue. An infected prosthesis is removed and a new one is implanted the same day or after resolution of the infection.

Some centers use hyperbaric oxygen to increase the activity of naturally occurring leukocytes. Free-tissue transfers and local muscle flaps are also used to fill in dead space and increase blood supply.

Special considerations

Your major concerns are to control infection, protect the bone from injury, and offer meticulous supportive care.

♦ Use strict sterile technique when changing dressings and irrigating wounds. If the patient is in skeletal traction for compound fractures, cover insertion points of pin tracks with small, dry dressings, and instruct not to touch the skin around the pins and wires.

♦ Administer I.V. fluids to maintain adequate hydration as necessary. Provide a diet high in protein and vitamin C.

♦ Assess vital signs, wound appearance, and new pain, which may indicate secondary infection, daily.

♦ Carefully monitor suctioning equipment and the amount of solution it instills and suctions.

♦ Support the affected limb with firm pillows. Keep the limb level with the body; *don't* let it sag. Turn the patient gently every 2 hours and watch for signs of developing pressure ulcers. Report any signs of pressure ulcer formation immediately.

♦ Support the cast with firm pillows and smooth rough cast edges by petaling with pieces of adhesive tape or moleskin. Check circulation and drainage; if a wet spot appears on the cast, circle it with a marking pen, and note the time of appearance (on the cast). Be aware of how much drainage is expected. Check the circled spot at least every 4 hours and report any enlargement immediately.

♦ Protect the patient from mishaps, such as jerky movements and falls, which may threaten bone integrity. Report sudden pain, crepitus, or deformity immediately. Watch for any sudden malposition of the limb, which may indicate fracture.

♦ Provide emotional support and appropriate diversions. Before discharge, teach the patient how to protect and clean the wound and, most importantly, how to recognize signs of recurring infection (increased temperature, redness, localized heat, and swelling). Stress the need for follow-up examinations. Instruct the patient to seek prompt treatment for possible sources of recurrence—blisters, boils, styes, and impetigo.

OSTEOPOROSIS

Osteoporosis is a metabolic bone disorder in which the rate of bone resorption accelerates while the rate of bone formation slows down, causing a loss of bone mass. Bones affected by this disease lose calcium and phosphate salts and thus become porous, brittle, and abnormally vulnerable to fractures. Osteoporosis may be primary or secondary to an underlying disease. Primary osteoporosis is commonly called *postmenopausal osteoporosis* because it typically develops in postmenopausal women. (See *What is osteoporosis,* page 309.)

PATHOPHYSIOLOGY
What is osteoporosis?

Osteoporosis is a metabolic disease of the skeleton that reduces the amount of bone tissue. Bones weaken as local cells resorb, or take up, bone tissue. Trabecular bone at the core becomes less dense, and cortical bone on the perimeter losses thickness.

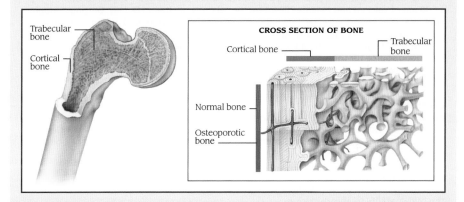

Causes and incidence

The cause of primary osteoporosis is unknown; however, a mild but prolonged negative calcium balance, resulting from an inadequate dietary intake of calcium, may be an important contributing factor—as may declining gonadal or adrenal function, faulty protein metabolism due to estrogen deficiency, and sedentary lifestyle. (See *Preventing osteoporosis*, page 310.) Causes of secondary osteoporosis are many: prolonged therapy with steroids or heparin, cigarette smoking, total immobilization or disuse of a bone (as with hemiplegia, for example), alcoholism, malnutrition, malabsorption, celiac disease, scurvy, lactose intolerance, osteogenesis imperfecta, Sudeck atrophy (localized to hands and feet, with recurring attacks), and endocrine disorders (hypopituitarism, acromegaly, thyrotoxicosis, long-standing diabetes mellitus, hyperthyroidism).

The incidence of osteoporosis is high, with an estimated 10 million U.S. residents suffering from osteoporosis and another 18 million suffering from low bone mass, or osteopenia. Incidence is higher in women than in men, with women older than 50 years accounting for 20% of cases. Another 30% of women have osteopenia, which can deteriorate into osteoporosis.

Pathophysiology

In normal bone, the rates of bone formation and resorption are constant; replacement follows resorption immediately, and the amount of bone replaced equals the amount of bone resorbed. Osteoporosis develops when the remodeling cycle is interrupted, and new bone formation falls behind resorption.

When bone is resorbed faster than it forms, the bone becomes less dense. Men have about 30% greater bone mass than women, which may explain why osteoporosis develops later in men.

Complication

◆ Bone fractures, especially in vertebrae, femoral neck, and distal radius

Signs and symptoms

Osteoporosis is usually discovered incidentally on X-ray; the patient may have been asymptomatic for years. Vertebral collapse, causing a backache with pain that radiates around the trunk, is the most common presenting feature. Any movement or jarring aggravates the backache.

In another common pattern, osteoporosis can develop insidiously, with increasing deformity, kyphosis, and loss of height. Sometimes a dowager hump is present. As bones weaken, spontaneous wedge fractures, pathologic fractures of the neck or femur, Colles fractures after a minor fall, and hip fractures become increasingly common.

ELDER TIP *Osteoporosis usually affects older people and is a major risk factor in vertebral compression fractures and hip fractures.*

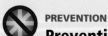

PREVENTION
Preventing osteoporosis

To help prevent osteoporosis, tell the patient to follow these guidelines.

Maintain adequate calcium and vitamin D intake
Postmenopausal women and all men and women older than 65 years should consume 1,500 mg of calcium and at least 800 international units of vitamin D daily. Getting enough vitamin D is as important as getting enough calcium because vitamin D aids in absorption of calcium and improves muscle strength.

Most people get adequate amounts of vitamin D from sunlight; however, this may not be a good source for those who live in high latitudes, are housebound, or regularly use sunscreen or avoid the sun entirely because of the risk of skin cancer. Calcium supplements with added vitamin D are a good alternative.

Exercise
Exercise can help build strong bones and slow bone loss. Strength-training exercises should be combined with weight-bearing exercises. Strength training helps strengthen muscles and bones in the arms and upper spine, and weight-bearing exercises mainly affect the bones in the legs, hips, and lower spine.

Limit alcohol intake
Consuming more than two alcoholic drinks a day may decrease bone formation and reduce the body's ability to absorb calcium.

Limit caffeine
Limit the amount of caffeinated beverages to about two to three cups of coffee a day. If the diet contains adequate calcium, moderate caffeine consumption won't harm you. Don't forget to count caffeine-containing beverages such as colas and teas.

Osteoporosis primarily affects the weight-bearing vertebrae. Only when the condition is advanced or severe, as in Cushing syndrome or hyperthyroidism, do comparable changes occur in the skull, ribs, and long bones.

Diagnosis
Differential diagnosis must exclude other causes of rarefying bone disease, especially those affecting the spine, such as metastatic cancer and advanced multiple myeloma. The differential diagnosis should also exclude osteomalacia, osteogenesis imperfecta tarda, skeletal hyperparathyroidism, and hyperthyroidism. Initial evaluation attempts to identify the specific cause of osteoporosis through the patient history.

♦ Bone mineral density testing is performed in dual-energy X-ray absorptiometry (DEXA) and measures the mineralization of bones. It's the gold standard for evaluating osteoporosis.
♦ A spine CT scan shows demineralization. Quantitative CT can evaluate bone density but is less available and more expensive than DEXA.
♦ X-rays show fracture or vertebral collapse in severe cases.

♦ Urine calcium can provide evidence of bone turnover but is limited in value. Newer tests include urinary N-telopeptide to help diagnose osteoporosis.

Treatment
Treatment aims to slow down or prevent bone loss, prevent additional fractures, and control pain. A physical therapy program that emphasizes gentle exercise and activity is an important part of the treatment. Medications may include bisphosphonates, such as alendronate and risedronate, to prevent bone loss and reduce the risk of fractures. The physician may also recommend adequate calcium and vitamin D intake. Raloxifene and calcitonin have also been prescribed. Weakened vertebrae should be supported, usually with a back brace. Surgery can correct pathologic fractures of the femur by open reduction and internal fixation. Colles fracture requires reduction with casting immobilization for 4 to 10 weeks.

The incidence of primary osteoporosis may be reduced through adequate intake of dietary calcium and regular exercise. Fluoride treatments may also offer some preventive benefit.

Hormone replacement therapy (HRT) with estrogen and progesterone may retard bone loss and prevent the occurrence of fractures; however, this therapy remains controversial. HRT decreases bone reabsorption and increases bone mass. Secondary osteoporosis can be prevented through effective treatment of the underlying disease as well as corticosteroid therapy, early mobilization after surgery or trauma, careful observation for signs of malabsorption, and prompt treatment of hyperthyroidism. Men with osteoporosis, hypogonadism, and low libido may benefit from testosterone replacement therapy. Decreased alcohol consumption and caffeine use, as well as smoking cessation, are also helpful preventive measures.

Special considerations

Your care plan should focus on the patient's fragility, stressing careful positioning, ambulation, and prescribed exercises.

◆ Check the patient's skin daily for redness, warmth, and new sites of pain, which may indicate new fractures. Encourage activity; help the patient walk several times daily. As appropriate, perform passive ROM exercises or encourage the patient to perform active exercises. Make sure the patient regularly attends scheduled physical therapy sessions.

◆ Impose safety precautions. Keep the side rails of the patient's bed in raised position. Move the patient gently and carefully always. Explain to the patient's family and ancillary health care personnel how easily an osteoporotic patient's bones can fracture.

◆ Provide a balanced diet, high in nutrients that support skeletal metabolism: vitamin D, calcium, and protein. Administer analgesics and heat to relieve pain.

◆ Make sure the patient and the family clearly understand the prescribed drug regimen. Tell them how to recognize significant adverse effects and to report them immediately. The patient should also report any new pain sites immediately, especially after trauma, no matter how slight. Advise the patient to sleep on a firm mattress and avoid excessive bed rest. Ensure the patient knows how to wear the back brace.

◆ Thoroughly explain osteoporosis to the patient and the family. If the patient/family don't understand the nature of this disease, they may feel the fractures could have been prevented if they had been more careful.

◆ Teach the patient to use good body mechanics—to stoop before lifting anything and to avoid twisting movements and prolonged bending.

LEGG–CALVÉ–PERTHES DISEASE

Legg–Calvé–Perthes disease (also called *coxa plana*) is ischemic necrosis that leads to eventual flattening of the head of the femur caused by vascular interruption. The disease occurs in five stages.

◆ Growth arrest: Avascular phase; may last 6 to 12 months. Early changes include inflammation and synovitis of the hip and ischemic changes in the ossific nucleus of the femoral head.

◆ Subchondral fracture: Radiographic visualization of the fracture varies with the age of the child at clinical onset and the extent of epiphyseal involvement; may last 3 to 8½ months.

◆ Reabsorption, also called *fragmentation* or *necrosis:* The necrotic bone beneath the subchondral fracture is gradually and irregularly reabsorbed; lasts 6 to 12 months.

◆ Reossification, or healing stage: Ossification of the primary bone begins irregularly in the subchondral area and progresses centrally; takes 6 to 24 months.

◆ Healed stage, also called *residual stage:* Complete ossification of the epiphysis of the femoral head, with or without residual deformity.

Although this disease usually runs its course in 3 to 4 years, it may lead to premature osteoarthritis later in life from misalignment of the acetabulum and flattening of the femoral head.

Causes and incidence

The exact vascular obstructive changes that initiate Legg–Calvé–Perthes disease are unknown. Current etiologic theories include venous obstruction with secondary intraepiphyseal thrombosis, trauma to retinacular vessels, vascular irregularities (congenital or developmental), vascular occlusion secondary to increased intracapsular pressure from acute transient synovitis, and increased blood viscosity resulting in stasis and decreased blood flow.

Legg–Calvé–Perthes disease occurs most frequently in boys 4 to 10 years old and tends to occur in families. Although typically unilateral, it occurs bilaterally in 20% of patients.

Pathophysiology

The disease occurs in four stages. The first stage, synovitis, is characterized by synovial inflammation and increased joint fluid, and typically lasts 1 to 3 weeks. In the second (avascular) stage, vascular interruption causes necrosis of the ossification center of the femoral head (usually in several months to 1 year). In the third stage (which ordinarily lasts 2 to 4 years), revascularization, a new blood supply causes bone resorption and deposition of immature bone cells. New bone replaces necrotic bone and the femoral head gradually reforms. The final, or residual, stage involves healing and regeneration. Immature bone cells are replaced by normal bone cells, thereby fixing the joint's shape. There may or may not be residual deformity, based on the degree of necrosis that occurred in stage two.

Complications
◆ Permanent disability
◆ Premature osteoarthritis

Signs and symptoms
The first indication of Legg–Calvé–Perthes disease is usually a persistent thigh pain or limp that becomes progressively severe. This symptom appears during the second stage, when bone resorption and deformity begin. Other effects may include mild pain in the hip, thigh, or knee that's aggravated by activity and relieved by rest; muscle spasm; atrophy of muscles in the upper thigh; slight shortening of the leg; and severely restricted abduction and internal rotation of the hip.

Diagnosis
CONFIRMING DIAGNOSIS *A thorough physical examination and clinical history suggest Legg–Calvé–Perthes disease. Hip X-rays confirm the diagnosis, with findings that vary according to the stage of the disease. Anterior–posterior X-ray and MRI enhance early diagnosis of necrosis and visualization of articular surface.*

Diagnostic evaluation must also differentiate between Legg–Calvé–Perthes disease (restriction of only the abduction and rotation of the hip) and infection or arthritis (restriction of all motion). Aspiration and culture of synovial fluid rule out joint sepsis.

Treatment
The aim of treatment is to protect the femoral head from further stress and damage by containing it within the acetabulum. After 1 to 2 weeks of bed rest, therapy may include reduced weight bearing by means of bed rest in bilateral split counterpoised traction, then application of hip abduction splint or cast, or weight bearing while a splint, cast, or brace holds the leg in abduction. Braces may remain in place for 6 to 18 months. Analgesics help relieve pain. Physical therapy with passive and active ROM exercises after cast removal helps restore motion.

For a young child in the early stages of the disease, osteotomy and subtrochanteric derotation provide maximum confinement of the epiphysis within the acetabulum to allow return of the femoral head to normal shape and full ROM. Proper placement of the epiphysis thus allows remolding with ambulation. Postoperatively, the patient requires a spica cast for about 2 months.

Special considerations
When caring for the hospitalized child, do the following.
◆ Monitor the patient's fluid intake and output. Maintain sufficient fluid balance. Provide a diet sufficient for growth without causing excessive weight gain, which might necessitate cast change and loss of the corrective position.
◆ Provide cast care. Turn the child every 2 to 3 hours to expose the cast to air. When the cast is still wet, turn the child with your palms because depressions in the plaster may lead to pressure ulcers. After the cast dries, petal it with pieces of adhesive tape or moleskin, changing them as they become soiled. Protect the cast with a plastic covering during each bowel movement.
◆ Watch for circulatory or neurologic changes in the leg. Check toes for color, temperature, swelling, sensation, and motion; report dusky, cool, numb toes immediately. Check the skin under the cast with a flashlight every 4 hours while the patient is awake. Follow a consistent plan of skin care to prevent skin breakdown. *Never* use oils or powders under the cast because they increase skin breakdown and soften the cast. Check under the cast daily for odors, particularly after surgery, to detect skin breakdown or wound problems. Report persistent soreness.
◆ Relieve itching by using a hair dryer (set on cool) at the cast edges; this also decreases dampness from perspiration. If itching becomes excessive, get an order for an antipruritic. *Never* insert an object under the cast to scratch.
◆ Provide continuous emotional support. Explain all procedures and the need for bed rest, cast, or braces to the child; encourage the child to verbalize fears and anxiety. Encourage parents to participate in their child's care. Teach them proper cast care and how to recognize signs of skin breakdown. Offer tips for making home management of the bedridden child easier. Tell them what special supplies are needed: pajamas and trousers a size larger (open the side seam, and attach Velcro fasteners to close it), bedpan, adhesive tape, moleskin and, possibly, a hospital bed.
◆ When the cast is removed, debride dry, scaly skin *gradually* by applying lotion after bathing.
◆ Stress the need for follow-up care to monitor rehabilitation. Also stress home tutoring and

socialization to promote normal mental and emotional growth and development.

OSGOOD–SCHLATTER DISEASE

Osgood–Schlatter disease, also called *osteochondrosis*, is a painful, incomplete separation of the epiphysis of the tibial tubercle from the tibial shaft. This is the common cause of knee pain in an adolescent. Severe disease may cause permanent tubercle enlargement.

Causes and incidence

Osgood–Schlatter disease probably results from trauma before the complete fusion of the epiphysis to the main bone has occurred (between ages 10 and 15). Other causes include locally deficient blood supply and genetic factors. It's most common in active adolescent boys, generally affecting one or both knees. It may occur in girls, typically between ages 10 and 11.

Pathophysiology

The proximal tibia has two ossification centers, the proximal tibial epiphysis and the tibial tuberosity, which are separated by a cartilage bridge. Before ossification, the tibial tuberosity is composed of fibrocartilage that has good tensile strength. However, during ossification, columnated cartilaginous cells with poor tensile strength replace the fibrocartilage, and it is within this small window between fibrocartilage and ossified matrix that the tibial tuberosity is at risk of avulsion fractures.

Complications

◆ Irregular growth
◆ Partial avascular necrosis of proximal tibial epiphysis

Signs and symptoms

The patient complains of constant aching and pain and tenderness over the tibial tubercle, which worsens during any activity that causes forceful contraction of the patellar tendon on the tubercle, such as ascending or descending stairs, running, squatting, jumping, or forced flexion. The pain may be associated with some obvious soft-tissue swelling and localized heat and tenderness.

Diagnosis

Physical examination supports the diagnosis: the examiner forces the tibia into internal rotation while slowly extending the patient's knee from 90 degrees of flexion; at about 30 degrees, flexion produces pain that subsides immediately with external rotation of the tibia. Visible

soft-tissue edema may be present over proximal tibial tuberosity with tenderness to palpation. Some patients' quadriceps may atrophy.

X-rays may be normal or show epiphyseal separation and soft-tissue swelling for up to 6 months after onset; eventually, they may show bone fragmentation. Bone scan may show increased uptake in the tibial tuberosity—even greater than the typical increased uptake in the normal epiphysis of the unaffected side.

Treatment

Osteochondrosis is usually self-limiting, and conservative treatment designed to reduce pain and decrease stress to the affected knee is usually adequate. Avoid strenuous exercises that involve the knee; use frequent ice applications after exercise for pain. Rest and quadriceps strengthening, hip extension, adductor strengthening, and hamstring and quadriceps-stretching exercises are recommended. Knee immobilization in extension for 6 to 8 weeks may be necessary. Analgesics and NSAIDs may be given for pain relief and reduction of local swelling.

Rarely, conservative measures fail, and surgery may be necessary. Such surgery includes removal or fixation of the epiphysis or drilling holes through the tubercle to the main bone to form channels for rapid revascularization.

Special considerations

The following special considerations should be observed for patients with Osgood–Schlatter disease:
◆ Monitor the patient's circulation, sensation, and pain, and watch for excessive bleeding after surgery.
◆ Assess daily for limitation of motion. Administer analgesics as needed.
◆ Make sure knee support or splint isn't too tight. Keep the cast dry and clean, and petal it around the top and bottom margins to avoid skin irritation. Teach proper use of crutches. Tell the patient to protect the injured knee with padding and to avoid trauma and repeated flexion (running, contact sports).
◆ Monitor for muscle atrophy.
◆ Give reassurance and emotional support because disruption of normal activities is difficult for an active teenager. Emphasize that restrictions are temporary.

PAGET DISEASE

Paget disease, also called *osteitis deformans*, is a slowly progressive metabolic bone disease characterized by an initial phase of excessive bone resorption (osteoclastic phase), followed by a reactive phase of excessive abnormal bone formation (osteoblastic phase). The new bone structure, which is chaotic, fragile, and weak, causes painful deformities of both external contour and internal structure. Paget disease usually localizes in one or more areas of the skeleton, but occasionally skeletal deformity is widely distributed. The bones most frequently affected are pelvis, leg, spine, arm, collar, and skull. It can be fatal, particularly when it's associated with heart failure (widespread disease creates a continuous need for high cardiac output), bone sarcoma, or giant-cell tumors.

Causes and incidence

The disease occurs worldwide, but is more common in Europe, Australia, and New Zealand, where it's seen in up to 5% of the elderly population. The incidence is higher in men than in women and usually occurs in patients older than 40 years. Although its exact cause is unknown, one theory holds that early viral infection causes a dormant skeletal infection that erupts many years later as Paget disease. Genetic factors are also suspected.

Pathophysiology

Repeated episodes of accelerated osteoclastic resorption of spongy bone occur. The trabeculae diminish, and vascular fibrous tissue replaces marrow. This is followed by short periods of rapid, abnormal bone formation. The collagen fibers in this new bone are disorganized, and glycoprotein levels in the matrix decrease. The partially resorbed trabeculae thicken and enlarge because of excessive bone formation, and the bone becomes soft and weak.

Eventually, Paget disease progresses to an inactive phase in which abnormal remodeling is minimal or absent.

Complications

◆ Fractures
◆ Vertebral collapse
◆ Paraplegia
◆ Blindness and hearing loss (impingement on cranial nerves)
◆ Osteoarthritis
◆ Sarcoma
◆ Hypertension
◆ Renal calculi
◆ Hypercalcemia
◆ Gout

Signs and symptoms

Clinical effects of Paget disease vary. Early stages may be asymptomatic, but when pain does develop, it's usually severe and persistent and may coexist with impaired movement resulting from

impingement of abnormal bone on the spinal cord or sensory nerve root. Such pain intensifies with weight bearing.

The patient with skull involvement shows characteristic cranial enlargement over frontal and occipital areas (hat size may increase) and may complain of headaches. Other deformities include kyphosis (spinal curvature due to compression fractures of pagetic vertebrae), accompanied by a barrel-shaped chest and asymmetrical bowing of the tibia and femur, which commonly reduces height. Pagetic sites are warm and tender and are susceptible to pathologic fractures after minor trauma. Pagetic fractures heal slowly and usually incompletely.

Bony impingement on the cranial nerves may cause blindness and hearing loss with tinnitus and vertigo. Other complications include hypertension, renal calculi, hypercalcemia, gout, heart failure, a waddling gait (from softening of pelvic bones), and hearing loss.

Diagnosis

X-rays taken before overt symptoms develop show increased bone expansion and density. A bone scan, which is more sensitive than X-rays, clearly shows early pagetic lesions (radioisotope collects around areas of active disease). CT scan or MRI shows extra bony extension if sarcomatous degeneration occurs. Bone biopsy reveals characteristic mosaic pattern.

Other laboratory findings include:
◆ elevated serum alkaline phosphatase levels (an index of osteoblastic activity and bone formation)
◆ elevated serum calcium

Increasing use of routine chemistry screens (including serum alkaline phosphatase) is making early diagnosis more common. Serum osteocalcin and N-telopeptide are usually increased.

Treatment

Primary treatment consists of drug therapy and includes one of the following:
◆ Calcitonin (subcutaneously or intranasally) is used to retard bone resorption (which relieves bone lesions) and reduce levels of serum alkaline phosphate and urinary hydroxyproline secretion. Although calcitonin therapy requires long-term maintenance, improvement is noticeable after the first few weeks of treatment.
◆ Bisphosphonates, such as alendronate, ibandronate, pamidronate, risedronate, and zoledronic acid, produce rapid reduction in bone turnover and relieve pain. They also reduce serum alkaline phosphate and urinary hydroxyproline secretion. Therapy produces noticeable improvement after 1 to 3 months.

◆ Plicamycin, a cytotoxic antibiotic, is used to decrease calcium, urinary hydroxyproline, and serum alkaline phosphatase. It produces remission of symptoms within 2 weeks and biochemical improvement in 1 to 2 months. Plicamycin is used to control the disease and is reserved for severe cases with neurologic compromise and for those resistant to other therapies. However, it may destroy platelets or compromise renal function.

Orthopedic surgery is used to correct specific deformities in severe cases, reduce or prevent pathologic fractures, correct secondary deformities, or relieve neurologic impairment. Joint replacement is difficult because bonding material (methyl methacrylate) doesn't set properly on pagetic bone.

Other treatment varies according to symptoms. Analgesics or NSAIDs may be given to control pain.

Special considerations

Patients with Paget disease require the following special considerations:
◆ To evaluate the effectiveness of analgesics, assess level of pain daily. Watch for new areas of pain or restricted movements, which may indicate new fracture sites, and sensory or motor disturbances, such as difficulty in hearing, seeing, or walking.
◆ Monitor serum calcium and alkaline phosphatase levels.
◆ If the patient is confined to prolonged bed rest, prevent pressure ulcers by providing good skin care. Reposition the patient frequently and use a flotation mattress. Provide high-topped sneakers to prevent footdrop.
◆ Monitor intake and output. Encourage adequate fluid intake to minimize renal calculi formation.
◆ Demonstrate how to inject calcitonin and rotate injection sites properly or how to perform nasal inhalation of the drug if that's the form prescribed. Warn the patient that adverse effects may occur (nausea, vomiting, local inflammatory reaction at injection site, facial flushing, itching of hands, and fever). Give reassurance that these adverse effects are usually mild and infrequent.
◆ To help the patient adjust to the changes in lifestyle imposed by this disease, teach how to pace activities and, if necessary, how to use assistive devices. Encourage the patient to follow a recommended exercise program, avoiding both immobilization and excessive activity. Suggest a firm mattress or a bed board to minimize spinal deformities. Warn against imprudent use of analgesics because diminished sensitivity to

pain resulting from analgesic use may make the patient unaware of new fractures. To prevent falls at home, advise removal of throw rugs and other obstacles.
◆ Help the patient and family make use of community support resources, such as a visiting nurse or home health agency. For more information, refer them to the Paget's Disease Foundation.

HALLUX VALGUS

Hallux valgus is a lateral deviation of the great toe at the metatarsophalangeal joint. It occurs with medial enlargement of the first metatarsal head and bunion formation (bursa and callus formation at the bony prominence).

Causes and incidence

Hallux valgus may be acquired or congenital. Acquired hallux valgus results from degenerative arthritis or prolonged pressure on the foot, especially from narrow-toed or high-heeled shoes that compress the forefoot. Bony alignment is normal at the outset of the disorder. This form typically occurs more frequently in women.

In congenital hallux valgus, abnormal bony alignment—increased space between first and second metatarsal (metatarsus primus varus)—causes bunion formation. This form is usually first observed in childhood.

Pathophysiology

During the gait cycle, the hallux and digits generally remain parallel to the long axis of the foot, regardless of the degree of forefoot abduction (or pronation) occurring. This is because of the pull of the conjoined adductor tendon, extensor hallucis longus, and flexor hallucis longus tendons. The tendons gain greater mechanical advantage the further the joint is displaced, with tension created in the medial aspect of the joint and compression laterally.

Line of pull of extensor hallucis longus causing metatarsal to deviate medially and hallux to deviate laterally.

Medial tension causes the medial collateral ligaments to pull on the dorsomedial aspect of the first metatarsal head, causing bone proliferation. Lateral tension causes the sesamoid apparatus to fixate in a laterally dislocated position. Remodeling also occurs laterally in addition to medially, as evidenced by the increase in the proximal articular set angle or structural remodeling of the cartilage. Therefore, without correction of the biomechanical factors, excessive pronation continues, with propagation of the deformity.

Complications
◆ Foot deformity
◆ Difficulty walking

Signs and symptoms
Hallux valgus characteristically begins as a tender bunion covered by deformed, hard, erythematous skin and palpable bursa, typically distended with fluid. The first indication of hallux valgus may be pain over the bunion from shoe pressure. Pain can also stem from traumatic arthritis, bursitis, or abnormal stresses on the foot because hallux valgus changes the body's weight-bearing pattern. In an advanced stage, a flat, splayed forefoot may occur, with severely curled toes (*hammer toes*) and formation of a small bunion on the fifth metatarsal. (See *Hammer toe*.)

Diagnosis

℞ CONFIRMING DIAGNOSIS A red, tender bunion makes hallux valgus obvious. X-rays confirm the diagnosis by showing medial deviation of the first metatarsal and lateral deviation of the great toe.

Treatment
In the very early stages of acquired hallux valgus, good foot care and wide-toed shoes may eliminate the need for further treatment. Other useful measures for early management include felt pads to protect the bunion, foam pads or other devices to separate the first and second toes at night, and a supportive pad and exercises to strengthen the metatarsal arch. Early treatment is vital in patients predisposed to foot problems, such as those with rheumatoid arthritis or diabetes mellitus. If the disease progresses to severe deformity with disabling pain, bunionectomy is necessary.

After surgery, the toe is immobilized in its corrected position in one of two ways: with a soft compression dressing that may cover the entire foot or just the great toe and the second toe, thereby serving as a splint, or with a short cast such as a light slipper spica cast.

The patient may need crutches or controlled weight bearing. Depending on the extent of the surgery, some patients walk on their heels a few days after surgery; others must wait 4 to 6 weeks to bear weight on the affected foot. Supportive treatment may include physical therapy, such as warm compresses, soaks, and exercises, and analgesics to relieve pain and stiffness.

Special considerations
Before surgery, obtain a patient history and assess the neurovascular status of the foot (temperature, color, sensation, and blanching sign). If necessary, teach the patient how to walk with crutches.

After bunionectomy:
◆ Apply ice to reduce swelling. Support the patient's foot with pillows, elevate the foot of the bed, or put the bed in Trendelenburg position.
◆ Record the neurovascular status of the toes, including the patient's ability to move the toes (dressing may inhibit movement), every hour for the first 24 hours and then every 4 hours. Report any change in neurovascular status to the surgeon immediately.
◆ Prepare the patient for walking by instructing to dangle the affected foot over the side of the bed for a short time before standing, allowing a

Hammer toe

In hammer toe, the toe assumes a clawlike appearance from hyperextension of the metatarsophalangeal joint, flexion of the proximal interphalangeal joint, and hyperextension of the distal interphalangeal joint, usually under pressure from hallux valgus displacement. A painful corn forms on the back of the interphalangeal joint and on the bone end, and a callus forms on the sole of the foot, both of which make walking painful. Hammer toe may be mild or severe and can affect one toe or all five, as in clawfoot (which also causes a very high arch).

Hammer toe can be congenital (and familial) or acquired from constantly wearing short, narrow shoes, which put pressure on the end of the long toe. Acquired hammer toe is commonly bilateral and often develops in children who rapidly outgrow shoes and socks.

In young children, or adults with early deformity, repeated foot manipulation and splinting of the affected toe relieve discomfort and may correct the deformity. Other treatment includes protection of protruding joints with felt pads, corrective footwear (open-toed shoes and sandals or special shoes that conform to the shape of the foot), the use of a metatarsal arch support, and exercises, such as passive manual stretching of the proximal interphalangeal joint. Severe deformity requires surgical fusion of the proximal interphalangeal joint in a straight position.

gradual increase in venous pressure. If crutches are needed, supervise the patient in using them, and make sure this skill is mastered before discharge. The patient should have a proper cast shoe or boot to protect the cast or dressing.

◆ Before discharge, instruct the patient to limit activities, to rest frequently with feet elevated, to elevate feet whenever pain or swelling is experienced, and to wear wide-toed shoes and sandals after the dressings are removed. Urge female patients not to resume wearing high-heeled, pointy-toed shoes.

◆ Teach proper foot care, such as cleanliness, massages, and cutting toenails straight across to prevent ingrown nails and infection.

◆ Suggest exercises to do at home to strengthen foot muscles, such as standing at the edge of a step on the heel and then raising and inverting the top of the foot.

◆ Stress the importance of follow-up care and prompt medical attention for painful bunions, corns, and calluses.

KYPHOSIS

Kyphosis, also called *roundback* or *hunchback*, is an anteroposterior curving of the spine that causes a bowing of the back, commonly at the thoracic, but sometimes at the thoracolumbar or sacral, level. The normal spine displays some convexity, but excessive thoracic kyphosis is pathologic.

Causes and incidence

Kyphosis occurs in children and adults. Although congenital kyphosis is rare, it's usually severe, with resultant cosmetic deformity and reduced pulmonary function.

Adolescent kyphosis (also called *Scheuermann disease*, *juvenile kyphosis*, and *vertebral epiphysitis*), the most common form of this disorder, may result from growth retardation or a vascular disturbance in the vertebral epiphysis (usually at the thoracic level) during periods of rapid growth or from congenital deficiency in the thickness of the vertebral plates. Other causes include infection, inflammation, aseptic necrosis, and disk degeneration. The subsequent stress of weight bearing on the compromised vertebrae may result in the thoracic hump commonly seen in adolescents with kyphosis. Symptomatic adolescent kyphosis is more prevalent in girls than in boys and occurs most commonly between ages 12 and 16.

Adult kyphosis (adult roundback) may result from aging and associated degeneration of intervertebral disks, atrophy, and osteoporotic collapse of the vertebrae; from endocrine disorders, such as hyperparathyroidism and Cushing disease; and from prolonged steroid therapy. Adult kyphosis may also result from conditions such as arthritis, Paget disease, polio, compression fracture of the thoracic vertebrae, metastatic tumor, plasma cell myeloma, or tuberculosis (TB). In both children and adults, kyphosis may also result from poor posture.

Disk lesions called *Schmorl nodes* may develop in anteroposterior curving of the spine and are localized protrusions of nuclear material through the cartilage plates and into the spongy bone of the vertebral bodies. If the anterior portions of the cartilage are destroyed, bridges of new bone may transverse the intervertebral space, causing ankylosis.

Pathophysiology

The pathophysiology of kyphosis depends on the etiologic factor. The exact cause of Scheuermann disease is still imprecisely defined. Scheuermann postulated that the condition resulted from avascular necrosis of the apophyseal ring. Other theories include histologic abnormalities at the endplate, osteoporosis, and mechanical factors that affect spinal growth. A Danish study demonstrated an important genetic component to the entity.

Postural kyphosis is present when accentuated kyphosis is observed without the characteristic 5 degrees of wedging over three consecutive vertebral segments that defines Scheuermann kyphosis. This is felt to be due to muscular imbalance leading to the roundback appearance of these individuals.

When focal kyphosis occurs after a fracture, more height is lost in the anterior aspect than in the posterior aspect; this is the typical fracture pattern. The angulation can increase as the fracture heals, placing pressure on the spinal cord. Patients with fractures have historically been treated with laminectomy alone, especially in the thoracic spine, and they often had progressive kyphosis at the fracture site.

Postinfectious kyphosis occurs in a manner similar to that just described. The mechanical integrity of the anterior column is lost as a consequence of the infectious process. Bending forces then accentuate the normal sagittal contour.

Complications

◆ Debilitating back pain
◆ Leg weakness or paralysis
◆ Decreased lung capacity

Signs and symptoms

Development of adolescent kyphosis is usually insidious and may be asymptomatic except for the obvious curving of the back (sometimes more than 90 degrees). In some adolescents, kyphosis may produce mild pain at the apex of the curve (about 50% of patients), fatigue, tenderness or stiffness in the involved area or along the entire spine, and prominent vertebral spinous processes at the lower dorsal and upper lumbar levels, with compensatory increased lumbar lordosis, and hamstring tightness. Rarely, kyphosis may cause neurologic damage: spastic paraparesis secondary to spinal cord compression or herniated nucleus pulposus. In both adolescent and adult forms of kyphosis that aren't due to poor posture alone, the spine won't straighten when the patient assumes a recumbent position.

Adult kyphosis produces a characteristic roundback appearance, possibly associated with pain, weakness of the back, and generalized fatigue. Unlike the adolescent form, adult kyphosis rarely produces local tenderness, except in osteoporosis with a recent compression fracture.

Diagnosis

Physical examination reveals curvature of the thoracic spine in varying degrees of severity. X-rays may show vertebral wedging, Schmorl nodes, irregular end plates, and possibly mild scoliosis of 10 to 20 degrees. MRI should be used to distinguish adolescent kyphosis from TB and other inflammatory or neoplastic diseases that cause vertebral collapse; the severe pain, bone destruction, or systemic symptoms associated with these diseases help rule out a diagnosis of kyphosis. Other sites of bone disease, primary sites of malignancy, and infection must also be evaluated, possibly through vertebral biopsy.

Treatment

For kyphosis caused by poor posture alone, treatment may consist of therapeutic exercises, bed rest on a firm mattress (with or without traction), and a brace to straighten the kyphotic curve until spinal growth is complete. Corrective exercises include pelvic tilt to decrease lumbar lordosis, hamstring stretch to overcome muscle contractures, and thoracic hyperextension to flatten the kyphotic curve. These exercises may be performed in or out of the brace. Lateral X-rays taken every 4 months evaluate correction. Gradual weaning from the brace can begin after maximum correction of the kyphotic curve and after vertebral wedging has decreased and the spine has reached full skeletal maturity. Loss of correction indicates that weaning from the brace has been too rapid, and time out of the brace is decreased accordingly.

Treatment for both adolescent and adult kyphosis also includes appropriate measures for the underlying cause and, possibly, spinal arthrodesis for relief of symptoms. Although rarely necessary, surgery may be recommended when kyphosis causes neurologic damage, a spinal curve greater than 60 degrees, or intractable and disabling back pain in a patient with full skeletal maturity. Preoperative measures may include halo-femoral traction. Corrective surgery includes a posterior spinal fusion with spinal instrumentation, iliac bone grafting, and plaster immobilization. Anterior spinal fusion followed by immobilization in plaster may be necessary when kyphosis produces a spinal curve greater than 70 degrees.

Special considerations

Effective management of kyphosis necessitates first-rate supportive care for patients in traction or a brace, skillful patient teaching, and sensitive emotional support.

◆ Teach the patient with adolescent kyphosis caused by poor posture alone the prescribed therapeutic exercises and the fundamentals of good posture. Suggest bed rest when pain is severe. Encourage use of a firm mattress, preferably with a bed board. If the patient needs a brace, explain its purpose, how and when to wear it.

◆ Teach good skin care. Tell the patient not to use lotions, ointments, or powders where the brace contacts the skin. Provide instructions that only the physician or orthotist should adjust the brace.

◆ If corrective surgery is needed, explain all preoperative tests thoroughly as well as the need for postoperative traction or casting, if applicable. After surgery, check neurovascular status every 2 to 4 hours for the first 48 hours, and report any changes immediately. Turn the patient often by logrolling and teach the patient how to logroll independently. Provide meticulous skin care. Check the skin at the cast edges several times a day; use heel and elbow protectors to prevent skin breakdown. Remove antiembolism stockings, if ordered, at least three times a day for at least 30 minutes. Change dressings as ordered.

◆ Provide emotional support. The adolescent patient is likely to exhibit mood changes and periods of depression. Maintain communication and offer frequent encouragement and reassurance.

◆ Assist during removal of sutures and application of a new cast (usually about 10 days after surgery). Encourage gradual ambulation (usually with the use of a tilt table in the physical therapy department).

◆ At discharge, provide detailed, written cast care instructions. Tell the patient to immediately report pain, burning, skin breakdown, loss of feeling, tingling, numbness, or cast odor. Advise the patient to drink plenty of liquids to avoid constipation and to report any illness immediately. Arrange for home visits by a social worker and a home care nurse, as needed.

HERNIATED DISK

Herniated disk, also called *ruptured* or *slipped disk* and *herniated nucleus pulposus*, occurs when all or part of the nucleus pulposus—the soft, gelatinous, central portion of an intervertebral disk—is forced through the disk's weakened or torn outer ring (anulus fibrosus). When this happens, the extruded disk may impinge on spinal nerve roots as they exit from the spinal canal or on the spinal cord itself, resulting in back pain and other signs of nerve root irritation.

Causes and incidence

Herniated disks may result from severe trauma or strain or may be related to intervertebral joint degeneration. Although herniated disks usually occur in adults (mostly men) younger than 45 years old, elderly people are also at risk because minor trauma may cause herniation in disks that have begun to deteriorate due to age. Ninety percent of herniation occurs in the lumbar and lumbosacral regions of the spine; 8% in the cervical region; and 1% to 2% in the thoracic region. Patients with a congenitally small lumbar spinal canal or with osteophyte formation on the vertebrae may be more susceptible to nerve root compression by a herniated disk and more likely to have neurologic symptoms.

Pathophysiology

An intervertebral disk has two parts: the soft center called the *nucleus pulposus* and the tough, fibrous surrounding ring called the *anulus fibrosus*. The nucleus pulposus acts as a shock absorber, distributing the mechanical stress applied to the spine when the body moves.

Physical stress, usually a twisting motion, can tear or rupture the anulus fibrosus so that the nucleus pulposus herniates into the spinal canal. When this happens, the extruded disk may impinge on spinal nerve roots as they exit from the spinal canal or on the spinal cord itself, resulting in back pain and other signs of nerve root irritation. The vertebrae move closer together and in turn exert pressure on the nerve roots as they exit between the vertebrae. Pain and possibly sensory and motor loss follow. A herniated disk can also follow intervertebral joint degeneration; minor trauma may cause herniation.

Herniation occurs in three steps:
◆ *protrusion*—nucleus pulposus presses against the anulus fibrosus

◆ *extrusion*—nucleus pulposus bulges forcibly through the anulus fibrosus, pushing against the nerve root
◆ *sequestration*—anulus fibrosis gives way as the disk's core bursts and presses against the nerve root.

Complications
◆ Long-term back pain
◆ Rarely, spinal cord injuries, resulting in loss of movement or sensation in legs and feet or loss of bowel and bladder function

Signs and symptoms

The overriding symptom of lumbar herniated disk is severe low back pain that radiates to the buttocks, legs, and feet, usually unilaterally. When herniation follows trauma, the pain may begin suddenly, subside in a few days, and then recur at shorter intervals and with progressive intensity. Sciatic pain follows, beginning as a dull pain in the buttocks. Valsalva's maneuver, coughing, sneezing, or bending intensifies the pain, which is commonly accompanied by muscle spasms. Herniated disk may also cause paresthesias or hyperesthesias, as well as sensory and motor loss in the area innervated by the compressed spinal nerve root and, in later stages, weakness and atrophy of leg muscles.

Diagnosis

Obtaining a careful patient history is vital because the events that intensify disk pain are diagnostically significant. The straight-leg–raising test and its variants are perhaps the best tests for herniated disk but may still be negative.

For the straight-leg–raising test, the patient lies in a supine position while the examiner places one hand on the patient's ilium, to stabilize the pelvis, and the other hand under the ankle, then slowly raises the patient's leg. The test is positive only if the patient complains of posterior leg (sciatic) pain, not back pain. In Lasègue's test, the patient lies flat while the thigh and knee are flexed to a 90-degree angle. Resistance and pain as well as loss of ankle or knee-jerk reflex indicate spinal root compression.

X-rays of the spine are essential to rule out other abnormalities but may not diagnose herniated disk because marked disk prolapse can be present despite a normal X-ray. A thorough check of the patient's peripheral vascular status—including posterior tibial and dorsalis pedis pulses and skin temperature of limbs—helps rule out ischemic disease, another cause of leg pain or numbness. After physical examination and X-rays, myelography, CT scans, and MRI provide the most specific diagnostic information, showing spinal canal compression by herniated disk material. MRI is the method of choice to confirm the diagnosis and determine the exact level of herniation. A myelogram can define the size and location of disk herniation. An electromyogram can determine the exact nerve root involved. A nerve conduction velocity test may also be performed.

Treatment

Unless neurologic impairment progresses rapidly, treatment is initially conservative and consists of several weeks of bed rest (possibly with pelvic traction), administration of NSAIDs, heat applications, and an exercise program. Epidural corticosteroids, short-term oral corticosteroids, nerve root blocks, or physical therapy may be used to decrease pain. Muscle relaxants, such as diazepam, methocarbamol, or cyclobenzaprine, may relieve associated muscle spasms.

A herniated disk that fails to respond to conservative treatment may necessitate surgery. The most common procedure, laminectomy, involves excision of a portion of the lamina and removal of the protruding disk. If laminectomy doesn't alleviate pain and disability, a spinal fusion may be necessary to overcome segmental instability. Laminectomy and spinal fusion are sometimes performed concurrently to stabilize the spine. Microdiskectomy can also be used to remove fragments of nucleus pulposus.

Injection of the enzyme chymopapain into the herniated disk produces a loss of water and proteoglycans from the disk, thereby reducing both the disk's size and the pressure in the nerve root.

Special considerations

Herniated disk requires supportive care, careful patient teaching, and strong emotional support to help the patient cope with the discomfort and frustration of chronic low back pain.

◆ If the patient requires myelography, question carefully about allergies to iodides, iodine-containing substances, or seafood because such allergies may indicate sensitivity to the test's radiopaque dye. Reinforce previous explanations of the need for this test and tell the patient to expect some pain. Provide assurance that a sedative will be provided before the test, if needed, to promote comfort and lessen anxiety. After the test, urge the patient to remain in bed with the head elevated (especially if metrizamide was used) and to drink plenty of fluids. Monitor intake and output. Watch for seizures and allergic reaction.

◆ During conservative treatment, watch for any deterioration in neurologic status (especially during the first 24 hours after admission), which may indicate an urgent need for surgery.

Use antiembolism stockings as prescribed, and encourage the patient to move the legs, as allowed. Provide high-topped sneakers to prevent footdrop. Work closely with the physical therapy department to ensure a consistent regimen of leg- and back-strengthening exercises. Give plenty of fluids to prevent renal stasis, and remind the patient to cough, deep breathe, and use blow bottles or an incentive spirometer to preclude pulmonary complications. Provide good skin care. Assess for bowel and bladder functions. Use a fracture bedpan for the patient on complete bed rest.

◆ After laminectomy, microdiskectomy, or spinal fusion, enforce bed rest, as indicated. If a blood drainage system (Hemovac or Jackson–Pratt drain) is in use, check the tubing frequently for kinks and a secure vacuum. Empty the Hemovac at the end of each shift and record the amount and color of drainage. Report colorless moisture on dressings (possible cerebrospinal fluid leakage) or excessive drainage immediately. Observe neurovascular status of the legs (color, motion, temperature, and sensation).

◆ Monitor vital signs and check for bowel sounds and abdominal distention. Use logrolling technique to turn the patient. Administer analgesics as ordered, especially 30 minutes before initial attempts at sitting or walking. Give the patient assistance during the first attempt to walk. Provide a straight-backed chair for limited sitting.

◆ Teach the patient who has undergone spinal fusion how to wear a brace. Assist with straight-leg–raising and toe-pointing exercises, as indicated. Before discharge, teach proper body mechanics—bending at the knees and hips (never at the waist), standing straight, and carrying objects close to the body. Advise the patient to lie down when tired and to sleep on either side (never on abdomen) on an extra-firm mattress or a bed board. Urge maintenance of proper weight to prevent lordosis caused by obesity.

◆ After chemonucleolysis, enforce bed rest as ordered. Administer analgesics and apply heat, as needed. Urge the patient to cough and deep breathe. Assist with physical therapy as necessary and advise the patient to continue these exercises after discharge.

◆ Tell the patient who must receive a muscle relaxant of possible adverse effects, especially drowsiness. Provide instruction to avoid activities that require alertness until the effects to the medication are known, and a tolerance has been built up.

◆ Provide emotional support. Try to cheer the patient up during periods of frustration and depression. Provide reassurance of progress, and offer encouragement. (See *Preventing a herniated disk*, page 321.)

PREVENTION
Preventing a herniated disk

To prevent a herniated disk, tell your patient to follow these guidelines.

Exercise
Getting regular exercise can slow the degeneration of the disks related to aging. Muscle strength gained through exercising can strengthen and stabilize the spine. If the patient has previously had a herniated disk, he should remember to avoid high-impact activities such as jogging, tennis, and high-impact aerobics for the first few months after a herniated disk.

Maintain good posture
Good posture reduces the pressure on the spine and disks. Keeping the back straight and aligned is essential, particularly when sitting for longer periods. Also, heavy objects should be lifted properly by letting the legs—not the back—do most of the work.

Maintain a healthy weight
Excess weight puts more pressure on the spine and disks, making them more susceptible to a herniation.

SCOLIOSIS

Scoliosis is a lateral curvature of the spine that may occur in the thoracic, lumbar, or thoracolumbar spinal segment. The curve may be convex to the right (more common in thoracic curves) or to the left (more common in lumbar curves). Rotation of the vertebral column around its axis occurs and may cause rib cage deformity. Scoliosis is commonly associated with kyphosis (*roundback*) and lordosis (*swayback*).

Causes and incidence

Scoliosis may be functional, structural, or idiopathic. Functional (postural) scoliosis usually results from a discrepancy in leg lengths rather than from a fixed deformity of the spinal column; it corrects when the patient bends toward the convex side. Structural scoliosis results from a deformity of the vertebral bodies, and it doesn't correct when the patient bends to the side. Structural scoliosis may be:

◆ *congenital:* usually related to a congenital defect, such as wedge vertebrae, fused ribs or vertebrae, or hemivertebrae; may result from trauma to zygote or embryo
◆ *paralytic or musculoskeletal:* develops several months after asymmetrical paralysis of the trunk muscles due to polio, cerebral palsy, or muscular dystrophy
◆ *idiopathic (the most common form):* may be transmitted as an autosomal dominant or multifactorial trait. This form appears in a previously straight spine during the growing years. Brainstem dysfunction, possibly due to a lesion of the posterior columns or the inner ear, may be the cause

PEDIATRIC TIP *Idiopathic scoliosis can be classified as infantile, which affects mostly male infants between birth and age 3 and causes left thoracic and right lumbar curves; juvenile, which affects both sexes between ages 4 and 10 and causes varying types of curvature; or adolescent, which generally affects girls between age 10 and achievement of skeletal maturity and causes varying types of curvature.*

Pathophysiology

Differential stress on vertebral bone causes an imbalance of osteoblastic activity; thus, the curve progresses rapidly during adolescent growth spurt. Without treatment, the imbalance continues into adulthood.

Complications
◆ Debilitating back pain
◆ Reduced pulmonary function
◆ Cor pulmonale

Signs and symptoms

The most common curve in functional or structural scoliosis arises in the thoracic segment, with convexity to the right, and compensatory curves (S curves) in the cervical segment above and the lumbar segment below, both with convexity to the left. (See *Cobb method for measuring angle of curvature,* page 322.) As the spine curves laterally, compensatory curves develop to maintain body balance and mark the deformity. Scoliosis rarely produces subjective symptoms until it's well established; when symptoms do occur, they include backache, fatigue, and dyspnea.

Cobb method for measuring angle of curvature

The Cobb method measures the angle of curvature in scoliosis. The top vertebra in the curve (T6 in the illustration) is the uppermost vertebra whose upper face tilts toward the curve's concave side. The bottom vertebra in the curve (T12) is the lowest vertebra whose lower face tilts toward the curve's concave side. The angle at which perpendicular lines drawn from the upper face of the top vertebra and the lower face of the bottom vertebra intersect is the angle of the curve.

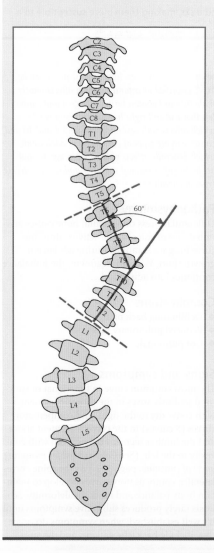

Because many teenagers are shy about their bodies, their parents suspect that something is wrong only after they notice uneven hemlines, pant legs that appear unequal in length, or subtle physical signs like one hip appearing higher than the other. Untreated scoliosis may result in pulmonary insufficiency (curvature may decrease lung capacity), back pain, degenerative arthritis of the spine, disk disease, and sciatica.

Diagnosis

CONFIRMING DIAGNOSIS *Anterior, posterior, and lateral spinal X-rays, taken with the patient standing upright and bending, confirm scoliosis and determine the degree of curvature (Cobb method) and flexibility of the spine.*

A scoliometer can also be used to measure the angle of trunk rotation. Physical examination reveals unequal shoulder heights, elbow levels, and heights of the iliac crests. Muscles on the convex side of the curve may be rounded and those on the concave side flattened, producing asymmetry of paraspinal muscles.

Treatment

Only two treatments effectively treat scoliosis: spinal bracing and surgery. If monitored closely, a properly constructed and fitted brace can successfully halt progression of a curve in approximately 70% of cooperative patients. Most braces should be worn over a long T-shirt or similar article of clothing for 23 hours a day. However, mild curvatures may require wearing the brace for fewer hours a day. Exercises must be done daily both in and out of the brace to maintain muscle strength. Patients should be seen for follow-up and brace adjustment every 3 months. Radiographs should be repeated at 6-month intervals. As the skeleton matures, as seen radiographically, brace wear should be gradually decreased until it's worn only at night.

The primary indications for surgery are relentless curve progression (usually curves over 40 degrees) or significant curve progression despite bracing. Surgery corrects lateral curvature by posterior spinal fusion and internal stabilization with metal rods. A distraction rod on the concave side of the curve "jacks" the spine into a straight position and provides an internal splint. An alternative procedure, anterior spinal fusion, corrects curvature with vertebral staples and an anterior stabilizing cable. Some spinal fusions may require postoperative immobilization in a brace. Postoperatively, periodic checkups are required for several months to monitor stability of the correction.

Special considerations

It's important to provide emotional support in addition to meticulous skin care and patient teaching.

If the patient needs a brace:

◆ Enlist the help of a physical therapist, a social worker, and an orthotist. Before the patient goes home, explain what the brace does and how to care for it (how to check the screws for tightness and pad the uprights to prevent excessive wear on clothing). Suggest that loose-fitting, oversized clothes be worn for greater comfort.

◆ Tell the patient to wear the brace 23 hours/day and to remove it only for bathing and exercise. While still adjusting to the brace, instruct to lie down and rest several times per day.

◆ Suggest a soft mattress if a firm one is uncomfortable.

◆ To prevent skin breakdown, advise the patient not to use lotions, ointments, or powders on areas where the brace contacts the skin. Instruct keeping the skin dry and clean and to wear a snug T-shirt under the brace.

◆ Advise the patient to increase activities gradually and avoid vigorous sports. Emphasize the importance of conscientiously performing prescribed exercises.

◆ Instruct the patient to turn the whole body, instead of just the head, when looking to the side. To make reading easier, instruct to hold the book so it will be straight ahead at it instead of down. Prism glasses may be beneficial if this is difficult.

If the patient needs traction or a cast before surgery:

◆ Explain these procedures to the patient and the family. Remember that application of a body cast can be traumatic because it's done on a special frame and the patient's head and face are covered throughout the procedure.

◆ Check the skin around the cast edge daily. Keep the cast clean and dry and the edges of the cast petaled. Warn the patient not to insert or let anything get under the cast and to immediately report cracks in the cast, pain, burning, skin breakdown, numbness, or odor.

After corrective surgery:

◆ **ALERT** *Check sensation, movement, color, and blood supply in all limbs every 2 to 4 hours for the first 48 hours and then several times a day, for signs of neurovascular deficit, a serious complication following spinal surgery. Logroll the patient often.*

◆ Measure intake, output, and urine specific gravity to monitor effects of blood loss, which is usually substantial.

◆ Monitor abdominal distention and bowel sounds.

◆ Encourage deep-breathing exercises to avoid pulmonary complications.

◆ Medicate for pain, especially before any activity.

◆ Promote active ROM arm exercises to help maintain muscle strength. Remember that any exercise, even brushing the hair or teeth, is helpful. Encourage the patient to perform quadriceps-setting, calf-pumping, and active ROM exercises of the ankles and feet.

◆ Watch for skin breakdown and signs of cast syndrome. Teach the patient how to recognize these signs. (See *Cast syndrome*.)

◆ Offer emotional support to help prevent depression that may result from altered body image and immobility. Encourage the patient to wear his or her own clothes, wash hair, and use makeup.

◆ If the patient is being discharged with a rod and cast and must have bed rest, arrange for a social worker and a visiting nurse to provide home care. Before discharge, check with the surgeon about activity limitations, and make sure the patient understands them.

◆ If you work in a school, screen children routinely for scoliosis during physical examinations.

Cast syndrome

Cast syndrome is a serious complication that sometimes follows spinal surgery and application of a body cast. Characterized by nausea, abdominal pressure, and vague abdominal pain, cast syndrome probably results from hyperextension of the spine. This hyperextension accentuates lumbar lordosis, compressing the third portion of the duodenum between the superior mesenteric artery anteriorly and the aorta and vertebral column posteriorly. High intestinal obstruction produces nausea, vomiting, and ischemic infarction of the mesentery.

After removal of the cast, treatment includes gastric decompression and I.V. fluids, with nothing by mouth. Antiemetics should be given sparingly because they may mask symptoms of cast syndrome, which, if untreated, may be fatal.

Teach patients who are discharged in body jackets, localizer casts, or high hip-spica casts how to recognize cast syndrome, which may manifest several weeks or months after application of the cast.

Muscle and connective tissue

TENDINITIS AND BURSITIS

Tendinitis is a painful inflammation of tendons and of tendon-muscle attachments to bone, usually in the shoulder rotator cuff, hip, Achilles tendon, or hamstring. *Bursitis* is a painful inflammation of one or more of the bursae—closed sacs lubricated with small amounts of synovial fluid that facilitate the motion of muscles and tendons over bony prominences. Bursitis usually occurs in the subdeltoid, olecranon, trochanteric, calcaneal, or prepatellar bursae.

Causes and incidence

Tendinitis commonly results from overuse or injury (such as strain during sports activity), another musculoskeletal disorder (such as rheumatic diseases or congenital defects), or aging.

Bursitis can occur at any age but usually occurs in older individuals due to an inflammatory joint disease (such as rheumatoid arthritis or gout) or recurring trauma that stresses or pressures a joint. Chronic bursitis follows attacks of acute bursitis or repeated trauma and infection. Septic bursitis may result from wound infection or from bacterial invasion of skin over the bursa.

Pathophysiology

In tendinitis, fluid from inflammation accumulates, causing swelling of the tendon and its enclosing sheath. Inflammatory changes cause thickening of the sheath, which limits movements and causes pain. Microtears cause bleeding, edema, and pain in the involved tendon or tendons. At times, after repeated inflammations, calcium may be deposited in the tendon origin area, causing a calcific tendinitis.

The usual bursitis is an inflammation that is reactive to overuse or excessive pressure. The inflamed bursal sac becomes engorged, and the inflammation can spread to adjacent tissues. The inflammation may decrease with rest, heat, and aspiration of the fluid.

Complications

◆ Contractures of the tendon
◆ Scarring
◆ Muscle wasting
◆ Disability

Signs and symptoms

The patient with tendinitis of the shoulder complains of restricted shoulder movement, especially abduction, and localized pain, which is most severe at night and usually interferes with

sleep. The pain extends from the acromion (the shoulder's highest point) to the deltoid muscle insertion, predominantly in the so-called painful arc—that is, when the patient abducts the arm between 50 and 130 degrees. Fluid accumulation causes swelling. In calcific tendinitis, calcium deposits in the tendon cause proximal weakness and, if calcium erodes into adjacent bursae, acute calcific bursitis.

In bursitis, fluid accumulation in the bursae causes irritation, inflammation, sudden or gradual pain, and limited movement. Other symptoms vary according to the affected site. Subdeltoid bursitis impairs arm abduction, prepatellar bursitis (housemaid's knee) produces pain when the patient climbs stairs, and hip bursitis makes crossing the legs painful.

Diagnosis

In tendinitis, X-rays may be normal at first but later show bony fragments, osteophyte sclerosis, or calcium deposits. Arthrography is usually normal, with occasional small irregularities on the undersurface of the tendon. CT scan and MRI have replaced X-ray and even arthrography of the shoulder as diagnostic tools. An MRI will usually identify tears, partial tears, inflammation, or tumor but cannot reveal irregularities of the tendon sheath itself. Diagnosis of tendinitis must rule out other causes of shoulder pain, such as myocardial infarction, cervical spondylosis, degenerative changes, and tendon tear or rupture. Significantly, in tendinitis, heat aggravates shoulder pain; in other painful joint disorders, heat usually provides relief.

Localized pain and inflammation and a history of unusual strain or injury 2 to 3 days before onset of pain are the bases for diagnosing bursitis. During early stages, X-rays are usually normal, except in calcific bursitis, where X-rays may show calcium deposits.

Treatment

Treatment to relieve pain includes resting the joint (by immobilization with a sling, splint, or cast, or via activity modification), NSAIDs, analgesics, application of cold or heat, ultrasound, or local injection of an anesthetic and corticosteroids to reduce inflammation. A mixture of a corticosteroid and an anesthetic such as lidocaine generally provides immediate pain relief. Extended-release injections of a corticosteroid, such as triamcinolone or prednisolone, offer long-term pain relief. Until the patient is free of pain and able to perform ROM exercises easily, treatment also includes oral NSAIDs, such as ibuprofen, naproxen, indomethacin, or oxaprozin. Short-term analgesics include propoxyphene, codeine, acetaminophen with codeine and, occasionally, oxycodone.

Supplementary treatment includes fluid removal by aspiration and heat therapy; for calcific tendinitis, ice packs, physical therapy, ultrasonography, or hydrotherapy generally helps maintain or regain ROM. It may be necessary to delay treatment until the acute attack is over to ensure maximum patient compliance. Rarely, calcific tendinitis requires surgical removal of calcium deposits. Long-term control of chronic bursitis and tendinitis may require changes in lifestyle to prevent recurring joint irritation.

Special considerations

When treating patients with tendinitis or bursitis, remember to consider the following:
◆ Assess the severity of pain and the ROM to determine the effectiveness of the treatment.
◆ Before injecting corticosteroids or local anesthetics, ask the patient about drug allergies.
◆ Assist with intra-articular injection. Scrub the patient's skin thoroughly with povidone–iodine or a comparable solution. After the injection, massage the area to ensure penetration through the tissue and joint space. Apply ice intermittently for about 4 hours to minimize pain. Avoid applying heat to the area for 2 days.
◆ Tell the patient to take anti-inflammatory agents with milk to minimize GI distress and to report any signs of distress immediately.
◆ Advise the patient to perform strengthening exercises and avoid activities that aggravate the joint.
◆ Remind the patient to wear a splint or sling during the first few days of an attack of subdeltoid bursitis or tendinitis to support the arm and protect the shoulder, particularly at night. Demonstrate how to wear the sling so it won't put too much weight on the shoulder.
◆ Advise the patient to maintain joint mobility and prevent muscle atrophy by performing exercises or physical therapy when free of pain.

PEDIATRIC TIP *A common form of tendinitis in adolescents (both males and females) is patellar tendinitis associated with inflammation of the tibial epiphysis in Osgood–Schlatter disease.*

EPICONDYLITIS

Lateral epicondylitis of the elbow (tennis elbow) is inflammation of the extensor tendons of the forearm. Medial epicondylitis (golfer's elbow) is inflammation at the origin of the flexor muscles of the wrist.

Causes and incidence

Epicondylitis probably begins as a partial tear and is common among tennis players or persons whose activities require a forceful grasp, wrist extension against resistance, or frequent rotation of the forearm, such as using a screwdriver. Untreated epicondylitis may become disabling as adherent fibers form between the tendons and the elbow capsule.

Pathophysiology

Epicondylitis is the result of irritation and inflammation where the tendon attaches to a bone. Overuse and excessive pressure are factors.

Complications

◆ Recurrence of injury
◆ Tendon rupture

Signs and symptoms

The patient's initial symptom is elbow pain that gradually worsens and commonly radiates to the forearm and back of the hand whenever an object is grasped, or the elbow is twisted. Other associated signs and symptoms include tenderness over the involved lateral or medial epicondyle or over the head of the radius and a weak grasp. In rare instances, epicondylitis may cause local heat, swelling, or restricted ROM.

Diagnosis

Because X-rays are almost always negative, diagnosis typically depends on clinical signs and symptoms and a patient history of playing tennis or engaging in similar activities. The pain can be reproduced by wrist extension and supination with lateral epicondyle involvement or by flexion and pronation with medial epicondyle involvement.

Treatment

Treatment aims to relieve pain, usually by NSAIDs or local injection of corticosteroids and an anesthetic. Supportive treatment includes an immobilizing splint from the distal forearm to the elbow or wrist splint, which generally relieves pain in 2 to 3 weeks; heat therapy, such as warm compresses, short-wave diathermy, and ultrasound (alone or in combination with diathermy); and physical therapy, such as manipulation and massage to detach the tendon from the chronically inflamed periosteum. A "tennis elbow strap" or counterface brace has helped many patients. This strap, which is wrapped snugly around the forearm approximately 1 (2.5 cm) below the epicondyle, helps relieve the strain on affected forearm muscles and tendons. If these measures prove ineffective, surgical release of the tendon at the epicondyle may be necessary.

Special considerations

The following special considerations accompany diagnosis and treatment of epicondylitis:
◆ Assess the patient's level of pain, ROM, and sensory function. Monitor heat therapy to prevent burns.
◆ Advise the patient to take anti-inflammatory drugs with food to avoid GI irritation.
◆ Instruct the patient to rest the elbow, wrist, or both until inflammation subsides.
◆ Remove the support daily, and gently move the arm to prevent stiffness and contracture.
◆ Instruct the patient to follow the prescribed exercise program. For example, the arm may be stretched and the wrist flexed to the maximum then press the back of the hand against a wall until a pull can be felt in the forearm and hold this position for 1 minute.
◆ Advise the patient to warm up for 15 to 20 minutes before beginning any sports activity.
◆ Urge the patient to wear an elastic support or splint during any activity that stresses the forearm or elbow.
◆ Tell the patient to check the equipment. For example, a tennis racquet may not be the right size or weight. Also, changing surfaces may help to reduce stress.

ACHILLES TENDON CONTRACTURE

Achilles tendon contracture is a shortening of the Achilles tendon (*tendo calcaneus* or *heel cord*) that causes foot pain and strain and limits ankle dorsiflexion.

Causes and incidence

Achilles tendon contracture may reflect a congenital structural anomaly or a muscular reaction to chronic poor posture, especially in women who wear high-heeled shoes or joggers who land on the balls of their feet instead of their heels. Other causes include paralytic conditions of the legs, such as poliomyelitis or cerebral palsy.

Pathophysiology

The Achilles tendon spans two joints and connects the calcaneus to the gastrocnemius and soleus muscles, comprising the largest and strongest muscle complex in the calf. The tendon is vulnerable to injury because of its limited blood supply, especially when subjected to strong forces.

The blood supply to the tendon is provided by longitudinal arteries that run the length of the muscle complex. The area of the tendon with the poorest blood supply is approximately 2 to 6 cm above the insertion into the calcaneus. The blood supply diminishes with age,

predisposing this area of the tendon to chronic inflammation and possible rupture.

Complication
◆ Permanent weakness

Signs and symptoms

Sharp, spasmodic pain during dorsiflexion of the foot characterizes the reflex type of Achilles tendon contracture. In footdrop (fixed equinus), contracture of the flexor foot muscle prevents placing the heel on the ground.

Diagnosis

Physical examination and patient history suggest Achilles tendon contracture.

℞ **CONFIRMING DIAGNOSIS** *A simple test confirms Achilles tendon contracture: While the patient keeps the knee flexed, the examiner places the foot in dorsiflexion; gradual knee extension forces the foot into plantar flexion.*

Treatment

Conservative treatment aims to correct Achilles tendon contracture by raising the inside heel of the shoe in the reflex type; by gradually lowering the heels of shoes (sudden lowering can aggravate the problem) and stretching exercises if the cause is high heels; or by using support braces or casting to prevent footdrop in a paralyzed patient. Alternative therapy includes using wedged plaster casts or stretching the tendon by manipulation. Analgesics may be given to relieve pain.

With fixed footdrop, treatment may include surgery. Although this procedure may weaken the tendon, it allows further stretching by cutting the tendon. After surgery, a short leg cast maintains the foot in 90-degree dorsiflexion for 6 weeks. Some surgeons allow partial weight bearing on a walking cast after 2 weeks.

Special considerations

After surgery to lengthen the Achilles tendon:
◆ Elevate the casted foot to decrease venous pressure and edema by raising the foot of the bed or supporting the foot with pillows.
◆ Record the neurovascular status of the toes (temperature, color, sensation, capillary refill time, and toe mobility) every hour for the first 24 hours and then every 4 hours. If any changes are detected, increase the elevation of the patient's legs and notify the surgeon immediately.
◆ Prepare the patient for ambulation by dangling the foot over the side of the bed for short periods (5 to 15 minutes) before getting out of bed, allowing for a gradual increase in

venous pressure. Assist the patient in walking, as ordered (usually within 24 hours of surgery), using crutches and a nonweight-bearing or touch-down gait.

◆ Protect the patient's skin with moleskin or by petaling the edges of the cast. Before discharge, teach the patient how to care for the cast, and advise to elevate the foot regularly when sitting or whenever the foot throbs or becomes edematous. Also, make sure the patient understands how much exercise and walking are recommended after discharge.

◆ To prevent Achilles tendon contracture in paralyzed patients, apply support braces, universal splints, casts, or high-topped sneakers. Make sure the weight of the sheets doesn't keep paralyzed feet in plantar flexion. For other patients, teach good foot care and urge them to seek immediate medical care for foot problems. Warn women against wearing high heels constantly and suggest regular foot (dorsiflexion) exercises.

CARPAL TUNNEL SYNDROME

Carpal tunnel syndrome, a form of repetitive stress injury, is the most common of the nerve entrapment syndromes. It results from compression of the median nerve at the wrist, within the carpal tunnel. This compression neuropathy causes sensory and motor changes in the median distribution of the hand.

Causes and incidence

The carpal tunnel is formed by the carpal bones and the transverse carpal ligament. (See *The carpal tunnel.*) Inflammation or fibrosis of the tendon sheaths that pass through the carpal tunnel commonly causes edema and compression of the median nerve. Many conditions can cause the contents or structure of the carpal tunnel to swell and press the median nerve against the transverse carpal ligament, including rheumatoid arthritis, flexor tenosynovitis (commonly associated with rheumatic disease), nerve compression, pregnancy, renal failure, menopause, diabetes mellitus, acromegaly, edema following Colles fracture, hypothyroidism, amyloidosis, myxedema, benign tumors, TB, and other granulomatous diseases. Another source of damage to the median nerve is dislocation or acute sprain of the wrist.

Carpal tunnel injury is five times more common in women than in men. It usually occurs in women between ages 30 and 60 and poses a serious occupational health problem. Assembly-line workers and packers and people who repeatedly use poorly designed tools are most likely to develop this disorder. Any

The carpal tunnel

The carpal tunnel is clearly visible in this palmar view and cross section of a right hand. Note the median nerve, flexor tendons of fingers, and blood vessels passing through the tunnel on their way from the forearm to the hand.

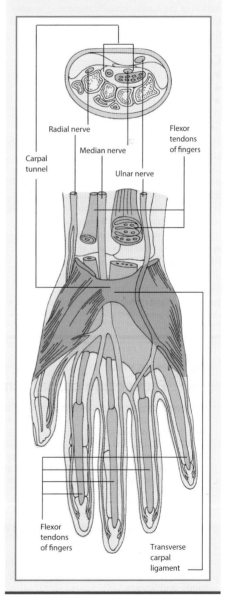

Radial nerve

Flexor tendons of fingers

Median nerve

Carpal tunnel

Ulnar nerve

Flexor tendons of fingers

Transverse carpal ligament

strenuous use of the hands—sustained grasping, twisting, or flexing—aggravates this condition. (See *Preventing carpal tunnel syndrome.*)

Pathophysiology

The carpal bones and the transverse carpal ligament form the carpal tunnel. Inflammation or fibrosis of the tendon sheaths that pass through the carpal tunnel usually causes edema and compression of the median nerve. (See *Cross section of the wrist with carpal tunnel syndrome*, page 327.) This compression neuropathy causes sensory and motor changes in the median distribution of the hands, initially impairing sensory transmission to the thumb, index finger, second finger, and inner aspect of the third finger.

Complications

◆ Decreased wrist function
◆ Permanent nerve damage
◆ Loss of movement and sensation

Signs and symptoms

The patient with carpal tunnel syndrome usually complains of weakness, pain, burning, numbness, or tingling in one or both hands. This paresthesia affects the thumb, forefinger, middle finger, and half of the fourth finger. The patient is unable to clench the hand into a fist; the nails may be atrophic, the skin dry and shiny.

Because of vasodilatation and venous stasis, symptoms are typically worse at night and in the morning. The pain may spread to the forearm and, in severe cases, as far as the shoulder or neck. The patient can usually relieve such pain by shaking or rubbing hands vigorously or dangling his arms.

Diagnosis

Physical examination reveals decreased sensation to light touch or pinpricks in the affected fingers. Thenar muscle atrophy occurs in about half of all cases of carpal tunnel syndrome, but it's usually a late sign. The patient exhibits a positive Tinel's sign (tingling over the median nerve on light percussion) and responds positively to Phalen's wrist-flexion test (holding the forearms vertically and allowing both hands to drop into complete flexion at the wrists for 1 minute reproduces symptoms of carpal tunnel syndrome). A compression test supports this diagnosis: A blood pressure cuff inflated above systolic pressure on the forearm for 1 to 2 minutes provokes pain and paresthesia along the distribution of the median nerve.

Electromyography and nerve conduction velocity detect a median nerve motor conduction delay of more than 5 ms. Other laboratory tests may identify the underlying disease.

Treatment

Conservative treatment should be tried first, including resting the hands by splinting the wrist in neutral extension for 1 to 2 weeks. NSAIDs usually provide symptomatic relief. Injection of the carpal tunnel with hydrocortisone and lidocaine may provide significant but temporary relief. If a definite link has been established between the patient's occupation and the development of repetitive stress injury, seeking another type of work may be recommended.

 PREVENTION

Preventing carpal tunnel syndrome

To prevent carpal tunnel syndrome, advise your patients to make these lifestyle changes.

Take frequent breaks
Gently stretching and bending the hands and wrists every 15 to 20 minutes gives the hands and wrists a break, especially when using equipment that vibrates or exerts a great amount of force. Tasks should also be alternated to avoid repetitive movements, which can contribute to tendinitis and carpal tunnel syndrome.

Watch hand and wrist positioning
When using a keyboard, bending the wrist all the way up or down should be avoided. A relaxed middle position is best. The keyboard should be kept at elbow height or slightly lower.

Improve posture
Poor posture can cause the shoulders to roll forward, allowing the neck and shoulder muscles to shorten, which can compress the nerves in the neck. This position can affect the wrists, hands, and fingers.

Keep hands warm
Hand stiffness and pain develops more frequently in a cold environment. Using fingerless gloves may help if the temperature can't be adjusted at work.

Effective treatment may also require correction of an underlying disorder. When conservative treatment fails, the only alternative is surgical decompression of the nerve by resecting the entire transverse carpal tunnel ligament or by using endoscopic surgical techniques. Neurolysis (freeing of the nerve fibers) may also be necessary.

Special considerations

Patient care for carpal tunnel syndrome includes the following:

◆ Administer mild analgesics as needed. Encourage the patient to use the hands as much as possible. If the dominant hand has been impaired, you may have to help with eating and bathing.

◆ Teach the patient how to apply a splint. Instruct to not to make it too tight. Demonstrate how to remove the splint to perform gentle ROM exercises, which should be done daily. Make sure the patient knows how to do these exercises before discharge.

◆ After surgery, monitor vital signs, and regularly check the color, sensation, and motion of the affected hand.

◆ Advise the patient who's about to be discharged to occasionally exercise the hands in warm water. If the arm is in a sling, instruct to remove the sling several times a day to do exercises for the elbow and shoulder.

◆ Suggest occupational counseling for the patient who must change jobs because of repetitive stress injury.

TORTICOLLIS

Torticollis, sometimes called *wryneck*, is a neck deformity in which the sternocleidomastoid (SCM) neck muscles are spastic or shortened, causing bending of the head to the affected side and rotation of the chin to the opposite side.

Causes and incidence

Torticollis may be congenital or acquired. The three types of acquired torticollis—acute, spasmodic, and hysterical—have differing causes. The acute form results from muscular damage caused by inflammatory diseases, such as myositis, lymphadenitis, or TB; from cervical spinal injuries that produce scar tissue contracture; and, less commonly, from tumor or medication. The spasmodic form results from rhythmic muscle spasms caused by an organic central nervous system disorder (probably due to irritation of the nerve root by arthritis or osteomyelitis). Hysterical torticollis is due to a psychogenic inability to control neck muscles.

Acquired torticollis usually develops during the first 10 years of life or between ages 30 and 60. The incidence of congenital (muscular) torticollis is highest in infants after difficult delivery (breech presentation), in firstborn infants, and in girls. Possible causes of congenital torticollis include malposition of the head in utero, prenatal injury, fibroma, interruption of blood supply, or fibrotic rupture of the SCM muscle, with hematoma and scar formation.

Pathophysiology
Congenital torticollis

Congenital muscular torticollis is rare (<2%) and is believed to be caused by local trauma to the soft tissues of the neck just before or during delivery. The most common explanation involves birth trauma to the SCM muscle, resulting in fibrosis or that intrauterine malpositioning leads to unilateral shortening of the SCM. There may be resultant hematoma formation followed by muscular contracture. These children often have undergone breech or difficult forceps delivery.

The fibrosis in the muscle may be due to venous occlusion and pressure on the neck in the birth canal because of cervical and skull position. Another hypothesis includes malposition in utero resulting in intrauterine or perinatal compartment syndrome. Other causes of congenital torticollis include postural torticollis, pterygium colli (webbed neck), SCM cysts, vertebral anomalies, odontoid hyperplasia, spina bifida, hypertrophy or absence of cervical musculature, and Arnold–Chiari syndrome. It can also be seen with clavicular fractures, especially in neonates secondary to birth trauma. Up to 20% of children with congenital muscular torticollis have congenital dysplasia of the hip as well.

Acquired torticollis

The pathophysiology of acquired torticollis depends on the underlying disease process. Cervical muscle spasm causing torticollis can result from any injury or inflammation of the cervical muscles or cranial nerves from different disease processes.

Acute torticollis can be the result of blunt trauma to head and neck, or from simply sleeping in an awkward position. Acute torticollis may be self-limited in days to weeks or the result of idiosyncrasy to certain medications (e.g., traditional dopamine receptor blockers, metoclopramide, phenytoin, or carbamazepine). After stopping medication, it quickly resolves without further action. After the resolution of acute traumatic torticollis, a chronic or persistent form may reappear after days or weeks of a quiescent interval. This situation often has legal implications regarding liability associated with the acute traumatic incident.

Complication
◆ Permanent contracture

Signs and symptoms

PEDIATRIC TIP *The first sign of congenital torticollis is commonly a firm, nontender, palpable enlargement of the SCM muscle that's visible at birth and for several weeks afterward. It slowly regresses during a period of 6 months, although incomplete regression can cause permanent contracture. If the deformity is severe, the infant's face and head flatten from sleeping on the affected side; this asymmetry gradually worsens. The infant's chin turns away from the side of the shortened muscle, and the head tilts to the shortened side. The shoulder may elevate on the affected side, restricting neck movement.*

The first sign of acquired torticollis is usually recurring unilateral stiffness of neck muscles followed by a drawing sensation and a momentary twitching or contraction that pulls the head to the affected side. This type of torticollis commonly produces severe neuralgic pain throughout the head and neck.

Diagnosis

A history of painless neck deformity from birth suggests congenital torticollis; gradual onset of painful neck deformity suggests acquired torticollis. Diagnosis must rule out TB of the cervical spine, pharyngeal or tonsillar inflammations, spinal accessory nerve damage, ruptured transverse ligaments, subdural hematoma, tumors of soft tissue or bone, dislocations and fractures, scoliosis, congenital abnormalities of the cervical spine and base of the skull, rheumatoid arthritis, and osteomyelitis. In acquired torticollis, cervical spine X-rays are negative for bone or joint disease but may reveal an associated disorder (such as TB, scar tissue formation, tumor, deformities, or arthritis). CT scan or MRI may help rule out pathogenic causes.

Treatment

Treatment of congenital torticollis aims to stretch the shortened muscle. Nonsurgical treatment includes passive neck stretching and proper positioning during sleep for an infant and active stretching exercises for an older child—for example, touching the ear opposite the affected side to the shoulder and touching the chin to the same shoulder.

Surgical correction involves sectioning the SCM muscle; this should be done during preschool years and only if other therapies fail.

Treatment of acquired torticollis aims to control pain and correct the underlying cause of the disease. In the acute form, application of heat, cervical traction, and gentle massage may help relieve pain; analgesics may also be helpful. Stretching exercises and a neck brace may relieve symptoms of the spasmodic and hysterical forms. Drug treatment includes anticholinergic drugs such as baclofen. Botulinum toxin injections are effective in temporarily relieving torticollis, but injections must be repeated every 3 months.

Special considerations

Patient care for torticollis includes the following:
◆ To aid early diagnosis of congenital torticollis, observe the infant for limited neck movement, and thoroughly assess the degree of discomfort.
◆ Teach the parents of an affected child how to perform stretching exercises with the infant. Suggest placing toys or mobiles on the side of the crib opposite the affected side of the child's neck to encourage the child to move the head and stretch the neck.
◆ If surgery is necessary, prepare the patient by shaving the neck to the hairline on the affected side.

After corrective surgery:
◆ Monitor the patient closely for nausea or signs of respiratory complications, especially if in cervical traction. Keep suction equipment available to prevent aspiration.
◆ The patient may be in a cast or in traction day and night or at night only. Monitor the skin around the chin, ears, and back of the head if the patient is in cervical traction. Monitor for problems related to clenching of teeth. If the patient is in a cast, give meticulous cast care, including the monitoring of circulation, sensation, and color around the cast. Protect the cast around the patient's chin and mouth with waterproof material. Check for skin irritation, pressure areas, or softening of cast pad.
◆ Provide emotional support for the patient and the family to relieve their anxiety due to fear, pain, limitations from the brace or traction, and an altered body image.
◆ Begin stretching exercises as soon as the patient can tolerate them.
◆ Before discharge, explain to the patient or the parents the importance of continuing daily heat applications, massages, and stretching exercises, as prescribed, and of keeping the cast clean and dry. Emphasize that physical therapy is essential for a successful rehabilitation after the cast is removed.

RHABDOMYOLYSIS

Rhabdomyolysis is the breakdown of muscle fibers that results in the release of muscle fiber content into the circulation. It results from the toxicity of destroyed muscle cells, causing kidney damage or failure. Predisposing factors include trauma, ischemia, polymyositis, and drug overdose. Toxins and environmental, infectious, and metabolic factors may induce it. Rhabdomyolysis accounts for 8% to 15% of cases of acute renal failure; about 5% of cases result in death.

Causes and incidence

Rhabdomyolysis follows direct injury to the skeletal muscle fibers, specifically the sarcolemma, which then release myoglobin into the bloodstream. Myoglobin is an oxygen-binding protein pigment found in skeletal muscle. When this muscle is damaged, myoglobin is released into the bloodstream. It's then filtered by the kidneys.

Myoglobin may occlude the structures of the kidney causing damage, such as acute tubular necrosis or kidney failure. Myoglobin can also cause kidney failure because it breaks down into potentially toxic compounds. Necrotic skeletal muscle may cause massive fluid shifts from the bloodstream into the muscle, reducing the relative fluid volume of the body and leading to shock and reduced blood flow to the kidneys.

The disorder may be caused by any condition that results in damage to skeletal muscle. Rhabdomyolysis may result from blunt trauma; extensive burn injury; viral, bacterial, or fungal infection (such as Legionnaires' disease or, especially, influenza type A or B); prolonged immobilization; near electrocution or near drowning; metabolic or genetic factors; drug therapy; or toxins. Heavy exercise may result in rhabdomyolysis. Other causes include shaken baby syndrome, exposure to extreme cold, heatstroke, and snakebite.

In the United States, rhabdomyolysis affects about 8% to 15% of people with acute renal failure and has a slightly higher incidence in men than in women. The overall mortality rate is 5%. It can occur in infants, toddlers, and adolescents who inherited enzyme deficiencies of carbohydrate and lipid metabolism or those with inherited myopathies, such as Duchenne muscular dystrophy, and malignant hyperthermia.

Pathophysiology

Muscle trauma that compresses tissue causes ischemia and necrosis. The ensuing local edema further increases compartment pressure and tamponade; pressure from severe swelling causes blood vessels to collapse, leading to

tissue hypoxia, muscle infarction, neural damage in the area of the fracture, and release of myoglobin from the necrotic muscle fibers into the circulation. Myoglobin may occlude the structures of the kidney, causing such damage as acute tubular necrosis or kidney failure. Myoglobin can also cause kidney failure because it breaks down into potentially toxic compounds.

Complications

◆ Acute tubular necrosis
◆ Kidney failure

Signs and symptoms

Signs and symptoms of rhabdomyolysis include myalgias or muscle pain (especially in the thighs, calves, or lower back), weakness, tenderness, malaise, fever, dark urine, nausea, and vomiting. The patient may also experience weight gain, seizures, joint pain, and fatigue. Symptoms may be subtle initially. Rhabdomyolysis can result in acute renal failure.

Diagnosis

A serum or urine myoglobin test is positive. Creatine kinase levels 100 times above normal or higher suggest rhabdomyolysis. A urinalysis may reveal casts and may be positive for hemoglobin without evidence of red blood cells on microscopic examination. Serum potassium may be very high (potassium is released from cells into the bloodstream when cell breakdown occurs).

Treatment

Early, aggressive hydration may prevent complications from rhabdomyolysis by rapidly eliminating the myoglobin from the kidneys. I.V. hydration and diuretics promote diuresis. Diuretic medications, such as mannitol or furosemide, may aid in flushing the pigment out of the kidneys. If urine output is sufficient, bicarbonate may be given to maintain an alkaline urine state, thereby helping to prevent the dissociation of myoglobin into toxic compounds. Hyperkalemia should be treated if present. Kidney failure should be treated as appropriate. Dialysis may be necessary and, in severe cases, kidney transplantation.

Special considerations

◆ Monitor the patient's intake and output, vital signs, electrolyte levels, daily weight, and laboratory results.

▼ ALERT *Watch for signs of renal failure (such as decreasing urine output and increasing urine specific gravity), fluid overload (such as dyspnea and tachycardia), pulmonary edema, and electrolyte imbalances (such as serum potassium).*

◆ Provide reassurance and emotional support for the patient and the family.

◆ To help prevent rhabdomyolysis from occurring, ensure adequate hydration, monitor the patient for adverse reactions to any prescribed medications, and monitor blood transfusion administration carefully.

SELECTED REFERENCES

Goodman, S. B. (2017). Inflammation and the musculoskeletal system. *Journal of Orthopaedic Translation, 10,* A1–A2. doi:10.1016/j.jot.2017.07.001

Mehdipour, F. (2017). Pediatric musculoskeletal imaging guidelines, pediatric musculoskeletal imaging age considerations. *Iranian Journal of Radiology, 14*(Special issue), e48347. doi:10.5812/iranjradiol.48347

Oliveira, P. R., et al. (2017). Optimizing the treatment of osteomyelitis with antimicrobial drugs: Current concepts. *Current Orthopaedic Practice, 28*(2), 208–212. doi:10.1097/BCO.0000000000000477

Qaseem, A., et al. (2017). Treatment of low bone density or osteoporosis to prevent fractures in men and women: A clinical practice guideline update from the American College of Physicians. *Annals of Internal Medicine, 166*(11), 818–839. doi:10.7326/M15-1361

Winzenberg, T., et al. (2015). Musculoskeletal chest wall pain. *Australian Family Physician, 44*(8), 540–544. Retrieved from https://www.racgp.org.au/afp/2015/august/musculoskeletal-chest-wall-pain/

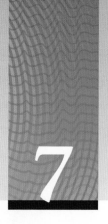

RENAL AND UROLOGIC DISORDERS

Introduction

The kidneys are located retroperitoneally in the lumbar area, with the right kidney a little lower than the left because of the liver above it. The left kidney is slightly longer than the right and closer to the midline. The kidneys move as body position changes. They're covered by the fibrous capsule, perirenal fat, renal fascia, and pararenal fat. (See *Structure of the kidneys*, page 334.)

Renal arteries branch into five segmental arteries that supply different areas of the kidneys. The segmental arteries then branch into several divisions from which the afferent arterioles and vasa recta arise. Renal veins follow a similar branching pattern, characterized by stellate vessels and segmental branches, and empty into the inferior vena cava. The tubular system receives its blood supply from a peritubular capillary network of vessels.

The gross structure of each kidney includes the lateral and medial margins, the hilus, the renal sinus, and renal parenchyma. The hilus, located at the medial margin, is the indentation where the blood and lymph vessels enter the kidney and the ureter emerges. The hilus leads to the renal sinus, which is a spacious cavity filled with adipose tissue, branches of the renal vessels, calyces, the renal pelvis, and the ureter. The renal sinus is surrounded by parenchyma, which consists of a cortex and a medulla.

The cortex (outermost layer of the kidney) contains glomeruli (parts of the nephron),

cortical arches (areas that separate the medullary pyramids from the renal surface), columns of Bertin (areas that separate the pyramids from one another), and medullary rays of Ferrein (long, delicate processes from the bases of the pyramids that mix with the cortex). The medulla contains pyramids (cone-shaped structures of parenchymal tissue), papillae (apical ends of the pyramids through which urine oozes into the minor calyces), and papillary ducts of Bellini (collecting ducts in the pyramids that empty into the papillae).

URETERS

The ureters are a pair of retroperitoneally located, mucosa-lined, fibromuscular tubes that transport urine from the renal pelvis to the urinary bladder. Although the ureters have no sphincters, their oblique entrance into the bladder creates a mucosal fold that may produce a sphincterlike action.

The adult urinary bladder is a spherical, hollow muscular sac, with a normal capacity of 300 to 600 mL. It is located anterior and inferior to the peritoneal cavity, and posterior to the pubic bones. The gross structure of the bladder includes the fundus (large central, posterosuperior portion of the bladder), the apex (anterosuperior region), the body (posteroinferior region containing the ureteral orifices), and the urethral orifice, or neck (most inferior portion of the bladder). The three orifices comprise a triangular area called the *trigone*.

Structure of the kidneys

The major components of the kidneys are depicted below.

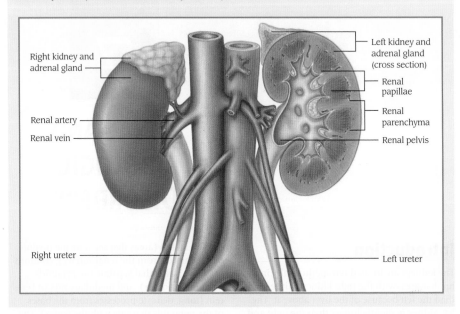

Right kidney and adrenal gland

Renal artery

Renal vein

Right ureter

Left kidney and adrenal gland (cross section)

Renal papillae

Renal parenchyma

Renal pelvis

Left ureter

NEPHRONS

The functional units of each kidney are its 1 to 3 million nephrons. Each nephron is composed of the renal corpuscle and the tubular system. The renal corpuscle includes the glomerulus (a network of minute blood vessels) and Bowman's capsule (an epithelial sac surrounding the glomerulus that's part of the tubular system). The renal corpuscle has a vascular pole, where the afferent arteriole enters and the efferent arteriole emerges, and a urinary pole that narrows to form the beginning of the tubular system. The tubular system includes the proximal convoluted tubule, the loop of Henle, and the distal convoluted tubule. The last portion of the nephron consists of the collecting duct.

INNERVATION AND VASCULATURE

The kidneys are innervated by sympathetic branches from the celiac plexus, upper lumbar splanchnic and thoracic nerves, and the intermesenteric and superior hypogastric plexuses, which form a plexus around the kidneys. Similar numbers of sympathetic and parasympathetic nerves from the renal plexus, superior hypogastric plexus, and intermesenteric plexus innervate the ureters. Nerves that arise from the

inferior hypogastric plexuses innervate the bladder. The parasympathetic nerve supply to the bladder controls micturition.

The ureters receive their blood supply from the renal, vesical, gonadal, and iliac arteries, and the abdominal aorta. The ureteral veins follow the arteries and drain into the renal vein. The bladder receives blood through vesical arteries. Vesical veins unite to form the pudendal plexus, which empties into the iliac veins. A rich lymphatic system drains the renal cortex, the kidneys, the ureters, and the bladder.

HOMEOSTASIS

Through the production and elimination of urine, the kidneys maintain homeostasis. These vital organs regulate the volume, electrolyte concentration, and acid–base balance of body fluids; detoxify the blood and eliminate wastes; regulate blood pressure; and aid in erythropoiesis. The kidneys eliminate wastes from the body through urine formation (by glomerular filtration, tubular reabsorption, and tubular secretion) and excretion. Glomerular filtration, the process of filtering the blood flowing through the kidneys, depends on the permeability of the capillary walls, vascular pressure, and filtration pressure. The normal glomerular filtration rate (GFR) is about 120 mL/minute.

CLEARANCE MEASURES FUNCTION

Clearance is the volume of plasma that can be cleared of a given substance per unit of time, and depends on how renal tubular cells handle the substance that has been filtered by the glomerulus:

◆ If the tubules don't reabsorb or secrete the substance, clearance equals the GFR.

◆ If the tubules reabsorb it, clearance is less than the GFR.

◆ If the tubules secrete it, clearance is greater than the GFR.

◆ If the tubules reabsorb and secrete it, clearance is less than, equal to, or greater than the GFR.

The most accurate measure of glomerular function is creatinine clearance, because this substance is filtered only by the glomerulus and isn't reabsorbed by the tubules.

The transport of filtered substances in tubular reabsorption or secretion may be active (requiring the expenditure of energy) or passive (requiring none). For example, energy is required to move sodium across tubular cells (active transport), but none is required to move urea (passive transport). The amount of reabsorption or secretion of a substance depends on the maximum tubular transport capacity for that substance; that is, the greatest amount of a substance that can be reabsorbed or secreted per minute without saturating the system.

ELDER TIP *After age 40, a person's renal function begins to diminish; if the person lives to age 90, it may have decreased by as much as 50%. This change is reflected in a decreased GFR; it's caused by age-related changes in the renal vasculature that disturb glomerular hemodynamics as well as by reduced cardiac output and atherosclerotic changes that reduce renal blood flow by more than 50%.*

WATER REGULATION

Hormones partially control water regulation by the kidneys. Hormonal control depends on the response of osmoreceptors to changes in osmolality. The two hormones involved are antidiuretic hormone (ADH), produced by the pituitary gland, and aldosterone, produced by the adrenal cortex. ADH alters the collecting tubules' permeability to water. When plasma concentration of ADH is high, the tubules are very permeable to water, so a greater amount of water is reabsorbed, creating a high concentration but small volume of urine. The reverse is true if ADH concentration is low.

Aldosterone regulates sodium and water reabsorption from the distal tubules. High plasma aldosterone concentration promotes sodium and water reabsorption from the tubules and decreases sodium and water excretion in the urine; low plasma aldosterone concentration promotes sodium and water excretion. Aldosterone also helps control the distal tubular secretion of potassium. Other factors that determine potassium secretion include the amount of potassium ingested, number of hydrogen ions secreted, level of intracellular potassium, amount of sodium in the distal tubule, and the GFR.

The countercurrent mechanism—composed of a multiplication system and an exchange system that occur in the renal medulla via the limbs of the loop of Henle and the vasa recta—is the method by which the kidneys concentrate urine. It achieves active transport of sodium and chloride between the loop of Henle and the medullary interstitial fluid. Failure of the countercurrent mechanism produces polyuria and nocturia.

To regulate acid–base balance, the kidneys secrete hydrogen ions, reabsorb sodium and bicarbonate ions, acidify phosphate salts, and synthesize ammonia—which keep the blood at its normal pH of 7.37 to 7.43.

The kidneys assist in regulating blood pressure by synthesizing and secreting renin in response to an actual, or perceived, decrease in the volume of extracellular fluid. Renin, in turn, acts on a substrate to form angiotensin I, which is converted to angiotensin II. Angiotensin II increases arterial blood pressure by peripheral vasoconstriction and stimulation of aldosterone secretion. The resulting increase in the aldosterone level promotes the reabsorption of sodium and water to correct the fluid deficit and renal ischemia.

The kidneys secrete erythropoietin in response to decreased oxygen tension in the renal blood supply. Erythropoietin then acts on the bone marrow to increase the production of red blood cells (RBCs).

Renal tubular cells synthesize active vitamin D and help regulate calcium balance and bone metabolism.

CLINICAL ASSESSMENT

Assessment of the renal and urologic systems begins with an accurate patient history and requires a thorough physical examination and certain laboratory data and test results from invasive and noninvasive procedures. When obtaining a patient history, ask about symptoms that pertain specifically to the pathology of the renal and urologic systems, such as frequency or urgency, and about the presence of any systemic diseases that can produce renal or urologic dysfunction, such as hypertension, diabetes mellitus, or bladder infections. Family history may also suggest a genetic predisposition to certain renal diseases, such as glomerulonephritis or polycystic kidney disease. Also, ask what medications the patient has been taking; abuse of analgesics or antibiotics may cause nephrotoxicity.

PHYSICAL EXAMINATION FOR RENAL DISEASE

The first step in physical examination is careful observation of the patient's overall appearance because renal disease affects all body systems. Examine the patient's skin for color, turgor, intactness, and texture; mucous membranes for color, secretions, odor, and intactness; eyes for periorbital edema and vision; general activity for motion, gait, and posture; muscle movement for motor function and general strength; and mental status for level of consciousness, orientation, and response to stimuli. (See *Common renal symptoms*.)

Common renal symptoms

Symptom	Possible cause
Dribbling	Prostatic enlargement, strictures
Dysuria	Infection, inflammation of bladder or urethra
Edema	Nephrotic syndrome, failure
Frequency	Infection, diabetes, bladder tumors, medications
Hematuria	Glomerular diseases, trauma, neoplasms, renal calculi
Hesitancy	Neurogenic bladder, infection
Incontinence	Infection, neoplasms, prolapsed uterus
Nocturia	Infection, nephrotic syndrome, diabetes, medications
Oliguria	Failure, insufficiency, neoplasms
Proteinuria	Glomerular diseases, infection
Pyuria	Infection
Renal colic	Calculi
Urgency	Infection, prostatic disease, medications

Renal disease causes distinctive changes in vital signs: hypertension due to fluid and electrolyte imbalances and hyperactivity of the renin–angiotensin system; a strong, fast, irregular pulse due to fluid and electrolyte imbalances; hyperventilation to compensate for metabolic acidosis; and an increased susceptibility to infection due to overall decreased resistance. Palpation and percussion may reveal little because the kidneys and bladder are difficult to palpate unless they are enlarged or distended.

NONINVASIVE TESTS AND MONITORING

Laboratory tests analyze serum levels of chemical substances such as uric acid, creatinine, and blood urea nitrogen; tests also determine urine characteristics, including the presence of RBCs, white blood cells (WBCs), casts, or bacteria; specific gravity and pH; and physical properties, such as clarity, color, and odor. (See *Serum and urine values in renal disease*, page 337.)

◆ Intake and output assessment: Fluid intake and output measurement helps determine the patient's hydration status but isn't a reliable method of evaluating renal function because urine output varies with different types of renal disorders. To provide the most useful and accurate information, use calibrated containers, establish baseline values for each patient, compare measurement patterns, and validate intake and output measurements by checking the patient's weight daily. Monitor all fluid losses—including blood, vomitus, and diarrhea. Also assess wound and stoma drainage daily.

◆ Specimen collection: Meticulous specimen collection is vital for valid laboratory data. If the patient is collecting the specimen, explain the importance of cleaning the meatal area thoroughly. The culture specimen should be caught midstream, in a sterile container; a specimen for urinalysis, in a clean container, preferably at the first voiding of the day. Begin a 24-hour specimen collection after discarding the first voiding; such specimens often necessitate special handling or preservatives. When obtaining a urine specimen from a catheterized patient, remember to avoid taking the specimen from the collection bag; instead, aspirate a sample through the collection port in the catheter, with a sterile needle and a syringe.

◆ Kidney–ureter–bladder radiography: This test assesses size, shape, position, and areas of calcification of these organs.

◆ Ultrasonography: This safe, painless procedure allows for visualization of the renal parenchyma, calyces, pelvis, ureters, and bladder. Because the test doesn't depend on renal

Serum and urine values in renal disease

	Normal serum value	Deviation	Normal urine value	Deviation
Sodium	135 to 145 mEq/L	↑ or N	30 to 280 mEq/L	V
Potassium	3.8 to 5.5 mEq/L	↑	25 to 100 mEq/L	↓
Chloride	100 to 108 mEq/L	↑	110 to 250 mEq/ 24 hour	↓
Calcium	8.9 to 10.1 mg/dL	↓	Female: <250 mg/ 24 hour	↓
			Male: <275 mg /24 hour	
Phosphorus	2.5 to 4.5 mg/dL	↑ or N	1 g/24 hour	V
Magnesium	1.7 to 2.1 mEq/L	↑	<150 mg/24 hour	↓
Carbon dioxide combining power	22 to 34 mEq/L	↓		
Specific gravity			1.005 to 1.035	↓
pH			4.5 to 8	↑
Blood urea nitrogen	8 to 20 mg/dL	↑	10 to 20 g/L	↓
Creatinine	Female: 0.6 to 0.9 mg/dL	↑	Female: 0 to 80 mg/24 hour	↓
	Male: 0.8 to 1.2 mg/dL		Male: 0 to 40 mg/ 24 hour	
Osmolality	280 to 295 mOsm/kg	V	500 to 1,400 mOsm/kg	↓
Uric acid	Female: 2.3 to 6 mg/dL	↑		
	Male: 4.3 to 8 mg/dL			
Glucose	70 to 100 mg/dL	N	0	N
Protein	6.9 to 7.9 g/dL	↓ or N	0	V
Hematocrit	Female: 38% to 46%	↓		
	Male: 42% to 54%			
Hemoglobin	Female: 12 to 16 g/dL	↓		
	Male: 14 to 18 g/dL			
White blood cells	4,000 to 10,000/µL		None	V
Red blood cells			None	V
Casts			None	V
Bacteria			None	V
Alkaline phosphatase	Female age 24 to 65: 82 to 282 U/L	↑		
	Male age 19 or older: 98 to 251 U/L			

Key: ↑, increased; ↓, decreased; N, normal; V, varies.

function, it's useful in patients with renal failure and in detecting complications after kidney transplantation.

◆ Invasive tests: See *Invasive diagnostic tests for assessing the renal and urologic systems*, pages 338 and 339.

Invasive diagnostic tests for assessing the renal and urologic systems

Several invasive tests are available to assist in the diagnosis of renal and urologic problems. The most serious complication that occurs with many of these procedures is hypersensitivity to the contrast media. Symptoms may include increased pulse rate, itching, hives, chills, fever, dyspnea, and shock.

Procedure	Purpose	Special considerations
Computed tomography scan (CT) or magnetic resonance imaging (MRI)	Although CT scan and MRI can be noninvasive, I.V. contrast material is often given to enhance the views obtained. These tests are especially helpful in evaluating renal or bladder mass lesions.	*Before:* Check for prior history of contrast sensitivity. *After:* After using I.V. contrast medium, observe for hypersensitivity reaction and hematoma at injection site.
Cystoscopy	A fiberoptic scope is used to visualize the inside of the bladder in cystoscopy.	*Before:* Give sedatives as ordered. *After:* Offer increased fluids; administer analgesics; watch for hematuria and signs of perforation, hemorrhage, and infection (chills, fever, increased pulse rate, shock).
Cystourethrography	In cystourethrography, X-rays and I.V. contrast material are used to determine size and shape of the bladder and urethra.	*Before:* Check for prior history of contrast sensitivity. *During:* Catheterize the patient. *After:* Offer increased fluids; observe for hypersensitivity reaction.
Cystometry	Cystometry is used to evaluate bladder pressure, sensation, and capacity. A catheter is introduced into the bladder, and saline solution is instilled. Results are shown on a computer at the time of testing.	*Before:* Observe voiding; catheterize for residual urine. *After:* Remove catheter; watch for stress incontinence when patient coughs; watch voiding; catheterize for residual urine.
Excretory urography	Excretory urography uses X-rays and I.V. contrast material to allow visualization of renal parenchyma, calyces, pelves, ureters, bladder, and stones.	*Before:* Check for prior history of contrast sensitivity. *After:* Observe for hypersensitivity reaction; watch for hematomas at injection site.
Nephrotomography	In nephrotomography, I.V. contrast material and tomography are used to visualize parenchyma, calyces, and pelves in layers.	*Before:* Check for prior history of contrast sensitivity. *After:* Observe for hypersensitivity reaction.

Invasive diagnostic tests for assessing the renal and urologic systems (*continued*)

Renal angiography	Renal angiography uses contrast material injected into a catheter in the femoral artery or vein to allow visualization of the arterial tree and capillaries as well as venous drainage of the kidney.	*Before:* Check for prior history of contrast sensitivity. *After:* Observe for hypersensitivity reaction, hematomas and hemorrhage at injection site, and nephrotoxicity. Offer increased fluids.
Renal scan	In renal scan, radioisotopes are administered I.V., and images of the kidney are taken at intervals to determine renal function.	*Before:* Check for prior history of sensitivity. *After:* Observe for hypersensitivity reaction.
Renal biopsy	The specimen obtained in renal biopsy is used to develop histologic diagnosis and determine therapy and prognosis.	*Before:* Make sure the patient's clotting times, prothrombin times, and platelet count are recorded on his or her chart. *After:* Apply gentle pressure to the bandage site. Watch for hemorrhage and hematoma at the biopsy site, and look for hematuria.

TREATMENT METHODS

Treatment of intractable renal or urinary system dysfunction may require urinary diversion, dialysis, or kidney transplantation. Urinary diversion is the surgical creation of an outlet for excreting urine. The types of urinary diversion include ileal conduit, cutaneous ureterostomy, ureterosigmoidostomy, and creation of a rectal bladder.

In dialysis, a semipermeable membrane, osmosis, and diffusion imitate normal renal function by eliminating excess body fluids, maintaining or restoring plasma electrolyte and acid–base balance, and removing waste products and dialyzable poisons from the blood. Dialysis is most often used for patients with acute or chronic renal failure. The two most common types of dialysis are peritoneal dialysis and hemodialysis.

In peritoneal dialysis, a dialysate solution is infused into the peritoneal cavity. Substances then diffuse through the peritoneal membrane. Waste products remain in the dialysate solution and are removed.

Hemodialysis separates solutes by differential diffusion through a cellophane membrane placed between the blood and the dialysate solution, in an external receptacle. Because the blood must actually pass out of the body into a dialysis machine, hemodialysis requires an access route to the blood supply by an arteriovenous fistula or cannula or by a bovine or synthetic graft. When caring for a patient with such an access route, monitor the patency of the access route, prevent infection, and promote safety and adequate function. After dialysis, watch for such complications as headache, vomiting, agitation, and twitching.

Patients with end-stage renal disease may benefit from kidney transplantation, despite its limitations: a shortage of donor kidneys, the chance of transplant rejection, and the need for lifelong medications and follow-up care. After kidney transplantation, maintain fluid and electrolyte balance, prevent infection, monitor for rejection, and promote psychological well-being.

Congenital anomalies

MEDULLARY SPONGE KIDNEY

In medullary sponge kidney, the collecting ducts in the renal pyramids dilate, and cavities, clefts, and cysts form in the medulla. This disease may affect only a single pyramid in one kidney or all pyramids in both kidneys. The kidneys are usually somewhat enlarged but may be of normal size; they appear spongy.

Because this disorder is usually asymptomatic and benign, it's often overlooked until the patient reaches adulthood. The prognosis is generally very good. Medullary sponge kidney is unrelated to medullary cystic disease; these conditions are similar only in the presence and location of the cysts.

Pathophysiology
Medullary sponge kidney may be transmitted as an autosomal dominant trait, but this remains unproven. Most nephrologists consider it a congenital abnormality.

Although medullary sponge kidney may be found in both sexes and in all age groups, it primarily affects males ages 40 to 70. It occurs in about 1 in every 5,000 to 20,000 persons.

Complications
◆ Calcium oxalate calculi
◆ Infection

Signs and symptoms
Symptoms usually appear only as a result of complications and are seldom present before adulthood. Complications include formation of calcium oxalate stones, which lodge in the dilated cystic collecting ducts or pass through a ureter, and infection secondary to dilation of the ducts. These complications, which occur in about 30% of patients, are likely to produce severe colic, hematuria, lower urinary tract infection ([UTI]; burning on urination, urgency, frequency), and pyelonephritis. Secondary impairment of renal function from obstruction and infection occurs in only about 10% of patients.

Diagnosis
Excretory urography is usually the key to diagnosis, often showing a characteristic flowerlike appearance of the pyramidal cavities when they fill with contrast material. It may also show renal calculi. Urinalysis is generally normal unless complications develop; however, it may show a slight reduction in concentrating ability or hypercalciuria. Diagnosis must distinguish medullary sponge kidney from renal tuberculosis, renal tubular acidosis, and papillary necrosis.

Treatment
Treatment focuses on preventing or treating complications caused by stones and infection.

Specific measures include increasing fluid intake and monitoring renal function and urine. New symptoms necessitate immediate evaluation.

Because medullary sponge kidney is a benign condition, surgery is seldom necessary, except to remove stones during acute obstruction. Only serious, uncontrollable infection or hemorrhage requires nephrectomy.

Special considerations
Patient care includes explaining the disease to the patient and family and reassuring them that the condition is benign and the prognosis good.
◆ To prevent infection, instruct the patient to bathe often and use proper toilet hygiene; this is especially important for a female patient because the proximity of the urinary meatus and the anus increases the risk of infection.
◆ If infection occurs, stress the importance of completing the prescribed course of antibiotic therapy.
◆ Emphasize the need for adequate fluid intake.
◆ Explain all diagnostic procedures, and provide emotional support. Teach the patient how to collect a clean-catch urine specimen for culture. Check for allergy to excretory urography dye.
◆ When the patient is hospitalized for a stone, strain all urine, administer analgesics as ordered, and force fluids. Before discharge, tell the patient to watch for and report any signs of stone passage and UTI.

POLYCYSTIC KIDNEY DISEASE
Polycystic kidney disease is an inherited disorder characterized by multiple, bilateral, grapelike clusters of fluid-filled cysts that grossly enlarge the kidneys, compressing and eventually replacing functioning renal tissue. (See *Polycystic kidney*, page 341.) The disease appears in two distinct forms: The infantile form typically causes stillbirth or early neonatal death, although some infants may survive for 2 years, then develop fatal renal, cardiac, or respiratory failure. The adult form begins insidiously but usually becomes obvious between ages 30 and 50 years old; rarely, it causes no symptoms until the patient is in his 70s. In the adult form, renal deterioration is more gradual but, as in the infantile form, progresses relentlessly to fatal uremia.

The prognosis in adults is extremely variable. Progression may be slow, even after symptoms of renal insufficiency appear. However, after uremic symptoms develop, polycystic kidney disease is usually fatal within 4 years, unless the patient receives treatment with dialysis, kidney transplantation, or both.

Polycystic kidney

In polycystic kidney disease, cysts are seen in grapelike clusters, as shown below.

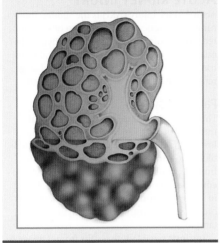

Pathophysiology

Although both types of polycystic kidney disease are genetically transmitted, the incidence in two distinct age groups and different inheritance patterns suggest two unrelated disorders. The infantile type appears to be inherited as an autosomal recessive trait, whereas the adult type seems to be an autosomal dominant trait. The gene has been located on chromosome 6, supporting the premise that this is a single genetic disease with variable phenotype presentation.

Polycystic kidney disease reportedly affects 1 in every 1,000 Americans; that number may be even higher because some cases from patients who aren't symptomatic go unreported. Both types of polycystic kidney disease affect males and females equally.

Complications

◆ Hypertension
◆ UTI
◆ Kidney infection
◆ End-stage kidney disease
◆ Kidney stones
◆ Ruptured cysts

Signs and symptoms

PEDIATRIC TIP *The neonate with infantile polycystic disease often has pronounced epicanthal folds, a pointed nose, a small chin, and floppy, low-set ears (Potter facies). At* birth, the child has huge bilateral masses on the flanks that are symmetrical, tense, and can't be transilluminated. The patient characteristically shows signs of respiratory distress and heart failure. Eventually, the patient develops uremia and renal failure. Accompanying hepatic fibrosis may cause portal hypertension and bleeding varices to develop, requiring sclerotherapy or portacaval shunting.

Adult polycystic kidney disease is commonly asymptomatic through the patient's 40s, but may induce nonspecific symptoms, such as hypertension, polyuria, and recurrent UTIs. Later, the patient develops overt symptoms related to the enlarging kidney mass, such as lumbar pain, widening girth, and swollen or tender abdomen. Abdominal pain is usually worsened by exertion and relieved by lying down. In advanced stages, this disease may cause recurrent hematuria, life-threatening retroperitoneal bleeding resulting from cyst rupture, proteinuria, and colicky abdominal pain from the ureteral passage of clots or calculi. Generally, about 10 years after symptoms appear, progressive compression of kidney structures by the enlarging mass produces renal failure and uremia. Hypertension is found in about 20% to 30% of children and up to 75% of adults due to intrarenal ischemia, which activates the renin–angiotensin system.

Diagnosis

A family history and a physical examination revealing large bilateral, irregular masses in the flanks strongly suggest polycystic kidney disease. In advanced stages, grossly enlarged and palpable kidneys make the diagnosis obvious. In patients with these findings, the following laboratory results are typical:
◆ Excretory urography reveals enlarged kidneys, with elongation of pelvis, flattening of the calyces, and indentations caused by cysts. Excretory urography of the neonate shows poor excretion of contrast medium.
◆ Ultrasound and computed tomography (CT) scan show kidney enlargement and the presence of cysts; tomography demonstrates multiple areas of cystic damage. Ultrasonography is the preferred imaging technique because it's less expensive, doesn't require contrast or radiation exposure, and is easily and safely performed on children and pregnant females.
◆ Urinalysis and creatinine clearance tests are nonspecific tests that evaluate renal function and reveal urine protein or blood in the urine.

Diagnosis must rule out the presence of renal tumors.

Treatment

Polycystic kidney disease can't be cured. The primary goal of treatment is preserving renal parenchyma and preventing infectious complications. Management of secondary hypertension will also help prevent rapid deterioration in function. Progressive renal failure requires treatment similar to that for other types of renal disease, including dialysis or, rarely, kidney transplantation.

When adult polycystic kidney disease is discovered in the asymptomatic stage, careful monitoring is required, including urine cultures and creatinine clearance tests every 6 months. Prompt and vigorous antibiotic treatment is needed when a urine culture reveals infection—even when the patient is asymptomatic. As renal impairment progresses, selected patients may undergo dialysis, transplantation, or both. Cystic abscess or retroperitoneal bleeding may require surgical drainage; intractable pain (a rare symptom) may also require surgery. However, because this disease affects both kidneys, nephrectomy usually isn't recommended because it increases the risk of infection in the remaining kidney.

Special considerations

Because polycystic kidney disease is usually relentlessly progressive, comprehensive patient teaching and emotional support are essential.
◆ Refer the young adult patient or the parents of infants with polycystic kidney disease for genetic counseling. Parents will probably have many questions about the risk to other offspring.
◆ Provide supportive care to minimize any associated symptoms. Carefully assess the patient's lifestyle and his physical and mental status; determine how rapidly the disease is progressing. Use this information to plan individualized patient care.
◆ Acquaint yourself with all aspects of end-stage renal disease, including dialysis and transplantation, so you can provide appropriate care and patient teaching as the disease progresses.
◆ Explain all diagnostic procedures to the patient or to the family if the patient is an infant. Before beginning excretory urography or other procedures that use an iodine-based contrast medium, determine whether the patient has ever had an allergic reaction to iodine or shellfish. Even if the patient has no history of allergy, watch for an allergic reaction after performing the procedures.
◆ Administer antibiotics as ordered for UTI. Stress to the patient the need to take the medication exactly as prescribed, even if symptoms are minimal or absent.

Acute renal disorders

ACUTE KIDNEY INJURY

Acute kidney injury (AKI) is the sudden interruption of kidney function due to obstruction, reduced circulation, or renal parenchymal disease. It's usually reversible with medical treatment; otherwise, it may progress to end-stage renal disease, uremic syndrome, and death.

Pathophysiology

The causes of AKI are classified as prerenal, intrinsic (or parenchymal), and postrenal. Prerenal failure is associated with diminished blood flow to the kidneys, possibly resulting from hypovolemia, shock, severe anaphylaxis, embolism, blood loss, sepsis, pooling of fluid in ascites or burns, or from cardiovascular disorders, such as heart failure, arrhythmias, and tamponade.

Intrinsic renal failure results from damage to the kidneys themselves, usually due to acute tubular necrosis (ATN), but possibly due to acute poststreptococcal glomerulonephritis (APSGN), systemic lupus erythematosus, periarteritis nodosa, vasculitis, sickle cell disease, bilateral renal vein thrombosis, nephrotoxins, chronic misuse of nonsteroidal anti-inflammatory drugs, radiopaque contrast agents, ischemia, renal myeloma, acute pyelonephritis, and exposure to heavy metals, such as lead or mercury.

Postrenal failure results from bilateral obstruction of urinary outflow. Its multiple causes include kidney stones, blood clots, papillae from papillary necrosis, tumors, benign prostatic hyperplasia (BPH), strictures, and urethral edema from catheterization.

In the United States, the annual incidence of AKI is 100 cases for every million people. It's diagnosed in 1% of hospital admissions. Hospital-acquired AKI occurs in 4% of all admitted patients and 20% of patients who are admitted to critical care units.

Complications

◆ Volume overload
◆ Pulmonary edema
◆ Electrolyte imbalance
◆ Metabolic acidosis

Signs and symptoms

AKI is a critical illness. Its early signs are oliguria, azotemia, and, rarely, anuria. Electrolyte imbalance, metabolic acidosis, and other severe effects follow, as the patient becomes increasingly uremic and renal dysfunction disrupts other body systems:

◆ *Gastrointestinal (GI):* anorexia, nausea, vomiting, diarrhea or constipation, stomatitis, bleeding, hematemesis, dry mucous membranes, uremic breath

◆ *Central nervous system (CNS):* headache, drowsiness, irritability, confusion, peripheral neuropathy, seizures, coma

◆ *Cutaneous:* dryness, pruritus, pallor, purpura and, rarely, uremic frost

◆ *Cardiovascular:* early in the disease, hypotension; later, hypertension, arrhythmias, fluid overload, heart failure, systemic edema, anemia, altered clotting mechanisms

◆ *Respiratory:* pulmonary edema, Kussmaul respirations.

Fever and chills indicate infection, a common complication.

Diagnosis

The patient's history may include a disorder that can cause renal failure. Blood test results indicating intrinsic renal failure include elevated blood urea nitrogen, serum creatinine, and potassium levels and low blood pH, bicarbonate, hematocrit (HCT), and hemoglobin (Hb) level. Urine specimens show casts, cellular debris, decreased specific gravity and, in glomerular diseases, proteinuria and urine osmolality close to serum osmolality. Urine sodium level is less than 20 mEq/L if oliguria is due to decreased perfusion; more than 40 mEq/L if due to an intrinsic problem. Other studies include renal ultrasonography, kidney–ureter–bladder X-rays, cautious use of excretory urography, renal scan, and nephrotomography.

Treatment

The goal of treatment is to correct or eliminate any reversible causes of kidney failure, such as obstructive uropathy, volume depletion, or the use of kidney-toxic medications. Supportive measures include a diet high in calories and low in protein, sodium, and potassium, with supplemental vitamins and restricted fluids. Meticulous electrolyte monitoring is essential to detect hyperkalemia. If hyperkalemia occurs, acute therapy may include dialysis, I.V. administration of hypertonic glucose, insulin infusion, and sodium bicarbonate, and administration of a potassium exchange resin (orally or by enema) to remove potassium from the body.

If measures fail to control uremic symptoms, hemodialysis or peritoneal dialysis may be necessary. Continuous arteriovenous hemodiafiltration and continuous venovenous hemodiafiltration are alternative hemodialysis techniques for the treatment of AKI. They're generally reserved for when intermittent dialysis fails to control hypervolemia or uremia, or for patients for whom peritoneal dialysis isn't possible.

Special considerations

Patient care includes careful monitoring and dietary education.

◆ Measure and record intake and output, including all body fluids, such as wound drainage, nasogastric tube output, and diarrhea. Weigh the patient daily.

◆ Assess Hb levels and HCT and replace blood components, as indicated. *Don't* use whole blood if the patient is prone to heart failure and can't tolerate extra fluid volume. Packed RBCs deliver the necessary blood components without added volume.

◆ Monitor vital signs. Watch for and report any signs of pericarditis (pleuritic chest pain, tachycardia, pericardial friction rub), inadequate renal perfusion (hypotension), and acidosis.

◆ Maintain proper electrolyte balance. Strictly monitor potassium levels. Watch for symptoms of hyperkalemia (malaise, anorexia, paresthesia, or muscle weakness) and electrocardiogram changes (tall, peaked T waves, widening QRS segment, and disappearing P waves), and report them immediately. Avoid administering medications containing potassium.

◆ **ALERT** *Assess the patient frequently, especially during emergency treatment to lower potassium levels. If the patient receives hypertonic glucose and insulin infusions, monitor potassium levels. If you give sodium polystyrene sulfonate rectally, make sure the patient doesn't retain it and become constipated, to prevent bowel perforation.*

◆ Maintain nutritional status. Provide a high-calorie, low-protein, low-sodium, and low-potassium diet, with vitamin supplements. Give the anorectic patient small, frequent meals.

◆ Use sterile technique, because the patient with AKI is highly susceptible to infection. Personnel with upper respiratory tract infections shouldn't provide care for the patient.

◆ Prevent complications of immobility by encouraging frequent coughing and deep breathing and by performing passive range-of-motion exercises. Help the patient walk as soon as possible.

◆ Provide good mouth care frequently because mucous membranes are dry. If stomatitis occurs, an antibiotic solution may be ordered. Have the patient swish the solution around in his mouth before swallowing.

◆ Monitor for GI bleeding by guaiac testing all stools for blood. Administer medications carefully, especially antacids and stool softeners. Use aluminum-hydroxide–based antacids; magnesium-based antacids can cause serum magnesium levels to rise to critical levels.

◆ Use appropriate safety measures, such as side rails and restraints, because the patient with CNS involvement may be dizzy or confused.

◆ Provide emotional support to the patient and his family. Reassure them by clearly explaining all procedures.

◆ If the patient requires hemodialysis, check the blood access site (arteriovenous fistula, subclavian or femoral catheter) as per facility protocol or every 2 hours for patency and signs of clotting. Don't use the arm with the shunt or fistula for taking blood pressures or drawing blood. Weigh the patient before beginning dialysis. During dialysis, monitor vital signs, clotting times, blood flow, the function of the vascular access site, and arterial and venous pressures. Watch for complications, such as septicemia, embolism, hepatitis, and rapid fluid and electrolyte loss. After dialysis, monitor vital signs and the vascular access site; weigh the patient; watch for signs of fluid and electrolyte imbalances.

◆ During peritoneal dialysis, position the patient carefully. Elevate the head of the bed to reduce pressure on the diaphragm and aid respiration. Be alert for signs of infection (cloudy drainage, elevated temperature) and, rarely, bleeding. If pain occurs, reduce the amount of dialysate. Monitor the diabetic patient's blood glucose periodically, and administer insulin as ordered. Watch for complications, such as peritonitis, atelectasis, hypokalemia, pneumonia, and shock.

◆ Use standard precautions when handling all blood and body fluids.

▒▒▒▒ PREVENTION
◆ *Evaluate all drugs the patient is taking and determine which drugs may be affected by or have an effect on renal function.*
◆ *Aggressively restore fluid volume after major surgery or trauma.*

ACUTE PYELONEPHRITIS

Acute pyelonephritis (also known as *acute infective tubulointerstitial nephritis*) is a sudden inflammation caused by bacteria that primarily affects the interstitial area and the renal pelvis or, less often, the renal tubules. It's one of the most common renal diseases. With treatment and continued follow-up care, the prognosis is good, and extensive permanent damage is rare. (See *Chronic pyelonephritis,* page 345.)

Pathophysiology

Acute pyelonephritis results from bacterial infection of the kidneys. Infecting bacteria usually are normal intestinal and fecal flora that grow readily in urine. The most common causative organism is *Escherichia coli,* but *Proteus, Pseudomonas, Staphylococcus aureus,* and *Enterococcus faecalis* (formerly *Streptococcus faecalis*) may also cause this infection.

Typically, the infection spreads from the bladder to the ureters, then to the kidneys, as in vesicoureteral reflux due to congenital weakness at the junction of the ureter and the bladder. Bacteria refluxed to intrarenal tissues may create colonies of infection within 24 to 48 hours. Infection may also result from instrumentation (such as catheterization, cystoscopy, or urologic surgery), from a hematogenic infection (as in septicemia or endocarditis), or possibly from lymphatic infection.

Pyelonephritis may also result from an inability to empty the bladder (e.g., in patients with neurogenic bladder), urinary stasis, or urinary obstruction due to tumors, strictures, or BPH.

Pyelonephritis occurs more commonly in women, probably because of a shorter urethra and the proximity of the urinary meatus to the vagina and the rectum—both of which allow bacteria to reach the bladder more easily—and a lack of the antibacterial prostatic secretions produced by men. Incidence increases with age and is higher in the following groups:

◆ *Sexually active women:* Intercourse increases the risk of bacterial contamination.

◆ *Pregnant women:* About 5% develop asymptomatic bacteriuria; if untreated, about 40% develop pyelonephritis.

◆ *Diabetics:* Neurogenic bladder causes incomplete emptying and urinary stasis; glycosuria may support bacterial growth in the urine.

◆ *Persons with other renal diseases:* Compromised renal function aggravates susceptibility.

Complications

◆ Recurrence of pyelonephritis
◆ Sepsis
◆ Perinephric abscess
◆ Renal failure

Signs and symptoms

Typical clinical features include urgency, frequency, burning during urination, dysuria, nocturia, and hematuria (usually microscopic but may be gross). Urine may appear cloudy and have an ammonia-like or fishy odor. Other common symptoms include a temperature of

102° F (38.9° C) or higher, shaking chills, flank pain, anorexia, and general fatigue.

These symptoms characteristically develop rapidly over a few hours or a few days. Although these symptoms may disappear within days, even without treatment, residual bacterial infection is likely and may cause symptoms to recur later.

🌀 ELDER TIP *Elderly patients may exhibit altered mental status or GI or pulmonary symptoms rather than the usual febrile responses to pyelonephritis.*

🕯 PEDIATRIC TIP *In children younger than age 2, fever, vomiting, nonspecific abdominal complaints, or failure to thrive may be the only signs of acute pyelonephritis.*

Diagnosis

Diagnosis requires urinalysis and culture. Typical findings include:

◆ Pyuria (pus in urine): Urine sediment reveals the presence of leukocytes singly, in clumps, and in casts; and, possibly, a few RBCs.

◆ Significant bacteriuria: Urine culture reveals more than 100,000 organisms/mL of urine.

◆ Low specific gravity and osmolality: These findings result from a temporarily decreased ability to concentrate urine.

◆ Slightly alkaline urine pH.

◆ Proteinuria, glycosuria, and ketonuria: These conditions are less common.

◆ Costovertebral angle tenderness.

Excretory urography or CT scan of the kidneys, ureters, and bladder also help in the evaluation of acute pyelonephritis by revealing calculi, tumors, or cysts in the kidneys and the urinary tract. In addition, excretory urography may show asymmetrical kidneys.

Treatment

Treatment centers on antibiotic therapy appropriate to the specific infecting organism after identification by urine culture and sensitivity studies. When the infecting organism can't be identified, therapy usually consists of a broad-spectrum antibiotic. Urinary analgesics are also appropriate.

⚠ ALERT *If a woman is pregnant, antibiotics must be prescribed cautiously.*

Symptoms may disappear after several days of antibiotic therapy. Although urine usually becomes sterile within 48 to 72 hours, the course of such therapy is 10 to 14 days. Follow-up treatment may include reculturing urine 1 week after drug therapy stops, then periodically for the next year to detect residual or recurring infection. Most patients with uncomplicated

---

Chronic pyelonephritis

Chronic pyelonephritis is a persistent kidney inflammation that can scar the kidneys and may lead to chronic renal failure. Its etiology may be bacterial, metastatic, or urogenous. This disease is most common in patients who are predisposed to recurrent acute pyelonephritis, such as those with urinary obstructions or vesicoureteral reflux.

Patients with chronic pyelonephritis may have a childhood history of unexplained fevers or bedwetting. Clinical effects may include flank pain, anemia, low urine specific gravity, proteinuria, waxy casts, leukocytes in urine and, especially in late stages, hypertension. Uremia rarely develops from chronic pyelonephritis unless structural abnormalities exist in the excretory system. Bacteriuria may be intermittent. When no bacteria are found in the urine, diagnosis depends on excretory urography (renal pelvis may appear small and flattened) and renal biopsy.

Effective treatment of chronic pyelonephritis requires control of hypertension, elimination of the existing obstruction (when possible), and long-term antimicrobial therapy.

---

infections respond well to therapy and don't suffer reinfection.

In infection from obstruction or vesicoureteral reflux, antibiotics may be less effective; treatment may then necessitate surgery to relieve the obstruction or correct the anomaly. Patients at high risk of recurring urinary tract and kidney infections, such as those with prolonged use of an indwelling catheter or maintenance antibiotic therapy, require long-term follow-up. Recurrent episodes of acute pyelonephritis can eventually result in chronic pyelonephritis.

Special considerations

Patient care is supportive during antibiotic treatment of the underlying infection.

◆ Administer antipyretics for fever.

◆ Encourage fluids to achieve urine output of more than 2,000 mL/day. This helps to empty the bladder of contaminated urine. Don't encourage intake of more than 2 to 3 qt (2 to 3 L) because this may decrease the effectiveness of the antibiotics.

◆ Provide an acid-ash diet to prevent stone formation.

◆ Teach proper technique for collecting a clean-catch urine specimen. Be sure to refrigerate or culture a urine specimen within 30 minutes of collection to prevent overgrowth of bacteria.

◆ Stress the need to complete prescribed antibiotic therapy, even after symptoms subside. Encourage long-term follow-up care for high-risk patients.

To prevent acute pyelonephritis:

!!!!!! **PREVENTION**

◆ *Observe strict sterile technique during catheter insertion and care.*

◆ *Instruct women to prevent bacterial contamination by wiping the perineum from front to back after defecation.*

◆ *Advise routine checkups for patients with a history of UTIs. Teach them to recognize signs of infection, such as cloudy urine, burning on urination, urgency, and frequency, especially when accompanied by a low-grade fever.*

ACUTE POSTSTREPTOCOCCAL GLOMERULONEPHRITIS

APSGN, also known as *acute glomerulonephritis*, is a relatively common bilateral inflammation of the glomeruli. It usually follows a streptococcal infection of the respiratory tract or, less often, a skin infection such as impetigo.

Pathophysiology

APSGN results from the entrapment and collection of antigen–antibody complexes (produced as an immunologic mechanism in response to streptococcus) in the glomerular capillary membranes, inducing inflammatory damage and impeding glomerular function. Sometimes, the immune complement further damages the glomerular membrane. The damaged and inflamed glomerulus loses the ability to be selectively permeable, and allows RBCs and proteins to filter through as the GFR falls. Uremic poisoning may result.

APSGN is most common in boys ages 3 to 7, but it can occur at any age. Incidence is rising in the United States and Europe, with epidemics occurring in developing countries in Africa, the West Indies, and the Middle East.

Up to 95% of children and up to 70% of adults with APSGN recover fully; the rest may progress to chronic renal failure within months.

Complications

◆ AKI or chronic kidney failure
◆ End-stage renal disease
◆ Hypertension
◆ Heart failure
◆ Pulmonary edema
◆ Chronic glomerulonephritis
◆ Nephrotic syndrome

Signs and symptoms

APSGN begins within 1 to 3 weeks after pharyngitis. Symptoms include mild to moderate edema, oliguria (<400 mL/24 hours), proteinuria, azotemia, hematuria, and fatigue. Mild to severe hypertension may result from either sodium or water retention (due to decreased GFR) or inappropriate renin release. Heart failure from hypervolemia leads to pulmonary edema.

PEDIATRIC TIP *The presenting features of APSGN in children may be encephalopathy with seizures and focal neurologic deficits.*

Diagnosis

Diagnosis requires a detailed patient history and assessment of clinical symptoms and laboratory tests.

Urinalysis typically reveals proteinuria and hematuria. RBCs, WBCs, and mixed cell casts are common in urinary sediment. Elevated serum creatinine levels and low creatinine clearance accompany impaired glomerular filtration. Elevated antistreptolysin-O titers (in 80% of patients), elevated streptozyme and anti-DNase B titers, and low serum complement levels verify recent streptococcal infection. A throat culture may also show group A beta-hemolytic streptococcus. Renal ultrasound may show a normal or slightly enlarged kidney. A renal biopsy may confirm the diagnosis or assess renal tissue status.

Treatment

The goals of treatment are relief of symptoms and prevention of complications. Vigorous supportive care includes bed rest, fluid and dietary sodium restrictions, and correction of electrolyte imbalances (possibly with dialysis, although this is rarely necessary). Therapy may include diuretics to reduce extracellular fluid overload and an antihypertensive. The use of antibiotics is recommended for 7 to 10 days if staphylococcal infection is documented. Otherwise, antibiotic use is controversial.

Special considerations

APSGN usually resolves within 2 weeks, so patient care is primarily supportive.

◆ Check vital signs and electrolyte values. Monitor intake and output and daily weight. Assess renal function daily through serum creatinine, blood urea nitrogen, and urine creatinine clearance levels. Watch for and immediately report signs of acute renal failure (oliguria, azotemia, and acidosis).

◆ Consult the dietitian to provide a diet high in calories and low in protein, sodium, potassium, and fluids.

◆ Protect the debilitated patient against secondary infection by providing good nutrition, using good hygienic technique, and preventing contact with infected persons.

◆ Bed rest is necessary during the acute phase. Allow the patient to *gradually* resume normal activities as symptoms subside.

◆ Provide emotional support for the patient and family. If the patient is on dialysis, explain the procedure fully.

◆ Advise the patient with a history of chronic upper respiratory tract infections to immediately report signs of infection (fever, sore throat).

◆ Tell the patient that follow-up examinations are necessary to detect chronic renal failure. Stress the need for regular blood pressure, urinary protein, and renal function assessments during the convalescent months to detect recurrence. After APSGN, gross hematuria may recur during nonspecific viral infections; abnormal urinary findings may persist for years.

◆ Encourage pregnant women with a history of APSGN to have frequent medical evaluations because pregnancy further stresses the kidneys and increases the risk of chronic renal failure.

ACUTE TUBULAR NECROSIS

ATN, also known as *acute tubulointerstitial nephritis*, accounts for about 75% of all cases of AKI and is the most common cause of AKI in critically ill patients. ATN injures the tubular segment of the nephron, causing renal failure and uremic syndrome. Mortality ranges from 40% to 70%, depending on complications from underlying diseases. Nonoliguric forms of ATN have a better prognosis.

Pathophysiology

ATN results from ischemic or nephrotoxic injury, most commonly in debilitated patients, such as the critically ill or those who have undergone extensive surgery. In ischemic injury, disruption of blood flow to the kidneys may result from circulatory collapse, severe hypotension, trauma, hemorrhage, dehydration, cardiogenic or septic shock, surgery, anesthetics, or reactions to transfusions. Nephrotoxic injury may follow ingestion of certain chemical agents or result from a hypersensitive reaction of the kidneys. (See *Rise in nephrotoxic injury.*) Because nephrotoxic ATN doesn't damage the basement membrane of the nephron, it's potentially reversible. However, ischemic ATN can damage the epithelial and basement membranes and

---

Rise in nephrotoxic injury

The incidence of acute tubular necrosis (ATN) due to ingestion or inhalation of toxic substances is rising. ATN may occur in hospitalized patients following exposure to toxic agents, such as antibiotics, chemotherapeutic agents, or contrast material. Other nephrotoxic agents include pesticides, fungicides, heavy metals (e.g., mercury, arsenic, lead, bismuth, uranium), and organic solvents containing carbon tetrachloride or ethylene glycol, such as cleaning fluids or industrial solvents. Ingestion of these substances may be accidental or intentional.

---

can cause lesions in the renal interstitium. ATN may result from:

◆ diseased tubular epithelium that allows leakage of glomerular filtrate across the membranes and reabsorption of filtrate into the blood

◆ obstruction of urine flow by the collection of damaged cells, casts, RBCs, and other cellular debris within the tubular walls

◆ ischemic injury to glomerular epithelial cells, resulting in cellular collapse and decreased glomerular capillary permeability

◆ ischemic injury to vascular endothelium, eventually resulting in cellular swelling and obstruction.

Complications
◆ Fluid and electrolyte imbalance
◆ Heart failure
◆ GI hemorrhage
◆ Pulmonary edema

Signs and symptoms
Nephrotoxic injury causes multiple symptoms similar to those of renal failure, particularly azotemia, anemia, acidosis, overhydration, and hypertension. Some patients may also experience fever, rash, and eosinophilia. However, ATN is usually difficult to recognize in its early stages because effects of the critically ill patient's primary disease may mask the symptoms of ATN. (See *A close look at acute tubular necrosis,* page 348.) The first recognizable effect may be decreased urine output. Generally, hyperkalemia and the characteristic uremic syndrome soon follow, with oliguria (or, rarely, anuria) and confusion, which may progress to uremic coma. Other possible complications may

PATHOPHYSIOLOGY
A close look at acute tubular necrosis

In acute tubular necrosis caused by ischemia, patches of necrosis occur, usually in the straight portion of the proximal tubules as shown. In areas without lesions, tubules are usually dilated.

In acute tubular necrosis caused by nephrotoxicity, the tubules have a more uniform appearance, as shown in the second illustration.

---

include heart failure, uremic pericarditis, pulmonary edema, uremic lung, anemia, anorexia, intractable vomiting, and poor wound healing due to debilitation.

⚠ **ALERT** *Fever and chills may signal the onset of an infection, which is the leading cause of death in ATN.*

Diagnosis

Diagnosis is usually delayed until the condition has progressed to an advanced stage. The most significant laboratory clues are urinary sediment containing RBCs and casts, and dilute urine of a low specific gravity (1.010), low osmolality (<400 mOsm/kg), and high sodium level (40 to 60 mEq/L). Blood studies reveal elevated blood urea nitrogen and serum creatinine levels, anemia, defects in platelet adherence, metabolic acidosis, and hyperkalemia. An electrocardiogram may show arrhythmias (due to electrolyte imbalances) and, with hyperkalemia, widening QRS segment, disappearing P waves, and tall, peaked T waves.

Treatment

Treatment consists of identifying the nephrotoxic substance, eliminating its use, and removing it from the body, possibly by hemodialysis or hemoperfusion in extreme cases. Initial treatment may include administration of diuretics and infusion of a large volume of fluids to flush tubules of cellular casts and debris and to replace fluid loss. However, this treatment carries a risk of fluid overload. Long-term fluid management requires daily replacement of projected and calculated losses (including insensible loss). Diet may be high in carbohydrates and low in protein, sodium, and potassium to minimize their buildup in the body. During the course of acute renal failure, treatment is supportive.

Other appropriate measures to control complications include transfusion of packed RBCs for anemia and administration of antibiotics for infection. Epoetin alfa may be given to stimulate RBC production as an alternative to blood transfusion. Hyperkalemia may require emergency I.V. administration of 50% glucose, regular insulin, and sodium bicarbonate. Sodium polystyrene sulfonate with sorbitol may be given by mouth or by enema to reduce extracellular potassium levels. Peritoneal dialysis or hemodialysis may be needed if the patient is catabolic.

Special considerations

Patient care is largely supportive.

♦ Maintain fluid balance. Watch for fluid overload, a common complication of therapy. Accurately record intake and output, including wound drainage, nasogastric tube output, and hemodialysis and peritoneal dialysis balances. Weigh the patient daily.

♦ Monitor Hb levels and HCT, and administer blood products as needed. Use fresh packed cells instead of whole blood to prevent fluid overload and heart failure.

♦ Maintain electrolyte balance. Monitor laboratory results and report imbalances. Enforce dietary restriction of foods containing sodium and potassium, such as bananas, orange juice, and baked potatoes. Check for potassium content in prescribed medications (e.g., potassium penicillin). Provide adequate calories and essential amino acids while restricting protein intake to maintain an anabolic state. Total parenteral nutrition may be indicated in the severely debilitated or catabolic patient.

♦ Use sterile technique, particularly when handling catheters, because the debilitated patient is vulnerable to infection. Immediately report fever, chills, delayed wound healing, or flank pain if the patient has an indwelling catheter in place.

♦ Watch for complications. If anemia worsens (pallor, weakness, lethargy with decreased Hb level), administer RBCs as ordered. For acidosis, give sodium bicarbonate or assist with dialysis in severe cases, as ordered. Watch for signs of diminishing renal perfusion (hypotension and decreased urine output). Encourage coughing and deep breathing to prevent pulmonary complications.

◆ Perform passive range-of-motion exercises. Provide good skin care; apply lotion or bath oil for dry skin. Help the patient to walk as soon as possible, but guard against exhaustion.

◆ Provide reassurance and emotional support. Encourage the patient and family to express their fears. Fully explain each procedure; repeat the explanation each time the procedure is done. Help the patient and family set realistic goals according to individual prognosis.

◆ To prevent ATN, make sure patients are well hydrated before surgery or after X-rays that use a contrast medium. Administer mannitol, as ordered, to high-risk patients before and during these procedures. Carefully monitor patients receiving blood transfusions to detect early signs of transfusion reaction (fever, rash, and chills), and discontinue such transfusion immediately.

▓▓▓▓ **PREVENTION**

◆ *Immediately treat disorders that cause a decrease in blood flow and oxygenation to the kidneys, such as severe hypotension and cardiogenic or septic shock.*

◆ *Proper hydration before surgery is very important. Adequate hydration after administration of radiocontrast dyes may allow for their excretion and reduce the risk of kidney damage.*

◆ *Proper typing and crossmatching before blood transfusions reduces the risk of incompatibility reactions.*

◆ *When a patient is exposed to drugs toxic to the renal system, monitor carefully by checking levels regularly.*

◆ *Patients with diseases, such as diabetes, liver disease, and cardiac disorders, are at higher risk for ATN. These patients need to be well controlled in order to prevent the risk of ATN.*

RENAL INFARCTION

Renal infarction is the formation of a coagulated, necrotic area in one or both kidneys that results from renal blood vessel occlusion. The location and size of the infarction depend on the site of vascular occlusion; most often, infarction affects the renal cortex, but it can extend into the medulla. Residual renal function after infarction depends on the extent of the damage from the infarction.

Pathophysiology

In 75% of patients, renal infarction results from renal artery embolism secondary to mitral stenosis, infective endocarditis, atrial fibrillation,

microthrombi in the left ventricle, rheumatic valvular disease, or recent myocardial infarction. The embolism reduces the rate of blood flow to renal tissue and leads to ischemia. The rate and degree of blood flow reduction determine whether or not the insult will be acute or chronic as arterial narrowing progresses. Less common causes of renal infarction are atherosclerosis, with or without thrombus formation, and thrombus from flank trauma, sickle cell anemia, scleroderma, polyarteritis nodosa, and arterionephrosclerosis.

Complications

◆ End-stage renal disease
◆ Granular kidneys
◆ Severe hypertension
◆ Cardiac hypertrophy
◆ Heart failure

Signs and symptoms

Although renal infarction may be asymptomatic, typical symptoms include severe upper abdominal pain or gnawing flank pain and tenderness, costovertebral tenderness, fever, anorexia, nausea, and vomiting. Gross hematuria may be present. When arterial occlusion causes infarction, the affected kidney is small and not palpable. Renovascular hypertension, a frequent complication that may occur several days after infarction, results from reduced blood flow, which stimulates the renin–angiotensin mechanism.

Diagnosis

A history of predisposing cardiovascular disease or other factors in a patient with typical clinical features strongly suggests renal infarction. Firm diagnosis requires appropriate laboratory tests:

◆ Urinalysis shows proteinuria and microscopic hematuria.

◆ Urine enzyme levels, especially lactate dehydrogenase (LDH) and alkaline phosphatase, are often elevated as a result of tissue destruction.

◆ Serum enzyme levels, especially aspartate aminotransferase, alkaline phosphatase, and LDH, are elevated. Blood studies may also show leukocytosis and increased erythrocyte sedimentation rate.

◆ Excretory urography shows diminished or absent excretion of contrast dye, indicating vascular occlusion or urethral obstruction.

◆ Isotopic renal scan, a benign, noninvasive technique, demonstrates absent or reduced blood flow to the kidneys.

℞ **CONFIRMING DIAGNOSIS** *Renal arteriography provides absolute proof of infarction but is used as a last resort because it's a high-risk procedure.*

Treatment

Infection in the infarcted area or significant hypertension may require surgical repair of the occlusion or nephrectomy. Surgery to establish collateral circulation to the area can relieve renovascular hypertension. Persistent hypertension may respond to antihypertensives and a low-sodium diet. Additional treatments may include administration of intra-arterial streptokinase, lysis of blood clots, and heparin therapy. For bilateral emboli, intra-arterial streptokinase or transluminal angioplasty is recommended. If effective renal blood flow is obtained, long-term anticoagulation is recommended.

Special considerations

Assess the degree of renal function and offer supportive care to maintain homeostasis.

◆ Monitor intake and output, vital signs (particularly blood pressure), electrolytes, and daily weight. Watch for signs of fluid overload, such as dyspnea, tachycardia, pulmonary edema, and electrolyte imbalances.

◆ Carefully explain all diagnostic procedures.

◆ Provide reassurance and emotional support for the patient and family.

◆ Encourage the patient to return for follow-up examination, which usually includes excretory urography or a renal scan to assess regained renal function.

RENAL CALCULI

Renal calculi or nephrolithiasis (commonly called *kidney stones*) may form anywhere in the urinary tract but usually develop in the renal pelvis or the calyces of the kidneys. Calculi formation follows precipitation of substances normally dissolved in the urine, such as calcium oxalate, calcium phosphate, magnesium ammonium phosphate, or, occasionally, urate or cystine. (See *How urine pH affects calculi formation.*) Renal calculi vary in size and may be solitary or multiple. They may remain in the renal pelvis or enter the ureter and may damage renal parenchyma; large calculi cause pressure necrosis. In certain locations, calculi cause obstruction, with resultant hydronephrosis, and tend to recur.

Pathophysiology

Although the exact cause of renal calculi is unknown, predisposing factors include:

◆ *Dehydration:* Decreased urine production concentrates calculus-forming substances.

◆ *Infection:* Infected, damaged tissue serves as a site for calculus development; pH changes provide a favorable medium for calculus formation (especially for magnesium ammonium phosphate or calcium phosphate calculi); infected calculi (usually magnesium ammonium phosphate or staghorn calculi) may develop if

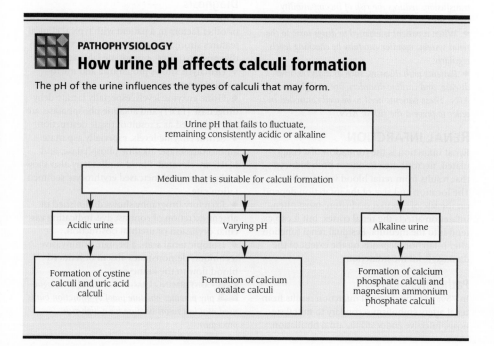

PATHOPHYSIOLOGY
How urine pH affects calculi formation

The pH of the urine influences the types of calculi that may form.

Urine pH that fails to fluctuate, remaining consistently acidic or alkaline

↓

Medium that is suitable for calculi formation

↓

Acidic urine	Varying pH	Alkaline urine
Formation of cystine calculi and uric acid calculi	Formation of calcium oxalate calculi	Formation of calcium phosphate calculi and magnesium ammonium phosphate calculi

bacteria serve as the nucleus in calculus formation. Infections may promote destruction of renal parenchyma.

◆ *Obstruction:* Urinary stasis (as in immobility from spinal cord injury) allows calculus constituents to collect and adhere, forming calculi. Obstruction also promotes infection, which, in turn, compounds the obstruction.

◆ *Metabolic factors:* These factors may predispose to renal calculi: hyperparathyroidism, renal tubular acidosis, elevated uric acid (usually with gout), defective metabolism of oxalate, genetic defect in metabolism of cystine, and excessive intake of vitamin D or dietary calcium.

Among Americans, renal calculi develop in 2% to 10% of the population, with people living in southeastern states having an increased risk. They're more common in men (especially those ages 30 to 40) than in women by a 3:1 ratio. They're rare in children.

Some types of calculi tend to be familial; some are associated with other conditions, such as bowel disease, bariatric surgery for obesity, or renal tubule defects. Calcium calculi are most common, accounting for more than 75% of all calculi, and are two to three times more common in males, usually appearing between 20 and 30 years old. The calcium may combine with other substances, such as oxalate (the most common substance), phosphate, or carbonate, to form the stone. Oxalate is present in certain foods. Diseases of the small intestine increase the tendency to form calcium oxalate calculi. Recurrence is likely.

Uric acid calculi are also more common in men and make up about 6% of all calculi. These calculi are associated with gout and chemotherapy. Cystine calculi, which make up about 2% of all calculi, may form in people with cystinuria, a hereditary disorder affecting both men and women. Struvite calculi, accounting for about 15% of all calculi, are mainly found in women as a result of a UTI. They can grow very large and may obstruct the kidney, ureter, or bladder.

Indinavir stones appear in patients with human immunodeficiency virus who are treated with the protease inhibitor indinavir.

Complications
◆ Damage or destruction of renal parenchyma
◆ Pressure necrosis
◆ Hydronephrosis
◆ Bleeding

Signs and symptoms
Clinical effects vary with size, location, and etiology of the calculi. Pain, the key symptom, usually results from obstruction; large, rough calculi occlude the opening to the ureter and increase the frequency and force of peristaltic contractions. The pain of classic renal colic travels from the costovertebral angle to the flank, to the suprapubic region and external genitalia. The intensity of this pain fluctuates and may be excruciating at its peak. If calculi are in the renal pelvis and calyces, pain may be more constant and dull. Back pain (from calculi that produce an obstruction within a kidney) and severe abdominal pain (from calculi traveling down a ureter) may also occur. (See *Types of renal calculi.*) Nausea and vomiting usually accompany severe pain.

Other associated signs include fever, chills, hematuria (when calculi abrade a ureter), abdominal distention, pyuria, and, rarely, anuria (from bilateral obstruction, or unilateral obstruction in the patient with one kidney).

Diagnosis
Diagnosis is based on the clinical picture and the following tests:
◆ CT scan (preferred study, non contrast) or magnetic resonance imaging (MRI) is highly sensitive for identifying hydronephrosis and detecting small renal and ureteral stones.
◆ Excretory urography may be used for diagnosis of obstruction by urinary calculus.
◆ Kidney–ureter–bladder X-rays reveal most renal calculi.
◆ Calculus analysis shows mineral content.

℞ **CONFIRMING DIAGNOSIS** *Excretory urography confirms the diagnosis, determines size and location of calculi, and is used only if noncontrast spiral CT is not confirmatory.*
◆ Kidney ultrasonography is an easily performed, noninvasive, nontoxic test to detect obstructive changes such as hydronephrosis.

Types of renal calculi

Multiple small calculi may vary in size; they may remain in the renal pelvis or pass down the ureter.

A staghorn calculus (a cast of the calyceal and pelvic collecting system) may form from a stone that stays in the kidney.

♦ Urine culture of midstream sample may indicate UTI.

♦ Urinalysis may be normal or may show increased specific gravity and acid or alkaline pH suitable for different types of stone formation. Other urinalysis findings include hematuria (gross or microscopic), crystals (urate, calcium, or cystine), casts, and pyuria with or without bacteria and WBCs.

♦ A 24-hour urine collection is evaluated for calcium oxalate, phosphorus, and uric acid excretion levels.

♦ Serial blood calcium and phosphorus levels detect hyperparathyroidism and show increased calcium level in proportion to normal serum protein.

Increased blood uric acid levels may indicate gout as the cause. Diagnosis must rule out appendicitis, cholecystitis, peptic ulcer, and pancreatitis as potential sources of pain.

Treatment

Because 90% of renal calculi are smaller than 5 mm in diameter, treatment usually consists of measures to promote their natural passage. Along with vigorous hydration, such treatment includes antimicrobial therapy (varying with the cultured organism) for infection, analgesics such as meperidine for pain, and diuretics to prevent urinary stasis and further calculus formation (thiazides decrease calcium excretion into the urine). Prophylaxis to prevent calculus formation includes a low-calcium diet for absorptive hypercalciuria, parathyroidectomy for hyperparathyroidism, allopurinol for uric acid calculi, and daily administration of ascorbic acid by mouth to acidify the urine. (See *Preventing renal calculi*.)

Calculi too large for natural passage may require surgical removal. When a calculus is in the ureter, a cystoscope or ureteroscope may be inserted through the urethra and the calculus manipulated with the ureteroscope, catheters, ultrasonic lithotripter, Holmium laser wire, or other retrieval instruments. Extraction of calculi from other areas (kidney calyx, renal pelvis) may necessitate a flank or lower abdominal approach. Percutaneous ultrasonic lithotripsy and extracorporeal shock wave lithotripsy shatter the calculus into fragments for removal by suction or natural passage.

Special considerations

Patient care includes confirming the diagnosis, facilitating passage of the stone, and prevention of future occurrences.

PREVENTION
Preventing renal calculi

The formation of kidney stones may be prevented by making certain lifestyle changes. If these lifestyles changes don't help in the prevention of kidney stone formation, drugs are needed. Advise your patient to make these changes.

Maintain hydration
The most important lifestyle change is drinking plenty of fluids, especially water. An adult needs to drink at least 3½ qt/day. Drinking plenty of fluids helps to flush out the kidneys.

Adjust diet
For a patient who tends to form calcium oxalate stones, suggest an oxalate-restricted diet. Foods that are high in oxalate should be avoided. These foods include rhubarb, star fruit, beets, beet greens, collards, okra, refried beans, spinach, Swiss chard, sweet potatoes, sesame seeds, almonds, and soy products. Restricting calcium in the diet doesn't seem to reduce the risk of kidney stones. Diets high in calcium actually help reduce the risk of oxalate stone formation. Calcium binds with oxalate so it can't be absorbed in the gastrointestinal tract and excreted by the kidneys.

All patients who form kidney stones should be on low-sodium diets. Sodium intake should be restricted to 3 to 4 g/day. Also, diets very low in animal proteins may help reduce the risk of stones.

Take prescribed drugs
Drugs can be helpful in preventing stone formation. The drugs prescribed depend on the type of stone. Some stones, such as calcium stones, develop more easily in more alkaline environments, and some stones, such as uric acid stones, develop in an acid environment. Patients with struvite stones are treated with antibiotics to prevent infection. Cystine stones are the hardest to treat, and they're treated with a urine alkalinizer and chelator (D-penicillamine and tiopronin).

◆ To aid diagnosis, maintain a 24- to 48-hour record of urine pH, with nitrazine pH paper; strain all urine through gauze or a tea strainer, and save all solid material recovered for analysis.

◆ To facilitate spontaneous passage, encourage the patient to walk if possible. Also promote sufficient intake of fluids to maintain a urine output of 3 to 4 L/day (urine should be very dilute and colorless). Addition of Flowmax (tamsulosin) 0.4 mg daily can also help facilitate the spontaneous passage of ureteral stones. To help acidify urine, offer fruit juices, particularly cranberry juice. If the patient can't drink the required amount of fluid, supplemental I.V. fluids may be given. Record intake and output and daily weight to assess fluid status and renal function.

◆ Stress the importance of proper diet and compliance with drug therapy. For example, if the patient's stone is caused by a hyperuricemic condition, advise the patient (or whoever prepares meals for the patient) to avoid foods high in purine. Restrict protein to 60 g/day to decrease calcium and uric acid, and limit sodium to 3 to 4 g/day. Oxalate foods are restricted.

◆ If surgery is necessary, give reassurance by supplementing and reinforcing what the surgeon has told the patient about the procedure. The patient is apt to be fearful, especially if surgery includes removal of a kidney, so emphasize the fact that the body can adapt well to one kidney. If he's to have an abdominal or flank incision, teach deep breathing and coughing exercises.

◆ After surgery, the patient will probably have an indwelling catheter or a nephrostomy tube. Unless one of his kidneys was removed, expect bloody drainage from the catheter. Never irrigate the catheter without a physician's order. Check dressings regularly for bloody drainage, and know how much drainage to expect. Immediately report suspected hemorrhage (excessive drainage, rising pulse rate). Use sterile technique when changing dressings or providing catheter care.

◆ Watch for signs of infection (rising fever, chills), and give antibiotics as ordered. To prevent pneumonia, encourage frequent position changes, and ambulate the patient as soon as possible. Have the patient hold a small pillow over the operative site to splint the incision and thereby facilitate deep breathing and coughing exercises.

◆ Before discharge, teach the patient and family the importance of following the prescribed dietary and medication regimens to prevent recurrence of calculi. Encourage increased fluid intake. If appropriate, show the patient how to check the urine pH, and instruct them to keep a daily record. Tell them to immediately report symptoms of acute obstruction (pain, inability to void).

RENAL VEIN THROMBOSIS

Renal vein thrombosis—clotting in the renal vein—results in renal congestion, engorgement and, possibly, infarction. Thrombosis may affect both kidneys and may occur in an acute or a chronic form. Chronic thrombosis usually impairs renal function, causing nephrotic syndrome. Abrupt onset of thrombosis that causes extensive damage may precipitate rapidly fatal renal infarction. If thrombosis affects both kidneys, the prognosis is poor. However, less severe thrombosis that affects only one kidney, or gradual progression that allows development of collateral circulation, may preserve partial renal function.

Pathophysiology

Renal vein thrombosis often results from a tumor that obstructs the renal vein (usually hypernephroma). Other causes include thrombophlebitis of the inferior vena cava (may result from abdominal trauma) or blood vessels of the legs, heart failure, and periarteritis.

🚼 PEDIATRIC TIP *In infants, renal vein thrombosis usually follows diarrhea that causes severe dehydration. Chronic renal vein thrombosis is often a complication of other glomerulopathic diseases, such as amyloidosis, systemic lupus erythematosus, diabetic nephropathy, and membranoproliferative glomerulonephritis.*

Complications

◆ Fatal renal infarction
◆ Disseminated intravascular coagulation

Signs and symptoms

Clinical features of renal vein thrombosis vary with speed of onset. Rapid onset of venous obstruction produces severe lumbar pain and tenderness in the epigastric region and the costovertebral angle. Other characteristic features include fever, leukocytosis, pallor, hematuria, proteinuria, peripheral edema, and, when the obstruction is bilateral, oliguria and other uremic signs. The kidneys enlarge and become easily palpable. Hypertension is unusual but may develop.

Gradual onset causes symptoms of nephrotic syndrome. Peripheral edema is possible, but pain is generally absent. Other clinical signs include proteinuria, hypoalbuminemia, and hyperlipidemia.

Infants with this disease have enlarged kidneys, oliguria, and renal insufficiency that may progress to acute or chronic renal failure.

Diagnosis

A variety of tests are used to confirm diagnosis of renal vein thrombosis.

◆ CT scan with contrast is the procedure of choice because it reveals enlargement and distention of the affected renal vein with visualization of the clots within the vein.

◆ Excretory urography provides reliable diagnostic evidence. In acute renal vein thrombosis, the kidneys appear enlarged and excretory function diminishes. Contrast medium seems to "smudge" necrotic renal tissue. In chronic thrombosis, it may show ureteral indentations that result from collateral venous channels.

℞ CONFIRMING DIAGNOSIS *Renal arteriography and biopsy may also confirm the diagnosis. Venography confirms thrombosis.*

◆ Urinalysis reveals gross or microscopic hematuria, proteinuria (>2 g/day in chronic disease), casts, and oliguria.

◆ Blood studies show leukocytosis, hypoalbuminemia, and hyperlipidemia.

◆ MRI, abdominal X-ray, or abdominal ultrasound may show occlusion of the renal vein.

Treatment

Treatment is most effective for gradual thrombosis that affects only one kidney. Anticoagulation therapy reduces the incidence of new thrombus formation and often reverses the deterioration of renal function. Heparin is the initial therapy of choice. After 5 to 7 days, warfarin (Coumadin) therapy can be instituted for long-term care. Streptokinase or urokinase infusion may be successful in early resolution of acute renal vein thrombosis. Surgery is rarely used; it must be performed within 24 hours of thrombosis but even then has limited success because thrombi often extend into the small veins. Extensive intrarenal bleeding may necessitate nephrectomy.

Patients who survive abrupt thrombosis with extensive renal damage develop nephrotic syndrome and require treatment for renal failure, such as dialysis and, possibly, transplantation.

👣 PEDIATRIC TIP *Some infants with renal vein thrombosis recover completely following heparin therapy or surgery; others suffer irreversible kidney damage.*

Special considerations

Patient care includes careful monitoring of symptoms for signs of improvement or worsening.

◆ Assess renal function regularly. Monitor vital signs, intake and output, daily weight, and electrolytes.

◆ Administer diuretics for edema as ordered, and enforce dietary restrictions of sodium and potassium intake.

◆ Monitor closely for signs of pulmonary emboli (chest pain, dyspnea).

◆ If heparin is given by constant I.V. infusion, frequently monitor partial thromboplastin time to determine the patient's response. Dilute the drug; administer it by infusion pump or controller, so the patient receives the least amount necessary.

❗ ALERT *During anticoagulant therapy, watch for and report signs of bleeding, such as tachycardia, hypotension, hematuria, bleeding from nose or gums, ecchymoses, petechiae, and tarry stools. Instruct the patient on maintenance warfarin therapy to use an electric razor and a soft toothbrush, and to avoid trauma. Suggest that the patient wear a medical identification bracelet, and to avoid aspirin, which aggravates bleeding tendencies. Stress the need for close follow-up.*

Chronic renal disorders

NEPHROTIC SYNDROME

Nephrotic syndrome is a condition characterized by marked proteinuria, hypoalbuminemia, hyperlipidemia, and edema. (See *What happens in nephrotic syndrome*, page 355.) Although nephrotic syndrome isn't a disease itself, it results from a specific glomerular defect and indicates renal damage. The prognosis is highly variable, depending on the underlying cause. Some forms may progress to end-stage renal failure.

Pathophysiology

About 75% of nephrotic syndrome cases result from primary (idiopathic) glomerulonephritis. Classifications include:

◆ In *lipid nephrosis* (*nil lesions*), the main cause of nephrotic syndrome in children, the glomerulus looks normal by light microscopy. Some tubules may contain increased lipid deposits.

◆ *Membranous glomerulonephritis*, the most common lesion in adult idiopathic nephrotic syndrome, is characterized by uniform thickening of the glomerular basement membrane containing dense deposits and eventually progresses to renal failure.

◆ *Focal glomerulosclerosis* can develop spontaneously at any age, follow renal transplantation, or result from heroin abuse. Reported incidence of this condition is 10% in children with nephrotic syndrome and up to 20% in adults. Lesions initially affect the deeper glomeruli, causing hyaline sclerosis, with later involvement of the superficial glomeruli. These lesions generally cause slowly progressive deterioration in renal function. Remissions occur occasionally.

◆ In *membranoproliferative glomerulonephritis,* slowly progressive lesions develop in the subendothelial region of the basement membrane. Lesions may follow infection, particularly streptococcal infection. This disease occurs primarily in children and young adults.

Other causes of nephrotic syndrome include metabolic diseases such as diabetes mellitus; collagen vascular disorders, such as systemic lupus erythematosus and periarteritis nodosa; circulatory diseases, such as heart failure, sickle cell anemia, and renal vein thrombosis; nephrotoxins, such as mercury, gold, and bismuth; allergic reactions; and infections, such as tuberculosis or enteritis. Other possible causes are pregnancy, hereditary nephritis, multiple myeloma, and other neoplastic diseases. These diseases increase glomerular protein permeability, leading to increased urinary excretion of

protein, especially albumin, and subsequent hypoalbuminemia.

Nephrotic patients have an increased risk of infection, particularly of peritonitis.

⬛ **PEDIATRIC TIP** *Black children appear to be at greater risk for peritonitis.*

Complications
◆ Atherosclerosis
◆ Renal vein thrombosis
◆ Acute renal failure
◆ Chronic renal failure
◆ Infections
◆ Malnutrition
◆ Fluid overload

Signs and symptoms
The dominant clinical feature of nephrotic syndrome is mild to severe dependent edema of the ankles or sacrum, or periorbital edema, especially in children. Edema may lead to ascites, pleural effusion, and swollen external genitalia. Accompanying symptoms may include

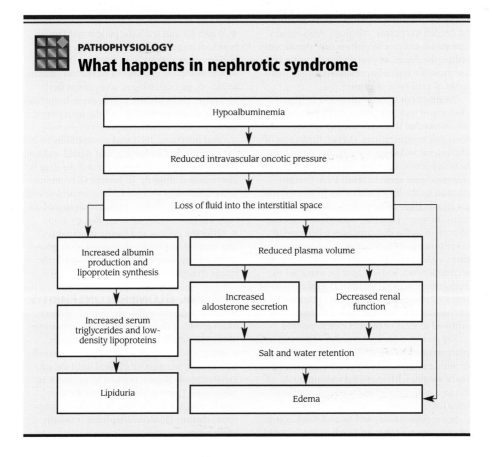

PATHOPHYSIOLOGY
What happens in nephrotic syndrome

Hypoalbuminemia → Reduced intravascular oncotic pressure → Loss of fluid into the interstitial space

Loss of fluid into the interstitial space → Increased albumin production and lipoprotein synthesis → Increased serum triglycerides and low-density lipoproteins → Lipiduria

Loss of fluid into the interstitial space → Reduced plasma volume → Increased aldosterone secretion → Salt and water retention → Edema

Reduced plasma volume → Decreased renal function → Salt and water retention

orthostatic hypotension, lethargy, anorexia, depression, and pallor. Major complications are malnutrition, infection, coagulation disorders, thromboembolic vascular occlusion, and accelerated atherosclerosis.

Diagnosis

Consistent proteinuria in excess of 3.5 g for 24 hours strongly suggests nephrotic syndrome; examination of urine also reveals increased number of hyaline, granular, and waxy, fatty casts, and oval fat bodies. Serum values that support the diagnosis are increased cholesterol, phospholipids, and triglycerides and decreased albumin levels. Histologic identification of the lesion requires kidney biopsy. Other tests may be done to rule out metabolic causes.

Treatment

The goals of treatment of nephrotic syndrome are to relieve symptoms, prevent complications, and delay progressive kidney damage. Treatment of the causative disorder—possibly lifelong—is necessary to control nephrotic syndrome. Corticosteroid, immunosuppressive, antihypertensive, and diuretic medications may help control symptoms. Antibiotics may be needed to control infections. Angiotensin-converting enzyme inhibitors may significantly reduce the degree of protein loss in urine and are therefore typically prescribed for the treatment of nephrotic syndrome.

Treatment of hypertension and of high cholesterol and triglyceride levels are also recommended to reduce the risk of atherosclerosis and complications. Dietary limitation of cholesterol and saturated fats may be of little benefit because the high levels that accompany this condition seem to result from overproduction by the liver rather than from excessive fat intake. High-protein diets are of debatable value. In many patients, reducing the amount of protein in the diet produces a decrease in urine protein. In most cases, a moderate-protein diet (1 g/kg of body weight per day) is usually recommended. Sodium may be restricted to help control edema. Vitamin D may need to be replaced if nephrotic syndrome is chronic and unresponsive to therapy. Blood thinners may be required to treat or prevent clot formation.

Supportive treatment consists of protein replacement with infusion of salt-poor albumin or with a nutritional diet of 1.5 g protein/kg of body weight, with restricted sodium intake of 0.5 to 1 g/day; diuretics for edema; and antibiotics for infection.

Some patients respond to an 8-week course of corticosteroid therapy (such as prednisone),

followed by a maintenance dose. Others respond better to a combination course of prednisone and azathioprine or cyclophosphamide.

Special considerations

Patient care includes identification and treatment of the underlying cause accompanied by supportive care during treatment.

◆ Frequently check urine protein. (Urine containing protein appears frothy.)

◆ Measure blood pressure while the patient is supine and also while he's standing; immediately report a drop in blood pressure that exceeds 20 mm Hg.

ALERT *After kidney biopsy, watch for bleeding and shock.*

◆ Monitor intake and output and check weight at the same time each morning—after the patient voids and before eating—and while they are wearing the same kind of clothing. Ask the dietitian to plan a high-protein, low-sodium diet.

◆ Provide good skin care because the patient with nephrotic syndrome usually has edema.

◆ To avoid thrombophlebitis, encourage activity and exercise, and provide antiembolism stockings as ordered.

◆ Watch for and teach the patient and family how to recognize adverse drug effects, such as bone marrow toxicity from cytotoxic immunosuppressants and cushingoid symptoms (muscle weakness, mental changes, acne, moon face, hirsutism, girdle obesity, purple striae, bone fractures, and amenorrhea) from long-term steroid therapy. Other steroid complications include masked infections, increased susceptibility to infections, ulcers, GI bleeding, and steroid-induced diabetes; a steroid crisis may occur if the drug is discontinued abruptly. To prevent GI complications, administer steroids with an antacid or with cimetidine or ranitidine. Explain that steroid adverse effects will subside when therapy stops.

◆ Offer the patient and family reassurance and support, especially during the acute phase, when edema is severe and the patient's body image changes.

CHRONIC GLOMERULONEPHRITIS

A slowly progressive disease, chronic glomerulonephritis is characterized by inflammation of the glomeruli, which results in sclerosis, scarring, and eventual renal failure. This condition usually remains subclinical until the progressive phase begins, marked by proteinuria, cylindruria (presence of granular tube casts), and hematuria. By the time it produces symptoms, chronic glomerulonephritis is usually irreversible.

Pathophysiology

Common causes of chronic glomerulonephritis include primary renal disorders, such as membranoproliferative glomerulonephritis, membranous glomerulopathy, focal glomerulosclerosis, rapidly progressive glomerulonephritis, and, less often, poststreptococcal glomerulonephritis. Systemic disorders that may cause chronic glomerulonephritis include lupus erythematosus, Goodpasture syndrome, and hemolytic-uremic syndrome.

Chronic glomerulonephritis is twice as common in men as it is in women.

Complications

◆ End-stage renal disease
◆ Severe hypertension
◆ Heart failure
◆ Increased susceptibility to infections
◆ Nephrotic syndrome

Signs and symptoms

Chronic glomerulonephritis typically develops insidiously and asymptomatically, usually over many years. At any time, however, it may suddenly become progressive, producing nephrotic syndrome, hypertension, proteinuria, and hematuria. In late stages of progressive chronic glomerulonephritis, it may accelerate to uremic symptoms, such as azotemia, nausea, vomiting, pruritus, dyspnea, malaise, and fatigability. Mild to severe edema and anemia may accompany these symptoms. Severe hypertension may cause cardiac hypertrophy, leading to heart failure, and may accelerate the development of advanced renal failure, eventually necessitating dialysis or transplantation.

Diagnosis

Patient history and physical assessment seldom suggest glomerulonephritis. Suspicion develops from urinalysis revealing proteinuria, hematuria, cylindruria (aka casts), and RBC casts. Rising blood urea nitrogen and serum creatinine levels indicate advanced renal insufficiency. X-ray or ultrasound shows smaller kidneys. Kidney biopsy identifies the underlying disease and provides data needed to guide therapy.

Treatment

Treatment is essentially nonspecific and symptomatic, with its goals to control hypertension with antihypertensives and a sodium-restricted diet, to correct fluid and electrolyte imbalances through restrictions and replacement, to reduce edema with diuretics such as furosemide, and to prevent heart failure. Treatment may also include antibiotics (for symptomatic UTIs), dialysis, or transplantation.

Special considerations

Patient care is primarily supportive, focusing on continual observation and sound patient teaching.

◆ Accurately monitor vital signs, intake and output, and daily weight to evaluate fluid retention. Observe for signs of fluid, electrolyte, and acid–base imbalances.
◆ Ask the dietitian to plan low-sodium, high-calorie meals with adequate protein.
◆ Administer medications as ordered, and provide good skin care (because of pruritus and edema) and oral hygiene. Instruct the patient to continue taking prescribed antihypertensives as scheduled, even if they are feeling better, and to report any adverse effects. Advise the patient to take diuretics in the morning, so they won't have to disrupt sleep to void. Teach them how to assess ankle edema.
◆ Warn the patient to report signs of infection, particularly UTI, and to avoid contact with persons who have infections. Urge follow-up examinations to assess renal function.
◆ Help the patient adjust to this illness by encouraging him or her to express his or her feelings. Explain all necessary procedures beforehand, and answer the patient's questions about them.

RENOVASCULAR HYPERTENSION

Renovascular hypertension is a rise in systemic blood pressure resulting from stenosis of the major renal arteries or their branches or from intrarenal atherosclerosis. This narrowing or sclerosis may be partial or complete, and the resulting blood pressure elevation, benign or malignant. (See *Mechanism of renovascular hypertension,* page 358.)

Pathophysiology

Stenosis or occlusion of the renal artery stimulates the affected kidney to release the enzyme renin, which converts angiotensinogen—a plasma protein—to angiotensin I. As angiotensin I circulates through the lungs and liver, it converts to angiotensin II, which causes peripheral vasoconstriction, increased arterial pressure and aldosterone secretion and, eventually, hypertension.

Atherosclerosis (especially in older men) and fibromuscular diseases of the renal artery wall layers—such as medial fibroplasia and, less commonly, intimal and subadventitial fibroplasia—are the primary causes in 95% of all patients with renovascular hypertension.

Mechanism of renovascular hypertension

(1) Renal artery stenosis causes a reduction in blood flow to the kidneys. (2) The kidneys secrete renin in response. (3) Renin combines with angiotensinogen in the liver to form angiotensin I. (4) In the lungs angiotensin I is converted to angiotensin II, a vasoconstrictor.

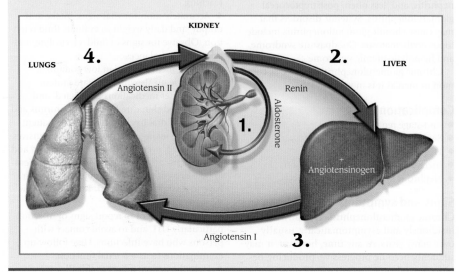

Other causes include arteritis, anomalies of the renal arteries, embolism, trauma, tumor, and dissecting aneurysm. Less than 5% of patients with high blood pressure display renovascular hypertension; it's most common in persons younger than 30 years old or older than 50.

PEDIATRIC TIP *Fibromuscular dysplasia is the most common cause of renovascular hypertension in children. The surgical cure rate is very high.*

Complications
◆ Heart failure
◆ Myocardial infarction
◆ Stroke
◆ Renal failure (occasionally)

Signs and symptoms
In addition to elevated systemic blood pressure, renovascular hypertension usually produces symptoms common to hypertensive states, such as headache, palpitations, tachycardia, anxiety, light-headedness, decreased tolerance of temperature extremes, retinopathy, and mental sluggishness. Significant complications include heart failure, myocardial infarction, stroke, and, occasionally, renal failure.

Diagnosis
CONFIRMING DIAGNOSIS *The gold standard for diagnosing renal artery stenosis is renal arteriography. However, there are a variety of less invasive tests used for screening.*
◆ Gadolinium-enhanced magnetic resonance angiography can identify turbulent blood flow indicative of renal stenosis. However, patients with moderate to end-stage kidney disease or AKI should not receive gadolinium contrast agents.
◆ Duplex Doppler ultrasonography scans the renal artery and will reveal stenosis, but results vary.
◆ Oral captopril renography is the simplest, most noninvasive test for detection of renovascular hypertension but has a relatively high false-positive rate.

Treatment
Surgery, the treatment of choice, is performed to restore adequate circulation and to control severe hypertension or severely impaired renal function by renal artery bypass, endarterectomy, arterioplasty, or, as a last resort, nephrectomy. Balloon catheter renal artery dilation is used in selected cases to correct renal artery stenosis

without the risks and morbidity of surgery. Symptomatic measures include antihypertensives, diuretics, and a sodium-restricted diet.

Medications that may be used in an attempt to control blood pressure include diuretics, beta-adrenergic blockers, calcium channel blockers, angiotensin-converting enzyme inhibitors, angiotensin receptor blockers, and alpha-adrenergic blockers. Diazoxide or nitroprusside may be given in the hospital if symptoms are acute. Response to medications is highly individual, and the dosage or specific drug used may need frequent adjustment.

Lifestyle changes may be recommended, including weight, exercise, and dietary adjustments; smoking cessation; and avoidance of alcohol. These habits add to the effects of hypertension in causing complications.

Special considerations

The care plan must emphasize helping the patient and family understand renovascular hypertension and the importance of following the prescribed treatment.

◆ Accurately monitor intake and output and daily weight. Check blood pressure in both arms regularly, with the patient lying down and standing. A drop of 20 mm Hg or more on arising may necessitate an adjustment in antihypertensive medications. Assess renal function daily.

◆ Maintain fluid and sodium restrictions. Explain the purpose of a low-sodium diet.

◆ Explain the diagnostic tests, and prepare the patient appropriately; for example, adequately hydrate the patient before tests that use contrast media. Make sure the patient isn't allergic to the dye used in diagnostic tests. After excretory urography or arteriography, watch for complications.

◆ If a nephrectomy is necessary, reassure the patient that the remaining kidney is adequate for renal function.

ALERT *Postoperatively, watch for bleeding and hypotension. If the sutures around the renal vessels slip, the patient can quickly go into shock because the kidneys receive 25% of cardiac output.*

◆ Provide a quiet, stress-free environment if possible. Urge the patient and family members to have regular blood pressure screenings.

PREVENTION *Preventing atherosclerosis can help prevent renovascular hypertension. To reduce the risk of atherosclerosis, give patients this advice:*

◆ *Stop smoking because smoking damages the arteries.*

◆ *Get regular exercise. Regular exercise improves circulation and helps develop collateral blood vessels.*

◆ *Eat a healthy diet. Eating a diet low in saturated fats, cholesterol, and sodium can help control weight, blood pressure, and cholesterol.*

◆ *Manage stress. Some stress reduction techniques include deep breathing and stretching exercises.*

HYDRONEPHROSIS

Hydronephrosis is an abnormal dilation of the renal pelvis and the calyces of one or both kidneys, caused by an obstruction of urine flow in the genitourinary tract. (See *Renal damage in hydronephrosis.*) Although partial obstruction and hydronephrosis may not produce symptoms initially, the pressure built up behind the area of obstruction eventually results in symptomatic renal dysfunction.

Pathophysiology

Almost any type of obstructive uropathy can result in hydronephrosis. The most common causes are BPH, urethral strictures, and calculi; less common causes include strictures or stenosis of the ureter or bladder outlet, congenital abnormalities, abdominal tumors, blood clots, and neurogenic bladder. If obstruction is in the urethra or bladder, hydronephrosis is usually bilateral; if obstruction is in a ureter, it's usually unilateral. Obstructions distal to the bladder cause the bladder to dilate and act as a buffer zone, delaying hydronephrosis. Total obstruction of urine flow with dilation of the collecting system ultimately causes complete cortical atrophy and cessation of glomerular filtration.

Hydronephrosis occurs in 1 of every 100 people.

PATHOPHYSIOLOGY
Renal damage in hydronephrosis

In hydronephrosis, the ureters dilate and kink, the renal pelvis dilates, and the parenchyma and papilla atrophy.

Complications
◆ Pyelonephritis
◆ Paralytic ileus
◆ Renal failure

Signs and symptoms
Clinical features of hydronephrosis vary with the cause of the obstruction. In some patients, hydronephrosis produces no symptoms or only mild pain and slightly decreased urinary flow; in others, it may produce severe, colicky renal pain or dull flank pain that may radiate to the groin, and gross urinary abnormalities, such as hematuria, pyuria, dysuria, alternating oliguria and polyuria, or complete anuria. Other symptoms of hydronephrosis include nausea, vomiting, abdominal fullness, pain on urination, dribbling, or hesitancy. Unilateral obstruction may cause pain on only one side, usually in the flank area.

The most common complication of an obstructed kidney is infection (pyelonephritis) due to stasis that exacerbates renal damage and may create a life-threatening crisis. Paralytic ileus frequently accompanies acute obstructive uropathy.

Diagnosis
CONFIRMING DIAGNOSIS *While the patient's clinical features may suggest hydronephrosis, excretory urography, isotope renography (radioisotope scan of the kidneys), CT scan of the kidneys or abdomen, abdominal MRI, renal ultrasound, and renal function studies are necessary to confirm it.*

Treatment
The goals of treatment are to preserve renal function and prevent infection through surgical removal of the obstruction, such as dilation for stricture of the urethra or prostatectomy for BPH.

If renal function has already been affected, therapy may include a diet low in protein, sodium, and potassium. This diet is designed to stop the progression of renal failure before surgery. Inoperable obstructions may necessitate decompression and drainage of the kidney using a nephrostomy tube placed temporarily or permanently in the renal pelvis or placement of a ureteral stent to allow the ureter to drain. Concurrent infection requires appropriate antibiotic therapy.

Special considerations
Explain hydronephrosis as well as the purpose of excretory urography and other diagnostic procedures. Check the patient for allergy to excretory urography dye.

◆ Administer medication for pain, as needed and prescribed.

◆ Postoperatively, closely monitor intake and output, vital signs, and fluid and electrolyte status. Watch for a rising pulse rate and cold, clammy skin, which indicate possible impending hemorrhage and shock. Monitor renal function studies daily.

◆ If a nephrostomy tube has been inserted, check it frequently for bleeding and patency. Irrigate the tube only as ordered, and don't clamp it.

◆ If the patient is to be discharged with a nephrostomy tube in place, teach them how to care for it properly.

PREVENTION *To prevent progression of hydronephrosis to irreversible renal disease, urge older men (especially those with family histories of BPH or prostatitis) to have routine medical checkups. Teach them to recognize and report symptoms of hydronephrosis (colicky pain, hematuria) or UTI.*

RENAL TUBULAR ACIDOSIS
Renal tubular acidosis (RTA)—a syndrome of persistent dehydration, hyperchloremia, hypokalemia, metabolic acidosis, and nephrocalcinosis—results from the kidneys' inability to conserve bicarbonate. This disorder occurs as distal RTA (Type I, or classic RTA) or proximal RTA (Type II). The prognosis is usually good but depends on the severity of renal damage that precedes treatment.

Pathophysiology
Metabolic acidosis usually results from renal excretion of bicarbonate. However, metabolic acidosis associated with RTA results from a defect in the kidneys' normal tubular acidification of urine.

Distal RTA results from an inability of the distal tubule to secrete hydrogen ions against established gradients across the tubular membrane. This results in decreased excretion of titratable acids and ammonium, increased loss of potassium and bicarbonate in the urine, and systemic acidosis. Prolonged acidosis causes mobilization of calcium from bone and, eventually, hypercalciuria, predisposing the kidney to the formation of renal calculi. Distal RTA may be classified as primary or secondary.

◆ *Primary distal RTA* may occur sporadically or through a hereditary defect and is most prevalent in women, older children, adolescents, and young adults.

◆ It can also be caused by certain drugs, such as amphotericin B, lithium, and analgesics.

◆ *Secondary distal RTA* has been linked to many renal or systemic conditions, such as starvation, malnutrition, hepatic cirrhosis, and several genetically transmitted disorders.

Proximal RTA results from defective reabsorption of bicarbonate in the proximal tubule. This causes bicarbonate to flood the distal tubule, which normally secretes hydrogen ions, and leads to impaired formation of titratable acids and ammonium for excretion. Ultimately, metabolic acidosis results. Proximal RTA occurs in two forms:

◆ In *primary proximal RTA*, the reabsorptive defect is idiopathic and is the only disorder present.

◆ In *secondary proximal RTA*, the reabsorptive defect may be one of several defects and is due to proximal tubular cell damage from a disease such as Fanconi syndrome.

Complications
◆ Pyelonephritis
◆ Hypercalciuria
◆ Renal calculi

Signs and symptoms
PEDIATRIC TIP *In infants, RTA produces anorexia, vomiting, occasional fever, polyuria, dehydration, growth retardation, apathy, weakness, tissue wasting, constipation, nephrocalcinosis, and rickets.*

In children and adults, RTA may lead to UTI, rickets, and growth problems. Possible complications of RTA include nephrocalcinosis and pyelonephritis.

Diagnosis
CONFIRMING DIAGNOSIS *Demonstration of impaired acidification of urine with systemic metabolic acidosis confirms distal RTA. Demonstration of bicarbonate wasting caused by impaired reabsorption confirms proximal RTA.*

Other relevant laboratory results show:
◆ decreased serum bicarbonate, pH, potassium, and phosphorus
◆ increased serum chloride and alkaline phosphatase
◆ alkaline pH, with low titratable acids and ammonium content in urine
◆ increased urinary bicarbonate and potassium
◆ low specific gravity

In later stages, X-rays may show nephrocalcinosis.

Treatment
Supportive treatment for patients with RTA requires replacement of those substances being abnormally excreted, especially bicarbonate, and may include sodium bicarbonate tablets or solution to control acidosis. Potassium may be given by mouth for dangerously low potassium levels. Vitamins D and calcium supplements are usually avoided because the tendency toward nephrocalcinosis persists even after bicarbonate therapy. If pyelonephritis occurs, treatment may include antibiotics as well.

Treatment for renal calculi secondary to nephrocalcinosis varies and may include supportive therapy until the calculi pass or until surgery for severe obstruction is performed.

Special considerations
Urge compliance with all medication instructions. Inform the patient and family that the prognosis for RTA and bone lesion healing is directly related to the adequacy of treatment.
◆ Monitor laboratory values, especially potassium, for hypokalemia.
◆ Test urine for pH, and strain it for calculi.
◆ If rickets develops, explain the condition and its treatment to the patient and family.
◆ Teach the patient how to recognize signs and symptoms of calculi (hematuria, low abdominal or flank pain). Tell the patient to immediately report signs and symptoms.
◆ Instruct the patient with low potassium levels to eat foods with high potassium content, such as bananas, leafy green vegetables, and baked potatoes. Orange juice is also high in potassium.
◆ Because RTA may be caused by a genetic defect, encourage family members to seek genetic counseling or screening for this disorder.

CHRONIC RENAL FAILURE
Chronic renal failure is usually the end result of a gradually progressive loss of renal function; occasionally, it's the result of a rapidly progressive disease of sudden onset. Few symptoms develop until after more than 75% of glomerular filtration is lost; then the remaining normal parenchyma deteriorates progressively, and symptoms worsen as renal function decreases.

If this condition continues unchecked, uremic toxins accumulate and produce potentially fatal physiologic changes in all major organ systems. If the patient can tolerate it, maintenance dialysis or kidney transplantation can sustain life. (See *Comparing peritoneal dialysis and hemodialysis,* page 362. Also see *Continuous ambulatory peritoneal dialysis,* page 363.)

Pathophysiology
Diabetes and hypertension are the primary causes of chronic renal failure, accounting for two-thirds of cases. Other causes of chronic renal failure include:
◆ chronic glomerular disease such as glomerulonephritis

Comparing peritoneal dialysis and hemodialysis

Advantages, disadvantages, and complications of peritoneal dialysis and hemodialysis are described below.

Type	Advantages	Disadvantages	Possible complications
Peritoneal dialysis			
	◆ Can be performed immediately ◆ Requires less complex equipment and less specialized personnel than hemodialysis ◆ Requires small amounts of heparin or none at all ◆ No blood loss; minimal cardiovascular stress ◆ Can be performed by patient anywhere (continuous ambulatory peritoneal dialysis), without assistance and with minimal patient teaching ◆ Allows patient independence without long interruptions in daily activities because exchange may be done at night while he or she sleeps ◆ Lower infection rate ◆ Lower cost	◆ Contraindicated within 72 hours of abdominal surgery ◆ Requires 48 to 72 hours for significant response to treatment ◆ Severe protein loss necessitates high-protein diet (up to 100 g/day) ◆ High risk of peritonitis; repeated bouts may cause scarring, preventing further treatments with peritoneal dialysis ◆ Urea clearance less than with hemodialysis (60%)	◆ Bacterial or chemical peritonitis ◆ Pain (abdominal, low back, shoulder) ◆ Shortness of breath or dyspnea ◆ Atelectasis and pneumonia ◆ Severe loss of protein into the dialysis solution in the abdominal cavity (10 to 20 g/day) ◆ Fluid overload ◆ Excessive fluid loss ◆ Constipation ◆ Catheter site inflammation, infection, or leakage ◆ Anorexia ◆ Hypertriglyceridemia ◆ Abdominal hernias
Hemodialysis			
	◆ Takes only 3 to 5 hours per treatment ◆ Faster results in an acute situation ◆ Total number of hours of maintenance treatment that's only half that of peritoneal dialysis ◆ In an acute situation, can use an I.V. route without a surgical access route	◆ Requires surgical creation of a vascular access between circulation and dialysis machine ◆ Requires complex water treatment, dialysis equipment, and highly trained personnel ◆ Requires administration of larger amounts of heparin ◆ Confines patient to special treatment unit	◆ Septicemia ◆ Air emboli ◆ Rapid fluid and electrolyte imbalance (disequilibrium syndrome) ◆ Hemolytic anemia ◆ Metastatic calcification ◆ Increased risk of hepatitis ◆ Hypotension or hypertension ◆ Itching ◆ Pain (generalized or in chest) ◆ Heparin overdose, possibly causing hemorrhage ◆ Leg cramps ◆ Nausea and vomiting ◆ Headache

Continuous ambulatory peritoneal dialysis

Continuous ambulatory peritoneal dialysis is a useful alternative to hemodialysis in patients with renal failure. Using the peritoneum as a dialysis membrane, it allows almost uninterrupted exchange of dialysis solution. With this method, four to six exchanges of fresh dialysis solution are infused each day. The approximate dwell-time for daytime exchanges is 5 hours; for overnight exchanges, the dwell-time is 8 to 10 hours. After each dwell-time, the patient removes the dialyzing solution by gravity drainage. This form of dialysis offers the unique advantages of a simple, easily taught procedure and patient independence from a special treatment center.

After applying a mask, the patient attaches a bag of dialysate to the tube entering his abdominal area so that the fluid flows into the peritoneal cavity. The patient can remove the mask when this step is completed.

After applying a mask, the patient unrolls the bag and suspends it below his pelvis to allow the dialysate to drain from the peritoneal cavity back into the bag.

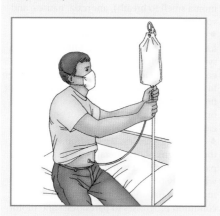

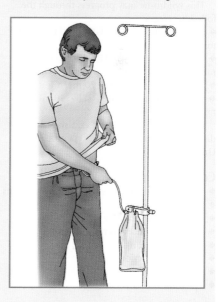

While the dialysate remains in the peritoneal cavity, the patient rolls up the bag, places it under his shirt, and goes about his normal activities.

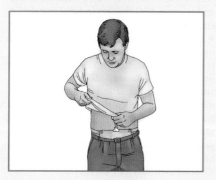

◆ chronic infections, such as chronic pyelonephritis or tuberculosis
◆ congenital anomalies such as polycystic kidneys
◆ vascular diseases such as renal nephrosclerosis
◆ obstructive processes such as calculi
◆ collagen diseases such as systemic lupus erythematosus
◆ nephrotoxic agents such as long-term aminoglycoside therapy.

These conditions gradually destroy the nephrons and eventually cause irreversible renal failure. Similarly, acute renal failure that fails to respond to treatment becomes chronic renal failure.

This syndrome may progress through the following stages:
◆ reduced renal reserve (GFR is 40 to 70 mL/minute)
◆ renal insufficiency (GFR 20 to 40 mL/minute)
◆ renal failure (GFR 10 to 20 mL/minute)
◆ end-stage renal disease (GFR < 10 mL/minute).

Chronic renal failure and end-stage renal disease affect about 2 of 1,000 people in the United States.

Complications
◆ Fatal physiologic changes in all major organs
◆ Anemia
◆ Peripheral neuropathy
◆ Cardiopulmonary complication
◆ GI complication
◆ Sexual dysfunction
◆ Dry skin
◆ Fractures

Signs and symptoms
Chronic renal failure produces major changes in all body systems:
◆ *Renal and urologic:* Initially, salt-wasting and consequent hyponatremia produce hypotension, dry mouth, loss of skin turgor, listlessness, fatigue, and nausea; later, somnolence and confusion develop. As the number of functioning nephrons decreases, so does the kidneys' capacity to excrete sodium, resulting in salt retention and overload. Accumulation of potassium causes muscle irritability, then muscle weakness as the potassium level continues to rise. Fluid overload and metabolic acidosis also occur. Urine output decreases; urine is very dilute and contains casts and crystals.
◆ *Cardiovascular:* Renal failure leads to hypertension, arrhythmias (including life-threatening ventricular tachycardia or fibrillation), cardiomyopathy, uremic pericarditis, pericardial effusion with possible cardiac tamponade, heart failure, and periorbital and peripheral edema.
◆ *Respiratory:* Pulmonary changes include reduced pulmonary macrophage activity with increased susceptibility to infection, pulmonary edema, pleuritic pain, pleural friction rub and effusions, crackles, thick sputum, uremic pleuritis and uremic lung (or uremic pneumonitis), dyspnea due to heart failure, and Kussmaul respirations as a result of acidosis.
◆ *GI:* Inflammation and ulceration of GI mucosa cause stomatitis, gum ulceration and bleeding and, possibly, parotitis, esophagitis, gastritis, duodenal ulcers, lesions on the small and large bowel, uremic colitis, pancreatitis, and proctitis. Other GI symptoms include a metallic taste in the mouth, uremic fetor (ammonia smell to breath), anorexia, nausea, and vomiting.
◆ *Cutaneous:* Typically, the skin is pallid, yellowish bronze, dry, and scaly. Other cutaneous symptoms include severe itching; purpura; ecchymoses; petechiae; uremic frost (most often in critically ill or terminal patients; thin, brittle fingernails with characteristic lines; and dry, brittle hair that may change color and fall out easily.
◆ *Neurologic:* Restless leg syndrome, one of the first signs of peripheral neuropathy, causes pain, burning, and itching in the legs and feet, which may be relieved by voluntarily shaking, moving, or rocking them. Eventually, this condition progresses to paresthesia and motor nerve dysfunction (usually bilateral footdrop) unless dialysis is initiated. Other signs and symptoms include muscle cramping and twitching, shortened memory and attention span, apathy, drowsiness, irritability, confusion, coma, and seizures. EEG changes indicate metabolic encephalopathy.
◆ *Endocrine:* Common endocrine abnormalities include stunted growth patterns in children (even with elevated growth hormone levels), infertility and decreased libido in both sexes, amenorrhea and cessation of menses in females, and impotence, decreased sperm production, and testicular atrophy in males. Increased aldosterone secretion (related to increased renin production) and impaired carbohydrate metabolism (increased blood glucose levels similar to diabetes mellitus) may also occur.
◆ *Hematopoietic:* Anemia, decreased RBC survival time, blood loss from dialysis and GI bleeding, mild thrombocytopenia, and platelet defects occur. Other problems include increased bleeding and clotting disorders, demonstrated by purpura, hemorrhage from body orifices, easy bruising, ecchymoses, and petechiae.

◆ *Skeletal:* Calcium-phosphorus imbalance and consequent parathyroid hormone imbalances cause muscle and bone pain, skeletal demineralization, pathologic fractures, and calcifications in the brain, eyes, gums, joints, myocardium, and blood vessels. Arterial calcification may produce coronary artery disease. In children, renal osteodystrophy (renal rickets) may develop.

Diagnosis

The diagnosis of chronic renal failure is based on clinical assessment, a history of chronic progressive debilitation, and gradual deterioration of renal function as determined by creatinine clearance tests. The following laboratory findings also aid in diagnosis:

◆ Blood studies show elevated blood urea nitrogen, serum creatinine, and potassium levels; decreased arterial pH and bicarbonate; and low Hb level and HCT.

◆ Urine specific gravity becomes fixed at 1.010; urinalysis may show proteinuria, glycosuria, RBCs, leukocytes, and casts, depending on the etiology.

◆ X-ray studies include kidney–ureter–bladder films, excretory urography, nephrotomography, renal scan, and renal arteriography.

◆ Renal or abdominal CT scan, MRI, or ultrasound indicates changes associated with chronic renal failure, including abnormally small size in both kidneys.

◆ Kidney biopsy allows histologic identification of the underlying pathology.

Treatment

Treatment focuses on controlling the symptoms, minimizing complications, and slowing the progression of the disease. Associated diseases that cause or result from chronic renal failure, such as hypertension, must be controlled. Conservative treatment aims to correct specific symptoms. A low-protein diet reduces the production of end products of protein metabolism that the kidneys can't excrete. (A patient receiving continuous peritoneal dialysis should have a high-protein diet.) A high-calorie diet prevents ketoacidosis and the negative nitrogen balance that results in catabolism and tissue atrophy, and restricts sodium and potassium.

Maintaining fluid balance requires careful monitoring of vital signs, weight changes, and urine volume (if present). If some renal function remains, administration of loop diuretics such as furosemide and fluid restriction can reduce fluid retention. Cardiac glycosides may be used to mobilize edema fluids; antihypertensives to control blood pressure and associated edema. Antiemetics taken before meals may relieve nausea and vomiting; cimetidine or ranitidine may decrease gastric irritation. Methylcellulose or docusate can help prevent constipation.

Treatment may also include regular stool analysis (guaiac test) to detect occult blood and, as needed, cleaning enemas to remove blood from the GI tract. Anemia necessitates iron and folate supplements; severe anemia requires infusion of fresh frozen packed cells or washed packed cells. However, transfusions relieve anemia only temporarily. Epoetin alfa (erythropoietin) increases RBC production.

Drug therapy often relieves associated symptoms: an antipruritic, such as trimeprazine or diphenhydramine, for itching and aluminum hydroxide gel to lower serum phosphate levels. The patient may also benefit from supplementary vitamins (particularly B vitamins and vitamin D) and essential amino acids.

ALERT *Careful monitoring of serum potassium levels is necessary to detect hyperkalemia. Emergency treatment for severe hyperkalemia includes dialysis therapy and administration of 50% hypertonic glucose I.V., regular insulin, calcium gluconate I.V., sodium bicarbonate I.V., and cation exchange resins such as sodium polystyrene sulfonate.*

ALERT *Cardiac tamponade resulting from pericardial effusion may require emergency pericardial tap or surgery.*

Blood gas measurements may indicate acidosis; intensive dialysis and thoracentesis can relieve pulmonary edema and pleural effusions.

Hemodialysis or peritoneal dialysis (particularly continuous ambulatory peritoneal dialysis and continuous cyclic peritoneal dialysis) can help control most manifestations of end-stage renal disease; altering dialyzing bath fluids can correct fluid and electrolyte disturbances. But anemia, peripheral neuropathy, cardiopulmonary and GI complications, sexual dysfunction, and skeletal defects may persist. Maintenance dialysis itself may produce complications, such as protein wasting, refractory ascites, and dialysis dementia. Kidney transplantation may eventually be the treatment of choice for some patients with end-stage renal disease.

PEDIATRIC TIP *Children require more dialysis in relation to their body weight than adults because their metabolic rates and, therefore, food intake, are higher.*

Special considerations

Because chronic renal failure has such widespread clinical effects, it requires meticulous and carefully coordinated supportive care.

◆ Good skin care is important. Bathe the patient daily, using superfatted soaps, oatmeal baths, and skin lotion without alcohol to ease pruritus. Don't use glycerin-containing soaps because they'll cause skin drying. Give good perineal care, using mild soap and water. Pad the side rails to guard against ecchymoses. Turn the patient often, and use a convoluted foam mattress to prevent skin breakdown.

◆ Provide good oral hygiene. Brush the patient's teeth often with a soft brush or sponge tip to reduce breath odor. Sugarless hard candy and mouthwash minimize bad taste in the mouth and alleviate thirst.

◆ Offer small, palatable meals that are also nutritious; try to provide favorite foods within dietary restrictions. Encourage intake of high-calorie foods. Instruct the outpatient to avoid high-sodium foods and high-potassium foods. Encourage adherence to fluid and protein restrictions. To prevent constipation, stress the need for exercise and sufficient dietary bulk.

◆ Watch for hyperkalemia. Observe for cramping of the legs and abdomen, and diarrhea. As potassium levels rise, watch for muscle irritability and a weak pulse rate. Monitor the electrocardiogram for tall, peaked T waves, widening QRS segment, prolonged PR interval, and disappearance of P waves, indicating hyperkalemia.

◆ Assess hydration status carefully. Check for jugular vein distention, and auscultate the lungs for crackles. Measure daily intake and output carefully, including all drainage, emesis, diarrhea, and blood loss. Record daily weight, presence or absence of thirst, axillary sweat, dryness of tongue, hypertension, and peripheral edema.

◆ Monitor for bone or joint complications. Prevent pathologic fractures by turning the patient carefully and ensuring his safety. Provide passive range-of-motion exercises for the bedridden patient.

◆ Encourage deep breathing and coughing to prevent pulmonary congestion. Listen often for crackles, rhonchi, and decreased breath sounds. Be alert for clinical effects of pulmonary edema (dyspnea, restlessness, and crackles). Administer diuretics and other medications, as ordered.

◆ Maintain strict sterile technique. Use a micropore filter during I.V. therapy. Watch for signs of infection (listlessness, high fever, and leukocytosis). Urge the outpatient to avoid contact with infected persons during the cold and flu season.

◆ Carefully observe and document seizure activity. Infuse sodium bicarbonate for acidosis, and sedatives or anticonvulsants for seizures, as ordered. Pad the side rails and keep an oral airway and suction setup at bedside. Assess neurologic status periodically, and check for Chvostek and Trousseau signs, indicators of low serum calcium levels.

◆ Observe for signs of bleeding. Watch for prolonged bleeding at puncture sites and at the vascular access site used for hemodialysis. Monitor Hb levels and HCT, and check stool, urine, and vomitus for blood.

◆ Report signs of pericarditis, such as a pericardial friction rub and chest pain.

⚠️ **ALERT** *Watch for the disappearance of friction rub, with a drop of 15 to 20 mm Hg in blood pressure during inspiration (paradoxical pulse)—an early sign of pericardial tamponade.*

◆ Schedule medications carefully. Give iron before meals, aluminum hydroxide gels after meals, and antiemetics, as necessary, a half hour before meals. Administer antihypertensives at appropriate intervals. If the patient requires a rectal infusion of sodium polystyrene sulfonate for dangerously high potassium levels, apply an emollient to soothe the perianal area. Be sure the sodium polystyrene sulfonate enema is expelled; otherwise, it will cause constipation and won't lower potassium levels. Recommend antacid cookies as an alternative to aluminum hydroxide gels needed to bind GI phosphate.

If the patient requires dialysis:

◆ Prepare the patient by fully explaining the procedure. Be sure that they understand how to protect and care for the arteriovenous shunt, fistula, or other vascular access. Check the vascular access site per facility protocol or every 2 hours for patency and check the limb for adequate blood supply and intact nervous function (temperature, pulse rate, capillary refill, and sensation). If a fistula is present, feel for a thrill and listen for a bruit. Use a gentle touch to avoid occluding the fistula. Report signs of possible clotting. Don't use the arm with the vascular access site to take blood pressure readings, draw blood, or give injections as these procedures may rupture the fistula or occlude blood flow.

◆ Withhold the 6 a.m. (or morning) dose of antihypertensive on the morning of dialysis, and instruct the outpatient to do the same.

◆ Use standard precautions when handling body fluids and needles.

◆ Monitor Hb levels and HCT. Assess the patient's tolerance of these levels. Some individuals are more sensitive to lower levels than others. Instruct the anemic patient to conserve energy and to rest frequently.

◆ After dialysis, check for disequilibrium syndrome, a result of sudden correction of blood chemistry abnormalities. Symptoms range from a headache to seizures. Also, check for excessive bleeding from the dialysis site. Apply pressure dressing or absorbable gelatin sponge, as indicated. Monitor blood pressure carefully after dialysis.

◆ A patient undergoing dialysis is under a great deal of stress, as is the family. Refer them to appropriate counseling agencies for assistance in coping with chronic renal failure.

Lower urinary tract disorders

LOWER URINARY TRACT INFECTION

Cystitis and urethritis, the two forms of lower UTI, are nearly 10 times more common in women than in men and affect about 10% to 20% of all women at least once. Lower UTI is also a prevalent bacterial disease in children, with girls again most commonly affected. In men and children, lower UTIs are frequently related to anatomic or physiologic abnormalities and therefore require extremely close evaluation. UTIs often respond readily to treatment, but recurrence and resistant bacterial flare-up during therapy are possible.

PEDIATRIC TIP *Have a workup done on all children with proven UTI to exclude an abnormality of the urinary tract that would predispose them to renal damage.*

Pathophysiology

Most lower UTIs result from ascending infection by a single, gram-negative, enteric bacterium, such as *E. coli, Klebsiella, Proteus, Enterobacter, Pseudomonas,* or *Serratia.* However, in a patient with neurogenic bladder, an indwelling catheter, or a fistula between the intestine and the bladder, lower UTI may result from simultaneous infection with multiple pathogens. Infection can result from a breakdown in local defense mechanisms in the bladder that allow bacteria to invade the bladder mucosa and multiply. These bacteria can't be readily eliminated by normal micturition.

Bacterial flare-up during treatment is generally caused by the pathogenic organism's resistance to the prescribed antimicrobial therapy. The presence of even a small number (<10,000/mL) of bacteria in a midstream urine sample obtained during treatment casts doubt on the effectiveness of treatment.

In 99% of patients, recurrent lower UTI results from reinfection by the same organism or from some new pathogen; in the remaining 1%, recurrence reflects persistent infection, usually from renal calculi, chronic bacterial prostatitis, or a structural anomaly that may become a source of infection.

The high incidence of lower UTI among women may result from the shortness of the female urethra (1¼" to 2" [3 to 5 cm]), which predisposes women to infection caused by bacteria from the vagina, perineum, rectum, or a sexual partner. (See *Preventing UTIs,* page 368.) Men are less vulnerable because their urethras are longer (7¼" [18.4 cm]) and because prostatic fluid serves as an antibacterial shield. However, in men older than age 60, incidence rates match those of women. In both men and women, infection usually ascends from the urethra to the bladder.

ELDER TIP *As a person ages, the bladder muscles weaken, which may result in incomplete bladder emptying and chronic urine retention—factors that predispose the older person to bladder infections.*

Complications

◆ Chronic or recurrent UTI
◆ Complicated UTI
◆ Kidney infection

Signs and symptoms

Lower UTI usually produces urgency, frequency, dysuria, cramps or spasms of the bladder, itching, a feeling of warmth during urination, nocturia, and possibly urethral discharge in males. Inflammation of the bladder wall also causes hematuria and fever. Other common features include low back pain, malaise, nausea, vomiting, abdominal pain or tenderness over the bladder area, chills, and flank pain.

ELDER TIP *The most common initial symptoms of lower UTI in elderly patients are lethargy and a change in mental status.*

Diagnosis

Characteristic clinical features and a microscopic urinalysis showing RBCs and WBCs greater than 10/high-power field suggest lower UTI.

CONFIRMING DIAGNOSIS *A clean-catch midstream urine specimen revealing a bacterial count above 100,000/mL confirms the diagnosis.*

Lower counts don't necessarily rule out infection, especially if the patient is voiding frequently because bacteria require 30 to 45 minutes to reproduce in urine. Careful midstream, clean-catch collection is preferred to catheterization, in men. In women catheterization is the preferred method of obtaining a truly representative sample of the bladder urine as clean catch, irrespective of how fastidiously it is performed, can show perineal bacteria and cellular material.

Culture identifies the infecting organism while sensitivity testing determines the

appropriate therapeutic antimicrobial. If patient
history and physical examination warrant, a
blood test or a stained smear of the discharge
rules out venereal disease. Voiding cystourethrography or excretory urography may detect
congenital anomalies that predispose the patient to recurrent UTIs.

Treatment

Appropriate antimicrobials are the treatment
of choice for most initial lower UTIs. A course
of antibiotic therapy lasting from 7 to 10 days
is standard, but recent studies suggest that a
single dose of an antibiotic or an antibiotic
regimen of 3 to 5 days length may be sufficient
to render the urine sterile. After 3 days of antibiotic therapy, urine culture should show no
organisms. If the urine isn't sterile, bacterial
resistance has probably occurred, making the
use of a different antimicrobial necessary. Single-dose antibiotic therapy with amoxicillin
or trimethoprim and sulfamethoxazole may
be effective in females with acute noncompli-
cated UTI. A urine culture taken 1 to 2 weeks
later indicates whether or not the infection has
been eradicated.

Recurrent infections due to infected renal
calculi, chronic prostatitis, or structural abnormality may necessitate surgery; prostatitis
also requires long-term antibiotic therapy. In
patients without these predisposing conditions,
long-term, low-dosage antibiotic therapy is the
treatment of choice.

PEDIATRIC TIP *Fluoroquinolones aren't used
for children because of possible adverse effects
on developing cartilage.*

Special considerations

The care plan should include careful patient
teaching, supportive measures, and proper specimen collection.

◆ Explain the nature and purpose of antimicrobial therapy. Emphasize the importance of
completing the prescribed course of therapy
or, with long-term prophylaxis, of adhering
strictly to the ordered dosage. Urge the patient
to drink plenty of water (at least eight glasses a
day). Stress the need to maintain a consistent
fluid intake of about 2 qt (2 L)/day. More or
less than this amount may alter the effect of the
prescribed antimicrobial. Fruit juices, especially
cranberry juice, and oral doses of vitamin C
may help acidify the urine and enhance the action of the medication.

◆ Watch for GI disturbances from antimicrobial
therapy. Nitrofurantoin macrocrystals, taken
with milk or a meal, prevent such distress. If
therapy includes phenazopyridine (might mention the new urinary analgesic Uribel and Uro-
gesic Blue which turn the urine blue), warn the
patient that this drug may turn urine red-orange.

◆ Suggest warm sitz baths for relief of perineal
discomfort. If baths aren't effective, apply heat
sparingly to the perineum but be careful not to
burn the patient. Apply topical antiseptics, such
as povidone-iodine ointment, on the urethral
meatus as necessary.

◆ Collect all urine samples for culture and
sensitivity testing carefully and promptly. Teach
a woman how to clean the perineum properly
and keep the labia separated during voiding. A
noncontaminated midstream specimen is essential for accurate diagnosis.

◆ To prevent recurrent lower UTIs, teach a woman to carefully wipe the perineum from front to back and to clean it thoroughly with soap and water after defecation. Advise an infection-prone woman to void immediately after sexual intercourse. Stress the need to drink plenty of fluids routinely and to avoid postponing urination. Recommend frequent comfort stops during long car trips. Also stress the need to completely empty the bladder. To prevent recurrent infections in men, urge prompt treatment of predisposing conditions such as chronic prostatitis. Have the patient use a commode rather than a bedpan to promote sitting up, which assists in emptying the bladder.

VESICOURETERAL REFLUX

In vesicoureteral reflux, urine flows from the bladder back into the ureters and eventually into the renal pelvis or the parenchyma. Because the bladder empties poorly, UTI may result, possibly leading to acute or chronic pyelonephritis with renal damage.

Vesicoureteral reflux is most common during infancy in boys and during early childhood (ages 3 to 7) in girls. Primary vesicoureteral reflux that results from congenital anomalies is most prevalent in females and is rare in blacks. Up to 25% of asymptomatic siblings of children with diagnosed primary vesicoureteral reflux also show reflux.

Pathophysiology

In patients with vesicoureteral reflux, incompetence of the ureterovesical junction and shortening of intravesical ureteral musculature allow backflow of urine into the ureter when the bladder contracts during voiding. Incompetence may result from congenital anomalies of the ureters or bladder, including short or absent intravesical ureter, ureteral ectopia lateralis (greater-than-normal lateral placement of ureters), and gaping ureteral orifice; inadequate detrusor muscle buttress in the bladder, stemming from congenital paraureteral bladder diverticulum; acquired diverticulum (from outlet obstruction); flaccid neurogenic bladder; and high intravesical pressure from outlet obstruction or an unknown cause. Vesicoureteral reflux may also result from cystitis, with inflammation of the intravesical ureter, which causes edema and fixation of the intramural ureter and usually leads to reflux in persons with congenital ureteral or bladder anomalies or other predisposing conditions.

Reflux nephropathy occurs in about 4 of 1,000 asymptomatic people. However, in infants and children who experience UTIs, its prevalence approaches 40% to 50%. Reflux nephropathy may lead to chronic renal failure and end-stage renal disease.

Complications
◆ Recurrent UTI
◆ Chronic pyelonephritis
◆ Renal scarring
◆ Hypertension

Signs and symptoms

Vesicoureteral reflux typically manifests itself as the signs and symptoms of UTI: frequency, urgency, burning on urination, hematuria, foul-smelling urine and, in infants, dark, concentrated urine. With upper urinary tract involvement, signs and symptoms usually include high fever, chills, flank pain, vomiting, and malaise.

PEDIATRIC TIP *In children, fever, nonspecific abdominal pain, and diarrhea may be the only clinical effects. Rarely, children with minimal symptoms remain undiagnosed until puberty or later, when they begin to exhibit clear signs of renal impairment (anemia, hypertension, and lethargy).*

Diagnosis

Symptoms of UTI provide the first clues to diagnosis of vesicoureteral reflux. In infants, hematuria or strong-smelling urine may be the first indication; palpation may reveal a hard, thickened bladder (hard mass deep in the pelvis) if posterior urethral valves are causing an obstruction in male infants.

Cystoscopy, with instillation of a solution containing methylene blue or indigo carmine dye, may confirm the diagnosis. After the bladder is emptied and refilled with clear sterile water, color-tinged efflux from either ureter positively confirms reflux.

Other pertinent laboratory studies include the following:
◆ Clean-catch urinalysis shows a bacterial count greater than 100,000/mL. Microscopic examination may reveal WBCs, RBCs, and an increased urine pH in the presence of infection. Specific gravity less than 1.010 demonstrates inability to concentrate urine.
◆ Laboratory studies reveal elevated creatinine levels (>1.2 mg/dL) and elevated blood urea nitrogen levels (>18 mg/dL), indicating advanced renal dysfunction.
◆ Excretory urography may show dilated lower ureter, ureter visible for its entire length, hydronephrosis, calyceal distortion, and renal scarring.
◆ Voiding cystourethrography (either fluoroscopic or radionuclide) identifies and

determines the degree of reflux and shows when reflux occurs. It may also pinpoint the causative anomaly. In this procedure, contrast material is instilled into the bladder, and X-rays are taken before, during, and after voiding. Nuclear cystography and renal ultrasound may also be used to detect reflux.

◆ Abdominal CT scan or ultrasound of the kidneys or abdomen shows hydronephrosis, reflux, a small kidney, or scarring.

◆ Catheterization of the bladder after the patient voids determines the amount of residual urine.

Treatment

The goal of treatment in a patient with vesicoureteral reflux is to prevent pyelonephritis and renal dysfunction with antibiotic therapy and, when necessary, vesicoureteral reimplantation. Appropriate surgical procedures create a normal valve effect at the junction by reimplanting the ureter into the bladder wall at a more oblique angle.

Antimicrobial therapy is usually effective for reflux that's secondary to infection, reflux related to neurogenic bladder and, in children, reflux related to a short intravesical ureter (which abates spontaneously with growth). Reflux related to infection generally subsides after the infection is cured. However, 80% of females with vesicoureteral reflux will have recurrent UTIs within a year. Recurrent infection requires long-term prophylactic antibiotic therapy and careful patient follow-up (cystoscopy and excretory urography every 4 to 6 months) to track the degree of reflux.

UTI that recurs despite adequate prophylactic antibiotic therapy necessitates vesicoureteral reimplantation or reconstructive repair. Bladder outlet obstruction in people with neurogenic bladder requires surgery only if renal dysfunction is present. After surgery, as after antibiotic therapy, close medical follow-up is necessary (excretory urography every 2 to 3 years and urinalysis once per month for 1 year), even if symptoms haven't recurred.

Special considerations

Patient care includes education and postoperative support.

◆ To ensure complete emptying of the bladder, teach the patient with vesicoureteral reflux to double void (void once and then try to void again in a few minutes). Because the natural urge to urinate may be impaired, advise them to void every 2 to 3 hours whether or not they feel the urge.

PEDIATRIC TIP *Because the diagnostic tests may frighten the child, encourage one of his*

parents to stay with the patient during all procedures. Explain the procedures to the parents and to the child, if he's old enough to understand.

◆ If surgery is necessary, explain postoperative care: suprapubic catheter in the male, indwelling catheter in the female; and, in both, one or two ureteral catheters or (stents) brought out of the bladder through a small abdominal incision. The suprapubic or indwelling catheter keeps the bladder empty and prevents pressure from stressing the surgical wound; ureteral catheters drain urine directly from the renal pelvis. After complicated reimplantations, all catheters remain in place for 7 to 10 days. Explain that the child will be able to move and walk with the catheters but must be very careful not to dislodge them.

◆ Postoperatively, closely monitor fluid intake and output. Give analgesics and antibiotics, as ordered. Make sure the catheters are patent and draining well. Maintain sterile technique during catheter care. Watch for fever, chills, and flank pain, which suggest a blocked catheter.

◆ Before discharging the patient, stress the importance of close follow-up care and adequate fluid intake throughout childhood.

◆ Instruct parents to watch for and report recurring signs of UTI (painful, frequent, burning urination; foul-smelling urine).

◆ If the child is taking antimicrobial drugs, make sure his parents understand the importance of completing the prescribed therapy or maintaining low-dose prophylaxis.

NEUROGENIC BLADDER

Neurogenic bladder (also known as *neuromuscular dysfunction of the lower urinary tract, neurologic bladder dysfunction,* and *neuropathic bladder*) refers to all types of bladder dysfunction caused by an interruption of normal bladder innervation. Subsequent complications include incontinence, residual urine retention, urinary infection, stone formation, and renal failure. A neurogenic bladder can be spastic (hypertonic, reflex, or automatic) or flaccid (hypotonic, atonic, nonreflex, or autonomous).

Pathophysiology

At one time, neurogenic bladder was thought to result primarily from spinal cord injury; now, it appears to stem from a host of underlying conditions:

◆ cerebral disorders, such as stroke, brain tumor (meningioma and glioma), Parkinson disease, multiple sclerosis, dementia, and incontinence caused by aging

◆ spinal cord disease or trauma, such as herniated vertebral disks, spina bifida, myelomeningocele, spinal stenosis (causing cord compression) or arachnoiditis (causing adhesions between the membranes covering the cord), cervical spondylosis, myelopathies from hereditary or nutritional deficiencies and, rarely, tabes dorsalis

◆ disorders of peripheral innervation, including autonomic neuropathies resulting from endocrine disturbances such as diabetes mellitus (most common)

◆ metabolic disturbances, such as hypothyroidism, porphyria, or uremia (infrequent)

◆ acute infectious diseases such as transverse myelitis

◆ heavy metal toxicity

◆ chronic alcoholism

◆ collagen diseases such as systemic lupus erythematosus

◆ vascular diseases such as atherosclerosis

◆ distant effects of cancer such as primary oat cell carcinoma of the lung

◆ herpes zoster

◆ syphilis

◆ sacral agenesis.

An upper motor neuron lesion causes spastic neurogenic bladder, with spontaneous contractions of detrusor muscles, elevated intravesical voiding pressure, bladder wall hypertrophy with trabeculation, and urinary sphincter spasms. A lower motor neuron lesion causes flaccid neurogenic bladder, with decreased intravesical pressure, increased bladder capacity and large residual urine retention, and poor detrusor contraction.

Complications

◆ Calculus formation

◆ Incontinence

◆ Renal failure

◆ Residual urine retention

◆ UTI

◆ Autonomic dysreflexia

Signs and symptoms

Neurogenic bladder produces a wide range of clinical effects, depending on the underlying cause and its effect on the structural integrity of the bladder. Usually, this disorder causes some degree of incontinence, changes in initiation or interruption of micturition, and the inability to empty the bladder completely. Other effects of neurogenic bladder include vesicoureteral reflux, deterioration or infection in the upper urinary tract, and ureteral dilatation with hydronephrosis.

Depending on the site and extent of the spinal cord lesion, spastic neurogenic bladder may produce involuntary or frequent scanty urination, without a feeling of bladder fullness, and possibly spontaneous spasms of the arms and legs. Anal sphincter tone may be increased. Tactile stimulation of the abdomen, thighs, or genitalia may precipitate voiding and spontaneous contractions of the arms and legs. With cord lesions in the upper thoracic (cervical) level, bladder distention can trigger hyperactive autonomic reflexes, resulting in severe hypertension, bradycardia, and headaches.

Flaccid neurogenic bladder may be associated with overflow incontinence, diminished anal sphincter tone, and a greatly distended bladder (evident on percussion or palpation), but without the accompanying feeling of bladder fullness due to sensory impairment.

Diagnosis

The patient's history may include a condition or disorder that can cause neurogenic bladder, incontinence, and disruptions of micturition patterns. Voiding cystourethrography evaluates bladder neck function, vesicoureteral reflux, and continence.

Urodynamic studies help evaluate how urine is stored in the bladder, how well the bladder empties, and the rate of movement of urine out of the bladder during voiding. These studies consist of five components:

◆ Urine flow study (uroflow) shows diminished or impaired urine flow.

◆ Cystometry evaluates bladder nerve supply, detrusor muscle tone, and intravesical pressures during bladder filling and contraction.

◆ Urethral pressure profile determines urethral function with respect to the length of the urethra and the outlet pressure resistance.

◆ Sphincter electromyelography correlates the neuromuscular function of the external sphincter with bladder muscle function during bladder filling and contraction. This evaluates how well the bladder and urinary sphincter muscles work together.

◆ Retrograde urethrography reveals the presence of strictures and diverticula. This test may not be performed on a routine basis.

Treatment

The goals of treatment are to maintain the integrity of the upper urinary tract, control infection, and prevent urinary incontinence through evacuation of the bladder, drug therapy, surgery or, less commonly, neural blocks and electrical stimulation.

Techniques of bladder evacuation include Credé's method, Valsalva's maneuver, and intermittent self-catheterization. Credé's method— application of manual pressure over the lower abdomen—promotes complete emptying of the bladder. After appropriate instruction, most patients can perform this maneuver themselves. Even when patients perform this maneuver properly, however, Credé's method isn't always successful and doesn't always eliminate the need for catheterization.

Intermittent self-catheterization—more effective than either Credé's method or Valsalva's maneuver—has proved to be a major advance in the treatment of neurogenic bladder because it allows complete emptying of the bladder without the risks that an indwelling catheter poses. Generally, men can perform this procedure more easily than women, but women can learn self-catheterization with the help of a mirror. Intermittent self-catheterization, in conjunction with a bladder-retraining program, is especially useful for patients with flaccid neurogenic bladder.

Drug therapy for neurogenic bladder may include bethanechol and phenoxybenzamine to facilitate bladder emptying and propantheline, methantheline, flavoxate, dicyclomine, and imipramine to facilitate urine storage.

When conservative treatment fails, surgery may correct the structural impairment through transurethral resection of the bladder neck, urethral dilatation, external sphincterotomy, or urinary diversion procedures. Implantation of an artificial urinary sphincter may be necessary if permanent incontinence follows surgery for neurogenic bladder.

Special considerations

Care for patients with neurogenic bladder varies according to the underlying cause and method of treatment.

◆ Explain all diagnostic tests clearly so the patient understands the procedure, time involved, and possible results. Assure the patient that the lengthy diagnostic process is necessary to identify the most effective treatment plan. After the treatment plan is chosen, explain it to the patient in detail.

◆ Use strict sterile technique during insertion of an indwelling catheter (a temporary measure to drain the incontinent patient's bladder). Don't interrupt the closed drainage system for any reason. Obtain urine specimens with a syringe and small-bore needle inserted through the aspirating port of the catheter itself (below the junction of the balloon instillation site). Irrigate in the same manner if ordered.

◆ Clean the catheter insertion site with soap and water at least twice a day. Don't allow the catheter to become encrusted. Use a sterile applicator to apply antibiotic ointment around the meatus after catheter care. Keep the drainage bag below the tubing, and don't raise the bag above the level of the bladder. Clamp the tubing, or empty the bag before transferring the patient to a wheelchair or stretcher to prevent accidental urine reflux. If urine output is considerable, empty the bag more frequently than once every 8 hours because bacteria can multiply in standing urine and migrate up the catheter and into the bladder.

◆ Watch for signs of infection (fever, cloudy or foul-smelling urine). Encourage the patient to drink plenty of fluids to prevent calculus formation and infection from urinary stasis. Try to keep the patient as mobile as possible. Perform passive range-of-motion exercises if necessary.

◆ If a urinary diversion procedure is to be performed, arrange for consultation with an enterostomal therapist, and coordinate the care plans.

◆ Before discharge, teach the patient and family evacuation techniques as necessary (Credé's method, intermittent catheterization). Counsel regarding sexual activities. Remember, the incontinent patient feels embarrassed and distressed. Provide emotional support.

CONGENITAL ANOMALIES OF THE URETER, BLADDER, AND URETHRA

The most common congenital malformations of the ureter, bladder, and urethra include duplicated ureter, retrocaval ureter, ectopic orifice of the ureter, stricture or stenosis of the ureter, ureterocele, exstrophy of the bladder, congenital bladder diverticulum, hypospadias, and epispadias. Some of these abnormalities are obvious at birth; others aren't apparent and are recognized only after they produce symptoms. (See *Congenital urologic anomalies*, page 373.)

Pathophysiology

Congenital anomalies of the ureter, bladder, and urethra are among the most common birth defects, occurring in about 5% of all births. Their causes are unknown; diagnosis and treatment vary.

Complications

◆ Calculi
◆ Hematuria
◆ Infections

Special considerations

PEDIATRIC TIP *Because these anomalies aren't always obvious at birth, carefully evaluate the newborn's urogenital function. Document the*

Congenital urologic anomalies

Duplicated ureter	Retrocaval ureter (preureteral vena cava)	Ectopic orifice of ureter
Pathophysiology ♦ Most common ureteral anomaly ♦ *Complete*, a double collecting system with two separate pelves, each with its own ureter and orifice ♦ *Incomplete* (*Y* type), two separate ureters join before entering bladder	**Pathophysiology** ♦ The right ureter passes behind the inferior vena cava before entering the bladder. Compression of the ureter between the vena cava and the spine causes dilation and elongation of the pelvis; hydroureter and hydronephrosis; and fibrosis and stenosis of the ureter in the compressed area. ♦ Relatively uncommon; higher incidence in males	**Pathophysiology** ♦ Ureters single or duplicated in females, ureteral orifice usually inserts in urethra or vaginal vestibule, beyond external urethral sphincter; in males, in prostatic urethra, or in seminal vesicles or vas deferens
Clinical features ♦ Persistent or recurrent infection ♦ Frequency, urgency, or burning on urination ♦ Diminished urine output ♦ Flank pain, fever, and chills	**Clinical features** ♦ Right flank pain ♦ Recurrent urinary tract infection ♦ Renal calculi ♦ Hematuria	**Clinical features** ♦ Symptoms rare when ureteral orifice opens between trigone and bladder neck ♦ Obstruction, reflux, and incontinence (dribbling) in 50% of females ♦ In males, flank pain, frequency, urgency
Diagnosis and treatment ♦ Excretory urography ♦ Voiding cystoscopy ♦ Cystourethrography ♦ Retrograde pyelography ♦ Surgery for obstruction, reflux, or severe renal damage	**Diagnosis and treatment** ♦ Excretory urography demonstrates superior ureteral enlargement with spiral appearance ♦ Surgical resection and anastomosis of ureter with renal pelvis, or reimplantation into bladder	**Diagnosis and treatment** ♦ Excretory urography ♦ Urethroscopy, vaginoscopy ♦ Voiding cystourethrography ♦ Resection and ureteral reimplantation into bladder for incontinence

Strictures or stenosis of ureter	Ureterocele	Exstrophy of bladder
Pathophysiology ♦ Most common site, the distal ureter above ureterovesical junction; less common, ureteropelvic junction; rare, the midureter ♦ Discovered during infancy in 25% of patients; before puberty in most ♦ More common in males	**Pathophysiology** ♦ Bulging of submucosal ureter into bladder can be 1 or 2 cm, or can almost fill entire bladder ♦ Unilateral, bilateral, ectopic with resulting hydroureter and hydronephrosis	**Pathophysiology** ♦ Absence of anterior abdominal and bladder wall allows the bladder to protrude onto abdomen ♦ In males, undescended testes and epispadias; in females, cleft clitoris, separated labia, or absent vagina ♦ Skeletal or intestinal anomalies possible
Clinical features ♦ Megaloureter or hydroureter (enlarged ureter), with hydronephrosis when stenosis occurs in distal ureter ♦ Hydronephrosis alone when stenosis occurs at ureteropelvic junction	**Clinical features** ♦ Obstruction ♦ Persistent or recurrent infection	**Clinical features** ♦ Obvious at birth, with urine seeping onto abdominal wall from abnormal ureteral orifices ♦ Surrounding skin excoriated; exposed bladder mucosa ulcerated; infection; related abnormalities

(continued)

Congenital urologic anomalies (*continued*)

Strictures or stenosis of ureter	Ureterocele	Exstrophy of bladder
Diagnosis and treatment ♦ Ultrasound ♦ Excretory urography ♦ Voiding cystography ♦ Surgical repair of stricture; nephrectomy for severe renal damage	**Diagnosis and treatment** ♦ Voiding cystourethrography ♦ Excretory urography and cystoscopy show thin, translucent mass ♦ Surgical excision or resection of ureterocele, with reimplantation of ureter	**Diagnosis and treatment** ♦ Excretory urography ♦ Surgical closure of defect, and bladder and urethra reconstruction during infancy to allow pubic bone fusion; alternative treatment: protective dressing and diapering; urinary diversion eventually necessary for most patients

Congenital bladder diverticulum	Hypospadias	Epispadias
Pathophysiology ♦ Circumscribed pouch or sac (diverticulum) of bladder wall ♦ Can occur anywhere in bladder, usually lateral to ureteral orifice. Large diverticulum at orifice can cause reflux.	**Pathophysiology** ♦ Urethral opening on ventral surface of penis or, in females (rare), within vagina ♦ Occurs in 1 in 300 live male births; genetic factor suspected in less severe cases	**Pathophysiology** ♦ Urethral opening on dorsal surface of penis; in females, a fissure of the upper wall of urethra ♦ A rare anomaly; usually more common in males; often accompanies bladder exstrophy
Clinical features ♦ Fever, frequency, and painful urination ♦ Urinary tract infection ♦ Cystitis, particularly in males ♦ Diagnosis and treatment-Excretory urography shows diverticulum ♦ Retrograde cystography shows vesicoureteral reflux in ureter ♦ Surgical correction for reflux	**Clinical features** ♦ Usually associated with chordee, making normal urination with penis elevated impossible ♦ Absence of ventral prepuce ♦ Vaginal discharge in females ♦ Diagnosis and treatment-Mild disorder requires no treatment ♦ Surgical repair of severe anomaly usually necessary before child reaches school age	**Clinical features** ♦ In mild cases, orifice appears along dorsum of glans; in severe cases, along dorsum of penis ♦ In females, bifid clitoris and short, wide urethra ♦ Diagnosis and treatment-Surgical repair, in several stages, almost always necessary

amount and color of urine, voiding pattern, strength of stream, and any indications of infection, such as fever and urine odor. Tell parents to watch for these signs at home. In all children, watch for signs of obstruction, such as dribbling, oliguria or anuria, abdominal mass, hypertension, fever, bacteriuria, or pyuria.

♦ Monitor renal function daily; record intake and output accurately.

♦ Follow strict sterile technique in handling cystostomy tubes or indwelling urinary catheters.

♦ Make sure that ureteral, suprapubic, or urethral catheters remain in place and don't become contaminated. Document the type, color, and amount of drainage.

♦ Apply sterile saline pads to protect the exposed mucosa of the newborn with bladder exstrophy. Don't use heavy clamps on the umbilical cord, and avoid dressing or diapering the infant. Place the infant in an incubator, and direct a stream of saline mist onto the bladder to keep it moist. Use warm water and mild soap to keep the surrounding skin clean. Rinse well, and keep the area as dry as possible to prevent excoriation.

◆ Infant boys diagnosed with hypospadias and epispadias should not be circumcised because the foreskin can and typically is used in the surgical repair.

◆ Provide reassurance and emotional support to the parents. When possible, allow them to participate in their child's care to promote normal bonding. As appropriate, suggest or arrange for genetic counseling.

Prostate and epididymis disorders

PROSTATITIS

Prostatitis, inflammation of the prostate gland, may be acute or chronic. Acute prostatitis most often results from gram-negative bacteria and is easy to recognize and treat. However, chronic prostatitis, the most common cause of recurrent UTIs in males, is less easy to recognize.

Pathophysiology

About 80% of bacterial prostatitis cases result from infection by *E. coli*; the rest are due to infection by *Klebsiella, Enterobacter, Proteus, Pseudomonas, Streptococcus,* or *Staphylococcus.* These organisms probably spread to the prostate by the bloodstream or from ascending urethral infection, invasion of rectal bacteria via lymphatics, reflux of infected bladder urine into the prostate ducts or, less commonly, infrequent or excessive sexual intercourse or such procedures as cystoscopy or catheterization. Chronic prostatitis usually results from bacterial invasion from the urethra.

It's estimated that 2 of every 10,000 people who seek outpatient care do so because of prostatitis. As many as 35% of males older than age 50 have chronic prostatitis; about 50% of males will be diagnosed with prostatitis at some point in their lives.

Complications

◆ UTI
◆ Prostatic abscess
◆ Pyelonephritis
◆ Epididymitis

Signs and symptoms

Acute prostatitis begins with fever, chills, low back pain, myalgia, perineal fullness, and arthralgia. Urination is frequent and urgent. Dysuria, nocturia, and urinary obstruction may also occur. The urine may appear cloudy. When palpated rectally, the prostate is tender, indurated, swollen, firm, and warm. If the patient has shaking chills and fever prostate manipulation should be deferred.

Chronic bacterial prostatitis sometimes produces no symptoms but usually elicits the same urinary symptoms as the acute form but to a lesser degree. UTI is a common complication. Other possible signs include painful ejaculation, hemospermia, persistent urethral discharge, and sexual dysfunction.

Diagnosis

Characteristic rectal examination findings suggest prostatitis (boggy, tender prostate). In some cases, a urine culture can identify the causative infectious organism which is most often *E. coli.* Expressed prostatic secretion (EPS) should be attempted during the prostate exam and any seminal fluid expressed should be examined microscopically looking for WBCs in clumps. Bacteria are seldom seen in an EPS.

℞ **CONFIRMING DIAGNOSIS** *A firm diagnosis depends on a comparison of urine cultures of specimens obtained by the Meares and Stamey technique. This test requires three urine specimens and one specimen of prostatic secretions. Urine is collected when the patient starts voiding (sample 1); then at midstream (sample 2), after which the patient is asked to stop voiding with some urine remaining in the bladder; the physician massages the prostate and a specimen of EPS is obtained; and, finally, the first-voided urine after this prostatic massage is collected (sample 3). A significant increase in colony count in sample 3 compared with samples 1 and 2 confirms prostatitis.*

Treatment

Systemic antibiotic therapy chosen according to the infecting organism is the treatment of choice for acute prostatitis. If sepsis is likely, I.V. antibiotics may be given until sensitivity test results are known. If test results and clinical response are favorable, parenteral therapy continues for 48 hours to 1 week, after which an oral agent is substituted for 30 days. For infections caused by a sexually transmitted disease, injection of ceftriaxone followed by a 10-day course of doxycycline or floxacin is effective.

Supportive therapy includes bed rest, adequate hydration, and administration of analgesics, antipyretics, sitz baths, and stool softeners as necessary. Diet therapy includes avoiding substances that irritate the bladder, such as alcohol, caffeinated food and beverages, citrus juices, and hot or spicy foods. Increasing the intake of fluids (1.5 to 4 L/day) encourages frequent urination that will help flush the bacteria from the bladder. In symptomatic chronic prostatitis, regular massage of the prostate is most effective. Regular ejaculation may help promote drainage of prostatic secretions. Anticholinergics and analgesics may help relieve nonbacterial prostatitis symptoms.

If drug therapy is unsuccessful, treatment may include transurethral resection of the prostate (TURP), which requires removal of all infected tissue. However, this procedure usually isn't performed on young adults because it may cause retrograde ejaculation and sterility. Total prostatectomy is curative but may cause impotence and incontinence.

Special considerations
Patient care is primarily supportive.
◆ Ensure bed rest and adequate hydration. Provide stool softeners and administer sitz baths, as ordered.
◆ As needed, prepare to assist with suprapubic needle aspiration of the bladder or a suprapubic cystostomy (rarely used).
◆ Emphasize the need for strict adherence to the prescribed drug regimen. Instruct the patient to drink at least eight glasses of water a day. Have the patient report adverse drug reactions (rash, nausea, vomiting, fever, chills, and GI irritation).
◆ Adding probiotics during prolonged antibiotic therapy can help prevent gut bacteria overgrowth.

EPIDIDYMITIS
This infection of the epididymis, the testicle's cordlike excretory duct, is one of the most common infections of the male reproductive tract. It usually affects adults and is rare before puberty. Epididymitis may spread to the testicle itself, causing orchitis; bilateral epididymitis may cause sterility. (See *Orchitis.*)

Pathophysiology
Epididymitis is usually a complication of pyogenic bacterial infection of the urinary tract (urethritis or prostatitis). The pyogenic organisms, such as staphylococci, *E. coli*, streptococci, *Chlamydia trachomatis*, and *Neisseria gonorrhoeae*, reach the epididymis through the lumen of the vas deferens. Rarely, epididymitis is secondary to a distant infection, such as pharyngitis or tuberculosis, that spreads through the lymphatics or, less commonly, the bloodstream. Other causes include trauma, gonorrhea, syphilis, or a chlamydial infection. Trauma may reactivate a dormant infection or initiate a new one. Epididymitis may be a complication of prostatectomy and may also result from chemical irritation by extravasation of urine through the vas deferens. The incidence is about 600,000 cases per year, with the highest prevalence in young males ages 19 to 35.

Complications
◆ Bilateral epididymitis can cause sterility
◆ Orchitis

Signs and symptoms
The key symptoms are pain, extreme tenderness, and swelling in the groin and scrotum with erythema, high fever, malaise, and a characteristic waddle—an attempt to protect the groin and scrotum during walking. An acute hydrocele may also result from inflammation.

Orchitis
Orchitis, an infection of the testicles, is a serious complication of epididymitis. It may also result from mumps, which may lead to sterility. Orchitis may, rarely, result from other systemic infections, testicular torsion, or severe trauma. Its typical effects include unilateral or bilateral tenderness, sudden onset of pain, and swelling of the scrotum and testicles. The affected testicle may be red. Nausea and vomiting also occur. Sudden cessation of pain indicates testicular ischemia, which may result in permanent damage to one or both testicles.

Treatment consists of immediate antibiotic therapy; in orchitis due to mumps, diethylstilbestrol may be given to relieve pain, swelling, and fever. Severe orchitis may require surgery to incise and drain the hydrocele and improve testicular circulation. Other treatment is similar to that for epididymitis. To prevent orchitis due to mumps, stress the need for prepubertal males to receive mumps vaccine (or gamma globulin injection after contracting mumps).

Diagnosis

Clinical features suggest epididymitis, but diagnosis is actually made with the aid of laboratory tests:

◆ urinalysis: increased WBC count indicates infection

◆ urine culture and sensitivity tests: may identify causative organism

◆ serum WBC count: more than 10,000/µL in infection.

! ALERT *Scrotal ultrasonography may help differentiate acute epididymitis from other conditions, such as testicular torsion, which is a surgical emergency.*

Testicular scan (nuclear medicine scan) may be done to rule out torsion. In epididymitis, increased blood flow is also demonstrated.

Treatment

The goal of treatment is to reduce pain and swelling and combat infection. Therapy must begin immediately, particularly in the patient with bilateral epididymitis because sterility is always a threat. During the acute phase, treatment consists of bed rest, scrotal elevation with towel rolls or adhesive strapping, broad-spectrum antibiotics, and analgesics. An ice bag applied to the area may reduce swelling and relieve pain (heat is contraindicated because it may damage germinal cells, which are viable only at or below normal body temperature). When pain and swelling subside and allow walking, an athletic supporter may prevent pain. Occasionally, corticosteroids may be prescribed to help counteract inflammation, but their use is controversial.

❀ ELDER TIP *In the older patient undergoing open prostatectomy, bilateral vasectomy may be necessary to prevent epididymitis as a postoperative complication; however, antibiotic therapy alone may prevent it. When epididymitis is refractory to antibiotic therapy, epididymectomy under local anesthetic is necessary.*

Special considerations

Patient care includes support and monitoring for worsening of symptoms.

◆ Watch closely for abscess formation (localized, hot, red, tender area) or extension of infection into the testes. Closely monitor temperature, and ensure adequate fluid intake.

◆ Because the patient is usually very uncomfortable, administer analgesics as necessary. During bed rest, check often for proper scrotum elevation.

◆ Before discharge, emphasize the importance of completing the prescribed antibiotic therapy, even after symptoms subside. Educate the patient regarding preventing the transmission of sexually transmitted diseases, as appropriate.

◆ If the patient faces the possibility of sterility, suggest supportive counseling as necessary.

BENIGN PROSTATIC HYPERPLASIA

Although most men older than age 50 have some prostatic enlargement, in BPH, also known as *benign prostatic hypertrophy*, the prostate gland enlarges sufficiently to compress the urethra and cause some overt urinary obstruction. Depending on the size of the enlarged prostate, the age and health of the patient, and the extent of obstruction, BPH is treated symptomatically or surgically.

Pathophysiology

Evidence suggests a link between BPH and hormonal activity. As men age, production of androgenic hormones decreases, causing an imbalance in androgen and estrogen levels, and high levels of dihydrotestosterone, the main prostatic intracellular androgen. Other causes include neoplasm, arteriosclerosis, diabetes, inflammation, and metabolic or nutritional disturbances.

Regardless of the cause, BPH begins with changes in periurethral glandular tissue. As the prostate enlarges, it may extend into the bladder and obstruct urinary outflow by compressing or distorting the prostatic urethra. BPH may also cause a pouch to form in the bladder that retains urine when the rest of the bladder empties. This retained urine may lead to calculus formation or cystitis.

The likelihood of developing an enlarged prostate increases with age. A small amount of prostate enlargement is present in many men older than age 40 (8%), up to 40% to 50% in men 51 to 60, and more than 80% to 90% of men older than age 80. Blacks, with an incidence of 224.3 cases per 100,000 people, are at the greatest risk, present with more advanced disease, and have a poorer prognosis. Whites, by comparison, have an incidence of 150.3 cases per 100,000 people, and Asians have an incidence of 82.2 cases per 100,000 people.

Complications

◆ Urinary stasis
◆ UTI
◆ Calculi (bladder and prostatic)
◆ Bladder wall trabeculation
◆ Detrusor muscle hypertrophy
◆ Bladder diverticula and saccules
◆ Urethral stenosis

◆ Hydronephrosis
◆ Paradoxical incontinence
◆ Acute or chronic renal failure
◆ Acute postobstructive diuresis

Signs and symptoms

Clinical features of BPH depend on the extent of prostatic enlargement and the lobes affected. Characteristically, the condition starts with a group of symptoms known as *prostatism*: reduced urine stream caliber and force, urinary hesitancy, and difficulty starting micturition (resulting in straining, feeling of incomplete voiding, and an interrupted stream). As the obstruction increases, it causes frequent urination with nocturia, dribbling, urine retention, incontinence, and possibly hematuria. Physical examination indicates a visible midline mass above the symphysis pubis that represents an incompletely emptied bladder; rectal palpation discloses an enlarged prostate. Examination may detect secondary anemia and, possibly, renal insufficiency secondary to obstruction.

As BPH worsens, complete urinary obstruction may follow infection or use of decongestants, tranquilizers, alcohol, antidepressants, or anticholinergics. Complications include infection, renal insufficiency, hemorrhage, and shock.

Diagnosis

Clinical features and a rectal examination are usually sufficient for diagnosis. Other findings help to confirm it:
◆ Excretory urography may indicate urinary tract obstruction, hydronephrosis, calculi or tumors, and filling and emptying defects in the bladder.
◆ Elevated blood urea nitrogen and serum creatinine levels suggest renal dysfunction.
◆ Urinalysis and urine culture show hematuria, pyuria and, when the bacterial count exceeds 100,000/mL, UTI.

When symptoms are severe, a cystourethroscopy is definitive, but this test is performed only immediately before surgery to help determine the best procedure. It can show prostate enlargement, bladder wall changes, and a raised bladder neck.

Treatment

Conservative therapy includes prostate massages, sitz baths, fluid restriction for bladder distention, and antimicrobials for infection. If symptoms are mild, methods for relief may include avoiding alcohol and caffeine, especially after dinner; urinating when the urge is first felt; avoiding over-the-counter cold and sinus medications that contain decongestants or antihistamines because they can increase BPH symptoms; keeping warm and exercising regularly because cold weather and lack of physical activity may worsen symptoms; performing pelvic strengthening exercises (Kegel exercises); and reducing stress because nervousness and tension can lead to more frequent urination. Some men have had success taking extracts of saw palmetto berries, a herb that has been used to ease prostate symptoms. Fat-soluble saw palmetto extract that has been standardized to contain 85% to 95% fatty acids and sterols is more effective. Regular ejaculation may help relieve prostatic congestion.

Urine flow rates can be improved with alpha₁-adrenergic blockers, which relieve bladder outlet obstruction by preventing contractions of the prostatic capsule and bladder neck. Finasteride (5-alpha reductase inhibitor) lowers levels of hormones produced by the prostate (dihydrotestosterone), reduces the size of the prostate gland, increases urine flow rate, and decreases symptoms of BPH. It may take 3 to 6 months before a significant improvement in symptoms occurs. Potential adverse effects related to finasteride include decreased sex drive and impotence. Recently Cialis 5 mg daily has shown some benefit in men who have failed alpha₁-adrenergic blockers such as Terazosin, Doxazosin, Tamsulosin, Alfuzosin, and/or Silodosin.

Surgery is the only effective therapy to relieve acute urine retention, hydronephrosis, severe hematuria, recurrent UTIs, and other intolerable symptoms. A transurethral resection may be performed if the prostate weighs less than 2 oz (56.7 g). In TURP, a resectoscope removes tissue with a wire loop and electric current. In high-risk patients, postoperative continuous drainage with a three-way indwelling urinary catheter alleviates urine retention caused by clotting. Transurethral needle ablation (transurethral microwave thermotherapy) may be used to heat and destroy prostate tissue by radiofrequency; this helps spare surrounding tissue. Laser prostate ablation can also be used but pathologic specimens are vaporized and destroyed during the procedure.

The following procedures involve open surgical removal:
◆ *suprapubic (transvesical) resection*: most common and useful when prostatic enlargement remains within the bladder and the prostate is bigger than 60 g
◆ *retropubic (extravesical) resection*: allows direct visualization; potency and continence are usually maintained.

Balloon dilatation of the prostate has been used with varying degrees of success. Prostate stenting has also been used, again with varying degrees of success.

Special considerations

Prepare the patient for diagnostic tests and surgery, as appropriate.

◆ Monitor and record the patient's vital signs, intake and output, and daily weight. Watch closely for signs of postobstructive diuresis (such as increased urine output and hypotension), which may lead to serious dehydration, lowered blood volume, shock, electrolyte loss, and anuria.

◆ Administer antibiotics, as indicated, for UTI, urethral instrumentation, and cystoscopy.

◆ If urine retention is present, insert an indwelling urinary catheter (although this is usually difficult in a patient with BPH). If the catheter can't be passed transurethrally, assist with suprapubic cystostomy (under local anesthetic). Avoid rapid bladder decompression.

After prostatic surgery:

◆ Maintain patient comfort, and watch for and prevent postoperative complications. Observe for immediate dangers of prostatic bleeding (shock and hemorrhage). Check the catheter often (every 15 minutes for the first 2 to 3 hours) for patency and urine color; check dressings for bleeding.

◆ Postoperatively, many urologists insert a three-way catheter and establish continuous bladder irrigation. Keep the catheter open at a rate sufficient to maintain returns that are clear and light pink. Watch for fluid overload from absorption of the irrigating fluid into systemic circulation. If a regular catheter is used, observe it closely. If drainage stops because of clots, irrigate the catheter, as indicated, usually with 80 to 100 mL of normal saline solution, while maintaining strict sterile technique.

▼ ALERT *Watch for septic shock, the most serious complication of prostatic surgery, which may cause severe chills, sudden fever, tachycardia, hypotension, or other signs of shock. Start rapid infusion of antibiotics I.V. as indicated. Watch for pulmonary embolus, heart failure, and renal shutdown. Monitor vital signs, central venous pressure, and arterial pressure continuously. The patient may need intensive supportive care in the intensive care unit.*

◆ Administer anticholinergics, as indicated, to relieve painful bladder spasms that often occur after transurethral resection.

◆ Provide patient comfort measures after an open procedure: suppositories (except after perineal prostatectomy), analgesic medication to control incisional pain, and frequent dressing changes.

◆ Continue infusing I.V. fluids until the patient can drink sufficient fluids (2 to 3 L/day) to maintain adequate hydration.

◆ Administer stool softeners and laxatives, as needed, to prevent straining. Don't check for fecal impaction because a rectal examination may precipitate bleeding.

◆ After the catheter is removed, the patient may experience frequency, dribbling, and occasional hematuria. Reassure the patient that he'll gradually regain urinary control.

◆ Reinforce prescribed limits on activity. Warn the patient against lifting, strenuous exercise, and long automobile rides because these increase the risk of bleeding. Also caution the patient to restrict sexual activity for at least several weeks after discharge from the hospital.

◆ Instruct the patient to follow the prescribed oral antibiotic drug regimen, and discuss the indications for using gentle laxatives. Urge the patient to seek medical care immediately if they can't void, pass bloody urine, or develop a fever.

SELECTED REFERENCES

Levinson, W. (2010). Antibacterial drugs: Mechanism of action. In W. Levinson, et al. (Eds.), *Review of medical microbiology & immunology: A guide to clinical infectious diseases* (15th ed., chap. 10). New York: McGraw-Hill. Retrieved from http://accessmedicine.mhmedical.com/content.aspx?bookid=2381&sectionid=187687177

Meng, M. V., et al. (2018). Urologic disorders. In M. A. Papadakis, et al. (Eds.), *Current medical diagnosis & treatment* (chap. 23). New York: McGraw-Hill. Retrieved from http://accessmedicine.mhmedical.com/content.aspx?bookid=2192&sectionid=168019217

Porten, S. P., & Greene, K. L. (2013). Urologic laboratory examination. In J. W. McAninch & T. F. Lue (Eds.), *Smith and Tanagho's general urology* (18th ed., chap. 5). New York: McGraw-Hill. Retrieved from http://accessmedicine.mhmedical.com/content.aspx?bookid=508&sectionid=41088082

Sharp, V. A., & Wilbur, J. K. (2016). Men's health. In J. K. Wilbur, et al. (Eds.), *Graber and Wilbur's family medicine examination & board review* (4th ed., chap. 16). New York: McGraw-Hill. Retrieved from http://accessmedicine.mhmedical.com/content.aspx?bookid=2359&sectionid=185016771

Stoller, M. L. (2013a). Retrograde instrumentation of the urinary tract. In J. W. McAninch & T. F. Lue (Eds.), *Smith and Tanagho's general urology* (18th ed., chap. 11). New York: McGraw-Hill. Retrieved from http://accessmedicine.mhmedical.com/content.aspx?bookid=508&sectionid=41088088

Stoller, M. L. (2013b). Urinary stone disease. In J. W. McAninch & T. F. Lue (Eds.), *Smith and Tanagho's general urology* (18th ed., chap. 17). New York: McGraw-Hill. Retrieved from http://accessmedicine.mhmedical.com/content.aspx?bookid=508&sectionid=41088094; https://www.davita.com/kidney-disease/overview/stages-of-kidney-disease7

8

IMMUNE
DISORDERS

Introduction

The environment contains thousands of pathogenic microorganisms—viruses, bacteria, fungi, and parasites. Ordinarily, we protect ourselves from infectious organisms and other harmful invaders through an elaborate network of safeguards—the host defense system. Understanding how this system functions provides the framework for studying various immune disorders.

HOST DEFENSE SYSTEM

The host defense system includes physical and chemical barriers to infection, the inflammatory response, and the immune response. Physical barriers, such as the skin and mucous membranes, prevent invasion by most organisms. Those organisms that penetrate this first line of defense simultaneously trigger the inflammatory and immune responses. Both responses involve cells derived from a hematopoietic stem cell in the bone marrow.

Chemical barriers include lysozymes (found in body secretions, such as tears, mucus, and saliva) and hydrochloric acid (found in the stomach). Lysozymes destroy bacteria by removing cell walls. Hydrochloric acid breaks down food and mucus that contains pathogens.

The inflammatory response involves polymorphonuclear leukocytes, basophils, mast cells, platelets, and, to some extent, monocytes and macrophages.

The immune response primarily involves the interaction of lymphocytes (T and B cells),

macrophages, and macrophage-like cells and their products. These cells may be circulating or may be localized in the immune system's tissues and organs, including the thymus, lymph nodes, spleen, and tonsils. The thymus participates in the maturation of T lymphocytes (cell-mediated immunity); here these cells are "educated" to differentiate "self" from "nonself." In contrast, B lymphocytes (humoral immunity) mature in the bone marrow. The key humoral effector mechanism is the production of immunoglobulin (Ig) by B cells and the subsequent activation of the complement cascade. The lymph nodes, spleen, liver, and intestinal lymphoid tissue help remove and destroy circulating antigens in the blood and lymph.

ANTIGENS

An antigen is any substance that can induce an immune response. T and B lymphocytes have specific receptors that respond to specific antigen molecular shapes (epitopes). In B lymphocytes, or B cells, this receptor is an Ig (antibody) cell: IgD or IgM, sometimes referred to as a surface Ig. The T-cell antigen receptor recognizes antigens only in association with specific cell-surface molecules known as the major histocompatibility complex (MHC). (See *The major histocompatibility complex,* page 381.) MHC molecules, which differ among individuals, identify substances as self or nonself. Slightly different antigen receptors can recognize a phenomenal number of distinct antigens, which are coded by distinct, variable region genes.

The major histocompatibility complex

The major histocompatibility complex (MHC) is a cluster of genes on human chromosome 6 that plays a pivotal role in the immune response. Also known as *human leukocyte antigen* (*HLA*) *genes*, these genes are inherited in an autosomal codominant manner. That is, each individual receives one set of MHC genes (haplotype) from each parent, and both sets of genes are expressed on the individual's cells. These genes play a role in the recognition of self versus nonself and in the interaction of immunologically active cells by coding for cell-surface proteins.

HLA genes are divided into three classes. Class I molecules appear on the surface of nearly all of the body's cells and include HLA-A, HLA-B, and HLA-C genes.

During tissue graft rejection, they're the chief antigens recognized by the host. When killer (CD8+) T cells detect a virally infected antigen, they recognize it in the context of a class I molecule. Class II molecules only appear on B cells, macrophages, and activated T cells. They include the HLA-D and HLA-DR genes. Class II molecules promote efficient collaboration between immunocompetent cells.

Helper (CD4+) T cells require that antigen be presented in the context of a class II molecule. Because these molecules also determine whether an individual responds to a particular antigen, they're also known as *immune response genes*. Class III molecules include certain complement proteins (C2, C4, and Factor B).

Groups, or clones, of lymphocytes exist with identical receptors for a specific antigen. The clone of a lymphocyte rapidly proliferates when exposed to the specific antigen. Some lymphocytes further differentiate, and others become memory cells, which allow a more rapid response—the memory or anamnestic response—to subsequent challenge by the antigen.

Many factors influence antigenicity. Among them are the antigen's physical and chemical characteristics, its relative foreignness, and the individual's genetic makeup, particularly the MHC molecules. Most antigens are large molecules, such as proteins or polysaccharides. (Smaller molecules such as drugs that aren't antigenic by themselves are known as *haptens*. These haptens can bind with larger molecules, or carriers, and become antigenic or immunogenic.) The antigen's relative foreignness influences the immune response's intensity. For example, little or no immune response may follow transfusion of serum proteins between humans; however, a vigorous immune response (serum sickness) commonly follows transfusion of horse serum proteins to a human. Genetic makeup may also determine why some individuals respond to certain antigens, whereas others don't. The genes responsible for this phenomenon encode the MHC molecules.

B LYMPHOCYTES

B lymphocytes and their products, Igs, contribute to humoral immunity. The binding of soluble antigen with B-cell antigen receptors initiates the humoral immune response. The activated B cells differentiate into plasma cells that secrete Igs or antibodies. This response is regulated by T lymphocytes and their products, lymphokines. These lymphokines, which include interleukin (IL)-2, IL-4, IL-5, and interferon (IFN) gamma, are important in determining the class of Igs made by B cells.

The Igs secreted by plasma cells are four-chain molecules with two heavy (H) and two light (L) chains. (See *Structure of the immunoglobulin molecule*, page 382.) Each chain has a variable (V) region and one or more constant (C) regions, which are coded by separate genes. The V regions of both L and H chains participate in the binding of antigens. The C regions of the H chain provide a binding site for crystallizable fragment (Fc) receptors on cells and govern other mechanisms.

Any clone of B lymphocytes has one antigen specificity determined by the V regions of its L and H chains. However, the clone can change the class of Ig that it makes by changing the association between its V region genes and H chain C region genes (a process known as *isotype switching*). For example, a clone of B lymphocytes genetically preprogrammed to recognize tetanus toxoid initially will make an IgM antibody against tetanus toxoid and later an IgG or other antibody against it.

The five known classes of Igs—IgG, IgM, IgA, IgE, and IgD—are distinguished by the constant portions of their H chains. However, each class has a kappa or a lambda L chain, which gives rise to many subtypes. The almost limitless combinations of L and H chains give Igs their specificity.

Structure of the immunoglobulin molecule

The immunoglobulin (Ig) molecule consists of four polypeptide chains—two heavy (H) and two light (L) chains—held together by disulfide bonds. The H chain has one variable (V) and at least three constant (C) regions. The L chain has one V and one C regions. Together, the V regions of the H and L chains form a pocket known as the antigen-binding site. This site is located within the antigen-binding fragment (Fab) region of the molecule. Part of the C region of the H chains forms the crystallizable fragment (Fc) region of the molecule. This region mediates effector mechanisms such as complement activation and is the portion of the Ig molecule bound by Fc receptors on phagocytic cells, mast cells, and basophils. Each Ig molecule also has two antibody-combining sites (except for the IgM molecule, which has 10, and IgA, which may have two or more).

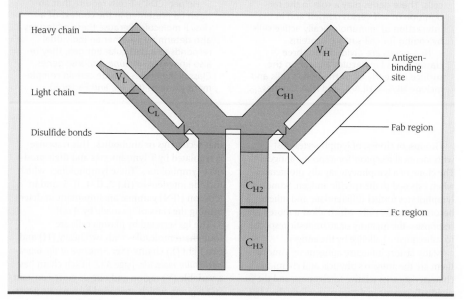

◆ *IgG*, the smallest Ig, appears in all body fluids because of its ability to move across membranes as a single structural unit (a monomer). It constitutes 75% of total serum Igs and is the major antibacterial and antiviral antibody.

◆ *IgM*, the largest Ig, appears as a pentamer (five monomers joined by a J-chain). Unlike IgG—which is produced mainly in the secondary, or recall, response—IgM dominates in the primary, or initial, immune response. However, like IgG, IgM is involved in classic antibody reactions, including precipitation, agglutination, neutralization, and complement fixation. Because of its size, IgM can't readily cross membrane barriers and is usually present only in the vascular system. IgM constitutes 5% of total serum Igs.

◆ *IgA* exists in serum primarily as a monomer; in secretory form, IgA exists almost exclusively as a dimer (two monomer molecules joined by a J-chain and a secretory component chain). As

a secretory Ig, IgA defends external body surfaces and is present in colostrum, saliva, tears, nasal fluids, and respiratory, gastrointestinal (GI), and genitourinary (GU) secretions. This antibody is considered important in preventing antigenic agents from attaching to epithelial surfaces. IgA makes up 20% of total serum Igs.

◆ *IgE*, present in trace amounts in serum, is involved in the release of vasoactive amines stored in basophils and tissue mast cell granules. When released, these bioamines cause the allergic effects characteristic of this type of hypersensitivity (erythema, itching, smooth-muscle contraction, secretions, and swelling).

◆ *IgD*, present as a monomer in serum in minute amounts, is the predominant antibody found on the surface of B lymphocytes and serves mainly as an antigen receptor. It may function in controlling lymphocyte activation or suppression.

T LYMPHOCYTES

T lymphocytes, or T cells, and macrophages are the chief participants in cell-mediated immunity. Immature T lymphocytes are derived from the bone marrow. Upon migration to the thymus, they undergo a maturation process that depends on the HLA genes. Thus, mature T cells can distinguish between self and nonself. T cells acquire certain surface molecules, or markers; these markers combined with the T-cell antigen receptor promote the particular activation of each type of T cell. T-cell activation requires presentation of antigens in the context of a specific HLA gene. Helper T cells require class II HLA genes; cytotoxic T cells require class I HLA genes. T-cell activation also involves IL-1, produced by macrophages, and IL-2, produced by T cells.

Natural killer (NK) cells are a discrete population of large lymphocytes, some of which resemble T lymphocytes. NK cells recognize surface changes on body cells infected with a virus; they then bind to and, in many cases, kill the infected cells.

MACROPHAGES

Important cells of the reticuloendothelial system, macrophages influence both immune and inflammatory responses. Macrophage precursors circulate in the blood. When they collect in various tissues and organs, they differentiate into macrophages with varying characteristics. Unlike B and T lymphocytes, macrophages lack surface receptors for specific antigens; instead, they have receptors for the C region of the H chain (Fc region) of Ig, for fragments of the third component of complement (C3), and for nonimmunologic factors such as carbohydrate molecules.

One of the most important functions of macrophages is the presentation of antigen to T lymphocytes. Macrophages ingest and process antigen, then deposit it on their own surfaces in association with HLA gene. T lymphocytes become activated upon recognizing this complex. Macrophages also function in the inflammatory response by producing IL-1, which generates fever. Additionally, macrophages synthesize complement proteins and other mediators that produce phagocytic, microbicidal, and tumoricidal effects.

CYTOKINES

Cytokines are low–molecular-weight proteins involved in communication between cells. Their purpose is to induce or regulate a variety of immune or inflammatory responses. However, disorders may occur if cytokine production or regulation is impaired. Cytokines are categorized as follows:

◆ *Colony-stimulating factors* function primarily as hematopoietic growth factors, guiding the division and differentiation of bone marrow stem cells. They also influence the functioning of mature lymphocytes, monocytes, macrophages, and neutrophils.

◆ *Interferons* act early to limit the spread of viral infections. They also inhibit tumor growth. Mainly, they determine how well tissue cells interact with cytotoxic cells and lymphocytes.

◆ *Interleukins* are a large group of cytokines. (Those produced primarily by T lymphocytes are called *lymphokines*. Those produced by mononuclear phagocytes are called *monokines*.) They have a variety of effects, but most direct other cells to divide and differentiate.

◆ *Tumor necrosis factor* is believed to play a major role in mediating inflammation and cytotoxic reactions (along with IL-1, IL-6, and IL-8).

◆ *Transforming growth factor* demonstrates both inflammatory and anti-inflammatory effects. It's believed to be partially responsible for tissue fibrosis associated with many diseases. It demonstrates immunosuppressive effects on T cells, B cells, and NK cells.

COMPLEMENT SYSTEM

The chief humoral effector of the inflammatory response, the complement system consists of more than 20 serum proteins that are synthesized primarily in the liver. When activated, these proteins interact in a cascadelike process that has profound biologic effects. Complement activation takes place through one of two pathways. In the classical pathway, binding of IgM or IgG and antigen forms antigen–antibody complexes that activate the first complement component, C1. This, in turn, activates C4, C2, and C3. In the alternative pathway, activating surfaces such as bacterial membranes directly amplify spontaneous cleavage of C3. Once C3 is activated in either pathway, activation of the terminal components—C5 to C9—follows.

The major biologic effects of complement activation include phagocyte attraction (chemotaxis) and activation, histamine release, viral neutralization, promotion of phagocytosis by opsonization, and lysis of cells and bacteria. Other mediators of inflammation derived from the kinin and coagulation pathways interact with the complement system.

POLYMORPHONUCLEAR LEUKOCYTES

Besides macrophages and complement, other key participants in the inflammatory response are the polymorphonuclear leukocytes (also known as *granulocytes*)—neutrophils, eosinophils, and basophils.

Neutrophils, the most numerous of these cells, derive from bone marrow and increase dramatically in number in response to infection and inflammation. Highly mobile cells, neutrophils are attracted to areas of inflammation (chemotaxis); in fact, they're the primary constituent of pus.

Neutrophils have surface receptors for Ig and complement fragments, and they avidly ingest opsonized particles such as bacteria. Ingested organisms are then promptly killed by toxic oxygen metabolites and enzymes such as lysozyme. Unfortunately, neutrophils not only kill invading organisms, but may also damage host tissues.

Also derived from bone marrow, *eosinophils* multiply in both allergic disorders and parasitic infestations. Although their phagocytic function isn't clearly understood, evidence suggests that they participate in host defense against parasites. Their products may also diminish the inflammatory response in allergic disorders.

Two other types of cells that function in allergic disorders are basophils and mast cells. (Mast cells, however, aren't blood cells.) *Basophils* circulate in peripheral blood, whereas *mast cells* accumulate in connective tissue, particularly in the lungs, intestines, and skin. Both types of cells have surface receptors for IgE. When cross-linked by an IgE–antigen complex, they release mediators characteristic of the allergic response.

IMMUNE DISORDERS

Because of their complexity, the processes involved in host defense and immune response may malfunction. When the body's defenses are exaggerated, misdirected, or either absent or depressed, the result may be a hypersensitivity disorder, autoimmunity, or immunodeficiency, respectively. Some forms of immunodeficiency are iatrogenic. (See *Iatrogenic immunodeficiency*.)

Iatrogenic immunodeficiency

Iatrogenic immunodeficiency may be a complicating adverse effect of chemotherapy or other treatments. At times, though, it's the goal of therapy—for example, to suppress immune-mediated tissue damage in autoimmune disorders or to prevent rejection of an organ transplant.

As explained below, iatrogenic immunodeficiency may be induced by immunosuppressive drugs, radiation therapy, or splenectomy.

Immunosuppressive drug therapy
Immunosuppressive drugs fall into several categories:
♦ Cytotoxic drugs. These drugs kill immunocompetent cells while they're replicating. However, most cytotoxic drugs aren't selective and thus interfere with all rapidly proliferating cells. As a result, they reduce the number of lymphocytes as well as phagocytes. Besides depleting their number, cytotoxic drugs interfere with lymphocyte synthesis and release of immunoglobulins (Igs) and lymphokines.

Cyclophosphamide, a potent and commonly used immunosuppressant, initially depletes the number of B cells, suppressing humoral immunity. However, chronic therapy also depletes T cells, suppressing cell-mediated immunity as well. Cyclophosphamide may be used in systemic lupus erythematosus, Wegener granulomatosis, other systemic vasculitides, and in certain autoimmune disorders. Because it nonselectively destroys rapidly dividing cells, this drug can cause severe bone marrow suppression with neutropenia, anemia, and thrombocytopenia; gonadal suppression with sterility; alopecia; hemorrhagic cystitis; and nausea, vomiting, and stomatitis. It may also increase the risk of lymphoproliferative neoplasms.

Among other cytotoxic drugs used for immunosuppression are azathioprine (commonly used in kidney transplantation) and methotrexate (occasionally used in rheumatoid arthritis [RA] and other autoimmune disorders).

If the patient is receiving cytotoxic drugs, monitor the white blood cell (WBC) count. If it falls too low, the drug dosage may need to be adjusted. Also monitor urine output and watch for signs of cystitis, especially if the patient is taking cyclophosphamide. Ensure adequate fluid intake (2 qt [about 2 L] daily). Give mesna as ordered to help prevent hemorrhagic cystitis. Provide antiemetics to relieve nausea and vomiting as ordered. Give meticulous oral hygiene and report signs of stomatitis.

Teach the patient about the early signs and symptoms of infection. If the WBC count falls too low, granulocyte colony-stimulating factor may be used to boost the count. Make sure the male patient understands the risk of sterility; advise sperm banking if appropriate.

Iatrogenic immunodeficiency (*continued*)

Young women may take hormonal contraceptives to minimize ovarian dysfunction and to prevent pregnancy during administration of these potentially teratogenic drugs.

♦ Corticosteroids. These adrenocortical hormones are used to treat immune-mediated disorders because of their potent anti-inflammatory and immunosuppressive effects. Corticosteroids stabilize the vascular membrane, blocking tissue infiltration by neutrophils and monocytes, thus inhibiting inflammation. They also "kidnap" T cells in the bone marrow, causing lymphopenia. Because these drugs aren't cytotoxic, lymphocyte concentration can return to normal within 24 hours after they're withdrawn. Corticosteroids also appear to inhibit Ig synthesis and to interfere with the binding of Ig to antigen or to cells with crystallizable fragment (Fc) receptors. These drugs have many other effects as well.

The most commonly used oral corticosteroid is prednisone. For long-term therapy, prednisone is best given early in the morning to minimize exogenous suppression of cortisol production and with food or milk to minimize gastric irritation. After the acute phase, it's usually reduced to an alternate-day schedule and then gradually withdrawn to minimize potentially harmful adverse effects. Other corticosteroids used for immunosuppression include hydrocortisone, methylprednisolone, and dexamethasone.

Chronic corticosteroid therapy can cause numerous adverse effects, which are sometimes more harmful than the disease itself. Neurologic adverse effects include euphoria, insomnia, or psychosis; cardiovascular effects include hypertension and edema; and GI effects include gastric irritation, ulcers, and increased appetite with weight gain. Other possible effects are cataracts, hyperglycemia, glucose intolerance, muscle weakness, osteoporosis, delayed wound healing, and increased susceptibility to infection.

During corticosteroid therapy, monitor the patient's blood pressure, weight, intake and output, and blood glucose. Instruct the patient to eat a well-balanced, low-salt diet or to follow the specially prescribed diet to prevent excessive weight gain. Remember that even though the patient is more susceptible to infection, the patient shows fewer or less dramatic signs of inflammation.

Cyclosporine. Cyclosporine selectively suppresses the proliferation and development of helper T cells, resulting in depressed cell-mediated immunity. This drug is used primarily to prevent rejection of kidney, liver, and heart transplants but is also being investigated for use in several other disorders. Significant toxic effects of cyclosporine primarily involve the liver and kidney, so treatment with this drug requires regular evaluation of renal and hepatic function. Adjusting the dose or the duration of therapy helps minimize certain adverse effects.

♦ Antilymphocyte serum or antithymocyte globulin (ATG). This anti–T-cell antibody reduces T-cell number and function, thus suppressing cell-mediated immunity. It has been used effectively to prevent cell-mediated rejection of tissue grafts or transplants. Usually, ATG is administered immediately before the transplant and continued for some time afterward. Potential adverse effects include anaphylaxis and serum sickness. Occurring 1 to 2 weeks after injection of ATG, serum sickness is characterized by fever, malaise, rash, arthralgias, and, occasionally, glomerulonephritis or vasculitis. It presumably results from the deposition of immune complexes throughout the body.

Radiation therapy

Because irradiation is cytotoxic to proliferating and intermitotic cells, including most lymphocytes, radiation therapy may induce profound lymphopenia, resulting in immunosuppression. Irradiation of all major lymph node areas—a procedure known as *total nodal irradiation*—is used to treat certain disorders such as Hodgkin lymphoma. Its effectiveness in severe RA, lupus nephritis, and the prevention of kidney transplant rejection is still under investigation.

Splenectomy

Splenectomy may be performed to manage various disorders, including splenic injury or trauma, tumor, Hodgkin lymphoma, hairy cell leukemia, Felty syndrome, Gaucher disease, idiopathic thrombocytopenic purpura, hereditary spherocytosis and hereditary elliptocytosis, thalassemia major, and chronic lymphocytic leukemia.

After splenectomy, the patient has increased susceptibility to infection. These patients should receive the pneumococcal vaccine polyvalent (Pneumovax) for prophylaxis and be warned to avoid exposure to infection and trauma.

HYPERSENSITIVITY DISORDERS

An exaggerated or inappropriate immune response may lead to various hypersensitivity disorders. Such disorders are classified as type I through type IV, although some overlap exists. (See *Classification of hypersensitivity reactions*, pages 386 and 387.)

Type I hypersensitivity (allergic disorders)

In individuals with type I hypersensitivity, certain antigens (allergens) activate T cells. These, in turn, induce B-cell production of IgE, which binds to the Fc receptors on the surface of mast cells. When these cells are re-exposed to the same antigen, the antigen binds with the surface IgE, cross-links the Fc receptors, and causes mast cell degranulation with release of various mediators. (Degranulation may also be triggered by complement-derived anaphylatoxins—C3a and C5a—or by certain drugs such as morphine.)

Some of these mediators are preformed, whereas others are newly synthesized upon activation of mast cells. Preformed mediators include heparin, histamine, proteolytic and other enzymes, and chemotactic factors for eosinophils and neutrophils. Newly synthesized mediators include prostaglandins and leukotrienes. Mast cells also produce a variety of cytokines. The effects of these mediators include smooth-muscle contraction, vasodilation, bronchospasm, edema, increased vascular permeability, mucus secretion, and cellular infiltration by eosinophils and neutrophils. Among classic associated signs and symptoms are hypotension, wheezing, swelling, urticaria, and rhinorrhea.

Examples of type I hypersensitivity disorders are anaphylaxis, atopy (an allergic reaction related to genetic predisposition), hay fever (allergic rhinitis), and, in some cases, asthma.

Type II hypersensitivity (antibody-dependent cytotoxicity)

In type II hypersensitivity, antibody is directed against cell-surface antigens. (Alternatively, though, antibody may be directed against small molecules adsorbed to cells or against cell-surface receptors rather than against cell constituents themselves.) Type II hypersensitivity then causes tissue damage through several mechanisms. Binding of antigen and antibody activates complement, which ultimately disrupts cellular membranes.

Another mechanism is mediated by various phagocytic cells with receptors for Ig (Fc region) and complement fragments. These cells envelop and destroy (phagocytize) opsonized targets, such as red blood cells (RBCs), white blood cells (WBCs), and platelets. Antibody against these cells may be visualized by immunofluorescence. Cytotoxic T lymphocytes and NK cells may contribute to tissue damage in type II hypersensitivity.

Examples of type II hypersensitivity include transfusion reactions, hemolytic disease of the neonate, autoimmune hemolytic anemia, Goodpasture syndrome, and myasthenia gravis.

Classification of hypersensitivity reactions

Type	Cause	Antibody or cell involved	Pathophysiology
I—Immediate hypersensitivity (anaphylaxis, atopy)	Foreign protein (antigen)	Immunoglobulin (Ig) E	IgE attaches to the surface of the mast cell and specific antigen, and triggers release of intracellular granules from mast cells
II—Cytotoxic hypersensitivity	Foreign protein (antigen)	IgG or IgM	IgG or IgM reacts with antigen, activates complement, and causes cytolysis or phagocytosis
III—Immune complex disease	Foreign protein (antigen) Endogenous antigens	IgG, IgM, IgA	Antigen–antibody complexes precipitate in tissue, activate complement, and cause inflammatory reaction
IV—Delayed cell-mediated	Foreign protein, cell, or tissue	T lymphocytes	Sensitized T cells react with specific antigen to induce inflammatory process by direct cell action or by activity of lymphokines

Type III hypersensitivity (immune complex disease)

In type III hypersensitivity, excessive circulating antigen–antibody complexes (immune complexes) result in the deposition of these complexes in tissue—most commonly in the kidneys, joints, skin, and blood vessels. (Normally, immune complexes are effectively cleared by the reticuloendothelial system.) These deposited immune complexes activate the complement cascade, resulting in local inflammation. They also trigger platelet release of vasoactive amines that increase vascular permeability, augmenting deposition of immune complexes in vessel walls.

Type III hypersensitivity may be associated with infections, such as hepatitis B and bacterial endocarditis; certain cancers in which a serum sickness-like syndrome may occur; and autoimmune disorders such as lupus erythematosus. This hypersensitivity reaction may also follow drug or serum therapy.

Type IV hypersensitivity (delayed hypersensitivity)

In type IV hypersensitivity, also known as *cell-mediated hypersensitivity*, antigen is processed by macrophages and presented to T cells. The sensitized T cells then release lymphokines, which recruit and activate other lymphocytes, monocytes, macrophages, and polymorphonuclear leukocytes. The coagulation, kinin, and complement pathways also contribute to tissue damage in this type of reaction.

Clinical examples

Extrinsic asthma, allergic rhinitis, anaphylaxis, reactions to stinging insects, some food and drug reactions

Transfusion reaction, hemolytic drug reaction, Goodpasture syndrome, hemolytic disease of the neonate

Rheumatoid arthritis, systemic lupus erythematosus, serum sickness to some drugs or viral hepatitis antigen, glomerulonephritis

Contact dermatitis, graft-versus-host disease, granulomatous diseases

Examples of type IV hypersensitivity include tuberculin reactions, contact hypersensitivity, and sarcoidosis.

AUTOIMMUNE DISORDERS

Autoimmunity is characterized by a misdirected immune response in which the body's defenses become self-destructive. Autoimmune diseases aren't transmitted from one person to another, and the causes of autoimmunity aren't clearly understood. However, the process of autoimmunity is related to genes or a combination of genes, hormones, and environmental stimuli. Individuals with specific genes or gene combinations may be at a higher risk for developing autoimmune disorders, which may be triggered by outside stimuli, such as sun exposure, infection, drugs, or pregnancy.

Recognition of self through the MHC is of primary importance in an immune response. However, how an immune response against self is prevented and which cells are primarily responsible isn't well understood.

Many autoimmune disorders are characterized by B-cell hyperactivity, marked by proliferation of B cells and autoantibodies and by hypergammaglobulinemia. B-cell hyperactivity is probably related to T-cell abnormalities, but the molecular basis of autoimmunity is poorly understood. Hormonal and genetic factors strongly influence the incidence of autoimmune disorders; for example, lupus erythematosus predominantly affects females of childbearing age, and certain HLA haplotypes are associated with an increased risk of specific autoimmune disorders.

Autoimmune diseases may not follow a clear pattern of symptoms; therefore, a definitive diagnosis may be delayed. Diagnosis may rely on the patient's medical history; family history; physical examination, including signs and symptoms; and laboratory tests. Autoantibodies are usually found with such disorders as rheumatoid arthritis (RA) or systemic lupus erythematosus (SLE), but confusion may occur because individuals with these disorders may have false-negative results on laboratory tests.

Treatment for autoimmune disorders focuses on relieving symptoms, preserving organ function, and providing medication that can target the immune system, such as cyclophosphamide and cyclosporine. Autoimmune and immunologic disorders are being researched. Websites for the National Institutes of Health (*www.nih.gov*) and other organizations offer substantial healthcare information relevant to both the patient and the physician.

IMMUNODEFICIENCY

In immunodeficiency, the immune response is absent or depressed, resulting in increased susceptibility to infection. This disorder may be primary or secondary. Primary immunodeficiency reflects a defect involving T cells, B cells, or lymphoid tissues. The National Primary Immunodeficiency Resource Center is a source of information on primary immunodeficiency syndromes.

Secondary immunodeficiency results from an underlying disease or factor that depresses or blocks the immune response. The most common forms of immunodeficiency are caused by viral infection (as in acquired immunodeficiency syndrome [AIDS]).

Allergy

ASTHMA

Asthma is a lung disease characterized by reversible obstruction or narrowing of the airways.

Causes and incidence

Asthma that results from sensitivity to specific external allergens is known as *extrinsic*. In cases in which the allergen isn't obvious, asthma is referred to as *intrinsic*. Allergens that cause extrinsic asthma include pollen, animal dander, house dust or mold, kapok or feather pillows, food additives containing sulfites, and any other sensitizing substance. Extrinsic (atopic) asthma usually begins in childhood and is accompanied by other manifestations of atopy (type I, IgE-mediated allergy), such as eczema and allergic rhinitis. In intrinsic (nonatopic) asthma, no extrinsic allergen can be identified. Most cases are preceded by a severe respiratory infection. Irritants, emotional stress, fatigue, exposure to noxious fumes as well as changes in endocrine function, temperature, and humidity may aggravate intrinsic asthma attacks. In many asthmatics, intrinsic and extrinsic asthma coexist.

Several drugs and chemicals may provoke an asthma attack without using the IgE pathway. Apparently, they trigger release of mast cell mediators by way of prostaglandin inhibition. Examples of these substances include aspirin, various nonsteroidal anti-inflammatory drugs (NSAIDs such as indomethacin and mefenamic acid), and tartrazine, a yellow food dye. Exercise may also provoke an asthma attack. In exercise-induced asthma, bronchospasm may follow heat and moisture loss in the upper airways.

The allergic response has two phases. When the patient inhales an allergenic substance, sensitized IgE antibodies trigger mast cell degranulation in the lung interstitium, releasing histamine, cytokines, prostaglandins, thromboxanes, leukotrienes, and eosinophil chemotactic factors. Histamine then attaches to receptor sites in the larger bronchi, causing irritation, inflammation, and edema. In the late phase, inflammatory cells flow in. The influx of eosinophils provides additional inflammatory mediators and contributes to local injury.

Although this common condition can strike at any age, half of all cases first occur in children younger than age 10; in this age group, asthma affects twice as many males as females. In the United States, 14 million adults and 6 million children have asthma. Emergency department visits, hospitalizations, and mortality from asthma have been increasing for more than 20 years, especially among children and blacks.

Pathophysiology

Asthma is characterized by reversible obstruction or narrowing of the airways, which are typically inflamed and hyperresponsive to a variety of stimuli. It may resolve spontaneously or with treatment. Its symptoms range from mild wheezing and dyspnea to life-threatening respiratory failure. (See *Determining asthma's severity,* page 389.) Symptoms of bronchial airway obstruction may persist between acute episodes.

Complications
◆ Status asthmaticus
◆ Respiratory failure

Signs and symptoms

An asthma attack may begin dramatically, with simultaneous onset of many severe symptoms, or insidiously, with gradually increasing respiratory distress. It typically includes progressively worsening shortness of breath, cough, wheezing, and chest tightness or some combination of these signs or symptoms.

During an acute attack, the cough sounds tight and dry. As the attack subsides, tenacious mucoid sputum is produced (except in young children, who don't expectorate). Characteristic wheezing may be accompanied by coarse rhonchi, but fine crackles aren't heard unless associated with a related complication. Between acute attacks, breath sounds may be normal.

The intensity of breath sounds in symptomatic asthma is typically reduced. A prolonged phase of forced expiration is typical of airflow obstruction. Evidence of lung hyperinflation

Determining asthma's severity

Asthma is classified by severity using these features:

♦ frequency, severity, and duration of symptoms

♦ degree of airflow obstruction (spirometry measure) or peak expiratory flow (PEF)

♦ frequency of nighttime symptoms and the degree to which the asthma interferes with daily activities

Severity can change over time, and even milder cases can become severe in an uncontrolled attack. Long-term therapy depends on whether the patient's asthma is classified as mild intermittent, mild persistent, moderate persistent, or severe persistent. For all patients, quick relief can be obtained by using a short-acting bronchodilator (2 to 4 puffs of short-acting inhaled beta$_2$-adrenergic agonists as needed for symptoms). However, the use of a short-acting bronchodilator more than twice a week in patients with intermittent asthma or daily or increasing use in patients with persistent asthma may indicate the need to initiate or increase long-term control therapy.

Mild intermittent asthma

The signs and symptoms of mild intermittent asthma include:

♦ daytime symptoms no more than twice a week

♦ nighttime symptoms no more than twice a month

♦ lung function testing (either PEF or forced expiratory volume in 1 second) is 80% of predicted value or higher

♦ PEF varies no more than 20%

Severe exacerbations, separated by long, symptomless periods of normal lung function, indicate mild intermittent asthma. A course of systemic corticosteroids is recommended for these exacerbations; otherwise, daily medication isn't required.

Mild persistent asthma

The signs and symptoms of mild persistent asthma include:

♦ daytime symptoms 3 to 6 days a week

♦ nighttime symptoms three to four times a month

♦ lung function testing 80% of predicted value or higher

♦ PEF between 20% and 30%

The preferred treatment for mild, persistent asthma is low-dose inhaled corticosteroids, but alternative treatments include cromolyn, a leukotriene modifier, nedocromil, or sustained-release theophylline.

Moderate persistent asthma

The signs and symptoms of moderate persistent asthma include:

♦ daily daytime symptoms

♦ at least weekly nighttime symptoms

♦ lung function testing 60% to 80% of predicted value

♦ PEF varying more than 30%

The preferred treatment for moderate persistent asthma is low- or medium-dose inhaled corticosteroids combined with a long-acting inhaled beta$_2$-adrenergic agonist. Alternative treatments include increasing inhaled corticosteroids within the medium-dose range or low- or medium-dose inhaled corticosteroids with either a leukotriene modifier or theophylline.

For recurring exacerbations, the preferred treatment is to increase inhaled corticosteroids within the medium-dose range and add a long-acting inhaled beta$_2$-adrenergic agonist. The alternative treatment is to increase inhaled corticosteroids within the medium-dose range and add either a leukotriene modifier or theophylline.

Severe persistent asthma

The signs and symptoms of severe persistent asthma include:

♦ continual daytime symptoms

♦ frequent nighttime symptoms

♦ lung function testing 60% of predicted value or lower

♦ PEF varying more than 30%

The preferred treatment for severe, persistent asthma includes high-dose inhaled corticosteroids combined with long-acting inhaled beta$_2$-adrenergic agonists. Long-term administration of corticosteroid tablets or syrup (2 mg/kg/day, not to exceed 60 mg/day) may be used to reduce the need for systemic corticosteroid therapy.

PATHOPHYSIOLOGY
How status asthmaticus progresses

A potentially fatal complication, status asthmaticus arises when impaired gas exchange and heightened airway resistance increase the work of breathing. This flow chart shows the stages of status asthmaticus.

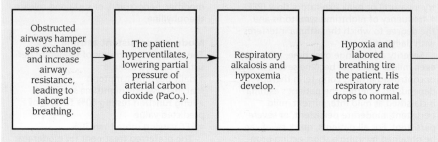

Obstructed airways hamper gas exchange and increase airway resistance, leading to labored breathing. → The patient hyperventilates, lowering partial pressure of arterial carbon dioxide ($PaCO_2$). → Respiratory alkalosis and hypoxemia develop. → Hypoxia and labored breathing tire the patient. His respiratory rate drops to normal.

(use of accessory muscles, for example) is particularly common in children. Acute attacks may be accompanied by tachycardia, tachypnea, and diaphoresis. In severe attacks, the patient may be unable to speak more than a few words without pausing for breath. Cyanosis, confusion, and lethargy indicate the onset of respiratory failure.

Diagnosis

Laboratory studies in patients with asthma commonly show these abnormalities:
◆ Pulmonary function studies reveal signs of airway obstruction (decreased peak expiratory flow rates and forced expiratory volume in 1 second), low-normal or decreased vital capacity, and increased total lung and residual capacity. However, pulmonary function studies may be normal between attacks.
◆ Pulse oximetry may reveal decreased arterial oxygen saturation (SaO_2).
◆ Arterial blood gas (ABG) analysis provides the best indications of an attack's severity. In acutely severe asthma, the partial pressure of arterial oxygen is less than 60 mm Hg, the partial pressure of arterial carbon dioxide ($PaCO_2$) is 40 mm Hg or more, and pH is usually decreased.
◆ Complete blood count (CBC) with differential reveals increased eosinophil count.
◆ Chest X-rays may show hyperinflation with areas of focal atelectasis.

Before initiating tests for asthma, rule out other causes of airway obstruction and wheezing. In children, such causes include cystic fibrosis, tumors of the bronchi or mediastinum, and acute viral bronchitis; in adults, other causes include obstructive pulmonary disease, heart failure, and epiglottitis.

Treatment

Treatment of acute asthma aims to decrease bronchoconstriction, reduce bronchial airway edema, and increase pulmonary ventilation. After an acute episode, treatment focuses on avoiding or removing precipitating factors, such as environmental allergens or irritants.

If asthma is known to be caused by a particular antigen, it may be treated by desensitizing the patient through a series of injections of limited amounts of the antigen. The aim is to curb the patient's immune response to the antigen.

If asthma results from an infection, antibiotics are prescribed. Drug therapy is most effective when begun soon after the onset of signs and symptoms. For relief of symptoms in adults and children older than age 5, short-acting inhaled beta₂-adrenergic agonists for bronchodilation may be used, and a course of systemic corticosteroids may be needed. Other control drugs that may be used are leukotriene inhibitors, theophylline, zileuton, omalizumab, or cromolyn sodium. The goal of therapy is asthma control with minimal or no adverse effects from medication.

Acute attacks that don't respond to self-treatment may require hospital care, beta₂-adrenergic agonists by inhalation or subcutaneous injection (in three doses over 60 to 90 minutes), and, possibly, oxygen for hypoxemia. If the patient responds poorly, systemic corticosteroids and, possibly, subcutaneous epinephrine may help. Beta₂-adrenergic agonist

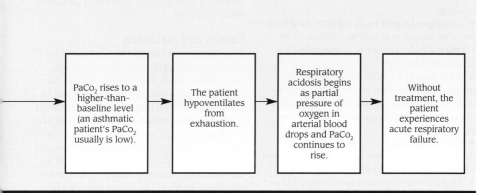

| PaCo$_2$ rises to a higher-than-baseline level (an asthmatic patient's PaCo$_2$ usually is low). | The patient hypoventilates from exhaustion. | Respiratory acidosis begins as partial pressure of oxygen in arterial blood drops and PaCo$_2$ continues to rise. | Without treatment, the patient experiences acute respiratory failure. |

inhalation continues hourly. I.V. theophylline, although rarely used, may be added to the regimen and I.V. fluid therapy is started. Patients who don't respond to this treatment, whose airways remain obstructed, and who have increasing respiratory difficulty are at risk for status asthmaticus and may require mechanical ventilation.

Treatment of status asthmaticus consists of aggressive drug therapy with a beta$_2$-adrenergic agonist by nebulizer every 30 to 60 minutes, possibly supplemented with subcutaneous epinephrine, I.V. corticosteroids, I.V. theophylline, oxygen administration, I.V. fluid therapy, and intubation and mechanical ventilation for hypercapnic respiratory failure (Paco$_2$ of 40 mm Hg or more). (See *How status asthmaticus progresses,* pages 390 and 391.)

Special considerations
During an acute attack, proceed as follows:
♦ First, assess the severity of asthma.
♦ Administer the prescribed treatments and assess the patient's response.
♦ Place the patient in high Fowler's position. Encourage pursed-lip and diaphragmatic breathing. Help the patient to relax.

ALERT *Monitor the patient's vital signs. Keep in mind that developing or increasing tachypnea may indicate worsening asthma or drug toxicity. Blood pressure readings may reveal pulsus paradoxus, indicating severe asthma. Hypertension may indicate asthma-related hypoxemia.*
♦ Administer prescribed humidified oxygen by nasal cannula at 2 L/minute to ease breathing and to increase Sao$_2$. Later, adjust oxygen

according to the patient's vital signs and ABG levels.
♦ Anticipate intubation and mechanical ventilation if the patient fails to maintain adequate oxygenation.
♦ Monitor serum theophylline levels to ensure they're in the therapeutic range. Observe your patient for signs and symptoms of theophylline toxicity (vomiting, diarrhea, and headache), as well as for signs of subtherapeutic dosage (respiratory distress and increased wheezing).
♦ Observe the frequency and severity of your patient's cough, and note whether it's productive. Then auscultate the lungs, noting adventitious or absent breath sounds. If the cough isn't productive and rhonchi are present, teach the patient effective coughing techniques. If the patient can tolerate postural drainage and chest percussion, perform these procedures to clear secretions. Suction an intubated patient as needed.
♦ Treat dehydration with I.V. fluids until the patient can tolerate oral fluids, which will help loosen secretions.
♦ If conservative treatment fails to improve the airway obstruction, anticipate bronchoscopy or bronchial lavage when a lobe or larger area collapses.

During long-term care, proceed as follows:
♦ Monitor the patient's respiratory status to detect baseline changes, to assess response to treatment, and to prevent or detect complications.
♦ Auscultate the lungs frequently, noting the degree of wheezing and quality of air movement.

◆ Review ABG levels, pulmonary function test results, and Sao$_2$ readings.

◆ If the patient is taking systemic corticosteroids, observe for complications, such as elevated blood glucose levels and friable skin and bruising.

◆ Cushingoid effects resulting from long-term use of corticosteroids may be minimized by alternate-day dosage or use of prescribed inhaled corticosteroids.

◆ If the patient is taking corticosteroids by inhaler, watch for signs of candidal infection in the mouth and pharynx. Using an extender device and rinsing the mouth afterward may prevent this.

◆ Observe the patient's anxiety level. Keep in mind that measures that reduce hypoxemia and breathlessness should help relieve anxiety.

◆ Keep the room temperature comfortable and use an air conditioner or a fan in hot, humid weather.

◆ Control exercise-induced asthma by instructing the patient to use a bronchodilator or cromolyn 30 minutes before exercise. Also instruct the patient to use pursed-lip breathing while exercising.

All patients should know the following:
◆ Teach the patient and family to avoid known allergens and irritants.

◆ Describe to the patient prescribed drugs, including their names, dosages, actions, adverse effects, and special instructions.

◆ Teach the patient how to use a metered-dose inhaler. If the patient has difficulty using an inhaler, the patient may need an extender device to optimize drug delivery and lower the risk of candidal infection with orally inhaled corticosteroids.

◆ If the patient has moderate to severe asthma, explain how to use a peak flow meter to measure the degree of airway obstruction. Tell the patient to keep a record of peak flow readings and to bring it to medical appointments. Explain the importance of calling the physician at once if the peak flow drops suddenly (may signal severe respiratory problems).

◆ Tell the patient to notify the physician if developing a fever above 100° F (37.8° C), chest pain, shortness of breath without coughing or exercising, or uncontrollable coughing. An uncontrollable asthma attack requires immediate attention.

◆ Teach the patient diaphragmatic and pursed-lip breathing as well as effective coughing techniques.

◆ Urge the patient to drink at least 3 qt (3 L) of fluids daily to help loosen secretions and maintain hydration.

ALLERGIC RHINITIS

Allergic rhinitis is a reaction to airborne (inhaled) allergens. Depending on the allergen, the resulting rhinitis and conjunctivitis may occur seasonally (hay fever) or year-round (perennial allergic rhinitis).

Causes and incidence

In most cases, it's induced by windborne pollens: in the spring by tree pollens (oak, elm, maple, alder, birch, and cottonwood), in the summer by grass pollens (sheep sorrel and English plantain), and in the fall by weed pollens (ragweed). Occasionally, hay fever is induced by allergy to fungal spores. In addition to individual sensitivity and geographic differences in plant population, the amount of pollen in the air can be a factor in determining whether symptoms develop. Hot, dry, windy days have more pollen than cool, damp, rainy days.

The major perennial allergens and irritants include dust mites, feather pillows, mold, cigarette smoke, upholstery, and animal dander. Seasonal pollen allergy may exacerbate signs and symptoms of perennial rhinitis.

Allergic rhinitis is the most common atopic allergic reaction, affecting more than 20 million Americans. It's most prevalent in young children and adolescents but can occur in all age groups.

Pathophysiology

Hay fever reflects an IgE-mediated type I hypersensitivity response to an environmental antigen (allergen) in a genetically susceptible individual.

In perennial allergic rhinitis, inhaled allergens provoke antigen responses that produce recurring symptoms year-round. The allergens trigger antibody production and histamine release, producing itching, swelling, and mucus.

Complications

◆ Secondary sinus and middle ear infections
◆ Nasal polyps
◆ Nasal obstruction

Signs and symptoms

In seasonal allergic rhinitis, the key signs and symptoms are paroxysmal sneezing, profuse watery rhinorrhea, nasal obstruction or congestion, and pruritus of the nose and eyes. It's usually accompanied by pale, cyanotic, edematous nasal mucosa; red and edematous eyelids and conjunctivae; excessive lacrimation; and headache or sinus pain. Some patients also complain of itching in the throat and malaise.

In perennial allergic rhinitis, conjunctivitis and other extranasal effects are rare, but chronic nasal obstruction is common. In many cases, this obstruction extends to eustachian tube obstruction, particularly in children.

In both types of allergic rhinitis, dark circles may appear under the patient's eyes ("allergic shiners") because of venous congestion in the maxillary sinuses. The severity of signs and symptoms may vary from season to season and from year to year.

Diagnosis

Microscopic examination of sputum and nasal secretions reveals large numbers of eosinophils. Blood chemistry shows normal or elevated IgE. A definitive diagnosis is based on the patient's personal and family history of allergies as well as physical findings during a symptomatic phase. Skin testing paired with tested responses to environmental stimuli can pinpoint the responsible allergens given the patient's history. In patients who can't tolerate skin testing, the radioallergosorbent test may be helpful in determining specific allergen sensitivity.

To distinguish between allergic rhinitis and other nasal mucosa disorders, remember these differences:

◆ In chronic vasomotor rhinitis, eye symptoms are absent, rhinorrhea is mucoid, and seasonal variation is absent.

◆ In infectious rhinitis (the common cold), the nasal mucosa is beet red; nasal secretions contain polymorphonuclear, not eosinophilic, exudate; and signs and symptoms include fever and sore throat. This condition isn't a recurrent seasonal phenomenon.

◆ In rhinitis medicamentosa, which results from excessive use of nasal sprays or drops, nasal drainage and mucosal redness and swelling disappear when such medication is withheld.

PEDIATRIC TIP *In children, differential diagnosis involves ruling out a nasal foreign body, such as a bean or a button.*

Treatment

Treatment aims to control symptoms by eliminating the environmental antigen, if possible, and providing drug therapy and immunotherapy.

Antihistamines block histamine effects but commonly produce anticholinergic adverse effects (sedation, dry mouth, nausea, dizziness, blurred vision, and nervousness). Antihistamines, such as cetirizine, loratadine, and fexofenadine, produce fewer adverse effects and are less likely to cause sedation.

Inhaled intranasal steroids produce local anti-inflammatory effects with minimal systemic adverse effects. The most commonly used intranasal steroids are beclomethasone, flunisolide, fluticasone, mometasone, and triamcinolone. These drugs are effective when symptoms aren't relieved by antihistamines alone.

Advise the patient to use intranasal steroids regularly as prescribed for optimal effectiveness. Oral or parenteral steroids may be used for 6 to 8 weeks when conventional therapy isn't working. Cromolyn may be helpful in treating hay fever, but this drug may take up to 4 weeks to produce a satisfactory effect and must be taken regularly during allergy season. Eye drop versions of cromolyn and antihistamines are available for itchy, bloodshot eyes.

Long-term management includes immunotherapy, or desensitization with injections of extracted allergens, administered before or during allergy season or perennially. Seasonal allergies require particularly close dosage regulation.

Special considerations

◆ Before desensitization injections, assess the patient's symptom status. Afterward, watch for adverse reactions, including anaphylaxis and severe localized erythema.

ALERT *Keep epinephrine and emergency resuscitation equipment available, and observe the patient for 30 minutes after the injection. Instruct the patient to call the physician if a delayed reaction should occur.*

The following protocol is recommended for allergic rhinitis:

◆ Monitor the patient's compliance with prescribed drug treatment regimens. Also, carefully note any changes in the control of symptoms or any signs of drug misuse.

◆ To reduce environmental exposure to airborne allergens, suggest that the patient sleep with the windows closed, avoid the countryside during pollination seasons, use air-conditioning to filter allergens and minimize moisture and dust, and eliminate dust-collecting items, such as wool blankets, deep-pile carpets, and heavy drapes, from the home.

◆ In severe and resistant cases, suggest that the patient consider drastic changes in lifestyle such as relocation to a pollen-free area either seasonally or year-round.

◆ Be aware that some patients may develop chronic complications, including sinusitis and nasal polyps.

ATOPIC DERMATITIS

Atopic dermatitis is a chronic type I immediate hypersensitivity skin disorder that's characterized by superficial skin inflammation and intense itching. Although this disorder may appear at any age, it typically begins during infancy or early childhood. It may then subside spontaneously, followed by exacerbations in late childhood, adolescence, or early adulthood. Atopic dermatitis affects 2.5% of the population.

Causes and incidence

The cause of atopic dermatitis is still unknown.

Exacerbating factors of atopic dermatitis include irritants, infections (commonly caused by *Staphylococcus aureus*), and some allergens. Although no reliable link exists between atopic dermatitis and exposure to inhalant allergens (such as house dust and animal dander), exposure to food allergens (such as soybeans, fish, or nuts) may coincide with flare-ups of atopic dermatitis.

Pathophysiology

Several theories attempt to explain its pathogenesis. One theory suggests an underlying metabolically or biochemically induced skin disorder that's genetically linked to elevated serum IgE levels. Another theory suggests defective T-cell function.

Complications

◆ Scarring
◆ Secondary infection

Signs and symptoms

Scratching the skin causes vasoconstriction and intensifies pruritus, resulting in erythematous, weeping lesions. Eventually, the lesions become scaly and lichenified. Usually, they're located in areas of flexion and extension, such as the neck, antecubital fossa, popliteal folds, and behind the ears. Patients with atopic dermatitis are prone to unusually severe viral infections, bacterial and fungal skin infections, ocular complications, and allergic contact dermatitis.

Diagnosis

Typically, the patient has a history of atopy, such as asthma, hay fever, or urticaria; the family may have a similar history. Laboratory tests reveal eosinophilia and elevated serum IgE levels. A skin biopsy may be performed, but it isn't always required to make the diagnosis.

Treatment

Measures to ease this chronic disorder include meticulous skin care, environmental control of offending allergens, and drug therapy. Because dry skin aggravates itching, frequent application of nonirritating topical lubricants is important, especially after bathing or showering. Minimizing exposure to allergens and irritants, such as wools and harsh detergents, also helps control symptoms.

Drug therapy involves corticosteroids and antipruritics. Atopic dermatitis responds well to topical corticosteroids, which should be applied immediately after bathing for optimal penetration. Oral antihistamines are commonly used to help control itching. A bedtime dose may reduce involuntary scratching during sleep. If secondary infection develops, antibiotics are necessary. Topical immunomodulatory agents are a steroid-free treatment for itching and rash and have demonstrated an 80% success rate in studies.

Special considerations

◆ Monitor the patient's compliance with drug therapy.
◆ Teach the patient when and how to apply topical corticosteroids.
◆ Emphasize the importance of regular personal hygiene using only water with little soap.
◆ Be alert for signs and symptoms of secondary infection; teach the patient how to recognize them as well.
◆ If the patient's diet is modified to exclude food allergens, monitor nutritional status.
◆ Offer support to help the patient and family cope with this chronic disorder.
◆ Discourage use of laundry additives.
◆ Dissuade the patient from scratching during urticaria to help prevent an infection.

LATEX ALLERGY

Latex is a substance found in an increasing number of products both on the job and in the home environment. Latex allergy is a hypersensitivity reaction to products that contain natural latex, which is derived from the sap of a rubber tree, not synthetic latex.

Causes and incidence

About 1% of the population has a latex allergy. Anyone who is in frequent contact with latex-containing products is at risk for developing a latex allergy. (See *Products that contain latex*, page 395.) The more frequent the exposure, the higher the risk. The populations at highest risk are medical and dental professionals, workers in latex companies, and patients with spina bifida.

Pathophysiology

There are two types of latex allergy. A type I hypersensitivity reaction involves mast cells releasing histamine and other secretory products. This leads to vasodilation and bronchoconstriction. A type IV delayed hypersensitivity reaction occurs as a reaction to chemicals involved in processing rather than to the latex itself. Sensitized T lymphocytes are triggered, which cause other lymphocytes and mononuclear cells to proliferate, resulting in tissue inflammation.

Other individuals at risk include:

◆ patients with a history of asthma or other allergies, especially to bananas, avocados, tropical fruits, or chestnuts

◆ patients with a history of multiple intra-abdominal or GU surgeries

◆ patients who require frequent intermittent urinary catheterization

Complications

◆ Respiratory obstruction
◆ Systemic vascular collapse

Signs and symptoms

Type I symptoms can include rhinitis, conjunctivitis, asthma, and anaphylaxis. Type IV symptoms may include contact dermatitis with vesicular skin lesions, pruritus, edema, and erythema. Although type IV hypersensitivity is not life-threatening, those who are sensitized to latex are at increased risk for development of type I reactions.

Diagnosis

A patient who describes even the mildest symptoms during a history and physical assessment should be suspected of having a latex allergy. The patient may describe dermatitis or mild respiratory distress when using latex gloves, inflating a balloon, or coming in contact with other latex products.

℞ CONFIRMING DIAGNOSIS *A blood test for latex sensitivity can confirm the diagnosis. This test, which measures specific IgE antibodies against latex, should be used only when latex allergy is suspected; it isn't recommended as a screening tool.*

Treatment

The best treatment of latex allergy is prevention; the more a latex-sensitive person is exposed to latex, the worse the symptoms will become. To avoid exposure, advise the patient to substitute products made of silicone and vinyl for those made of latex.

When a latex allergy is suspected or known, the patient may receive medications before and after surgery or other invasive procedures. Pre- and post-procedure medications may include corticosteroids, antihistamines, and H_2-receptor antagonists.

Products that contain latex

Many medical and everyday items contain latex, which can be a threat to the patient with latex allergy. The most common items that contain latex are listed below.

Medical products
◆ Adhesive bandages
◆ Airways, nasogastric tubes
◆ Blood pressure cuff, tubing, and bladder
◆ Catheters
◆ Catheter leg straps
◆ Dental devices
◆ Elastic bandages
◆ Electrode pads
◆ Fluid-circulating hypothermia blankets
◆ Handheld resuscitation bag
◆ Hemodialysis equipment
◆ I.V. catheters
◆ Latex or rubber gloves
◆ Medication vials
◆ Pads for crutches
◆ Protective sheets
◆ Reservoir breathing bags
◆ Rubber airway and endotracheal tubes
◆ Stethoscopes
◆ Tape
◆ Tourniquets

Nonmedical products
◆ Adhesive tape
◆ Balloons (excluding Mylar)
◆ Cervical diaphragms
◆ Condoms
◆ Dishwashing gloves
◆ Disposable diapers
◆ Elastic stockings
◆ Glue
◆ Latex paint
◆ Nipples and pacifiers
◆ Racquet handles
◆ Rubber bands
◆ Tires

There's no known treatment for an allergic reaction to latex. Care is supportive in nature. The patient's airway, breathing, and circulation must be monitored. An artificial airway, oxygen therapy, cardiopulmonary resuscitation, and fluid management may be necessary. During an acute reaction, epinephrine, diphenhydramine, and hydrocortisone are commonly administered by I.V. infusion.

Special considerations

◆ Urge the patient to wear an identification tag mentioning latex allergy.

♦ Teach the patient and family members how to use an epinephrine autoinjector.

♦ Teach the patient to be aware of all latex-containing products and to use vinyl or silicone products instead. Advise the patient that Mylar balloons don't contain latex.

▓▓▓▓ PREVENTION

♦ *Make sure that items that aren't available in a latex-free form, such as stethoscopes and blood pressure cuffs, are wrapped in cloth before they come in contact with a hypersensitive patient's skin.*

♦ *Place the patient in a private room or with another patient who requires a latex-free environment.*

♦ *When adding medication to an I.V. bag, inject the drug through the spike port, not the rubber latex port.*

ANAPHYLAXIS

Anaphylaxis is a dramatic, acute atopic reaction marked by the sudden onset of rapidly progressive urticaria and respiratory distress. A severe reaction may precipitate vascular collapse, leading to systemic shock, and, sometimes, death.

Causes and incidence

The source of anaphylactic reactions is ingestion of, or other systemic exposure to, sensitizing drugs or other substances. Such substances may include animal serums, vaccines, allergen extracts, enzymes (L-asparaginase), hormones, penicillin and other antibiotics, sulfonamides, local anesthetics, salicylates, polysaccharides, diagnostic chemicals (sulfobromophthalein, sodium dehydrocholate, and radiographic contrast media), foods (especially legumes, nuts, berries, seafood, and egg albumin) and sulfite-containing food additives, insect venom (honeybees, wasps, hornets, yellow jackets, fire ants, mosquitoes, and certain spiders), and, rarely, ruptured hydatid cyst.

A common cause of anaphylaxis is penicillin, which induces anaphylaxis in 1 to 4 of every 10,000 patients treated with it. Penicillin is most likely to induce anaphylaxis after parenteral administration or prolonged therapy and in atopic patients with an allergy to other drugs or foods. (See *Preventing allergic response to penicillin.*)

At the same time, two other chemical mediators, bradykinin and leukotrienes, induce vascular collapse by stimulating contraction of certain groups of smooth muscles and by increasing vascular permeability. In turn, increased vascular permeability leads to decreased peripheral resistance and plasma leakage from the circulation to extravascular tissues, which lowers blood volume, causing hypotension, hypovolemic shock, and cardiac dysfunction. (See *Understanding anaphylaxis*, page 397.)

Pathophysiology

An anaphylactic reaction requires previous sensitization or exposure to the specific antigen, resulting in the production of specific IgE antibodies by plasma cells. This antibody production takes place in the lymph nodes and is enhanced by helper T cells. IgE antibodies then bind to membrane receptors on mast cells (found throughout connective tissue) and basophils.

On re-exposure, the antigen binds to adjacent IgE antibodies or cross-linked IgE receptors, activating a series of cellular reactions that trigger degranulation—the release of powerful chemical mediators (such as histamine and eosinophil chemotactic factor of anaphylaxis) from mast cell stores. IgG or IgM enters into the reaction and activates the release of complement fractions.

PREVENTION
Preventing allergic response to penicillin

When administering penicillin or its derivatives, such as ampicillin or carbenicillin, follow these recommendations from the World Health Organization to prevent an allergic response:

♦ Have an emergency kit available to treat allergic reactions.

♦ Take a detailed patient history, including penicillin allergy and other allergies. In an infant younger than 3 months, check for penicillin allergy in the mother.

♦ Never give penicillin to a patient who has had an allergic reaction to it.

♦ Before giving penicillin to a patient with suspected penicillin allergy, refer the patient for skin and immunologic tests to confirm it.

♦ Always tell a patient he's going to receive penicillin before taking the first dose.

♦ Observe the patient carefully for adverse effects for at least half an hour after penicillin administration.

♦ Be aware that penicillin derivatives also may elicit an allergic reaction.

PATHOPHYSIOLOGY
Understanding anaphylaxis

The illustrations below teach the development of anaphylaxis.

Response to antigen
Immunoglobulins (Ig) M and G recognize and bind the antigen.

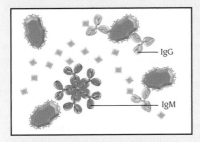

Release of chemical mediators
Activated IgE on basophils promotes the release of mediators: histamine, serotonin, and leukotrienes.

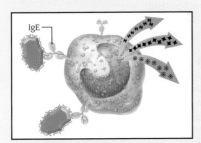

Intensified response
Mast cells release more histamine and eosinophil chemotactic factor of anaphylaxis.

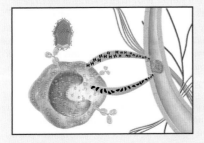

Respiratory distress
In the lungs, histamine causes endothelial cell destruction and allows fluid to leak into alveoli.

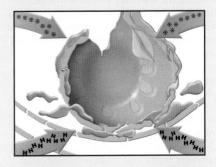

Deterioration
Meanwhile, mediators increase vascular permeability, causing fluid to leak from the vessels.

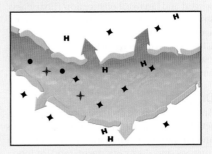

Failure of compensatory mechanisms
Endothelial cell damage causes basophils and mast cells to release heparin and mediator-neutralizing substances. However, anaphylaxis is now irreversible.

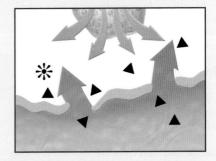

KEY	
Complement cascade ▨	Prostaglandins ✦
Histamine **H**	ECF-A ◗
Serotonin ✦	Bradykinin ●
Leukotrienes ✳	Heparin ▲

Complications

- ◆ Respiratory obstruction
- ◆ Systemic vascular collapse
- ◆ Death

Signs and symptoms

An anaphylactic reaction produces sudden physical distress within seconds or minutes (although a delayed or persistent reaction may occur for up to 24 hours) after exposure to an allergen. The reaction's severity is inversely related to the interval between exposure to the allergen and the onset of symptoms. Usually, the first symptoms include a feeling of impending doom or fright, weakness, sweating, sneezing, shortness of breath, nasal pruritus, urticaria, and angioedema, followed rapidly by symptoms in one or more target organs.

Cardiovascular symptoms include hypotension, shock, and, sometimes, cardiac arrhythmias. If untreated, arrhythmia may precipitate circulatory collapse. Respiratory symptoms can occur at any level in the respiratory tract and commonly include nasal mucosal edema, profuse watery rhinorrhea, itching, nasal congestion, and sudden sneezing attacks. Edema of the upper respiratory tract results in hypopharyngeal and laryngeal obstruction (hoarseness, stridor, and dyspnea). This is an early sign of acute respiratory failure, which can be fatal. GI and GU symptoms include severe stomach cramps, nausea, diarrhea, and urinary urgency and incontinence.

Diagnosis

Anaphylaxis can be diagnosed by the rapid onset of severe respiratory or cardiovascular signs and symptoms after ingestion or injection of a drug, vaccine, diagnostic agent, food, or food additive or after an insect sting. If these symptoms occur without a known allergic stimulus, rule out other possible causes of shock (acute myocardial infarction, status asthmaticus, or heart failure).

Tests that help determine a patient's risk of anaphylaxis include skin tests that may show hypersensitivity to a specific allergen and an elevated serum IgE level.

Treatment

Anaphylaxis is always an emergency. It requires an *immediate* injection of epinephrine 1:1,000 aqueous solution, 0.1 to 0.5 mL, repeated every 5 to 20 minutes as needed.

In the early stages of anaphylaxis, when the patient hasn't lost consciousness and is normotensive, give epinephrine I.M. or subcutaneously and help it move into circulation faster by massaging the injection site. In severe reactions, when the patient has lost consciousness and is hypotensive, give epinephrine I.V.

⚠️ **ALERT** *Maintain airway patency. Observe the patient for early signs of laryngeal edema (hoarseness, stridor, and dyspnea), which will probably require endotracheal tube insertion or a tracheotomy and oxygen therapy.*

In case of cardiac arrest, begin cardiopulmonary resuscitation, including closed-chest heart massage, assisted ventilation, and other therapies as indicated by clinical response.

Watch for hypotension and shock, and maintain circulatory volume with volume expanders (plasma, plasma expanders, saline, and albumin) as needed. Stabilize blood pressure with the I.V. vasopressors norepinephrine and dopamine. Monitor blood pressure, central venous pressure, and urine output as a response index.

After the initial emergency, administer other medications as ordered: subcutaneous epinephrine, longer-acting epinephrine, corticosteroids, and I.V. diphenhydramine for long-term management and an inhaled beta-agonist for bronchospasm.

Special considerations

▒▒▒▒ **PREVENTION**

- ◆ *Teach the patient to avoid exposure to known allergens. A person allergic to certain foods or drugs must learn to avoid the offending food or drug in all its forms. A person allergic to insect stings should avoid open fields and wooded areas during the insect season. An anaphylaxis kit (epinephrine, antihistamine, and tourniquet) should also be carried whenever the patient with known severe allergic reactions goes outdoors. In addition, every patient prone to anaphylaxis should wear a medical identification bracelet identifying allergies.*
- ◆ *If a patient must receive a drug to which he or she's allergic, prevent a severe reaction by making sure the patient receives careful desensitization with gradually increasing doses of the antigen or advance administration of steroids. Of course, a person with a known allergic history should receive a drug with a high anaphylactic potential only after cautious pretesting for sensitivity. Closely monitor the patient during testing, and make sure you have resuscitative equipment and epinephrine ready. When any patient needs a drug with a high anaphylactic potential (particularly parenteral drugs), make sure they received each dose under close medical observation.*
- ◆ *Closely monitor a patient undergoing diagnostic tests that use radiographic contrast media, such as excretory urography, cardiac catheterization, and angiography.*

URTICARIA AND ANGIOEDEMA

Urticaria, commonly known as *hives*, is an episodic, usually self-limited skin reaction characterized by local dermal wheals surrounded by an erythematous flare. Angioedema is a subcutaneous and dermal eruption that produces deeper, larger wheals (usually on the hands, feet, lips, genitals, and eyelids) and a more diffuse swelling of loose subcutaneous tissue. Urticaria and angioedema can occur simultaneously, but angioedema may last longer.

Causes and incidence

Urticaria and angioedema are common allergic reactions that may occur in 20% of the general population. The causes of these reactions include allergy to drugs, foods, insect bites and stings, and, occasionally, inhalant allergens (animal dander and cosmetics) that provoke an IgE-mediated response to protein allergens. However, certain drugs may cause urticaria without an IgE response. When urticaria and angioedema are part of an anaphylactic reaction, they almost always persist long after the systemic response has subsided. This occurs because circulation to the skin is the last to be restored after an allergic reaction, which results in slow histamine reabsorption at the reaction site.

Nonallergic urticaria and angioedema are also related to histamine release. External physical stimuli, such as cold (usually in young adults), heat, water, or sunlight, may also provoke urticaria and angioedema. *Dermographism urticaria*, which develops after stroking or scratching of the skin, occurs in as much as 20% of the population. Such urticaria develops with varying pressure, usually under tight clothing, and is aggravated by scratching.

Pathophysiology

Several different mechanisms and underlying disorders may provoke urticaria and angioedema. These include IgE-induced release of mediators from cutaneous mast cells; binding of IgG or IgM to antigen, resulting in complement activation; and such disorders as localized or secondary infections (such as respiratory infection), neoplastic diseases (such as Hodgkin lymphoma), connective tissue diseases (such as SLE), collagen vascular diseases, and psychogenic diseases.

Complications

◆ Infection from scratching
◆ Laryngeal edema (upper respiratory tract involvement)
◆ Severe abdominal colic (GI involvement)

Signs and symptoms

The characteristic features of urticaria are distinct, raised, evanescent (temporary) dermal wheals surrounded by an erythematous flare. These lesions may vary in size. In cholinergic urticaria, the wheals may be tiny and blanched, surrounded by erythematous flares.

Angioedema characteristically produces nonpitted swelling of deep subcutaneous tissue, usually on the eyelids, lips, genitalia, and mucous membranes. These swellings don't usually itch but may burn and tingle.

Diagnosis

An accurate patient history can help determine the cause of urticaria. Such a history should include:
◆ drug history, including over-the-counter preparations (vitamins, aspirin, and antacids)
◆ frequently ingested foods (strawberries, milk products, fish)
◆ environmental influences (pets, carpet, clothing, soap, inhalants, cosmetics, hair dye, and insect bites and stings)

Diagnosis also requires physical assessment to rule out similar conditions as well as a CBC, urinalysis, erythrocyte sedimentation rate (ESR), and a chest X-ray to rule out inflammatory infections. Skin testing, an elimination diet, and a food diary (recording time and amount of food eaten and circumstances) can pinpoint provoking allergens. The food diary may also suggest other allergies. For instance, a patient allergic to fish may also be allergic to iodine contrast materials.

Recurrent angioedema without urticaria, along with a familial history, points to hereditary angioedema. (See *Hereditary angioedema*, page 400.) Decreased serum levels of complement 4 and complement 1 esterase inhibitors confirm this diagnosis.

Treatment

Treatment aims to prevent or limit contact with triggering factors or, if this is impossible, to desensitize the patient to them and to relieve symptoms. During desensitization, progressively larger doses of specific antigens (determined by skin testing) are injected intradermally. After the triggering stimulus has been removed, urticaria usually subsides in a few days—except for drug reactions, which may persist as long as the drug is in the bloodstream.

Diphenhydramine, hydroxyzine, or another antihistamine can ease itching and swelling in every kind of urticaria. Corticosteroid therapy may be necessary for some patients.

Hereditary angioedema

A nonallergenic type of angioedema, hereditary angioedema results from an autosomal dominant trait—a hereditary deficiency of an alpha globulin, the normal inhibitor of C1 esterase (a component of the complement system). This deficiency allows uninhibited C1 esterase release, resulting in the vascular changes common to angioedema.

The clinical effects of hereditary angioedema usually appear in childhood with recurrent episodes of subcutaneous or submucosal edema at irregular intervals of weeks, months, or years, in many cases after trauma or stress. Hereditary angioedema is unifocal, without urticarial pruritus, but associated with recurrent edema of the skin and mucosa (especially of the GI and respiratory tracts). GI tract involvement may cause nausea, vomiting, and severe abdominal pain. Laryngeal angioedema may cause fatal airway obstruction.

Treatment of acute hereditary angioedema may require androgens such as danazol. Tracheotomy may be necessary to relieve airway obstruction resulting from laryngeal angioedema.

Special considerations

◆ Inform the patient receiving antihistamines of the possibility of drowsiness.
◆ Suggest cool compresses to reduce swelling and pain. A cool bath may be used for large areas. Calamine lotion may be soothing as well.
◆ Avoid hot baths, which can cause hives to return.
◆ Advise the patient to avoid tight-fitting clothing.

BLOOD TRANSFUSION REACTION

Mediated by immune or nonimmune factors, a transfusion reaction accompanies or follows I.V. administration of blood components. Its severity varies from mild (fever and chills) to severe (acute renal failure or complete vascular collapse and death), depending on the amount of blood transfused, the type of reaction, and the patient's general health.

Causes and incidence

◆ Mismatched blood
◆ Rh-incompatible blood
◆ Allergic reactions
◆ Febrile nonhemolytic reactions
◆ Transfusion-related acute lung injury (TRALI)
◆ Bacterial contamination

Pathophysiology

Acute hemolytic reactions follow transfusion of mismatched blood. Transfusion of serologically incompatible blood triggers the most serious reaction, marked by intravascular agglutination of RBCs. The recipient's antibodies (IgG or IgM) attach to the donated RBCs, leading to widespread clumping and destruction of the recipient's RBCs and, possibly, the development of disseminated intravascular coagulation (DIC) and other serious effects.

Transfusion of Rh-incompatible blood triggers a less serious reaction within several days to 2 weeks. Rh reactions are most common in females sensitized to RBC antigens by prior pregnancy or by unknown factors (such as bacterial or viral infection) and in people who have received more than five transfusions. (See *Understanding the Rh system.*)

Allergic reactions are fairly common but only occasionally serious. In this type of reaction, transfused soluble antigens react with surface IgE molecules on mast cells and basophils,

Understanding the Rh system

The Rh system contains more than 30 antibodies and antigens. Eighty-five percent of the world's population is Rh-positive, which means that the red blood cells of most people carry the D or Rh antigen. The remaining 15% of the population, who are Rh-negative, don't carry this antigen.

When Rh-negative people receive Rh-positive blood for the first time, they become sensitized to the D antigen but show no immediate reaction to it. If they receive Rh-positive blood a second time, they then develop a massive hemolytic reaction. For example, an Rh-negative mother who delivers an Rh-positive baby is sensitized by the baby's Rh-positive blood. During the next Rh-positive pregnancy, sensitized blood would cause a hemolytic reaction in fetal circulation. Thus, the Rh-negative mother should receive Rh₀(D) immune globulin (human) I.M. within 72 hours after delivering an Rh-positive baby to prevent the formation of antibodies against Rh-positive blood.

causing degranulation and release of allergic mediators. Antibodies against IgA in an IgA-deficient recipient can also trigger a severe allergic reaction (anaphylaxis).

Febrile nonhemolytic reactions, the most common type of reaction, apparently develop when cytotoxic or agglutinating antibodies in the recipient's plasma attack antigens on transfused lymphocytes, granulocytes, or plasma cells.

TRALI occurs when acutely increased permeability of the pulmonary microcirculation causes massive leakage of fluids and protein into the alveolar spaces and interstitium, usually within 6 hours of transfusion. In many cases, it is associated with the presence of granulocyte antibodies in the donor or recipient, causing complement and histamine release.

Although uncommon, *bacterial contamination* of donor blood can occur during donor phlebotomy. Offending organisms are usually gram-negative, especially *Pseudomonas* species, *Citrobacter freundii*, and *Escherichia coli*.

Contamination of donor blood with viruses, such as hepatitis, cytomegalovirus, and malaria, is also possible.

Complications

- Bronchospasm
- Respiratory failure
- Acute tubular necrosis
- Acute renal failure
- Anaphylactic shock
- Vascular collapse
- DIC

Signs and symptoms

Immediate effects of a hemolytic transfusion reaction develop within a few minutes or hours after the start of the transfusion and may include chills, fever, urticaria, tachycardia, dyspnea, nausea, vomiting, tightness in the chest, chest and back pain, hypotension, bronchospasm, angioedema, and signs and symptoms of anaphylaxis, shock, pulmonary edema, heart failure, and renal failure. In a surgical patient under anesthesia, these symptoms are masked, but blood oozes from mucous membranes or the incision site.

Delayed hemolytic reactions can occur up to several weeks after a transfusion, causing fever, an unexpected fall in serum hemoglobin (Hb) level, and jaundice.

Allergic reactions are typically afebrile and characterized by urticaria and angioedema, possibly progressing to cough, respiratory distress, nausea, vomiting, diarrhea, abdominal cramps, vascular instability, shock, and coma.

The hallmark of febrile nonhemolytic reactions is mild to severe fever that may begin at the start of transfusion or within 2 hours after its completion.

Symptoms of TRALI include severe respiratory distress within 6 hours of transfusion, fever, chills, cyanosis, and hypotension.

Bacterial contamination produces a high fever, nausea, vomiting, diarrhea, abdominal cramps, and, possibly, shock. Symptoms of viral contamination may not appear for several weeks after transfusion.

Diagnosis

℞ **CONFIRMING DIAGNOSIS** *Confirming a hemolytic transfusion reaction requires proof of blood incompatibility and evidence of hemolysis, such as hemoglobinuria, anti-A or anti-B antibodies in the serum, low serum Hb levels, and elevated bilirubin levels.*

If you suspect such a reaction, have the patient's blood retyped and crossmatched with the donor's blood. After a hemolytic transfusion reaction, laboratory tests will show increased indirect bilirubin levels, decreased haptoglobin levels, increased serum Hb levels, and Hb in the urine. As the reaction progresses, tests may show signs of DIC (thrombocytopenia, increased prothrombin time, and decreased fibrinogen level) and acute tubular necrosis (increased blood urea nitrogen [BUN] and serum creatinine levels).

A blood culture to isolate the causative organism should be done when bacterial contamination is suspected.

Treatment

At the first sign of a hemolytic reaction, *stop the transfusion immediately*. Depending on the nature of the patient's reaction, prepare to:

- monitor vital signs every 15 to 30 minutes, watching for signs of shock.
- maintain a patent I.V. line with normal saline solution; insert an indwelling catheter and monitor intake and output.
- cover the patient with blankets to ease chills, and explain what's happening.
- deliver supplemental oxygen at low flow rates through a nasal cannula or bag-valve-mask (handheld resuscitation bag).
- give drugs as ordered: an I.V. antihypotensive drug (like dopamine) and normal saline solution to combat shock, epinephrine to treat dyspnea and wheezing, diphenhydramine to combat cellular histamine released from mast cells, corticosteroids to reduce inflammation, and mannitol or furosemide to increase renal blood flow ensure 30 to 100 mL/hour of urine

output. Administer parenteral antihistamines and corticosteroids for allergic reactions. (Severe reactions such as anaphylaxis may require epinephrine.) Administer antipyretics for non-hemolytic febrile reactions and appropriate I.V. antibiotics for bacterial contamination.

♦ Treatment for TRALI usually requires aggressive respiratory support, which may include intubation and mechanical ventilation. Diuretics are not effective because the underlying pathology involves microvascular injury rather than fluid overload.

Special considerations

♦ Remember to fully document the transfusion reaction on the patient's chart, noting the transfusion's duration, the amount of blood absorbed, and a complete description of the reaction and of any interventions.

▓▓▓▓ **PREVENTION** *Make sure you know your hos-*
pital's policy about giving blood before you
give a transfusion. Then make sure you have the
right blood and the right patient. Check and
double-check the patient's name, hospital number,
ABO blood group, and Rh status. If you find even a
small discrepancy, don't give the blood. Notify the
blood bank immediately and return the unopened
unit.

Autoimmunity

RHEUMATOID ARTHRITIS

A chronic, systemic, inflammatory disease, RA primarily attacks peripheral joints and surrounding muscles, tendons, ligaments, and blood vessels. Spontaneous remissions and unpredictable exacerbations mark the course of this potentially crippling disease. RA usually requires lifelong treatment and, sometimes, surgery. In most patients, the disease follows an intermittent course and allows normal activity, although 10% suffer total disability from severe articular deformity, associated extra-articular symptoms, or both. The prognosis worsens with the development of nodules, vasculitis, and high titers of rheumatoid factor (RF).

Causes and incidence

RA occurs worldwide, striking three times more females than males. Although it can occur at any age, it begins most often between ages 25 and 55. This disease affects more than 7 million people in the United States alone.

What causes the chronic inflammation characteristic of RA isn't known, but various theories point to infectious, genetic, and endocrine factors.

Pathophysiology

It's believed that a genetically susceptible individual develops abnormal or altered IgG antibodies when exposed to an antigen. This altered IgG antibody isn't recognized as "self," and the individual forms an antibody against it—an antibody known as RF. By aggregating into complexes, RF generates inflammation. Eventually, cartilage damage by inflammation triggers additional immune responses, including activation of complement. This in turn attracts polymorphonuclear leukocytes and stimulates release of inflammatory mediators, which enhance joint destruction.

If unarrested, the inflammatory process within the joints occurs in four stages. First, synovitis develops from congestion and edema of the synovial membrane and joint capsule. Formation of pannus—thickened layers of granulation tissue—marks the second stage's onset. Pannus covers and invades cartilage and eventually destroys the joint capsule and bone. Progression to the third stage is characterized by fibrous ankylosis—fibrous invasion of the pannus and scar formation that occludes the joint space. Bone atrophy and malalignment cause visible deformities and disrupt the articulation of opposing bones, causing muscle atrophy and imbalance, and, possibly, partial dislocations or subluxations. In the fourth stage, fibrous tissue calcifies, resulting in bony ankylosis and total immobility. (See *The effects of rheumatoid arthritis on certain joints,* page 403.)

Complications

♦ Fibrous or bony ankylosis
♦ Soft-tissue contractures
♦ Joint deformities
♦ Subluxations
♦ Carpal tunnel syndrome
♦ Popliteal (Baker's) cysts
♦ Osteoporosis
♦ Vasculitis
♦ Amyloidosis
♦ Cardiac and pulmonary disorders

Signs and symptoms

RA usually develops insidiously and initially produces nonspecific signs and symptoms, such as fatigue, malaise, anorexia, persistent low-grade fever, weight loss, lymphadenopathy, and vague articular symptoms. Later, more specific localized articular symptoms develop, commonly in the fingers at the proximal interphalangeal, metacarpophalangeal, and metatarsophalangeal joints. These symptoms usually occur bilaterally and symmetrically and

PATHOPHYSIOLOGY
The effects of rheumatoid arthritis on certain joints

Many joints can be affected by rheumatoid arthritis, including the knee, hand and wrist, and hip.

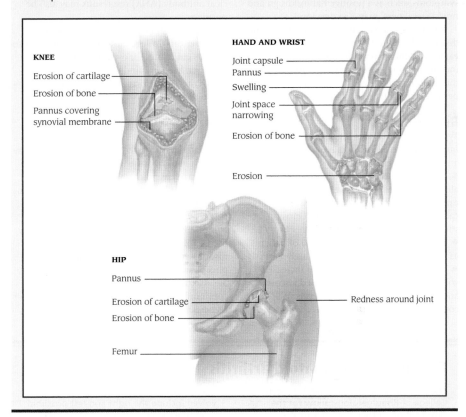

KNEE

Erosion of cartilage

Erosion of bone

Pannus covering synovial membrane

HAND AND WRIST

Joint capsule

Pannus

Swelling

Joint space narrowing

Erosion of bone

Erosion

HIP

Pannus

Erosion of cartilage

Erosion of bone

Femur

Redness around joint

---

may extend to the wrists, knees, hips, elbows, and ankles. The affected joints stiffen after inactivity, especially on rising in the morning. The fingers may assume a spindle shape from marked edema and joint congestion. The joints become tender and painful, at first only when the patient moves them, but eventually even at rest. They commonly feel hot to the touch. Ultimately, joint function is diminished.

Deformities are common if active disease continues. Proximal interphalangeal joints may develop flexion deformities or become hyperextended. Metacarpophalangeal joints may swell dorsally, and volar subluxation and stretching of tendons may pull the fingers to the ulnar side ("ulnar drift"). The fingers may become fixed in a characteristic "swan's neck" appearance, or "boutonnière" deformity. The hands appear foreshortened, the wrists boggy; carpal tunnel syndrome from synovial pressure on the median nerve causes tingling paresthesia in the fingers.

The most common extra-articular finding is the gradual appearance of rheumatoid nodules—subcutaneous, round or oval, non-tender masses—usually on pressure areas such as the elbows. Vasculitis can lead to skin lesions, leg ulcers, and multiple systemic complications. Peripheral neuropathy may produce numbness or tingling in the feet or weakness and loss of sensation in the fingers. Stiff, weak, or painful muscles are common. Other common extra-articular effects include pericarditis, pulmonary nodules or fibrosis, pleuritis, scleritis, and episcleritis.

Another complication is destruction of the odontoid process, part of the second cervical vertebra. Rarely, cord compression may occur, particularly in patients with long-standing deforming disease. Upper motor neuron signs and symptoms, such as a positive Babinski sign and muscle weakness, may also develop.

RA can also cause temporomandibular joint disease, which impairs chewing and causes earaches. Other extra-articular findings may include infection, osteoporosis, myositis, cardiopulmonary lesions, lymphadenopathy, and peripheral neuritis.

Diagnosis

Typical clinical features suggest this disorder, but a definitive diagnosis is based on laboratory and other test results:

♦ X-rays—in early stages, show bone demineralization and soft-tissue swelling; later, loss of cartilage and narrowing of joint spaces; finally, cartilage and bone destruction and erosion, subluxations, and deformities

♦ RF test—positive in 75% to 80% of patients, as indicated by a titer of 1:160 or higher

♦ Synovial fluid analysis—reveals increased volume and turbidity but decreased viscosity and complement (C3 and C4) levels; WBC count usually exceeds 10,000/μL

♦ ESR—elevated in 85% to 90% of patients (may be useful to monitor response to therapy because elevation commonly parallels disease activity)

♦ CBC—usually reveals moderate anemia and slight leukocytosis

A C-reactive protein test may be positive and can help monitor response to therapy. Antinuclear antibody (ANA) test results may also be positive.

The criteria for classifying RA developed by the American College of Rheumatology can also serve as guidelines for establishing a diagnosis. However, keep in mind that failure to meet these criteria—particularly early in the disease—doesn't exclude the diagnosis. (See *Classifying rheumatoid arthritis*.)

Treatment

Salicylates, particularly aspirin, are the mainstay of RA therapy because they decrease inflammation and relieve joint pain. Other useful medications include NSAIDs (such as indomethacin, fenoprofen, and ibuprofen), antimalarials (hydroxychloroquine), penicillamine (not as commonly used), gold salts (not as commonly used), Tofacitinib, and corticosteroids (prednisone). Immunosuppressants, such as cyclophosphamide, methotrexate, and azathioprine, are also therapeutic and are being used more commonly in early disease. (See *Drug therapy for rheumatoid arthritis*, pages 405 to 407.)

Classifying rheumatoid arthritis

The criteria established by the American College of Rheumatology allow for the classification of rheumatoid arthritis (RA).

Guidelines

A patient who meets four of the seven criteria is classified as having RA. The patient must experience the first four criteria for at least 6 weeks, and a physician must observe the second through fifth criteria.

A patient with two or more other clinical diagnoses can also be diagnosed with RA.

Criteria

♦ Morning stiffness in and around the joints that lasts for 1 hour before full improvement

♦ Arthritis in three or more joint areas, with at least three joint areas (as observed by a physician) exhibiting soft-tissue swelling or joint effusions, not just bony overgrowth (the 14 possible areas involved include the right and left proximal interphalangeal, metacarpophalangeal, wrist, elbow, knee, ankle, and metatarsophalangeal joints)

♦ Arthritis of hand joints, including the wrist, the metacarpophalangeal joint, or the proximal interphalangeal joint

♦ Arthritis that involves the same joint area on both sides of the body

♦ Subcutaneous rheumatoid nodules over bony prominences

♦ Demonstration of abnormal amounts of serum rheumatoid factor by any method that produces a positive result in less than 5% of patients without RA

♦ Radiographic changes, usually on posteroanterior hand and wrist X-rays; these changes must show erosions or unequivocal bony decalcification localized in or most notably adjacent to the involved joints

Drug therapy for rheumatoid arthritis

Drug and adverse effects	*Clinical considerations*

Analgesics

Aspirin

Prolonged bleeding time; gastrointestinal (GI) disturbances, including anorexia, nausea, dyspepsia, ulcers, and hemorrhage; hypersensitivity reactions ranging from urticaria to anaphylaxis; salicylism (mild toxicity: tinnitus, dizziness; moderate toxicity: restlessness, hyperpnea, delirium, marked lethargy; and severe toxicity: coma, seizures, severe hyperpnea)	♦ Don't use in patients with GI ulcers, bleeding, or hypersensitivity or in neonates. ♦ Tell the patient to take the drug with food, milk, antacid, or a large glass of water to reduce GI adverse effects. ♦ Monitor the patient's salicylate level. Remember that toxicity can develop rapidly in febrile, dehydrated children. ♦ Teach the patient to reduce the dose, one tablet at a time, if tinnitus occurs. ♦ Teach the patient to watch for signs of bleeding, such as bruising, melena, and petechiae.

Nonsteroidal anti-inflammatory drugs (NSAIDs)

Celecoxib, fenoprofen, ibuprofen, naproxen, piroxicam, sulindac, and tolmetin

Prolonged bleeding time; central nervous system (CNS) abnormalities (headache, drowsiness, restlessness, dizziness, and tremor); GI disturbances, including hemorrhage and peptic ulcer; increased blood urea nitrogen and liver enzyme levels	♦ Tell the patient taking NSAIDs that they may have a higher risk of having a heart attack or stroke than those not taking NSAIDs. ♦ Don't use in patients with renal disease, in patients with asthma who have nasal polyps, or in children. ♦ Use cautiously in patients with GI and cardiac disease or if a patient is allergic to other NSAIDs. ♦ Tell the patient to take the drug with milk or meals to reduce GI adverse effects. ♦ Tell the patient that the drug effect may be delayed for 2 to 3 weeks. ♦ Monitor the patient's kidney, liver, and auditory functions in long-term therapy. Stop the drug if abnormalities develop. ♦ Use cautiously in elderly patients; they may experience severe GI bleeding without warning.

Corticosteroids

Prednisone

Increased appetite, indigestion, GI irritation, nervousness, osteoporosis, easy bruising, fluid retention, weight gain, muscle weakness, onset or worsening of diabetes, cataracts, increased risk of infection, hypertension, arrhythmias, thromboembolism	♦ Use cautiously in patients with recent myocardial infarction (MI), GI ulcer, osteoporosis, diabetes mellitus, hypothyroidism, cirrhosis, diverticulitis, seizures, heart failure, ocular herpes simplex, emotional instability, and psychotic tendencies. ♦ Monitor patient's blood pressure, sleep patterns, and potassium level. ♦ Weigh patient daily; report sudden weight gain to prescriber. ♦ Monitor patient for cushingoid effects. ♦ Watch for depression or psychotic episodes, especially during high-dose therapy. ♦ Diabetic patients may need increased insulin; monitor level. ♦ Elderly patients may be more susceptible to osteoporosis with long-term use. ♦ Drug may mask or worsen infection. ♦ Gradually reduce dosage after long-term therapy.

(continued)

Drug therapy for rheumatoid arthritis (*continued*)

Drug and adverse effects	*Clinical considerations*
Disease-modifying antirheumatic drugs (DMARDs)	

Hydroxychloroquine and sulfasalazine

Blood dyscrasias, GI irritation, corneal opacities, and keratopathy or retinopathy	✦ Don't use in patients with retinal or visual field changes. ✦ Use cautiously in patients with hepatic disease, alcoholism, glucose-6-phosphate dehydrogenase deficiency, or psoriasis. ✦ Perform complete blood count (CBC) and liver function tests before therapy and during chronic therapy. The patient should also have regular ophthalmologic examinations. ✦ Tell the patient to take the drug with food or milk to minimize GI adverse effects. ✦ Warn the patient that dizziness may occur.

Gold (oral and parenteral)

Dermatitis, pruritus, rash, stomatitis, nephrotoxicity, blood dyscrasias and, with oral form, GI distress and diarrhea	✦ Watch for and report adverse effects. Observe for nitritoid reaction (flushing, fainting, and sweating). ✦ Check the patient's urine for blood and albumin before giving each dose. If positive, hold the drug and notify the physician. Stress to the patient the need for regular follow-up, including blood and urine testing. ✦ To avoid local nerve irritation, mix the drug well and give it via a deep I.M. injection in the buttock. ✦ Advise the patient not to expect improvement for 3 to 6 months. ✦ Tell the patient to report rash, bruising, bleeding, hematuria, or oral ulcers.

Methotrexate

Tubular necrosis, bone marrow depression, leukopenia, thrombocytopenia, pulmonary interstitial infiltrates, hyperuricemia, stomatitis, rash, pruritus, dermatitis, alopecia, diarrhea, dizziness, cirrhosis, and hepatic fibrosis	✦ Don't give to women who are pregnant or breast-feeding or to patients who are alcoholic. ✦ Monitor the patient's uric acid levels, CBC, and intake and output. ✦ Warn the patient to report any unusual bleeding (especially GI) or bruising promptly. ✦ Warn the patient to avoid alcohol, aspirin, and NSAIDs. ✦ Advise the patient to follow the prescribed regimen.

Biologic response modifiers	

Etanercept, golimumab, infliximab, and adalimumab

Headache, dizziness, peripheral edema, rhinitis, pharyngitis, mouth ulcers, dyspepsia, abdominal pain, upper respiratory tract infections, cough, rash, alopecia, infections	✦ Use cautiously in patients with chronic or invasive infections, malignancies, heart failure, or CNS demyelination. ✦ Monitor patient closely for signs and symptoms of infection. ✦ Evaluate patient for latent tuberculosis (TB) with tuberculin skin test before initiating treatment. Monitor for active TB during treatment. ✦ Monitor for new or worsening heart failure. ✦ Monitor patient for lymphomas and other malignancies. ✦ Monitor CBC regularly during therapy.

Drug therapy for rheumatoid arthritis (*continued*)

Drug and adverse effects	Clinical considerations
Anakinra Headache, sinusitis, abdominal pain, diarrhea, neutropenia, upper respiratory tract infection, ecchymosis, infection (cellulitis, pneumonia, bone and joint infection), flulike symptoms	◆ Use drug cautiously in immunosuppressed patients, those with chronic infections, the elderly, and breastfeeding women. ◆ Don't start treatment if patient has active infection. ◆ Monitor patient for infection and injection site reactions. ◆ Monitor patient for possible anaphylactic reactions. ◆ Obtain neutrophil count before treatment, monthly for the first 3 months of treatment, and then quarterly for up to 1 year.
Rituximab Asthenia, fever, headache, agitation, dizziness, insomnia, hypotension, arrhythmia, bradycardia, chest pain, edema, flushing, hypertension, tachycardia, conjunctivitis, sinusitis, abdominal pain or enlargement, anorexia, acute renal failure, leukopenia, neutropenia, thrombocytopenia, anemia, hyperglycemia, arthritis, bronchospasm, severe mucocutaneous reactions, angioedema, infusion reaction, tumor lysis syndrome	◆ Use cautiously in patients at high risk for hepatitis B viral infection. ◆ Monitor patient for infusion reaction complex, including hypoxia, pulmonary infiltrates, acute respiratory distress syndrome, MI, or cardiogenic shock. ◆ Monitor patient closely for signs of hypersensitivity. ◆ Monitor patient's blood pressure closely during infusion. If hypotension, bronchospasm, or angioedema occurs, stop infusion and restart at half the rate when symptoms resolve. ◆ Withhold antihypertensive 12 hours before infusion because transient hypotension may occur. ◆ If serious or life-threatening arrhythmias occur, stop infusion. ◆ Severe mucocutaneous reactions may occur 1 to 13 weeks after administration. Avoid further infusions and promptly start treatment of the skin reaction.
Abatacept Headache, dizziness, hypertension, nasopharyngitis, GI disturbances, including dyspepsia, nausea; urinary tract infection; back pain; respiratory system disturbances including upper respiratory infection, cough, exacerbation of chronic obstructive pulmonary disease (COPD); skin rash; infusion-related hypersensitivity reactions, infections, malignancy	◆ Don't give live vaccines during therapy and for 3 months after the end of treatment because it may decrease immune response to vaccine. ◆ Use cautiously in patients with active infections, history of chronic infection, or COPD or in women who are pregnant. ◆ Patients who test positive for TB should be treated before using abatacept. ◆ Contraindicated in patients taking a tumor necrosis factor antagonist.

Supportive measures include 8 to 10 hours of sleep every night, frequent rest periods between daily activities, and splinting to rest inflamed joints. A physical therapy program that includes range-of-motion (ROM) exercises and carefully individualized therapeutic exercises forestalls joint function loss; application of heat relaxes muscles and relieves pain. Moist heat usually works best for patients with chronic disease. Ice packs are effective during acute episodes.

Advanced disease may require synovectomy, joint reconstruction, or total joint arthroplasty.

Useful surgical procedures in RA include metatarsal head and distal ulnar resectional arthroplasty, insertion of a Silastic prosthesis between the metacarpophalangeal and proximal

When arthritis requires surgery

Arthritis severe enough to warrant total knee or total hip arthroplasty calls for comprehensive preoperative teaching and postoperative care.

Before surgery

♦ Explain preoperative and surgical procedures. Show the patient the prosthesis to be used if available.

♦ Teach the patient postoperative exercises such as isometrics, and supervise the practice. Also, teach deep-breathing and coughing exercises that will be necessary after surgery.

♦ Explain that total hip or knee arthroplasty requires frequent range-of-motion exercises of the leg after surgery; total knee arthroplasty requires frequent leg-lift exercises.

♦ Show the patient how to use a trapeze to move himself about in bed after surgery, and make sure there is a fracture bedpan handy.

♦ Tell the patient what kind of dressings to expect after surgery. After total knee arthroplasty, the patient's knee may be placed in a constant-passive-motion device to increase postoperative mobility and prevent emboli. After total hip arthroplasty, they'll have an abduction pillow between the legs to help keep the hip prosthesis in place.

After surgery

♦ Closely monitor and record vital signs. Watch for complications, such as steroid crisis and shock in patients receiving steroids. Monitor distal leg pulses often, marking them with a waterproof marker to make them easier to find.

♦ As soon as the patient awakens, encourage active dorsiflexion; if unable, report this immediately. Supervise isometric

exercises every 2 hours. After total hip arthroplasty, check traction for pressure areas and keep the bed's head raised between 30 and 45 degrees.

♦ Change or reinforce dressings, as needed, using sterile technique. Check wounds for hematoma, excessive drainage, color changes, or foul odor—all possible signs of hemorrhage or infection. (Wounds on rheumatoid arthritis patients may heal slowly.) Avoid contaminating dressings while helping the patient use the urinal or bedpan.

♦ Administer blood replacement products, antibiotics, and pain medication, as ordered. Monitor serum electrolyte and hemoglobin levels and hematocrit.

♦ Have the patient turn, cough, and deep-breathe every 2 hours; then percuss the chest.

♦ After total knee arthroplasty, keep the patient's leg extended and slightly elevated.

♦ After total hip arthroplasty, keep the patient's hip in abduction to prevent dislocation by using such measures as a wedge pillow. Prevent external rotation and avoid hip flexion greater than 90 degrees. Watch for and immediately report any inability to rotate the hip or bear weight on it, increased pain, or a leg that appears shorter—all may indicate dislocation.

♦ As soon as allowed, help the patient get out of bed and sit in a chair, keeping the weight on the unaffected side. When he's ready to walk, consult with the physical therapist for walking instruction and aids.

---

interphalangeal joints, and arthrodesis (joint fusion). Arthrodesis sacrifices joint mobility for stability and pain relief. Synovectomy (removal of destructive, proliferating synovium, usually in the wrists, knees, and fingers) may halt or delay the course of this disease. Osteotomy (the cutting of bone or excision of a wedge of bone) can realign joint surfaces and redistribute stresses. Tendons may rupture spontaneously, requiring surgical repair. Tendon transfers may prevent deformities or relieve contractures. (See *When arthritis requires surgery.*)

Special considerations

♦ Assess all joints carefully. Look for deformities, contractures, immobility, and inability to perform everyday activities.

♦ Monitor the patient's vital signs and note weight changes, sensory disturbances, and level of pain. Administer analgesics as ordered and watch for adverse effects.

♦ Provide meticulous skin care. Check for rheumatoid nodules as well as pressure ulcers and breakdowns due to immobility, vascular impairment, corticosteroid treatment, or improper splinting. Use lotion or cleansing oil, not soap, for dry skin.

◆ Explain all diagnostic tests and procedures. Tell the patient to expect multiple blood samples to allow firm diagnosis and accurate monitoring of therapy.

◆ Monitor the duration, not the intensity, of morning stiffness because duration more accurately reflects the disease's severity. Encourage the patient to take hot showers or baths at bedtime or in the morning to reduce the need for pain medication.

◆ Apply splints carefully and correctly. Observe for pressure ulcers if the patient is in traction or wearing splints.

◆ Explain the nature of the disease. Make sure the patient and family understand that RA is a chronic disease that requires major changes in lifestyle. Emphasize that there are no miracle cures, despite claims to the contrary.

◆ Encourage a balanced diet, but make sure the patient understands that special diets won't cure RA. Stress the need for weight control because obesity adds further stress to joints.

◆ Urge the patient to perform activities of daily living (ADLs), such as practicing good hygiene and dressing and feeding oneself. Suggest ADL aids, such as a long-handled shoehorn; elastic shoelaces; zipper-pulls; button hooks; easy-to-handle cups, plates, and silverware; elevated toilet seats; and battery-operated toothbrushes. Household cleaning devices such as long-handled dustpans are also available. Patients who have trouble maneuvering fingers into gloves should wear mittens.

◆ ADLs that can be done in a sitting position should be encouraged. Allow the patient enough time to calmly perform these tasks.

◆ Provide emotional support. Remember that the patient with chronic illness easily becomes depressed, discouraged, and irritable. Encourage the patient to discuss fears concerning dependency, sexuality, body image, and self-esteem. Refer the patient to an appropriate social service agency as needed.

◆ Discuss sexual aids: alternative positions, pain medication, and moist heat to increase mobility.

◆ Before discharge, make sure the patient knows how and when to take prescribed medication and how to recognize possible adverse effects.

◆ Teach the patient how to stand, walk, and sit correctly: upright and erect. Tell the patient to sit in chairs with high seats and armrests; the patient will find it easier to get up from a chair if the knees are lower than the hips. If the patient doesn't own a chair with a high seat, recommend putting blocks of wood under a favorite chair's legs. Suggest an elevated toilet seat.

◆ Mobility aids are very helpful. Many medical and commercial stores offer assistive and supportive devices that promote self-care, including an overhead grasping trapeze to get out of bed, easy-to-open drawers, handheld shower nozzles, handrails, and grab bars.

◆ Instruct the patient to pace daily activities, resting for 5 to 10 minutes out of each hour and alternating sitting and standing tasks. Adequate sleep and correct sleeping posture are important. The patient should sleep on their back on a firm mattress and should avoid placing a pillow under the knees, which encourages flexion deformity.

◆ Teach the patient to avoid putting undue stress on joints and to use the largest joint available for a given task, to support weak or painful joints as much as possible, to avoid positions of flexion and promote positions of extension, to hold objects parallel to the knuckles as briefly as possible, to always use hands toward the center of the body, and to slide—not lift—objects whenever possible. Enlist the aid of the occupational therapist to teach how to simplify activities and protect arthritic joints. Stress the importance of shoes with proper support.

◆ **ELDER TIP** *Reinforce safety precautions for elderly patients, such as the removal of throw rugs and the use of handrails and adequate night lighting. Recommend a step stool for elderly patients who need to reach in overhead cupboards. Suggest that the patient purchase medication without safety caps, if available, because these caps can be difficult to open. Medication administration should be designed to follow a standard regimen that fits with the patient's lifestyle.*

◆ Refer the patient to the Arthritis Foundation for more information on coping with the disease.

JUVENILE RHEUMATOID ARTHRITIS

Affecting children younger than age 16, juvenile rheumatoid arthritis (JRA) is an inflammatory disorder of the connective tissues, characterized by joint swelling and pain or tenderness. It may also involve organs such as the skin, heart, lungs, liver, spleen, and eyes, producing extra-articular signs and symptoms.

JRA has three major types: systemic (Still disease or acute febrile type), polyarticular, and pauciarticular. Depending on the type, this disease can occur as early as age 6 weeks—although rarely before 6 months—with peaks of onset at ages 1 to 3 and 8 to 12.

The prognosis for JRA is generally good, although disabilities can occur. Long periods of spontaneous remission are common. Improvement or remission may occur at puberty.

Causes and incidence

The cause of JRA remains puzzling. Research continues to test several theories, such as those linking the disease to genetic factors or to an abnormal immune response. Viral or bacterial (particularly streptococcal) infection, trauma, and emotional stress may be precipitating factors, but their relationship to JRA remains unclear.

Considered the major chronic rheumatic disorder of childhood, JRA affects an estimated 50 to 100 per 100,000 children in the United States; overall incidence is twice as high in females, with variation among the types of JRA.

Pathophysiology

The etiology and pathogenesis of JRA are not completely understood. Genetic susceptibility plays a major role, but there is significant overlap between loci associated with juvenile idiopathic arthritis and those associated with other autoimmune diseases.

Complications

◆ Ocular damage
◆ Loss of vision
◆ Growth disturbances

Signs and symptoms

Signs and symptoms vary with the type of JRA. Affecting boys and girls almost equally, *systemic JRA* accounts for about 10% of cases. The affected children may have mild, transient arthritis or frank polyarthritis with fever and rash. Joint involvement may not be evident at first, but the child's behavior may clearly suggest joint pain. Such a child may constantly want to sit in a flexed position, may not walk much, or may refuse to walk at all. Young children with JRA are noticeably irritable and listless.

Fever in systemic JRA occurs suddenly and spikes to 103° F (39.4° C) or higher once or twice daily, usually in the late afternoon, then rapidly returns to normal or subnormal. (This "sawtooth" or intermittent spiking fever pattern helps differentiate JRA from other inflammatory disorders.) When fever spikes, an evanescent rheumatoid rash commonly appears, consisting of small pale or salmon pink macules, usually on the trunk and proximal extremities and occasionally on the face, palms, and soles. Massaging or applying heat intensifies this rash. It's usually most conspicuous where the skin has been rubbed or subjected to pressure such as the areas of skin covered by underclothing.

Other signs and symptoms of systemic JRA may include hepatosplenomegaly, lymphadenopathy, pleuritis, pericarditis, myocarditis, and nonspecific abdominal pain.

Polyarticular JRA accounts for about 40% of cases and is three times more common in females than in males; affected children may be seronegative or seropositive for RF. It involves five or more joints and usually develops insidiously. Most commonly involved joints are the wrists, elbows, knees, ankles, and small joints of the hands and feet. Polyarticular JRA can also affect larger joints, including the temporomandibular joints, cervical spine, hips, and shoulders. These joints become swollen, tender, and stiff. Usually, the arthritis is symmetrical; it may be remittent or indolent. The patient may run a low-grade fever with daily peaks. Listlessness and weight loss can occur, possibly with lymphadenopathy and hepatosplenomegaly. Other signs of polyarticular JRA include subcutaneous nodules on the elbows or heels and noticeable developmental retardation.

Seropositive polyarticular JRA, the more severe type, usually occurs late in childhood and can cause destructive arthritis that mimics adult RA.

Pauciarticular JRA involves few joints (usually no more than four), typically affecting the knees and other large joints. This form accounts for 50% of cases and has major subtypes. The first, pauciarticular JRA with chronic iridocyclitis, most commonly strikes females younger than age 6 and involves the knees, elbows, ankles, or iris. Inflammation of the iris and ciliary body is commonly asymptomatic but may produce pain, redness, blurred vision, and photophobia.

The second subtype, pauciarticular JRA with sacroiliitis, usually strikes males (9:1) older than age 8, who tend to test positive for human leukocyte antigen (HLA)-B27. This subtype is characterized by lower-extremity arthritis that produces hip, sacroiliac, heel, and foot pain as well as Achilles tendinitis. These patients may later develop the sacroiliac and lumbar arthritis characteristic of ankylosing spondylitis. Some also experience acute iritis, but not as many as those with the first subtype.

The third subtype includes patients with joint involvement who are ANA and HLA-B27 negative and don't develop iritis. These patients have a better prognosis than those with the first or second subtype.

Common to all types of JRA is joint stiffness in the morning or after periods of inactivity. Back pain and limited ROM are common. Growth disturbances may also occur, resulting in uneven length of arms or legs due to overgrowth or undergrowth adjacent to inflamed joints.

Diagnosis

Persistent joint pain and the rash and fever clearly point to JRA. Laboratory tests are useful for ruling out other inflammatory or even malignant diseases that can mimic JRA. Disease activity and response to therapy can also be monitored through laboratory results.
◆ CBC shows decreased Hb levels, neutrophilia, and thrombocytosis.
◆ ESR and C-reactive protein, haptoglobin, Ig, and C3 complement levels may be elevated.
◆ ANA test may be positive in patients who have pauciarticular JRA with chronic iridocyclitis.
◆ RF is present in 15% of JRA cases, compared with 85% of RA cases.
◆ Positive HLA-B27 antigens may forecast later development of ankylosing spondylitis.
◆ X-rays in early stages reveal changes, including soft-tissue swelling, effusion, and periostitis in affected joints. Later, osteoporosis and accelerated bone growth may appear, followed by subchondral erosions, joint space narrowing, bone destruction, and fusion.

Treatment

Successful management of JRA usually involves administration of anti-inflammatory drugs, physical therapy, carefully planned nutrition and exercise, and regular eye examinations. Both child and parents must be involved in therapy.

NSAIDs, disease-modifying antirheumatic drugs (DMARDs), biologic agents, and corticosteroids are classifications of medications that may be used in treatment. Because of adverse effects, steroids are generally reserved for treatment of systemic complications, such as pericarditis or iritis, that are resistant to NSAIDs. Corticosteroids and mydriatic drugs are commonly used for iridocyclitis. If little relief is obtained from these drugs, biologic response modifiers may be used. These drugs work by blocking various actions of the inflammatory process.

Physical therapy promotes regular exercise to maintain joint mobility and muscle strength, thereby preventing contractures, deformity, and disability. Good posture, gait training, and joint protection are also beneficial. Splints help reduce pain, prevent contractures, and maintain correct joint alignment.

Surgery is usually limited to soft-tissue releases to improve joint mobility. Joint replacement is delayed until the child has matured physically and can handle vigorous rehabilitation.

Special considerations

◆ Parents and healthcare professionals should encourage the child to be as independent as possible and to develop a positive attitude toward school, social development, and vocational planning.
◆ Regular slit-lamp examinations help ensure early diagnosis and treatment of iridocyclitis. Children with pauciarticular JRA with chronic iridocyclitis should be checked every 3 months during periods of active disease and every 6 months during remissions.

PSORIATIC ARTHRITIS

Psoriatic arthritis is a rheumatoid-like joint disease associated with psoriasis of nearby skin and nails. Although the arthritis component of this syndrome may be clinically indistinguishable from RA, the rheumatoid nodules are absent, and serologic tests for RF are negative. Psoriatic arthritis is usually mild, with intermittent flare-ups, but in rare cases may progress to crippling arthritis mutilans. This disease affects males and females equally; onset usually occurs between ages 30 and 35.

Causes and incidence

Evidence suggests that predisposition to psoriatic arthritis is hereditary; 20% to 50% of patients are HLA-B27 positive. However, onset is usually precipitated by streptococcal infection or trauma.

About 5% to 8% of patients with psoriasis develop psoriatic arthritis. It occurs in up to 1% of the general population.

Signs and symptoms

Psoriatic lesions usually precede the arthritic component; however, after the full syndrome is established, joint and skin lesions recur simultaneously. Arthritis may involve one joint or several joints symmetrically. Spinal involvement occurs in some patients. Peripheral joint involvement is most common in the distal interphalangeal joints of the hands, which have a characteristic sausage-like appearance. Nail changes include pitting, transverse ridges, onycholysis, keratosis, yellowing, and destruction. The patient may experience general malaise, fever, and eye involvement.

Diagnosis

Inflammatory arthritis in a patient with psoriatic skin lesions suggests psoriatic arthritis.

℞ **CONFIRMING DIAGNOSIS** *X-rays confirm joint involvement and show:*
◆ *erosion of terminal phalangeal tufts*
◆ *"whittling" of the distal end of the terminal phalanges*

◆ *"pencil-in-cup" deformity of the distal interphalangeal joints*
◆ *relative absence of osteoporosis*
◆ *sacroiliitis*
◆ *atypical spondylitis with syndesmophyte formation. Hyperostosis and paravertebral ossification result, which may lead to vertebral fusion*

Blood studies indicate negative RF and elevated ESR and uric acid levels.

Treatment

In mild psoriatic arthritis, treatment is supportive and consists of immobilization through bed rest or splints, isometric exercises, paraffin baths, heat therapy, and aspirin and other NSAIDs. Some patients respond well to low-dose systemic corticosteroids; topical steroids may help control skin lesions. DMARDs such as sulfasalazine and methotrexate therapy are effective in treating both the articular and cutaneous effects of psoriatic arthritis. Antimalarials are contraindicated because they can provoke exfoliative dermatitis. Tumor necrosis factor inhibitors such as adalimumab, etanercept, and infliximab block proteins in the inflammatory process, helping to reduce inflammation.

Special considerations

◆ Explain the disease and its treatment to the patient and family.
◆ Encourage exercise, particularly swimming, to maintain strength and ROM.
◆ Teach the patient how to apply skin care products and medications correctly; explain possible adverse effects.
◆ Stress the importance of adequate rest and protection of affected joints.
◆ Encourage regular, moderate exposure to the sun.
◆ Refer the patient to the Arthritis Foundation for self-help and support groups.

ANKYLOSING SPONDYLITIS

A chronic, usually progressive inflammatory disease, ankylosing spondylitis primarily affects the sacroiliac, apophyseal, and costovertebral joints, along with adjacent soft tissue. The disease (also known as *rheumatoid spondylitis* and *Marie–Strümpell disease*) usually begins in the sacroiliac joints and gradually progresses to the spine's lumbar, thoracic, and cervical regions. Deterioration of bone and cartilage can lead to fibrous tissue formation with eventual fusion of the spine or peripheral joints.

Ankylosing spondylitis may be equally prevalent in both sexes. Progressive disease is well recognized in men, but the diagnosis is commonly overlooked or missed in females, who tend to have more peripheral joint involvement.

Pathophysiology

The pathophysiology remains quite unknown. However, new insights have been provided by the recent identification of susceptibility genes other than HLA-B27; evidence of a pivotal role for several proinflammatory cytokines including IL-23 and IL-17; and the recognition that inflammation and structural progression proceed separately from each other.

Causes and incidence

Evidence strongly suggests a familial tendency in ankylosing spondylitis. The presence of HLA-B27 (positive in >90% of patients with this disease) and circulating immune complexes suggests immunologic activity.

One of 10,000 people has ankylosing spondylitis. It affects more males than females and usually emerges between ages 20 and 40, although it may develop in children younger than age 10.

Complication

◆ Atlantoaxial subluxation

Signs and symptoms

The first indication of ankylosing spondylitis is intermittent low back pain that's usually most severe in the morning or after a period of inactivity. Other signs and symptoms depend on the disease stage and may include:
◆ hip deformity and associated limited ROM
◆ kyphosis in advanced stages, caused by chronic stooping to relieve symptoms
◆ mild fatigue, fever, anorexia, or weight loss; occasional iritis; aortic insufficiency and cardiomegaly; and upper lobe pulmonary fibrosis (mimics tuberculosis)
◆ pain and limited expansion of the chest due to involvement of the costovertebral joints
◆ peripheral arthritis involving shoulders, hips, and knees
◆ stiffness and limited motion of the lumbar spine
◆ tenderness over the inflammation site

These signs and symptoms progress unpredictably, and the disease can go into remission, exacerbation, or arrest at any stage.

Diagnosis

Typical symptoms, family history, and the presence of HLA-B27 strongly suggest ankylosing spondylitis.

Dx CONFIRMING DIAGNOSIS *Confirmation requires these characteristic X-ray findings:*
◆ *blurring of the bony margins of joints in the early stage*
◆ *bilateral sacroiliac involvement*
◆ *patchy sclerosis with superficial bony erosions*
◆ *eventual squaring of vertebral bodies*
◆ *bamboo spine with complete ankylosis*

ESR and alkaline phosphatase and serum IgG A levels may be elevated. A negative RF helps rule out RA, which produces similar symptoms.

Treatment

No treatment reliably stops progression of this disease, so management aims to delay further deformity through good posture, stretching and deep-breathing exercises and, in some patients, braces and lightweight supports. Anti-inflammatory analgesics, such as aspirin, indomethacin, sulfasalazine, and sulindac, control pain and inflammation.

Tumor necrosis factor inhibitors have been shown to improve symptoms. Corticosteroid therapy or medication to suppress the immune system may be prescribed to control various symptoms. DMARDs such as methotrexate and sulfasalazine have been used in patients who don't respond well to corticosteroids or those who are dependent on high doses of corticosteroids.

Severe hip involvement usually necessitates surgical hip replacement. Severe spinal involvement may require a spinal wedge osteotomy to separate and reposition the vertebrae. This surgery is performed only on selected patients because of the risk of spinal cord damage and the long convalescence involved.

Special considerations

Ankylosing spondylitis can be an extremely painful and crippling disease, so your main responsibility is to promote the patient's comfort. When dealing with such a patient, keep in mind that limited ROM makes simple tasks difficult. Offer support and reassurance.
◆ Administer medications as ordered. Apply local heat and provide massage to relieve pain. Assess mobility and degree of discomfort frequently. Teach and assist with daily exercises as needed to maintain strength and function. Stress the importance of maintaining good posture.
◆ If treatment includes surgery, provide good postoperative care. Because ankylosing spondylitis is a chronic, progressively crippling condition, a comprehensive treatment plan should also reflect counsel from a social worker, visiting nurse, and dietitian.

◆ To minimize deformities, advise the patient to:
   ◆ avoid any physical activity that places undue stress on the back, such as lifting heavy objects
   ◆ stand upright; to sit upright in a high, straight chair; and to avoid leaning over a desk
   ◆ sleep in a prone position on a hard mattress and to avoid using pillows under neck or knees
   ◆ avoid prolonged walking, standing, sitting, or driving
   ◆ perform regular stretching and deep-breathing exercises and to swim regularly, if possible
   ◆ have height measured every 3 to 4 months to detect any tendency toward kyphosis
   ◆ seek vocational counseling if work requires standing or prolonged sitting at a desk
   ◆ contact the local Arthritis Foundation chapter for a support group

SJÖGREN SYNDROME

The second most common autoimmune rheumatic disorder after RA, Sjögren syndrome is characterized by diminished lacrimal and salivary gland secretion (sicca complex). Sjögren syndrome may be a primary disorder or it may be associated with connective tissue disorders, such as RA, scleroderma, SLE, and polymyositis. In some patients, the disorder is limited to the exocrine glands (glandular Sjögren syndrome); in others, it also involves other organs, such as the lungs and kidneys (extraglandular Sjögren syndrome).

Causes and incidence

The cause of Sjögren syndrome is unknown, but genetic and environmental factors probably contribute to its development. Viral or bacterial infection or perhaps exposure to pollen may trigger Sjögren syndrome in a genetically susceptible individual. Tissue damage results from infiltration by lymphocytes or from the deposition of immune complexes. Lymphocytic infiltration may be classified as benign, malignant, or pseudolymphoma (nonmalignant, but tumorlike aggregates of lymphoid cells).

This syndrome occurs mainly in females (90% of patents); mean age of onset is 40 to 50.

Pathophysiology

The pathophysiology of Sjögren syndrome is not well understood. The presence of activated salivary gland epithelial cells expressing MHC class II molecules and the identification of inherited susceptibility markers suggest that environmental or endogenous antigens trigger a self-perpetuating inflammatory response in susceptible individuals. In addition, the continuing presence of active IFN pathways in Sjögren syndrome suggests ongoing activation of the innate immune system. Together, these findings suggest an ongoing interaction between the innate and acquired immune systems in Sjögren syndrome.

Complications

◆ Corneal ulceration
◆ Deafness
◆ Renal tubular necrosis
◆ Splenomegaly

Signs and symptoms

About 50% of patients with Sjögren syndrome have confirmed RA and a history of slowly developing sicca complex. However, some patients seek medical help for rapidly progressive and severe oral and ocular dryness, in many cases accompanied by periodic parotid gland enlargement. Ocular dryness (xerophthalmia) leads to foreign body sensation (gritty, sandy eye), redness, burning, photosensitivity, eye fatigue, itching, and mucoid discharge. The patient may also complain of a film across the field of vision.

Oral dryness (xerostomia) leads to difficulty swallowing and talking; abnormal taste or smell sensation or both; thirst; ulcers of the tongue, buccal mucosa, and lips (especially at the corners of the mouth); and severe dental caries. Dryness of the respiratory tract leads to epistaxis, hoarseness, chronic nonproductive cough, recurrent otitis media, and increased incidence of respiratory infections.

Other effects may include dyspareunia and pruritus (associated with vaginal dryness), generalized itching, fatigue, recurrent low-grade fever, and arthralgia or myalgia. Lymph node enlargement may be the first sign of malignant lymphoma or pseudolymphoma.

Specific extraglandular findings in Sjögren syndrome include interstitial pneumonitis; interstitial nephritis, which results in renal tubular acidosis in 25% of patients; Raynaud phenomenon (20%); and vasculitis, usually limited to the skin and characterized by palpable purpura on the legs (20%). About 50% of patients show signs of hypothyroidism related to autoimmune thyroid disease. A few patients develop systemic necrotizing vasculitis.

Diagnosis

The diagnosis of Sjögren syndrome rests on the detection of two of the following three conditions: xerophthalmia, xerostomia (with salivary gland biopsy showing lymphocytic infiltration), and an associated autoimmune or lymphoproliferative disorder. Diagnosis must rule out other causes of oral and ocular dryness, including sarcoidosis, endocrine disorders, anxiety or depression, and effects of therapy such as radiation to the head and neck. More than 200 commonly used drugs also produce dry mouth as an adverse effect. In patients with salivary gland enlargement and severe lymphoid infiltration, diagnosis must rule out cancer.

Laboratory values include elevated ESR in most patients, mild anemia and leukopenia in 30%, and hypergammaglobulinemia in 50%. Autoantibodies are also common, including anti-Sjögren syndrome-A (anti-Ro) and anti-Sjögren syndrome-B (anti-La), which are antinuclear and antisalivary duct antibodies. From 75% to 90% of patients test positive for RF; 90%, for antinuclear antibodies.

Other tests help support this diagnosis. Schirmer tearing test and slit-lamp examination with rose Bengal dye are used to measure eye involvement. Salivary gland involvement is evaluated by measuring the volume of parotid saliva and by secretory sialography and salivary scintigraphy. Lower-lip biopsy shows salivary gland infiltration by lymphocytes.

Treatment

Treatment is usually symptomatic and includes conservative measures to relieve ocular or oral dryness. Mouth dryness can be relieved by using a methylcellulose swab or spray and by drinking plenty of fluids, especially at mealtime. Meticulous oral hygiene is essential, including regular flossing, brushing, at-home fluoride treatment, and frequent dental checkups.

Instill artificial tears as often as every half hour to prevent eye damage (corneal ulcerations and corneal opacifications) from insufficient tear secretions. Some patients may also benefit from instillation of an eye ointment at bedtime or from twice-a-day use of sustained-release cellulose capsules (Lacrisert). If infection develops, antibiotics should be given immediately; topical steroids should be avoided. Other treatment measures vary with associated extraglandular findings. Parotid gland enlargement requires local heat and analgesics. Pulmonary and renal interstitial disease necessitate corticosteroid use. Accompanying lymphoma is treated with a combination of chemotherapy, surgery, or radiation.

Special considerations

◆ Stress the need to humidify home and work environments to help relieve respiratory dryness.

◆ Advise the patient to avoid drugs that decrease saliva production, such as atropine derivatives, antihistamines, anticholinergics, and antidepressants.

◆ If mouth lesions make eating painful, suggest high-protein, high-calorie liquid supplements to prevent malnutrition.

◆ Advise the patient to avoid sugar, which contributes to dental caries. Tobacco; alcohol; and spicy, salty, or highly acidic foods, which cause mouth irritation, should also be avoided.

◆ Suggest normal saline solution drops or aerosolized spray for nasal dryness.

◆ Advise the patient to avoid prolonged hot showers and baths and to use moisturizing lotions to help ease dry skin. Suggest K-Y lubricating jelly as a vaginal lubricant.

◆ Suggest the use of sunglasses to protect the patient's eyes from dust, wind, and strong light. Moisture chamber spectacles may also be helpful. Because dry eyes are more susceptible to infection, advise the patient to keep the face clean and to avoid rubbing the eyes.

◆ Refer the patient to the Sjögren's syndrome Foundation for additional information and support.

LUPUS ERYTHEMATOSUS

A chronic inflammatory disorder of the connective tissues, lupus erythematosus appears in two forms. *Discoid lupus erythematosus* (DLE) affects only the skin. (See *Discoid lupus erythematosus.*) SLE affects multiple organ systems as well as the skin and can be fatal. (See *Organs affected by systemic lupus erythematosus*, page 416.) Like RA, SLE is characterized by recurring remissions and exacerbations, especially common during the spring and summer. The prognosis improves with early detection and treatment, but remains poor for patients who develop cardiovascular, renal, or neurologic complications or severe bacterial infections.

Causes and incidence

The exact cause of SLE remains a mystery, but evidence points to interrelated immunologic, environmental, hormonal, and genetic factors. Autoimmunity is thought to be the prime causative mechanism.

Certain predisposing factors may make a person susceptible to SLE. Physical or mental stress, streptococcal or viral infections, exposure to sunlight or ultraviolet light, immunization, pregnancy, and abnormal estrogen metabolism may all affect this disease's development.

SLE may also be triggered or aggravated by treatment with certain drugs—for example, procainamide, hydralazine, anticonvulsants, and, less commonly, penicillins, sulfa drugs, and hormonal contraceptives.

Discoid lupus erythematosus

Discoid lupus erythematosus (DLE) is a form of lupus erythematosus marked by chronic skin eruptions that, if untreated, can lead to scarring and permanent disfigurement. About 1 of 20 patients with DLE later develops systemic lupus erythematosus (SLE). The exact cause of DLE is unknown, but some evidence suggests an autoimmune defect. An estimated 60% of patients with DLE are women in their late 20s or older. This disease is rare in children.

DLE lesions are raised, red, scaling plaques, with follicular plugging and central atrophy. The raised edges and sunken centers give them a coinlike appearance. Although these lesions can appear anywhere on the body, they usually erupt on the face, scalp, ears, neck, and arms or on any part of the body that's exposed to sunlight. Such lesions can resolve completely or may cause hypopigmentation or hyperpigmentation,

atrophy, and scarring. Facial plaques sometimes assume the butterfly pattern characteristic of SLE. Hair tends to become brittle or may fall out in patches.

As a rule, patient history and the appearance of the rash itself are diagnostic. Lupus erythematosus cell test is positive in fewer than 10% of patients. Skin biopsy of lesions reveals immunoglobulins or complement components. SLE must be ruled out.

Patients with DLE should avoid prolonged exposure to the sun, fluorescent lighting, or reflected sunlight. They should wear protective clothing, use sunscreening agents, avoid engaging in outdoor activities during periods of most intense sunlight (between 10 a.m. and 2 p.m.), and report any changes in the lesions. Drug treatment consists of topical, intralesional, or systemic medication, as in SLE.

Organs affected by systemic lupus erythematosus

Systemic lupus erythematosus affects multiple organ systems as well as the skin and can be fatal.

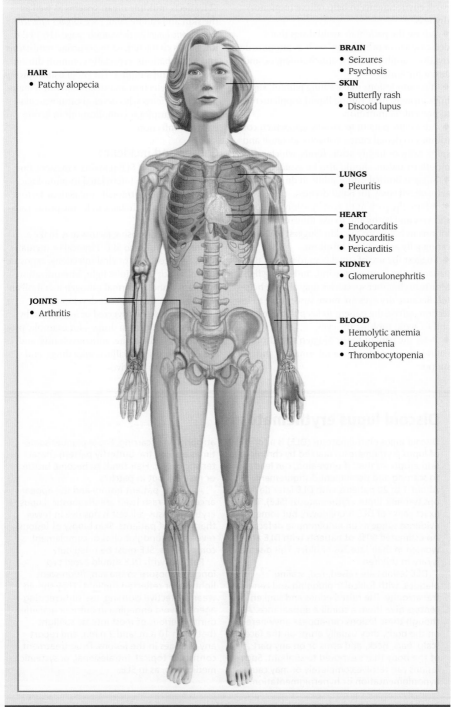

HAIR
- Patchy alopecia

BRAIN
- Seizures
- Psychosis

SKIN
- Butterfly rash
- Discoid lupus

LUNGS
- Pleuritis

HEART
- Endocarditis
- Myocarditis
- Pericarditis

KIDNEY
- Glomerulonephritis

JOINTS
- Arthritis

BLOOD
- Hemolytic anemia
- Leukopenia
- Thrombocytopenia

SLE strikes 9 times more women than men, increasing to 15 times more during childbearing years. It occurs worldwide but is most prevalent among Asians and Blacks.

Pathophysiology

Autoimmunity is felt to be the culprit. In autoimmunity, the body produces antibodies against its own cells, such as the ANA. The formed antigen–antibody complexes can suppress the body's normal immunity and damage tissues. Patients with SLE produce antibodies against many different tissue components, such as RBCs, neutrophils, platelets, lymphocytes, or almost any organ or tissue in the body.

Complications

◆ Pleurisy
◆ Pleural effusions
◆ Pneumonitis
◆ Pulmonary hypertension
◆ Pericarditis
◆ Endocarditis
◆ Coronary atherosclerosis
◆ Renal failure

Signs and symptoms

The onset of SLE may be acute or insidious and produces no characteristic clinical pattern. However, its symptoms commonly include fever, weight loss, malaise, and fatigue as well as rashes and polyarthralgia. SLE may involve every organ system. In 90% of patients, joint involvement is similar to that in RA. Skin lesions are most commonly erythematous rashes in areas exposed to light. The classic butterfly rash over the nose and cheeks occurs in fewer than 50% of the patients. (See *Butterfly rash.*) Ultraviolet rays often provoke or aggravate skin eruptions. Vasculitis can develop (especially in the digits), possibly leading to infarctive lesions, necrotic leg ulcers, or digital gangrene. Raynaud phenomenon appears in about 20% of patients. Patchy alopecia and painless ulcers of the mucous membranes are common.

Constitutional symptoms of SLE include aching, malaise, fatigue, low-grade or spiking fever, chills, anorexia, and weight loss. Lymph node enlargement (diffuse or local, and nontender), abdominal pain, nausea, vomiting, diarrhea, and constipation may occur. Females may experience irregular menstrual periods or amenorrhea during the active phase of SLE.

About 50% of SLE patients develop signs of cardiopulmonary abnormalities, such as pleuritis, pericarditis, and dyspnea. Myocarditis, endocarditis, tachycardia, parenchymal infiltrates, and pneumonitis may occur. Renal effects may

Butterfly rash

In the classic butterfly rash, lesions appear on the cheeks and the bridge of the nose, creating a characteristic butterfly pattern. The rash may vary in severity from malar erythema to discoid lesions (plaque).

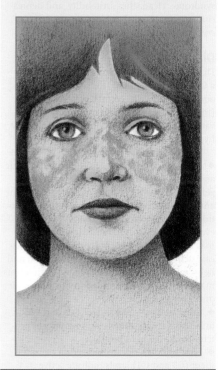

Signs of systemic lupus erythematosus

Diagnosing systemic lupus erythematosus (SLE) is difficult because SLE commonly mimics other diseases; symptoms may be vague and vary greatly from patient to patient.

The revised criteria for SLE must include four or more of the following signs:
◆ abnormal titer of antinuclear antibody
◆ hemolytic disorder
◆ malar rash
◆ discoid rash
◆ arthritis
◆ oral ulcerations
◆ photosensitivity
◆ serositis
◆ renal disorder
◆ neurologic disorder
◆ immunologic disorder

include hematuria, proteinuria, urine sediment, and cellular casts, which may progress to total kidney failure. Urinary tract infections may result from heightened susceptibility to infection. Seizure disorders and mental dysfunction may indicate neurologic damage. Central nervous system (CNS) involvement may produce emotional instability, psychosis, and organic mental syndrome. Headaches, irritability, and depression are common. (See *Signs of systemic lupus erythematosus*, page 417.)

Diagnosis

Diagnostic tests for patients with SLE include a CBC with differential (for signs of anemia and decreased WBC count); platelet count (may be decreased); ESR (commonly elevated); and serum electrophoresis (may show hypergammaglobulinemia).

Specific tests for SLE include:

◆ ANA panel, including anti-deoxyribonucleic acid (DNA) and anti-Smith antibodies—generally positive for lupus alone. (Because the anti-DNA test is rarely positive in other conditions, it's the most specific test for SLE. However, if the patient is in remission, anti-DNA may be reduced or absent [correlates with disease activity, especially renal involvement, and helps monitor response to therapy]. Other tests may be performed as needed to rule out other disorders.)

◆ urine studies—may show RBCs and WBCs, urine casts and sediment, and significant protein loss (>0.5 g/24 hours)

◆ blood studies—decreased serum complement (C3 and C4) levels indicate active disease

◆ chest X-ray—may show pleurisy or lupus pneumonitis

◆ electrocardiogram—may show conduction defect with cardiac involvement or pericarditis

◆ kidney biopsy—determines disease stage and extent of renal involvement

Some patients show a positive lupus anticoagulant test and a positive anticardiolipin test. Such patients are prone to antiphospholipid syndrome (thrombosis and thrombocytopenia).

Treatment

Patients with mild disease require little or no medication. NSAIDs, including aspirin, control arthritis symptoms in many patients. Skin lesions need topical treatment. Corticosteroid creams are recommended for acute lesions.

Refractory skin lesions are treated with intralesional corticosteroids or antimalarials such as hydroxychloroquine. Because hydroxychloroquine can cause retinal damage, such treatment

requires ophthalmologic examination every 6 months.

Corticosteroids remain the treatment of choice for systemic symptoms of SLE, for acute generalized exacerbations, or for serious disease related to vital organ systems, such as pleuritis, pericarditis, lupus nephritis, vasculitis, and CNS involvement. Initial doses equivalent to 60 mg or more of prednisone often bring noticeable improvement within 48 hours. As soon as symptoms are under control, steroid dosage is tapered slowly. (Rising serum complement levels and decreasing anti-DNA titers indicate patient response.) Diffuse proliferative glomerulonephritis, a major complication of SLE, requires treatment with large doses of steroids. If renal failure occurs, dialysis or kidney transplant may be necessary. In some patients, cytotoxic drugs may delay or prevent deteriorating renal status. Antihypertensive drugs and dietary changes may also be warranted in renal disease. Antimalarials are helpful in treating skin, musculoskeletal, and systemic effects. For more serious cases of SLE, immunosuppressants may aid patients who have not responded to other drugs.

The photosensitive patient should wear protective clothing (hat, sunglasses, long sleeves, and slacks) and use a screening agent, with a sun protection factor of at least 15, when outdoors. Because SLE usually strikes females of childbearing age, questions about pregnancy commonly arise. Available evidence indicates that a woman with SLE can have a safe, successful pregnancy if the patient has no serious renal or neurologic impairment.

Special considerations

Careful assessment, supportive measures, emotional support, and patient education are all important parts of the care plan for patients with SLE.

◆ Watch for constitutional symptoms: joint pain or stiffness, weakness, fever, fatigue, and chills. Observe for dyspnea, chest pain, and any edema of the extremities. Note the size, type, and location of skin lesions. Check urine for hematuria, scalp for hair loss, and skin and mucous membranes for petechiae, bleeding, ulceration, pallor, and bruising.

◆ Provide a balanced diet. Renal involvement may mandate a low-sodium, low-protein diet.

◆ Urge the patient to get plenty of rest. Schedule diagnostic tests and procedures to allow adequate rest. Explain all tests and procedures. Tell the patient that several blood samples are needed initially, then periodically, to monitor progress.

◆ Apply heat packs to relieve joint pain and stiffness. Encourage regular exercise to maintain full ROM and prevent contractures. Teach ROM exercises as well as body alignment and postural techniques. Arrange for physical therapy and occupational counseling as appropriate.

◆ Explain the expected benefit of prescribed medications. Watch for adverse effects, especially when the patient is taking high doses of corticosteroids.

◆ Advise the patient receiving cyclophosphamide to maintain adequate hydration. If prescribed, give mesna to prevent hemorrhagic cystitis and ondansetron to prevent nausea and vomiting.

◆ Monitor vital signs, intake and output, weight, and laboratory reports. Check pulse rates and observe for orthopnea. Check stools and GI secretions for blood.

◆ Observe for hypertension, weight gain, and other signs of renal involvement.

◆ Assess for signs of neurologic damage: personality change, paranoid or psychotic behavior, ptosis, or diplopia. Take seizure precautions. If Raynaud phenomenon is present, warm and protect the patient's hands and feet.

◆ Offer cosmetic tips such as suggesting the use of hypoallergenic makeup and refer the patient to a hairdresser who specializes in scalp disorders.

◆ Advise the patient to purchase medications in quantity, if possible. Warn against "miracle" drugs for relief of arthritis symptoms.

◆ Refer the patient to the Lupus Foundation of America and the Arthritis Foundation as needed.

FIBROMYALGIA SYNDROME

Fibromyalgia syndrome (FMS), previously called fibrositis, is a diffuse pain syndrome and one of the most common causes of chronic musculoskeletal pain. It's characterized by diffuse musculoskeletal pain, daily fatigue, and poor-quality sleep, along with multiple tender points on examination (in specific areas). More women than men are affected, and although FMS may occur at almost any age, the peak incidence is in patients between ages 20 and 60.

FMS has also been reported in children, who have more diffuse pain and a higher incidence of sleep disturbances than adult patients. They may have fewer tender points and typically improve after 2 to 3 years of follow-up.

Causes and incidence

The cause of FMS is unknown, but it may be a primary disorder or occur in association with an underlying disease, such as SLE, RA, osteoarthritis, and sleep apnea syndrome.

The pain is located mainly in muscle areas, but no distinct abnormalities have been documented on microscopic evaluation of biopsies of tender points when compared with normal muscle. One theory suggests that blood flow to the muscle is decreased (because of poor muscle aerobic conditioning, rather than other physiologic abnormalities); another suggests cerebral blood flow in the thalamus and caudate nucleus is decreased, leading to a lowered pain threshold. Still other theories suggest that the cause lies in endocrine dysfunction, such as abnormal pituitary–adrenal axis responses, or in abnormal levels of the neurotransmitter serotonin in brain centers, which affect pain and sleep. Abnormal functioning of other pain-processing pathways may also be involved.

Considerable overlap of symptoms with other pain syndromes, such as chronic fatigue syndrome (CFS), raises the question of association with microbial infection, such as parvovirus B19.

The development of FMS may be multifactorial and influenced by stress (physical and mental), physical conditioning, poor-quality sleep, neuroendocrine factors, psychiatric factors, and possibly, hormonal factors (explaining the predominance in women).

Pathophysiology

Fibromyalgia is currently understood to be a disorder of central pain processing or a syndrome of central sensitivity. Research has provided evidence for altered functional connectivity and chemistry in the pain-processing system of the brain.

Complications

◆ Mental fog
◆ Constant pain
◆ Fatigue
◆ Lack of sleep
◆ Depression
◆ Death from suicide or injury

Signs and symptoms

The primary symptom is diffuse, dull, aching pain that's typically concentrated across the neck and shoulders as well as in the lower back and proximal limbs. It can involve all body quadrants (bilateral upper trunk and arms, and bilateral lower trunk and legs) and typically is worse in the morning, when it's associated with stiffness. The pain can vary from day to day and can be exacerbated by stress, lack of sleep, weather changes, and inactivity.

Sleep disturbance and fatigue are commonly reported. The patient awakens feeling fatigued and remains so throughout the day. Fatigue is commonly present from a half hour to several hours after rising in the morning and can last for the rest of the day.

Other associated features that can occur with FMS include irritable bowel syndrome, tension headaches, puffy hands (sensation of hand swelling, especially in the morning), and paresthesia.

Diagnosis

FMS is diagnosed in a patient with characteristic symptoms, multiple tender points on examination, and exclusion of other illnesses that can cause similar features. Tender points are elicited by applying a moderate amount of pressure to specific locations. This examination can be fairly subjective, but many FMS patients with true tender points wince or withdraw when pressure is applied at a certain intensity. Nontender control points can also be tested to assess for conversion reactions (psychogenic rheumatism), in which patients hurt everywhere or exhibit other psychosomatic illnesses. (See *Tender points of fibromyalgia.*)

Treatment

NSAIDs and acetaminophen may help relieve the pain and stiffness of fibromyalgia. Antidepressants such as duloxetine and milnacipran may be used to lessen pain and fatigue. Antiseizure drugs, including gabapentin and pregabalin, may aid in reducing fibromyalgia pain.

Tender points of fibromyalgia

The patient with fibromyalgia may report specific areas of tenderness. These areas are indicated in the illustrations below.

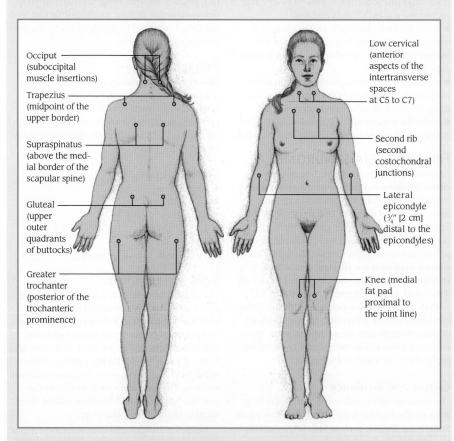

Occiput (suboccipital muscle insertions)

Trapezius (midpoint of the upper border)

Supraspinatus (above the medial border of the scapular spine)

Gluteal (upper outer quadrants of buttocks)

Greater trochanter (posterior of the trochanteric prominence)

Low cervical (anterior aspects of the intertransverse spaces at C5 to C7)

Second rib (second costochondral junctions)

Lateral epicondyle ($\frac{3}{4}$" [2 cm] distal to the epicondyles)

Knee (medial fat pad proximal to the joint line)

A physical therapist may assist in the management of FMS through the use of education, injection of tender points, massage therapy, and ultrasound treatments for particular problem areas. In a few studies, acupuncture, phototherapy, and mind-body exercises (such as yoga and tai chi) have been somewhat beneficial.

Special considerations

◆ The most important aspect of FMS management is patient education. Patients must understand that although FMS pain can be severe and is often chronic, the syndrome is common and doesn't lead to deforming or life-threatening complications.

◆ A regular, low-impact aerobic exercise can be effective in improving the patient's muscle conditioning, energy level, and overall sense of well-being. The FMS patient should be taught preexercise and postexercise stretching to minimize injury. Strongly encourage a low-intensity exercise program, such as walking, bicycling, or swimming, and to increase level of intensity as tolerated.

GOODPASTURE SYNDROME

In Goodpasture syndrome, hemoptysis and rapidly progressive glomerulonephritis follow the deposition of antibody against the alveolar and glomerular basement membrane (GBM). The prognosis improves with aggressive immunosuppressive and antibiotic therapy along with dialysis or renal transplantation.

Causes and incidence

The cause of Goodpasture syndrome is unknown. Although some cases have been associated with exposure to hydrocarbons or type 2 influenza, many have no precipitating events. The high incidence of HLA DRW2 in these patients suggests a genetic predisposition.

This syndrome may occur at any age but is most common in men between ages 20 and 30. A second peak incidence occurs between ages 50 and 70, with men and women in this age group affected equally.

Pathophysiology

Abnormal production and deposition of antibody against GBM and alveolar basement membrane activate the complement and inflammatory responses, resulting in glomerular and alveolar tissue damage.

Complications

◆ Renal failure
◆ Pulmonary edema and hemorrhage

Signs and symptoms

Goodpasture syndrome may initially cause malaise, fatigue, and pallor associated with severe iron deficiency anemia. Pulmonary findings range from slight dyspnea and cough with blood-tinged sputum to hemoptysis and frank pulmonary hemorrhage. Subclinical pulmonary bleeding may precede overt hemorrhage and renal disease by months or years. Usually, renal findings are subtler, although some patients note hematuria and peripheral edema.

Diagnosis

℞ CONFIRMING DIAGNOSIS *Confirmation of Goodpasture syndrome requires measurement of circulating anti-GBM antibody by radioimmunoassay and linear staining of GBM and alveolar basement membrane by immunofluorescence.*

Immunofluorescence of alveolar basement membrane shows linear deposition of Ig as well as complement 3 and fibrinogen. Immunofluorescence of GBM also shows linear deposition of Ig combined with detection of circulating anti-GBM antibody. This finding distinguishes Goodpasture from other pulmonary-renal syndromes, such as Wegener granulomatosis, polyarteritis, and SLE.

A lung biopsy reveals interstitial and intra-alveolar hemorrhage with hemosiderin-laden macrophages. Chest X-ray reveals pulmonary infiltrates in a diffuse, nodular pattern, and renal biopsy commonly shows focal necrotic lesions and cellular crescents.

Creatinine and BUN levels typically increase two to three times normal. Urinalysis may reveal RBCs and cellular casts, which typify glomerular inflammation. Granular casts and proteinuria may also be observed.

Treatment

Treatment aims to remove antibody by plasmapheresis and to suppress antibody production with immunosuppressive drugs, such as cyclophosphamide, to stop attacks by immune cells on the kidneys and lungs. Patients with renal failure may benefit from dialysis or transplantation. Aggressive ultrafiltration helps relieve pulmonary edema that may aggravate pulmonary hemorrhage. High-dose I.V. steroids also help control pulmonary hemorrhage.

Special considerations

◆ Promote adequate oxygenation by elevating the bed's head and administering humidified oxygen. Encourage the patient to conserve their energy. Assess respirations and breath sounds regularly; note sputum quantity and quality.

◆ Monitor vital signs, ABGs, hematocrit, and coagulation studies.

◆ Transfuse blood and administer steroids as ordered. Observe closely for drug adverse effects.

◆ Assess renal function by monitoring symptoms, intake and output, daily weights, creatinine clearance, and BUN and creatinine levels.

◆ Tell the patient and the family what signs and symptoms to expect and how to relieve them. Carefully describe other treatment measures such as dialysis.

REACTIVE ARTHRITIS

A self-limiting syndrome associated with polyarthritis (dominant feature), urethritis, balanitis (inflammation of the glans penis), conjunctivitis, and mucocutaneous lesions, reactive arthritis (ReA), previously known as *Reiter syndrome*, appears to be related to infection, either venereal or enteric.

Causes and incidence

The cause of ReA is unknown, but most cases follow venereal or enteric infection. Because 75% to 85% of patients with ReA test positive for the HLA-B27, genetic susceptibility is likely. ReA has followed infections caused by *Campylobacter*, *Salmonella*, *Yersinia*, and *Chlamydia* organisms.

This disease usually affects young males (ages 20 to 40); it's rare in females and children. However, due to the uncertainty of diagnosis and variations in the definition of this disorder, incidence is estimated at approximately 3.5 per 100,000 people. About 1% to 3% of all patients with nonspecific urethritis develop an episode of arthritis.

Pathophysiology

ReA is usually triggered by a GU or GI infection. Evidence indicates that a preceding *Chlamydia* respiratory infection may also trigger ReA. The frequency of ReA after enteric infection averages 1% to 4% but varies greatly, even among outbreaks of the same organism. Although severely symptomatic GI infections are associated with an increased risk of ReA, asymptomatic venereal infections more frequently cause this disease.

Complications

◆ Chronic heel pain

◆ Ankylosing spondylitis

◆ Persistent joint pain and swelling

Signs and symptoms

The patient with ReA may complain of dysuria, hematuria, urgent and frequent urination, and mucopurulent penile discharge, with swelling and reddening of the urethral meatus. Small painless ulcers may erupt on the glans penis (balanitis). These coalesce to form irregular patches that cover the penis and scrotum. The patient may also experience suprapubic pain, fever, anorexia with weight loss, and other GU complications, such as prostatitis and hemorrhagic cystitis.

Arthritic symptoms usually follow GU or enteric symptoms and last from 2 to 4 months. Asymmetrical and extremely variable polyarticular arthritis is most common, with a tendency to develop in weight-bearing joints of the legs and sometimes in the low back or sacroiliac joints. The arthritis is usually acute, with warm, erythematous, and painful joints, but it may be mild, with minimal synovitis. Muscle wasting is common near affected joints. Fingers and toes may swell and appear sausagelike.

Ocular symptoms include mild bilateral conjunctivitis, possibly complicated by keratitis, iritis, retinitis, or optic neuritis. In severe cases, burning, itching, and profuse mucopurulent discharge are possible.

In 30% of patients, skin lesions (keratoderma blennorrhagica) develop 4 to 6 weeks after onset of other symptoms and may last for several weeks. These macular to hyperkeratotic lesions commonly resemble those of psoriasis. They usually occur on the palms and soles but can develop anywhere on the trunk, extremities, or scalp. Nails become thick, opaque, and brittle; keratic debris accumulates under the nails. In many patients, painless, transient ulcerations erupt on the buccal mucosa, palate, and tongue.

Diagnosis

Nearly all patients with ReA test positive for HLA-B27 and have an elevated WBC count and ESR. Mild anemia may develop. Urethral discharge and synovial fluid contain many WBCs, mostly polymorphonuclear leukocytes. Synovial fluid is high in complement and protein and is grossly purulent. Cultures of discharge and synovial fluid rule out other causes such as gonococci.

During the first few weeks, X-rays are normal and may remain so, but some patients may show osteoporosis in inflamed areas. If inflammation persists, X-rays may show erosions of the small joints, periosteal proliferation (new bone formation) of involved joints, and calcaneal spurs.

Treatment

No specific treatment exists for ReA. Most patients recover in 2 to 16 weeks. About 50% of patients have recurring acute attacks, whereas the rest follow a chronic course, experiencing continued synovitis and sacroiliitis. In acute stages, limited weight bearing or complete bed rest may be necessary.

Any underlying infection should be treated with antibiotics. Arthritis is treated with nonsteroidal anti-inflammatory agents and pain relievers. Local administration of corticosteroids may help relieve persistent inflammation in one joint. Physical therapy includes ROM and strengthening exercises and the use of padded or supportive shoes to prevent contractures and foot deformities. Therapy to suppress the immune system may be considered in severe cases but is limited due to toxic adverse effects.

Special considerations

◆ Explain ReA. Discuss the medications and their possible adverse effects. Warn the patient to take medications with meals or milk to prevent GI bleeding.

◆ Encourage normal daily activity and moderate exercise. Suggest a firm mattress and encourage good posture and body mechanics.

◆ Arrange for occupational counseling if the patient has severe or chronic joint impairment.

SCLERODERMA

Scleroderma, also known as *systemic sclerosis*, is a diffuse connective tissue disease characterized by fibrotic, degenerative, and occasionally inflammatory changes in skin, blood vessels, synovial membranes, skeletal muscles, and internal organs (especially the esophagus, intestinal tract, thyroid, heart, lungs, and kidneys).

This disease can be classified as systemic (involving skin, blood vessels, and internal organs) or localized (limited to skin and tissues). Each classification has distinctive forms.

Systemic forms include:

◆ *limited cutaneous systemic sclerosis* (*or CREST syndrome*)—a benign form characterized by calcinosis, Raynaud phenomenon, esophageal dysfunction, sclerodactyly, and telangiectasia

◆ *diffuse cutaneous systemic sclerosis*—characterized by generalized skin thickening and invasion of internal organs

◆ *systemic sine scleroderma*—a rare form of the disease, includes involvement of internal organs but does not have skin involvement

Localized forms include:

◆ *morphea*—characterized by patchy skin changes with a droplike appearance

◆ *linear scleroderma*—characterized by a band of thickened skin on the face or extremities that severely damages underlying tissues, causing atrophy and deformity (most common in childhood)

Other forms include *chemically induced localized scleroderma, eosinophilia myalgia syndrome* (recently associated with ingestion of L-tryptophan), *toxic oil syndrome* (associated with contaminated oil), and *graft-versus-host disease*.

Causes and incidence

The cause of scleroderma is unknown. Risk factors include exposure to silica dust and polyvinyl chloride.

Scleroderma affects 300,000 people in the United States, more women than men, especially between ages 30 and 50. About 30% of patients with scleroderma die within 5 years of onset.

Complications

◆ Arrhythmias
◆ Dyspnea
◆ Malignant hypertension

Pathophysiology

The pathogenesis of systemic sclerosis is complex. Increasing evidence suggests an interaction between environmental and genetic factors, with a regulatory epigenetic mechanism involving changes in the expression of DNA and microRNA.

The clinical and pathologic manifestations result from three distinct processes: (1) severe fibroproliferative vascular lesions of small arteries and arterioles, (2) excessive and often progressive deposition of collagen and other extracellular matrix macromolecules in skin and various internal organs, and (3) alterations in humoral and cellular immunity. It is not clear which of these processes is of primary importance or how they are temporally related during the development and progression of the disease.

Complications

◆ Compromised circulation due to thickened vessels
◆ Decreased food intake or weight loss due to GI symptoms
◆ Arrhythmias
◆ Dyspnea
◆ Malignant hypertension

Signs and symptoms

Scleroderma typically begins with Raynaud phenomenon—blanching, cyanosis, and erythema of the fingers and toes in response to stress or exposure to cold. Progressive phalangeal resorption may shorten the fingers.

Compromised circulation, which results from abnormal thickening of the arterial intima, may cause slowly healing ulcerations on the tips of the fingers or toes that may lead to gangrene. Raynaud phenomenon may precede scleroderma by months or years.

Later symptoms include pain, stiffness, and finger and joint swelling. Skin thickening produces taut, shiny skin over the entire hand and forearm. Facial skin also becomes tight and inelastic, causing a masklike appearance and "pinching" of the mouth. As tightening progresses, contractures may develop.

GI dysfunction causes frequent reflux, heartburn, dysphagia, and bloating after meals. These symptoms may cause the patient to decrease food intake and lose weight. Other GI effects include abdominal distention, diarrhea, constipation, and malodorous floating stools.

Diagnosis

Typical cutaneous changes provide the first clue to diagnosis. Results of diagnostic tests include:
◆ blood studies—slightly elevated ESR, positive RF in 25% to 35% of patients, and positive ANA test
◆ chest X-rays—bilateral basilar pulmonary fibrosis
◆ electrocardiogram—possible nonspecific abnormalities related to myocardial fibrosis
◆ GI X-rays—distal esophageal hypomotility and stricture, duodenal loop dilation, small-bowel malabsorption pattern, and large diverticula
◆ hand X-rays—terminal phalangeal tuft resorption, subcutaneous calcification, and joint space narrowing and erosion
◆ pulmonary function studies—decreased diffusion and vital capacity and restrictive lung disease
◆ skin biopsy—may show changes consistent with the disease's progress, such as marked thickening of the dermis and occlusive vessel changes
◆ urinalysis—proteinuria, microscopic hematuria, and casts (with renal involvement)

Treatment

Currently, no cure exists for scleroderma. Treatment aims to preserve normal body functions and minimize complications. Use of an immunosuppressant is a common palliative measure. Corticosteroids, NSAIDs, cyclooxygenose-2 inhibitors, and analgesics help to alleviate joint pain and stiffness. Blood platelet levels need to be monitored throughout drug therapy.

Other treatments vary according to symptoms:
◆ chronic digital ulcerations—a digital plaster cast to immobilize the area, minimize trauma, and maintain cleanliness; possibly surgical debridement
◆ esophagitis with stricture—antacids, histamine-2 (H_2) receptor agonists, proton pump inhibitors, periodic esophageal dilation, and a soft, bland diet
◆ hand debilitation—physical therapy to maintain function and promote muscle strength, heat therapy to relieve joint stiffness, and patient teaching to make performance of daily activities easier
◆ Raynaud phenomenon—various vasodilators and antihypertensive agents (such as calcium channel blockers, angiotensin II receptor antagonists, or angiotensin-converting enzyme inhibitors), intermittent cervical sympathetic blockade, or, rarely, thoracic sympathectomy
◆ scleroderma kidney (with malignant hypertension and impending renal failure)—dialysis, antihypertensives, and calcium channel blockers
◆ small-bowel involvement (diarrhea, pain, malabsorption, and weight loss)—broad-spectrum antibiotics, such as erythromycin or tetracycline, to counteract bacterial overgrowth in the duodenum and jejunum related to hypomotility

Special considerations

◆ Assess the patient's motion restrictions, pain, vital signs, intake and output, respiratory function, and daily weight.
◆ Because of compromised circulation, warn against finger-stick blood tests.
◆ Remember that air-conditioning may aggravate Raynaud phenomenon.
◆ Help the patient and family adjust to the patient's new body image and to the limitations and dependence that these changes cause.
◆ Teach the patient to avoid fatigue by pacing activities and organizing schedules to include necessary rest.
◆ Stress to the patient and family the need to accept the fact that this condition is incurable. Encourage them to express their feelings and help them cope with their fears and frustrations by offering information about the disease, its treatment, and relevant diagnostic tests.
◆ Whenever possible, let the patient participate in treatment by measuring their own intake and output, planning their own diet, assisting in dialysis, performing their own heat therapy, and doing prescribed exercises.
◆ Direct the patient to seek out support groups, which can be found in every state. Instruct the patient to call 1-800-722-HOPE or go to *www.scleroderma.org*.

VASCULITIS

Vasculitis includes a broad spectrum of disorders characterized by inflammation and necrosis of blood vessels. Its clinical effects, which reflect tissue ischemia caused by blood flow obstruction, and confirming laboratory procedures depend on the vessels involved. The prognosis is variable. For example, hypersensitivity vasculitis is usually a benign disorder limited to the skin, but more extensive polyarteritis nodosa can be rapidly fatal. Vasculitis can occur at any age, except for mucocutaneous lymph node syndrome, which occurs only during childhood. Vasculitis may be a primary disorder or occur secondary to other disorders, such as RA or SLE.

Causes and incidence

How vascular damage develops in vasculitis isn't well understood. It has been associated with a history of serious infectious disease, such as hepatitis B or bacterial endocarditis, and high-dose antibiotic therapy.

Pathophysiology

Current theory holds that it's initiated by excessive circulating antigen, which triggers the formation of soluble antigen–antibody complexes. These complexes can't be effectively cleared by the reticuloendothelial system, so they're deposited in blood vessel walls (type III hypersensitivity). Increased vascular permeability associated with the release of vasoactive amines by platelets and basophils enhances such deposition. The deposited complexes activate the complement cascade, resulting in chemotaxis of neutrophils, which release lysosomal enzymes. In turn, these enzymes cause vessel damage and necrosis, which may precipitate thrombosis, occlusion, hemorrhage, and ischemia.

Another mechanism that may contribute to vascular damage is the cell-mediated (T-cell) immune response. In this response, circulating antigen triggers the release of soluble mediators by sensitized lymphocytes, which attracts macrophages. The macrophages release intracellular enzymes, which cause vascular damage. They can also transform into the epithelioid and multinucleated giant cells that typify the granulomatous vasculitides. Phagocytosis of immune complexes by macrophages enhances granuloma formation.

Complications

- Renal failure
- Renal hypertension
- Glomerulitis
- Fibrous scarring of lung tissue
- Stroke
- GI bleeding
- Necrotizing vasculitis
- Spontaneous hemorrhage
- Intestinal obstruction
- Myocardial infarction
- Pericarditis
- Rupture of mesenteric aneurysms

Signs and symptoms

The clinical effects of vasculitis vary according to the blood vessels involved.

Diagnosis

Laboratory tests performed to confirm a diagnosis of vasculitis depend on the blood vessels involved. (See *Types of vasculitis,* pages 426 to 428.)

Treatment

Treatment of vasculitis aims to minimize irreversible tissue damage associated with ischemia. In primary vasculitis, treatment may involve removal of an offending antigen or use of anti-inflammatory or immunosuppressant drugs. For example, antigenic drugs, food, and other environmental substances should be identified and eliminated, if possible.

Drug therapy in primary vasculitis commonly involves low-dose cyclophosphamide (2 mg/kg orally daily) with daily corticosteroids. In rapidly fulminant vasculitis, cyclophosphamide dosage may be increased to 4 mg/kg daily for the first 2 to 3 days, followed by the regular dose. Prednisone should be given in a dose of 1 mg/kg/day in divided doses for 7 to 10 days, with consolidation to a single morning dose by 2 to 3 weeks. When the vasculitis appears to be in remission or when prescribed cytotoxic drugs take full effect, corticosteroids are tapered down to a single daily dose. Finally, an alternate-day schedule of steroids may continue for 3 to 6 months before slow discontinuation of steroids.

In secondary vasculitis, treatment focuses on the underlying disorder.

Special considerations

- Assess patients with Wegener granulomatosis for dry nasal mucosa. Instill nose drops to lubricate the mucosa and help diminish crusting, or irrigate the nasal passages with warm normal saline solution.
- Monitor vital signs. Use a Doppler ultrasonic flowmeter, if available, to auscultate blood pressure in patients with Takayasu arteritis, whose peripheral pulses are generally difficult to palpate.

Types of vasculitis

Vasculitis occurs in various forms; diagnosis depends on the presenting signs and symptoms.

Type	Vessels involved	Signs and symptoms	Diagnosis
Polyarteritis nodosa	Small to medium arteries throughout the body (Lesions tend to be segmental, occur at bifurcations and branchings of arteries, and spread distally to arterioles. In severe cases, lesions circumferentially involve adjacent veins.)	Hypertension, abdominal pain, myalgias, headache, joint pain, and weakness	History of symptoms; elevated erythrocyte sedimentation rate (ESR) and blood urea nitrogen and creatinine levels; leukocytosis; anemia; thrombocytosis; depressed C3 complement; rheumatoid factor > 1:60; circulating immune complexes; tissue biopsy showing necrotizing vasculitis
Allergic angiitis and granulomatosis (Churg–Strauss syndrome)	Small to medium arteries (including arterioles, capillaries, and venules), mainly of the lungs, kidneys, but also other organs	Resembles polyarteritis nodosa with hallmark of severe pulmonary involvement	History of asthma; eosinophilia; increased immunoglobulin (Ig) E level; tissue biopsy showing granulomatous inflammation with eosinophilic infiltration
Polyangiitis overlap syndrome (microscopic polyangiitis)	Small to medium arteries (including arterioles, capillaries, and venules) of the lungs and other organs	Combines symptoms of polyarteritis nodosa, allergic angiitis, and granulomatosis	Possible history of allergy; eosinophilia; tissue biopsy showing granulomatous inflammation with eosinophilic infiltration
Wegener granulomatosis	Medium to large vessels of the respiratory tract and kidney; may also involve small arteries and veins	Fever, pulmonary congestion, cough, malaise, anorexia, weight loss, and mild to severe hematuria	Tissue biopsy showing necrotizing vasculitis with granulomatous inflammation; leukocytosis; elevated ESR and immunoglobulin IgA and IgG levels; low titer rheumatoid factor; circulating immune complexes; antineutrophil cytoplasmic antibody in >90% of patients
Temporal arteritis (giant cell arteritis)	Medium to large arteries, most commonly branches of the carotid artery	Fever, myalgia, jaw claudication, visual changes, and headache (associated with polymyalgia rheumatica syndrome)	Decreased hemoglobin (Hb) level; elevated ESR; tissue biopsy showing panarteritis with infiltration of mononuclear cells, giant cells within vessel wall, fragmentation of internal elastic lamina, and proliferation of intima

Types of vasculitis (*continued*)

Type	Vessels involved	Signs and symptoms	Diagnosis
Takayasu arteritis (aortic arch syndrome)	Medium to large arteries, particularly the aortic arch, its branches and, possibly, the pulmonary artery	Malaise, pallor, nausea, night sweats, arthralgias, anorexia, weight loss, pain or paresthesia distal to affected area, bruits, loss of distal pulses, syncope and, if a carotid artery is involved, diplopia and transient blindness; may progress to heart failure or stroke	Decreased Hb level; leukocytosis; positive lupus erythematosus cell preparation and elevated ESR; arteriography showing calcification and obstruction of affected vessels; tissue biopsy showing inflammation of adventitia and intima of vessels, and thickening of vessel walls
Hypersensitivity vasculitis	Small vessels, especially of the skin	Palpable purpura, papules, nodules, vesicles, bullae, ulcers, or chronic or recurrent urticaria	History of exposure to antigen, such as a microorganism or drug; tissue biopsy showing leukocytoclastic angiitis, usually in postcapillary venules, with infiltration of polymorphonuclear leukocytes, fibrinoid necrosis, and extravasation of erythrocytes
Mucocutaneous lymph node syndrome (Kawasaki disease)	Small to medium vessels, primarily of the lymph nodes; may progress to involve coronary arteries	Fever; nonsuppurative cervical adenitis; edema; congested conjunctivae; erythema of oral cavity, lips, and palms; and desquamation of fingertips; may progress to arthritis, myocarditis, pericarditis, myocardial infarction, and cardiomegaly	History of symptoms; elevated ESR; tissue biopsy showing intimal proliferation and infiltration of vessel walls with mononuclear cells; echocardiography necessary
Behçet disease	Small vessels, primarily of the mouth and genitalia, but also of the eyes, skin, joints, GI tract, and central nervous system	Recurrent oral ulcers, eye lesions, genital lesions, and cutaneous lesions	History of symptoms

(continued)

Types of vasculitis (continued)

Type	Vessels involved	Signs and symptoms	Diagnosis
Henoch–Schön-lein purpura	Any blood vessel in the skin	Red to purple papule skin lesions, pain, infarction, joint pain, numbness, weakness, fever, fatigue, dys-menorrhea, heart-burn, dysphonia, and dysphagia	History of symptoms; biopsy showing leuko-cytoclastic vasculitis; abdominal imaging studies demonstrating decreased motility and dilated loops of bowel; and elevated ESR
Rheumatoid vasculitis	Small and medium vessels, especially of the eyes, skin, hands, and feet	Digital ischemia of fingers and toes, scleritis, fever, weight loss, wrist drop	History of rheumatoid arthritis, symptoms; elevated ESR or C-reac-tive protein and rheu-matoid factors; low antinuclear antibody

◆ Monitor intake and output. Check daily for edema. Keep the patient well hydrated (3 L daily) to reduce the risk of hemorrhagic cystitis associated with cyclophosphamide therapy.
◆ Provide emotional support to help the patient and family cope with an altered body image— the result of the disorder or its therapy (e.g., Wegener granulomatosis may be associated with saddle nose, steroids may cause weight gain, and cyclophosphamide may cause alopecia).
◆ Teach the patient how to recognize drug ad-verse effects. Monitor the patient's WBC count during cyclophosphamide therapy to prevent severe leukopenia.

POLYMYOSITIS AND DERMATOMYOSITIS

Diffuse, inflammatory myopathies of unknown cause, polymyositis and dermatomyositis pro-duce symmetrical weakness of striated muscle— primarily proximal muscles of the shoulder and pelvic girdles, neck, and pharynx. In dermato-myositis, such muscle weakness is accompanied by cutaneous involvement. These diseases usually progress slowly, with frequent exacer-bations and remissions. They occur in twice as many females as males (except dermatomyositis with malignant tumor, which is most common in males older than age 40).

The prognosis usually worsens with age. Death commonly occurs from associated can-cer, respiratory disease, or heart failure or from the adverse effects of drug therapy. On the other hand, 80% to 90% of affected children regain normal function with proper treatment. How-ever, if untreated, childhood dermatomyositis

may progress rapidly to disabling contractures and muscle atrophy.

Causes and incidence

Although the cause of polymyositis remains puzzling, researchers believe that it may result from an autoimmune reaction. Polymyositis and dermatomyositis may be associated with other disorders, such as allergic reactions; SLE; scleroderma; RA; Sjögren syndrome; carcino-mas of the lung, breast, or other organs; and systemic viral infection; or D-penicillamine administration.

Annual incidence is 5 to 10 in 100,000 people.

Pathophysiology

Presumably, the patient's T cells inappropriately recognize muscle fiber antigens as foreign and attack muscle tissue, causing diffuse or focal muscle fiber degeneration. (Regeneration of new muscle cells then follows, producing remission.)

Complications
◆ Rhabdomyolysis
◆ Interstitial lung disease
◆ Cardiovascular disease
◆ Infection
◆ Dysphagia
◆ Overlapping autoimmune diseases

Signs and symptoms

Polymyositis begins acutely or insidiously with muscle weakness, tenderness, and discomfort. It affects proximal muscles more than distal muscles and impairs performance of ordinary activities. The patient may have trouble getting up from a chair, combing their hair, reaching into a high cupboard, climbing stairs, or even raising their head from a pillow. Other muscular symptoms include inability to move against resistance, proximal dysphagia, dysphonia, and difficulty breathing.

In dermatomyositis, an erythematous rash usually erupts on the face, neck, upper back, chest, and arms as well as around the nail beds. A characteristic heliotrope rash appears on the eyelids, accompanied by periorbital edema. Gottron papules (violet, flat-topped lesions) may appear on the interphalangeal joints.

Diagnosis

CONFIRMING DIAGNOSIS *Diagnosis requires a muscle biopsy that shows necrosis, degeneration, regeneration, and interstitial chronic lymphocytic infiltration. Magnetic resonance imaging and an electrocardiogram, as well as the use of electromyography, aid in diagnosis.*

Other tests differentiate polymyositis from diseases that cause similar muscular or cutaneous symptoms, such as muscular dystrophy, advanced trichinosis, psoriasis, seborrheic dermatitis, and SLE.

Typical laboratory results in polymyositis include elevated ESR, elevated WBC count, and elevated muscle enzyme levels (creatine kinase, aldolase, and serum aspartate aminotransferase) not attributable to hemolysis of RBCs or hepatic or other diseases. Other laboratory results include increased urine creatine level (>150 mg/24 hours), decreased creatinine level, and positive antinuclear antibodies. Electromyography shows polyphasic short-duration potentials, fibrillation (positive spike waves), and bizarre high-frequency repetitive changes.

Treatment

High-dose corticosteroid therapy relieves inflammation and lowers muscle enzyme levels. Within 2 to 6 weeks after treatment, serum muscle enzyme levels usually return to normal, and muscle strength improves, permitting a gradual tapering down of corticosteroid dosage. If the patient responds poorly to corticosteroids, treatment may include cytotoxic or immunosuppressant drugs. Supportive therapy includes bed rest during the acute phase, ROM exercises to prevent contractures, analgesics and application of heat to relieve painful muscle spasms, and diphenhydramine to relieve itching. Patients older than age 40 need thorough assessment for coexisting cancer.

Special considerations

◆ Assess level of pain, muscle weakness, and ROM daily. Give analgesics as needed.

◆ If the patient is confined to bed, prevent pressure ulcers by giving good skin care. To prevent footdrop and contractures, apply high-topped sneakers, and assist with passive ROM exercises at least four times daily. Teach the patient's family how to perform these exercises on the patient.

◆ If 24-hour urine collection for creatine or creatinine is necessary, make sure your coworkers understand the procedure. When you assist with muscle biopsy, make sure the biopsy isn't taken from an area of recent needle insertion.

◆ If the patient has a rash, warn the patient not to scratch, as it may cause infection. If antipruritic medication doesn't relieve severe itching, apply tepid sponges or compresses.

◆ Encourage the patient to feed and dress to the best of their ability but to ask for help when needed. Advise the patient to pace activities to counteract muscle weakness. Encourage the patient to express anxiety. Ease the fear of dependence by reassuring the patient that muscle weakness is probably temporary.

◆ Explain the disease to the patient and family. Prepare them for diagnostic procedures and possible adverse effects of corticosteroid therapy (weight gain, hirsutism, hypertension, edema, amenorrhea, purplish striae, glycosuria, acne, and easy bruising). Advise a low-sodium diet to prevent fluid retention. Emphatically warn against abruptly discontinuing corticosteroids. Reassure the patient that steroid-induced weight gain will diminish when the drug is discontinued.

Immunodeficiency

AGAMMAGLOBULINEMIA

Agammaglobulinemia is a recessive, congenital disorder in which all five Igs—IgM, IgG, IgA, IgD, and IgE—and circulating B cells are absent or deficient but T cells are intact. It's also called *Bruton agammaglobulinemia* and *X-linked agammaglobulinemia*. Affecting males almost exclusively, this disorder causes severe, recurrent infections during infancy. Prognosis is good with early treatment, except in infants who develop polio or persistent viral infection. Infection usually causes some permanent damage, especially in the neurologic or respiratory system.

Causes and incidence

Humoral (B-cell) immune deficiencies account for 50% of all primary immunodeficiencies. IgA deficiency is the most common antibody deficiency syndrome, followed by common variable immunodeficiency (CVID). The incidence of these two disorders is 1 in 700 persons.

Selective IgM deficiency is rare. IgG4 deficiency occurs in 10% to 15% of the population.

Pathophysiology
B cells and B-cell precursors may be present in the bone marrow and peripheral blood, but a mutation in the B-cell protein tyrosine kinase keeps B cells from maturing and secreting Ig. Without protective Igs, the affected person develops repeated infections.

Complications
◆ Chronic otitis media
◆ Chronic sinusitis
◆ Encephalitis
◆ Failure to thrive
◆ Hepatitis
◆ Enteroviral infections
◆ Meningitis

Signs and symptoms
Typically, the infant with agammaglobulinemia is asymptomatic until age 6 months, when transplacental maternal Igs that provided immunity have been depleted. The patient then develops recurrent bacterial otitis media, pneumonia, dermatitis, bronchitis, and meningitis—usually caused by pneumococci, streptococci, *Haemophilus influenzae*, or other gram-negative organisms. Purulent conjunctivitis, abnormal dental caries, and polyarthritis resembling RA may also occur. Severe malabsorption associated with infestation by *Giardia lamblia* may retard development. Despite recurrent infections, lymphadenopathy and splenomegaly are usually absent.

Diagnosis
The diagnosis of agammaglobulinemia can be especially difficult because recurrent infections are common even in normal infants (many of whom don't start producing their own antibodies until age 18 to 20 months). Immunoelectrophoresis and quantitative Igs (nephelometry) confirm decreased levels, or a total absence, of IgM, IgA, and IgG in the serum. IgG is usually less than 200 mg/dL, and IgA and IgM are almost unmeasurable. However, diagnosis by this method usually isn't possible until the infant is 9 months old. Antigenic stimulation confirms an inability to produce specific antibodies, although cellular immunity remains intact. Flow cytometry may be helpful in measuring circulating B lymphocytes.

Treatment
Treatment aims to prevent or control infections and to boost the patient's immune response.

Injection of immune serum globulin (gamma globulin, IV Ig) helps maintain immune response. Because these injections are painful, give them deep into a large muscle mass, such as the gluteal or thigh muscles, and massage well. If the dosage is more than 1.5 mL, divide it and inject it into more than one site; for frequent injections, rotate the injection sites. Because immune globulin is composed primarily of IgG, the patient may also need fresh frozen plasma infusions to provide IgA and IgM. Mucosal secretory IgA can't be replaced by therapy, resulting in crippling pulmonary disease in many patients.

The judicious use of antibiotics also helps combat infection; in some cases, chronic broad-spectrum antibiotics may be indicated. During acute infection, monitor the patient closely. Maintain adequate nutrition and hydration. Perform chest physiotherapy if required.

Special considerations
◆ Carefully explain all treatment measures, and make sure the patient and family understand the disorder.
◆ Teach the patient and family how to recognize early signs of infection and counsel them to report such signs promptly. Advise them to have cuts and scrapes cleaned immediately. Warn them to avoid crowds and people who have active infections.
◆ Advise parents that live-virus vaccines are contraindicated due to the potential to cause infections.
◆ Suggest genetic counseling if parents have questions about vulnerability of future offspring.

COMMON VARIABLE IMMUNODEFICIENCY
CVID is characterized by progressive deterioration of B-cell (humoral) immunity, resulting in increased susceptibility to infection.

Causes and incidence
The cause of CVID is unknown.

Unlike agammaglobulinemia, this disorder (also known as *acquired hypogammaglobulinemia*) usually causes symptoms after infancy and childhood, between ages 25 and 40. It affects males and females equally and usually doesn't interfere with normal life span or normal pregnancy and offspring.

Pathophysiology
Most patients have a normal circulating B-cell count but defective synthesis or release of Igs.

Many also exhibit progressive deterioration of T-cell (cell-mediated) immunity revealed by delayed hypersensitivity skin testing.

Complications
◆ Conjunctivitis
◆ Chronic sinusitis
◆ *Giardia lamblia* GI infestation
◆ Upper and lower respiratory tract infections
◆ Encephalitis
◆ Meningitis
◆ Hemolytic anemia

Signs and symptoms
In CVID, pyogenic bacterial infections are characteristic but tend to be chronic rather than acute (as in agammaglobulinemia). Recurrent sinopulmonary infections, chronic bacterial conjunctivitis, and malabsorption (associated with infestation by *G. lamblia*) are usually the first clues to immunodeficiency.

CVID may be associated with autoimmune diseases, such as SLE, RA, hemolytic anemia, and pernicious anemia, and with cancers, such as leukemia and lymphoma.

Diagnosis
Characteristic diagnostic markers in this disorder are decreased serum Ig (IgM, IgA, and IgG) levels detected by immunoelectrophoresis, along with a normal circulating B-cell count. Antigenic stimulation confirms an inability to produce specific antibodies; cell-mediated immunity may be intact or delayed. X-rays usually show signs of chronic lung disease or sinusitis.

Treatment
Treatment and care of patients with CVID are essentially the same as for those with agammaglobulinemia.

Injection of immune globulin (usually weekly to monthly) helps maintain the immune response. Because these injections are painful, give them deep into a large muscle mass, such as the gluteal or thigh muscles, and massage well. If the dosage is more than 1.5 mL, divide the dose and inject it into more than one site; for frequent injections, rotate the injection sites. Because immune globulin is composed primarily of IgG, the patient may also need fresh frozen plasma infusions to provide IgA and IgM.

Antibiotics are the mainstay for combating infection. Regular X-rays and pulmonary function studies help monitor lung infection; chest physiotherapy may be ordered to forestall or help clear such infection.

Special considerations
◆ Teach the patient and family how to recognize early signs of infection and counsel them to report such signs promptly. Advise the patient to avoid crowds and people who have active infections.
◆ Stress the importance of good nutrition and regular follow-up care.

IgA DEFICIENCY
Total absence or severe deficiency of IgA, also known as *selective IgA deficiency*, is the most common primary Ig deficiency, appearing in as many as 1 in 400 to 1,000 people. IgA—the major Ig in human saliva, nasal and bronchial fluids, and intestinal secretions—guards against bacterial and viral reinfections. Consequently, IgA deficiency leads to chronic sinopulmonary infections, allergies, chronic diarrhea, GI diseases, and other disorders. The prognosis is good for patients who receive correct treatment, especially if they have no associated disorders.

Causes and incidence
IgA deficiency seems to be linked to autosomal dominant or recessive inheritance. The disorder has familial trends and occurs frequently in immediate relatives of individuals with CVID. Congenital intrauterine infection with rubella, toxoplasmosis, or cytomegalovirus can result in selective IgA deficiency. Treatment for seizures with phenytoin and hydantoin, as well as Wilson disease (an inherited disorder treated with penicillamine), can result in temporarily acquired selective IgA deficiency. When the medications are stopped, the IgA level returns to normal. Some drugs, such as anticonvulsants, may cause transient IgA deficiency.

Pathophysiology
The presence of normal numbers of peripheral blood lymphocytes carrying IgA receptors and of normal amounts of other Igs suggests that B cells may not be secreting IgA, as they haven't matured into IgA-producing plasma cells.

Signs and symptoms
Some IgA-deficient patients have no symptoms, possibly because they have extra amounts of low–molecular-weight IgM. This Ig takes over IgA function and helps maintain immunologic defenses. Among patients who develop symptoms, chronic sinopulmonary infection is the most common. Other effects are respiratory allergy, often triggered by infection; GI tract diseases, such as celiac disease, ulcerative colitis, and regional enteritis; autoimmune diseases,

such as RA, SLE, immunohemolytic anemia, and chronic hepatitis; and malignant tumors, such as squamous cell carcinoma of the lungs, reticulum cell sarcoma, and thymoma.

Age of onset varies. Some IgA-deficient children with recurrent respiratory disease and middle ear inflammation may begin to synthesize IgA spontaneously as recurrent infections subside and their condition improves.

Diagnosis

Serum immunoelectrophoresis and quantitative immunologic analyses of patients with IgA deficiency show serum IgA levels below 7 mg/dL. Although IgA is usually absent from secretions in patients with IgA deficiency, levels may be normal in rare cases. IgE is normal, whereas IgM may be normal or elevated in serum and secretions. Normally absent low–molecular-weight IgM may be present.

Tests may also indicate autoantibodies and antibodies against IgG (RF), IgM, and bovine milk. Cell-mediated immunity and secretory piece (the glycopeptide that transports IgA) are usually normal, and most circulating B cells appear normal.

Treatment

Selective IgA deficiency has no known cure. Treatment aims to control symptoms of associated diseases, such as respiratory and GI infections, and is generally the same as for a patient with normal IgA.

⚠ ALERT *Don't give an IgA-deficient patient immune globulin (IV Ig) because sensitization may lead to anaphylaxis during future administration of blood products.*

If transfusion with blood products is necessary, minimize the risk of adverse reaction by using washed RBCs or avoid the reaction completely by crossmatching the patient's blood with that of an IgA-deficient donor.

Special considerations

Because this is a lifelong disorder, teach the patient to prevent infection, to recognize its early signs, and to seek treatment promptly.

DiGEORGE SYNDROME

DiGeorge syndrome (DGS), also called *22q11.2 deletion syndrome*, is a disorder caused by a large deletion from chromosome 22. This deletion means that several genes from this region are not present in DGS patients. The variation in the symptoms of the disease appears to be related to the amount of genetic material lost in the chromosomal deletion. DGS can affect a few or many body systems. Problems that

---

> ## Role of the thymus in immune response
>
> The thymus provides an environment in which T cells develop and learn to distinguish self from nonself during fetal and early postnatal stages. Most cells that enter the thymus are destroyed. T-cell clones that react strongly to self and those that don't recognize self are deleted (negative selection). T-cell clones that recognize self but don't react strongly against self are positively selected.
>
> After early life, mature T cells reside primarily in peripheral lymph organs and recirculate in blood and lymph.

---

are commonly associated with this syndrome include heart defects, cleft palate, and developmental and behavioral disorders.

In addition, some neonates may present with immunologic problems. Errors during fetal development of the third and fourth pharyngeal pouches interfere with thymus formation; the thymus may be completely absent or partially present in an abnormal location, causing deficient T-cell (cell-mediated) immunity. (See *Role of the thymus in immune response.*) As a result, recurrent infections or difficulty with vaccinations may occur. Many children outgrow these problems by age 1 year. However, some continue with problems throughout childhood and into adulthood. These immunodeficiency problems include Graves disease, idiopathic thrombocytopenia, and juvenile arthritis.

Causes and incidence

DGS is caused by a genetic defect on chromosome 22. This syndrome is present in 1 in 4,000 live births. It may also be found in 1 in 68 children with congenital heart defects, and 5% to 8% of children born with a cleft palate.

Pathophysiology

The 22q11.2 deletion results in a range of embryonic developmental disruptions involving the head, neck, brain, skeleton, and kidneys. Portions of the heart, head and neck, thymus, and parathyroids derive from the third and fourth pharyngeal pouches, and this developmental field is disrupted due to the chromosomal microdeletion. This, in turn, leads to hypocalcemia and variable T-cell deficiency. A combined T- and B-cell deficiency in part results from lack of T-helper cell function as seen in cases of complete 22q11.2DS.

Complications
- Hypocalcemia (life-threatening)
- Seizures
- CNS damage
- Failure to thrive
- Anorexia
- Diarrhea
- Weight loss
- Cardiac failure

Signs and symptoms
Symptoms are usually obvious at birth or shortly thereafter. An infant with DGS may have low-set prominent ears, notched ear pinnae, a mouth without the usual bow-shaped lip, an undersized jaw, and abnormally wide-set eyes (hypertelorism) that are low-set and posteriorly angulated. Additionally, an infant may have a bifid uvula and a high, arched palate. Congenital heart anomalies are common. Cardiovascular abnormalities include great blood vessel anomalies (these may also develop soon after birth) and tetralogy of Fallot.

An infant with thymic hypoplasia (rather than aplasia) may experience a spontaneous return of cell-mediated immunity but can develop severe T-cell deficiencies later in life. This allows exaggerated susceptibility to viral, fungal, or bacterial infections, which may be overwhelming. Hypoparathyroidism, usually associated with DGS, typically causes tetany, hyperphosphatemia, and hypocalcemia. Hypocalcemia (calcium levels <7 mg/dL) develops early and is unusually resistant to treatment. It can lead to tetany, seizures, CNS damage, and early heart failure.

Diagnosis
Immediate diagnosis is difficult unless the infant has typical facial anomalies—normally the first clues to the disorder. A definitive diagnosis depends on successful treatment of hypocalcemia and other life-threatening birth defects during the first few weeks of life. Such diagnosis rests on proof of decreased or absent T lymphocytes (sheep cell test, lymphopenia), partial B-cell immunodeficiency, and of an absent thymus (chest X-ray). Fluorescent in situ hybridization test can reveal the chromosomal 22 deletion.

Additional tests showing low serum calcium level, elevated serum phosphorus level, and missing parathyroid hormone confirm hypoparathyroidism.

Treatment
⚠ ALERT *Life-threatening hypocalcemia must be treated immediately, but it's unusually resistant and requires aggressive treatment, for example, with rapid I.V. infusion of a 10% solution of calcium gluconate.*

During such an infusion, monitor heart rate and watch carefully to avoid infiltration. Remember that calcium supplements *must* be given with vitamin D, or sometimes also with parathyroid hormone, to ensure effective calcium utilization. After hypocalcemia is under control, a fetal thymus transplant or hematopoietic cell transplant may restore normal cell-mediated immunity. Cardiac anomalies require surgical repair when possible.

Special considerations
- Instruct the patient with DGS to follow a low-phosphorus diet, and educate about measures to prevent infection.
- Teach the parents of an infant with DGS to watch for signs of infection and have it treated immediately, to keep the infant away from crowds or any other potential sources of infection, and to provide good hygiene and adequate nutrition and hydration.
- Advise the parents to schedule and keep regular follow-up visits to the infant's pediatrician.

ACQUIRED IMMUNODEFICIENCY SYNDROME
AIDS is a serious secondary immunodeficiency disorder caused by the human immunodeficiency virus (HIV). Immunodeficiency makes the patient susceptible to opportunistic infections, unusual cancers, and other abnormalities. (See *Common infections and neoplasms in HIV and AIDS*, page 434.)

The Centers for Disease Control and Prevention (CDC) first described AIDS in 1981. Since then, the CDC has declared a case surveillance definition for AIDS and modified it several times, most recently in 2008.

Causes and incidence
AIDS results from infection with HIV, which has two forms: HIV-1 and HIV-2. Both forms of HIV have the same modes of transmission and similar opportunistic infections associated with AIDS, but studies indicate that HIV-2 develops more slowly and presents with milder symptoms than HIV-1.

Transmission occurs through contact with infected blood or body fluids and is associated with identifiable high-risk behaviors. It's disproportionately represented in:
- homosexual and bisexual men
- persons who use illicit I.V. drugs
- neonates of infected females

Common infections and neoplasms in HIV and AIDS

This is a list of commonly seen disorders with human immunodeficiency virus (HIV) and acquired immunodeficiency syndrome (AIDS). AIDS is diagnosed when a patient diagnosed with HIV has a CD4+ T-cell count of less than 200 cells/µL.

♦ Common infections in a patient with a CD4+ count less than 350 cells/µL include:
  ♦ herpes simplex virus
  ♦ herpes zoster
  ♦ *Mycobacterium tuberculosis*
  ♦ non-Hodgkin lymphoma
  ♦ oral or vaginal thrush
♦ Common infections in a patient with a CD4+ count less than 200 cells/µL include:
  ♦ esophagitis
  ♦ *Pneumocystis jiroveci* (*carinii*) pneumonia
♦ Common infections in a patient with a CD4+ count less than 100 cells/µL include:
  ♦ AIDS dementia
  ♦ cryptococcal meningitis
  ♦ progressive multifocal leukoencephalopathy
  ♦ toxoplasmosis encephalitis
  ♦ wasting syndrome
♦ Common infections in a patient with a CD4+ count less than 50 cells/µL include:
  ♦ *Cytomegalovirus* infection
  ♦ *Mycobacterium avium*
♦ Common neoplasms in patients with HIV and AIDS include:
  ♦ Hodgkin lymphoma
  ♦ Kaposi sarcoma
  ♦ malignant lymphoma

♦ recipients of contaminated blood or blood products (incidence dramatically decreased since mid-1985)
♦ heterosexual partners of persons in the former groups

Pathophysiology

The disease is characterized by the progressive destruction of cell-mediated (T-cell) immunity with subsequent effects on humoral (B-cell) immunity because of the pivotal role of the CD4+ helper T cells in immune reactions.

Complications

♦ Opportunistic infections
♦ Certain cancers

Signs and symptoms

A person with HIV may remain asymptomatic for months or years. Initially, laboratory evidence of seroconversion to HIV antibodies may be the only clinical evidence of infection. However, as the disease progresses, the patient may develop generalized adenopathy and nonspecific signs and symptoms, such as weight loss, fatigue, night sweats, and fevers. As the patient's T-cell count lowers further, neurologic symptoms, opportunistic infections, and certain normally rare cancers may develop. (See *Manifestations of HIV infection and AIDS*, page 435.) HIV also destroys lymph nodes and immunologic organs, leading to major dysfunctions of the immunologic system. Eventually, HIV advances to AIDS. (Some individuals, termed *nonprogressors*, develop AIDS very slowly or not at all. They seem to have genetic differences that prevent the virus from attaching to certain immune receptors.)

PEDIATRIC TIP *The clinical course varies slightly in children, who have a shorter incubation time (mean, 17 months). Signs and symptoms resemble those in adults, except for findings related to sexually transmitted disease (STD). Children show virtually all of the opportunistic infections observed in adults, with a higher incidence of bacterial infections: otitis media, pneumonias other than that caused by Pneumocystis carinii, sepsis, chronic salivary gland enlargement, and lymphoid interstitial pneumonia.*

Diagnosis

CONFIRMING DIAGNOSIS *Signs and symptoms may occur at any time after infection with HIV, but AIDS isn't officially diagnosed until the patient's CD4+ T-cell count falls below 200 cells/µL or the associated clinical conditions or disease are present.*

The most commonly performed tests, antibody tests, indicate HIV infection indirectly by revealing HIV antibodies. The recommended protocol requires initial screening of individuals and blood products with an enzyme-linked immunosorbent assay (ELISA). A positive ELISA should be repeated and then confirmed by an alternate method, usually the Western blot or an immunofluorescence assay. The radioimmunoprecipitation assay is considered more sensitive and specific than the Western blot, but because it requires radioactive materials, it's a poor choice for routine screening. In addition, antibody testing isn't reliable. Because people produce detectable levels of antibodies at different rates—a "window" varying from a few weeks to as long as 35 months in one documented case—an HIV-infected person can test

PATHOPHYSIOLOGY
Manifestations of HIV infection and AIDS

A person infected with human immunodeficiency virus (HIV) may remain asymptomatic for months or years. However, if the disease progresses, it will eventually advance to acquired immunodeficiency syndrome (AIDS).

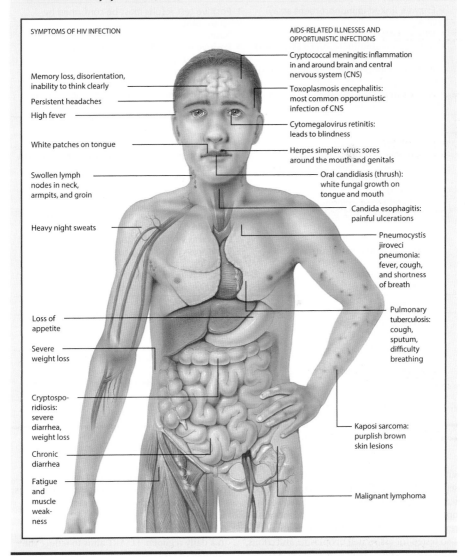

SYMPTOMS OF HIV INFECTION

Memory loss, disorientation, inability to think clearly

Persistent headaches

High fever

White patches on tongue

Swollen lymph nodes in neck, armpits, and groin

Heavy night sweats

Loss of appetite

Severe weight loss

Cryptosporidiosis: severe diarrhea, weight loss

Chronic diarrhea

Fatigue and muscle weakness

AIDS-RELATED ILLNESSES AND OPPORTUNISTIC INFECTIONS

Cryptococcal meningitis: inflammation in and around brain and central nervous system (CNS)

Toxoplasmosis encephalitis: most common opportunistic infection of CNS

Cytomegalovirus retinitis: leads to blindness

Herpes simplex virus: sores around the mouth and genitals

Oral candidiasis (thrush): white fungal growth on tongue and mouth

Candida esophagitis: painful ulcerations

Pneumocystis jiroveci pneumonia: fever, cough, and shortness of breath

Pulmonary tuberculosis: cough, sputum, difficulty breathing

Kaposi sarcoma: purplish brown skin lesions

Malignant lymphoma

negative for HIV antibodies. Antibody tests are also unreliable in neonates because transferred maternal antibodies persist for 6 to 10 months. To overcome these problems, direct tests are used, including antigen tests (p24 antigen), HIV cultures, nucleic acid probes of peripheral blood lymphocytes, and the polymerase chain reaction. (See *Laboratory tests for diagnosing and tracking HIV and assessing immune status,* page 436.)

Additional tests to support the diagnosis and help evaluate the severity of immunosuppression include CD4+ and CD8+ T-lymphocyte

Laboratory tests for diagnosing and tracking HIV and assessing immune status

Test	Findings in HIV infection
HIV antibody tests	
◆ Enzyme-linked immunosorbent assay (ELISA)	◆ Positive test results must be confirmed by Western blot
◆ Western blot	◆ Positive
◆ Indirect immunofluorescence assay (IFA)	◆ Positive test results must be confirmed by Western blot
◆ Radioimmunoprecipitation assay (RIPA)	◆ Positive, more sensitive and specific than Western blot
◆ Home sample collection (dried blood spot, oral mucosa fluid, urine)	◆ Findings confirmed with ELISA or Western blot
HIV tracking	
◆ p24 antigen	◆ Positive for free viral protein
◆ Polymerase chain reaction (PCR)	◆ Detection of HIV ribonucleic acid (RNA) or DNA
◆ Branch deoxyribonucleic acid (bDNA)	◆ Detection of HIV RNA
◆ Nucleic acid sequence-based amplification (NASBA)	◆ Detection of HIV RNA
◆ Peripheral blood mononuclear cell (PBMC) culture for HIV-1	◆ Positive when two consecutive assays detect reverse transcriptase or p24 antigen in increasing magnitude
◆ Quantitative cell culture	◆ Measures viral load within cells
◆ Quantitative plasma culture	◆ Measures viral load by free infectious virus in the plasma
◆ Beta2–microglobulin	◆ Protein is increased with disease progression
◆ Serum neopterin	◆ Increased levels seen with disease progression
Immune status	
◆ Number of CD4+ cells	◆ Decreased
◆ Percentage of CD4+ cells	◆ Decreased
◆ CD4+:CD8+ ratio	◆ Decreased
◆ White blood cell count	◆ Normal to decreased
◆ Immunoglobulin levels	◆ Increased
◆ CD4+ cell function tests	◆ CD4+ T cells have decreased ability to respond to antigen
◆ Skin test sensitivity reaction	◆ Decreased to absent

subset counts, ESR, complete blood cell count, serum beta$_2$-microglobulin, p24 antigen, neopterin levels, and anergy testing. Because many opportunistic infections in AIDS patients are reactivations of previous infections, patients are also tested for associated neoplasms, infections, and STDs.

Treatment

There is no cure for either HIV or AIDS. However, significant advances have been made to help patients control signs and symptoms and impair disease progression. Because HIV can become resistant to any drug, healthcare professionals use combination treatments and multiple drug regimens to suppress the virus. Patients receiving medication remain infectious.

An effective method of treatment is highly active antiretroviral therapy (HAART), which combines three or more anti-HIV medications in a daily regimen. HAART aims to reduce the number of HIV particles in the blood as measured by viral load, thus increasing T-cell counts and improving the immunologic system's functioning. A regular and vigilant medication regimen is critical or resistance will develop because HIV strains mutate and can become resistant to HAART relatively easily.

The *nucleoside reverse transcriptase inhibitors* have been the mainstay of AIDS therapy in recent years. These drugs interfere with viral reverse transcriptase, which impairs HIV's ability to turn its ribonucleic acid into DNA for insertion into the host cell.

Antiretroviral therapy typically begins when the patient's CD4+ T-cell count drops to less than 500/µL or when the patient develops an opportunistic infection. Most clinicians recommend starting the patient on a combination of these drugs in an attempt to gain the maximum benefit and to inhibit the production of resistant mutant strains of HIV. The drug combinations and dosages are then altered, depending on the patient's response.

Increasingly, physicians are basing changes in therapy on the patient's viral load rather than on the CD4+ T-cell count. Because the CD4+ count is influenced by the total WBC count, changes in the CD4+ count may have nothing to do with changes in the patient's HIV status. Many physicians suggest that patients on antiretroviral therapy have their viral load checked every 3 months.

The increasing use of protease inhibitors (PIs) has greatly increased the life expectancy of patients with AIDS. These drugs block the enzyme protease, which HIV needs to produce virions, the viral particles that spread the virus to other cells. The use of PIs dramatically reduces viral load—sometimes to undetectable levels—while producing a corresponding increase in the CD4+ T-cell count and, because they act at a different site than nucleoside analogues, the PIs don't produce additional adverse effects when added to a patient's regimen.

Antiviral therapy includes the use of multiple combined drug therapies that suppress the replication of the HIV virus in the body. Entry/fusion inhibitors are a class of antiviral drugs that work by blocking HIV entry into cells and can be used as part of the HAART regimen. In addition, integrase inhibitors, which stop the protein integrase from allowing HIV to place its genetic material into an infected cell, may also be added to the treatment regimen. After antiviral therapy is initiated, treatment should be aggressive. Initially, HAART, consisting of a triple-drug therapy regimen—a PI and two non-nucleoside reverse transcriptase inhibitors—is recommended. In addition to these primary treatments, anti-infectives are used to combat opportunistic infections (some are used prophylactically to help patients resist opportunistic infections), and antineoplastic drugs are used to fight associated neoplasms. Supportive treatments help maintain nutritional status and relieve pain and other distressing physical and psychological symptoms.

Special considerations

♦ Advise healthcare workers and the public to use precautions in all situations that risk exposure to blood, body fluids, and secretions. Diligently practicing standard precautions can prevent the inadvertent transmission of AIDS and other infectious diseases that are transmitted by similar routes. (See *Preventing AIDS transmission*.)

♦ Recognize that a diagnosis of AIDS is profoundly distressing because of the disease's social impact and discouraging prognosis. The patient may lose his or her job and financial security as well as the support of family and friends. Do your best to help the patient cope with an altered body image, the emotional burden of serious illness, and the threat of death, and encourage and assist the patient in learning about AIDS societies and support programs.

CHRONIC MUCOCUTANEOUS CANDIDIASIS

Chronic mucocutaneous candidiasis is a form of candidiasis (moniliasis) that usually develops during the first year of life but occasionally occurs as late as the 20s, affecting males and females. In some patients, an autoimmune response affecting the endocrine system may induce various endocrinopathies.

Despite chronic candidiasis, these patients seldom die of systemic infection. Instead, they usually die of hepatic or endocrine failure. The prognosis for chronic mucocutaneous candidiasis depends on the severity of the associated endocrinopathy. Patients with associated endocrinopathy seldom live beyond their 30s.

Causes and incidence

No characteristic immunologic defects have been identified in this infection, but many patients have a diminished response to various antigens or to *Candida* alone. In some patients, anergy may result from deficient migration inhibition factor, a mediator normally produced by lymphocytes.

Candida species infections are the most common causes of fungal infections in patients who are immunocompromised. About three of every four females have at least one bout of vulvovaginal candidiasis during their lifetimes. In individuals who are HIV-positive, more than 90% experience oropharyngeal candidiasis and 10% have at least one episode of esophageal candidiasis.

Pathophysiology

Chronic mucocutaneous candidiasis is characterized by repeated infection with *Candida albicans* that may result from an inherited defect in cell-mediated (T-cell) immunity. (Humoral [B-cell] immunity remains intact and provides a normal antibody response to *C. albicans*.)

Complications

♦ Addison disease
♦ Nephrotoxicity
♦ Hypoparathyroidism
♦ Hypocalcemia with seizures
♦ Diabetes mellitus
♦ Pernicious anemia
♦ Corticotropin deficiency
♦ Ovarian failure

Signs and symptoms

Chronic candidal infections can affect the skin, mucous membranes, nails, and vagina, usually causing large, circular lesions. These infections seldom produce systemic symptoms but in late stages may be associated with recurrent respiratory tract infections. Other associated conditions include severe viral infections that may precede the onset of endocrinopathy and, sometimes, hepatitis. Involvement of the mouth, nose, and palate may cause speech and eating difficulties.

Symptoms of endocrinopathy are peculiar to the organ involved. Tetany and hypocalcemia are most common and are associated with hypoparathyroidism. Addison disease, hypothyroidism, diabetes, and pernicious anemia are also connected with chronic mucocutaneous candidiasis. Psychiatric disorders are likely because of disfigurement and multiple endocrine aberrations.

Diagnosis

Laboratory findings usually show a normal circulating T-cell count, although it may be decreased. Skin tests don't usually show delayed hypersensitivity to *Candida*, even during the infectious stage. Migration inhibiting factor that indicates the presence of activated T cells may not respond to *Candida*.

Nonimmunologic abnormalities resulting from endocrinopathy may include hypocalcemia, abnormal hepatic function studies, hyperglycemia, iron deficiency, and abnormal vitamin B_{12} absorption (pernicious anemia). Diagnosis must rule out other immunodeficiency disorders associated with chronic *Candida* infection, especially DGS, ataxia-telangiectasia, and severe combined immunodeficiency disease (SCID), all of which produce severe immunologic defects. After diagnosis, the patient needs evaluation of adrenal, pituitary, thyroid, gonadal, pancreatic, and parathyroid function as well as careful follow-up. The disease is progressive, and most patients eventually develop endocrinopathy.

Treatment

Treatment aims to control infection but isn't always successful. Topical antifungal agents, such as clotrimazole, miconazole, and nystatin, are useful. They may be prescribed as mouthwashes or troches (lozenges) for 5 to 10 days.

Systemic infections may not be fatal, but they're serious enough to warrant vigorous treatment. Ketoconazole and fluconazole have had some positive effect. Oral or I.M. iron replacement may also be necessary. Treatment may also include plastic surgery of the lesions, when possible, and counseling to help patients cope with their disfigurement.

Special considerations
Teach the patient about the disease's progressive manifestations and emphasize the importance of seeing an endocrinologist for regular checkups.

CHRONIC FATIGUE SYNDROME
Sometimes called *chronic Epstein-Barr virus* or *myalgic encephalomyelitis*, chronic fatigue and immune dysfunction syndrome is typically marked by debilitating fatigue, neurologic abnormalities, and persistent symptoms that suggest chronic mononucleosis. It commonly occurs in adults younger than age 45, primarily in women.

Causes and incidence
The cause of CFS is unknown, but researchers suspect that it may be found in human herpes virus-6 or in other herpesviruses, enteroviruses, or retroviruses. Recent studies have shown that inflammation of nervous system pathways, acting as an immune or autoimmune response, may play a role as well. CFS may also be associated with a reaction to viral illness that's complicated by dysfunctional immune response and by other factors that may include gender, age, genetic disposition, prior illness, stress, and environment.

Of the 4 million people with CFS in the United States, less than 20% have been diagnosed.

Pathophysiology
The immune system is upregulated in CFS and the levels of antibodies to various previously encountered antigens are increased. Although increased titers do not indicate a causal relationship in CFS, the titers are nonetheless useful as laboratory clues, which, when taken together, are common in patients with CFS.

Signs and symptoms
CFS has specific symptoms and signs, based on the exclusion of other possible causes. Its characteristic symptom is prolonged, often overwhelming fatigue that's commonly associated with a varying complex of other symptoms that are similar to those of many infections, including myalgia and cephalgia. It may develop within a few hours and can last for 6 months or more. Fatigue isn't relieved by rest and is severe enough to restrict ADLs by at least 50%.

Diagnosis
Because the cause and nature of CFS are still unknown, no single test unequivocally confirms its presence. Therefore, physicians base this diagnosis on the patient's history and the CDC criteria. (See *Criteria for diagnosing chronic fatigue syndrome,* page 440.) Because the CDC's criteria are admittedly a working concept that may not include all forms of this disease and are based on symptoms that can result from other diseases, diagnosis is difficult and uncertain.

Treatment
No treatment is known to cure CFS. Symptomatic treatment may involve the use of medications to treat depression, anxiety, pain, discomfort, and fever. Hidden yeast infections may be present and should be treated. Endocrine abnormalities should be treated with replacement therapy when possible.

Special considerations
◆ Some patients may benefit from avoiding environmental irritants and certain foods.
◆ Because patients with CFS may benefit from supportive contact with others who share this disease, refer the patient to the CFS Association for information and to local support groups. Patients may also benefit from psychological counseling.

CHRONIC GRANULOMATOUS DISEASE
Patients with chronic granulomatous disease (CGD) may develop granulomatous inflammation, which leads to ischemic tissue damage.

Causes and incidence
CGD is inherited as a recessive X-linked trait in 50% to 60% of affected patients. Males are more likely to be affected. The genetic defect may be linked to deficiency of the enzyme nicotinamide adenine dinucleotide phosphate oxidase. The inability of phagocytic cells to kill certain bacteria and fungi leads to long-term and repeated infections.

Pathophysiology
Abnormal neutrophil metabolism impairs phagocytosis—one of the body's chief defense mechanisms—resulting in increased susceptibility to low-virulent or nonpathogenic organisms, such as *Staphylococcus epidermidis, E. coli, Aspergillus,* and *Nocardia.* Phagocytes attracted to sites of infection can engulf these invading organisms but are unable to destroy them.

Criteria for diagnosing chronic fatigue syndrome

There is no blood test, brain scan, or other laboratory test to diagnose chronic fatigue syndrome (CFS); it's a diagnosis of exclusion. Following a detailed patient history, review of medications, and laboratory screening tests, the physician should consider a diagnosis of CFS if two of these criteria are met:

1. Unexplained, persistent fatigue that's not due to ongoing exertion, isn't substantially relieved by rest, is of new onset (not lifelong), and results in a significant reduction in previous levels of activity.

2. Four or more of the following symptoms are present for 6 months or more:
   ◆ Impaired memory or concentration
   ◆ Postexertional malaise (extreme, prolonged exhaustion and sickness following physical or mental activity)
   ◆ Unrefreshing sleep
   ◆ Muscle pain
   ◆ Multijoint pain without swelling or redness
   ◆ Headaches of a new type or severity
   ◆ Sore throat that's frequent or recurring
   ◆ Tender cervical or axillary lymph nodes

From: Centers for Disease Control and Prevention. *Myalgic encephalomyelitis/chronic fatigue syndrome.* Retrieved April 19, 2011 from www.cdc.gov/cfs/cfsdiagnosis.htm.

Complications

◆ Bone damage and infections
◆ Pneumonia
◆ Lung damage
◆ Skin damage
◆ Chronic infections

Signs and symptoms

Usually, the patient with CGD displays signs and symptoms associated with infections of the skin, lymph nodes, lung, liver, and bone by age 2. Skin infection is characterized by small, well-localized areas of tenderness. Seborrheic dermatitis of the scalp and axilla is also common. Lymph node infection typically causes marked lymphadenopathy with draining lymph nodes and hepatosplenomegaly. Many patients develop liver abscess, which may be recurrent and multiple; abdominal tenderness, fever, anorexia, and nausea point to abscess formation. Other common infections include osteomyelitis, which causes localized pain and fever, pneumonia, and gingivitis with severe periodontal disease.

Diagnosis

Clinical features of osteomyelitis, pneumonia, liver abscess, or chronic lymphadenopathy in a young child provide the first clues to CGD diagnosis.

℞ CONFIRMING DIAGNOSIS *An important tool for confirming this diagnosis is the nitroblue tetrazolium (NBT) test. A clear yellow dye, NBT is normally reduced by neutrophil metabolism, resulting in a color change from yellow to blue. Quantifying this color change estimates the degree of neutrophil metabolism.*

Patients with CGD show impaired NBT reduction, indicating abnormal neutrophil metabolism. Another test measures the rate of intracellular killing by neutrophils; in CGD, killing is delayed or absent.

Other laboratory values may support the diagnosis or help monitor disease activity. Osteomyelitis typically causes elevated WBC count and ESR; bone scans help locate and size such infections. Recurrent liver or lung infection may eventually cause abnormal function studies. Cell-mediated and humoral immunity are usually normal in CGD, although some patients have hypergammaglobulinemia.

Treatment

Early, aggressive treatment of infection is the chief goal in caring for a patient with CGD. Areas of suspected infection should be biopsied or cultured, and broad-spectrum antibiotics are usually started immediately—without waiting for results of cultures. Confirmed abscesses may be drained or surgically removed. Provide meticulous wound care after such treatment, including irrigation or packing.

Many patients with CGD receive a combination of I.V. antibiotics, in many cases extended beyond the usual 10- to 14-day course. However, for fungal infections with *Aspergillus* or *Nocardia*, treatment involves amphotericin B in gradually increasing doses to achieve a maximum cumulative dose. During I.V. drug therapy, monitor vital signs frequently and rotate the I.V. site every 48 to 72 hours.

To help treat antibiotic-resistant or life-threatening infection, or to help localize infection, the patient may receive granulocyte transfusions—usually once daily until the crisis has passed. During such transfusions, watch for fever and chills (these effects can sometimes be prevented by premedication with acetaminophen). Transfusions shouldn't be given for 6 hours before or after amphotericin B to avoid severe pulmonary edema and, possibly, respiratory arrest.

IFN-gamma may help reduce the number of severe infections. Bone marrow transplantation is also promising.

Special considerations
◆ If prophylactic antibiotics are ordered, teach the patient and family how to administer them properly and how to recognize adverse effects. Advise them to promptly report any signs or symptoms of infection.
◆ Stress the importance of good nutrition and hygiene, especially meticulous skin and mouth care.
◆ During hospitalizations, encourage the patient to continue ADLs as much as possible.
◆ If the patient is a child, arrange for a tutor to help them keep up with schoolwork.

SEVERE COMBINED IMMUNODEFICIENCY DISEASE
In SCID, both cell-mediated (T-cell) and humoral (B-cell) immunity are deficient or absent, resulting in susceptibility to infection from all classes of microorganisms during infancy. It's the most severe form of T-cell and B-cell deficiency.

Pathophysiology
At least three types of SCID exist: reticular dysgenesis, the most severe type, in which the hematopoietic stem cell fails to differentiate into lymphocytes and granulocytes; Swiss-type agammaglobulinemia, in which the hematopoietic stem cell fails to differentiate into lymphocytes alone; and enzyme deficiency, such as adenosine deaminase (ADA) deficiency, in which the buildup of toxic products in the lymphoid tissue causes damage and subsequent dysfunction.

Causes and incidence
SCID is usually transmitted as an autosomal recessive trait, although it may be X-linked. In most cases, the genetic defect seems associated with failure of the stem cell to differentiate into T and B lymphocytes. Many molecular defects, such as mutation of the kinase ZAP-70, can cause SCID. X-linked SCID is due to a mutation of a subunit of the IL-2, IL-4, and IL-7 receptors. Less commonly, it results from an enzyme deficiency.

SCID affects more males than females. Its estimated incidence is 1 in every 100,000 to 500,000 births. Most untreated patients die from infection within 1 year of birth.

Complications
◆ Infection
◆ Pneumonia
◆ Oral ulcers
◆ Failure to thrive
◆ Dermatitis

Signs and symptoms
An extreme susceptibility to infection becomes obvious in the infant with SCID in the first months of life. The infant fails to thrive and develops chronic otitis; sepsis; watery diarrhea (associated with *Salmonella* or *E. coli*); recurrent pulmonary infections (usually caused by *Pseudomonas*, cytomegalovirus, or *P. jiroveci* [formerly *carinii*]); persistent oral candidiasis, sometimes with esophageal erosions; and possibly fatal viral infections such as chickenpox.

Pneumocystis jiroveci pneumonia usually strikes a severely immunodeficient infant in the first 3 to 5 weeks after birth. Onset is typically insidious, with gradually worsening cough, low-grade fever, tachypnea, and respiratory distress. Chest X-ray characteristically shows bilateral pulmonary infiltrates.

Diagnosis
Diagnosis is generally made clinically because most SCID infants suffer recurrent overwhelming infections within 1 year of birth. Some infants are diagnosed after a severe reaction to vaccination.

Defective humoral immunity is difficult to detect before age 5 months. Before that period, even normal infants have very small amounts of serum IgM and IgA. Normal IgG levels merely reflect maternal IgG.

℞ CONFIRMING DIAGNOSIS *Severely diminished or absent T-cell number and function, as well as lymph node biopsy showing absence of lymphocytes, can confirm the diagnosis of SCID.*

Treatment
Treatment aims to restore the immune response and prevent infection. Histocompatible bone marrow transplantation is the only satisfactory treatment available to correct immunodeficiency. Because bone marrow cells must be HLA and mixed leukocyte culture matched, the most common donors are histocompatible siblings. However, because bone marrow transplant can produce a potentially fatal graft-versus-host (GVH) reaction, newer methods of bone

marrow transplant that eliminate GVH reaction (such as lectin separation and the use of mono-clonal antibodies) are being evaluated.

Fetal thymus and liver transplants have achieved limited success. Immune globulin administration may also play a role in treatment. Some SCID infants have received long-term protection by being isolated in a completely sterile environment. However, this approach isn't effective if the infant already has had recurring infections.

The standard treatment for ADA deficiency is enzyme therapy. The enzyme used, PEG-ADA, is 90% effective in children. Gene therapy is also being used to treat ADA deficiency.

Special considerations
Patient care is primarily preventive and supportive.
◆ Constantly monitor the infant for early signs of infection. If infection develops, provide prompt and aggressive drug therapy as ordered. Watch for adverse effects of any medications given.
◆ Avoid vaccinations and give only irradiated blood products if a transfusion is ordered.
◆ Although SCID infants must remain in strict protective isolation, try to provide a stimulating atmosphere to promote growth and development. Encourage the parents to visit their child often, to hold the child, and to bring toys that can be easily sterilized. If the parents can't visit, call them often to report on the infant's condition. Explain all procedures, medications, and precautions to them. Maintain a normal day and night routine for the child and talk to the child as much as possible.
◆ Because the parents will have questions about the vulnerability of future offspring, refer them for genetic counseling.
◆ Arrange for psychological and spiritual support for the parents and siblings to help them cope with the child's inevitable long-term illness and early death.

COMPLEMENT DEFICIENCIES
Complement is a series of circulating enzymatic serum proteins with nine functional components, labeled C1 through C9. (The first four complement components are numbered out of sequence, in order of their discovery—C1, C4, C2, and C3—but the remaining five are numbered sequentially.)

Complement deficiency or dysfunction may increase susceptibility to infection and also seems related to certain autoimmune disorders. Theoretically, any complement component may be deficient or dysfunctional, and many such disorders are under investigation. Inherited or primary complement deficiencies are rare. The most common are C2, C4, C6, and C8 deficiencies and C5 familial dysfunction. More common secondary complement abnormalities have been confirmed in patients with lupus erythematosus, in some with dermatomyositis, in some with scleroderma, and in a few with gonococcal and meningococcal infections. The prognosis varies with the abnormality and the severity of associated diseases.

Pathophysiology
When IgG or IgM reacts with antigens as part of an immune response, it activates C1, which then combines with C4, initiating the classic complement pathway, or cascade. (An alternative complement pathway involves the direct activation of C3 by the serum protein properdin, bypassing the initial components [C1, C4, and C2] of the classic pathway.) Complement then combines with the antigen–antibody complex and undergoes a sequence of reactions that amplify the immune response against the antigen. This complex process, which is vital to normal immune response, is called *complement fixation;* it's necessary to promote chemotaxis, opsonization, phagocytosis, bacteriolysis, and anaphylaxis reactions.

Causes and incidence
Primary complement deficiencies are inherited as autosomal recessive traits, except for deficiency of C1 esterase inhibitor, which is autosomal dominant. Secondary deficiencies may follow complement-fixing (complement-consuming) immunologic reactions, such as drug-induced serum sickness, acute streptococcal glomerulonephritis, and acute active SLE.

Inherited deficiency is rare in the general population, with an incidence of 0.03%. C2 protein deficiency disorder occurs in 1 in 10,000 persons.

Complications
◆ Systemic lupus erythematosus
◆ Glomerulonephritis
◆ JRA

Signs and symptoms
Clinical effects vary with the specific deficiency. C2 and C3 deficiencies and C5 familial dysfunction increase susceptibility to bacterial infection (which may involve several body systems simultaneously). C2 and C4 deficiencies are also associated with collagen vascular disease such as lupus erythematosus and with chronic renal failure. C5 dysfunction, a familial defect

in infants, causes failure to thrive, diarrhea, and seborrheic dermatitis. C1 esterase inhibitor deficiency (hereditary angioedema) may cause periodic swelling in the face, hands, abdomen, or throat, with potentially fatal laryngeal edema.

Diagnosis

Diagnosis of a complement deficiency is difficult, requiring careful interpretation of both clinical features and laboratory results. Total serum complement level (CH50) is low in various complement deficiencies. In addition, specific assays may be done to confirm deficiency of specific complement components. For example, detection of complement components and IgG by immunofluorescent examination of glomerular tissues in glomerulonephritis strongly suggests complement deficiency.

Treatment

Primary complement deficiencies have no known cure. Associated infection, collagen vascular disease, or renal disease requires prompt, appropriate treatment. Transfusion of fresh frozen plasma to provide replacement of complement components is controversial because replacement therapy doesn't cure complement deficiencies, and any beneficial effects are transient. A bone marrow transplant may be helpful but can cause a potentially fatal reaction (graft-versus-host-rejection). Anabolic steroids such as danazol and antifibrinolytic agents are often used to reduce acute swelling in patients with C1 esterase inhibitor deficiency.

Special considerations

◆ Teach the patient (or his/her family, if the patient is a child) the importance of avoiding infection, how to recognize its early signs and symptoms, and the need for prompt treatment if it occurs.
◆ After a bone marrow transplant, monitor the patient closely for signs of a transfusion reaction or GVH reaction.
◆ Meticulous patient care can speed recovery and prevent complications. For example, a patient with renal infection needs careful monitoring of intake and output, tests for serum electrolytes and acid–base balance, and observation for signs of renal failure.
◆ When caring for a patient with hereditary angioedema, be prepared for emergency management of laryngeal edema; keep airway equipment on hand.

SELECTED REFERENCES

Abbas, A., & Lichtman, A. (2010). *Basic immunology: Functions and disorders of the immune system* (3rd ed.). Philadelphia: WB Saunders, Co.

Arthritis Foundation. (2017). *Rheumatoid arthritis treatment.* Retrieved from https://www.arthritis.org/about-arthritis/types/rheumatoid-arthritis/treatment.php

Bawle, E. (2017). *DiGeorge syndrome.* Retrieved from https://emedicine.medscape.com/article/886526-overview#a3

Boomershine, C. (2017). *Fibromyalgia.* Retrieved from https://emedicine.medscape.com/article/329838-overview#a2

Chatterjee, K. (2010). Host genetic factors in susceptibility to HIV-1 infection and progression to AIDS. *Journal of Genetics, 89*(1), 109–116.

Corbridge, S., & Corbridge, T. (2010). Asthma in adolescents and adults. *Journal of Nursing, 110*(5), 28–38.

Cunha, B. (2017). *Chronic fatigue syndrome.* Retrieved from https://emedicine.medscape.com/article/235980-overview#a4

Grigoriadou, S., & Longhurst, H. (2009). Clinical immunology review series: An approach to the patient with angio-oedema. *Clinical and Experimental Immunology, 155*(3), 367–377.

Jacques, P., et al. (2010). Interactions between gut inflammation and arthritis/spondylitis. *Current Opinion in Rheumatology, 22*(4), 368–374.

Jimenez, S. (2017). *Scleroderma.* Retrieved from https://emedicine.medscape.com/article/331864-overview#a3

Pham, T. (2008). Pathophysiology of ankylosing spondylitis: What's new? *Joint Bone Spine, 75*(6), 656. doi:10.1016/j.jbspin.2008.09.003

Pullen, R., & Hall, D. (2010). Sjogren syndrome: More than just dry eyes. *Nursing, 40*(8), 36–41.

Ranatunga, S. (2018). *Sjogren syndrome.* Retrieved from https://emedicine.medscape.com/article/332125-overview#a5

Sandler, G. (2017). *Transfusion reactions.* Retrieved from https://emedicine.medscape.com/article/206885-overview

Sherry, D. (2017). *Juvenile idiopathic arthritis.* Retrieved from https://emedicine.medscape.com/article/1007276-overview#a4

US Department of Health and Human Services. (2012). *Asthma quick care reference.* Retrieved from https://www.nhlbi.nih.gov/files/docs/guidelines/asthma_qrg.pdf

9

HEMATOLOGIC DISORDERS

Introduction

Blood, one of the body's major fluid tissues, continuously circulates through the heart and blood vessels, carrying vital elements to every part of the body.

Blood basics

Blood performs several vital functions through its special components: the liquid portion (plasma) and the formed constituents (erythrocytes, leukocytes, and thrombocytes) that are suspended in it. Erythrocytes (red blood cells [RBCs]) carry oxygen to the tissues and remove carbon dioxide from them. Leukocytes (white blood cells [WBCs]) act in inflammatory and immune responses. Plasma (a clear, straw-colored fluid) carries antibodies and nutrients to tissues and carries waste away; plasma coagulation factors and thrombocytes (platelets) control clotting. (See *Coagulation factors*.)

Typically, the average person has 5 to 6 L of circulating blood, which constitutes 5% to 7% of body weight (as much as 10% in premature neonates). Blood is three to five times more viscous than water, with an alkaline pH of 7.35 to 7.45, and is either bright red (arterial blood) or dark red (venous blood), depending on the degree of oxygen saturation and the hemoglobin (Hb) level.

Coagulation factors

Factor	Synonym
Factor I	Fibrinogen
Factor II	Prothrombin
Factor III	Tissue thromboplastin
Factor IV	Calcium ion
Factor V	Labile factor
Factor VII	Stable factor
Factor VIII	Antihemophilic globulin or antihemophilic factor A
Factor IX	Plasma thromboplastin component, Christmas factor
Factor X	Stuart–Prower factor
Factor XI	Plasma thromboplastin antecedent
Factor XII	Hageman factor
Factor XIII	Fibrin-stabilizing factor

Formation and characteristics

Hematopoiesis, the process of blood formation, occurs primarily in the bone marrow of the femur, sternum, and vertebrae, where primitive blood cells (stem cells) produce the precursors of erythrocytes (normoblasts), leukocytes, and thrombocytes. During embryonic development, blood cells are derived from mesenchyma and form in the yolk sac. As the fetus matures, blood cells are produced in the liver, the spleen, and the thymus; by the fifth month of gestation, blood cells also begin to form in bone marrow. After birth, blood cells are usually produced only in the marrow.

Blood's function

The most important function of blood is to *transport oxygen* (bound to RBCs inside Hb) from the lungs to the body tissues and to *return carbon dioxide* from these tissues to the lungs. Blood also performs the following functions:
◆ production and delivery of antibodies (by WBCs) formed by plasma cells and lymphocytes
◆ transportation of granulocytes and mono- cytes to defend the body against pathogens by phagocytosis
◆ immunity against viruses and cancer cells through sensitized lymphocytes
◆ provision of complement, a group of im- munologically important protein substances in plasma essential for immune and inflammatory responses

Blood's other functions include control of hemostasis by platelets, plasma, and coagu- lation factors that repair tissue injuries and prevent or halt bleeding; acid–base and fluid balance; regulation of body temperature by carrying off excess heat generated by the in- ternal organs for dissipation through the skin; and transportation of nutrients and regulatory hormones to body tissues and of metabolic wastes to the organs of excretion (kidneys, lungs, and skin).

Blood dysfunction

Because of the rapid reproduction of bone mar- row cells and the short life span and minimal storage in the bone marrow of circulating cells, bone marrow cells and their precursors are particularly vulnerable to physiologic changes that can affect cell production, or *hematopoiesis*. Resulting blood disorders may be primary or secondary, quantitative or qualitative, or both; they may involve some or all blood compo- nents. Quantitative blood disorders result from increased or decreased cell production or cell destruction; qualitative blood disorders stem from intrinsic cell abnormalities or plasma component dysfunction. Specific causes of

blood disorders include trauma, chronic dis- ease, surgery, malnutrition, drugs, exposure to toxins and radiation, and genetic and congeni- tal defects that disrupt production and function. For example, depressed bone marrow produc- tion or mechanical destruction of mature blood cells can reduce the number of RBCs, platelets, and granulocytes, resulting in pancytopenia (anemia, thrombocytopenia, and granulocyto- penia). Increased production of multiple bone marrow components can follow myeloprolifer- ative disorders.

Erythropoiesis

The tissues' demand for oxygen and the blood cells' ability to deliver it regulate RBC produc- tion, or *erythropoiesis*. Consequently, hypoxia (or tissue anoxia) stimulates RBC production by triggering the formation and release of erythropoietin, a hormone (produced by the kidneys) that activates bone marrow to produce RBCs. Erythropoiesis may also be stimulated by androgens (which accounts for the higher RBC counts in men). RBCs have a life span of approximately 120 days.

The actual formation of an erythrocyte be- gins with an uncommitted stem cell that may eventually develop into an RBC or a WBC. Such formation requires certain vitamins—B_{12} and folic acid—and minerals, such as copper, cobalt, and especially iron, which is vital to Hb's oxygen-carrying capacity. Iron is obtained from various foods and is absorbed in the du- odenum and upper jejunum, leaving the excess for temporary storage in reticuloendothelial cells, especially those in the liver. Iron excess is stored as ferritin and hemosiderin until it's released for use in the bone marrow to form new RBCs.

ELDER TIP *In older adults, fatty bone marrow replaces some active cell-forming marrow— first in the long bones and later in the flat bones. The altered bone marrow can't increase erythrocyte production as readily as before in response to such stimuli as hormones, anoxia, hemorrhage, and hemolysis.*

RBC disorders

RBC disorders include quantitative and quali- tative abnormalities. Deficiency of RBCs (ane- mia) can follow any condition that destroys or inhibits the formation of these cells. Common factors leading to this deficiency include:
◆ chronic illnesses, such as renal disease, can- cer, and chronic infections, chronic inflamma- tion (rheumatoid arthritis)

◆ congenital or acquired defects that cause bone marrow aplasia and suppress general hematopoiesis (aplastic anemia) or erythropoiesis
◆ deficiencies of vitamins (vitamin B_{12} deficiency or pernicious anemia) or minerals (iron, folic acid, copper, and cobalt deficiency anemias) that cause inadequate RBC production
◆ drugs, toxins, and ionizing radiation
◆ excessive chronic or acute blood loss (posthemorrhagic anemia)
◆ intrinsically or extrinsically defective RBCs (sickle cell anemia and hemolytic transfusion reaction)
◆ metabolic abnormalities (sideroblastic anemia)

Comparatively few conditions lead to excessive numbers of RBCs:
◆ abnormal proliferation of all bone marrow elements (polycythemia vera), especially RBC mass
◆ a single-element abnormality (for instance, an increase in RBCs that results from erythropoietin excess, which in turn results from hypoxemia, hypertension, or pulmonary disease)
◆ decreased plasma cell volume, which produces a corresponding relative increase in RBC concentration (such as through the use of drugs)

Function of WBCs

WBCs, or leukocytes, protect the body against harmful bacteria and infection and are classified as granular leukocytes (basophils, neutrophils, and eosinophils) or nongranular leukocytes (lymphocytes, monocytes, and plasma cells). (See *Two types of leukocytes,* page 447.) Usually, WBCs are produced in bone marrow; lymphocytes and plasma cells are produced in lymphoid tissue as well. Neutrophils have a circulating half-life of less than 6 hours; some lymphocytes may survive for weeks or months. Normally, WBCs number between 5,000 and 10,000/μL.

There are six types of WBCs:
◆ *Neutrophils,* the predominant form of granulocyte, make up about 60% of WBCs; they help devour invading organisms by phagocytosis.
◆ *Eosinophils,* minor granulocytes, may defend against parasites and lung and skin infections and act in allergic reactions. They account for 1% to 5% of the total WBC count.
◆ *Basophils,* minor granulocytes, may release heparin and histamine into the blood and participate in delayed hypersensitivity reactions. They account for 0% to 1% of the total WBC count.
◆ *Monocytes,* along with neutrophils, help devour invading organisms by phagocytosis. They

help process antigens for lymphocytes and form macrophages in the tissues; they account for 1% to 6% of the total WBC count.
◆ *Lymphocytes* occur as B cells and T cells. B cells aid antibody synthesis; T cells regulate cell-mediated immunity. They account for 20% to 40% of the total WBC count.
◆ *Plasma cells* develop from lymphocytes, reside in the tissue, and produce antibodies. Plasma cells do not normally circulate in the blood.

A temporary increase in production and release of mature WBCs (leukemic reaction) is a normal response to infection. However, an excessive number of immature WBC precursors and their accumulation in bone marrow or lymphoid tissue are characteristic of leukemia. These nonfunctioning WBCs (blasts) provide no protection against infection; crowd out RBCs, platelets, and mature WBCs; and spill into the bloodstream, sometimes infiltrating organs and impairing function.

WBC deficiencies may reflect inadequate cell production, drug reactions, ionizing radiation, infiltrated bone marrow (cancer), congenital defects, aplastic anemia, folic acid deficiency, or hypersplenism. The major WBC deficiencies are granulocytopenia, lymphocytopenia, and monocytopenia.

Platelets, plasma, and clotting

Platelets are small (2 to 4 μm in diameter), colorless, disk-shaped cytoplasmic fragments split from cells in bone marrow called *megakaryocytes.* The normal platelet concentration is 150,000 to 400,000/μL. These fragments, which have a life span of approximately 10 days, perform three vital functions:
◆ initiate vasoconstriction of damaged blood vessels to minimize blood loss
◆ form hemostatic plugs in injured blood vessels
◆ with plasma, provide materials that accelerate blood coagulation—notably platelet factor III

Plasma consists mainly of proteins (chiefly albumin, globulin, and fibrinogen) held in aqueous suspension. Other components of plasma include glucose, lipids, amino acids, electrolytes, pigments, hormones, respiratory gases (oxygen and carbon dioxide), and products of metabolism, such as urea, uric acid, creatinine, and lactic acid. Its fluid characteristics—including osmotic pressure, viscosity, and suspension qualities—depend on its protein content. Plasma components regulate

Two types of leukocytes

Leukocytes vary in size, shape, and number.

GRANULAR LEUKOCYTES

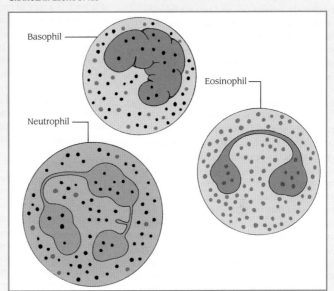

Granular leukocytes
Granular leukocytes (granulocytes) are the most numerous and include basophils, containing cytoplasmic granules that stain readily with alkaline dyes; eosinophils, which stain with acidic dyes; and neutrophils, which are finely granular and recognizable by their multinucleated appearance.

NONGRANULAR LEUKOCYTES

Nongranular leukocytes
Lymphocytes and monocytes have few, if any, granulated particles in the cytoplasm.

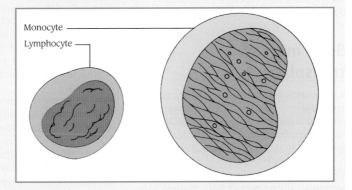

acid–base balance and immune responses and mediate coagulation and nutrition.

In a complex process called *hemostasis*, platelets, plasma, and coagulation factors interact to control bleeding.

Hemostasis and the clotting mechanism

Hemostasis is the complex process by which the body controls bleeding. When a blood vessel ruptures, local vasoconstriction and platelet clumping (aggregation) at the injury site initially help prevent hemorrhage. This activation of the coagulation system, called *extrinsic cascade*, requires release of tissue thromboplastin from the damaged cells. However, formation of a more stable clot requires initiation of the complex clotting mechanism known as the *intrinsic cascade system*. When endothelial vessel injury or a foreign body in the bloodstream activates this system, *activating factor XII* triggers clotting. In the final common pathway, prothrombin is converted to thrombin. Thrombin acts on fibrinogen to form fibrin, the basis of a clot.

Therapy with blood components

Because of improved methods of collection, component separation, and storage, blood transfusions are being used more effectively than ever. Separating blood into components permits a single unit of blood to benefit several patients with different hematologic abnormalities. Component therapy allows replacement of a specific blood component without risking reactions from other components.

Blood typing, crossmatching, and human leukocyte antigen (HLA) typing are compatibility tests used to ensure safe, effective replacement therapy and minimize the risk of transfusion reactions. Blood typing determines the antigens present in the patient's RBCs by reaction with standardized sera. (Critical antigen groups are those of ABO and Rh factor.) Crossmatching the patient's blood with transfusion blood provides some assurance that the patient doesn't have antibodies against donor red cells. HLA typing may be helpful for the patient who needs long-term transfusion therapy or frequent platelet transfusions, but usually, only family members can provide an appropriate match because antigenic properties are genetically determined.

Bone marrow transplantation

Bone marrow transplantation is used to treat acute leukemia, aplastic anemia, severe combined immunodeficiency disease (SCID), Nezelof syndrome, and Wiskott–Aldrich syndrome. In this procedure, marrow from a twin or another HLA-identical donor (usually a sibling) is transfused in an attempt to repopulate the recipient's bone marrow with normal cells.

A hematologic disorder can affect nearly every aspect of the patient's life, perhaps resulting in life-threatening emergencies that require prompt medical treatment. This is particularly true of patients with such diseases as hemophilia and thalassemia major, diseases for which no cure is available. Astute, sensitive care founded on a firm understanding of hematologic basics can help the patient survive such illnesses. In situations with poor prognoses, the patient may need to make many adjustments to maintain an optimal quality of life.

Anemias
PERNICIOUS ANEMIA
Pernicious anemia, also known as *vitamin B$_{12}$ deficiency*, is a type of megaloblastic anemia characterized by decreased gastric production of hydrochloric acid and deficiency of intrinsic factor (IF), a substance normally secreted by the parietal cells of the gastric mucosa that's essential for vitamin B$_{12}$ absorption in the ileum. The resulting deficiency of vitamin B$_{12}$ causes serious neurologic, gastric, and intestinal abnormalities. Untreated pernicious anemia may lead to permanent neurologic disability and death. (See *Peripheral blood smear in pernicious anemia*, page 449.)

Pathophysiology
Familial incidence of pernicious anemia suggests a genetic predisposition. (It may involve an inherited single dominant autosomal factor.) Significantly higher incidence in patients with immunologically related endocrine diseases, such as thyroiditis, myxedema, and Graves disease, seems to support a widely held theory that an inherited autoimmune response causes gastric mucosal atrophy and, therefore, deficiency of hydrochloric acid and IF. IF deficiency impairs vitamin B$_{12}$ absorption. The resultant vitamin B$_{12}$ deficiency inhibits cell growth, particularly of RBCs, leading to insufficient and deformed RBCs with poor oxygen-carrying capacity. It also impairs myelin formation, causing neurologic damage. Iatrogenic induction can follow partial gastrectomy and/or bypass for obesity.

PEDIATRIC TIP *Juvenile pernicious anemia, occurring in children younger than age 10, stems from a congenital stomach disorder that causes secretion of abnormal IF.*

ELDER TIP *With age, vitamin B$_{12}$ absorption may also diminish, resulting in reduced erythrocyte mass and decreased Hb levels and hematocrit (HCT).*

Pernicious anemia primarily affects people of northern European ancestry. It's rare in children and infants. Onset typically occurs after age 35, and incidence increases with age. It affects about 2% of people older than age 60.

Complications
◆ Paralysis
◆ Psychotic behavior
◆ Loss of bowel and bladder sphincter control

Signs and symptoms
Characteristically, pernicious anemia has an insidious onset but eventually causes an

Peripheral blood smear in pernicious anemia

Pernicious anemia is caused by malabsorption of vitamin B$_{12}$.

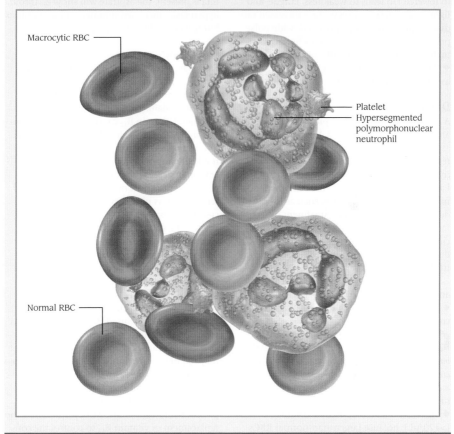

Macrocytic RBC

Platelet
Hypersegmented
polymorphonuclear
neutrophil

Normal RBC

unmistakable triad of symptoms: weakness, sore tongue, and numbness and tingling in the extremities. The lips, gums, and tongue appear markedly bloodless. Hemolysis-induced hyperbilirubinemia may cause faintly jaundiced sclera and pale to bright yellow skin. In addition, the patient may become highly susceptible to infection, especially of the genitourinary (GU) tract.

Other systemic symptoms of pernicious anemia include the following:

◆ *Gastrointestinal* (*GI*)—Gastric mucosal atrophy and decreased hydrochloric acid production disturb digestion and lead to nausea, vomiting, anorexia, weight loss, flatulence, diarrhea, and constipation. Gingival bleeding and tongue inflammation may hinder eating and intensify anorexia.

◆ *Central nervous system* (*CNS*)—Demyelination caused by vitamin B$_{12}$ deficiency initially affects the peripheral nerves but gradually extends to the spinal cord. Consequently, the neurologic effects of pernicious anemia may include neuritis; weakness in extremities; peripheral numbness and paresthesia; disturbed position sense; lack of coordination; ataxia; impaired fine finger movement; positive Babinski and Romberg signs; light-headedness; altered vision (diplopia and blurred vision), taste, and hearing (tinnitus); optic muscle atrophy; loss of bowel and bladder control; and, in males, impotence. Its effects on the nervous system may also produce irritability, poor memory, headache, depression, and delirium. Although some of these symptoms are temporary, irreversible CNS changes may have occurred before treatment.

♦ *Cardiovascular*—Increasingly fragile cell membranes induce widespread destruction of RBCs, resulting in low Hb levels. The impaired oxygen-carrying capacity of the blood secondary to lowered Hb leads to weakness, fatigue, and light-headedness. Compensatory increased cardiac output results in palpitations, wide pulse pressure, dyspnea, orthopnea, tachycardia, premature beats and, eventually, heart failure.

♦ *Musculoskeletal*—Scissors gait can also occur as a late sign of untreated anemia.

Diagnosis

A positive family history, typical ethnic heritage, and results of blood studies, bone marrow aspiration, gastric analysis, and the Schilling test establish the diagnosis. (See *Tests for blood composition, production, and function*, page 451.) Laboratory screening must rule out other anemias with similar symptoms, such as folic acid deficiency anemia, because treatment differs. Diagnosis must also rule out vitamin B_{12} deficiency resulting from malabsorption due to GI disorders, gastric surgery including obesity gastric bypass surgery, radiation, or drug therapy.

Blood study results that suggest pernicious anemia include:

♦ decreased Hb levels (4 to 5 g/dL) and decreased RBC count

ELDER TIP *Hb levels drop 1 to 2 g/dL in elderly men, and HCT may decrease slightly in both men and women. These changes reflect decreased bone marrow and hematopoiesis and (in men) decreased androgen levels; they aren't an indicator of pernicious anemia.*

♦ increased mean corpuscular volume (>120/µL); because larger-than-normal RBCs *each* contain increased amounts of Hb, mean corpuscular Hb concentration is also increased

♦ possible low WBC and platelet counts and large, malformed platelets

♦ serum vitamin B_{12} assay levels less than 0.1 µg/mL

♦ elevated serum lactate dehydrogenase levels

Bone marrow aspiration reveals erythroid hyperplasia (crowded red bone marrow), with increased numbers of megaloblasts but few normally developing RBCs. Gastric analysis shows absence of free hydrochloric acid after histamine or pentagastrin injection.

CONFIRMING DIAGNOSIS *The Schilling test was once the definitive diagnostic test for pernicious anemia. It is rarely used now because it involves the injection of radioactive vitamin B_{12}. Now, vitamin B_{12} levels are measured along with tests for the presence of IF and antiparietal cell antibodies.*

In addition, a complete blood count (CBC) with decreased Hb level and RBC count will reveal anemia. Elevated homocysteine and methylmalonic acid levels may indicate pernicious anemia. In some cases, bone marrow aspiration may be performed. If pernicious anemia is present, the aspirate will show erythroid hyperplasia, increased numbers of megaloblasts but few normally developing RBCs.

Treatment

Early parenteral vitamin B_{12} replacement can reverse pernicious anemia, minimize complications and, possibly, prevent permanent neurologic damage. An initial high dose of parenteral vitamin B_{12} causes rapid RBC regeneration. Within 2 weeks, Hb levels should rise to normal, and the patient's condition should markedly improve. Because rapid cell regeneration increases the patient's iron and folate requirements, concomitant iron and folic acid replacement is necessary to prevent iron deficiency anemia.

After the patient's condition improves, the vitamin B_{12} dosage can be decreased to maintenance levels and given monthly. Because such injections must be continued for life, the patient should learn self-administration of vitamin B_{12}.

A new vitamin B_{12} nasal gel that is applied once a week may be used in place of injections to maintain vitamin B_{12} levels.

If anemia causes extreme fatigue, the patient may require bed rest until Hb levels rise. If Hb levels are dangerously low, the patient may need blood transfusions. Digoxin, a diuretic, and a low-sodium diet may be necessary for a patient with heart failure. Most important is the replacement of vitamin B_{12} to control the condition that led to this failure. Antibiotics help combat accompanying infections.

Special considerations

Supportive measures minimize the risk of complications and speed recovery. Patient and family teaching can promote compliance with lifelong vitamin B_{12} replacement.

♦ If the patient has severe anemia, plan activities, rest periods, and necessary diagnostic tests to conserve his energy. Monitor pulse rate often; tachycardia means activities are too strenuous.

♦ To ensure accurate Schilling test results, make sure that all urine over a 24-hour period is collected and that the specimens are uncontaminated.

♦ Warn the patient to guard against infections and tell them to report signs of infection promptly, especially pulmonary and urinary tract infections, because the patient's weakened condition may increase susceptibility.

Tests for blood composition, production, and function

Overall composition

♦ Peripheral blood smear shows maturity and morphologic characteristics of blood elements and determines qualitative abnormalities.

♦ Complete blood count (CBC) determines the actual number of blood elements in relation to volume and quantifies abnormalities.

♦ Bone marrow aspiration or biopsy allows evaluation of hematopoiesis by showing blood elements and precursors, and abnormal or malignant cells.

Red blood cell function

♦ Hematocrit, or packed cell volume, measures the percentage of red blood cells (RBCs) per fluid volume of whole blood.

♦ Hemoglobin (Hb) measures the amount (grams) of Hb per deciliter of blood, to determine oxygen-carrying capacity.

♦ Reticulocyte count assesses RBC production by determining concentration of this erythrocyte precursor.

♦ Schilling test determines absorption of vitamin B_{12} (necessary for erythropoiesis) by measuring excretion of radioactive B_{12} in the urine.

♦ Mean corpuscular volume describes the RBC in terms of size.

♦ Mean corpuscular Hb determines the average amount of Hb per RBC.

♦ Mean corpuscular Hb concentration establishes the average Hb concentration in 1 dL of packed RBCs.

♦ Sucrose hemolysis test assesses the susceptibility of RBCs to hemolyze with complement.

♦ Direct Coombs test demonstrates the presence of immunoglobulin G (IgG) antibodies (such as antibodies to Rh factor) or, possibly, complement on circulating RBCs.

♦ Indirect Coombs test, a two-step test, detects the presence of IgG antibodies in the serum.

♦ Sideroblast test detects stainable iron (available for Hb synthesis) in normoblastic RBCs.

♦ Hb electrophoresis demonstrates abnormal Hb such as sickle cell anemia.

Hemostasis

♦ Platelet count determines the number of platelets.

♦ Bleeding time (Ivy bleeding time) assesses the capacity for platelets to stop bleeding in capillaries and small vessels.

♦ Prothrombin time (Quick test, pro time) assists in evaluation of thrombin generation (extrinsic clotting mechanism).

♦ Partial thromboplastin time aids evaluation of the adequacy of plasma-clotting factors (intrinsic clotting mechanism).

♦ International normalized ratio normalizes ratios between labs.

♦ Fibrin degradation products (fibrin split products, FDPs) test the amount of clot breakdown products in serum.

♦ Thrombin time detects abnormalities in thrombin fibrinogen reaction.

♦ Fibrinogen (factor I) measures this coagulation factor in plasma.

♦ D-dimer test determines if FDPs are from normal mechanisms or excessive fibrinolysis and is commonly used to diagnose disseminated intravascular coagulation (DIC).

White blood cell function

♦ White blood cell (WBC) count and differential establishes quantity and maturity of WBC elements (neutrophils [called polymorphonuclear granulocytes or bands], basophils, eosinophils, lymphocytes, monocytes).

♦ Quantified $CD4^+$:$CD8^+$ T lymphocytes determines helper:suppressor ratio, which is important to immune function and is decreased in HIV infection.

Plasma

♦ Erythrocyte sedimentation rate measures the rate of RBCs settling from plasma and may reflect infection.

♦ Electrophoresis of serum proteins determines the amount of various serum proteins (classified by mobility in response to an electrical field). It's commonly used to diagnose plasma cell myeloma.

♦ Immunoelectrophoresis of serum proteins separates and classifies serum antibodies (immunoglobulins) through specific antisera.

♦ Provide a well-balanced diet, including foods high in vitamin B_{12} (meat, liver, fish, eggs, and milk). Offer between-meal snacks and encourage the family to bring favorite foods from home.

♦ Because a sore mouth and tongue make eating painful, ask the dietitian to avoid giving the patient irritating foods. If these symptoms make talking difficult, supply a pad and pencil or some other aid to facilitate nonverbal communication; explain this problem to the family. Provide diluted mouthwash or, with severe conditions, swab the patient's mouth with tap water or warm saline solution or use topical anesthetic mouthwash.

♦ Warn the patient with a sensory deficit not to use a heating pad, because it may cause burns.

♦ If the patient is incontinent, establish a regular bowel and bladder routine. After the patient is discharged, a home healthcare nurse should follow up on this schedule and make adjustments, as needed.

♦ If neurologic damage causes behavioral problems, assess mental and neurologic status often; if needed, give tranquilizers, as ordered, and apply wrist or jacket restraint and utilize bed alert alarm at night.

♦ Stress that vitamin B_{12} replacement isn't a permanent cure and that these injections *must* be continued for life, even after symptoms subside.

▦ PREVENTION *To prevent vitamin B_{12} deficiency, emphasize the importance of vitamin B_{12} supplements for patients who have had extensive gastric resections or who follow strict vegetarian or vegan diets.*

FOLIC ACID DEFICIENCY ANEMIA

Folic acid is a water-soluble vitamin that is rapidly excreted; body stores are limited to a few weeks. It is therefore relatively easy to develop a folic acid deficiency.

Folic acid deficiency anemia is a common, slowly progressive, megaloblastic anemia. It usually occurs in infants, adolescents, pregnant and lactating females, alcoholics, elderly people, and people with malignant or intestinal diseases.

Pathophysiology

Folic acid deficiency anemia may result from:

♦ alcohol abuse (alcohol may suppress metabolic effects of folate)

♦ poor diet (common in alcoholics, elderly people living alone, and infants, especially those with infections or diarrhea)

♦ impaired absorption (due to intestinal dysfunction from disorders such as celiac disease, tropical sprue, regional jejunitis, or bowel resection and bariatric surgery)

♦ bacteria competing for available folic acid

♦ excessive cooking, which can destroy a high percentage of folic acids in foods (See *Preventing folic acid deficiency anemia.*)

♦ limited storage capacity in infants

♦ prolonged drug therapy (anticonvulsants and estrogens)

♦ increased folic acid requirements during pregnancy; during rapid growth in infancy (common because of recent increase in survival of premature infants); during childhood and adolescence (because of general use of folate-poor cow's milk); and in patients with neoplastic diseases and some skin diseases (chronic exfoliative dermatitis)

It's estimated that 10% of the United States population has low folate stores.

Signs and symptoms

Folic acid deficiency anemia gradually produces clinical features characteristic of other megaloblastic anemias, without the neurologic manifestations: progressive fatigue, shortness of

PREVENTION

Preventing folic acid deficiency anemia

Folic acid (pteroylglutamic acid, folacin) is found in most body tissues, where it acts as a coenzyme in metabolic processes involving one carbon transfer. It's essential for formation and maturation of red blood cells and for synthesis of deoxyribonucleic acid. Although its body stores are relatively small (about 70 mg), this vitamin is plentiful in most well-balanced diets.

However, because folic acid is water-soluble and heat-labile, it's easily destroyed by cooking. Also, approximately 20% of folic acid intake is excreted unabsorbed. Insufficient daily folic acid intake (<50 µg/day) usually induces folic acid deficiency within 4 months. To prevent folic acid deficiency anemia, foods high in folic acid content should be chosen, such as those listed below:

Food	µg/100 g
Asparagus spears	109
Beef liver	294
Broccoli spears	54
Collards (cooked)	102
Mushrooms	24
Oatmeal	133
Peanut butter	57
Red beans	180
Wheat germ	305

breath, palpitations, weakness, glossitis, mouth ulcers, nausea, anorexia, headache, fainting, irritability, forgetfulness, pallor, and slight jaundice. Folic acid deficiency anemia doesn't cause neurologic impairment unless it's associated with vitamin B_{12} deficiency, as in pernicious anemia.

Diagnosis

℞ CONFIRMING DIAGNOSIS *A CBC with significant findings including macrocytosis, decreased reticulocyte count, abnormal platelets, low Hb level, normal or high vitamin B_{12} level, and serum folate less than 3 ng/mL confirm the diagnosis.*

Treatment

Treatment consists primarily of folic acid supplements and elimination of contributing causes. Folic acid supplements may be given orally or parenterally (to patients who are severely ill, have malabsorption, or are unable to take oral medication). Many patients respond favorably to a well-balanced diet. Vitamin B_{12} deficiency should be ruled out before administering folic acid. If the patient has combined B_{12} and folate deficiencies, folic acid replenishment alone may aggravate neurologic dysfunction.

Special considerations

◆ Teach the patient to meet daily folic acid requirements by including a food from each food group in every meal. If they have a severe deficiency, explain that diet only reinforces folic acid supplementation and isn't therapeutic by itself. Urge compliance with the prescribed course of therapy. Advise them not to stop taking the supplements when they begin to feel better.

◆ If the patient has glossitis, emphasize the importance of good oral hygiene. Suggest regular use of mild or diluted mouthwash and a soft toothbrush.

◆ Watch fluid and electrolyte balance, particularly in the patient who has severe diarrhea and is receiving parenteral fluid replacement therapy.

◆ Because anemia causes severe fatigue, schedule regular rest periods until the patient is able to resume normal activity.

PREVENTION *Emphasize the importance of a well-balanced diet high in folic acid. Identify alcoholics with poor dietary habits and try to arrange for appropriate counseling. Tell mothers who aren't breast-feeding to use commercially prepared formulas.*

APLASTIC ANEMIAS

Aplastic, or hypoplastic, anemias result from injury to or destruction of stem cells in bone marrow or the bone marrow matrix, causing pancytopenia (anemia, granulocytopenia, and thrombocytopenia) and bone marrow hypoplasia. (See *Peripheral blood smear in aplastic anemia*, page 454.) Although commonly used interchangeably with other terms for bone marrow failure, *aplastic anemia* properly refers to pancytopenia resulting from the decreased functional capacity of a hypoplastic, fatty bone marrow. These disorders generally produce fatal bleeding or infection, particularly when they're idiopathic or stem from chloramphenicol or from infectious hepatitis. Mortality for aplastic anemias with severe pancytopenia is 80% to 90%.

Pathophysiology

Aplastic anemias usually develop when damaged or destroyed stem cells (which develop into RBCs, WBCs, and platelets) inhibit RBC production. Less commonly, they develop when damaged bone marrow microvasculature creates an unfavorable environment for cell growth and maturation. About one-half of such anemias result from drugs (antibiotics, anticonvulsants, anti-inflammatory drugs, antineoplastics, diuretics, phenothiazines, antidiabetics, and antithyroid drugs), toxic agents (such as benzene and chloramphenicol), or radiation. The rest may result from immunologic factors (unconfirmed), severe disease (especially hepatitis), viral infection (especially in children), or preleukemic and neoplastic infiltration of bone marrow.

Idiopathic anemias may be congenital. Two such forms of aplastic anemia have been identified: Congenital hypoplastic anemia (Blackfan–Diamond anemia) develops between ages 2 and 3 months; Fanconi syndrome, between birth and age 10. In Fanconi syndrome, chromosomal abnormalities are usually associated with multiple congenital anomalies, such as dwarfism, and hypoplasia of the kidneys and spleen. In the absence of a consistent familial or genetic history of aplastic anemia, researchers suspect that these congenital abnormalities result from an induced change in the fetus' development.

Incidence is 0.6 to 6.1 cases per 1 million people in the United States. There is no racial predilection.

Complications

◆ Life-threatening hemorrhage
◆ Secondary opportunistic infections

Signs and symptoms

Clinical features of aplastic anemias vary with the severity of pancytopenia but develop insidiously in many cases. Anemic symptoms include

Peripheral blood smear in aplastic anemia

Aplastic anemia results from injury to or destruction of stem cells in the bone marrow or the bone marrow matrix, causing pancytopenia.

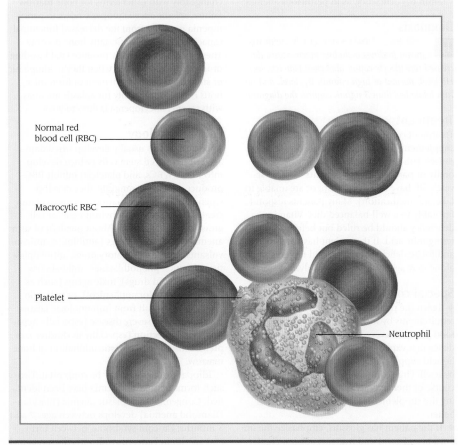

Normal red blood cell (RBC)

Macrocytic RBC

Platelet

Neutrophil

progressive weakness and fatigue, shortness of breath, headache, pallor and, ultimately, tachycardia and heart failure. Thrombocytopenia leads to ecchymosis, petechiae, and hemorrhage, especially from the mucous membranes (nose, gums, rectum, and vagina) or into the retina or CNS. Neutropenia may lead to infection (fever, oral and rectal ulcers, and sore throat) but without characteristic inflammation.

Diagnosis

Confirmation of aplastic anemia requires a series of laboratory tests:

◆ RBCs are usually normochromic and normocytic (although macrocytosis [larger-than-normal erythrocytes] and anisocytosis [excessive variation in erythrocyte size]

may exist), with a total count of 1 million/µL or less. Absolute reticulocyte count is very low.

◆ Serum iron level is elevated (unless bleeding occurs), but total iron-binding capacity is normal or slightly reduced. Hemosiderin (a derivative of Hb) is present, and tissue iron storage is visible microscopically.

◆ Platelet, neutrophil, and WBC counts fall.

◆ Coagulation tests (bleeding time), reflecting decreased platelet count, are abnormal.

◆ Bone marrow aspiration from several sites may yield a "dry tap," and biopsy will show severely hypocellular or aplastic marrow with varied amounts of fat, fibrous tissue, or gelatinous replacement; absence of tagged iron (because iron is deposited in the liver rather than bone marrow) and megakaryocytes (platelet precursors); and depression of erythroid elements.

Differential diagnosis must rule out paroxysmal nocturnal hemoglobinuria and other diseases in which pancytopenia is common.

Treatment

Effective treatment must eliminate any identifiable cause and provide vigorous supportive measures, such as packed RBCs, platelets, and experimental histocompatibility locus antigen-matched leukocyte transfusions. Even after

elimination of the cause, recovery can take months. Bone marrow or stem cell transplantation is the treatment of choice for anemia due to severe aplasia and for patients who need constant RBC transfusions. (See *Bone marrow transplantation*, pages 455 and 456.)

Patients with low leukocyte counts need special measures to prevent infection. The infection itself may require specific antibiotics; however, these aren't given prophylactically because they tend to encourage resistant strains of organisms. Patients with low Hb levels may need

---

Bone marrow transplantation

In bone marrow transplantation, usually 500 to 700 mL of marrow is aspirated from the pelvic bones of a human leukocyte antigen (HLA)-compatible donor (allogeneic) or of the recipient himself during complete remission (autologous). The aspirated marrow is filtered and then infused into the recipient in an attempt to repopulate the patient's marrow with normal cells. This procedure has effected long-term, healthy survival in about 50% of patients with severe aplastic anemia. Bone marrow transplantation may also be effective in patients with acute leukemia, certain immunodeficiency diseases, and solid tumor neoplasms.

Because bone marrow transplantation carries serious risks, it requires strict adherence to infection control and strict sterile techniques, and a primary nurse to provide consistent care and continuous monitoring of the patient's status.

Before transplantation

♦ Explain that the success rate depends on the stage of the disease and an HLA-identical match.

♦ After bone marrow aspiration is completed under a local anesthetic, apply pressure dressings to the donor's aspiration sites. Observe the sites for bleeding. Relieve pain with analgesics and ice packs, as needed.

♦ Assess the patient's understanding of bone marrow transplantation. If necessary, correct any misconceptions about this procedure and provide additional information, as appropriate. Prepare the patient to expect an extended hospital stay. Explain that chemotherapy and possible radiation treatments are necessary to destroy cells that may cause the body to reject the transplant.

♦ Various treatment protocols are used. For example, I.V. cyclophosphamide may

be used with additional chemotherapeutic agents or total body irradiation. This treatment requires aggressive hydration to prevent hemorrhagic cystitis. Control nausea and vomiting with an antiemetic, such as ondansetron (Zofran) or metoclopramide (Reglan), as needed. Give allopurinol, as prescribed, to prevent hyperuricemia resulting from tumor breakdown products. Because alopecia is a common adverse effect of high-dose cyclophosphamide therapy, encourage the patient to choose a wig or scarf before treatment begins.

♦ Total body irradiation may follow chemotherapy, inducing total marrow aplasia. Warn the patient that cataracts, GI disturbances, and sterility are possible adverse effects.

♦ Assess venous access. If necessary, the patient may have an indwelling central venous catheter inserted.

During marrow infusion

♦ Monitor vital signs every 15 minutes.

♦ Watch for complications of marrow infusion, such as pulmonary embolus, hypersensitivity reactions, and volume overload.

♦ Reassure the patient throughout the procedure.

After the infusion

♦ Continue to monitor the patient's vital signs every 15 minutes for 2 hours after infusion, then every 4 hours. Watch for fever and chills, which may be the only signs of infection. Give prophylactic antibiotics as prescribed. To reduce the possibility of bleeding, don't administer medications rectally or I.M.

♦ Administer methotrexate or cyclosporine, as prescribed, to prevent graft-versus-host (GVH) reaction, a potentially fatal complication of allogeneic transplantation. Watch for signs or symptoms of GVH reaction, such

(continued)

Bone marrow transplantation (continued)

as maculopapular rash, pancytopenia, jaundice, joint pain, and generalized edema.
♦ Administer vitamins, steroids, and iron and folic acid supplements, as appropriate. Administration of blood products, such as platelets and packed red blood cells, may also be indicated, depending on the results of daily blood studies.

♦ Provide good mouth care every 2 hours. Use hydrogen peroxide and nystatin mouthwash or oral fluconazole, for example, to prevent candidiasis and other mouth infections. Also provide meticulous skin care, paying special attention to pressure points and open sites, such as those from the marrow aspiration and I.V. insertion.

---

respiratory support with oxygen in addition to blood transfusions.

For older patients, or for those who don't have a matched bone marrow donor, antithymocyte globulin (ATG) is an alternative treatment. ATG is a horse serum that contains antibodies against human T cells. It may be used in an attempt to suppress the body's immune system, allowing the bone marrow to resume its blood cell-generating function. Other immunosuppressant agents, such as cyclosporine, may also be used.

Other treatments may include corticosteroids to stimulate erythroid production, marrow-stimulating agents such as androgens (which remain controversial), and colony stimulation factors to encourage growth of specific cellular components.

Special considerations

♦ If the platelet count is low (<20,000/µL), prevent bleeding by avoiding I.M. injections, suggesting the use of an electric razor and a soft toothbrush, humidifying oxygen to prevent drying of mucous membranes, avoiding enemas and rectal temperatures, and promoting regular bowel movements through the use of a stool softener and a proper diet to prevent constipation. Also, apply pressure to venipuncture sites until bleeding stops. Detect bleeding early by checking for blood in urine and stool, and assessing skin for petechiae.

♦ Take safety precautions to prevent falls that could lead to prolonged bleeding or hemorrhage.

♦ Help prevent infection by washing your hands thoroughly before entering the patient's room, by making sure they are receiving a nutritious diet (high in vitamins and proteins) to improve resistance, and by encouraging meticulous mouth and perianal care.

♦ Watch for life-threatening hemorrhage, infection, adverse effects of drug therapy, or blood transfusion reaction. Make sure routine throat, urine, nose, rectal, and blood cultures are done regularly and correctly to check for infection. Teach the patient to recognize signs of

infection, and tell to report any abnormal signs immediately.

♦ If the patient has a low Hb level, which causes fatigue, schedule frequent rest periods. Administer oxygen therapy as needed. If blood transfusions are necessary, assess for a transfusion reaction by checking the patient's temperature and watching for the development of other signs and symptoms, such as rash, hives, itching, back pain, restlessness, and shaking chills.

♦ Reassure and support the patient and their family by explaining the disease and its treatment, particularly if they have recurring acute episodes. Explain the purpose of all prescribed drugs and discuss possible adverse effects, including which ones they should report promptly. Encourage the patient who doesn't require hospitalization to continue their normal lifestyle, with appropriate restrictions (such as regular rest periods), until remission occurs.

♦ To prevent aplastic anemia, monitor blood studies carefully in the patient receiving anemia-inducing drugs.

♦ Support efforts to educate the public about the hazards of toxic agents. Tell parents to keep toxic agents out of the reach of children. Encourage people who work with radiation to wear protective clothing and a radiation-detecting badge, and to observe plant safety precautions. Those who work with benzene (solvent) should know that 10 parts per million is the highest safe environmental level and that a delayed reaction to benzene may develop.

SIDEROBLASTIC ANEMIAS

Sideroblastic anemias are a group of heterogeneous disorders with a common defect; they fail to use iron in Hb synthesis, despite the availability of adequate iron stores. These anemias may be hereditary or acquired; the acquired form, in turn, can be primary or secondary. Hereditary sideroblastic anemia may respond to treatment with pyridoxine. Correction of the secondary acquired form depends on the causative disorder; the primary acquired (idiopathic) form, however, resists treatment and usually proves fatal within 10 years after onset of complications or a concomitant disease.

Pathophysiology

Hereditary sideroblastic anemia appears to be transmitted by X-linked inheritance, occurring mostly in young males; females are carriers and usually show no signs of this disorder.

The acquired form may be secondary to ingestion of or exposure to toxins, such as alcohol and lead, or to certain drugs, such as isoniazid used to treat tuberculosis. It can also occur as a complication of other diseases, such as rheumatoid arthritis, lupus erythematosus, multiple myeloma, tuberculosis, and severe infections.

The primary acquired form, known as *refractory anemia with ringed sideroblasts*, is most common in elderly people. It's commonly associated with thrombocytopenia or leukopenia as part of a myelodysplastic syndrome.

In sideroblastic anemia, normoblasts fail to use iron to synthesize Hb. As a result, iron is deposited in the mitochondria of normoblasts, which are then termed *ringed sideroblasts*. (See *Ringed sideroblast*.)

Complications

◆ Severe cardiac, hepatic, and pancreatic disease
◆ Respiratory complications

Signs and symptoms

Sideroblastic anemias usually produce nonspecific clinical effects, which may exist for several years before being identified. Such effects include anorexia, fatigue, weakness, dizziness, pale skin and mucous membranes and, occasionally, enlarged lymph nodes. Heart and liver failure may develop due to excessive iron accumulation in these organs, causing dyspnea, exertional angina, slight jaundice, and hepatosplenomegaly. Hereditary sideroblastic anemia is associated with increased GI absorption of iron, causing signs of hemosiderosis. Additional symptoms in secondary sideroblastic anemia depend on the underlying cause.

Diagnosis

CONFIRMING DIAGNOSIS *Ringed sideroblasts on microscopic examination of bone marrow aspirate, stained with Prussian blue or alizarin red dye, confirm this diagnosis.*

Microscopic examination of blood shows erythrocytes to be hypochromic or normochromic and slightly macrocytic. Red cell precursors may be megaloblastic, with anisocytosis (abnormal variation in RBC size) and poikilocytosis (abnormal variation in RBC shape). Unlike iron deficiency anemia, sideroblastic anemia lowers Hb levels and raises serum iron and transferrin levels. In turn, faulty Hb production raises urobilinogen and bilirubin levels. Platelets and leukocytes remain normal, but, occasionally, thrombocytopenia or leukopenia occurs.

Treatment

Treatment of sideroblastic anemias depends on the underlying cause. The hereditary form usually responds to several weeks of treatment with high doses of pyridoxine (vitamin B_6). The acquired secondary form generally subsides after the causative drug or toxin is removed or the underlying condition is adequately treated. Folic acid supplements may also be beneficial when concomitant megaloblastic nuclear changes in RBC precursors are present. Elderly patients with sideroblastic anemia (usually the primary acquired form) are less likely to improve quickly and are more likely to develop serious complications. Deferoxamine may be used to treat chronic iron overload in selected patients.

Carefully crossmatched transfusions (providing needed Hb) or high doses of androgens are effective palliative measures for some patients with the primary acquired form of sideroblastic anemia. However, this form is essentially refractory to treatment and usually leads to death from acute leukemia or from respiratory or cardiac complications.

Some patients with sideroblastic anemia may benefit from phlebotomy to prevent hemochromatosis (the accumulation of iron in body tissues). Phlebotomy steps up the rate of

Ringed sideroblast

Electron microscopy shows large iron deposits in the mitochondria that surround the nucleus, forming the characteristic ringed sideroblast.

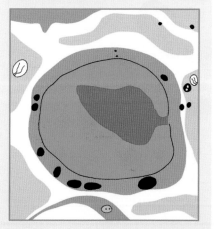

erythropoiesis and uses up excess iron stores; thus, it reduces serum and total body iron levels.

Special considerations

◆ Administer medications as indicated. Teach the patient the importance of continuing prescribed therapy, even after they begin to feel better.

◆ Provide frequent rest periods if the patient becomes easily fatigued.

◆ If phlebotomy is scheduled, explain the procedure thoroughly to help reduce anxiety. If this procedure must be repeated frequently, provide a high-protein diet to help replace the protein lost during phlebotomy. Encourage the patient to follow a similar diet at home.

◆ Always inquire about the possibility of exposure to lead in the home (especially for children) or on the job.

◆ Identify patients who abuse alcohol; refer them for appropriate therapy.

THALASSEMIA

Thalassemia, a hereditary group of hemolytic anemias, is characterized by defective synthesis in the polypeptide chains necessary for Hb production. Consequently, RBC synthesis is also impaired. (See *Peripheral blood smear in thalassemia major.*)

Beta-thalassemia is the most common form of this disorder. It results from defective beta polypeptide chain synthesis and occurs in three clinical forms: major, intermedia, and minor. The resulting anemia's severity depends on whether the patient is homozygous or heterozygous for the thalassemic trait. The prognosis

---

Peripheral blood smear in thalassemia major

Thalassemia major is a hereditary group of hemolytic anemias. It is characterized by defective synthesis in the polypeptide chains necessary for hemoglobin production that results in impairment of red blood cell production.

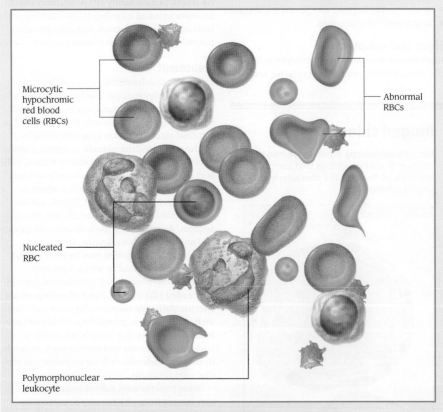

Microcytic hypochromic red blood cells (RBCs)

Abnormal RBCs

Nucleated RBC

Polymorphonuclear leukocyte

for beta-thalassemia varies. People with thalassemia major seldom survive to adulthood; children with thalassemia intermedia develop normally into adulthood, although puberty is usually delayed; people with thalassemia minor can expect a normal life span.

Pathophysiology

Thalassemia major and *thalassemia intermedia* result from homozygous inheritance of the partially dominant autosomal gene responsible for this trait. *Thalassemia minor* results from heterozygous inheritance of the same gene. In these disorders, total or partial deficiency of beta polypeptide chain production impairs Hb synthesis and results in continual production of fetal Hb, lasting even past the neonatal period.

Thalassemia is most common in people of Mediterranean ancestry (especially Italian and Greek) but also occurs in blacks and people from southern China, Southeast Asia, and India.

Complications

◆ Pathologic fractures
◆ Cardiac arrhythmias
◆ Heart failure

Signs and symptoms

In thalassemia major (also known as *Cooley anemia, Mediterranean disease,* and *erythroblastic anemia*), the neonate is well at birth but develops severe anemia, bone abnormalities, failure to thrive, and life-threatening complications. (See *Thalassemia major.*) In many cases, the first signs are pallor and yellow skin and sclera in infants ages 3 to 6 months. Later clinical features, in addition to severe anemia, include splenomegaly or hepatomegaly, with abdominal enlargement, frequent infections, bleeding tendencies (especially toward epistaxis), and anorexia.

Children with thalassemia major typically have small bodies and large heads and may also be mentally retarded. Infants may have mongoloid features because bone marrow hyperactivity has thickened the bone at the base of the nose. As these children grow older, they become susceptible to pathologic fractures as a result of expansion of the marrow cavities with thinning of the long bones. They're also subject to cardiac arrhythmias, heart failure, and other complications that result from iron deposits in the heart and in other tissues from repeated blood transfusions.

Thalassemia intermedia comprises moderate thalassemic disorders in homozygotes. Patients with this condition show some degree of anemia, jaundice, and splenomegaly and, possibly,

Thalassemia major

X-ray shows a characteristic skull abnormality in thalassemia major: diploetic fibers extending from the internal lamina.

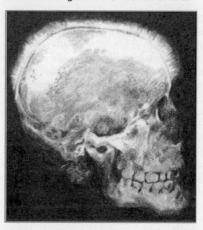

signs of hemosiderosis due to increased intestinal absorption of iron.

Thalassemia minor may cause mild anemia but usually produces no symptoms and is commonly overlooked. It should be differentiated from iron deficiency anemia.

Diagnosis

In the infant, the development of anemia with the characteristic bone abnormalities suggests the diagnosis of thalassemia major. Laboratory results show lowered RBC count and Hb level, microcytosis, and elevated reticulocyte, bilirubin, and urinary and fecal urobilinogen levels. A low serum folate level indicates increased folate utilization by the hypertrophied bone marrow. A peripheral blood smear reveals target cells, microcytes, pale nucleated RBCs, and marked anisocytosis. X-rays of the skull and long bones show thinning and widening of the marrow space because of overactive bone marrow. The bones of the skull and vertebrae may appear granular; long bones may show areas of osteoporosis. The phalanges may also be deformed (rectangular or biconvex). Quantitative Hb studies show a significant rise in HbF and a slight increase in HbA_2. Diagnosis must rule out iron deficiency anemia, which also produces hypochromia (slightly lowered Hb level) and microcytic (notably small) RBCs.

In thalassemia intermedia, laboratory results show hypochromia and microcytic RBCs, but the anemia is less severe than that in thalassemia major. In thalassemia minor, laboratory results show hypochromia and microcytic RBCs. Quantitative Hb studies show a significant increase in HbA_2 levels and a moderate rise in HbF levels.

Treatment

Treatment of thalassemia major is essentially supportive. For example, infections require prompt treatment with appropriate antibiotics. Folic acid supplements help maintain folic acid levels in the face of increased requirements. Transfusions of packed RBCs raise Hb levels but must be used judiciously to minimize iron overload. In addition, patients who receive blood transfusions should avoid iron supplements and oxidative drugs because iron levels can become toxic. Those who receive significant numbers of blood transfusions may require chelation therapy to remove iron from the body. Bone marrow transplantation is performed only in severe cases due to riskiness of the procedure and difficulty finding a good donor match.

Thalassemia intermedia and thalassemia minor generally don't require treatment.

Iron supplements are contraindicated in all forms of thalassemia.

Special considerations

◆ During and after RBC transfusions for thalassemia major, watch for adverse reactions—shaking chills, fever, rash, itching, and hives.
◆ Stress the importance of good nutrition, meticulous wound care, periodic dental checkups, and other measures to prevent infection.
◆ Discuss with the parents of a young patient various options for healthy physical and creative outlets. Such a child must avoid strenuous athletic activity because of increased oxygen demand and the tendency toward pathologic fractures, but may participate in less stressful activities.
◆ Teach parents to watch for signs of hepatitis and iron overload, which are always possible with frequent transfusions.
◆ Because parents may have questions about the vulnerability of future offspring, refer them for genetic counseling. Also refer adult patients with thalassemia minor and thalassemia intermedia for genetic counseling; they need to recognize the risk of transmitting thalassemia major to their children if they marry another person with thalassemia. If such people choose to marry and have children, their children should be evaluated for thalassemia by age 1. Be sure to tell people with thalassemia minor that their condition is benign.

IRON DEFICIENCY ANEMIA

Iron deficiency anemia is caused by an inadequate supply of iron for optimal formation of RBCs, resulting in smaller (microcytic) cells with less color on staining. (See *Peripheral blood smear in iron deficiency anemia*, page 461.) Body stores of iron, including plasma iron, decrease, as do levels of transferrin, which binds with and transports iron. Insufficient body stores of iron lead to a depleted RBC mass and, in turn, to a decreased Hb concentration (hypochromia) and decreased oxygen-carrying capacity of the blood. (See *Absorption and storage of iron*, page 461.)

Pathophysiology

Iron deficiency anemia may result from:
◆ inadequate dietary intake of iron (<1 to 2 mg/day), such as in prolonged unsupplemented breast-feeding or bottle-feeding of infants or during periods of stress such as rapid growth in children and adolescents
◆ iron malabsorption, such as in chronic diarrhea, partial or total gastrectomy, chronic diverticulosis, and malabsorption syndromes, such as celiac disease and pernicious anemia. Can also see iron deficiency in patient who have had bariatric surgery
◆ blood loss secondary to drug-induced GI bleeding (from anticoagulants, aspirin, and steroids) or due to heavy menses, hemorrhage from trauma, GI ulcers, esophageal varices, or cancer
◆ pregnancy, which diverts maternal iron to the fetus for erythropoiesis
◆ intravascular hemolysis-induced hemoglobinuria or paroxysmal nocturnal hemoglobinuria
◆ mechanical erythrocyte trauma caused by a prosthetic heart valve or vena cava filters
◆ anemia of chronic inflammation (as in rheumatoid arthritis)

A common disease worldwide, iron deficiency anemia affects 10% to 30% of the adult population of the United States. It occurs most commonly in premenopausal women, infants (particularly premature or low–birth-weight neonates), children, and adolescents (especially girls). Persons who are at increased risk for iron deficiency include those of low socioeconomic status who don't get a well-balanced diet that includes iron-rich foods.

Complications

◆ Infection
◆ Pneumonia
◆ Pica (in children)
◆ Bleeding
◆ Hemochromatosis (from excess iron treatment in children)

Peripheral blood smear in iron deficiency anemia

Iron deficiency anemia is caused by an inadequate supply of iron for the formation of red blood cells, resulting in smaller (microcytic) cells with less color on staining.

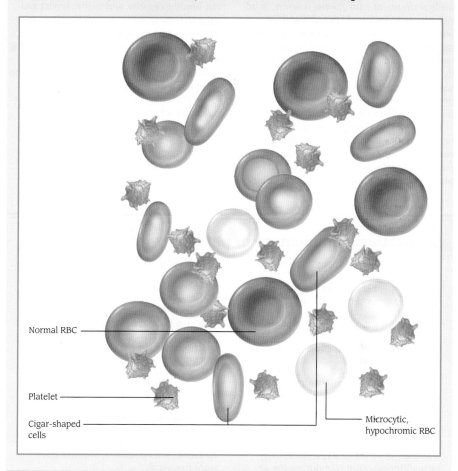

Normal RBC

Platelet

Cigar-shaped cells

Microcytic, hypochromic RBC

Absorption and storage of iron

Iron, which is essential to erythropoiesis, is abundant throughout the body. Two-thirds of total body iron is found in hemoglobin (Hb); the other third, mostly in the reticuloendothelial system (liver, spleen, bone marrow), with small amounts in muscle, blood serum, and body cells.

Adequate dietary ingestion of iron and recirculation of iron released from disintegrating red cells maintain iron supplies.

The duodenum and upper part of the small intestine absorb dietary iron. Such absorption depends on gastric acid content, the amount of reducing substances (e.g., ascorbic acid) present in the alimentary canal, and dietary iron intake. If iron intake is deficient, the body gradually depletes its iron stores, causing decreased Hb levels and, eventually, symptoms of iron deficiency anemia.

Signs and symptoms

Because of the gradual progression of iron deficiency anemia, many patients are initially asymptomatic except for symptoms of any underlying condition. They tend not to seek medical treatment until anemia is severe. At advanced stages, decreased Hb levels and the consequent decrease in the blood's oxygen-carrying capacity cause the patient to develop dyspnea on exertion, fatigue, listlessness, pallor, inability to concentrate, irritability, headache, and a susceptibility to infection. Decreased oxygen perfusion causes the heart to compensate with increased cardiac output and tachycardia.

In chronic iron deficiency anemia, nails become spoon-shaped and brittle, the mouth's corners crack, the tongue turns smooth, and the patient complains of dysphagia or may develop pica. Associated neuromuscular effects include vasomotor disturbances, numbness and tingling of the extremities, and neuralgic pain.

Diagnosis

Blood studies (serum iron levels, total iron-binding capacity, and ferritin levels) and stores in bone marrow may confirm iron deficiency anemia. However, the results of these tests can be misleading because of complicating factors, such as infection, pneumonia, blood transfusion, or iron supplements. Characteristic blood test results include:

◆ low Hb levels (in males, <12 g/dL; in females, <10 g/dL)
◆ low HCT (in males, <39%; in females, <35%)
◆ low serum iron levels, with elevated total iron-binding capacity
◆ low serum ferritin levels

Supportive management of patients with anemia

To meet the anemic patient's nutritional needs:
◆ If the patient is fatigued, urge them to eat small, frequent meals throughout the day.
◆ If the patient has oral lesions, suggest soft, cool, bland foods.
◆ If the patient has dyspepsia, eliminate spicy foods, and include milk and dairy products in his diet.
◆ If the patient is anorexic and irritable, encourage the family to bring their favorite foods from home (unless the diet is restricted) and to keep them company during meals, if possible.
  To set limitations on activities:
◆ Assess the effect of a specific activity by monitoring pulse rate during the activity. If the patient's pulse accelerates rapidly and the patient develops hypotension with hyperpnea, diaphoresis, light-headedness, palpitations, shortness of breath, or weakness, the activity is too strenuous.
◆ Tell the patient to pace his activities and to allow for frequent rest periods.
  To decrease susceptibility to infection:
◆ Use strict sterile technique.
◆ Isolate the patient from infectious persons.
◆ Instruct the patient to avoid crowds and other sources of infection. Encourage them to practice good hand-washing technique. Stress the importance of receiving necessary immunizations and prompt medical treatment for any sign of infection.

To prepare the patient for diagnostic testing:
◆ Explain erythropoiesis, the function of blood, and the purpose of diagnostic and therapeutic procedures.
◆ Tell the patient how they can participate in diagnostic testing. Give them an honest description of the pain or discomfort they will probably experience.
◆ If possible, schedule all tests to avoid disrupting the patient's meals, sleep, and visiting hours.
  To prevent complications:
◆ Observe for signs of bleeding that may exacerbate anemia. Check stool for occult bleeding. Assess for ecchymoses, gingival bleeding, and hematuria. Monitor vital signs frequently.
◆ If the patient is confined to strict bed rest, assist with range-of-motion exercises and frequent turning, coughing, and deep breathing.
◆ If blood transfusions are needed for severe anemia (hemoglobin level <5 g/dL), give washed red blood cells, as ordered, in partial exchange if evidence of pump failure is present. Carefully monitor for signs of circulatory overload or transfusion reaction. Watch for a change in pulse rate, blood pressure, or respiratory rate, or onset of fever, chills, pruritus, or edema. If any of these signs develop, stop the transfusion and notify the physician.
◆ Warn the patient to move about or change positions slowly to minimize dizziness induced by cerebral hypoxia.

How to inject iron solutions

For deep I.M. injections of iron solutions, use the Z-track technique to avoid subcutaneous irritation and discoloration from leaking medication.

Choose a 19G to 20G, 2" to 3" needle. After drawing up the solution, change to a fresh needle to avoid tracking the solution through to subcutaneous tissue. Draw 0.5 mL of air into the syringe as an "air lock."

Displace the skin and fat at the injection site (in the upper outer quadrant of the buttocks or the ventrogluteal site only) firmly to one side. Clean the area and insert the needle. Aspirate to check for entry into a blood vessel. Inject the solution slowly, followed by the 0.5 mL of air in the syringe. Wait 10 seconds, then pull the needle straight out, and release tissues.

Apply direct pressure to the site but don't massage it. Caution the patient against vigorous exercise for 15 to 30 minutes.

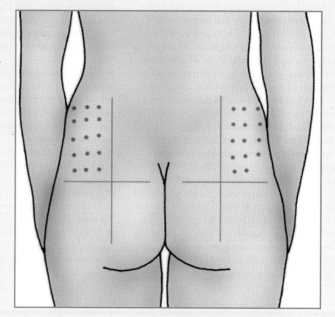

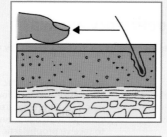

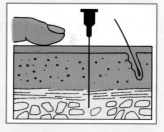

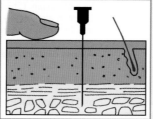

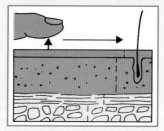

◆ low RBC count, with microcytic and hypochromic cells (in early stages, RBC count may be normal, except in infants and children)
◆ decreased mean corpuscular volume in severe anemia

Although rarely used, bone marrow studies provide a definitive diagnosis by revealing depleted or absent iron stores (done by staining) and normoblastic hyperplasia.

Diagnosis must rule out other forms of anemia, such as those that result from thalassemia minor, cancer, and chronic inflammatory, hepatic, and renal disease.

Treatment

The first priority of treatment is to determine the underlying cause of anemia. Once this is determined, iron replacement therapy can begin. Treatment of choice is an oral preparation of iron or a combination of iron and ascorbic acid (which enhances iron absorption). However, in some cases, iron may have to be administered parenterally—for instance, if the patient is noncompliant to the oral preparation, needs more iron than can be taken orally, if malabsorption prevents adequate iron absorption, or if a maximum rate of Hb regeneration is desired.

Because total dose I.V. infusion of supplemental iron is painless and requires fewer injections, it's usually preferred to I.M. administration. Pregnant patients and geriatric patients with severe anemia, for example, should receive a total dose infusion of iron dextran in normal saline solution over 8 hours. To minimize the risk of an allergic reaction to iron, an I.V. test dose of 0.5 mL should be given first. For more patient care information, see *Supportive management of patients with anemia*, above.

Special considerations

◆ Monitor the patient's compliance with the prescribed iron supplement therapy. Advise the patient not to stop therapy even if they feel better, because replacement of iron stores takes time. Iron supplementation must be continued for at least 1 year after Hb has risen to normal levels.

◆ Tell the patient they may take iron supplements with a meal to decrease gastric irritation. Advise them to avoid fiber, milk, and milk products, and antacids because they interfere with iron absorption; however, vitamin C can increase absorption.

◆ Warn the patient that iron supplements may result in dark green or black stools and can cause constipation.

◆ Instruct the patient to drink liquid supplemental iron through a straw to prevent staining his teeth.

◆ Tell the patient to report reactions, such as nausea, vomiting, diarrhea, constipation, fever, or severe stomach pain, which may require a dosage adjustment.

 PREVENTION

Preventing iron deficiency anemia

Play a vital role in preventing iron deficiency anemia in your patients by encouraging the following actions:

Include iron-rich foods in diet
Teach the basics of a nutritionally balanced diet by having your patients include foods rich in iron, such as those listed below, in their diet:
◆ Meat (especially liver)
◆ Egg yolks
◆ Dried beans or peas
◆ Green leafy vegetables
◆ Dried fruits
◆ Cream of wheat cereal
◆ Molasses

Include vitamin C-rich foods in diet
Encourage your patients to consume foods high in vitamin C (ascorbic acid) at the same time they're eating iron-rich foods. The vitamin C aids in the absorption of the iron. These foods are rich in vitamin C:
◆ Citrus fruit or juice
◆ Tomatoes
◆ Broccoli
◆ Melons
◆ Strawberries
◆ Red peppers

Include prophylactic oral iron
Emphasize the need for high-risk individuals, such as premature infants, children younger than age 2, and pregnant women, to receive prophylactic oral iron, as ordered by a physician. (Children younger than age 2 should also receive supplemental cereals and formulas high in iron.)

Assess dietary habits
Assess a family's dietary habits for iron intake and note the influence of childhood eating patterns, cultural food preferences, and family income on adequate nutrition.

Assess medication history
Carefully assess your patients' drug histories because certain drugs, such as pancreatic enzymes and vitamin E, may interfere with iron metabolism and absorption and because aspirin, steroids, and other drugs may cause GI bleeding. (Teach patients who must take medications that are gastric irritants to take these medications with meals or milk.)

ALERT *If the patient receives I.V. iron, monitor the infusion rate carefully and observe for an allergic reaction. Stop the infusion and begin supportive treatment immediately if the patient shows signs of an adverse reaction. Also, watch for dizziness and headache and for thrombophlebitis around the I.V. site.*

◆ Use the Z-track injection method when administering iron I.M. to prevent skin discoloration, scarring, and irritating iron deposits in the skin. (See *How to inject iron solutions,* page 463.)

◆ Because an iron deficiency may recur, advise regular checkups and blood studies. (See *Preventing iron deficiency anemia,* page 464.)

Polycythemias

POLYCYTHEMIA VERA

Polycythemia vera is a chronic, myeloproliferative disorder characterized by increased RBC mass. In addition, there may also be leukocytosis, thrombocytosis, and increased Hb concentration, with normal or increased plasma volume. This disease is also known as *primary polycythemia, erythremia, polycythemia rubra vera, splenomegalic polycythemia,* and *Vaquez–Osler disease.* (See *Peripheral blood smear in polycythemia vera.*)

Peripheral blood smear in polycythemia vera

Polycythemia vera is a chronic, myeloproliferative disorder characterized by increased red blood cell mass, leukocytosis, thrombocytosis, and increased hemoglobin concentration, with normal or increased plasma volume.

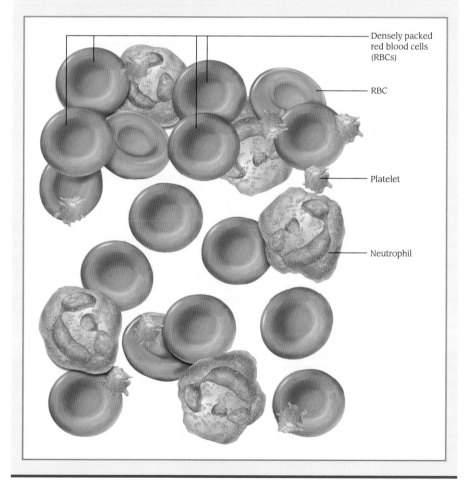

Densely packed red blood cells (RBCs)

RBC

Platelet

Neutrophil

Clinical features of polycythemia vera

Signs and symptoms	Causes
Eye, ear, nose, and throat	
◆ Visual disturbances (blurring, diplopia, scotoma, engorged veins of fundus and retina) and congestion of conjunctiva, retina, retinal veins, oral mucous membrane	◆ Hypervolemia and hyperviscosity
◆ Epistaxis or gingival bleeding	◆ Engorgement of capillary beds
Central nervous system	
◆ Headache or fullness in the head, lethargy, weakness, fatigue, syncope, tinnitus, paresthesia of digits, and impaired mentation	◆ Hypervolemia and hyperviscosity leading to decreased cerebral blood flow
Cardiovascular system	
◆ Hypertension	◆ Hypervolemia and hyperviscosity
◆ Intermittent claudication, thrombosis and emboli, angina, thrombophlebitis	◆ Hypervolemia, thrombocytosis, and vascular disease
◆ Hemorrhage	◆ Engorgement of capillary beds
Skin	
◆ Pruritus (especially after hot bath)	◆ Basophilia (secondary histamine release)
◆ Urticaria	◆ Altered histamine metabolism
◆ Ruddy cyanosis	◆ Hypervolemia and hyperviscosity due to congested vessels, increased oxyhemoglobin, and reduced hemoglobin
◆ Night sweats	◆ Hypermetabolism
◆ Ecchymosis	◆ Hemorrhage
GI system	
◆ Epigastric distress	◆ Hypervolemia and hyperviscosity
◆ Early satiety and fullness	◆ Hepatosplenomegaly
◆ Peptic ulcer pain	◆ Gastric thrombosis and hemorrhage
◆ Hepatosplenomegaly	◆ Congestion, extramedullary hematopoiesis, and myeloid metaplasia
◆ Weight loss	◆ Hypermetabolism
Respiratory system	
◆ Dyspnea	◆ Hypervolemia and hyperviscosity
Musculoskeletal system	
◆ Joint symptoms	◆ Increased urate production secondary to nucleoprotein turnover

The prognosis depends on the patient's age at diagnosis, the type of treatment used, and complications. Mortality is high if polycythemia is untreated or progresses to leukemia or myeloid metaplasia.

Pathophysiology

In polycythemia vera, uncontrolled and rapid cellular reproduction and maturation cause proliferation or hyperplasia of all bone marrow cells (panmyelosis). The cause of such uncontrolled cellular activity is unknown but it's probably due to a mutation in the protein *JAK2*.

Polycythemia vera usually occurs between ages 40 and 60, most commonly among males and those with a family history; it seldom affects children or blacks and doesn't appear to be familial. The disease may manifest itself in women after menopause.

Complications

- Thrombosis of small vessels
- Ruddy cyanosis of nose
- Clubbing
- Splenomegaly
- Renal calculus formation
- Abdominal thrombosis
- Hemorrhage

Signs and symptoms

Increased RBC mass results in hyperviscosity and retards blood flow to microcirculation. Subsequently, increased viscosity, diminished velocity, and thrombocytosis promote intravascular thrombosis. In early stages, polycythemia vera usually produces no symptoms. (Increased HCT may be an incidental finding.) However, as altered circulation secondary to increased RBC mass produces hypervolemia and hyperviscosity, the patient may complain of a feeling of fullness in the head, headache, dizziness, and other symptoms, depending on the body system affected. The patient may also complain of severe itching after a warm or hot shower. Hyperviscosity may lead to thrombosis of smaller vessels with ruddy cyanosis of the nose and clubbing of the digits. Splenomegaly is present in about one-third of patients at the time of diagnosis.

Paradoxically, hemorrhage is a complication of polycythemia vera. It may be due to defective platelet function or to hyperviscosity and the local effects from excess RBCs exerting pressure on distended venous and capillary walls. (See *Clinical features of polycythemia vera*, page 466.)

Diagnosis

Laboratory studies confirm polycythemia vera by showing increased RBC mass and normal arterial oxygen saturation in association with splenomegaly or two of the following: thrombocytosis, leukocytosis, elevated leukocyte alkaline phosphatase level, or elevated serum vitamin B_{12} level or unbound B_{12}-binding capacity. A low serum erythropoietin level will also confirm diagnosis.

Another common finding is increased uric acid production, leading to hyperuricemia and hyperuricuria. Other laboratory results include increased blood histamine levels, decreased serum iron concentration, and decreased or absent urinary erythropoietin. Bone marrow biopsy reveals panmyelosis and possibly a genetic mutation of *JAK2*.

Treatment

Phlebotomy can reduce RBC mass promptly. The frequency of phlebotomy and the amount of blood removed each time depend on the patient's condition. Typically, 350 to 500 mL of blood can be removed every other day until the HCT is reduced to the low-normal range. After repeated phlebotomies, the patient develops iron deficiency, which stabilizes RBC production and reduces the need for phlebotomy. Pheresis permits the return of plasma to the patient, diluting the blood and reducing hypovolemic symptoms.

Phlebotomy doesn't reduce the WBC or platelet count and won't control the hyperuricemia associated with marrow cell proliferation. For severe symptoms, myelosuppressive therapy may be used. Chemotherapeutic agents may be used to suppress the bone marrow, but these agents may cause leukemia and should be reserved for older patients and those with problems uncontrolled by phlebotomy. The current preferred myelosuppressive agent is hydroxyurea, which isn't associated with leukemia. Patients who have had previous thrombotic problems should be considered for myelosuppressive therapy. The use of antiplatelet therapy is controversial because it may cause gastric bleeding. Allopurinol may be given for hyperuricemia.

Special considerations

If the patient requires phlebotomy, explain the procedure, and provide reassurance that it will relieve distressing symptoms. Check blood pressure, pulse rate, and respiratory rate. During phlebotomy, make sure the patient is lying down comfortably to prevent vertigo and syncope. Stay alert for tachycardia, clamminess, or complaints of vertigo. If these effects occur, the procedure should be stopped.

- Immediately after phlebotomy, check blood pressure and pulse rate. Have the patient sit up for about 5 minutes before allowing them to walk; this prevents vasovagal attack or orthostatic hypotension. Also, have them drink 24 oz (710 mL) of juice or water.
- Tell the patient to watch for and report signs or symptoms of iron deficiency (pallor, weight loss, asthenia [weakness], and glossitis).
- Keep the patient active and ambulatory to prevent thrombosis. If bed rest is absolutely necessary, prescribe a daily program of both active and passive range-of-motion exercises.
- Watch for complications: hypervolemia, thrombocytosis, and signs or symptoms of an impending stroke (decreased sensation, numbness, transitory paralysis, fleeting blindness, headache, and epistaxis).
- Regularly examine the patient closely for bleeding. Tell them which are the most

common bleeding sites (such as the nose, gingiva, and skin) so they can check for bleeding. Advise them to report any abnormal bleeding promptly.

◆ To compensate for increased uric acid production, give additional fluids, administer allopurinol, and alkalinize the urine to prevent uric acid calculi.

◆ If the patient has symptom-producing splenomegaly, suggest or provide small, frequent meals, followed by a rest period, to prevent nausea and vomiting.

◆ Report acute abdominal pain immediately; it may signal splenic infarction, renal calculi, or abdominal organ thrombosis.

During myelosuppressive treatment:

◆ Monitor CBC and platelet count before and during therapy. Warn the outpatient who develops leukopenia that his resistance to infection is low; advise the patient to avoid crowds and watch for the symptoms of infection. If leukopenia develops in a hospitalized patient who needs reverse isolation, follow hospital guidelines. If thrombocytopenia develops, tell the patient to watch for signs of bleeding (blood in urine, nosebleeds, and black stool).

◆ Tell the patient about possible reactions (nausea, vomiting, and risk of infection) to alkylating agents. Alopecia may follow the use of busulfan, cyclophosphamide, and uracil mustard; sterile hemorrhagic cystitis may follow the use of cyclophosphamide (forcing fluids can prevent it). Watch for and report all reactions. If nausea and vomiting occur, begin antiemetic therapy and adjust the patient's diet.

SPURIOUS POLYCYTHEMIA

Spurious polycythemia, also known as *relative polycythemia, stress erythrocytosis, stress polycythemia, benign polycythemia, Gaisböck syndrome,* and *pseudopolycythemia,* is characterized by increased HCT and normal or decreased RBC total mass; it results from decreasing plasma volume and subsequent hemoconcentration.

Pathophysiology

There are three possible causes of spurious polycythemia:

◆ Dehydration—Conditions that promote severe fluid loss decrease plasma levels and lead to hemoconcentration. Such conditions include persistent vomiting or diarrhea, burns, adrenocortical insufficiency, aggressive diuretic therapy, decreased fluid intake, diabetic acidosis, and renal disease.

◆ Hemoconcentration due to stress—Nervous stress leads to hemoconcentration by some unknown mechanism (possibly by temporarily

decreasing circulating plasma volume or vascular redistribution of erythrocytes). This form of erythrocytosis (chronically elevated HCT) is particularly common in the middle-aged man who's a chronic smoker and a type A personality (tense, hard driving, and anxious).

◆ High normal RBC mass and low-normal plasma volume—In many patients, an increased HCT merely reflects a normally high RBC mass and low plasma volume. This is particularly common in patients who don't smoke, aren't obese, and have no history of hypertension.

Other factors that may be associated with spurious polycythemia include hypertension, thromboembolic disease, elevated serum cholesterol and uric acid levels, and familial tendency. It usually affects middle-aged people and occurs more commonly in men than in women.

Complications

◆ Hypercholesterolemia
◆ Hyperlipidemia
◆ Hyperuricemia

Signs and symptoms

The patient with spurious polycythemia usually has no specific symptoms but may have vague complaints, such as headaches, dizziness, and fatigue. Less commonly, the patient may develop diaphoresis, dyspnea, and claudication.

Typically, the patient has a ruddy appearance, a short neck, slight hypertension, and a tendency to hypoventilate when recumbent. The patient shows no associated hepatosplenomegaly but may have cardiac or pulmonary disease.

Diagnosis

Hb levels, HCT, and RBC count are elevated; RBC mass, arterial oxygen saturation, and bone marrow are normal. Plasma volume may be decreased or normal. Hypercholesterolemia, hyperlipidemia, or hyperuricemia may be present.

℞ CONFIRMING DIAGNOSIS *Spurious polycythemia is distinguishable from true polycythemia vera by its characteristic normal RBC mass, elevated HCT, and the absence of leukocytosis and thrombocytosis.*

Treatment

The principal goals of treatment are to prevent life-threatening thromboembolism and to correct dehydration. Rehydration with appropriate fluids and electrolytes is the primary therapy for spurious polycythemia secondary to dehydration. Therapy must also include appropriate measures to prevent further fluid loss such as antidiarrheals, if needed, and avoiding dietary diuretics.

Special considerations
◆ During rehydration, carefully monitor intake and output to maintain fluid and electrolyte balance.
◆ Whenever appropriate, suggest counseling about the patient's work habits and lack of relaxation. If the patient smokes, make sure they understand how important it is to stop. Refer the patient to a smoking-cessation program if necessary.
◆ Emphasize the need for follow-up examinations every 3 to 4 months after leaving the hospital.
◆ Thoroughly explain spurious polycythemia, diagnostic measures, and therapy. The hard-driving person predisposed to spurious polycythemia is likely to be more inquisitive and anxious than the average patient. Answer questions honestly, but take care to reassure that they can effectively control symptoms by complying with the prescribed treatment.

▦ **PREVENTION** *To prevent thromboemboli in predisposed patients, suggest regular exercise and a low-cholesterol diet. Antilipemics may also be necessary. Reduced calorie intake may be required for the obese patient.*

SECONDARY POLYCYTHEMIA
Secondary polycythemia (also called *reactive polycythemia* or *secondary erythrocytosis*) is a disorder characterized by excessive production of circulating RBCs due to hypoxia, tumor, or disease.

Pathophysiology
Secondary polycythemia may result from increased production of erythropoietin. This hormone, which is possibly produced and secreted in the kidneys, stimulates bone marrow production of RBCs. Increased production may be a compensatory physiologic response to hypoxemia, which may result from:
◆ chronic obstructive pulmonary disease
◆ Hb abnormalities (such as carboxyhemoglobinemia, which is seen in heavy smokers)
◆ heart failure (causing a decreased ventilation–perfusion ratio)
◆ right-to-left shunting of blood in the heart (as in transposition of the great vessels)
◆ central or peripheral alveolar hypoventilation (as in barbiturate intoxication or pickwickian syndrome)
◆ low oxygen content at high altitudes
Increased production of erythropoietin may also be an inappropriate (pathologic) response to renal disease (such as renal vascular impairment, renal cysts, or hydronephrosis), to CNS disease (such as encephalitis and

parkinsonism), to neoplasms (such as liver tumors, adrenal adenoma, renal tumors, uterine myomas, or cerebellar hemangiomas), or to endocrine disorders (such as Cushing syndrome, Bartter syndrome, or pheochromocytomas). Rarely, secondary polycythemia results from a recessive genetic trait.

Secondary polycythemia occurs in about 2 out of every 100,000 people living at or near sea level; incidence rises among those living at high altitudes.

Complications
◆ Hemorrhage
◆ Thromboemboli

Signs and symptoms
In the hypoxic patient, suggestive physical findings include ruddy cyanotic skin, emphysema, and hypoxemia without hepatosplenomegaly or hypertension. Clubbing of the fingers may occur if the underlying disease is cardiovascular. When secondary polycythemia isn't caused by hypoxemia, it's usually an incidental finding during treatment of an underlying disease.

Diagnosis
℞ **CONFIRMING DIAGNOSIS** *Laboratory values for secondary polycythemia include increased RBC mass (increased HCT, Hb levels, and mean corpuscular volume and mean corpuscular Hb values) and serum and urinary erythropoietin and blood histamine levels, with decreased or normal arterial oxygen saturation. Bone marrow biopsies reveal hyperplasia confined to the erythroid series.*

Unlike polycythemia vera, secondary polycythemia isn't associated with leukocytosis or thrombocytosis.

Treatment
The goal of treatment is correction of the underlying disease or environmental condition. In severe secondary polycythemia in which altitude is a contributing factor, relocation may be advisable. If secondary polycythemia has produced hazardous hyperviscosity or if the patient doesn't respond to treatment of the primary disease, reduction in blood volume by phlebotomy or pheresis may be effective. Emergency phlebotomy is indicated for prevention of impending vascular occlusion or before emergency surgery. In the latter case, it's usually advisable to remove excess RBCs and reinfuse the patient's plasma.

⚠ **ALERT** *Because a patient with polycythemia has an increased risk of hemorrhage during and after surgery, elective surgery should be avoided until polycythemia is controlled.*

Typically, secondary polycythemia disappears when the primary disease is corrected.

Special considerations

◆ Keep the patient as active as possible to decrease the risk of thrombosis due to increased blood viscosity.

◆ Reduce calorie and sodium intake to counteract the tendency toward hypertension.

◆ Before and after phlebotomy, check blood pressure with the patient lying down. After the procedure, have the patient drink 24 oz (710 mL) of water or juice. To prevent syncope, have them sit upright for about 5 minutes before walking.

◆ Emphasize the importance of regular blood studies (every 2 to 3 months), even after the disease is controlled.

◆ Teach the patient and their family about the underlying disorder. Help them understand its relationship to polycythemia and the measures needed to control both.

◆ Teach the patient to recognize symptoms of recurring polycythemia and the importance of reporting them promptly.

Hemorrhagic disorders

ALLERGIC PURPURAS

Allergic purpura, a nonthrombocytopenic purpura, is an acute or chronic vascular inflammation affecting the skin, joints, and GI and GU tracts, in association with allergy symptoms. When allergic purpura primarily affects the GI tract, with accompanying joint pain, it's called *Henoch–Schönlein syndrome*, or *anaphylactoid purpura*. However, the term *allergic purpura* applies to purpura associated with many other conditions, such as erythema nodosum. An acute attack of allergic purpura can last for several weeks and is potentially fatal (usually from renal failure); however, most patients do recover.

Fully developed allergic purpura is persistent and debilitating, possibly leading to chronic glomerulonephritis (especially following a streptococcal infection).

Pathophysiology

The most common identifiable cause of allergic purpura is probably an autoimmune reaction directed against vascular walls, triggered by a bacterial infection (particularly streptococcal infection). Typically, upper respiratory tract infection occurs 1 to 3 weeks before the onset of symptoms. Other possible causes include allergic reactions to some drugs and vaccines, to insect bites, and to some foods (such as wheat, eggs, milk, and chocolate).

Purpuric lesions

Lesions of allergic purpura, such as those pictured on the foot and leg below, characteristically vary in size.

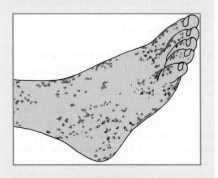

Allergic purpura affects males more than females and is most prevalent in children ages 3 to 7. The prognosis is more favorable for children than adults.

Complications

◆ Renal failure
◆ Acute glomerulonephritis

Signs and symptoms

Characteristic skin lesions of allergic purpura are purple, macular, ecchymotic, and of varying size. They're caused by vascular leakage into the skin and mucous membranes. (See *Purpuric lesions.*) The lesions usually appear in symmetric patterns on the arms, legs, and buttocks and are accompanied by pruritus, paresthesia and, occasionally, angioneurotic edema. In children, skin lesions are generally urticarial and expand and become hemorrhagic. Scattered petechiae may appear on the legs, buttocks, and perineum.

Henoch–Schönlein syndrome commonly produces transient or severe colic, tenesmus (spasmodic contraction of the anal sphincter) and constipation, vomiting, and edema or hemorrhage of the mucous membranes of the bowel, resulting in GI bleeding, occult blood in the stool and, possibly, intussusception. Such GI abnormalities may *precede* overt, cutaneous signs of purpura. Musculoskeletal symptoms, such as rheumatoid pains and periarticular effusions, mostly affect the legs and feet.

In 25% to 50% of patients, allergic purpura is associated with GU signs and symptoms: nephritis; renal hemorrhages that may cause microscopic hematuria and disturb renal function; bleeding from the mucosal surfaces of the ureters, bladder, or urethra; and, occasionally, glomerulonephritis. Also possible are moderate and irregular fever, headache, anorexia, and localized edema of the hands, feet, or scalp.

Diagnosis

No laboratory test clearly identifies allergic purpura (although WBC count and erythrocyte sedimentation rate may be elevated). Diagnosis therefore necessitates careful clinical observation, in many cases during the second or third attack. Except for a positive tourniquet test (a test to assess the capillaries' ability to withstand increased pressure), coagulation and platelet function tests are usually normal. Small-bowel X-rays may reveal areas of transient edema; in many cases, tests for blood in the urine and stool are positive. Increased blood urea nitrogen and creatinine levels may indicate renal involvement. Diagnosis must rule out other forms of nonthrombocytopenic purpura.

Treatment

Treatment is generally symptomatic; for example, severe allergic purpura may require steroids to relieve edema and analgesics to relieve joint and abdominal pain. Some patients with chronic renal disease may benefit from immunosuppressive therapy with azathioprine along with identification of the provocative allergen. *An accurate allergy history is essential.*

Special considerations

◆ Encourage maintenance of an elimination diet to help identify specific allergenic foods so these foods can be eliminated from the patient's diet.
◆ Monitor skin lesions and level of pain. Provide analgesics as needed.
◆ Watch carefully for complications: GI and GU tract bleeding, edema, nausea, vomiting, headache, hypertension (with nephritis), abdominal rigidity and tenderness, and absence of stool (with intussusception).
◆ To prevent muscle atrophy in the bedridden patient, provide passive or active range-of-motion exercises.
◆ Provide emotional support and reassurance, especially if florid skin lesions temporarily disfigure the patient.
◆ After the acute stage, stress the need for the patient to *immediately* report *any* recurrence of symptoms (recurrence is most common about 6 weeks after initial onset) and to return for follow-up urinalysis as scheduled.

HEREDITARY HEMORRHAGIC TELANGIECTASIA

Hereditary hemorrhagic telangiectasia (also called *Osler–Weber–Rendu syndrome*) is an inherited vascular disorder in which venules and capillaries dilate and form fragile masses of thin convoluted vessels (telangiectases), resulting in an abnormal tendency to hemorrhage. This disorder affects both sexes but may cause less severe bleeding in girls and women.

Complication

◆ Secondary iron deficiency anemia

Pathophysiology

Hereditary hemorrhagic telangiectasia is transmitted by autosomal dominant inheritance. It seldom skips generations. In its homozygous state, it may be lethal. It affects 1 in 5,000 to 1 in 10,000 people worldwide.

Signs and symptoms

Signs of hereditary hemorrhagic telangiectasia are present in childhood but increase in severity with age. Localized aggregations of dilated capillaries appear on the skin of the face, ears, scalp, hands, arms, and feet; under the nails; and on the mucous membranes of the nose, mouth, and stomach. These dilated capillaries cause frequent epistaxis, hemoptysis, and GI bleeding, usually leading to iron deficiency anemia. (In children, epistaxis is usually the first symptom.)

Characteristic telangiectases are violet, bleed spontaneously, may be flat or raised, blanch on pressure, and are nonpulsatile. They may be associated with vascular malformations such as arteriovenous fistulas. Visceral telangiectases are common in the liver, bladder, respiratory tract, and stomach. The type and distribution of these lesions are generally similar among family members.

Generalized capillary fragility, as evidenced by spontaneous bleeding, petechiae, ecchymoses, and spider hemangiomas of varying sizes, may exist without overt telangiectasia. (See *Typical lesions of hereditary hemorrhagic telangiectasia,* page 472.) Rarely, vascular malformation may cause pulmonary arteriovenous fistulas; then, shunting of blood through the fistulas may lead to hypoxemia, recurring cerebral embolism, brain abscess, and clubbing of digits.

Diagnosis

Diagnosis is based principally on an established familial pattern of bleeding disorders and on clinical evidence of telangiectasia and

Typical lesions of hereditary hemorrhagic telangiectasia

Dilated capillaries, either flat or raised, appear in localized aggregations, as on the fingers.

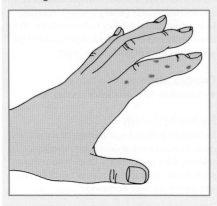

On the face, spider hemangiomas reflect capillary fragility.

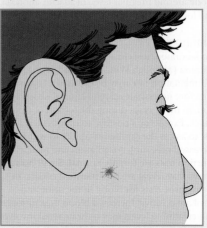

hemorrhage. Hypochromic, microcytic anemia is common; abnormal platelet function may also be found.

Treatment

Supportive therapy includes blood transfusions for acute hemorrhage and supplemental iron administration to replace iron lost in repeated mucosal bleeding. Ancillary treatments consist of applying pressure and topical hemostatic agents to bleeding sites, using electrocautery or laser surgery on bleeding sites not readily accessible, and protecting the patient from trauma and unnecessary bleeding. Endovascular embolization may be used to treat abnormal blood vessels in the brain and other parts of the body.

Oral and, rarely, parenteral administration of supplemental iron enhances absorption to maintain adequate iron stores and prevents gastric irritation. Administering antipyretics or antihistamines before blood transfusions, and using saline-washed cells, frozen blood, or other types of leukocyte-poor blood instead of whole blood may prevent febrile transfusion reactions.

The administration of estrogen has proved effective in some patients, especially when used to control epistaxis.

Special considerations

⚠ **ALERT** *During the first 15 minutes of a blood transfusion, stay with the patient to* *watch for adverse reactions. Afterward, check again every 15 minutes for signs and symptoms of a febrile or an allergic transfusion reaction (flushing, shaking chills, fever, headache, rash, tachycardia, and hypertension) because patients with this disorder are quite susceptible to this type of reaction.*

◆ Observe the patient for indications of GI bleeding, such as hematemesis and melena. Instruct them to watch for and report such signs as well.

◆ If the patient requires an iron supplement, stress the importance of following dosage instructions and of taking oral iron with meals to minimize gastric irritation. Warn them that iron turns stools dark green or black and may cause constipation.

◆ Provide emotional and psychological support. Encourage the patient to express concerns they may have about the disease and its treatment. As much as possible, include them in care decisions.

◆ Encourage fluid intake, when possible, if the patient is experiencing a bleeding episode or is hypovolemic. Monitor intake and output.

◆ Provide good skin care and hygiene, and use sterile technique when caring for the patient. Lesions bleed easily, which may result in infection and skin breakdown.

◆ Monitor the patient's organ function through physical examination and the comparison of laboratory tests to detect renal, hepatic, or respiratory failure.

◆ Teach the patient and their family how to manage minor bleeding episodes, especially recurrent epistaxis, and how to recognize major episodes that necessitate emergency intervention.

◆ Teach the patient and their family about the disease's hereditary nature. Refer for genetic counseling, as appropriate, and to the Hereditary Hemorrhagic Telangiectasia Foundation International for support and information.

THROMBOCYTOPENIA

The most common cause of hemorrhagic disorders, thrombocytopenia is characterized by deficiency of circulating platelets. Because platelets play a vital role in coagulation, this deficiency poses a serious threat to hemostasis. (See *What happens in thrombocytopenia*, page 474.) The prognosis is excellent in drug-induced thrombocytopenia if the offending drug is withdrawn; in such cases, recovery may be immediate. In other types, the prognosis depends on the patient's response to treatment of the underlying cause.

Causes

Thrombocytopenia may be congenital or acquired; the acquired form is more common. In either case, it usually results from decreased or defective production of platelets in the marrow (such as occurs in leukemia, aplastic anemia, or toxicity with certain drugs) or from increased destruction outside the marrow caused by an underlying disorder (such as cirrhosis of the liver, disseminated intravascular coagulation [DIC], or severe infection). Less commonly, it results from sequestration (hypersplenism and hypothermia) or platelet loss. Acquired thrombocytopenia may result from certain drugs, such as sulfonamides, antibiotics, gold salts, estrogens, or chemotherapeutic agents. (See *Causes of decreased circulating platelets*.)

⬡ **ELDER TIP** *In older adults, platelet characteristics change. Granular constituents decrease and platelet-release factors increase. These changes may reflect diminished bone marrow and increased fibrinogen levels.*

An idiopathic form of thrombocytopenia commonly occurs in children. A transient form may follow viral infection (such as Epstein–Barr virus or infectious mononucleosis).

Complication
◆ Acute hemorrhage

Signs and symptoms
Thrombocytopenia typically produces a sudden onset of petechiae or ecchymoses in the skin or bleeding into any mucous membrane.

Nearly all patients are otherwise asymptomatic, although some may complain of malaise, fatigue, and general weakness. In adults, large, blood-filled bullae characteristically appear in the mouth. In severe thrombocytopenia, hemorrhage may lead to tachycardia, shortness of breath, loss of consciousness, and death.

Causes of decreased circulating platelets

Diminished or defective platelet production
Congenital
◆ Wiskott–Aldrich syndrome
◆ Maternal ingestion of thiazides
◆ Neonatal rubella
◆ Polycythemia

Acquired
◆ Aplastic anemia
◆ Marrow infiltration (acute and chronic leukemias, tumor)
◆ Nutritional deficiency (vitamin B_{12}, folic acid)
◆ Myelosuppressive agents
◆ Drugs that directly influence platelet production (thiazides, alcohol, hormones)
◆ Radiation
◆ Viral infections (measles, dengue)

Increased peripheral platelet destruction
Congenital
◆ Nonimmune (prematurity, erythroblastosis fetalis, infection)
◆ Immune (drug sensitivity, maternal idiopathic thrombocytopenic purpura [ITP])

Acquired
◆ Nonimmune (infection, disseminated intravascular coagulation, thrombotic thrombocytopenic purpura)
◆ Immune (drug-induced, especially with quinine and quinidine; posttransfusion purpura; acute and chronic ITP; sepsis; alcohol)
◆ Invasive lines and devices
◆ Intra-aortic balloon pump
◆ Prosthetic heart valves
◆ Heparin

Platelet sequestration
◆ Hypersplenism
◆ Hypothermia

Platelet loss
◆ Hemorrhage
◆ Extracorporeal perfusion

PATHOPHYSIOLOGY
What happens in thrombocytopenia

Thrombocytopenia is the most common cause of bleeding disorders and is characterized by a severe decrease in platelets. This platelet decrease can result from hematologic malignancy, radiation or drug therapy, idiopathic causes, blood transfusions, disseminated intravascular coagulation (DIC), or splenomegaly. Excessive hemorrhaging can lead to shock if interventions are delayed. This chart shows how these conditions and treatments develop into thrombocytopenic hemorrhage.

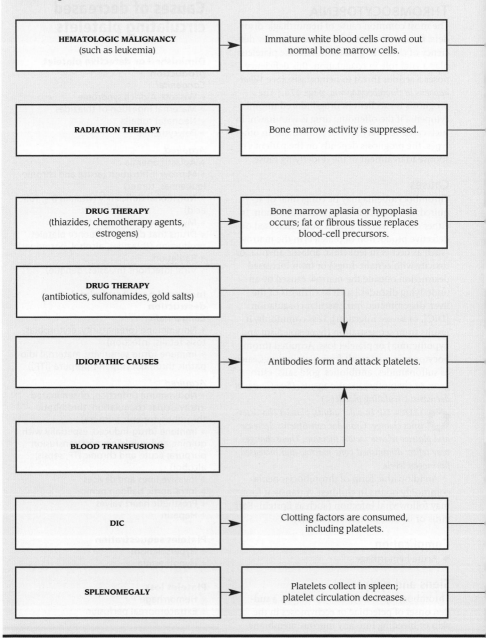

HEMATOLOGIC MALIGNANCY (such as leukemia)	Immature white blood cells crowd out normal bone marrow cells.
RADIATION THERAPY	Bone marrow activity is suppressed.
DRUG THERAPY (thiazides, chemotherapy agents, estrogens)	Bone marrow aplasia or hypoplasia occurs; fat or fibrous tissue replaces blood-cell precursors.
DRUG THERAPY (antibiotics, sulfonamides, gold salts)	
IDIOPATHIC CAUSES	Antibodies form and attack platelets.
BLOOD TRANSFUSIONS	
DIC	Clotting factors are consumed, including platelets.
SPLENOMEGALY	Platelets collect in spleen; platelet circulation decreases.

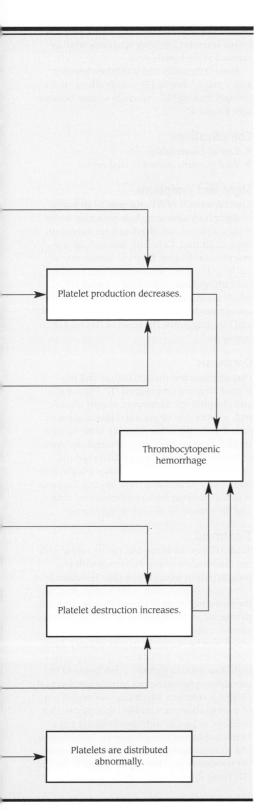

Platelet production decreases.

Thrombocytopenic hemorrhage

Platelet destruction increases.

Platelets are distributed abnormally.

Diagnosis

Diagnosis is based on the results of the patient history (especially a drug history), physical examination, and laboratory tests. Coagulation tests and CBC reveal a decreased platelet count (in adults, <100,000/μL), prolonged bleeding time (although this doesn't always indicate platelet quality), and normal prothrombin time and partial thromboplastin time. If increased destruction of platelets is causing thrombocytopenia, bone marrow studies will reveal a greater number of megakaryocytes (platelet precursors) and shortened platelet survival (several hours or days rather than the usual 7 to 10 days).

Treatment

Treatment varies with the underlying cause and severity and may include corticosteroids or immune globulin to increase platelet production. The treatment of choice is removal of the offending agents in drug-induced thrombocytopenia or treatment of the underlying cause. Platelet transfusions are helpful only in treating complications of severe hemorrhage. In cases of severe thrombocytopenia where medications fail to work, a splenectomy may be performed.

Special considerations

When caring for the patient with thrombocytopenia, take every possible precaution against bleeding.
◆ Protect the patient from trauma. Keep the side rails up and pad them, if possible. Promote the use of an electric razor and a soft toothbrush. Avoid invasive procedures, such as venipuncture or urinary catheterization, if possible. When venipuncture is unavoidable, be sure to exert pressure on the puncture site for at least 20 minutes or until the bleeding stops.
◆ Monitor platelet count daily.
◆ Test stool for guaiac; dipstick urine and vomitus for blood.
◆ Watch for bleeding (petechiae, ecchymoses, surgical or GI bleeding, and menorrhagia).
◆ Warn the patient to avoid aspirin in any form and other drugs that impair coagulation. Teach them how to recognize aspirin or ibuprofen compounds on labels of over-the-counter remedies.
◆ Advise the patient to avoid straining at stool or coughing, as both can lead to increased intracranial pressure, possibly causing cerebral hemorrhage in the patient with thrombocytopenia. Provide a stool softener to avoid constipation.
◆ During periods of active bleeding, maintain the patient on strict bed rest if necessary.

♦ When administering platelet concentrate, remember that platelets are extremely fragile, so infuse them quickly. Don't give platelets to a patient with a fever.

⚠ ALERT *During platelet transfusion, monitor the patient for febrile reaction (flushing, chills, fever, headache, tachycardia, and hypertension).*

♦ Histocompatibility locus antigen-typed platelets may be ordered to prevent febrile reaction. A patient with a history of minor reactions may benefit from acetaminophen and diphenhydramine before transfusion.

♦ If thrombocytopenia is drug-induced, stress the importance of avoiding the offending drug.

♦ If the patient must receive long-term steroid therapy, teach them to watch for and report cushingoid signs (acne, moon face, hirsutism, buffalo hump, hypertension, girdle obesity, thinning arms and legs, glycosuria, and edema). Emphasize that steroid doses must be discontinued gradually. During steroid therapy, monitor fluid and electrolyte balance, and watch for infection, pathologic fractures, and mood changes.

IDIOPATHIC THROMBOCYTOPENIC PURPURA

Idiopathic thrombocytopenic purpura (ITP), thrombocytopenia that results from immunologic platelet destruction, may be acute (post viral thrombocytopenia) or chronic (Werlhof disease, purpura hemorrhagica, essential thrombocytopenia, and autoimmune thrombocytopenia). The prognosis for acute ITP is excellent; nearly four out of five patients recover without treatment. The prognosis for chronic ITP is good; remissions lasting weeks or years are common, especially among women. Other names for ITP include immune thrombocytopenic purpura and autoimmune thrombocytopenic purpura.

Pathophysiology

ITP may be an autoimmune disorder, because antibodies that reduce the life span of platelets have been found in nearly all patients. The spleen probably helps to remove platelets modified by the antibody. Acute ITP usually follows a viral infection, such as rubella or chickenpox, and can follow immunization with a live-virus vaccine. Chronic ITP seldom follows infection and is commonly linked to immunologic disorders such as systemic lupus erythematosus. It's also linked to drug reactions. ITP frequently occurs in patients who have abused alcohol,

heroin, or morphine, and in patients with acquired immunodeficiency syndrome who are exposed to the rubella virus.

Acute ITP usually affects children between ages 2 and 6; chronic ITP mainly affects adults younger than age 50, especially women between ages 20 and 40.

Complications
♦ Cerebral hemorrhage
♦ Fatal purpuric lesions in vital organs

Signs and symptoms

Clinical features of ITP common to all forms of thrombocytopenia include petechiae, ecchymoses, and mucosal bleeding from the mouth, nose, or GI tract. Generally, hemorrhage is a rare physical finding. Purpuric lesions may occur in vital organs, such as the lungs, kidneys, or brain, and may prove fatal. In acute ITP, which commonly occurs in children, onset is usually sudden, causing easy bruising, epistaxis, and bleeding gums. The onset of chronic ITP is insidious.

Diagnosis

Platelet count less than 20,000/µL and prolonged bleeding time suggest ITP. Platelet size and morphologic appearance may be abnormal; anemia may be present if bleeding has occurred. As in thrombocytopenia, bone marrow studies show an abundance of megakaryocytes and a shortened circulating platelet survival time (hours or days). Occasionally, platelet antibodies may be found in vitro, but this diagnosis is usually inferred from platelet survival data and the absence of an underlying disease.

Treatment

Acute ITP may be allowed to run its course without intervention or may be treated with glucocorticoids or immune globulin. For chronic ITP, corticosteroids such as prednisone may be the initial treatment of choice. Patients who fail to respond within 4 months or who need high steroid dosage are candidates for splenectomy, which may be successful in 50% of cases. Alternative treatments include immunosuppression, high-dose gamma globulin injections, and immunoabsorption apheresis using staphylococcal protein-A columns, which filter antibodies out of the bloodstream. Anti-RhD therapy can also be useful in people with specific blood types. Eltrombopag and romiplostim are thrombopoietin receptor agonists that are used to increase the number of platelets in patients with chronic ITP. These drugs should only be used in those who have not responded to other treatments, including splenectomy.

Before splenectomy, the patient may require blood, blood components, and vitamin K to correct anemia and coagulation defects. After splenectomy, they may need blood and component replacement and platelet concentrate. Normally, platelet counts increase spontaneously after splenectomy.

Special considerations

Patient care for ITP is essentially the same as for other types of thrombocytopenia, with emphasis on teaching the patient to observe for petechiae, ecchymoses, and other signs of recurrence. Monitor patients receiving immunosuppressants for signs of bone marrow depression, infection, mucositis, GI ulcers, and severe diarrhea or vomiting. Tell the patient to avoid aspirin, ibuprofen, and warfarin, as these drugs interfere with platelet function and blood clotting.

PLATELET FUNCTION DISORDERS

Platelet function disorders are similar to thrombocytopenia but result from platelet dysfunction rather than platelet deficiency. They characteristically cause defects in platelet adhesion or procoagulation activity (ability to bind coagulation factors to their surface to form a stable fibrin clot). Such disorders may also create defects in platelet aggregation and thromboxane A_2 and may produce abnormalities by preventing the release of adenosine diphosphate (defective platelet-release reaction). The prognosis varies widely.

Pathophysiology

Abnormal platelet function disorders may be inherited (autosomal recessive) or acquired. Inherited disorders cause bone marrow production of platelets that are ineffective in the clotting mechanism. Acquired disorders result from the effects of such drugs as aspirin, nonsteroidal anti-inflammatory drugs, or carbenicillin; from such systemic diseases as uremia; or from other hematologic disorders such as myelofibrosis or polycythemia vera.

Complication

♦ Hemorrhage

Signs and symptoms

Generally, the sudden appearance of petechiae or purpura or excessive bruising and bleeding of the nose and gums are the first overt signs of platelet function disorders. More serious signs are external hemorrhage, internal hemorrhage into the muscles and visceral organs, or excessive bleeding during surgery.

Diagnosis

Prolonged bleeding time in a patient with both a normal platelet count and normal clotting factors suggests this diagnosis. Determination of the defective mechanism requires a blood film and a platelet function test to measure platelet-release reaction and aggregation. Depending on the type of platelet dysfunction, some or all of the test results may be abnormal.

Other typical laboratory findings are poor clot retraction and decreased prothrombin conversion. Baseline testing includes CBC and differential and appropriate tests to determine hemorrhage sites. In platelet function disorders, plasma-clotting factors, platelet counts, prothrombin and partial thromboplastin times, and thrombin times are usually normal.

Treatment

Platelet replacement is the only satisfactory treatment for inherited platelet dysfunction. However, acquired platelet function disorders respond to adequate treatment of the underlying disease or discontinuation of damaging drug therapy. Plasmapheresis effectively controls bleeding caused by a plasma element that's inhibiting platelet function. During this procedure, one or more units of whole blood are removed from the patient; the plasma is removed from the whole blood, and the remaining

---

Facts about platelet concentrate

Contents
♦ Platelets, white blood cells, some plasma
♦ Random platelets (ABO matched)
♦ Human leukocyte antigen (HLA) platelets (HLA-typed for multiple transfusions)

Amount
♦ 30 to 50 mL per donor
♦ 4 to 8 donor units given each time (each unit should raise the platelet count by 5,000/µL)

Shelf life
♦ 6 to 72 hours (best used within 24 hours)

packed RBCs are reinfused. (See *Facts about platelet concentrate*, page 477.)

Special considerations

◆ Obtain an accurate patient history, including onset of bleeding, use of drugs (especially aspirin), and family history of bleeding disorders.
◆ Watch closely for bleeding from skin, nose, gums, GI tract, or an injury site.
◆ Help the patient avoid unnecessary trauma. Advise them to tell the dentist about this condition before undergoing oral surgery. (Also stress the need for good oral hygiene to help prevent the need for such surgery.)
◆ Alert other care team members to the patient's hemorrhagic potential, especially before they undergo diagnostic tests or surgery that may cause trauma and bleeding.
◆ Observe the patient undergoing plasmapheresis for hypovolemia, hypotension, tachycardia, and other signs of volume depletion.
◆ If platelet dysfunction is inherited, help the patient and family understand and accept the disorder's nature. Teach them how to manage potential bleeding episodes. Warn them that petechiae, ecchymoses, and bleeding from the nose, gums, and GI tract signal abnormal bleeding and should be reported immediately.
◆ Tell the patient with a known coagulopathy or hepatic disease to avoid aspirin, aspirin compounds, and other agents that impair coagulation.
◆ Advise the patient to wear a medical identification bracelet or to carry a card identifying them as a potential bleeder.

VON WILLEBRAND DISEASE

von Willebrand disease is a hereditary bleeding disorder characterized by prolonged bleeding time; moderate deficiency of von Willebrand factor (VWF), clotting factor VIII (antihemophilic factor) and, possibly, factor VIII coagulant protein (VIII:C); and impaired platelet function. This disease commonly causes bleeding from the skin or mucosal surfaces and, in females, excessive uterine bleeding. Bleeding may range from mild and asymptomatic to severe, potentially fatal hemorrhage. The prognosis, however, is usually good.

The three types of von Willebrand disease are:
◆ *Type 1:* the most common form; there's decreased VWF, and factor VIII may be below normal; this is the mildest form
◆ *Type 2:* the VWF contains a defect causing it to not function properly; there are four subtypes: 2A, 2B, 2M, and 2N; it's important to

know which subtype is present because each is treated differently
◆ *Type 3:* this is the rarest and most severe form; there's no VWF and factor VIII is at low levels

Pathophysiology

Unlike hemophilia, von Willebrand disease is inherited as an autosomal dominant trait that affects males and females equally. One theory of pathophysiology holds that mild to moderate deficiency of factor VIII and defective platelet adhesion prolong coagulation time. Specifically, this results from a deficiency of the VWF, which stabilizes the factor VIII molecule and is needed for proper platelet function.

Defective platelet function is characterized by:
◆ decreased agglutination and adhesion at the bleeding site
◆ reduced platelet retention when filtered through a column of packed glass beads
◆ diminished ristocetin-induced platelet aggregation

Recently, an acquired form has been identified in patients with cancer and immune disorders.

von Willebrand disease, which doesn't have any racial or ethnic associations, affects about 1% of the population.

Complication

◆ Severe, potentially life-threatening hemorrhage

Signs and symptoms

von Willebrand disease produces easy bruising, epistaxis, and bleeding from the gums. Petechiae are rarely seen. Severe forms of this disease may cause hemorrhage after laceration or surgery, menorrhagia, and GI bleeding. Excessive postpartum bleeding is uncommon because factor VIII levels and bleeding time abnormalities become less pronounced during pregnancy. Massive soft-tissue hemorrhage and bleeding into joints seldom occur. Severity of bleeding may lessen with age, and bleeding episodes occur sporadically—a patient may bleed excessively after one dental extraction but not after another.

Diagnosis

Diagnosis is difficult because symptoms are mild, laboratory values are borderline, and factor VIII levels fluctuate. However, a positive family history and characteristic bleeding patterns and laboratory values help establish the diagnosis. Typical laboratory data include:
◆ prolonged bleeding time (>6 minutes)
◆ slightly prolonged partial thromboplastin time (>45 seconds)

♦ absent or reduced levels of factor VIII-related antigens and low factor VIII activity level
♦ defective in vitro platelet aggregation (using the ristocetin coagulation factor assay test)
♦ normal platelet count and normal clot retraction

Treatment

The goals of treatment are to shorten bleeding time by local measures and to replace factor VIII (and, consequently, VWF) by infusion of cryoprecipitate or blood fractions that are rich in factor VIII.

During bleeding and before surgery, I.V. infusion of cryoprecipitate or fresh frozen plasma (in quantities sufficient to raise factor VIII levels to 50% of normal) shortens bleeding time. Desmopressin given parenterally or intranasally is effective in raising serum levels of VWF in type 1 disease by releasing stores of VWF for 8 to 10 hours. Repeat doses are less effective unless stores of VWF are allowed to reaccumulate (about 48 hours). DDAVP is not effective in the other types of von Willebrand disease and may even be harmful.

For women with menorrhagia, oral contraceptives may be ordered to control heavy menstrual bleeding. Another treatment for menorrhagia is the intrauterine placement of a progesterone-containing contraceptive device. Antifibrinolytic medications, which help slow down clotting factor breakdown, may be given before or after surgical procedures.

Special considerations

The care plan should include local measures to control bleeding and patient teaching to prevent bleeding, unnecessary trauma, and complications.
♦ After surgery, monitor bleeding time for 24 to 48 hours, and watch for signs of new bleeding.
♦ During a bleeding episode, elevate and apply cold compresses and gentle pressure to the bleeding site.
♦ Refer parents of affected children for genetic counseling.
♦ Advise the patient to consult the physician after even minor trauma and before all surgery to determine if replacement of blood components is necessary.
♦ Instruct the patient to watch for signs of hepatitis within 6 weeks to 6 months after transfusion.
♦ Warn the patient against using aspirin and other drugs that impair platelet function.
♦ Advise the patient who has a severe form to avoid contact sports.

DISSEMINATED INTRAVASCULAR COAGULATION

DIC occurs as a life-threatening complication of diseases and conditions that accelerate clotting, causing small blood vessel occlusion, organ necrosis, depletion of circulating clotting factors and platelets, and activation of the fibrinolytic system. This, in turn, can provoke severe hemorrhage. (See *Three mechanisms of DIC*, page 480.) Clotting in the microcirculation usually affects the kidneys and extremities but may occur in the brain, lungs, pituitary and adrenal glands, and GI mucosa. Other conditions, such as vitamin K deficiency, hepatic disease, and anticoagulant therapy, may cause a similar hemorrhage. DIC, also called *consumption coagulopathy* or *defibrination syndrome*, is generally an acute condition but may be chronic in cancer patients. The prognosis depends on early detection and treatment, the hemorrhage's severity, and treatment of the underlying disease or condition.

Causes

DIC may result from:
♦ infection—gram-negative or gram-positive septicemia; viral, fungal, or rickettsial infection; protozoal infection
♦ obstetric complications—abruptio placentae, amniotic fluid embolism, retained dead fetus, septic abortion, and eclampsia
♦ neoplastic disease—acute leukemia, metastatic carcinoma, and aplastic anemia
♦ disorders that produce necrosis—extensive burns and trauma, brain tissue destruction, transplant rejection, and hepatic necrosis
♦ other factors—heatstroke, shock, poisonous snakebite, cirrhosis, fat embolism, incompatible blood transfusion, cardiac arrest, surgery necessitating cardiopulmonary bypass, giant hemangioma, severe venous thrombosis, and purpura fulminans

It isn't clear why such disorders lead to DIC, nor is it certain that they lead to it through a common mechanism. In many patients, the triggering mechanisms may be the entrance of foreign protein into the circulation and vascular endothelial injury. Regardless of how DIC begins, the typical accelerated clotting results in generalized activation of prothrombin and a consequent excess of thrombin. Excess thrombin converts fibrinogen to fibrin, producing fibrin clots in the microcirculation. This process consumes exorbitant amounts of coagulation factors (especially fibrinogen, prothrombin, platelets, and factor V and factor VIII), causing hypofibrinogenemia, hypoprothrombinemia, thrombocytopenia,

PATHOPHYSIOLOGY
Three mechanisms of DIC

However disseminated intravascular coagulation (DIC) begins, accelerated clotting (characteristic of DIC) usually results in excess thrombin, which in turn causes fibrinolysis with excess fibrin formation and fibrin degradation products (FDP), activation of fibrin-stabilizing factor (factor XIII), consumption of platelet and clotting factors and, eventually, hemorrhage.

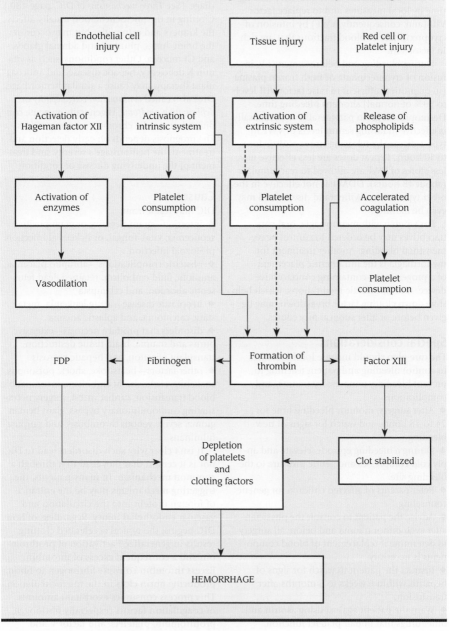

and deficiencies in factor V and factor VIII. Circulating thrombin activates the fibrinolytic system, which lyses fibrin clots into fibrin degradation products (FDPs). The hemorrhage that occurs may be due largely to the anticoagulant activity of FDPs, as well as depletion of plasma coagulation factors.

Complications
◆ Ischemia of legs, arms, or organs
◆ Severe bleeding
◆ Stroke

Signs and symptoms
The most significant feature of DIC is abnormal bleeding, *without* a history of a serious hemorrhagic disorder. Almost always, this complication occurs in the setting of a serious underlying illness. Principal signs of such bleeding include cutaneous oozing, petechiae, ecchymoses, and hematomas caused by bleeding into the skin. Bleeding from surgical or I.V. sites and from the GI tract are equally significant signs, as are acrocyanosis (cyanosis of the extremities) and signs of acute tubular necrosis. Related signs, symptoms, and other effects include nausea, vomiting, dyspnea, oliguria, seizures, coma, shock, major organ failure, confusion, epistaxis, hemoptysis, and severe muscle, back, abdominal, and chest pain.

Diagnosis
Abnormal bleeding in a patient with severe illness and in the absence of a known hematologic disorder suggests DIC. Initial laboratory findings reflect coagulation factor deficiencies:
◆ decreased platelet count: less than 100,000/μL
◆ decreased fibrinogen level: less than 150 mg/dL

As the excessive clot breaks down, hemorrhagic diathesis occurs, and test results reflect coagulation abnormalities:
◆ prolonged prothrombin time: more than 15 seconds
◆ prolonged partial thromboplastin time: more than 60 seconds
◆ increased FDPs: commonly more than 45 μg/mL

Other supportive data include positive fibrin monomers, diminished levels of factors V and VIII, fragmentation of RBCs, and decreased Hb level (<10 g/dL). Assessment of renal status demonstrates reduction in urine output (<30 mL/hour) and elevated blood urea nitrogen (>25 mg/dL) and serum creatinine (>1.3 mg/dL) levels.

A positive D-dimer test (results < 1:8 dilution and decreased levels of factors V and VIII) is specific for DIC. Confirming the diagnosis may be difficult because many of these test results also occur in other disorders (e.g., primary fibrinolysis).

Treatment
Successful management of DIC necessitates prompt recognition and adequate treatment of the underlying disorder. Treatment may be supportive when the underlying disorder is self-limiting or highly specific. If the patient isn't bleeding, supportive care alone may reverse DIC. However, bleeding may require administration of blood, fresh frozen plasma, platelets, or packed RBCs to support hemostasis. Cryoprecipitate may also be used if fibrinogen is significantly decreased. Heparin is used in the early stages to prevent microclotting and is sometimes used in combination with replacement therapy.

Special considerations
Patient care must focus on early recognition of abnormal bleeding, prompt treatment of the underlying disorders, and prevention of further bleeding.
◆ To avoid dislodging clots and causing fresh bleeding, don't scrub bleeding areas. Use pressure, cold compresses, and topical hemostatic agents to control bleeding.
◆ To prevent injury, enforce complete bed rest during bleeding episodes. If the patient is agitated, pad the side rails.
◆ Check all I.V. and venipuncture sites frequently for bleeding. Apply pressure to injection sites for at least 20 minutes. Alert other personnel to his tendency to hemorrhage.
◆ Monitor intake and output hourly in acute DIC, especially when administering blood products. Watch for transfusion reactions and signs of fluid overload. To measure the amount of blood lost, weigh dressings and linen, and record drainage. Weigh the patient daily, particularly if there's renal involvement.
◆ Watch for bleeding from the GI and GU tracts. If you suspect intra-abdominal bleeding, measure the patient's abdominal girth at least every 4 hours, and monitor closely for signs of shock.
◆ Monitor the results of serial blood studies (particularly HCT, Hb levels, and coagulation times).
◆ Explain all diagnostic tests and procedures. Allow time for questions.
◆ Inform the patient's family of the progress. Prepare them for the presence of I.V. lines, nasogastric tubes, bruises, and dried blood. Provide emotional support for the patient and family. As needed, enlist the aid of a social worker,

chaplain, and other members of the healthcare team in providing such support.

Miscellaneous disorders

NEUTROPENIA AND LYMPHOCYTOPENIA

Granulocytopenia (commonly referred to as *neutropenia*) is characterized by a marked reduction in the number of circulating granulocytes. Although this implies all the granulocytes (neutrophils, basophils, and eosinophils) are reduced, granulocytopenia usually refers to decreased neutrophils. (See *Understanding neutropenia*, page 483.) This disorder, which can occur at any age, is associated with infections and ulcerative lesions of the throat, GI tract, other mucous membranes, and skin. The severest form is known as *agranulocytosis*.

Lymphocytopenia (sometimes called *lymphopenia*), a rare disorder, is a deficiency of circulating lymphocytes (leukocytes produced mainly in lymph nodes).

In both granulocytopenia and lymphocytopenia, the total leukocyte count (WBC count) may reach dangerously low levels, leaving the body unprotected against infection. The prognosis in both disorders depends on the underlying cause and whether it can be treated. Untreated, severe granulocytopenia can be fatal in 3 to 6 days.

Causes

Granulocytopenia may result from diminished production of granulocytes in bone marrow, increased peripheral destruction of granulocytes, or greater utilization of granulocytes. Diminished production of granulocytes in bone marrow generally stems from radiation or drug therapy; it's a common adverse effect of antimetabolites and alkylating agents and may occur in the patient who is hypersensitive to phenothiazine, sulfonamides (and some sulfonamide derivatives), antibiotics, and antiarrhythmic drugs. Drug-induced granulocytopenia usually develops slowly and typically correlates with the dosage and duration of therapy. Production of granulocytes also decreases in conditions such as aplastic anemia and bone marrow malignancies and in some hereditary disorders (infantile genetic agranulocytosis).

The growing loss of peripheral granulocytes is due to increased splenic sequestration, diseases that destroy peripheral blood cells (viral and bacterial infections), and drugs that act as haptens (carrying antigens that attack blood cells and causing acute idiosyncratic or non–dose–related drug reactions). Infections such as infectious mononucleosis may result in granulocytopenia because of increased utilization of granulocytes.

Similarly, lymphocytopenia may result from decreased production, increased destruction, or loss of lymphocytes. Decreased production of lymphocytes may be secondary to a genetic or a thymic abnormality or to immunodeficiency disorders, such as thymic dysplasia or ataxia-telangiectasia. Increased destruction of lymphocytes may be secondary to radiation, chemotherapy, or human immunodeficiency virus infection. Loss of lymphocytes may follow postsurgical thoracic duct drainage, intestinal lymphangiectasia, or impaired intestinal lymphatic drainage (as in Whipple disease).

Lymphocyte depletion can also result from elevated plasma corticoid levels (due to stress, corticotropin or steroid treatment, or heart failure). Other disorders associated with lymphocyte depletion include Hodgkin disease, leukemia, aplastic anemia, sarcoidosis, myasthenia gravis, lupus erythematosus, protein-calorie malnutrition, renal failure, terminal cancer, tuberculosis and, in infants, SCID.

Complication
◆ Infection

Signs and symptoms

Patients with granulocytopenia, if the disease is associated with anemia, experience slowly progressive fatigue and weakness; however, if they develop an infection, they can exhibit sudden onset of fever and chills and mental status changes. Overt signs of infection (pus formation) are usually absent. Localized infection can quickly become systemic (bacteremia) or spread throughout an organ (pneumonia). All patients should be meticulously evaluated for even subtle signs of infection because untreated infections can lead to septic shock in 8 to 24 hours. If granulocytopenia results from an idiosyncratic drug reaction, signs of infection develop abruptly, without slowly progressive fatigue and weakness.

Patients with lymphocytopenia may exhibit enlarged lymph nodes, spleen, and tonsils and signs of an associated disease.

Diagnosis

Diagnosis of granulocytopenia necessitates a thorough patient history to check for precipitating factors. Physical examination for clinical effects of underlying disorders is also essential.

PATHOPHYSIOLOGY
Understanding neutropenia

Neutropenia, a deficiency in the number of mature neutrophils, is the most common immune system deficiency. It can result from a disease or from radiation or drug therapy. Common infections that occur secondary to neutropenia include aerobic gram-negative bacilli and *Staphylococcus aureus* and certain fungal infections, such as candidiasis and aspergillosis.

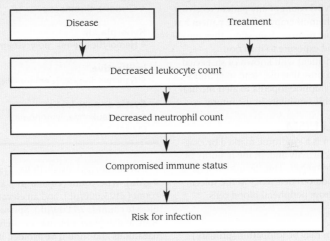

Disease   Treatment

Decreased leukocyte count

Decreased neutrophil count

Compromised immune status

Risk for infection

℞ **CONFIRMING DIAGNOSIS** *A markedly decreased absolute neutrophil count (<500/μL leads to severe bacterial infections) and a WBC count lower than 2,000/μL, with few observable granulocytes on CBC, confirm granulocytopenia.*

Bone marrow examination shows a scarcity of granulocytic precursor cells beyond the most immature forms, but this may vary, depending on the cause.

A lymphocyte count below 1,500/μL in adults or below 3,000/μL in children indicates lymphocytopenia. Identifying the cause by evaluation of clinical status, bone marrow and lymph node biopsies, or other appropriate diagnostic tests helps establish the diagnosis.

Treatment

Effective management of granulocytopenia must identify and eliminate the cause and control infection until the bone marrow can generate more leukocytes. In many cases, this means drug or radiation therapy must be stopped and antibiotic treatment begun immediately, even while awaiting test results. Treatment may also include antifungal preparations. Administration of granulocyte colony-stimulating factor (CSF) or granulocyte-macrophage CSF is a newer treatment used to stimulate bone marrow

production of neutrophils. Spontaneous restoration of leukocyte production in bone marrow generally occurs within 1 to 3 weeks.

Treatment of lymphocytopenia includes eliminating the cause and managing any underlying disorders. For infants with SCID, therapy may include bone marrow transplantation.

Special considerations

◆ Monitor vital signs frequently. Obtain cultures from blood, throat, urine, mouth, nose, rectum, vagina, and sputum, as ordered. Give antibiotics as scheduled.

◆ Explain the necessity of infection protection procedures to the patient and their family. Teach proper hand-washing technique and the correct use of gowns and masks. Prevent patient contact with staff or visitors with respiratory infections.

◆ Maintain adequate nutrition and hydration because malnutrition aggravates immunosuppression. Make sure the patient with mouth ulcerations receives a high-calorie liquid diet. Offer a straw to make drinking less painful.

◆ Provide warm saline water gargles and rinses, analgesics, and anesthetic lozenges. Good oral hygiene promotes comfort and facilitates healing.

♦ Ensure adequate rest, which is essential to the mobilization of the body's defenses against infection. Provide good skin and perineal care.

♦ Monitor CBC and differential, blood culture results, serum electrolyte levels, intake and output, and daily weight.

♦ To help detect granulocytopenia and lymphocytopenia in the early, most treatable stages, monitor the WBC count of any patient receiving radiation or chemotherapy. After the patient has developed bone marrow depression, they must zealously avoid exposure to infection.

♦ Advise the patient with known or suspected sensitivity to a drug that may lead to granulocytopenia or lymphocytopenia to alert medical personnel to this sensitivity in the future.

HYPERSPLENISM

Hypersplenism is a syndrome marked by exaggerated splenic activity and, in the majority of patients, splenomegaly. This disorder results in peripheral blood cell deficiency as the spleen traps and destroys peripheral blood cells.

Causes

Hypersplenism may be idiopathic (primary) or secondary to an extrasplenic disorder, such as chronic malaria, polycythemia vera, rheumatoid arthritis, or liver disease. (See *Causes of splenomegaly*.) In hypersplenism, the spleen's normal filtering and phagocytic functions accelerate indiscriminately, automatically removing antibody-coated, aging, and abnormal cells, even though some cells may be functionally normal. The spleen may also temporarily sequester normal platelets and RBCs, withholding them from circulation. In this manner, the enlarged spleen may trap as much as 90% of the body's platelets and up to 45% of its RBC mass.

Signs and symptoms

Most patients with hypersplenism develop anemia, leukopenia, or thrombocytopenia, in many cases with splenomegaly. They may contract bacterial infections frequently, bruise easily, hemorrhage spontaneously from the mucous membranes and GI or GU tract, and suffer ulcerations of the mouth, legs, and feet. They commonly develop fever, weakness, and palpitations. Patients with secondary hypersplenism may have other clinical abnormalities, depending on the underlying disease.

Diagnosis

Diagnosis requires evidence of abnormal splenic destruction or sequestration of RBCs or platelets and splenomegaly.

Causes of splenomegaly

Infectious
♦ Acute (abscesses, subacute infective endocarditis), chronic (tuberculosis, malaria, Felty syndrome)

Congestive
♦ Cirrhosis, thrombosis

Hyperplastic
♦ Hemolytic anemia, polycythemia vera

Infiltrative
♦ Gaucher disease, Niemann–Pick disease

Cystic or neoplastic
♦ Cysts, leukemia, lymphoma, myelofibrosis

CBC shows decreased Hb level (as low as 4 g/dL), WBC count (<4,000/μL), and platelet count (<125,000/μL), and an elevated reticulocyte count (>75,000/μL). Splenic biopsy, scan, and angiography may be useful; biopsy is hazardous and should be avoided if possible. In sequestration, the spleen is palpable. Use abdominal palpation cautiously because it may create injury, bleeding, or rupture.

Treatment

Splenectomy is indicated only in transfusion-dependent patients who are refractory to medical therapy. Splenectomy seldom cures the patient, but it does correct the effects of cytopenia. Postoperative complications may include infection and thromboembolic disease. Occasionally, splenectomy may result in accelerated blood cell destruction in the bone marrow and liver. Secondary hypersplenism necessitates treatment of the underlying disease.

Special considerations

♦ If splenectomy is scheduled, administer preoperative transfusions of blood or blood products (fresh frozen plasma and platelets) to replace deficient blood elements. Also treat symptoms or complications of any underlying disorder.

♦ Postoperatively, monitor vital signs. Check for any excessive drainage or apparent bleeding. Watch for infection, thromboembolism, and abdominal distention. Keep the nasogastric tube patent; listen for bowel sounds. Instruct the patient to perform deep-breathing exercises, and encourage early ambulation to prevent respiratory complications and venous stasis.

ELDER TIP *Older adults may be at higher risk for infection because of decreased leuko-cyte and lymphocyte production. Fewer and weaker lymphocytes and immune system changes diminish the antigen–antibody response in older adults.*

SELECTED REFERENCES

Adamson, J. W., & Longo, D. L. (2014). Anemia and poly-cythemia. In D. Kasper, et al. (Eds.), *Harrison's principles of internal medicine* (19th ed.). New York: McGraw-Hill. Retrieved from http://accessmedicine.mhmedical.com/content.aspx?bookid=1130&sectionid=79727787

Hink, A. B., et al. (2012). Surgical management of obesity. In S. C. McKean, et al. (Eds.), *Principles and practice of hospital medicine* (2nd ed.). New York: McGraw-Hill. Retrieved from http://accessmedicine.mhmedical.com/content.aspx?bookid=1872&sectionid=147024798

von Willebrand Disease. (2017). In M. A. Papadakis & S. J. McPhee (Eds.), *Quick medical diagnosis & treatment*. New York: McGraw-Hill. Retrieved from http://accessmedicine.mhmedical.com/content.aspx?bookid=2033&sectionid=152420265

10

METABOLIC AND NUTRITIONAL DISORDERS

Introduction

Metabolism is the physiologic process that allows cells to transform food into energy and continually rebuild body cells. Metabolism has two phases: catabolism and anabolism. In *catabolism*, the energy-producing phase of metabolism, the body breaks down large food molecules into smaller ones; in *anabolism*, the tissue-building phase, the body converts small molecules into larger ones (such as antibodies to keep the body capable of fighting infection). Both phases are accomplished by means of a chemical process using energy. A wide range of nutrients is metabolized to meet the body's needs. (See *Essential nutrients and their functions*, page 487.)

⬡ **ELDER TIP** *A person's protein, vitamin, and mineral requirements usually remain the same as they age, although calorie needs decline. Diminished activity may lower energy requirements by almost 200 calories/day for men and women ages 51 to 75, 400 calories/day for women older than age 75, and 500 calories/day for men older than age 75.*

CARBOHYDRATES: PRIMARY ENERGY SOURCE

The body gets most of its energy by metabolizing carbohydrates, especially glucose. Glucose catabolism proceeds in three phases:

♦ *Glycolysis*, a series of chemical reactions, converts glucose molecules into pyruvic or lactic acid.
♦ The *citric acid cycle* removes ionized hydrogen atoms from pyruvic acid and produces carbon dioxide.
♦ *Oxidative phosphorylation* traps energy from the hydrogen electrons and combines the hydrogen ions and electrons with oxygen to form water and the common form of biological energy, adenosine triphosphate (ATP).

Other essential processes in carbohydrate metabolism include glycogenesis—the formation of glycogen, a storage form of glucose—which occurs when cells become saturated with glucose-6-phosphate (an intermediate product of glycolysis); glycogenolysis, the reverse process, which converts glycogen into glucose-6-phosphate in muscle cells and liberates free glucose in the liver; and gluconeogenesis, or "new" glucose formation from protein amino acids or fat glycerols.

A complex interplay of hormonal and neural controls regulates glucose metabolism. Hormone secretions of five endocrine glands dominate this regulatory function:
♦ Alpha cells of the islets of Langerhans secrete glucagon, which increases the blood glucose level by stimulating phosphorylase activity to accelerate liver glycogenolysis.
♦ Beta cells of the islets of Langerhans secrete the glucose-regulating hormone insulin, which

Essential nutrients and their functions

Nutrients are required for the body to work properly and avoid disease.

Nutrients	Functions
Carbohydrates	◆ Energy source
Fats and essential fatty acids	◆ Energy source; essential for growth, normal skin, and membranes
Proteins and amino acids	◆ Synthesis of all body proteins, growth, and tissue maintenance
Water-soluble vitamins	
◆ Ascorbic acid (C)	◆ Collagen synthesis, wound healing, antioxidation
◆ Thiamine (B1)	◆ Coenzyme in carbohydrate metabolism
◆ Riboflavin (B2)	◆ Coenzyme in energy metabolism
◆ Niacin	◆ Coenzyme in carbohydrate, fat, energy metabolism, and tissue metabolism
◆ Vitamin B12	◆ Deoxyribonucleic acid (DNA) and ribonucleic acid synthesis; erythrocyte formation
◆ Folic acid	◆ Coenzyme in amino acid metabolism; heme and hemoglobin formation; DNA synthesis; lowering homocysteine levels
Fat-soluble vitamins	
◆ Vitamin A	◆ Vision in dim light, mucosal epithelium integrity, tooth development, endocrine function
◆ Vitamin D	◆ Regulation of calcium and phosphate absorption and metabolism; renal phosphate clearance; musculoskeletal function
◆ Vitamin E	◆ Antioxidation; essential for muscle, liver, and red blood cell integrity
◆ Vitamin K	◆ Blood clotting (catalyzes synthesis of prothrombin by liver); skeletal function

assists in glucose transport across cell membranes and storage of excess glucose as fat.

◆ The adrenal medulla, as a physiologic response to stress, secretes epinephrine, which stimulates liver and muscle glycogenolysis to increase the blood glucose level.

◆ Corticotropin and glucocorticoids also increase blood glucose levels. Glucocorticoids accelerate gluconeogenesis by promoting the flow of amino acids to the liver, where they're synthesized into glucose.

◆ Human growth hormone (hGH) limits the fat storage and favors fat catabolism; consequently, it inhibits carbohydrate catabolism and thus raises blood glucose levels.

◆ Thyroid-stimulating hormone and thyroid hormone have mixed effects on carbohydrate metabolism and may raise or lower blood glucose levels.

FATS: CATABOLISM AND ANABOLISM

The breaking up of triglycerides—*lipolysis*—yields fatty acids and glycerol. Beta oxidation breaks down fatty acids into acetyl coenzyme A,

which can then enter the citric acid cycle; glycerol can also undergo gluconeogenesis or enter the glycolytic pathways to produce energy. Conversely, *lipogenesis* is the chemical formation of fat from excess carbohydrates and proteins or from the fatty acids and glycerol products of lipolysis. Adipose tissue is the primary storage site for excess fat and thus is the greatest source of energy reserve. Certain unsaturated fatty acids are necessary for the synthesis of vital body compounds. Because the body can't produce these essential fatty acids, they must be provided through diet. Insulin, hGH, catecholamines, corticotropin, and glucocorticoids control fat metabolism in an inverse relationship with carbohydrate metabolism; large amounts of carbohydrates promote fat storage, and deficiency of available carbohydrates promotes fat breakdown for energy needs.

PROTEINS: ANABOLISM

The primary process in protein metabolism is anabolism. Catabolism is relegated to a supporting role in protein metabolism—a reversal of the roles played by these two processes in carbohydrate and fat metabolisms. By synthesizing proteins—the tissue-building foods—the body derives substances essential for life (such as plasma proteins) and can reproduce, control cell growth, and repair itself. However, when carbohydrates or fats are unavailable as energy sources, or when energy demands are exceedingly high, protein catabolism converts protein into an available energy source. Protein metabolism consists of many processes, including:

◆ *Deamination*—a catabolic and energy-producing process occurring in the liver with the splitting off of the amino acid to form ammonia and a keto acid

◆ *Transamination*—anabolic conversion of keto acids to amino acids

◆ *Urea formation*—a catabolic process occurring in the liver, producing urea, the end product of protein catabolism

The male hormone testosterone and hGH stimulate protein anabolism; corticotropin prompts secretion of glucocorticoids, which, in turn, facilitate protein catabolism. Normally, the rate of protein anabolism equals the rate of protein catabolism—a condition known as *nitrogen balance* (because ingested nitrogen equals nitrogen waste excreted in urine, feces, and sweat). When excessive catabolism causes the amount of nitrogen excreted to exceed the amount ingested, a state of *negative nitrogen balance* exists—usually the result of starvation and cachexia or surgical stress.

FLUID AND ELECTROLYTE BALANCE

A critical component of metabolism is fluid and electrolyte balance. Water is an essential body substance and constitutes almost 60% of an adult's body weight and more than 75% of a neonate's body weight. In both older and obese adults, the ratio of water to body weight drops; children and lean people have a higher proportion of water in their bodies.

Body fluids can be classified as intracellular (or cellular) or extracellular. Intracellular fluid constitutes about 40% of total body weight and 60% of all body fluid; it contains large quantities of potassium and phosphates but very little sodium and chloride. Conversely, extracellular fluid (ECF) contains mostly sodium and chloride but very little potassium and phosphates. Incorporating interstitial, cerebrospinal, intraocular, and gastrointestinal (GI) fluids and plasma, ECF supplies cells with nutrients and other substances needed for cellular function. The many components of body fluids have the important function of preserving osmotic pressure and acid–base and anion–cation balance.

Homeostasis is a stable state—the equilibrium of chemical and physical properties of body fluid. Body fluids contain two kinds of dissolved substances: those that dissociate in solution (electrolytes) and those that don't. For example, glucose, when dissolved in water, doesn't break down into smaller particles; but sodium chloride dissociates in solution into sodium cations (+) and chloride anions (–). The composition of these electrolytes in body fluids is electrically balanced so the positively charged ions (cations: sodium, potassium, calcium, and magnesium) equal the negatively charged ions (anions: chloride, bicarbonate, sulfate, phosphate, proteinate, and carbonic and other organic acids). Although these particles are present in relatively low concentrations, any deviation from their normal levels can have profound physiologic effects.

ELDER TIP *Institutionalized older people are at particularly high risk for dehydration because of their diminished thirst perception and any combination of physical, cognitive, speech, mobility, and visual impairment.*

In homeostasis—an ever-changing but balanced state—water and electrolytes and other solutes move continually between cellular and extracellular compartments. Such motion is made possible by semipermeable membranes that allow diffusion, filtration, and active transport. *Diffusion* refers to the movement of particles or molecules from an area of greater concentration to one of lesser concentration. Normally, particles move randomly and constantly until the concentrations within given solutions are equal. Diffusion also depends on permeability, electrical gradient, and pressure gradient. Particles, however, can't diffuse against any of these gradients without energy and a carrier substance (active transport). ATP is released from cells to aid particles needing energy to pass through the cell membrane.

The diffusion of water from a solution of low concentration to one of high concentration is called *osmosis*. The pressure that develops when a selectively permeable cell membrane separates solutions of different strengths of concentrations is known as *osmotic pressure*, expressed in terms of osmoles or milliosmoles (mOsm). Osmotic activity is described in terms of *osmolality*—the osmotic pull exerted by all particles per unit of water, expressed in mOsm/kg of water—or *osmolarity*, when expressed in mOsm/L of solution.

The normal range of body fluid osmolality is 285 to 295 mOsm/kg. Solutions of 50 mOsm above or below the high and low points of this normal range exert little or no osmotic effect (iso-osmolality). A solution below 240 mOsm contains a lower particle concentration than plasma (hypo-osmolar), whereas a solution over 340 mOsm has a higher particle concentration than plasma (hyperosmolar).

Rapid I.V. administration of iso-osmolar solutions to patients who are debilitated, are very old or very young, or have cardiac or renal insufficiency could lead to ECF volume overload and induce pulmonary edema and heart failure because particulate concentration is the same as plasma, so fluid shifting into and out of cells will occur.

Continuous I.V. administration of hypo-osmolar solutions decreases serum osmolality and leads to excess intracellular fluid volume (water intoxication), whereas continuous I.V. administration of hyperosmolar solutions results in intracellular dehydration, increased serum osmolality and, eventually, ECF volume deficit due to excessive urinary excretion. These states occur because of fluid diffusion and the cell's attempt to balance the particulate concentrations inside and outside the cell.

REGULATION OF pH

Primarily through the complex chemical regulation of carbonic acid by the lungs and of base bicarbonate by the kidneys, the body maintains the hydrogen ion concentration to keep the ECF pH between 7.35 and 7.45. Nutritional deficiency or excess, disease, injury, or metabolic disturbance can interfere with normal homeostatic mechanisms and raise pH (acidosis) or lower it (alkalosis).

ASSESSING HOMEOSTASIS

The goal of metabolism and homeostasis is to maintain the complex environment of ECF—the plasma—which nourishes and supports every body cell. This special environment is subject to multiple interlocking influences and readily reflects any disturbance in nutrition, chemical or fluid content, and osmotic pressure. Such disturbances can be detected by various laboratory tests. For example, measurements of albumin, prealbumin, and other blood proteins; electrolyte concentration; enzyme and antibody levels; and urine and blood chemistry levels (lipoproteins, glucose, blood urea nitrogen [BUN], creatinine, and creatinine-height index [CHI]) reflect the state of metabolism, homeostasis, and nutrition throughout the body. (See *Laboratory tests: Assessing nutritional status,* page 490.) Results of such laboratory tests, of course, supplement the information obtained from dietary history and physical examination—which offer gross clinical information about the quality, quantity, and efficiency of metabolic processes. To support clinical information, anthropometry, height-weight ratio, and skinfold thickness determinations specifically define tissue nutritional status.

The following measures can help you maintain your patient's homeostasis:
◆ Obtain a complete dietary history and nutritional assessment, including weight history and GI symptoms, to determine if carbohydrate, fat, protein, vitamin, mineral, and water intake are adequate for energy production and for tissue repair and growth. Remember that during periods of rapid tissue synthesis (growth, pregnancy, healing), protein needs increase.
◆ Consult a dietitian about any patient who may be malnourished because of malabsorption syndromes, renal or hepatic disease, or clear-liquid diets or who may possibly receive nothing by mouth for more than 5 days. Planned meals that provide adequate carbohydrates, fats, and protein are necessary for convalescence. Supplementary carbohydrates are often needed to spare protein and achieve a positive nitrogen balance.
◆ Accurately record intake and output to assess fluid balance (this includes intake of oral liquids or I.V. solutions and urine, gastric, and stool output).
◆ Weigh the patient daily—at the same time, with the same-type clothing, and on the same scale. Remember, a weight loss of 2.2 lb (1 kg) is equivalent to the loss of 1 L of fluid.
◆ Observe the patient closely for insensible water or unmeasured fluid losses (such as through diaphoresis). Remember, fluid loss from the skin and lungs (normally 900 mL/day) can reach as high as 2,000 mL/day from hyperventilation or tachypnea, thus increasing insensible water losses.

ELDER TIP *Teach elderly patients and others vulnerable to fluid imbalances the importance of maintaining adequate fluid intake.*
◆ Recognize I.V. solutions that are hypo-osmolar, such as 0.45% NaCl (half-normal saline solution). Iso-osmolar solutions include normal saline solution (0.9% NaCl), 5% dextrose in 0.2% NaCl, Ringer solutions, and 5% dextrose in water. (The latter acts like a hypotonic solution because dextrose is quickly metabolized, leaving only free water.) Hyperosmolar solutions include 5% dextrose in normal saline solution, 10% dextrose in water, and 5% dextrose in Ringer lactate solution.
◆ When continuously administering hypo-osmolar solutions, watch for signs of

Laboratory tests: Assessing nutritional status

Blood and urine tests provide the most precise data about nutritional status, often revealing nutritional problems before they're clinically apparent. The list below explains some common tests and what their results mean.

Serum vitamins and minerals
Vitamin and mineral deficiencies commonly screened for include deficiencies in A, B, B_{12}, folic acid, ascorbic acid, beta-carotene, riboflavin and, sometimes, zinc, calcium, magnesium, iron, and other minerals.

Serum nutrients
Glucose levels help assess suspected diabetes or hypoglycemia. Glucose may be elevated with stress, acromegaly, Cushing syndrome, corticosteroid use, liver disease, sepsis, or overfeeding. Glucose may be decreased with fluid overload, adrenal insufficiency, liver disease, severe sepsis, insulinoma, or pancreatic disorders. Cholesterol and triglyceride levels help differentiate the type of hyperlipoproteinemia.

Nitrogen balance
A negative nitrogen balance indicates inadequate intake of protein or calories.

Hemoglobin and hematocrit
Decreased levels can occur in protein-calorie malnutrition, iron deficiency, overhydration, hemorrhage, and hemolytic disease; elevated levels in dehydration, polycythemia, and folate and vitamin B_{12} deficiency.

Serum albumin
Reduced levels may indicate overhydration or visceral protein depletion because of GI disease, liver disease, or nephrotic syndrome. Elevated levels occur in dehydration.

Creatinine-height index (CHI)
This calculated value reflects muscle mass and estimates muscle protein depletion. Reduced CHI may indicate protein-calorie malnutrition or impaired renal function.

Serum prealbumin
This carrier protein for thyroxine is a sensitive indicator of visceral protein.

Total lymphocyte count
This provides an indication of immune status. Counts are low in malnutrition and acquired immunodeficiency syndrome.

---

water intoxication: headaches, behavior changes (confusion or disorientation), nausea, vomiting, rising blood pressure, and falling pulse rate.
◆ When continuously administering hyperosmolar solutions, be alert for signs of hypovolemia: thirst, dry mucous membranes, slightly falling blood pressure, rising pulse rate and respirations, low-grade fever (99° F [37.2° C]), and elevated hematocrit, hemoglobin, and BUN levels.
◆ Administer fluid cautiously, especially to the patient with cardiopulmonary or renal disease, and watch for signs of overhydration: constant and irritating cough, dyspnea, moist crackles, rising central venous pressure, and pitting edema (late sign). When the patient is in an upright position, neck and hand vein engorgement is a sign of fluid overload.

ELDER TIP *Many older patients take drugs to treat a variety of conditions. Remember that drugs can affect the patient's nutritional status by altering nutrient absorption, metabolism, utilization, or excretion. Likewise, various foods, beverages, and mineral or vitamin supplements can affect the absorption and effectiveness of drugs. Be aware of*

these potential interactions when evaluating the patient's medication regimen and nutritional status.

Nutritional imbalance

VITAMIN A DEFICIENCY
A fat-soluble vitamin absorbed in the GI tract, vitamin A maintains epithelial tissue and retinal function. Consequently, deficiency of this vitamin may result in night blindness, decreased color adjustment, keratinization of epithelial tissue, and poor bone growth. Healthy adults have adequate vitamin A reserves to last up to a year; children often don't.

Causes and incidence
Vitamin A deficiency usually results from inadequate intake of foods high in vitamin A (liver, kidney, butter, milk, cream, cheese, and fortified margarine) or carotene, a precursor of vitamin A found in dark green leafy vegetables and yellow or orange fruits and vegetables. (Six milligrams of beta-carotene is equal to 1 mg of vitamin A.) The recommended daily allowance for

vitamin A is 3,000 IU for adult males and 2,310 IU for adult females.

Less common causes of vitamin A deficiency include:

◆ malabsorption due to celiac disease, sprue, cirrhosis, obstructive jaundice, cystic fibrosis, giardiasis, or habitual use of mineral oil as a laxative

◆ massive urinary excretion caused by cancer, tuberculosis, pneumonia, nephritis, or urinary tract infection

◆ decreased storage and transport of vitamin A due to hepatic disease

Each year, more than 80,000 people worldwide—mostly children in underdeveloped countries—lose their sight from severe vitamin A deficiency. This condition is rare in the United States, although many disadvantaged children have substandard levels of vitamin A. With therapy, the chance of reversing symptoms of night blindness and milder conjunctival changes is excellent. When corneal damage is present, emergency treatment is necessary.

Pathophysiology

Once ingested, provitamins A are released from proteins in the stomach. These retinyl esters are then hydrolyzed to retinol in the small intestine, because retinol is more efficiently absorbed. Carotenoids are cleaved in the intestinal mucosa into molecules of retinaldehyde, which is subsequently reduced to retinol and then esterified to retinyl esters. The retinyl esters of retinoid and carotenoid origin are transported via micelles in the lymphatic drainage of the intestine to the blood and then to the liver as components of chylomicrons. In the body, 50% to 80% of vitamin A is stored in the liver, where it is bound to the cellular retinol-binding protein (RBP). The remaining vitamin A is deposited into adipose tissue, the lungs, and the kidneys as retinyl esters, most commonly as retinyl palmitate.

Vitamin A can be mobilized from the liver to peripheral tissue by a process of deesterification of the retinyl esters. In blood, vitamin A is bound to RBP, which transports it as a complex with transthyretin. The hepatic synthesis of RBP is dependent on the presence of zinc and amino acids to maintain its narrow serum range of 40 to 50 µg/dL. Through a receptor-mediated process, the retinol is taken up by the peripheral tissues from the RBP-transthyretin complex.

Complication

◆ Corneal damage

Signs and symptoms

Typically, the first symptom of vitamin A deficiency is night blindness (nyctalopia), which usually becomes apparent when the patient enters a dark place or is caught in the glare of oncoming headlights while driving at night. This condition can progress to xerophthalmia, or drying of the conjunctivas, with development of gray plaques (Bitot spots); if unchecked, perforation, scarring, and blindness may result. Keratinization of epithelial tissue causes dry, scaly skin; follicular hyperkeratosis; and shrinking and hardening of the mucous membranes, possibly leading to infections of the eyes and the respiratory or genitourinary tract. An infant with severe vitamin A deficiency shows signs of failure to thrive and apathy, along with dry skin and corneal changes, which can lead to ulceration and rapid destruction of the cornea.

Diagnosis

Dietary history and typical ocular lesions suggest vitamin A deficiency. Carotene levels less than 40 µg/dL also suggest vitamin A deficiency, but they vary with seasonal ingestion of fruits and vegetables.

℞ **CONFIRMING DIAGNOSIS** *A serum level of vitamin A that falls below 10 µg/dL confirms the diagnosis. Levels between 10 and 19 µg/dL are also considered low, but the patient isn't likely to have developed significant symptoms.*

Treatment

Mild conjunctival changes or night blindness requires vitamin A replacement in the form of cod liver oil or halibut liver oil. Acute deficiency requires aqueous vitamin A solution I.M., or oral tablets, especially when corneal changes have occurred. Therapy for underlying biliary obstruction consists of administration of bile salts; for pancreatic insufficiency, pancreatin, or pancrelipase. Dry skin responds well to cream-based or petroleum-based products.

In patients with chronic malabsorption of fat-soluble vitamins, and in those with low dietary intake, prevention of vitamin A deficiency requires aqueous I.V. supplements or an oral water-miscible preparation.

Special considerations

◆ Administer oral vitamin A supplements with or after meals or parenterally, as indicated. Watch for signs of hypercarotenemia (orange coloration of the skin and eyes) and hypervitaminosis A (rash, hair loss, anorexia, transient hydrocephalus, and vomiting in children;

bone pain, hepatosplenomegaly, diplopia, and irritability in adults). If these signs occur, discontinue supplements and notify the physician immediately. (Hypercarotenemia is relatively harmless; hypervitaminosis A may be toxic.)

▒▒▒▒ PREVENTION *Because vitamin A deficiency usually results from dietary insufficiency, provide nutritional counseling. Tell the patient that vitamin A comes from animal sources, such as eggs, meat, milk, cheese, cream, liver, kidney, and cod and halibut fish oil, but that healthier choices, such as carrots, pumpkins, sweet potatoes, and most dark green, leafy vegetables are good sources of beta-carotene, vitamin A's precursor form. Instruct the patient to choose intense-colored fruit or vegetables, which have high beta-carotene content. Provide referrals to appropriate community agencies if necessary.*

VITAMIN B DEFICIENCIES

Vitamin B complex is a group of water-soluble vitamins essential to normal metabolism, cell growth, and blood formation. (See *Recommended daily allowance of B complex vitamins.*) The most common deficiencies involve thiamine (B_1), riboflavin (B_2), niacin (B_3), pyridoxine (B_6), and cobalamin (B_{12}).

Causes and incidence

Thiamine deficiency results from malabsorption or inadequate dietary intake of vitamin B_1. It also results from alcoholism, prolonged diarrhea, or from increased requirement, which can occur in pregnancy, lactation, and hyperthyroidism. Beriberi, a serious thiamine deficiency disease, is most prevalent in Asians, who subsist mainly on diets of unenriched rice and wheat. Although this disease is uncommon in the United States, alcoholics may develop cardiac (wet) beriberi with high-output heart

failure, neuropathy, and cerebral disturbances. In times of stress (e.g., pregnancy), malnourished young adults may develop beriberi; infantile beriberi may appear in infants on low-protein diets or in those breast-fed by thiamine-deficient mothers.

Riboflavin deficiency (ariboflavinosis) results from a diet deficient in milk, meat, fish, legumes, and green, leafy vegetables. Alcoholism or prolonged diarrhea may also induce riboflavin deficiency. Exposure of milk to sunlight or treatment of legumes with baking soda can destroy riboflavin.

Niacin deficiency, in its advanced form, produces pellagra, which affects the skin, central nervous system (CNS), and GI tract. (See *Recognizing pellagra,* page 493.) Although this deficiency is now seldom found in the United States, it was once common among Southerners who subsisted mainly on corn and consumed minimal animal protein. (Corn is low in niacin and in available tryptophan, the amino acid from which the body synthesizes niacin.) Niacin deficiency is still common in parts of Egypt, Romania, Africa, Serbia, and Montenegro, where corn is the dominant staple food. Niacin deficiency can also occur secondary to carcinoid syndrome or Hartnup disease.

Pyridoxine deficiency usually results from destruction of pyridoxine in infant formulas by autoclaving. A frank deficiency is uncommon in adults, except in patients taking pyridoxine antagonists, such as isoniazid and penicillamine.

Cobalamin deficiency most commonly results from an absence of intrinsic factor in gastric secretions, or an absence of receptor sites after ileal resection. Other causes include malabsorption syndromes associated with sprue, intestinal worm infestation, regional ileitis, and gluten enteropathy, and a diet low in animal protein.

Recommended daily allowance of B complex vitamins

Vitamin	Men (age 23 to 70)	Women (age 23 to 70)	Infants	Children (age 1 to 18)
B1*	1.2 mg	1.1 mg	0.2 to 0.3 mg	0.5 to 1.2 mg
B2*	1.3 mg	1.1 mg	0.3 to 0.4 mg	0.5 to 1.3 mg
Niacin*	16 mg	14 mg	2 to 4 mg	6 to 16 mg
B6	1.3 mg	1.3 mg	0.1 to 0.3 mg	0.5 to 1.3 mg
B12	2.4 µg	2.4 µg	0.4 to 0.5 µg	0.9 to 2.4 µg

*Requirements per 1,000 kcal of dietary intake.

Recognizing pellagra

This patient with pellagra shows dark, scaly, advanced dermatitis. In advanced niacin deficiency, such dermatitis usually occurs on areas exposed to the sun.

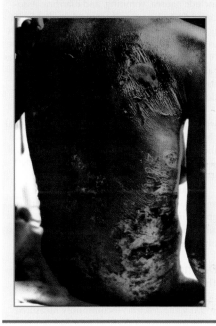

Pathophysiology

Thiamine deficiency (B_1)—when healthy individuals are deprived of thiamine, thiamine stores are depleted within 1 month. However, within a week after thiamine intake stops, healthy people develop a resting tachycardia, weakness, and decreased deep tendon reflexes; some people develop a peripheral neuropathy.

Riboflavin deficiency (B_2)—riboflavin deficiency can alter iron absorption and cause an anemia that leads to fatigue. Riboflavin is involved in red blood cell (RBC) production and transportation of oxygen to the cells. Improving the amount of riboflavin in the body can increase circulating hemoglobin levels and increase red cell production. Collagen is a protein found in most skin and hair, so riboflavin is necessary to maintain a good collagen level. Taking supplements of riboflavin is also a cure for migraines. Research showed that 400 mg of riboflavin a day had demonstrated efficacy in prevention of a migraine in adults, but it must be taken for a minimum of 3 months for good results. This is most likely because

mitochondrial dysfunction has been shown to play a role in migraines, and riboflavin is a precursor of flavin cofactors of the electron transport chain.

Niacin deficiency (B_3)—niacin is essential for adequate cellular function because of its required roles in two similar but distinct coenzymes (i.e., nicotinamide adenine dinucleotide [NAD] and nicotinamide adenine dinucleotide phosphate [NADP]). Both of these are cofactors that can be recycled by serving as both oxidizing (NAD, NADP) and reducing (NADH, NADPH) agents.

During the oxidation of glucose and other intermediary metabolites, a substantial amount of chemical energy is released. NAD/NADH are able to transfer electrons in a process that captures the energy by generating high-energy phosphate bonds. The synthesized ATP then provides the energy necessary for other reactions of intermediary metabolism that simultaneously regenerate NAD from the reduced NADH. A portion of this cofactor is also converted to NADP/NADPH, which plays several distinct roles. Reduced NADPH is used in reactions that detoxify reactive oxygen species, that metabolize drugs in a cytochrome P450 system, and that support lipid biosynthesis.

Pyridoxine deficiency (B_6)—after absorption, pyridoxine, pyridoxamine, and pyridoxal are transported into hepatic cells by facilitated diffusion. Pyridoxal kinase phosphorylates pyridoxine and pyridoxamine, after which they are converted to pyridoxal 5'-phosphate (PLP) by a flavin-dependent enzyme. PLP either remains in the hepatocyte, where it is bound to an apoenzyme, or it is released into the serum, where it is tightly bound to albumin. Free pyridoxal is degraded by alkaline phosphatase, hepatic and renal aldehyde oxidases, and pyridoxal dehydrogenase.

Pyridoxine 5'-phosphate is an essential cofactor in various transamination, decarboxylation, and synthesis pathways involving carbohydrates, sphingolipids, sulfur-containing amino acids, heme, and neurotransmitters. PLP is a coenzyme of tryptophan, methionine, and gamma aminobutyric acid (GABA) metabolism. With methionine deficiency, S-adenosylmethionine accumulates, resulting in the inhibition of sphingolipid and myelin synthesis. Tryptophan is a precursor to several neurotransmitters and is required for niacin production. Thus, pyridoxine deficiency can cause a syndrome indistinguishable from pellagra. PLP is a cofactor for glutamic acid decarboxylase, the enzyme that produces GABA, such that PLP deficiency results in insufficient GABA. Since GABA is the major inhibitor cortical neurotransmitter, PLP deficiency can lead to seizures. Interestingly, pyridoxine-dependent seizures are not caused by a pyridoxine deficiency per se but rather due to an increased depletion of PLP.

The neurotransmitters dopamine, serotonin, epinephrine, norepinephrine, glycine, glutamate, and GABA also require PLP for their production. Homocysteine metabolism is dependent on pyridoxine, and high homocysteine levels can result from pyridoxine deficiency.

Cobalamin deficiency (B_{12})—cobalamin deficiency is caused by the failure of gastric parietal cells to produce sufficient IF (a gastric protein secreted by parietal cells) to permit the absorption of adequate quantities of dietary vitamin B_{12}. Other disorders that interfere with the absorption and metabolism of vitamin B_{12} can produce cobalamin deficiency, with the development of a macrocytic anemia and neurologic complications.

Complications

◆ heart failure
◆ neuropathy
◆ pellagra
◆ anemia
◆ seizures

Signs and symptoms

Thiamine deficiency causes polyneuritis and, possibly, Wernicke encephalopathy and Korsakoff psychosis. In infants (infantile beriberi), this deficiency produces edema, irritability, abdominal pain, pallor, vomiting, loss of voice and, possibly, seizures. In wet beriberi, severe edema starts in the legs and moves up through the body; dry beriberi causes multiple neurologic symptoms and an emaciated appearance. Thiamine deficiency may also cause cardiomegaly, palpitations, tachycardia, dyspnea, and circulatory collapse. Constipation and indigestion are common; ataxia, nystagmus, and ophthalmoplegia are also possible.

Riboflavin deficiency characteristically causes cheilosis (cracking of the lips and corners of the mouth) and glossitis. It may also cause seborrheic dermatitis in the nasolabial folds, scrotum, and vulva and, possibly, generalized dermatitis involving the arms, legs, and trunk. This deficiency can also affect the eyes, producing burning, itching, light sensitivity, tearing, and vascularization of the corneas. Late-stage riboflavin deficiency causes neuropathy, mild anemia and, in children, growth retardation.

Niacin deficiency in its early stages produces fatigue, anorexia, muscle weakness, headache,

indigestion, mild skin eruptions, weight loss, and backache. In advanced stages (pellagra), it produces dark, scaly dermatitis, especially on exposed body parts, that makes the patient appear to be severely sunburned. The mouth, tongue, and lips become red and sore, which may interfere with eating. Common GI symptoms include nausea, vomiting, and diarrhea. Associated CNS aberrations—confusion, disorientation, and neuritis—may become severe enough to induce hallucinations and paranoia. Because of this triad of symptoms, pellagra is sometimes called a "3-D" syndrome—dementia, dermatitis, and diarrhea. If not reversed by therapeutic doses of niacin, pellagra can be fatal.

Pyridoxine deficiency in infants causes a wide range of symptoms: dermatitis, occasional cheilosis or glossitis unresponsive to riboflavin therapy, abdominal pain, vomiting, ataxia, and seizures. This deficiency can also lead to CNS disturbances.

Cobalamin deficiency causes pernicious anemia, which produces anorexia, weight loss, abdominal discomfort, constipation, diarrhea, and glossitis; peripheral neuropathy; and, possibly, ataxia, spasticity, and hyperreflexia.

Diagnosis

The following values confirm vitamin B deficiency.

◆ *Thiamine deficiency*—commonly measured as micrograms per deciliter in a 24-hour urine collection. Deficiency levels are age-related: 1 to 3 years, less than 120; 4 to 6 years, less than 85; 7 to 9 years, less than 70; 10 to 12 years, less than 60; 13 to 15 years, less than 50; adults, less than 27; pregnant women, less than 23 (second trimester), less than 21 (third trimester).

◆ *Riboflavin deficiency*—measured as micrograms per gram of creatinine in a 24-hour urine collection. Deficiency levels are age-related: 1 to 3 years, less than 150; 4 to 6 years, less than 100; 7 to 9 years, less than 85; 10 to 15 years, less than 70; adults, less than 27; pregnant women, less than 39 (second trimester), less than 30 (third trimester).

◆ *Niacin deficiency*—measured by N-methyl nicotinamide in a 24-hour urine collection as micrograms per gram of creatinine. Deficiency levels in adults are less than 0.5; in pregnant women, less than 0.5 (first trimester), less than 0.6 (second trimester), and less than 0.8 (third trimester).

◆ *Pyridoxine deficiency*—xanthurenic acid more than 50 mg/day in 24-hour urine collection after administration of 10 g of L-tryptophan; decreased levels of serum and RBC transaminases; reduced excretion of pyridoxic acid in urine.

◆ *Cobalamin deficiency*—cobalamin serum levels less than 170 pg/mL. Tests to discover the deficiency's cause include gastric analysis and hemoglobin studies. In addition, the Schilling test measures absorption of radioactive cobalamin with and without intrinsic factor; however, it is rarely used.

Treatment

Diet and supplementary vitamins can correct or prevent vitamin B deficiencies, as follows.

◆ *Thiamine deficiency*—a high-protein diet, with adequate calorie intake, possibly supplemented by B complex vitamins for early symptoms. Thiamine-rich foods include pork, peas, wheat bran, oatmeal, and liver. Alcoholic beriberi may require thiamine supplements or thiamine hydrochloride as part of a B complex concentrate.

◆ *Riboflavin deficiency*—supplemental riboflavin in patients with intractable diarrhea or increased need for riboflavin related to growth, pregnancy, lactation, or wound healing. Good sources of riboflavin are meats, enriched flour, milk and dairy products, eggs, cereal, and green, leafy vegetables. Acute riboflavin deficiency requires daily oral doses of riboflavin alone or with other B complex vitamins. Riboflavin phosphate can also be administered I.V. or I.M.

◆ *Niacin deficiency*—supplemental B complex vitamins and dietary enrichment in patients at risk because of marginal diets or alcoholism. Meats, fish, peanuts, brewer's yeast, enriched breads, and cereals are rich in niacin; milk and eggs, in tryptophan. Confirmed niacin deficiency requires daily doses of niacinamide orally or I.V.

◆ *Pyridoxine deficiency*—prophylactic pyridoxine therapy in infants and in children with a seizure disorder; supplemental B complex vitamins in patients with anorexia, malabsorption, or those taking isoniazid or penicillamine. Some women who take hormonal contraceptives may have to supplement their diets with pyridoxine. Confirmed pyridoxine deficiencies require oral or parenteral pyridoxine. Children with seizures stemming from metabolic dysfunction may require daily doses of 200 to 600 mg pyridoxine.

◆ *Cobalamin deficiency*—parenteral cobalamin in patients with reduced gastric secretion of hydrochloric acid, lack of intrinsic factor, some malabsorption syndromes, or ileum resections. Strict vegetarians may have to supplement their diets with oral vitamin B_{12}. Depending on the deficiency's severity, supplementary cyanocobalamin or methylcobalamin is usually given parenterally for 5 to 10 days, followed by monthly or daily vitamin B_{12} supplements.

Special considerations

An accurate dietary history provides a baseline for effective dietary counseling.

◆ Identify and observe patients who are at risk for vitamin B deficiencies—alcoholics, the elderly, pregnant women, oral hormonal contraceptive users (vitamins B_6 and B_{12}), and people on limited diets.

◆ Administer prescribed supplements. Make sure patients understand how important it is that they adhere strictly to their prescribed treatment for the rest of their lives. Watch for adverse effects from large doses of niacinamide, such as a flushed sensation or hot flashes, in patients with niacin deficiency. Remember, prolonged intake of niacin can cause hepatic dysfunction. Caution patients with Parkinson disease receiving pyridoxine that this drug can impair response to levodopa therapy.

◆ Explain all tests and procedures. Reassure patients that, with treatment, the prognosis is good. Refer patients to appropriate assistance agencies if their diets are inadequate due to adverse socioeconomic conditions.

⁞⁞⁞⁞⁞ **PREVENTION**
◆ *Encourage the patient to follow a well-balanced diet.*
◆ *Vitamin B_{12} injections can prevent anemia after surgeries known to cause vitamin B_{12} deficiency.*

VITAMIN C DEFICIENCY

Vitamin C (ascorbic acid) deficiency leads to scurvy or inadequate production of collagen, an extracellular substance that binds the cells of the teeth, bones, and capillaries. It's essential for wound healing and burn recovery. Vitamin C is also an important factor in metabolizing such amino acids as tyrosine and phenylalanine. It also acts as a reductant, activating enzymes in the body, as well as converting folic acid into useful components.

Severe vitamin C deficiency results in scurvy, evidenced by hemorrhagic tendencies and abnormal osteoid and dentin formation.

Causes and incidence

This deficiency's primary cause is a diet lacking in vitamin C-rich foods, such as citrus fruits, tomatoes, cabbage, broccoli, spinach, and berries. Because the body can't store this water-soluble vitamin in large amounts, the supply needs to be replenished daily. Other causes include:

◆ destruction of vitamin C in foods by overexposure to air or by overcooking

◆ excessive ingestion of vitamin C during pregnancy, which causes the neonate to require large amounts of the vitamin after birth

◆ marginal intake of vitamin C during periods of physiologic stress—caused by infectious disease, for example—which can deplete tissue saturation of vitamin C

Historically common among sailors and others deprived of fresh fruits and vegetables for long periods of time, vitamin C deficiency is uncommon today in the United States, except in alcoholics, people on restricted-residue diets, and infants weaned from breast milk to cow's milk without a vitamin C supplement.

Pathophysiology

Humans, other primates, and guinea pigs are unable to synthesize L-ascorbic acid (vitamin C); therefore, they require it in their diet. The enzyme L-gulonolactone oxidase, which would usually catalyze the conversion of L-gluconogammalactone to L-ascorbic acid, is defective due to a mutation or inborn error in carbohydrate metabolism.

Ascorbic acid is metabolized in the liver by oxidation and sulfation. The renal threshold for excretion by the kidney in urine is approximately 1.4 mg/100 mL plasma. Excess amounts of ascorbic acid are excreted unchanged or as metabolites. When body tissue or plasma concentrations of vitamin C are low, excretion of the vitamin is decreased. Scurvy occurs after vitamin C has been eliminated from the diet for at least 3 months and when the body pool falls below 350 mg.

Complication

◆ Scurvy

Signs and symptoms

Clinical features of vitamin C deficiency appear as capillaries become increasingly fragile. In an adult, it produces petechiae, ecchymoses, follicular hyperkeratosis (especially on the buttocks and legs), anemia, anorexia, limb and joint pain (especially in the knees), pallor, weakness, swollen or bleeding gums, loose teeth, lethargy, insomnia, poor wound healing, and ocular hemorrhages in the bulbar conjunctivae. (See *Scurvy's effect on gums and legs.*) Vitamin C deficiency can also cause beading, fractures of the costochondral junctions of the ribs or epiphysis, and such psychological disturbances as irritability, depression, hysteria, and hypochondriasis.

In a child, vitamin C deficiency produces tender, painful swelling in the legs, causing the child to lie with the legs partially flexed. Other symptoms include fever, diarrhea, and vomiting.

Scurvy's effect on gums and legs

In adults, scurvy causes swollen or bleeding gums and loose teeth.

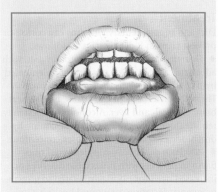

It also causes follicular hyperkeratosis, usually on the legs.

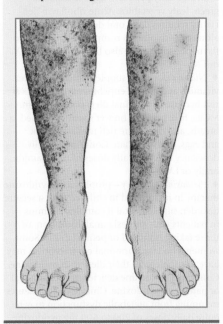

Diagnosis

℞ **CONFIRMING DIAGNOSIS** *Serum ascorbic acid levels less than 0.2 mg/dL and white blood cell ascorbic acid levels less than 30 mg/dL help confirm the diagnosis.*

Dietary history revealing an inadequate intake of ascorbic acid suggests vitamin C deficiency. A capillary fragility test may be performed on the patient's forearm with a blood pressure cuff; it's positive if more than 10 petechiae form after 5 minutes of pressure.

Treatment

Because scurvy may be fatal, treatment begins immediately to restore adequate vitamin C intake with daily doses of 100 to 200 mg synthetic vitamin C or orange juice in mild disease and with doses as high as 500 mg/day in severe disease. Symptoms usually subside in 2 to 3 days; hemorrhages and bone disorders, in 2 to 3 weeks.

Special considerations

◆ Administer ascorbic acid orally or by slow I.V. infusion, as indicated. Avoid moving the patient unnecessarily to avoid irritating painful joints and muscles. Encourage the patient to drink orange juice.
◆ Explain the importance of supplemental ascorbic acid. Counsel the patient and family about good dietary sources of vitamin C.
◆ Advise against taking too much vitamin C. Explain that excessive doses of ascorbic acid may cause nausea, diarrhea, and renal calculi formation and may also interfere with anticoagulant therapy.

:::::::: **PREVENTION** *Patients unable or unwilling to consume foods rich in vitamin C or those facing surgery should take daily supplements of ascorbic acid. The recommended daily allowance is 75 to 90 mg/day. Vitamin C supplementation may also prevent this deficiency in recently weaned infants or those drinking formula not fortified with vitamin C.*

VITAMIN D DEFICIENCY

Vitamin D deficiency, commonly called *rickets*, causes failure of normal bone calcification, which occurs through several mechanisms: decreased calcium and phosphorus (the major components of bone) from the intestines, increased excretion of calcium from renal tubules, and increased parathyroid secretion resulting in increased release of calcium from the bone. The deficiency results in rickets in infants and young children and osteomalacia in adults. With treatment, the prognosis is good. However, in rickets, bone deformities usually persist, whereas in osteomalacia, such deformities may disappear.

Causes and incidence

Vitamin D deficiency results from inadequate dietary intake of preformed vitamin D, malabsorption of vitamin D, or too little exposure to sunlight.

Once a common childhood disease, rickets is now rare in the United States but occasionally appears in breast-fed infants who don't receive a vitamin D supplement or in infants receiving a formula with a nonfortified milk base. This deficiency may also occur in overcrowded urban areas in which smog limits sunlight penetration. Incidence is highest in black children who, because of their skin color, absorb less sunlight. (Solar ultraviolet rays irradiate 7-dehydrocholesterol, a precursor of vitamin D, to form calciferol.)

Osteomalacia, also uncommon in the United States, is most prevalent in Asia, among young multiparas who eat a cereal diet and have minimal exposure to sunlight. Other causes include:
◆ vitamin D-resistant rickets (refractory rickets, familial hypophosphatemia) from an inherited impairment of renal tubular reabsorption of phosphate (from vitamin D insensitivity)
◆ conditions that lower absorption of fat-soluble vitamin D, such as chronic pancreatitis, celiac disease, Crohn disease, cystic fibrosis, gastric or small-bowel resections, fistulas, colitis, and biliary obstruction
◆ hepatic or renal disease, which interferes with the formation of hydroxylated calciferol, necessary to initiate the formation of a calcium-binding protein in intestinal absorption sites
◆ malfunctioning parathyroid gland (decreased secretion of parathyroid hormone [PTH]), which contributes to calcium deficiency (normally, vitamin D controls calcium and phosphorus absorption through the intestine) and interferes with activation of vitamin D in the kidneys

Pathophysiology

Inadequate circulation of 25(OH)D is associated with elevated PTH; this condition is called secondary hyperparathyroidism. The rise in PTH may result in increased mobilization of calcium from the bone, which leads to decreased mineralization of the bone.

Of note, prolonged exposure to the sun does not cause vitamin D toxicity. This is because after prolonged UVB radiation exposure, the vitamin D made in the skin is further degraded to the inactive vitamin D metabolites tachysterol and lumisterol.

Complications

◆ Chronic skeletal pain
◆ Skeletal deformities
◆ Skeletal fractures

Signs and symptoms

Early indications of vitamin D deficiency are profuse sweating, restlessness, and irritability. Chronic deficiency induces numerous bone malformations due to softening of the bones:

Recognizing bowlegs

This infant with rickets shows characteristic bowing of the legs.

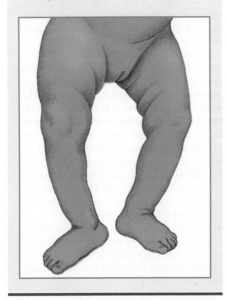

bowlegs, knock-knees, rachitic rosary (beading of ends of ribs), enlargement of wrists and ankles, pigeon breast, delayed closing of the fontanels, softening of the skull, and bulging of the forehead. (See *Recognizing bowlegs.*)

Other rachitic features are poorly developed muscles (potbelly) and infantile tetany. Bone deformities may cause difficulty in walking and in climbing stairs, spontaneous multiple fractures, and lower back and leg pain.

Diagnosis

Physical examination, dietary history, and laboratory tests establish the diagnosis. Test results that suggest vitamin D deficiency include plasma calcium serum levels less than 7.5 mg/dL, serum inorganic phosphorus levels less than 3 mg/dL, serum citrate levels less than 2.5 mg/dL, and alkaline phosphatase levels less than 4 Bodansky U/dL.

℞ CONFIRMING DIAGNOSIS *X-rays confirm the diagnosis by showing characteristic bone deformities and abnormalities such as Looser zones (pseudofractures).*

Treatment

For osteomalacia and rickets—except when caused by malabsorption—treatment consists of oral doses of vitamin D or sources such as fish, liver, and processed milk. Exposure to sunlight is encouraged. For rickets refractory to vitamin D or in rickets accompanied by hepatic or renal disease, treatment includes 25-hydroxycholecalciferol, 1,25-dihydroxycholecalciferol, or a synthetic analog of active vitamin D. Replacement of deficient calcium and phosphorus also helps to eliminate most symptoms of rickets. Positioning or bracing may be used to reduce or prevent deformities; some skeletal deformities may require corrective surgery.

Special considerations

◆ Obtain a dietary history to assess the patient's current vitamin D intake. Encourage the patient to eat foods high in vitamin D—fortified milk, fish liver oils, herring, liver, and egg yolks—and get sufficient sun exposure. If deficiency is due to socioeconomic conditions, refer the patient to appropriate community agencies.
◆ If the patient must take vitamin D for a prolonged period, tell the patient to watch for signs of vitamin D toxicity (headache, nausea, constipation and, after prolonged use, renal calculi).

░░░░░ PREVENTION
◆ *Administer supplementary aqueous preparations of vitamin D for chronic fat malabsorption, hydroxylated cholecalciferol for refractory rickets, and supplemental vitamin D for breast-fed infants.*
◆ *Consider genetic counseling for a patient with a family history of inherited disorders that can cause rickets.*

VITAMIN E DEFICIENCY

Vitamin E (tocopherol) appears to act primarily as an antioxidant, preventing intracellular oxidation of polyunsaturated fatty acids and other lipids. It protects body tissue from damage caused by unstable substances called *free radicals*, which can harm cells, tissues, and organs and are believed to be one of the causes of aging's degenerative process. Vitamin E is also important in the formation of RBCs and helps the body to use vitamin K. Vitamin E deficiency usually manifests as hemolytic anemia in low–birth-weight or premature neonates. With treatment, prognosis is good.

Causes and incidence

Vitamin E deficiency in infants usually results from consuming formulas high in polyunsaturated fatty acids that are fortified with iron but not vitamin E. Such formulas increase the need for antioxidant vitamin E because the iron supplement catalyzes the oxidation of RBC lipids. A neonate has low tissue concentrations of vitamin E to begin with because only a small amount passes through the placenta; the mother retains most of it. Because vitamin E is a fat-soluble vitamin, deficiency develops in conditions associated with fat malabsorption, such as kwashiorkor, celiac disease, or cystic fibrosis. These conditions may induce megaloblastic or hemolytic anemia and creatinuria, all of which are reversible with vitamin E administration.

Vitamin E deficiency is uncommon in adults but is possible in people whose diets are high in polyunsaturated fatty acids, which increase vitamin E requirements, and in people with vitamin E malabsorption, which impairs RBC survival.

Complication
◆ Hemolytic anemia

Signs and symptoms
Vitamin E deficiency is difficult to recognize, but its early symptoms include edema and skin lesions in infants and muscle weakness or intermittent claudication in adults. In premature neonates, vitamin E deficiency produces hemolytic anemia, thrombocythemia, and erythematous papular skin eruption, followed by desquamation.

Diagnosis
CONFIRMING DIAGNOSIS *Dietary and medical histories suggest vitamin E deficiency. Serum alpha-tocopherol levels below 0.5 mg/dL in adults and below 0.2 mg/dL in infants confirm it. Creatinuria, increased creatine kinase levels, hemolytic anemia, and an elevated platelet count generally support the diagnosis.*

Treatment
Replacement of vitamin E with a water-soluble supplement, either oral or parenteral, is the only appropriate treatment.

Special considerations
◆ As indicated, prevent deficiency by providing vitamin E supplements for low–birth-weight neonates receiving formulas not fortified with vitamin E and for adults with vitamin E malabsorption. Many commercial multivitamin supplements are easily absorbed by patients with vitamin E malabsorption.
◆ If vitamin E deficiency is related to socioeconomic conditions, refer the patient to appropriate community agencies.

PREVENTION
◆ *Inform new mothers who plan to breastfeed that human milk provides adequate vitamin E.*
◆ *Encourage adult patients to eat foods high in vitamin E; good sources include vegetable oils (corn, safflower, soybean, cottonseed); whole grains; dark green, leafy vegetables; nuts; and legumes. Tell them that heavy consumption of polyunsaturated fatty acids increases the need for vitamin E.*

VITAMIN K DEFICIENCY
Deficiency of vitamin K, an element necessary for formation of prothrombin and other clotting factors in the liver, produces abnormal bleeding. If the deficiency is corrected, the prognosis is excellent.

Causes and incidence
Vitamin K deficiency is common among neonates in the first few days postpartum due to poor placental transfer of vitamin K and inadequate production of vitamin K-producing intestinal flora. Its other causes include prolonged use of drugs, such as the anticoagulant warfarin and antibiotics that destroy normal intestinal bacteria; decreased flow of bile to the small intestine from obstruction of the bile duct or bile fistula; malabsorption of vitamin K due to sprue, pellagra, bowel resection, ileitis, or ulcerative colitis; chronic hepatic disease, with impaired response of hepatic ribosomes to vitamin K; and cystic fibrosis, with fat malabsorption. Vitamin K deficiency seldom results from insufficient dietary intake of this vitamin.

Pathophysiology
Vitamin K is necessary for the formation of prothrombin and other blood-clotting factors in the liver, and it also plays a role in bone metabolism. A form of the vitamin is produced by bacteria in the colon and can be utilized to some degree. Vitamin K deficiency causes impaired clotting of the blood and internal bleeding, even without injury.

Complications
◆ Hemorrhagic disease
◆ Osteoporosis

Signs and symptoms
The cardinal sign of vitamin K deficiency is an abnormal bleeding tendency, accompanied by prolonged prothrombin time (PT); these signs disappear with vitamin K administration. Without treatment, bleeding may be severe and, possibly, fatal.

Diagnosis
CONFIRMING DIAGNOSIS *A PT that's 25% longer than the normal range of 10 to 20 seconds, measured by the Quick method, confirms the diagnosis of vitamin K deficiency after other causes of prolonged PT (such as anticoagulant therapy or*

hepatic disease) have been ruled out. The international normalized ratio (normal value, 0.8 to 1.2) is the more common method of assessing PT adequacy.

Repetition of testing in 24 hours (and regularly during treatment) monitors the therapy's effectiveness.

Treatment

Administration of vitamin K I.V. or I.M. corrects abnormal bleeding tendencies.

Special considerations

▓▓▓▓ PREVENTION

◆ *Administer vitamin K to neonates and patients with fat malabsorption or with prolonged diarrhea from colitis, ileitis, or long-term antibiotic drug therapy.*

◆ *If the deficiency has a dietary cause, help the patient and family plan a diet that includes important sources of vitamin K, such as cauliflower, tomatoes, cheese, egg yolks, liver, and green, leafy vegetables.*

◆ *Warn against self-medication with or overuse of antibiotics, because these drugs destroy the intestinal bacteria needed to generate significant amounts of vitamin K.*

HYPERVITAMINOSES A AND D

Hypervitaminosis A is excessive accumulation of vitamin A; hypervitaminosis D, of vitamin D. Although these are toxic conditions, they usually respond well to treatment. They're most prevalent in infants and children, usually as a result of accidental or misguided overdosage by parents. A related, benign condition called *hypercarotenemia* results from excessive consumption of carotene, a chemical precursor of vitamin A.

Causes and incidence

Vitamins A and D are fat-soluble vitamins that accumulate in the body because they aren't dissolved and excreted in the urine. (See *Important facts about vitamins A and D.*) In most cases, hypervitaminoses A and D result from ingestion of excessive amounts of supplemental vitamin preparations. A single dose of more than 1 million units of vitamin A can cause acute toxicity; daily doses of 15,000 to 25,000 U taken over weeks or months have proven toxic in infants and children. For the same dose to produce toxicity in adults, ingestion over years is necessary. Doses of 100,000 IU of vitamin D daily for several months can cause toxicity in adults. Individuals who are at risk include those with hyperparathyroidism, kidney disease, sarcoidosis, tuberculosis, or histoplasmosis.

Pathophysiology

Vitamin A—The bioavailability of retinol is generally more than 80%, whereas the bioavailability and bioconversion of carotenes (i.e., provitamin A) are lower. These may be affected by species, molecular linkage, amount of carotene, nutritional status, genetic factors, and other interactions.

While in general the body absorbs retinoids and vitamin A very efficiently, it lacks the mechanisms to destroy excessive loads. Thus, the possibility of toxicity exists unless intake is carefully regulated. It has been suggested that earlier estimates of daily human requirements of vitamin A be revised downward.

Vitamin D—The acute toxic dose for vitamin D has not been established. The chronic toxic dose is more than 50,000 IU/day in adults. In infants younger than 6 months,

---

Important facts about vitamins A and D

This table illustrates good sources of vitamins A and D, their recommended daily allowances, and the actions they produce.

Vitamin	Sources	Recommended dietary allowance	Action
Vitamin A	◆ Carrots; sweet potatoes; dark green, leafy vegetables; butter; margarine; liver; egg yolk	◆ Ages 1 to 13: 1,000 to 2,000 IU ◆ Ages ≥14: 2,300 to 3,000 IU ◆ Lactating women: 4,000 to 4,300 IU	◆ Produces retinal pigment and maintains epithelial tissue
Vitamin D	◆ Ultraviolet light; fortified foods (especially milk)	◆ 600 IU daily	◆ Promotes absorption and regulates metabolism of calcium and phosphorus

1,000 IU/day may be considered unsafe. However, a wide variance in potential toxicity exists for vitamin D.

PEDIATRIC TIP In infants, giving 40,000 IU daily of vitamin D can cause toxicity in 1 to 4 months.

Hypervitaminosis A may occur in patients receiving pharmacologic doses of vitamin A for dermatologic disorders. Hypervitaminosis D may occur in patients receiving high doses of the vitamin as treatment for hypoparathyroidism, rickets, and the osteodystrophy of chronic renal failure, and in infants who consume fortified milk and cereals plus a vitamin supplement. Concentrations of vitamin A in common foods are generally too low to pose a danger of excessive intake. However, hypercarotenemia results from excessive consumption of vegetables high in carotene (a protovitamin that the body converts into vitamin A), such as carrots, sweet potatoes, and dark green, leafy vegetables.

Complications
◆ Liver damage
◆ Osteoporosis
◆ Excess calcium buildup (which could cause kidney damage)

Signs and symptoms
Chronic hypervitaminosis A produces anorexia, irritability, headache, hair loss, malaise, itching, vertigo, bone pain, bone fragility, and dry, peeling skin. It may also cause hepatosplenomegaly and emotional lability. Acute toxicity may also produce transient hydrocephalus and vomiting. (Hypercarotenemia produces yellow or orange skin coloration.)

Hypervitaminosis D causes anorexia, headache, nausea, vomiting, weight loss, polyuria, and polydipsia. Because vitamin D promotes calcium absorption, severe toxicity can lead to hypercalcemia, including calcification of soft tissues, as in the heart, aorta, and renal tubules. Lethargy, confusion, and coma may accompany severe hypercalcemia.

Diagnosis
A thorough patient history suggests hypervitaminosis A.

CONFIRMING DIAGNOSIS An elevated serum vitamin A level (over 90 µg/dL) confirms hypervitaminosis A.

Patient history and an elevated serum calcium level (over 10.5 µg/dL) suggest hypervitaminosis D.

CONFIRMING DIAGNOSIS An elevated serum vitamin D level confirms hypervitaminosis D.

In children, X-rays showing calcification of tendons, ligaments, and subperiosteal tissues support this diagnosis.

CONFIRMING DIAGNOSIS An elevated serum carotene level (over 250 µg/dL) confirms hypercarotenemia.

Treatment
Withholding vitamin supplements usually corrects hypervitaminosis A quickly and hypervitaminosis D gradually. Hypercalcemia may persist for weeks or months after the patient stops taking vitamin D. Treatment for severe hypervitaminosis D may include glucocorticoids to control hypercalcemia and prevent renal damage. In the acute stage, diuretics or other emergency measures for severe hypercalcemia may be necessary. Hypercarotenemia responds well to a diet free of high-carotene foods.

Special considerations
◆ Keep the patient comfortable, and reassure the patient that symptoms will subside after they stop taking the vitamin.
◆ Make sure the patient or the parents of a child with these conditions understand that vitamins aren't innocuous. Explain the hazards associated with excessive vitamin intake. Point out that vitamin A and D requirements can easily be met with a diet containing dark green, leafy vegetables; fruits; and fortified milk or milk products.

PREVENTION Monitor serum vitamin A levels in patients receiving doses above the recommended daily allowance and serum calcium levels in patients receiving pharmacologic doses of vitamin D.

IODINE DEFICIENCY
Iodine deficiency is the absence of sufficient levels of iodine to satisfy daily metabolic requirements. Because the thyroid gland uses most of the body's iodine stores, iodine deficiency is apt to cause hypothyroidism and thyroid gland hypertrophy (endemic goiter). Other effects of deficiency range from dental caries to cretinism in neonates born to iodine-deficient mothers. Iodine deficiency is most common in pregnant or lactating women due to their exaggerated metabolic need for this element. Iodine deficiency responds readily to treatment with iodine supplements.

Causes and incidence
Iodine deficiency usually results from insufficient intake of dietary sources of iodine, such as iodized table salt, seafood, and dark green, leafy vegetables. (Normal iodine requirements range from 35 µg/day for infants to 150 µg/day for

lactating women; the average adult needs 1 µg/kg of body weight.) Iodine deficiency may also result from an increase in metabolic demands during pregnancy, lactation, and adolescence.

Pathophysiology
Dietary iodine is taken up readily through the gut in the form of iodide. From the circulation, it is concentrated in the thyroid gland by means of an energy-dependent sodium iodide symporter. In the follicle cells of the thyroid gland, four atoms of iodine are incorporated into each molecule of thyroxine (T_4) and three atoms into each molecule of triiodothyronine (T_3).

Complications
◆ Hypothyroidism
◆ Goiter

Signs and symptoms
Clinical features of iodine deficiency depend on the degree of hypothyroidism that develops (in addition to the development of a goiter). Mild deficiency may produce only mild, nonspecific symptoms, such as lassitude, fatigue, and loss of motivation. Severe deficiency usually generates the typically overt and unmistakable features of hypothyroidism: bradycardia; decreased pulse pressure and cardiac output; weakness; hoarseness; dry, flaky, inelastic skin; puffy face; thick tongue; delayed relaxation phase in deep tendon reflexes; poor memory; hearing loss; chills; anorexia; and nystagmus. In women, iodine deficiency may also cause menorrhagia and amenorrhea.

Cretinism—hypothyroidism that develops in utero or in early infancy—is characterized by failure to thrive, neonatal jaundice, and hypothermia. By age 3 to 6 months, the infant may display spastic diplegia and signs and symptoms similar to those seen in infants with Down syndrome.

Diagnosis
CONFIRMING DIAGNOSIS *Abnormal laboratory test results include low thyroxine (T_4) levels with high radioactive iodine (^{131}I) uptake, low 24-hour urine iodine levels, and high thyroid-stimulating hormone levels. Radioiodine uptake test traces ^{131}I in the thyroid 24 hours after administration; triiodothyronine-resin or T_4-resin uptake test shows values 25% below normal.*

Treatment
Severe iodine deficiency requires administration of iodine supplements (potassium iodide [SSKI]). Mild deficiency may be corrected by increasing iodine intake through the use of iodized table salt and consumption of iodine-rich foods (seafood and green, leafy vegetables).

Special considerations
◆ Administer SSKI preparation in milk or juice to reduce gastric irritation and mask its metallic taste. To prevent tooth discoloration, tell the patient to drink the solution through a straw. Store the solution in a light-resistant container.

▓▓▓ PREVENTION
◆ *Recommend the use of iodized salt and consumption of iodine-rich foods for high-risk patients—especially adolescents and pregnant or lactating women.*
◆ *Advise pregnant women that severe iodine deficiency may produce cretinism in neonates, and instruct them to watch for early signs of iodine deficiency, such as fatigue, lassitude, weakness, and decreased mental function.*

ZINC DEFICIENCY
Zinc, an essential trace element that's present in the bones, teeth, hair, skin, testes, liver, and muscles, is also a vital component of many enzymes. The prognosis is good with correction of the deficiency.

Causes and incidence
Zinc deficiency usually results from excessive intake of foods (containing iron, calcium, vitamin D, and the fiber and phytates in cereals) that bind zinc to form insoluble chelates that prevent its absorption. Occasionally, it results from blood loss due to parasitism and low intake of foods containing zinc. Alcohol and corticosteroids increase renal excretion of zinc.

Zinc deficiency is most common in people from underdeveloped countries, especially in the Middle East. Children are most susceptible to this deficiency during periods of rapid growth.

Pathophysiology
Zinc promotes synthesis of deoxyribonucleic acid, ribonucleic acid and, ultimately, protein, and maintains normal blood concentrations of vitamin A by mobilizing it from the liver.

Complications
◆ Mental lethargy
◆ Decreased wound healing
◆ Impaired immune function

Signs and symptoms
Zinc deficiency produces hepatosplenomegaly, sparse hair growth, soft and misshapen nails, poor wound healing, anorexia,

hypogeusesthesia (decreased taste acuity), dysgeusia (unpleasant taste), hyposmia (decreased odor acuity), dysosmia (unpleasant odor in nasopharynx), severe iron deficiency anemia, bone deformities and, when chronic, hypogonadism, dwarfism, and hyperpigmentation.

Diagnosis

CONFIRMING DIAGNOSIS *Fasting serum zinc levels below 70 µg/dL confirm zinc deficiency and indicate altered phosphate metabolism, imbalance between aerobic and anaerobic metabolism, and decreased pancreatic enzyme levels.*

Treatment

Treatment consists of correcting the deficiency's underlying cause and administering zinc supplements, as necessary.

Special considerations

◆ Advise the patient to take zinc supplements with milk or meals to prevent gastric distress and vomiting.

PREVENTION *Encourage a balanced diet that includes seafood, oatmeal, bran, meat, eggs, nuts, and dry yeast and the correct use of calcium and iron supplements.*

OBESITY

Obesity is an excess of body fat, generally 20% above ideal body weight. The prognosis for correction of obesity is poor: Fewer than 30% of patients succeed in losing 20 lb (9 kg), and only half of these maintain the loss over a prolonged period.

Causes and incidence

Obesity results from excessive calorie intake and inadequate expenditure of energy. Rates of obesity are climbing, and the percentage of children and adolescents who are obese has doubled in the past 20 years.

Pathophysiology

Theories to explain this condition include hypothalamic dysfunction of hunger and satiety centers, genetic predisposition, abnormal absorption of nutrients, and impaired action of GI and growth hormones and of hormonal regulators such as insulin. An inverse relationship between socioeconomic status and the prevalence of obesity has been documented, especially in women. Obesity in parents increases the probability of obesity in children, from genetic or environmental factors, such as activity levels and learned patterns of eating. Psychological factors, such as stress or emotional eating, may also contribute to obesity.

Complications

◆ Respiratory difficulties
◆ Hypertension
◆ Cardiovascular disease
◆ Diabetes mellitus
◆ Renal disease
◆ Gallbladder disease
◆ Psychosocial difficulties
◆ Premature death

Signs and symptoms

Obesity is a problem of too much weight typically resulting in a body mass index (BMI) of 30 or higher. (See *Diagnostic aids.*)

Diagnostic aids

Weight categories, overweight and obesity, are determined by using a person's height and weight to calculate the BMI. *Overweight* is defined as a BMI between 25.0 and 29.9. *Obesity* is defined as a BMI of 30 or higher. Measurement of the thickness of subcutaneous fat folds with calipers provides an approximation of total body fat. Although this measurement is reliable and isn't subject to daily fluctuations, it has little meaning for the patient in monitoring subsequent weight loss.

Treatment

Successful management of obesity must decrease the patient's daily calorie intake while increasing their activity level. Effective treatment must be based on a balanced, low-calorie diet that eliminates foods high in fat or sugar. Lifelong maintenance of these improved eating and exercise patterns is necessary to achieve long-term benefits.

The popular low-carbohydrate diets offer no long-term advantage; rapid early weight reduction is due to loss of water, not fat. These and other crash or fad diets have the overwhelming drawback that they don't teach the patient long-term modification of eating patterns and often lead to the "yo-yo syndrome"—episodes of repeated weight loss followed by weight gain. This can be more detrimental than the obesity itself because of the severe stress it can place on the body.

Total fasting is an effective method of rapid weight reduction but requires close monitoring and supervision to minimize risks of ketonemia, electrolyte imbalance, hypotension, and loss of lean body mass. Prolonged fasting and very-low-calorie diets have been associated with sudden death, possibly resulting from cardiac arrhythmias caused by electrolyte abnormalities. These methods also neglect patient re-education, which is necessary for long-term weight maintenance. The best way to lose weight is to do so slowly, losing 1 to 2 lb/week.

Treatment may also include behavior modification techniques, which promote fundamental changes in eating habits and activity patterns.

Food and Drug Administration (FDA)-approved medications for chronic weight loss include Alli (orlistat), Qsymia (phentermine and topiramate), Belviq (lorcaserin), Contrave (naltrexone/bupropion), and Saxenda (liraglutide). These drugs promote weight loss by decreasing the absorption of dietary fat. They need to be combined with healthy eating and physical activity to be most effective.

Obesity may be treated surgically with restriction or malabsorptive procedures. Those with a BMI greater than 40 or with a BMI between 35 and 39.9 along with a weight-related health problem may qualify for weight-loss surgery. Vertical banded gastroplasty, gastric banding, and the sleeve procedure represent restrictive surgical procedures that aid in weight loss by decreasing the volume of food that the stomach can accommodate. Gastric bypass with a Roux-en-Y procedure produces weight loss by both restricting stomach capacity and inducing malabsorption; food is rerouted to bypass part of the small intestine. Nutrition counseling before and after these procedures is recommended to enhance safe weight loss, educate the patient about proper diet advancement, and monitor for nutritional deficiencies. Psychological and social support are also beneficial before and after surgery.

Special considerations

◆ Obtain an accurate diet history to identify the patient's eating patterns and the importance of food to their lifestyle. Ask the patient to keep a careful record of what, where, and when they eat to help identify situations that normally provoke overeating.
◆ Explain the prescribed diet carefully, and encourage compliance to improve health status.
◆ To increase calorie expenditure, promote increased physical activity, including an exercise program. Recommend varying activity levels according to the patient's general condition and cardiovascular status.
◆ Teach the grossly obese patient the importance of good skin care to prevent breakdown in moist skin folds. Recommend the regular use of powder to keep skin dry.

⋮⋮⋮⋮⋮ **PREVENTION**
◆ *Teach parents to avoid overfeeding their infants and to familiarize themselves with actual nutritional needs and optimum growth rates.*

Discourage parents from using food to reward or console their children, from emphasizing the importance of "clean plates," and from allowing eating to prevent hunger rather than to satisfy it.
◆ *Encourage physical activity and exercise, especially in children and young adults, to establish lifelong patterns. Suggest low-calorie snacks such as raw vegetables.*

PROTEIN-CALORIE MALNUTRITION

One of the most prevalent and serious depletion disorders, protein-calorie malnutrition (PCM) occurs as marasmus (protein-calorie deficiency), characterized by growth failure and wasting, and as kwashiorkor (protein deficiency), characterized by tissue edema and damage. Both forms vary from mild to severe and may be fatal, depending on the accompanying stress (particularly sepsis or injury) and duration of deprivation. PCM increases the risk of death from pneumonia, chickenpox, or measles.

Causes and incidence

Both kwashiorkor (edematous PCM) and marasmus (nonedematous PCM) are common in underdeveloped countries and in areas in which dietary amino acid content is insufficient to satisfy growth requirements. Kwashiorkor typically occurs at about age 1, after infants are weaned from breast milk to a protein-deficient diet of starchy gruels or sugar water, but it can develop at any time during the formative years. Marasmus affects infants ages 6 to 18 months as a result of breast-feeding failure, or a debilitating condition such as chronic diarrhea.

In industrialized countries, PCM may occur secondary to chronic metabolic disease that decreases protein and calorie intake or absorption, or trauma that increases protein and calorie requirements.

✿ **ELDER TIP** *In the United States, PCM is estimated to occur to some extent in 50% of elderly people in nursing homes.*

Those who aren't allowed anything by mouth for an extended period are at high risk of developing PCM. Conditions that increase protein-calorie requirements include severe burns and injuries, systemic infections, and cancer (accounts for the largest group of hospitalized patients with PCM). Conditions that cause defective utilization of nutrients include malabsorption syndrome, short-bowel syndrome, and Crohn disease.

Pathophysiology

Marasmus is an insufficient energy intake to match the body's requirements. As a result, the body draws on its own stores, resulting in emaciation. In kwashiorkor, adequate carbohydrate consumption and decreased protein intake lead to decreased synthesis of visceral proteins. The resulting hypoalbuminemia contributes to extravascular fluid accumulation. Impaired synthesis of B-lipoprotein produces a fatty liver.

Protein-energy malnutrition also involves an inadequate intake of many essential nutrients.

Complications
◆ Mental and physical disabilities
◆ Coma
◆ Shock

Signs and symptoms
Children with chronic PCM are small for their chronological age and tend to be physically inactive, mentally apathetic, and susceptible to frequent infections. Anorexia and diarrhea are common.

In acute PCM, children are small, gaunt, and emaciated, with no adipose tissue. Skin is dry and "baggy," and hair is sparse and dull brown or reddish-yellow. Temperature is low; pulse rate and respirations are slowed. Such children are weak, irritable, and usually hungry, although they may have anorexia, with nausea and vomiting.

Unlike marasmus, chronic kwashiorkor allows the patient to grow in height, but adipose tissue diminishes as fat metabolizes to meet energy demands. Edema often masks severe muscle wasting; dry, peeling skin and hepatomegaly are common. Patients with secondary PCM show signs similar to marasmus, primarily loss of adipose tissue and lean body mass, lethargy, and edema. Severe secondary PCM may cause loss of immunocompetence.

Diagnosis
CONFIRMING DIAGNOSIS *Clinical appearance, dietary history, and anthropometry confirm PCM. If the patient doesn't suffer from fluid retention, weight change over time is the best index of nutritional status.*

The following factors support the diagnosis:
◆ height and weight less than 80% of standard for the patient's age and sex, and below-normal arm circumference and triceps skinfold
◆ serum albumin level less than 2.8 g/dL (normal: 3.3 to 4.3 g/dL)
◆ urinary creatinine (24-hour) level used to show lean body mass status by relating creatinine excretion to height and ideal body weight, to yield CHI.

Treatment
The aim of treatment is to provide sufficient proteins, calories, and other nutrients for nutritional rehabilitation and maintenance. When treating severe PCM, restoring fluid and electrolyte balance parentally is the initial concern. Nutrition provision should not be increased until laboratory values, such as electrolyte level, stabilize. A patient who shows normal absorption may receive enteral nutrition after anorexia has subsided. When possible, the preferred treatment is oral feeding. Foods are introduced slowly due to the risk of refeeding syndrome. Carbohydrates are given first to supply energy, and then high-quality protein foods, especially milk, and protein-calorie supplements are given. A patient who's unwilling or unable to eat may require supplementary feedings through a nasogastric (NG) tube or total parenteral nutrition (TPN), which is given through a central venous catheter because of its higher osmolality. Peripheral parenteral nutrition, which has a lower osmolality than TPN and can be given through a peripheral I.V. line, is an alternative to TPN, but it's given less commonly. Accompanying infection must also be treated, preferably with antibiotics that don't inhibit protein synthesis. Cautious realimentation is essential to prevent complications from overloading the compromised metabolic system.

Special considerations
◆ Encourage the patient with PCM to consume as much nutritious food and beverage as possible. (It's often helpful to "cheer the patient on" as he or she eats.) Assist the patient with eating if necessary. Cooperate closely with the dietitian to monitor intake, and provide acceptable meals and snacks.
◆ If TPN is necessary, observe strict sterile technique when handling catheters, tubes, and solutions and during dressing changes.

!!!!!! PREVENTION
◆ *Watch for PCM in patients who have been hospitalized for a prolonged period, have had no oral intake for several days, or have cachectic disease.*
◆ *To help eradicate PCM in developing countries, encourage prolonged breast-feeding, educate mothers about their children's needs, and provide supplementary foods, as needed.*

ELDER TIP *If the older patient is anorexic, consider asking family members and other visitors to bring in special foods from home that may improve the patient's appetite. In addition, encouraging the family to collaborate on feeding a dependent patient can help promote recovery, enhance feelings of well-being, and stimulate the patient to eat more.*

Metabolic disorders

GALACTOSEMIA

Galactosemia is any disorder of galactose metabolism. It produces symptoms ranging from cataracts and liver damage to mental retardation and occurs in two forms: classic galactosemia and galactokinase deficiency galactosemia. Although a galactose-free diet relieves most symptoms, galactosemia-induced mental impairment is irreversible; some residual vision impairment may also persist.

Causes and incidence

Both forms of galactosemia are inherited as autosomal recessive defects and occur in about 1 in 60,000 births in the United States. Up to 1.25% of the population is heterozygous for the classic galactosemia gene. Classic galactosemia results from a defect in the enzyme galactose-1-phosphate uridyl transferase. (See *Metabolic pathway in galactosemia*.) Galactokinase deficiency galactosemia, the rarer form of this disorder, stems from a deficiency of the enzyme galactokinase. In both forms of galactosemia, the inability to normally metabolize the sugar galactose (which is mainly formed by digestion of the disaccharide lactose that's present in milk) causes galactose accumulation.

Pathophysiology

An elevated blood galactose concentration is the result of altered metabolism of galactose due to a genetic deficiency in enzyme activity or secondary hypergalactosemia due to liver disease (congenital hepatitis, patent ductus venosus, congenital hepatic arteriovenous malformation).

Complications

- ◆ Ovarian dysfunction
- ◆ Cataracts
- ◆ Abnormal speech
- ◆ Cognitive impairment
- ◆ Motor delay
- ◆ Growth retardation

Signs and symptoms

In children who are homozygous for the classic galactosemia gene, signs are evident at birth or begin within a few days after milk ingestion, and include failure to thrive, vomiting, and diarrhea. Other clinical effects include liver damage (which causes jaundice, hepatomegaly, cirrhosis, and ascites), splenomegaly, galactosuria, proteinuria, and aminoaciduria. Cataracts may also be present at birth or develop later. Pseudotumor cerebri may occur.

Metabolic pathway in galactosemia

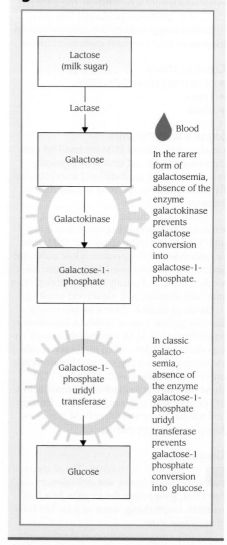

In the rarer form of galactosemia, absence of the enzyme galactokinase prevents galactose conversion into galactose-1-phosphate.

In classic galactosemia, absence of the enzyme galactose-1-phosphate uridyl transferase prevents galactose-1 phosphate conversion into glucose.

Continued ingestion of galactose- or lactose-containing foods may cause mental retardation, malnourishment, progressive hepatic failure, and death—from the still-unknown process of galactose metabolites accumulating in body tissues. Although treatment may prevent mental impairment, galactosemia can produce a short attention span, difficulty with spatial and mathematical relationships, and apathetic, withdrawn behavior. Cataracts may be the only sign of galactokinase deficiency, resulting from the accumulation of galactitol, a metabolic by-product of galactose, in the lens.

Diagnosis

℞ **CONFIRMING DIAGNOSIS** *Deficiency of the enzyme galactose-1-phosphate uridyl transferase in RBCs confirms classic galactosemia; decreased RBC levels of galactokinase confirm galactokinase deficiency. Prenatal diagnosis may be made by direct measurement of galactose-1-phosphate uridyl transferase.*

Related laboratory results include increased galactose levels in blood (normal value in children is <20 mg/dL) and urine (must use galactose oxidase to avoid confusion with other reducing sugars). Galactose measurements in blood and urine must be interpreted carefully because some children who consume large amounts of milk have elevated plasma galactose concentrations and galactosuria but aren't galactosemic. Also, neonates excrete galactose in their urine for about a week after birth; premature infants, even longer.

Other test results include:
◆ liver biopsy—typical acinar formation
◆ liver enzymes (aspartate aminotransferase, alanine aminotransferase levels)—elevated
◆ urinalysis—albumin in urine
◆ ophthalmoscopy—punctate lesions in the fetal lens nucleus (with treatment, cataracts regress)
◆ amniocentesis—prenatal diagnosis of galactosemia (recommended for heterozygous and homozygous parents)

Treatment

Elimination of galactose and lactose from the diet causes most effects to subside. The infant is fed soy formula, meat-base formula, protein hydrolysate formula, or another lactose-free formula. The infant gains weight; liver anomalies, nausea, vomiting, galactosemia, proteinuria, and aminoaciduria disappear; and cataracts regress. As the child grows, a balanced, galactose-free diet must be maintained. Hormone replacement is sometimes necessary for puberty. A pregnant woman who's heterozygous or homozygous for galactosemia should also follow a galactose-restricted diet. Such a diet supports normal growth and development and may delay symptoms in the neonate.

Special considerations

◆ To eliminate galactose and lactose from an infant's diet, replace cow's milk formula or breast milk with a meat-base or soybean formula.
◆ Teach the parents about dietary restrictions and stress the importance of compliance.

Diet for galactosemia

A patient with galactosemia must follow a lactose-free diet. It's important for the patient to carefully read food labels to avoid milk and milk products, including dry milk products. The patient may eat these foods:
◆ fish and animal products (except brains and mussels)
◆ fresh fruits and vegetables (except peas and lima beans)
◆ only bread and rolls made from cracked wheat.
  He should avoid these foods:
◆ dairy products
◆ puddings, cookies, cakes, pies
◆ food coloring
◆ instant potatoes
◆ canned and frozen foods (if lactose is listed as an ingredient)

(See *Diet for galactosemia.*) Warn them to read medication labels carefully and avoid giving any medication that contains lactose fillers.
◆ If the child has a learning disability, help parents secure educational assistance. Refer parents who want to have other children for genetic counseling. In some states, screening of all neonates for galactosemia is required by law.
◆ Instruct the parents to contact support groups, such as Parents of Galactosemic Children, for further information and support if appropriate.

GLYCOGEN STORAGE DISEASES

Glycogen storage diseases consist of at least eight distinct errors of metabolism, all inherited, that alter the synthesis or degradation of glycogen, the form in which glucose is stored in the body. Normally, muscle and liver cells store glycogen. Muscle glycogen is used in muscle contraction; liver glycogen can be converted into free glucose, which can then diffuse out of the liver cells to increase blood glucose levels. Glycogen storage diseases manifest as dysfunctions of the liver, heart, or musculoskeletal system. Symptoms vary from mild and easily controlled hypoglycemia to severe organ involvement that may lead to heart failure and respiratory failure.

Causes and incidence

Almost all glycogen storage diseases (types I through V and type VII) are transmitted as autosomal recessive traits. The transmission mode of type VI is unknown; type VIII may be an X-linked trait.

Pathophysiology

The most common glycogen storage disease is type I—von Gierke, or hepatorenal glycogen storage disease—which results from a deficiency of the liver enzyme glucose-6-phosphatase. This enzyme converts glucose-6-phosphate into free glucose and is necessary for the release of stored glycogen and glucose into the bloodstream, to relieve hypoglycemia. Infants may die of acidosis before age 2; if they survive past this age, with proper treatment, they may grow normally and live to adulthood, with only minimal hepatomegaly. However, there's a danger of adenomatous liver nodules, which may be premalignant.

Complications

◆ Heat intolerance
◆ Easy bruising
◆ Slowed growth
◆ Incomplete sexual development
◆ Hepatic adenomas
◆ Multiple organ failure

Signs and symptoms

Primary clinical features of the liver glycogen storage diseases (types I, III, IV, VI, and VIII) are hepatomegaly and rapid onset of hypoglycemia and ketosis when food is withheld. Symptoms of the muscle glycogen storage diseases (types II, V, and VII) include poor muscle tone; type II may result in death from heart failure. (See *Rare forms of glycogen storage disease*, pages 508 and 509.)

Rare forms of glycogen storage disease

Type	Clinical features	Diagnostic test results
II (Pompe)		
Absence of alpha-1,4-glucosidase (acid maltase)	◆ *Infants:* cardiomegaly, profound hypotonia and, occasionally, endocardial fibroelastosis (usually fatal before age 1 due to cardiac or respiratory failure) ◆ *Some infants and young children:* muscle weakness and wasting, variable organ involvement (slower progression, usually fatal by age 19) ◆ *Adults:* muscle weakness without organomegaly (slowly progressive but not fatal)	◆ *Muscle biopsy:* increased concentration of glycogen with normal structure; alpha-1,4-glucosidase deficiency ◆ *Electrocardiogram (in infants):* large QRS complexes in all leads; inverted T waves; shortened PR interval ◆ *Electromyography (in adults):* muscle fiber irritability; myotonic discharges ◆ *Amniocentesis:* alpha-1,4-glucosidase deficiency ◆ *Placenta or umbilical cord examination:* alpha-1,4-glucosidase deficiency
III (Cori)		
Absence of debranching enzyme (amylo-1,6-glucosidase) (*Note:* predominant cause of glycogen storage disease in Israel)	◆ *Young children:* massive hepatomegaly, which may disappear by puberty; growth retardation; moderate splenomegaly; hypoglycemia ◆ *Adults:* progressive myopathy ◆ Occasionally, moderate cardiomegaly, cirrhosis, muscle wasting, hypoglycemia	◆ *Liver biopsy:* deficient debranching activity; increased glycogen concentration ◆ *Laboratory tests (in children only):* elevated aspartate aminotransferase or alanine aminotransferase levels; increased erythrocyte glycogen levels
IV (Andersen)		
Deficiency of branching enzyme (amylo-1,4-1,6-transglucosidase) (*Note:* extremely rare)	◆ *Infants:* hepatosplenomegaly, ascites, muscle hypotonia; usually fatal before age 2 from progressive cirrhosis	◆ *Liver biopsy:* deficient branching enzyme activity; glycogen molecule has longer outer branches

Rare forms of glycogen storage disease (*continued*)

Type	Clinical features	Diagnostic test results
V (McArdle)		
Deficiency of muscle phosphorylase	◆ *Children:* mild or no symptoms ◆ *Adults:* muscle cramps and pain during strenuous exercise, possibly resulting in myoglobinuria and renal failure ◆ *Older patients:* significant muscle weakness and wasting	◆ *Serum lactate:* no increase in venous levels in sample drawn from extremity after ischemic exercise ◆ *Muscle biopsy:* lack of phosphorylase activity; increased glycogen content
VI (Hers)		
Possible deficiency of hepatic phosphorylase	Mild symptoms (similar to those of type I), requiring no treatment	*Liver biopsy:* decreased phosphorylase b activity, increased glycogen concentration
VII (Tarui)		
Deficiency of muscle phosphofructokinase	◆ Muscle cramps during strenuous exercise, resulting in myoglobinuria and possible renal failure ◆ Reticulocytosis	◆ *Serum lactate:* no increase in venous levels in sample drawn from extremity after ischemic exercise ◆ *Muscle biopsy:* deficient phosphofructokinase; marked rise in glycogen concentration ◆ *Blood studies:* low erythrocyte phosphofructokinase activity; reduced half-life of red blood cells
VIII		
Deficiency of hepatic phosphorylase kinase	◆ Mild hepatomegaly ◆ Mild hypoglycemia	◆ *Liver biopsy:* deficient phosphorylase b kinase activity; increased glycogen concentration ◆ *Blood study:* deficient phosphorylase b kinase in leukocytes

In addition, type I may produce these symptoms:
◆ infants—acidosis, hyperlipidemia, GI bleeding, coma
◆ children—low resistance to infection and, without proper treatment, short stature
◆ adolescents—gouty arthritis and nephropathy; chronic tophaceous gout; bleeding (especially epistaxis); small superficial vessels visible in skin due to impaired platelet function; fat deposits in cheeks, buttocks, and subcutaneous tissues; poor muscle tone; enlarged kidneys; xanthomas over extensor surfaces of arms and legs; steatorrhea; multiple, bilateral, yellow lesions in fundi; and osteoporosis, probably secondary to negative calcium balance. Correct treatment of glycogen storage disease should prevent all of these effects.

Diagnosis

CONFIRMING DIAGNOSIS *Liver biopsy confirms the diagnosis by showing normal glycogen synthetase and phosphorylase enzyme activities but reduced or absent glucose-6-phosphatase activity. Glycogen structure is normal but amounts are elevated. Spectroscopy may be used to show abnormal muscle metabolism with the use of magnetic resonance imaging in specialized centers.*

◆ Laboratory studies of plasma demonstrate low glucose levels but high levels of free fatty acids, triglycerides, cholesterol, and uric acid. Serum analysis reveals high pyruvic acid levels and high lactic acid levels. Prenatal diagnoses are available for types II, III, and IV.
◆ Injection of glucagon or epinephrine increases pyruvic and lactic acid levels but doesn't increase blood glucose levels. Glucose tolerance test curve typically shows depletional

hypoglycemia and reduced insulin output. Intrauterine diagnosis is possible.

Treatment

For type I, treatment aims to maintain glucose homeostasis and prevent secondary consequences of hypoglycemia through frequent feedings and constant nocturnal enteral feeding with Polycose or Vivonex. Treatment includes a low-fat diet, with normal amounts of protein and calories; carbohydrates should contain glucose or glucose polymers only. Physically modified cornstarch is also used to prevent hypoglycemia.

Therapy for type III includes frequent feedings (every 3 to 4 hours) and a high-protein diet. Type IV requires a high-protein, high-calorie diet; bed rest; diuretics; sodium restriction; and paracentesis, if necessary, to relieve ascites. Ultimately treat with liver transplant. Types V and VII require no treatment except avoidance of strenuous exercise. No treatment is necessary for types VI and VIII; no effective treatment exists for type II.

Special considerations

When managing type I disease:
◆ Advise the patient or parents to include carbohydrate foods containing mainly starch in the diet and to sweeten foods with glucose only.
◆ Before discharge, teach the patient or family member how to use the enteral feeding equipment, monitor blood glucose levels with glucose reagent strips, and recognize symptoms of hypoglycemia.
◆ Watch for and report signs of infection (fever, chills, myalgia) and of hepatic encephalopathy (mental confusion, stupor, asterixis, coma) due to increased blood ammonia levels.

When managing other types, do the following.
◆ *Type II:* Explain test procedures, such as electromyography and electroencephalography (EEG), thoroughly.
◆ *Type III:* Instruct the patient to eat a high-protein diet (eggs, nuts, fish, meat, poultry, and cheese).
◆ *Type IV:* Watch for signs of hepatic failure (nausea, vomiting, irregular bowel function, clay-colored stools, right upper quadrant pain, jaundice, dehydration, electrolyte imbalance, edema, and changes in mental status, progressing to coma).

When caring for patients with types II, III, and IV glycogen storage disease, offer the patient and parents reassurance and emotional support. Recommend and arrange for genetic counseling, if appropriate.

◆ *Types V through VIII:* Care for these patients is minimal. Explain the disorder to the patient and his/her family, and help them accept the limitations imposed by the patient's particular type of glycogen storage disease.

HYPOGLYCEMIA

Hypoglycemia is an abnormally low glucose level in the bloodstream. It occurs when glucose burns up too rapidly, when the glucose release rate falls behind tissue demands, or when excessive insulin enters the bloodstream. Hypoglycemia is classified as reactive or fasting. *Reactive hypoglycemia* results from the reaction to the disposition of meals or the administration of excessive insulin. *Fasting hypoglycemia* causes discomfort during long periods of abstinence from food, for example, in the early morning before breakfast. Although hypoglycemia is a specific endocrine imbalance, its symptoms are often vague and depend on how quickly the patient's glucose levels drop. If not corrected, severe hypoglycemia may result in coma and irreversible brain damage.

Causes and incidence

Reactive hypoglycemia may take several forms. In a diabetic patient, it may result from administration of too much insulin or too much oral antidiabetic medication. In a mildly diabetic patient (or one in the early stages of diabetes mellitus), reactive hypoglycemia may result from delayed and excessive insulin production after carbohydrate ingestion. Similarly, a nondiabetic patient may develop reactive hypoglycemia from a sharp increase in insulin output after a meal. Sometimes called *postprandial hypoglycemia,* this type of reactive hypoglycemia usually disappears when the patient eats something sweet. In some patients, reactive hypoglycemia has no known cause (idiopathic reactive) or may result from gastric dumping syndrome and from impaired glucose tolerance.

Hypoglycemia is at least as common in neonates and children as it is in adults and affects 1 out of 1,000 people. Usually, infants develop hypoglycemia because of an increased number of cells per unit of body weight and because of increased demands on stored liver glycogen to support respirations, thermoregulation, and muscular activity. In full-term neonates, hypoglycemia may occur 24 to 72 hours after birth and is usually transient. In neonates who are premature or small for gestational age, the onset of hypoglycemia is much more rapid (it can occur as soon as 6 hours after birth) because of their small, immature livers, which produce much less glycogen. Maternal disorders that can produce hypoglycemia in neonates within 24 hours after birth include diabetes mellitus, toxemia, erythroblastosis, and glycogen storage disease.

Pathophysiology

Fasting hypoglycemia usually results from an excess of insulin or insulin-like substance or from a decrease in counterregulatory hormones. It can be *exogenous*, resulting from external factors such as alcohol or drug ingestion, or *endogenous*, resulting from organic problems.

Endogenous hypoglycemia may result from tumors or liver disease. Insulinomas, small islet cell tumors in the pancreas, secrete excessive amounts of insulin, which inhibit hepatic glucose production. They're generally benign (in 90% of patients). Extrapancreatic tumors, though uncommon, can also cause hypoglycemia by increasing glucose utilization and inhibiting glucose output. Such tumors occur primarily in the mesenchyma, liver, adrenal cortex, GI system, and lymphatic system. They may be benign or malignant. Among nonendocrine causes of fasting hypoglycemia are severe liver diseases, including hepatitis, cancer, cirrhosis, and liver congestion associated with heart failure. All of these conditions reduce the uptake and release of glycogen from the liver. Some endocrine causes include adrenocortical insufficiency, which contributes to hypoglycemia by reducing the production of cortisol and cortisone needed for gluconeogenesis; and pituitary insufficiency, which reduces corticotropin and growth hormone levels.

Complication

◆ Permanent brain damage

Signs and symptoms

Signs and symptoms of reactive hypoglycemia include fatigue, malaise, nervousness, irritability, trembling, tension, headache, hunger, cold sweats, and rapid heart rate. These same clinical effects usually characterize fasting hypoglycemia. In addition, fasting hypoglycemia may also cause CNS disturbances; for example, blurry or double vision, confusion, motor weakness, hemiplegia, seizures, or coma.

In infants and children, signs and symptoms of hypoglycemia are vague. A neonate's refusal to feed may be the primary clue to underlying hypoglycemia. Associated CNS effects include tremors, twitching, weak or high-pitched cry, sweating, limpness, seizures, and coma.

Diagnosis

A blood glucose monitor or glucose reagent strips provide quick screening methods for determining the blood glucose level. A reading less than 50 mg/dL indicates the need for a venous blood sample. (See *Diagnosing hypoglycemia,* page 512.)

 CONFIRMING DIAGNOSIS *Laboratory testing confirms the diagnosis by showing decreased blood glucose levels. The following values indicate hypoglycemia:*
◆ *Full-term infants*
  ◆ less than 30 mg/dL before feeding
  ◆ less than 40 mg/dL after feeding
◆ *Preterm infants*
  ◆ less than 20 mg/dL before feeding
  ◆ less than 30 mg/dL after feeding
◆ *Children and adults*
  ◆ less than 40 mg/dL before meal
  ◆ less than 50 mg/dL after meal

In addition, a 5-hour glucose tolerance test may be administered to provoke reactive hypoglycemia. Following a 12-hour fast, laboratory testing to detect plasma insulin and plasma glucose levels may identify fasting hypoglycemia.

Treatment

Effective treatment of reactive hypoglycemia requires dietary modification to help delay glucose absorption and gastric emptying. Usually this includes small, frequent meals; ingestion of complex carbohydrates, fiber, and fat; and avoidance of simple sugars, alcohol, and fruit drinks. The patient may also receive anticholinergic drugs to slow gastric emptying and intestinal motility and to inhibit vagal stimulation of insulin release.

For fasting hypoglycemia, surgery and drug therapy are usually required. In patients with insulinoma, tumor removal is the treatment of choice. Drug therapy may include nondiuretic thiazides such as diazoxide to inhibit insulin secretion; streptozocin; and hormones, such as glucocorticoids and long-acting glycogen.

Therapy for neonates who have hypoglycemia or who are at risk of developing it includes preventive measures. A hypertonic solution of 10% dextrose, calculated at 5 to 10 mL/kg of body weight administered I.V. over 10 minutes and followed by 4 to 8 mg/kg/minute for maintenance, should correct a severe hypoglycemic state in neonates. To reduce the chance of hypoglycemia in high-risk neonates, they should receive feedings (either breast milk or a solution of 5% to 10% glucose and water) as soon after birth as possible.

Diagnosing hypoglycemia

This flowchart lists possible diagnostic findings and interpretations to assist with treatment of the patient with hypoglycemia.

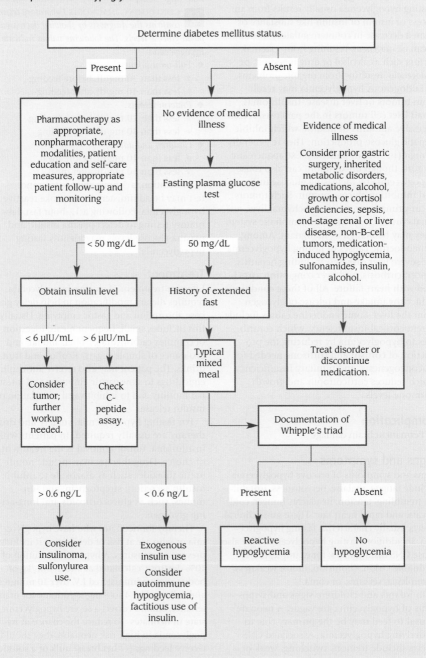

Determine diabetes mellitus status.

Present → Pharmacotherapy as appropriate, nonpharmacotherapy modalities, patient education and self-care measures, appropriate patient follow-up and monitoring

Absent
- No evidence of medical illness
  - Fasting plasma glucose test
    - < 50 mg/dL → Obtain insulin level
      - < 6 µIU/mL → Consider tumor; further workup needed.
      - > 6 µIU/mL → Check C-peptide assay.
        - > 0.6 ng/L → Consider insulinoma, sulfonylurea use.
        - < 0.6 ng/L → Exogenous insulin use. Consider autoimmune hypoglycemia, factitious use of insulin.
    - 50 mg/dL → History of extended fast
      - Typical mixed meal
        - Documentation of Whipple's triad
          - Present → Reactive hypoglycemia
          - Absent → No hypoglycemia
- Evidence of medical illness

  Consider prior gastric surgery, inherited metabolic disorders, medications, alcohol, growth or cortisol deficiencies, sepsis, end-stage renal or liver disease, non-B-cell tumors, medication-induced hypoglycemia, sulfonamides, insulin, alcohol.
  - Treat disorder or discontinue medication.

Special considerations

◆ Watch for and report signs of hypoglycemia, such as poor feeding, in high-risk neonates.

◆ Monitor infusion of hypertonic glucose in the neonate to avoid hyperglycemia, circulatory overload, and cellular dehydration. Terminate glucose solutions gradually to prevent hypoglycemia caused by hyperinsulinemia.

◆ Explain the purpose and procedure for any diagnostic tests. Collect blood samples at the appropriate times, as ordered.

◆ Monitor the effects of drug therapy and watch for the development of any adverse effects.

◆ Teach the patient or family which foods to include in the diet (complex carbohydrates, fiber, fat) and which foods to avoid (simple sugars, alcohol). Refer the patient and family for dietary counseling as appropriate.

HEREDITARY FRUCTOSE INTOLERANCE

Hereditary fructose intolerance is an inability to metabolize fructose. After fructose is eliminated from the diet, symptoms subside within weeks. Older children and adults with hereditary fructose intolerance have normal intelligence and apparently normal liver and kidney function.

Causes and incidence

Transmitted as an autosomal recessive trait, hereditary fructose intolerance results from a deficiency in the enzyme fructose-1-phosphate aldolase. The enzyme operates at only 1% to 10% of its normal biological activity, thus preventing rapid uptake of fructose by the liver after ingestion of fruit or foods containing cane sugar.

In some European countries, hereditary fructose intolerance may have an incidence as high as 1 in 20,000 people.

Pathophysiology

Affected individuals are completely asymptomatic until they ingest fructose. Thus, homozygous neonates remain clinically well until confronted with dietary sources of fructose. Although lactose is the carbohydrate base in most infant formulas, some (e.g., soy formulas) contain sucrose, a fructose-glucose disaccharide that may cause symptoms. The biochemistry of hereditary fructose intolerance is complex for two reasons: (1) Three isozymes of aldolase (A, B, C) exist, of which aldolase B is expressed exclusively in the liver, kidney, and intestine; and (2) aldolase B mediates three separate reactions (i.e., cleavage of fructose 1-phosphate [F-1-P]; cleavage of fructose 1,6-diphosphate; and

condensation of the triose phosphates, glyceraldehyde phosphate, and dihydroxyacetone phosphate to form fructose 1,6-diphosphate).

In normal cellular conditions, the primary enzymatic activity of aldolase B is to cleave fructose diphosphate, which forms rather than condenses the triose phosphate compounds. Here, the enzyme is central to the glycolytic pathway. Because the reaction is reversible, aldolase B is an essential enzyme in the process of gluconeogenesis (which is, in some respects, a reversal of glycolysis). The absence of the latter function readily explains the clinical hypoglycemia in individuals with hereditary fructose intolerance.

Reduced cleavage of F-1-P leads to its cellular accumulation and fructokinase inhibition, causing free fructose accumulation in the blood. A generally accepted consequence of this sequence is a dramatic change in the ATP-adenosine monophosphate cellular ratio, with a resultant acceleration in production of uric acid. This accounts for the hyperuricemia observed during an acute episode. Competition between urate and lactate for renal tubule excretion accounts for the lactic acidemia.

The cause of severe hepatic dysfunction remains unknown but may be a manifestation of focal cytoplasmic degeneration and cellular fructose toxicity. The cause of renal tubular dysfunction also remains unclear; patients with renal tubular dysfunction primarily present with a proximal tubular acidosis complicated by aminoaciduria, glucosuria, and phosphaturia. Thus, in an infant who is homozygous for fructose 1-aldolase deficiency, fructose ingestion triggers a cascade of biochemical events that result in severe clinical disease.

Complications

◆ Kidney dysfunction
◆ Liver dysfunction
◆ Infants—failure to thrive

Signs and symptoms

Typically, clinical features of hereditary fructose intolerance appear shortly after dietary introduction of foods containing fructose or sucrose. Symptoms are more severe in infants than in older people and include hypoglycemia, nausea, vomiting, pallor, excessive sweating, cyanosis, and tremor. In neonates and young children, continuous ingestion of foods containing fructose may result in failure to thrive, hypoglycemia, jaundice, hyperbilirubinemia, ascites, hepatomegaly, vomiting, dehydration, hypophosphatemia, albuminuria, aminoaciduria, seizures, coma, febrile episodes, substernal pain, and anemia.

Diagnosis

A dietary history often suggests hereditary fructose intolerance.

📴 CONFIRMING DIAGNOSIS *A fructose tolerance test (using glucose oxidase or paper chromatography to measure glucose levels) usually confirms the diagnosis. However, liver biopsy showing a deficiency in fructose-1-phosphate aldolase may be necessary for a definitive diagnosis.*

Supportive values may include decreased serum inorganic phosphorus levels. Urine studies may show fructosuria and albuminuria.

Treatment

Treatment of hereditary fructose intolerance consists of exclusion of fructose and sucrose (cane sugar or table sugar) from the diet. Otherwise, treatment is supportive as the patient's progress is monitored.

Special considerations

◆ Tell the patient to avoid fruits containing fructose and vegetables containing sucrose (sugar beets, sweet potatoes, and peas), because sucrose is digested to glucose and fructose in the intestine. Fruits containing the least amount of fructose include strawberries, blackberries, blueberries, oranges, and grapefruits; others low in fructose are cherries, pears, bananas, grapes, and apples.

◆ Refer the patient and family for genetic and dietary counseling as appropriate.

HYPERLIPOPROTEINEMIA

Hyperlipoproteinemia occurs as five distinct metabolic disorders, all of which may be inherited.

Causes and incidence

This disorder affects lipid transport in serum and produces varied clinical changes, from relatively mild symptoms that can be corrected by dietary management to potentially fatal pancreatitis.

Pathophysiology

Types I and III are transmitted as autosomal recessive traits; types II, IV, and V are transmitted as autosomal dominant traits. (See *Types of hyperlipoproteinemia,* page 515.) About one in five persons with elevated plasma lipid and lipoprotein levels has hyperlipoproteinemia. It's marked by increased plasma concentrations of one or more lipoproteins. Hyperlipoproteinemia may also occur secondary to other conditions, such as diabetes, pancreatitis, hypothyroidism, or renal disease.

Complications

◆ Coronary artery disease
◆ Pancreatitis

Signs and symptoms

◆ *Type I:* recurrent attacks of severe abdominal pain similar to pancreatitis, usually preceded by fat intake; abdominal spasm, rigidity, or rebound tenderness; hepatosplenomegaly, with liver or spleen tenderness; papular or eruptive xanthomas (pinkish-yellow cutaneous deposits of fat) over pressure points and extensor surfaces; lipemia retinalis (reddish-white retinal vessels); malaise; anorexia; and fever
◆ *Type II:* tendinous xanthomas (firm masses) on the Achilles tendons and tendons of the hands and feet, tuberous xanthomas, xanthelasma, juvenile corneal arcus (opaque ring surrounding the corneal periphery), accelerated atherosclerosis and premature coronary artery disease, and recurrent polyarthritis and tenosynovitis
◆ *Type III:* peripheral vascular disease manifested by claudication or tuboeruptive xanthomas (soft, inflamed, pedunculated lesions) over the elbows and knees; palmar xanthomas on the hands, particularly the fingertips; premature atherosclerosis
◆ *Type IV:* predisposition to atherosclerosis and early coronary artery disease, exacerbated by excessive calorie intake, obesity, diabetes, and hypertension
◆ *Type V:* abdominal pain (most common), pancreatitis, peripheral neuropathy, eruptive xanthomas on extensor surfaces of the arms and legs, lipemia retinalis, and hepatosplenomegaly

Treatment

The first goal is to identify and treat any underlying problem such as diabetes. If no underlying problem exists, the primary treatment of types II, III, and IV is dietary management, especially restriction of cholesterol intake, possibly supplemented by drug therapy (cholestyramine, fenofibrate, gemfibrozil, atorvastatin, niacin) to lower plasma triglyceride or cholesterol level when diet alone is ineffective.

Type I hyperlipoproteinemia requires long-term weight reduction, with fat intake restricted to less than 20 g/day. A 20- to 40-g/day medium-chain triglyceride diet may be ordered to supplement calorie intake. The patient should also avoid alcoholic beverages, to decrease plasma triglyceride levels. The prognosis is good with treatment; without treatment, death can result from pancreatitis.

For type II, dietary management to restore normal lipid levels and decrease the risk of

Types of hyperlipoproteinemia

Type	Causes and incidence	Diagnostic findings
I		
(Frederickson's hyperlipo-proteinemia, fat-induced hyperlipemia, idiopathic familial)	◆ Deficient or abnormal lipoprotein lipase, result-ing in decreased or absent post-heparin lipolytic activity ◆ Relatively rare ◆ Present at birth	◆ Chylomicrons (very-low-density lipoprotein [VLDL], low-density lipoprotein [LDL], high-density lipopro-tein), in plasma 14 hours or more after last meal ◆ Highly elevated serum chylomicrons and triglycer-ide levels; slightly elevated serum cholesterol levels ◆ Lower serum lipoprotein lipase levels ◆ Leukocytosis
II		
(familial hyperbetalipopro-teinemia, essential familial hypercholesterolemia)	◆ Deficient cell surface receptor that regulates LDL degradation and choles-terol synthesis, resulting in increased levels of plasma LDL over joints and pres-sure points ◆ Onset between ages 10 and 30	◆ Increased plasma concen-trations of LDL ◆ Increased serum LDL and cholesterol levels ◆ Amniocentesis shows in-creased LDL levels
III		
(familial broad-beta disease, dysbetalipopro-teinemia, remnant re-moval disease, xanthoma tuberosum)	◆ Unknown underlying defect results in deficient conversion of triglycer-ide-rich VLDL to LDL ◆ Uncommon; usually oc-curs after age 20 but can occur earlier in men	◆ Abnormal serum betalipoprotein ◆ Elevated cholesterol and triglyceride levels ◆ Slightly elevated glucose tolerance ◆ Hyperuricemia
IV		
(endogenous hy-pertriglyceridemia, hyperbetalipoproteinemia)	◆ Usually occurs secondary to obesity, alcoholism, diabetes, or emotional disorders ◆ Relatively common, es-pecially in middle-age men	Elevated VLDL levels ◆ Abnormal levels of triglycerides in plasma; variable increase in serum ◆ Normal or slightly elevated serum cholesterol levels ◆ Mildly abnormal glucose tolerance ◆ Family history ◆ Early coronary artery disease
V		
(mixed hypertri-glyceridemia, mixed hyperlipidemia)	◆ Defective triglyceride clearance causes pancre-atitis; usually secondary to another disorder, such as obesity or nephrosis ◆ Uncommon; onset usu-ally occurs in late adoles-cence or early adulthood	◆ Chylomicrons in plasma ◆ Elevated plasma VLDL levels ◆ Elevated serum choles-terol and triglyceride levels

atherosclerosis includes restriction of cholesterol intake to less than 300 mg/day for adults and less than 150 mg/day for children; triglycerides must be restricted to less than 100 mg/day for children and adults. Diet should also be high in polyunsaturated fats. In familial hypercholesterolemia, nicotinic acid with a bile acid usually normalizes low-density lipoprotein (LDL) levels. For severely affected children, a portacaval shunt is a last resort to reduce plasma cholesterol levels. The prognosis remains poor regardless of treatment; in homozygotes, myocardial infarction usually causes death before age 30.

For type III, dietary management includes restriction of cholesterol intake to less than 300 mg/day; carbohydrates must also be restricted, while polyunsaturated fats are increased. Statins, fibrates, estrogens (in women) and niacin help lower blood lipid levels. Weight reduction is helpful. With strict adherence to prescribed diet, the prognosis is good.

For type IV, weight reduction may normalize blood lipid levels without additional treatment. Long-term dietary management includes restricted cholesterol intake, increased polyunsaturated fats, and avoidance of alcoholic beverages. Fenofibrate, gemfibrozil, and niacin may lower plasma lipid levels. The prognosis remains uncertain, however, because of predisposition to premature coronary artery disease.

The most effective treatment for type V is weight reduction and long-term maintenance of a low-fat diet. Alcoholic beverages must be avoided. Niacin, fenofibrate, gemfibrozil, and a 20- to 40-g/day medium-chain triglyceride diet may prove helpful. The prognosis is uncertain

because of the risk of pancreatitis. Increased fat intake may cause recurrent bouts of illness, possibly leading to pseudocyst formation, hemorrhage, and death.

Special considerations
Nursing care for hyperlipoproteinemia emphasizes careful monitoring for adverse drug effects and teaching the importance of long-term dietary management.

◆ Administer cholestyramine before meals or before bedtime. This drug must not be given with other medications. (See *Using bile acid sequestrants*.) Watch for adverse effects, such as nausea, vomiting, constipation, steatorrhea, rashes, and hyperchloremic acidosis. Also watch for malabsorption of other medications and fat-soluble vitamins.

⚠ **ALERT** *Don't administer niacin to patients with active peptic ulcers or hepatic disease. Use with caution in patients with diabetes. In other patients, watch for adverse effects, such as flushing, pruritus, hyperpigmentation, and exacerbation of inactive peptic ulcers.*

◆ Urge the patient to adhere to the ordered diet (usually 1,000 to 1,500 calories/day) and to avoid excess sugar and alcoholic beverages, to minimize the intake of saturated fats (higher in meats, coconut oil), and to increase the intake of polyunsaturated fats (vegetable oils).

◆ Instruct the patient, for the 2 weeks preceding serum cholesterol and serum triglyceride tests, to maintain a steady weight and to adhere strictly to the prescribed diet. The patient should also fast for 12 hours preceding the test.

GAUCHER DISEASE
Gaucher disease, the most common lysosomal storage disease, causes an abnormal accumulation of glucocerebrosides in reticuloendothelial cells. It occurs in three forms: type I (adult); type II (infantile); and type III (juvenile). Type II can prove fatal within 9 months of onset, usually from pulmonary involvement.

Causes and incidence
The three forms of Gaucher disease are classified by age of onset and the presence or absence of neurologic involvement. Type I, characterized by lack of neurologic involvement, is the most common form affecting both children and adults and is most prevalent in the Ashkenazi Jewish population, affecting anywhere from 1 of 500 to 1,000 births. Type II usually presents in infancy with severe neurologic involvement, resulting in seizures and CNS damage. Type II

Using bile acid sequestrants

Before giving the patient a bile acid sequestrant, such as cholestyramine, to lower cholesterol levels, make certain the patient isn't taking a drug whose absorption is affected by bile acid sequestrants. For example, bile acid sequestrants decrease the absorption of diuretics such as chlorothiazide. Other drugs affected besides diuretics include:
◆ beta-adrenergic blockers
◆ digitoxin
◆ fat-soluble vitamins
◆ folic acid
◆ thiazides
◆ thyroxine
◆ warfarin

also presents with spleen and bone marrow damage. Type III typically has mild neurologic involvement and runs a slower, more favorable course. The incidence of types II and III is 1 of 50,000 to 100,000 births. The juvenile form can begin in childhood, typically in the teenage years, and causes spleen, bone marrow, and neurologic damage.

Pathophysiology

Gaucher disease results from an autosomal recessive inheritance, which causes decreased activity of the enzyme glucocerebrosidase. Glucocerebrosidase deficiency leads to an accumulation of glucosylceramide in the storage compartments (lysosomes) of certain body cells. Glucosylceramide buildup occurs in the liver, spleen, bones, and bone marrow, eventually leading to decreased production of RBCs (anemia) and thinning of the bones (osteopenia).

Complications

◆ Neurologic impairment
◆ Portal hypertension
◆ Pathologic fractures
◆ Anemia
◆ Respiratory failure (type II)

Signs and symptoms

The key signs of all types of Gaucher disease are hepatosplenomegaly and bone lesions. In type I, bone lesions lead to thinning of cortices, pathologic fractures, collapsed hip joints and, eventually, vertebral compression. Severe episodic pain may develop in the legs, arms, and back but usually not until adolescence. (The adult form of Gaucher disease is generally diagnosed while the patient is in their teens; the word "adult" is used loosely here.) Other clinical effects of type I are fever, abdominal distention (from hypotonicity of the large bowel), respiratory problems (pneumonia or, rarely, cor pulmonale), easy bruising and bleeding, anemia and, rarely, pancytopenia. Older patients may develop a yellow pallor and brown-yellow pigmentation on the face and legs.

In type II, motor dysfunction and spasticity occur at age 6 to 7 months. Other signs of the infantile form of Gaucher disease include abdominal distention, strabismus, muscle hypertonicity, retroflexion of the head, neck rigidity, dysphagia, laryngeal stridor, hyperreflexia, seizures, respiratory distress, and easy bruising and bleeding.

Clinical effects of type III after infancy include seizures, hypertonicity, strabismus, poor coordination and mental ability and, possibly, easy bruising and bleeding.

Diagnosis

℞ CONFIRMING DIAGNOSIS *Bone marrow aspiration showing Gaucher cells and direct assay of glucocerebrosidase activity, which can be performed on venous blood, confirms this diagnosis.*

Supportive laboratory results include increased serum acid phosphatase level, decreased platelets and serum iron level and, in type III, abnormal EEG after infancy.

Treatment

Treatment is mainly supportive and consists of vitamins, supplemental iron or liver extract to prevent anemia caused by iron deficiency and to alleviate other hematologic problems, blood transfusions for anemia, splenectomy for thrombocytopenia, and strong analgesics for bone pain. Injections of a replacement synthetic enzyme have proven helpful. Imiglucerase, a recombinant form of acid beta-glucosidase has been used to treat symptomatic Gaucher disease. The FDA has recently approved velaglucerase alfa for injection to treat children and adults as a long-term enzyme replacement therapy for type I Gaucher disease. Patients receiving imiglucerase can safely be switched to velaglucerase alfa.

Special considerations

◆ In the patient confined to bed, prevent pathologic fractures by turning the patient carefully. If the patient is ambulatory, make sure that he's assisted when getting out of bed or walking.
◆ Observe closely for changes in pulmonary status.
◆ Explain all diagnostic tests and procedures to the patient or parents. Help the patient accept the limitations imposed by this disorder.
◆ Recommend genetic counseling for patients with a family history of Gaucher disease. Prenatal testing can determine if a fetus has the syndrome.

PORPHYRIAS

Classification of porphyrias depends on the site of excessive porphyrin production; they may be erythropoietic (erythroid cells in bone marrow), hepatic (in the liver), or erythrohepatic (in bone marrow and liver). (See *Types of porphyria*, pages 518 and 519.) An acute episode of intermittent hepatic porphyria may cause fatal respiratory paralysis. In the other forms of porphyrias, the prognosis is good with proper treatment.

Causes and incidence

Porphyrias are inherited as autosomal dominant traits, except for Günther disease (autosomal recessive trait) and toxic-acquired

Types of porphyria

Porphyria	Signs and symptoms	Treatment
Erythropoietic porphyria		
Günther disease ♦ Usual onset before age 5	♦ Red urine (earliest, most characteristic sign); severe cutaneous photosensitivity, leading to vesicular or bullous eruptions on exposed areas and, eventually, scarring and ulceration ♦ Hypertrichosis ♦ Brown-stained or red-stained teeth ♦ Splenomegaly, hemolytic anemia	♦ Oral beta-carotene to prevent photosensitivity reactions ♦ Anti-inflammatory ointments ♦ Oral activated charcoal to absorb excess porphyrins ♦ Packed red cells to inhibit erythropoiesis and excreted porphyrins ♦ Heme therapy for recurrent attacks ♦ Splenectomy for hemolytic anemia ♦ Topical dihydroxyacetone and lawsone sunscreen filter
Erythrohepatic porphyria		
Protoporphyria ♦ Usually affects children ♦ Occurs most often in males	♦ Photosensitive dermatitis ♦ Hemolytic anemia ♦ Chronic hepatic disease	♦ Avoidance of causative factors ♦ Beta-carotene to reduce photosensitivity
Toxic-acquired porphyria ♦ Usually affects children ♦ Significant mortality	♦ Acute colicky pain ♦ Anorexia, nausea, vomiting ♦ Neuromuscular weakness ♦ Behavioral changes ♦ Seizures, coma	♦ Chlorpromazine I.V. to relieve pain and GI symptoms ♦ Avoidance of lead exposure
Hepatic porphyria		
Acute intermittent porphyria ♦ Most common form ♦ Affects females most often, usually between ages 15 and 40	♦ Colicky abdominal pain with fever, general malaise, and hypertension ♦ Peripheral neuritis, behavioral changes, possibly leading to frank psychosis ♦ Possible respiratory paralysis	♦ Chlorpromazine I.V. to relieve abdominal pain and control psychic abnormalities ♦ Avoidance of barbiturates, sulfonamides, infections, alcohol, and fasting ♦ Heme therapy for recurrent attacks ♦ High-carbohydrate diet
Variegate porphyria ♦ Usual onset between ages 30 and 50 ♦ Occurs almost exclusively among South African whites ♦ Affects males and females equally	♦ Skin lesions, extremely fragile skin in exposed areas ♦ Hypertrichosis ♦ Hyperpigmentation ♦ Abdominal pain during acute attack ♦ Neuropsychiatric manifestations	♦ Avoidance of sunlight, or wearing protective clothing when avoidance isn't possible ♦ Heme therapy for recurrent attacks

Types of porphyria (continued)

Porphyria	Signs and symptoms	Treatment
Porphyria cutanea tarda ◆ Most frequent in men ages 40 to 60 ◆ Highest incidence in South Africans	◆ Facial pigmentation ◆ Red-brown urine ◆ Photosensitive dermatitis ◆ Hypertrichosis	◆ Avoidance of precipitating factors, such as alcohol and estrogens ◆ Phlebotomy at 2-week intervals to lower serum iron level
Hepatic porphyria		
Hereditary coproporphyria ◆ Rare ◆ Affects males and females equally	◆ Asymptomatic or mild neurologic, abdominal, or psychiatric symptoms	◆ High-carbohydrate diet ◆ Avoidance of barbiturates ◆ Heme therapy for recurrent attacks

porphyria (usually from ingestion of or exposure to lead). Menstruation often precipitates acute porphyria in premenopausal women. (See *Preventing porphyria*.)

Pathophysiology

Porphyrias are inborn errors of metabolism that affect the biosynthesis of heme (a component of hemoglobin) and cause excessive production and excretion of porphyrins or their precursors. Porphyrins, which are present in all protoplasm, figure prominently in energy storage and utilization.

Complications

◆ Neurologic and hepatic dysfunction (hepatic)
◆ Cholelithiasis
◆ Coma
◆ Flaccid paralysis, respiratory paralysis, and death (acute intermittent)
◆ Hemolytic anemia (erythropoietic)

Signs and symptoms

Porphyrias are generally marked by photosensitivity, acute abdominal pain, and neuropathy. Hepatic porphyrias may produce a complex syndrome marked by distinct neurologic and hepatic dysfunction:
◆ Neurologic symptoms include chronic brain syndrome, peripheral neuropathy and autonomic effects, tachycardia, labile hypertension, severe colicky lower abdominal pain, and constipation.
◆ During an acute attack, fever, leukocytosis, and fluid and electrolyte imbalance may occur.
◆ Structural hepatic effects include fatty infiltration of the liver, hepatic sclerosis, and focal hepatocellular necrosis.
◆ Skin lesions may cause itching and burning, erythema, and altered pigmentation and edema in areas exposed to light. Some chronic skin changes include milia (white papules on the hands' dorsal aspects) and hirsutism on the upper cheeks and periorbital areas.

PREVENTION

Preventing porphyria

Precipitating factors may lead to signs and symptoms of porphyria. Encourage the patient to avoid:
◆ crash dieting
◆ fasting
◆ specific drugs, including alcohol, barbiturates, and estrogens
◆ stress
◆ infection

Helpful hints
◆ Stress management techniques may help because emotional stress may also precipitate an attack.
◆ Reduce infection risk with proper handwashing and avoiding people with known infection.
◆ Genetic counseling may also be of benefit to prospective parents with a family history of porphyria.

Diagnosis

℞ **CONFIRMING DIAGNOSIS** *Generally, diagnosis requires screening tests for porphyrins or their precursors (such as aminolevulinic acid [ALA] and porphobilinogen [PBG]) in urine, stool, blood or, occasionally, skin biopsy. A urinary lead level of 0.2 mg/L confirms toxic-acquired porphyria.*

Other laboratory values may include increased serum iron levels in porphyria cutanea tarda; leukocytosis, syndrome of inappropriate antidiuretic hormone (SIADH), and elevated bilirubin and alkaline phosphatase levels in acute intermittent porphyria.

Treatment

Treatment for porphyrias includes avoiding overexposure to the sun and using beta-carotene to reduce photosensitivity, as well as support for acute and long-term management. Heme therapy (panhematin) is given to control recurrent attacks of acute intermittent porphyria, Günther disease, variegate porphyria, and hereditary coproporphyria. A high-carbohydrate diet decreases urinary excretion of ALA and PBG, with restricted fluid intake to inhibit release of antidiuretic hormone (ADH).

Special considerations

♦ Warn the patient to avoid excessive sun exposure, use a sunscreen when outdoors, and take a beta-carotene supplement to reduce photosensitivity.
♦ Encourage a high-carbohydrate diet.
♦ Administer beta-carotene and hemin, as ordered.
♦ Advise the patient to avoid drugs that may precipitate signs and symptoms of porphyrias. (See *Drugs that aggravate porphyria*.)

METABOLIC SYNDROME

Metabolic syndrome—also called *syndrome X, insulin resistance syndrome, dysmetabolic syndrome,* and *obesity syndrome*—is a cluster of conditions characterized by abdominal obesity, high blood glucose (type 2 diabetes mellitus), insulin resistance, high blood cholesterol and triglycerides, low levels of high-density lipoprotein (HDL); and high blood pressure. More than 22% of people in the United States meet three or more of these criteria, raising their risk of heart disease and stroke and placing them at high risk for dying of myocardial infarction.

Causes and incidence

Abdominal obesity is a strong predictor of metabolic syndrome because abdominal fat tends to be more resistant to insulin than fat in other areas. This increases the release of free fatty acids into the portal system, leading to increased apolipoprotein B, increased LDL, decreased HDL, and increased triglyceride levels. As a result, the risk of cardiovascular disease is increased.

Type 2 diabetes mellitus is a risk factor because a hallmark for metabolic syndrome is a fasting glucose level greater than 100 mg/dL. People with diabetes develop atherosclerotic heart disease at a younger age than other people. They're also at increased risk of macrovascular disease (ischemic heart disease, stroke, and peripheral vascular disease). Diabetes is a coronary artery disease risk equivalent.

Insulin resistance and dyslipidemia are also risk factors because insulin resistance leads to hyperinsulinemia, hyperglycemia, abnormal glucose and lipid metabolism, damaged endothelium, and cardiovascular disease. Insulin is also responsible for reducing the amount of free fatty acids in the liver. However, people with insulin resistance have an increased amount of free fatty acids reaching the liver, resulting in high triglycerides and LDLs and producing an abnormal endothelium and atherosclerosis.

High blood pressure is a risk factor because the combination of insulin resistance, hyperinsulinemia, and abdominal obesity leads to

---

Drugs that aggravate porphyria

Make sure the patient with porphyria doesn't receive any of the following drugs, which are known to precipitate signs and symptoms of porphyria:
♦ Alcohol
♦ Barbiturates
♦ Carbamazepine
♦ Carisoprodol
♦ Chloramphenicol
♦ Chlordiazepoxide
♦ Diazepam
♦ Ergot alkaloids
♦ Estrogens
♦ Griseofulvin
♦ Imipramine
♦ Meprobamate
♦ Methsuximide
♦ Methyldopa
♦ Pentazocine
♦ Phenytoin
♦ Progesterones
♦ Sulfonamides
♦ Tolbutamide

hypertension and its harmful cardiovascular effects. Moreover, insulin resistance promotes salt sensitivity in people with high blood pressure.

Women who have a history of polycystic ovarian syndrome are also at increased risk for developing metabolic syndrome.

Research also indicates that there may be a genetic predisposition to metabolic syndrome.

Pathophysiology

In the normal digestion process, the intestines break down food into its basic components, one of which is glucose. Glucose provides energy for cellular activity, while excess glucose is stored in cells for future use. Insulin, a hormone secreted in the pancreas, guides glucose into storage cells. However, in people with metabolic syndrome, glucose is insulin-resistant and doesn't respond to insulin's attempt to guide it into storage cells. Excess insulin is then required to overcome this resistance. This excess in quantity and force of insulin causes damage to the lining of the arteries, promotes fat storage deposits, and prevents fat breakdown. This series of events can lead to diabetes, blood clots, and coronary events.

Complications

◆ Coronary artery disease
◆ Diabetes mellitus
◆ Hyperlipidemia

Signs and symptoms

Assessment commonly reveals a history of hypertension, abdominal obesity, sedentary lifestyle, poor diet, and a family history of metabolic syndrome. Physical findings include abdominal obesity (evidenced by a waist of more than 40″ [101.6 cm] in men and 35″ [88.9 cm] in women), blood pressure 130/85 mm Hg or higher, and a fasting blood glucose level that's 100 mg/dL or higher. The patient may feel tired, especially after eating, and may have difficulty losing weight. If left untreated, such complications as coronary artery disease, diabetes, hyperlipidemia, and premature death may develop.

Diagnosis

Blood studies commonly indicate elevated blood glucose levels, hyperinsulinemia, and elevated serum uric acid. Lipid profile studies reveal elevated LDL levels, low HDL levels, and elevated triglycerides. Further diagnostic procedures are nonspecific, but may be performed to detect hypertension, diabetes, hyperlipidemia, and hyperinsulinemia.

Treatment

Lifestyle modification, focusing on weight reduction and exercise, is an important part of the treatment regimen. Modest weight reduction through diet and exercise considerably improves hemoglobin A_{1c} levels, reduces insulin resistance, improves blood lipid levels, and decreases blood pressure—all elements of metabolic syndrome. Recent studies have shown that in patients with impaired glucose tolerance, losing an average of 7% of body weight reduced the risk of developing type 2 diabetes by 58%. A long-term target goal for BMI should aim for less than 25 kg/m^2.

To improve cardiovascular health, a diet rich in vegetables, fruits, whole grains, fish, and low-fat dairy products combined with regular exercise is recommended. Moreover, nutrient-dense, low-energy foods should replace low-nutrient, high-calorie foods. A healthy diet should also be low in saturated fat, trans fat, cholesterol, and sodium. (See *Therapeutic lifestyle-change diet*, page 522.)

A regular exercise program of moderate physical activity, in addition to dietary modifications, promotes weight loss, improves insulin sensitivity, and reduces blood glucose levels. According to the Surgeon General's Report on Physical Activity and Health, a person should exercise moderately for a minimum of 30 minutes on most (if not all) days of the week. The selected exercise program should improve cardiovascular conditioning, increase strength through resistance training, and improve flexibility.

Medications may be used in the treatment of metabolic syndrome for patients who have a BMI of 27 kg/m^2 or greater in the presence of other risk factors (such as diabetes, hypertension, and hyperlipidemia) or for patients with a BMI of 30 kg/m^2 or greater without other risk factors. Weight-loss drugs may also be added to lifestyle changes if the patient hasn't achieved significant weight loss after 12 weeks.

Pharmacologic treatment may also be indicated. Phentermine is used for short-term treatment of obesity in conjunction with diet and exercise.

Surgical treatment of obesity, such as through gastric bypass procedures, produces a greater degree and duration of weight loss than other therapies and improves or resolves most of the factors of metabolic syndrome. Candidates for surgical intervention include patients with a BMI greater than 40 kg/m^2 or those with a BMI greater than 35 kg/m^2 with obesity-related medical conditions. Gastric bypass procedures produce permanent weight loss in the majority of patients.

Special considerations

◆ Monitor the patient's blood pressure, blood glucose, blood cholesterol, and insulin levels.
◆ Because research indicates that longer lifestyle modification programs are associated with improved weight-loss maintenance, encourage patients with metabolic syndrome to begin an exercise and weight-loss program with a friend or family member. Assist the patient in exploring options and support their efforts.

Therapeutic lifestyle-change diet

The therapeutic lifestyle-change diet is low in saturated fats and cholesterol to reduce blood cholesterol levels and prevent development of heart disease and its complications.

Nutrient	Recommended intake
Saturated fat*	<7% of total calories
Polyunsaturated fat	Up to 10% of total calories
Monounsaturated fat	Up to 20% of total calories
Total fat	25% to 35% of total calories
Carbohydrate**	50% to 60% of total calories
Fiber	20 to 30 g/day
Protein	~15% of total calories
Cholesterol < 200 mg/day	Sodium ≤2,400 mg/day
Total calories***	Balance energy intake and expenditure to maintain desirable body weight and prevent weight gain

* Trans fatty acids are another low-density lipoprotein–raising fat that should be minimized or avoided.
** Carbohydrates should be derived predominantly from foods rich in complex carbohydrates, including grains—especially whole grains, fruits, and vegetables.
*** Daily expenditure should include at least moderate physical activity (contributing about 200 kcal/day).

Source: From National Heart, Lung, and Blood Institute; National Institutes of Health; U.S. Department of Health and Human Services.

◆ To improve compliance, schedule frequent follow-up appointments with the patient. At that time, review food diaries and exercise logs. Be positive and promote active participation and partnership in the treatment plan.
◆ A patient planning gastric bypass surgery should receive psychological and nutritional counseling before and after the surgery to assist with diet and lifestyle changes.

Homeostatic imbalance
POTASSIUM IMBALANCE

Potassium, a cation that's the dominant cellular electrolyte, facilitates contraction of both skeletal and smooth muscles—including myocardial contraction—and figures prominently in nerve impulse conduction, acid–base balance, enzyme action, and cell membrane function. Because serum potassium level has such a narrow range (3.5 to 5 mEq/L), a slight deviation in either direction can produce profound clinical consequences.

Causes and incidence

Because many foods contain potassium, hypokalemia seldom results from a dietary deficiency. Instead, potassium loss may result from:
◆ excessive GI losses, such as diarrhea, dehydration, anorexia, or chronic laxative abuse (Vomiting and gastric suction cause dehydration, resulting in hyperaldosteronism [sodium retention and potassium excretion occur].)
◆ trauma (injury, burns, or surgery), in which damaged cells release potassium, which enters serum or ECF, to be excreted in the urine
◆ chronic renal disease, with tubular potassium wasting
◆ certain drugs, especially potassium-wasting diuretics, steroids, and certain sodium-containing antibiotics (carbenicillin)
◆ acid–base imbalances, which cause potassium shifting into cells without true depletion in alkalosis
◆ prolonged potassium-free I.V. therapy
◆ hyperglycemia, causing osmotic diuresis and glycosuria
◆ Cushing syndrome, primary hyperaldosteronism, excessive licorice ingestion, and severe serum magnesium deficiency
◆ refeeding syndrome

Hyperkalemia results from the kidneys' inability to excrete excessive amounts of potassium infused I.V. or administered orally; from decreased urine output, renal dysfunction, or renal failure; or the use of potassium-sparing diuretics, such as triamterene, by patients with renal disease. It may also result from

Clinical effects of potassium imbalance

Dysfunction	Hypokalemia	Hyperkalemia
Acid–base balance	◆ Metabolic alkalosis	◆ Metabolic acidosis
Cardiovascular	◆ Dizziness, hypotension, arrhythmias, electrocardiogram (ECG) changes (flattened T waves, elevated U waves, depressed ST segment), cardiac arrest (with serum potassium levels <2.5 mEq/L)	◆ Tachycardia and later bradycardia, ECG changes (tented and elevated T waves, widened QRS complex, prolonged PR interval, flattened or absent P waves, depressed ST segment), cardiac arrest (with levels >7 mEq/L)
Gastrointestinal	◆ Nausea, vomiting, anorexia, diarrhea, abdominal distention, paralytic ileus, or decreased peristalsis	◆ Nausea, diarrhea, abdominal cramps
Genitourinary	◆ Polyuria	◆ Oliguria, anuria
Musculoskeletal	◆ Muscle weakness and fatigue, leg cramps	◆ Muscle weakness, flaccid paralysis
Neurologic	◆ Malaise, irritability, confusion, mental depression, speech changes, decreased reflexes, respiratory paralysis	◆ Hyperreflexia progressing to weakness, numbness, tingling, flaccid paralysis

any injuries or conditions that release cellular potassium or favor its retention, such as burns, crushing injuries, failing renal function, adrenal gland insufficiency, dehydration, or diabetic acidosis.

Pathophysiology
Paradoxically, both hypokalemia (potassium deficiency) and hyperkalemia (potassium excess) can lead to muscle weakness and flaccid paralysis, because both create an ionic imbalance in neuromuscular tissue excitability. Both conditions also diminish excitability and conduction rate of the heart muscle, which may lead to cardiac arrest. (See *Clinical effects of potassium imbalance.*)

Complications
◆ Muscle weakness
◆ Flaccid paralysis
◆ Cardiac arrest

Signs and symptoms
Usually symptoms of low potassium are mild, sometimes vague. These include weakness, numbness/tingling, nausea/vomiting, abdominal cramps, hypotension, palpitations, and changes in behavior.

Patients with high potassium may be asymptomatic or have mild symptoms. They may report vague symptoms, such as nausea, tingling, muscle weakness, and fatigue. Symptoms may

be more significant, such as slow and weak pulse, and cardiac standstill. Patients may not recognize symptoms until potassium is very high (>7.0 mEq/L). A slow rise is often better tolerated than a rapid rise.

Diagnosis
℞ CONFIRMING DIAGNOSIS *Serum potassium levels less than 3.5 mEq/L confirm hypokalemia; serum levels greater than 5 mEq/L confirm hyperkalemia.*

Additional tests may be necessary to determine the imbalance's underlying cause. Hypokalemia is also associated with hypomagnesemia, so further study of other electrolytes is warranted.

Treatment
For hypokalemia, replacement therapy with potassium chloride (I.V. or orally) is the primary treatment. When diuresis is necessary, spironolactone, a potassium-sparing diuretic, may be administered concurrently with a potassium-wasting diuretic to minimize potassium loss. Hypokalemia can be prevented by giving a maintenance dose of potassium I.V. to patients who may not take anything by mouth and to others predisposed to potassium loss.

For hyperkalemia, rapid infusion of 10% calcium gluconate decreases myocardial irritability and temporarily prevents cardiac arrest but doesn't correct serum potassium excess; it's also contraindicated in patients receiving cardiac glycosides. As an emergency measure, sodium bicarbonate I.V. increases pH and causes potassium to shift back into the cells. Insulin and 10% to 50% glucose I.V. also move potassium back into cells. Infusions should be followed by dextrose 5% in water because infusion of 10% to 15% glucose will stimulate endogenous insulin secretion. Sodium polystyrene sulfonate with 70% sorbitol produces exchange of sodium ions for potassium ions in the intestine. Hemodialysis or peritoneal dialysis also aids in removal of excess potassium.

Special considerations

For hypokalemia:

◆ Check serum potassium and other electrolyte levels in patients apt to develop potassium imbalance and in those requiring potassium replacement; they risk overcorrection to hyperkalemia.

◆ Assess intake and output carefully. Remember, the kidneys excrete 80% to 90% of ingested potassium. Never give supplementary potassium to a patient whose urine output is below 600 mL/day. Also, measure GI loss from suctioning or vomiting.

◆ Administer slow-release potassium or dilute oral potassium supplements in 4 oz (118 mL) or more of water or other fluid to reduce gastric and small-bowel irritation. Determine the patient's chloride level. As ordered, give a potassium chloride supplement if the level is low and potassium gluconate if it's normal.

◆ Give potassium I.V. only after it's diluted in solution (usually, 10 mEq/100 mL of fluid); potassium is very irritating to vascular, subcutaneous, and fatty tissues and may cause phlebitis or tissue necrosis if it infiltrates. Infuse slowly (no more than 20 mEq/L/hour through central administration or 10 mEq/hour through peripheral administration) to prevent hyperkalemia.

ALERT *Never administer by I.V. push or bolus; it may cause cardiac arrest.*

◆ Carefully monitor patients receiving cardiac glycosides because hypokalemia enhances the action of these drugs and may produce signs of digoxin toxicity (anorexia, nausea, vomiting, blurred vision, and arrhythmias).

◆ To prevent hypokalemia, instruct patients (especially those predisposed to hypokalemia due to long-term diuretic therapy) to include in their diet foods rich in potassium—oranges, bananas, tomatoes, milk, dried fruits, apricots, peanuts, and dark green, leafy vegetables.

ALERT *Monitor the patient's cardiac rhythm and respond to any irregularities immediately.*

For hyperkalemia:

◆ As in hypokalemia, frequently monitor serum potassium and other electrolyte levels, and carefully record intake and output.

◆ Administer sodium polystyrene sulfonate orally or rectally (by retention enema) in patients with significant potassium elevations because of intravascular sodium shifting. Watch for signs of hypokalemia with prolonged use and for clinical effects of hypoglycemia (muscle weakness, syncope, hunger, and diaphoresis) with repeated insulin and glucose treatment.

◆ Watch for signs of hyperkalemia in predisposed patients, especially those with poor urine output or those receiving potassium supplements orally or I.V. Administer no more than 10 to 20 mEq/L of potassium chloride per hour; check the I.V. infusion site for signs of phlebitis or infiltration of potassium into tissues. Also, before giving a blood transfusion, check to see how long ago the blood was donated; cell hemolysis in older blood releases potassium. Infuse only *fresh* blood for patients with average to high serum potassium levels.

◆ Watch for and report cardiac arrhythmias.

SODIUM IMBALANCE

Although the body requires only 2 to 4 g of sodium daily, most Americans consume 6 to 10 g daily (mostly sodium chloride, as table salt), excreting excess sodium through the kidneys and skin.

A low-sodium diet or excessive use of diuretics may induce hyponatremia (decreased serum sodium concentration); dehydration may induce hypernatremia (increased serum sodium concentration).

Causes and incidence

Hyponatremia can result from:

◆ excessive GI loss of water and electrolytes due to vomiting, suctioning, or diarrhea; excessive perspiration or fever; use of potent diuretics; or tap-water enemas (When such losses decrease circulating fluid volume, increased secretion of ADH promotes maximum water reabsorption, which further dilutes serum sodium. These factors are especially likely to cause hyponatremia when combined with excessive intake of free water.)

◆ excessive drinking of water, infusion of I.V. dextrose in water without other solutes, malnutrition or starvation, or a low-sodium diet, usually in combination with one of the other causes

◆ trauma, surgery (wound drainage), or burns, which cause sodium to shift into damaged cells

◆ adrenal gland insufficiency (Addison disease) or hypoaldosteronism

◆ cirrhosis of the liver with ascites

◆ SIADH, resulting from brain tumor, stroke, pulmonary disease, or neoplasm with ectopic ADH production. Certain drugs, such as chlorpropamide and clofibrate, may produce an SIADH-like syndrome

Causes of hypernatremia include:
◆ decreased water intake (When severe vomiting and diarrhea cause water loss that exceeds sodium loss, serum sodium levels rise, but overall ECF volume decreases.)
◆ excess adrenocortical hormones, as in Cushing syndrome
◆ ADH deficiency (diabetes insipidus)
◆ salt intoxication (less common), which may be produced by excessive ingestion of table salt

Pathophysiology
Sodium is the major cation (90%) in ECF; potassium, the major cation in intracellular fluid. During repolarization, the sodium–potassium pump continually shifts sodium into the cells and potassium out of the cells; during depolarization, it does the reverse. Sodium cation functions include maintaining tonicity and concentration of ECF, acid–base balance (reabsorption of sodium ion and excretion of hydrogen ion), nerve conduction and neuromuscular function, glandular secretion, and water balance.

Complications
◆ Seizures
◆ Coma
◆ Permanent neurologic damage

Signs and symptoms
Sodium imbalance has profound physiologic effects and can induce severe CNS, cardiovascular, and GI abnormalities. For example, hyponatremia may cause renal dysfunction or, if serum sodium loss is abrupt or severe, seizures; hypernatremia may produce pulmonary edema, circulatory disorders, and decreased level of consciousness. (See *Clinical effects of sodium imbalance.*)

Diagnosis
Hyponatremia is defined as a serum sodium level less than 135 mEq/L; hypernatremia, as a serum sodium level greater than 145 mEq/L. However, additional laboratory studies are necessary to determine etiology and to differentiate between a true deficit and an apparent deficit due to sodium shift or to hypervolemia or hypovolemia. In true hyponatremia, supportive values include urine sodium greater than 100 mEq/24 hours, with low serum osmolality; in true hypernatremia, urine sodium level is less than 40 mEq/24 hours, with high serum osmolality. (See *Diagnosing hyponatremia*, page 526.)

Treatment
Therapy for mild hyponatremia usually consists of restricted free water intake when it's due to hemodilution, SIADH, or such conditions as heart failure, cirrhosis of the liver, and renal failure. If fluid restriction alone fails to normalize serum sodium levels, demeclocycline or lithium, which blocks ADH action in the renal tubules, can be used to promote water excretion. In extremely rare instances of severe symptomatic hyponatremia, when serum sodium levels fall below 110 mEq/L, treatment may include infusion of 3% or 5% saline solution.

Treatment with saline infusion requires careful monitoring of venous pressure to prevent

Clinical effects of sodium imbalance

Dysfunction	Hyponatremia	Hypernatremia
Cardiovascular	◆ Hypotension; tachycardia; with severe deficit, vasomotor collapse, thready pulse	◆ Hypertension, tachycardia, pitting edema, excessive weight gain
Cutaneous	◆ Cold, clammy skin; decreased skin turgor	◆ Flushed skin; dry, sticky mucous membranes
Gastrointestinal	◆ Nausea, vomiting, abdominal cramps	◆ Rough, dry tongue; intense thirst
Genitourinary	◆ Oliguria or anuria	◆ Oliguria
Neurologic	◆ Anxiety, headaches, muscle twitching and weakness, confusion, seizures	◆ Fever, agitation, restlessness, seizures
Respiratory	◆ Cyanosis with severe deficiency	◆ Dyspnea, respiratory arrest, and death (from dramatic rise in osmotic pressure)

Diagnosing hyponatremia

This flowchart lists possible diagnostic findings and interpretations to assist in treating a patient with hyponatremia.

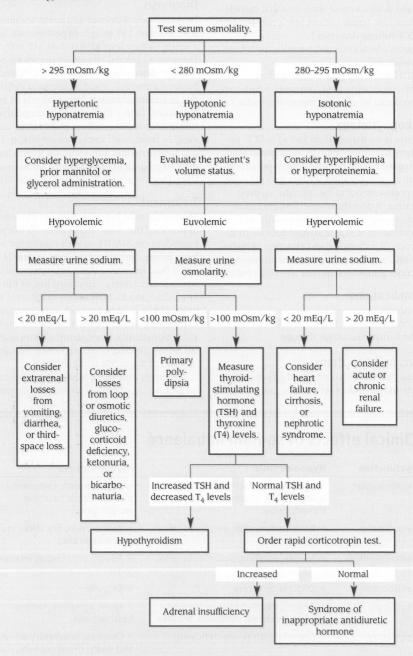

potentially fatal circulatory overload. The aim of treatment of secondary hyponatremia is to correct the underlying disorder.

Primary treatment of hypernatremia is administration of salt-free solutions (such as dextrose in water) to return serum sodium levels to normal, followed by infusion of half-normal saline solution to prevent hyponatremia. Other measures include a sodium-restricted diet and discontinuation of drugs that promote sodium retention.

Special considerations

When managing the patient with hyponatremia:
◆ Watch for and report extremely low serum sodium and accompanying serum chloride levels. Monitor urine specific gravity and other laboratory results. Record fluid intake and output accurately, and weigh the patient daily.
◆ During administration of iso-osmolar or hyperosmolar saline solution, watch closely for signs of hypervolemia (dyspnea, crackles, engorged jugular or hand veins). Report conditions that may cause excessive sodium loss (diaphoresis or prolonged diarrhea or vomiting, and severe burns).
◆ Refer the patient on maintenance dosage of diuretics to a dietitian for instruction about dietary sodium intake.

▦▦▦▦ PREVENTION *To prevent hyponatremia, administer iso-osmolar solutions.*

When managing the patient with hypernatremia:
◆ Measure serum sodium levels at least every 6 hours until stabilized. Monitor vital signs for changes, especially for rising pulse rate. Watch for signs of hypervolemia, especially in the patient receiving I.V. fluids.
◆ Record fluid intake and output accurately, checking for body fluid loss. Weigh the patient daily.
◆ Obtain a drug history to check for drugs that promote sodium retention.
◆ Explain the importance of sodium restriction and teach the patient how to plan a low-sodium diet. Closely monitor the serum sodium levels of high-risk patients.

CALCIUM IMBALANCE

Calcium plays an indispensable role in cell permeability, bone and teeth formation, blood coagulation, transmission of nerve impulses, and normal muscle contraction. Nearly all (99%) of the body's calcium is found in the bones. The remaining 1% exists in the blood, with 50% of the remainder bound to plasma proteins and 40% ionized or free.

Causes and incidence

Common causes of hypocalcemia include:
◆ inadequate intake of calcium and vitamin D, in which inadequate levels of vitamin D inhibit intestinal absorption of calcium
◆ hypoparathyroidism as a result of injury, disease, or surgery that decreases or eliminates secretion of PTH, which is needed for calcium absorption and normal serum calcium levels
◆ malabsorption or loss of calcium from the GI tract, caused by increased intestinal motility from severe diarrhea or laxative abuse; can also

Clinical effects of calcium imbalance

Dysfunction	Hypocalcemia	Hypercalcemia
Cardiovascular	◆ Arrhythmias, hypotension	◆ Signs of heart block, cardiac arrest in systole, hypertension
Gastrointestinal	◆ Increased GI motility, diarrhea	◆ Anorexia, nausea, vomiting, constipation, dehydration, polydipsia
Musculoskeletal	◆ Paresthesia (tingling and numbness of the fingers), tetany or painful tonic muscle spasms, facial spasms, abdominal cramps, muscle cramps, spasmodic contractions	◆ Weakness, muscle flaccidity, bone pain, osteoporosis, pathologic fractures
Neurologic	◆ Anxiety, irritability, twitching around mouth, laryngospasm, seizures, Chvostek sign, Trousseau sign	◆ Drowsiness, lethargy, headaches, depression or apathy, irritability, confusion
Other	◆ Blood-clotting abnormalities	◆ Renal polyuria, flank pain and, eventually, azotemia

result from inadequate levels of vitamin D or PTH, or a reduction in gastric acidity, decreasing the solubility of calcium salts

◆ severe infections or burns, in which diseased and burned tissue traps calcium from the ECF

◆ overcorrection of acidosis, resulting in alkalosis, which causes decreased ionized calcium and induces symptoms of hypocalcemia

◆ pancreatic insufficiency, which may cause malabsorption of calcium and subsequent calcium loss in feces. In pancreatitis, participation of calcium ions in saponification contributes to calcium loss

◆ renal failure, resulting in excessive excretion of calcium secondary to increased retention of phosphate

◆ hypomagnesemia, which causes decreased PTH secretion and blocks the peripheral action of that hormone

Causes of hypercalcemia include the following:

◆ hyperparathyroidism, which increases serum calcium levels by promoting calcium absorption from the intestine, resorption from bone, and reabsorption from the kidneys

◆ hypervitaminosis D, which can promote increased absorption of calcium from the intestine

◆ tumors, which raise serum calcium levels by destroying bone or by releasing PTH or a PTH-like substance, osteoclast-activating factor, prostaglandins and, perhaps, a vitamin D-like sterol

◆ multiple fractures and prolonged immobilization, which release bone calcium and raise the serum calcium level

◆ multiple myeloma, which promotes loss of calcium from bone

Other causes include milk-alkali syndrome, sarcoidosis, hyperthyroidism, adrenal insufficiency, thiazide diuretics, and loss of serum albumin secondary to renal disease.

Complications

◆ Laryngeal spasm, tetany, seizures and, possibly, respiratory arrest (hypocalcemia)

◆ Coma and cardiac arrest (hypercalcemia)

Pathophysiology

The ionized calcium in the serum is critical to healthy neurologic function. The parathyroid glands regulate ionized calcium and determine its resorption into bone, absorption from the GI mucosa, and excretion in urine and feces. Severe calcium imbalance requires emergency treatment because a deficiency (hypocalcemia) can lead to tetany and seizures; an excess (hypercalcemia), to cardiac arrhythmias and coma. (See *Clinical effects of calcium imbalance*, page 527.)

Complications

◆ Laryngeal spasm, tetany, seizures and, possibly, respiratory arrest (hypocalcemia)

◆ Coma and cardiac arrest (hypercalcemia)

Signs and symptoms

Calcium deficit causes nerve fiber irritability and repetitive muscle spasms. Consequently, characteristic symptoms of hypocalcemia include perioral paresthesia, twitching, carpopedal spasm, tetany, seizures and, possibly, cardiac arrhythmias. Chvostek sign and Trousseau sign are reliable indicators of hypocalcemia. (See *Trousseau sign*. Also see *Chvostek sign*, page 529.)

Clinical effects of hypercalcemia include muscle weakness, decreased muscle tone, lethargy, anorexia, constipation, nausea, vomiting, dehydration, polydipsia, and polyuria. Severe hypercalcemia (serum levels that exceed 15 mg/dL) may produce cardiac arrhythmias and, eventually, coma.

Diagnosis

℞ CONFIRMING DIAGNOSIS *A serum calcium level less than 8.5 mg/dL confirms hypocalcemia; a level more than 10.5 mg/dL confirms*

Trousseau sign

To check for Trousseau sign, apply a blood pressure cuff to the patient's arm. A carpopedal spasm that causes thumb adduction and phalangeal extension, as shown, confirms tetany.

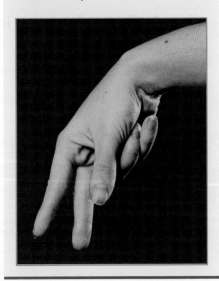

Chvostek sign

To check for Chvostek sign, tap the facial nerve above the mandibular angle, adjacent to the earlobe. A facial muscle spasm that causes the patient's upper lip to twitch, as shown, confirms tetany.

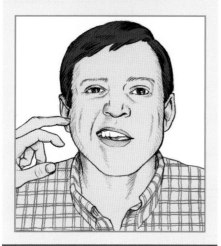

hypercalcemia. (However, because approximately one-half of serum calcium is bound to albumin, changes in serum protein must be considered when interpreting serum calcium levels. A common conversion formula is calcium corrected = calcium actual + 0.8 × [4.0 − albumin level]. Ionized calcium levels are 4.65 to 5.28 mg/dL and are a measure of the fraction of serum calcium in ionized form.)

The Sulkowitch urine test shows increased calcium precipitation in hypercalcemia. In hypocalcemia, an electrocardiogram (ECG) reveals lengthened QT interval, prolonged ST segment, and arrhythmias; in hypercalcemia, shortened QT interval and heart block. (See *Diagnosing hypercalcemia*, pages 530 and 531.)

Treatment

Treatment varies and requires correction of the acute imbalance, followed by maintenance therapy and correction of the underlying cause. Mild hypocalcemia may require nothing more than an adjustment in diet to allow adequate intake of calcium, vitamin D, and protein, possibly with oral calcium supplements. Acute hypocalcemia is an emergency that needs immediate correction by I.V. administration of calcium gluconate or calcium chloride. Chronic hypocalcemia also requires vitamin D supplements to facilitate GI absorption

of calcium. To correct mild deficiency states, the amounts of vitamin D in most multivitamin preparations are adequate. For severe deficiency, vitamin D is used in four forms: ergocalciferol (vitamin D$_2$), cholecalciferol (vitamin D$_3$), calcitriol, and dihydrotachysterol, a synthetic form of vitamin D$_2$.

Treatment of hypercalcemia primarily eliminates excess serum calcium through hydration with normal saline solution, which promotes calcium excretion in the urine. Loop diuretics, such as ethacrynic acid and furosemide, also promote calcium excretion. (Thiazide diuretics are contraindicated in hypercalcemia because they inhibit calcium excretion.) Corticosteroids, such as prednisone and hydrocortisone, are helpful in treating sarcoidosis, hypervitaminosis D, and certain tumors. Plicamycin can also lower serum calcium levels and is especially effective against hypercalcemia secondary to certain tumors. Calcitonin may also be helpful in certain instances. Drugs that stop bone breakdown and reabsorption by the body, such as bisphosphonates, may be administered I.V.

Special considerations

Watch for hypocalcemia in patients receiving massive transfusions of citrated blood; in those with chronic diarrhea, severe infections, and insufficient dietary intake of calcium and protein (especially in elderly patients); and in those who are hyperventilating.

◆ Check serum calcium level every 12 to 24 hours, and report a calcium level less than 8.5 mg/dL immediately. When giving calcium supplements, frequently check the pH level because a pH lower than 7.45 inhibits calcium ionization. Check for Trousseau and Chvostek signs.

◆ Administer calcium gluconate slow I.V. in 5% dextrose in water or in normal saline solution. Don't add calcium gluconate I.V. to solutions containing bicarbonate; it will precipitate. When administering calcium solutions, watch for anorexia, nausea, and vomiting—possible signs of overcorrection to hypercalcemia. Never infuse more than 1 g/hour, except in an emergency. Use a volume-control device to ensure proper flow rate.

◆ If the patient is receiving calcium chloride, watch for abdominal discomfort.

ALERT *Don't confuse calcium chloride with calcium gluconate in administration; 1 g of calcium chloride has three times the calcium as 1 g of calcium gluconate.*

◆ Monitor the patient closely for a possible drug interaction if he's receiving cardiac glycosides with large doses of oral calcium

DIFFERENTIAL DIAGNOSIS

Diagnosing hypercalcemia

This flowchart lists possible diagnostic findings and interpretations to assist with treatment of the patient with hypercalcemia.

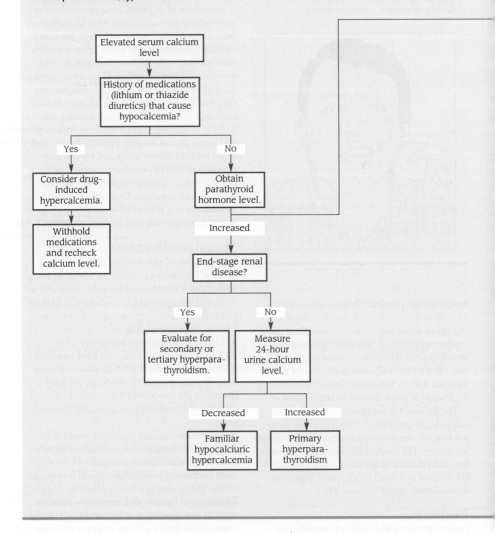

supplements; watch for signs of digoxin toxicity (anorexia, nausea, vomiting, yellow vision, and cardiac arrhythmias). Administer oral calcium supplements 1 to 1½ hours after meals or with milk.

◆ Provide a quiet, stress-free environment for the patient with tetany. Observe seizure precautions for patients with severe hypocalcemia.

⁞⁞⁞⁞⁞⁞ **PREVENTION** *To prevent hypocalcemia, advise all patients—especially elderly patients—to eat foods rich in calcium, vitamin D, and protein, such*

as fortified milk and cheese. Explain how important calcium is for normal bone formation and blood coagulation. Discourage chronic use of laxatives. Also, warn hypocalcemic patients not to overuse antacids, because these may aggravate the condition.

If the patient has hypercalcemia:
◆ Check serum calcium level frequently. Watch for cardiac arrhythmias if serum calcium levels exceed their normal values of 8.5 to 10.5 mg/dL. Increase fluid intake to dilute calcium in serum and urine, and to prevent renal damage

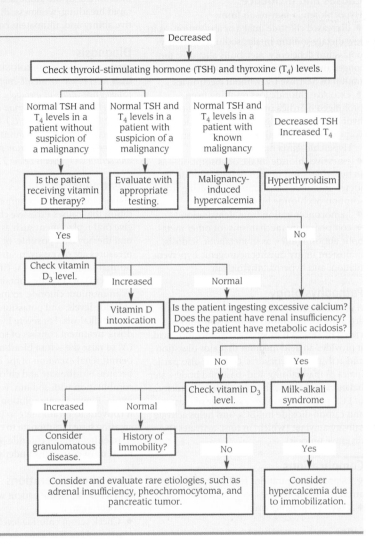

and dehydration. Watch for signs of heart failure in patients receiving normal saline diuresis.
◆ Administer loop diuretics (not thiazide diuretics), as ordered. Monitor intake and output, and check urine for renal calculi and acidity. Provide acid-ash drinks, such as cranberry or prune juice, because calcium salts are more soluble in acid than in alkali.
◆ Check ECG and vital signs frequently. In the patient receiving cardiac glycosides, watch for signs of toxicity, such as anorexia, nausea, vomiting, and bradycardia (often with arrhythmia).
◆ Ambulate the patient as soon as possible. Handle the patient with chronic hypercalcemia *gently* to prevent pathologic fractures. If the patient is bedridden, reposition the patient frequently and encourage range-of-motion exercises to promote circulation and prevent urinary stasis and calcium loss from bone.
◆ To prevent recurrence, suggest a low-calcium diet, with increased fluid intake.

CHLORIDE IMBALANCE

Hypochloremia and hyperchloremia are, respectively, conditions of deficient or excessive serum levels of the chloride anion.

Causes and incidence

Hypochloremia may result from:

◆ decreased chloride intake or absorption, as in low dietary sodium intake, sodium deficiency, potassium deficiency, metabolic alkalosis; prolonged use of mercurial diuretics; or administration of dextrose I.V. without electrolytes

◆ excessive chloride loss resulting from prolonged diarrhea or diaphoresis; loss of hydrochloric acid in gastric secretions due to vomiting, gastric suctioning, or gastric surgery.

Hyperchloremia may result from:

◆ excessive chloride intake or absorption—as in hyperingestion of ammonium chloride, or ureterointestinal anastomosis—allowing reabsorption of chloride by the bowel

◆ hemoconcentration from dehydration

◆ compensatory mechanisms for other metabolic abnormalities, as in metabolic acidosis, brainstem injury causing neurogenic hyperventilation, and hyperparathyroidism

Pathophysiology

A predominantly extracellular anion, chloride accounts for two-thirds of all serum anions. Secreted by stomach mucosa as hydrochloric acid, it provides an acid medium that aids digestion and activation of enzymes. Chloride also participates in maintaining acid–base and body water balances, influences the osmolality or tonicity of ECF, plays a role in the exchange of oxygen and carbon dioxide in RBCs, and helps activate salivary amylase (which, in turn, activates the digestive process).

Complications

◆ Depressed respirations leading to respiratory arrest (hypochloremia)

◆ Coma (hyperchloremia)

Signs and symptoms

Hypochloremia is usually associated with hyponatremia and its characteristic muscle weakness and twitching because renal chloride loss always accompanies sodium loss, and sodium reabsorption isn't possible without chloride. However, if chloride depletion results from metabolic alkalosis secondary to loss of gastric secretions, chloride is lost independently from sodium; typical symptoms are muscle hypertonicity, tetany, and shallow, depressed breathing.

Because of the natural affinity of sodium and chloride ions, hyperchloremia usually produces

clinical effects associated with hypernatremia and resulting ECF volume excess (agitation, tachycardia, hypertension, pitting edema, dyspnea). Hyperchloremia associated with metabolic acidosis is due to excretion of base bicarbonate by the kidneys, and induces deep, rapid breathing; weakness; diminished cognitive ability and, ultimately, coma.

Diagnosis

℞ **CONFIRMING DIAGNOSIS** *A serum chloride level below 97 mEq/L confirms hypochloremia. (Supportive values in metabolic alkalosis include serum pH above 7.45 and serum carbon dioxide [CO_2] level above 32 mEq/L.) A serum chloride level above 108 mEq/L confirms hyperchloremia; with metabolic acidosis, serum pH is below 7.35 and serum CO_2 level is below 22 mEq/L.*

Treatment

Hypochloremia therapy aims to correct the condition that causes excessive chloride loss and to give oral replacement such as salty broth. When oral therapy isn't possible, or when emergency measures are necessary, treatment may include normal saline solution I.V. (if hypovolemia is present) or chloride-containing drugs, such as ammonium chloride, to increase serum chloride levels, and potassium chloride for metabolic alkalosis. For severe hyperchloremic acidosis, treatment consists of sodium bicarbonate I.V. to raise the serum bicarbonate level and permit renal excretion of the chloride anion, because bicarbonate and chloride compete for combination with sodium. For mild hyperchloremia, Ringer lactate solution is administered; it converts to bicarbonate in the liver, thus increasing base bicarbonate to correct acidosis.

In either kind of chloride imbalance, treatment must correct the underlying disorder.

Special considerations

When managing the patient with hypochloremia:

◆ Check serum chloride level frequently, particularly during I.V. therapy.

◆ Watch for signs of hyperchloremia or hypochloremia. Be alert for respiratory difficulty.

◆ To prevent hypochloremia, monitor laboratory results (serum electrolyte levels and blood gas values) and fluid intake and output of patients who are vulnerable to chloride imbalance, particularly those recovering from gastric surgery. Record and report excessive or continuous loss of gastric secretions. Also report prolonged infusion of dextrose in water without saline.

When managing the patient with hyperchloremia:

◆ Check serum electrolyte levels every 3 to 6 hours. If the patient is receiving high doses of sodium bicarbonate, watch for signs of overcorrection (metabolic alkalosis, respiratory depression) or lingering signs of hyperchloremia, which indicate inadequate treatment.

▓▓▓▓ **PREVENTION** *To prevent hyperchloremia, check laboratory results for elevated serum chloride levels or potassium imbalance if the patient is receiving I.V. solutions containing sodium chloride, and monitor fluid intake and output. Also, watch for signs of metabolic acidosis. When administering I.V. fluids containing Ringer lactate solution, monitor flow rate according to the patient's age, physical condition, and bicarbonate level. Report any irregularities promptly.*

MAGNESIUM IMBALANCE

Magnesium is the second most common cation in intracellular fluid.

Because many common foods contain magnesium, a dietary deficiency is rare. Hypomagnesemia generally follows impaired absorption, too-rapid excretion, or inadequate intake during TPN. It frequently coexists with other electrolyte imbalances, especially low calcium and potassium levels. Magnesium excess (hypermagnesemia) is common in patients with renal failure and excessive intake of magnesium-containing antacids.

Causes and incidence

Hypomagnesemia usually results from impaired absorption of magnesium in the intestines or excessive excretion in urine or stool. Possible causes include:
◆ decreased magnesium intake or absorption, as in malabsorption syndrome, chronic diarrhea, or postoperative complications after bowel resection; chronic alcoholism; prolonged diuretic therapy, NG suctioning, or administration of parenteral fluids without magnesium salts; and starvation or malnutrition
◆ excessive loss of magnesium, as in severe dehydration and diabetic acidosis; hyperaldosteronism and hypoparathyroidism, which result in hypokalemia and hypocalcemia; hyperparathyroidism and hypercalcemia; excessive release of adrenocortical hormones; drugs such as cisplatin and amphotericin; and diuretic therapy
◆ refeeding syndrome

Hypermagnesemia results from the kidneys' inability to excrete magnesium that was either absorbed from the intestines or infused. Common causes of hypermagnesemia include:
◆ chronic renal insufficiency
◆ use of laxatives (magnesium sulfate, milk of magnesia, and magnesium citrate solutions), especially with renal insufficiency

◆ overuse of magnesium-containing antacids
◆ severe dehydration (resulting oliguria can cause magnesium retention)
◆ overcorrection of hypomagnesemia

Pathophysiology

Magnesium's major function is to enhance neuromuscular integration; it also stimulates PTH secretion, thus regulating intracellular fluid calcium levels. Therefore, magnesium deficiency (hypomagnesemia) may result in transient hypoparathyroidism or interference with the peripheral action of PTH. Magnesium may also regulate skeletal muscles through its influence on calcium utilization by depressing acetylcholine release at synaptic junctions. In addition, magnesium activates many enzymes for proper carbohydrate and protein metabolism, aids in cell metabolism and the transport of sodium and potassium across cell membranes, and influences sodium, potassium, calcium, and protein levels.

About one-third of magnesium taken into the body is absorbed through the small intestine and is eventually excreted in the urine; the remaining unabsorbed magnesium is excreted in the stool.

Complications
◆ Cardiac arrhythmias, hypoparathyroidism, seizures, confusion, and coma (hypomagnesemia)
◆ Complete heart block and respiratory paralysis (hypermagnesemia)

Signs and symptoms

Hypomagnesemia causes neuromuscular irritability and cardiac arrhythmias. Hypermagnesemia causes CNS and respiratory depression, in addition to neuromuscular and cardiac effects. (See *Signs and symptoms of magnesium imbalance,* page 534.)

Diagnosis

℞ **CONFIRMING DIAGNOSIS** *Serum magnesium level less than 1.5 mEq/L confirms hypomagnesemia; a level greater than 2.5 mEq/L confirms hypermagnesemia.*

Low levels of other serum electrolytes (especially potassium and calcium) often coexist with hypomagnesemia. In fact, unresponsiveness to correct treatment for hypokalemia strongly suggests hypomagnesemia. Similarly, elevated levels of other serum electrolytes are associated with hypermagnesemia.

Treatment

Therapy for magnesium imbalance aims to identify and correct the underlying cause.

Treatment of mild hypomagnesemia consists of daily magnesium supplements I.M. or orally;

Signs and symptoms of magnesium imbalance

Dysfunction	Hypomagnesemia	Hypermagnesemia
Cardiovascular	◆ Arrhythmias (such as torsades de pointes), vasomotor changes (vasodilation and hypotension) and, occasionally, hypertension	◆ Bradycardia, weak pulse, hypotension, heart block, cardiac arrest (common with serum levels of 25 mEq/L)
Neurologic	◆ Confusion, delusions, hallucinations, seizures	◆ Drowsiness, flushing, lethargy, confusion, diminished sensorium
Neuromuscular	◆ Hyperirritability, tetany, leg and foot cramps, Chvostek sign (facial muscle spasms induced by tapping the branches of the facial nerve)	◆ Diminished reflexes, muscle weakness, flaccid paralysis, respiratory muscle paralysis that may cause respiratory insufficiency

of severe hypomagnesemia, magnesium sulfate I.V. (10 to 40 mEq/L diluted in I.V. fluid). Magnesium intoxication (a possible adverse effect) requires calcium gluconate I.V.

Therapy for hypermagnesemia includes increased fluid intake and loop diuretics (such as furosemide) with impaired renal function; calcium gluconate (10%), a magnesium antagonist, for temporary relief of symptoms in an emergency; and peritoneal dialysis or hemodialysis if renal function fails or if excess magnesium can't be eliminated.

Special considerations

For patients with hypomagnesemia:
◆ Monitor serum electrolyte levels (including magnesium, calcium, and potassium) daily for mild deficits and every 6 to 12 hours during replacement therapy.
◆ Measure intake and output frequently. (Urine output shouldn't fall below 0.5 to 1 mL/kg/day in patients with healthy body weight; in heavier patients, <50 mL/hour is a cause for concern.) Remember, the kidneys excrete excess magnesium, and hypermagnesemia could occur with renal insufficiency.

▮ ALERT *Monitor vital signs during I.V. therapy. Infuse magnesium replacement slowly and watch for bradycardia, heart block, and decreased respiratory rate. Have calcium gluconate I.V. available to reverse hypermagnesemia from overcorrection. In patients with torsade de pointes, elevated magnesium levels are therapeutic.*
◆ Advise patients to eat foods high in magnesium, such as fish and green vegetables.
◆ Watch for and report signs of hypomagnesemia in patients with predisposing diseases or conditions, especially those not permitted anything by mouth or who receive I.V. fluids without magnesium.

For patients with hypermagnesemia:
◆ Frequently assess level of consciousness, muscle activity, and vital signs.
◆ Keep accurate intake and output records. Provide sufficient fluids for adequate hydration and maintenance of renal function.
◆ Report abnormal serum electrolyte levels immediately.
◆ Monitor and report ECG changes (peaked T waves, increased PR intervals, widened QRS complex).
◆ Watch patients receiving cardiac glycosides and calcium gluconate simultaneously, because calcium excess enhances digoxin action, predisposing the patient to digoxin toxicity.
◆ Advise patients, particularly elderly patients and patients with compromised renal function, not to abuse laxatives and antacids containing magnesium.
◆ Watch for signs of hypermagnesemia in predisposed patients. Observe closely for respiratory distress if magnesium serum levels rise above 10 mEq/L.

PHOSPHORUS IMBALANCE

Phosphorus exists primarily in inorganic combination with calcium in teeth and bones. The incidence of hypophosphatemia varies with the underlying cause; hyperphosphatemia occurs most often in children who tend to consume more phosphorus-rich foods and beverages than adults, and in children and adults with renal insufficiency. The prognosis for both conditions depends on the underlying cause.

Causes and incidence

Hypophosphatemia is usually the result of inadequate dietary intake; it's often related to malnutrition resulting from a prolonged catabolic state or chronic alcoholism. It may also stem from intestinal malabsorption, chronic diarrhea, hyperparathyroidism with resultant hypercalcemia, hypomagnesemia, or deficiency of vitamin D, which is necessary for intestinal phosphorus absorption. Other causes include chronic use of antacids containing aluminum hydroxide, use of parenteral nutrition solution with inadequate phosphate content, renal tubular defects, tissue damage in which phosphorus is released by injured cells, refeeding syndrome, and diabetic acidosis.

Hyperphosphatemia is generally secondary to hypocalcemia, hypervitaminosis D, hypoparathyroidism, or renal failure (often due to stress or injury). It may also result from overuse of laxatives with phosphates or phosphate enemas.

Pathophysiology

In ECF, the phosphate ion supports several metabolic functions: utilization of B vitamins, acid–base homeostasis, bone formation, nerve and muscle activity, cell division, transmission of hereditary traits, and metabolism of carbohydrates, proteins, and fats. Renal tubular reabsorption of phosphate is inversely regulated by calcium levels—an increase in phosphorus causes a decrease in calcium. An imbalance causes hypophosphatemia or hyperphosphatemia.

Complications

◆ *Hypophosphatemia*—heart failure, shock, arrhythmias, rhabdomyolysis, seizures, and coma
◆ *Hyperphosphatemia*—soft-tissue complications

Signs and symptoms

Hypophosphatemia produces anorexia, muscle weakness, tremor, paresthesia and, when persistent, osteomalacia, causing bone pain. Impaired RBC functions may occur in hypophosphatemia due to alterations in oxyhemoglobin dissociation, which may result in peripheral hypoxia. Hyperphosphatemia usually remains asymptomatic unless it results in hypocalcemia, with tetany and seizures.

Diagnosis

℞ **CONFIRMING DIAGNOSIS** *Serum phosphorus levels less than 1.7 mEq/L or 2.5 mg/dL confirm hypophosphatemia. Urine phosphorus levels above 1.3 g/24 hours support this diagnosis. Serum phosphorus levels above 2.6 mEq/L or 4.5 mg/dL confirm hyperphosphatemia. Supportive values include decreased levels of serum calcium (<9 mg/dL) and urine phosphorus (<0.9 g/24 hours).*

Foods high in phosphorus

Food	Portion	Amount (mg)
Almonds	1 oz	134
Beef	3 oz	173
Egg	1 large	104
Carbonated cola beverages	12 oz	40
Milk (skim)	8 oz	247
Turkey (roasted)	3 oz	173

Treatment

Treatment aims to correct the underlying cause of phosphorus imbalance. Until this is done, the management of hypophosphatemia consists of phosphorus replacement with a high-phosphorus diet and oral administration of phosphate salt tablets or capsules. (See *Foods high in phosphorus*.) Severe hypophosphatemia requires I.V. infusion of potassium phosphate. Severe hyperphosphatemia may require peritoneal dialysis or hemodialysis to lower the serum phosphorus level.

Special considerations

◆ Carefully monitor serum electrolyte, calcium, magnesium, and phosphorus levels. Report any changes immediately.

To manage hypophosphatemia:
◆ Record intake and output accurately. Administer potassium phosphate via slow I.V. to prevent overcorrection to hyperphosphatemia. Assess renal function and be alert for hypocalcemia when giving phosphate supplements. If phosphate salt tablets cause nausea, use capsules instead.
◆ To prevent recurrence, advise the patient to follow a high-phosphorus diet containing milk and milk products, kidney, liver, turkey, and dried fruits.

To manage hyperphosphatemia:
◆ Monitor intake and output. If urine output falls below 25 mL/hour or 600 mL/day, notify the physician immediately, because decreased output can seriously affect renal clearance of excess serum phosphorus.
◆ Watch for signs of hypocalcemia, such as muscle twitching and tetany, which often accompany hyperphosphatemia.
◆ To prevent recurrence, advise the patient to eat foods with low phosphorus content such

as vegetables. Obtain dietary consultation if the condition results from chronic renal insufficiency.

SYNDROME OF INAPPROPRIATE ANTIDIURETIC HORMONE

SIADH, also known as *dilutional hyponatremia*. The prognosis depends on the underlying disorder and response to treatment.

Causes and incidence

The most common cause of SIADH (80% of patients) is oat cell carcinoma of the lung, which secretes excessive ADH or vasopressor-like substances. Other neoplastic diseases, such as pancreatic and prostatic cancer, Hodgkin lymphoma, and thymoma, may also trigger SIADH.

Less common causes include:
◆ CNS disorders: brain tumor or abscess, stroke, head injury, Guillain–Barré syndrome, and lupus erythematosus
◆ pulmonary disorders: pneumonia, tuberculosis, lung abscess, and positive-pressure ventilation
◆ drugs: chlorpropamide, vincristine, cyclophosphamide, carbamazepine, clofibrate, and morphine
◆ miscellaneous conditions: myxedema and psychosis

Pathophysiology

SIADH is marked by excessive release of ADH, which disturbs fluid and electrolyte balance. Such disturbances result from the inability to excrete dilute urine, free water retention, ECF volume expansion, and hyponatremia. SIADH occurs secondary to diseases that affect the osmoreceptors (supraoptic nucleus) of the hypothalamus.

Complications

◆ Water intoxication
◆ Cerebral edema
◆ Severe hyponatremia
◆ Coma

Signs and symptoms

SIADH may produce weight gain despite anorexia, nausea, and vomiting; muscle weakness; restlessness; and, possibly, coma and seizures. Edema is rare unless water overload exceeds 4 L because much of the free water excess is within cellular boundaries.

Diagnosis

A complete medical history revealing positive water balance may suggest SIADH.

℞ **CONFIRMING DIAGNOSIS** *Serum osmolality less than 280 mOsm/kg of water and a serum sodium level below 123 mEq/L confirm the diagnosis (normal urine osmolality is 11/2 times serum values).*

Supportive laboratory values include high urine sodium secretion (>20 mEq/L) without diuretics and high urine osmolality. In addition, diagnostic studies show normal renal function and no evidence of dehydration.

Treatment

Treatment for SIADH is symptomatic and begins with restricted water intake (500 to 1,000 mL/day). For chronic treatment, fluid restriction, vasopressin receptor antagonist, loop diuretics, increased salt intake, urea, mannitol, and demeclocycline.

With acute severe water intoxication, fluid restriction, vasopressin receptor antagonist, furosemide, hypertonic saline to replace excreted sodium.

When possible, treatment should include correction of the underlying cause of SIADH. If SIADH is due to cancer, success in alleviating water retention may be obtained by surgical resection, irradiation, or chemotherapy.

Special considerations

◆ Closely monitor and record intake and output, vital signs, and daily weight. Watch for hyponatremia.
◆ Observe the patient for restlessness, irritability, seizures, heart failure, and unresponsiveness due to hyponatremia and water intoxication.
◆ To prevent water intoxication, explain to the patient and family why they must restrict intake.

METABOLIC ACIDOSIS

Symptoms result from the body's attempts to correct the acidotic condition through compensatory mechanisms in the lungs, kidneys, and cells. Metabolic acidosis is more prevalent among children, who are vulnerable to acid–base imbalance because their metabolic rates are faster and their ratios of water to total body weight are lower. Severe or untreated metabolic acidosis can be fatal.

Causes and incidence

Metabolic acidosis usually results from excessive fat burning in the absence of usable carbohydrates. This can be caused by diabetic ketoacidosis, chronic alcoholism, malnutrition, or a low-carbohydrate, high-fat diet—all of which produce more keto acids than the metabolic process can handle. Other causes include:

◆ anaerobic carbohydrate metabolism: a decrease in tissue oxygenation or perfusion (as occurs with pump failure after myocardial infarction, or with pulmonary or hepatic disease, shock, or anemia) forces a shift from aerobic to anaerobic metabolism, causing a corresponding rise in lactic acid level
◆ renal insufficiency and failure (renal acidosis): underexcretion of metabolized acids or inability to conserve base
◆ diarrhea and intestinal malabsorption: loss of sodium bicarbonate from the intestines, causing the bicarbonate buffer system to shift to the acidic side. For example, ureteroenterostomy and Crohn disease can also induce metabolic acidosis.

Less often, metabolic acidosis results from salicylate intoxication (overuse of aspirin), exogenous poisoning, or Addison disease with an increased excretion of sodium and chloride, and retention of potassium ions.

Pathophysiology
Metabolic acidosis is a physiologic state of excess acid accumulation and deficient base bicarbonate produced by an underlying pathologic disorder.

Complications
◆ Coma
◆ Arrhythmias
◆ Cardiac arrest

Signs and symptoms
In mild acidosis, the underlying disease's symptoms may obscure any direct clinical evidence. Metabolic acidosis typically begins with headache and lethargy, progressing to drowsiness, CNS depression, Kussmaul respirations (as the lungs attempt to compensate by "blowing off"

carbon dioxide), stupor and, if the condition is severe and goes untreated, coma and death. Associated GI distress usually produces anorexia, nausea, vomiting, and diarrhea, and may lead to dehydration. Underlying diabetes mellitus may cause fruity breath from catabolism of fats and excretion of accumulated acetone through the lungs.

Diagnosis
CONFIRMING DIAGNOSIS *Arterial pH below 7.35 confirms metabolic acidosis. In severe acidotic states, pH may fall to 7.10, and the partial pressure of arterial carbon dioxide may be normal or below 34 mm Hg as compensatory mechanisms take hold. Bicarbonate may be below 22 mEq/L.*

A metabolic panel can help reveal the cause and severity of metabolic acidosis. A complete blood count can be done to help assess possible causes as well. Supportive findings include:
◆ urine pH: below 4.5 in the absence of renal disease
◆ serum potassium levels: above 5.5 mEq/L from chemical buffering
◆ glucose levels: above 150 mg/dL in diabetes
◆ serum ketone bodies: elevated levels in diabetes mellitus
◆ serum osmolarity: increased levels, as in hyperosmolar hyperglycemic nonketotic acidosis or dehydration
◆ plasma lactic acid: elevated levels in lactic acidosis
◆ anion gap: greater than 14 mEq/L indicating metabolic acidosis (diabetic ketoacidosis, aspirin overdose, alcohol poisoning)
(See *Anion gap.*)

Treatment
In metabolic acidosis, treatment consists of administration of sodium bicarbonate I.V. for

Anion gap
The anion gap is the difference between concentrations of serum cations and anions—determined by measuring one cation (sodium) and two anions (chloride and bicarbonate). The normal concentration of sodium is 140 mEq/L; of chloride, 102 mEq/L; and of bicarbonate, 26 mEq/L. Thus, the anion gap between *measured* cations (actually sodium alone) and *measured* anions is about 12 mEq/L (140 minus 128).

Concentrations of potassium, calcium, and magnesium (*unmeasured* cations), or proteins, phosphate, sulfate, and organic acids (*unmeasured* anions) aren't needed

to measure the anion gap. Added together, the concentration of unmeasured cations would be about 11 mEq/L; of unmeasured anions, about 23 mEq/L. Thus, the normal anion gap between unmeasured cations and anions is about 12 mEq/L (23 minus 11)—plus or minus 2 mEq/L for normal variation. An anion gap over 14 mEq/L indicates *metabolic acidosis*. It may result from accumulation of excess organic acids or from retention of hydrogen ions, which chemically bond with bicarbonate and decrease bicarbonate levels.

severe cases, evaluation and correction of electrolyte imbalances and, ultimately, correction of the underlying cause. For example, in diabetic ketoacidosis, a low-dose continuous I.V. infusion of insulin is recommended.

Special considerations

◆ Keep sodium bicarbonate ampules handy for emergency administration. Monitor vital signs, laboratory results, and level of consciousness frequently because changes can occur rapidly.

◆ In diabetic acidosis, watch for secondary changes due to hypovolemia, such as decreasing blood pressure.

◆ Record intake and output accurately to monitor renal function. Watch for signs of excessive serum potassium—weakness, flaccid paralysis, and arrhythmias, possibly leading to cardiac arrest. After treatment, check for overcorrection to hypokalemia.

◆ Because metabolic acidosis commonly causes vomiting, position the patient to prevent aspiration. Prepare for possible seizures with seizure precautions.

◆ Provide good oral hygiene. Use sodium bicarbonate washes to neutralize mouth acids, and lubricate the patient's lips with lemon and glycerin swabs as indicated.

▦▦▦▦ **PREVENTION** *Carefully observe patients receiv-*
▲▲▲ *ing I.V. therapy or who have intestinal tubes in place as well as those suffering from shock, hyperthyroidism, hepatic disease, circulatory failure, or dehydration. Teach the patient with diabetes how to routinely test urine for glucose and acetone, and encourage strict adherence to insulin or oral hypoglycemic therapy.*

METABOLIC ALKALOSIS

With early diagnosis and prompt treatment, prognosis is good; however, untreated metabolic alkalosis may lead to coma and death.

Causes and incidence

Metabolic alkalosis results from loss of acid, retention of base, or renal mechanisms associated with decreased serum levels of potassium and chloride.

Causes of critical acid loss include vomiting, NG tube drainage or lavage without adequate electrolyte replacement, fistulas, and the use of steroids and certain diuretics (furosemide, thiazides, and ethacrynic acid). Hyperadrenocorticism is another cause of severe acid loss. Cushing disease, primary hyperaldosteronism, and Bartter syndrome, for example, all lead to retention of sodium and chloride, and urinary loss of potassium and hydrogen.

Excessive base retention can result from excessive intake of bicarbonate of soda or other

antacids (usually for treatment of gastritis or peptic ulcer), excessive intake of absorbable alkali (as in milk-alkali syndrome, often seen in patients with peptic ulcers), administration of excessive amounts of I.V. fluids with high concentrations of bicarbonate or lactate, or respiratory insufficiency—all of which cause chronic hypercapnia from high levels of plasma bicarbonate.

Pathophysiology

A clinical state marked by decreased amounts of acid or increased amounts of base bicarbonate, metabolic alkalosis causes metabolic, respiratory, and renal responses, producing characteristic symptoms (most notably hypoventilation). This condition is always secondary to an underlying cause.

Complications

◆ Coma
◆ Atrioventricular arrhythmias

Signs and symptoms

Clinical features of metabolic alkalosis result from the body's attempt to correct the acid–base imbalance, primarily through hypoventilation. Other manifestations include irritability, picking at bedclothes (carphology), twitching, confusion, nausea, vomiting, and diarrhea (which aggravates alkalosis). Cardiovascular abnormalities (such as atrial tachycardia) and respiratory disturbances (such as cyanosis and apnea) also occur. In the alkalotic patient, diminished peripheral blood flow during repeated blood pressure checks may provoke carpopedal spasm in the hand—a possible sign of impending tetany (Trousseau sign). Uncorrected metabolic alkalosis may progress to seizures and coma.

Diagnosis

℞ **CONFIRMING DIAGNOSIS** *Blood pH level greater than 7.45 and bicarbonate levels above 29 mEq/L confirm the diagnosis. A partial pressure of carbon dioxide above 45 mm Hg indicates attempts at respiratory compensation. Serum electrolyte studies show low potassium, calcium, and chloride levels.*

Other characteristic findings include:
◆ Urine pH is usually about 7.0.
◆ Urinalysis reveals alkalinity after the renal compensatory mechanism begins to excrete bicarbonate.
◆ ECG may show low T wave, merging with a U wave (secondary to hypocalcemia from metabolic alkalosis), and atrial or sinus tachycardia.

Treatment

Treatment aims to correct the underlying cause of metabolic alkalosis. Therapy for severe alkalosis may include cautious administration of ammonium chloride I.V. or hydrochloric acid to release hydrogen chloride and restore concentration of ECF and chloride levels. Potassium chloride and normal saline solution (except in the presence of heart failure) are usually sufficient to replace losses from gastric drainage. Electrolyte replacement with potassium chloride and discontinuing diuretics correct metabolic alkalosis resulting from potent diuretic therapy.

Oral or I.V. acetazolamide, which enhances renal bicarbonate excretion, may be prescribed to correct metabolic alkalosis without rapid volume expansion. Because acetazolamide also enhances potassium excretion, potassium may have to be administered before giving this drug.

Special considerations

Structure the care plan around cautious I.V. therapy, keen observation, and strict monitoring of the patient's status.

◆ Dilute potassium when giving I.V. containing potassium salts. Monitor the infusion rate to prevent damage to blood vessels; watch for signs of phlebitis. When administering ammonium chloride 0.9%, limit the infusion rate to 1 L in 4 hours; faster administration may cause hemolysis of RBCs. Avoid overdosage because it may cause overcorrection to metabolic acidosis. Don't give ammonium chloride to patients with signs of hepatic or renal disease; instead, use hydrochloric acid.

◆ Watch closely for signs of muscle weakness, tetany, or decreased activity. Monitor vital signs frequently and record intake and output to evaluate respiratory, fluid, and electrolyte status. Remember, respiratory rate usually decreases in an effort to compensate for alkalosis. Hypotension and tachycardia may indicate electrolyte imbalance, especially hypokalemia.

◆ Observe seizure precautions.

▓▓▓▓ PREVENTION *To prevent metabolic alkalosis, warn patients against overusing alkaline agents. Irrigate NG tubes with isotonic saline solution instead of plain water to prevent loss of gastric electrolytes. Monitor I.V. fluid concentrations of bicarbonate or lactate. Teach patients with ulcers to recognize signs of milk-alkali syndrome: a distaste for milk, anorexia, weakness, and lethargy.*

SELECTED REFERENCES

AACE Obesity Resource Center. (n.d.). *Section 3.3 weight-loss medications.* Retrieved from http://obesity.aace.com/weight-loss-medications

Akobeng, A., & Thomas, A. (2010). Refeeding syndrome following exclusive enteral nutritional treatment in Crohn disease. *Journal of Pediatric Gastroenterology & Nutrition, 51*(3), 364–366.

Ansstas, G. (2016). *Vitamin A deficiency.* Retrieved from https://emedicine.medscape.com/article/126004-overview#a5

Banks, S. (2017). *Riboflavin deficiency.* Retrieved from https://www.ncbi.nlm.nih.gov/books/NBK470460/#_article-28577_s2_

Bermudez, V., et al. (2010). Lipoprotein(a): From molecules to therapeutics. *American Journal of Therapeutics, 17*(3), 263–273.

Coman, D., et al. (2010). Galactosemia, a single gene disorder with epigenetic consequences. *Pediatric Research, 67*(3), 286–292.

Frye, R. (2016). *Pyridoxine deficiency.* Retrieved from https://emedicine.medscape.com/article/124947-overview#a5

Goebel, L. (2017). *Scurvy.* Retrieved from https://emedicine.medscape.com/article/125350-overview#a4

Lee, S. (2017). *Iodine deficiency.* Retrieved from https://emedicine.medscape.com/article/122714-overview#a4

Leiter, L., et al. (2008). How to reach LDL targets quickly in patients with diabetes or metabolic syndrome. *Journal of Family Practice, 57*(3), 661–668.

Luder, E. (2010). Early-life influences in the inception of obesity and asthma. *Topics in Clinical Nutrition, 25*(3), 128–135.

Nutritional Disease. (2018). In *Encyclopaedia Britannica.* Retrieved from https://www.britannica.com/science/nutritional-disease/Vitamin-K#ref414345

Rabinowitz, S. (2016). *Pediatric pellagra.* Retrieved from https://emedicine.medscape.com/article/985427-overview#a5

Rosenbloom, M. (2017). *Vitamin toxicity.* Retrieved from https://emedicine.medscape.com/article/819426-overview#a4

Roth, K. (2017). *Hereditary fructose intolerance.* Retrieved from https://reference.medscape.com/article/944548-overview#a5

Schick, P. (2017). *Pernicious anemia.* Retrieved from https://emedicine.medscape.com/article/204930-overview

Schneidfeld, N. (2016). *Protein-energy malnutrition.* Retrieved from https://emedicine.medscape.com/article/1104623-overview#a5

Tangpricha, V. (2017). *Vitamin D deficiency and related disorders.* Retrieved from https://emedicine.medscape.com/article/128762-overview#a4

The University of Chicago. (2013). *Galactosemia.* Retrieved from https://pedclerk.bsd.uchicago.edu/page/galactosemia

Thomas, C. (2017). *Syndrome of inappropriate antidiuretic hormone secretion treatment & management.* Retrieved from https://emedicine.medscape.com/article/246650-treatment#d11

Winfield, R., et al. (2010). Traditional resuscitative practices fail to resolve metabolic acidosis in morbidly obese patients after severe blunt trauma. *Journal of Trauma-Injury Infection & Critical Care, 68*(3), 317–330.

Zinn, A. (2010). Unconventional wisdom about the obesity epidemic. *American Journal of the Medical Sciences, 340*(3), 481–491.

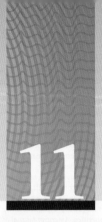

ENDOCRINE
DISORDERS

Introduction

Together with the nervous system, the endocrine system regulates and integrates the body's metabolic activities. The endocrine system meets the nervous system at the hypothalamus. The hypothalamus, the main integrative center for the endocrine and autonomic nervous systems, controls the function of endocrine organs by neural and hormonal pathways. A *hormone* is a chemical transmitter released from specialized cells into the bloodstream, which carries it to specialized organ receptor cells that respond to it.

Neural pathways connect the hypothalamus to the posterior pituitary, or neurohypophysis. Neural stimulation to the posterior pituitary provokes the secretion of two effector hormones: antidiuretic hormone (ADH) and oxytocin, and influences thyroid-stimulating hormone (TSH), corticotropin, prolactin, and gonadotropin-releasing hormone.

HYPOTHALAMIC CONTROL

The hypothalamus also exerts hormonal control at the anterior pituitary through releasing and inhibiting factors, which arrive by a portal system. Hypothalamic hormones stimulate the pituitary to release trophic hormones, such as corticotropin, TSH, luteinizing hormone (LH), and follicle-stimulating hormone (FSH), and to release or inhibit effector hormones, such as the growth hormone (GH) and prolactin. In turn, secretion of trophic hormones stimulates the adrenal cortex, thyroid, and gonads. In a patient whose clinical condition suggests endocrine pathology, this complex hormonal sequence requires careful evaluation at each level to identify the dysfunction; dysfunction may result from defects of releasing, trophic, or effector hormones or of the target tissue. Hyperthyroidism, for example, may result from an excess of thyrotropin-releasing hormone (TRH), TSH, or thyroid hormone.

In addition to hormonal and neural controls, a negative feedback system regulates the endocrine system. (See *Feedback mechanism of the endocrine system*, page 541.) The mechanism of feedback may be simple or complex. Simple feedback occurs when the level of one substance regulates secretion of a hormone. For example, low serum calcium levels stimulate parathyroid hormone (PTH) secretion; high serum calcium levels inhibit it. Complex feedback occurs through the hypothalamic–pituitary–target organ axis; for example, secretion of the hypothalamic corticotropin-releasing hormone (CRH) releases pituitary corticotropin, which, in turn, stimulates adrenal cortisol secretion. Subsequently, a rise in serum cortisol level inhibits corticotropin by decreasing CRH secretion. Steroid therapy disrupts the hypothalamic–pituitary–adrenal (HPA) axis by suppressing hypothalamic–pituitary secretion. Because abrupt withdrawal of steroids doesn't allow time for recovery of the HPA axis to stimulate cortisol secretion, it can induce a life-threatening adrenal crisis.

Feedback mechanism of the endocrine system

The hypothalamus receives regulatory information from its own circulating hormones (short feedback) and also from target glands (long feedback).

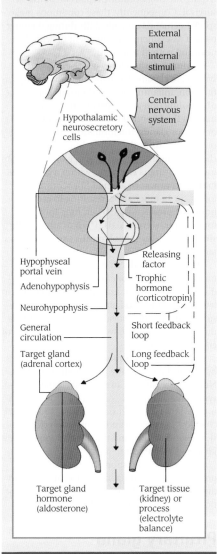

External and internal stimuli

Central nervous system

Hypothalamic neurosecretory cells

Hypophyseal portal vein

Adenohypophysis

Neurohypophysis

General circulation

Target gland (adrenal cortex)

Releasing factor

Trophic hormone (corticotropin)

Short feedback loop

Long feedback loop

Target gland hormone (aldosterone)

Target tissue (kidney) or process (electrolyte balance)

HORMONAL EFFECTS

In response to the hypothalamus, the *posterior pituitary* secretes oxytocin and ADH. Oxytocin stimulates contraction of the uterus and is responsible for the milk let-down reflex in lactating females. ADH controls the concentration of body fluids by altering the permeability of the distal convoluted tubules and collecting ducts of the kidneys to conserve water. The secretion of ADH depends on plasma volume and osmolality as monitored by hypothalamic neurons. Circulatory shock and severe hemorrhage are the most powerful stimulators of ADH; other stimulators include pain, emotional stress, trauma, morphine, tranquilizers, certain anesthetics, and positive pressure breathing.

The syndrome of inappropriate ADH secretion is a disorder that produces hyponatremia with water overload. Generally, however, overhydration suppresses ADH secretion (as does alcohol). ADH deficiency causes diabetes insipidus (DI), a condition of high urine output.

The *anterior pituitary* secretes prolactin, which stimulates milk production, and human growth hormone (hGH), which stimulates growth by increasing protein synthesis and fat mobilization and by decreasing carbohydrate utilization. Hyposecretion of hGH results in dwarfism; hypersecretion causes gigantism in children and acromegaly in adults.

The *thyroid gland* secretes the iodinated hormones thyroxine (T_4) and triiodothyronine (T_3). Thyroid hormones, necessary for normal growth and development, act on many tissues to increase metabolic activity and protein synthesis. Deficiency of thyroid hormone causes varying degrees of hypothyroidism, from a mild, clinically insignificant form to life-threatening myxedema coma. Congenital hypothyroidism causes cretinism. Hypersecretion causes hyperthyroidism and, in extreme cases, thyrotoxic crisis. Excessive secretion of TSH causes thyroid gland hyperplasia, resulting in goiter.

The *parathyroid glands* secrete PTH, which regulates calcium and phosphate metabolism. PTH elevates serum calcium levels by stimulating resorption of calcium and phosphate from bone, reabsorption of calcium and excretion of phosphate by the kidneys and, by combined action with vitamin D, absorption of calcium and phosphate from the gastrointestinal (GI) tract. PTH also stimulates conversion of vitamin D to its metabolically active form. Thyrocalcitonin, a secretion from the thyroid, opposes the effect of PTH and therefore decreases serum calcium levels. Hyperparathyroidism results in hypercalcemia, and hypoparathyroidism causes hypocalcemia. Altered calcium levels may also result from nonendocrine causes such as metastatic bone disease or nutritional vitamin D deficiency.

The *endocrine* part of the *pancreas* produces glucagon from the alpha cells and insulin from the beta cells. Glucagon, the hormone of the fasting state, releases stored glucose to raise the blood glucose level. Insulin, the hormone of the nourished state, facilitates glucose transport, promotes glucose storage, stimulates protein synthesis, and enhances free fatty acid uptake and storage. Absolute or relative insulin deficiency causes diabetes mellitus (DM). Insulin excess can result from an insulinoma (a tumor of the beta cells).

✿ **ELDER TIP** *A common and important endocrine change in elderly individuals is a decreased ability to tolerate stressors, as demonstrated by glucose metabolism. Normally, fasting blood glucose levels aren't significantly different in young and old adults. However, when stress stimulates an older person's pancreas, the blood glucose concentration increases and remains elevated longer than in a young adult.*

The *adrenal cortex* secretes mineralocorticoids, glucocorticoids, and sex steroids. Aldosterone, a mineralocorticoid, regulates the reabsorption of sodium and the excretion of potassium by the kidneys. Although affected by corticotropin, aldosterone is regulated by angiotensin II, which, in turn, is regulated by renin and plasma volume. Together, aldosterone, angiotensin, and renin may be implicated in the pathogenesis of hypertension. An excess of aldosterone (aldosteronism) can result primarily from hyperplasia or from adrenal adenoma or secondarily from many conditions, including heart failure and cirrhosis.

Cortisol, a glucocorticoid, stimulates gluconeogenesis, increases protein breakdown and free fatty acid mobilization, suppresses the immune response, and provides for an appropriate response to stress. Hyperactivity of the adrenal cortex results in Cushing syndrome; hypoactivity of the adrenal cortex causes Addison disease and, in extreme cases, adrenal crisis. Adrenogenital syndromes may result from overproduction of sex steroids.

The *adrenal medulla* is an aggregate of nervous tissue that produces the catecholamines epinephrine and norepinephrine, both of which cause vasoconstriction. Epinephrine also causes the fight-or-flight response—dilation of bronchioles and increased blood pressure, blood glucose levels, and heart rate. Pheochromocytoma, a tumor of the adrenal medulla, causes hypersecretion of catecholamines and results in characteristic sustained or paroxysmal hypertension.

The *testes* synthesize and secrete testosterone in response to gonadotropic hormones, especially LH, from the anterior pituitary gland; spermatogenesis occurs in response to FSH.

The *ovaries* produce sex steroid hormones, primarily estrogen and progesterone, in response to LH and FSH.

ENDOCRINE DYSFUNCTION

Chronic endocrine abnormalities are common health problems. For example, deficiencies of cortisol, thyroid hormone, or insulin may require lifelong hormone replacement for survival. Consequently, these conditions make special demands on your skills during ongoing patient assessment, management of acute illness, and patient teaching.

Common dysfunctions of the endocrine system are classified as hypofunction and hyperfunction, inflammation, and tumor. The source of hypofunction and hyperfunction may originate in the hypothalamus or in the pituitary or effector glands. Inflammation may be acute or subacute, as in thyroiditis, but is usually chronic, commonly resulting in glandular hypofunction. Tumors can occur within a gland—as in thyroid cancer or adrenal pheochromocytoma—or in other areas, resulting in ectopic hormone production. Certain lung tumors, for example, secrete ADH, PTH, or structurally similar substances that have the same effects on target tissues.

The study of endocrine function focuses on measuring the level or effect of a hormone. Radioimmunoassay, for example, measures insulin levels; a fasting blood glucose test measures insulin's effects. Sophisticated techniques of hormone measurement have improved diagnosis of endocrine disorders.

Diagnostic tests confirm endocrine disorders, but clinical data usually provide the first clues. Nursing assessment can reveal such signs and symptoms as excessive or delayed growth, wasting, weakness, polydipsia, polyuria, and mental changes. The quality and distribution of hair, skin pigmentation, and the distribution of body fat are also significant.

Nurses are also responsible for patient preparation, including instruction and support during testing, and for specimen collection, particularly of timed blood and urine specimens.

Pituitary gland

The pituitary (hypophysis) is a bean-sized glad suspended from the hypothalamus by a stalk called the infundibulum. The hypothalamus and pituitary function together—the hypothalamic–pituitary complex—to integrate and regulate the metabolic activities of the body in response to feedback from the nervous and endocrine systems.

The pituitary gland is made up of an anterior segment (adenohypophysis) and a posterior segment (neurohypophysis). The anterior pituitary responds primarily to hypothalamic signals to secrete or inhibit secretion of the trophic and tropic hormones produced in the anterior pituitary. *Tropic hormones* are secreted to influence the secretion of hormones from other endocrine glands/cells. *Trophic hormones* are secreted for a growth effect: hyperplasia or hypertrophy, on the target tissue. The four tropic hormones of the anterior pituitary are: Corticotropin (ACTH), thyrotropin (TSH), and the gonadotropins LH and FSH. Prolactin and GH are not tropic—their target tissues being nonendocrine.

The posterior pituitary doesn't actually produce any hormones; rather, in response to signals from the hypothalamus, it stores or secretes two hormones produced in the hypothalamus: oxytocin and vasopressin (also called ADH).

HYPOPITUITARISM

Hypopituitarism, which includes panhypopituitarism and dwarfism, results from dysfunction or disease affecting either the pituitary or the hypothalamus. It is a complex clinical syndrome marked by metabolic dysfunction, sexual immaturity, and growth delays (when it occurs in childhood), resulting from a deficiency or absence of one or more of the eight hormones secreted by the pituitary gland. Panhypopituitarism refers to a rare condition caused by partial or total failure of ALL of the anterior pituitary's vital hormones—corticotropin (ACTH), TSH, LH, FSH, hGH, and prolactin—plus vasopressin and oxytocin from the posterior pituitary. Depending on the level of insufficiency, hypopituitarism may be partial or complete. Both partial and complete hypopituitarism occur in adults and children; in children, these diseases may cause dwarfism and delayed puberty. The prognosis may be good with adequate replacement therapy and correction of the underlying causes.

Causes and incidence

The incidence of hypopituitarism is 12 to 42 per 1,000,000 per year with a prevalence of 300 to 455 per 1,000,000 patients per year. Approximately 30% to 70% of patients with traumatic brain injury have symptoms of partial hypopituitarism. Hypopituitarism secondary to Sheehan syndrome occurs in 10 of every 100,000 completed pregnancies. Hypopituitarism occurs in both men and women equally and can be diagnosed in adults and children.

The most common causes of primary hypopituitarism in adults are pituitary adenoma

and complications of surgery and treatment for pituitary adenoma, although more cases are being recognized posttraumatic brain injury. Other causes include congenital defects (hypoplasia or aplasia of the pituitary gland); pituitary infarction—most often from postpartum hemorrhage (Sheehan syndrome); or partial or total hypophysectomy by surgery, irradiation, or chemical agents; and, rarely, infectious (e.g., tuberculosis) or infiltrative disease (e.g., hemochromatosis). Occasionally, hypopituitarism may have no identifiable cause, or it may be related to autoimmune destruction of the gland. Secondary hypopituitarism stems from pituitary hormone deficiency secondary to hypothalamic or pituitary stalk dysfunction—either idiopathic or possibly resulting from infection, trauma, or a tumor.

Primary hypopituitarism usually develops in a predictable pattern of hormonal failures. It generally starts with hypogonadism from gonadotropin failure (decreased FSH and LH levels). In adults, it causes cessation of menses in females and impotence in men. GH deficiency follows; in adults, it causes osteoporosis, decreased lean-to-fat body mass index, adverse lipid changes, and subtle emotional dysphoria and lethargy. Subsequent failure of thyrotropin (decreased TSH levels) causes hypothyroidism; finally, adrenocorticotropic failure (decreased corticotropin levels) results in adrenal insufficiency. However, when hypopituitarism follows surgical ablation or trauma, the pattern of hormonal events may not necessarily follow this sequence. Sometimes, damage to the hypothalamus or neurohypophysis from one of the above leads to DI. Hypopituitarism may develop years after pituitary radiation treatment.

Pathophysiology

The normal hypothalamic–pituitary complex responds to a variety of stimulus to maintain the metabolic function of the body. In the presence of low levels of hormone in one of the target glands, negative feedback to the pituitary gland would induce increased trophic hormone secretion. However, hypopituitarism results in absent, insufficient, or inappropriate secretion of pituitary hormones. This results in low target gland hormone levels in conjunction with low or inappropriately normal levels of tropic pituitary hormones.

Complication

◆ The complications of hypopituitarism are secondary diseases that develop as a result of hormone deficiencies.

Signs and symptoms

Clinical features of hypopituitarism develop slowly and vary with the age of onset, the cause of the hypopituitarism, the severity of hormone loss, and the number of deficient hormones. Signs and symptoms of hypopituitarism in adults may include gonadal failure (secondary amenorrhea, impotence, infertility, decreased libido), DI, hypothyroidism (fatigue, lethargy, sensitivity to cold, menstrual disturbances), and adrenocortical insufficiency (hypoglycemia, anorexia, nausea, abdominal pain, orthostatic hypotension).

Sheehan syndrome characteristically causes failure of lactation, menstruation, and growth of pubic and axillary hair; and symptoms of thyroid and adrenocortical failure.

Pediatric hypopituitarism is not common, occurring at a frequency of 1 in 3,500 children. Rarely, hypopituitarism in children results from a genetic mutation or deletion affecting the proteins that code for the development and differentiation of the pituitary cells, such as Kallmann syndrome. Currently there are at least eight known genes wherein mutations or deletions can result in pituitary hormone deficiency; most commonly the PIT-1, GH, beta-LH, GHRH-R, and *PROP-1* genes. In children the most common effects of hypopituitarism are related to GH deficiency: slow growth, short stature, delayed development, and delayed or absent puberty. Pituitary dwarfism usually isn't apparent at birth but early signs begin to appear during the first few months of life; by age 6 months, growth delay is obvious. Although these children generally enjoy good health, pituitary dwarfism may cause central obesity due to fat deposits in the lower trunk, delayed secondary tooth eruption, and, possibly, hypoglycemia. Growth continues at less than half the normal rate—sometimes extending into the patient's 20s or 30s—to an average height of 4' (122 cm), with normal proportions.

When hypopituitarism strikes before puberty, it prevents development of secondary sex characteristics (including facial and body hair). In males, it produces undersized testes, penis, and prostate gland; absent or minimal libido; and the inability to initiate and maintain an erection. In females, it usually causes immature development of the breasts, sparse or absent pubic and axillary hair, and primary amenorrhea.

Panhypopituitarism may induce a host of mental and physiologic abnormalities, including lethargy, psychosis, orthostatic hypotension, bradycardia, anemia, and anorexia. However, clinical manifestations of hormonal deficiencies resulting from pituitary destruction don't become apparent until 75% of the gland is destroyed. Total loss of all hormones released by the anterior pituitary is fatal unless treated.

Neurologic signs associated with hypopituitarism and produced by pituitary tumors include headache, bilateral temporal hemianopia, loss of visual acuity, and, possibly, blindness. Acute hypopituitarism resulting from surgery or infection is often associated with fever, hypotension, vomiting, and hypoglycemia—all characteristic of adrenal insufficiency.

Diagnosis

In suspected hypopituitarism, evaluation must confirm hormonal deficiency due to impairment or destruction of the anterior pituitary gland and rule out disease of the target organs (adrenals, gonads, and thyroid) or the hypothalamus. Low serum levels of T_4, for example, indicate diminished thyroid gland function, but further tests are necessary to identify the source of this dysfunction as the thyroid, pituitary, or hypothalamus.

Serum insulin-like growth factor 1 (IGF-1) and its precursor insulin-like growth factor-binding protein 3 (IGFBP-3) are measured when abnormal GH production is suspected. Cranial computed tomography (CT) scan or magnetic resonance imaging (MRI) of the hypothalamus, pituitary and sellar space may reveal a structural abnormality, abnormally positioned pituitary, or abnormal mass. Fasting, morning immunoassays can reliably be used to measure basal levels of GH, prolactin, LH, FSH, TSH, and ACTH and their target hormones—decreased plasma levels of some or all pituitary hormones, accompanied by end-organ hypofunction, suggests pituitary failure, and eliminates target gland disease. Failure of TRH administration to increase TSH or prolactin concentrations rules out hypothalamic dysfunction as the cause of hormonal deficiency.

Provocative tests are helpful in pinpointing the source of low cortisol levels as adrenal insufficiency or pituitary ACTH deficiency. There are several tests that can be used to assess the integrity of the hypothalamic–pituitary axis. Oral metyrapone can be administered to block cortisol synthesis, which should stimulate pituitary secretion of corticotropin and the adrenal precursors of cortisol; the results are measured via radioimmunoassay of 11-deoxycortisol. Insulin-induced hypoglycemia also stimulates corticotropin secretion—insulin tolerance testing is considered the gold standard. (See *Confirming diagnosis.*) Persistently low levels of corticotropin indicate pituitary or hypothalamic failure. These tests require careful medical supervision because they may precipitate an adrenal crisis.

CONFIRMING DIAGNOSIS *Definitive diagnosis of ACTH deficiency and GH deficiency require measurement of GH levels in the blood after stimulation—most commonly done using the insulin tolerance test. Regular insulin is administered, inducing hypoglycemia which should provoke increased secretion of GH. After provocative testing—GH levels less than 3 µg/L are indicative of severe GH deficiency, levels between 3.0 and 4.9 µg/L are indicative of partial GH deficiency, and GH levels of 5.0 µg/L or more are normal. In patients where hypoglycemia is contraindicated alternate stimulation testing can be undertaken. CT scan, MRI, or cerebral angiography confirms the presence of intrasellar or extrasellar tumors. Provocative testing using insulin must only be carried out under close supervision of a healthcare provider secondary to the risk of severe hypoglycemia.*

Treatment

In the majority of cases hypopituitarism is irreversible; therefore, treatment is centered on hormone replacement. With the exception of GH and ADH, replacement of hormones secreted by the target glands versus the hypothalamic or pituitary hormone is the most convenient and cost-effective treatment for hypopituitarism. Hormone replacement therapy includes cortisol, T_4, and androgen or cyclic estrogen. Prolactin and oxytocin need not be replaced. The patient of reproductive age may benefit from administration of FSH and human chorionic gonadotropin to boost fertility. ADH is replaced using a synthetic vasopressin preparation such as intranasal desmopressin to stabilize the fluid balance.

GH replacement is recommended in children with short stature due to GH deficiency, but the treatment for adults is not well established. Replacement is done via daily subcutaneous injections of one of several biosynthetic GH preparations, the dose is titrated based on serum IGF-1 levels. Lean body mass increases, whereas adipose tissue—particularly in the abdomen—decreases. The risk of cardiovascular disease and osteoporosis also decreases with treatment. Many patients also notice an improved sense of well-being. Somatropin, a biosynthetic substitute for hGH with the same sequence of 191 amino acids achieved using recombinant DNA technology, has replaced GHs derived from human sources. Biosynthetic hGH is effective for treating GH deficiency and stimulates growth in children resulting in a linear increase in height until the epiphyses close. After pubertal changes have occurred, the effects of hGH therapy are limited. Children with hypopituitarism may also need replacement of adrenal and thyroid hormones and, as they approach puberty, sex hormones.

Special considerations

Caring for patients with hypopituitarism requires an understanding of hormonal effects and skilled physical and psychological support.

◆ Monitor the results of all laboratory tests for hormonal deficiencies, and understand the parameters. Until hormone replacement therapy is complete, check for signs of thyroid deficiency (increasing lethargy, slow pulse, constipation, dry hair and skin), adrenal deficiency (weakness, orthostatic hypotension, hypoglycemia, fatigue, and weight loss), and gonadotropin deficiency (decreased libido, lethargy, and apathy).

◆ Monitor patients on hGH replacement for signs of insulin resistance and impaired glucose tolerance (IGT). Glucose metabolism can be monitored via the oral glucose tolerance test or glycosylated hemoglobin (HbA_{1c}).

◆ Watch for anorexia in the patient with panhypopituitarism. Help plan a menu containing favorite foods—ideally, high-calorie foods. Monitor for weight loss or gain.

◆ If the patient has trouble sleeping, encourage exercise during the day.

◆ Record temperature, blood pressure, and heart rate every 4 to 8 hours. Check eyelids, nail beds, and skin for pallor, which indicates anemia.

◆ Prevent infection by giving meticulous skin care. Because the patient's skin is probably dry, use oil or lotion instead of soap. If body temperature is low, provide additional clothing and covers, as needed, to keep the patient warm.

◆ Darken the room if the patient has a tumor that's causing headaches and visual disturbances. Help with any activity that requires good vision such as reading the menu. The patient with bilateral hemianopia has impaired peripheral vision, so be sure to stand where the patient can see you, and advise the family to do the same.

◆ During insulin testing, monitor closely for signs of hypoglycemia (initially, slow cerebration, tachycardia, diaphoresis, and nervousness, progressing to seizures). Keep dextrose 50% in water available for I.V. administration to correct hypoglycemia rapidly.

◆ To prevent orthostatic hypotension, be sure to keep the patient supine during levodopa testing.

◆ Instruct the patient to wear a medical identification bracelet. Teach the individual and family members how to administer steroids rectally or parenterally in case of an emergency.

◆ Refer the family of a child with pituitary dwarfism to the appropriate community resources for psychological counseling because the emotional stress caused by this disorder increases as the child becomes more aware of their condition.

HYPERPITUITARISM

Hyperpituitarism is excess secretion of one or more of the hormones produced by the anterior pituitary gland. This excessive production is usually secondary to hyperplasia of one of the secretory cell types that result in a pituitary tumor called an adenoma. Pituitary adenomas are classified by size as microadenomas (<10 mm) or macroadenomas (>10 mm). Though the prognosis is dependent on the age at onset, the hormone effect, and the causative factor, most individuals respond well to medical or surgical treatment. The most common tumors are prolactinoma, corticotropinoma, and somatotropinoma.

Causes and incidence

Typically, the over-secretion of GH is caused by a pituitary adenoma (somatotropinoma), and referred to as *acromegaly* in adults and *gigantism* in children. Very rarely, elevated GH occurs as a result of a genetic mutation such as microduplications in *Xp26.3*—causing early onset gigantism. Gigantism begins before epiphyseal closure and causes proportional overgrowth of all body tissues. Proportional overgrowth of all body tissues causes remarkable height increases of as much as 6″ (15 cm) per year. Gigantism affects infants and children, causing them to attain as much as three times the normal height for their age. As adults, they may ultimately reach a height of more than 80″ (203 cm). Gigantism is rare; there have only been 100 reported cases.

Acromegaly occurs after epiphyseal closure. Pituitary adenoma is responsible for 98% of all cases. The tumor causes primary elevation in GH levels and as it grows, can cause secondary hypopituitarism or compression of surrounding tissue such as the optic nerve. The most common presenting features are coarsening facial features secondary to thickening of the skin and skeletal overgrowth of the mandible and forehead, enlargement of the hands and feet, arthritis, and excessive sweating. Acromegaly occurs equally among males and females, and among all racial and ethnic backgrounds. Annually, it affects three to four people per every million. As the disease progresses, loss of other trophic hormones, such as TSH, LH, FSH, and corticotropin, may cause dysfunction of the target organs.

Pathophysiology

The majority of pituitary adenomas are functional and secrete the hormone according to their cell of origin. Current research shows that most pituitary adenomas are monoclonal (stemming from the abnormal cloning of a single cell) and growth is stimulated from a spontaneous intrinsic genetic disruption within the pituitary itself. This spontaneous mutation results in increased in cell division and hormone secretion. Less commonly, the increased hormone is a result of a neuroendocrine tumor found elsewhere in the body.

Complications

◆ *Increased hGH secretion*—arthritis, carpal tunnel syndrome, osteoporosis, kyphosis, hypertension, arteriosclerosis, cardiomyopathy, cardiac hypertrophy, kidney failure, colorectal cancer
◆ *Acromegaly*—blindness, changes in the visual field, neurologic disturbances
◆ *Acromegaly and gigantism*—IGT, frank DM, obstructive sleep apnea, peripheral neuropathy

Signs and symptoms

Acromegaly develops slowly and typically produces diaphoresis, oily skin, hypermetabolism, and hypertrichosis. Severe headache, central nervous system (CNS) impairment, bitemporal hemianopia, loss of visual acuity, and blindness may result from the intrasellar tumor compressing the optic chiasm or nerves.

Hypersecretion of hGH produces cartilaginous and connective tissue overgrowth, resulting in a characteristic hulking appearance, with an enlarged supraorbital ridge and thickened ears and nose. Prognathism, projection of the jaw, becomes marked and may interfere with chewing. Laryngeal hypertrophy, paranasal sinus enlargement, and thickening of the tongue cause the voice to sound deep and hollow. Distal phalanges display an arrowhead appearance on X-rays, and the fingers are thickened. Irritability, hostility, and various psychological disturbances may occur.

Prolonged effects of excessive hGH secretion include bowlegs, barrel chest, arthritis, osteoporosis, kyphosis, hypertension, and arteriosclerosis. Both gigantism and acromegaly may also cause signs of IGT and clinically apparent DM because of the insulin-antagonistic character of hGH. If acromegaly is left untreated, the patient is at risk for cardiovascular failure, kidney failure, and colorectal cancer.

Gigantism develops abruptly, producing some of the same skeletal abnormalities seen in acromegaly. As the disease progresses, the pituitary tumor enlarges and invades normal tissue, resulting in the loss of other trophic hormones, such as TSH, LH, FSH, and corticotropin, thus causing the target organ to stop functioning.

Diagnosis

The most reliable testing for elevated GH is a glucose suppression test. Glucose normally suppresses hGH secretion; therefore, a glucose infusion that doesn't suppress the hormone level to below the accepted normal value of 5 ng/mL, when combined with characteristic clinical features, strongly suggests hyperpituitarism. Radioimmunoassays for serum total and free IGF-1 and IGFBP-3 can also be useful. Typically, elevated IGF-1 and IGFBP-3 correlate with excessive GH production, but results may be misleading in adolescents and therefore must be matched with a control of the same age, gender, and Tanner stage. Because hGH secretion is pulsatile, random GH levels are not clinically relevant and are not recommended.

In addition, skull X-rays, CT scan, arteriography, and MRI determine the presence and extent of the pituitary lesion. Bone X-rays showing a thickening of the cranium (especially of frontal, occipital, and parietal bones) and of the long bones, as well as osteoarthritis in the spine, support this diagnosis.

Treatment

Treatment aims to curb overproduction of hGH through removal of the underlying tumor by cranial or transsphenoidal hypophysectomy or pituitary radiation therapy. In acromegaly, surgery is mandatory when a tumor causes blindness or other severe neurologic disturbances. Postoperative therapy often requires replacement of thyroid, cortisone, and gonadal hormones. Adjunctive treatment may include administration of bromocriptine or cabergoline and octreotide and postoperative conventional proton beam radiation, which inhibit hGH synthesis. The therapeutic goal is to reach and maintain hGH levels less than 1 ng/mL and IGF-1 to normal range for age and gender, because at that level, life expectancy is restored to that of age-matched controls.

Special considerations

The extreme body changes characteristic of this disorder can cause severe psychological stress; therefore, emotional support to help the patient cope with their altered body image is an integral part of patient care.

◆ Assess for skeletal manifestations, such as arthritis of the hands and osteoarthritis of the spine. Administer medications as ordered. To promote maximum joint mobility, perform or assist with range-of-motion exercises.

◆ Evaluate muscle weakness, especially in the patient with late-stage acromegaly. Check the strength of the patient's handclasp. If it's very weak, help with tasks such as cutting food.

◆ Keep the skin dry. Avoid using an oily lotion because the skin is already oily.

◆ Test blood for glucose. Check for signs of hyperglycemia (fatigue, polyuria, and polydipsia).

◆ Be aware that the tumor may cause visual problems. If the patient has hemianopia, stand where they can see you. Remember, this disease can also cause inexplicable mood changes. Reassure the family that these mood changes result from the disease and can be modified with treatment.

◆ Before surgery, reinforce what the surgeon has told the patient, and try to allay the patient's fear with a clear and honest explanation of the scheduled operation.

PEDIATRIC TIP *If the patient is a child, explain to the parents that such surgery prevents permanent soft-tissue deformities but won't correct bone changes that have already taken place. Arrange for counseling, if necessary, to help the child and the parents cope with these permanent defects.*

ALERT *After surgery, diligently monitor vital signs and neurologic status. Immediately report increased urine output lasting longer than 2 hours, alteration in level of consciousness, unequal pupil size, changes in visual acuity, vomiting, falling pulse rate, or rising blood pressure. These changes may signal an increase in intracranial pressure due to intracranial bleeding or cerebral edema.*

◆ Check blood glucose level often. Remember, hGH levels usually fall rapidly after surgery, removing an insulin-antagonist effect in many patients and possibly precipitating hypoglycemia. Measure intake and output hourly, and report large increases. Transient DI, which sometimes occurs after surgery for hyperpituitarism, can cause such increases in urine output.

◆ If the transsphenoidal approach is used, a large nasal packing is kept in place for several days. Because the patient must breathe through the mouth, give good mouth care. Pay special attention to the mucous membranes—which usually become dry—and the incision site under the upper lip, at the top of the gum line. The surgical site is packed with a piece of tissue generally taken from a midthigh donor site. Watch for cerebrospinal fluid leaks from the packed site, which may necessitate additional surgery to repair the leak. Look for increased external nasal drainage or drainage into the nasopharynx.

◆ Encourage the patient to walk as soon as possible after surgery.

◆ Before discharge, emphasize the importance of continuing hormone replacement therapy, if ordered. Make sure the patient and their family understand which hormones are to be taken and why as well as the correct times and dosages. Warn against stopping the hormones suddenly.

◆ Advise the patient to wear a medical identification bracelet at all times and to bring their hormone replacement schedule with them whenever they return to the healthcare facility.

◆ Instruct the patient to have follow-up examinations for the rest of his or her life because a slight chance exists that the tumor that caused their condition may recur.

DIABETES INSIPIDUS

DI (also called *pituitary DI*) is a disorder of fluid metabolism; characterized by polydipsia and dilute polyuria resulting from deficient ADH (also called arginine vasopressin) from the pituitary gland (central DI) or decreased response to ADH in the renal tubules of the kidney (nephrogenic DI). Deficient ADH causes imbalances in the fluid and electrolyte levels in the body secondary to lack of regulation of water excretion and reabsorption. (See *Mechanism of ADH deficiency*, page 549.)

Pathophysiology

Fluid balance in humans is primarily regulated via thirst, ADH and kidney function. ADH regulates fluid balance—mainly via the excretion or reabsorption of water in the kidneys. Hypothalamic neurosecretory cells (osmoreceptors) mediate the amount of circulating ADH—they are stimulated by high osmotic pressure or inhibited by low osmotic pressure.

In a normally functioning individual, water conservation occurs when a state of dehydration resulting in increased plasma osmolarity triggers the osmoreceptors of the hypothalamus to stimulate the nerve impulses that release ADH from where it is stored in the posterior pituitary, increasing systemic circulation of ADH. Increased circulating ADH has three major outcomes:

◆ The membranes of the renal tubules become increasingly permeable resulting in a higher rate of solute free water reabsorption (decreasing plasma osmolarity) and increased circulating fluid volume, and decreased urine output (increasing urine osmolarity).

◆ The smooth muscle cells in the arterioles of the body constrict in reaction to vasopressin resulting in an increase in arterial blood pressure.

◆ The number of surface sweat glands decreases resulting in decreased loss of water via perspiration.

Causes and incidence

DI is rare, with a prevalence of 1 in 25,000 people. It can present at any age, dependent on the etiology, but is most often seen in 10 to 20 year olds. Males and females are affected equally. The disorder may start in childhood or early adulthood; however, fewer than 10% of cases are hereditary. There is no significant difference in prevalence between ethnic groups. In uncomplicated DI, the prognosis is good with adequate water replacement and replacement of ADH by tablet or nasal spray, and patients usually lead normal lives.

DI results centrally from intracranial neoplastic or metastatic lesions, hypophysectomy or other neurosurgery, a skull fracture, or head trauma that damages the neurohypophyseal structures. It can also result nephrogenically from infection, granulomatous disease, and vascular lesions; it may be idiopathic and, rarely, hereditary. (*Note:* Pituitary DI shouldn't be confused with nephrogenic DI, a rare congenital disturbance of water metabolism that results from renal tubular resistance to vasopressin.)

Normally, the hypothalamus synthesizes vasopressin. The posterior pituitary gland (or neurohypophysis) stores vasopressin and releases it into general circulation, where it causes the kidneys to reabsorb water by making the distal tubules and collecting duct cells water-permeable. The absence of vasopressin in DI allows the filtered water to be excreted in the urine instead of being reabsorbed.

Nephrogenic DI involves a defect in the parts of the kidneys that reabsorb water back into the bloodstream. It occurs less commonly than central DI. Nephrogenic DI may occur as autosomal dominant, autosomal recessive, but most commonly is an X-linked recessive inherited disorder. This is most frequently caused by mutations in the *AQP2* or *Xq28* genes. Nephrogenic DI may also be caused by diseases of the kidney (such as polycystic kidney disease) and the effects of certain drugs (such as lithium and amphotericin B) and as a result of hypercalcemia and hypokalemia.

Gestational DI occurs during pregnancy when an enzyme made by the placenta destroys

Mechanism of ADH deficiency

Diabetes insipidus (DI) is a disorder of water metabolism resulting from a deficiency of vasopressin (also called antidiuretic hormone, ADH). DI is characterized by excessive fluid intake and hypotonic polyuria.

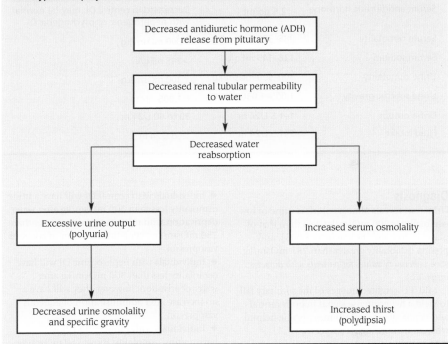

ADH in the mother. It occurs in about 1 in 30,000 pregnancies and typically presents in the third trimester and spontaneously resolves 2 to 3 weeks after delivery.

Complications
◆ Hypovolemia
◆ Hyperosmolality
◆ Circulatory collapse
◆ Loss of consciousness
◆ CNS damage

Signs and symptoms
The patient's history typically shows an abrupt onset of extreme polyuria (usually 8 to 16 L/day of dilute urine but sometimes as much as 30 L/day). As a result, the patient experiences extreme thirst which results in polydipsia (excessive fluid intake of up to 20 L/day). This disorder may also result in nocturia (usually presents as enuresis in children). In severe cases, it may lead to extreme

fatigue from inadequate rest caused by frequent voiding and excessive thirst.

Other characteristic features of DI include signs and symptoms of dehydration (poor tissue turgor, dry mucous membranes, constipation, muscle weakness, dizziness, and hypotension, dry skin, and weight loss), fever, tachycardia, and altered level of consciousness. These symptoms usually begin abruptly, commonly appearing within 1 to 2 days after a basal skull fracture, a stroke, or surgery; or gradually due to tumor or idiopathic causes. Relieving cerebral edema or increased intracranial pressure may cause all of these symptoms to subside just as rapidly as they began.

PEDIATRIC TIP *Pediatric patients may present with severe dehydration, vomiting, constipation, fever, failure to thrive, sleep disturbances, developmental delay, and irritability. Intellectual development can be affected secondary to untreated repetitive bouts of dehydration.*

Laboratory values for patients with diabetes insipidus

Diagnosis of diabetes insipidus requires evidence of vasopressin deficiency resulting in the kidneys' inability to concentrate urine. Evidence of this can be seen in the patient's laboratory values.

Value	Normal	Diabetes insipidus (DI)
Serum antidiuretic hormone	<2.5 pg/mL	Decreased in central DI; may be normal with nephrogenic or psychogenic DI
Serum osmolality	285–300 mOsm/kg	>300 mOsm/kg
Serum sodium	136–145 mEq/L	>145 mEq/L
Urine osmolality	300–900 mOsm/kg	<300 mOsm/kg
Urine specific gravity	1.005–1.030	<1.005
Urine output	1–1.5 L/24 hr	30 to 40 L/24 hr
Fluid intake	1–1.5 L/24 hr	>50 L/24 hr

Diagnosis

Urinalysis reveals almost colorless urine of low osmolality (<200 mOsm/kg, less than that of plasma), low specific gravity (<1.005), and plasma osmolality greater than 287 mOsm/kg. (See *Laboratory values for patients with diabetes insipidus.*)

MRI-T1-weighted images of the pituitary fail to yield a hyperintense signal in both central and nephrogenic DI. MRI may also be helpful wherein hemorrhage is suspected.

℞ CONFIRMING DIAGNOSIS *Diagnosis requires evidence of vasopressin deficiency, resulting in the kidneys' inability to concentrate urine during a water deprivation test (the Miller-Moses test).*

In this test, after baseline vital signs, weight, and urine and plasma osmolalities are obtained, the patient is deprived of fluids for up to 7 hours. Hourly measurements then record the total volume of urine output, body weight, urine osmolality or specific gravity, plasma arginine vasopressin, and plasma osmolality. Throughout the test, blood pressure and pulse rate must be monitored for signs of orthostatic hypotension. When two sequential urine osmolality results have less than 30 mOsm/kg difference or weight decreases by more than 3% to 5%, patients receive 5 units of aqueous vasopressin subcutaneously. Sixty minutes after administration of aqueous vasopressin, a final urine osmolality measurement is obtained.

◆ Individuals with normal functionality will have urine osmolality two to four times greater than plasma osmolality.

◆ Individuals with central DI will have a urine osmolality less than 300 mOsm/kg after water deprivation with urine osmolality greater than 750 mOsm/kg after administration of aqueous vasopressin.

◆ Individuals with nephrogenic DI will have osmolality less than 300 mOsm/kg after water deprivation; however, they will have no increase after administration of aqueous vasopressin.

◆ Individuals with primary polydipsia will have a urine osmolality above 750 mOsm/kg after water deprivation.

Treatment

Mild cases require no treatment other than fluid intake to replace fluid lost. Until the cause of more severe cases of DI can be identified and eliminated, administration of various forms of vasopressin or of a vasopressin stimulant can control fluid balance and prevent dehydration. Desmopressin acetate is the drug of choice for patients with central DI and is available as an oral preparation, a nasal spray, or by injection given subcutaneously or I.V.; this drug is effective for 8 to 20 hours, depending on the dosage. Hydrochlorothiazide can be used in both central and nephrogenic DI. Indomethacin and amiloride are alternative medications used in nephrogenic DI when hormone replacement with desmopressin is not available. If nephrogenic DI is caused by medication (such as lithium [Eskalith]), stopping the medicine can lead to kidney recovery.

Special considerations

Patient care includes monitoring symptoms to ensure that fluid balance is restored and maintained.

◆ Record fluid intake and output carefully. Maintain fluid intake that's adequate to prevent severe dehydration. Watch for signs of hypovolemic shock, and monitor blood pressure and heart and respiratory rates regularly, especially during the water deprivation test. Check the patient's weight daily.

◆ If the patient is dizzy or has muscle weakness, keep the side rails up and assist with walking.

◆ If the patient is unable to adequately replace his or her fluids orally, then fluid replacement should be dextrose and water via I.V. Do not replace without dextrose as it can result in hemolysis.

◆ To avoid hyperglycemia and fluid overload, fluid replacement should not exceed a rate of 500 to 750 mL/hour.

◆ For patients receiving initial treatment with desmopressin, frequent monitoring of electrolyte levels and fluid retention should be performed.

◆ Monitor urine specific gravity between doses. Watch for a decrease in specific gravity accompanied by increasing urine output, indicating the recurrence of polyuria and necessitating administration of the next dose of medication or a dosage increase.

◆ Institute safety precautions for the patient who is dizzy or who has muscle weakness.

◆ If constipation develops, add more high-fiber foods and fruit juices to the patient's diet. If necessary, obtain an order for a mild laxative such as milk of magnesia.

◆ Provide meticulous skin and mouth care; apply petroleum jelly, as needed, to cracked or sore lips.

◆ Before discharge, teach the patient how to monitor intake and output.

◆ Instruct the patient to administer desmopressin by nasal spray only after the onset of polyuria—not before—to prevent excess fluid retention and water intoxication.

◆ Tell the patient to report weight gain, which may indicate that their medication dosage is too high. Recurrence of polyuria, as reflected on the intake and output sheet, indicates that the dosage is too low.

◆ Teach the parents of a child with DI about normal growth and development. Discuss how their child may differ from others at this developmental stage.

◆ Encourage the parents to help identify the child's strengths and to use them in developing coping strategies.

◆ Refer the family for counseling if necessary.

◆ Advise the patient with DI to wear a medical identification bracelet and to carry needed medication at all times.

◆ Patients should receive follow-up monitoring every 6 to 12 months.

Thyroid gland

The thyroid gland is butterfly shaped, weighs approximately 15 g, and is located in the anterior section of the neck between the second and fourth tracheal cartilages. The thyroid produces and secretes T_4 and T_3. This process is controlled via the hypothalamic–pituitary thyroid axis. T_3 and T_4 primarily influence the metabolic processes in the body as well as certain aspects of growth and development. The normal thyroid gland releases approximately 100 µg of T_4 into the body's circulation each day. Approximately 30 µg of T_3 is also produced, as T_4 is converted to T_3 in the body's peripheral tissues (about 80% of the T_3 produced daily) via removal of an iodine molecule. The thyroid gland requires approximately 100 µg of iodide daily in order to make sufficient thyroid hormone. Iodide is turned into iodine via an oxidation process by the enzyme thyroid peroxidase. T_3 is the more biologically potent of the two thyroid hormones. The secretion of these hormones is regulated via thyrotropin (TSH) from the anterior pituitary which is in turn governed via TRH via the hypothalamus. The release of TSH and TRH is regulated via a negative feedback from T_3 and T_4—primarily T_3. The majority of T_3 and T_4 circulating in the body are bound to carrier proteins such as thyroid binding globulin. There is only a small amount of unbound circulating T_3 and T_4 (0.3% and 0.03%, respectively). However, it is this very small unbound portion that is responsible for the majority of the physiologic and biologic activities of thyroid hormone in the body.

HYPOTHYROIDISM IN ADULTS

Hypothyroidism, a state of low serum thyroid hormone, results from hypothalamic, pituitary, or thyroid insufficiency. The disorder can progress to life-threatening myxedema coma.

Causes and incidence

Hypothyroidism results from inadequate production of thyroid hormone—usually because of dysfunction of the thyroid gland due to surgery (thyroidectomy), irradiation therapy (particularly with ^{131}I), inflammation, chronic autoimmune thyroiditis (Hashimoto disease), or, rarely, conditions such as amyloidosis and sarcoidosis. It may also result from pituitary failure to produce TSH, hypothalamic failure to produce TRH, inborn errors of thyroid hormone synthesis, the inability to synthesize thyroid hormone because of iodine deficiency (usually dietary), or the use of antithyroid medications such as propylthiouracil, lithium, and amiodarone. In patients with hypothyroidism, infection, exposure to cold, and sedatives may precipitate myxedema coma.

Hypothyroidism is five to eight times more prevalent in females than in males, and frequency increases with age; in the United States, the incidence is rising significantly in people ages 40 to 50. Approximately 20 million Americans have thyroid dysfunction, and an estimated 12% of the adult population will have thyroid dysfunction at some point in their life.

Pathophysiology

In hypothyroidism there is an insufficient amount of circulating unbound thyroid hormone and conversely in hyperthyroidism there are elevated concentrations of unbound T_4 and unbound T_3. On occasions (such as pregnancy, certain medications, and certain bacterial and viral infections), serum concentrations of thyroid binding proteins fluctuate but the levels of unbound T_3 and T_4 remain constant and so the individual continues to be euthyroid.

Complications

◆ *Cardiovascular*—bradycardia, poor peripheral circulation, masked hypertension, and pericardial effusion
◆ *Gastrointestinal*—achlorhydria, pernicious anemia, megacolon, and intestinal obstruction
◆ Iron deficiency anemia
◆ Bleeding tendencies
◆ Emotional lability, depression, impaired memory and inability to concentrate
◆ Carpal tunnel syndrome
◆ Impaired fertility
◆ Benign intracranial hypertension
◆ Conductive or sensorineural deafness
◆ Myxedema coma
◆ Arteriosclerosis, ischemic heart disease, cardiomegaly, heart failure, and pleural and pericardial effusion
◆ Altered mental status
◆ Hypothermia

Facial signs of myxedema

Characteristic myxedematous signs in adults include dry, flaky, inelastic skin; puffy face; and upper eyelid droop.

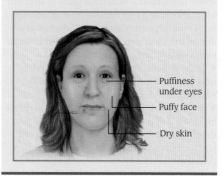

Puffiness under eyes
Puffy face
Dry skin

◆ Hypercarbia
◆ Hyponatremia

Signs and symptoms

Typically, the early clinical features of hypothyroidism are vague: fatigue, menstrual changes, hypercholesterolemia, forgetfulness, sensitivity to cold, unexplained weight gain, and constipation. As the disorder progresses, characteristic myxedematous signs and symptoms appear: decreasing mental stability; dry, flaky, inelastic skin; puffy face, hands, and feet; hoarseness; periorbital edema; upper eyelid droop; dry, sparse hair; and thick, brittle nails. (See *Facial signs of myxedema*.)

Cardiovascular involvement leads to decreased cardiac output, slow pulse rate, signs of poor peripheral circulation, and, occasionally, an enlarged heart. Other common effects include anorexia, abdominal distention, menorrhagia, decreased libido, infertility, ataxia, intention tremor, and nystagmus. Reflexes show delayed relaxation time (especially in the Achilles tendon).

⚠ **ALERT** *Progression to myxedema coma is usually gradual but when stress (such as hip fracture, infection, or myocardial infarction) aggravates severe or prolonged hypothyroidism, coma may develop abruptly. Clinical effects include progressive stupor, hypoventilation, hypoglycemia, hyponatremia, hypothermia, hypotension, hypoxia, seizures, and shock.*

Diagnosis

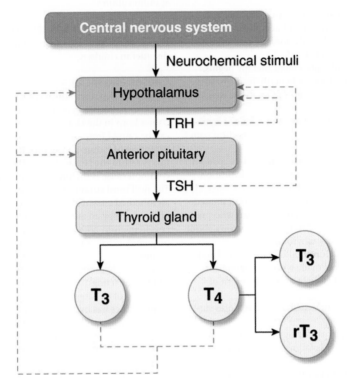

℞ **CONFIRMING DIAGNOSIS** *Elevated serum* *TSH in conjunction with low free T₄ or low free T₄ index is considered hypothyroid. The American Thyroid Association recommends against using T₃ levels to diagnose patients with hypothyroidism as patients can be severely hypothyroid and have a normal serum T₃.*

Supportive laboratory findings include:
◆ Elevated third-generation TSH level when hypothyroidism is due to thyroid insufficiency; decreased TSH level when hypothyroidism is due to hypothalamic or pituitary insufficiency (normal range 0.40 to 4.2 mIU/L)
◆ Thyroid antibody testing for two common antibodies that can cause hypothyroidism: antithyroid peroxidase and antithyroglobulin antibodies
◆ Radioactive iodine uptake (RAIU)—a low RAIU is seen when the thyroid is underactive
◆ Thyroid ultrasound—may show nodularity
◆ Elevated levels of serum cholesterol, alkaline phosphatase, and triglycerides
◆ Normocytic normochromic anemia

In myxedema coma, laboratory tests may also show low serum sodium levels, as well as decreased pH and increased partial pressure of carbon dioxide, indicating respiratory acidosis.

Treatment

Therapy for hypothyroidism consists of gradual thyroid replacement with levothyroxine (for low T₄ levels) and, occasionally, liothyronine (for inadequate T₃ levels).

During myxedema coma, effective treatment supports vital functions while restoring euthyroidism. To support blood pressure and pulse rate, treatment includes I.V. administration of levothyroxine and hydrocortisone to correct possible pituitary or adrenal insufficiency. Hypoventilation requires oxygenation and respiratory support. Other supportive measures include fluid replacement and antibiotics for infection.

Special considerations

To manage the hypothyroid patient:
◆ Thyroid function testing should be monitored routinely to keep TSH at a steady state but thyroid function should be reassessed upon initiation of estrogen or androgen therapies

or any other medications that could affect T_4 metabolism.

◆ Provide a high-bulk, low-calorie diet and encourage activity to combat constipation and promote weight loss. Administer cathartics and stool softeners, as needed.

◆ After thyroid replacement therapy begins, watch for symptoms of hyperthyroidism, such as restlessness, sweating, and excessive weight loss.

◆ Tell the patient to report any signs of aggravated cardiovascular disease, such as chest pain and tachycardia.

◆ To prevent myxedema coma, tell the patient to continue the course of thyroid medication even if symptoms subside.

◆ Warn the patient to report infection immediately and to make sure any physician who prescribes medications for the patient knows about the underlying hypothyroidism.

◆ Thyroid function should be reassessed and dose adjustments made with any significant changes in body weight and in the event of pregnancy.

Treatment of myxedema coma requires supportive care:

◆ Check frequently for signs of decreasing cardiac output such as falling urine output.

◆ Monitor temperature until stable. Provide extra blankets and clothing and a warm room to compensate for hypothermia. Rapid rewarming may cause vasodilation and vascular collapse.

◆ Record intake and output and daily weight. As treatment begins, urine output should increase and body weight decrease; if not, report this immediately.

◆ Turn the edematous bedridden patient every 2 hours, and provide skin care, particularly around bony prominences.

◆ Avoid sedation when possible or reduce dosage because hypothyroidism delays metabolism of many drugs.

◆ Maintain a patent I.V. line. Monitor serum electrolyte levels carefully when administering I.V. fluids.

⚠ **ALERT** *Monitor vital signs carefully when administering levothyroxine because rapid correction of hypothyroidism can cause adverse cardiac effects. Report chest pain or tachycardia immediately. Watch for hypertension and heart failure in the elderly patient.*

◆ Check arterial blood gas values for hypercapnia and hypoxia to determine whether the patient who's severely myxedematous requires ventilatory assistance.

◆ Because myxedema coma may have been precipitated by an infection, check possible sources

of infection, such as blood or urine, and obtain sputum cultures.

HYPOTHYROIDISM IN CHILDREN
Hypothyroidism is the most common thyroid disorder in children.

Causes and incidence
Congenital hypothyroidism (previously called cretinism) affects 1 in every 1,500 to 3,000 babies born in the United States each year. It can be caused from inadequate maternal consumption of iodine during pregnancy although this is rare in the United States. The most common cause is thyroid dysgenesis in utero. The next most common cause can be traced to an inherited enzymatic defect in the synthesis of T_4 caused by an autosomal recessive gene. Less frequently, antithyroid drugs taken during pregnancy cause congenital hypothyroidism in infants.

Acquired hypothyroidism is common in children affecting 1 in every 1,250 children. In fact, 4.6% of children aged 12 and older in the United States has hypothyroidism according to the National Health and Nutrition Examination Survey. The most common acquired hypothyroidism in children and teens is Hashimoto thyroiditis.

Untreated hypothyroidism is characterized in infants by respiratory difficulties, persistent jaundice, and hoarse crying; in older children, by growth delay (dwarfism), bone and muscle dystrophy, and intellectual disability. Hypothyroidism is three times more common in females than in males. Early diagnosis and treatment allow the best prognosis; infants treated before age 3 months usually grow and develop normally. As there are no immediate symptoms, most newborns in the United States have this detected during the newborn screen which is mandatory at all U.S. hospitals. Children who remain untreated beyond age 3 months and children with acquired hypothyroidism who remain untreated beyond age 2 suffer irreversible intellectual disability; however, skeletal abnormalities may be reversible with treatment.

Pathophysiology
In children hypothyroidism can be congenital or acquired. Congenital hypothyroidism results from agenesis or dysgenesis of the thyroid, defects in thyroid hormone synthesis and release, or insufficiency of the hypothalamus or pituitary. Congenital hypothyroidism generally presents at birth or over the first few months of life. Acquired hypothyroidism in children is usually a result of thyroid destruction caused

by autoimmune thyroid disease such as Hashimoto thyroiditis or chronic lymphocytic thyroiditis.

Complications
◆ Severe intellectual disability
◆ Skeletal malformations (dwarfism, epiphyseal degeneration, and bone and muscle dystrophy)

Signs and symptoms
The weight and length of an infant with infantile hypothyroidism appear normal at birth, but characteristic signs of hypothyroidism develop by the time the infant is 3 to 6 months old. In a breast-fed infant the onset of most symptoms may be delayed until weaning because breast milk contains small amounts of thyroid hormone.

Typically, an infant with hypothyroidism sleeps excessively, seldom cries (except for occasional hoarse crying), and is inactive. Because of this, the parents may describe the infant as a "good baby—no trouble at all." However, such behavior actually results from lowered metabolism and progressive mental impairment. The infant with hypothyroidism also exhibits abnormal deep tendon reflexes, hypotonic abdominal muscles, a protruding abdomen, and slow, awkward movements. The infant has feeding difficulties, develops constipation and, because the immature liver can't conjugate bilirubin, becomes jaundiced.

The infant may have a large, protruding tongue which obstructs respiration, making breathing loud and noisy and forcing open mouth breathing. The infant may have dyspnea on exertion, anemia, abnormal facial features—such as a short forehead; puffy, wide-set eyes (periorbital edema); wrinkled eyelids; and a broad, short, upturned nose. The infant's skin may be cold and mottled because of poor circulation and hair may be dry, brittle, and dull. Teeth erupt late and tend to decay early; body temperature is below normal; and pulse rate is slow.

In the child who acquires hypothyroidism after age 2, appropriate treatment can prevent intellectual delay. However, growth delay becomes apparent in short stature (due to delayed epiphyseal maturation, particularly in the legs), obesity, and a head that appears abnormally large because the arm and leg length are less than expected on an age-appropriate growth curve. An older child may show delayed or accelerated sexual development.

Diagnosis
A high serum level of TSH, associated with low T_3 and T_4 levels, points to hypothyroidism.

Because early detection and treatment can minimize the effects of hypothyroidism, thyroid screening is included in the mandatory routine newborn screening at all U.S. hospitals and birth centers.

Thyroid scan and RAIU tests show decreased uptake levels and confirm the absence of thyroid tissue in athyroidic children. Increased gonadotropin levels are compatible with sexual precocity in older children and may coexist with hypothyroidism.

Electrocardiogram (ECG) shows bradycardia and flat or inverted T waves in untreated infants. Hip, knee, and thigh X-rays reveal absence of the femoral or tibial epiphyseal line and delayed skeletal development that's markedly inappropriate for the child's chronological age. A low T_4 level associated with a normal TSH level suggests hypothyroidism secondary to hypothalamic or pituitary disease, a rare condition.

Treatment
Early detection is mandatory to prevent irreversible intellectual disability and permit normal physical development. Treatment of infants younger than age 1 consists of replacement therapy with oral levothyroxine, beginning with moderate doses. Dosage gradually increases to levels sufficient for lifelong maintenance. (Rapid increase in dosage may precipitate thyrotoxicity.) Doses are proportionately higher in children than in adults because children metabolize thyroid hormone more quickly. Therapy in older children includes hormone replacement with levothyroxine.

Special considerations
Prevention, early detection, comprehensive parent teaching, and psychological support are essential. Know the early signs. Be especially wary if parents emphasize how good and how quiet their new baby is.
◆ If parents opt to have a home delivery, they should be encouraged to get a newborn screen as soon as possible as it tests for hypothyroidism as well as a number of other congenital diseases.
◆ Synthetic thyroid hormone replacement should be given as a crushed pill in a small amount of breast milk or formula as the liquid formulation is unstable. It should also no be given with soy formula or with iron or calcium supplements as it will decrease the absorption of the hormone replacement.
◆ During early management of infantile hypothyroidism, monitor blood pressure and pulse rate; report hypertension and tachycardia immediately. But remember—normal infant heart

rate is approximately 120 beats/minute. If the infant's tongue is unusually large, position the infant on his or her side and observe frequently to prevent airway obstruction. Check rectal temperature every 2 to 4 hours. Keep the infant warm and skin hydrated.

◆ Inform parents that the child will require lifelong treatment with thyroid supplements. Teach them to recognize signs of overdose: rapid pulse rate, irritability, insomnia, fever, sweating, and weight loss. Stress the need to comply with the treatment regimen to prevent further mental impairment.

◆ Provide support to help parents deal with a child who may be intellectually disabled. Help them adopt a positive but realistic attitude, and focus on their child's strengths rather than the child's weaknesses. Encourage them to provide stimulating activities to help the child reach his or her maximum potential. Refer them to the appropriate community resources for support.

▩▩▩▩▩ **PREVENTION** *To prevent congenital hypothy-roidism, emphasize the importance of adequate nutrition during pregnancy, including iodine-rich foods and the use of iodized salt or, in case of sodium restriction, an iodine supplement.*

THYROIDITIS
Causes and incidence and pathophysiology

Thyroiditis is a broad descriptor for inflammatory processes affecting the thyroid. Thyroiditis is more common in people with human leukocyte antigen Bw35. The types of thyroiditis are autoimmune thyroiditis (Hashimoto thyroiditis), silent thyroiditis, postpartum thyroiditis, acute thyroiditis (suppurative), subacute thyroiditis (de Quervain thyroiditis or granulomatous thyroiditis), drug-induced thyroiditis, and radiation-induced thyroiditis. Hashimoto thyroiditis is caused by antithyroid antibody activity related to autoimmune disease and generally results in thyrotoxicosis followed by usually permanent hypothyroidism. Riedel thyroiditis (RT), a rare variant of Hashimoto thyroiditis, is caused by inflammation followed by replacement of the normal thyroid parenchyma with dense fibrotic tissue. The fibrotic tissue of RT differs from Hashimoto in that the fibrotic tissue changes extend beyond the capsule of the thyroid gland. Hypothyroidism is noted in approximately 30% of cases with rare cases of hyperthyroidism occurring. Silent thyroiditis can occur in men and women; the initial inflammation causes high thyroid levels (thyrotoxicosis) followed by transient hypothyroidism that resolves within 12 to 18 months (only

20% of cases result in permanent hypothyroidism). It is called silent thyroiditis because it is generally painless. In postpartum thyroiditis there is an autoimmune-related thyroid inflammation within 6 months of giving birth. It causes transient thyrotoxicosis but within a few weeks the thyroid becomes depleted resulting in symptoms of transient hypothyroidism in most women. It usually resolves within 12 months of giving birth; however, in 20% of cases, it can result in permanent hypothyroidism. Acute thyroiditis is generally seen as a result of a bacterial infection and causes generalized illness, occasionally causes thyroid pain, and rarely causes mild hypothyroidism, but all symptoms should resolve with treatment of the infectious agent. However, it should be noted that acute thyroiditis can cause extremely severe symptoms. Subacute thyroiditis generally results from viral infection causing thyroid pain and thyrotoxicosis followed by transient hypothyroidism that resolves in 12 to 18 months in 95% of cases. de Quervain thyroiditis is usually caused by a viral infection such as mumps, measles, influenza, coxsackievirus, mononucleosis, sarcoidosis, or malaria and causes fever and pain in the neck and jaw. The inflammation usually results in transient thyrotoxicosis followed by hypothyroidism that usually resolves within 12 to 18 months with 5% chance of permanent hypothyroidism. Drug-induced thyroiditis is usually caused by medications such as amiodarone, lithium, interferons, and cytokines, and they can cause thyrotoxicosis and hypothyroidism in certain individuals. The symptoms will usually persist until the drug is discontinued. Radiation-induced thyroiditis is seen following radiation therapy for specific cancers or radioactive iodine treatment for hypothyroidism. Occasionally this results in transient thyrotoxicosis; however, the most common affect is permanent hypothyroidism. Thyroiditis is most prevalent among people ages 30 to 50 and is more common in women than in men. The incidence is highest in the Appalachian region of the United States.

Complications
◆ *Hashimoto*—compression of surrounding tissues
◆ *Subacute*—permanent hypothyroid or hyperthyroid condition
◆ *Pyrogenic*—rupture of abscess into mediastinum, trachea, or esophagus
◆ *Riedel*—hypothyroidism, tracheal or esophageal compression, and necrosis or hemorrhage of compressed tissue

Signs and symptoms

The symptoms of thyroiditis are dependent on the type of thyroiditis. In autoimmune thyroiditis the destruction of thyroid tissue is slow and chronic. It eventually leads to a fall in thyroid hormone levels but until then is usually asymptomatic. It's the most prevalent cause of spontaneous hypothyroidism. In cases of thyroiditis that cause rapid cell damage causing excessive secretion of thyroid hormone and thyrotoxicosis, patients experience symptoms such as tachycardia, palpitations, anxiety, insomnia, weight loss, and irritability. In subacute granulomatous thyroiditis, moderate thyroid enlargement may follow an upper respiratory tract infection or a sore throat. The thyroid may be painful and tender, and dysphagia may occur. In patients with silent (painless) and postpartum thyroiditis, there is no pain but they may transiently experience hyperthyroid symptoms until the hormone is depleted.

Individuals with acute infectious thyroiditis may experience thyroid pain or painless enlargement of the thyroid accompanied by the symptoms of the specific systemic illness that precipitated the thyroiditis. Thyroid symptoms usually resolve once the infection resolves.

In RT, the gland enlarges slowly as it's replaced by hard, fibrous tissues. This fibrosis may compress the trachea or the esophagus. The thyroid feels firm.

Clinical effects of miscellaneous thyroiditis are characteristic of pyogenic infection: fever, pain, tenderness, and reddened skin over the gland.

Diagnosis

Precise diagnosis depends on the type of thyroiditis; however, an assessment of serum thyroid function studies including TSH, free T_4, free T_4 index, and possibly T_3 levels will help determine the stage of the disease:

◆ *Autoimmune:* elevated levels of antithyroglobulin antibody and antithyroid peroxidase antibodies are present in serum
◆ *Subacute granulomatous:* elevated erythrocyte sedimentation rate, increased thyroid hormone levels, decreased thyroidal radioiodine uptake
◆ *Chronic infective and noninfective:* varied findings, depending on underlying infection or other disease

Treatment

Appropriate treatment varies with the type of thyroiditis. Drug therapy includes levothyroxine for accompanying hypothyroidism, analgesics and anti-inflammatory drugs for mild subacute granulomatous thyroiditis, beta-blockers such as propranolol for the symptoms of hyperthyroidism such as palpitations and anxiety, and steroids for severe episodes of acute inflammation. Suppurative thyroiditis requires antibiotic therapy. A partial thyroidectomy may be necessary to relieve tracheal or esophageal compression in RT.

Special considerations

Before treatment, obtain a patient history to identify underlying diseases that may cause thyroiditis, such as tuberculosis or a recent viral infection.
◆ Check the patient's vital signs and examine the neck for unusual swelling, enlargement, or redness. Provide a liquid diet if the patient has difficulty swallowing, especially when due to fibrosis. If the neck is swollen, measure and record the circumference daily to monitor progressive enlargement.
◆ Administer antibiotics as indicated, and report and record elevations in temperature.
◆ Instruct the patient to watch for and report signs of hypothyroidism (lethargy, restlessness, sensitivity to cold, forgetfulness, and dry skin), especially if the patient has Hashimoto thyroiditis, which often causes hypothyroidism.
◆ Check for signs of hyperthyroidism (nervousness, tachycardia, tremor, and weakness), which commonly occurs in subacute thyroiditis.
◆ After thyroidectomy, check vital signs every 15 to 30 minutes until the patient's condition stabilizes. Stay alert for signs of tetany secondary to accidental parathyroid injury during surgery. Keep 10% calcium gluconate available for I.V. use if needed. Assess dressings frequently for excessive bleeding. Watch for signs of airway obstruction, such as difficulty in talking or increased swallowing; keep tracheotomy equipment handy.
◆ Explain to the patient that they'll need lifelong thyroid hormone replacement therapy if hypothyroidism occurs. Tell the patient to watch for signs of overdose, such as nervousness and palpitations.

SIMPLE GOITER

Simple (or nontoxic) goiter is a thyroid gland enlargement that isn't caused by inflammation or a neoplasm, and is commonly classified as endemic or sporadic. Endemic goiter usually results from inadequate dietary intake of iodine associated with such factors as iodine-depleted soil or malnutrition. Sporadic goiter follows ingestion of certain drugs or foods.

Simple goiter affects more females than males, especially during adolescence, pregnancy, and menopause, when the body's demand for thyroid hormone increases. Sporadic goiter affects no particular population segment. With appropriate treatment, the prognosis is good for either type of goiter.

Causes and incidence

Simple goiter occurs when the thyroid gland can't secrete enough thyroid hormone to meet metabolic requirements. As a result, the thyroid gland enlarges to compensate for inadequate hormone synthesis, a compensation that usually overcomes mild to moderate hormonal impairment. Because TSH levels are generally within normal limits in patients with simple goiter, goitrogenicity probably results from impaired intrathyroidal hormone synthesis and depletion of glandular iodine, which increases the thyroid gland's sensitivity to TSH. However, increased levels of TSH may be transient and therefore missed.

Endemic goiter usually results from inadequate dietary intake of iodine, which leads to inadequate secretion of thyroid hormone. Since the introduction of iodized salt in the United States, cases of endemic goiter have virtually disappeared.

Sporadic goiter commonly results from the ingestion of large amounts of goitrogenic foods or the use of goitrogenic drugs. Goitrogenic foods, such as rutabagas, cabbage, soybeans, peanuts, peaches, peas, strawberries, spinach, and radishes, contain agents that decrease T_4 production. Goitrogenic drugs include propylthiouracil, iodides, phenylbutazone, para-aminosalicylic acid, cobalt, and lithium. In a pregnant woman, these substances may cross the placenta and affect the fetus.

Inherited defects may be responsible for insufficient T_4 synthesis or impaired iodine metabolism. Because families tend to congregate in a single geographic area, this familial factor may contribute to the incidence of both endemic and sporadic goiters.

Females are more commonly affected than males. Incidence increases after age 40.

Pathophysiology

There are multiple factors that can interfere with the hypothalamic–pituitary–thyroid axis. Significant changes in that feedback axis can result in structural and functional changes in the thyroid gland. The hypothalamus produces thyrotropin-releasing hormone (TRH) which stimulates the pituitary to produce TSH. TSH regulates the production and secretion of thyroid hormone from the thyroid gland. The thyroid gland synthesizes thyroid hormone by combining iodine and the amino acid tyrosine. These hormones, T_4 and T_3, regulate the body's growth and metabolic functions. In turn, feedback from serum levels of those thyroid hormones regulates TRH and TSH production. Insufficient levels of T_3 and T_4 in the body trigger increased TSH production. If this increased TSH production continues untreated, it can lead to increased cellular differentiation in the thyroid tissue resulting in hypertrophy and goiter.

Complications

◆ Dysphagia
◆ Respiratory distress

Signs and symptoms

Thyroid enlargement may range from a mildly enlarged gland to a massive, multinodular goiter. (See *Massive goiter.*) The presence of goiter does not guarantee thyroid dysfunction; patients with goiter can be euthyroid, hyperthyroid, or hypothyroid. However, the presence of goiter does indicate the presence of an underlying condition causing hyperplasia of the thyroid

Massive goiter

Massive multinodular goiter causes gross distention and swelling of the neck.

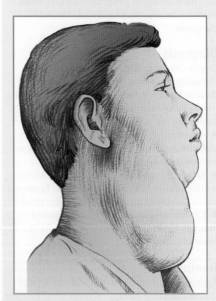

tissue. Because simple goiter doesn't alter the patient's metabolic state, clinical features arise solely from enlargement of the thyroid gland. The patient may complain of respiratory distress and dysphagia from compression of the trachea and esophagus, and swelling and distention of the neck. In addition, large goiters may obstruct venous return, produce venous engorgement and, in rare cases, induce development of collateral venous circulation in the chest. Obstruction may cause dizziness or syncope (Pemberton sign) when the patient raises their arms above their head.

Diagnosis
Diagnosis of simple goiter requires a thorough patient history and physical examination to rule out disorders with similar clinical effects, such as Graves disease, Hashimoto thyroiditis, and thyroid carcinoma. A detailed patient history may also reveal goitrogenic medications or foods or endemic influence. The results of diagnostic laboratory tests include the following.
◆ TSH: high or normal levels
◆ Serum T_4 and free T_4 concentrations: low normal or normal
◆ RAIU: normal or increased (50% of the dose at 24 hours)
◆ Ultrasound of thyroid: nodules may be present, necessitating biopsy for further evaluation

Treatment
The treatment will depend on the cause of the goiter. The goal of treatment is to reduce thyroid hyperplasia. Exogenous thyroid hormone replacement with levothyroxine is the treatment of choice; it inhibits TSH secretion and allows the gland to rest. Small doses of iodide (Lugol or potassium iodide solution) commonly relieve goiter that's due to iodine deficiency. Sporadic goiter requires avoidance of known goitrogenic drugs and foods. Treatment will reduce the size of the goiter but frequently it may not completely resolve. A large goiter that is unresponsive to treatment may require subtotal thyroidectomy.

Special considerations
Patient care includes measuring the patient's neck circumference daily to check for progressive thyroid gland enlargement and checking for the development of hard nodules in the gland, which may indicate carcinoma.
◆ To maintain constant hormone levels, instruct the patient to take the prescribed thyroid hormone preparations at the same time each day. Advise the patient to avoid taking the medicine at the same time as any calcium- or iron-containing supplements (including prenatal vitamins), or with Metamucil, grapefruit, or grapefruit juice. Also advise the patient that they cannot eat within 30 minutes of taking their medication.
◆ Teach the patient and the patient's family to identify and immediately report signs of thyrotoxicosis, including increased pulse rate, palpitations, diarrhea, sweating, tremors, agitation, and shortness of breath.
◆ Instruct the patient with endemic goiter to use iodized salt to supply the daily 150 to 300 µg of iodine necessary to prevent goiter.
◆ Monitor the patient taking goitrogenic drugs for signs of sporadic goiter.

HYPERTHYROIDISM
Causes and incidence
Hyperthyroidism may result from both genetic and immunologic factors. An increased incidence of this disorder in monozygotic twins, for example, points to an inherited factor, probably an autosomal recessive gene. This disease occasionally coexists with abnormal iodine metabolism and other endocrine abnormalities, such as DM, hyperparathyroidism, and thyroiditis. Autoimmune hyperthyroidism such as Graves disease triggers the body to produce thyrotropin receptor antibodies and thyroid-stimulating immunoglobulins that bind to the receptors of the thyroid cells and stimulate them to overproduce, frequently resulting in goiter, and release excessive thyroid hormone. The incidence of Graves disease is highest between ages 30 and 40, especially in people with family histories of thyroid abnormalities; only 5% of hyperthyroid patients are younger than age 15.

In a patient with latent hyperthyroidism, excessive dietary intake of iodine and, possibly, stress can precipitate clinical hyperthyroidism. In a person with inadequately treated hyperthyroidism, stress—including surgery, infection, toxemia of pregnancy, and diabetic ketoacidosis—can precipitate thyroid storm. Thyroid storm—an acute exacerbation of hyperthyroidism—is an emergent hypermetabolic state caused by excessive levels of thyroid hormone that may lead to life-threatening cardiac, hepatic, or renal failure. (See *Other forms of hyperthyroidism*, page 560.)

Pathophysiology
Hyperthyroidism (thyrotoxicosis) results from overactive thyroid hormone production and secretion, resulting in increased serum levels of unbound thyroid hormones and an increase

Other forms of hyperthyroidism

◆ *Toxic adenoma*—a small, benign nodule in the thyroid gland that secretes thyroid hormone—is the second most common cause of hyperthyroidism. The cause of toxic adenoma is unknown; incidence is highest in the elderly. Clinical effects are essentially similar to those of Graves disease, except that toxic adenoma doesn't induce ophthalmopathy, pretibial myxedema, or acropachy. Presence of adenoma is confirmed by radioactive iodine (^{131}I) uptake and thyroid scan, which show a single hyperfunctioning nodule suppressing the rest of the gland. Treatment includes ^{131}I therapy or surgery to remove adenoma after antithyroid drugs achieve a euthyroid state.

◆ *Thyrotoxicosis factitia* results from chronic ingestion of thyroid hormone for thyrotropin suppression in patients with thyroid carcinoma or from thyroid hormone abuse by people who are trying to lose weight.

◆ *Functioning metastatic thyroid carcinoma* is a rare disease that causes excessive production of thyroid hormone.

◆ *Thyroid-stimulating hormone–secreting pituitary tumor* causes overproduction of thyroid hormone.

◆ *Subacute thyroiditis* is a virus-induced granulomatous inflammation of the thyroid, producing transient hyperthyroidism associated with fever, pain, pharyngitis, and tenderness in the thyroid gland.

◆ *Silent thyroiditis* is a self-limiting, transient form of hyperthyroidism, with histologic thyroiditis but no inflammatory symptoms.

◆ Osteoporosis
◆ Vitiligo and hyperpigmentation
◆ Corneal ulcers
◆ Graves ophthalmopathy
◆ Graves dermopathy (pretibial myxedema)
◆ Myasthenia gravis
◆ Impaired fertility
◆ Decreased libido
◆ Gynecomastia

Signs and symptoms

The classic features of hyperthyroidism are an enlarged thyroid (goiter), nervousness, heat intolerance, weight loss despite increased appetite, sweating, frequent stools or diarrhea, tremor, and palpitations. Exophthalmos is considered most characteristic but is absent in many patients with hyperthyroidism. Many other symptoms are common because hyperthyroidism profoundly affects virtually every body system.

◆ *Central nervous system*—difficulty in concentrating because increased T_4 secretion accelerates cerebral function; excitability or nervousness due to increased basal metabolic rate; fine tremor, shaky handwriting, and clumsiness from increased activity in the spinal cord area that controls muscle tone; emotional instability and mood swings, ranging from occasional outbursts to overt psychosis

◆ *Skin, hair, and nails*—smooth, warm, flushed skin (patient sleeps with minimal covers and little clothing); fine, soft hair; premature graying and increased hair loss in both sexes; friable nails and onycholysis (distal nail separated from the bed); pretibial myxedema (dermopathy), producing thickened skin, accentuated hair follicles, raised red patches of skin that are itchy and sometimes painful, with occasional nodule formation. (Microscopic examination shows increased mucin deposits.)

◆ *Cardiovascular system*—tachycardia; full, bounding pulse; wide pulse pressure; cardiomegaly; increased cardiac output and blood volume; visible point of maximal impulse; paroxysmal supraventricular tachycardia and atrial fibrillation (especially in the elderly); and, occasionally, systolic murmur at the left sternal border

◆ *Respiratory system*—dyspnea on exertion and at rest, possibly from cardiac decompensation and increased cellular oxygen utilization

◆ *GI system*—possible anorexia; nausea and vomiting due to increased GI motility and peristalsis; increased defecation; soft stools or, with severe disease, diarrhea; and liver enlargement

◆ *Musculoskeletal system*—weakness, fatigue, and muscle atrophy; rare coexistence with

in the body's basal metabolic rate. It can be caused by a disturbance at any point in the hypothalamic–pituitary–thyroid feedback axis. The most common type of hyperthyroidism (70% of cases) is Graves disease (diffuse toxic goiter), followed by toxic multinodular goiter (Plummer disease), toxic thyroid adenoma, and thyroiditis. With treatment, most patients can lead normal lives.

Complications

◆ *Cardiovascular* (most common in elderly)—arrhythmias, especially atrial fibrillation, cardiac insufficiency, cardiac decompression, and resistance to usual dosages of cardiac glycosides
◆ Muscle weakness and atrophy
◆ Paralysis

myasthenia gravis; generalized or localized paralysis associated with hypokalemia may occur; and occasional *acropachy*—soft-tissue swelling, accompanied by underlying bone changes where new bone formation occurs

♦ *Reproductive system*—in women, oligomenorrhea or amenorrhea, decreased fertility, higher incidence of spontaneous abortions; in men, gynecomastia due to increased estrogen levels; in both sexes, diminished libido

♦ *Eyes*—exophthalmos (from the combined effects of accumulation of mucopolysaccharides and fluids in the retro-orbital tissues that force the eyeball outward, and of lid retraction that produces the characteristic staring gaze); occasional inflammation of conjunctivae, corneas, or eye muscles; diplopia; and increased tearing

ALERT *When hyperthyroidism escalates to thyroid storm, these symptoms can be accompanied by extreme irritability, hypertension, tachycardia, congestive heart failure, vomiting, temperature up to 106° F (41.1° C), delirium, and coma.*

Diagnosis

The diagnosis of hyperthyroidism is usually straightforward and depends on a careful clinical history and physical examination, a high index of suspicion, and routine hormone determinations.

CONFIRMING DIAGNOSIS *The following tests confirm the disorder:*

♦ *Radioimmunoassay shows increased serum T_4 and T_3 concentrations.*

♦ *Thyroid scan reveals increased uptake of radioactive iodine (^{131}I). This test is contraindicated if the patient is pregnant.*

♦ *TSH levels are decreased.*

♦ *Ultrasonography confirms subclinical ophthalmopathy.*

♦ *Thyroid-stimulating immunoglobulin is positive in Graves disease.*

Treatment

A number of approaches are used to treat hyperthyroidism, primarily antithyroid drugs (propylthiouracil and methimazole), beta-blockers, radioactive iodine (^{131}I), and surgery. Appropriate surgical treatment depends on the size of the goiter, the causes, the patient's age and parity, and if the patient is an appropriate candidate for surgery.

Antithyroid drug therapy is used for children, young adults, pregnant females, and patients who refuse surgery or radioactive iodine treatment. Thyroid hormone antagonists are given to block thyroid hormone synthesis. Although hypermetabolic symptoms subside within 4 to

8 weeks after such therapy begins, the patient must continue the medication for 6 months to 2 years, depending on the clinical circumstances. Beta-adrenergic blockers may be given concomitantly to manage tachycardia and other peripheral effects of excessive hypersympathetic activity.

During pregnancy, antithyroid medication should be kept at the minimum dosage required to keep maternal thyroid function within the high-normal range until delivery and to minimize the risk of fetal hypothyroidism—even though most infants of hyperthyroid mothers are born with mild and transient hyperthyroidism.

PEDIATRIC TIP *Neonatal hyperthyroidism may even necessitate treatment with antithyroid medications and propranolol for 2 to 3 months.*

Because hyperthyroidism is sometimes exacerbated in the puerperal period, continuous control of maternal thyroid function is essential. About 3 to 6 months postpartum, antithyroid drug administration can be gradually tapered and thyroid function reassessed. The mother receiving low-dose antithyroid treatment may breast-feed as long as the infant's thyroid function is checked periodically. Small amounts of the drug can be found in breast milk.

A single oral dose of ^{131}I is the treatment of choice for patients not planning to have children. (Patients of reproductive age must not be pregnant and should give informed consent for this treatment because small amounts of ^{131}I concentrate in the gonads. However, there have been no reports of damage to subsequently conceived children in >50 years of ^{131}I use.) During treatment with radioactive iodine, the thyroid gland picks up the radioactive element as it would regular iodine. Subsequently, the radioactivity destroys some of the cells that normally concentrate iodine and produce T_4, thus decreasing thyroid hormone production and normalizing thyroid size and function. In most patients, hypermetabolic symptoms diminish from 6 to 8 weeks after such treatment. However, some patients may require a second dose. Radioactive iodine permanently cures hyperthyroidism by destroying the thyroid tissue, so patients who receive this treatment will then have to take thyroid replacement hormones for the rest of their lives.

Subtotal (partial) thyroidectomy, which decreases the thyroid gland's capacity for hormone production, is indicated for patients with a large goiter whose hyperthyroidism has repeatedly relapsed after drug therapy or patients who refuse or aren't candidates for ^{131}I treatment.

Preoperatively, the patient may receive iodides (Lugol solution or saturated solution of potassium iodide), antithyroid drugs, or high doses of propranolol to help prevent thyroid storm. If euthyroidism isn't achieved, surgery should be delayed and propranolol administered to decrease the systemic effects (cardiac arrhythmias) caused by hyperthyroidism. After ablative treatment with ^{131}I or surgery, patients require regular medical supervision for the rest of their lives because they usually develop hypothyroidism, sometimes as long as several years after treatment.

Therapy for hyperthyroid ophthalmopathy includes local applications of topical medications but may require high doses of corticosteroids. A patient with severe exophthalmos that causes pressure on the optic nerve may require external beam radiation therapy or surgical decompression to lessen pressure on the orbital contents.

Treatment of thyroid storm includes administration of an antithyroid drug, propranolol I.V. to block sympathetic effects, a corticosteroid to inhibit the conversion of T_4 to T_3 and to replace depleted cortisol levels, and an iodide to block the release of thyroid hormone. Supportive measures include administration of nutrients, vitamins, fluids, and sedatives.

Special considerations

Patients with hyperthyroidism require vigilant care to prevent acute exacerbations and complications.

♦ Record vital signs and weight.
♦ Monitor serum electrolyte levels, and check periodically for hyperglycemia and glycosuria.

✿ **ELDER TIP** *Carefully monitor cardiac function if the patient is elderly or has coronary artery disease. If the heart rate is more than 100 beats/minute, check blood pressure and pulse rate often.*

♦ *Check level of consciousness and urine output.*

ALERT *If the patient is pregnant, tell her to watch closely during the first trimester for signs of spontaneous abortion and to report such signs immediately.*

♦ Encourage bed rest, and keep the patient's room cool, quiet, and dark. The patient with dyspnea will be most comfortable sitting upright or in high Fowler position.
♦ Remember, extreme nervousness may produce erratic behaviors. Reassure the patient and their family that such behavior will probably subside with treatment. Provide sedatives as necessary.
♦ To promote weight gain, provide a balanced diet, with six meals a day. If the patient has edema, suggest a low-sodium diet.

♦ If iodide is part of the treatment, mix it with milk, juice, or water to prevent GI distress, and administer it through a straw to prevent tooth discoloration.

ALERT *Watch for signs of thyroid storm, such as tachycardia, hyperkinesis, fever, vomiting, and hypertension.*

♦ Check intake and output carefully to ensure adequate hydration and fluid balance.
♦ Closely monitor blood pressure, cardiac rate and rhythm, and temperature. If the patient has a high fever, reduce it with appropriate hypothermic measures. Maintain an I.V. line and give drugs, as ordered.
♦ If the patient has exophthalmos or other ophthalmopathy, suggest sunglasses or eye patches to protect their eyes from light. Moisten the conjunctivae often with isotonic eye drops. Warn the patient with severe lid retraction to avoid sudden physical movements that might cause the lid to slip behind the eyeball. The patient should avoid potential eye irritants such as cigarette smoke.
♦ Avoid excessive palpation of the thyroid to avoid precipitating thyroid storm.

Thyroidectomy necessitates meticulous postoperative care to prevent complications:
♦ Watch for evidence of hemorrhage into the neck, such as a tight dressing with no blood on it. Change dressings and perform wound care, as ordered; check the *back* of the dressing for drainage. Keep the patient in semi-Fowler position, and support the head and neck to ease tension on the incision.
♦ Check for dysphagia or hoarseness from possible laryngeal nerve injury.
♦ Watch for signs of hypoparathyroidism (tetany, numbness), a complication that results from accidental removal of the parathyroid glands during surgery.
♦ Stress the importance of regular medical follow-up after discharge because hypothyroidism may develop from 2 to 4 weeks postoperatively.

ALERT *Check often for respiratory distress, and keep a tracheotomy tray at bedside.*

Drug therapy and ^{131}I therapy require careful monitoring and comprehensive patient teaching:
♦ After ^{131}I therapy, tell the patient not to expectorate or cough freely because their saliva will be radioactive for 24 hours. Stress the need for repeated measurement of serum T_4 levels.
♦ If the patient is taking propylthiouracil and methimazole, monitor complete blood count periodically to detect leukopenia, thrombocytopenia, and agranulocytosis. Instruct the patient to take these medications with meals to minimize GI distress and to avoid over-the-counter

cough preparations because many contain iodine. Monitor hepatic function. Stop drug if liver abnormality occurs.

◆ Tell the patient to report fever, enlarged cervical lymph nodes, sore throat, mouth sores, and other signs of blood dyscrasias and any rash or skin eruptions—signs of hypersensitivity.

◆ Watch the patient taking propranolol for signs of hypotension (dizziness, decreased urine output). Tell the patient to rise slowly after sitting or lying down to prevent orthostatic syncope.

◆ Instruct the patient receiving antithyroid drugs or ^{131}I therapy to report any symptoms of hypothyroidism.

Parathyroid glands

PATHOPHYSIOLOGY

Humans generally have four parathyroid glands located in the neck just posterior to the thyroid gland. The primary function of these glands is the production and secretion of PTH which regulates homeostasis of calcium in the blood. Secretion of PTH stimulates osteoclast activity causing the bones to release calcium, inhibits osteoblasts sparing existent blood calcium, and increases reabsorption of calcium and magnesium in the renal tubules as well as stimulating the kidneys to produce calcitriol (the active form of vitamin D_3) resulting in increased absorption of dietary calcium in the gut. PTH is secreted when low blood calcium levels are detected; conversely, rising levels inhibit further release via stimulation of release of calcitonin from the thyroid gland.

HYPOPARATHYROIDISM

Causes and incidence

Hypoparathyroidism may be acute or chronic and is classified as idiopathic or acquired. The acquired form may also be reversible. *Idiopathic hypoparathyroidism* may result from an autoimmune genetic disorder or the congenital absence of the parathyroid glands. Congenital hypoparathyroid disorders can have an autosomal recessive, autosomal dominant, X-linked, or mitochondrial inheritance pattern. *Acquired hypoparathyroidism* commonly results from accidental removal of or injury to one or more parathyroid glands during thyroidectomy or other neck surgery (incidence 0.12% to 4.6%); rarely it results from massive thyroid irradiation. It may also result from ischemic infarction of the parathyroids during surgery or from hemochromatosis, sarcoidosis, amyloidosis, tuberculosis, neoplasms, or trauma. An *acquired,*

reversible hypoparathyroidism may result from hypomagnesemia-induced impairment of hormone synthesis, from suppression of normal gland function due to hypercalcemia, or from delayed maturation of parathyroid function. Most patients with acquired hypoparathyroidism recover; to be classified as a chronic disorder, symptoms must persist for greater than 6 months. (See *What happens in acute hypoparathyroidism,* page 564.)

PTH isn't regulated by the pituitary or hypothalamus. It normally maintains blood calcium levels by increasing bone resorption and GI absorption of calcium. It also maintains an inverse relationship between serum calcium and phosphate levels by inhibiting phosphate reabsorption in the renal tubules. Abnormal PTH production disrupts this balance. The incidence is 4 of 100,000 people. The incidence of the idiopathic and reversible forms is highest in children; that of the irreversible acquired form, in older patients who have undergone surgery for hyperthyroidism or other head and neck conditions. The prevalence in the United States is 60,000 to 115,000, most of whom are greater than 45 years of age. Frequency is greater in females than in males at a rate of 3:1.

Pathophysiology

Hypoparathyroidism is a deficiency of PTH caused by disease, injury (usually surgical), or congenital malfunction of the parathyroid glands. PTH deficiency can lead to extremely low levels of blood calcium (hypocalcemia), the physiologic effects of which are decreased absorption of dietary calcium, renal calcium absorption, alteration in phosphate concentration, and decreased skeletal bone resorption. Hypocalcemia usually produces neuromuscular, cardiac, cognitive, and muscular symptoms. The clinical effects of hypoparathyroidism are usually correctable with replacement therapy. However, some complications of this disorder, such as cataracts and basal ganglion calcifications, are irreversible.

Complications

◆ Tetany
◆ Loss of consciousness
◆ Osteoporosis
◆ Developmental delay in children
◆ Cataracts
◆ Arrhythmias

Signs and symptoms

Although mild hypoparathyroidism may be asymptomatic, it usually produces hypocalcemia and high serum phosphate levels that affect the

PATHOPHYSIOLOGY
What happens in acute hypoparathyroidism

Causes of acute hypoparathyroidism include injury to the glands, accidental removal of the parathyroid glands during thyroidectomy or other neck surgery, autoimmune disease, tumor, tuberculosis, sarcoidosis, hemochromatosis, and severe magnesium deficiency associated with alcoholism and intestinal malabsorption. These disorders and conditions cause a cascade of effects that result in severe hypocalcemia and hyperphosphatemia, which can lead to seizures, tetany, laryngospasm, and central nervous system (CNS) abnormalities, as shown in the flow chart below.

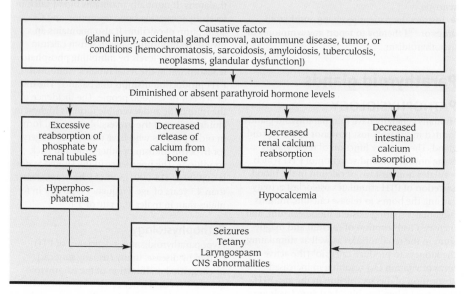

CNS as well as other body systems. Chronic hypoparathyroidism typically causes neuromuscular irritability, increased deep tendon reflexes, Chvostek sign (hyperirritability of the facial nerve, producing a characteristic spasm when it's tapped), dysphagia, organic brain syndrome, psychosis, intellectual disability in children, and tetany.

Acute (overt) tetany begins with a tingling in the fingertips, around the mouth, and, occasionally, in the feet. This tingling spreads and becomes more severe, producing muscle tension and spasms and consequent adduction of the thumbs, wrists, and elbows. Pain varies with the degree of muscle tension but seldom affects the face, legs, or feet. Chronic tetany is usually unilateral and less severe; it may cause difficulty in walking and a tendency to fall. Both forms of tetany can lead to laryngospasm, stridor, and, eventually, cyanosis. They may also cause seizures. These CNS abnormalities tend to be exaggerated during hyperventilation, pregnancy, infection, withdrawal of thyroid hormone, therapy with loop diuretics, and before menstruation.

Other clinical effects include abdominal pain; dry, lusterless hair; spontaneous hair loss; brittle fingernails that develop ridges or fall out; dry, scaly skin; cataracts; and weakened tooth enamel, which causes teeth to stain, crack, and decay easily. Hypocalcemia may induce cardiac arrhythmias and may eventually lead to heart failure.

Postsurgically hypoparathyroidism can present with acute tachycardia, tetany, cramping, and altered mental status.

Diagnosis
An evaluation for hypoparathyroidism requires a complete family history for potential genetic mutations or deletions and autoimmune disorders, complete medical history and surgical history for prior thyroid, parathyroid, or neck surgery. Physical examination is completed to evaluate for any scarring around the neck, cataracts, signs of tetany, short stature, and intellectual delay.

℞ **CONFIRMING DIAGNOSIS** *Primary hypoparathyroidism is characterized by hypocalcemia with concomitant absent or low PTH level. Patients with pseudohypoparathyroidism will have elevated PTH concentrations. In secondary hypoparathyroidism the PTH concentration is low but the serum calcium level is elevated.*

♦ *PTH assay: absent or inappropriately low PTH concentration*
  ♦ *PTH can be screened using second- or third-generation assay*
♦ *Albumin adjusted calcium concentration: decreased*
  ♦ *Confirmed on at least two occasions separated by at least 2 weeks*
  ♦ *25-hydroxy-vitamin D should be measured to exclude vitamin D deficiency as the causative factor for hypocalcemia*
♦ *Serum phosphorus: upper normal or frankly elevated*
♦ *Urine calcium: increased*
♦ *Serum magnesium: decreased*
  ♦ *Hypomagnesemia can cause PTH deficiency followed by hypocalcemia*
♦ *Electrocardiogram: prolonged QT and ST intervals due to hypocalcemia*
♦ *Genetic studies should be done if there is an appropriate family history, multiple endocrine gland failure, or hypoparathyroidism is diagnosed at a young age*

Inflating a blood pressure cuff on the upper arm to between diastolic and systolic blood pressure and maintaining this inflation for 3 minutes elicits Trousseau sign (carpal spasm), thereby provoking clinical evidence of hypoparathyroidism.

Treatment

Because calcium absorption from the small intestine requires the presence of vitamin D, treatment includes vitamin D and calcium supplements. Therapy is usually lifelong, except for the reversible form of the disease. If the patient can't tolerate the pure form of vitamin D, alternatives include dihydrotachysterol, if hepatic and renal function is adequate, and calcitriol, if it's severely compromised. In patients with preexisting hypomagnesemia, this condition must be corrected to treat the resulting hypocalcemia. A high-calcium, low-phosphorus diet is recommended.

Acute life-threatening tetany requires immediate I.V. administration of calcium salts followed by calcium gluconate to raise serum calcium levels. The patient who's awake and able to cooperate can help raise serum calcium levels by breathing into a paper bag and then inhaling their own carbon dioxide; this produces hypoventilation and mild respiratory acidosis. Sedatives and anticonvulsants may control spasms until calcium levels rise. Chronic tetany requires maintenance therapy with oral calcium and vitamin D supplements.

Special considerations

⚠ **ALERT** *While awaiting diagnosis of hypoparathyroidism in a patient with a history of tetany, maintain a patent I.V. line and keep I.V. calcium available. Because the patient is vulnerable to seizures, maintain seizure precautions. Also, keep a tracheotomy tray and endotracheal tube at the bedside because laryngospasm may result from hypocalcemia.*

♦ Instruct the patient to follow a high-calcium, low-phosphorus diet.
♦ When caring for a patient on thiazide diuretics used to manage hypercalciuria, encourage low salt diet.
♦ When caring for the patient with chronic disease, particularly a child, stay alert for minor muscle twitching and for signs of laryngospasm because these effects may signal the onset of tetany.
♦ For the patient on drug therapy, emphasize the importance of checking serum and 24-hour urine calcium levels at least three times a year. Instruct the patient to watch for signs of hypercalcemia and to keep medications away from light and heat.
♦ Dental changes, cataracts, and brain calcifications are permanent. These can be prevented with early detection and periodic calcium determinations.

⚠ **ALERT** *Because the patient with chronic disease has prolonged QT intervals on ECG, watch for heart block and signs of decreasing cardiac output. Because calcium potentiates the effect of cardiac glycosides, closely monitor the patient receiving both a cardiac glycoside and calcium. Stay alert for signs of digoxin toxicity, such as arrhythmias, nausea, fatigue, and vision changes.*

♦ Instruct the patient with scaly skin to use creams to soften their skin. Also, tell the patient to keep their nails trimmed to prevent them from splitting.
♦ Hyperventilation or recent blood transfusions may worsen tetany. (Anticoagulant in stored blood binds calcium.)
♦ For the patient with tetany, administer 10% calcium gluconate by slow I.V. infusion (1 mL/minute), and maintain a patent airway. The patient may also require intubation and sedation. Monitor vital signs often after sedation to make certain that blood pressure and heart rate return to normal.

HYPERPARATHYROIDISM

Causes and incidence

Hyperparathyroidism can be categorized as primary or secondary. Primary hyperparathyroidism (PHPT) is characterized by hypercalcemia and elevated levels of serum PTH. Less commonly a variant of hyperparathyroidism results in hypercalcemia in conjunction with normal PTH levels. Eighty percent of cases of PHPT are caused by a single parathyroid adenoma followed by rare cases of multiple parathyroid gland involvement, inherited hyperparathyroidism, and parathyroid cancer. PHPT usually occurs between ages 30 and 50 but can also occur in children and the elderly. It affects two to three times more females than males. It's a common disorder, affecting 1 in 1,000 people.

Secondary hyperparathyroidism is caused by a disease outside of the parathyroid glands which causes enlargement in all four parathyroid glands. It is an excessive compensatory production of PTH stemming from a hypocalcemia-producing abnormality outside the parathyroid gland, which causes a resistance to the metabolic action of PTH. The most common cause is kidney failure with resultant elevations in elevated phosphorus, decreased calcitriol, and hypocalcemia. The chronic nature of that imbalance causes constant stimulation of the parathyroid glands resulting in enlargement and excessive secretion of PTH. Less commonly secondary hyperparathyroidism is caused by long-term use of the medication Lithium, severe vitamin D deficiency, malnutrition, malabsorptive syndromes of the GI tract, and hypermagnesemia.

Pathophysiology

Hyperparathyroidism is characterized by overactivity of one or more of the parathyroid glands resulting in excessive secretion of PTH. Hypersecretion of PTH promotes excessive bone resorption and leads to hypercalcemia and hypophosphatemia resulting in decreased bone density, spontaneous fractures, bone deformities, and increased formation of renal calculi as a result of increased renal and GI absorption of calcium.

Complications

◆ Osteoporosis
◆ Renal calculi
◆ Renal failure
◆ Hypertension
◆ Peptic ulcers
◆ Cardiac arrhythmias
◆ Heart failure
◆ Diabetes mellitus

Signs and symptoms

Clinical effects of PHPT result from hypercalcemia and are typically present in several body systems.

◆ *Renal system*—nephrocalcinosis due to elevated levels of calcium and, possibly, recurring nephrolithiasis, which may lead to renal insufficiency. Renal manifestations, including polyuria, are the most common effects of hyperparathyroidism.

◆ *Skeletal and articular system*—chronic low back pain and easy fracturing due to bone degeneration; bone tenderness; chondrocalcinosis; occasional severe osteopenia, especially on the vertebrae; erosions of the juxta-articular surface; subchondral fractures; traumatic synovitis; and pseudogout

◆ *GI system*—pancreatitis, causing constant, severe epigastric pain radiating to the back; peptic ulcers, causing abdominal pain, anorexia, nausea, and vomiting

◆ *Neuromuscular system*—marked muscle weakness and atrophy, particularly in the legs

◆ *Central nervous system*—psychomotor and personality disturbances, depression, overt psychosis, stupor, and, possibly, coma

◆ *Other*—skin necrosis, cataracts, calcium microthrombi to lungs and pancreas, polyuria, anemia, and subcutaneous calcification

Similarly, in secondary hyperparathyroidism, decreased serum calcium levels may produce the same features as calcium imbalance, with skeletal deformities of the long bones (e.g., rickets) as well as symptoms of the underlying disease.

Diagnosis

Requires a careful history for objective renal and skeletal manifestation, such as nephrolithiasis, fragility fractures and osteoporosis, as well as subjective symptoms such as neuropsychiatric, cognitive, musculoskeletal, and GI complaints.

℞ CONFIRMING DIAGNOSIS *To establish diagnosis in primary disease, a persistently elevated concentration of second- or third-generation assay PTH with concomitant elevated total serum calcium on more than one occasion should be measured as normo-calcemic primary hyperparathyroid variant may be present.*

Laboratory tests: serum total calcium, 24-hour urinary calcium and creatinine, PTH, serum creatinine, 5-hydroxy-vitamin D, chloride, and alkaline phosphatase levels and a decreased phosphatase level.

Hyperparathyroidism may also raise uric acid and creatinine levels and increase basal acid secretion and serum immunoreactive gastrin. Increased serum amylase levels may indicate acute pancreatitis.

Laboratory findings in secondary hyperparathyroidism show normal or slightly decreased serum calcium levels and variable serum phosphorus levels. Phosphorus can be quite elevated, especially in osteomalacia or renal disease. Patient history may reveal familial renal disease, seizure disorders, or drug ingestion. Other laboratory values and physical examination findings identify the cause of secondary hyperparathyroidism.

The American Association of Endocrine Surgeons Guidelines 2016 recommend:
◆ Bone mineral density screening at the lumbar spine, hip, and distal radius using DXA
◆ Genetic counseling for patients younger than 40 diagnosed with hyperparathyroidism or multiglandular disease

Treatment

Treatment varies, depending on the cause of the disease. The only definitive treatment of PHPT is parathyroidectomy. Recent meta-analyses show that observational and pharmacologic therapies are less effective even when the patient is asymptomatic. Surgery is indicated for all symptomatic patients and for asymptomatic patients when the serum calcium level is greater than 1 mg/dL above normal. Surgery may relieve bone pain within 3 days. Development of new kidney stones should decrease significantly; however, renal damage such as insufficiency and nephrocalcinosis may be irreversible, though declining glomerular filtration rate should be stabilized.

Preoperatively—or if surgery isn't feasible or necessary—other treatments can decrease calcium levels. These include forcing fluids; limiting dietary intake of calcium; promoting sodium and calcium excretion through forced diuresis using normal saline solution (up to 6 L in life-threatening circumstances), furosemide, or ethacrynic acid; and administering oral sodium or potassium phosphate, subcutaneous calcitonin, I.V. plicamycin, or I.V. bisphosphonates.

Therapy for potential postoperative magnesium and phosphate deficiencies includes I.V. administration of magnesium and phosphate, or sodium phosphate solution given orally or by retention enema. In addition, during the first 4 to 5 days after surgery, when serum calcium falls to low normal levels, supplemental calcium may be necessary; vitamin D or calcitriol may also be used to raise serum calcium levels.

Treatment of secondary hyperparathyroidism must correct the underlying cause of parathyroid hypertrophy. Vitamin D therapy or, in the patient with renal disease, administration of an oral calcium preparation (calcium acetate, if possible) for hyperphosphatemia is typically used, although surgical excision may be necessary. In the patient with renal failure, dialysis is necessary to lower calcium levels and may have to continue for the remainder of the patient's life. A new class of drugs, the calcimimetics, has been approved for secondary hyperparathyroidism. These drugs act by turning off the secretion of PTH. In the patient with chronic secondary hyperparathyroidism, the enlarged glands may not revert to normal size and function even after calcium levels have been controlled.

Special considerations

Care emphasizes prevention of complications from the underlying disease and its treatment.
◆ Obtain pretreatment baseline serum potassium, calcium, phosphate, and magnesium levels because these values may change abruptly during treatment.
◆ During hydration to reduce serum calcium level, record intake and output accurately. Strain urine to check for calculi. Provide at least 3 qt (3 L) of fluid a day, including cranberry or prune juice to increase urine acidity and help prevent calculus formation. As ordered, obtain blood and urine samples to measure sodium, potassium, and magnesium levels, especially for the patient taking furosemide.
◆ Auscultate for breath sounds often. Listen for signs of pulmonary edema in the patient receiving large amounts of saline solution I.V., especially if the patient has pulmonary or cardiac disease. Monitor the patient on cardiac glycosides carefully because elevated calcium levels can rapidly produce toxic effects.
◆ Because the patient is predisposed to pathologic fractures, take safety precautions to minimize the risk of injury. Assist the patient with walking, keep the bed at its lowest position, and raise the side rails. Lift the immobilized patient carefully to minimize bone stress. Schedule care to allow the patient with muscle weakness as much rest as possible.
◆ Watch for signs of peptic ulcer and administer antacids, as appropriate.

After parathyroidectomy:
◆ Check frequently for respiratory distress, and keep a tracheotomy tray at the bedside. Watch for postoperative complications, such as cervical hematoma, laryngeal nerve damage, or, rarely, hemorrhage. Monitor intake and output carefully.
◆ Check for swelling at the operative site. Place the patient in semi-Fowler position, and support their head and neck to decrease edema, which may cause pressure on the trachea.

◆ Watch for signs of mild tetany, such as complaints of tingling in the hands and around the mouth. These symptoms should subside quickly but may be prodromal signs of tetany, so keep calcium gluconate or calcium chloride I.V. available for emergency administration. Watch for increased neuromuscular irritability and other signs of severe tetany, and report them immediately. Ambulate the patient as soon as possible postoperatively, even though the patient may find this uncomfortable, because pressure on bones speeds up bone recalcification.

◆ Check laboratory results for low serum calcium, magnesium, and vitamin D levels.

◆ Monitor mental status and watch for listlessness. In the patient with persistent hypercalcemia, check for muscle weakness and psychiatric symptoms.

◆ Before discharge, advise the patient of the possible adverse effects of drug therapy. Emphasize the need for periodic follow-up through laboratory blood tests (calcium, PTH, 25-hydroxy-vitamin D, and magnesium). If hyperparathyroidism wasn't corrected surgically, warn the patient to avoid calcium-containing antacids and thiazide diuretics.

⁞⁞⁞⁞⁞ PREVENTION *Secondary hyperparathyroidism may be prevented by adequate intake of calcium in the diet or by the addition of calcium supplements and adequate vitamin D supplements.*

Adrenal glands

ADRENAL HYPOFUNCTION

Causes and incidence

Adrenal hypofunction occurs when more than 90% of both adrenal glands are destroyed, an occurrence that typically results from an autoimmune process in which circulating antibodies react specifically against the adrenal tissue. Other causes include tuberculosis (once the chief cause; now responsible for <20% of adult cases), bilateral adrenalectomy, hemorrhage into the adrenal gland, neoplasms, and infections (acquired immunodeficiency syndrome, histoplasmosis, and cytomegalovirus). Rarely, a familial tendency to autoimmune disease predisposes the patient to adrenal hypofunction and other endocrinopathies.

Secondary adrenal hypofunction that results in glucocorticoid deficiency can stem from hypopituitarism (causing decreased corticotropin secretion), abrupt withdrawal of long-term corticosteroid therapy (long-term exogenous corticosteroid stimulation suppresses pituitary corticotropin secretion and results in adrenal gland atrophy), or removal of a nonendocrine, corticotropin-secreting tumor. Adrenal crisis (addisonian crisis), a critical deficiency of mineralocorticoids and glucocorticoids, generally follows acute stress, sepsis, trauma, surgery, or omission of steroid therapy in patients who have chronic adrenal insufficiency. A medical emergency, adrenal crisis necessitates immediate, vigorous treatment.

A relatively uncommon disorder, adrenal hypofunction can occur at any age and in both sexes. Adrenal hypofunction affects 1 in 16,000 neonates congenitally. In adults, it affects 8 in 100,000 people, and males and females are affected equally. There's no racial predilection.

Pathophysiology

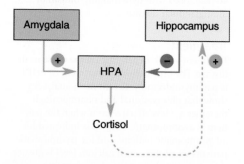

Adrenal insufficiency is an endocrine disorder resulting from insufficient production of hormones from the adrenal gland. The hypothalamic–pituitary–adrenal axis governs the production and secretion of ACTH in the anterior pituitary as well as aldosterone and cortisol in the adrenal cortex via negative feedback loops.

Adrenal insufficiency can be primary or secondary. Primary adrenal insufficiency, also called Addison disease, is characterized by a deficiency of the glucocorticoid hormone cortisol. This deficiency results from hypofunction of the adrenal cortex secondary to idiopathic atrophy, granulomatous disease, or certain medications that suppress cortisol synthesis. There may also be a deficiency of the mineralocorticoid aldosterone. Secondary adrenal insufficiency results from deficient production of adrenocorticotropin hormone (ACTH) in the pituitary gland. A normally functioning pituitary secretes ACTH to stimulate production of glucocorticoids and mineralocorticoids in the adrenal gland. Lack of stimulation via ACTH causes the adrenal glands to decrease hormone production and eventually atrophy. Secondary adrenal insufficiency is more common than primary adrenal insufficiency.

Complication

◆ Adrenal crisis

Signs and symptoms

Adrenal hypofunction typically produces such effects as hypovolemia, hypotension, hyponatremia, hypokalemia, fever, abdominal pain, weakness, fatigue, weight loss, and various GI disturbances, such as nausea, vomiting, anorexia, and chronic diarrhea. When primary, the disorder usually causes hyperpigmentation—a conspicuous bronze coloration of the skin. The patient appears to be deeply suntanned, especially in the creases of the hands and over the metacarpophalangeal joints, the elbows, and the knees. The patient may also exhibit a darkening of scars, areas of vitiligo (absence of pigmentation), and increased pigmentation of the mucous membranes, especially the gingival mucosa. Abnormal skin and mucous membrane coloration results from decreased secretion of cortisol (one of the glucocorticoids), which causes the pituitary gland to simultaneously secrete excessive amounts of corticotropin and melanocyte-stimulating hormone (MSH). Children with unexplained hypoglycemia should be screened for primary adrenal insufficiency.

Associated cardiovascular abnormalities in adrenal hypofunction include orthostatic hypotension, decreased cardiac size and output, and a weak, irregular pulse. Other clinical effects include decreased tolerance for even minor stress, poor coordination, fasting hypoglycemia (due to decreased *gluconeogenesis*), and a craving for salty food. Adrenal hypofunction may also delay axillary and pubic hair growth in females, decrease the libido (from decreased androgen production), and, in severe cases, cause amenorrhea.

Secondary adrenal hypofunction produces similar clinical effects but without hyperpigmentation because corticotropin and MSH levels are low. Because aldosterone secretion may continue at fairly normal levels in secondary adrenal hypofunction, this condition doesn't necessarily cause accompanying hypotension and electrolyte abnormalities.

ALERT *Adrenal crisis produces profound weakness, fatigue, nausea, vomiting, hypovolemia, hyponatremia, hyperkalemia, hypotension, dehydration, and, occasionally, high fever followed by hypothermia. If untreated, this condition can ultimately lead to vascular collapse, renal shutdown, coma, and death.*

Diagnosis

Diagnosis requires demonstration of decreased corticosteroid concentrations in plasma and an accurate classification of adrenal hypofunction as primary or secondary. If secondary adrenal hypofunction is suspected, the metyrapone test is indicated. This test requires oral or I.V. administration of metyrapone, which blocks cortisol production and should stimulate the release of corticotropin from the hypothalamic–pituitary system. In adrenal hypofunction, the hypothalamic–pituitary system responds normally, and plasma reveals high levels of corticotropin; however, plasma levels of cortisol precursor and urinary concentrations of 17-hydroxycorticosteroids don't rise.

The Endocrine Society's 2016 Guidelines recommend confirming diagnosis of primary adrenal insufficiency with a corticotropin stimulation test if the patient's condition is suitable. The corticotropin stimulation test involves injecting 250 µg of synthetic ACTH and the amount of cortisol and aldosterone produced by the adrenal glands in response is measured. This test allows the provider to distinguish between primary and secondary adrenal insufficiency.

- Primary adrenal insufficiency—low cortisol (levels <18 µg/dL at 30 to 60 minutes), low aldosterone, elevated plasma renin
- Secondary adrenal insufficiency—low ACTH

If both corticotropin and cortisol are low, the long corticotropin test may be done. The test involves I.V. administration of corticotropin over 6 to 8 hours, after samples have been obtained to determine baseline plasma cortisol and 24-hour urine cortisol levels. In adrenal hypofunction, plasma and urine cortisol levels fail to rise normally in response to corticotropin; in secondary hypofunction, repeated doses of corticotropin over successive days produce a gradual increase in cortisol levels until normal values are reached.

In a patient with typical addisonian symptoms, the following laboratory findings strongly suggest acute adrenal hypofunction:

- Decreased cortisol levels in plasma (<10 µg/dL in the morning, with lower levels in the evening); however, this test is time-consuming, and emergency therapy shouldn't be postponed for test results
- Decreased serum sodium and fasting blood glucose levels
- Increased serum potassium and blood urea nitrogen levels
- Elevated hematocrit and lymphocyte and eosinophil counts
- X-rays showing a small heart and adrenal calcification

Treatment

For all patients with primary or secondary adrenal hypofunction, glucocorticoid replacement, usually with cortisone or hydrocortisone (both of which also have a mineralocorticoid effect), is the primary treatment and must continue throughout life. Adrenal hypofunction with confirmed aldosterone deficiency necessitates treatment with oral fludrocortisone, a synthetic mineralocorticoid, which prevents dangerous dehydration and hypotension.

Adrenal crisis requires prompt I.V. bolus administration of hydrocortisone and fluid resuscitation. Later, doses are given I.M. or are diluted with dextrose in saline solution and given I.V. until the patient's condition stabilizes.

With proper treatment, adrenal crisis usually subsides quickly; the patient's blood pressure should stabilize, and water and sodium levels should return to normal. After the crisis, maintenance doses of hydrocortisone preserve physiologic stability.

Special considerations

In adrenal crisis, monitor vital signs carefully, especially for hypotension, volume depletion, and other signs of shock (decreased level of consciousness and urine output). Watch for hyperkalemia before treatment and for hypokalemia after treatment (from excessive mineralocorticoid effect).

◆ If the patient also has diabetes, check blood glucose levels periodically because steroid replacement may require adjustment of insulin dosage.

◆ Record weight and intake and output carefully because the patient may have volume depletion. Until onset of mineralocorticoid effect, force fluids to replace excessive fluid loss.

To manage the patient receiving maintenance therapy:

◆ Arrange for a diet that maintains sodium and potassium balances.

◆ If the patient is anorexic, suggest six small meals a day to increase calorie intake. Ask the dietitian to provide a diet high in protein and carbohydrates. Keep a late-morning snack available in case the patient becomes hypoglycemic.

◆ Observe the patient receiving steroids for cushingoid signs such as fluid retention around the eyes and face. Watch for fluid and electrolyte imbalance, especially if the patient is receiving mineralocorticoids. Monitor weight and check blood pressure to assess body fluid status. Remember, steroids administered in the late afternoon or evening may cause stimulation of the CNS and insomnia in some patients. Check for petechiae because the patient bruises easily.

◆ Patients receiving mineralocorticoid replacement should be assessed for electrolyte imbalances, hypertension, postural hypotension, and edema. Patients with uncontrolled hypertension

should be started on a dehypertensive treatment and instructed not to stop their fludrocortisone.

◆ If the patient receives glucocorticoids alone, monitor for orthostatic hypotension or electrolyte abnormalities, which may indicate a need for mineralocorticoid therapy.

◆ Explain that lifelong steroid therapy is necessary.

◆ Teach the patient the symptoms of too great or too little a dose.

◆ Tell the patient that dosage may need to be increased during times of stress (e.g., when they have a cold).

◆ Warn that infection, injury, or profuse sweating in hot weather may precipitate adrenal crisis.

◆ Warn the patient that any stress may necessitate additional cortisone to prevent adrenal crisis.

◆ Instruct the patient to always carry a medical identification card stating that they take a steroid and giving the name of the drug and the dosage.

◆ Tell the patient to keep an emergency kit available containing hydrocortisone in a prepared syringe for use in times of stress.

◆ Teach the patient how to give himself or herself an injection of hydrocortisone.

◆ Pregnant women with primary adrenal insufficiency (PAI) should be monitored for signs of over or under replacement of glucocorticoids via routine measurements of weight, blood pressure for postural hypotension or hypertension, hyperglycemia, and fatigue each trimester. Increased hydrocortisone dosage may be needed during the third trimester.

◆ Women with low libido and depressive symptoms in PAI may benefit from a 6-month trial of dehydroepiandrosterone (DHEA). DHEA replacement can be measured via morning serum DHEA sulfate levels.

CUSHING SYNDROME

Cushing syndrome is a cluster of clinical abnormalities caused by excessive levels of adrenocortical hormones (particularly cortisol) or related corticosteroids and, to a lesser extent, androgens and aldosterone. Its unmistakable signs include rapidly developing adiposity of the face (moon face), neck, and trunk and purple striae on the skin. (See *Symptoms of cushingoid syndrome,* page 571.) The prognosis depends on the underlying cause; it's poor in untreated people and in those with untreatable ectopic corticotropin-producing carcinoma.

Causes and incidence

In approximately 70% of patients, Cushing syndrome results from excessive production of corticotropin and consequent hyperplasia of the adrenal cortex. Overproduction of corticotropin may stem from pituitary hypersecretion

Symptoms of cushingoid syndrome

Chronic depression, alcoholism, and long-term treatment with corticosteroids may produce an adverse effect called *cushingoid syndrome*—a condition marked by obvious fat deposits between the shoulders and around the waist, and widespread systemic abnormalities.

Differentiating between cushingoid syndrome and Cushing syndrome can be difficult, so in addition to the symptoms shown in the illustration on the right, observe for signs of hypertension, renal disorders, hyperglycemia, tissue wasting, muscle weakness, and labile emotional state. The patient may also have amenorrhea and glycosuria.

Resolution of the underlying disorder results in disappearance of cushingoid symptoms.

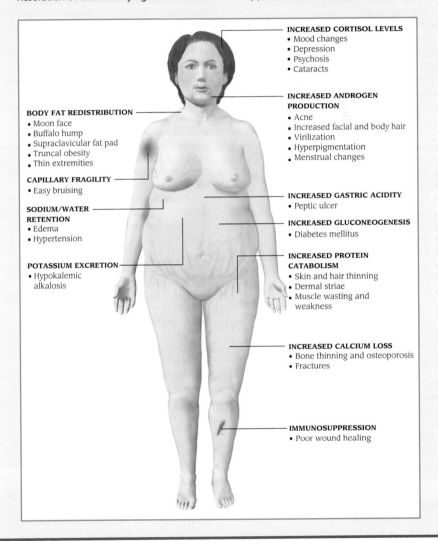

INCREASED CORTISOL LEVELS
- Mood changes
- Depression
- Psychosis
- Cataracts

INCREASED ANDROGEN PRODUCTION
- Acne
- Increased facial and body hair
- Virilization
- Hyperpigmentation
- Menstrual changes

BODY FAT REDISTRIBUTION
- Moon face
- Buffalo hump
- Supraclavicular fat pad
- Truncal obesity
- Thin extremities

CAPILLARY FRAGILITY
- Easy bruising

SODIUM/WATER RETENTION
- Edema
- Hypertension

POTASSIUM EXCRETION
- Hypokalemic alkalosis

INCREASED GASTRIC ACIDITY
- Peptic ulcer

INCREASED GLUCONEOGENESIS
- Diabetes mellitus

INCREASED PROTEIN CATABOLISM
- Skin and hair thinning
- Dermal striae
- Muscle wasting and weakness

INCREASED CALCIUM LOSS
- Bone thinning and osteoporosis
- Fractures

IMMUNOSUPPRESSION
- Poor wound healing

(Cushing disease), a corticotropin-producing tumor in another organ (particularly bronchogenic or pancreatic cancer), or excessive administration of exogenous glucocorticoids.

In the remaining 30% of patients, Cushing syndrome results from a cortisol-secreting adrenal tumor, which is usually benign. In infants, the usual cause of Cushing syndrome is adrenal carcinoma.

Cushing syndrome affects 13 of every 1 million people. It's more common in women than in men and occurs primarily between ages 25 and 40.

Pathophysiology

Secretion of CRH from the hypothalamus stimulates production and secretion of ACTH from the anterior pituitary. ACTH stimulates the adrenal glands to produce and secrete cortisol. When cortisol levels rise, negative feedback is initiated for both CRH from the hypothalamus and ACTH from the anterior pituitary.

Endogenous Cushing syndrome can be dependent on or independent from ACTH from the anterior pituitary. In endogenous ACTH-independent Cushing syndrome, the ACTH level is low secondary to negative feedback from elevated serum cortisol. Conversely, ACTH is elevated in ACTH-dependent Cushing syndrome; usually due to an anterior pituitary tumor. ACTH-dependent Cushing syndrome comprises 60% to 70% of cases. Rarely, ectopic non-pituitary tumors producing ACTH or CRH are the causative factor.

Complications

- ◆ Osteoporosis
- ◆ Pathologic fractures
- ◆ Peptic ulcer
- ◆ Impaired glucose tolerance and insulin resistance
- ◆ Dyslipidemia
- ◆ Frequent infections
- ◆ Slow wound healing
- ◆ Venous thrombosis
- ◆ Obesity
- ◆ Arterial hypertension
- ◆ Ischemic heart disease
- ◆ Heart failure
- ◆ Menstrual disturbances
- ◆ Sexual dysfunction
- ◆ Impaired linear growth in children

Signs and symptoms

Like other endocrine disorders, Cushing syndrome induces changes in multiple body systems, depending on the adrenocortical hormone involved. The symptoms of Cushing syndrome can be rapid or gradual but regardless of how they present they will all worsen if not treated. Clinical effects may include the following.

- ◆ *Endocrine and metabolic systems*—DM, with decreased glucose tolerance, fasting hyperglycemia, and glycosuria
- ◆ *Musculoskeletal system*—muscle weakness due to hypokalemia or to loss of muscle mass from increased catabolism, pathologic fractures due to decreased bone mineral, and impaired linear growth in children
- ◆ *Skin*—purplish striae; fat pads above the clavicles, over the upper back (buffalo hump), on the face (moon face), and throughout the trunk,

with slender arms and legs; little or no scar formation; poor wound healing; skin bruises easily; acne and hirsutism in females

- ◆ *GI system*—peptic ulcer, resulting from increased gastric secretions and pepsin production, and decreased gastric mucus
- ◆ *Central nervous system*—irritability and emotional lability, ranging from euphoric behavior to depression or psychosis; insomnia
- ◆ *Cardiovascular system*—hypertension due to sodium and water retention; left ventricular hypertrophy; capillary weakness due to protein loss, which leads to bleeding, petechiae, and ecchymosis
- ◆ *Immune system*—increased susceptibility to infection due to decreased lymphocyte production and suppressed antibody formation; decreased resistance to stress. (Suppressed inflammatory response may mask even a severe infection.)
- ◆ *Renal and urologic systems*—sodium and secondary fluid retention, increased potassium excretion, inhibited ADH secretion, ureteral calculi from increased bone demineralization with hypercalciuria
- ◆ *Reproductive system*—increased androgen production with clitoral hypertrophy, mild virilism, infertility, and amenorrhea or oligomenorrhea in women. Sexual dysfunction also occurs

Diagnosis

Recommended diagnostic testing from the Endocrine Society's Clinical Practice Guideline (2015)

- ◆ Late-night salivary cortisol—elevated (normal is <0.10 to 0.15 µg/dL)
- ◆ 24-hour urine free cortisol—elevated (normal is <40 to 50 µg/dL)
- ◆ Overnight low-dose dexamethasone suppression test (1 mg dexamethasone at 2,300 and obtain a serum cortisol before 09.00 am the following day)—elevated (normal is <1.8 µg/dL)

Initially, diagnosis of Cushing syndrome requires determination of plasma steroid levels. In people with normal hormone balance, plasma cortisol levels are higher in the morning and decrease gradually throughout the day (diurnal variation). In patients with Cushing syndrome, cortisol levels don't fluctuate and typically remain consistently elevated; 24-hour urine sample demonstrates elevated free cortisol levels.

Ⓡ **CONFIRMING DIAGNOSIS** *A low-dose dexamethasone suppression test confirms the diagnosis of Cushing syndrome. Salivary cortisol levels collected at midnight (usually performed on an outpatient basis) are elevated and are the most sensitive confirmatory test. (See Diagnosing Cushing syndrome, page 573.)*

DIFFERENTIAL DIAGNOSIS
Diagnosing Cushing syndrome

The flow chart below aids in differential diagnosis of Cushing syndrome.

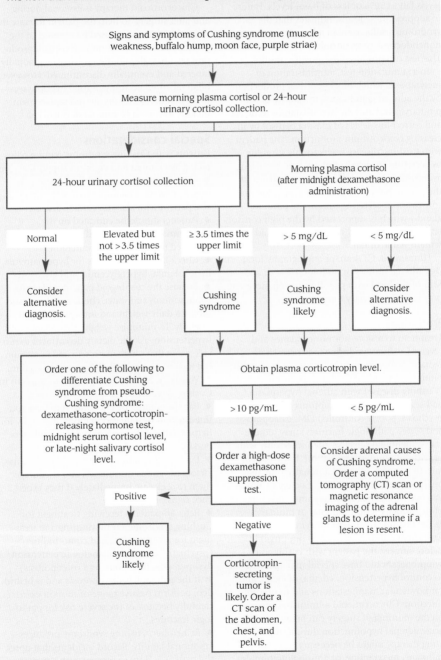

Signs and symptoms of Cushing syndrome (muscle weakness, buffalo hump, moon face, purple striae)

↓

Measure morning plasma cortisol or 24-hour urinary cortisol collection.

24-hour urinary cortisol collection

- Normal → Consider alternative diagnosis.
- Elevated but not >3.5 times the upper limit
- ≥3.5 times the upper limit → Cushing syndrome

Morning plasma cortisol (after midnight dexamethasone administration)

- >5 mg/dL → Cushing syndrome likely
- <5 mg/dL → Consider alternative diagnosis.

Order one of the following to differentiate Cushing syndrome from pseudo-Cushing syndrome: dexamethasone–corticotropin-releasing hormone test, midnight serum cortisol level, or late-night salivary cortisol level.

Obtain plasma corticotropin level.

- >10 pg/mL → Order a high-dose dexamethasone suppression test.
- <5 pg/mL → Consider adrenal causes of Cushing syndrome. Order a computed tomography (CT) scan or magnetic resonance imaging of the adrenal glands to determine if a lesion is resent.

High-dose dexamethasone suppression test:
- Positive → Cushing syndrome likely
- Negative → Corticotropin-secreting tumor is likely. Order a CT scan of the abdomen, chest, and pelvis.

A high-dose dexamethasone suppression test can determine if Cushing syndrome results from pituitary dysfunction (Cushing disease). In this test, dexamethasone suppresses plasma cortisol levels, and urinary 17-hydroxycorticosteroid (17-OHCS) and 17-ketogenic steroid levels fall to 50% or less of basal levels. Failure to suppress these levels indicates that the syndrome results from an adrenal tumor or a nonendocrine, corticotropin-secreting tumor. This test can produce false-positive results.

In a stimulation test, administration of metyrapone, which blocks cortisol production by the adrenal glands, tests the ability of the pituitary gland and the hypothalamus to detect and correct low levels of plasma cortisol by increasing corticotropin production. The patient with Cushing disease reacts to this stimulus by secreting an excess of plasma corticotropin, as measured by levels of urinary 17-OHCS. If the patient has an adrenal or a nonendocrine corticotropin-secreting tumor, the pituitary gland—which is suppressed by the high cortisol levels—can't respond normally, so steroid levels remain stable or fall.

Ultrasound, CT scan, or angiography localizes adrenal tumors or nodules; CT scan and MRI of the head with gadolinium enhancement may identify pituitary tumors.

Treatment

Treatment to restore hormone balance and reverse Cushing syndrome may necessitate radiation, drug therapy, or surgery. For example, pituitary-dependent Cushing syndrome (Cushing disease) with adrenal hyperplasia and severe cushingoid symptoms (such as psychosis, poorly controlled DM, osteoporosis, and severe pathologic fractures) may require transsphenoidal selective adenomectomy with or without pituitary irradiation. If the patient fails to respond, bilateral adrenalectomy may be performed. The Endocrine Society's Clinical Practice Guideline (2015) recommends surgery of the primary lesion (adrenal or pituitary) as the first-line treatment for symptomatic Cushing syndrome, unless it is not possible. Before surgery, the patient with cushingoid symptoms should have special management to control hypertension, edema, diabetes, and cardiovascular manifestations and to prevent infection. Glucocorticoid administration on the morning of surgery can help prevent acute adrenal hypofunction during surgery. Drug therapy might be necessary (e.g., with mitotane, metyrapone, or aminoglutethimide) to decrease cortisol levels if symptoms persist.

Steroidogenesis inhibitors (metyrapone and ketoconazole) decrease cortisol levels and have beneficial effects for many cushingoid patients; they may also be useful for symptom control in metastatic adrenal carcinoma with or without radiotherapy.

Glucocorticoid therapy is essential during and after surgery, to help the patient tolerate the physiologic stress imposed by removal of the pituitary or adrenals. If normal cortisol production resumes, steroid therapy may be gradually tapered and eventually discontinued. However, bilateral adrenalectomy or total hypophysectomy mandates lifelong steroid replacement therapy to correct hormonal deficiencies.

Special considerations

Patients with Cushing syndrome require painstaking assessment and vigorous supportive care.
◆ Frequently monitor vital signs, especially blood pressure. Carefully observe the hypertensive patient who also has cardiac disease.
◆ Patients should be educated on the long-term risk if myocardial infarction and encouraged to have routine evaluation.
◆ Check laboratory reports for hypernatremia, hypokalemia, hyperglycemia, and glycosuria.
◆ Because the cushingoid patient is likely to retain sodium and water, check for edema, and monitor daily weight and intake and output carefully. To minimize weight gain, edema, and hypertension, ask the dietary department to provide a diet that's high in protein and potassium but low in calories, carbohydrates, and sodium.
◆ Watch for infection—a particular problem in Cushing syndrome.
◆ Patients should be encouraged to have routine age-appropriate vaccinations, especially for herpes zoster, influenza, and pneumonia secondary to increased risk of infection.
◆ Evaluate and educate patients regarding risk factors of venous thrombosis and encourage them to seek care immediately if they experience signs or symptoms.
◆ Refer all patients receiving treatment for Cushing syndrome for monitoring and treatment for all cortisol-related comorbidities (psychiatric disorders, diabetes, hypertension, dyslipidemia, infections, and osteoporosis).
◆ If the patient has osteoporosis and is bedridden, perform passive range-of-motion exercises carefully because of the severe risk for pathologic fractures.
◆ Remember, Cushing syndrome produces emotional lability. Record incidents that upset the patient and try to prevent such situations from occurring if possible. Help the patient get the physical and mental rest they need—by

sedation if necessary. Offer support to the emotionally labile patient throughout the difficult testing period. In addition, encourage ongoing follow-up with a mental health provider.

After bilateral adrenalectomy and pituitary surgery:

◆ Report wound drainage or temperature elevation to the patient's physician immediately. Use strict sterile technique in changing the patient's dressings.

◆ Administer analgesics and replacement steroids, as ordered.

◆ Monitor urine output, and check vital signs carefully, watching for signs of shock (decreased blood pressure, increased pulse rate, pallor, and cold, clammy skin). To counteract shock, give vasopressors and increase the rate of I.V. fluids, as ordered. Because mitotane, aminoglutethimide, etomidate, and metyrapone decrease mental alertness and produce physical weakness, assess neurologic and behavioral status, and warn the patient of adverse CNS effects. Also watch for severe nausea, vomiting, and diarrhea.

◆ Check laboratory reports for hypoglycemia due to removal of the source of cortisol, a hormone that maintains blood glucose levels.

◆ Check for abdominal distention and return of bowel sounds after adrenalectomy.

◆ Check regularly for signs of adrenal hypofunction—orthostatic hypotension, apathy, weakness, fatigue—indicators that steroid replacement is inadequate.

◆ In the patient undergoing pituitary surgery, check for and immediately report signs of increased intracranial pressure (confusion, agitation, changes in level of consciousness, nausea, hypotension, and vomiting). Watch for hypopituitarism.

Provide comprehensive teaching to help the patient cope with lifelong treatment:

◆ Advise the patient to take replacement steroids with antacids or meals, to minimize gastric irritation. (Usually it's helpful to take two-thirds of the dosage in the morning and the remaining third in the early afternoon to mimic diurnal adrenal secretion.)

◆ Tell the patient to carry a medical identification card and to immediately report physiologically stressful situations such as infections, which necessitate increased dosage.

◆ Instruct the patient to watch closely for signs of inadequate steroid dosage (fatigue, weakness, dizziness) and of overdosage (severe edema, weight gain). Emphatically warn against abrupt discontinuation of steroid dosage because this may produce a fatal adrenal crisis.

◆ Teach the patient about using I.M. hydrocortisone if they can't tolerate oral steroids.

HYPERALDOSTERONISM

In hyperaldosteronism (Conn syndrome), hypersecretion of the mineralocorticoid aldosterone by the adrenal cortex causes excessive reabsorption of sodium and water, and excessive renal excretion of potassium.

Causes and incidence

Hyperaldosteronism may be primary (uncommon) or secondary. The majority of hyperaldosterone cases result from bilateral idiopathic adrenal hyperplasia (IAH) or a benign aldosterone-producing adrenal adenoma. It is important to distinguish between aldosteronomas and bilateral IAH because the treatments are quite different. The treatment of choice for aldosteronomas is surgical while the treatment for IAH is medical therapy with an aldosterone antagonist. In rare cases, the cause is an intermediate variant with histologic features of both adenoma and hyperplasia or carcinoma. There are also three genetic variants of primary aldosteronism:

◆ Type 1—glucocorticoid-remediable aldosteronism (GRA). It is due to a mutation that causes a chimeric gene that combines *CYP11B1* and *CYP11B2* leading to increased synthesis and secretion of aldosterone.

◆ Type 2—non-glucocorticoid sensitive form of primary aldosteronism. The exact genetic mutation has not been identified; however, it is located on band *7p22*. It can manifest as hyperplasia or adenoma.

◆ Type 3—potassium channel mutation at *KCNJ5*.

The incidence of primary hyperaldosteronism caused by adenomas is higher in females than in males with a ratio of 2:1 and is highest between ages 30 and 50. Primary hyperaldosteronism caused by IAH is four times more prevalent in men than in women with the highest incidence between ages 50 and 60.

In primary hyperaldosteronism, chronic aldosterone excess is independent of the renin–angiotensin system and, in fact, suppresses plasma renin activity (PRA). This aldosterone excess enhances sodium reabsorption by the kidneys, which leads to mild hypernatremia and, simultaneously, hypokalemia and increased extracellular fluid (ECF) volume. Expansion of intravascular fluid volume also occurs and results in volume-dependent hypertension and increased cardiac output. Excessive ingestion of English black licorice or licorice-like substances can produce a syndrome similar to primary hyperaldosteronism due to the mineralocorticoid action of glycyrrhizic acid.

Secondary hyperaldosteronism results from an extra-adrenal abnormality that stimulates the adrenal gland to increase production of aldosterone. For example, conditions that reduce renal blood flow (renal artery stenosis) and ECF volume or produce a sodium deficit activate the renin–angiotensin system and, subsequently, increase aldosterone secretion. Thus, secondary hyperaldosteronism may result from conditions that induce hypertension through increased renin production (such as Wilms tumor), ingestion of hormonal contraceptives, and pregnancy.

However, secondary hyperaldosteronism may also result from disorders unrelated to hypertension, which may or may not cause edema. For example, nephrotic syndrome, hepatic cirrhosis with ascites, and heart failure commonly induce edema, whereas Bartter syndrome and salt-losing nephritis don't.

Pathophysiology

Aldosterone is a mineralocorticoid produced in the zona glomerulosa of the adrenal cortex. The primary action of aldosterone is regulation of sodium, potassium, and hydrogen ions in the kidney. Secondary sites of action include the GI tract and the sweat glands. Aldosterone production and secretion is predominantly controlled via the renin–angiotensin system and the circulating concentration of potassium ions. Excessive secretion of aldosterone causes increased sodium reabsorption and excessive loss of both potassium and hydrogen ions.

Complications

◆ Neuromuscular irritability
◆ Treatment-resistant hypertension
◆ Seizures
◆ Hypokalemia
◆ Cardiac arrhythmias
◆ Myocardial infarction
◆ Hypertensive nephropathy
◆ Hypertensive retinopathy
◆ Ischemic heart disease
◆ Left ventricular hypertrophy
◆ Congestive heart failure

Signs and symptoms

Most clinical effects of hyperaldosteronism result from hypokalemia, which increases neuromuscular irritability and produces muscle weakness; intermittent, flaccid paralysis; fatigue; headaches; paresthesia; and, possibly, tetany (resulting from metabolic alkalosis), which can lead to hypocalcemia.

DM is common, perhaps because hypokalemia interferes with normal insulin secretion. Hypertension and its accompanying complications

are also common. Other characteristic findings include visual disturbances and loss of renal concentrating ability, resulting in nocturnal polyuria and polydipsia. Azotemia indicates chronic potassium depletion nephropathy.

Diagnosis

Persistently low serum potassium levels (<3.6 mEq/L) and bicarbonate levels indicative of mild metabolic alkalosis (>31 mEq/L) in a nonedematous patient who isn't taking diuretics, who doesn't have obvious GI losses (from vomiting or diarrhea), and who has a normal sodium intake, suggest hyperaldosteronism. In addition, serum sodium and magnesium levels will show mild hypernatremia and mild hypomagnesemia. If hypokalemia develops in a hypertensive patient shortly after starting treatment with potassium-wasting diuretics (such as thiazides), and if it persists after the diuretic has been discontinued and potassium replacement therapy has been instituted, evaluation for hyperaldosteronism is necessary.

CONFIRMING DIAGNOSIS *A low PRA level that fails to increase appropriately during volume depletion (upright posture, sodium depletion) and a high plasma aldosterone level during volume expansion by salt loading confirm primary hyperaldosteronism in a hypertensive patient without edema. In primary aldosteronism PRA is less than 1 ng/mL/hour and fails to rise about 2 ng/mL/hour following salt and water depletion, furosemide administration, or 4 hours of erect posture.*

The serum bicarbonate level is often elevated, with ensuing alkalosis due to hydrogen and potassium ion loss in the distal renal tubules. Other tests show markedly increased urinary aldosterone levels, increased plasma aldosterone levels, and, in secondary hyperaldosteronism, increased plasma renin levels.

A suppression test is useful to differentiate between primary and secondary hyperaldosteronism. During this test, the patient receives oral desoxycorticosterone for 3 days while plasma aldosterone levels and urinary metabolites are continuously measured. These levels decrease in secondary hyperaldosteronism but remain the same in primary hyperaldosteronism. Simultaneously, renin levels are low in primary hyperaldosteronism and high in secondary hyperaldosteronism.

To determine if the primary hyperaldosteronism is being caused by an IAH versus aldosteronoma, there is a standard postural test protocol wherein baseline values of serum aldosterone and PRA levels are measured and then rechecked after the patient has assumed an erect posture for 2 hours. In patients with aldosteronomas, serum aldosterone levels typically do not rise and might even drop. In healthy persons or patients with IAH serum aldosterone levels typically rise 50% above baseline.

Other helpful diagnostic evidence includes an increase in plasma volume of 30% to 50% above normal, ECG signs of hypokalemia (ST-segment depression and U waves), chest X-ray showing left ventricular hypertrophy from chronic hypertension, and localization of the tumor by adrenal angiography, MRI, or CT scan.

Treatment

The appropriate treatment for hyperaldosteronism depends on its cause. The treatment of primary hyperaldosteronism caused by aldosteronoma is unilateral adrenalectomy. The treatment for patients with primary hyperaldosteronism due to IAH is medical management primarily using diuretics and antihypertensives. In patients with secondary aldosteronism, mineralocorticoid antagonists, such as spironolactone, and selective aldosterone receptor antagonists, such as eplerenone, can be useful. In addition, sodium restriction may help control hyperaldosteronism. The treatment of secondary hyperaldosteronism must include correction of the underlying cause. In patients with GRA the preferred treatment is low-dose glucocorticoid treatment using prednisone or hydrocortisone.

Special considerations

Patient care includes careful monitoring and recording of urine output, blood pressure, weight, and serum potassium levels.

◆ Watch for signs of tetany (muscle twitching, Chvostek sign) and for hypokalemia-induced cardiac arrhythmias, paresthesia, or weakness. Give potassium replacement, as ordered, and keep calcium gluconate I.V. available.

◆ Ask the dietitian to provide a low-sodium, high-potassium diet.

◆ After adrenalectomy, watch for weakness, hyponatremia, rising serum potassium levels, and signs of adrenal hypofunction, especially hypotension.

◆ If the patient is taking spironolactone, advise the patient to watch for signs of hyperkalemia. If the patient is male, inform him that impotence and gynecomastia may follow long-term use.

◆ Tell the patient who must take steroid hormone replacement to wear a medical identification bracelet.

ADRENOGENITAL SYNDROME

Adrenogenital syndrome results from disorders of adrenocortical steroid biosynthesis. This syndrome may be inherited (congenital adrenal hyperplasia [CAH]) or acquired, usually as a result of an adrenal tumor (adrenal virilism). Salt-wasting CAH may cause fatal adrenal crisis in neonates.

Causes and incidence

CAH is transmitted as an autosomal recessive trait that causes deficiencies in the enzymes needed for adrenocortical secretion of cortisol and, possibly, aldosterone. Compensatory secretion of corticotropin produces varying degrees of adrenal hyperplasia. In simple virilizing CAH, deficiency of the enzyme 21-hydroxylase results in underproduction of cortisol. In turn, this cortisol deficiency stimulates increased secretion of corticotropin, producing large amounts of cortisol precursors and androgens that don't require 21-hydroxylase for synthesis.

In salt-wasting CAH, 21-hydroxylase is almost completely absent. Corticotropin secretion increases, causing excessive production of cortisol precursors, including salt-wasting compounds. However, plasma cortisol and aldosterone levels—both dependent on 21-hydroxylase—fall precipitously and, in combination with the excessive production of salt-wasting compounds, precipitate acute adrenal crisis. Corticotropin hypersecretion stimulates adrenal androgens, possibly even more than in simple virilizing CAH, and produces masculinization.

Adrenal hyperplasia caused by 11-hydroxylase and 17-hydroxylase deficiency cause sodium retention and hypertension secondary to elevated concentration of deoxycorticosterone. Other rare CAH enzyme deficiencies exist and lead to increased or decreased production of affected hormones.

CAH is the most prevalent adrenal disorder in infants and children; simple virilizing CAH and salt-wasting CAH are the most common forms. Acquired adrenal virilism is rare and affects twice as many females as males. About 1 in 10,000 to 18,000 is born with CAH.

Pathophysiology

Genetic mutations and deletions in the *CYP21A2*, *CYP11B1*, *CYP17A1*, *HSD3B2*, *CYP11A1*, *StAR*, and *CYPOR* genes result in enzymatic deficiencies causing disruption of the biochemical processes involved in steroidogenesis by the adrenal glands resulting in deficient mineralocorticoid and glucocorticoid production and excessive synthesis of sex steroids. Less frequently an adrenal tumor can cause similar symptoms.

Complications
◆ Cardiovascular collapse and cardiac arrest (in neonates)
◆ Hypertension
◆ Hyperkalemia
◆ Infertility
◆ Adrenal tumor
◆ Altered growth, external genitalia, and sexual maturity

Signs and symptoms
The neonatal female with simple virilizing CAH has ambiguous genitalia (enlarged clitoris, with urethral opening at the base; some labioscrotal fusion) but normal genital tract and gonads. As she grows older, signs of progressive virilization develop: early appearance of pubic and axillary hair, deep voice, acne, and facial hair. The neonatal male with this condition has no obvious abnormality; however, at prepuberty, he shows accentuated masculine characteristics, such as deepened voice and an enlarged phallus, with frequent erections. At puberty, females fail to begin menstruation, and males have small testes. Both males and females with this condition may be taller than other children their age as a result of rapid bone and muscle growth, but because excessive androgen levels hasten epiphyseal closure, abnormally short adult stature results. (See *Acquired adrenal virilism*, page 581.)

Salt-wasting CAH in females causes more complete virilization than the simple form and results in development of male external genitalia without testes. Because males with this condition have no external genital abnormalities, immediate neonatal diagnosis is difficult, and is commonly delayed until the infant develops severe systemic symptoms. Characteristically, such an infant is apathetic, fails to eat, and has diarrhea; he develops symptoms of adrenal crisis in the first week of life (vomiting, dehydration from hyponatremia, hyperkalemia). Unless this condition is treated promptly, dehydration and hyperkalemia may lead to cardiovascular collapse and cardiac arrest.

Diagnosis
The diagnosis of CAH depends on the enzymatic mutation and resultant excess concentrations of precursor hormones in addition to inadequate cortisol, aldosterone, or both.

Physical examination is needed for determining the presence of clinical features suggesting CAH; clitoromegaly or ambiguous genitalia, precocious pubic hair, hirsutism, and excessive growth.

℞ **CONFIRMING DIAGNOSIS** *The following laboratory findings confirm the diagnosis of 21-hydroxylaze deficiency: elevated plasma 17-KS, which can be suppressed by administering oral dexamethasone; elevated urinary levels of hormone metabolites, particularly pregnanetriol; elevated plasma 17-hydroxyprogesterone level; and normal or decreased urinary levels of 17-hydroxycorticosteroids. Elevated dehydroepiandrosterone sulfate is present.*

Adrenal hypofunction or adrenal crisis in the first week of life suggests salt-wasting CAH. Low serum aldosterone, hyperkalemia, hyponatremia, elevated PRA levels, and hypochloremia with elevated 24-hour urinary 17-ketosteroids (17-KS) and pregnanetriol and decreased urinary aldosterone levels confirm it.

Treatment
Simple virilizing CAH requires correction of the cortisol deficiency and inhibition of excessive pituitary corticotropin production by daily administration of cortisol. Treatment returns androgen production to normal levels. Measurement of urinary 17-KS levels determines the initial dose of cortisone or hydrocortisone; this dose is usually large and is given I.M. Later dosage is modified according to decreasing urinary 17-KS levels. Infants must continue to receive cortisone or hydrocortisone I.M. until age 18 months; thereafter, they may take it orally.

PEDIATRIC TIP *The infant with salt-wasting CAH in adrenal crisis requires immediate I.V. sodium chloride and glucose infusion to maintain fluid and electrolyte balance and to stabilize vital signs. If saline and glucose infusion doesn't control symptoms while the diagnosis is being established, hydrocortisone I.V. is necessary. Later, maintenance includes mineralocorticoid (fludrocortisone) and glucocorticoid (cortisone or hydrocortisone) replacement.*

Pelvic ultrasound may be helpful to identify the presence of gonads/streak gonadal tissue or renal anomalies that can be associated with other conditions that present with ambiguous genitalia. A karyotype is essential in evaluating an infant with abnormal or ambiguous genitalia in order to determine the chromosomal sex of the child, as the phenotypic sex may be indeterminate. Children with ambiguous or abnormally developed genitalia may require reconstructive surgery; for example, females with virilization may undergo correction of the labial fusion and of the urogenital sinus. Surgery is usually scheduled between ages 1 and 3, after the effect of cortisone therapy has been assessed.

Special considerations

◆ Suspect CAH in infants hospitalized for failure to thrive, dehydration, or diarrhea, as well as in tall, sturdy-looking children with a record of numerous episodic illnesses.

◆ When caring for an infant with adrenal crisis, keep the I.V. line patent, infuse fluids, and give steroids, as ordered. Monitor body weight, blood pressure, and serum electrolyte levels carefully, especially sodium and potassium levels. Watch for cyanosis, hypotension, tachycardia, tachypnea, and signs of shock. Minimize external stressors.

◆ If the child is receiving maintenance therapy with steroid injections, rotate I.M. injection sites to prevent atrophy; tell parents to do the same. Teach them the possible adverse effects (cushingoid symptoms) of long-term therapy. Explain that maintenance therapy with hydrocortisone, cortisone, or the mineralocorticoid fludrocortisone is essential for life. Warn parents not to withdraw these drugs suddenly because potentially fatal adrenal hypofunction will result. Instruct parents to report stress and infection, which require increased steroid dosages.

◆ Monitor the patient receiving fludrocortisone for edema, weakness, and hypertension. Be alert for significant weight gain and rapid changes in height because normal growth is an important indicator of adequate therapy.

◆ Instruct the patient to wear a medical identification bracelet indicating that they are on prolonged steroid therapy and providing information about dosage.

◆ Help the parents of a female infant with male genitalia to understand that she's physiologically a female and that reconstructive surgery is available should that prove to be in the best interest of the child. Arrange for supportive counseling if necessary. Genetic counseling should also be arranged if appropriate.

PHEOCHROMOCYTOMA

Pheochromocytomas and extra-adrenal paragangliomas (PPGL) are catecholamine-secreting chromaffin cell tumors that may result in excess circulating levels of the catecholamines epinephrine and norepinephrine and occasionally dopamine; adrenal hormones help regulate blood glucose levels, heart rate, blood pressure, and stress response. Excess levels of these hormones can result in severe hypertension, increased metabolism, and hyperglycemia. This disorder is potentially fatal if left untreated, but the prognosis is generally good with treatment. However, pheochromocytoma-induced kidney damage is irreversible.

Causes and incidence

A pheochromocytoma may result from an inherited autosomal dominant trait (about 30%); however, the majority originate spontaneously. Classically, PPGL is associated with three hereditary syndromes

◆ von Hippel-Lindau syndrome

◆ multiple endocrine neoplasia type 2 (MEN2A and MEN2B)

◆ neurofibromatosis type 1

Research regarding genetic involvement is ongoing and currently there are 10 genes wherein associated mutations can lead to PPGL. The incidence of PPGL is increased in inherited syndromes, occurring in approximately 70% of MEN2 cases. The overall prevalence of PPGL is low (1.5 to 1.6/10,000 persons), though the prevalence is higher in patients who present with hypertension (approximately 20 to 60 per 10,000 persons). In patients with incidental finding of an adrenal mass, it can be as high as 500 per 10,000 persons. It is frequently missed though because about 5 per 10,000 persons are found to have a PPGL upon autopsy. While this tumor is usually benign, it may be malignant in as many as 10% of these patients. It affects all races and both sexes, occurring primarily between ages 30 and 50. Only 10% of incidents occur in children.

Pathophysiology

The majority of pheochromocytomas (85%) originate in the adrenal glands. The remaining 15% are extra-adrenal and originate in the parangliar cells of the nervous system and are called paragangliomas. Common sites for extra-adrenal pheochromocytomas are the paraganglion chromaffin tissue of the nervous system (nerve pathways) in the urinary bladder, brain, organ of Zuckerkandl, heart, mediastinum, and carotid. There are two subtypes: adrenergic and noradrenergic. Adrenergic pheochromocytomas are located in the adrenal medulla and produce epinephrine, metanephrine, and norepinephrine. Noradrenergic tumors can be located in either the adrenal medulla or be extra-adrenal and they either exclusively produce norepinephrine, or they produce norepinephrine and normetanephrine and rarely dopamine. Secretion from either subtype can occur intermittently or continuously. The biochemical phenotype can help determine the type of genetic mutation that caused the tumor to originate and can also contribute to treatment strategy as patients with adrenergic tumors are more likely to have paroxysmal symptoms than those with noradrenergic tumors. Pheochromocytomas are not innervated; therefore, the secretion of catecholamine is unregulated. Catecholamine stimulation of alpha-adrenergic receptors causes increased cardiac contractility, hypertension, gluconeogenesis, and glycogenolysis. Catecholamine stimulation of the beta-adrenergic receptors causes increased cardiac contractility and increased heart rate. Only 10% of pheochromocytomas are malignant but the secretion of norepinephrine, epinephrine, and dopamine from these tumors can cause life-threatening hypertensive crisis.

Complications
◆ Stroke
◆ Retinopathy
◆ Heart failure
◆ Irreversible kidney damage
◆ Myocardial infarction

Signs and symptoms
The cardinal sign of pheochromocytoma is persistent or paroxysmal hypertension. Common clinical effects include palpitations, tachycardia, headache, diaphoresis, pallor, warmth or flushing, paresthesia, tremor, excitation, fright, nervousness, feelings of impending doom, abdominal pain, tachypnea, nausea, and vomiting. Orthostatic hypotension and paradoxical response to antihypertensive drugs are common, as are associated glycosuria, hyperglycemia, and hypermetabolism. Patients with hypermetabolism may show marked weight loss, but some patients with pheochromocytomas are obese. Symptomatic episodes may recur as seldom as once every 2 months or as often as 25 times a day. They may occur spontaneously or may follow certain precipitating events, such as postural change, exercise, laughing, smoking, induction of anesthesia, urination, or a change in environmental or body temperature.

Pheochromocytoma is commonly diagnosed during pregnancy, when uterine pressure on the tumor induces more frequent attacks; such attacks can prove fatal for both mother and fetus as a result of a stroke, acute pulmonary edema, cardiac arrhythmias, or hypoxia. In such patients, the risk of spontaneous abortion is high but most fetal deaths occur during labor or immediately after birth. However, if the diagnosis is made antenatally, then fetal mortality is reduced to 15% and maternal mortality is virtually eliminated.

Diagnosis
The classic triad of symptoms is pounding heading, sweating, and palpitations that occur paroxysmally and can last several minutes to 1 hour; symptoms resolve completely between spells. The frequency varies from patient to patient and can happen as frequently as several times a day to one to two times a month. The symptoms can be spontaneous or triggered by physical or chemical stimuli such as medications like beta-adrenergic inhibitors, glucocorticoids, and anesthesia. So, 35% of patients with PPGL have paroxysmal hypertension while others might have sustained hypertension with superimposed peaks of severely high blood pressure or even hypertensive crisis. The most common clinical presentation for pheochromocytoma is hypertension. Current guidelines do not recommend biochemical screening for all patients who present with hypertension; however, a history of acute episodes of hypertension, headache, sweating, and tachycardia—particularly in a patient with hyperglycemia, glycosuria, and hypermetabolism—strongly suggests PPGL and screening is advised. Generally, diagnosis depends on biochemical laboratory findings.

℞ **CONFIRMING DIAGNOSIS** *For high-risk patients (patients having a family history of pheochromocytomas and those with predisposing genetic conditions), plasma-free metanephrine testing is suggested. For low-risk patients, the increased urinary excretion of total free catecholamines and their metabolites, vanillylmandelic acid (VMA) and metanephrine, as measured by analysis of a 24-hour urine specimen, confirms pheochromocytoma. The diagnostic accuracy is similar in the plasma-free or 24-hour urine fractionated metanephrine testing but those for plasma or urinary catecholamines, VMA and urinary chromogranin A are not as accurate. Biochemical testing should be avoided in critically ill patients due to elevated false-positive results.*

Patients with normal testing while symptomatic can have a definitive exclusionary diagnosis; however, testing done on patients who are asymptomatic requires repeat testing prior to excluding a diagnosis of PPGL. Labile blood pressure necessitates urine collection during a hypertensive episode and comparison of this specimen with a baseline specimen. Plasma-free metanephrine levels of more than three times the reference limit or 24-hour urinary fractionated metanephrine levels greater than two times the upper limit indicate PPGL. If feasible, patients should rest in the supine position for 30 minutes prior to a plasma-free metanephrine test because sitting can cause a mildly elevated false positive in some patients. If repeat testing is necessary, both a 24-hour urinary fractionated and metanephrine and plasma chromogranin A should be done because this allows the

Acquired adrenal virilism

Acquired adrenal virilism results from virilizing adrenal tumors, carcinomas, or adenomas. This rare disorder is twice as common in females as in males. Although acquired adrenal virilism can develop at any age, its clinical effects vary with age at onset:

♦ Prepubescent females: pubic hair, clitoral enlargement; at puberty, delayed breast development, delayed or absent menses
♦ Prepubescent males: hirsutism, macrogenitosomia praecox (excessive body development, with marked enlargement of genitalia). Occasionally, the penis and prostate equal those of an adult male in size; however, testicular maturation fails to occur
♦ Females (especially middle-aged): dark hair on legs, arms, chest, back, and face; pubic hair extending toward navel; oily skin, sometimes with acne; menstrual irregularities; muscular hypertrophy (masculine resemblance); male pattern baldness; and atrophy of breasts and uterus
♦ Males: no overt signs; discovery of tumor usually accidental

♦ All patients: good muscular development; taller than average during childhood and adolescence; short stature as adults due to early closure of epiphyses

Diagnosis and treatment
♦ Diagnostic tests for this disorder include:
♦ Urinary total 17-ketosteroids (17-KS): greatly elevated but levels vary daily; dexamethasone P.O. doesn't suppress 17-KS
♦ Plasma levels of dehydroepiandrosterone: greatly elevated
♦ Serum electrolyte levels: normal
♦ X-ray of kidneys: may show downward displacement of kidneys by tumor

Treatment requires surgical excision of tumor and metastases (if present), when possible, or radiation therapy and chemotherapy. Preoperative treatment may include glucocorticoids. With treatment, the prognosis is very good in patients with slow-growing and nonrecurring tumors. Periodic follow-up urine testing (for increased 17-KS levels) to check for tumor recurrence is essential.

---

exclusion of a false positive. An alternative test, the clonidine suppression test will cause decreased plasma catecholamine levels in normal patients but no change in those with pheochromocytoma. After demonstrating biochemical evidence of pheochromocytoma, CT scan or MRI of the abdomen (where 95% of pheochromocytomas are located) is warranted. If a tumor isn't located—or if there is more than one—a radioactive iodine metaiodobenzylguanidine scintiscan or nuclear scan usually confirms the diagnosis in unclear cases. Angiography and excretory urography are no longer used; adrenal venography is used, but rarely.

Treatment
Surgical removal of the tumor is the treatment of choice. Preoperatively, care must be taken to manage to control blood pressure and correct fluid volume in order to avoid intraoperative hypertensive crisis. Alpha blockade with phenoxybenzamine should be started 10 to 14 days prior to surgery and beta blockade initiated once alpha blockade has been achieved with the final doses given the morning of surgery. Also, preoperatively a high-sodium diet with supplemental fluid intake should be followed

to prevent severe hypotension after tumor removal. Postoperatively, I.V. fluids, plasma volume expanders, vasopressors, and, possibly, transfusions may be required for hypotension. Persistent hypertension in the immediate postoperative period can occur. If surgery isn't feasible, alpha-adrenergic blockers and beta-adrenergic blockers—such as phenoxybenzamine and propranolol, respectively—are beneficial in controlling catecholamine effects and preventing attacks. Management of an acute attack or hypertensive crisis requires I.V. phentolamine (push or drip) or nitroprusside to normalize blood pressure.

In rare cases the tumor is cancerous; treatment would include radiation or chemotherapy.

If pheochromocytoma is diagnosed during the first two trimesters of pregnancy, termination is not necessary; however, there is a high chance of spontaneous abortion. Alpha-adrenergic blockers should be started immediately with laparoscopic removal of the tumor as soon as possible. If diagnosed during the third trimester, the patient should be managed medically until fetal lung development is confirmed at which point delivery by cesarean sections is recommended due to decreased fetal mortality versus vaginal delivery. The pheochromocytoma may be removed during the cesarean section or postpartum.

Special considerations

To ensure the reliability of urine catecholamine measurements, make sure the patient avoids foods high in vanillin (such as coffee, nuts, chocolate, and bananas) for 2 days before urine collection of VMA. Also, be aware of possible drug therapy that may interfere with the accurate determination of VMA (such as guaifenesin and salicylates). Collect the urine in a special container, with hydrochloric acid, that has been prepared by the laboratory.

◆ Obtain blood pressure readings often because transient hypertensive attacks are possible. Tell the patient to report headaches, palpitations, nervousness, or other symptoms of an acute attack. If hypertensive crisis develops, monitor blood pressure and heart rate every 2 to 5 minutes until blood pressure stabilizes at an acceptable level.

◆ Hourly blood glucose checks should be performed for at least the first 12 to 24 hours postoperatively because the sudden catecholamine withdrawal after tumor removal can lead to rebound hyperinsulinemia resulting in hypoglycemia.

◆ After surgery, blood pressure may rise or fall sharply. Keep the patient quiet; provide a private room, if possible, because excitement may trigger a hypertensive episode. Postoperative hypertension is common because the stress of surgery and manipulation of the adrenal gland stimulate secretion of catecholamines. Because this excess secretion causes profuse sweating, keep the room cool, and change the patient's clothing and bedding often. If the patient receives phentolamine, monitor blood pressure closely. Observe and record adverse effects: dizziness, hypotension, and tachycardia. The first 24 to 48 hours immediately after surgery are the most critical because blood pressure can drop drastically.

◆ If the patient is receiving vasopressors I.V., check blood pressure as per facility protocol or every 15 minutes while titrating, and regulate the drip to maintain a safe pressure. Arterial pressure lines facilitate constant monitoring.

◆ Watch for abdominal distention and return of bowel sounds.

◆ Immediately postadrenalectomy, observe patients for signs of shock secondary to drastic drop in catecholamine levels; blood pressure changes, clammy skin, paleness, changes in level of consciousness.

◆ For patients with bilateral adrenalectomy, provide patient teaching regarding the possibility of lifelong steroid replacement and to wear a medical alert bracelet.

⚠ **ALERT** *Check dressings and vital signs for indications of hemorrhage (increased pulse rate, decreased blood pressure, cold and clammy skin, pallor, and unresponsiveness).*

◆ Give analgesics for pain, as ordered, but monitor blood pressure carefully because many analgesics can cause hypotension.

◆ If autosomal dominant transmission of pheochromocytoma is suspected, the patient's family should receive genetic counseling for this condition and testing if appropriate.

Pancreatic and multiple disorders

MULTIPLE ENDOCRINE NEOPLASIA

Multiple endocrine neoplasia (MEN) is a hereditary disorder in which two or more endocrine glands develop hyperplasia, adenoma, or carcinoma, concurrently or consecutively. There are three types: MEN1, MEN2 (two subtypes: 2A and 2B), and MEN4. MEN1 is the most common form.

Causes and incidence

MEN mutations usually follow an autosomal dominant inheritance; however, they can also occur sporadically. MEN1 is caused by inactivating mutations of the MEN1 tumor suppressor gene at the 11q13 and also as a result of mutations in cyclin-dependent kinase inhibitor genes *CD-KN1A, CDKN2B,* and *CDKN2C. MEN2* is caused by germline mutations in the *RET proto-oncogene 10q11.2. MEN4* is due to inactivating mutations in the *CDKN1B gene 12p13.1-p12.* The reported age range for MEN mutations is infancy to greater than 81 years with equal female to male incidence; however, the peak incidence of symptoms is typically seen by women in their 30s and men in their 40s. The typical onset of MEN2B is childhood but it only accounts for 5% to 10% of all cases of MEN2 syndrome. There's no racial predilection.

Pathophysiology

MEN is a group of disorders that typically involves hyperplasia or tumor growth in multiple endocrine glands resulting in overproduction and secretion of hormone. The tumors can be malignant or benign. The two most common forms are MEN1 and MEN2. The majority of cases are inherited and result from genetic mutation. MEN1 generally involves tumor development in the pancreas, parathyroid, and pituitary glands. MEN2 has three subtypes; MEN2A, MEN2B, and familial medullary thyroid carcinoma. The majority of people with MEN2 regardless of subtype will develop medullary thyroid cancer and 50% will develop pheochromocytomas. MEN2A also involves primary mild hyperparathyroidism resulting from hyperplasia or adenoma. MEN2B increases the likelihood of ganglioneuromas and mucosal neuromas with a marfanoid habitus. MEN4 is characterized by the development of tumors in the parathyroid glands and anterior pituitary.

Complications

The possible complications of MEN types 1 and 2 include:

♦ Metastasis of the medullary thyroid cancer
♦ Renal failure
♦ Recurrent tumors
♦ Recurrent gastric and duodenal ulcers
♦ Pathological fractures, due to weak bones
♦ Kidney stones
♦ Vision disturbances

Signs and symptoms

Clinical effects of MEN may develop in various combinations and orders, depending on the glands involved. The most common manifestation of MEN1 is hyperparathyroidism, followed by peptic ulcer and steatorrhea due to Zollinger–Ellison syndrome (marked by increased gastrin production from nonbeta islet cell tumors of the pancreas). Hypoglycemia may result from pancreatic beta islet cell tumors, with increased insulin production. They may also have severe diarrhea and dehydration secondary to excessive production of vasoactive intestinal polypeptide. When MEN1 affects the parathyroid glands, it produces signs of hyperparathyroidism, including hypercalcemia (because the parathyroid glands are primarily responsible for the regulation of calcium and phosphorus levels). When MEN causes pituitary tumor, it's most commonly a prolactinoma, but can be a GH or corticotropin, or even a nonsecretory adenoma.

Characteristic features of MEN2 with medullary carcinoma of the thyroid include enlarged thyroid mass, with resultant increased calcitonin and, occasionally, ectopic corticotropin, causing Cushing syndrome. With tumors of the adrenal medulla, symptoms include headache, tachyarrhythmias, and hypertension; with adenomatosis or hyperplasia of the parathyroid glands, symptoms result from renal calculi. MEN2B typically presents with medullary

thyroid cancer, pheochromocytomas, and neuromas, in addition, 5% have Hirschsprung disease (congenital megacolon). Of note, the majority of MEN2B cases are de novo and resultant medullary cancer has been found in patients as young as 3 months of age.

Diagnosis

Investigating symptoms of pituitary tumor, hypoglycemia, hypercalcemia, or GI hemorrhage may lead to a diagnosis of MEN. Testing is done via radioimmune assay of hormone levels in blood and urine secondary to the presenting symptoms. Diagnostic tests must be used to carefully evaluate each affected endocrine gland. For example, radioimmunoassay showing increased levels of gastrin in patients with peptic ulceration and Zollinger–Ellison syndrome suggests the need for follow-up studies for MEN I because 50% of patients with Zollinger–Ellison syndrome have MEN. If a MEN variant is suspected, genetic screening must be done to verify the specific germline mutation; once a mutation is confirmed, family members should receive genetic counseling and testing as appropriate for this inherited syndrome. Because MEN has an autosomal dominant inheritance pattern, antenatal genetic screening and potential preimplantation genetic diagnosis with in vitro fertilization may be appropriate for people prior to starting a family.

Imaging tests such as ultrasonography, MRI, or CT may be helpful in determining the location of tumors or hyperplasia.

Treatment

There is no known cure for MEN. The goal of treatment is to correct the resultant hormone imbalance; therefore, changes in each gland must be treated individually. Tumors are generally treated by surgical removal whenever possible. Subsequent therapy controls residual symptoms. In MEN1, peptic ulceration is usually the most urgent clinical feature, so primary treatment emphasizes control of bleeding or resection of necrotic tissue. In hypoglycemia caused by insulinoma, oral administration of glucose can keep blood glucose levels within acceptable limits. Subtotal (partial) pancreatectomy is required to remove the tumor. Because all parathyroid glands have the potential for neoplastic enlargement, subtotal parathyroidectomy may also be required along with transsphenoidal hypophysectomy. In MEN2, treatment of an adrenal medullary tumor includes antihypertensives and resection of the tumor. In patients diagnosed with MEN2A or 2B, preventive thyroidectomy may be performed secondary to the high incidence of aggressive medullary thyroid cancer in this population. Bromocriptine and cabergoline may be used for pituitary tumors that secrete prolactin. Hormonal replacement therapy is necessary when glands are removed or secretion is inadequate.

Special considerations

Supportive care depends on the body system involved (see special considerations listed for each endocrine system in this chapter).

◆ If MEN involves the pancreas, monitor blood glucose levels frequently. If it affects the adrenal glands, monitor blood pressure closely, especially during drug therapy.

◆ Manage peptic ulcers, hypoglycemia, and other complications, as needed.

◆ If pituitary tumor is suspected, watch for signs of pituitary trophic hormone dysfunction, which may affect any of the endocrine glands. Also, be aware that pituitary apoplexy (sudden severe headache, altered level of consciousness, visual disturbances) may occur.

DIABETES MELLITUS

DM is a group of chronic metabolic disorders characterized by hyperglycemia and deficient or ineffective endogenous insulin.

Pathophysiology

Diabetes mellitus type 1

DM type 1 is a chronic autoimmune disease. An external stimulus, such as a virus, activates an autoimmune change in the body of susceptible individuals stimulating lymphocytic infiltration into the pancreatic islets of Langerhans. The subsequent inflammatory process, called insulitis, causes destruction of the insulin-secreting pancreatic beta cells. Once the initial inflammation recedes the islets atrophy and the resultant deficient or absent beta-cell function causes insulin deficiency. Hyperglycemia develops when 80% to 90% of the pancreatic beta cells are destroyed as there is no longer enough available insulin to maintain normal blood glucose levels.

Diabetes mellitus type 2

DM type 2 results from inadequate secretion of insulin from the pancreatic beta cells in combination with insulin resistance in the peripheral tissue (primarily the muscle, liver, and fat cells). In normally functioning glucose metabolism, there is a feedback loop between the insulin-secreting beta cells of the pancreas and insulin-sensitive tissue in the body. If insulin resistance alone is present, the body compensates by increasing insulin output. However, when pancreatic beta cells cannot secrete sufficient insulin in the presence of peripheral insulin resistance, hyperglycemia results.

Causes and incidence

DM is a chronic disease of absolute or relative insulin deficiency or resistance characterized by disturbances in carbohydrate, protein, and fat metabolism. Insulin transports glucose into the cell for use as energy and storage as glycogen. It also stimulates protein synthesis and free fatty acid storage in the fat deposits. Insulin deficiency compromises the body tissues' access to essential nutrients for fuel and storage.

Diabetes is the seventh leading cause of death in the United States. Approximately 30 million Americans (9.5% of the population) have diabetes. Of those 30 million only 1.25 million have type 1 DM. Twenty-five percent of Americans age 65 and older have DM. The risk by race and ethnicity is higher in Hispanic, Black, American Indian, and Alaskan Native populations. Diabetes is a contributing factor in about 50% of myocardial infarctions and about 75% of strokes as well as in renal failure and peripheral vascular disease. It's also the leading cause of new blindness.

DM occurs in four forms classified by etiology.

Type 1 diabetes mellitus

In type 1 diabetes, pancreatic beta-cell destruction or a primary defect in beta-cell function results in failure to release insulin and ineffective glucose transport. Type 1 immune-mediated diabetes is caused by cell-mediated destruction of pancreatic beta cells. The rate of beta-cell destruction is usually higher in children than in adults. The idiopathic form of type 1 diabetes has no known cause. Patients with this form have no evidence of autoimmunity and don't produce insulin.

Type 1 is further subdivided into immune-mediated diabetes and idiopathic diabetes. Those who were previously in the type 1 diabetes group fall into this group. Children and adolescents with type 1 immune-mediated diabetes rapidly develop ketoacidosis, but most adults with this type experience only modest fasting hyperglycemia unless they develop an infection or experience another stressor. Patients with type 1 idiopathic diabetes are prone to ketoacidosis.

Type 2 diabetes mellitus

In type 2 diabetes, beta cells release insulin, but receptors are insulin-resistant and glucose transport is variable and ineffective. Most patients with type 2 diabetes are obese.

Risk factors for type 2 diabetes include:
◆ Overweight and obesity (even an increased percentage of body fat primarily in the abdominal region); risk decreases with weight and drug therapy
◆ Lack of physical activity
◆ History of GDM
◆ Hypertension
◆ Black, Hispanic, Pacific Islander, Asian American, Native American origin
◆ Strong family history of diabetes
◆ Older than age 45
◆ High-density lipoprotein cholesterol of less than 35 mg/dL or triglyceride of greater than 250 mg/dL
◆ Cigarette smoking
◆ Seriously impaired glucose tolerance

Other specific types

The "other specific types" of DM result from various conditions (such as a genetic defect of the beta cells or endocrinopathies) or from use of, or exposure to, certain drugs or chemicals. Some of these are:
◆ Maturity onset diabetes of the young (MODY)
  ◆ Single gene mutation (HNF1-alpha, HNF1-beta, HNF4-alpha, glucokinase) with an autosomal dominant inheritance pattern. Regardless of weight, lifestyle, ethnicity, or sex diagnosis by age 25.
◆ Neonatal diabetes
  ◆ Diagnosed prior to age 6 months, is not an autoimmune condition, caused by a genetic mutation (KCNJ11 or ABCC8) that affects insulin production, may occur with concurrent epilepsy, can be transient or permanent; however, even if transient, can reoccur later in life
◆ Wolfram syndrome (also known as DIDMOAD syndrome)
  ◆ Four most common features are DI, DM, optic atrophy, and deafness, prevalence—1 in 770,000 persons
◆ Alstrom syndrome
  ◆ There are only 950 people diagnosed worldwide, autosomal recessive genetic inheritance pattern, caused by a mutation in the ALMS1 gene, causes cone-rod dystrophy, hearing loss, obesity, insulin resistance, hyperinsulinemia, type 2 DM, dilated cardiomyopathy, and progressive hepatic and renal dysfunction.

Gestational diabetes mellitus

GDM is considered present whenever a patient has any degree of abnormal glucose during pregnancy. This form may result from weight gain, increased levels of estrogen and progesterone, and placental factors such as human placental lactogen and placental tumor necrosis factor alpha, which antagonize insulin. In this type of diabetes, glucose tolerance levels usually return to normal after delivery. Women who had GDM have a 40% to 60% chance of developing type 2 diabetes within 5 to 10 years.

ELDER TIP *As the body ages, the cells become more resistant to insulin, thus reducing the older adult's ability to metabolize glucose. In addition, the release of insulin from the pancreatic beta cells is reduced and delayed. These combined processes result in hyperglycemia. In the older patient, sudden concentrations of glucose cause increased and more prolonged hyperglycemia.*

Complications

◆ Cardiovascular disease
◆ Peripheral vascular disease
◆ Retinopathy
◆ Nephropathy
◆ Susceptibility to skin and urinary tract infections (UTIs) and vaginitis

Signs and symptoms

Diabetes may begin dramatically with ketoacidosis or insidiously. Its most common symptom is fatigue from energy deficiency and a catabolic state. Insulin deficiency causes hyperglycemia, which pulls fluid from body tissues, causing osmotic diuresis, polyuria, dehydration, polydipsia, dry mucous membranes, poor skin turgor, blurred vision, nausea, and, in most patients, unexplained weight loss.

ELDER TIP *Because their thirst mechanism functions less effectively, older adults may not report polydipsia, a hallmark of diabetes in younger adults.*

In ketoacidosis and hyperosmolar hyperglycemic nonketotic syndrome, dehydration may cause hypovolemia and shock. Wasting of glucose in the urine usually produces weight loss and hunger in type 1 diabetes, even if the patient eats voraciously. (See *Understanding ketoacidosis and hyperosmolar coma,* pages 586 and 587.)

The long-term effects of diabetes may include retinopathy, nephropathy, atherosclerosis,

PATHOPHYSIOLOGY
Understanding ketoacidosis and hyperosmolar coma

Ketoacidosis and hyperosmolar coma are acute complications of hyperglycemic crisis that may occur in a patient with diabetes. If not treated properly, either may result in coma or death.

Ketoacidosis is most common in patients with type 1 diabetes; in fact, it may be the first evidence of previously unrecognized type 1 diabetes. Although hyperosmolar coma is most common in patients with type 2 diabetes, it may also occur in anyone whose insulin tolerance is stressed and in patients who have undergone certain therapeutic procedures, such as peritoneal dialysis, hemodialysis, tube feedings, or total parenteral nutrition.

Acute insulin deficiency (absolute in ketoacidosis; relative in hyperosmolar coma) precipitates both conditions. Causes include illness, stress, infection, and failure to take insulin (only in a patient with ketoacidosis).

Buildup of glucose
Inadequate insulin hinders glucose uptake by fat and muscle cells. Because the cells can't take in glucose to convert to energy, glucose accumulates in the blood. At the same time, the liver responds to the demands of the energy-starved cells by converting glycogen to glucose and releasing glucose into the blood, *further* increasing the blood glucose level. When this level exceeds the renal threshold, excess glucose is excreted in the urine.

Still, the insulin-deprived cells can't use glucose. Their response is rapid metabolism of protein, which results in loss of intracellular potassium and phosphorus and in excessive liberation of amino acids. The

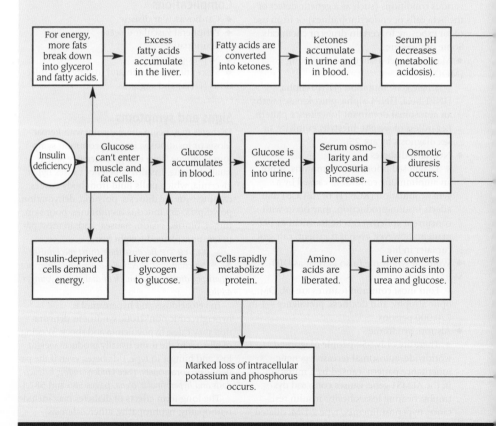

liver converts these amino acids into urea and glucose.

As a result of these processes, the blood glucose level is grossly elevated. The aftermath is increased serum osmolarity and glycosuria (higher in patients with hyperosmolar coma than in those with ketoacidosis because the blood glucose level is higher in those with hyperosmolar coma), leading to osmotic diuresis.

A deadly cycle
The massive fluid loss from osmotic diuresis causes fluid and electrolyte imbalances and dehydration. Water loss exceeds electrolyte loss, contributing to hyperosmolarity. This, in turn, perpetuates dehydration, decreasing the glomerular filtration rate and reducing the amount of glucose excreted in the urine, leading to a deadly cycle:

Diminished glucose excretion *further* raises the blood glucose level, producing severe hyperosmolarity and dehydration and finally causing shock, coma, and death.

Further ketoacidosis complication
All these steps hold true for both ketoacidosis and hyperosmolar coma. But ketoacidosis has an additional simultaneous process that leads to metabolic acidosis. The absolute insulin deficiency causes cells to convert fats into glycerol and fatty acids for energy. The fatty acids can't be metabolized as quickly as they're released, so they accumulate in the liver, where they're converted into ketones (ketoacids). These ketones accumulate in the blood and urine and cause acidosis. Acidosis leads to more tissue breakdown, more ketosis, more acidosis, and eventually shock, coma, and

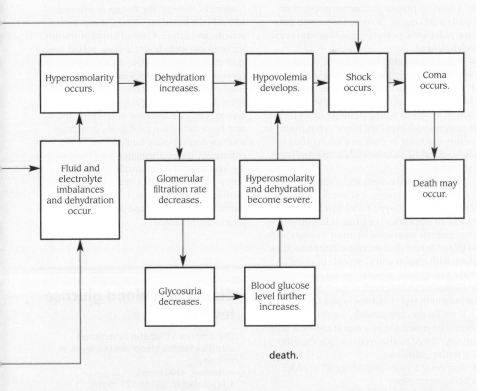

death.

and peripheral and autonomic neuropathy. Peripheral neuropathy usually affects the hands and feet and may cause numbness or pain. Autonomic neuropathy may manifest itself in several ways, including gastroparesis (leading to delayed gastric emptying and a feeling of nausea and fullness after meals), nocturnal diarrhea, impotence, and orthostatic hypotension.

Because hyperglycemia impairs the patient's resistance to infection, diabetes may result in skin and UTIs and vaginitis. Glucose content of the epidermis and urine encourages bacterial growth.

Diagnosis

According to the American Diabetes Association (ADA), DM can be diagnosed if any of the following exist:

◆ A fasting (no caloric intake for at least 8 hours) plasma blood glucose level greater than or equal to 126 mg/dL or

◆ A plasma glucose value in the 2-hour sample of the oral glucose tolerance test greater than or equal to 200 mg/dL. This test should be performed after an oral glucose load dose of 75 g of anhydrous glucose or

◆ A random plasma glucose greater than or equal to 200 mg/dL in conjunction with polyuria, polydipsia, polyphagia, and unexplained weight loss or

◆ If DM is suspected but polyuria, polydipsia, polyphagia, a random glucose level of 200 mg/dL and unexplained weight loss are absent a hemoglobin A_{1c} of 6.5% or higher with confirmation by repeat testing (testing cannot be used in patients with rapid red blood cell turnover or infants and must be done at a lab certified by the National Glycohemoglobin Standardization Program).

Because there has been an increase in type 2 diabetes in the young, it is important to differentiate between type 1 and type 2 DM. The American Association of Clinical Endocrinologists suggests measuring immune markers such as glutamic acid decarboxylase autoantibodies along with insulin and C-peptide in order to make a diagnosis. In addition, anti-insulin autoantibodies and islet cell autoantibodies may be present in type 1 but not type 2 DM.

If results are questionable, the diagnosis should be confirmed by a repeat test on a different day. The ADA also recommends the following testing guidelines:

◆ Test every 3 years: people age 45 or older without symptoms

◆ Test immediately: people with the classic symptoms

◆ High-risk groups should be tested frequently: Individuals with IGT usually have normal blood levels unless challenged by a glucose load, such as a piece of pie or glass of orange juice. Two hours after a glucose load, the glucose level ranges from 140 to 199 mg/dL. These individuals have an abnormal fasting glucose level between 110 and 125 mg/dL. Because the fasting plasma glucose test is sufficient to make the diagnosis of diabetes, it replaces the oral glucose tolerance test. (See *Classifying blood glucose levels*.)

An ophthalmologic examination may show diabetic retinopathy. Other diagnostic and monitoring tests include urinalysis for acetone and blood testing for HbA_{1c}, which reflects recent glucose cortisol.

◆ Fructosamine levels reflect glucose control in the previous 1 to 3 weeks and can be useful for monitoring intensive therapies or short-term changes (e.g., in GDM)

Treatment

Effective treatment normalizes blood glucose and decreases complications using insulin replacement, diet, and exercise. Patients with type 1 DM will require lifelong insulin replacement therapy. The dosage is adjusted individually based on blood glucose testing, activity, and intake. Current forms of insulin replacement include single-dose, mixed-dose, split-mixed dose, multiple-dose regimens, and continuous subcutaneous insulin infusion. Insulin may be rapid acting, short acting, intermediate acting, long acting, and ultra-long acting; it may be standard or purified, and it may be derived from beef, pork, or human sources. Recombinant human insulin is used commonly today. The majority of insulins are injectable or infused subcutaneously via pump but there is also a rapid acting inhaled insulin powder available. Pancreas transplantation is experimental and requires chronic immunosuppression.

Classifying blood glucose levels

The American Diabetes Association classifies fasting blood glucose levels as follows.

◆ Normal: <100 mg/dL
◆ Prediabetes: 100 to 125 mg/dL
◆ Diabetes: ≥126 mg/dL

Successful insulin replacement requires routine monitoring of blood glucose levels. This can be done at home by patients using glucometers and testing at set times, such as fasting and pre- and postprandial, as well as when they are symptomatic for hyper- or hypoglycemia. There are also devices that allow for continuous glucose monitoring (CGM). They are subcutaneous sensors that measure interstitial glucose levels every 1 to 5 minutes and they alarm if the parameters are over or under the specified range or if they are rapidly rising or falling. They will transmit to a receiver which patients have—either a pager-like device or it is integrated into their insulin pump. The 2018 ADA recommendations suggest CGM usage for all persons aged 18 or over with type 1 DM. A very useful mechanism in the CGM is that if the sensor detects levels below the preset value and a patient doesn't respond to the alarms, the pump will automatically stop basal insulin delivery. There is research and development in process for closed loop electronic systems called artificial pancreases.

Successful treatment requires an extensive dietary education. The patient's diet is specifically tailored to include the right amount and combination of foods. Almost all foods may be eaten occasionally. The diet should address dietary prescriptions as well as personal and cultural preferences to improve adherence and control. For the obese patient with type 2 diabetes, weight reduction is a goal. In type 1 diabetes, the calorie allotment may be high, depending on growth stage and activity level.

Type 2 diabetes may require oral antidiabetic drugs to stimulate endogenous insulin production, increase insulin sensitivity at the cellular level, and suppress hepatic gluconeogenesis.

Many types of drugs have been used to treat diabetes. Sulfonylureas stimulate pancreatic insulin release, increase tissue sensitivity to insulin, and require insulin's presence to work. Meglitinides cause immediate, brief release of insulin and are taken immediately before meals. Biguanides decrease hepatic glucose production and increase tissue sensitivity to insulin. Hypoglycemia antidotes elevate blood glucose by promoting hepatic gluconeogenesis and inhibiting glycogen synthesis. Alpha-glucosidase inhibitors slow the breakdown of glucose and decrease postprandial glucose peaks. Glucagon-like peptide-1 agonists improve glycemic control by reducing glucagon, slowing gastric emptying, and improving glucose-dependent insulin secretion by pancreatic beta cells. Dipeptidyl peptidase IV inhibitors help improve glucose homeostasis by increasing insulin release and decreasing circulating glucagon levels. Selective sodium-glucose transporter-2 inhibitors lower the renal glucose threshold, thereby increasing urinary glucose excretion thus lowering the reabsorption of glucose in the renal tubules and increasing glucose excretion in the urine. Bile acid sequestrants improve glycemic control in type 2 diabetes but their exact action is unknown. Dopamine agonists improve glycemic control in insulin-resistant patients by decreasing the hypothalamic drive for increased fasting and postprandial plasma glucose, triglyceride, and free fatty acid levels. The thiazolidinediones increase insulin sensitivity in peripheral tissue such as muscle and fat; however, insulin must be present for them to work. These drugs also reduce insulin resistance by decreasing hepatic glucose production and increasing glucose uptake. They have also been shown to lower blood pressure in diabetic hypertensive patients. Cholesterol and triglyceride levels may also be reduced.

A new class of antihyperglycemics—amylinomimetics—a synthetic analogue of human amylin called pramlintide acetate, helps control glucose. Amylin is absent in patients with diabetes. When used with insulin, this synthetic hormone can improve glycemic control by delaying gastric emptying and decreasing the release of postprandial glucagon thus decreasing postprandial glucose level peaks.

Combination drugs, such as glyburide and metformin (Glucotrol), are also available that combine varying doses of two types of diabetes drugs, allowing the patient to take fewer pills. These are frequently prescribed once the patient is stable on individual drugs for a while.

Treatment of long-term diabetic complications may include transplantation or dialysis for renal failure, photocoagulation for retinopathy, and vascular surgery for large-vessel disease. Meticulous blood glucose control is essential.

⚠ ALERT *Any patient with a wound that has lasted more than 8 weeks and who has tried standard wound care and revascularization without improvement should consider hyperbaric oxygen therapy. This treatment may speed healing by allowing more oxygen to get to the wound and may therefore result in fewer amputations.*

Keeping glucose at near-normal levels for 5 years or more reduces both the onset and progression of retinopathy, nephropathy, and neuropathy. In type 2 diabetes, blood pressure control as well as smoking cessation reduces the onset and progression of complications, including cardiovascular disease. (See *Insulin therapy,* page 590.)

Insulin therapy

Insulin is administered as prescribed. There are several routes of administration and devices for injection.

Subcutaneous route

Insulin is usually given by subcutaneous (Subcut) injection with a standard insulin syringe. Subcut insulin can also be given with a penlike injection device that uses a disposable needle and replaceable insulin cartridges or in disposable pens, eliminating the need to draw insulin into a syringe.

Jet-injection devices

Jet-injection devices are expensive and require special cleaning procedures, but they disperse insulin more rapidly and speed absorption. These devices draw up insulin from standard containers, which enables the patient to mix insulins, if necessary, but requires a special procedure for drawing it up. After the insulin is drawn up, it's delivered into the subcutaneous tissue with a pressure jet.

Insulin pumps

Multiple-dose regimens may use an insulin pump to deliver insulin continuously into subcutaneous tissue. The infusion rate selector automatically releases about half of the total daily insulin requirement evenly over 24 hours. The patient releases the remainder in bolus amounts before meals and snacks.

Site rotation

When insulin injections are administered subcutaneously, the injection sites should be rotated. Because absorption rates differ at each site, diabetic educators recommend rotating the injection site within a specific area, such as the abdomen.

I.V. and I.M. routes

Regular insulin or insulin lispro may also be administered I.M. or I.V. during severe episodes of hyperglycemia. These are the only types of insulin that should ever be administered by these routes.

Special considerations

Stress the importance of complying with the prescribed treatment program. Tailor your teaching to the patient's needs, abilities, and developmental stage. Include diet; purpose, administration, and possible adverse effects of medication; exercise; monitoring; hygiene; and the prevention and recognition of hypoglycemia and hyperglycemia. Stress the effect of blood glucose control on long-term health. (See *Preventing diabetes complications*, page 591.)

⚠ ALERT *Watch for acute complications of diabetic therapy, especially hypoglycemia (vagueness, slow cerebration, dizziness, weakness, pallor, tachycardia, diaphoresis, seizures, and coma); immediately give carbohydrates, ideally in the form of glucose tablets, honey, or fruit juice. If the patient is unconscious, give glucagon or dextrose I.V. Check glucose level every 20 minutes and repeat glucose tablets until glucose level exceeds 120 mg/dL or meets institutional policy.*

⚠ ALERT *Be alert for signs of ketoacidosis (acetone breath, dehydration, weak and rapid pulse, and Kussmaul respirations) and hyperosmolar coma (polyuria, thirst, neurologic abnormalities, and stupor). These hyperglycemic crises require I.V. fluids, insulin and, usually, potassium replacement.*

♦ Monitor diabetes control by obtaining blood glucose, HbA_{1c}, lipid levels, and blood pressure measurements regularly.

♦ Ensure patients keep a blood glucose log and bring them to their follow-up visits.

♦ Advise the patient to ensure that they are aware of the difference in the U-500 versus U-100 strengths of insulin so they can ensure the correct self-dosing at home as it is a potential safety issue.

♦ Patients should be taught that insulin is reactive to heat and oxygen therefore a vial of insulin should be used for no longer than 28 days before it is discarded (even if there is insulin remaining in the vial).

♦ The ADA recommends that pregnant women with preexisting type 1 or type 2 DM commence low-dose daily aspirin at the end of the first trimester to decrease the risk of preeclampsia.

♦ Adolescents and children who are overweight or obese and have at least one additional diabetes risk factor should be screened routinely for prediabetes and type 2 diabetes.

♦ Because of the increased risks of infection in this population, individuals with type 1 and type 1 diabetes should be encouraged to have routine vaccinations, especially for influenza and pneumonia.

PREVENTION
Preventing diabetes complications

Although diabetes mellitus itself cannot be prevented, several things can be done to prevent serious complications, such as blindness, kidney damage, and limb amputations.

Managing glucose
◆ Managing glucose level is important for preventing complications because wildly fluctuating blood glucose levels place the patient at much higher risk. High levels of glucose can cause arteriosclerosis, which can lead to heart attack and stroke. By exercising and maintaining blood glucose at or near-normal levels, the risk can be reduced.
◆ High glucose level can cause blockage of the small blood vessels that supply the limbs with blood. This can cause nerve damage with a loss of sensation. In addition, the patient with diabetes has slow tissue repair, which makes them more prone to infections and amputation of the limbs. The patient with diabetes should never walk around barefoot. Even the smallest cut can cause problems.
◆ Following the prescribed diet (with weight loss if needed), medication regimen (if prescribed), and the recommended exercise program should be the keys to controlling glucose levels.

Managing blood pressure
◆ The patient with diabetes who also has hypertension is at greater risk for developing cardiovascular and kidney disease. Continuing high blood pressure can damage the kidney's filtration mechanism and cause kidney failure.
◆ Blood pressure control can reduce heart disease and stroke by about one-third to one-half and can reduce eye, kidney, and nerve disease by about a third.

Preventive care
◆ The patient with diabetes should check his or her feet every day for swelling, redness, and warmth. These are signs that the patient should notify the practitioner immediately. In addition, the patient should have his or her feet checked at least once a year by the practitioner.
◆ Diabetes can damage the retina of the eye, producing *retinal neuropathy*, which can lead to blindness. Eye examinations should be done once a year and any blurred vision should be reported to the practitioner immediately.

◆ Watch for diabetic effects on the cardiovascular system, such as cerebrovascular, coronary artery, and peripheral vascular impairment, and on the peripheral and autonomic nervous systems. Treat all injuries, cuts, and blisters (particularly on the legs or feet) meticulously. Be alert for signs of UTI and renal disease.
◆ Urge regular ophthalmologic examinations to detect diabetic retinopathy.
◆ Assess for signs of diabetic neuropathy (numbness or pain in hands and feet, footdrop, neurogenic bladder). Stress the need for personal safety precautions because decreased sensation can mask injuries. Minimize complications by maintaining strict blood glucose control.
◆ Teach the patient to care for the feet by washing them daily, drying carefully between toes, and inspecting for corns, calluses, redness, swelling, bruises, and breaks in the skin. Urge the patient to report changes to the physician. Advise the patient to wear nonconstricting shoes and to avoid walking barefoot. Instruct the patient to use over-the-counter athlete's foot remedies and seek professional care should athlete's foot not improve.
◆ Teach the patient how to manage diabetes when they have a minor illness, such as a cold, flu, or upset stomach.
◆ To delay the clinical onset of diabetes, teach people at high risk to avoid risk factors. Advise genetic counseling for young adult diabetics who are planning families.
◆ Further information may be obtained from the Juvenile Diabetes Foundation, the ADA, and the American Association of Diabetes Educators.

SELECTED REFERENCES
Akhtar, S. (2012). Diseases of the endocrine system. In L. A. Fleisher, eds. *Anesthesia and uncommon diseases* (6th ed., pp. 401–432). Philadelphia: W.B. Saunders.

American Diabetes Association. (2015). Standards of medical care in diabetes—2015: Abridged for primary care providers. *Clinical Diabetes, 33*(2), 97–111.

Baz, B., et al. (2016). Endocrinology of pregnancy: Gestational diabetes mellitus: Definition, aetiological and clinical aspects. *European Journal of Endocrinology, 174*(2), R43–R51. doi:10.1530\EJE-15-0378

Bilezikian, J., et al. (2011). Hypoparathyroidism in the adult: Epidemiology, diagnosis, pathophysiology, target organ involvement, treatment, and challenges for future research. *Journal of Bone and Mineral Research, 26*(10), 2317–2337. doi:10.1002/jbmr.483

Bilezikian, J. P., et al. (2018). Hyperparathyroidism. *The Lancet, 391*(10116), 168–178. doi:10.1016/S0140-6736(17)31430-7

Bornstein, S. R., et al. (2015). Diagnosis and treatment of primary adrenal insufficiency: An Endocrine Society Clinical Practice Guideline. *The Journal of Clinical Endocrinology and Metabolism, 101*(2), 364–389. doi:10.1210/jc.2015-1710

Brandi, M. L., et al. (2016). Management of hypoparathyroidism: Summary statement and guidelines. *The Journal of Clinical Endocrinology and Metabolism, 101*(6), 2273–2283. doi:10.1210/jc.2015-3907

Caon, M. (2008). Osmoles, osmolality and osmotic pressure: Clarifying the puzzle of solution concentration. *Contemporary Nurse, 29*, 92–99. doi:10.5172/conu.673.29.1.92

Carroll, T., & Findling, J. (2009). Cushing's syndrome of nonpituitary causes. *Current Opinion in Endocrinology, Diabetes and Obesity, 16*(4), 308–315.

Cavalier, E., et al. (2015). Considerations in parathyroid hormone testing. *Clinical Chemistry and Laboratory Medicine, 53*(12), 1913–1919.

Centers for Disease Control and Prevention. (2017). *National diabetes statistics report: 2017.* Atlanta: Centers for Disease Control and Prevention, U.S. Department of Health and Human Services. Retrieved from http://www.diabetes.org/assets/pdfs/basics/cdc-statistics-report-2017.pdf

Di Iorgi, N., et al. (2012). Diabetes insipidus—Diagnosis and management. *Hormone Research in Paediatrics, 77*(2), 69–84. doi:10.1159/000336333

Ferreira, V. M., et al. (2016). Pheochromocytoma is characterized by catecholamine-mediated myocarditis, focal and diffuse myocardial fibrosis, and myocardial dysfunction. *Journal of the American College of Cardiology, 67*(20), 2364–2374.

Funder, J. W., et al. (2016). The management of primary aldosteronism: Case detection, diagnosis, and treatment: An Endocrine Society Clinical Practice Guideline. *Journal of Clinical Endocrinology and Metabolism, 101*(5), 1889–1916.

Galati, S. J., et al. (2013). Primary aldosteronism: Emerging trends. *Trends in Endocrinology and Metabolism, 24*(9):421–430.

Gibney, J., et al. (2008). A simple and cost-effective approach to assessment of pituitary adrenocorticotropin and growth hormone reserve: Combined use of the overnight metyrapone test and insulin-like growth factor-I standard deviation scores. *Journal of Clinical Endocrinology and Metabolism, 93*, 3763.

Gounden, V., & Jialal, I. (2017). Hypopituitarism (Panhypopituitarism). In *StatPearls* [Internet]. Treasure Island: StatPearls Publishing. Retrieved from https://www.ncbi.nlm.nih.gov/books/NBK470414

Graversen, D., et al. (2012). Mortality in Cushing's syndrome: A systematic review and meta-analysis. *European Journal of Internal Medicine, 23*(3), 278–282.

Hannah-Shmouni, F., et al. (2016). Cortisol in the evaluation of adrenal insufficiency. *JAMA, 316*(5), 535–536. doi:10.1001/jama.2016.8360

Harvey, A. M. (2014). Hyperaldosteronism: Diagnosis, lateralization, and treatment. *Surgical Clinics of North America, 94*(3), 643–656.

Jonklaas, J., et al. (2014). Guidelines for the treatment of hypothyroidism: Prepared by the American Thyroid Association Task Force on Thyroid Hormone Replacement. *Thyroid, 24*(12), 1670–1751. doi:10.1089/thy.2014.0028

Judson, B., & Shaha, A. (2008). Nuclear imaging and minimally invasive surgery in the management of hyperparathyroidism. *Journal of Nuclear Medicine, 49*(11), 1813–1818.

Kahn, S. E., et al. (2014). Pathophysiology and treatment of type 2 diabetes: Perspectives on the past, present and future. *Lancet, 383*(9922), 1068–1083. doi:10.1016/S0140-6736(13)62154-6

Kalra, S., et al. (2016). Diabetes insipidus: The other diabetes. *Indian Journal of Endocrinology and Metabolism, 20*(1), 9–21. doi:10.4103/2230-8210.172273

Kapustin, J. (2010). Hypothyroidism: An evidenced-based approach to a complex disorder. *The Nurse Practitioner, 35*(8), 44–53.

Katabathina, V. S., et al. (2016). Immunoglobulin G4-related disease: Recent advances in pathogenesis and imaging findings. *Radiology Clinics of North America, 54*(3), 535–551.

Kim, S. Y. (2015). Diagnosis and treatment of hypopituitarism. *Endocrinology and Metabolism, 30*(4), 443–455. doi:10.3803/EnM.2015.30.4.443

Klonoff, D. C., et al. (2011) Continuous glucose monitoring: An Endocrine Society Clinical Practice Guideline. *Journal of Clinical Endocrinology and Metabolism, 96*(10), 2968–2979.

LaVan, J. T., et al. (2017). *Essential evidence PLUS: Hypopituitarism.* Hoboken: John Wiley & Sons. Retrieved from https://www.essentialevidenceplus.com/

Lenders, J. W., et al. (2014). Pheochromocytoma and paraganglioma: An Endocrine Society clinical practice guideline. *Journal of Clinical Endocrinology and Metabolism, 99*(6), 1915–1942.

Lerner, N., et al. (2013). Predicting type 2 diabetes mellitus using haemoglobin A1c: A community-based historic cohort study. *European Journal of General Practice, 20*(2), 100–106.

Mulatero, P., et al. (2010). Evaluation of primary aldosteronism. *Current Opinion in Endocrinology, Diabetes and Obesity, 17*(3), 188–193.

Nieman, L. K., et al. (2015). Treatment of Cushing's syndrome: An Endocrine Society clinical practice guideline. *The Journal of Clinical Endocrinology & Metabolism, 100*(8), 2807–2831. doi:10.1210/jc.2015-1818

O'Keefe, J., et al. (2011). Strategies for optimizing glycemic control and cardiovascular prognosis in patients with type 2 diabetes mellitus. *Mayo Clinic Proceedings, 86*(2), 128–138.

Parikh, P. P., et al. (2017). Nationwide review of hormonally active adrenal tumors highlights high morbidity in pheochromocytoma. *Journal of Surgical Research, 215*, 204–210.

Piantanida, E., et al. (2016). Masked hypertension in newly diagnosed hypothyroidism: A pilot study. *Journal of Endocrinology Investigation, 39*(10), 1131–1138.

Ramachandran, R., & Rewari, V. (2017). Current perioperative management of pheochromocytomas. *Indian Journal of Urology: IJU: Journal of the Urological Society of India, 33*(1), 19–25. doi:10.4103/0970-1591.194781

Salehi, F., et al. (2008). Pituitary tumor-transforming gene in endocrine and other neoplasms: A review and update. *Endocrine-Related Cancer, 15*(3), 721–743.

Schlegel, A. (2015). Metyrapone stimulation test to diagnose central adrenal insufficiency. *Lancet Diabetes and Endocrinology, 3*, 407.

Simmons, S. (2010). Flushing out the truth about diabetes insipidus. *Nursing, 40*(1), 55–59.

Speiser, P. W., et al. Congenital adrenal hyperplasia due to steroid 21-hydroxylase deficiency: An Endocrine Society Clinical Practice Guideline. *Journal of Clinical Endocrinology and Metabolism, 95*(9), 4133–4160.

Wang, D., et al. (2015). Recombinant human growth hormone in treatment of diabetes: Report of three cases and review of relative literature. *International Journal of Clinical and Experimental Medicine, 8*(5), 8243–8248.

Wilhelm, S. M., et al. (2016). The American Association of Endocrine Surgeons Guidelines for definitive management of primary hyperparathyroidism. *JAMA Surgery, 151*(10), 959–968. doi:10.1001/jamasurg.2016. 2310

Winther, K. H., et al. Disease-specific as well as generic quality of life is widely impacted in autoimmune hypothyroidism and improves during the first six months of levothyroxine therapy. *PLoS One, 11*(6), e0156925.

Witchel, S. (2012). Nonclassic congenital adrenal hyperplasia. *Current Opinions in Endocrinology, Diabetes and Obesity, 19*(3), 151–158.

Young, W. F., et al. (2017). Screening for endocrine hypertension: An Endocrine Society scientific statement. *Endocrine Reviews, 38*, 103–122.

Yuen, K. C., et al. (2013). Influence of glucocorticoids and growth hormone on insulin sensitivity in humans. *Diabetic Medicine, 30*, 651–663.

12

EYE DISORDERS

Introduction

Vision, the most complex sense, has been the focus of significant medical and surgical innovations. Disorders that affect the eye can lead to vision loss or impairment; routine ophthalmic examinations and early treatment can help prevent it.

REVIEW OF ANATOMY

The visual system consists mainly of the eyeball, optic nerves, extraocular muscles, cranial nerves, blood vessels, orbital fat, and lacrimal system, which are all housed within the bony orbit, and the eyelid, which covers the eye, moistens it, and protects it from injury.

The orbit (also called the *socket*) encloses the eye in a protective recess in the skull. Its seven bones—frontal, sphenoid, zygomatic, maxillary, palatine, ethmoid, and lacrimal—form a cone. The apex of this cone points toward the brain, and the cone's base forms the orbital rim.

Extraocular muscles hold the eyes in place and control their movement, as described below:

◆ *superior rectus:* elevates the eye upward; adducts and rotates the eye inward
◆ *inferior rectus:* depresses the eye downward; adducts and rotates the eye outward
◆ *lateral rectus:* abducts or turns the eye outward (laterally)
◆ *medial rectus:* adducts or turns the eye inward (medially)
◆ *superior oblique:* rotates the eye inward; abducts and depresses the eye
◆ *inferior oblique:* rotates the eye outward; abducts and elevates the eye

The actions of these muscles are mutually antagonistic: As one contracts, its opposing muscle relaxes.

❂ **ELDER TIP** *Eye structure and activity change with age. The eyes set deeper in their sockets and the eyelids lose their elasticity, allowing the orbital fat to protrude forward. Eyelids appear more saggy and wrinkled.*

OCULAR LAYERS

The eye has three structural layers: the sclera and cornea, the uveal tract, and the retina. (See *Cross section of the eye*, page 595.)

The sclera is the dense, white, fibrous outer protective coat of the eye. It meets the cornea at the limbus (corneoscleral junction) anteriorly and the dural sheath of the optic nerve posteriorly. The lamina cribrosa is a sievelike structure composed of a few strands of scleral tissue through which the optic nerve bundles pass. The sclera is covered by the episclera, a thin layer of fine elastic tissue.

❂ **ELDER TIP** *In older adults, lens changes occur typically with the formation of a cataract. The vitreous body liquefies and pulls away from the retina, generating floating vitreous debris and vitreous detachments.*

The cornea is the transparent, avascular, dome-shaped layer of the eye that's continuous with the sclera. The cornea consists of five layers: the epithelium, which contains sensory nerves; Bowman's membrane, the basement membrane for the epithelial cells; the stroma, or supporting tissue (90% of the corneal structure); Descemet's membrane, containing many elastic fibers; and the endothelium, a single

PATHOPHYSIOLOGY
Cross section of the eye

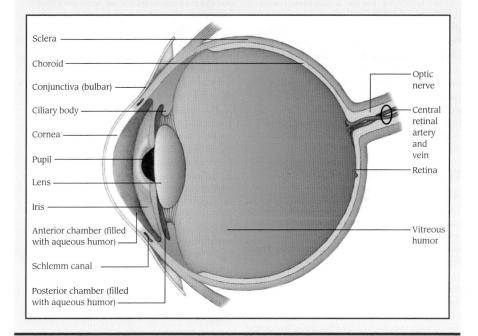

Sclera

Choroid

Conjunctiva (bulbar)

Ciliary body

Cornea

Pupil

Lens

Iris

Anterior chamber (filled with aqueous humor)

Schlemm canal

Posterior chamber (filled with aqueous humor)

Optic nerve

Central retinal artery and vein

Retina

Vitreous humor

---

layer of cells that acts as a pump to maintain proper dehydration or detumescence of the cornea. Aqueous humor bathes the posterior surface of the cornea, providing it with nutrients, and maintaining intraocular pressure (IOP) by volume and rate of outflow. The anterior cornea is kept moist by the tear film.

ELDER TIP Dry eye syndrome is more common in the elderly. Certain medications, such as histamines, some antidepressants, and antihypertensives, as well as systemic conditions (such as menopause, diabetes, and thyroid disorders), can exacerbate dry eyes, which may result in decreased vision, eye redness, and discomfort.

The middle layer of the eye, the uveal tract, is pigmented and vascular. It consists of the iris and the ciliary body in the anterior portion and the choroid in the posterior portion. In the center of the iris is the pupil. The sphincter and dilator muscles control the amount of light that enters the eye by changing the size of the pupil.

ELDER TIP It is believed that atrophy of the dilator muscle fibers and increased rigidity of the blood vessels of the iris reduce pupil size, decreasing the amount of light that reaches the retina. Consequently, higher levels of illumination may be

needed to improve uncorrected visual acuity in the older adult.

The angle formed by the anterior iris surface and the posterior corneal structures contains the many minute collecting channels of the trabecular meshwork. Aqueous humor drains through these channels into an encircling venous system called *the canal of Schlemm.*

The ciliary body, which extends from the root of the iris to the peripheral retina, produces aqueous humor and controls lens accommodation through its action on the zonular fibers. The choroid, the largest part of the uveal tract, is made up of blood vessels bound externally by the suprachoroid and internally by the retina.

The retina is the innermost coat of the eye. It receives visual images in the form of light and converts the images into neural impulses. The photoreceptor cells (rods and cones) are the light-sensitive cells. These and other retina cell types are interconnected by synapses and organized in layers that transmit the neural signals to the brain. Although both rods and cones are light receptors, they respond to light differently. Rods, scattered throughout the retina, respond to low levels of light and detect moving objects;

cones, located in the fovea centralis, function best in brighter light and perceive finer details.

Three types of cones contain different visual pigments and react to specific light wavelengths: one type reacts to red light, one to green, and one to blue-violet. The eye mixes these colors into various shades.

✿ **ELDER TIP** *Many elderly patients lose their ability to discriminate blue-greens, and white objects appear yellowish; these patients may also have difficulty discriminating among pastels, violets, and yellow-greens. The retinal pigmented epithelium layer, which is just posterior to the photoreceptors, has multiple support functions, including phagocytosis of photoreceptor segments, vitamin A metabolism, and regulation of molecule transport to the retina.*

THE LENS AND ACCOMMODATION

The lens of the eye is biconvex, avascular, and transparent; the lens capsule is a semipermeable membrane that encloses the lens and allows water and nutrients to reach the lens cells. The lens changes shape (accommodation) for near and far vision. For near vision, the ciliary body contracts and relaxes the zonules, the lens becomes steeper, the pupil constricts, and the eyes converge; for far vision, the ciliary body relaxes, the zonules tighten, the lens becomes flatter, the eyes straighten, and the pupils dilate. The lens refines the refraction necessary to focus a clear image on the retina.

✿ **ELDER TIP** *In older adults, lens changes occur, typically with the formation of a cataract. Symptoms of a cataract include glare, decreased vision, and the need for increased illumination. The purpose of cataract surgery is to remove the opacified lens (cataract) and to sharpen vision.*

The vitreous body, which is 99% water and a small amount of insoluble protein, constitutes two thirds of the eye's volume. This transparent, gelatinous body gives the eye its shape and contributes to the refraction of light rays. The vitreous is firmly attached to the peripheral retina near the ciliary body (anteriorly) and to the optic disk (posteriorly). The vitreous face contacts the lens; the vitreous gel rests against the retina.

LACRIMAL APPARATUS AND EYELIDS

The lacrimal apparatus consists of the lacrimal glands, upper and lower canaliculi, lacrimal sac, and nasolacrimal duct. The main gland, located in a shallow fossa beneath the superior temporal orbital rim, secretes reflex tears. Small

lacrimal glands throughout the conjunctiva are responsible for basal tear production. Multiple sebaceous glands in the eyelids produce an oily secretion that prevents tears from evaporating. With every blink, the eyelids direct the flow to the inner canthus, where the tears pool and then drain through a tiny opening called the *punctum*. The tears then pass through the canaliculi and lacrimal sac and down the nasolacrimal duct, which opens into the nasal cavity. The integrity of the lacrimal system is critical for moisturizing and also removing excess tears from the corneal surface.

The eyelids (palpebrae) consist of tarsal plates that are composed of dense connective tissue. The orbital septum—the fascia behind the orbicularis oculi muscle—acts as a barrier between the lids and the orbit. The levator palpebrae muscle elevates the upper lid. The eyelids contain three types of glands:
◆ glands of Zeis—modified sebaceous glands connected to the follicles of the eyelashes
◆ meibomian glands—sebaceous glands in the tarsal plates that secrete an oily substance as a tear film component (About 25 of these glands are found in the upper lid and about 20 in the lower lid.)
◆ Moll glands—ordinary sweat glands

The conjunctiva is the thin mucous membrane that lines the eyelids (palpebral conjunctiva), folds over at the fornix, and covers the surface of the eyeball (bulbar conjunctiva). The conjunctiva produces mucin, another component of the tear film. The ophthalmic, lacrimal, and multiple anastomoses of facial arteries supply blood to the lids. The space between the open lids is the palpebral fissure; the juncture of the upper and lower lids is the canthus. The junction near the nose is called the nasal, medial, or inner canthus; the junction on the temporal side, the lateral or external canthus.

OPTIC NERVE

The optic nerve is composed of the nerve fibers (axons) that originate in the retina and synapse at the lateral geniculate nucleus in the brain. Approximately 1 million nerve axons are contained in the optic nerve. The nerve from each eye exits the eye posteriorly and courses through the orbit to the optic canal. Both nerves meet at the optic chiasm, located intracranially near the pituitary gland. In the optic chiasm, part of the nerve fibers from one eye cross to the other side, and vice versa. From the synapse at the lateral geniculate nucleus, nerves carry visual information to the visual cortex, located in the majority of the occipital lobe of the brain. Some axons from the optic nerve synapse at other parts of the brain to regulate pupil responses, eye movements, and the sleep–wake cycle.

⬡ **ELDER TIP** *Age-related vision changes are usually first noticed during the fifth decade of life and may include the inability to focus, narrowing of the visual field, reduced peripheral vision, and loss of iris elasticity producing decreased response to light and dark. In addition, as people age, production of any of the three tear film components may decrease, causing dry eyes.*

DEPTH PERCEPTION

In normal binocular vision, a perceived image is projected onto the two foveae. Impulses then travel along the optic pathways to the occipital cortex, which perceives a single image. However, the cortex receives two images—each from a slightly different angle—giving the images perspective and providing depth perception.

VISION TESTING

Several tests assess visual acuity and identify visual defects:

♦ Ishihara test determines color blindness by using a series of plates composed of a colored background, with a letter, number, or pattern of a contrasting color located in the center of each plate. The patient with deficient color perception can't perceive the differences in color or, consequently, the designs formed by the color contrasts.

♦ The Snellen chart or other eye charts evaluate visual acuity. Such charts use progressively smaller letters or symbols to determine central vision on a numerical scale. A person with normal acuity should be able to read the letters or recognize the symbols on the 20/20 line of the eye chart at a distance of 20′.

SUBJECTIVE TESTING

Several tests accomplish objective testing of the eyes.

♦ B-mode ultrasonography delineates retinal tumors, detachments, and vitreous hemorrhages—even in the presence of opacities of the cornea and lens. A handheld B-scanner has simplified ultrasonic examination of the eye, making it possible to perform such studies in the eye care practitioner's office.

♦ The cover-uncover test assesses eye muscle misalignment or tendency toward misalignment. In this test, the patient stares at a small, fixed object—first from a distance of 20′ (6.1 m) and then from 1′ (0.3 m). The examiner covers the patient's eyes one at a time, noting any movement of the uncovered eye and the direction of any deviation. In exotropia

the eyes are naturally deviated outward. In the cover-uncover test, the eyes recover by moving inward to focus. The reverse is true in esotropia.

♦ Duction test checks eye movement in all directions of gaze. While one eye is covered, the other eye follows a moving light. This test detects weakness of rotation due to muscle paralysis or structural dysfunction.

♦ Fluorescein angiography evaluates the blood vessels in the choroid and retina after I.V. injection of fluorescein dye; images of the dye-enhanced vasculature are recorded by rapid-sequence photographs of the fundus.

♦ Goldmann applanation, Tonopen tonometry, and pneumotonometry all measure IOP. After instilling a local anesthetic in the patient's eye, the examiner touches the Tonopen tonometer tip to the surface of the cornea. The IOP reading is displayed and measured in mm Hg. Applanation tonometry gauges the force required to flatten a small area of the central cornea, and is the most accurate method of measuring IOP. For this test, a patient must be seated at a slit lamp and the cornea stained with fluorescein dye before the prism of the applanation tonometer touches the cornea and the examiner adjusts the controls until the two lines form an "S."

♦ Gonioscopy allows for direct visualization of the anterior chamber angle.

♦ The Maddox rod test assesses muscle dysfunction; it's especially useful in disclosing and measuring heterophoria (the tendency of the eyes to deviate). It can reveal horizontal, vertical, and, especially, torsional deviations.

♦ Ophthalmoscopy—direct ophthalmoscopy or binocular indirect ophthalmoscopy allows examination of the interior of the eye after the pupil has been dilated with a mydriatic. A light source and lenses are used by the examiner to focus on the posterior ocular structures (such as the retina and optic nerve).

♦ Refraction tests may be performed with or without cycloplegics. In cycloplegic refraction, eyedrops weaken the accommodative power of the ciliary muscle. Lenses placed in front of the eye direct light rays onto the retina, thus focusing the image so that it can be transmitted along the visual pathway. A retinoscope may be used in the same way by directing a beam of light through the pupil onto the retina; the light's shadow is neutralized by placing the appropriate lens in front of the eye.

♦ Slit-lamp biomicroscopic examination allows a well-illuminated examination of the eyelids and the anterior segment of the eyeball using a specialized microscope.

◆ Visual field tests assess the function of the retina, the optic nerve, and the optic pathways by recording the responses of the patient to light impulses directed to various areas of the visual field.

Eyelid and lacrimal ducts

BLEPHARITIS

A common inflammation, blepharitis produces a red-rimmed appearance of the margins of the eyelids. It's frequently chronic and bilateral and can affect both upper and lower lids. Seborrheic blepharitis is characterized by formation of waxy scales on the eyelashes and eyelid margins, and symptoms of burning and foreign body sensation.

Pathophysiology

Seborrheic blepharitis may be seen in conjunction with seborrhea of the scalp, eyebrows, and ears. It's common in elderly people and in people with red hair. Staphylococcal (ulcerative) blepharitis is characterized by the formation of dry scales along the inflamed lid margins, which also have ulcerated areas and may be associated with keratoconjunctivitis sicca, a dry eye syndrome. Staphylococcal blepharitis is associated with *Staphylococcus aureus* infection and is more common in females than in males. Both types may coexist. Blepharitis tends to recur and become chronic. It can be controlled if treatment begins before the onset of ocular involvement.

Allergies and eyelash infestations with lice are less common causes of blepharitis. Blepharitis may also be associated with repeated styes and chalazion.

Complications
◆ Keratitis
◆ Conjunctivitis
◆ Dry eyes

Signs and symptoms

Clinical features of blepharitis include itching, burning, foreign body sensation, and sticky, crusted eyelids on waking. This constant irritation results in unconscious rubbing of the eyes (causing reddened rims) or continual blinking. Other signs include waxy scales in seborrheic blepharitis; and flaky scales on lashes, loss of lashes, and ulcerated areas on lid margins in ulcerative blepharitis.

Diagnosis

Diagnosis depends on patient history and characteristic symptoms. In staphylococcal blepharitis, culture of ulcerated lid margin shows *S. aureus*.

Treatment

The goals of therapy are to control the disease and its underlying causes, maintain vision, and avoid secondary complications. Treatment depends on the type of blepharitis:
◆ blepharitis resulting from pediculosis—removal of nits (with forceps) or application of ophthalmic physostigmine or other ointment as an insecticide (This may cause pupil constriction and, possibly, headache, conjunctival irritation, and blurred vision from the film of ointment on the cornea.)
◆ seborrheic blepharitis—daily lid hygiene (using a mild shampoo on a damp applicator stick or a washcloth) and hot compresses to remove scales from the lid margins; also, frequent shampooing of the scalp and eyebrows
◆ staphylococcal blepharitis—warm compresses and an antibiotic, such as tetracycline or erythromycin eye ointment, may be used. For some patients, systemic antibiotics are indicated

Special considerations
◆ Instruct the patient to gently remove scales from the lid margins daily, with an applicator stick or a clean washcloth.
◆ Teach the patient the following method for applying warm compresses: First, run warm water into a clean bowl. Then, immerse a clean cloth in the water and wring it out. Place the warm cloth against the closed eyelid (be careful not to burn the skin). Hold the compress in place until it cools. Continue this procedure for 15 minutes.
◆ Antibiotic ophthalmic ointment should be applied after 15-minute application of warm compresses.
◆ Treatment for seborrheic blepharitis also requires attention to the face and scalp.

EXOPHTHALMOS

Exophthalmos (also called *proptosis*) is the unilateral or bilateral bulging or protrusion of the eyeballs or their apparent forward displacement (with lid retraction). The prognosis depends on the underlying cause.

Pathophysiology and incidence

Exophthalmos commonly results from hyperthyroidism, particularly ophthalmic Graves disease, in which the eyeballs are displaced forward and the lids retract. Unilateral exophthalmos may also result from trauma (such as fracture of the ethmoid bone, which allows

Recognizing exophthalmos

This photograph shows the characteristic forward protrusion of the eyes from the orbit associated with exophthalmos.

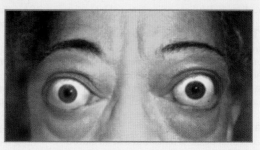

air from the sinus to enter the orbital tissue, displacing soft tissue and the eyeball forward). Exophthalmos may also stem from hemorrhage, varicosities, thrombosis, and edema, all of which similarly displace one or both eyeballs forward.

Other systemic and ocular causes include:
◆ infection—orbital cellulitis, panophthalmitis, and infection of the lacrimal gland or orbital tissues
◆ parasitic cysts—in surrounding tissue
◆ tumors and neoplastic diseases—in children, rhabdomyosarcomas, leukemia, gliomas of the optic nerve, dermoid cysts, teratomas, metastatic neuroblastomas, and lymphoma; in adults, lacrimal gland tumors, mucoceles, cavernous hemangioma, meningiomas, metastatic carcinomas, and lymphoma

Signs and symptoms

The obvious sign is a bulging eyeball, commonly with diplopia, due to eyeball misalignment or extraocular muscle dysfunction. (See *Recognizing exophthalmos*.) A rim of the sclera may be visible below the upper lid as lid retraction occurs. Other symptoms depend on the cause: pain may accompany traumatic exophthalmos; a tumor may produce conjunctival hyperemia or chemosis; retraction of the upper lid predisposes to exposure keratitis. If exophthalmos is associated with cavernous sinus thrombosis, the patient may exhibit paresis of the muscles supplied by cranial nerves III, IV, and VI; limited ocular movement; and a septic-type (high) fever.

Diagnosis

Exophthalmos is usually obvious on physical examination; exophthalmometer readings confirm diagnosis by showing the degree of anterior projection and asymmetry between the eyes (normal bar readings range from 12 to 20 mm).

The following diagnostic measures identify the cause:
◆ Computed tomography scan or magnetic resonance imaging detects swollen extraocular muscles or lesions within the orbit.
◆ Culture of discharge determines the infecting organism; sensitivity testing indicates appropriate antibiotic therapy.
◆ Biopsy of orbital tissue may be necessary if initial treatment fails.

Treatment

Eye trauma may require cold compresses for the first 24 hours, followed by warm compresses, and prophylactic antibiotic therapy. After edema subsides, surgery may be necessary in a small percentage of cases. It is important to counsel patients with acute orbital fractures not to blow their nose, to avoid air entering the orbit, which may cause acute exophthalmos. Eye infection requires treatment with broad-spectrum antibiotics during the 24 hours preceding positive identification of the organism, followed by specific antibiotics. A patient with exophthalmos resulting from an orbital tumor may initially benefit from antibiotic or corticosteroid therapy. Eventually, surgical exploration of the orbit and excision of the tumor, enucleation, or exenteration may be necessary. Radiation and chemotherapy may be used when primary orbital tumors can't be fully excised as encapsulated lesions, such as in rhabdomyosarcoma lesions.

Treatment for Graves disease may include antithyroid drug therapy or partial or total thyroidectomy to control hyperthyroidism; initial high doses of systemic corticosteroids, such as prednisone, for optic neuropathy and, if lid retraction is severe, protective lubricants.

Surgery may include orbital decompression (removal of any of the orbital walls) if vision is threatened, followed by muscle surgery and then lid surgery (eyelid retraction repair).

Special considerations

◆ It is critical to protect the exposed cornea with lubricants to prevent corneal drying until the disease stabilizes or is corrected by surgery.

PTOSIS

Ptosis (drooping of the upper eyelid) may be congenital or acquired, unilateral or bilateral, and constant or intermittent. Severe ptosis usually responds well to treatment; slight ptosis may require no treatment at all.

Pathophysiology

Congenital ptosis is transmitted as an autosomal dominant trait or results from a congenital anomaly in which the levator muscles of the eyelids fail to develop. This condition is usually unilateral.

Acquired ptosis may result from any of the following:

◆ advanced age (involutional ptosis, the most common form, usually seen in older patients)

◆ mechanical factors that make the eyelid heavy, such as swelling caused by a foreign body on the palpebral surface of the eyelid or by edema, inflammation produced by a tumor or pseudotumor, or an extra fatty fold

◆ myogenic factors, such as muscular dystrophy or myasthenia gravis (in which the defect appears to be in humoral transmission at the myoneural junction)

◆ neurogenic (paralytic) factors from interference in innervation of the eyelid by the oculomotor nerve (cranial nerve III), most commonly due to trauma, diabetes, or carotid aneurysm (Ptosis due to oculomotor nerve damage produces a fixed, dilated pupil, divergent strabismus, and slight depression of the eyeball.)

◆ nutritional factors, such as thiamine deficiency in chronic alcoholism, hyperemesis gravidarum, and other malnutrition-producing states

Risk factors for ptosis include aging, diabetes, stroke, Horner syndrome, myasthenia gravis, and cancer that affects nerve or muscle response.

◆ In myasthenia gravis, ptosis results from fatigue and characteristically appears in the evening but is relieved by rest.

The child with unilateral ptosis that covers the pupil can develop an amblyopic eye from disuse or lack of eye stimulation. In bilateral ptosis, the child may elevate the brow in an attempt to compensate, wrinkling the forehead in an effort to raise the upper lid. Additionally, the child may tip the head backward to see.

Complication

◆ Lazy eye in children (amblyopia)

Signs and symptoms

PEDIATRIC TIP *An infant with congenital ptosis has a smooth, flat upper eyelid, without the eyelid fold normally caused by the pull of the levator muscle; associated weakness of the superior rectus muscle isn't uncommon.*

Diagnosis

Examination includes measurement of the position of the upper eyelid margin relative to the pupil, degree of eyelid excursion, presence or absence of lagophthalmos, Bell phenomenon, and eyelid crease. Diagnosis may also include these tests to determine any underlying cause:

◆ digital subtraction angiography or magnetic resonance imaging—aneurysm

◆ glucose tolerance test—diabetes

◆ ophthalmologic examination—foreign bodies

◆ patient history—chronic alcoholism

◆ Tensilon test—myasthenia gravis (in acquired ptosis with no history of trauma)

Treatment

Slight ptosis that doesn't produce deformity or loss of vision requires no treatment. Severe ptosis that interferes with vision or is cosmetically undesirable usually necessitates reattachment of a stretched levator aponeurosis. Surgery to correct congenital ptosis is usually performed at age 3 or 4, but it may be done earlier if amblyopia is a concern. The surgical approach depends on the degree of ptosis. If surgery is contraindicated, special glasses with an attached suspended crutch on the frames may elevate the eyelid.

Effective treatment for ptosis also requires treatment for any underlying cause. For example, in patients with myasthenia gravis, neostigmine or steroids may be prescribed to increase the effect of acetylcholine and aid transmission of nerve impulses to muscles.

Special considerations

◆ After surgery to correct ptosis, watch for blood on the pressure patch. (Some surgical procedures may not require a patch.) Apply ointment to the sutures as prescribed.

◆ Emphasize to the patient and family the need to prevent accidental trauma to the surgical site until healing is complete (6 weeks). Suture line damage can precipitate recurrence of ptosis.

ORBITAL CELLULITIS

Orbital cellulitis is an acute infection of the orbital tissues and eyelids that doesn't involve the eyeball. With treatment, the prognosis is good;

if untreated, the infection may spread intracranially to the cavernous sinus or the meninges, where it can be life-threatening.

Pathophysiology

Orbital cellulitis may result from bacterial, fungal, or parasitic infection. It can develop from direct inoculation, via the bloodstream, or spread from adjacent structures (e.g., the sinuses or eyelids). Periorbital tissues may be inoculated as a result of surgery, foreign body trauma, and even animal or insect bites.

PEDIATRIC TIP *The most common pathogens in children are* Haemophilus influenzae, Streptococcus pneumoniae, *and* S. aureus. *In young children, infection spreads from adjacent sinuses (especially the ethmoid air cells) and accounts for the majority of postseptal cellulitis cases. The incidence has decreased because of the use of the H. influenzae b (Hib) vaccine.*

Immunosuppressed patients are also susceptible.

Complications

◆ Cavernous sinus thrombosis
◆ Hearing loss
◆ Septicemia
◆ Meningitis
◆ Optic nerve damage

Signs and symptoms

Orbital cellulitis generally produces unilateral eyelid edema, reddened eyelids, and matted lashes. Although the eyeball is initially unaffected, proptosis develops later (because of edematous tissues within the bony confines of the orbit). Other indications include extreme orbital pain, impaired eye movement, chemosis, purulent discharge from indurated areas, decreased vision, and an afferent pupillary defect. The severity of associated systemic symptoms (chills, fever, and malaise) varies according to the cause.

Complications include posterior extension, causing cavernous sinus thrombosis, panophthalmitis, meningitis, or brain abscess and, rarely, atrophy and subsequent loss of vision secondary to optic neuritis.

Diagnosis

Typical clinical features establish diagnosis. Computed tomography scan or magnetic resonance imaging of the sinuses and orbit tissues will determine if the cause of the cellulitis is preseptal or if deeper structures are involved, or if a tumor is the cause of swelling. Usually the patient will also be febrile with this type of infection. Wound culture and sensitivity testing determine the causative organism and specific antibiotic therapy. Other tests include white blood cell count and ophthalmologic examination.

Treatment

Prompt treatment is necessary to prevent complications. Primary treatment consists of antibiotic therapy. Systemic antibiotics (I.V. or oral) and eyedrops or ointment will be ordered. Supportive therapy consists of fluids; warm, moist compresses; and bed rest. The patient should be monitored closely. If during the initial 48 to 72 hours of treatment no improvement is seen, adjustment of antibiotics guided by drug sensitivity should be considered. If an orbital abscess is present, surgical incision and drainage may be necessary.

Special considerations

◆ Monitor vital signs at least every 4 hours, and maintain fluid and electrolyte balance.
◆ Have the patient instill antibiotic eyedrops frequently during the day and apply ointment at night.
◆ Apply compresses every 3 to 4 hours to localize inflammation and relieve discomfort. Teach the patient to apply these compresses. Give pain medication, as ordered, after assessing pain level.
◆ Before discharge, stress the importance of completing prescribed antibiotic therapy. To prevent orbital cellulitis, tell the patient to maintain good general hygiene and to carefully clean abrasions and cuts that occur near the orbit.
◆ Ensure patient has appropriate follow-up.

PREVENTION
◆ *Use Hib vaccination to prevent Haemophilus infection in children.*
◆ *Treat sinus and dental infections early to decrease spread to the eye.*

DACRYOCYSTITIS

Dacryocystitis is an infection of the lacrimal sac. It can be acute, chronic, or congenital. In infants, dacryocystitis results from congenital atresia of the nasolacrimal duct; in adults, it results from an obstruction (dacryostenosis) of the nasolacrimal duct (most common in women older than age 40).

Pathophysiology

Atresia of the nasolacrimal ducts results from failure of canalization or, in the first few months of life, from blockage when the membrane that separates the lower part of the nasolacrimal duct and the inferior nasal meatus fails to open spontaneously before tear secretion. Bony obstruction of the duct may also occur.

In acute dacryocystitis, *S. aureus* and, occasionally, beta-hemolytic streptococci are the cause. In chronic dacryocystitis, *S. pneumoniae* or, sometimes, a fungus—such as *Actinomyces* or *Candida albicans*—is the causative organism. Primary lumps and secondary tumors from sinuses, nose, and orbits have also been reported as causes.

Complication
◆ Orbital cellulitis

Signs and symptoms
The hallmark of both the acute and chronic forms of dacryocystitis is constant tearing. Other symptoms of dacryocystitis include inflammation and tenderness over the nasolacrimal sac; pressure over this area may fail to produce purulent discharge from the punctum. Acute dacryocystitis is painful for the patient.

Diagnosis
Clinical features and a physical examination suggest dacryocystitis. Culture of the discharged material demonstrates *S. aureus* and, occasionally, beta-hemolytic streptococci in acute dacryocystitis, and *S. pneumoniae* or *C. albicans* in the chronic form. The white blood cell count may be elevated in the acute form; in the chronic form, it's generally normal. An X-ray after injection of a radiopaque medium (dacryocystography) locates the atresia in infants.

Treatment
Treatment for acute dacryocystitis consists of warm compresses, topical and systemic antibiotic therapy, and, occasionally, incision and drainage. Chronic dacryocystitis may eventually require dacryocystorhinostomy. Laser-assisted endoscopic dacryocystorhinostomy and balloon dilatation or probing of the nasolacrimal system may also be used.

Therapy for nasolacrimal duct obstruction in an infant consists of careful massage of the area over the lacrimal sac four times a day for 6 to 9 months. If this fails to open the duct, dilation of the punctum and probing of the duct are necessary.

Special considerations
◆ Check the patient history for possible allergy to antibiotics before administration. Emphasize the importance of precise compliance with the prescribed antibiotic regimen.

◆ Tell the adult patient what to expect after surgery. The patient should expect to have ice compresses over the surgical site and will have bruising and swelling.
◆ Monitor blood loss by counting dressings used to collect the blood.
◆ Apply ice compresses postoperatively. A small adhesive bandage may be placed over the suture line to protect it from damage.

CHALAZION
A chalazion is a chronic granulomatous inflammation of a meibomian gland or gland of Zeis in the upper or lower eyelid. (There are ~100 of these glands located near the eyelashes.) This common eye disorder is characterized by localized swelling within the tarsal plate, or it may break through the conjunctival or skin side. Mild irritation and blurred vision usually develop slowly over several weeks. (See *Recognizing chalazion.*) A chalazion may become large enough to press on the eyeball, causing astigmatism. A large chalazion seldom subsides spontaneously. It's generally benign and chronic, and can occur at any age. In some patients, it's apt to recur.

Pathophysiology
Obstruction of the meibomian (sebaceous) gland duct causes a chalazion.

Complication
◆ Astigmatism

Signs and symptoms
A chalazion occurs as a painless, hard lump that usually points toward the conjunctival side of

Recognizing chalazion

A chalazion is a nontender granulomatous inflammation of a meibomian gland on the upper or lower eyelid.

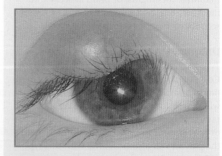

the eyelid. Eversion of the lid reveals a red or red-yellow elevated area on the conjunctival surface. Otherwise, it's seen as an indurated bump under the skin of the upper eyelid.

Diagnosis

Diagnosis requires visual examination and palpation of the eyelid, revealing a small bump or nodule. Persistently recurrent chalazions, especially in an adult, necessitate biopsy to rule out sebaceous cell carcinoma.

Treatment

Initial treatment consists of application of warm compresses for 10 to 15 minutes at least four times a day to open the lumen of the gland, soften the hardened oils blocking the duct, and promote drainage and healing. If such therapy fails, or if the chalazion presses on the eyeball or causes a severe cosmetic problem, steroid injection or incision and curettage under local anesthetic may be necessary. After such surgery, a pressure eye patch applied for 4 to 6 hours controls bleeding and swelling. After removal of the patch, treatment again consists of warm compresses. Antibiotic eyedrops are occasionally prescribed before and after cyst removal, but otherwise are of little value.

Special considerations

◆ Instruct the patient how to properly apply warm compresses: Educate the patient to take special care to avoid burning the skin, to always use a clean cloth, and to discard used compresses. In addition, instruct the patient to start applying warm compresses at the first sign of lid irritation to increase the blood supply and keep the lumen open.
◆ Teach the patient how to instill antibiotic eyedrops.

STYE

A localized, purulent staphylococcal infection, a stye (or hordeolum) can occur externally (in the lumen of the smaller glands of Zeis or in Moll glands) or internally (in the larger meibomian gland). A stye can occur at any age. Generally, styes are self-limiting and respond well to hot, moist compresses. More than one may occur at the same time. If untreated, a stye can eventually lead to cellulitis of the eyelid. Styes can also develop into a chalazion if gland ducts are fully blocked.

Pathophysiology

Skin bacteria that enter eyelash hair follicles and cause inflammation can result in stye formation. Risk factors include blepharitis,

Recognizing a stye

A stye is a localized red, swollen, and tender abscess of the lid glands.

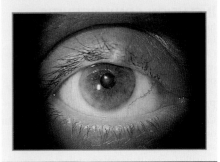

diabetes and other chronic debilitating illnesses, and seborrhea.

Complication

◆ Cellulitis of the eyelid

Signs and symptoms

Typically, a stye produces redness, swelling, and pain. An abscess frequently forms at the lid margin, with an eyelash pointing outward from its center. (See *Recognizing a stye*.)

Diagnosis

Visual examination generally confirms this infection. Culture of purulent material from the abscess usually reveals a staphylococcal organism.

Treatment

Treatment consists of warm compresses applied for 10 to 15 minutes, four times a day for 3 to 4 days, to facilitate drainage of the abscess, to relieve pain and inflammation, and to promote suppuration. Drug therapy includes antibiotic eyedrops or ointment and, occasionally, a systemic antibiotic for secondary eyelid cellulitis. If conservative treatment fails, incision and drainage may be necessary.

Special considerations

◆ Instruct the patient to use a clean cloth for each application of warm compresses and to dispose of it or launder it separately.
◆ Warn against squeezing the stye; this spreads the infection and may cause cellulitis.
◆ Teach the patient or family members the proper technique for instilling eyedrops or ointments into the cul-de-sac of the lower eyelid.

▓▓▓▓ **PREVENTION** *Teach proper eye hygiene, such*
░▒▓ *as washing hands and using clean towels, to*
prevent recurrent infections.

Conjunctival disorders

INCLUSION CONJUNCTIVITIS

Inclusion conjunctivitis is an acute ocular
inflammation resulting from infection by
Chlamydia trachomatis. Although inclusion conjunctivitis occasionally becomes chronic, the
prognosis is usually good.

Pathophysiology

Chlamydia trachomatis is an obligate intracellular
organism of the lymphogranuloma venereum
serotype group. Serotypes D through K are
sexually transmitted, and secondary eye involvement in adults occurs in about 1 in 300 genital
cases. Because contaminated cervical secretions
infect the eyes of the neonate during birth,
inclusion conjunctivitis is an important cause
of ophthalmia neonatorum. Ocular chlamydial
disease occurs most frequently in adults between ages 18 and 30.

Complications

♦ Otitis media
♦ Blindness

Signs and symptoms

Inclusion conjunctivitis develops 5 to 12 days
after contamination (it takes longer to develop
than gonococcal ophthalmia). In a neonate,
reddened eyelids and tearing with moderate
mucoid discharge are presenting symptoms. In
neonates, pseudo membranes may form, which
can lead to conjunctival scarring. In adults,
follicles appear inside the lower eyelids; such
follicles don't form in infants because the lymphoid tissue isn't yet well developed. Children
and adults also develop preauricular lymphadenopathy, and children may develop otitis media
as a complication. Inclusion conjunctivitis may
persist for weeks or months, possibly with superficial corneal involvement.

Diagnosis

Clinical features and a history of sexual contact
with an infected individual suggest inclusion
conjunctivitis.

℞ **CONFIRMING DIAGNOSIS** *Examination of
Giemsa-stained conjunctival scraping reveals
cytoplasmic inclusion bodies in conjunctival epithelial cells and is effective in detecting chlamydial infection in infants. The direct fluorescent monoclonal
antibody and enzyme-linked immunosorbent assay
are most effective in adults.*

Treatment

Because infection isn't limited to the eye in neonates, infants, or adults, systemic antimicrobial
treatment is necessary. In infants, effective therapy is achieved with erythromycin. Adults may be
given tetracycline, doxycycline, or erythromycin.

Prophylactic tetracycline or erythromycin
ointment is applied once, 1 hour after delivery.
However, this treatment hasn't been found to
be significantly more effective than Credé procedure (1% silver nitrate).

Special considerations

♦ Keep the patient's eyes as clean as possible,
using sterile technique. Clean the eyes from the
inner to the outer canthus. Apply warm soaks as
needed. Record the amount and color of drainage.
♦ Remind the patient not to rub the eyes,
which can irritate them.
♦ If the patient's eyes are sensitive to light, keep
the room dark or suggest wearing dark glasses.

▓▓▓▓ **PREVENTION** *Take these actions to prevent
░▒▓ further spread of inclusion conjunctivitis:*
♦ *Wash hands thoroughly before and after administering eye medications.*
♦ *Suggest genital examination of the mother of
an infected neonate or of any adult with inclusion
conjunctivitis.*
♦ *Obtain a history of recent sexual contacts, so they
can be examined for chlamydial infection.*

CONJUNCTIVITIS

Conjunctivitis is characterized by hyperemia
of the conjunctiva due to infection, allergy, or
chemical reactions. (See *Recognizing conjunctivitis.*) This disorder usually occurs as benign,

---

Recognizing conjunctivitis

Itching is the hallmark of allergy. Giant
papillae resembling cobblestones may
be seen on the palpebral conjunctiva, as
shown here.

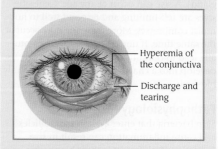

Hyperemia of
the conjunctiva

Discharge and
tearing

self-limiting pinkeye; it may also be chronic, possibly indicating degenerative changes or damage from repeated acute attacks.

Pathophysiology

The most common causative organisms include:
◆ bacterial—*S. aureus, S. pneumoniae, Neisseria gonorrhoeae, Neisseria meningitidis*
◆ chlamydial—*C. trachomatis* (inclusion conjunctivitis)
◆ viral—adenovirus types 3, 7, and 8; herpes simplex virus, type 1

Other causes include allergic reactions to pollen, grass, topical medications, air pollutants, smoke, or unknown seasonal allergens (vernal conjunctivitis); environmental (wind, dust, and smoke) and occupational irritants (acids and alkalies); and a hypersensitivity to contact lenses or solutions.

Vernal conjunctivitis (so-called because symptoms tend to be worse in the spring) is a severe form of immunoglobulin E-mediated mast cell hypersensitivity reaction. This form of conjunctivitis is bilateral. It usually begins at age 3 to 5 years and persists for about 10 years. It's sometimes associated with other signs of allergy commonly related to pollens, asthma, and allergic rhinitis.

Epidemic keratoconjunctivitis is an acute, highly contagious viral conjunctivitis caused by adenovirus types 8 and 19. On occasion it is complicated by visual loss due to corneal subepithelial infiltrates. Healthcare providers must be careful to wash their hands and sterilize equipment to prevent the spread of this disease.

In the Western hemisphere, conjunctivitis is probably the most common eye disorder.

Complications

◆ Corneal infiltrates
◆ Corneal ulcers
◆ Reinfection

Signs and symptoms

Conjunctivitis commonly produces hyperemia of the conjunctiva, sometimes accompanied by discharge, tearing and, with corneal involvement, pain and photophobia. It generally doesn't affect vision. Conjunctivitis usually begins in one eye and rapidly spreads to the other by contamination of towels, washcloths, or the patient's own hand.

Acute bacterial conjunctivitis (pinkeye) usually lasts only 2 weeks. The patient typically complains of itching, burning, and the sensation of a foreign body in the eye. The eyelids show a crust of sticky, mucopurulent discharge. If the disorder is due to *N. gonorrhoeae*, however,

the patient exhibits a profuse, purulent discharge. In that case, treatment is required to avoid severe complications, including corneal perforation and endophthalmitis.

Viral conjunctivitis produces copious tearing with minimal exudate, and enlargement of the preauricular lymph node. Some viruses follow a chronic course; others last 2 to 3 weeks and are self-limiting.

Diagnosis

Examination includes inspection of the eyelids, conjunctiva, and cornea. Regional lymph nodes should also be palpated. In children, possible systemic symptoms include sore throat or fever, if the conjunctivitis is suspected of being of adenoviral origin.

Lymphocytes are predominant in stained smears of conjunctival scrapings if conjunctivitis is caused by a virus. Polymorphonuclear cells (neutrophils) predominate if conjunctivitis is due to bacteria; eosinophils, if it's allergy-related. Culture and sensitivity tests identify the causative bacterial organism and indicate appropriate antibiotic therapy.

Treatment

Treatment for conjunctivitis varies with the cause. Bacterial conjunctivitis requires topical application of the appropriate broad-spectrum antibiotic. Although viral conjunctivitis resists treatment, a sulfonamide or broad-spectrum antibiotic eyedrops may prevent a secondary infection. Patients may be contagious for several weeks after onset. The most important aspect of treatment is preventing transmission. Herpes simplex infection generally responds to treatment with trifluridine drops or vidarabine ointment or oral acyclovir, but the infection may persist for 2 to 3 weeks. Treatment for vernal (allergic) conjunctivitis includes administration of corticosteroid drops followed by cromolyn sodium, cold compresses to relieve itching, and, occasionally, oral antihistamines.

Instillation of a one-time dose of erythromycin or 1% silver nitrate solution (Credé procedure) into the eyes of neonates prevents gonococcal conjunctivitis.

Special considerations

◆ Apply compresses and therapeutic ointment or drops, as ordered. Don't irrigate the eye, as this will spread the infection. Have the patient wash hands before using the medication. Instruct the patient to use clean washcloths or towels frequently to avoid infecting the other eye. (See *Preventing conjunctivitis*, page 606.)

Preventing conjunctivitis

To prevent conjunctivitis from occurring or recurring, teach your patient to practice good hygiene. Encourage the following prevention tips.

Practice good hygiene
To encourage good eye hygiene, teach proper hand-washing technique because bacterial and viral conjunctivitis are highly contagious. Stress the risk of spreading infection to family members by sharing washcloths, towels, and pillows. Suggest the use of tissues or disposable wipes to reduce the risk of transmission from contaminated linens. Caution the patient against rubbing the infected eye, which could spread infection to the other eye.

Use cosmetics carefully
If the patient uses eye cosmetics, instruct the patient not to share them. Also, encourage the patient to replace eye cosmetics regularly.

Keep contact lenses clean
If the patient wears contact lenses, teach the patient to handle and clean contact lenses properly. Also, advise the patient to stop wearing contact lenses until the infection clears.

Avoid contact with contagious people
Because conjunctivitis is highly contagious, particularly among children, infected children should avoid close contact with other children. Warn the patient with "cold sores" to avoid kissing others on the eyelids to prevent the spread of the disease.

◆ Teach the patient to instill eyedrops and ointments correctly—without touching the bottle tip to the eye or lashes.
◆ Remind the patient that the ointment will cause blurred vision.
◆ Stress the importance of safety glasses for the patient who works near chemical irritants.
◆ Notify public health authorities if cultures show *N. gonorrhoeae*.
◆ Ensure appropriate follow-up (e.g., patients on corticosteroid drops should have their IOP monitored periodically).

TRACHOMA

The most common cause of preventable blindness in underdeveloped areas of the world, trachoma is a chronic form of keratoconjunctivitis. This infection is usually confined to the eye but may have a systemic component. Although trachoma itself is self-limiting, it causes permanent damage to the cornea and conjunctiva by scarring the lids, and it results in secondary infections that can lead to blindness. (See *What happens in trachoma*, page 607.) Early diagnosis and treatment (before trachoma results in scar formation) ensure recovery but without immunity to reinfection.

Pathophysiology

Trachoma results from infection with *C. trachomatis*, a gram-negative obligate intracellular bacterium. These organisms are transmitted from eye to eye by flies and gnats and through hand-to-eye contact in endemic areas.

Trachoma is spread by close contact between family members or among schoolchildren. It's prevalent in Africa, Latin America, and Asia, particularly in children. Other predisposing factors include poverty and poor hygiene due to lack of water. Patients in hot, dusty climates are at greater risk.

Complications

◆ Conjunctival and corneal scarring
◆ Deformities of the eyelid
◆ Vision loss

Signs and symptoms

Trachoma begins with a mild infection resembling bacterial conjunctivitis (visible conjunctival follicles, red and edematous eyelids, pain, photophobia, tearing, and exudation).

After about 1 month, if the infection is untreated, conjunctival follicles enlarge into inflamed papillae that later become yellow or gray. At this stage, small blood vessels invade the superior cornea under the upper lid.

Eventually, severe scarring and contraction of the eyelids cause entropion; the eyelids turn inward and the lashes rub against the cornea, producing corneal scarring and visual distortion. In late stages, severe conjunctival scarring may obstruct the lacrimal ducts and cause dry eyes.

PATHOPHYSIOLOGY
What happens in trachoma

Trachoma results from infection with *C. trachomatis* and in its early stages resembles bacterial conjunctivitis. If untreated, this chronic infection can spread to the cornea and lead to scarring and, eventually, to blindness.

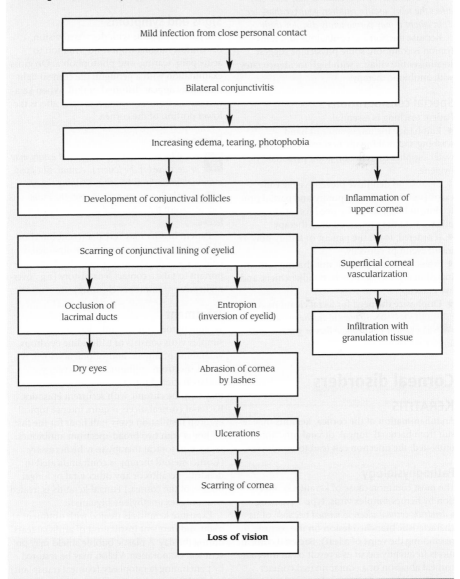

Diagnosis

Follicular conjunctivitis with corneal infiltration, and upper lid or conjunctival scarring suggest trachoma, especially in endemic areas, when these symptoms persist longer than 3 weeks.

CONFIRMING DIAGNOSIS *Microscopic examination of a Giemsa-stained conjunctival scraping confirms the diagnosis by showing cytoplasmic inclusion bodies, some polymorphonuclear reaction, plasma cells, and large macrophages containing phagocytosed debris.*

Treatment

Primary treatment for trachoma consists of topical or systemic antibiotic therapy with erythromycin (and its derivatives), doxycycline, or sulfonamides. Severe entropion requires surgical correction.

⚠ ALERT *Tetracycline is contraindicated in pregnant women, because it may adversely affect the fetus, and in children younger than age 7, in whom it may permanently discolor teeth.*

Because trachoma is contagious and reinfection is common, some physicians suggest treating entire villages with high incidence rates with antibiotic therapy.

Special considerations

Patient teaching is essential:

◆ Emphasize the importance of hand washing and making the best use of available water supplies to maintain good personal hygiene.

◆ Because no definitive preventive measure exists (vaccines offer temporary and partial protection, at best), stress the need for strict compliance with the prescribed drug therapy.

◆ If ordered, teach the patient or family how to instill eyedrops correctly.

◆ Stress the importance of not sharing contaminated items, such as towels, handkerchiefs, and eye makeup.

◆ Emphasize the need for facial cleanliness.

▓ PREVENTION *To prevent trachoma, warn the patient not to allow flies or gnats to settle around the eyes.*

Corneal disorders

KERATITIS

An inflammation of the cornea, keratitis may result from bacterial, fungal, or viral infection. If untreated, the infection can lead to blindness.

Pathophysiology

The most common cause of keratitis is infection by herpes simplex virus, type 1 (causing a *dendritic corneal ulcer, so named* because of its characteristic branched lesion on the cornea resembling the veins of a leaf). Bacterial corneal ulcers frequently occur as a result of an infected corneal abrasion or a contaminated contact lens. Fungal keratitis is more frequently encountered in tropical climates, after trauma, or in the elderly. Poor lid closure can result in exposure keratitis. Chemicals accidentally splashed into the eye and exposure to ultraviolet light (sunlamps, sunlight, or welding arcs) also can produce keratitis.

⚠ ALERT *An ocular chemical burn is an ophthalmic emergency. Patients need copious irrigation of the affected eye until the pH of the tears is back to physiologic levels.*

Complications

◆ Irregular astigmatism
◆ Corneal scarring or perforation

Signs and symptoms

The patient presents with decreased vision, discomfort ranging from mild irritation to acute pain, tearing, and photophobia. On gross examination with a penlight, the corneal light reflex may appear distorted or dull. When keratitis results from exposure, it usually affects the lower portion of the cornea.

Diagnosis

℞ CONFIRMING DIAGNOSIS *Visual acuity may be decreased if the lesion is central. Slit-lamp examination confirms keratitis. Staining the eye with a sterile fluorescein strip enables the examiner to discern the extent and depth of any corneal lesion.*

Patient history may reveal a recent infection of the upper respiratory tract accompanied by cold sores, if the etiology is herpetic. It is important to take a contact lens history (e.g., overnight wear or improper cleaning).

Treatment

Treatment for acute keratitis due to herpes simplex virus consists of trifluridine eyedrops, vidarabine ointment, and/or oral acyclovir. A broad-spectrum antibiotic may prevent secondary bacterial infection. Dendritic keratitis may become chronic with recurrent episodes. Bacterial corneal ulcers require intense topical eyedrop instillation every half hour for the first 48 hours with two broad-spectrum antibiotics. Long-term topical therapy may be necessary. (Corticosteroid therapy is contraindicated in dendritic keratitis or any other viral or fungal disease of the cornea.) Fungal keratitis is treated with polyhexamethylene biguanide.

Exposure keratitis is treated with ointment at night and frequent instillation of artificial tears during the day. A plastic bubble shield may prevent tear evaporation. Vision may be restored by penetrating keratoplasty (corneal transplant) in blindness resulting from corneal scarring.

Special considerations

◆ Protect the exposed corneas of unconscious patients by cleaning the eyes daily, applying moisturizing ointment, or covering the eyes with an eye shield.

◆ Be aware that the patient with a red eye may have keratitis. Check for a history of contact lens wear, cold sores, or recent foreign body sensation. Refer the patient for slit-lamp examination as soon as possible for intense treatment.

CORNEAL ABRASION

A corneal abrasion is a scratch on the surface epithelium of the cornea. With treatment, the prognosis is usually good.

Pathophysiology

Eye trauma or a foreign body (such as a cinder or a piece of dust, dirt, or grit) on the cornea or under the lid are the most common causes of an abrasion.

A corneal scratch produced by a fingernail, a piece of paper, or other organic substance may cause a persistent lesion. The epithelium doesn't always heal properly, and a recurrent corneal erosion may develop, with delayed effects more severe than the original injury.

In the United States, corneal abrasions are a common ophthalmologic cause of emergency department visits. Incidence is highest among younger, physically active individuals; corneal abrasions are rare in elderly people.

Complications

◆ Corneal erosion
◆ Corneal ulceration
◆ Permanent vision loss

Signs and symptoms

A corneal abrasion typically produces redness, increased tearing, discomfort with blinking, a sensation of "something in the eye" and, because the cornea is richly endowed with nerve endings from the trigeminal nerve (cranial nerve V), pain disproportionate to the size of the injury. It may also affect visual acuity, depending on the size and location of the injury.

Diagnosis

History of eye trauma or prolonged wearing of contact lenses and typical symptoms suggest corneal abrasion.

CONFIRMING DIAGNOSIS *Staining the cornea with fluorescein stain confirms the diagnosis: The injured area appears green when examined with a cobalt blue light. Slit-lamp examination discloses depth and allows measurement of the abrasion.*

Examining the eye with a flashlight may reveal a foreign body on the cornea; the eyelid must be everted to check for a foreign body embedded under the lid.

Before beginning treatment, a test to determine visual acuity provides a medical baseline and a legal safeguard.

Treatment

Topical anesthetic eyedrops are instilled in the affected eye before removal of a superficial foreign body, using a foreign body spud. A rust ring on the cornea must be removed with an ophthalmic burr.

Treatment includes instillation of broad-spectrum antibiotic eyedrops in the affected eye every 3 to 4 hours. Application of a pressure patch prevents further corneal irritation when the patient blinks. If the patient wears contact lenses, advise the patient to abstain from wearing the lenses until the corneal abrasion heals.

Special considerations

◆ Assist with examination of the eye. Check visual acuity before beginning treatment.
◆ If a foreign body is visible, carefully irrigate with normal saline solution.
◆ Tell the patient with an eye patch to leave it in place as directed. Warn that a patch alters depth perception, so advise caution in daily activities, such as climbing stairs or stepping off a curb.
◆ Reassure the patient that the corneal epithelium usually heals in 24 to 48 hours.
◆ Stress the importance of instilling antibiotic eyedrops, as ordered, because an untreated corneal abrasion, if infected, can lead to a corneal ulcer and permanent vision loss. Teach the patient the proper way to instill eye medications.

PREVENTION *Emphasize the importance of wearing safety glasses to protect a worker's eyes from flying fragments. Also review instructions for wearing and caring for contact lenses, to prevent further trauma. Encourage use of sunglasses.*

CORNEAL ULCERS

A major cause of blindness worldwide, ulcers produce corneal scarring or perforation. They occur in the central or marginal areas of the cornea, vary in shape and size, and may be singular or multiple. Marginal ulcers are the most common form. Prompt treatment (within hours of onset) can prevent visual impairment.

Pathophysiology

Corneal ulcers generally result from bacterial, viral, fungal, or protozoan infections. Common bacterial sources include *S. aureus, Pseudomonas aeruginosa, Streptococcus viridans, S. (Diplococcus) pneumoniae*, and *Moraxella liquefaciens*; viral sources comprise herpes simplex type 1, variola, vaccinia, and varicella-zoster viruses; and common fungal sources are *Candida, Fusarium*, and *Cephalosporium*.

Other causes include trauma, exposure, reactions to bacterial infections, toxins, trichiasis, entropion, allergens, and wearing of contact lenses. (See *What happens in corneal ulceration.*) Tuberculoprotein causes a classic phlyctenular keratoconjunctivitis, vitamin A deficiency results in xerophthalmia, and fifth cranial nerve lesions lead to neurotropic ulcers.

Complications
◆ Corneal scarring
◆ Loss of the eye
◆ Vision loss
◆ Irregular astigmatism
◆ Corneal perforation

Signs and symptoms
Typically, corneal ulceration begins with pain and foreign body sensation (aggravated by blinking) and photophobia, followed by increased tearing. The eye may appear injected. If a bacterial ulcer is present, purulent discharge is possible.

Diagnosis
A history of trauma or use of contact lenses and flashlight examination that reveals irregular corneal surface suggest corneal ulcer. Exudate may be present on the cornea, and a hypopyon (accumulation of white cells in the anterior chamber) may appear as a white crescent moon inside the eye that moves when the head is tilted.

PATHOPHYSIOLOGY
What happens in corneal ulceration

Corneal ulcers can be caused by infection (protozoan, bacterial, viral, or fungal), trauma, exposure, toxins, contact lenses, or allergens. Scarring or perforation can cause changes in the eye structure and can lead to partial or total vision loss.

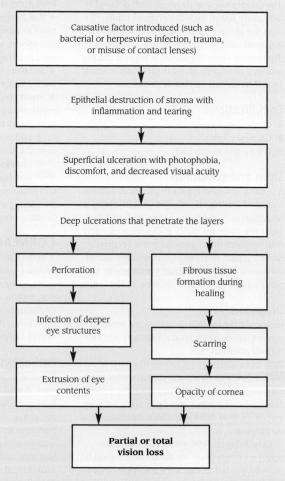

℞ **CONFIRMING DIAGNOSIS** *Fluorescein dye, instilled in the conjunctival sac, stains the outline of the ulcer and confirms the diagnosis.*

Culture and sensitivity testing of corneal scrapings may identify the causative bacteria or fungus, and may indicate appropriate antibiotic or antifungal therapy.

Treatment

Prompt treatment is essential for all forms of corneal ulcer to prevent complications and permanent visual impairment. Treatment usually consists of topical broad-spectrum antibiotics until culture results identify the causative organism. The goals of treatment are to eliminate the underlying cause of the ulcer and to relieve pain:
- Fungi—topical instillation of polyhexamethylene biguanide for *Fusarium, Cephalosporium,* and *Candida.*
- Herpes simplex virus type 1—topical application of trifluridine drops or vidarabine ointment. Corneal ulcers resulting from a viral infection often recur, requiring further treatment with trifluridine.
- Hypovitaminosis A—correction of dietary deficiency or gastrointestinal (GI) malabsorption of vitamin A.
- Infection by *P. aeruginosa*—fluoroquinolones, administered topically and by subconjunctival injection, tobramycin I.V. Because this type of corneal ulcer spreads so rapidly, it can cause corneal perforation and loss of the eye within 48 hours. Immediate treatment and isolation of hospitalized patients are required.

⚠ **ALERT** *Treatment for a corneal ulcer due to bacterial infection should never include an eye patch because patching creates the dark, warm, moist environment ideal for bacterial growth.*
- Neurotropic ulcers or exposure keratitis—frequent instillation of artificial tears or lubricating ointments and use of a plastic bubble eye shield.
- Varicella-zoster virus—topical erythromycin ointment applied three to four times daily to prevent secondary infection. These lesions are unilateral, following the pathway of the fifth cranial nerve, and are typically quite painful. Give analgesics and oral acyclovir as ordered. Associated anterior uveitis requires cycloplegic eyedrops. Watch for signs of secondary glaucoma (transient vision loss and halos around lights).

Special considerations
- Keep the room darkened and orient the patient as necessary.
- Teach the patient how to properly clean and wear contact lenses to prevent a recurrence.

▦ **PREVENTION** *Encourage your patient to:*
- seek treatment early for eye infections
- wash hands before handling contact lenses
- avoid wearing contact lenses overnight

Uveal tract, retinal, and lens disorders

UVEITIS

Uveitis is inflammation of the uveal tract. It occurs as anterior uveitis, which affects the iris (iritis) or both the iris and the ciliary body (iridocyclitis); as posterior uveitis, which affects the choroid (choroiditis) or both the choroid and the retina (chorioretinitis); or as panuveitis, which affects the entire uveal tract. Although clinical distinction isn't always possible, anterior uveitis occurs in two forms—granulomatous and nongranulomatous. (See *The uveal tract and causes of uveitis,* page 612.)

Granulomatous uveitis was once thought to be caused by tuberculosis bacilli; nongranulomatous uveitis, by streptococci. Although this isn't true, the terms are still used. Untreated anterior uveitis may result in elevated IOP, leading to vision loss. With immediate treatment, anterior uveitis usually subsides after a few days to several weeks; however, recurrence can occur. Posterior uveitis may lead to vision loss if the macula is involved.

Pathophysiology

Typically, uveitis is idiopathic. However, it can result from allergy, bacteria, viruses, fungi, chemicals, trauma, or surgery; or it may be associated with systemic diseases, such as rheumatoid arthritis, ankylosing spondylitis, and toxoplasmosis.

Uveitis occurs in 15 of every 100,000 people.

Complications
- Cataracts
- Glaucoma
- Retinal detachment
- Vision loss

Signs and symptoms

Anterior uveitis produces moderate to severe unilateral eye pain; severe ciliary injection; photophobia; tearing; a small, nonreactive pupil; and blurred vision (due to the increased number of cells in the aqueous humor). It sometimes produces deposits called *keratic precipitates* on the back of the cornea. The iris may adhere to the lens, causing posterior synechiae and pupillary distortion. Onset may be acute or insidious.

The uveal tract and causes of uveitis

Uveitis is the inflammation of the uveal tract. It occurs as anterior uveitis, posterior uveitis, or panuveitis (affects the entire uveal tract).

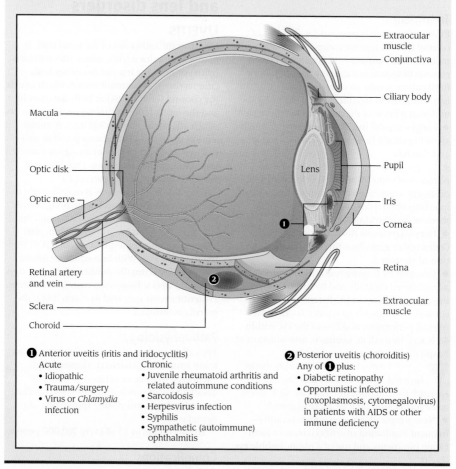

❶ Anterior uveitis (iritis and iridocyclitis)

Acute	Chronic
• Idiopathic	• Juvenile rheumatoid arthritis and related autoimmune conditions
• Trauma/surgery	• Sarcoidosis
• Virus or *Chlamydia* infection	• Herpesvirus infection
	• Syphilis
	• Sympathetic (autoimmune) ophthalmitis

❷ Posterior uveitis (choroiditis)
Any of ❶ plus:
• Diabetic retinopathy
• Opportunistic infections (toxoplasmosis, cytomegalovirus) in patients with AIDS or other immune deficiency

Posterior uveitis begins insidiously, with complaints of slightly decreased or blurred vision or floating spots. Posterior uveitis may be acute or chronic, and it may affect one or both eyes. Retinal damage caused by lesions from toxoplasmosis and retinal detachments may occur. Refer the patient to an eye care practitioner for dilated fundus examination and treatment for systemic diseases.

Diagnosis

℞ **CONFIRMING DIAGNOSIS** *In anterior and posterior uveitis, a slit-lamp examination shows a "flare and cell" pattern, which looks like particles dancing in a sunbeam. With a special lens, slit-lamp and ophthalmoscopic examination can also identify active inflammatory fundus lesions involving the retina and choroid, although a hazy vitreous may obscure the view.*

In posterior uveitis, serologic tests may be used to rule out toxoplasmosis, other infections, or inflammatory etiologies.

Treatment

Uveitis requires vigorous and prompt management, which includes treatment for any known underlying cause—corticosteroids with antibiotic therapy for infectious diseases and immune suppression therapy for autoimmune diseases—and application of a topical cycloplegic, such as

1% atropine sulfate, and of topical corticosteroids applied three to four times daily. For severe uveitis, therapy includes oral systemic corticosteroids.

⚠ **ALERT** *Long-term steroid therapy can cause a rise in IOP and cataracts. Carefully monitor IOP during acute inflammation. If IOP rises, therapy should include an antiglaucoma medication, such as brimonidine, an alpha2-adrenergic agonist, dorzolamide, a sulfonamide, or timolol (a beta-adrenergic blocker).*

Occasionally, posterior uveitis requires systemic immunosuppression.

Special considerations
◆ Encourage rest during the acute phase.
◆ Teach the patient the proper method of instilling eyedrops.
◆ Suggest the use of dark glasses to ease the discomfort of photophobia.
◆ Instruct the patient to watch for and report adverse effects of systemic corticosteroid therapy (e.g., edema or muscle weakness).
◆ Stress the importance of follow-up care for IOP checks while the patient is taking steroids. Tell the patient to seek treatment immediately at the first sign of iritis.

RETINAL DETACHMENT
Retinal detachment occurs when the outer retinal pigment epithelium splits from the neural retina, creating subretinal space. This space then fills with fluid, called *subretinal fluid*. Retinal detachment usually involves only one eye, but may later involve the other eye. Surgical reattachment is usually successful. However, the prognosis for good vision depends on which area of the retina has been affected.

Pathophysiology
Any retinal tear or hole allows the liquid vitreous to seep between the retinal layers, separating the retina from its choroidal blood supply. Predisposing factors include myopia, intraocular surgery, and trauma. In adults, retinal detachment usually results from degenerative changes of aging, which cause a spontaneous retinal hole. Perhaps the influence of trauma explains why retinal detachment is twice as common in males. Retinal detachment may also result from seepage of fluid into the subretinal space (because of inflammation, tumors, or systemic diseases) or from traction that's placed on the retina by vitreous bands or membranes (due to proliferative diabetic retinopathy, posterior uveitis, or a traumatic intraocular foreign body).

Retinal detachment is rare in children, but occasionally can develop as a result of retinopathy of prematurity, tumors (retinoblastomas), trauma, or myopia (which tends to run in families).

In the United States, about 10,000 people per year are affected by retinal detachments.

Complications
◆ Severe vision impairment
◆ Blindness

Signs and symptoms
Initially, the patient may complain of floating spots and recurrent flashes of light (photopsia). However, as detachment progresses, gradual, painless vision loss may be described as a veil, curtain, or cobweb that obscures a portion of the visual field.

Diagnosis
℞ **CONFIRMING DIAGNOSIS** *Diagnosis depends on ophthalmoscopy after full pupil dilation. Examination shows the usually transparent retina as gray and opaque; in severe detachment, it reveals folds in the retina and ballooning out of the area. Indirect ophthalmoscopy is used to search for retinal tears. Ultrasound is performed if the lens is opaque.*

Treatment
Treatment depends on the location and severity of the detachment. It may include restriction of eye movements and complete bed rest until surgical reattachment is done. A hole in the peripheral retina can be treated with cryotherapy; in the posterior portion, with laser therapy. Retinal detachment usually requires a scleral buckling procedure or a vitrectomy to reattach the retina. Basic salt solution is used to reposition the retina while the vitreous is removed.

Certain types of uncomplicated retinal detachment may be treated by pneumatic retinopexy, in which an expansile gas is initially injected into the vitreous cavity and the patient's head is positioned to facilitate retina reattachment. This procedure can be performed under local anesthesia.

Special considerations
◆ Provide emotional support because the patient may be understandably distraught about loss of vision.
◆ During transportation, position the patient's head so that the detached portion of the retina will fall back with the aid of gravity.
◆ To prepare for surgery, wash the patient's face with no-tears shampoo. Give antibiotics and cycloplegic-mydriatic eyedrops.
◆ Postoperatively, position the patient as recommended by the surgeon. Discourage

straining at stool, bending down, hard coughing, sneezing, or vomiting, which can raise IOP. Antiemetics may be indicated.

♦ Protect the patient's eye with a shield or glasses.

♦ To reduce edema and discomfort, apply ice packs as ordered. Administer pain medication, as ordered, for eye pain.

♦ After removing the eye shield, gently clean the eye and administer steroid-antibiotic eyedrops, as ordered. Use cold compresses to decrease swelling and pain.

♦ Administer analgesics as needed, and report persistent pain. Teach the patient how to properly instill eyedrops, and emphasize compliance and follow-up care. Suggest dark glasses to compensate for light sensitivity caused by cycloplegia.

VASCULAR RETINOPATHIES

Vascular retinopathies are noninflammatory retinal disorders that result from interference with the blood supply to the eyes. The five most common types of vascular retinopathy are central retinal artery occlusion, central retinal vein occlusion, diabetic retinopathy, hypertensive retinopathy, and sickle cell retinopathy.

Pathophysiology

When one of the arteries maintaining blood circulation in the retina becomes obstructed, the diminished blood flow causes visual deficits. (See *Anatomy of vascular retinopathy*.)

Central retinal artery occlusion may be idiopathic or may result from embolism, atherosclerosis, infection, or conditions that retard blood flow, such as temporal arteritis, carotid occlusion, and heart failure. This occlusion is rare, occurs unilaterally, and usually affects elderly patients. However, if it occurs in a younger person, the obstruction may have originated in the heart (such as embolization from plaque material from valve vegetations) and should be investigated accordingly.

Causes of central retinal vein occlusion include atherosclerosis, hypertension, optic disk edema, hypercoagulable states (polycythemia, leukemia, or sickle cell disease), glaucoma, retrobulbar compression (such as an orbital tumor), and drugs such as hormonal contraceptives. This form of vascular retinopathy is most prevalent in elderly patients and is characterized by impaired venous outflow.

Diabetic retinopathy results from type 1 or type 2 diabetes. Microcirculatory changes occur more rapidly when diabetes is poorly controlled. About 90% of patients with type 1 diabetes develop retinopathy within 20 years of onset of diabetes. In adults with diabetes, incidence increases with the duration of diabetes; 80% of patients who have had diabetes for 20 to 25 years develop retinopathy. This condition is a leading cause of acquired adult blindness.

Anatomy of vascular retinopathy

Vascular changes that occur with retinopathy, as seen by an ophthalmoscope, are depicted below.

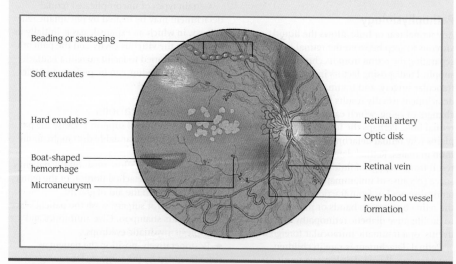

Beading or sausaging

Soft exudates

Hard exudates

Boat-shaped hemorrhage

Microaneurysm

Retinal artery

Optic disk

Retinal vein

New blood vessel formation

Hypertensive retinopathy results from prolonged hypertensive disease, producing retinal vasospasm, and consequent damage and arteriolar narrowing.

Sickle cell retinopathy results from impaired ability of the sickled cell to pass through microvasculature, producing vaso-occlusion. This leads to microaneurysms, chorioretinal infarction, and retinal detachment.

Complications
◆ Blindness
◆ Secondary glaucoma

Signs and symptoms
Central retinal artery occlusion produces sudden, painless, unilateral loss of vision (partial or complete). It may follow amaurosis fugax or transient episodes of unilateral loss of vision lasting from a few seconds to minutes, probably due to vasospasm. This condition typically causes permanent blindness. However, some patients experience spontaneous resolution within hours and regain partial vision.

Central retinal vein occlusion causes reduced visual acuity, allowing perception of only hand movement and light. This condition is painless, except when it results in secondary neovascular glaucoma (uncontrolled proliferation of weak blood vessels). The prognosis is poor—some patients with this condition develop secondary glaucoma within 3 to 4 months after occlusion.

Nonproliferative diabetic retinopathy produces changes in the lining of the retinal blood vessels that cause the vessels to leak plasma or fatty substances, which decrease or block blood flow (nonperfusion) within the retina. This disorder may also produce microaneurysms and small hemorrhages. Nonproliferative retinopathy causes no symptoms in some patients; in others, leakage of fluid into the macular region causes significant loss of central visual acuity (necessary for reading and driving) and diminished night vision.

Proliferative diabetic retinopathy produces fragile new blood vessels on the disk (neovascularization) and elsewhere in the fundus. These vessels can grow into the vitreous and then rupture, causing vitreous hemorrhage with corresponding sudden vision loss. Scar tissue that may form along the new blood vessels can pull on the retina, causing it to tear or even detach.

Symptoms of hypertensive retinopathy include blurred vision, often accompanied by headache. Ophthalmoscopic examination may reveal diffuse arteriolar narrowing, venular tortuosity, silver wire reflexes, macular stars, and swelling of the head of the optic nerve (disk edema). Severe, prolonged disease eventually produces blindness; mild, prolonged disease produces visual defects.

Symptoms of sickle cell retinopathy include peripheral arteriolar occlusions, peripheral arteriovenous anastomoses, sea fan neurovascular fronds, vitreous hemorrhage as tractional forces and vitreous collapse tear fragile neovascular membranes and, with advanced disease, severe vitreous traction and retinal detachment.

Diagnosis
Check visual acuity and then vital signs, including blood pressure. Diagnosis is made on fundal examination with an ophthalmoscope. Determine if female patients are pregnant; hypertensive retinopathy may be an early sign of preeclampsia. (See *Diagnostic tests for vascular retinopathies*, page 616.)

Treatment
No treatment has been shown to improve or resolve central retinal artery occlusion. However, an attempt is made to release the occlusion into the peripheral circulation. To reduce IOP, therapy includes acetazolamide I.V., eyeball massage, thrombolysis by intra-arterial injection or I.V., high concentrations of inhaled oxygen, and anterior chamber paracentesis (to try to move the arterial obstruction into the peripheral field).

Therapy for central retinal vein occlusion may include aspirin, which acts as a mild anticoagulant. Patients with central retinal vein occlusion have reported improved vision after direct injection of tissue plasminogen activator into the retinal venous system. Laser photocoagulation can reduce the risk of neovascular glaucoma for some patients whose eyes have widespread capillary nonperfusion.

Treatment for nonproliferative diabetic retinopathy is prophylactic. Careful control of blood glucose levels reduces the severity of the retinopathy or may delay its onset. Patients with early symptoms of microaneurysms should have frequent eye examinations; children with diabetes should have an annual eye examination.

Treatment for proliferative diabetic retinopathy or severe macular edema is laser photocoagulation, which cauterizes the leaking blood vessels. Laser treatment may be focal (aimed at new blood vessels) or panretinal (placing burns throughout the peripheral retina). Despite treatment, neovascularization continues to proliferate, and vitreous hemorrhage, with or without retinal detachment, may follow. If the blood isn't absorbed in 6 weeks to 3 months, vitrectomy may restore partial vision. New agents, such as vascular endothelial growth factor inhibitors,

Diagnostic tests for vascular retinopathies

Central retinal artery occlusion
♦ Ophthalmoscopy (direct or indirect): shows blockage of retinal arterioles during a transient attack.
♦ Retinal examination: within 2 hours of onset, shows clumps or segmentation in the artery; later, milky white retina around the disk due to swelling and necrosis of ganglion cells caused by reduced blood supply; also shows a cherry-red spot in the macula that subsides after several weeks.
♦ Color Doppler tests: evaluate carotid occlusion with no need for arteriography.
♦ Physical examination: reveals the underlying cause of vascular retinopathy, for example, diabetes or hypertension.

Central retinal vein occlusion
♦ Ophthalmoscopy (direct or indirect): shows flame-shaped hemorrhages, retinal vein engorgement, white patches among hemorrhages, and edema around the disk.
♦ Color Doppler tests: confirm or rule out occlusion of blood vessels.
♦ Physical examination: reveals the underlying cause.

Diabetic retinopathy
♦ Ophthalmoscopic examination: shows retinal changes such as microaneurysms

(earliest change), retinal hemorrhages and edema, venous dilation and beading, lipid exudates, fibrous bands in the vitreous, and growth of new blood vessels. Infarcts of the nerve fiber layer are observed.
♦ Fluorescein angiography: shows leakage of fluorescein from weak-walled vessels and "lights up" microaneurysms, differentiating them from true hemorrhages.
♦ History: of diabetes.

Hypertensive retinopathy
♦ Ophthalmoscopy (direct or indirect): in early stages, shows hard, shiny deposits; flame-shaped hemorrhages; silver wire appearance of narrowed arterioles; and nicking of veins where arteries cross them (atrioventricular nicking). In late stages, shows cotton wool patches, lipid exudates, retinal edema, papilledema due to ischemia and capillary insufficiency, hemorrhages, and microaneurysms in both eyes.
♦ Physical examination: reveals elevated blood pressure.
♦ History: of decreased vision, headache, and nausea.
♦ History: of hypertension, usually acute or malignant.

---

can cause temporary regression of the abnormal blood vessels. This would be followed by panretinal laser treatment to prevent recurrence.

Treatment for hypertensive retinopathy includes control of blood pressure with appropriate drugs, diet, and exercise. Treating the systemic hypertension should improve the condition of the eyes. If left untreated, hypertensive retinopathy results in severe vision loss.

The treatment goal of sickle cell retinopathy is to reduce the risk of, or prevent or eliminate, retinal neovascularization. Patients with symptoms should receive follow-up care twice a year with ocular examinations and dilated retinal evaluation. Proliferative disease should be evaluated with fluorescein angiography and treated with panretinal photocoagulation. Cryotherapy hasn't been proven to be effective and has a high complication rate.

Special considerations
♦ Monitor a patient's blood pressure if there are complaints of occipital headache and blurred vision.

⚠ ALERT *Arrange for immediate evaluation when a patient complains of sudden, unilateral loss of vision. Blindness may be permanent if treatment is delayed.*
♦ Encourage a diabetic patient to comply with the prescribed regimen.
♦ For a patient with hypertensive retinopathy, stress the importance of complying with antihypertensive therapy.

AGE-RELATED MACULAR DEGENERATION

Macular degeneration is the atrophy or degeneration of the macular region of the retina. Two types of age-related macular degeneration occur. The dry, or atrophic, form (which is the most common) is characterized by atrophic pigment epithelial changes and is most often associated with a slow, progressive, and mild vision loss. The wet, exudative form causes progressive visual distortion leading to vision loss. It's characterized by subretinal neovascularization that causes leakage, hemorrhage, and fibrovascular scar formation, which produce significant loss of central vision.

Pathophysiology

Age-related macular degeneration results from underlying pathologic changes that occur primarily at the level of the retinal pigment epithelium and the adjacent structures (Bruch membrane and the choriocapillaris) in the macular region. Drusen, which are common in elderly people, appear as yellow deposits beneath the pigment epithelium and may be prominent in the macula. No predisposing conditions have been identified; however, some forms of the disorder are hereditary.

Macular degeneration is the most common cause of legal blindness in adults, accounting for about 12% of blindness cases in the United States and for about 17% of new blindness cases. It's also one of the causes of severe irreversible loss of central vision in elderly people—by age 75, almost 15% of people have this condition. Whites have the highest incidence. Other risk factors are family history and cigarette smoking.

Complications

◆ Blindness
◆ Metamorphopsia

Signs and symptoms

The patient notices a change in central vision. Initially, straight lines (e.g., of buildings) become distorted; later, a blank area appears in the center of a printed page (central scotoma).

Diagnosis

◆ Ophthalmoscopy—fundus examination through a dilated pupil may reveal gross macular changes.
◆ I.V. fluorescein angiography—sequential photographs may show leaking vessels as fluorescein dye flows into the tissues from the subretinal neovascular net.
◆ Amsler grid—used to monitor metamorphopsia and the appearance of new scotomas.

Treatment

Recent studies have shown that the dry form of age-related macular degeneration can be prevented and treated with daily vitamin therapy that includes lutein and zeaxanthin.

Laser photocoagulation reduces the incidence of severe vision loss in the patient with noncentral subretinal neovascularization, halting its progression. Injection of an antivascular endothelial growth factor agent into the vitreous is the most common treatment for serous (wet) age-related macular degeneration. Timely treatment (before the formation of fibrovascular scars and retinal atrophy) can result in vision recovery. Recurrence may occur. Injections are repeated periodically, depending on the retinal evaluation.

Special considerations

◆ Inform the patient with bilateral central vision loss of the visual rehabilitation services available.
◆ Special devices, such as low-vision optical aids, are available to improve the quality of life in the patient with good peripheral vision.
▓▓▓▓ **PREVENTION** *Encourage early detection through regular eye examinations.*

CATARACT

The most common cause of correctable vision loss, a cataract is a gradually developing opacity of the lens or lens capsule of the eye. Cataracts commonly occur bilaterally, with each progressing independently. Exceptions are traumatic cataracts, which are usually unilateral, and congenital cataracts, which may remain stationary. The prognosis is generally good; surgery improves vision in 95% of affected people.

Pathophysiology

Cataracts have various causes:
◆ Senile cataracts develop in elderly patients, probably because of degenerative changes in the chemical state of lens proteins.
◆ Congenital cataracts occur in neonates as genetic defects or as a sequela of maternal infections during the first trimester. Some cataracts are inherited in an autosomal dominant pattern.
◆ Traumatic cataracts develop after a foreign body injures the lens with sufficient force to allow aqueous or vitreous humor to enter the lens capsule. Trauma may also dislocate the lens.
◆ Complicated cataracts develop as secondary effects in patients with uveitis, glaucoma, or retinitis pigmentosa, or in the course of a systemic disease, such as diabetes, hypoparathyroidism, or atopic dermatitis. They can also result from exposure to ionizing radiation or infrared rays.
◆ Toxic cataracts result from drug or chemical toxicity with prednisone, ergot alkaloids, dinitrophenol, naphthalene, phenothiazines, or pilocarpine or from extended exposure to ultraviolet rays.

Cataracts occur as part of the aging process and are most prevalent in people older than age 70.

Complication

◆ Vision loss

Signs and symptoms
Characteristically, a patient with a cataract experiences painless, gradual blurring and loss of vision. As the cataract progresses, the normally black pupil appears hazy, and when a mature cataract develops, the white lens may be seen through the pupil. Some patients complain of blinding glare from headlights when they drive at night; others complain of poor reading vision, and of an unpleasant glare and poor vision in bright sunlight. Patients with central opacities report better vision in dim light than in bright light because the cataract is nuclear and, as the pupils dilate, patients can see around the lens opacity.

Diagnosis
On examination, visual acuity is decreased.

℞ CONFIRMING DIAGNOSIS *Ophthalmoscopy or slit-lamp examination confirms the diagnosis by revealing a dark area in the normally homogeneous red reflex.*

Treatment
Treatment consists of surgical extraction of the cataractous lens opacity and insertion of an intraocular artificial lens. Surgery is a same-day procedure. Surgical procedures include the following:

◆ Extracapsular cataract extraction (ECCE) removes the anterior lens capsule and cortex, leaving the posterior capsule intact. With this procedure, a posterior chamber intraocular lens (IOL) is implanted where the patient's own lens used to be. (A posterior chamber IOL is currently the most common type used in the United States.) This procedure is appropriate for use in patients of all ages.

◆ Phacoemulsification uses ultrasonic vibrations to fragment and then emulsify the lens, which is then aspirated through a small incision.

◆ Intracapsular cataract extraction removes the entire lens within the intact capsule. This procedure is seldom performed today. ECCE with phacoemulsification has replaced it as the most commonly performed procedure.

◆ Discission and aspiration can still be used for children with soft cataracts, but this procedure has largely been replaced by phacoemulsification.

Infection is the most serious complication of intraocular surgery. Wound dehiscence can occur but is seldom a complication because of the small incision and minute sutures that are used. Hyphema, pupillary block glaucoma, and retinal detachment still occasionally occur.

The patient with an IOL implant may experience improved vision shortly after surgery if there's no corneal or retinal pathology. Most IOLs correct for distance vision, but new IOLs are multifocal. However, the majority of patients will need either corrective reading glasses or a corrective contact lens, which will be fitted sometime between 4 and 6 weeks after surgery.

Where no IOL has been implanted, the patient may be given temporary aphakic cataract glasses; in about 4 to 8 weeks, he'll be refracted for glasses.

Some patients who have an ECCE develop a secondary membrane in the posterior lens capsule (which has been left intact), which causes decreased visual acuity. This membrane can be removed by the Nd:YAG laser, which cuts an area out of the center of the membrane, thereby restoring vision. Laser therapy isn't used to remove a cataract.

Posterior capsular opacification occurs in approximately 15% to 20% of all patients within 2 years after cataract surgery.

Special considerations
After surgery to extract a cataract:

◆ Because the patient will be discharged after recovering from anesthesia, remind the patient to return for a checkup the next day, and advise avoidance of activities that increase IOP such as straining.

◆ Urge the patient to protect the eye from accidental injury at night by wearing a plastic or metal shield with perforations; a shield or glasses should be worn for protection during the day.

◆ Before discharge, teach the patient to administer antibiotic ointment or drops to prevent infection and steroids to reduce inflammation; combination steroid-antibiotic eyedrops can also be used.

◆ Advise the patient to watch for the development of complications, such as a pain in the eye uncontrolled by analgesics, eye or eyelid redness, or decreased vision, and to report them immediately. These symptoms may indicate an infection.

◆ Caution the patient about activity restrictions, and advise that it will take several weeks to receive corrective reading glasses or lenses.

▓ PREVENTION *Encourage your patient to:*
◆ *quit smoking*
◆ *wear sunglasses*

RETINITIS PIGMENTOSA
Retinitis pigmentosa is a group of hereditary disorders whose common feature is a gradual deterioration of the light-sensitive cells of the

retina. Postmortem examination of the eyes reveals pigment cells that have clumped together as a result of the pigment epithelium budding off and settling within the layers of the retina. Retinitis pigmentosa often accompanies other hereditary disorders in several distinct syndromes—including Usher syndrome, in which sight and hearing are both affected; and Laurence–Moon–Biedl syndrome (most common), which is typified by visual destruction from retinitis pigmentosa, with obesity, mental retardation, polydactyly, hypogenitalism, and spastic paraplegia.

Pathophysiology
Retinitis pigmentosa can be classified according to its inheritance pattern: autosomal dominant, autosomal recessive, and X-linked. Typically, in all forms of retinitis pigmentosa, the retinal rods slowly deteriorate. Clumps of pigment resembling bone corpuscles aggregate in the peripheral region of the retina and later involve the macular areas. Visual symptoms usually appear between ages 10 and 30, though some children may become blind within the first year of life.

Retinitis pigmentosa affects 1 of every 4,000 people in the United States.

Signs and symptoms
Typically, night blindness occurs during the teen years. As the disease progresses, the visual field gradually constricts, causing tunnel or "gun-barrel" vision. Many people retain this tunnel of useful vision until quite late in life. The speed of vision loss varies considerably from person to person. However, blindness follows invasion of the macular region.

Diagnosis
A detailed family history may imply predisposition to retinitis pigmentosa. In the patient whose history suggests this condition, the following tests help confirm diagnosis.
◆ Electroretinography shows a slower than normal or absent retinal response time.
◆ Fluorescein angiography visualizes white dots (areas of depigmentation) in the retina.
◆ Ophthalmoscopy may initially show normal fundi but later shows black pigmentary disturbance and white dots (depigmentation) in the retina.
◆ Visual field testing detects ring scotomata.

Treatment
No cure exists for retinitis pigmentosa. However, vitamin A and E supplementation may slow degeneration. Researchers are working on the potential for tissue transplant, but research is still in its infancy.

Special considerations
◆ Teach the patient and family about retinitis pigmentosa.
◆ Encourage the patient to use sunglasses to protect the retina from ultraviolet light and to help preserve vision.
◆ Explain that the disorder is hereditary, and suggest genetic counseling for adults who risk transmitting it to their children.
◆ Encourage annual eye examinations to monitor the progress of the disease.
◆ Warn the patient of the potential for not being able to drive a car safely at night.
◆ Refer the patient to a social service agency or to the National Retinitis Pigmentosa Foundation for information and for counseling to prepare for eventual blindness.
◆ Because the prospect of blindness is frightening, it's important that you provide emotional support and guidance.

▓▓ *PREVENTION Encourage the patient to seek genetic counseling.*

Miscellaneous disorders
OPTIC ATROPHY
Optic atrophy, or degeneration of the optic nerve, can develop spontaneously (primary) or can follow inflammation or edema of the nerve head (secondary). Some forms of this condition may subside without treatment, but degeneration of the optic nerve is irreversible.

Pathophysiology
Optic atrophy usually results from central nervous system disorders (such as chiasmal tumors, syphilis, ischemic optic neuropathy, drugs, retinal vascular disease, or degenerative disease) or from end-stage glaucoma. Other causes include retinitis pigmentosa; chronic papilledema and papillitis; trauma; central retinal artery or vein occlusion that interrupts the blood supply to the optic nerve, causing degeneration of ganglion cells; ingestion of toxins, such as methanol and quinine; and deficiencies of vitamin B_{12}, amino acids, and zinc.

Several rare forms of hereditary optic atrophy can affect children and young adults.

Complications
◆ Central vision loss
◆ Peripheral vision loss
◆ Loss of contrast
◆ Loss of color vision
◆ Loss of visual field

Signs and symptoms

Optic atrophy causes abrupt or gradual painless loss of visual field or visual acuity, with changes in color vision.

Diagnosis

℞ CONFIRMING DIAGNOSIS *Visual acuity testing reveals poor vision. An afferent pupillary defect is noted when pupils are examined. Fundus examination through a dilated pupil with an ophthalmoscope shows pallor of the nerve head from loss of microvascular circulation in the disk and deposit of fibrous or glial tissue. Visual field testing reveals a scotoma and, possibly, major visual field impairment.*

Treatment

Optic atrophy is irreversible, so treatment aims to correct the underlying cause and prevent further vision loss. If a space-occupying lesion is the cause, neurosurgery may be required. In multiple sclerosis, optic neuritis often subsides spontaneously but may recur and improve repeatedly.

Special considerations

◆ Provide symptomatic care during diagnostic procedures and treatment. Assist the patient who's visually compromised to perform daily activities.

◆ Explain procedures, to minimize anxiety. Offer emotional support to help the patient deal with loss of vision.

EXTRAOCULAR MOTOR NERVE PALSIES

Extraocular motor nerve palsies are dysfunctions of the third, fourth, and sixth cranial nerves. The oculomotor (third cranial) nerve innervates the inferior, medial, and superior rectus muscles; the inferior oblique extraocular muscles; the pupilloconstrictor muscles; and the levator palpebrae muscles. The trochlear (fourth cranial) nerve innervates the superior oblique muscles. The abducens (sixth cranial) nerve innervates the lateral rectus muscles.

Pathophysiology

Causes of these disorders vary, depending on the cranial nerve involved:

◆ Third nerve (oculomotor) palsy (acute ophthalmoplegia) may be congenital or acquired. Causes include intracranial tumors or aneurysms, diabetic neuropathy, and trauma.

◆ Fourth nerve (trochlear) palsy is most commonly caused by trauma.

◆ Sixth nerve (abducens) palsy commonly has an unknown etiology. Strokes are a common cause. Brainstem lesions, elevated intracranial pressure, inflamed petrous pyramid due to otitis media, cavernous sinus, orbital involvement with tumor and inflammation, or thyroid eye disease may be responsible for sixth nerve palsy.

Complications

◆ Loss of eye muscle control (strabismus)
◆ Double vision (diplopia)
◆ Ptosis
◆ Dilated pupil (mydriasis)

Signs and symptoms

The most characteristic clinical symptom of extraocular motor nerve palsies is diplopia of recent onset, which varies in different visual fields, depending on the muscles affected.

Typically, the patient with third nerve palsy exhibits ptosis, exotropia (eye looks outward), pupil dilation, and unresponsiveness to light; the eye is unable to move and can't accommodate.

The patient with fourth nerve palsy displays diplopia and an inability to rotate the eye downward or upward. The head is usually turned to the side opposite the involved eye in superior oblique palsy to compensate for the diplopia.

Sixth nerve palsy causes one eye to turn; the eye can't abduct beyond the midline. To compensate for diplopia, the patient turns the head to the unaffected side and can develop torticollis.

Diagnosis

Diagnosis necessitates an orthoptic examination to isolate the involved muscle, a complete neuro-ophthalmologic examination, and a thorough patient history. Differential diagnosis of third, fourth, or sixth nerve palsy depends on the specific motor defect exhibited by the patient.

For all extraocular motor nerve palsies, a computed tomography scan or magnetic resonance imaging rules out tumors and may help detect the cause of the palsy, such as the cause of increased intracranial pressure. The patient is also evaluated for an aneurysm or diabetes. If sixth nerve palsy results from infection, culture and sensitivity tests identify the causative organism, and specific antibiotic therapy can be determined.

Treatment

Identification of the underlying cause is essential because treatment for extraocular motor nerve palsies varies accordingly. Neurosurgery is necessary if the cause is a brain tumor or an

Normal flow of aqueous humor

Aqueous humor, a plasmalike fluid produced by the ciliary epithelium of the ciliary body, flows from the posterior chamber to the anterior chamber through the pupil. Here it flows peripherally and filters through the trabecular meshwork to the canal of Schlemm, through which the fluid ultimately enters venous circulation.

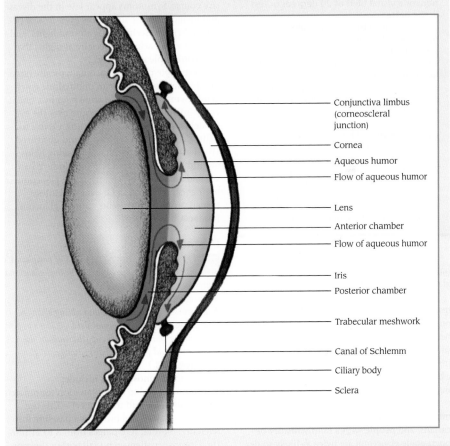

- Conjunctiva limbus (corneoscleral junction)
- Cornea
- Aqueous humor
- Flow of aqueous humor
- Lens
- Anterior chamber
- Flow of aqueous humor
- Iris
- Posterior chamber
- Trabecular meshwork
- Canal of Schlemm
- Ciliary body
- Sclera

aneurysm. For infection, massive I.V. doses of antibiotics may be appropriate.

Special considerations
◆ If the palsy results from thyroid eye disease, the patient must have normal thyroid levels before eye muscle surgery is attempted.

GLAUCOMA
Glaucoma is a group of disorders characterized by damage to the optic nerve, most commonly associated with high IOP. If untreated, it can lead to gradual peripheral vision loss and, ultimately, blindness. (See *Blindness*, page 622.) Glaucoma occurs in several forms: chronic open-angle (primary), acute angle-closure, congenital (inherited as an autosomal recessive trait), and secondary to other causes. The prognosis for maintaining vision is good with early treatment.

Pathophysiology
Chronic open-angle glaucoma results from overproduction of aqueous humor or obstruction to its outflow through the trabecular meshwork or the canal of Schlemm. (See *Normal flow of aqueous humor*.) This form of glaucoma, which is estimated to be present in 1% to 2% of people older than age 40, is frequently familial in origin and affects 90% of all patients with glaucoma. Diabetes and systemic hypertension

Blindness

Blindness affects 28 million people worldwide. In the United States, blindness is legally defined as visual acuity of 20/200 or less in the better eye after best correction, or a visual field of 20 degrees or less in the better eye.

According to the World Health Organization, the most common causes of preventable blindness worldwide are trachoma, cataracts, onchocerciasis (microfilarial infection transmitted by a blackfly and other species of *Simulium*), and xerophthalmia (dryness of conjunctiva and cornea from vitamin A deficiency).

In the United States, the most common causes of acquired blindness are glaucoma, age-related macular degeneration, and diabetic retinopathy. However, the incidence of blindness from glaucoma is decreasing owing to early detection and treatment. Rarer causes of acquired blindness include herpes simplex keratitis, cataracts, and retinal detachment.

have also been associated with this form of glaucoma.

Acute angle-closure (narrow-angle) glaucoma results from obstruction to the outflow of aqueous humor due to anatomically narrow angles between the anterior iris and the posterior corneal surface, shallow anterior chambers, a thickened iris that causes angle closure on pupil dilation, or a bulging iris that presses on the trabeculae, closing the angle (peripheral anterior synechiae).

Persons of African descent are four times more likely to have this disorder than Caucasians, and people with a family history of open-angle glaucoma are twice as likely to develop it than people without a family history of this disorder. The use of systemic anticholinergic medications, such as atropine or eye dilation drops, in a person who's already at high risk for acute glaucoma increases the risk. Other risk factors include farsightedness and age-related changes that create an increase in IOP.

Congenital glaucoma occurs when there is an abnormal fluid drainage angle of the eye. It may be caused by congenital infections such as TORCH virus (*t*oxoplasmosis, *o*ther [varicella, mumps, parvovirus, human immunodeficiency virus], *r*ubella, *c*ytomegalovirus, and *h*erpes), Sturge–Weber syndrome, or retinopathy of prematurity.

Secondary glaucoma can result from uveitis, trauma, or drugs (such as steroids). Neovascularization in the angle can result from vein occlusion or diabetes.

Complications
◆ Blindness
◆ Vision loss

Signs and symptoms

Chronic open-angle glaucoma is usually bilateral, with insidious onset and a slowly progressive course. Symptoms appear late in the disease and include mild aching in the eyes, loss of peripheral vision, seeing halos around lights, and reduced visual acuity (especially at night) that isn't correctable with glasses.

Acute angle-closure glaucoma typically has a rapid onset, constituting an ophthalmic emergency. Symptoms include acute pain in a unilaterally inflamed eye, with pressure over the eye, moderate pupil dilation that's nonreactive to light, a cloudy cornea, blurring and decreased visual acuity, photophobia, and seeing halos around lights. Increased IOP may induce nausea and vomiting, which may cause glaucoma to be misinterpreted as GI distress. Unless treated promptly, this acute form of glaucoma produces blindness in 3 to 5 days.

Diagnosis

CONFIRMING DIAGNOSIS *Loss of peripheral vision and disk changes confirm that glaucoma is present. Diagnosis is made by:*
◆ *testing IOP*
◆ *measuring the visual field and noting changes, such as loss of peripheral visual field*
◆ *observing changes in the cup/disk ratio of the optic nerve head (See Optic disk changes in glaucoma, page 623.)*

Relevant diagnostic tests include:
◆ Tonometry (using an applanation tonometer [Tonopen] or air puff tonometer)—This test measures the IOP and provides a baseline for reference. Normal IOP ranges from 8 to 21 mm Hg. However, patients who fall within this normal range can develop signs and symptoms of glaucoma, and patients who have abnormally high pressure may have no clinical effects. Fingertip tension is another way to measure IOP. On gentle palpation of closed eyelids, one eye feels harder than the other in acute angle-closure glaucoma.
◆ Slit-lamp examination—The slit lamp facilitates examination of the anterior structures of the eye: the cornea, iris, and lens.
◆ Gonioscopy—By determining the angle of the anterior chamber of the eye, this test enables differentiation between chronic open-angle glaucoma and acute angle-closure glaucoma. The angle is normal in chronic open-angle glaucoma. However, in older patients, partial closure of the angle may occur, so that two forms of glaucoma may coexist.

PATHOPHYSIOLOGY
Optic disk changes in glaucoma

Diagnosis of glaucoma is confirmed with a loss of peripheral vision and disk changes.

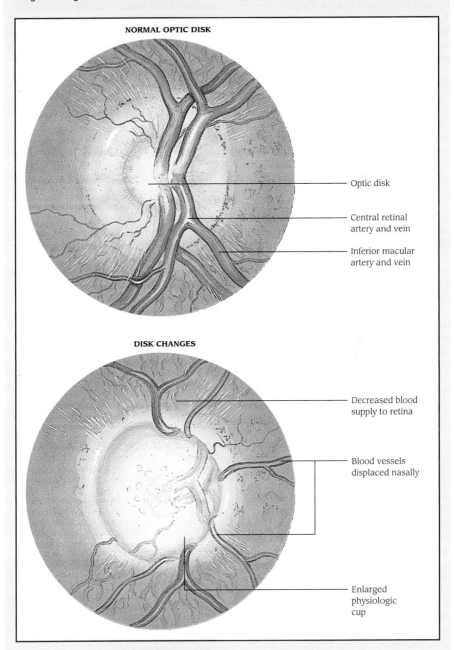

NORMAL OPTIC DISK

Optic disk

Central retinal artery and vein

Inferior macular artery and vein

DISK CHANGES

Decreased blood supply to retina

Blood vessels displaced nasally

Enlarged physiologic cup

◆ Ophthalmoscopy—This test enables the examiner to look at the fundus to establish if there are any cup/disk ratio changes. These changes appear later in chronic glaucoma if the disease isn't brought under control.

◆ Fundus photography—Pictures of the optic nerve head are made to track changes.

◆ Perimetry or visual field tests—These reveal the extent of damage to the optic neurons, signaled by an enlarged blind spot and loss of peripheral vision.

Treatment

For chronic open-angle glaucoma, treatment initially decreases IOP through the use of one of five classes of drops; alpha antagonists such as brimonidine tartrate, beta blockers such as timolol (contraindicated for asthmatics or patients with bradycardia), prostaglandin analogs (such as latanoprost), carbonic anhydrase inhibitors (topical or oral), or miotics (such as pilocarpine).

Patients who are unresponsive to drug therapy may be candidates for argon laser trabeculoplasty (ALT) or a surgical filtering procedure called *trabeculectomy*, which creates an opening for aqueous outflow. In ALT, an argon laser beam is focused on the trabecular meshwork of an open angle. This produces a thermal burn that changes the surface of the meshwork and increases the outflow of aqueous humor. In trabeculectomy, a flap of sclera is dissected free to expose the trabecular meshwork. Then this discrete tissue block is removed and a peripheral iridectomy is performed. This produces an opening for aqueous outflow under the conjunctiva, creating a filtering bleb. In chronic refractory glaucoma, a tube shunt or valve is used to keep IOP within normal limits.

Acute angle-closure glaucoma is an ocular emergency requiring immediate treatment to lower the high IOP. Drug therapy to lower IOP includes I.V. acetazolamide, pilocarpine (constricts the pupil, forcing the iris away from the trabeculae, allowing fluid to escape), timolol, and a topical steroid to quiet the inflammatory response, along with I.V. mannitol (20%) or oral glycerin (50%) to force fluid from the eye by making the blood hypertonic. Oral medication or topical drops may be prescribed separately or in combination. Severe pain may necessitate administration of opioid analgesics. If pressure doesn't decrease with drug therapy, laser iridotomy or surgical peripheral iridectomy must be performed promptly to save the patient's vision. Iridectomy relieves pressure by excising part of the iris to reestablish aqueous humor outflow. A prophylactic iridectomy is performed a few days later on the other eye to prevent an acute episode of glaucoma in the normal eye.

Special considerations

◆ Stress the importance of meticulous compliance with prescribed drug therapy to prevent an increase in IOP, resulting in disk changes and loss of vision.

◆ For the patient with acute angle-closure glaucoma, give medications as ordered, and prepare the patient physically and psychologically for laser iridotomy or surgery.

◆ Postoperative care after peripheral iridectomy includes cycloplegic eyedrops to relax the ciliary muscle and to decrease inflammation, thus preventing adhesions.

⚠ ALERT *Cycloplegics must be used only in the affected eye. The use of these drops in the normal eye may precipitate an attack of acute angle-closure glaucoma in this eye, threatening the patient's residual vision.*

◆ Encourage ambulation immediately after surgery.

◆ Postoperative care after surgical filtering includes dilation and topical steroids to rest the pupil and topical steroids.

◆ Stress the importance of glaucoma screening for early detection and prevention. All people older than age 35, especially those with family histories of glaucoma, should have an annual tonometric examination.

SELECTED REFERENCES

Bagheri, N., & Wajda, B. N. (Eds.). (2016). *The wills eye manual: Office and emergency room diagnosis and treatment of eye disease* (7th ed.). Philadelphia: Lippincott Williams & Wilkins.

Eisenhauer, B., et al. (2017). Lutein and zeaxanthin: Food sources, bioavailability and dietary variety in age-related macular degeneration protection. *Nutrition, 9*(120), 1–14. doi:10.3390/nu9020120

Farahani, M., et al. (2017). Infectious corneal ulcers. *Disease-a-Month, 63*, 33–37.

Hoogewoud, F., et al. (2016). Traumatic retinal detachment the difficulty and importance of correct diagnosis. *Survey of Ophthalmology, 61*, 156–163.

Imburgia, A., et al. (2016). Treatment of exophthalmos and strabismus surgery in thyroid-associated orbitopathy. *International Journal of Oral Maxillofacial Surgery, 45*, 743–749. doi:10.1016/j.ijom.2015.12.002

Jonas, J. B., et al. (2017). Glaucoma. *Lancet, 390*, 2083–2093. doi:10.1016/S0140-6736(17)31469-1

Lai, H. P., et al. (2014). Clinical outcomes of cataract surgery in very elderly adults. *Journal of the American Geriatric Society, 62*, 165–170.

Mostovoy, D., et al. (2017). The association of keratoconus with blepharitis. *Clinical and Experimental Optometry, 101*, 339–344. doi:10.1111/cxo.12643

National Guidelines Clearinghouse: Agency for Healthcare Research and Quality. (2018). Retrieved from https://www.guideline.gov

Taylor, H. R., et al. (2014). Trachoma. *Lancet, 384*, 2142–2152.

13

EAR, NOSE, AND THROAT DISORDERS

Introduction

Ear, nose, and throat disorders rarely prove fatal (except for those resulting from neoplasms, epiglottitis, and neck trauma), but they may cause serious social, cosmetic, and communication problems. Untreated hearing loss or deafness can drastically impair the ability to interact with society. Ear disorders also can cause impaired equilibrium. Nasal disorders can cause changes in facial features and interfere with breathing and tasting. Diseases arising in the throat may threaten airway patency and interfere with speech. In addition, these disorders can cause considerable discomfort and pain for the patient and require thorough assessment and prompt treatment.

THE EAR

Hearing begins when sound waves reach the tympanic membrane, which then vibrates the ossicles, incus, malleus, and stapes in the middle ear cavity. The stapes transmits these vibrations to the perilymphatic fluid in the inner ear by vibrating against the oval window. The vibrations then pass across the cochlea's fluid receptor cells in the basilar membrane, stimulating movement of the hair cells of the organ of Corti. The axons of the cochlear nerve terminate around the bases of those hair cells. Sound waves, which initiate impulses, travel over the auditory nerve (made up of the cochlear nerve

and the vestibular nerve) to the temporal lobe of the brain.

The inner ear structures also maintain the body's equilibrium and balance through the fluid in the semicircular canals. This fluid is set in motion by body movement and stimulates nerve cells that line the canals. These cells, in turn, transmit impulses to the cerebellum of the brain by way of the vestibular branch of the eighth cranial nerve (the acoustic nerve).

Although the ear can respond to sounds that vibrate at frequencies from 20 to 20,000 Hz, the range of normal speech is from 250 to 4,000 Hz, with 70% falling between 500 and 2,000 Hz. The ratio between sound intensities, the decibel (dB) is the unit for expressing the relative intensity (loudness) of sounds. A faint whisper registers 10 to 15 dB; average conversation, 50 to 60 dB; a shout, 85 to 90 dB. Hearing damage may follow exposure to sounds louder than 90 dB.

ASSESSMENT

After obtaining a thorough patient history of any ear disease, inspect the auricle and surrounding tissue for deformities, lumps, and skin lesions. (See *Structures of the external ear*, page 626.) Ask the patient if they have ear pain. If you see inflammation, check for tenderness by moving the auricle and pressing on the tragus and the mastoid process. Check the ear canal for excessive cerumen, discharge, or foreign bodies.

Structures of the external ear

The structures of the external ear are depicted below.

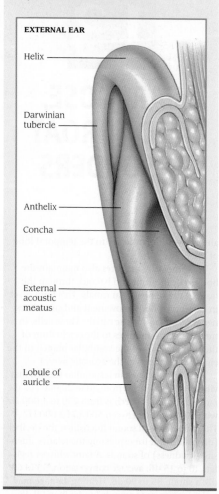

EXTERNAL EAR

- Helix
- Darwinian tubercle
- Anthelix
- Concha
- External acoustic meatus
- Lobule of auricle

Ask the patient if they have had episodes of vertigo or blurred vision. To test for vertigo, have the patient stand on one foot and close their eyes, or have them walk a straight line with their eyes closed. Ask them if they always fall to the same side and if the room seems to be spinning.

AUDIOMETRIC TESTING

Audiometric testing evaluates hearing and determines the type and extent of hearing loss. The simplest but least reliable method for judging hearing acuity consists of covering one of the patient's ears, standing 18″ to 24″ (46 to 61 cm) from the uncovered ear, and whispering a short phrase or series of numbers. (Block the patient's vision to prevent lip reading.) Then ask the patient to repeat the phrase or series of numbers. To test hearing at both high and low frequencies, repeat the test in a normal speaking voice. (As an alternative, you can hold a ticking watch to the patient's ear.)

If you identify a hearing loss, further testing is necessary to determine if the loss is conductive or sensorineural. A conductive loss can result from faulty bone conduction (inability of the eighth cranial nerve to respond to sound waves traveling through the skull) or faulty air conduction (impaired transmission of sound through ear structures to the auditory nerve and, ultimately, the temporal lobe of the brain).

Sensorineural hearing loss results from damage to the cochlear or vestibulocochlear nerve, which can result from aging and prolonged exposure to high frequency or loud noises.

The following tests assess bone and air conduction:

◆ Impedance audiometry detects middle ear pathology, precisely determining the degree of tympanic membrane and middle ear mobility. One end of the impedance audiometer, a probe with three small tubes, is inserted into the external canal; the other end is attached to an oscillator. One tube delivers a low tone of variable intensity, the second contains a microphone, and the third, an air pump. A mobile tympanic membrane reflects minimal sound waves and produces a low-voltage curve on the graph. A tympanic membrane with decreased mobility reflects maximal sound waves and produces a high-voltage curve.

◆ Pure tone audiometry uses an audiometer to produce a series of pure tones of calibrated decibels of loudness at different frequencies (125 to 8,000 Hz). These test tones are conveyed to the patient's ears through headphones or a bone conduction (sound) vibrator. Speech threshold represents the loudness at which a person with normal hearing can perceive the tone. Both air conduction and bone conduction are measured for each ear, and the results are plotted on a graph. If hearing is normal, the line is plotted at 0 dB. In adults, normal hearing may range from 0 to 25 dB.

◆ In the Rinne test, the base of a lightly vibrating tuning fork is placed on the mastoid process (bone conduction). Then the fork is moved to the front of the meatus, where the patient should continue to hear the vibrations (air conduction). The patient must determine which sounds are heard longer. In a positive Rinne test, sounds heard through air conduction are heard relatively longer than those heard through bone conduction. This may suggest sensorineural hearing loss. In a negative Rinne test, sounds heard through bone conduction are heard longer than those heard through air conduction, which may suggest a conductive loss.

◆ Speech audiometry uses the same technique as pure tone audiometry, but with speech, instead of pure tones, transmitted through the headset. (A person with normal hearing can hear and repeat 88% to 100% of transmitted words.)

◆ Tympanometry, using the impedance audiometer, measures tympanic membrane compliance with air pressure variations in the external canal and determines the degree of negative pressure in the middle ear.

◆ In Weber test (used for testing unilateral hearing loss), the handle of a lightly vibrating tuning fork is placed on the midline of the forehead. Normally, the patient should hear sounds equally in both ears. With conductive hearing loss, sound lateralizes (localizes) to the ear with the poorest hearing. With sensorineural loss, sound lateralizes to the better functioning ear.

THE NOSE

As air travels between the septum and the turbinates, it touches sensory hairs (cilia) in the mucosal surface, which then add, retain, or remove moisture and particles in the air to ensure delivery of humid, bacteria-free air to the pharynx and lungs. In addition, when air touches the mucosal cilia, the resultant stimulation of the first cranial nerve sends nerve impulses to the olfactory area of the frontal cortex, providing the sense of smell.

ASSESSMENT

Check the external nose for redness, edema, masses, or poor alignment. Marked septal cartilage depression may indicate saddle deformity because of septal destruction from trauma or congenital syphilis; extreme lateral deviation may result from injury. Red nostrils may indicate frequent nose blowing caused by allergies or infectious rhinitis. Dilated, engorged blood vessels may suggest alcoholism or constant exposure to the elements. A bulbous, discolored nose may be a sign of rosacea.

With a nasal speculum and adequate lighting, check nasal mucosa for pallor and edema or redness and inflammation, dried mucous plugs, furuncles, and polyps. Also, look for abnormal appearance of the capillaries, boggy turbinates, and a deviated or perforated septum.

Check for nasal discharge (assess color, consistency, and odor) and blood. Profuse, thin, watery discharge may indicate allergy or cold; excessive, thin, purulent discharge may indicate cold or chronic sinus infection.

Check for sinus inflammation by applying pressure to the nostrils, orbital rims, and cheeks. Pain after pressure applied above the upper orbital rims indicates frontal sinus irritation; pain after pressure applied to the cheeks, maxillary sinus irritation.

THE THROAT

Parts of the throat include the pharynx, epiglottis, and larynx. The pharynx is the passageway for food to the esophagus and air to the larynx. The epiglottis (the lid of the larynx) diverts material away from the glottis during swallowing. The larynx produces sounds by vibrating expired air through the vocal cords. Changes in vocal cord length and air pressure affect pitch and voice intensity. The larynx also stimulates the vital cough reflex when a foreign body touches its sensitive mucosa.

ASSESSMENT

Using a bright light and a tongue blade, inspect the patient's mouth and throat. Look for inflammation or white patches, and any irregularities on the tongue or throat. Make sure the patient's airway isn't compromised and also assess vital signs. Watch for and immediately report signs of respiratory distress (dyspnea, tachycardia, tachypnea, inspiratory stridor, restlessness, and nasal flaring) and changes in voice or in skin color, such as circumoral or nail bed cyanosis. Assess symmetry of the tongue as well as function of the soft palate. The main diagnostic test used in throat assessment is a culture to identify the infective organism.

External ear

OTITIS EXTERNA

Otitis externa, inflammation of the skin of the external ear canal and auricle, may be acute or chronic. Also known as *external otitis* and *swimmer's ear*, it's most common in the summer. With treatment, acute otitis externa usually subsides within 7 days—although it may become chronic—and tends to recur.

Causes and incidence

Otitis externa usually results from bacteria, such as *Pseudomonas*, *Proteus vulgaris*, *Staphylococcus aureus*, and streptococci and, sometimes, from fungi, such as *Aspergillus niger* and *Candida albicans* (fungal otitis externa is most common in tropical regions). Occasionally, chronic otitis externa results from dermatologic conditions, such as seborrhea or psoriasis. Allergic reactions stemming from nickel or chromium earrings, chemicals in hair spray, cosmetics, hearing aids, and medications (such as sulfonamide and neomycin, which is commonly used to treat otitis externa) can also cause otitis externa.

Predisposing factors include:
◆ Swimming in contaminated water. (Cerumen creates a culture medium for the waterborne organism.)
◆ Cleaning the ear canal with a cotton swab, bobby pin, finger, or other foreign object. (This irritates the ear canal and, possibly, introduces the infecting microorganism.)
◆ Exposure to dust or hair-care products (such as hair spray or other irritants), which causes the patient to scratch the ear, excoriating the auricle and canal.
◆ Regular use of earphones, earplugs, or earmuffs, which trap moisture in the ear canal, creating a culture medium for infection (especially if earplugs don't fit properly).
◆ Chronic drainage from a perforated tympanic membrane.
◆ Perfumes or self-administered eardrops.

Pathophysiology

Otitis externa can take an acute or a chronic form. Acute disease commonly results from bacterial or fungal overgrowth in an ear canal subjected to excess moisture or to local trauma. Chronic disease often is part of a more generalized dermatologic or allergic problem. Symptoms of early acute and most chronic disease include pruritus and local discomfort. If left untreated, acute disease can be followed by canal edema, discharge, and pain, and eventually by extra-canal manifestations. Topical application of an acidifying solution is usually adequate in treating early disease. An antimicrobial-containing ototopical is the preferred treatment for later-stage acute disease, and oral antibiotic therapy is reserved for advanced disease or those who are immunocompromised. Preventive measures reduce recurrences and typically involve minimizing ear canal moisture, trauma, or exposure to materials that incite local irritation or contact dermatitis.

Complications

◆ Complete closure of the ear canal
◆ Significant hearing loss
◆ Otitis media
◆ Cellulitis
◆ Abscesses
◆ Stenosis

Signs and symptoms

Acute otitis externa characteristically produces moderate to severe pain that's exacerbated by manipulating the auricle or tragus, clenching the teeth, opening the mouth, or chewing. Its other clinical effects may include fever, foul-smelling discharge, crusting in the external ear, regional cellulitis, partial hearing loss, and itching. It's usually difficult to view the tympanic membrane because of pain in the external canal. Hearing acuity is normal unless complete occlusion has occurred.

Fungal otitis externa may be asymptomatic, although *A. niger* produces a black or gray, blotting, paper-like growth in the ear canal. In chronic otitis externa, pruritus replaces pain, and scratching may lead to scaling and skin thickening. Aural discharge may also occur.

Diagnosis

℞ **CONFIRMING DIAGNOSIS** *Physical examination confirms otitis externa. In acute otitis externa, otoscopy reveals a swollen external ear canal (sometimes to the point of complete closure), preauricular lymphadenopathy (tender nodes anterior to the tragus, posterior to the ear, or in the upper neck), and, occasionally, regional cellulitis.*

In fungal otitis externa, removal of the growth reveals thick red epithelium. Microscopic examination or culture and sensitivity tests can identify the causative organism and determine antibiotic treatment. Pain on palpation of the tragus or auricle distinguishes acute otitis externa from acute otitis media. (See *Differentiating acute otitis externa from acute otitis media*, page 629.)

In chronic otitis externa, physical examination reveals thick red epithelium in the ear canal. Severe chronic otitis externa may reflect underlying diabetes mellitus, hypothyroidism, or nephritis. Microscopic examination or culture and sensitivity tests can identify the causative organism and help in the determination of antibiotic treatment.

Treatment

To relieve the pain of acute otitis externa, treatment includes heat therapy to the preauricular region (heat lamp; hot, damp compresses; or a heating pad), aspirin or acetaminophen, and codeine. Instillation of antibiotic eardrops (with or without hydrocortisone) follows cleaning of the ear and removal of debris. However, a corticosteroid helps reduce the inflammatory response.

If fever persists or regional cellulitis or tender postauricular adenopathy develops, a systemic antibiotic is necessary.

Differentiating acute otitis externa from acute otitis media

Use the assessment findings shown below to help differentiate acute otitis externa from acute otitis media.

ACUTE OTITIS EXTERNA (OCCURS PRIMARILY IN SUMMER)

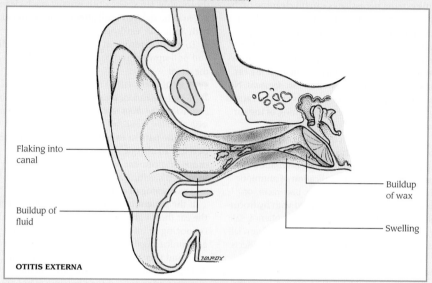

Flaking into canal

Buildup of fluid

Buildup of wax

Swelling

OTITIS EXTERNA

ACUTE OTITIS MEDIA (OCCURS PRIMARILY IN WINTER)

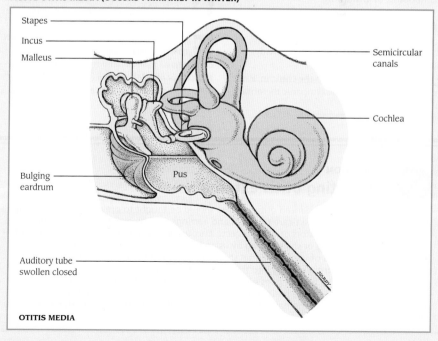

Stapes

Incus

Malleus

Semicircular canals

Cochlea

Bulging eardrum

Pus

Auditory tube swollen closed

OTITIS MEDIA

If the ear canal is too edematous for the instillation of eardrops, an ear wick may be used for the first few days.

Topical treatment is generally required for otitis externa, as systemic antibiotics alone aren't sufficient. Analgesics, such as acetaminophen or ibuprofen, may be required temporarily.

As with other forms of this disorder, fungal otitis externa necessitates careful cleaning of the ear. Application of a keratolytic or 2% salicylic acid in cream-containing nystatin may help treat otitis externa resulting from candidal organisms. Instillation of slightly acidic eardrops creates an unfavorable environment in the ear canal for most fungi as well as *Pseudomonas*. No specific treatment exists for otitis externa caused by *A. niger*, except repeated cleaning of the ear canal with baby oil.

In chronic otitis externa, primary treatment consists of cleaning the ear and removing debris. Supplemental therapy includes instillation of antibiotic eardrops or application of antibiotic ointment or cream (neomycin, bacitracin, or polymyxin B, possibly combined with hydrocortisone). Another ointment contains phenol, salicylic acid, precipitated sulfur, and petroleum jelly and produces exfoliative and antipruritic effects.

For mild chronic otitis externa, treatment may include instillation of antibiotic eardrops once or twice weekly and wearing of specially fitted earplugs while the patient is showering, shampooing, or swimming.

Special considerations

If the patient has acute otitis externa:
♦ The patient shouldn't participate in any swimming activity.
♦ Have the patient return to the clinic in 1 week for evaluation of the tympanic membrane to make sure it's intact.

♦ Monitor vital signs, particularly temperature. Watch for and record the type and amount of aural drainage.
♦ Remove debris and gently clean the ear canal with mild Burow solution (aluminum acetate). Place a wisp of cotton soaked with solution into the ear, and apply a saturated compress directly to the auricle. Afterward, dry the ear gently but thoroughly. (In severe otitis externa, such cleaning may be delayed until after initial treatment with antibiotic eardrops.)
♦ To instill eardrops in an adult, grasp the helix and pull upward and backward to straighten the canal.

PEDIATRIC TIP *To instill eardrops in a child, pull the earlobe downward and backward. To ensure that the drops reach the epithelium, insert a wisp of cotton moistened with eardrops.*

♦ Tell the patient to notify the physician if they develop an allergic reaction to the antibiotic drops or ointment, which may be indicated by increased swelling and discomfort of the area and worsening of other symptoms.

If the patient has chronic otitis externa, clean the ear thoroughly. Use wet soaks intermittently on oozing or infected skin. If the patient has a chronic fungal infection, clean the ear canal well, and then apply an exfoliative ointment.
♦ Urge prompt treatment for otitis media to prevent perforation of the tympanic membrane. (See *Preventing otitis externa*.)

ELDER TIP *If the patient is an elderly person or has diabetes, evaluate for malignant otitis externa.*

PEDIATRIC TIP *Children who have an intact tympanic membrane but are predisposed to otitis externa from swimming should instill two to three drops of a 1:1 solution of white vinegar and 70% ethyl alcohol into their ears before and after swimming.*

PREVENTION

Preventing otitis externa

Any patient who has experienced otitis externa should be taught to prevent a recurrence by avoiding irritants, such as hair-care products and earrings, and by avoiding cleaning the ears with cotton-tipped applicators or other objects. Encourage the patient to keep water out of the ears when showering or shampooing by using lamb's wool earplugs, coated with petroleum jelly. Also, parents of young children should be told that modeling clay makes a tight seal to prevent water from getting into the external ear canal.

In addition, when the patient goes swimming, keep their head above water or wear earplugs. After swimming, the patient should instill one or two drops of a mixture that is one-half 70% alcohol and one-half white vinegar to toughen the skin of the external ear canal.

BENIGN TUMORS OF THE EAR CANAL

Benign tumors may develop anywhere in the ear canal. Common types include keloids, osteomas, and sebaceous cysts; their causes vary. (See *Causes and characteristics of benign ear tumors.*) These tumors seldom become malignant; with proper treatment, the prognosis is excellent.

Signs and symptoms

A benign ear tumor is usually asymptomatic, unless it becomes infected, in which case pain, fever, or inflammation may result. (Pain is usually a sign of a malignant tumor.) If the tumor grows large enough to obstruct the ear canal by itself or through accumulated cerumen and debris, it may cause hearing loss and the sensation of pressure.

Diagnosis

℞ **CONFIRMING DIAGNOSIS** *Clinical features and patient history suggest a benign tumor of the ear canal; otoscopy confirms it. To rule out cancer, a biopsy may be necessary.*

Treatment

Generally, a benign tumor requires surgical excision if it obstructs the ear canal, is cosmetically undesirable, or becomes malignant.

Treatment for keloids may include surgery followed by repeated injections of long-acting steroids into the suture line. Excision must be complete, but even this may not prevent recurrence.

Surgical excision of an osteoma consists of elevating the skin from the surface of the bony growth and shaving the osteoma with a mechanical burr or drill.

Before surgery, a sebaceous cyst requires preliminary treatment with antibiotics, to reduce inflammation. To prevent recurrence, excision must be complete, including the sac or capsule of the cyst.

Special considerations

Because treatment for benign ear tumors generally doesn't require hospitalization, focus care on emotional support and on providing appropriate patient education so that the patient follows the therapeutic plan properly when he's at home.

♦ Thoroughly explain diagnostic procedures and treatment to the patient and family. Reassure them and answer any questions they may have.

♦ After surgery, instruct the patient in good aural hygiene. Until the ear is completely healed, advise the patient not to insert anything into their ear or allow water to get into it. Suggest that they cover their ears with a cap when showering.

♦ Teach the patient how to recognize signs of infection, such as pain, fever, localized redness, and swelling. If the patient detects any of these signs, instruct to report them immediately.

Causes and characteristics of benign ear tumors

Tumor	Causes and incidence	Characteristics
Keloid	♦ Surgery or trauma such as ear piercing ♦ Most common in blacks	♦ Hypertrophy and fibrosis of scar tissue ♦ Commonly recurs
Osteoma	♦ Idiopathic growth ♦ Predisposing factor: swimming in cold water ♦ Three times more common in males than in females ♦ Seldom occurs before adolescence	♦ Bony outgrowth from wall of external auditory meatus ♦ Usually bilateral and multiple (exostoses) ♦ May be circumscribed or diffuse, nondisplaceable, nontender
Sebaceous cyst	♦ Obstruction of a sebaceous gland	♦ Painless, circumscribed, round mass of variable size filled with oily, fatty, glandular secretions ♦ May occur on external ear and outer third of external auditory canal

Middle ear

OTITIS MEDIA

Otitis media, inflammation of the middle ear, may be suppurative or secretory, acute, persistent, unresponsive, or chronic. With prompt treatment, the prognosis for acute otitis media is excellent; however, prolonged accumulation of fluid within the middle ear cavity causes chronic otitis media and, possibly, perforation of the tympanic membrane. (See *Site of otitis media*.)

Chronic suppurative otitis media may lead to scarring, adhesions, and severe structural or functional ear damage. Chronic secretory otitis media, with its persistent inflammation and pressure, may cause conductive hearing loss.

Recurrent otitis media is defined as three near-acute otitis media episodes within 6 months or four episodes of acute otitis media within 1 year.

Otitis media with complications involves damage to middle ear structures (such as adhesions, retraction, pockets, cholesteatoma, and intratemporal and intracranial complications).

Causes and incidence

Otitis media results from disruption of eustachian tube patency. In the suppurative form, respiratory tract infection, allergic reaction, nasotracheal intubation, or positional changes allow nasopharyngeal flora to reflux through the eustachian tube and colonize the middle ear. Suppurative otitis media usually results from bacterial infection with pneumococcus, *Haemophilus influenzae* (the most common cause in children younger than age 6), *Moraxella catarrhalis*, beta-hemolytic streptococci, staphylococci (most common cause in children age 6 or older), or gram-negative bacteria. Predisposing factors include the normally wider, shorter, more horizontal eustachian tubes and increased lymphoid tissue in children, as well as anatomic anomalies. Chronic suppurative otitis media results from inadequate treatment for acute otitis episodes or from infection by resistant strains of bacteria or, rarely, tuberculosis.

Secretory otitis media results from obstruction of the eustachian tube. This causes a buildup of negative pressure in the middle ear

Site of otitis media

The common site of otitis media is shown below.

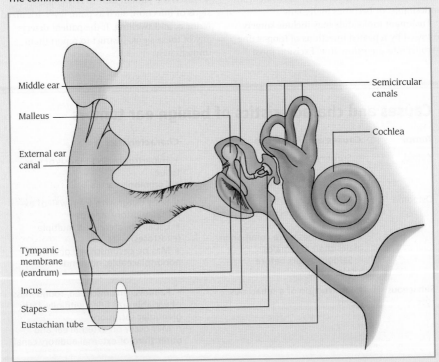

- Middle ear
- Malleus
- External ear canal
- Tympanic membrane (eardrum)
- Incus
- Stapes
- Eustachian tube
- Semicircular canals
- Cochlea

that promotes transudation of sterile serous fluid from blood vessels in the membrane of the middle ear. Such effusion may be secondary to eustachian tube dysfunction from viral infection or allergy. It may also follow barotrauma (pressure injury caused by the inability to equalize pressures between the environment and the middle ear), as occurs during rapid aircraft descent in a person with an upper respiratory tract infection (URTI) or during rapid underwater ascent in scuba diving (barotitis media).

Chronic secretory otitis media follows persistent eustachian tube dysfunction from mechanical obstruction (adenoidal tissue overgrowth or tumors), edema (allergic rhinitis or chronic sinus infection), or inadequate treatment for acute suppurative otitis media.

Acute otitis media is common in children; its incidence rises during the winter months, paralleling the seasonal rise in nonbacterial respiratory tract infections. Chronic secretory otitis media most commonly occurs in children with tympanostomy tubes or those with a perforated tympanic membrane.

Pathophysiology

Acute otitis media is an acute infection of the middle ear, usually lasting less than 6 weeks. The primary cause of acute otitis media is usually *Streptococcus pneumoniae, H. influenzae*, and *M. catarrhalis*, which enter the middle ear after eustachian tube dysfunction caused by obstruction related to upper respiratory infections, inflammation of surrounding structures (e.g., sinusitis, adenoid hypertrophy), or allergic reactions (e.g., allergic rhinitis). Bacteria can enter the eustachian tube from contaminated secretions in the nasopharynx and the middle ear from a tympanic membrane perforation. A purulent exudate is usually present in the middle ear, resulting in a conductive hearing loss.

Complications

- Spontaneous rupture of the tympanic membrane
- Persistent perforation
- Chronic otitis media
- Mastoiditis
- Abscesses
- Vertigo
- Permanent hearing loss

Signs and symptoms

Clinical features of acute suppurative otitis media include severe, deep, throbbing pain (from pressure behind the tympanic membrane); signs of URTI (sneezing or coughing); mild to very high fever; hearing loss (usually mild and conductive); tinnitus; dizziness; nausea; and vomiting. Other possible effects include bulging of the tympanic membrane, with concomitant erythema, and purulent drainage in the ear canal from tympanic membrane rupture. However, many patients are asymptomatic.

Acute secretory otitis media produces a severe conductive hearing loss—which varies from 15 to 35 dB, depending on the thickness and amount of fluid in the middle ear cavity—and, possibly, a sensation of fullness in the ear and popping, crackling, or clicking sounds on swallowing or with jaw movement. Accumulation of fluid may also cause the patient to hear an echo when the patient speaks and to experience a vague feeling of top-heaviness.

The cumulative effects of chronic otitis media include thickening and scarring of the tympanic membrane, decreased or absent tympanic membrane mobility, cholesteatoma (a cystlike mass in the middle ear), and, in chronic suppurative otitis media, a painless, purulent discharge. The extent of associated conductive hearing loss varies with the size and type of tympanic membrane perforation and ossicular destruction.

If the tympanic membrane has ruptured, the patient may state that the pain has suddenly stopped. Complications may include abscesses (brain, subperiosteal, and epidural), sigmoid sinus or jugular vein thrombosis, septicemia, meningitis, suppurative labyrinthitis, facial paralysis, and otitis externa.

PEDIATRIC TIP *The following factors increase a child's risk of developing otitis media:*
- *acute otitis media in the first year after birth (recurrent otitis media)*
- *day care*
- *family history of middle ear disease*
- *formula feeding*
- *male gender*
- *sibling history of otitis media*
- *smoking in the household*

Acute otitis media may not produce any symptoms in the first few months of life; irritability may be the only indication of earache.

Diagnosis

In acute suppurative otitis media, otoscopy reveals obscured or distorted bony landmarks of the tympanic membrane. Pneumatoscopy can show decreased tympanic membrane mobility, but this procedure is painful with an obviously bulging, erythematous tympanic membrane. The pain pattern is diagnostically significant: For example, in acute suppurative otitis media, pulling the auricle *doesn't* exacerbate the pain. A culture of the ear drainage identifies the causative organism.

In acute secretory otitis media, otoscopic examination reveals tympanic membrane retraction, which causes the bony landmarks to appear more prominent.

Examination also detects clear or amber fluid behind the tympanic membrane. If hemorrhage into the middle ear has occurred, as in barotrauma, the tympanic membrane appears blue-black.

In chronic otitis media, patient history discloses recurrent or unresolved otitis media. Otoscopy shows thickening, sometimes scarring, and decreased mobility of the tympanic membrane; pneumatoscopy shows decreased or absent tympanic membrane movement. A history of recent air travel or scuba diving suggests barotitis media.

Tympanocentesis for microbiologic diagnosis is recommended for treatment failures and may be followed by myringotomy. Tympanometry, acoustic reflex measurement, or acoustic reflexometry may be needed to document the presence of fluid in the middle ear. White blood cell count is higher in bacterial otitis media than in sterile otitis media. Mastoid X-rays or computed tomography (CT) scan of the head or mastoids may show the spreading of the infection beyond the middle ear.

Treatment

In acute suppurative otitis media, antibiotic therapy includes amoxicillin. In areas with a high incidence of beta-lactamase–producing *H. influenzae* and in patients who aren't responding to ampicillin or amoxicillin, amoxicillin/ clavulanate potassium may be used. For those who are allergic to penicillin derivatives, therapy may include cefaclor or trimethoprim and sulfamethoxazole. Severe, painful bulging of the tympanic membrane usually necessitates myringotomy. Broad-spectrum antibiotics can help prevent acute suppurative otitis media in high-risk patients. A single dose of ceftriaxone 50 mg/kg is effective against major pathogens but is expensive and is reserved for very sick infants. In the patient with recurring otitis media, antibiotics must be used with discretion to prevent the development of resistant strains of bacteria.

In acute secretory otitis media, inflation of the eustachian tube using Valsalva maneuver several times a day may be the only treatment required. Otherwise, nasopharyngeal decongestant therapy may be helpful. It should continue for at least 2 weeks and, sometimes, indefinitely, with periodic evaluation. If decongestant therapy fails, myringotomy and aspiration of middle ear fluid are necessary, followed by insertion of a polyethylene tube into the tympanic membrane, for immediate and prolonged equalization of pressure. The tube falls out spontaneously after 9 to 12 months. Concomitant treatment for the underlying cause (such as elimination of allergens, or adenoidectomy for hypertrophied adenoids) may also be helpful in correcting this disorder.

Treatment for chronic otitis media includes broad-spectrum antibiotics, such as amoxicillin/ clavulanate potassium or cefuroxime, for exacerbations of acute otitis media; elimination of eustachian tube obstruction; treatment for otitis externa; myringoplasty and tympanoplasty to reconstruct middle ear structures when thickening and scarring are present; and, possibly, mastoidectomy. Cholesteatoma requires excision.

Special considerations

◆ Explain all diagnostic tests and procedures. After myringotomy, maintain drainage flow. Don't place cotton or plugs deeply into the ear canal; however, sterile cotton may be placed loosely in the external ear to absorb drainage. To prevent infection, change the cotton whenever it gets damp, and wash hands before and after giving ear care. Watch for and report headache, fever, severe pain, or disorientation.

◆ After tympanoplasty, reinforce dressings and observe for excessive bleeding from the ear canal. Administer analgesics as needed. Warn the patient against blowing the nose or getting the ear wet when bathing.

◆ Encourage the patient to complete the prescribed course of antibiotic treatment. If nasopharyngeal decongestants are ordered, teach correct instillation.

◆ Suggest application of heat to the ear to relieve pain. (See *Preventing otitis media*, page 635.)

◆ Advise the patient with acute secretory otitis media to watch for and immediately report pain and fever—signs of secondary infection.

◆ Identify and treat allergies.

MASTOIDITIS

Mastoiditis is a bacterial infection and inflammation of the air cells of the mastoid antrum. Although the prognosis is good with early treatment, possible complications include meningitis, facial paralysis, brain abscess, and suppurative labyrinthitis.

Causes and incidence

Bacteria that cause mastoiditis include pneumococci, *H. influenzae*, *M. catarrhalis*, beta-hemolytic streptococci, staphylococci, and gram-negative organisms. Mastoiditis is usually a complication of chronic otitis media; less frequently, it develops after acute otitis media. An accumulation of pus under pressure in the middle ear cavity results in necrosis of adjacent tissue and extension of the infection into the mastoid cells. Chronic systemic diseases or immunosuppression may also lead to mastoiditis. Anaerobic organisms play a role in chronic mastoiditis.

PEDIATRIC TIP *Acute otitis media increases a child's risk of developing mastoiditis. If mastoiditis does occur in infants younger than age 1, the swelling occurs superior to the ear and pushes the auricle downward instead of outward. I.V. antibiotic treatment choice includes ampicillin or cefuroxime. Before antibiotics, mastoiditis was one of the leading causes of death in children; now, it's uncommon and less dangerous.*

Pathophysiology

Mastoiditis, inflammation of the mastoid process, a projection of the temporal bone just behind the ear. Mastoiditis, which primarily affects children, usually results from an infection of the middle ear (otitis media). Symptoms include pain and swelling behind the ear and over the side of the head and fever. An abscess may develop; this indicates that the infection has eroded the bone and destroyed its outer layer. Mastoiditis may affect other structures within the cranium and produce complications including meningitis, abscesses of the dura mater covering the brain; infection or blood clots of the lateral sinus (the large blood channel emptying into the internal jugular vein); and infection of the labyrinth (the inner ear) containing the balance and hearing apparatus. Mastoiditis is a rare condition that is treated by the early

administration of antibiotics. Surgical drainage and removal of diseased bone may be necessary if antibiotics are not successful.

Complications
- Destruction of the mastoid bone
- Facial paralysis
- Meningitis
- Partial or complete hearing loss

Signs and symptoms

Primary clinical features include a dull ache and tenderness in the area of the mastoid process, low-grade fever, headache, and a thick, purulent discharge that gradually becomes more profuse, possibly leading to otitis externa. Postauricular erythema and edema may push the auricle out from the head; pressure within the edematous mastoid antrum may produce swelling and obstruction of the external ear canal, causing conductive hearing loss.

Diagnosis

X-rays or CT scan of the mastoid area reveal hazy mastoid air cells; the bony walls between the cells appear decalcified. Audiometric testing may reveal a conductive hearing loss. Physical examination shows a dull, thickened, and edematous tympanic membrane, if the membrane isn't concealed by obstruction. During examination, the external ear canal is cleaned; persistent oozing into the canal indicates perforation of the tympanic membrane.

Treatment

Treatment for mastoiditis consists of intense parenteral antibiotic therapy. Reasonable initial antibiotic choices include ceftriaxone with nafcillin or clindamycin. If bone damage is minimal, myringotomy or tympanocentesis drains purulent fluid and provides a specimen of discharge for culture and sensitivity testing. Recurrent or persistent infection or signs of intracranial complications necessitate simple mastoidectomy. This procedure involves removal of the diseased bone and cleaning of the affected area, after which a drain is inserted.

A chronically inflamed mastoid requires radical mastoidectomy (excision of the posterior wall of the ear canal, remnants of the tympanic membrane, and the malleus and incus, although these bones are usually destroyed by infection before surgery). The stapes and facial nerve remain intact. Radical mastoidectomy, which is seldom necessary because of antibiotic therapy, doesn't drastically affect the patient's hearing because significant hearing loss precedes surgery. With either surgical procedure, the patient continues oral antibiotic therapy for several weeks after surgery and facility discharge. The prognosis is good if treatment is started early.

Indications for immediate surgical intervention include meningitis, brain abscess, cavernous sinus thrombosis, acute suppurative labyrinthitis, and facial palsy.

Special considerations

◆ After simple mastoidectomy, give pain medication as needed. Check wound drainage and reinforce dressings (the surgeon usually changes the dressing daily and removes the drain in 72 hours). Check the patient's hearing, and watch for signs of complications, especially infection (either localized or extending to the brain); facial nerve paralysis, with unilateral facial drooping; bleeding; and vertigo, especially when the patient stands.
◆ After radical mastoidectomy, the wound is packed with petroleum gauze or gauze treated with an antibiotic ointment. Give pain medication before the packing is removed, on the fourth or fifth postoperative day.
◆ Because of stimulation to the inner ear during surgery, the patient may feel dizzy and nauseated for several days afterward. Keep the side rails up, and assist the patient with ambulation. Also, give antiemetics as needed.
◆ Before discharge, teach the patient and family how to change and care for the dressing. Urge compliance with the prescribed antibiotic treatment and promote regular follow-up care.
◆ If the patient is an elderly person or diabetic, evaluate for malignant otitis externa.

 ELDER TIP *Encourage the patient to seek early treatment for ear infections.*

OTOSCLEROSIS

The most common cause of chronic, progressive conductive hearing loss, otosclerosis is the slow formation of spongy bone in the otic capsule, particularly at the oval window. With surgery, the prognosis is good.

Causes and incidence

Otosclerosis appears to result from a genetic factor transmitted as an autosomal dominant trait; many patients report family histories of hearing loss (excluding presbycusis). Pregnancy may trigger onset of this condition.

Otosclerosis occurs in at least 10% of the U.S. population. It's three times more prevalent in females than in males, usually affecting people between ages 15 and 30. Whites are most susceptible.

Pathophysiology

Otosclerosis is a localized disease of bone remodeling within the otic capsule of the human temporal bone. Unlike other similar bone diseases, it does not occur outside of the temporal bone. These lesions seem to begin by resorption of stable otic capsule bone in adults, followed by a reparative phase with bone deposition. There are clearly genetic factors that lead to this disease, but measles virus infection and autoimmunity also may play contributing roles. Surgical correction of the conductive hearing loss is highly effective, but nonsurgical intervention has not yet been shown to prevent or slow the disease.

Complications

◆ Bilateral conductive hearing loss
◆ Taste disturbance

Signs and symptoms

Spongy bone in the otic capsule immobilizes the footplate of the normally mobile stapes, disrupting the conduction of vibrations from the tympanic membrane to the cochlea. This causes progressive unilateral hearing loss, which may advance to bilateral deafness. Other symptoms include tinnitus and paracusis of Willis (hearing conversation better in a noisy environment than in a quiet one).

Diagnosis

Early diagnosis is based on a Rinne test that shows bone conduction lasting longer than air conduction (normally, the reverse is true). As otosclerosis progresses, bone conduction also deteriorates. Audiometric testing reveals hearing loss ranging from 60 dB in early stages to total loss. Weber test detects sound lateralizing to the more affected ear. Physical examination reveals a normal tympanic membrane. Head CT scan and X-ray help distinguish otosclerosis from other causes of hearing loss.

Treatment

Treatment consists of stapedectomy (removal of the stapes) and insertion of a prosthesis to restore partial or total hearing. This procedure is performed on only one ear at a time, beginning with the ear that has suffered greater damage. Alternative surgery includes stapedotomy (creation of a small hole in the stapes' footplate), through which a wire and piston are inserted. (See *Types of stapedectomy*.) Recent procedural innovations involve laser surgery. Postoperatively, treatment includes antibiotics to prevent infection. If surgery isn't possible, a hearing aid (air conduction aid with molded ear insert receiver) enables the patient to hear conversation in normal surroundings, although this therapy isn't as effective as stapedectomy.

Special considerations

◆ During the first 24 hours after surgery, keep the patient supine, with the affected ear facing upward (to maintain the position of the graft). Enforce bed rest with bathroom privileges for 48 hours. Because the patient may be dizzy, keep the side rails up, and assist them with ambulation. Assess for pain and vertigo, which may be relieved with repositioning or prescribed medication.

⚠ ALERT *Watch for and report postoperative facial drooping, which may indicate swelling of or around the facial nerve.*

◆ Tell the patient that hearing won't return until edema subsides and packing is removed.

◆ Before discharge, instruct the patient to avoid loud noises and sudden pressure changes (such as those that occur while diving or flying) until healing is complete (usually 6 months). Advise the patient not to blow their nose for at least 1 week to prevent contaminated air and bacteria from entering the eustachian tube.

◆ Stress the importance of protecting the ears against cold; avoiding any activities that provoke dizziness, such as straining, bending, or heavy lifting and, if possible, avoiding contact with anyone who has an URTI. Teach the patient and family how to change the external ear dressing (eye or gauze pad) and care for the incision. Emphasize the need to complete the prescribed antibiotic regimen and to return for scheduled follow-up care.

Types of stapedectomy

Surgery may remove part or all of the stapes, depending on the extent of otosclerotic growth. It may be performed using various techniques. Two techniques used to implant prostheses are depicted below.

NORMAL MIDDLE EAR

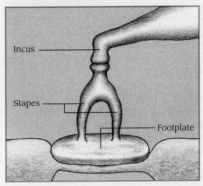

PARTIAL STAPEDECTOMY
Wire-Teflon prosthesis

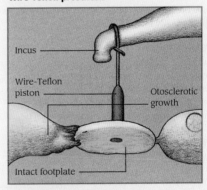

TOTAL STAPEDECTOMY
Vein graft and strut prosthesis

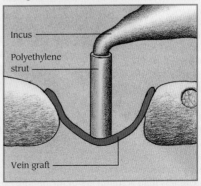

INFECTIOUS MYRINGITIS

Acute infectious myringitis is characterized by inflammation, hemorrhage, and effusion of fluid into the tissue at the end of the external ear canal and the tympanic membrane. This self-limiting disorder (resolving spontaneously within 3 days to 2 weeks) commonly follows acute otitis media or URTI.

Chronic granular myringitis, a rare inflammation of the squamous layer of the tympanic membrane, causes gradual hearing loss. Without specific treatment, this condition can lead to stenosis of the ear canal, as granulation extends from the tympanic membrane to the external ear.

Causes and incidence

Acute infectious myringitis usually follows viral infection but may also result from infection with bacteria (pneumococcus, *H. influenzae,* beta-hemolytic streptococci, staphylococci) or any other organism that can cause acute otitis media. Myringitis is a rare sequela of atypical pneumonia caused by *Mycoplasma pneumoniae.* The cause of chronic granular myringitis is unknown.

Acute infectious myringitis frequently occurs epidemically in children.

Pathophysiology

Bullous myringitis is a common condition characterized by vesicular eruptions of the tympanic membrane. In the majority of cases the condition is self-limited, although serious complications have been reported. The disease is primarily one of childhood, but is frequently seen in adults. Bullous myringitis is generally thought to be of viral origin, although several investigations have failed to establish this. Recent studies suggest a relationship to influenza virus and the Eaton agent, a pleuropneumonia-like organism (*M. pneumoniae*) known to be capable of producing primary atypical pneumonia.

Complications

◆ Gradual hearing loss
◆ Stenosis of the ear canal

Signs and symptoms

Acute infectious myringitis begins with severe ear pain, commonly accompanied by tenderness over the mastoid process. Small, reddened, inflamed blebs form in the canal, on the tympanic membrane, and, with bacterial invasion, in the middle ear. Fever and hearing loss are rare unless fluid accumulates in the middle ear or a large bleb totally obstructs the external auditory meatus. Spontaneous rupture of these blebs may cause bloody discharge. Chronic granular myringitis produces pruritus, purulent discharge, and gradual hearing loss.

Diagnosis

CONFIRMING DIAGNOSIS *Diagnosis of acute infectious myringitis is based on physical examination showing characteristic blebs and a typical patient history. Culture and sensitivity testing of exudate identifies secondary infection. In chronic granular myringitis, physical examination may reveal granulation extending from the tympanic membrane to the external ear.*

Treatment

Hospitalization usually isn't required for acute infectious myringitis. Treatment consists of measures to relieve pain: analgesics, such as aspirin or acetaminophen, and application of heat to the external ear are usually sufficient, but severe pain may necessitate the use of codeine.

ALERT *Aspirin and combination aspirin products aren't recommended for people younger than age 19 during episodes of fever-causing illnesses because the use of aspirin has been linked to Reye syndrome.*

Systemic or topical antibiotics prevent or treat secondary infection. Incision of blebs and evacuation of serum and blood may relieve pressure and help drain exudate but don't speed recovery.

Treatment for chronic granular myringitis consists of systemic antibiotics or local anti-inflammatory/antibiotic combination eardrops, and surgical excision and cautery. If stenosis is present, surgical reconstruction is necessary.

Special considerations

◆ Stress the importance of completing the prescribed antibiotic therapy.
◆ Teach the patient how to instill topical antibiotics (eardrops). When necessary, explain incision of blebs.

PREVENTION *Advise early treatment for acute otitis media.*

Inner ear

MÉNIÈRE DISEASE

Ménière disease, a labyrinthine dysfunction also known as *endolymphatic hydrops*, produces severe vertigo, sensorineural hearing loss, and tinnitus. After multiple attacks over several years, this disorder leads to residual tinnitus and hearing loss. Usually, only one ear is involved.

Causes and incidence

The exact cause of Ménière disease is unknown. It may result from overproduction or decreased absorption of endolymph, which causes endolymphatic hydrops or endolymphatic hypertension, with consequent degeneration of the vestibular and cochlear hair cells. This condition may also stem from autonomic nervous system dysfunction that produces a temporary constriction of blood vessels supplying the inner ear. In some cases, Ménière disease may be related to otitis media, syphilis, or head injury. Risk factors include recent viral illness, respiratory infection, stress, fatigue, use of prescription or nonprescription drugs (such as aspirin), and a history of allergies, smoking, and alcohol use. There also may be genetic risk factors: In some women, premenstrual edema may precipitate attacks of Ménière disease.

In the United States, about 100,000 people per year develop Ménière disease.

Pathophysiology

The pathophysiology of Ménière disease is not clearly understood. It was previously thought that Ménière was closely correlated with endolymphatic hydrops, a condition in which endolymph builds up because of an obstruction in the endolymphatic sac. Other possible origins of the disease are perisaccular fibrosis, atrophy of the endolymphatic sac and loss of epithelial integrity, hypoplasia of the vestibular aqueduct, and narrowing of the lumen of the endolymphatic duct.

Complications

◆ Tinnitus
◆ Partial to total hearing loss
◆ Permanent balance disability

Signs and symptoms

Ménière disease produces three characteristic effects: severe episodic vertigo, tinnitus, and sensorineural hearing loss. A feeling of fullness or blockage in the ear is also common. Violent paroxysmal attacks last from 10 minutes to several hours. During an acute attack, other symptoms include severe nausea, vomiting, sweating, giddiness, and nystagmus. Vertigo may cause loss of balance and falling to the affected side. Symptoms tend to wax and wane as the endolymphatic pressure rises and falls. To lessen these symptoms, the patient may assume a characteristic posture—lying on the side of the unaffected ear and looking in the direction of the affected ear.

Initially, the patient may be asymptomatic between attacks, except for residual tinnitus that worsens during an attack. Such attacks may occur several times a year, or remissions may last as long as several years. These attacks become less frequent as hearing loss progresses (usually unilaterally); they may cease when hearing loss is total. All symptoms are aggravated by motion.

Diagnosis

The presence of all three typical symptoms suggests Ménière disease. Audiometric studies indicate a sensorineural hearing loss and loss of discrimination and recruitment. Selected studies such as electronystagmography, electrocochleography, CT scan, magnetic resonance imaging, or X-rays of the internal meatus may be necessary for differential diagnosis.

Laboratory studies, including thyroid and lipid studies, may be performed to rule out other conditions such as *Treponema pallidum*.

Caloric testing may reveal loss or impairment of thermally induced nystagmus on the involved side. However, it's important not to overlook an acoustic tumor, which produces an identical clinical picture.

Treatment

Treatment with atropine may stop an attack in 20 to 30 minutes. Epinephrine or diphenhydramine may be necessary in a severe attack; dimenhydrinate, meclizine, diphenhydramine, or diazepam may be effective in a milder attack.

Long-term management includes use of a diuretic or vasodilator and restricted sodium intake (<2 g/day). A typical diuretic regime is hydrochlorothiazide 50 to 100 mg daily. Prophylactic antihistamines or mild sedatives (phenobarbital, diazepam) may also be helpful. If Ménière disease persists after 2 years of treatment, produces incapacitating vertigo, or resists medical management, surgery may be necessary. Destruction of the affected labyrinth permanently relieves symptoms but results in irreversible hearing loss. Systemic streptomycin is reserved for the patient with bilateral disease for whom no other treatment can be considered. If a patient fails medical therapy and remains disabled by vertigo, surgical decompression of the endolymphatic sac may bring relief.

Special considerations

If the patient is in the hospital during an attack of Ménière disease:
◆ Advise the patient against reading and exposure to glaring lights, to reduce dizziness.
◆ Keep the side rails of the patient's bed up to prevent falls. Tell the patient not to get out of bed or walk without assistance.

◆ Instruct the patient to avoid sudden position changes and any tasks that vertigo makes hazardous because an attack can begin quite rapidly. Hazardous activities, such as driving and climbing, should be avoided until 1 week after symptoms disappear.

◆ Before surgery, if the patient is vomiting, record fluid intake and output and characteristics of vomitus. Administer antiemetics as needed, and give small amounts of fluid frequently.

◆ After surgery, record intake and output carefully. Tell the patient to expect dizziness and nausea for 1 or 2 days after surgery. Give prophylactic antibiotics and antiemetics, as ordered.

LABYRINTHITIS

Labyrinthitis, an inflammation of the labyrinth of the inner ear, frequently incapacitates the patient by producing severe vertigo that lasts for 3 to 5 days; symptoms gradually subside over a 3- to 6-week period. Viral labyrinthitis is commonly associated with URTI.

Causes

Labyrinthitis is usually caused by viral infection. It may be a primary infection, the result of trauma, or a complication of influenza, otitis media, or meningitis. In chronic otitis media, cholesteatoma formation erodes the bone of the labyrinth, allowing bacteria to enter from the middle ear. Toxic drug ingestion is another possible cause of labyrinthitis and neuronitis.

Pathophysiology

Labyrinthitis is an inflammatory response within the membranous inner ear structures in response to infection. It is a generally short-lived minor illness that has the potential to cause temporary or permanent disablement in terms of hearing loss. Other symptoms include nausea and vomiting, pain in the affected ear, vertigo, and fever.

Complications

◆ Meningitis
◆ Permanent hearing loss
◆ Permanent balance disability

Signs and symptoms

Because the inner ear controls both hearing and balance, this infection typically produces severe vertigo (with any movement of the head) and sensorineural hearing loss. Vertigo begins gradually but peaks within 48 hours, causing loss of balance and falling in the direction of the affected ear. Other associated signs and symptoms include spontaneous nystagmus, with jerking

movements of the eyes toward the unaffected ear, and nausea, vomiting, and giddiness. With cholesteatoma, signs of middle ear disease may appear. With severe bacterial infection, purulent drainage, increased salivation, generalized malaise, and perspiration can occur. To minimize symptoms such as giddiness and nystagmus, the patient may assume a characteristic posture—lying on the side of the unaffected ear and looking in the direction of the affected ear.

Diagnosis

A typical clinical picture and a history of URTI suggest labyrinthitis. Typical diagnostic measures include culture and sensitivity testing to identify the infecting organism, if purulent drainage is present, and audiometric testing. When an infectious etiology can't be found, additional testing must be done to rule out a brain lesion or Ménière disease.

Differentiation from other causes of dizziness or vertigo may include head CT scan or magnetic resonance imaging, audiology or audiometry testing, caloric stimulation tests, electronystagmography, electroencephalogram, and auditory-evoked potential studies.

Treatment

Symptomatic treatment includes bed rest, with the head immobilized between pillows, and antibiotics to combat diffuse purulent labyrinthitis. Oral fluids can prevent dehydration caused by vomiting. For severe nausea and vomiting, I.V. fluids may be necessary. Medications that help reduce symptoms include antihistamines, anticholinergics, sedative-hypnotics, and antiemetics; benzodiazepines help control vertigo.

When conservative management fails, treatment necessitates surgical excision of the cholesteatoma and drainage of the infected areas of the middle and inner ear. Prevention is possible by early and vigorous treatment for predisposing conditions, such as otitis media and any local or systemic infection.

Special considerations

◆ Keep the side rails up to prevent falls. Tell the patient to keep still and rest during attacks and to avoid sudden position changes.

◆ If vomiting is severe, administer antiemetics as ordered. Record intake and output, and give I.V. fluids as ordered.

◆ During an attack, dim the lighting and tell the patient to avoid reading.

◆ Tell the patient that recovery may take as long as 6 weeks. During this time, they should limit activities that vertigo may make hazardous. Hazardous activities, such as driving and climbing, should be avoided until 1 week after symptoms disappear.

◆ If recovery doesn't occur within 4 to 6 weeks, a CT scan should be performed to rule out an intracranial lesion.

HEARING LOSS

Hearing loss results from a mechanical or nervous impediment to the transmission of sound waves. The major forms of hearing loss are classified as *conductive loss* (interrupted passage of sound from the external ear to the junction of the stapes and oval window), *sensorineural loss* (impaired cochlea or acoustic [eighth cranial] nerve dysfunction, causing failure of transmission of sound impulses within the inner ear or brain), or *mixed loss* (combined dysfunction of conduction and sensorineural transmission). Hearing loss may be partial or total and is calculated from this American Medical Association formula: Hearing is 1.5% impaired for every decibel that the pure tone average exceeds 25 dB.

Causes and incidence

Congenital hearing loss may be transmitted as a dominant, autosomal dominant, autosomal recessive, or sex-linked recessive trait. Hearing loss in neonates may also result from trauma, toxicity, or infection during pregnancy or delivery. Predisposing factors include a family history of hearing loss or known hereditary disorders (e.g., otosclerosis), maternal exposure to rubella or syphilis during pregnancy, use of ototoxic drugs during pregnancy, prolonged fetal anoxia during delivery, and congenital abnormalities of the ears, nose, or throat. Premature or low-birth-weight neonates are most likely to have structural or functional hearing impairment; those with serum bilirubin levels above 20 mg/dL also risk hearing impairment from the toxic effect of high-serum bilirubin levels on the brain. In addition, trauma during delivery may cause intracranial hemorrhage and may damage the cochlea or the acoustic nerve.

Sudden deafness refers to sudden hearing loss in a person with no prior hearing impairment. This condition is considered a medical emergency because prompt treatment may restore full hearing. Its causes and predisposing factors may include:

◆ acute infections, especially mumps (most common cause of unilateral sensorineural hearing loss in children), and other bacterial and viral infections, such as rubella, rubeola, influenza, herpes zoster, and infectious mononucleosis; and mycoplasma infections

◆ blood dyscrasias (leukemia, hypercoagulation)
◆ head trauma or brain tumors
◆ metabolic disorders (diabetes mellitus, hypothyroidism, hyperlipoproteinemia)
◆ neurologic disorders (multiple sclerosis, neurosyphilis)
◆ ototoxic drugs (tobramycin, streptomycin, quinine, gentamicin, furosemide, ethacrynic acid)
◆ vascular disorders (hypertension, arteriosclerosis)

Noise-induced hearing loss, which may be transient or permanent, may follow prolonged exposure to loud noise (85 to 90 dB) or brief exposure to extremely loud noise (>90 dB). Such hearing loss is common in workers subjected to constant industrial noise and in military personnel, hunters, and rock musicians.

Presbycusis, an otologic effect of aging, results from a loss of hair cells in the organ of Corti. This disorder causes progressive, symmetrical, bilateral sensorineural hearing loss, usually of high-frequency tones.

Minor decreases in hearing are common after age 20. Some deafness due to nerve damage occurs in one of every five people by age 55.

Complications
◆ Tympanic membrane perforation
◆ Cholesteatoma
◆ Permanent hearing loss

Signs and symptoms
PEDIATRIC TIP *Although congenital hearing loss may produce no obvious signs of hearing impairment at birth, a deficient response to auditory stimuli generally becomes apparent within 2 to 3 days. As the child grows older, hearing loss impairs speech development.*

Sudden deafness may be conductive, sensorineural, or mixed, depending on etiology. Associated clinical features depend on the underlying cause.

Noise-induced hearing loss causes sensorineural damage, the extent of which depends on the duration and intensity of the noise. Initially, the patient loses perception of certain frequencies (around 4,000 Hz) but, with continued exposure, eventually loses perception of all frequencies.

ELDER TIP *Presbycusis usually produces tinnitus and the inability to understand the spoken word.*

PEDIATRIC TIP *The behavior of an infant who's deaf may appear normal and mislead the parents as well as the professional, especially if the infant has autosomal recessive deafness and is the first child of carrier parents.*

Diagnosis

℞ **CONFIRMING DIAGNOSIS** *Patient, family, and occupational histories and a complete audiologic examination usually provide ample evidence of hearing loss and suggest possible causes or predisposing factors.*

The Weber, Rinne, and specialized audiologic tests differentiate between conductive and sensorineural hearing loss.

Treatment

After the underlying cause is identified, therapy for congenital hearing loss refractory to surgery consists of developing the patient's ability to communicate through sign language, speech reading, or other effective means. Measures to prevent congenital hearing loss include aggressively immunizing children against rubella to reduce the risk of maternal exposure during pregnancy; educating pregnant women about the dangers of exposure to drugs, chemicals, or infection; and careful monitoring during labor and delivery to prevent fetal anoxia.

Treatment for sudden deafness requires prompt identification of the underlying cause. Prevention necessitates educating patients and healthcare professionals about the many causes of sudden deafness and the ways to recognize and treat them.

Hyperbilirubinemia can be controlled by phototherapy and exchange transfusions. Children need the appropriate immunizations. Medications that may be ototoxic should be used judiciously in children and monitored closely. Reduction of exposure to loud noises generally prevents high-frequency hearing loss.

In people with noise-induced hearing loss, overnight rest usually restores normal hearing in those who have been exposed to noise levels greater than 90 dB for several hours, but not in those who have been exposed to such noise repeatedly. As hearing deteriorates, treatment must include speech and hearing rehabilitation, because hearing aids are seldom helpful. Prevention of noise-induced hearing loss requires public recognition of the dangers of noise exposure and insistence on the use, as mandated by law, of protective devices such as earplugs during occupational exposure to noise.

Amplifying sound, as with a hearing aid, helps some patients with presbycusis, but many patients have an intolerance to loud noise and wouldn't be helped by a hearing aid.

Special considerations

◆ When speaking to a patient with hearing loss who can read lips, stand directly in front of them, with the light on your face, and speak slowly and distinctly. If possible, speak to the patient at eye level. Approach the patient within their visual range, and elicit their attention by raising your arm or waving; touching them may be unnecessarily startling.

◆ Make other staff members and facility personnel aware of the patient's disability and their established method of communication. Carefully explain diagnostic tests and facility procedures in a way the patient understands.

◆ Make sure the patient with a hearing loss is in an area where activity can be observed and approaching persons can be seen because such a patient depends totally on visual clues.

◆ When addressing an older patient, speak slowly and distinctly in a low tone; avoid shouting.

◆ Provide emotional support and encouragement to the patient learning to use a hearing aid. Teach them how the aid works and how to maintain it.

◆ Refer children with suspected hearing loss to an audiologist or otolaryngologist for further evaluation. Any child who fails a language screening examination should be referred to a speech pathologist for language evaluation. The child with a mild language delay may be involved with a home language-enrichment program.

PREVENTION *Watch for signs of hearing impairment in the patient receiving ototoxic drugs. Emphasize the danger of excessive exposure to noise; stress the danger to pregnant women of exposure to drugs, chemicals, and infection (especially rubella); and encourage the use of protective devices in a noisy environment.*

MOTION SICKNESS

Motion sickness is characterized by loss of equilibrium associated with nausea and vomiting that results from irregular or rhythmic movements or from the sensation of motion. Removal of the stimulus restores normal equilibrium. Motion sickness also can be induced when patterns of motion differ from what the patient has previously experienced.

Causes and incidence

Motion sickness may result from excessive stimulation of the labyrinthine receptors of the inner ear by certain motions, such as those experienced in a car, boat, plane, or swing. The disorder may also be caused by confusion in the cerebellum from conflicting sensory input—the visual stimulus (a moving horizon) conflicts with labyrinthine perception. Predisposing factors include tension or fear, offensive odors, or sights and sounds associated with a previous attack. Motion sickness from cars, elevators, trains, and swings is most common in children; from boats and airplanes, in adults. People who suffer from one kind of motion sickness aren't necessarily susceptible to other types.

Pathophysiology

Motion sickness is a syndrome that occurs when a patient is exposed to certain types of motion and usually resolves soon after its cessation. It is a common response to motion stimuli during travel. Although nausea is a hallmark symptom, the syndrome includes symptoms ranging from vague malaise to completely incapacitating illness. These symptoms, which can affect the patient's recreation, employment, and personal safety, can occur within minutes of experiencing motion and can last for several hours after its cessation.

Signs and symptoms

Typically, motion sickness induces nausea, vomiting, headache, dizziness, fatigue, diaphoresis, and, occasionally, difficulty in breathing, leading to a sensation of suffocation. These symptoms usually subside when the precipitating stimulus is removed, but they may persist for several hours or days.

Treatment

The best way to treat the disorder is to stop the motion that's causing it. If this isn't possible, the patient will benefit from lying down, closing their eyes, and trying to sleep. Antiemetics, such as dimenhydrinate, cyclizine, meclizine, and scopolamine (transdermal patch), may prevent or relieve motion sickness.

Special considerations

◆ Tell the patient to avoid exposure to precipitating motion whenever possible.

PEDIATRIC TIP *An elevated car seat may help prevent motion sickness in a child by allowing the patient to see out of the front window.*

◆ Instruct the patient to avoid eating or drinking for at least 4 hours before traveling and to take an antiemetic 30 to 60 minutes before traveling or to apply a transdermal scopolamine patch at least 4 hours before traveling. Tell the patient with prostate enlargement or glaucoma to consult a physician or pharmacist before taking antiemetics.

PREVENTION *The traveler can minimize motion sickness by sitting where motion is least apparent (near the wing section in an aircraft, in the center of a boat, or in the front seat of an automobile). Instruct the patient to keep the head still and eyes closed or focused on a distant and stationary object.*

Nose

EPISTAXIS

Epistaxis, commonly known as a *nosebleed,* may be a primary disorder or may occur secondary to another condition. Such bleeding in children generally originates in the anterior nasal septum and tends to be mild. In adults, such bleeding is most likely to originate in the posterior septum and can be severe enough to warrant nasal packing. (See *Inserting an anterior–posterior nasal pack,* pages 644 and 645.) Epistaxis is twice as common in children as in adults.

Causes

Epistaxis usually follows trauma from external or internal causes: a blow to the nose, nose picking, or insertion of a foreign body; low humidity; or allergies, colds, or sinusitis. Less commonly, it follows polyps; acute or chronic infections such as sinusitis or rhinitis, which cause congestion and eventual bleeding of the capillary blood vessels; or inhalation of chemicals that irritate the nasal mucosa.

Predisposing factors include anticoagulant therapy, hypertension, long-term use of aspirin, overuse of decongestant nasal sprays, high altitudes and dry climates, sclerotic vessel disease, Hodgkin disease, hereditary hemorrhagic telangiectasia, neoplastic disorders (such as juvenile nasopharyngeal angiofibromas [JNAs]), scurvy, vitamin K deficiency, rheumatic fever, and blood dyscrasias (hemophilia, purpura, leukemia, and anemias).

Pathophysiology

Nosebleeds are due to the rupture of a blood vessel within the richly perfused nasal mucosa. Rupture may be spontaneous or initiated by trauma. An increase in blood pressure (e.g., due to general hypertension) tends to increase the duration of spontaneous epistaxis. Anticoagulant medication and disorders of blood clotting can promote and prolong bleeding. Spontaneous epistaxis is more common in the elderly as the nasal mucosa (lining) becomes dry and thin and blood pressure tends to be higher. The elderly are also more prone to prolonged nose bleeds as their blood vessels are less able to constrict and control the bleeding. Sometimes blood flowing from other sources of bleeding passes through the nasal cavity and exits the nostrils. It is thus blood coming from the nose but is not a true nosebleed, that is, not truly originating from the nasal cavity.

Complications

◆ Aspiration
◆ Shock

Inserting an anterior–posterior nasal pack

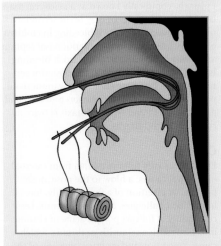 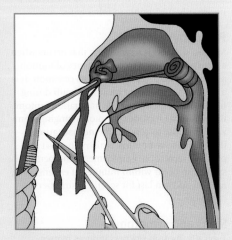

The first step in the insertion of an anterior–posterior nasal pack is the insertion of catheters into the nostrils. After the catheters are drawn through the mouth, a suture from the pack is tied to each (as shown above).

This positions the pack in place as the catheters are drawn back through the nostrils. Although the sutures are held tightly, packing is inserted into the anterior nose (as shown above).

Signs and symptoms

Blood oozing from the nostrils usually originates in the anterior nose and is bright red. Blood from the back of the throat originates in the posterior area and may be dark or bright red (commonly mistaken for hemoptysis due to expectoration). Epistaxis is generally unilateral, except when it's because of dyscrasia or severe trauma. In severe epistaxis, blood may seep behind the nasal septum; it may also appear in the middle ear and in the corners of the eyes.

Associated clinical effects depend on the severity of bleeding. Moderate blood loss may produce light-headedness, dizziness, and slight respiratory difficulty; severe hemorrhage causes hypotension, rapid and bounding pulse, dyspnea, and pallor. Bleeding is considered severe if it persists longer than 10 minutes after pressure is applied and causes blood loss as great as 1 L/hour in adults. Exsanguination (bleeding to death) from epistaxis is rare.

Diagnosis

CONFIRMING DIAGNOSIS *Although simple observation confirms epistaxis, inspection with a bright light and a nasal speculum is necessary to locate the site of bleeding.*

Relevant laboratory values include:
- gradual reduction in hemoglobin levels and hematocrit (HCT; usually inaccurate immediately following epistaxis because of hemoconcentration)
- decreased platelet count in the patient with blood dyscrasia
- prothrombin time and partial thromboplastin time showing a coagulation time twice the control, because of a bleeding disorder or anticoagulant therapy

Diagnosis must rule out underlying systemic causes of epistaxis, especially disseminated intravascular coagulation and rheumatic fever. Bruises or concomitant bleeding elsewhere probably indicates a hematologic disorder.

PEDIATRIC TIP *Bleeding tests are indicated if any of the following are present:*
- *family history of a bleeding disorder*
- *medical history of easy bleeding*
- *spontaneous bleeding at other sites*
- *onset before age 2 or a drop in HCT due to epistaxis*
- *bleeding that won't clot with direct pressure by the physician*
- *bleeding that lasts longer than 30 minutes*

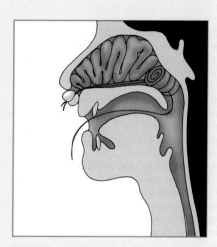

The sutures are then secured around a dental roll; the middle suture extends from the mouth (as shown above) and is taped to the cheek.

Treatment

Mild nosebleeds that occur spontaneously may be treated by gently squeezing the soft portion of the nose between the thumb and finger for 5 to 10 minutes while the patient leans forward slightly (to avoid swallowing the blood) and breathes through the mouth.

For anterior bleeding, treatment consists of application to the bleeding site of a cotton ball saturated with epinephrine, and external pressure, followed by cauterization with electrocautery or a silver nitrate stick. If these measures don't control the bleeding, petroleum gauze nasal packing may be needed.

For posterior bleeding, therapy includes gauze packing inserted through the nose, or postnasal packing inserted through the mouth, depending on the bleeding site. (Gauze packing generally remains in place for 24 to 48 hours; postnasal packing, 3 to 5 days.) An alternate method, the nasal balloon catheter, also controls bleeding effectively. Antibiotics may be appropriate if packing must remain in place for longer than 24 hours. If local measures fail to control bleeding, additional treatment may include supplemental vitamin K and, for severe bleeding, blood transfusions and surgical ligation or embolization of a bleeding artery.

Special considerations

To control epistaxis:
◆ Elevate the patient's head to 45 degrees.
◆ Continuously compress the soft portion of the nares against the septum for 5 to 10 minutes. Apply an ice collar or cold, wet compresses to the nose. If bleeding continues after 10 minutes of pressure, notify the physician.
◆ Administer oxygen as needed, and monitor saturation levels.
◆ Monitor vital signs and skin color; record blood loss.
◆ Tell the patient to breathe through their mouth and not to swallow blood, talk, or blow their nose.
◆ Keep vasoconstrictors, such as phenylephrine, handy.
◆ Reassure the patient and their family that epistaxis usually looks worse than it is.

░░░░░ **PREVENTION**
◆ *Instruct the patient not to pick their nose or insert foreign objects into it, and to avoid bending or lifting. Emphasize the need for follow-up examinations and periodic blood studies after an episode of epistaxis. Advise prompt treatment for nasal infection or irritation.*
◆ *Suggest humidifiers for people who live in dry climates or at high elevations, or whose homes are heated with circulating hot air.*

SEPTAL PERFORATION AND DEVIATION

Perforated septum, a hole in the nasal septum between the two air passages, usually occurs in the anterior cartilaginous septum but may occur in the bony septum. Deviated septum, a shift from the midline, is common in most adults. This condition may be severe enough to obstruct the passage of air through the nostrils. With surgical correction, the prognosis for either perforated or deviated septum is good.

Causes and incidence

Generally, perforated septum is caused by traumatic irritation, most commonly resulting from excessive nose picking; less frequently, it results from repeated cauterization for epistaxis or from penetrating septal injury. It may also result from perichondritis, an infection that gradually erodes the perichondrial layer and cartilage, finally forming an ulcer that perforates the septum. Other causes of septal perforation include syphilis, tuberculosis, untreated septal hematoma, inhalation of irritating chemicals, cocaine snorting, use of nasal sprays, chronic nasal infections, nasal carcinoma, granuloma, and chronic sinusitis.

Deviated septum commonly develops during normal growth, as the septum shifts from one side to the other. Consequently, few adults have perfectly straight septa. Nasal trauma resulting from a fall, a blow to the nose, or surgery further exaggerates the deviation. Congenital deviated septum is rare.

Complications

◆ Hemorrhage
◆ Infections
◆ Deformity

Signs and symptoms

A small septal perforation is usually asymptomatic but may produce a whistle on inspiration. A large perforation causes rhinitis, epistaxis, nasal crusting, and watery discharge.

The patient with a deviated septum may develop a crooked nose, as the midline deflects to one side. The predominant symptom of severe deflection, however, is nasal obstruction. Other manifestations include a sensation of fullness in the face, shortness of breath, stertor (snoring or laborious breathing), nasal discharge, recurring epistaxis, infection, sinusitis, and headache.

Diagnosis

Although clinical features suggest septal perforation or deviation, confirmation requires inspection of the nasal mucosa with a bright light and a nasal speculum.

Treatment

Symptomatic treatment for perforated septum includes decongestants to reduce nasal congestion by local vasoconstriction, local application of lanolin or petroleum jelly to prevent ulceration and crusting, and antibiotics to combat infection. Surgery may be necessary to graft part of the perichondrial layer over the perforation. Also, a plastic or Silastic "button" prosthesis may be used to close the perforation.

Symptomatic treatment for deviated septum usually includes analgesics to relieve headache, decongestants to minimize secretions, and, as necessary, vasoconstrictors, nasal packing, or cautery to control hemorrhage. Manipulation of the nasal septum at birth can correct congenital deviated septum.

Corrective surgical procedures include:
◆ reconstruction of the nasal septum by submucous resection to reposition the nasal septal cartilage and relieve nasal obstruction

◆ rhinoplasty to correct nasal structure deformity by intranasal incisions
◆ septoplasty to relieve nasal obstruction and enhance cosmetic appearance

Special considerations

◆ In the patient with perforated septum, use a cotton applicator to apply petroleum jelly to the nasal mucosa to minimize crusting and ulceration.
◆ Warn the patient with perforation or severe deviation against blowing their nose. To relieve nasal congestion, instill saline nose drops and suggest use of a humidifier. Give decongestants as ordered.
◆ Prevention and patient education are the first lines of treatment for perforations caused by nasal sprays. Proper technique (aiming away from the nasal septum) should be reviewed. Medication should be withheld when scabs are noted on the septum.
◆ To treat epistaxis, have the patient sit upright, provide an emesis basin, and instruct the patient to expectorate any blood. Compress the outer portion of the nose against the septum for 10 to 15 minutes, and apply ice packs. If bleeding persists, notify the physician.
◆ If corrective surgery is scheduled, prepare the patient to expect postoperative facial edema, periorbital bruising, and nasal packing, which remains in place for 12 to 24 hours. The patient must breathe through the mouth. After surgery for deviated septum, the patient may also have a splint on their nose.
◆ To reduce or prevent edema and promote drainage, place the patient in semi-Fowler position, and use a cool-mist vaporizer to liquefy secretions and facilitate normal breathing. To lessen facial edema and pain, place crushed ice in a rubber glove or a small ice bag, and apply the glove or ice bag intermittently over the eyes and nose for 24 hours.
◆ Because the patient is breathing through the mouth, provide frequent mouth care.
◆ Change the mustache dressing or drip pad as needed. Record the color, consistency, and amount of drainage. While nasal packing is in place, expect slight, bright red drainage, with clots. After packing is removed, watch for purulent discharge, an indication of infection.
◆ Watch for and report excessive swallowing, hematoma, or a falling or flapping septum (depressed, or soft and unstable septum). Intranasal examination is necessary to detect hematoma formation. Any of these complications requires surgical correction.
◆ Administer sedatives and analgesics as needed. Because of its anticoagulant properties,

aspirin is contraindicated after surgery for septal deviation or perforation.

◆ Nose blowing may cause bruising and swelling even after nasal packing is removed. After surgery, the patient must limit physical activity for 2 or 3 days and, if they are a smoker, they must stop smoking for at least 2 days.

◆ Instruct the patient to sneeze with their mouth open and to avoid bending over at the waist. (Advise the patient to stoop to pick up fallen objects.)

SINUSITIS

Sinusitis—inflammation of the paranasal sinuses—may be acute, subacute, chronic, allergic, or hyperplastic. Acute sinusitis usually results from the common cold and lingers in subacute form in only about 10% of patients. Chronic sinusitis follows persistent bacterial infection; allergic sinusitis accompanies allergic rhinitis; hyperplastic sinusitis is a combination of purulent acute sinusitis and allergic sinusitis or rhinitis. The prognosis is good for all types.

Causes and incidence

Sinusitis usually results from viral or bacterial infection. The bacteria responsible for acute sinusitis are usually pneumococci, other streptococci, *H. influenzae*, and *M. catarrhalis*. Staphylococci and gram-negative bacteria are more likely to cause sinusitis in chronic cases or in intensive care patients.

Predisposing factors include any condition that interferes with drainage and ventilation of the sinuses, such as chronic nasal edema, deviated septum, viscous mucus, nasal polyps, allergic rhinitis, nasal intubation, or debilitation due to chemotherapy, malnutrition, diabetes, blood dyscrasias, cystic fibrosis, human immunodeficiency virus or other immunodeficiency disorders, or chronic use of steroids. Bacterial invasion commonly occurs as a result of the conditions listed above or after a viral infection. It may also result from swimming in contaminated water.

Other risk factors for developing sinusitis include a history of asthma, overuse of nasal decongestants, presence of a foreign body in the nose, frequent swimming or diving, dental work, pregnancy, changes in altitude (flying or climbing), air pollution and smoke, gastroesophageal reflux disease (GERD), and having a deviated nasal septum, nasal bone spur, or polyp.

Each year, more than 30 million adults and children get sinusitis.

PEDIATRIC TIP *The incidence of both acute and chronic sinusitis increases in later childhood. Sinusitis may be more prevalent in children who have had tonsils and adenoids removed.*

Complications
◆ Meningitis
◆ Cavernous and sinus thrombosis
◆ Bacteremia or septicemia
◆ Brain abscess
◆ Osteomyelitis
◆ Mucocele
◆ Orbital cellulitis abscess

Pathophysiology

The most common cause of acute sinusitis is an URTI of viral origin. The viral infection can lead to inflammation of the sinuses that usually resolves without treatment in less than 14 days. If symptoms worsen after 3 to 5 days or persist for longer than 10 days and are more severe than normally experienced with a viral infection, a secondary bacterial infection is diagnosed. The inflammation can predispose to the development of acute sinusitis by causing sinus ostial blockage. Although inflammation in any of the sinuses can lead to blockade of the sinus ostia, the most commonly involved sinuses in both acute and chronic sinusitis are the maxillary and the anterior ethmoid sinuses. The nasal mucosa responds to the virus by producing mucus and recruiting mediators of inflammation, such as white blood cells, to the lining of the nose, which cause congestion and swelling of the nasal passages. The resultant sinus cavity hypoxia and mucus retention cause the cilia—which move mucus and debris from the nose—to function less efficiently, creating an environment for bacterial growth. If the acute sinusitis does not resolve, chronic sinusitis can develop from mucus retention, hypoxia, and blockade of the ostia. This promotes mucosal hyperplasia, continued recruitment of inflammatory infiltrates, and the potential development of nasal polyps.

Signs and symptoms

The primary indication of acute sinusitis is nasal congestion, followed by a gradual buildup of pressure in the affected sinus. For 24 to 48 hours after onset, nasal discharge may be present and later may become purulent. Associated symptoms include malaise, sore throat, headache, and low-grade fever of 99° to 99.5° F (37.2° to 37.5° C).

Characteristic pain depends on the affected sinus: maxillary sinusitis causes pain over the cheeks and upper teeth; ethmoid sinusitis, pain over the eyes; frontal sinusitis, pain over the eyebrows; and sphenoid sinusitis (rare), pain behind the eyes. (See *Locating the paranasal sinuses*, page 648.)

Locating the paranasal sinuses

The location of a patient's sinusitis pain indicates the affected sinus. For example, an infected maxillary sinus can cause tooth pain. (*Note:* The sphenoid sinus, which lies under the eye and above the soft palate, isn't depicted here.)

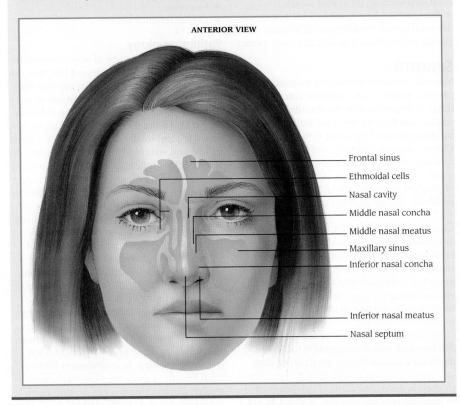

ANTERIOR VIEW

Frontal sinus

Ethmoidal cells

Nasal cavity

Middle nasal concha

Middle nasal meatus

Maxillary sinus

Inferior nasal concha

Inferior nasal meatus

Nasal septum

Purulent nasal drainage that continues for longer than 3 weeks after an acute infection subsides suggests *subacute sinusitis*. Other clinical features of the subacute form include nasal congestion, vague facial discomfort, fatigue, and a nonproductive cough.

Chronic sinusitis is defined as infection lasting longer than 8 weeks. The effects of chronic sinusitis are similar to those of acute sinusitis, but the chronic form causes continuous mucopurulent discharge.

The effects of *allergic sinusitis* are the same as those of allergic rhinitis. In both conditions, the prominent symptoms are sneezing, frontal headache, watery nasal discharge, and a stuffy, burning, itchy nose.

In *hyperplastic sinusitis*, bacterial growth on the diseased tissue causes pronounced tissue edema; thickening of the mucosal lining and the development of mucosal polyps combine to produce chronic stuffiness of the nose, in addition to headaches.

Diagnosis

The following measures are useful:

◆ Antral puncture promotes drainage of purulent material. It may also be used to provide a specimen for culture and sensitivity testing of the infecting organism, but it's seldom performed.

◆ Nasal examination reveals inflammation and pus.

◆ Palpation and percussion reveal tenderness of the frontal and maxillary sinuses.

◆ Sinus X-rays reveal cloudiness in the affected sinus, air and fluid, and any thickening of the mucosal lining.

◆ Transillumination is a simple diagnostic tool that involves shining a light into the patient's mouth with the lips closed around it. Infected sinuses look dark and normal sinuses transilluminate.

◆ Ultrasound, CT scan, magnetic resonance imaging, and X-rays aid in diagnosing suspected complications.

Treatment

Local decongestants usually are tried before systemic decongestants; steam inhalation may also be helpful. Antibiotics are necessary to combat purulent or persistent infection. Amoxicillin and amoxicillin/clavulanate potassium are usually the antibiotics of choice. Other possible therapy includes cefixime for responsive infections or if beta-lactamase-producing bacteria are present. Because sinusitis is a deep-seated infection, antibiotics should be given for 10 days to 2 weeks. Azithromycin is given for 5 days and may need to be repeated immediately. Local applications of heat may help to relieve pain and congestion. In subacute sinusitis, antibiotics and decongestants may be helpful.

Treatment for allergic sinusitis must include treatment for allergic rhinitis—avoidance measures, administration of antihistamines, identification of allergens by skin testing, and desensitization by immunotherapy. Severe allergic symptoms may require treatment with corticosteroids and epinephrine.

In both chronic sinusitis and hyperplastic sinusitis, using antihistamines, antibiotics, and a steroid nasal spray may relieve pain and congestion. If subacute infection persists, the sinuses may be irrigated. If irrigation fails to relieve symptoms, endoscopic sinus surgery may be required to obtain a histologic diagnosis, remove polyps, and provide adequate ventilation of the infected sinuses. Partial or total resection of the middle turbinate as well as more radical procedures, such as total sphenoethmoidectomy, may be performed.

Special considerations

◆ Enforce bed rest, and encourage the patient to drink plenty of fluids to promote drainage. Don't elevate the head of the bed by more than 30 degrees.

◆ To relieve pain and promote drainage, apply warm compresses continuously, or four times daily for 2-hour intervals. Also, give analgesics and antihistamines as needed.

◆ Watch for and report complications, such as vomiting, chills, fever, edema of the forehead or eyelids, blurred or double vision, and personality changes.

◆ If surgery is necessary, tell the patient what to expect postoperatively: nasal packing will be in place for 12 to 24 hours following surgery; he'll have to breathe through the mouth and won't be able to blow the nose. After surgery, monitor for excessive drainage or bleeding and watch for complications.

◆ To prevent edema and promote drainage, place the patient in semi-Fowler position. To relieve edema and pain and to minimize bleeding, apply ice compresses or a rubber glove filled with ice chips over the nose and iced saline gauze over the eyes. Continue these measures for 24 hours.

◆ Frequently change the mustache dressing or drip pad, and record the consistency, amount, and color of drainage (expect scant, bright red, and clotty drainage).

◆ Because the patient will be breathing through their mouth, provide meticulous mouth care.

◆ Tell the patient that even after the packing is removed, nose blowing may cause bleeding and swelling. If the patient is a smoker, instruct them not to smoke for at least 2 or 3 days after surgery.

◆ Tell the patient to finish the prescribed antibiotics, even if their symptoms disappear.

NASAL POLYPS

Benign and edematous growths, nasal polyps are usually multiple, mobile, and bilateral. Nasal polyps may become large and numerous enough to cause nasal distention and enlargement of the bony framework, possibly occluding the airway.

Causes and incidence

Nasal polyps are usually produced by the continuous pressure resulting from a chronic allergy that causes prolonged mucous membrane edema in the nose and sinuses. Other predisposing factors include chronic sinusitis, chronic rhinitis, and recurrent nasal infections.

Nasal polyps are more common in adults than in children and tend to recur. They're also commonly seen in patients with long-term allergic rhinitis and in patients with the aspirin triad (aspirin sensitivity, asthma, and nasal polyps). About 1 in 4 people with cystic fibrosis have nasal polyps.

Complication

◆ Airway obstruction

Signs and symptoms

Nasal obstruction is the primary indication of nasal polyps. Such obstruction causes anosmia, a sensation of fullness in the face, nasal discharge, headache, and shortness of breath. Associated clinical features are usually the same as those of allergic rhinitis.

Diagnosis

Diagnosis of nasal polyps is aided by the following tests.

◆ Examination with a nasal speculum shows a dry, red surface, with clear or gray growths. Large growths may resemble tumors.

◆ X-rays of sinuses and nasal passages reveal soft-tissue shadows over the affected areas.

PEDIATRIC TIP *Nasal polyps in children require further testing to rule out cystic fibrosis and Peutz–Jeghers syndrome.*

Treatment

Intranasal glucocorticoids are the treatment of choice. Direct injection into the polyps may temporarily reduce the polyp. A short course of oral corticosteroids (such as prednisone) may be beneficial. Treatment for the underlying cause may include nasal antihistamines to control allergy, and antibiotic therapy if infection is present. Local application of an astringent shrinks hypertrophied tissue.

Surgical treatment should be considered after medical management has failed. A polypectomy is usually performed under a local anesthetic and the use of surgical lasers is becoming more popular; however, patients should be warned that nasal polyps have high recurrence rates. Continued recurrence may require surgical opening of the ethmoid, sphenoid, and maxillary sinuses and evacuation of diseased tissue.

Special considerations

◆ Administer antihistamines, as ordered, for the patient with allergies. Prepare the patient for scheduled surgery by telling them what to expect postoperatively, such as nasal packing for 1 to 2 days after surgery.

After surgery:

◆ Watch for excessive bleeding or other drainage, and promote patient comfort.

◆ Elevate the head of the bed to facilitate breathing, reduce swelling, and promote adequate drainage. Change the mustache dressing or drip pad, as needed, and record the consistency, amount, and color of nasal drainage.

◆ Intermittently apply ice compresses over the nostrils to lessen swelling, prevent bleeding, and relieve pain.

◆ If nasal bleeding occurs—most likely after packing is removed—sit the patient upright, monitor vital signs, and advise not to swallow blood. Compress the outside of the nose against the septum for 10 to 15 minutes. If bleeding persists, nasal packing may be necessary.

PREVENTION *Instruct patients with allergies to avoid exposure to allergens and to take antihistamines at the first sign of an allergic reaction.*

Also, advise them to avoid overuse of nose drops and sprays.

NASAL PAPILLOMAS

A papilloma is a benign epithelial tissue overgrowth within the intranasal mucosa. Inverted papillomas grow into the underlying tissue, usually at the junction of the antrum and the maxillary sinus; they generally occur singly but sometimes are associated with squamous cell cancer. Exophytic papillomas, which also tend to occur singly, arise from epithelial tissue, commonly on the surface of the nasal septum.

Pathophysiology

Inverted papilloma is a benign epithelial growth in the underlying stroma of the nasal cavity and paranasal sinuses. The pathogenesis of this lesion remains unclear, although allergy, chronic sinusitis, and viral infections have been suggested as possible causes.

Causes and incidence

A papilloma may arise as a benign precursor of a neoplasm or as a response to tissue injury or viral infection, but its cause is unknown. Both types of papillomas are most prevalent in males. Recurrence is common, even after surgical excision.

Complications

◆ Severe respiratory distress (rare)
◆ Nasal drainage
◆ Infection

Signs and symptoms

Both inverted and exophytic papillomas typically produce symptoms related to unilateral nasal obstruction—congestion, postnasal drip, headache, shortness of breath, dyspnea, and, rarely, severe respiratory distress, nasal drainage, and infection. Epistaxis is most likely to occur with exophytic papillomas. Occasionally hemorrhage may be the presenting symptom.

Diagnosis

On examination of the nasal mucosa, inverted papillomas usually appear large, bulky, highly vascular, and edematous; color varies from dark red to gray; and consistency, from firm to friable. Exophytic papillomas are usually raised, firm, and rubbery; pink to gray; and securely attached by a broad or pedunculated base to the mucous membrane.

PEDIATRIC TIP *Juvenile angiofibroma is a benign vascular tumor that arises in the nasopharynx and occurs most commonly in adolescent males. Nasal obstruction and hemorrhage may occur* as with nasal papillomas. *Any adolescent male who continues to have recurrent episodes of epistaxis should be assessed for juvenile angiofibroma. Medical management involves surgical excision, with preoperative embolization to reduce bleeding.*

℞ CONFIRMING DIAGNOSIS *Tissue biopsy followed by histologic examination of excised tissue confirms the diagnosis.*

Treatment

The most effective treatment is wide surgical excision or diathermy, with careful inspection of adjacent tissues and sinuses to rule out extension. The use of surgical lasers is becoming more popular. Ibuprofen or acetaminophen and decongestants may relieve symptoms.

Special considerations

◆ If bleeding occurs, have the patient sit upright, and expectorate blood into an emesis basin. Compress both sides of the nose against the septum for 10 to 15 minutes, and apply ice compresses to the nose. If the bleeding doesn't stop, notify the physician.

⚠ ALERT *Check for airway obstruction. Place your hand under the patient's nostrils to assess air exchange and watch for signs of mild shortness of breath.*

◆ If surgery is scheduled, tell the patient what to expect postoperatively. Instruct the patient not to blow the nose. (Packing is usually removed 12 to 24 hours after surgery.)

◆ Postoperatively, monitor vital signs and respiratory status. Use pulse oximetry to monitor oxygen saturation levels. As needed, administer analgesics and facilitate breathing with a cool-mist vaporizer. Provide mouth care.

◆ Frequently change the mustache dressing or drip pad, to ensure proper absorption of drainage. Record the type and amount of drainage. While the nasal packing is in place, expect scant, usually bright red, clotted drainage. Remember that the amount of drainage typically increases for a few hours after the packing is removed.

◆ Because papillomas tend to recur, tell the patient to seek medical attention at the first sign of nasal discomfort, discharge, or congestion that doesn't subside with conservative treatment.

◆ Encourage regular follow-up visits to detect early signs of recurrence.

ADENOID HYPERPLASIA

A fairly common childhood condition, adenoid hyperplasia (also known as *adenoid hypertrophy*) is enlargement of the lymphoid tissue of the nasopharynx. Normally, adenoidal tissue is small at birth (¾″ to 1¼″ [2 to 3 cm]), grows until the child reaches adolescence, and then begins to slowly atrophy. In adenoid hyperplasia, however, this tissue continues to grow. Enlarged adenoids commonly accompany tonsillitis.

Causes and incidence

The cause of adenoid hyperplasia is unknown, but contributing factors may include heredity, chronic infection, chronic nasal congestion, persistent allergy, insufficient aeration, and inefficient nasal breathing. Inflammation resulting from repeated infection increases the patient's risk of respiratory obstruction.

Complications

◆ Otitis media
◆ Conductive hearing loss
◆ Sinusitis
◆ Cor pulmonale
◆ Pulmonary arterial hypertension

Signs and symptoms

Typically, adenoid hyperplasia produces symptoms of respiratory obstruction, especially mouth breathing, snoring at night, and frequent, prolonged nasal congestion. Persistent mouth breathing during the formative years produces voice alteration and distinctive changes in facial features—a slightly elongated face, open mouth, highly arched palate, shortened upper lip, and vacant expression.

PEDIATRIC TIP *Occasionally, the child is incapable of mouth breathing, snores loudly at night, and may eventually show effects of nocturnal respiratory insufficiency (sleep apnea), such as intercostal retractions and nasal flaring.*

Diagnosis

℞ CONFIRMING DIAGNOSIS *Nasopharyngoscopy or rhinoscopy confirms adenoid hyperplasia by allowing visualization of abnormal tissue. Lateral pharyngeal X-rays show an obliterated nasopharyngeal air column.*

Treatment

Adenoidectomy is the treatment of choice for adenoid hyperplasia and is commonly recommended for the patient with prolonged mouth breathing, nasal speech, adenoid facies, recurrent otitis media, constant nasopharyngitis, and nocturnal respiratory distress. This procedure usually eliminates recurrent nasal infections and ear complications, and reverses any secondary hearing loss.

Special considerations

Care requires sympathetic preoperative care and diligent postoperative monitoring.

Before surgery, do the following.

◆ Describe the facility routine, and arrange for the patient and their parents to tour relevant areas.

◆ Explain adenoidectomy to the child, using illustrations if necessary, and detail the recovery process. Advise them that they'll probably need to be hospitalized. If facility protocol allows, encourage one parent to stay with the child and participate in their care.

After surgery, take these steps.

🚩 **ALERT** *Maintain a patent airway. Position the child on their side, with their head down, to prevent aspiration of draining secretions. Frequently check the throat for bleeding. Be alert for vomiting of old, partially digested blood (coffee-ground vomitus). Closely monitor vital signs, and report excessive bleeding, rise in pulse rate, drop in blood pressure, tachypnea, and restlessness.*

◆ If no bleeding occurs, offer cracked ice or water when the patient is fully awake.

◆ Tell the parents that their child may temporarily have a nasal voice.

VELOPHARYNGEAL INSUFFICIENCY

Velopharyngeal insufficiency results from failure of the velopharyngeal sphincter to close properly during speech, giving the voice a hypernasal quality and permitting nasal emission (air escape during pronunciation of consonants).

Causes and incidence

Velopharyngeal insufficiency can result from an inherited palate abnormality, or it can be acquired from tonsillectomy, adenoidectomy, or palatal paresis. It commonly occurs in people who undergo cleft palate surgery and those with submucous cleft palates. Middle ear disease and hearing loss frequently accompany this disorder.

Pathophysiology

Velopharyngeal dysfunction (VPD) is a generic term, which describes a set of disorders resulting in the leakage of air into the nasal passages during speech production. As a result, speech samples can demonstrate hypernasality, nasal emissions, and poor intelligibility. The finding of VPD can be secondary to several causes: anatomic, musculoneuronal, or behavioral/mislearning. To identify the etiology of VPD, patients must undergo a thorough velopharyngeal assessment comprised of perceptual speech evaluation and functional imaging, including video nasendoscopy and speech videofluoroscopy. These studies are then evaluated by a multidisciplinary team of specialists, who can decide on an optimal course for patient management. A treatment plan is developed and may include speech therapy, use of a prosthetic device, and/or surgical intervention. Different surgical options are discussed, including posterior pharyngeal flap, sphincter pharyngoplasty, Furlow palatoplasty, palatal re-repair, and posterior pharyngeal wall augmentation.

Complication

◆ Airway obstruction

Signs and symptoms

Generally, this condition causes unintelligible speech, marked by hypernasality, nasal emission, poor consonant definition, and a weak voice. The patient experiences dysphagia and, if velopharyngeal insufficiency is severe, may regurgitate through the nose.

Diagnosis

Fiberoptic nasopharyngoscopy, which permits monitoring of velopharyngeal patency during speech, suggests this diagnosis. Ultrasound scanning, which shows air-tissue overlap, reflects the degree of velopharyngeal sphincter incompetence (an opening >20 mm^2 results in unintelligible speech). Videofluoroscopy simultaneously records the movement of the velopharyngeal sphincter and the patient's speech.

Treatment

Treatment consists of corrective surgery, usually at age 6 or 7. The preferred surgical method is the pharyngeal flap procedure, which diverts a tissue flap from the pharynx to the soft palate. Children with velopharyngeal insufficiency shouldn't have adenoidectomy except in cases of life-threatening obstruction.

Other appropriate surgical procedures include:

◆ augmentation pharyngoplasty, which narrows the velopharyngeal opening by enlarging the pharyngeal wall with a retropharyngeal implant

◆ palatal push-back, which separates the hard and soft palates to allow insertion of an obturator, thus lengthening the soft palate

◆ pharyngoplasty, which rotates pharyngeal flaps to lengthen the soft palate and narrow the pharynx

◆ velopharyngeal sphincter reconstruction, which uses free muscle implantation to reconstruct the sphincter

Surgery eliminates hypernasality and nasal emission, but speech abnormalities persist and usually necessitate speech therapy. Immediate postoperative therapy includes antibiotics and a clear, liquid diet for the first 3 days, followed by a soft diet for 2 weeks.

Special considerations
◆ After surgery for velopharyngeal insufficiency, maintain a patent airway (nasopharynx edema may obstruct the airway). Position the patient on their side, and suction the dependent side of their mouth, avoiding the pharynx.
◆ Control postoperative agitation, which may provoke pharyngeal bleeding, with sedation, as ordered.
◆ Administer high-humidity oxygen as ordered.
◆ Monitor vital signs frequently, and report any changes immediately. Observe for bleeding from the mouth or nose. Check intake and output, and watch for signs of dehydration.
◆ Advise the patient that preoperative and postoperative speech therapy require time and effort, but with persistence and practice, speech will improve. Before discharge, emphasize the importance of completing the prescribed antibiotic therapy.

Throat

PHARYNGITIS
The most common throat disorder, pharyngitis is an acute or chronic inflammation of the pharynx. It frequently accompanies the common cold.

Causes and incidence
Pharyngitis is usually caused by a virus. The most common bacterial cause is group A beta-hemolytic streptococci. Other common causes include *Mycoplasma* and *Chlamydia*. In up to 30% of cases, no organism is identified.

Pharyngitis is widespread among adults who live or work in dusty or very dry environments, use their voices excessively, habitually use tobacco or alcohol, or suffer from chronic sinusitis, persistent coughs, or allergies.

Pathophysiology
Pharyngitis is an inflammatory illness of the mucous membranes and underlying structures of the throat (pharynx). Inflammation usually involves the nasopharynx, uvula, soft palate, and tonsils. The illness can be caused by bacteria, viruses, mycoplasmas, fungi, and parasites and by recognized diseases of uncertain causes. Infection by *Streptococcus* bacteria may be a complication arising from a common cold. The symptoms of streptococcal pharyngitis (commonly known as strep throat) are generally redness and swelling of the throat, a pustulant fluid on the tonsils or discharged from the mouth, extremely sore throat that is felt during swallowing, swelling of lymph nodes, and a slight fever; sometimes in children there are abdominal pain, nausea, headache, and irritability. Diagnosis is established by a detailed medical history and by physical examination; the cause of pharyngeal inflammation can be determined by throat culture. Usually only the symptoms can be treated—with throat lozenges to control sore throat and acetaminophen or aspirin to control fever. If a diagnosis of streptococcal infection is established by culture, appropriate antibiotic therapy, usually with penicillin, is instituted. Within approximately 3 days the fever leaves; the other symptoms may persist for another 2 to 3 days.

Complications
◆ Otitis media
◆ Sinusitis
◆ Mastoiditis
◆ Rheumatic fever
◆ Nephritis

Signs and symptoms
Pharyngitis produces a sore throat and slight difficulty in swallowing. Swallowing saliva is usually more painful than swallowing food. Pharyngitis may also cause the sensation of a lump in the throat as well as a constant, aggravating urge to swallow. Associated features may include mild fever, headache, muscle and joint pain, coryza, and rhinorrhea. Uncomplicated pharyngitis usually subsides in 3 to 10 days.

PEDIATRIC TIP *More than 90% of cases of sore throat and fever in children are of viral origin. Associated symptoms usually include runny nose and nonproductive cough.*

Diagnosis
Physical examination of the pharynx reveals generalized redness and inflammation of the posterior wall, and red, edematous mucous membranes studded with white or yellow follicles. Exudate is usually confined to the lymphoid areas of the throat, sparing the tonsillar pillars. Bacterial pharyngitis usually produces a large amount of exudate.

A throat culture may be performed to identify bacterial organisms that may be the cause of the inflammation.

Treatment
Treatment for acute viral pharyngitis is usually symptomatic and consists mainly of rest, warm saline gargles, throat lozenges containing a mild anesthetic, plenty of fluids, and analgesics as

needed. If the patient can't swallow fluids, I.V. hydration may be required.

Suspected bacterial pharyngitis requires rigorous treatment with penicillin or another broad-spectrum antibiotic because *Streptococcus* is the chief infecting organism. Antibiotic therapy should continue for 48 hours until culture results are back. If the culture (or a rapid strep test) is positive for group A beta-hemolytic streptococci, or if bacterial infection is suspected despite negative culture results, penicillin therapy should be continued for 10 days. This is to prevent the sequelae of acute rheumatic fever.

Chronic pharyngitis requires the same supportive measures as acute pharyngitis but with greater emphasis on eliminating the underlying cause, such as an allergen. Preventive measures include adequate humidification and avoiding excessive exposure to air-conditioning. In addition, the patient should be urged to stop smoking.

Special considerations

◆ Administer analgesics and warm saline gargles, as ordered and as appropriate.
◆ Encourage the patient to drink plenty of fluids. Scrupulously monitor intake and output, and watch for signs of dehydration.
◆ Provide meticulous mouth care to prevent dry lips and oral pyoderma, and maintain a restful environment.
◆ Obtain throat cultures, and administer antibiotics as needed. If the patient has acute bacterial pharyngitis, emphasize the importance of completing the full course of antibiotic therapy.
◆ Teach the patient with chronic pharyngitis how to minimize sources of throat irritation in the environment, such as by using a bedside humidifier.
◆ Refer the patient to a self-help group to stop smoking if appropriate.
◆ Children attending school should receive at least 24 hours of therapy before being allowed to return to school.
◆ If the patient has exhibited three or more documented bacterial infections within 6 months, consider daily penicillin prophylaxis during the winter months. Also, consider treatment of carriers who live in closed or semi-closed communities.

TONSILLITIS

Tonsillitis—inflammation of the tonsils—can be acute or chronic. The uncomplicated acute form usually lasts 4 to 6 days. The presence of proven chronic tonsillitis justifies tonsillectomy, the only effective treatment. Tonsils tend to hypertrophy during childhood and atrophy after puberty.

Causes and incidence

Tonsillitis generally results from infection with group A beta-hemolytic streptococci but can result from other bacteria or viruses or from oral anaerobes. It commonly affects children between ages 5 and 10.

Pathophysiology

Tonsillitis is an inflammatory infection of the tonsils caused by invasion of the mucous membrane by microorganisms, usually hemolytic streptococci or viruses. The symptoms are sore throat, difficulty in swallowing, fever, malaise, and enlarged lymph nodes on both sides of the neck. The infection lasts about 5 days. The treatment includes bed rest until the fever has subsided, isolation to protect others from the infection, and warm throat irrigations or gargles with a mild antiseptic solution. Antibiotics or sulfonamides or both are prescribed in severe infections to prevent complications.

Complications

◆ Chronic upper airway obstruction
◆ Sleep apnea
◆ Cor pulmonale
◆ Failure to thrive
◆ Eating or swallowing disorders
◆ Febrile seizures
◆ Otitis media
◆ Cardiac valvular disease
◆ Peritonsillar abscesses
◆ Bacterial endocarditis
◆ Cervical lymph node abscesses

Signs and symptoms

Acute tonsillitis commonly begins with a mild to severe sore throat. A very young child, unable to describe a sore throat, may stop eating. Tonsillitis may also produce dysphagia, fever, swelling and tenderness of the lymph glands in the submandibular area, muscle and joint pain, chills, malaise, headache, and pain (frequently referred to the ears). Excess secretions may elicit the complaint of a constant urge to swallow; the back of the throat may feel constricted. Such discomfort usually subsides after 72 hours.

Chronic tonsillitis produces a recurrent sore throat and purulent drainage in the tonsillar crypts. Frequent attacks of acute tonsillitis may also occur. Complications include obstruction from tonsillar hypertrophy and peritonsillar abscess.

Diagnosis

℞ **CONFIRMING DIAGNOSIS** *Diagnostic confirmation requires a thorough throat examination that reveals:*

- *generalized inflammation of the pharyngeal wall*
- *swollen tonsils that project from between the pillars of the fauces and exude white or yellow follicles*
- *purulent drainage when pressure is applied to the tonsillar pillars*
- *possible edematous and inflamed uvula*

Culture may determine the infecting organism and indicate appropriate antibiotic therapy. Leukocytosis is also usually present. Differential diagnosis rules out infectious mononucleosis and diphtheria.

Treatment

Treatment for acute tonsillitis requires rest, adequate fluid intake, administration of ibuprofen or acetaminophen, and, for bacterial infection, antibiotics. When the causative organism is group A beta-hemolytic streptococcus, penicillin is the drug of choice (another broad-spectrum antibiotic may be substituted). Most oral anaerobes also respond to penicillin. To prevent complications, antibiotic therapy should continue for 10 to 14 days.

Chronic tonsillitis or the development of complications (obstructions from tonsillar hypertrophy, peritonsillar abscess) may require a tonsillectomy, but only after the patient has been free from tonsillar or respiratory tract infections for 3 to 4 weeks.

Special considerations

- Despite dysphagia, urge the patient to drink plenty of fluids, especially if the patient has a fever. Offer a child ice cream and flavored drinks and ices. Suggest gargling with warm salt water to soothe the throat, unless it exacerbates pain. Make sure the patient and parents understand the importance of completing the prescribed course of antibiotic therapy.
- Before tonsillectomy, explain to the adult patient that a local anesthetic prevents pain but allows a sensation of pressure during surgery. Warn the patient to expect considerable throat discomfort and some bleeding postoperatively. Watch for continuous swallowing, a sign of heavy bleeding.

PEDIATRIC TIP *For the pediatric patient, keep your explanation simple and nonthreatening. Show the patient the operating and recovery areas, and briefly explain the facility routine. Most facilities allow one parent to stay with the child.*

- Postoperatively, maintain a patent airway. To prevent aspiration, place the patient on their side. Monitor vital signs frequently, and check

for bleeding. Immediately report excessive bleeding, increased pulse rate, or dropping blood pressure. After the patient is fully alert and the gag reflex has returned, allow them to drink water. Later, urge them to drink plenty of nonirritating fluids, to ambulate, and to take frequent deep breaths to prevent pulmonary complications. Give pain medication as needed.

- Before discharge, provide the patient or their parents with written instructions on home care. Tell them to expect a white scab to form in the throat between 5 and 10 days postoperatively, and to report bleeding, ear discomfort, or a fever that lasts longer than 3 days.

THROAT ABSCESSES

Throat abscesses may be peritonsillar (quinsy) or retropharyngeal. Peritonsillar abscesses form in the connective tissue space between the tonsil capsule and the constrictor muscle of the pharynx. Retropharyngeal abscesses, or abscesses of the potential space, form between the posterior pharyngeal wall and the prevertebral fascia. With treatment, the prognosis for both types of abscesses is good.

Causes and incidence

Peritonsillar abscess is a complication of acute tonsillitis, usually after streptococcal or staphylococcal infection. It occurs more commonly in adolescents and young adults than in children.

Acute retropharyngeal abscess results from infection in the retropharyngeal lymph glands, which may follow an upper respiratory tract bacterial infection. Most common pathogens are beta-hemolytic *Streptococcus* and *S. aureus*. These lymph glands begin to atrophy after age 2. Acute retropharyngeal abscess most commonly affects infants and children younger than age 2.

Chronic retropharyngeal abscess may result from tuberculosis of the cervical spine (Pott disease) and may occur at any age.

Pathophysiology

Peritonsillar abscess, the most common deep infection of the head and neck that occurs in adults, is typically formed by a combination of aerobic and anaerobic bacteria. The presenting symptoms include fever, throat pain, and trismus. Ultrasonography and computed tomographic scanning are useful in confirming a diagnosis. Needle aspiration remains the gold standard for diagnosis and treatment of peritonsillar abscess. After performing aspiration, appropriate antibiotic therapy (including penicillin, clindamycin, cephalosporins, or metronidazole) must be initiated. In advanced cases, incision and drainage or immediate tonsillectomy may be required.

Complications
◆ Airway obstruction
◆ Cellulitis
◆ Endocarditis
◆ Pericarditis
◆ Pleural effusion
◆ Pneumonia

Signs and symptoms
Key symptoms of peritonsillar abscess include severe throat pain, occasional ear pain on the same side as the abscess, and tenderness of the submandibular gland. Dysphagia causes drooling. Trismus may occur as a result of the spread of edema and infection from the peritonsillar space to the pterygoid muscles. Other effects include fever, chills, malaise, rancid breath, nausea, muffled speech, dehydration, cervical adenopathy, and localized or systemic sepsis.

Clinical features of retropharyngeal abscess include pain, dysphagia, fever, and, when the abscess is located in the upper pharynx, nasal obstruction; with a low-positioned abscess, dyspnea, progressive inspiratory stridor (from laryngeal obstruction), neck hyperextension, and, in children, drooling and muffled crying occur. Other symptoms in children may include gurgling respirations, dyspnea and dysphagia, respiratory symptoms, and fever. A very large abscess may press on the larynx, causing edema, or may erode into major vessels, causing sudden death from asphyxia or aspiration.

Diagnosis
Diagnosis of peritonsillar abscess usually begins with a patient history of bacterial pharyngitis. Examination of the throat shows swelling of the soft palate on the abscessed side, with displacement of the uvula to the opposite side; red, edematous mucous membranes; and tonsil displacement toward the midline. Culture may reveal streptococcal or staphylococcal infection.

Diagnosis of retropharyngeal abscess is based on patient history of nasopharyngitis or pharyngitis and on physical examination revealing a soft, red bulging of the posterior pharyngeal wall. X-rays show the larynx pushed forward and a widened space between the posterior pharyngeal wall and vertebrae. If neck pain or stiffness occurs, look for extension to the epidural space or the cervical vertebrae. Culture and sensitivity tests isolate the causative organism and reveal the appropriate antibiotic.

Treatment
For early-stage peritonsillar abscess, large doses of penicillin or another broad-spectrum antibiotic is necessary. If the patient is immunocompromised or has been repeatedly hospitalized, antibiotic therapy should include coverage for staphylococci and gram-negative organisms. For late-stage abscess, with cellulitis of the tonsillar space, primary treatment is usually incision and drainage under a local anesthetic, followed by antibiotic therapy for 7 to 10 days. Tonsillectomy, scheduled no sooner than 1 month after healing, prevents recurrence but is recommended only after several episodes.

In acute retropharyngeal abscess, the primary treatment is incision and drainage through the pharyngeal wall. It's considered a surgical emergency. In chronic retropharyngeal abscess, drainage is performed through an external incision behind the sternomastoid muscle. During incision and drainage, strong, continuous mouth suction is necessary to prevent aspiration of pus, and the head should be kept down. Postoperative drug therapy includes I.V. antibiotics (usually penicillin or clindamycin) and analgesics.

Special considerations
⚠ **ALERT** *Be alert for signs of respiratory obstruction (inspiratory stridor, dyspnea, retractions and nasal flaring, increasing restlessness, and cyanosis). Keep emergency airway equipment nearby.*
◆ Explain the drainage procedure to the patient and their parents. Because the procedure is usually done under local anesthesia, the patient may be apprehensive.
◆ Assist with incision and drainage. To allow easy expectoration and suction of pus and blood, place the patient in a semirecumbent or sitting position.

After incision and drainage:
◆ Give antibiotics, analgesics, and antipyretics, as ordered. Stress the importance of completing the full course of prescribed antibiotic therapy.
◆ Monitor vital signs, and report significant changes or bleeding. Assess pain, and treat accordingly.
◆ If the patient is unable to swallow, ensure adequate hydration with I.V. therapy. Monitor fluid intake and output, and watch for dehydration.
◆ Provide meticulous mouth care. Apply petroleum jelly to the patient's lips. Promote healing with warm saline gargles or throat irrigations for 24 to 36 hours after incision and drainage. Encourage adequate rest.

▓ **PREVENTION** *Encourage early treatment of tonsillitis.*

VOCAL CORD PARALYSIS
Vocal cord paralysis results from disease of, or injury to, the superior or, most commonly, the recurrent laryngeal nerve. It may also be congenital.

Causes and incidence

Vocal cord paralysis commonly results from the accidental severing of the recurrent laryngeal nerve, or of one of its extralaryngeal branches, during thyroidectomy. Other causes include pressure from a thoracic aortic aneurysm or from an enlarged atrium (in patients with mitral stenosis), bronchial or esophageal carcinoma, hypertrophy of the thyroid gland, trauma (such as neck injuries) and intubation, and neuritis due to infections or metallic poisoning. Vocal cord paralysis can also result from hysteria and, rarely, lesions of the central nervous system.

Pathophysiology

Unilateral vocal fold paralysis occurs from a dysfunction of the recurrent laryngeal or vagus nerve innervating the larynx. It causes a characteristic breathy voice often accompanied by swallowing disability, a weak cough, and the sensation of shortness of breath. This is a common cause of neurogenic hoarseness.

Complications

- ◆ Airway obstruction
- ◆ Respiratory failure

Signs and symptoms

Unilateral paralysis, the most common form, may cause vocal weakness and hoarseness. Bilateral paralysis typically produces vocal weakness and incapacitating airway obstruction if the cords become paralyzed in the adducted position.

PEDIATRIC TIP *Children may present with hoarseness, aspiration, and stridor. If the paralysis is unilateral, it typically involves the left recurrent laryngeal nerve. In unilateral paralysis, airway intervention involving intubation and tracheostomy is rarely indicated; it's usually required if the paralysis is bilateral.*

Diagnosis

The patient history and characteristic features suggest vocal cord paralysis.

CONFIRMING DIAGNOSIS *Visualization by indirect laryngoscopy shows one or both cords fixed in an adducted or partially abducted position and confirms the diagnosis.*

X-ray or CT scan detect abnormalities in the mediastinum that may be responsible for the injury.

Treatment

Treatment for unilateral vocal cord paralysis consists of injection of Teflon into the paralyzed cord, under direct laryngoscopy. This procedure enlarges the cord and brings it closer to the other cord, which usually strengthens the voice and protects the airway from aspiration. Thyroplasty also serves to reposition the vocal cord, but in this procedure an implant is placed through a neck incision. The ansa cervicalis nerve transfer allows for reinnervation of the muscles of the vocal cord. Bilateral cord paralysis in an adducted position necessitates a tracheostomy.

Alternative treatments for adults include endoscopic arytenoidectomy to open the glottis, and lateral fixation of the arytenoid cartilage through an external neck incision. Excision or fixation of the arytenoid cartilage improves airway patency but produces residual voice impairment.

Treatment for hysterical aphonia may include psychotherapy and hypnosis.

Special considerations

If the patient chooses direct laryngoscopy and Teflon injection, explain these procedures thoroughly. Tell the patient these measures will improve their voice but won't restore it to normal. Patients are sometimes placed on voice rest for 24 to 48 hours to reduce stress on the vocal cords, which would increase the edema and might lead to airway obstruction.

Many patients with bilateral cord paralysis prefer to keep a tracheostomy instead of having an arytenoidectomy; voice quality is generally better with a tracheostomy alone than after corrective surgery.

If the patient is scheduled to undergo a tracheostomy:

- ◆ Explain the procedure thoroughly, and offer reassurance. Because the procedure is performed under a local anesthetic, the patient may be apprehensive.
- ◆ Teach the patient how to suction, clean, and change the tracheostomy tube.
- ◆ Reassure the patient that they can still speak by covering the lumen of the tracheostomy tube with a finger or a tracheostomy plug.

If the patient elects to have an arytenoidectomy, explain the procedure thoroughly. Advise the patient that the tracheostomy will remain in place until the edema has subsided and the airway is patent.

VOCAL CORD NODULES AND POLYPS

Vocal cord nodules result from hypertrophy of fibrous tissue and form at the point where the cords come together forcibly. Vocal cord polyps are chronic, subepithelial, edematous masses. Both nodules and polyps have a good prognosis unless continued voice abuse causes recurrence, with subsequent scarring and permanent hoarseness.

Causes and incidence

Vocal cord nodules and polyps usually result from voice abuse, especially in the presence of infection. Consequently, they're most common in teachers, singers, and sports fans, and in energetic children (ages 8 to 12) who continually shout while playing. Polyps are common in adults who smoke, live in dry climates, or have allergies.

🎐 **PEDIATRIC TIP** *In children, papillomas of the larynx (benign warty growths) are the most common laryngeal neoplasm. Suspected causes include human papillomavirus types 6, 11, and 16. The virus may be acquired during birth because many mothers have a history of condylomata acuminata at the time of delivery.*

Complication

◆ Permanent hoarseness

Signs and symptoms

Nodules and polyps inhibit the approximation of vocal cords and produce painless hoarseness. The voice may also develop a breathy or husky quality.

Diagnosis

Persistent hoarseness suggests vocal cord nodules and polyps; visualization by indirect laryngoscopy confirms it. In the patient with vocal cord nodules, laryngoscopy initially shows small red nodes and, later, white solid nodes on one or both cords. (See *Vocal cord nodules.*) In the patient with polyps, laryngoscopy reveals unilateral or, occasionally, bilateral, sessile or pedunculated polyps of varying size, anywhere on the vocal cords.

Treatment

Conservative management of small vocal cord nodules and polyps includes humidification, speech therapy (voice rest, training to reduce the intensity and duration of voice production), and treatment for any underlying allergies.

When conservative treatment fails to relieve hoarseness, nodules or polyps require removal under direct laryngoscopy. Microlaryngoscopy may be done for small lesions, to avoid injuring the vocal cord surface. If nodules or polyps are bilateral, excision may be performed in two stages: one cord is allowed to heal before excision of polyps on the other cord. Two-stage excision prevents laryngeal web, which occurs when epithelial tissue is removed from adjacent cord surfaces, and these surfaces grow together.

🎐 **PEDIATRIC TIP** *For children, treatment consists of speech therapy. If possible, surgery should be delayed until the child is old enough to benefit from voice training, or until the patient can understand the need to abstain from voice abuse.*

Special considerations

◆ Postoperatively, stress the importance of resting the voice for 10 to 14 days while the vocal cords heal. Provide an alternative means of communication—Magic Slate, pad and pencil, or alphabet board. Place a sign over the bed to

---

Vocal cord nodules

The most common site of vocal cord nodules is the point of maximal vibration and impact (junction of the anterior one third and the posterior two thirds of the vocal cord).

VOCAL CORDS OPEN

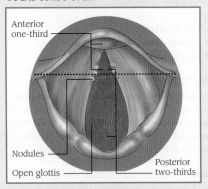

Anterior one-third

Nodules

Open glottis

Posterior two-thirds

Vocal cord nodules affect the voice by inhibiting proper closure of the vocal cords during phonation.

VOCAL CORDS CLOSED

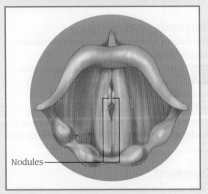

Nodules

remind visitors that the patient shouldn't talk. Mark the intercom so other facility personnel are aware that the patient can't answer. Minimize the need to speak by trying to anticipate the patient's needs.

◆ If the patient is a smoker, encourage them to stop smoking entirely or, at the very least, to refrain from smoking during recovery from surgery.

◆ Use a vaporizer to increase humidity and decrease throat irritation.

◆ Make sure the patient receives speech therapy after healing if necessary, because continued voice abuse causes recurrence of growths.

LARYNGITIS

A common disorder, laryngitis is an acute or chronic inflammation of the vocal cords. Acute laryngitis may occur as an isolated infection or as part of a generalized bacterial or viral URTI. Repeated attacks of acute laryngitis produce inflammatory changes associated with chronic laryngitis.

ALERT *Several forms of laryngitis occur in children and can lead to significant or fatal respiratory obstruction, such as croup and epiglottitis.*

Causes and incidence

Acute laryngitis usually results from infection (primarily viral) or excessive use of the voice, an occupational hazard in certain vocations (e.g., teaching, public speaking, or singing). It may also result from leisure activities (such as cheering at a sports event), inhalation of smoke or fumes, or aspiration of caustic chemicals. Chronic laryngitis may be caused by chronic upper respiratory tract disorders (sinusitis, bronchitis, nasal polyps, or allergy), mouth breathing, smoking, constant exposure to dust or other irritants, and alcohol abuse.

Pathophysiology

Acute laryngitis is an inflammation of the vocal fold mucosa and larynx that lasts less than 3 weeks. When the etiology of acute laryngitis is infectious, white blood cells remove microorganisms during the healing process. The vocal folds then become more edematous, and vibration is adversely affected.

Complications

◆ Permanent hoarseness
◆ Airway obstruction in severe laryngitis

Signs and symptoms

Acute laryngitis typically begins with hoarseness, ranging from mild to complete loss of voice. Associated clinical features include pain (especially when swallowing or speaking), a persistent dry cough, fever, laryngeal edema, and malaise. In chronic laryngitis, persistent hoarseness is usually the only symptom.

Diagnosis

CONFIRMING DIAGNOSIS *Indirect laryngoscopy confirms the diagnosis by revealing red, inflamed, and, occasionally, hemorrhagic vocal cords, with rounded rather than sharp edges and exudate. Bilateral swelling may be present.*

In severe cases or if toxicity is a concern, a culture of the exudate is obtained. Consider 24-hour pH probe testing in chronic laryngitis and GERD. Also consider biopsy in chronic laryngitis in an adult with a history of smoking or alcohol abuse.

Treatment

Primary treatment consists of resting the voice. For viral infection, symptomatic care includes analgesics and throat lozenges for pain relief. Bacterial infection requires antibiotic therapy. Severe, acute laryngitis may necessitate hospitalization. When laryngeal edema results in airway obstruction, a tracheostomy may be necessary. In chronic laryngitis, effective treatment must eliminate the underlying cause. Antacids or histamine-2 blockers may be used if GERD is the cause. Steam inhalation may also prove beneficial as are smoking cessation, reducing alcohol intake, and job change or modification if warranted.

Special considerations

◆ Explain to the patient why they shouldn't talk, and place a sign over the bed to remind others of this restriction. Provide a Magic Slate or a pad and pencil for communication. Mark the intercom panel so other facility personnel are aware that the patient can't answer. Minimize the need to talk by trying to anticipate the patient's needs.

◆ For the patient with a bacterial infection, stress the importance of completing the full course of antibiotic therapy.

◆ Suggest that the patient maintain adequate humidification by using a vaporizer or humidifier during the winter, by avoiding air-conditioning during the summer (because it dehumidifies), by using medicated throat lozenges, and by not smoking.

◆ Obtain a detailed patient history to help determine the cause of chronic laryngitis. Encourage the patient to modify predisposing habits, especially to stop smoking.

◆ Provide the patient with assistance for smoking cessation as well as for modification of other predisposing habits or occupational hazards.

JUVENILE ANGIOFIBROMA

An uncommon disorder, juvenile angiofibroma is a highly vascular, nasopharyngeal tumor made up of masses of fibrous tissue that contain many thin-walled blood vessels. The prognosis is good with treatment.

Causes and incidence

A type of hemangioma, this tumor grows on one side of the posterior nares and may completely fill the nasopharynx, nose, paranasal sinuses, and, possibly, the orbit. More commonly sessile than polypoid, juvenile angiofibroma is nonencapsulated; it invades surrounding tissue.

Juvenile angiofibroma is typically found in adolescent males and is extremely rare in females. It's associated with nasal obstruction and epistaxis.

Pathophysiology

JNA is a rare benign tumor arising predominantly in the nasopharynx of adolescent males. It is an aggressive neoplasm and shows a propensity for destructive local spread often extending to the base of the skull and into the cranium. Clinically, however, it is obscure with painless, progressive unilateral nasal obstruction being the common presenting symptom with or without epistaxis and rhinorrhea. Diagnosis of JNA is made by complete history, clinical examination, radiography, nasal endoscopy and by using specialized imaging techniques such as arteriography, CT, and magnetic resonance imaging. Early diagnosis, accurate staging, and adequate treatment are essential in the management of this lesion.

Complication

◆ Secondary anemia

Signs and symptoms

Juvenile angiofibroma produces unilateral or bilateral nasal obstruction and severe recurrent epistaxis, usually between ages 7 and 21. Recurrent epistaxis eventually causes secondary anemia. Associated effects include purulent rhinorrhea, facial deformity, and nasal speech. Serous otitis media and hearing loss may result from eustachian tube obstruction.

Diagnosis

A nasopharyngeal mirror or nasal speculum permits visualization of the tumor. X-rays show a bowing of the posterior wall of the maxillary sinus. Three-plane magnetic resonance imaging and CT scans determine the extent of the tumors, which are seldom limited to the nasopharynx. Angiography determines the size and location of the tumor and shows the source of vascularization.

 ALERT *Tumor biopsy is contraindicated because of the risk of hemorrhage.*

Treatment

Surgical procedures range from avulsion to cryosurgical techniques. Surgical excision is preferred after embolization with Teflon or an absorbable gelatin sponge to decrease vascularization. Whichever surgical method is used, this tumor must be removed in its entirety and not in pieces.

Preoperative hormonal therapy may decrease the tumor's size and vascularity. Blood transfusions may be necessary during avulsion. Radiation therapy produces only a temporary regression in an angiofibroma but is the treatment of choice if the tumor has expanded into the cranium or orbit. Because the tumor is multilobular and locally invasive, it recurs in about 30% of patients during the first year after treatment, but rarely after 2 years.

Special considerations

◆ Explain all diagnostic and surgical procedures. Provide emotional support; severe epistaxis frightens many people to the point of panic. Monitor hemoglobin levels and HCT for anemia.
◆ After surgery, immediately report excessive bleeding. Make sure an adequate supply of typed and crossmatched blood is available for transfusion.
◆ Monitor for any change in vital signs. Provide good oral hygiene, and use a bedside vaporizer to raise humidity.
◆ During blood transfusion, watch for transfusion reactions, such as fever, pruritus, chills, or a rash. If any of these reactions occur, discontinue the blood transfusion and notify the physician immediately.
◆ Teach the patient's family how to apply pressure over the affected area, and instruct them to seek immediate medical attention if bleeding occurs after discharge. Stress the importance of providing adequate humidification at home to keep the nasal mucosa moist.

SELECTED REFERENCES

Guideline on acute otitis media published by NICE. (2018). *Guidelines in Practice, 21*(4), 6.

Heining, C., et al. (2017). Audiological outcome of stapes surgery for far advanced cochlear otosclerosis. *Journal of Laryngology and Otology, 131*(11), 961–964. doi:10.1017/S0022215117001815

Loh, R., et al. (2018). Management of paediatric acute mastoiditis: Systematic review. *Journal of Laryngology and Otology, 132*(2), 96–104. doi:10.1017/S0022215117001840

Rosenfeld, R. M. (2016). Clinical practice. Acute sinusitis in adults. *New England Journal of Medicine, 375*(10), 962–970. doi:10.1056/NEJMcp1601749

14

SKIN DISORDERS

Introduction

Skin is the body's front-line protective barrier between internal structures and the external environment. It's tough, resilient, and virtually impermeable to aqueous solutions, bacteria, or toxic compounds. It also performs many vital functions. Skin protects against trauma, regulates body temperature, serves as an organ of excretion and sensation, and synthesizes vitamin D in the presence of ultraviolet (UV) light. Skin varies in thickness and other qualities from one part of the body to another, which often accounts for the distribution of skin diseases.

Skin has three primary layers: epidermis, dermis, and subcutaneous tissue. The epidermis (the outermost layer) produces keratin as its primary function. This layer is generally thin but is thicker in areas subject to constant pressure or friction, such as the soles and palms. The epidermis contains two sublayers: the stratum corneum, an outer horny layer of keratin that protects the body against harmful environmental substances and restricts water loss, and the cellular stratum, where keratin cells are synthesized. The basement membrane lies beneath the cellular stratum and serves to attach the epidermis to the dermis.

The cellular stratum, the deepest layer of the epidermis, consists of the basal layer, where mitosis takes place; the stratum spinosum, where cells begin to flatten, and fibrils—precursors of keratin—start to appear; and the stratum granulosum, made up of cells containing deeply staining granules of keratohyalin, which are generally thought to become the keratin that forms the stratum corneum. A skin cell moves from the basal layer of the cellular stratum to the stratum corneum in about 14 days. After another 14 days, normal wear and tear on the skin causes it to slough off. The epidermis also contains melanocytes, which produce the melanin that gives the skin its color, and Langerhans cells, which are involved in a variety of immunologic reactions.

The dermis, the second primary layer of the skin, consists of two fibrous proteins, fibroblasts, and an intervening ground substance. The proteins are collagen, which strengthens the skin to prevent it from tearing, and elastin to give it resilience. The ground substance, which makes the skin soft and compressible, contains primarily jellylike mucopolysaccharides. Two distinct layers constitute the dermis: the papillary dermis (top layer) and the reticular dermis (bottom layer).

Subcutaneous tissue, the third primary layer of the skin, consists mainly of fat (containing mostly triglycerides), which provides heat, insulation, shock absorption, and a reserve of calories. Both sensory and motor nerves (autonomic fibers) are found in the dermis and the subcutaneous tissue.

NAILS, GLANDS, AND HAIR

Nails are epidermal cells converted to hard keratin. The bed on which the nail rests is highly vascular, making the nail appear pink; the whitish, crescent-shaped area extending beyond the proximal nail fold, called the *lunula*—most visible in the thumbnail—marks the end of the matrix, the site of mitosis and of nail growth.

Sebaceous glands, found everywhere on the body (but mostly on the face and scalp) except the palms and soles, serve as appendages of the dermis. These glands generally excrete sebum into hair follicles, but in some cases, they empty directly onto the skin surface. Sebum is an oily substance that helps keep the skin and hair from drying out and prevents water and heat loss. Sebaceous glands abound on the scalp, forehead, cheeks, chin, back, and genitalia and may be stimulated by sex hormones—primarily testosterone.

The dermis and subcutaneous tissue contain eccrine and apocrine glands and hair. Eccrine sweat glands open directly onto the skin and regulate body temperature. Innervated by sympathetic nerves, these sweat glands are distributed throughout the body, except for the lips, ears, and parts of the genitalia. They secrete a hypertonic solution made up mostly of water and sodium chloride; the prime stimulus for eccrine gland secretion is heat. Other stimuli include muscular exertion and emotional stress.

Apocrine sweat glands appear chiefly in the axillae and genitalia; they're responsible for producing body odor and are stimulated by emotional stress. The sweat produced is sterile but undergoes bacterial decomposition on the skin surface. These glands become functional after puberty. (Ceruminous glands, located in the external ear canal, appear to be modified sweat glands and secrete a waxy substance known as *cerumen*.)

Hair grows on most of the body, except for the palms, the soles, and parts of the genitalia. An individual hair consists of a shaft (a column of keratinized cells), a root (embedded in the dermis), the hair follicle (the root and its covering), and the hair papilla (a loop of capillaries at the base of the follicle). Mitosis at the base of the follicle causes the hair to grow; the papilla provides nourishment for mitosis. Small bundles of involuntary muscles known as *arrectores pilorum* cling to hair follicles. When these muscles contract, usually during moments of cold, fear, or shock, the hairs stand on end, and the person is said to have goose bumps or gooseflesh. Melanocytes in the matrix (inner core) of the hair bulb produce melanin, which passes into the innermost layers of the hair and is responsible for hair color. Dark hair contains mostly true melanin. Blond and red hair contains variants of melanin that have iron and more sulfur. Gray hair results from pigment loss because of a decline of tyrosinase, which is required for melanin synthesis. White hair occurs when air bubbles accumulate in the center of the hair shaft.

VASCULAR INFLUENCE

The skin is served by a vast arteriovenous network, extending from subcutaneous tissue to the dermis. These blood vessels provide oxygen and nutrients to sensory nerves (which control touch, temperature, and pain), motor nerves (which control the activities of sweat glands, the arterioles, and smooth muscles of the skin), and skin appendages. Blood flow also influences skin coloring because the amount of oxygen carried to capillaries in the dermis can produce transient changes in color. For example, decreased oxygen supply can turn the skin pale or bluish; increased oxygen can turn it pink or ruddy.

ASSESSING SKIN DISORDERS

Assessment begins with a thorough patient history to determine whether a skin disorder is an acute flare-up, a recurrent problem, or a chronic condition. Ask the patient how long they have had the disorder; how a typical flare-up or attack begins; whether or not it itches; and what medications—systemic or topical—have been used to treat it. Also, find out if any family members, friends, or contacts have the same disorder, and if they live or work in an environment that could cause the condition. Also ask about hobbies.

When examining a patient with a skin disorder, be sure to look everywhere—mucous membranes, hair, scalp, axillae, groin, palms, soles, and nails. Note moisture, temperature, texture, thickness, mobility, edema, turgor, and any irregularities in skin color. Look for skin lesions; if you find a lesion, record its color, shape, size, and location. (See *Differentiating among skin lesions*.) Try to determine which is the primary lesion—the one that appeared first—which always starts in normal skin. The patient might be able to point it out.

If more than one lesion is in evidence, note the pattern of distribution. Lesions can be localized (isolated), regional, general, or universal (total), involving the entire skin, hair, and nails. Also, observe whether the lesions are unilateral or bilateral and symmetrical or asymmetrical; also note the arrangement of the lesions (clustered or linear configuration, for example).

DIAGNOSTIC AIDS

After simple observation, and examination of the affected area of the skin with a dermatoscope for morphologic detail, the following clinical diagnostic techniques may help to identify skin disorders:

Differentiating among skin lesions

The illustrations below depict the most common primary and secondary skin lesions.

Primary lesions

Bulla: Fluid-filled lesions more than 2 cm in diameter (also called blister), as occurs in severe poison oak or ivy dermatitis, bullous pemphigoid, and second-degree burns

Comedo: Plugged, exfoliative pilosebaceous duct formed from sebum and keratin—for example, blackhead (open comedo) and whitehead (closed comedo)

Cyst: Semisolid or fluid-filled encapsulated mass extending deep into dermis—for example, acne

Macule: Flat, pigmented, circumscribed area less than 1 cm in diameter—for example, freckle or rash that occurs in rubella

Nodule: Firm, raised lesion, 0.5 to 2 cm in diameter, that's deeper than a papule and extends into dermal layer—for example, intradermal nevus

Papule: Firm, inflammatory raised lesion up to 0.5 cm in diameter that may be the same color as skin or pigmented—for example, acne papule and lichen planus

Patch: Flat, pigmented, circumscribed area more than 1 cm in diameter—for example, herald patch (pityriasis rosea)

Plaque: Circumscribed, solid, elevated lesion more than 1 cm in diameter that is elevated above skin surface and occupies larger surface area in comparison with height, as occurs in psoriasis.

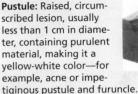

Pustule: Raised, circumscribed lesion, usually less than 1 cm in diameter, containing purulent material, making it a yellow-white color—for example, acne or impetiginous pustule and furuncle.

Tumor: Elevated, solid lesion larger than 2 cm in diameter that extends into dermal and subcutaneous layers—for example, dermatofibroma.

Vesicle: Raised, circumscribed, fluid-filled lesion less than 0.5 cm in diameter, as occurs in chickenpox or herpes simplex infection.

Wheal: Raised, firm lesion with intense localized skin edema that varies in size, shape, and color (from pale pink to red) and that disappears in hours—for example, hives and insect bites.

Secondary lesions

Atrophy: Thinning of skin surface at site of disorder—for example, striae and aging skin.

Crust: Dried sebum or serous, sanguineous, or purulent exudate, overlying an erosion or a weeping vesicle, bulla, or pustule, as occurs in impetigo.

(continued)

Differentiating among skin lesions (continued)

Erosion: Circumscribed lesion that involves loss of superficial epidermis—for example, abrasion.

Scale: Thin, dry flakes of shedding skin, as occurs in psoriasis, dry skin, or neonatal desquamation.

Excoriation: Linear scratched or abraded areas, often self-induced—for example, abraded acne lesions or eczema.

Scar: Fibrous tissue caused by trauma, deep inflammation, or surgical incision, which can be red and raised (recent) pink and flat (6 weeks), or pale and depressed (old)—for example, a healed surgical incision.

Fissure: Linear cracking of the skin that extends into the dermal layer—for example, hand dermatitis (chapped skin).

Ulcer: Epidermal and dermal destruction that may extend into subcutaneous tissue and that usually heals with scarring—for example, pressure ulcer or stasis ulcer.

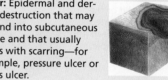

Lichenification: Thickened, prominent skin markings caused by constant rubbing, as occurs in chronic dermatitis.

♦ Biopsy determines histology of cells and may be diagnostic, confirmatory, or inconclusive, depending on the disease.

♦ Diascopy, in which a lesion is covered with a microscopic slide or piece of clear plastic, helps determine whether dilated capillaries or extravasated blood is causing the redness of a lesion.

♦ Gram stains and exudate cultures help identify the organism responsible for an underlying infection.

♦ Microscopic immunofluorescence identifies immunoglobulins and elastic tissue in detecting skin manifestations of immunologically mediated disease.

♦ Patch tests identify contact sensitivity (usually with dermatitis).

♦ Potassium hydroxide preparations permit examination for mycelia in fungal infections.

♦ Side-lighting shows minor elevations or depressions in lesions; it also helps determine the configuration and degree of eruption.

♦ Subdued lighting highlights the difference between normal skin and circumscribed lesions that are hypopigmented or hyperpigmented.

♦ Wood's light examination reveals yellow, green, or blue-green fluorescence when an area is infected with certain dermatophytes (fungi).

SPECIAL CONSIDERATIONS

When assessing a skin disorder, keep in mind its distressing social and psychological implications. Unlike internal disorders, such as cardiac disease or diabetes mellitus, a skin condition is usually obvious and disfiguring. Understandably, the psychological implications are most acute when skin disorders affect the face—especially during adolescence, an emotionally turbulent time of life. However, such disorders can also create tremendous psychological problems for adults. A skin disease usually interferes with a person's ability to work because the condition affects the hands or because it distresses the patient to such an extent that they can't function.

For these reasons, be empathetic and accepting. Above all, don't be afraid to touch such a patient; most skin disorders aren't contagious. Touching the patient naturally and without hesitation helps show your acceptance of the dermatologic condition. Such acceptance is no less important than your patient teaching about the disease and your guidance and help with carrying out prescribed treatment.

Bacterial infections

IMPETIGO

A contagious, superficial skin infection, impetigo occurs in nonbullous and bullous forms. This vesiculopustular eruptive disorder spreads most easily among infants, young children, and elderly people. Predisposing factors, such as poor hygiene, anemia, malnutrition, and a warm climate, favor outbreaks of this infection, most of which occur during the late summer and early fall. Impetigo can complicate chickenpox, eczema, or other skin conditions marked by open lesions.

Causes and incidence

Coagulase-positive *Staphylococcus aureus* and, less commonly, group A beta-hemolytic streptococci usually produce nonbullous impetigo; *S. aureus* (especially phage type 71) generally causes bullous impetigo.

In the United States, impetigo occurs most often in southern states. It often causes deeper dermal inflammation in persons of color, such as Hispanics, African Americans, and Asians, and may result in postinflammatory hypopigmentation or hyperpigmentation.

Pathophysiology

Disruption of the skin barrier by injury or other skin conditions allows the invasion of *S. aureus*, most commonly around mouth and nose. Bacterial toxins cause loss of cell adhesion in the epidermis leading to blisters and lesions in a localized area.

Complications

◆ Ecthyma
◆ Glomerulonephritis
◆ Permanent scarring

Signs and symptoms

Common nonbullous impetigo typically begins with a small red macule that turns into a vesicle or pustule. When the vesicle breaks, a thick yellow crust forms from the exudate. (See *Recognizing impetigo*.) Autoinoculation may cause satellite lesions. Although it can occur anywhere, impetigo usually occurs around the mouth and nose and on the knees and elbows. Other features include pruritus, burning, and regional lymphadenopathy.

Recognizing impetigo

In impetigo, when the vesicles break, crust forms from the exudate. This infection is especially contagious among young children.

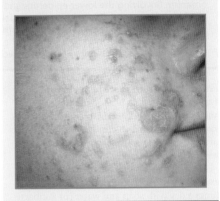

A rare but serious complication of streptococcal impetigo is glomerulonephritis, which is more likely to occur when many members of the same family have impetigo.

🛏 **PEDIATRIC TIP** *Infants and young children may develop aural impetigo or otitis externa; the lesions usually clear without treatment in 2 to 3 weeks, unless an underlying disorder such as eczema is present. Scarlet fever also may occur.*

In bullous impetigo, a thin-walled vesicle opens, and a thin, clear crust forms from the exudate. The lesion consists of a central clearing, circumscribed by an outer ring—much like a ringworm lesion—and commonly appears on the face or other exposed areas. Both forms usually produce painless itching; they may appear simultaneously and be clinically indistinguishable.

Ecthyma is a skin infection that resembles impetigo but extends into the dermis and takes longer to resolve. These lesions are painful and more common on distal extremities. (See *Ecthyma,* page 666.)

Diagnosis

Culture and sensitivity testing of fluid or denuded skin may indicate the most appropriate antibiotic, but therapy shouldn't be delayed for laboratory results, which can take 3 days. White blood cell count may be elevated in the presence of infection.

Treatment

Topical mupirocin and retapamulin are the treatments of choice if the lesions aren't too

Ecthyma

Ecthyma is a superficial skin infection that usually causes scarring. It commonly occurs in persons with poor hygiene or in those living in crowded conditions and generally results from infection by *S. aureus* or group A beta-hemolytic streptococci. Ecthyma differs from impetigo in that its characteristic ulcer results from deeper penetration of the skin by the infecting organism (involving the lower epidermis and dermis), and the overlying crust tends to be piled high (1 to 3 cm). These lesions are usually found on the legs after a scratch or bug bite. Autoinoculation can transmit ecthyma to other parts of the body, especially to sites that have been scratched open. Therapy is basically the same as for impetigo, but response may be slower. Parenteral antibiotics (usually a penicillinase-resistant penicillin) are also used.

extensive. These drugs are highly effective against group A beta-hemolytic streptococci and *S. aureus*, including methicillin-resistant *S. aureus*. Mupirocin also eliminates nasal carriers of these organisms. Extensive or nonresolving lesions require systemic antibiotics.

Therapy may also include removal of the exudate by washing the lesions two or three times a day with soap and water (or antibacterial soap) or, for stubborn crusts, warm soaks or compresses of normal saline or a diluted soap solution.

Special consideration

◆ Urge the patient not to scratch, because this spreads impetigo.

PEDIATRIC TIP *Advise parents to cut their child's fingernails and cover hands with socks or mittens to prevent scratching.*

◆ Give medications as indicated. Remember to check for medication allergy. Stress the need to continue prescribed medications for 7 to 10 days, even after lesions have healed.

◆ Teach the patient and family how to care for impetiginous lesions.

PREVENTION
◆ *To prevent further spread of this highly contagious infection, encourage frequent bathing using a bactericidal soap. Tell the patient not to share towels, washcloths, or bed linens with family members. Emphasize the importance of following proper hand-washing technique.*
◆ *Check family members for impetigo. If this infection is present in a school-age child, notify their school.*

FOLLICULITIS, FURUNCULOSIS, AND CARBUNCULOSIS

Folliculitis is a bacterial infection of the hair follicle that causes the formation of a pustule. The infection can be superficial (follicular impetigo or Bockhart's impetigo) or deep (sycosis barbae). Folliculitis may also lead to the development of furuncles (furunculosis), commonly known as *boils*, or carbuncles (carbunculosis), which involve multiple contiguous hair follicles. The prognosis depends on the severity of the infection and on the patient's physical condition and ability to resist infection.

Causes and incidence

The most common cause of folliculitis, furunculosis, or carbunculosis is coagulase-positive *S. aureus*. Predisposing factors include an infected wound, poor hygiene, debilitation, diabetes, alcoholism, occlusive cosmetics, tight clothes, friction, chafing, exposure to chemicals, and treatment for skin lesions with tar or with occlusive therapy, using steroids. Furunculosis often follows folliculitis exacerbated by irritation, pressure, friction, or perspiration. Carbunculosis follows persistent *S. aureus* infection and furunculosis.

Pathophysiology

The infectious agent, typically *S. aureus*, invades the hair follicle creating an inflammatory response. The inflammation obstructs the hair follicle causing a papulopustular area. A furuncle has the same pathogenesis but is a deeper infection creating a pustular nodule around a hair follicle and a carbuncle is the infection of multiple contiguous hair follicles.

Complications

◆ Cellulitis
◆ Septicemia
◆ Scarring

Signs and symptoms

Pustules of folliculitis usually appear in a hair follicle on the scalp, arms, and legs in children; on the face of bearded men (sycosis barbae); and on the eyelids (styes). Deep folliculitis may be painful.

Folliculitis may progress to the hard, painful nodules of furunculosis, which commonly develop on the neck, face, axillae, and buttocks. For several days these nodules enlarge, and then

Follicular skin infections

Degree of hair follicle involvement in bacterial skin infection ranges from superficial erythema and pustule of a single follicle to deep abscesses (carbuncles) involving several follicles.

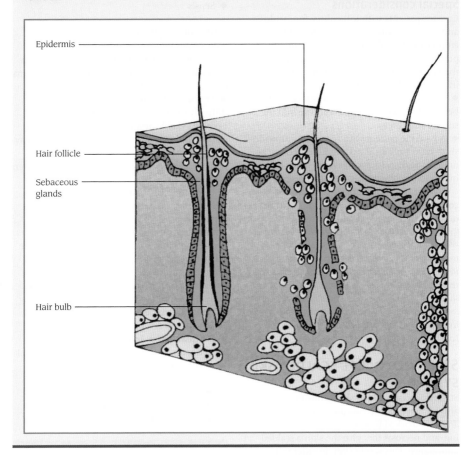

Epidermis

Hair follicle

Sebaceous glands

Hair bulb

rupture, discharging pus and necrotic material. After the nodules rupture, pain subsides, but erythema and edema may persist for days or weeks.

Carbunculosis is marked by extremely painful, deep abscesses that drain through multiple openings onto the skin surface, usually around several hair follicles. Fever and malaise may accompany these lesions. (See *Follicular skin infections*.)

Diagnosis

CONFIRMING DIAGNOSIS *The obvious skin lesion confirms folliculitis, furunculosis, or carbunculosis. Wound culture shows S. aureus; sensitivity will help guide antibiotic therapy.*

In carbunculosis, patient history reveals preexistent furunculosis. A complete blood count may reveal an elevated white blood cell count (leukocytosis).

Treatment

Treatment for folliculitis consists of cleaning the infected area thoroughly with antibacterial soap and water; applying warm, wet compresses to promote vasodilation and drainage from the lesions; topical antibiotics such as mupirocin ointment and, in extensive infection or if a furuncle or carbuncle has developed, systemic antibiotics. Use sensitivity results to guide therapy but begin treatment before receiving results.

Furunculosis and carbunculosis may also require incision and drainage of ripe lesions if the lesions don't drain after the application of warm, wet compresses. They may also require topical antibiotics after drainage.

Special considerations

Care for patients with folliculitis, furunculosis, and carbunculosis is basically supportive and emphasizes teaching the patient scrupulous personal and family hygiene measures. Taking the necessary precautions to prevent spreading infection is also an important part of care.

◆ Caution the patient never to squeeze a boil because this may cause it to rupture into the surrounding area.

◆ Advise the patient with recurrent furunculosis to have a physical examination because an underlying disease, such as diabetes or human immunodeficiency virus, may be present.

Trauma resulting from such hairstyles as cornrowing (gathering the hair into tight braids or tufts) can cause folliculitis.

▦ PREVENTION *To avoid spreading bacteria to family members, urge the patient not to share towels and washcloths. Tell the patient that these items should be laundered in hot water before being reused. The patient should change clothes and bedsheets daily, and these also should be washed in hot water. Encourage the patient to change dressings frequently and to discard them promptly in paper bags.*

STAPHYLOCOCCAL SCALDED SKIN SYNDROME

Staphylococcal scalded skin syndrome (SSSS), also known as *Ritter's disease* or *Ritter–Lyell syndrome,* is marked by epidermal erythema, peeling, and necrosis that give the skin a scalded appearance. This severe skin disorder follows a consistent pattern of progression, and most patients recover fully. Mortality is 2% to 3%.

Causes and incidence

The causative organism in SSSS is group 2 *S. aureus,* primarily phage type 71, which produces exotoxins that cause detachment of the epidermis. Predisposing factors may include impaired immunity and renal insufficiency—present to some extent in the normal neonate because of immature development of these systems.

SSSS is most prevalent in infants aged 1 to 3 months but may develop in children. It's uncommon in adults.

Pathophysiology

The bacteria, *S. aureus,* invades the skin releasing an exfoliative toxin. Initially, the toxin causes a red rash then progresses to the separation of the epidermis beneath the granular cell layer.

Complications

◆ Fluid and electrolyte loss
◆ Sepsis

Signs and symptoms

SSSS can usually be traced to a prodromal upper respiratory tract infection, possibly with concomitant purulent conjunctivitis. Cutaneous changes progress through three stages:

◆ Erythema: Erythema, which may begin diffusely or as a scarlatiniform rash, usually becomes visible around the mouth and other orifices and may spread in widening circles over the entire body surface. The skin becomes tender; Nikolsky's sign (sloughing of the skin when friction is applied) may appear.

◆ Exfoliation (24 to 48 hours later): In the more common, localized form of this disease, superficial erosions with a red, moist base and minimal crusting occur, generally around body orifices, and may spread to exposed areas of the skin. (See *Identifying SSSS.*) In the more severe forms of this disease, large, flaccid bullae erupt and may spread to cover extensive areas of the body. These bullae eventually rupture, revealing sections of denuded skin; mucous membranes are spared.

◆ Desquamation: In this final stage, affected areas dry up, and powdery scales form. Normal skin replaces these scales in 5 to 7 days.

Diagnosis

Diagnosis requires careful observation of the three-stage progression of this disease.

Identifying SSSS

SSSS is a severe skin disorder that commonly affects infants and children. The photo below shows the typical scalded skin appearance, with areas of denuded skin, found in an infant.

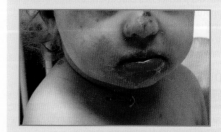

Results of exfoliative cytology and biopsy aid in differential diagnosis, ruling out erythema multiforme and drug-induced toxic epidermal necrolysis (TEN), both of which resemble SSSS. Sometimes it is mistaken for a possible sign of child abuse because of its similar appearance to scald-type burns.

℞ **CONFIRMING DIAGNOSIS** *Isolation of group 2 S. aureus on cultures of skin lesions confirms the diagnosis. However, skin lesions sometimes appear sterile.*

Treatment

Treatment includes systemic antibiotics, usually penicillinase-resistant penicillin. Severe cases require hospitalization and I.V. antibiotics. Oral antibiotics should be adequate for milder cases. Skin lubrication with a non–alcohol-based preparation is beneficial. Washing or bathing should be done sparingly. Replacement measures to maintain fluid and electrolyte balance are necessary.

PEDIATRIC TIP *Hospital admission is appropriate for neonates and young children with extensive sloughing.*

Special considerations

◆ Carefully monitor intake and output to assess fluid and electrolyte balance. In severe cases, I.V. fluid replacement may be necessary.
◆ Check vital signs. Be especially alert for a sudden rise in temperature, indicating sepsis, which requires prompt, aggressive treatment.
◆ Maintain skin integrity. Use strict sterile technique to preclude secondary infection, especially during the exfoliative stage, because of open lesions. To prevent friction and sloughing of the skin, leave affected areas uncovered or loosely covered. Place cotton between severely affected fingers and toes to prevent webbing.
◆ Gently debride exfoliated areas, especially those that have become necrotic.
◆ Reassure the parents that complications are rare and residual scars are unlikely.

PEDIATRIC TIP *Provide special care for the neonate, if required, including placement in a warming infant incubator to maintain body temperature and provide isolation.*

Fungal infections

TINEA VERSICOLOR

A chronic, superficial, fungal infection, tinea versicolor (also known as *pityriasis versicolor*) may produce a multicolored rash, commonly on the upper trunk. Recurrence is common.

Causes and incidence

The agent that causes tinea versicolor is *Pityrosporum orbiculare*, also known as *Pityrosporum ovale* and *Malassezia furfur*. Whether this condition is infectious or merely a proliferation of normal skin fungi is uncertain. Tinea versicolor is more common in hot climates—tropical countries or in those with high humidity—and is associated with increased sweating. It usually affects adolescents and young men when sebaceous gland activity is at its highest.

Pathophysiology

Normal skin flora that contains the causative organism is present on the outer layers of the epidermis. The fungi are present on the affected skin in the forms of yeast and filament. The organism is opportunistic and will innervate the skin and tissue and convert to the parasitic stage when certain circumstances are present such as humidity, immunosuppression, malnutrition, and pregnancy.

Complication

◆ Secondary bacterial infections

Signs and symptoms

Tinea versicolor typically produces raised or macular, round or oval, slightly scaly lesions on the upper trunk, which may extend to the lower abdomen, neck, arms, groin, thigh, genitalia, and, rarely, the face. These lesions are usually tawny but may range from hypopigmented (white) patches in dark-skinned patients to hyperpigmented (brown) patches in fair-skinned patients. Some areas don't tan when exposed to sunlight, causing the cosmetic defect for which most people seek medical help. Inflammation, burning, and itching are possible but are usually absent.

Diagnosis

Visualization of blue-green fluorescent lesions during Wood's light examination strongly suggests tinea versicolor. However, if the patient has recently showered, this fluorescence may not show because the chemical that causes fluorescence is water-soluble.

℞ **CONFIRMING DIAGNOSIS** *Microscopic examination of skin scrapings prepared in potassium hydroxide solution confirms the disorder by showing hyphae, clusters of yeast, and large numbers of variously sized spores (a combination referred to as "spaghetti and meatballs").*

Treatment

The most economical and effective treatment is selenium sulfide lotion 2.5% applied once a day for 7 days. It's left on the skin for 10 minutes, then rinsed off thoroughly. In persistent cases, therapy may require a single 12- or 24-hour application of this lotion, repeated once a week for 4 weeks. Either treatment may cause temporary redness and irritation.

Other treatments include sodium thiosulfate 25% solution, applied twice daily to affected areas for 2 to 4 weeks; sulfur salicylic shampoo applied as a lotion at bedtime each night and washed off each morning for 2 weeks; zinc pyrithione shampoo 1% lathered into affected areas for 5 minutes before showering, and repeated every day for 2 weeks; or imidazole antifungal agents applied twice daily for 2 weeks.

Ketoconazole and other azole-based creams, such as topical ketoconazole, may be applied once or twice daily for 2 weeks. Oral ketoconazole or another oral azole-based medication, such as fluconazole, may be used if the patient has extensive disease that fails to respond to other therapies.

Special considerations
◆ Instruct the patient to apply selenium sulfide lotion as ordered. Tell the patient that this medication may cause temporary adverse effects.
◆ Assure the patient that once the fungal infection is cured; discolored areas will gradually blend in after exposure to the sun or UV light.
◆ Because recurrence of tinea versicolor is common, advise the patient to watch for new areas of discoloration.
◆ Teach the patient proper hand-washing technique and encourage good personal hygiene.
◆ Provide written instructions for using prescribed medications. Tell the patient to contact the physician if adverse reactions occur.

:::::: PREVENTION
◆ *Stress the importance of not scratching or picking lesions to avoid the risk of skin breaks and secondary bacterial infections.*
◆ *Encourage the patient to avoid overexposure to heat and humidity.*

DERMATOPHYTOSIS
Dermatophytosis, commonly called *tinea*, may affect the scalp (tinea capitis), body (tinea corporis), nails (tinea unguium), hands (tinea manuum), feet (tinea pedis), groin (tinea cruris), and bearded skin (tinea barbae). With effective treatment, the cure rate is very high, although about 20% of infected people develop chronic conditions.

Causes and incidence
Tinea infections (except for tinea versicolor) result from dermatophytes (fungi) of the genera *Trichophyton*, *Microsporum*, and *Epidermophyton*. Transmission can occur through contact with infected lesions, household cats and dogs, and soiled or contaminated articles, such as shoes, towels, or shower stalls.

Tinea infections are prevalent in the United States. They're more common in males than in females.

Pathophysiology
Dermatophytes invade the superficial keratin layer of skin using enzymes called keratinases where the infection remains limited to this outer layer. The body's immune response is inhibited by mannans contained in the dermaphyte cell wall. Mannans reduce keratinocyte propagation, which can then decrease the rate of sloughing and creating a state of chronic infection.

Complications
◆ Hair or nail loss
◆ Secondary bacterial or candidal infections

Signs and symptoms
Lesions vary in appearance depending on the site of invasion (inside or outside the hair shaft), duration of infection, level of host resistance, and amount of inflammatory response. Tinea capitis ranges in appearance from broken-off hairs with little scaling to severe painful, inflammatory, pus-filled masses

Athlete's foot
Dermatophytosis of the feet (tinea pedis) is popularly called *athlete's foot*. This infection causes macerated, scaling lesions, which may spread from the interdigital spaces to the sole. Diagnosis must rule out other possible causes, such as eczema, psoriasis, contact dermatitis, and maceration by tight, ill-fitting shoes.

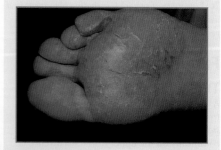

(kerions) covering the entire scalp. Partial hair loss occurs in all cases. The cardinal clue is broken-off hairs.

Tinea corporis produces flat lesions on the skin at any site except the scalp, bearded skin, hands, or feet. These lesions may be dry and scaly or moist and crusty; as they enlarge, their centers heal, causing the classic ring-shaped appearance. In tinea unguium (onychomycosis), infection typically starts at the tip of one or more toenails (fingernail infection is less common) and produces gradual thickening, discoloration, and crumbling of the nail, with accumulation of subungual debris. Eventually, the nail may be destroyed completely.

Tinea pedis, or *athlete's foot*, causes scaling and blisters between the toes. Severe infection may result in inflammation, with severe itching and pain on walking. A dry, squamous inflammation may affect the entire sole. (See *Athlete's foot*, page 670.) Tinea manuum produces scaling patches and hyperkeratosis on the palmar surface. It's usually unilateral and is associated with tinea pedis. Tinea cruris (jock itch) produces red, raised, sharply defined, itchy or burning lesions in the groin that may extend to the buttocks, inner thighs, and the external genitalia. Warm weather, obesity, and tight clothing encourage fungus growth. Tinea barbae is an uncommon infection that affects the bearded facial area of men.

Diagnosis

CONFIRMING DIAGNOSIS *Microscopic examination of lesion scrapings prepared in potassium hydroxide solution will reveal branching fungal hyphae. Gently heating the slide helps separate epithelial cells and hyphae. Lowering the microscope condenser and dimming the light make hyphae easier to identify, as does adding a drop of ink to the potassium hydroxide.*

Other diagnostic procedures include Wood's light examination (useful in only about 5% of cases of tinea capitis) and culture of the infecting organism, which is important for identifying hair and nail fungal infections.

Treatment

Tinea infections respond to a wide variety of medications. Typically, infections of the skin (hands, body, feet, and groin) require only topical therapy. Infections of the hair and nails, skin infections causing chronic thickening of the skin, and other unresolving infections require oral antifungal therapy.

Topical preparations are commonly azole-based, though other preparations are available. Oral therapy includes azole-based

medications and terbinafine. Griseofulvin is falling out of favor because newer products are easier to use and have a shorter duration of therapy.

ALERT *Caution must be taken when using systemic antifungals: liver enzyme levels must be monitored before and throughout treatment if therapy is expected to extend more than 2 months, and chronic medications must be monitored because of the antifungal's potential effect on blood levels.*

Treatment should continue from several days to 2 weeks after lesions have resolved. Topical agents with soothing and cooling effects may be used with systemic therapy for infections with severe itching and burning; they may be discontinued when the immediate discomfort resolves.

Special considerations

Management of tinea infections requires medication compliance, observation for sensitivity reactions, observation for secondary bacterial infections, and patient teaching. Specific care varies by site of infection.

◆ For tinea barbae: Suggest that the patient let their beard grow (whiskers may be trimmed with scissors, not a razor). If the patient insists that they must shave, advise them to use an electric razor instead of a blade.

◆ For tinea capitis: If the condition worsens, discontinue medications and notify the physician. Use good hand-washing technique and teach the patient to do the same. Spores of tinea capitis are shed in the air around an infected patient or may spread on contaminated clothing and other personal articles. To prevent spread of infection to others, advise to wash towels, bedclothes, and combs frequently in hot water and to avoid sharing them. Suggest that family members be checked for tinea capitis.

◆ For tinea corporis: Use abdominal pads between skin folds for the patient with excessive abdominal girth; change pads frequently. Check the patient daily for excoriated, newly denuded areas of skin. Apply wet Burow's compresses two or three times daily to decrease inflammation and help remove scales.

◆ For tinea cruris: Instruct the patient to dry the affected area thoroughly after bathing and to evenly apply antifungal powder after applying the topical antifungal agent. Advise them to wear loose-fitting clothing, which should be changed frequently and washed in hot water.

◆ For tinea pedis: Encourage the patient to expose feet to air whenever possible, and to wear sandals or leather shoes and clean, white cotton socks. Instruct the patient to wash their feet twice daily and, after drying them thoroughly, to apply antifungal cream followed by antifungal powder to absorb perspiration and prevent excoriation. Tell them to allow shoes to dry out by alternating pairs every other day. Also instruct them to wear shower shoes when using public facilities.

◆ For tinea unguium: Keep nails short and straight. Gently remove debris under the nails with an emery board. Prepare the patient for prolonged therapy.

Parasitic infestations

SCABIES

A common skin infection, scabies results from infestation with *Sarcoptes scabiei* var. *hominis* (itch mite), which provokes a sensitivity reaction. It's transmitted through skin or sexual contact.

Causes and incidence

Mites can live their entire life cycles in the skin of humans, causing chronic infection. (The adult mite can survive without a human host for only 2 or 3 days.) The female mite burrows into the skin to lay its eggs, from which larvae emerge to copulate and then reburrow under the skin. (See *Scabies: Cause and effect.*)

Scabies occurs worldwide, primarily in environments marked by overcrowding and poor hygiene, and can be endemic.

Pathophysiology

The female scabies mite lay its eggs, which hatch to the larvae stage and burrow into the epidermis. They molt twice before achieving adulthood and able to mate. The pregnant female makes a snake-like burrow using an enzyme to dissolve the stratum corneum while laying her eggs thus continuing the cycle. The subsequent rash and irritation is the result of an inflammatory response to the scabies mite's eggs, saliva, and fecal matter. The host may not get the pruritic rash on initial exposure but will have progressively worsening allergic response with subsequent exposures.

Complications

◆ Excoriation
◆ Tissue trauma
◆ Secondary bacterial infection

Signs and symptoms

Typically, scabies causes itching, which intensifies at night. Characteristic lesions are usually excoriated and may appear as erythematous nodules. These threadlike lesions are approximately 1 cm long and generally occur between

Scabies: Cause and effect

Infestation with *S. scabiei*—the itch mite—causes scabies. This mite (shown enlarged below) has a hard shell and measures a microscopic 0.1 mm. The illustration below shows the erythematous nodules with excoriation that appear in patients with scabies. These lesions are usually highly pruritic.

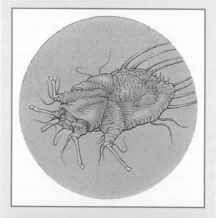

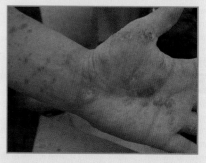

fingers, on flexor surfaces of the wrists, on elbows, in axillary folds, at the waistline, on nipples and buttocks in females, and on genitalia in males.

PEDIATRIC TIP *In infants, the burrows (lesions) may appear on the head and neck.*

Diagnosis

CONFIRMING DIAGNOSIS *Visual examination of the contents of the scabietic burrow may reveal the itch mite. If not, a drop of mineral oil placed over the burrow, followed by superficial scraping and examination of expressed material under a low-power microscope, may reveal ova or mite feces. However, excoriation or inflammation of* *the burrow often makes such identification difficult. If diagnostic tests offer no positive identification of the mite and if scabies is still suspected (e.g., if family members and close contacts of the patient also report itching), skin clearing that occurs after a therapeutic trial of a pediculicide confirms the diagnosis.*

Treatment

Generally, treatment for scabies consists of application of a pediculicide—permethrin, lindane cream, or crotamiton—in a thin layer over the entire skin surface from the neck down. Lindane and permethrin are left on the skin for 8 to 12 hours. Crotamiton is applied nightly for two consecutive nights and washed off 24 hours after the second application. To make certain that all areas have been treated, this application should be repeated in about 1 week. Oral ivermectin is also an effective treatment for scabies.

Lindane is an effective scabicide and, when used properly, may be applied safely to children, but shouldn't be used in children younger than age 2 or pregnant or nursing mothers because of potential neurologic toxicity. It also shouldn't be applied immediately after a shower. A 6% to 10% solution of sulfur in petrolatum may be used if patients object to using lindane, but they should be advised that sulfur is messy and odorous.

Persistent pruritus (from mite sensitization or contact dermatitis) may develop from repeated use of pediculicides rather than from continued infection. An antipruritic emollient, topical steroid, or oral antihistamine can reduce itching; intralesional steroids may resolve erythematous nodules.

Special considerations

◆ Instruct the patient to apply permethrin, crotamiton, or lindane cream or lotion from the neck down, covering the entire body. Then wait 15 minutes before dressing and avoid bathing for 8 to 12 hours or longer, depending on the treatment used. Contaminated clothing and linens must be washed in hot water or dry cleaned.
◆ Tell the patient not to apply lindane cream if skin is raw or inflamed. Advise them that if skin irritation or hypersensitivity reaction develops, they should notify the physician immediately, discontinue using the drug, and thoroughly wash it off their skin.
◆ Suggest to the patient that their family members and other close personal contacts be checked for possible symptoms.

▦ **PREVENTION** *If a hospitalized patient has scabies, prevent transmission to other patients. Practice good hand-washing technique or wear gloves when touching the patient; observe wound and skin precautions for 24 hours after treatment with a pediculicide; gas autoclave blood pressure cuffs before using them on other patients; isolate linens until the patient is noninfectious; and thoroughly disinfect the patient's room after discharge.*

CUTANEOUS LARVA MIGRANS

Cutaneous larva migrans (CLM), also known as *creeping eruption,* is a skin reaction to infestation by nematodes (hookworms or roundworms) that usually infect dogs and cats. Eruptions associated with CLM clear completely with treatment.

Causes and incidence

Under favorable conditions—warmth, moisture, sandy soil—hookworm or roundworm ova present in feces of affected animals (such as dogs and cats) and hatch into larvae, which can then burrow into human skin on contact. After penetrating its host, the larva becomes trapped under the skin, unable to reach the intestines to complete its normal life cycle.

The parasite then begins to move, producing the peculiar, tunnel-like lesions that are alternately meandering and linear, reflecting the nematode's persistent and unsuccessful attempts to escape its host.

In the United States, CLM is second to pinworm in infestation.

Pathophysiology

The larvae penetrate the corneum and begin to burrow and migrate. In the human host, the larvae are limited to the skin because they lack collagenase to move through the epidermal layer. The pruritic irritation is the immune response to the parasites and their products.

Complications

◆ Cellulitis
◆ Excoriation
◆ Secondary bacterial infection

Signs and symptoms

A transient rash, tingling, or, possibly, a small vesicle appears at the point of penetration, usually on an exposed area that has come in contact with the ground, such as the feet, legs, or buttocks. The incubation period is typically 1 to 6 days. The parasite may be active almost as soon as it enters the skin. Local pruritus begins within hours following penetration.

As the parasite migrates, it etches a noticeable thin, raised, red line on the skin, which may become vesicular and encrusted. Pruritus quickly develops, often with crusting and secondary infection following excoriation. Onset is usually characterized by slight itching that develops into intermittent stinging pain as the thin, red lines develop. The larva's apparently random path can cover from 1 mm to 1 cm a day. Penetration of more than one larva may involve a much larger area of the skin, marking it with many tracks.

Diagnosis
Characteristic migratory lesions strongly suggest CLM. A thorough patient history usually reveals contact with warm, moist soil within the past several months. A skin biopsy may reveal larva in the subbasal layer.

Treatment
Topical application of thiabendazole, ivermectin, or albendazole is effective. The suspension is applied to lesions and the immediate surrounding areas four times daily for 1 week. Oral thiabendazole given in two divided doses for 3 to 5 days is effective. Oral ivermectin and albendazole are equally effective. Tell the patient that adverse effects of systemic thiabendazole include nausea, vomiting, abdominal pain, and dizziness.

Special considerations
◆ Reassure the patient, especially if they are sensitive about their appearance, that larva

migrans lesions usually clear 1 to 2 weeks after treatment. Stress the importance of adhering to the treatment regimen exactly as ordered.
◆ Have the patient's nails cut short to prevent skin breaks and secondary bacterial infection from scratching. Apply cool, moist compresses to alleviate itching.
◆ Be alert for possible adverse reactions associated with systemic treatment, including nausea, vomiting, abdominal pain, and dizziness.
◆ Encourage the patient to verbalize feelings about the infestation, including embarrassment, fear of rejection by others, and body image disturbance.

⁞⁞⁞⁞⁞⁞ PREVENTION
◆ *Teach the patient that these parasites exist and about sanitation of beaches and sandboxes and about proper pet care.*
◆ *Instruct the patient and their family in good hand-washing technique, and stress the importance of preventing the spread of the infection among family members.*

PEDICULOSIS
Pediculosis is caused by parasitic forms of lice: *Pediculus humanus capitis* causes pediculosis capitis (head lice), *Pediculus humanus corporis* causes pediculosis corporis (body lice), and *Phthirus pubis* causes pediculosis pubis (crab lice). (See *Types of lice,* pages 674 and 675.)

Types of lice

Head louse
Pediculus humanus capitis (head louse) is similar in appearance to *P. humanus corporis.*

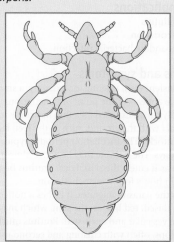

Body louse
Pediculus humanus corporis (body louse) has a long abdomen and all its legs are about the same length.

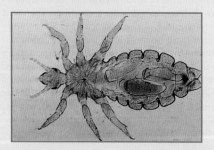

These lice feed on human blood and lay their eggs (nits) on body hairs or clothing fibers. After the nits hatch, the lice must feed within 24 hours or die; they mature in about 2 to 3 weeks. Treatment can effectively eliminate lice.

Causes and incidence

Pediculus humanus capitis (most common species) feeds on the scalp and, rarely, the eyebrows, eyelashes, and beard. It's most commonly seen on the back of the head and neck and behind the ears. This form of pediculosis is caused by overcrowded conditions and poor personal hygiene, and commonly affects children, especially girls. It spreads through shared clothing, hats, combs, and hairbrushes.

Pediculus humanus corporis lives in the seams of clothing, next to the skin, leaving only to feed on blood. Common causes include prolonged wearing of the same clothing (which might occur in cold climates), overcrowding, and poor personal hygiene. It spreads through shared clothing and bedsheets.

Phthirus pubis is primarily found in pubic hairs, but this species may extend to the eyebrows, eyelashes, and axillary or body hair. Pediculosis pubis is transmitted through sexual intercourse or by contact with clothes, bedsheets, or towels harboring lice.

In the United States, 6 to 12 million people are affected each year by pediculosis.

Pubic louse
Phthirus pubis (pubic or "crab lice") is slightly translucent; its first set of legs is shorter than its second and third.

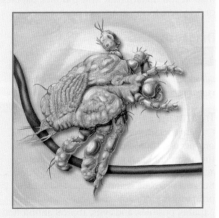

Pathophysiology

When a louse bites, it injects a toxin into the skin that produces mild irritation and a purpuric spot. Repeated bites cause sensitization to the toxin, leading to more serious inflammation.

Complications

◆ Excoriation
◆ Secondary bacterial infection

Signs and symptoms

Clinical features of pediculosis capitis include itching; excoriation (with severe itching); matted, foul-smelling, lusterless hair (in severe cases); occipital and cervical lymphadenopathy (posterior cervical lymphadenopathy without obvious disease is characteristic); and a rash on the trunk, probably because of sensitization. Adult lice migrate from the scalp and deposit oval, gray-white nits on the proximal one third of hair shafts.

Pediculosis corporis initially produces small, red papules (usually on the shoulders, trunk, or buttocks). Later, wheals (probably a sensitivity reaction) may develop. Untreated pediculosis corporis may lead to vertical excoriations and ultimately to dry, discolored, thickly encrusted, scaly skin, with bacterial infection and scarring. In severe cases, headache, fever, and malaise may accompany cutaneous symptoms.

Pediculosis pubis causes skin irritation from scratching, which is usually more obvious than the bites. Small gray-blue spots (maculae caeruleae) may appear on the thighs or upper body. Small red spots are often seen in the underclothing.

Diagnosis

Pediculosis is visible on physical examination.
◆ In pediculosis capitis—oval, grayish nits that can't be shaken loose like dandruff. (The closer the nits are to the end of the hair shaft, the longer the infection has been present, because the ova are laid close to the scalp.)
◆ In pediculosis corporis—characteristic skin lesions; nits found on clothing.
◆ In pediculosis pubis—nits attached to pubic hairs, which feel coarse and grainy to the touch.

Treatment

Lindane, pyrethrin, permethrin, and malathion, in shampoo or lotion preparations, are all effective against lice. Shampoos should be applied to the infected skin or hair, lathered, then washed off in 5 minutes. Lotions should be applied over the entire affected area, and then washed off after 10 minutes. Treatments should be repeated in 7 to 10 days.

Permethrin may be used for treating head lice. Saturate the hair and scalp and rinse after 10 minutes. Malathion lotion is also effective when applied to dry hair and washed out in 8 to 10 hours. After treatment, all nits (louse eggs) should be combed out of the hair with a metal nit comb. Nit removal may be aided by prerinsing with a prerinse solution containing formic acid or dipping the comb in vinegar. Normal laundering of clothes and bedclothes in hot water after treatment is sufficient to remove adult lice as well as nits.

Special considerations

◆ Teach the patient how to use the creams, ointments, powders, and shampoos that eliminate lice.
◆ Ask the patient with pediculosis pubis for a history of recent sexual contacts, so that they can be examined and treated.
◆ The patient should be tested for other sexually transmitted diseases, including human immunodeficiency virus.

PREVENTION
◆ *To prevent the spread of pediculosis to other hospitalized persons, examine all high-risk patients on admission, especially elderly people who depend on others for care, those admitted from nursing homes, and people who live in crowded conditions.*
◆ *To prevent your own infestation, avoid prolonged contact with the patient's hair, clothing, and bedsheets.*

Follicular and glandular disorders

ACNE VULGARIS

Acne vulgaris is an inflammatory disease of the sebaceous follicles. The prognosis is good with treatment.

Causes and incidence

The cause of acne is multifactorial, but theories regarding dietary influences appear to be groundless. Predisposing factors include heredity; hormonal contraceptives (many females experience an acne flare-up during their first few menstrual cycles after starting or discontinuing hormonal contraceptives); androgen stimulation; certain drugs, including corticosteroids, corticotropin, androgens, iodides, bromides, trimethadione, phenytoin, isoniazid, lithium, and halothane; cobalt irradiation; and hyperalimentation. Other possible factors are exposure to heavy oils, greases, or tars; trauma or rubbing from tight clothing; cosmetics; emotional stress; and unfavorable climate.

Pathophysiology

More is known about the pathogenesis of acne. (See *What happens in acne*, page 677.) Androgens stimulate sebaceous gland growth and production of sebum, which is secreted into dilated hair follicles that contain bacteria. The bacteria, usually *Propionibacterium acnes* and *Staphylococcus epidermidis* (which are normal skin flora), secrete lipase. This enzyme interacts with sebum to produce free fatty acids, which provoke inflammation. Also, the hair follicles produce more keratin, which joins with the sebum to form a plug in the dilated follicle.

Acne vulgaris primarily affects adolescents (usually between ages 15 and 18), although lesions can appear as early as age 8. Although acne strikes boys more often and more severely than girls, it usually occurs in girls at an earlier age and tends to last longer in girls as well, sometimes into adulthood.

Complications

◆ Abscess formation
◆ Permanent scarring
◆ Secondary bacterial infection

Signs and symptoms

The acne plug may appear as a closed comedo, or whitehead (if it doesn't protrude from the follicle and is covered by the epidermis), or as an open comedo, or blackhead (if it does protrude and isn't covered by the epidermis). The black coloration is caused by the melanin or pigment of the follicle. Rupture or leakage of an enlarged plug into the dermis produces inflammation and characteristic acne pustules, papules, or, in severe forms, acne cysts or abscesses.

Diagnosis

R **CONFIRMING DIAGNOSIS** *The appearance of characteristic acne lesions, especially in an adolescent patient, confirms the presence of acne vulgaris.*

Treatment

Current therapy for acne includes topical and oral agents. Topical retinoic acid (tretinoin) is the treatment of choice for noninflammatory acne consisting of open and closed comedones. Benzoyl peroxide is antibacterial and is used primarily for inflammatory acne, including papules, pustules, and cysts. Topical antibiotics are effective for mild pustular and comedone acne. Tetracycline, erythromycin, clindamycin,

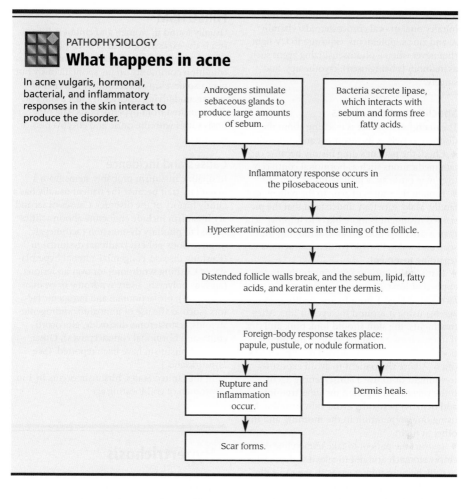

PATHOPHYSIOLOGY
What happens in acne

In acne vulgaris, hormonal, bacterial, and inflammatory responses in the skin interact to produce the disorder.

Androgens stimulate sebaceous glands to produce large amounts of sebum.

Bacteria secrete lipase, which interacts with sebum and forms free fatty acids.

Inflammatory response occurs in the pilosebaceous unit.

Hyperkeratinization occurs in the lining of the follicle.

Distended follicle walls break, and the sebum, lipid, fatty acids, and keratin enter the dermis.

Foreign-body response takes place: papule, pustule, or nodule formation.

Rupture and inflammation occur.

Dermis heals.

Scar forms.

meclocycline, and benzamycin are all available in topical forms. Systemic antibiotics, such as tetracycline, minocycline, clindamycin, erythromycin, ampicillin, cephalosporins, trimethoprim, and sulfamethoxazole, and systemic retinoids may help reduce the effects of acne.

Systemic therapy consists primarily of antibiotics, usually tetracycline (which also exhibits an anti-inflammatory effect), to decrease bacterial growth until the patient is in remission; then a lower dosage is used for long-term maintenance.

ALERT *Tetracycline is contraindicated during pregnancy because it discolors the teeth of the fetus. Erythromycin and ampicillin are alternatives for these patients. Exacerbation of pustules or abscesses during either type of antibiotic therapy requires a culture to identify a possible secondary bacterial infection.*

Oral isotretinoin combats acne by inhibiting sebaceous gland function and keratinization.

ALERT *Because of its severe adverse effects, the 16- to 20-week course of isotretinoin is limited to those with severe papulopustular or cystic acne who don't respond to conventional therapy. Because this drug is known to cause birth defects, the manufacturer, with Food and Drug Administration approval, recommends the following precautions: pregnancy testing before dispensing; dispensing of only a 30-day supply; repeat pregnancy testing throughout the treatment period; effective contraception during treatment; and informed consent of the patient or parents regarding the drug's adverse effects.*

A serum triglyceride level should be measured before therapy with isotretinoin begins and at intervals throughout its course.

Females may benefit from the administration of estrogens to inhibit androgen activity. Improvement rarely occurs before 2 to 4 months, and exacerbations may follow its discontinuation. Unfortunately, the high estrogen doses that are required present a major risk of severe adverse effects.

Other treatments for acne vulgaris include intralesional or oral corticosteroids, vitamin A, and zinc supplements, exposure to UV light (but never when a photosensitizing agent such as tretinoin is being used), cryotherapy, and surgery.

Special considerations

The main focus of care is teaching about the disorder as well as its treatment and prevention.

◆ Check the patient's drug history because certain medications such as hormonal contraceptives may cause an acne flare-up.

◆ Explain the causes of acne to the patient and family. Make sure they understand that the prescribed treatment is more likely to improve acne than a strict diet and fanatical scrubbing with soap and water. Provide written instructions regarding treatment.

◆ Instruct the patient receiving tretinoin to apply it at least 30 minutes after washing face and at least 1 hour before bedtime. Warn against using it around the eyes or lips. After treatments, the skin should look pink and dry. If it appears red or starts to peel, the preparation may have to be weakened or applied less often. Advise the patient to avoid exposure to sunlight or to use a sunscreening agent. If the prescribed regimen includes tretinoin and benzoyl peroxide, avoid skin irritation by using one preparation in the morning and the other at night.

◆ Instruct the patient to take tetracycline on an empty stomach and not to take it with antacids or milk because it interacts with their metallic ions and is then poorly absorbed.

◆ Tell the patient who's taking isotretinoin to avoid vitamin A supplements, which can worsen any adverse effects. Also, teach how to deal with the dry skin and mucous membranes that usually occur during treatment. Tell the female patient about the severe risk of teratogenicity. Monitor liver function and lipid levels.

◆ Inform the patient that acne takes a long time to clear—even years for complete resolution. Encourage continued local skin care even after acne clears. Explain the adverse effects of all drugs.

◆ Pay special attention to the patient's perception of their physical appearance and offer emotional support.

::::: **PREVENTION**

◆ *Try to identify predisposing factors that may be eliminated or modified.*

◆ *Teach the patient and family techniques to maintain a well-balanced diet, get adequate rest, and manage stress.*

HIRSUTISM

Usually found in women and children, hirsutism is the excessive growth of body hair, typically in an adult male distribution pattern. This condition commonly occurs spontaneously but may also develop as a secondary disorder of various underlying diseases. It must always be distinguished from hypertrichosis. The prognosis varies with the cause and effectiveness of treatment.

Causes and incidence

Idiopathic hirsutism probably stems from a hereditary trait because the patient usually has a family history of the disorder. Causes of secondary hirsutism include endocrine abnormalities related to pituitary dysfunction (acromegaly or precocious puberty), adrenal dysfunction (Cushing disease, congenital adrenal hyperplasia, or Cushing syndrome), or ovarian lesions (such as polycystic ovary syndrome or ovarian neoplasm); prolactinoma; and iatrogenic factors (such as the use of minoxidil, androgenic steroids, testosterone, diazoxide, glucocorticoids, and hormonal contraceptives). Other kinds of hirsutism have been reported. (See *Hypertrichosis.*)

In the United States, hirsutism occurs in 1 in 20 women of childbearing age.

Hypertrichosis

Hypertrichosis is a localized or generalized condition in males and females that's marked by excessive hair growth in areas that aren't androgen-sensitive. Localized hypertrichosis usually results from local trauma, chemical irritation, or hormonal stimulation; pigmented nevi (e.g., Becker nevus) may also contain hairs. Generalized hypertrichosis results from neurologic or psychiatric disorders, such as encephalitis, multiple sclerosis, concussion, anorexia nervosa, or schizophrenia; contributing factors include juvenile hypothyroidism, porphyria cutanea tarda, and the use of drugs such as phenytoin.

Hypertrichosis lanuginosa is a generalized proliferation of fine, lanugo-type hair (sometimes called *down* or *woolly hair*). Such hair may be present at birth but generally disappears shortly thereafter. This condition may become chronic, with persistent lanugo-type hair growing over the entire body, or may develop suddenly later in life; it is very rare and usually results from malignancy.

Pathophysiology

The quality of hair growth is influenced by hormones and the intrinsic characteristics of the hair follicle. During puberty, the hormone dihydrotestosterone converts fine vellus hairs into coarse pigmented terminal hairs. The production of this androgen is determined by 5-alpha-reductase activity in the skin, which can also affect the degree of hirsutism.

Complication

◆ Varies depending on the cause

Signs and symptoms

Hirsutism typically produces enlarged hair follicles as well as enlargement and hyperpigmentation of the hairs themselves. Excessive facial hair growth is the complaint for which most patients seek medical help. Generally, hirsutism involves appearance of thick, pigmented hair in the beard area, upper back, shoulders, sternum, axillae, and pubic area. Frontotemporal scalp hair recession is often a coexisting condition. Patterns of hirsutism vary widely, depending on the patient's race and age.

> **ELDER TIP** *Elderly women commonly show increased hair growth on the chin and upper lip.*

In secondary hirsutism, signs of masculinization may appear—deepening of the voice, increased muscle mass, increased size of genitalia, menstrual irregularity, and decreased breast size.

Diagnosis

A family history of hirsutism, absence of menstrual abnormalities or signs of masculinization, and a normal pelvic examination strongly suggest idiopathic hirsutism. Tests for secondary hirsutism depend on associated symptoms that suggest an underlying disorder. About 90% of women with hirsutism have an elevated free testosterone level.

Treatment

At the patient's request, treatment for idiopathic hirsutism consists of eliminating excess hair by scissors, shaving, or depilatory creams, or removal of the entire hair shaft with tweezers or wax. However, removal with laser is the most effective method. Bleaching with hydrogen peroxide may also be satisfactory. Electrolysis can destroy hair bulbs permanently, but it works best when only a few hairs need to be removed. (A history of keloid formation contraindicates this procedure.) Hirsutism due to elevated androgen levels may require low-dose dexamethasone or prednisone, hormonal contraceptives, or androgen receptor–competitive inhibitors—such as spironolactone or cimetidine—however, these drugs vary in effectiveness. Eflornithine hydrochloride cream is effective for slowing the growth of facial hair and is frequently used in combination with laser treatment.

Treatment for secondary hirsutism varies, depending on the nature of the underlying disorder.

Special considerations

Care for patients with idiopathic hirsutism focuses on emotional support and patient teaching; care for patients with secondary hirsutism depends on the treatment for the underlying disease.

◆ Provide emotional support by being sensitive to the patient's feelings about their appearance.
◆ Watch for signs of contact dermatitis in patients being treated with depilatory creams, especially elderly people. Also, watch for infection of hair follicles after hair removal with tweezers or wax.
◆ Suggest consulting a cosmetologist about makeup or bleaching agents.

ALOPECIA

Alopecia, or hair loss, usually occurs on the scalp but can also occur on bearded areas, eyebrows, and eyelashes. Hair loss elsewhere on the body is less common and less conspicuous. In the nonscarring form of this disorder (noncicatricial alopecia), the hair follicle can generally regrow hair. However, scarring alopecia involves tissue destruction, such as inflammation, scarring, and atrophy, and usually destroys the hair follicle, making hair loss irreversible.

Causes and incidence

The most common form of nonscarring alopecia is male-pattern alopecia, which appears to be related to androgen levels and to aging. Genetic predisposition commonly influences the time of onset, degree of baldness, speed with which it spreads, and pattern of hair loss. Women may experience diffuse thinning over the top of the scalp.

Other forms of nonscarring alopecia include:
◆ physiologic alopecia (usually temporary): sudden hair loss in infants, loss of straight hairline in adolescents, and diffuse hair loss after childbirth
◆ alopecia areata (idiopathic form): generally reversible and self-limiting; occurs most frequently in young and middle-age adults of both sexes (See *Alopecia areata*, page 680.)
◆ trichotillomania: compulsive pulling out of one's own hair; most common in children
◆ traction alopecia: localized areas of hair loss due to chronic use of tight braids (such as

Alopecia areata

"Exclamation point" hairs often border new patches of alopecia areata. Not seen in any other type of alopecia, these hairs indicate the patch is expanding.

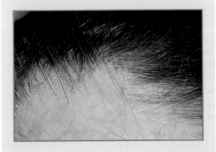

cornrows) or other hair styles. This condition may also result in scarring alopecia.

Pathophysiology

Multiple factors are involved in the pathophysiology of alopecia, scarring and nonscarring. An autoimmune response involving T lymphocytes can cause the production of cytotoxic substances. These toxins affect the pigmentation and keratinization of the hair shaft by shrinking the dermal papilla. This activity increases the resting phase of the hair growth cycle called telogen. When the telogen phase is longer than the anagen (growth) phase, there are fewer intact hairs remaining in the follicles. In scarring alopecia, physical damage can destroy the hair follicle and inhibit hair growth permanently.

Predisposing factors of nonscarring alopecia also include radiation, many types of drug therapies and drug reactions, bacterial and fungal infections, psoriasis, seborrhea, and endocrine disorders, such as thyroid, parathyroid, and pituitary dysfunctions.

Scarring alopecia causes irreversible hair loss. It may result from physical or chemical trauma and chronic tension on a hair shaft, as occurs in braiding. Diseases that produce alopecia include destructive skin tumors, granulomas, lupus erythematosus, scleroderma, follicular lichen planus, and severe fungal, bacterial, or viral infections, such as kerion, folliculitis, or herpes simplex.

Signs and symptoms

In male-pattern alopecia, hair loss is gradual and usually affects the thinner, shorter, and less pigmented hairs of the frontal and parietal portions of the scalp. In women, hair loss is generally more diffuse; completely bald areas are uncommon but may occur.

Alopecia areata affects small patches of the scalp but may also occur as alopecia totalis, which involves the entire scalp and eyebrows, or as alopecia universalis, which involves the entire body. Although mild erythema may occur initially, affected areas of scalp or skin appear normal. "Exclamation point" hairs (loose hairs with dark, rough, brushlike tips on narrow, less pigmented shafts) occur at the periphery of new patches. Regrowth hairs are thin and may be white or gray. They're usually replaced by normal hair.

In trichotillomania, patchy, incomplete areas of hair loss with many broken hairs appear on the scalp but may occur on other areas, such as the eyebrows.

Diagnosis

CONFIRMING DIAGNOSIS *Physical examination is usually sufficient to confirm alopecia. In trichotillomania, an occlusive dressing can establish the diagnosis by allowing new hair to grow, revealing that the hair is being pulled out. Diagnosis must also identify any underlying disorder.*

Treatment

Topical application of minoxidil, a peripheral vasodilator more typically used as an oral antihypertensive, has limited success in treating male-pattern alopecia. An alternative treatment is surgical redistribution of hair follicles by autografting. Oral finasteride has been shown to reverse androgenic loss, but it's approved only for use in men.

In alopecia areata, minoxidil is effective, although treatment is often unnecessary because spontaneous regrowth is common. Intralesional corticosteroid injections are beneficial for small patches and may produce regrowth in 4 to 6 weeks. Anthralin, topical high-potency corticosteroids, systemic corticosteroids, topical cyclosporine, and topical nitrogen mustard all have been used in treating alopecia areata. Hair loss that persists for more than a year has a poor prognosis for regrowth. In trichotillomania, an occlusive dressing encourages normal hair growth, simply by identifying the cause of hair loss; clomipramine may be effective for short-term treatment. Treatment for other types of alopecia varies according to the underlying cause.

Special considerations

◆ Reassure a woman with female-pattern alopecia that it doesn't lead to total baldness. Suggest that she wear a wig.

◆ If the patient has alopecia areata, explain the disorder and give reassurance that complete regrowth is possible.

ROSACEA

A chronic skin eruption, rosacea produces flushing and dilation of the small blood vessels in the face, especially the nose and cheeks. Papules and pustules may also occur, but without the characteristic comedones of acne vulgaris. Ocular involvement may result in blepharitis, conjunctivitis, uveitis, or keratitis. Rosacea usually spreads slowly and rarely subsides spontaneously.

Causes and incidence

Although the cause of rosacea is unknown, stress, infection, vitamin deficiency, menopause, and endocrine abnormalities can aggravate this condition. Anything that produces flushing—for example, hot beverages, such as tea or coffee, tobacco, alcohol, spicy foods, physical activity, sunlight, and extreme heat or cold—can also aggravate rosacea.

Rosacea is most common in white women between ages 30 and 50. When it occurs in men, however, it's usually more severe and often associated with rhinophyma, which is characterized by dilated follicles and thickened, bulbous skin on the nose.

Pathophysiology

Several factors are involved in the pathophysiology of rosacea including dysregulation of the immune system, genetic components, neural, and vascular dysfunction. The impairment of the skin barrier leads to excessive transepidermal water loss creating dry, scaly, and peeling facial skin. Higher numbers of blood vessels and increased blood flow are also the suggested cause for the characteristic facial flushing.

Complications

◆ Blepharitis
◆ Conjunctivitis
◆ Keratitis
◆ Uveitis

Signs and symptoms

Rosacea generally begins with periodic flushing across the central oval of the face, accompanied later by telangiectasia, papules, pustules, and nodules. Rhinophyma is commonly associated with severe untreated rosacea but may occur alone. Rhinophyma usually appears first on the lower half of the nose, and produces red, thickened skin and follicular enlargement. It's found almost exclusively in men older than age 40. Related ocular lesions are uncommon.

Diagnosis

℞ **CONFIRMING DIAGNOSIS** *Typical vascular and acneiform lesions—without the comedones characteristically associated with acne vulgaris—and rhinophyma in severe cases confirm rosacea.*

Treatment

Treatment for the acneiform component of rosacea consists of oral tetracycline or erythromycin in gradually decreasing doses over 1 to 2 months as symptoms subside. Resistant cases can be treated with oral minocycline or doxycycline. Isotretinoin is also effective, but its use is limited to those with severe disease. Topical metronidazole gel helps the papules, pustules, and erythema. Other treatments include electrolysis to destroy large, dilated blood vessels and removal of excess tissue in patients with rhinophyma. Topical hydrocortisone preparations worsen the condition.

Special considerations

Assess the effect of rosacea on body image. Because it's always apparent on the face, support is essential.

 PREVENTION
◆ *Instruct the patient to avoid spicy foods, hot beverages, alcohol, extended sun exposure, and other possible causes of flushing.*
◆ *Encourage the use of sunscreen.*

Pigmentation disorders

VITILIGO

Marked by stark-white skin patches that may cause a serious cosmetic problem, vitiligo results from the destruction and loss of pigment cells. It shows no racial preference, but the distinctive patches are most noticeable in blacks. Repigmentation therapy, which is widely used in treating vitiligo, may necessitate several summers of exposure to sunlight; the effects of this treatment may not be permanent.

Causes and incidence

Although the cause of vitiligo is unknown, inheritance seems to be a definite etiologic factor because about 30% of patients with vitiligo have family members with the same condition. Other theories implicate enzymatic self-destructing mechanisms, autoimmune mechanisms, and abnormal neurogenic stimuli.

Some link exists between vitiligo and many other disorders that it often accompanies—thyroid dysfunction, pernicious anemia, Addison disease, aseptic meningitis, diabetes mellitus, photophobia, hearing defects, alopecia areata, uveitis, chronic mucocutaneous candidiasis, and halo nevi.

The most frequently reported precipitating factor is a stressful physical or psychological event—severe sunburn, surgery, pregnancy, loss of a job, bereavement, or some other source of distress. Chemical agents, such as phenols and catechols, may also cause this condition.

Vitiligo affects about 1 to 2 million people in the United States, usually people between ages 10 and 30, with peak incidence around age 20. It affects men and women equally, but women are more likely to seek treatment.

Pathophysiology

Vitiligo pathogenesis is not definitively known but there are several widely accepted theories. The autoimmune and cytotoxic hypothesis suggests alterations in humoral and cellular immunity and destruction of melanocytes cause vitiligo symptoms. Additional evidence includes the presence of circulating antibodies against melanocyte proteins. Another theory is the intrinsic defect of melanocytes where genetic defects inhibit melanocyte growth and differentiation. The neural hypothesis suggests a neurochemical mediator prevents melanin production or destroys melanocytes. Oxidant/antioxidant mechanism proposes melanocyte disruption results from an intermediate or metabolic product of melanin synthesis.

Complications

◆ Sunburn
◆ Skin cancer

Signs and symptoms

Vitiligo produces depigmented or stark-white patches on the skin; on fair-skinned whites, these are almost imperceptible. Lesions are usually bilaterally symmetrical with sharp borders, which occasionally are hyperpigmented. Lesions that are small initially can enlarge and even progress to total depigmentation (universal vitiligo).

These unique patches generally appear over bony prominences on the back of the hands; on the face, the axillae, genitalia, nipples, or umbilicus; around orifices (such as the eyes, mouth, and anus); within body folds; and at sites of trauma. The hair within these lesions may also turn white. Because hair follicles and certain parts of the eyes also contain pigment

Recognizing vitiligo

This illustration shows characteristic depigmented skin patches in vitiligo. These patches are usually bilaterally symmetrical, with distinct borders.

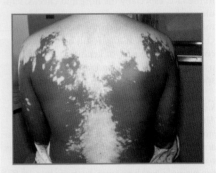

cells, vitiligo may be associated with premature gray hair and ocular pigmentary changes. (See *Recognizing vitiligo*.)

Diagnosis

Diagnosis requires an accurate history of onset and of associated illnesses, a family history, and observation of characteristic lesions. Other skin disorders such as tinea versicolor must be ruled out.

℞ CONFIRMING DIAGNOSIS *In fair-skinned patients, Wood's light examination in a darkened room detects vitiliginous patches; depigmented skin reflects the light, and pigmented skin absorbs it. Biopsy will show normal skin except for the absence of melanocytes. If autoimmune or endocrine disturbances are suspected, laboratory studies (such as thyroid studies) are appropriate.*

Treatment

Repigmentation therapy combines systemic or topical psoralen compounds (trimethylpsoralen or 8-methoxypsoralen) with exposure to sunlight or artificial UV light, wavelength A (UVA), a treatment known as PUVA. New pigment rises from hair follicles and appears on the skin as small freckles, which gradually enlarge and coalesce. Body parts containing few hair follicles (such as the fingertips) may resist this therapy.

Because PUVA affects the entire skin surface, systemic therapy enhances the contrast between normal skin, which turns darker than usual, and white, vitiliginous skin. Use of sunscreen on normal skin may minimize contrast while preventing sunburn.

Topical class I glucosteroid ointments may be used for single or small macules. Monitor patients on this therapy for skin atrophy or telangiectasia development.

Depigmentation therapy is suggested for patients with vitiligo affecting more than 50% of the body surface. A cream containing 20% monobenzone permanently destroys pigment cells in unaffected areas of the skin and produces a uniform skin tone. This medication is applied initially to a small area of normal skin once daily to test for unfavorable reactions such as contact dermatitis. In the absence of adverse effects, the patient begins applying the cream twice daily to those areas they wishes to depigment first. Eventually, the entire skin may be depigmented to achieve a uniform color. *Note:* Depigmentation is permanent and results in extreme photosensitivity. Patients may wish to take daily beta-carotene to impart an off-white color to the chalk-white skin.

Commercial cosmetics may also help de-emphasize vitiliginous skin. Some patients prefer dyes because these remain on the skin for several days, although the results aren't always satisfactory. Although often impractical, complete avoidance of exposure to sunlight through the use of screening agents and protective clothing may minimize vitiliginous lesions in whites.

Special considerations

◆ Instruct the patient to use psoralen medications three or four times weekly. (*Note:* Systemic psoralens should be taken 2 hours before exposure to sun; topical solutions should be applied 30 to 60 minutes before exposure.) Warn them to use a sunscreen (sun protection factor [SPF] 8 to 10) to protect both affected and normal skin during exposure and to wear sunglasses after taking the medication. If periorbital areas require exposure, tell the patient to keep eyes closed during treatment.

◆ Suggest that the patient receiving depigmentation therapy wear protective clothing and use a sunscreen (SPF 15). Explain the therapy thoroughly and allow the patient plenty of time to decide whether to undergo this treatment. Make sure they understand that the results of depigmentation are permanent and they must thereafter protect their skin from the adverse effects of sunlight.

◆ Caution the patient about buying commercial cosmetics or dyes without trying them first because some may not be suitable.

PEDIATRIC TIP *For the child with vitiligo, modify repigmentation therapy to avoid unnecessary restrictions. Tell parents to give the initial dose of psoralen medication at 1 p.m. and then let the child go out to play as usual. After this, medication should be given 30 minutes earlier each day of treatment, provided the child's skin doesn't turn more than slightly pink from exposure. If marked erythema develops, parents should discontinue treatment and notify the physician. Eventually, the child should be able to take the medication at 9:30 a.m. and play outdoors the rest of the day without adverse effects. Tell the parents the child should wear clothing that permits maximum exposure of vitiliginous areas to the sun.*

◆ Remind patients undergoing repigmentation therapy that exposure to sunlight also darkens normal skin. After being exposed to UVA for the prescribed amount of time, the patient should apply a sunscreen if they plan to be exposed to sunlight also. If sunburn occurs, advise the patient to discontinue therapy temporarily and to apply open wet dressings (using thin sheeting) to affected areas for 15 to 20 minutes, four or five times daily or as necessary for comfort. After application of wet dressings, allow the skin to air dry. Suggest application of a soothing lubricating cream or lotion while the skin is still slightly moist.

◆ Reinforce patient teaching with written instructions.

◆ Be sensitive to the patient's emotional needs but avoid promoting unrealistic hope for a total cure.

MELASMA

A patchy, hypermelanotic skin disorder, melasma (also known as *chloasma* or *mask of pregnancy*) can pose a serious cosmetic problem. It may be chronic but is never life threatening.

Causes and incidence

The cause of melasma is unknown, but onset is most common in young adults. Histologically, hyperpigmentation results from increased melanin production, although the number of melanocytes remains normal. Melasma may be related to the increased hormonal levels associated with pregnancy, menopause, ovarian cancer, and the use of hormonal contraceptives. Progestational agents, phenytoin, and mephenytoin may also contribute to this disorder. Exposure to sunlight stimulates melasma, but it may develop without any apparent predisposing factor. Patients with acquired immunodeficiency syndrome have an increased incidence of similar hyperpigmentation.

Melasma affects females more commonly than males. Although it tends to occur equally in all races, the light-brown color characteristic of melasma is most evident in dark-skinned whites.

Pathophysiology

Melasma is more common in women and thought to be directly related to hormones with the increased amounts of estrogen receptors in melasma lesions. The primary factor in the development of this condition is the exposure to UV radiation or sunlight. This increases the production of alpha melanocyte (hormone), interleukin-1, and endothelin-1, which cause intraepidermal melanocytes to increase melanin production.

Complication

◆ Negative cosmetic implications

Signs and symptoms

Typically, melasma produces large, brown, irregular patches, symmetrically distributed on the forehead, cheeks, and sides of the nose. Less commonly, these patches may occur on the neck, upper lip, temples and, occasionally, on the dorsa of the forearms.

Diagnosis

℞ **CONFIRMING DIAGNOSIS** *Observation of characteristic dark patches on the face usually confirms melasma. The patient history may reveal predisposing factors. Wood's lamp examination accentuates the hyperpigmentation.*

Treatment

Treatment consists primarily of application of bleaching agents containing 2% to 4% hydroquinone in combination with tretinoin or glycolic acid to inhibit melanin synthesis. This medication is applied twice daily for up to 8 weeks. Adjunctive measures include avoidance of exposure to sunlight, use of opaque sunscreens, and discontinuation of hormonal contraceptives.

Special considerations

◆ Tell the patient that melasma associated with pregnancy usually clears within a few months after delivery and may not return with subsequent pregnancies.

◆ Bleaching agents may help but may require repeated treatments to maintain the desired effect. Cosmetics may help mask deep pigmentation.

◆ Reassure the patient that melasma is treatable. It may fade spontaneously with protection from sunlight, postpartum, and after discontinuing hormonal contraceptives. Serial photographs help show the patient that patches are improving.

PREVENTION *Advise the patient to avoid sun exposure as much as possible by using sunscreens and wearing protective clothing.*

PHOTOSENSITIVITY REACTIONS

A photosensitivity reaction is a skin eruption that can be a toxic or allergic response to light alone or to light and chemicals. A phototoxic reaction is a dose-related primary response. A photoallergic reaction is an uncommon, acquired immune response that isn't dose-related—even slight exposure can cause a severe reaction.

Causes and incidence

Certain chemicals, including dyes, coal tar, and furocoumarin compounds found in plants, can cause a photosensitivity reaction. The list of drugs that can cause photosensitivity reactions is extensive and includes many drugs within each of the following general categories: antibiotics (especially tetracycline), antidepressants, antihistamines, anticancer agents, antiparasitic agents, antipsychotic agents, diuretics, hypoglycemics, nonsteroidal anti-inflammatories, sunscreens, and miscellaneous agents, such as cardiac glycosides, hormonal contraceptives, and acne medications.

Berlock dermatitis, a specific photosensitivity reaction, results from the use of oil of bergamot—a common component of perfumes, colognes, and pomades.

Pathophysiology

A cell-mediated immune response is a photoallergic reaction to a light-activated drug or compound. The development of antigens then is taken up by Langerhans cells and other antigen-presenting cells and move to the local lymph nodes. They are then involved in the activation of a T lymphocyte–mediated immune response leading to localized skin irritation or systemic response depending on how the causative agent was administered.

Complications

◆ Premature skin aging
◆ Skin cancer

Signs and symptoms

Immediately after sun exposure, a phototoxic reaction causes a burning sensation followed by erythema (sunburn-type reaction), edema, desquamation, and hyperpigmentation. Berlock dermatitis produces an acute reaction with erythematous vesicles that later become hyperpigmented.

Photoallergic reactions may take one of two forms. Developing 2 hours to 5 days after light exposure, polymorphous light eruption (PMLE) produces erythema, papules, vesicles, urticaria, and eczematous lesions on exposed areas;

pruritus may persist for 1 to 2 weeks. Solar urticaria begins minutes after exposure and lasts about an hour; erythema and wheals follow itching and burning sensations.

Diagnosis

Characteristic skin eruptions in sun-exposed areas and a patient history of recent exposure to light or certain chemicals suggest a photosensitivity reaction. A photopatch test for UVA and UVB done while the patient is on the drug may aid diagnosis and identify the causative light wavelength. Other studies must rule out connective tissue disease, such as lupus erythematosus and porphyrias.

Treatment

For many patients, treatment involves a sunscreen, protective clothing, and minimal exposure to sunlight while the patient continues the drug. For others, progressive exposure to sunlight can thicken the skin and produce a tan that interferes with photoallergens and prevents further eruptions.

Withdrawal of the causative agent and treatment with oral steroids usually provides relief. The patient should be advised not to use the causative agent again if it's known, even though this may limit the patient's treatment options.

Antimalarial drugs, beta-carotene, and PUVA (psoralen and UVA) may be used to treat PMLE. Treatment for solar urticaria may also require PUVA. Although hyperpigmentation usually fades in several months, hydroquinone preparations can hasten the process.

Special considerations

Tell the patient to inform their physician about sensitivity to any drugs.

⚏ PREVENTION *To prevent reactions, advise the patient to avoid prolonged exposure to light.*

Inflammatory reactions

DERMATITIS

Inflammation of the skin, dermatitis occurs in several forms: atopic (discussed here), seborrheic, nummular, contact, chronic, localized neurodermatitis, exfoliative, and stasis. (See *Types of dermatitis*, pages 686 to 689.) Atopic dermatitis (atopic or infantile eczema, neurodermatitis constitutionalis, or Besnier's prurigo) is a chronic inflammatory response often associated with other atopic diseases, such as bronchial asthma and allergic rhinitis.

Causes and incidence

The cause of atopic dermatitis is unknown, but a genetic predisposition may be exacerbated by factors such as food allergies, infections, irritating chemicals, temperature and humidity, and emotions. Approximately 10% of childhood cases are due to allergy to certain foods, particularly eggs, peanuts, milk, fish, soy, and wheat. Atopic dermatitis tends to flare up in response to extremes in temperature and humidity. Other causes of flare-ups are sweating and psychological stress.

An important secondary cause of atopic dermatitis is irritation, which seems to change the epidermal structure, allowing immunoglobulin (Ig) E activity to increase. Consequently, chronic skin irritation usually continues even after exposure to the allergen has ended or after the irritation has been systemically controlled.

⬛ PEDIATRIC TIP *Atopic dermatitis is most common in infants, usually developing between ages 1 month and 1 year, commonly in those with strong family histories of atopic disease. At least half of those cases clear by age 36 months. These children often acquire other atopic disorders as they grow older. Typically, this form of dermatitis flares and subsides repeatedly before finally resolving during adolescence. However, it can persist into adulthood.*

In adults, atopic dermatitis is generally chronic or recurring.

Pathophysiology

The barrier dysfunction theory suggests that antigens enter through an opening in the skin triggering the production of inflammatory cytokines. In the immune dysfunction theory there is an unbalanced relationship between the T-cell subsets resulting in the production of type 2 cytokines, which leads to the increase in IgE plasma cells and the development of atopic dermatitis.

Complications

◆ Altered pigmentation
◆ Lichenification
◆ Scarring

Signs and symptoms

Atopic skin lesions generally begin as erythematous areas on excessively dry skin.

⬛ PEDIATRIC TIP *In children, lesions typically appear on the forehead, cheeks, and extensor surfaces of the arms and legs.*

In adults, lesions appear at flexion points (antecubital fossa, popliteal area, and neck).

During flare-ups, pruritus and scratching cause edema, crusting, and scaling. Eventually, chronic atopic lesions lead to multiple areas of dry, scaly skin, with white dermatographia, blanching, and lichenification.

Types of dermatitis

Type	Causes	Signs and symptoms
Seborrheic dermatitis		
An acute or subacute skin disease that affects areas where sebaceous glands are most active—such as the scalp and face—and occasionally other areas, and is characterized by lesions covered with yellow or brownish gray scales	◆ Unknown; stress and neurologic conditions may be predisposing factors; may be related to the yeast *Pityrosporum ovale*	◆ Eruptions in areas with many sebaceous glands (usually scalp, face, and trunk) and in skin folds ◆ Itching, redness, and inflammation of affected areas; lesions may appear greasy; fissures may occur ◆ Indistinct, occasionally yellowish, scaly patches from excess stratum corneum (dandruff may be mild seborrheic dermatitis) ◆ Generally worse in winter
Nummular dermatitis (discoid eczema, nummular eczema)		
A chronic form of dermatitis characterized by inflammation of coin-shaped, vesicular, crusted scales and, possibly, pruritic lesions	◆ Possibly precipitated by stress, skin dryness, irritants, scratching, or bathing with hot water	◆ Round, nummular (coin-shaped) lesions, usually on arms and legs, with distinct borders of crusts and scales ◆ Possible oozing and severe itching ◆ Summertime remissions common, with wintertime recurrence
Contact dermatitis		
Often sharply demarcated inflammation and irritation of the skin caused by contact with substances to which the skin is sensitive, such as perfumes, soaps, plants, or chemicals	◆ Mild irritants: chronic exposure to detergents or solvents ◆ Strong irritants: damage on contact with acids or alkalis ◆ Allergens: sensitization after repeated exposure	◆ Mild irritants and allergens: erythema and small vesicles that ooze, scale, and itch ◆ Strong irritants: blisters and ulcerations ◆ Classic allergic response: clearly defined lesions, with straight lines following points of contact ◆ Severe allergic reaction: marked edema of affected areas
Chronic dermatitis		
Characterized by inflammatory eruptions of the hands and feet	◆ Usually unknown but may result from progressive contact dermatitis ◆ Secondary (possibly perpetuating) factors: trauma, infections, redistribution of normal flora, photosensitivity, and food sensitivity	◆ Thick, lichenified, single or multiple lesions on any part of body (often on hands) ◆ Inflammation and scaling ◆ Recurrence following long remissions

Diagnosis	Treatment and intervention
♦ Patient history and physical findings, especially distribution of lesions in sebaceous gland areas, confirm seborrheic dermatitis ♦ Diagnosis must rule out psoriasis	♦ Removal of scales with frequent washing and shampooing with selenium sulfide suspension (most effective), zinc pyrithione, or tar and salicylic acid shampoo ♦ Application of a topical steroid and an antifungal to nonhairy areas
♦ Physical findings and patient history confirm nummular dermatitis; a middle-age or older patient may have a history of atopic dermatitis ♦ Diagnosis must rule out fungal infections, atopic or contact dermatitis, and psoriasis	♦ Elimination of known irritants ♦ Measures to relieve dry skin: increased humidification, limited frequency of baths and use of mild soap and bath oils, and application of emollients ♦ Application of wet dressings in acute phase ♦ Topical steroids (occlusive dressings or intralesional injections) for persistent lesions ♦ Tar preparations and antihistamines to control itching ♦ Antibiotics for secondary infection ♦ Other interventions as for atopic dermatitis
♦ Patient history, patch testing to identify allergens, and shape and distribution of lesions suggest contact dermatitis	♦ Elimination of known allergens and decreased exposure to irritants, wearing protective clothing such as gloves, and washing immediately after contact with irritants or allergens ♦ Topical anti-inflammatory agents (including steroids); systemic corticosteroids for edema, bullae, or very extensive outbreaks; antihistamines; and local applications of Burow's solution (for blisters) ♦ Sensitization to topical medications may occur ♦ Other interventions as for atopic dermatitis
♦ No characteristic pattern or course; diagnosis relies on detailed patient history and physical findings	♦ Antibiotics for secondary infection ♦ Avoidance of excessive washing and drying of hands and of accumulation of soaps and detergents under rings ♦ Use of emollients with topical steroids ♦ Elimination of known allergens and decreased exposure to irritants, wearing protective clothing, and washing immediately after contact with irritants or allergens

(continued)

Types of dermatitis (continued)

Localized neurodermatitis (lichen simplex chronicus, essential pruritus)

Superficial inflammation of the skin characterized by itching and papular eruptions that appear on thickened, hyperpigmented skin	♦ Chronic scratching or rubbing of primary lesion or insect bite, or other skin irritation	♦ Intense, sometimes continual scratching ♦ Thick, sharp-bordered, possibly dry, scaly lesions with raised papules ♦ Usually affects easily reached areas, such as ankles, lower legs, anogenital area, back of neck, and ears

Exfoliative dermatitis

Severe, chronic skin inflammation characterized by redness and widespread erythema and scaling	♦ Usually, preexisting skin lesions progress to exfoliative stage, such as in contact dermatitis, drug reaction, lymphoma, or leukemia	♦ Generalized dermatitis, with acute loss of stratum corneum, and erythema and scaling ♦ Sensation of tight skin ♦ Hair loss ♦ Possible fever, sensitivity to cold, shivering, gynecomastia, and lymphadenopathy

Stasis dermatitis

A condition caused by impaired venous circulation and characterized by eczema of the legs with edema, hyperpigmentation, and persistent inflammation	♦ Secondary to peripheral vascular diseases affecting legs, such as recurrent thrombophlebitis and resultant chronic venous insufficiency	♦ Varicosities and edema common, but obvious vascular insufficiency not always present ♦ Usually affects the lower leg, just above internal malleolus, or sites of trauma or irritation ♦ Early signs: dusky red deposits of hemosiderin in skin, with itching and dimpling of subcutaneous tissue; later signs: edema, redness, and scaling of large area of legs ♦ Possible fissures, crusts, and ulcers

Common secondary conditions associated with atopic dermatitis include viral, fungal, or bacterial infections and ocular disorders.

Because of intense pruritus, the upper eyelid is commonly hyperpigmented and swollen, and a double fold occurs under the lower lid (Morgan–Dennie folds, Morgan folds, Dennie pleats, or Mongolian lines). Atopic cataracts are unusual but may develop between ages 20 and 40.

Kaposi's varicelliform eruption, a potentially fatal, generalized viral infection, may develop if the patient with atopic dermatitis comes in contact with a person who's infected with herpes simplex.

Diagnosis

A family history of allergy and chronic inflammation suggests atopic dermatitis. Typical distribution of skin lesions rules out other inflammatory skin lesions, such as diaper rash (lesions are confined to the diapered area), seborrheic dermatitis (no pigmentation changes, or lichenification occurs in chronic lesions), and chronic contact dermatitis (lesions affect hands and forearms, sparing antecubital and popliteal areas). Serum IgE levels are usually elevated.

Treatment

Effective treatment for atopic lesions consists of eliminating allergens and avoiding irritants,

◆ Physical findings confirm diagnosis	◆ Scratching must stop; then lesions will disappear in about 2 weeks ◆ Fixed dressing or Unna's boot to cover affected area ◆ Topical steroids under occlusion or by intralesional injection ◆ Antihistamines and open wet dressings ◆ Emollients ◆ Inform patient about underlying cause
◆ Diagnosis requires identification of the underlying cause	◆ Severe cases: may require hospitalization with protective isolation and hygienic measures to prevent secondary bacterial infection ◆ Open wet dressings, with colloidal baths ◆ Mild lotions over topical steroids ◆ Maintenance of constant environmental temperature to prevent chilling or overheating ◆ Careful monitoring of renal and cardiac status ◆ Systemic antibiotics and steroids ◆ Other interventions as for atopic dermatitis
◆ Diagnosis requires positive history of venous insufficiency and physical findings such as varicosities	◆ Measures to prevent venous stasis: avoidance of prolonged sitting or standing, use of support stockings, weight reduction in obese patients, and increasing of activity ◆ Corrective surgery for underlying cause ◆ After ulcer develops, encourage rest periods, with legs elevated; open wet dressings; Unna's boot (zinc gelatin dressing provides continuous pressure to affected areas); and antibiotics for secondary infection after wound culture

extreme temperature and humidity changes, and other precipitating factors; local and systemic measures relieve itching and inflammation. Antihistamines relieve itching and induce more restful sleep. Topical application of a corticosteroid ointment, especially after bathing, often alleviates inflammation. Between steroid doses, application of a moisturizing cream can help retain moisture. Systemic corticosteroid therapy should be used only during extreme exacerbations. Topical tacrolimus and pimecrolimus (an immunosuppressant known as a *topical immunomodulator*) are new agents used in patients older than age 2 who are intolerant of or unresponsive to conventional therapy. Weak tar preparations and UVB light therapy are used to increase the thickness of the stratum corneum. Antibiotics are appropriate if a bacterial agent has been cultured.

Special considerations

◆ Warn the patient that drowsiness is possible with the use of antihistamines to relieve daytime itching. If nocturnal itching interferes with sleep, suggest methods for inducing natural sleep, such as drinking a glass of warm milk, to prevent overuse of sedatives.
◆ Complement medical treatment by helping the patient set up an individual schedule and plan for daily skin care. Instruct the patient to bathe in plain water, according to the severity of

the lesions, and to bathe with a special nonfatty soap and tepid water (96° F [35.6° C]) but to avoid using any soap when lesions are acutely inflamed. Advise the patient to shampoo frequently and apply corticosteroid solution to the scalp afterward, to keep fingernails short to limit excoriation and secondary infections caused by scratching, and to lubricate skin after a tub bath. Advise the patient to avoid using any perfume or makeup that causes burning or itching.

◆ To help clear lichenified skin, apply occlusive dressings (such as plastic film) intermittently. This treatment requires a physician's order, experience in dermatologic treatment, and can't be used in all treatment modalities.

◆ Inform the patient that irritants, such as detergents and wool, and emotional stress, exacerbate atopic dermatitis.

◆ Be careful not to show any anxiety or revulsion when touching the lesions during treatment. Help the patient accept their altered body image and encourage them to verbalize feelings. Remember, coping with disfigurement is extremely difficult, especially for children and adolescents. Arrange for counseling, if necessary, to help the patient deal with this distressing condition more effectively.

Miscellaneous disorders

TOXIC EPIDERMAL NECROLYSIS

TEN is a rare, severe skin disorder that causes epidermal erythema, superficial necrosis, and skin erosions. Mortality is high (30%), especially among debilitated and elderly patients. Re-epithelialization is slow, and residual scarring is common. TEN primarily affects adults. Some experts consider TEN to be a maximal form of Stevens–Johnson syndrome (SJS), with SJS being a maximal variant of erythema multiforme major.

Causes and incidence

In 80% of cases, TEN is determined to result from a drug reaction—most commonly to sulfonamides, penicillins, barbiturates, hydantoins, procainamide, isoniazid, nonsteroidal anti-inflammatory drugs, or allopurinol. Numerous other drugs have also been implicated, although 5% of patients with TEN report no drug use. It may also result from chemical exposure, viral infection, mycoplasma pneumonia, or immunization.

TEN may reflect an immune response, or it may be related to overwhelming physiologic stress (coexisting sepsis, neoplastic diseases, and drug treatment).

The annual worldwide incidence of TEN is 1 to 3 cases for every 1 million people.

Pathophysiology

TEN pathogenesis is not precisely known but there are several accepted theories, one suggests that an immune-related cytotoxic reaction triggers the destruction of keratinocytes. This also results in extensive blistering, epidermolysis, and finally cell death.

Complications

◆ Bronchopneumonia
◆ Pulmonary edema
◆ Gastrointestinal and esophageal hemorrhage
◆ Shock
◆ Renal failure
◆ Sepsis
◆ Disseminated intravascular coagulation

Signs and symptoms

Early symptoms include inflammation of the mucous membranes, a burning sensation in the conjunctivae, malaise, fever, and generalized skin tenderness. After such prodromal symptoms, TEN erupts in three phases:

◆ diffuse, erythematous rash
◆ vesiculation and blistering
◆ large-scale epidermal necrolysis and desquamation

Large, flaccid bullae that rupture easily expose extensive areas of denuded skin, permitting both loss of tissue fluids and electrolytes and widespread systemic involvement.

Diagnosis

℞ **CONFIRMING DIAGNOSIS** *Early diagnosis is very important and is based on the patient's clinical status at the peak stage of the disease. Nikolsky's sign (skin sloughs off with slight friction) is present in erythematous areas. Culture and Gram stain of lesions determine whether infection is present. Supportive findings include leukocytosis, elevated levels of alanine aminotransferase and aspartate aminotransferase, albuminuria, and fluid and electrolyte imbalances.*

Exfoliative cytology and biopsy aid in ruling out erythema multiforme and exfoliative dermatitis.

Treatment

Treatment consists of transferring the patient to a burn center or an intensive care unit and providing I.V. fluid replacement to maintain fluid and electrolyte balance. Xenografts should be used to prevent pain and infection and to provide the framework for re-epithelialization. High doses of I.V. immunoglobulins may halt progression if given early in the course of illness. Steroids may be appropriate initially but should be discontinued as soon as healing occurs. Use of steroids may decrease survival rates only secondary to increased incidence of infections and other complications. Necrotic skin should be debrided. The patient also should stop using suspected drugs.

Special considerations
◆ Frequently assess hematocrit and hemoglobin, electrolyte, serum protein, and blood gas levels.
◆ Monitor vital signs, central venous pressure, and urine output. Watch for signs of renal failure (decreased urine output) and bleeding. Report fever immediately and obtain blood cultures and sensitivity tests promptly to detect and treat septic infection.
◆ Maintain skin integrity as much as possible. The patient shouldn't wear clothing and should be covered loosely to prevent friction and sloughing of skin. A low air-loss or air-fluidized bed is helpful.
◆ Administer analgesics as needed. Wounds will be virtually pain-free after the dermis is covered by the xenograft.
◆ Provide eye care hourly to remove exudate. Because ocular lesions are common, the ophthalmologist should examine the patent's eyes daily.
◆ Encourage the patient to wear a medical alert bracelet.

:::::: PREVENTION
◆ *Prevent secondary infection with appropriate precautions. Use systemic antibiotics for specific identified infections only.*
◆ *Ensure that suspected drugs are never administered.*

WARTS

Warts, also known as *verrucae*, are common, benign, viral infections of the skin and adjacent mucous membranes. The prognosis varies: Some warts disappear readily with treatment; others necessitate more vigorous and prolonged treatment. Some warts demonstrate spontaneous resolution.

Causes and incidence

Warts are caused by infection with the human papillomavirus, a group of ether-resistant, deoxyribonucleic acid-containing papovaviruses. Mode of transmission is probably through direct contact, but autoinoculation is possible.

Although their incidence is highest in children and young adults, warts may occur at any age.

Pathophysiology

In nongenital warts, the HPV virus infects the epithelium through an opening in the skin or contact with a mucous membrane. The virus replicates in the differentiated epithelial cells. In genital warts the virus enters into the basal layer of the epidermis through microabrasions in the genital mucosa. Genital warts result from the infected host cell infected and develop the morphologic atypical koilocytosis.

Complications
◆ Scarring
◆ Secondary infection

Signs and symptoms

Clinical manifestations depend on the type of wart and its location:
◆ common (verruca vulgaris): rough, elevated, rounded surface; appears most frequently on extremities, particularly hands and fingers; most prevalent in children and young adults
◆ condyloma acuminatum (moist wart or genital wart): usually small, pink to red, moist, and soft; may occur singly or in large cauliflower-like clusters on the penis, scrotum, vulva, cervix, vagina, and anus; can also occur on oral mucosa following oral–genital exposure; considered a sexually transmitted disease
◆ digitate: fingerlike, horny projection arising from a pea-shaped base; occurs on scalp or near hairline
◆ filiform: single, thin, threadlike projection; commonly occurs around the face and neck
◆ flat (also known as *juvenile* or *verruca plana*): multiple groupings of up to several hundred slightly raised lesions with smooth, flat, or slightly rounded tops; common on the face, neck, chest, knees, dorsa of hands, wrists, and flexor surfaces of the forearms; usually occur in children but can affect adults; often linear distribution because of spread from scratching or shaving
◆ periungual: rough, irregularly shaped, elevated surface; occurs around edges of fingernails and toenails; when severe, may extend under nail and lift it off nail bed, causing pain
◆ plantar: slightly elevated or flat; occur singly or in large clusters (mosaic warts), primarily at pressure points of feet

Diagnosis

℞ CONFIRMING DIAGNOSIS *Visual examination usually confirms the diagnosis. Plantar warts can be differentiated from corns and calluses by certain distinguishing features. Plantar warts obliterate natural lines of the skin, may contain red or black capillary dots that are easily discernible if the surface of the wart is shaved down with a scalpel, and are painful on application of pressure. Both plantar warts and corns have a soft, pulpy core surrounded by a thick callous ring; plantar warts and calluses are flush with the skin surface.*

Anal warts require anoscopy or sigmoidoscopy to rule out internal involvement, which may necessitate surgery. Women with vulvar lesions require examination of the vagina and cervix, including a Papanicolaou smear.

Treatment

Treatment for warts varies according to the location, size, number, pain level (present and projected), history of therapy, the patient's age, and compliance with treatment. Most persons eventually develop an immune response that causes warts to disappear spontaneously and require no treatment.

Treatment may include:
◆ Electrodesiccation and curettage—High-frequency electric current destroys the wart and is followed by surgical removal of dead tissue at the base and application of an antibiotic ointment (such as polysporin), covered with a bandage, for 48 hours. This method is effective for common, filiform, and, occasionally, plantar warts.
◆ Cryotherapy—Liquid nitrogen kills the wart; the resulting dried blister is peeled off several days later. If initial treatment isn't successful, it can be repeated at 2- to 4-week intervals. This method is useful either for periungual warts or for common warts on the face, extremities, penis, vagina, or anus.
◆ Acid therapy (primary or adjunctive)—The patient applies plaster patches impregnated with acid (such as 40% salicylic acid plasters) or acid drops (such as 5% to 16.7% salicylic acid in flexible collodion or trichloroacetic or dichloroacetic acids), every 12 to 24 hours for 2 to 4 weeks. This method isn't recommended for areas where perspiration is heavy, for those parts that are likely to get wet, or for exposed body parts where patches are cosmetically undesirable.
◆ Twenty-five percent podophyllin in compound with tincture of benzoin (for venereal warts)—The podophyllin solution is applied on moist warts. The patient must lie still while it dries, leave it on for 4 hours, and then wash it off with soap and water. Treatment may be repeated every 3 to 4 days and, in some cases, must be left on a maximum of 24 hours, depending on the patient's tolerance. Avoid using this drug on pregnant patients.

During acid or podophyllin therapy, the patient should protect the surrounding area with petroleum jelly or sodium bicarbonate (baking soda). A small amount of 25% to 50% trichloroacetic acid (for venereal warts) is applied to the wart. After the wart turns white, the acid is neutralized with baking soda or water.
◆ Carbon dioxide laser therapy—This treatment has successfully treated genital warts.

The use of antiviral drugs is under investigation; suggestion and hypnosis are occasionally successful, especially with children. Patients can apply topical imiquimod cream to sites that aren't thickly keratinized. It's applied at bedtime three times per week. Imiquimod can be used alternately with a topical retinoid such as tazarotene, which may increase effectiveness.

Occlusion may be beneficial to persistent warts.

Special considerations

Conscientious adherence to prescribed therapy is essential. The patient's sexual partner may also require treatment. Encourage the patient to seek counseling if applicable.

PSORIASIS

Psoriasis is a chronic, recurrent disease marked by epidermal proliferation. Its lesions, which appear as erythematous papules and plaques covered with silvery scales, vary widely in severity and distribution. Psoriasis is characterized by recurring partial remissions and exacerbations. Flare-ups are usually related to specific systemic and environmental factors but may be unpredictable; they can usually be controlled with therapy.

Causes and incidence

The tendency to develop psoriasis is genetically determined. Researchers have discovered a significantly higher-than-normal incidence of certain human leukocyte antigens (HLAs) in families with psoriasis, suggesting a possible immune disorder. Onset of the disease is also influenced by environmental factors. Trauma can trigger the isomorphic effect or Koebner's phenomenon, in which lesions develop at sites of injury. Infections, especially those resulting from beta-hemolytic streptococci, may cause a flare of guttate (drop-shaped) lesions. Other contributing factors include pregnancy, endocrine changes, climate (cold weather tends to exacerbate psoriasis), and emotional stress.

Generally, a skin cell takes 14 days to move from the basal layer to the stratum corneum, where, after 14 days of normal wear and tear, it's sloughed off. The life cycle of a normal skin cell is 28 days, compared with only 4 days for a psoriatic skin cell. This markedly shortened

Psoriatic plaques

In this patient with psoriasis, plaques consisting of silver scales cover the area behind the ear.

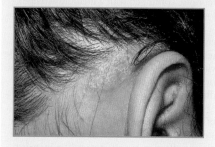

cycle doesn't allow time for the cell to mature. Consequently, the stratum corneum becomes thick and flaky, producing the cardinal manifestations of psoriasis.

Psoriasis affects approximately 2% of the population in the United States, and incidence is higher in whites than other races. Although this disorder is most common in young adults, it may strike at any age, including infancy.

Pathophysiology

A dysregulation in the immune system triggers a hyperproliferation of the epidermis. Erythema to the affected area is secondary to an increase in vascular endothelial growth factor expression thus increasing the formation of capillaries. The premature maturation of keratinocytes and incomplete cornification result in the characteristic scaling.

Complications

◆ Depression
◆ Infection

Signs and symptoms

The most common complaint of the patient with psoriasis is itching and, occasionally, pain from dry, cracked, encrusted lesions. Psoriatic lesions are erythematous and usually form well-defined plaques, sometimes covering large areas of the body. (See *Psoriatic plaques*.) Such lesions most commonly appear on the scalp, chest, elbows, knees, shins, back, and buttocks. The plaques consist of characteristic silver scales that either flake off easily or can thicken, covering the lesion. Removal of psoriatic scales frequently produces fine bleeding points (Auspitz sign). Occasionally, small guttate lesions

appear, either alone or with plaques; these lesions are typically thin and erythematous, with few scales.

Widespread shedding of scales is common in exfoliative or erythrodermic psoriasis and may also develop in chronic psoriasis.

Rarely, psoriasis becomes pustular, taking one of two forms. In localized pustular (Barber's) psoriasis, pustules appear on the palms and soles and remain sterile until opened. In generalized pustular (von Zumbusch's) psoriasis, which often occurs with fever, leukocytosis, and malaise, groups of pustules coalesce to form lakes of pus on red skin. These pustules also remain sterile until opened and commonly involve the tongue and oral mucosa.

In about 30% of patients, psoriasis spreads to the fingernails, producing small indentations and yellow or brown discoloration. In severe cases, the accumulation of thick, crumbly debris under the nail causes it to separate from the nail bed.

Some patients with psoriasis develop arthritic symptoms (psoriatic arthritis), usually in one or more joints of the fingers or toes, or sometimes in the sacroiliac joints, which may progress to spondylitis. Such patients may complain of morning stiffness. Joint symptoms show no consistent linkage to the course of the cutaneous manifestations of psoriasis; they demonstrate remissions and exacerbations similar to those of rheumatoid arthritis.

Diagnosis

Diagnosis depends on patient history, appearance of the lesions and, if needed, the results of skin biopsy. Typically, serum uric acid level is elevated as a result of accelerated nucleic acid degradation, but indications of gout are absent. HLA-Cw6, B13, and Bw57 may be present in early-onset psoriasis. Sudden onset of psoriasis may be associated with human immunodeficiency virus.

Treatment

Treatment depends on the type of psoriasis, the extent of the disease and the patient's response to it, and what effect the disease has on the patient's lifestyle. No permanent cure exists, and all methods of treatment are merely palliative. Ideally, all patients should see a dermatologist at least once.

Removal of psoriatic scales necessitates application of occlusive ointment bases, such as petroleum jelly, salicylic acid preparations, or preparations containing urea. Baker P & S liquid (phenol, sodium chloride, and liquid paraffin), applied to the scalp at bedtime, or liquor carbonis detergens in Nivea oil applied for 6 to 8 hours, is also effective. Shampoo or tar-based preparations are also used. These medications soften the scales, which can then be removed by scrubbing them carefully with a soft brush while bathing. Some preparations, such as tar-based preparations, can be used in whirlpools for extensively involved areas.

Methods to retard rapid cell production include exposure to UV light (UVB or natural sunlight) to the point of minimal erythema. Tar preparations or crude coal tar itself may be applied to affected areas about 15 minutes before exposure or may be left on overnight and wiped off the next morning. A thin layer of petroleum jelly may be applied before UVB exposure (the most common treatment for generalized psoriasis). Exposure time can increase gradually. Outpatient or day treatment with UVB prevents long hospitalizations and prolongs remission. Excimer laser is used for mild to moderate psoriasis. It provides a controlled beam of UVB light directly to the psoriasis plaques and is more effective than traditional phototherapy.

Steroid creams and ointments are useful to control psoriasis. A potent fluorinated steroid works well, except on the face and intertriginous areas. These creams require application twice daily, preferably after bathing to facilitate absorption, and overnight use of occlusive dressings, such as plastic wrap, plastic gloves or booties, or a vinyl exercise suit (under direct medical or nursing supervision). Small, stubborn plaques may require intralesional steroid injections. Anthralin, combined with a paste mixture, may be used for well-defined plaques but must not be applied to unaffected areas because it causes injury and stains normal skin. Apply petroleum jelly around the affected skin before applying anthralin. Commonly used concurrently with steroids, anthralin is applied at night and steroids during the day.

In a patient with severe chronic psoriasis, the Goeckerman regimen—which combines tar baths and UVB treatments—may help achieve the longest remission and clear the skin in 3 to 5 weeks. The Ingram technique is a variation of this treatment, using anthralin instead of tar. PUVA combines administration of psoralens with exposure to high-intensity UVA. Cytotoxin, usually methotrexate or cyclosporine, an immunosuppressant, may help severe, refractory psoriasis. For people who have failed to respond to traditional therapy, biologic agents such as alefacept, etanercept, infliximab, and ustekinumab may be used. The drugs must be used with caution because of their effect on the immune system and the risk of infection.

Etretinate, a retinoid compound, is effective in treating extensive cases of psoriasis. However, because this drug is a strong teratogen, it's unsafe for use in women of childbearing age. It also has numerous adverse effects that many patients find intolerable. Tazarotene, a topical retinoid, combined with a medium-strength topical corticosteroid, is also effective.

Low-dose antihistamines, oatmeal baths, emollients, and open wet dressings may help relieve pruritus. Aspirin and local heat help alleviate the pain of psoriatic arthritis; severe cases may require nonsteroidal anti-inflammatory drugs.

Therapy for psoriasis of the scalp consists of a tar shampoo followed by application of a steroid lotion; ketoconazole and anthralin may also be effective. No effective treatment exists for psoriasis of the nails.

Special considerations

Design your patient's care plan to include patient teaching and careful monitoring for adverse effects of therapy.

◆ Make sure the patient understands their prescribed therapy; provide written instructions to avoid confusion. Teach correct application of prescribed ointments, creams, and lotions. A steroid cream, for example, should be applied in a thin film and rubbed gently into the skin until the cream disappears. All topical medications, especially those containing anthralin and tar, should be applied with a downward motion to avoid rubbing them into the follicles. Gloves must be worn because anthralin stains and injures the skin. After application, the patient may dust themself with powder to prevent anthralin from rubbing off on their clothes. Warn the patient never to put an occlusive dressing over anthralin. Suggest use of mineral oil, then soap and water, to remove anthralin. Caution the patient to avoid scrubbing skin vigorously, to prevent Koebner's phenomenon. If a medication has been applied to the scales to soften them, suggest the patient use a soft brush to remove them.

◆ Watch for adverse effects, especially allergic reactions to anthralin, atrophy and acne from steroids, and burning, itching, nausea, and squamous cell epitheliomas from PUVA. Initially, evaluate the patient on methotrexate weekly, then monthly for red blood cell, white blood cell, and platelet counts because cytotoxins may cause hepatic or bone marrow toxicity. Liver biopsy may be done to assess the effects of methotrexate.

◆ Caution the patient receiving PUVA therapy to stay out of the sun on the day of treatment and to protect eyes with sunglasses that screen UVA for 24 hours after treatment. Tell them to wear goggles during exposure to this light.

◆ Be aware that psoriasis can cause psychological problems. Assure the patient that psoriasis isn't contagious and, although exacerbations and remissions occur, they're controllable with treatment. However, be sure they understand there's no cure. Also, because stressful situations tend to exacerbate psoriasis, help the patient learn to cope with these situations. Explain the relationship between psoriasis and arthritis but point out that psoriasis causes no other systemic disturbances. Refer all patients to the National Psoriasis Foundation, which provides information and directs patients to local chapters.

LICHEN PLANUS

A benign but pruritic skin eruption, lichen planus is a relatively rare disorder that usually produces scaling, purple papules marked by white lines or spots. The features of these lesions are called the "4 Ps"—purple, polygonal, pruritic, and papule.

In most patients, lichen planus resolves spontaneously in 6 to 18 months. In a few, chronic lichen planus may persist for several years.

Causes and incidence

The cause of lichen planus is unknown. Eruptions similar to lichen planus have been induced by arsenic, bismuth, gold, quinidine, propranolol, statins, and naproxen. Exposure to developers used in color photography may likewise cause an eruption that's indistinguishable from lichen planus.

Lichen planus is found in all geographic areas, with equal distribution among races. Eruptions of lesions with features characteristic of lichen planus occur most often in middle-age people and are uncommon in young and elderly people.

Pathophysiology

Lichen planus is a T-cell-mediated autoimmune condition where the auto-cytotoxic CD8 and T-cells trigger apoptosis of basal cells of the epithelium. Basal cell keratinocytes degenerate and disrupt the anchoring elements of the epithelium basement membrane and basal keratinocytes. This weakening of the epithelial connective tissue results in lesions and blisters on the oral mucosa.

Complications

◆ pain
◆ itching

◆ nail pitting
◆ genital or oral ulcerations
◆ hyperkeratosis

Signs and symptoms

Lichen planus may develop suddenly or insidiously. Initial lesions commonly appear on the arms or legs (generally on the wrist and medial sides of the thighs) and evolve into the generalized eruption of flat, glistening, purple papules marked with white lines or spots (Wickham's striae). These lesions may be linear from scratching or may coalesce into plaques. Lesions often affect the mucous membranes (especially the buccal mucosa), male genitalia, and, less often, the nails. These lesions are painful, especially when ulcers develop. Mild to severe pruritus is common.

Diagnosis

℞ CONFIRMING DIAGNOSIS *Although characteristic skin lesions usually establish the diagnosis of lichen planus, confirmation may require a skin biopsy.*

Treatment

Treatment is essentially symptomatic. The goal of therapy is to relieve itching with topical fluorinated steroids and occlusive dressings, intralesional injections of steroids, oatmeal baths, and antihistamines. Erosive oral lesions should be treated with triamcinolone acetonide in Orabase twice daily. Generalized severely pruritic skin lesions may be treated with systemic corticosteroids. An initial dosage of oral prednisone may be prescribed; thereafter, the dosage is decreased by approximately one third each week. If the patient experiences a recurrence of itching after the drug is discontinued, they will be given a low dose every other morning. If a drug is suspected as the cause, it should be discontinued.

Special considerations

◆ Administer medications as indicated, and inform the patient of possible adverse effects, especially drowsiness produced by antihistamines.
◆ Provide emotional support and reassure the patient that lichen planus, although annoying, is usually a benign, self-limiting condition, although lesions may persist for months or years.

CORNS AND CALLUSES

Usually located on areas of repeated trauma (especially the feet), corns and calluses are acquired skin conditions marked by hyperkeratosis of the stratum corneum. The prognosis is good with proper foot care.

Causes and incidence

A corn (also known as a *clavus*) is a hyperkeratotic area that usually results from external pressure, such as that from ill-fitting shoes or, less commonly, from internal pressure, such as that caused by a protruding underlying bone (e.g., due to arthritis). A callus is an area of thickened skin, generally found on the foot or hand, produced by external pressure or friction. Persons whose activities produce repeated trauma (e.g., manual laborers or guitarists) commonly develop calluses.

The severity of a corn or callus depends on the degree and duration of trauma.

Pathophysiology

The body's protective response to abnormal shearing, pressure, or friction results in an increase of keratinocyte activity, creating an accumulation of the horny layer of epithelium. These hyperkeratotic lesions protect irritated skin.

Complication

◆ Secondary infection

Signs and symptoms

Both corns and calluses cause pain through pressure placed on underlying tissue by localized thickened skin. Corns contain a central keratinous core, are smaller and more clearly defined than calluses, and are usually more painful. The pain they cause may be dull and constant or sharp when pressure is applied. "Soft" corns are caused by the pressure of a bony prominence. They appear as whitish thickenings and are commonly found between the toes, most often in the fourth interdigital web. "Hard" corns are sharply delineated and conical and appear most frequently over the dorsolateral aspect of the fifth toe.

Calluses have indefinite borders and may be quite large. They usually produce dull pain on pressure, rather than constant pain. Although calluses commonly appear over plantar warts, they're distinguished from these warts by normal skin markings.

Diagnosis

Diagnosis depends on careful physical examination of the affected area and on patient history revealing chronic trauma.

Treatment

Surgical debridement may be performed to remove the nucleus of a corn, usually under a local anesthetic. In intermittent debridement, keratolytics—usually 40% salicylic acid

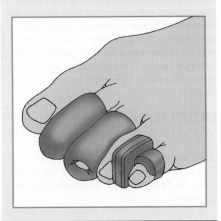
plasters—are applied to affected areas. Injections of corticosteroids beneath the corn may be necessary to relieve pain. However, the simplest and best treatment is essentially preventive—avoidance of trauma. Corns and calluses disappear after the source of trauma has been removed. Metatarsal pads may redistribute the weight-bearing areas of the foot; corn pads may prevent painful pressure. (See *Aids for relieving painful pressure*.)

Patients with persistent corns or calluses require referral to a podiatrist or dermatologist; those with corns or calluses caused by a bony malformation, as in arthritis, require orthopedic consultation.

Special considerations

◆ Teach the patient how to apply salicylic acid plasters. Make sure the plaster is large enough to cover the affected area. Place the sticky side down on the foot; then cover the plaster with adhesive tape. Plasters are usually taken off after an overnight application but may be left in place for as long as 7 days.

◆ After removing the plaster, the patient should soak the area in water and abrade the soft, macerated skin with a towel or pumice stone. The patient should then reapply the plaster and repeat the entire procedure until it has removed all the hyperkeratotic skin.

◆ Warn the patient against removing corns or calluses with a sharp instrument such as a razor blade.

!!!!! PREVENTION

◆ *Advise the patient to wear properly fitted shoes. Suggest the use of metatarsal or corn pads to relieve pressure. Refer to a podiatrist, dermatologist, or orthopedist, if necessary.*

◆ *Assure the patient that good foot care can correct this condition.*

◆ *Wear padded gloves when using hand tools.*

◆ *Keep hands and feet soft by applying moisturizer.*

PITYRIASIS ROSEA

An acute, self-limiting, inflammatory skin disease, pityriasis rosea usually produces a "herald" patch—which usually goes undetected—followed by a generalized eruption of papulosquamous lesions.

Causes and incidence

The cause of pityriasis rosea is unknown, but the brief course of the disease and the virtual absence of recurrence suggest a viral agent (herpes virus 7 is suspected) or an autoimmune disorder.

Although this noncontagious disorder may develop at any age, it's most apt to occur in adolescents and young adults. Incidence rises in the spring and fall. In the United States, less than 3% of people have this disease.

Pathophysiology

The pathophysiology of pityriasis rosea is not definitive but is thought to be a self-limiting papulosquamous disorder. An increase in CD4 lymphocytes and Langerhans cells in the dermis suggest a viral etiology.

Complication

◆ Secondary infection

Signs and symptoms

Pityriasis typically begins with an erythematous "herald" patch, which may appear anywhere on the body, although it occurs most commonly on the trunk. Although this slightly raised, oval lesion is about 2 to 6 cm in diameter, approximately 25% of patients don't notice it. A few days to several weeks later, yellow-tan or erythematous patches with scaly edges (about 0.5 to 1 cm in diameter) erupt on the trunk and extremities—and, rarely, on the face, hands, and feet in adolescents. Eruption continues for 7 to 10 days, and the patches persist for 2 to 6 weeks. Occasionally, these patches are macular, vesicular, or urticarial. A characteristic of this disease is the arrangement of lesions, which produces

Pressure points: Common sites of pressure ulcers

Pressure ulcers may develop in any of these pressure points. To prevent sores, reposition the patient every 1 to 2 hours, and carefully check for any change in the patient's skin tone.

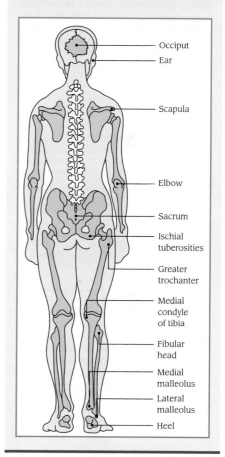

a pattern similar to that of a pine tree. Accompanying pruritus, if present, is usually mild but may be severe.

Diagnosis

Characteristic skin lesions support the diagnosis. Differential diagnosis must also rule out secondary syphilis (through serologic testing), dermatophytosis, and drug reaction.

Treatment

Treatment focuses on relief of pruritus, with emollients, oatmeal baths, antihistamines,

Pressure ulcer staging

The National Pressure Ulcer Advisory Panel has updated the staging of pressure ulcers to include the original four stages but also has added two other stages called *suspected deep tissue injury* and *unstageable.*

Suspected deep tissue injury

Suspected deep tissue injury involves maroon or purple intact skin or a blood-filled blister because of damage from shearing or pressure on the underlying soft tissue. Before the discoloration occurs, the area may be painful, mushy or firm or boggy, warmer or cooler as compared with other tissue.

Stage II

A stage II pressure ulcer is a superficial partial-thickness wound that presents clinically a shallow and open ulcer without slough and with a red and pink wound bed. This term shouldn't be used to describe perineal dermatitis, maceration, tape burns, skin tears or excoriation—only an abrasion, a blister, or a shallow crater that involves the epidermis and dermis.

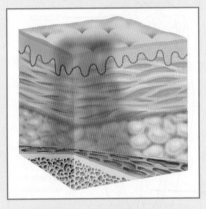

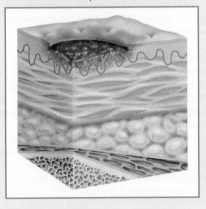

Stage I

A stage I pressure ulcer is an area of intact skin that does not blanch and is usually over a bony prominence. Skin that is darkly pigmented may not show blanching, but its color may differ from surrounding area. The area may be painful, firm or soft, or warmer or cooler when compared with the surrounding tissue.

Stage III

A stage III pressure ulcer is a full-thickness wound with tissue loss. The subcutaneous tissue may be visible, but muscle, tendon, and bone are not exposed. Slough may be present but it does not hide the depth of the tissue loss. Undermining and tunneling may be present.

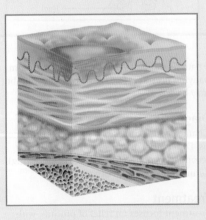

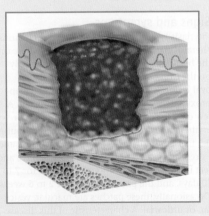

Stage IV
A stage IV pressure ulcer involves full-thickness skin loss with exposed muscle, bone, and tendon. Eschar and sloughing may be present as well as undermining and tunneling.

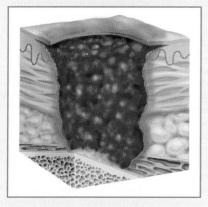

Unstageable
An unstageable pressure ulcer involves full-thickness tissue loss. The base of the ulcer is covered by yellow, tan, gray, green, or brown, slough or tan, brown, or black eschar. Some may have both slough and eschar. The pressure cannot be staged until enough eschar or slough is removed to expose the base of the wound.

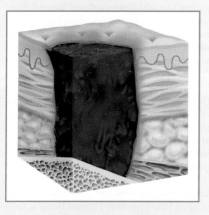

topical steroids, and occasionally exposure to UV light or sunlight. Rarely, if inflammation is severe, systemic corticosteroids may be required.

Special considerations
◆ Reassure the patient that pityriasis rosea isn't contagious, spontaneous remission usually occurs in 4 to 12 weeks, and lesions generally don't recur.
◆ Urge the patient not to scratch. Advise them to avoid hot baths because it may intensify itching. Encourage the use of antipruritics.

HYPERHIDROSIS
Primary hyperhidrosis is the excessive secretion of sweat from the eccrine glands. It usually occurs in the axillae (typically after puberty) and · on the palms and soles (often starting during infancy or childhood). Abnormal and excessive heat loss can occur, causing most patients to have body temperatures less than 98.6° F (37° C). In addition, secondary hyperhidrosis commonly occurs as a clinical manifestation of an underlying disorder.

Causes and incidence
Genetic factors may contribute to the development of primary hyperhidrosis and, in susceptible individuals, emotional stress appears to be the most prominent cause, although most patients aren't anxious. Increased central nervous system (CNS) impulses may provoke excessive release of acetylcholine, producing a heightened sweat response. Exercise and a hot climate can cause profuse sweating in these patients. Certain drugs (such as antipyretics, emetics, meperidine, and anticholinesterases) and certain foods (such as tomato sauce, chocolate, coffee, and spicy foods) have been known to increase sweating.

Secondary hyperhidrosis may be a result of infections; chronic diseases, such as tuberculosis, malaria, or lymphoma, may cause excessive nighttime sweating. A person with diabetes commonly demonstrates hyperhidrosis during a hypoglycemic crisis. Other predisposing conditions include hyperthyroidism; pheochromocytomas; cardiovascular disorders, such as shock or heart failure; CNS disturbances (generally lesions of the hypothalamus); withdrawal from drugs or alcohol; menopause; and Graves' disease.

Primary hyperhidrosis occurs in 2% to 3% of people in the United States.

Pathophysiology
In the anterior hypothalamus and preoptic areas in the brain are neurons that are sensitive to

temperatures. Sympathetic postganglionic fibers innervate through sweat glands with the chemical mediator acetylcholine triggering excessive sweating or hyperhidrosis.

Complication
◆ Fungal infections

Signs and symptoms
Axillary hyperhidrosis frequently produces such extreme sweating that patients often ruin their clothes in 1 day and develop contact dermatitis from clothing dyes; similarly, hyperhidrosis of the soles can easily damage a pair of shoes. Profuse sweating from both the soles and palms hinders the patient's ability to work and interact socially. Patients with this condition often report increased emotional strain.

Diagnosis
CONFIRMING DIAGNOSIS *Clinical observations and patient history confirm hyperhidrosis.*

Treatment
The treatment of choice is application of 20% aluminum chloride in absolute ethanol. (Most antiperspirants contain a 5% solution.) Formaldehyde may also be used but may lead to allergic contact sensitization. Glutaraldehyde produces less contact sensitivity than formaldehyde but stains the skin; it's used more often on the feet than on the hands, as a soak or applied directly several times a week and then weekly as needed. Botulinum toxin type A is helpful in temporarily blocking the nerves that stimulate sweating. It's injected in small doses in the axillae. It may cause side effects, such as pain at the injection site or flulike symptoms.

Iontophoresis (low-level electric current applied locally to skin surfaces) reduces sweat secretion at the site. Repeated treatments will be necessary for sustained relief.

Therapy sometimes includes anticholinergics, except in patients with glaucoma or prostatic hypertrophy. Severe hyperhidrosis unresponsive to conservative therapy may require local axillary removal of sweat glands or, as a last resort, an endoscopic thoracic sympathectomy, which stops the signal for excessive sweating. The procedure is performed under general anesthesia.

Special considerations
◆ Provide support and reassurance because hyperhidrosis may be socially embarrassing.
◆ Tell the patient to apply aluminum chloride in absolute ethanol nightly to dry axillae, soles, or palms. The area should be covered with plastic wrap for 6 to 8 hours, preferably overnight, then washed with soap and water. Tell him to repeat this procedure for several nights, until profuse daytime sweating subsides. Frequency of treatments can then be reduced.
◆ Advise the patient with hyperhidrosis of the soles to wear leather sandals and white or colorfast cotton socks.

PRESSURE ULCERS
Pressure ulcers, commonly called *pressure sores* or *bedsores*, are localized areas of cellular necrosis that occur most often in the skin and subcutaneous tissue over bony prominences. These ulcers may be superficial, caused by local skin irritation with subsequent surface maceration, or deep, originating in underlying tissue. Deep lesions typically go undetected until they penetrate the skin; but, by then, they've usually caused subcutaneous damage.

Causes and incidence
Most pressure ulcers are caused by pressure, particularly over bony prominences, that interrupts normal circulatory function, leading to ischemia of the underlying structures of skin, fat, and muscles. (See *Pressure points: Common sites of pressure ulcers,* page 697.) The intensity and duration of such pressure govern the severity of the ulcer; pressure exerted over an area for a moderate period (1 to 2 hours) produces tissue ischemia and increased capillary pressure, leading to edema and multiple small-vessel thrombosis. An inflammatory reaction gives way to ulceration and necrosis of ischemic cells. In turn, necrotic tissue predisposes to bacterial invasion and subsequent infection.

The patient's position determines the pressure exerted on the tissues. For example, if the head of the bed is elevated, or the patient assumes a slumped position, gravity pulls the patient's weight downward and forward. This shearing force causes deep ulcers because of ischemic changes in the muscles and subcutaneous tissues and occurs most often over the sacrum and ischial tuberosities.

Predisposing conditions for pressure ulcers include altered mobility, inadequate nutrition (leading to weight loss, subsequent reduction of subcutaneous tissue and muscle bulk and, possibly, a poorly functioning immune system), and a breakdown in skin or subcutaneous tissue (as a result of edema, incontinence, fever, pathologic conditions, or obesity).

Pressure ulcers occur in 10% to 17% of all hospitalized patients and 20% to 40% of all nursing home patients. Patients living at home aren't free from risk, either: 20% of all pressure

PREVENTION

Preventing pressure ulcers

Prevent pressure ulcers by repositioning the bedridden patient at least every 2 hours around the clock. To minimize the effects of a shearing force, use a footboard and raise the head of the bed to an angle not exceeding 60°. Also, use a draw or pull sheet to turn the patient or to pull the patient up. Keep the patient's knees slightly flexed for short periods. Perform passive range-of-motion exercises or encourage the patient to do active exercises if possible.

Pressure relief aids

To prevent pressure ulcers in immobilized patients, use pressure relief aids on their beds.

♦ *Gel flotation pads* disperse pressure over a greater skin surface area; they are convenient and adaptable for home and wheelchair use.

♦ *Alternating pressure mattress* contains tubelike sections, running lengthwise, that deflate and reinflate, changing areas of pressure. Use mattress with a single untucked sheet because layers of linen decrease its effectiveness.

♦ *Convoluted foam mattress* minimizes area of skin pressure with its alternating areas of depression and elevation: soft, elevated foam areas cushion skin; depressed areas relieve pressure. This mattress should be used with a single, loosely tucked sheet and is adaptable for home and wheelchair use. If the patient is incontinent, cover the mattress with the provided plastic sleeve.

♦ *Spenco mattress* has polyester fibers with silicone tubes to decrease pressure without limiting the patient's position. It has no weight limitations.

♦ *Sheepskin* is soft, dry, absorbent, and easy to clean. It should be in direct contact with the patient's skin. It's available in sizes to fit elbows and heels and is adaptable for home use.

♦ *Air-fluidized bed* supports the patient at a subcapillary pressure point and provides a warm, relaxing, therapeutic airflow. It eliminates friction and maceration.

♦ *Low air-loss beds*, such as Flexicare and Accucare, slow the drying of any saline soaks, and elderly patients often experience less disorientation than with high air-loss beds. The head of the bed can be elevated so there's less chance of aspiration, especially in patients who require tube feeding. Patients can get out of bed more easily on low air-loss surfaces.

Skin care

Provide meticulous skin care. Keep the skin clean and dry without the use of harsh soaps. Gently massaging the skin around the affected area—not on it—promotes healing. Thoroughly rub moisturizing lotions into the skin to prevent maceration

of the skin surface. Change bed linens frequently for patients who are diaphoretic or incontinent. Use a fecal incontinence bag for incontinent patients.

Skin-damaging agents to avoid include:
♦ harsh alkaline soaps
♦ alcohol-based products (can cause vasoconstriction)
♦ tincture of benzoin (may cause painful erosions)
♦ hexachlorophene (may irritate the CNS)
♦ petroleum gauze.

Topical dressings

Types of topical dressings that aid in prevention and treatment of pressure ulcers include:
♦ transparent films
♦ hydrocolloid dressings
♦ hydrogel dressings
♦ foam dressings
♦ calcium alginate dressings
♦ gauze dressings.

Special considerations

♦ During each shift, check the skin of bedridden patients for possible changes in color, turgor, temperature, and sensation. Examine an existing ulcer for any change in size or degree of damage. When using pressure relief aids or topical agents, explain their function to the patient.

♦ Clean open lesions with normal saline solution. Dressings, if needed, should be porous and lightly taped to healthy skin. Debridement of necrotic tissue may be necessary to allow healing. One method is to apply open wet dressings and allow them to dry on the ulcer. Removal of the dressings mechanically debrides exudate and necrotic tissue. Other methods include surgical debridement with a fine scalpel blade and chemical debridement using proteolytic enzyme agents.

♦ Encourage adequate intake of food and fluids to maintain body weight and promote healing. Consult with the dietary department to provide a diet that promotes granulation of new tissue. Encourage the debilitated patient to eat frequent, small meals that are rich in protein, iron, calories, and vitamin C to promote healing. Assist weakened patients with their meals.

ulcers occur in the home. In the United States, there are approximately 2 million new cases of pressure ulcers diagnosed every year.

Pathophysiology

When immobility is a factor for an extended period, external pressure on bony prominences can cause a disruption in circulation to tissues. The decrease in circulation to a particular area creates hypoxic tissue damage and eventually necrosis. The duration of pressure to cause tissue ischemia varies greatly for each patient depending on their overall state of health.

Complications

◆ Bacteremia
◆ Fluid and electrolyte loss
◆ Septicemia

Signs and symptoms

Pressure ulcers commonly develop over bony prominences. Early features of superficial lesions are shiny, erythematous changes over the compressed area, caused by localized vasodilation when pressure is relieved. Superficial erythema progresses to small blisters or erosions and, ultimately, to necrosis and ulceration.

An inflamed area on the skin's surface may be the first sign of underlying damage when pressure is exerted between deep tissue and bone. Bacteria in a compressed site cause inflammation and, eventually, infection, which leads to further necrosis. A foul-smelling, purulent discharge may seep from a lesion that penetrates the skin from beneath. Infected, necrotic tissue prevents healthy granulation of scar tissue; a black eschar may develop around and over the lesion. (See *Pressure ulcer staging*, pages 698 and 699.)

Diagnosis

Pressure ulcers are obvious on physical examination. Wound culture and sensitivity testing of the exudate in the ulcer identify infecting organisms and antibiotics that may be needed. If severe hypoproteinemia is suspected, total serum protein values and serum albumin studies may be appropriate.

Treatment

Successful treatment must relieve pressure on the affected area, keep the area clean and dry, and promote healing. (See *Preventing pressure ulcers*.)

SELECTED REFERENCES

Asai, Y., et al. (2016, February 2). Management of acne: Canadian clinical practice guideline. *Canadian Medical Association Journal, 188*(2), 118–126. doi:10.1503/cmaj.140665

Atkin, L. (2016). Cellulitis of the lower limbs: Incidence, diagnosis and management. *Wounds UK, 12*(2), 38–41.

Baldwin, H., et al. (2018, February). Best practices in the treatment of rosacea. *Dermatology Times*, 3–12.

Banasikowska, A. K. (2017). *Rosacea.* Retrieved from https://emedicine.medscape.com/article/1071429-overview

Bohl, B., et al. (2015, September–October). Clinical practice update: Pediculosis capitis. *Pediatric Nursing, 41*(5), 227–234.

Brodsky, J. (2009). Management of benign skin lesions commonly affecting the face: Actinic keratosis, seborrheic keratosis, and rosacea. *Current Opinion in Otolaryngology and Head and Neck Surgery, 17*(4), 315–320.

Cabrera, G., & Karakashian, A. L. (2017, October 27). Pediculosis (Lice infestation). *CINAHL Nursing Guide.*

Cantrell, W. (2017, July). Psoriasis & psoriatic therapies. *The Nurse Practitioner, 42*(7), 35–39. doi:10.1097/01.NPR.0000520419.09460.ad

Casey, G. (2016, April). Disorders of the skin. *Kai Tiaki Nursing New Zealand, 22*(20–24), 20–24.

Cohen, V. (2017). *Toxic epidermal necrolysis (TEN).* Retrieved from https://emedicine.medscape.com/article/229698-overview

Crouse, L. N. (2017). *Tinea versicolor.* Retrieved from https://emedicine.medscape.com/article/1091575-overview#a5

Dowsett, C., & Hallern, B. V. (2017). The triangle of wound assessment: A holistic framework from wound assessment to management goals and treatments. *Wounds International, 8*(4), 34–39.

Dressler, C., et al. (2016). The treatment of scabies a systemic review of randomized controlled trials. *Deutsches Arzteblatt International, 113*, 757–762. doi:10.3238/arztebl.2016.0757

Dudley, M., & Parsh, B. (2016, December). Recognizing staphylococcal scalded skin syndrome. *Nursing, 46*(12), 68. doi:10.1097/01.NURSE.0000504683.43755.18

Ely, J. W., et al. (2014, November 15). Diagnosis and management of tinea infections. *American Family Physician, 90*, 702–711.

Gawkrodger, D., et al. (2010). Vitiligo: Concise evidence based guidelines on diagnosis and management. *Postgraduate Medical Journal, 86*(1018), 466–471.

Ghadishah, D. (2016). *Genital warts.* Retrieved from https://emedicine.medscape.com/article/763014-overview

Goman, T. (2017). Identifying the different clinical presentation of psoriasis. *Journal of Community Nursing, 31*(2), 57–60.

Goman, T. (2017). Use of emollients in psoriasis management. *Journal of Community Nursing, 31*(3), 43–48.

Goman, T. (2017). Use of topical treatments in psoriasis management. *Journal of Community Nursing, 31*(5), 58–67.

Guenther, L. C. (2018). *Pediculosis and pthiriasis (lice infestation).* Retrieved from https://emedicine.medscape.com/article/225013-overview

Gupta, S., & Jawanda, M. K. (2015). Oral lichen planus: An update on etiology, pathogenesis, clinical presentation, diagnosis and management. *Indian Journal of Dermatology, 60*(3), 222–229. doi:10.4103/0019-5154.156315

Hashmi, F., et al. (2016). The evaluation of three treatments for plantar callus: A three-armed randomized comparative trial using biophysical outcome measures. *Trials, 17*, 1–11. doi:10.1186/s13063-016-1377-2

Ibler, K. S., & Kromann, C. B. (2014, February 18). Recurrent furunculosis—Challenges and management: A review. *Clinical, Cosmetic and Investigational Dermatology, 7*, 59–64. doi:10.2147/CCID.S35302

Kim, S. Y., & Ochsendorf, F. R. (2016, October 3). New Developments in acne treatment: Role of combination adapalene-benzoylperoxide. *Therapeutics and Clinical Risk Management, 12*, 1497–1506. doi:10.2147/TCRM.S49062

King, R. W. (2017). *Staphylococcal scaled skin syndrome (SSSS)*. Retrieved from https://emedicine.medscape.com/article/788199-overview#a5

Kong, Y. L., et al. (2017). Retrospective study on the characteristics and treatment of late-onset vitiligo. *Indian Journal of Dermatology, Venereology, and Leprology, 83,* 624. doi:10.4103/ijdvl.IJDVL_650_16

Lawton, S. (2017, May). Fungal skin infections: When patients present with a skin infection, it is important to correctly identify the condition through detailed history taking, thorough examination and appropriate investigations to ensure they are offered the right treatment. *Practice Nurse, 47*(5), 12–16.

Lewis, L. S. (2017). *Impetigo*. Retrieved from https://emedicine.medscape.com/article/965254-overview#a1

Lyford, W. H. (2017). *Melasma*. Retrieved from https://emedicine.medscape.com/article/1068640-overview

McPherson, T. (2016). Current understanding in pathogenesis of atopic dermatitis. *Indian Journal of Dermatology, 61*(6), 649–655. doi:10.4103/0019-5154.193674

Nalluri, R., & Harries, M. (2016). Alopecia in general medicine. *Royal College of Physicians, 16*(1), 74–78.

Nguyen, J., et al. (2016, September). Laser treatment of nongenital verrucae. *JAMA Dermatology, 152,* 1025–1033. doi:10.1001/jamadermatol.2016.0826

Nolan, J., et al. (2010). A review of home phototherapy for psoriasis. *Dermatology Online Journal, 16*(2), 1.

Norbury, W. (2010). Neonate twin with staphylococcal scalded skin syndrome from a renal source. *Pediatric Critical Care Medicine, 11*(2), e20–e23.

Pate, C. (2015). Issues faced by women with hirsutism: State of the science. *Health Care for Women International, 37,* 636–645. doi:10.1080/07399332.2015.1078805

Payne, D. (2017, August). Not just a childhood disease: Treating atopic dermatitis in older people. *British Journal of Community Nursing, 22,* 370–373. doi:10.12968/bjcn.2017.22.8.370

Plensdorf, S., et al. (2017). Pigmentation disorders: Diagnosis and management. *American Family Physician, 96*(12), 797–804.

Robles, D. T. (2017). *Cutaneous larva migrans*. Retrieved from https://emedicine.medscape.com/article/1108784-overview#a5

Roncone, K. (2017). *Vitiligo*. Retrieved from https://emedicine.medscape.com/article/1068962

Sacchidanand, S. A., et al. (2017, July–August). Synchronizing pharmacotherapy in acne with review of clinical care. *Indian Journal of Dermatology, 62,* 341–357. doi:10.4103/ijd.IJD_41_17

Satter, E. K. (2017). *Folliculitis*. Retrieved from https://emedicine.medscape.com/article/1070456-overview#a5

Sharma, J., et al. (2018, January–February). A comparative study of efficacy and safety of eberconazole versus terbinafine in patients of tinea versicolor. *Indian Journal of Dermatology, 63*(1), 53–56. doi:10.4103/ijd.IJD_126_17

Shenefelt, P. D. (2017). *Nongenital warts*. Retrieved from https://emedicine.medscape.com/article/1133317-overview

Siddalingappa, K., et al. (2015, September/October). Cutaneous larva migrans in early infancy. *Indian Journal of Dermatology, 60*(5), 49. doi:10.4103/0019-5154.164436

Sinha, S., et al. (2015). Immunomodulators in warts: Unexplored or ineffective. *Indian Journal of Dermatology, 60*(2), 118–129. doi:10.4103/0019-5154.152502

Teo, Y. X., & Walsh, S. A. (2016). Severe adverse drug reactions. *Clinical Medicine, 16*(1), 79–83.

van Zuuren, E. J., & Fedorowicz, Z. (2015). Interventions for hirsutism. *JAMA: Journal of the American Medical Association, 314,* 1863–1864. doi:10.1001/jama.2015.11743

VanRavenstein, K., & Edlund, B. J. (2017). Diagnosis and management of pityriasis rosacea. *Nurse Practitioner, 42*(1), 8–11. doi:10.1097/01.NPR.0000511012.21714.66

Walker, S., et al. (2010). Pressure ulcer prevention: Utilizing unlicensed assistive personnel. *Critical Care Nursing Quarterly, 33*(4), 348–355.

Watkins, J. (2015). Understanding and treating hyperhidrosis. *Practice Nursing, 26*(6), 295–297.

Zhang, A. Y. (2017). *Drug-induced photosensitivity*. Retrieved from https://emedicine.medscape.com/article/1049648-overview

15

MALIGNANT NEOPLASMS

Introduction

Mainly a disease of older adults, cancer is second to cardiovascular disease as the leading cause of death in the United States (>600,920 deaths annually). More than 70% of patients who die of cancer are older than age 65. The most common cancers in men in the United States are prostate, lung, and colorectal, and the leading causes of cancer death are lung, prostate, colorectal, and liver. The most common cancers in women in the United States are breast, lung, and colorectal, and the leading causes of cancer death are lung, breast, and colorectal.

Cancer results from a malignant transformation (carcinogenesis) of normal cells. (See *Histologic characteristics of cancer cells*, page 705.) Cancer cells proliferate uncontrollably, thus establishing themselves at other tissues to form secondary foci (metastasis). Cancer cells in malignant tumors differ from those in benign tumors, and they serve no useful purpose. (See *Comparing benign and malignant tumors*, page 705.) Cancer cells metastasize via circulation through the blood or lymphatics, by unintentional transplantation from one site to another during surgery, and by local extension. (See *How cancer metastasizes*, page 706.)

Classified by their histologic origin, tumors derived from epithelial tissues are called *carcinomas*; from epithelial and glandular tissues, *adenocarcinomas*; from connective, muscle, and bone tissues, *sarcomas*; from glial cells, *gliomas*; from pigmented cells, *melanomas*; and from plasma cells, *myelomas*. Cancer cells derived from erythrocytes are known as *erythroleukemia*; from lymphocytes, *leukemia*; and from lymphatic tissue, *lymphoma*.

WHAT CAUSES CANCER?

Cancer develops from mutations within the genes of cells. Thus, cancer is a genetic disease. Cancer susceptibility genes are of two types. Some are *oncogenes*, which activate cell division and influence embryonic development, and some are *tumor suppressor genes*, which halt cell division.

These genes are typically found in normal human cells, but certain kinds of mutations may transform the normal cells. Inherited defects may cause a *genetic mutation*, whereas repeated exposure to a carcinogen may cause an *acquired mutation*. Current evidence indicates that carcinogenesis results from a complex interaction of carcinogens and accumulated mutations in several genes.

In animal studies of the ability of viruses to transform cells, some human viruses exhibit carcinogenic potential. For example, the Epstein–Barr virus (EBV), the cause of infectious mononucleosis, has been linked to Burkitt lymphoma and nasopharyngeal cancer.

High-frequency radiation, such as ultraviolet and ionizing radiation, damages *deoxyribonucleic acid (DNA)*, possibly inducing genetically transferable abnormalities. Other factors, such as a person's tissue type and hormonal status,

Histologic characteristics of cancer cells

Cancer is a destructive (malignant) growth of cells, which invades nearby tissues and may metastasize to other areas of the body. Dividing rapidly, cancer cells tend to be extremely aggressive.

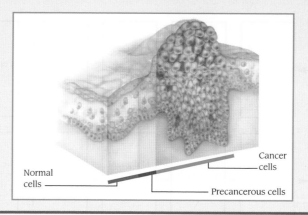

Normal cells

Precancerous cells

Cancer cells

Comparing benign and malignant tumors

Factor	Benign	Malignant
Differentiation	Well differentiated	Variable
Effect on body	Cachexia rare; usually not fatal but may obstruct vital organs, exert pressure, produce excess hormones; can become malignant	Cachexia typical, with such symptoms as anemia, loss of weight, and weakness; fatal if untreated
Growth	Slow expansion; push aside surrounding tissue but don't infiltrate	Usually infiltrate surrounding tissues rapidly, expanding in all directions
Limitation	Commonly encapsulated	Seldom encapsulated; in many cases poorly delineated
Mitotic activity	Variable	Extensive
Morphology	Cells closely resemble cells of tissue of origin	Cells may differ considerably from those of tissue of origin
Recurrence	Rare after surgical removal	When removed only by surgery, commonly recur due to infiltration into surrounding tissues
Spread	No metastasis	Spread via blood and lymph systems; establish secondary tumors
Tissue destruction	Usually slight	Extensive due to infiltration and metastatic lesion

PATHOPHYSIOLOGY
How cancer metastasizes

Metastasis usually occurs through the bloodstream to other organs and tissues, as shown here.

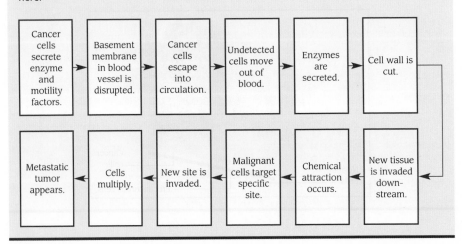

interact to potentiate radiation's carcinogenic effect. Examples of substances that may damage DNA and induce carcinogenesis include:
◆ alkylating agents—leukemia
◆ aromatic hydrocarbons and benzopyrene (from polluted air)—lung cancer
◆ asbestos—mesothelioma of the lung
◆ tobacco—cancer of the lung, oral cavity and upper airways, esophagus, pancreas, kidneys, and bladder
◆ vinyl chloride—angiosarcoma of the liver

Diet can also be a factor, especially in the development of gastrointestinal (GI) cancer as a result of a high animal fat diet. Additives composed of nitrates and certain methods of food preparation—particularly charbroiling—are also recognized factors.

The role of hormones in carcinogenesis is still controversial, but it seems that excessive use of some hormones, especially estrogen, produces cancer in animals. Also, the synthetic estrogen diethylstilbestrol (DES) causes vaginal cancer in some daughters of women who were treated with it. It's unclear, however, whether changes in human hormonal balance retard or stimulate cancer development.

Some forms of cancer and precancerous lesions result from genetic predisposition either directly (as in Wilms tumor and retinoblastoma) or indirectly (in association with inherited conditions such as Down syndrome

or immunodeficiency diseases). Expressed as autosomal recessive, X-linked, or autosomal dominant disorders, their common characteristics include:
◆ early onset of malignant disease
◆ increased incidence of bilateral cancer in paired organs (breasts, adrenal glands, kidneys, and eighth cranial nerve [acoustic neuroma])
◆ increased incidence of multiple primary malignancies in nonpaired organs
◆ abnormal chromosome complement in tumor cells

IMMUNE RESPONSE

Other factors that interact to increase susceptibility to carcinogenesis are immunologic competence, age, nutritional status, hormonal balance, and response to stress. Presumably, the body develops cancer cells continuously, but the immune system recognizes them as foreign cells and destroys them. This defense mechanism, known as *immunosurveillance*, has two major components: humoral immune response and cell-mediated immune response. Their interaction promotes antibody production, cellular immunity, and immunologic memory. Thus, the intact human immune system is responsible for spontaneous regression of tumors.

Theoretically, the *cell-mediated immune response* begins when T lymphocytes become sensitized by contact with a specific antigen.

After repeated contacts, sensitized T cells release chemical factors called *lymphokines*, some of which begin to destroy the antigen. This reaction triggers the transformation of an additional population of T lymphocytes into "killers" of antigen-specific cells—in this case, cancer cells.

Similarly, the *humoral immune response* reacts to an antigen by triggering the release of antibodies from plasma cells and activating the serum complement system, which destroys the antigen-bearing cell. However, an opposing immune factor, a "blocking antibody," enhances tumor growth by protecting malignant cells from immune destruction.

Cancer may arise when any one of several factors disrupts the immune system:

◆ Aging cells, when copying their genetic material, may begin to err, giving rise to mutations. The aging immune system may not recognize these mutations as foreign and thus may allow them to proliferate and form a malignant tumor.

◆ Cytotoxic drugs decrease antibody production and destroy circulating lymphocytes.

◆ Extreme stress or certain viral infections can depress the immune system.

◆ Increased susceptibility to infection commonly results from radiation, cytotoxic drug therapy, and lymphoproliferative and myeloproliferative diseases, such as lymphatic and myelocytic leukemia. These cause bone marrow depression, which can impair leukocyte function.

◆ Acquired immunodeficiency syndrome (AIDS) weakens cell-mediated immunity.

◆ Cancer itself is immunosuppressive; advanced cancer exhausts the immune response. (The absence of immune reactivity is known as *anergy*.)

DIAGNOSTIC METHODS

A thorough medical history and physical examination should be done before diagnostic procedures. Useful tests for the early detection and staging of tumors include X-ray, endoscopy, isotope scan, computed tomography (CT) scan, and magnetic resonance imaging (MRI), but the single most important diagnostic tool is a biopsy for direct histologic study of tumor tissue. Biopsy tissue samples can be taken by curettage, fluid aspiration (pleural effusion), fine needle aspiration biopsy (breast), dermal punch (skin or mouth), endoscopy (rectal polyps), and surgical excision (visceral tumors and nodes).

An important tumor marker, carcinogenic embryonic antigen (CEA), although nonspecific and not diagnostic by itself, can signal malignancies of the large bowel, stomach, pancreas, lungs, and breasts. CEA titers range from normal (<5 ng) to suspicious (5 to 10 ng) to suspect (>10 ng). CEA serves many valuable purposes:

◆ as a baseline during chemotherapy to evaluate the extent of tumor spread

◆ to regulate drug dosage

◆ to prognosticate after surgery or radiation

◆ to detect tumor recurrence

Although no more specific than CEA, alpha-fetoprotein—a fetal antigen uncommon in adults—can suggest testicular, ovarian, gastric, and hepatocellular cancers. Beta-human chorionic gonadotropin may point to testicular cancer or choriocarcinoma. Other commonly used tumor markers include prostate-specific antigen (PSA) to detect and monitor prostatic cancer, and CA-125, useful for monitoring ovarian, colorectal, and gastric cancers.

STAGING AND GRADING

Choosing effective therapeutic options depends on correct *staging* of malignant disease, commonly with the TNM staging system (*t*umor size, *n*odal involvement, *m*etastatic progress). This classification system provides an accurate tumor description that's adjustable as the disease progresses. TNM staging allows reliable comparison of treatments and survival rates among large population groups; it also identifies nodal involvement and metastasis to other areas.

Grading, another way to define a tumor, classifies the lesion according to corresponding normal cells, such as lymphoid or mucinous lesions; it compares tumor tissue to normal cells (differentiation); and it estimates the tumor's growth rate. For example, a low-grade tumor typically has cells more closely resembling normal cells, whereas a high-grade tumor has poorly differentiated cells.

FIVE MAJOR THERAPIES

Cancer treatments include surgery, radiation, chemotherapy, biotherapy (also called *immunotherapy*), and hormonal therapy. Therapies may be used alone or in combination, depending on the type, stage, localization, and responsiveness of the tumor and on limitations imposed by the patient's clinical status.

Surgery, the mainstay of cancer treatment, is often combined with other therapies. Surgery may be performed as a biopsy to obtain tissue for study; as continued surgery to remove the bulk of the tumor; or before chemotherapy or radiation to debulk the tumor in hope of a better outcome. Surgery can be curative as well. Other therapies may be used later to discourage proliferation of residual cells.

Surgery can also relieve pain, correct obstruction, and alleviate pressure. Current, less radical surgical procedures (such as lumpectomy instead of radical mastectomy) are often as effective as radical procedures and are better tolerated by patients.

Radiation therapy aims to destroy the dividing cancer cells while damaging nonmalignant cells as little as possible. Therapeutic radiation is either particulate or electromagnetic. Both types ionize matter and have cellular DNA as their target.

Radiation treatment approaches include external beam radiation and intracavitary and interstitial implants. The latter therapy requires personal radiation protection for all staff members who come in contact with the patient.

Normal and malignant cells respond to radiation differently, depending on blood supply, oxygen saturation, previous irradiation, and immune status. Generally, normal cells recover from radiation faster than malignant cells. The success of the treatment and damage to normal tissue also vary with the intensity of the radiation. Although a large single dose of radiation has greater cellular effects than fractions of the same amount delivered sequentially, a protracted schedule allows time for normal tissue to recover in the intervals between individual sublethal doses.

Radiation may be used palliatively to relieve or reduce pain, obstruction, malignant effusions, cough, dyspnea, ulcerations, and hemorrhage; it can also promote the repair of pathologic fractures after surgical stabilization and delay tumor spread.

Combining radiation and surgery can minimize radical surgery, prolong survival, and preserve anatomic function. For example, preoperative doses of radiation shrink a tumor, making it operable, while preventing further spread of the disease during surgery. After the wound heals, postoperative doses prevent residual cancer cells from multiplying or metastasizing.

Systemic adverse effects, such as weakness, fatigue, anorexia, nausea, vomiting, and anemia, may subside with antiemetics, steroids, frequent small meals, fluid maintenance, and rest. They are seldom severe enough to require discontinuing radiation but may require a dosage adjustment. (For localized adverse effects, see *Radiation's adverse effects*, page 709.)

Radiation therapy requires frequent blood counts (particularly of white blood cells [WBCs] and platelets), especially if the target site involves areas of bone marrow production. Radiation also requires special skin care, such as covering the irradiated area with loose cotton clothing and avoiding deodorants, colognes, and other topical agents during treatment. (See *How to prepare the patient for external radiation therapy*, page 709.)

Chemotherapy includes a wide array of drugs, which may induce regression of a tumor and its metastasis. It's particularly useful in controlling residual disease and, as an adjunct to surgery or radiation therapy, it can induce long remissions and sometimes effect cures, especially in patients with childhood leukemia, Hodgkin lymphoma (HL), choriocarcinoma, or testicular cancer. As a palliative treatment, chemotherapy aims to improve the patient's quality of life by temporarily relieving pain and other symptoms.

Some major chemotherapeutic agents include:

◆ alkylating agents and nitrosoureas, which inhibit cell growth and division by reacting with DNA

◆ antimetabolites, which prevent cell growth by competing with metabolites in the production of nucleic acid

◆ antitumor antibiotics, which block cell growth by binding with DNA and interfering with DNA-dependent ribonucleic acid synthesis

◆ plant alkaloids, which prevent cellular reproduction by disrupting cell mitosis

◆ steroid hormones, which inhibit the growth of hormone-susceptible tumors by changing their chemical environment

The adverse effects of chemotherapy vary. Antineoplastic agents, toxic to cancer cells, can also cause transient changes in normal tissues, especially among proliferating body cells. Antineoplastic agents typically suppress bone marrow, causing anemia, leukopenia, and thrombocytopenia; irritate GI epithelial cells, causing nausea and vomiting; and destroy the cells of the hair follicles and skin, causing alopecia and dermatitis. Some chemotherapy drugs can also have permanent effects such as peripheral neuropathy.

Some I.V. chemotherapy drugs are irritants; others are vesicants. Irritants can cause pain at the injection site and along the vein but usually don't cause tissue necrosis. However, vesicants, when extravasated, may cause deep cutaneous necrosis requiring debridement and skin grafting. (*Note:* Most drugs with the potential for direct tissue injury are now given through a central venous catheter.)

Therefore, all patients undergoing chemotherapy need special care:

▼ ALERT *Watch for signs of infection, especially if the patient is receiving simultaneous radiation treatment. Take the patient's temperature often*

Radiation's adverse effects

Area radiated	Effect	Management
Abdomen and pelvis	Cramps, diarrhea, nausea	Administer loperamide and diphenoxylate with atropine. Provide a low-residue diet. Maintain fluid and electrolyte balance. Administer antiemetics as ordered.
Chest	Esophagitis	Give pain medication. Provide total parenteral nutrition or tube feedings. Maintain fluid balance.
	Lung tissue irritation, persistent nonproductive cough	Explain the importance of not smoking and of avoiding people with upper respiratory infections. Provide steroid therapy as indicated. Provide humidifier if necessary. Administer cough suppressants as indicated.
	Pericarditis, myocarditis	Give antiarrhythmics, such as procainamide, disopyramide, and phosphate, as indicated. Monitor for heart failure.
Head and neck	Alopecia	Gently comb and groom scalp. Use a soft head covering.
	Dental caries	Apply fluoride to teeth prophylactically, encourage use of fluoride mouth rinses, and provide gingival care.
	Mucositis	Provide a nonalcohol-based mouthwash with viscous lidocaine; cool carbonated drinks; ice pops; and a soft, nonirritating diet. Use soft toothbrushes or swabs. Avoid spicy food and alcohol.
	Xerostomia (dry mouth)	Encourage good oral hygiene. Consider prescribing an oral saliva replacement. Moist foods are better tolerated than dry foods.
Kidneys	Nephritis, lassitude, headache, edema, dyspnea, hypertensive nephropathy, azotemia, anemia	Maintain fluid and electrolyte balance, and watch for signs of renal failure (such as decreased urine output, peripheral edema). Consider prescribing erythropoietin.

How to prepare the patient for external radiation therapy

✦ Show the patient where radiation therapy takes place, and introduce the patient to the radiation therapist.

✦ Tell the patient to remove all metal objects (pens, buttons, and jewelry) that may interfere with therapy. Explain that the areas to be treated will be marked with indelible ink and that *they must not scrub these areas* because it's important to radiate the same areas each time.

✦ Reinforce the practitioner's explanation of the procedure, and answer any questions as honestly as you can. If you don't know the answer to a question, refer the patient to the practitioner.

✦ Teach the patient to watch for and report any adverse effects. Because radiation therapy may increase susceptibility to infection, warn the patient to avoid people with colds or other infections during therapy. However, emphasize the benefits (such as outpatient treatment) instead of the adverse effects.

✦ Reassure the patient that treatment is painless and won't make the patient radioactive. Stress that he or she will be under constant surveillance during radiation administration and should call out if they need anything.

and be alert for even a low-grade fever when the granulocyte count falls below 500/µL.

◆ Increase the patient's fluid intake before and throughout chemotherapy.

◆ Inform the patient of possible temporary hair loss, and reassure the patient that hair should grow back after therapy ends. Suggest a wig or other head covering, and encourage the patient to purchase it before the hair loss.

◆ Check skin for petechiae, ecchymosis, chemical cellulitis, and secondary infection during treatment.

◆ Minimize tissue irritation and damage by checking needle placement before and during infusion if you administer the drug by a peripheral vein. Tell the patient to report any discomfort during infusion. If a vesicant extravasates, stop the infusion, aspirate the drug from the needle, and give the appropriate antidote if available.

Chemotherapeutic drugs can be given orally, subcutaneously, I.M., I.V., intracavitarily, intrathecally, intraperitoneally, topically, intralesionally, and by arterial infusion, depending on the drug and its pharmacologic action; usually, administration is intermittent to allow for bone marrow recovery between doses. Dosages are calculated according to the patient's body surface area, with adjustments for general condition, degree of myelosuppression, and weight changes.

Because many patients approach chemotherapy with apprehension, allow them to express their concerns, and provide simple, truthful information. Explain that not all patients who undergo chemotherapy experience nausea and vomiting and, for those who do, antiemetic drugs, relaxation therapy, and diet can minimize these problems.

Biotherapy (also known as *immunotherapy*) utilizes agents called *biological response modifiers*. Biological agents are usually combined with chemotherapeutic drugs or radiation therapy. Much of the work done in biotherapy is still experimental. However, the Food and Drug Administration (FDA) has approved several new drugs, which are providing promising results. For example, rituximab—a monoclonal antibody—is effective for treatment of relapsed or refractory B-cell non-Hodgkin lymphoma.

The main biotherapy agent classifications include *interferons, interleukins, hematopoietic growth factors,* and *monoclonal antibodies.* Interferons have antiviral, antiproliferative, and immunomodulatory effects. The interleukins exert their effects on the T lymphocytes. Monoclonal antibodies such as rituximab provide the most tumor-specific therapy for cancer by selectively binding to tumor cell surfaces.

Although not used to treat cancer directly, hematopoietic growth factors are used to increase the patient's blood counts when chemotherapy or radiation causes a decrease.

The adverse effects of biotherapeutic agents mimic the body's normal immune response with flulike symptoms being the most common.

Hormonal therapy is based on studies showing that certain hormones affect the growth of certain cancer types. For example, the gonadotropin-releasing hormone analogue leuprolide is used to treat prostate cancer. With long-term use, this hormone inhibits testosterone release and tumor growth; tamoxifen, an antiestrogen hormonal agent, blocks estrogen receptors in breast tumor cells that require estrogen to thrive. Additionally, tamoxifen can be given prophylactically to women at high risk for breast cancer.

Hormone-receptive tumors may be treated with aromatase inhibitors (anastrozole, exemestane, letrozole, and testolactone), which inhibit the conversion of adrenal androgens to estrogens, thereby inhibiting the growth of hormone-dependent tumors.

Some adverse effects of these hormonal agents include hot flashes, sweating, impotence, decreased libido, nausea and vomiting, and blood dyscrasias (with tamoxifen).

MAINTAINING NUTRITION AND FLUID BALANCE

Tumors grow at the expense of normal tissue by competing for nutrients; consequently, the cancer patient commonly suffers protein deficiency. Cancer treatments themselves produce fluid and electrolyte disturbances, such as vomiting and anorexia. Maintaining adequate nutrition, fluid intake, and electrolyte balance should be a major focus in cancer care.

◆ Obtain a comprehensive dietary history to pinpoint nutritional problems and their past causes such as diabetes; help plan the diet accordingly.

◆ Ask the dietitian to provide a liquid diet high in proteins, carbohydrates, and calories if the patient can't tolerate solid foods. If the patient has stomatitis, provide soft, bland, nonirritating foods.

◆ Encourage the patient's family to bring foods from home, if the patient requests.

◆ Make mealtime as relaxed and pleasant as possible. Encourage the patient to dine with visitors or other patients. Allow choices from a varied menu.

◆ With the practitioner's approval, you may suggest that the patient drink a glass of wine before dinner to stimulate the appetite and aid relaxation.

◆ Encourage the patient to drink eight 8-oz (236.6 mL) glasses of noncaffeinated liquids per day. Urge the patient to drink juice or other caloric beverages instead of water.

◆ Suggest frequent, small meals if the patient can't tolerate normal ones.

◆ Avoid strong-smelling foods.

IF THE PATIENT CAN'T EAT

The patient who has had recent head, neck, or GI surgery or who has pain when swallowing can receive nourishment through a nasogastric (NG) tube. If the patient still needs to use the tube after he or she is discharged, teach the patient how to insert it, how to test its position in the stomach by aspirating stomach contents, and how to use it to feed himself.

If an NG tube isn't appropriate, other alternatives are gastrostomy, jejunostomyzs, and, occasionally, esophagostomy. These procedures make it possible for you to feed the patient prescribed protein formulas and semiliquids, such as cream soups and eggnog; they also make it easier for the patient to feed himself.

Warn the patient that if spilled gastric or intestinal juices come in contact with the abdominal skin, they'll cause excoriation if they aren't washed off immediately. Always flush the tube well with water following each feeding.

Also, to provide adequate hydration, instill about 4 to 6 oz (118 to 177.5 mL) of water or another clear liquid between meals.

After jejunostomy, begin with small feedings, slowly and carefully increasing the amounts. Provide additional fluids and calories during these days of limited food intake by supplementing jejunostomy feedings with I.V. fat emulsions.

TOTAL PARENTERAL NUTRITION

Commonly considered an important component of cancer care if the patient can't tolerate enteral nutrition, total parenteral nutrition (TPN) can improve a severely debilitated patient's protein balance. In doing so, TPN characteristically strengthens and conditions the patient, allowing the patient to better tolerate treatment.

TPN can produce a slight weight gain in the patient receiving radiation therapy, provide optimum nutrition for wound healing, and help the patient combat infection after radical surgery.

PAIN CONTROL

Typically, cancer patients have a great fear of pain. Therefore, pain control is critical at every stage of managing cancer—from localized cancer to advanced metastasis. In cancer patients, pain may result from inflammation of or pressure on pain-sensitive structures, tumor infiltration of nerves or blood vessels, or metastatic extension to bone. Chronic and unrelenting pain can wear down the patient's tolerance to treatment, interfere with eating and sleeping, and cause anger, despair, and anxiety.

Opioid analgesics—either alone or in combination with nonopioid analgesics, antianxiety agents, or tricyclic antidepressants—are the mainstay of pain relief in patients with advanced cancer. In terminal stages of cancer, effective opioid dosages may be quite high because drug tolerance invariably develops. Provide such analgesics generously. Anticipate the need for pain relief, and provide it on a schedule that doesn't allow pain to break through. Don't wait to relieve pain until it becomes severe. Reassure the patient that you'll provide pain medication whenever they need it. (See *Patient-controlled analgesia system*, page 712.)

Nonpharmacologic pain relief techniques can be used alone or, more commonly, in combination with drug therapy. Popular techniques include cutaneous stimulation, relaxation, biofeedback, distraction, and guided imagery.

Surgical excision of the tumor can relieve pressure on sensitive tissues and pain caused by inflamed necrotic tissue; treatment with antibiotics can combat inflammation; radiation therapy can shrink metastatic tissue and control bone pain. When a tumor invades nerve tissue, effective pain control requires anesthetics, destructive nerve blocks, electronic nerve stimulation with a dorsal column or transcutaneous electrical nerve stimulator, rhizotomy, or chordotomy.

THE HOSPICE APPROACH

A holistic approach to patient care modeled after St. Christopher's Hospice in London, hospice care provides comprehensive physical, psychological, social, and spiritual care for terminally ill patients. Although some hospices are located in inpatient settings, most hospice programs serve terminally ill patients in the more familiar and relaxed surroundings of their own home.

The goal of the hospice care team is to help the patient achieve as full a life as possible, with minimal pain, discomfort, and restriction. Of the many medications provided for pain control, morphine is considered the drug of choice.

Hospice care also emphasizes a coordinated team effort to help the patient and family members overcome the severe anxiety, fear, and depression that occur with terminal illness.

Patient-controlled analgesia system

The patient-controlled analgesia (PCA) system is an option for pain treatment in cancer care. It's typically used in the postoperative clinical setting, where I.V. pain management is needed for acute intervention, and is also used in nonsurgical cancer patients to control severe pain. This system permits the patient to self-administer a premeasured dose of analgesic by pressing a button at the bedside that activates a pump fitted with a prefilled syringe containing the analgesic. Small, intermittent doses of the analgesic administered I.V. maintain blood levels that ensure comfort and minimize the risk of oversedation. The practitioner or the nursing staff presets doses and time intervals (usually 8 to 10 minutes) that allow the patient to determine his or her comfort level. The syringe is locked inside the pump as a safety feature, and the system will only dispense the analgesic when the correct (preset) time interval has elapsed.

Clinical studies report that patients on PCA tend to titrate analgesic drugs effectively and maintain comfort without oversedation. They also tend to use less of the drug than the amount normally given by I.M. injection.

PCA provides other significant advantages:
♦ Patients are alert and active during the day.
♦ Patients no longer need to suffer pain while awaiting their injections.
♦ Patients are free from pain caused by injections.
♦ The nursing staff is free for other clinical duties.

To that end, hospice staff encourage family members to help with the patient's care, thereby providing the patient with warmth and security and helping the family caregivers begin the grieving process before the patient dies.

Everyone involved in this method of care must be committed to high-quality patient care, unafraid of emotional involvement, and comfortable with personal feelings about death and dying. Good hospice care also requires open communication among team members, not just for evaluating patient care, but also for helping the staff cope with their own feelings.

PSYCHOLOGICAL ASPECTS

The diagnosis of cancer evokes a profound emotional response, which patients express in different ways. Some face this difficult reality from the outset of diagnosis and treatment. Many use denial as a coping mechanism and simply refuse to accept the truth, but this stance becomes increasingly difficult for them to maintain. As evidence of the tumor becomes inescapable, the patient may develop clinical depression. Family members may express denial in attempts to cope by encouraging unproven methods of cancer treatment, which can delay effective care. Some patients cope by intellectualizing about their disease, enabling them to obscure the reality of the cancer and regard it as unrelated to themselves. Generally, intellectualization is a more productive coping behavior than denial because the patient is receiving

treatment. Be aware of the possible behavioral responses so you can identify them and then interact supportively with the patient and family. For many malignancies, you can offer realistic hope for long-term survival or remission; even in advanced disease, you can offer short-term achievable goals. To help a patient cope with cancer, make sure you understand your own feelings about it. Then listen sensitively to the patient so you can offer genuine understanding and support. When caring for a patient with terminal cancer, increase your effectiveness by seeking out someone to help you through your own grieving.

Head, neck, and spine

MALIGNANT BRAIN TUMORS

Primary malignant brain tumors account for about 10% to 30% of adult cancers. These tumors may occur at any age. The most common tumor types in adults are gliomas and meningiomas, which usually occur supratentorially (above the covering of the cerebellum). In children, incidence is generally highest before age 12, affecting 3 of every 100,000 children; more than 1,200 new cases occur each year. The most common types in children are astrocytomas, medulloblastomas, ependymomas, and brainstem gliomas. In children, brain tumors of the central nervous system (CNS) account for 20% of all childhood cancers; they're similar in incidence to leukemias.

Causes and incidence

The cause of most brain tumors is unknown, but exposure to ionizing radiation is a known environmental risk. Additionally, most malignant tumors of the brain are of metastatic origin; 20% to 40% of patients with nonbrain primary cancer develop brain metastasis. (See *Comparing brain tumors*, pages 713 to 715.)

Pathophysiology

Brain tumors may originate from neural elements within the brain, or they may represent spread of distant cancers. Primary brain tumors arise from CNS tissue and account for roughly half of all cases of intracranial neoplasms. The remainder of brain neoplasms are caused by metastatic lesions.

Comparing brain tumors

Tumor	Clinical features
Astrocytoma	
♦ Second most common malignant glioma (about 10% of all gliomas) ♦ Occurs at any age; incidence higher in males ♦ Usually occurs in white matter of cerebral hemispheres; may originate in any part of the central nervous system ♦ Cerebellar astrocytomas usually confined to one hemisphere	*General* ♦ Headache; mental activity changes ♦ Decreased motor strength and coordination ♦ Seizures; scanning speech ♦ Altered vital signs *Localizing* ♦ Third ventricle: changes in mental activity and level of consciousness, nausea, pupillary dilation and sluggish light reflex; later—paresis or ataxia ♦ Brainstem and pons: early—ipsilateral trigeminal, abducens, and facial nerve palsies; later—cerebellar ataxia, tremors, other cranial nerve deficits ♦ Third or fourth ventricle or aqueduct of Sylvius: secondary hydrocephalus ♦ Thalamus or hypothalamus: various endocrine, metabolic, autonomic, and behavioral changes
Ependymoma	
♦ Rare glioma ♦ Most common in children and young adults ♦ Usually locates in fourth and lateral ventricles	*General* ♦ Similar to oligodendroglioma ♦ Increased intracranial pressure (ICP) and obstructive hydrocephalus, depending on tumor size
Glioblastoma multiforme (spongioblastoma multiforme)	
♦ Peak incidence at 50 to 60 years; twice as common in males; most common glioma (accounts for 60% of all gliomas) ♦ Unencapsulated, highly malignant; grows rapidly and infiltrates the brain extensively; may become enormous before diagnosed ♦ Usually occurs in cerebral hemispheres, especially frontal and temporal lobes (rarely in brainstem and cerebellum) ♦ Occupies more than one lobe of affected hemisphere; may spread to opposite hemisphere by corpus callosum; may metastasize into cerebrospinal fluid (CSF), producing tumors in distant parts of the nervous system	*General* ♦ Increased ICP (nausea, vomiting, headache, papilledema) ♦ Mental and behavioral changes ♦ Altered vital signs (increased systolic pressure, widened pulse pressure, respiratory changes) ♦ Speech and sensory disturbances ♦ In children, irritability, projectile vomiting *Localizing* ♦ Midline: headache (bifrontal or bioccipital); worse in the morning; intensified by coughing, straining, or sudden head movements ♦ Temporal lobe: psychomotor seizures ♦ Central region: focal seizures ♦ Optic and oculomotor nerves: visual defects ♦ Frontal lobe: abnormal reflexes, motor responses

(*continued*)

Comparing brain tumors (*continued*)

Tumor	Clinical features
Medulloblastoma	
♦ Rare glioma ♦ Incidence highest in children ages 4 to 6 ♦ Affects males more commonly than females ♦ Commonly metastasizes via CSF	*General* ♦ Increased ICP *Localizing* ♦ Brainstem and cerebrum: papilledema, nystagmus, hearing loss, flashing lights, dizziness, ataxia, paresthesia of face, cranial nerve palsies (V, VI, VII, IX, X, primarily sensory), hemiparesis, suboccipital tenderness; compression of supratentorial area produces other general and focal signs and symptoms
Meningioma	
♦ Most common nongliomatous brain tumor (15% of primary brain tumors) ♦ Peak incidence among 50-year-olds; rare in children; more common in females (ratio 3:2) ♦ Arises from the meninges ♦ Common locations include parasagittal area, sphenoidal ridge, anterior part of the base of the skull, cerebellopontine angle, spinal canal ♦ Benign, well-circumscribed, highly vascular tumors that compress underlying brain tissue by invading overlying skull	*General* ♦ Headache ♦ Seizures (in two thirds of patients) ♦ Vomiting ♦ Changes in mental activity ♦ Similar to schwannomas *Localizing* ♦ Skull changes (bony bulge) over tumor ♦ Sphenoidal ridge, indenting optic nerve: unilateral visual changes and papilledema ♦ Prefrontal parasagittal: personality and behavioral changes ♦ Motor cortex: contralateral motor changes ♦ Anterior fossa compressing both optic nerves and frontal lobes: headaches and bilateral vision loss ♦ Pressure on cranial nerves causing varying symptoms
Oligodendroglioma	
♦ Third most common glioma (accounts for <5% of all gliomas) ♦ Occurs in middle adult years; more common in women ♦ Slow growing	*General* ♦ Mental and behavioral changes ♦ Decreased visual acuity and other vision disturbances ♦ Increased ICP *Localizing* ♦ Temporal lobe: hallucinations, psychomotor seizures ♦ Central region: seizures (confined to one muscle group or unilateral) ♦ Midbrain or third ventricle: pyramidal tract symptoms (dizziness, ataxia, paresthesia of the face) ♦ Brainstem and cerebrum: nystagmus, hearing loss, dizziness, ataxia, paresthesia of the face, cranial nerve palsies, hemiparesis, suboccipital tenderness, loss of balance

Comparing brain tumors (*continued*)

Tumor	Clinical features
Schwannoma (acoustic neurinoma, neurilemoma, cerebellopontine angle tumor)	
♦ Accounts for about 10% of all intracranial tumors ♦ Higher incidence in women ♦ Onset of symptoms between ages 30 and 60 ♦ Affects the craniospinal nerve sheath, usually cranial nerve (CN) VIII; also, CN V and VII and, to a lesser extent, CN VI and X on the same side as the tumor ♦ Benign, but commonly classified as malignant because of its growth patterns; slow growing—may be present for years before symptoms occur	*General* ♦ Unilateral hearing loss with or without tinnitus ♦ Stiff neck and suboccipital discomfort ♦ Secondary hydrocephalus ♦ Ataxia and uncoordinated movements of one or both arms due to pressure on brainstem and cerebellum *Localizing* ♦ CN V: early—facial hypoesthesia or paresthesia on side of hearing loss; unilateral loss of corneal reflex ♦ CN VI: diplopia or double vision ♦ CN VII: paresis progressing to paralysis (Bell palsy) ♦ CN X: weakness of palate, tongue, and nerve muscles on same side as tumor

Complications
♦ Hypercalcemia
♦ Brain herniation
♦ Coma
♦ Respiratory or cardiac arrest
♦ Seizures

Signs and symptoms
Brain tumors cause CNS changes by invading and destroying tissues and by secondary effect—mainly compression of the brain, cranial nerves, and cerebral vessels; cerebral edema; and increased intracranial pressure (ICP). Generally, clinical features result from increased ICP; these features vary with the type of tumor, its location, and the degree of invasion. (See *What happens in increased ICP*, page 716.) Onset of symptoms is usually insidious, and brain tumors are commonly misdiagnosed.

Diagnosis
CONFIRMING DIAGNOSIS *In many cases, a definitive diagnosis follows a tissue biopsy performed by stereotactic surgery. In this procedure, a head ring is affixed to the skull, and an excisional device is guided to the lesion by a CT scan or MRI.*

Other diagnostic tools include a patient history, a neurologic assessment, skull X-rays, a brain scan, a CT scan, MRI, and cerebral angiography. An electroencephalogram may reveal focal abnormalities. Lumbar puncture shows increased pressure and protein levels, decreased glucose levels, and, occasionally, tumor cells in cerebrospinal fluid (CSF).

Treatment
Treatment includes surgical excision of a resectable tumor; surgical reduction of a nonresectable tumor; relief of cerebral edema, decrease of ICP, and other symptoms; and prevention of further neurologic damage.

The mode of therapy depends on the tumor's histologic type, radiosensitivity, and location and may include surgery, radiation, chemotherapy, or decompression of increased ICP with diuretics, corticosteroids, or possibly ventriculoatrial or ventriculoperitoneal shunting of CSF.

A glioma usually requires resection by craniotomy, followed by radiation therapy and chemotherapy. The combination of nitrosoureas (carmustine [BCNU], lomustine [CCNU], or procarbazine), or methylating agents such as temozolomide, and postoperative radiation is more effective than radiation alone. Concurrent temozolomide and radiation therapy daily for 6 weeks has been shown to substantially improve survival.

Surgical resection of low-grade cystic cerebellar astrocytomas brings long-term survival. Treatment of other astrocytomas includes repeated surgery, radiation therapy, and shunting of fluid from obstructed CSF pathways. Some astrocytomas are highly radiosensitive, but others are radioresistant.

Treatment of oligodendrogliomas and ependymomas includes resection and radiation therapy; for medulloblastomas, resection and possibly intrathecal infusion of methotrexate or another antineoplastic drug. Meningiomas

PATHOPHYSIOLOGY
What happens in increased ICP

Intracranial pressure (ICP) is the force exerted within the intact skull by intracranial volume: about 10% blood, 10% cerebrospinal fluid (CSF), and 80% brain tissue and water. The rigid skull allows little space for expansion of these substances. When ICP increases dramatically, brain damage can result.

The brain compensates for increases by regulating the volume of the three substances by limiting blood flow to the head, displacing CSF into the spinal canal, and increasing absorption or decreasing production of CSF. When compensatory mechanisms become overworked, small changes in volume lead to large changes in pressure.

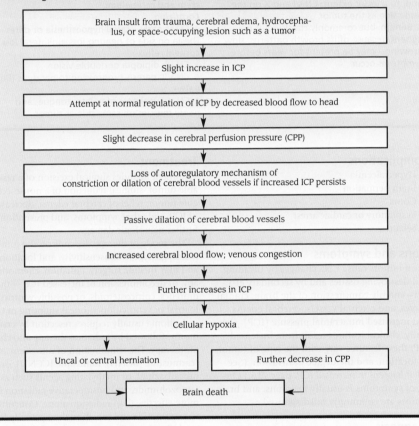

Brain insult from trauma, cerebral edema, hydrocephalus, or space-occupying lesion such as a tumor

↓

Slight increase in ICP

↓

Attempt at normal regulation of ICP by decreased blood flow to head

↓

Slight decrease in cerebral perfusion pressure (CPP)

↓

Loss of autoregulatory mechanism of constriction or dilation of cerebral blood vessels if increased ICP persists

↓

Passive dilation of cerebral blood vessels

↓

Increased cerebral blood flow; venous congestion

↓

Further increases in ICP

↓

Cellular hypoxia

↓   ↓

Uncal or central herniation   Further decrease in CPP

Brain death

require resection, including dura mater and bone (operative mortality may reach 10% because of large tumor size).

For schwannomas, microsurgical technique allows complete resection of the tumor and preservation of facial nerves. Although schwannomas are moderately radioresistant, postoperative radiation therapy is necessary.

The breakdown of the blood–brain barrier allows chemotherapeutic drugs to penetrate the cerebrum. Intrathecal and intra-arterial administration of drugs maximizes drug actions.

Palliative measures for gliomas, astrocytomas, oligodendrogliomas, and ependymomas include dexamethasone for cerebral edema; osmotic diuretics, such as urea and mannitol, to reduce brain swelling; analgesics to control pain; and antacids and histamine receptor antagonists for stress ulcers. These tumors and schwannomas may also require anticonvulsants such as phenytoin to prevent or control seizures.

Special considerations

A patient with a brain tumor requires comprehensive neurologic assessment, teaching, and supportive care. During your first contact with the patient, perform a comprehensive assessment (including a complete neurologic evaluation) to provide baseline data and to help develop your care plan. Obtain a thorough health history concerning onset of symptoms. Help the patient and family cope with the treatment, potential disabilities, and changes in lifestyle resulting from the tumor.

Throughout hospitalization:
◆ Carefully document seizure activity (occurrence, nature, and duration).
◆ Maintain airway patency.
◆ Monitor patient safety.
◆ Administer anticonvulsive drugs as ordered. Encourage the patient to wear a medical identification bracelet or necklace that identifies their risk for seizures.
◆ Check continuously for changes in neurologic status, and watch for an increase in ICP.

⚠ **ALERT** *Watch for and immediately report sudden unilateral pupillary dilation with loss of light reflex; this is an ominous change that indicates imminent transtentorial herniation.*

⚠ **ALERT** *Monitor respiratory changes carefully (abnormal respiratory rate and depth may point to rising ICP or herniation of the cerebellar tonsils from expanding infratentorial mass).*

◆ Monitor temperature carefully. Fever commonly follows hypothalamic anoxia but might also indicate meningitis. Use hypothermia blankets preoperatively and postoperatively to keep the patient's temperature down and minimize cerebral metabolic demands.
◆ Administer steroids and osmotic diuretics such as mannitol as ordered to reduce cerebral edema. Fluids may be restricted to 1,500 mL/24 hours. Monitor fluid and electrolyte balance to avoid dehydration.
◆ Observe and report signs and symptoms of stress ulcers: abdominal distention, pain, vomiting, and tarry stools. Administer antacids as ordered.

Surgery requires additional nursing care. After craniotomy, continue to monitor general neurologic status and watch for signs of increased ICP, such as an elevated bone flap and typical neurologic changes. To reduce the risk of increased ICP, restrict fluids to 1,500 mL/24 hours. To promote venous drainage and reduce cerebral edema after supratentorial craniotomy, elevate the head of the patient's bed about 30 degrees. Position the patient on the side to allow drainage of secretions and prevent aspiration. As appropriate, instruct the patient to avoid Valsalva maneuver or isometric muscle contractions when moving or sitting up in bed; these can increase intrathoracic pressure and thereby increase ICP. Withhold oral fluids, which may provoke vomiting and consequently raise ICP.

After infratentorial craniotomy, keep the patient flat for 48 hours, but logroll the patient every 2 hours to minimize complications of immobilization. Prevent other complications by paying careful attention to ventilatory status and to cardiovascular, GI, and musculoskeletal functions.
◆ Radiation therapy is usually delayed until after the surgical wound heals, but it can induce wound breakdown even then, so observe the wound carefully for infection and sinus formation. Because radiation may cause brain inflammation, watch for signs of rising ICP.
◆ Because chemotherapy—BCNU, CCNU, procarbazine, and temozolomide—used as adjuncts to radiotherapy and surgery can cause delayed bone marrow depression, tell the patient to watch for and immediately report any signs of infection or bleeding that appear within 4 weeks after the start of chemotherapy. Before chemotherapy, give ondansetron or another antiemetic, as ordered, to minimize nausea and vomiting.
◆ Teach the patient and family signs of recurrence; urge compliance with treatment regimen.
◆ Because brain tumors may cause residual neurologic deficits that disable the patient physically or mentally, begin rehabilitation early. Changes in cognitive function may also be observed and affect daily functional activities. Consult with occupational and physical therapists to encourage independence in daily activities and improve the quality of life. As necessary, provide aids for self-care and mobilization, such as bathroom rails for the wheelchair patient. If the patient is aphasic, arrange for consultation with a speech pathologist.
◆ Legal advice is helpful in forming advance directives such as power of attorney in cases where continued physical or intellectual decline is likely.
◆ Refer the patient for counseling and to national and local support groups to help the patient cope with this disorder.

PITUITARY TUMORS

Pituitary tumors, which constitute 10% of intracranial malignant neoplasms, usually originate in the anterior pituitary (adenohypophysis). They occur in adults of both sexes, usually during the third and fourth decades of life. The three tissue types of pituitary tumors are chromophobe adenoma (90%), basophil adenoma, and eosinophil adenoma.

The prognosis for patients depends on the extent to which the tumor spreads beyond the sella turcica.

Causes and incidence

Although the exact cause is unknown, a predisposition to pituitary tumors may be inherited through an autosomal dominant trait. Pituitary tumors aren't malignant in the strict sense but, because their growth is invasive, they're considered a neoplastic disease.

Chromophobe adenoma may be associated with the production of corticotropin, melanocyte-stimulating hormone, growth hormone (GH), and prolactin; basophil adenoma, with evidence of excess corticotropin production and, consequently, with signs of Cushing syndrome; eosinophil adenoma, with excessive GH.

Pituitary tumors develop in 1 in 10,000 people. About 15% of tumors located within the skull are pituitary tumors.

Complications

◆ Endocrine abnormalities
◆ Diabetes insipidus

Signs and symptoms

As pituitary adenomas grow, they replace normal glandular tissue and enlarge the sella turcica, which houses the pituitary gland. The resulting pressure on adjacent intracranial structures produces these typical clinical manifestations:

Neurologic:
◆ frontal headache
◆ visual symptoms, beginning with blurring and progressing to field cuts (hemianopsias) and then unilateral blindness
◆ cranial nerve (III, IV, VI) involvement from lateral extension of the tumor, resulting in strabismus; double vision, with compensating head tilting and dizziness; conjugate deviation of gaze; nystagmus; lid ptosis; and limited eye movements
◆ increased ICP (secondary hydrocephalus)
◆ personality changes or dementia, if the tumor breaks through to the frontal lobes
◆ seizures
◆ rhinorrhea, if the tumor erodes the base of the skull
◆ pituitary apoplexy secondary to hemorrhagic infarction of the adenoma. Such hemorrhage may lead to both cardiovascular and adrenocortical collapse

Endocrine:
◆ hypopituitarism, to some degree, in all patients with adenoma, becoming more obvious as the tumor replaces normal gland tissue (signs and symptoms include amenorrhea, decreased libido and impotence in men, skin changes [waxy appearance, decreased wrinkles, and pigmentation], loss of axillary and pubic hair, lethargy, weakness, increased fatigability, intolerance to cold, and constipation [because of decreased production of corticotropin and thyroid-stimulating hormone {TSH}])
◆ addisonian crisis, precipitated by stress and resulting in nausea, vomiting, hypoglycemia, hypotension, and circulatory collapse
◆ diabetes insipidus, resulting from extension to the hypothalamus
◆ prolactin-secreting adenomas (in 70% to 75%), with amenorrhea and galactorrhea
◆ GH-secreting adenomas, with acromegaly
◆ corticotropin-secreting adenomas, with Cushing syndrome

Diagnosis

◆ Skull X-rays with tomography show enlargement of the sella turcica or erosion of its floor; if GH secretion predominates, X-rays show enlarged paranasal sinuses and mandible, thickened cranial bones, and separated teeth.
◆ Carotid angiogram shows displacement of the anterior cerebral and internal carotid arteries if the tumor mass is enlarging; it also rules out intracerebral aneurysm.
◆ CT scan may confirm the existence of the adenoma and accurately depict its size.
◆ CSF analysis may show increased protein levels.
◆ Endocrine function tests may contribute helpful information, but results are commonly ambiguous and inconclusive.
◆ MRI differentiates healthy, benign, and malignant tissues as well as arteries and veins. MRI is an excellent modality for viewing the pituitary. (See *MRI of the pituitary*.)

MRI of the pituitary

MRI is an excellent imaging modality for the assessment of pituitary lesions. One advantage of MRI over computed tomography is the absence of bony artifact with MRI.

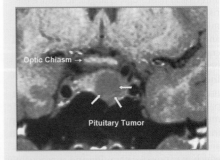

Treatment

Surgical options include transfrontal removal of large tumors impinging on the optic apparatus and transsphenoidal resection for smaller tumors confined to the pituitary fossa.

Radiation is the primary treatment for small, nonsecretory tumors that don't extend beyond the sella turcica or for patients who may be a poor surgical candidate; otherwise, it's an adjunct to surgery.

Postoperative treatment includes hormone replacement with cortisone, thyroid, and sex hormones; correction of electrolyte imbalance; and, as necessary, insulin therapy.

Drug therapy may include bromocriptine, an ergot derivative that shrinks prolactin- and GH-secreting tumors. Cyproheptadine, an antiserotonin drug, can reduce increased corticosteroid levels in the patient with Cushing syndrome.

Adjuvant radiation therapy is used when only partial removal of the tumor is possible. Cryohypophysectomy (freezing the area with a probe inserted by transsphenoidal route) is a promising alternative to surgical dissection of the tumor.

Special considerations

◆ Conduct a comprehensive health history and physical assessment to establish the onset of neurologic and endocrine dysfunction and provide baseline data for later comparison.

◆ Establish a supportive, trusting relationship with the patient and family to assist them in coping with the diagnosis, treatment, and potential long-term changes. Make sure they understand that the patient needs lifelong evaluations and, possibly, hormone replacement.

◆ Reassure the patient that some of the distressing physical and behavioral signs and symptoms caused by pituitary dysfunction (e.g., altered sexual drive, impotence, infertility, loss of hair, and emotional instability) will disappear with treatment.

◆ Maintain a safe, clutter-free environment for the visually impaired or acromegalic patient. Reassure the patient that he or she will probably recover sight.

▼ **ALERT** *Position patients who have undergone supratentorial or transsphenoidal hypophysectomy with the head of the bed elevated about 30 degrees to promote venous drainage from the head and reduce cerebral edema. Place the patient on the side to allow drainage of secretions and prevent aspiration.*

◆ Prevent vomiting, which increases ICP. Don't allow a patient who has had transsphenoidal surgery to blow his or her nose. Watch for CSF

Postcraniotomy care

◆ Monitor vital signs (especially level of consciousness), and perform a baseline neurologic assessment from which to plan further care and assess the patient's progress.
◆ Maintain the patient's airway; suction as necessary.
◆ Monitor intake and output carefully.
◆ Prevent aspiration and vomiting, which increases intracranial pressure.
◆ Observe for cerebral edema, bleeding, and leakage of cerebrospinal fluid.
◆ Provide a restful, quiet environment.
◆ Monitor for postoperative pain or headache

---

drainage from the nose. Monitor for signs of infection from the contaminated upper respiratory tract. Make sure the patient understands that he or she will lose sense of smell.

◆ Regularly compare the patient's postoperative neurologic status with your baseline assessment. (See *Postcraniotomy care.*)

◆ Monitor intake and output to detect fluid and electrolyte imbalances.

◆ Before discharge, encourage the patient to wear a medical identification bracelet or necklace that identifies hormone deficiencies and proper treatment.

LARYNGEAL CANCER

The most common form of laryngeal cancer is squamous cell cancer (95%); rare forms include adenocarcinoma, sarcoma, and others. Such cancer may be intrinsic or extrinsic. An *intrinsic* tumor is on the true vocal cord and doesn't tend to spread because underlying connective tissues lack lymph nodes. An *extrinsic* tumor is on some other part of the larynx and tends to spread early.

Causes and incidence

In laryngeal cancer, major predisposing factors include smoking and alcoholism; minor factors include chronic inhalation of noxious fumes and familial tendency. Cancer of the larynx rarely occurs in nonsmokers.

Laryngeal cancer is classified according to its location:

◆ supraglottis (false vocal cords)
◆ glottis (true vocal cords)
◆ subglottis (downward extension from vocal cords [rare])

The ratio of male to female incidence is 10:1. Most victims are between ages 50 and 65. The 5-year survival rate is 65%.

Pathophysiology

Pathological diagnosis for laryngeal cancer is achieved after biopsy which is obtained at direct laryngoscopy under general anesthesia. The vast majority of all laryngeal malignancies (95%) are conventional squamous cell carcinomas (SCC) and they vary according to their degree of differentiation to well, moderate, and poor carcinomas. Glottic cancers are generally well differentiated and have a less aggressive behavior in comparison with carcinomas at the other sites of the larynx. SCC often arises in a background of mucosal squamous dysplasia or carcinoma in situ and typically presents islands, tongues, and clusters of atypical cells invading the laryngeal stroma. Features of squamous differentiation also comprise individual cell keratinization, intercellular bridges, and keratin pearls.

Complications

◆ Airway obstruction
◆ Metastasis
◆ Pain
◆ Difficulty swallowing

Signs and symptoms

In intrinsic laryngeal cancer, the dominant and earliest symptom is hoarseness that persists longer than 3 weeks; in extrinsic cancer, it's a lump in the throat or pain or burning in the throat when drinking citrus juice or hot liquid. Later clinical effects of metastasis include dysphagia, dyspnea, cough, enlarged cervical lymph nodes, and pain radiating to the ear.

Diagnosis

Any hoarseness that lasts longer than 2 weeks requires visualization of the larynx by laryngoscopy.

℞ CONFIRMING DIAGNOSIS *Firm diagnosis also requires xeroradiography, biopsy, laryngeal tomography, CT scan, or laryngography to define the borders of the lesion and chest X-ray to detect metastasis.*

Treatment

Early lesions are treated with surgery or radiation; advanced lesions with surgery, radiation, and chemotherapy. In early stages, laser surgery can excise precancerous lesions; in advanced stages, it can help relieve obstruction caused by tumor growth. Surgical procedures vary with tumor size and can include cordectomy, partial or total laryngectomy, supraglottic laryngectomy, or total laryngectomy with laryngoplasty. Primary systemic therapy may be administered concurrently with radiation. Principal agents

include cisplatin, fluorouracil, carboplatin, and the taxanes. The goal is to eliminate the cancer and preserve speech. If speech preservation isn't possible, speech rehabilitation may include esophageal speech or prosthetic devices; surgical techniques to construct a new voice box are still experimental.

Special considerations

Provide psychological support and good preoperative and postoperative care to minimize complications and speed recovery.

Before partial or total laryngectomy:
◆ Instruct the patient to maintain good oral hygiene. If appropriate, instruct the patient to shave off beard.
◆ Encourage the patient to express his or her concerns before surgery. Help the patient choose a temporary nonspeaking communication method (such as writing).
◆ If appropriate, arrange for a laryngectomee to visit the patient. Explain postoperative procedures (suctioning, NG feeding, laryngectomy tube care) and their results (breathing through neck, speech alteration). Also prepare the patient for other functional losses: He or she won't be able to smell, blow his or her nose, whistle, gargle, sip, or suck on a straw.

After partial laryngectomy:
◆ Give I.V. fluids and, usually, tube feedings in the initial postoperative period; then resume oral fluids. Keep the tracheostomy tube (inserted during surgery) in place until edema subsides.
◆ Keep the patient from using his or her voice until he or she has medical permission (usually 2 to 3 days postoperatively). Then caution the patient to whisper until healing is complete.

After total laryngectomy:
◆ As soon as the patient returns to bed, place the patient on his or her side and elevate his or her head 30 to 45 degrees. When you move the patient, remember to support his or her neck.
◆ The patient will probably have a laryngectomy tube in place until their stoma heals (about 7 to 10 days). This tube is shorter and thicker than a tracheostomy tube but requires the same care. Watch for crusting and secretions around the stoma, which can cause skin breakdown. To prevent crust formation, provide adequate room humidification. Remove crusting with petroleum jelly, antimicrobial ointment, and moist gauze.
◆ Teach stoma care.
◆ Watch for and report complications: fistula formation (redness, swelling, secretions on suture line), carotid artery rupture (bleeding), and tracheostomy stenosis (constant shortness of

breath). A fistula may form between the reconstructed hypopharynx and the skin. This eventually heals spontaneously but may take weeks or months. Carotid artery rupture usually occurs in patients who have had preoperative radiation, particularly those with a fistula that constantly bathes the carotid artery with oral secretions.

⚠ **ALERT** *If carotid rupture occurs, apply pressure to the site; call for help immediately and take the patient to the operating room for carotid ligation.*

Tracheostomy stenosis occurs weeks to months after laryngectomy; treatment includes fitting the patient with successively larger tracheostomy tubes until he or she can tolerate insertion of a large one. If the patient has a fistula, feed through an NG tube; otherwise, food will leak through the fistula and delay healing. Monitor vital signs (be especially alert for fever, which indicates infection). Record fluid intake and output, and watch for dehydration.

◆ Give frequent mouth care.

◆ Suction gently, unless ordered otherwise. Don't attempt deep suctioning, which could penetrate the suture line. Suction through both the tube and the patient's nose because the patient can no longer blow air through his or her nose; suction his or her mouth gently.

◆ After insertion of a drainage catheter (usually connected to a wound drainage system or a GI drainage system), don't stop suction without the practitioner's consent. After catheter removal, check dressings for drainage.

◆ Give analgesics as ordered.

◆ If the patient has an NG feeding tube, check tube placement and elevate the patient's head to prevent aspiration.

◆ Reassure the patient that speech rehabilitation may help him or her speak again. Encourage contact with the International Association of Laryngectomees and other sources of support.

◆ Support the patient through the grieving process. If the depression seems severe, consider a psychiatric referral.

THYROID CANCER

Papillary and follicular carcinomas are the most common types of thyroid cancer and are usually associated with a longer survival. Papillary carcinoma accounts for half of all thyroid cancers in adults; it's most common in young adult females and metastasizes slowly. It's the least virulent form of thyroid cancer. Follicular carcinoma is less common but more likely to recur and metastasize to the regional nodes and through blood vessels into the bones, liver, and lungs. Medullary carcinoma originates in the parafollicular cells derived from the last branchial pouch and contains amyloid and calcium deposits. It can produce calcitonin, histaminase, corticotropin (producing Cushing syndrome), and prostaglandin E_2 and F_3 (producing diarrhea). Of the three types of medullary carcinoma, sporadic is the most common and isn't inherited. Multiple endocrine neoplasia, type II is familial; it's associated with pheochromocytoma and parathyroid gland tumors and is completely curable when detected before it causes symptoms. Untreated, it progresses rapidly. Seldom curable by resection, anaplastic tumors resist radiation and metastasize rapidly. The familial type of medullary cancer is also inherited but only affects the thyroid gland. Thyroid lymphoma begins in the lymphocytes and can move to the thyroid gland.

Causes and incidence

Predisposing factors to thyroid cancer include radiation exposure (especially childhood radiation therapy), prolonged TSH stimulation (through radiation or heredity), familial predisposition, or chronic goiter.

Thyroid cancer occurs in all age groups with peak ages of 45 to 49 years in women and 65 to 69 years in men. It is more common in people who have had radiation treatment of the neck area. Thyroid nodules are four times more common in women with thyroid carcinomas, occurring two to three times more often in women than in men.

Pathophysiology

The majority of thyroid cancers arise from the follicular epithelium, are usually well differentiated, and thus many have a follicular architecture with varying amounts of colloid present. Medullary carcinoma constitutes a minority of thyroid cancers and arises from the C cells.

Complications

◆ Dysphagia
◆ Stridor
◆ Low calcium levels
◆ Metastasis

Signs and symptoms

The primary sign of thyroid cancer is a painless nodule, a hard nodule in an enlarged thyroid gland, or palpable lymph nodes with thyroid enlargement. (See *Early, localized thyroid cancer*, page 722.) Eventually, the pressure of such a nodule or enlargement causes hoarseness, dysphagia, dyspnea, and pain on palpation. If the tumor is large enough to destroy the gland, hypothyroidism follows, with its typical symptoms of low metabolism (mental apathy and sensitivity to cold). However, if the tumor stimulates excess thyroid hormone production, it induces symptoms of hyperthyroidism (sensitivity to heat, restlessness, and hyperactivity). Other clinical features include diarrhea, anorexia, irritability, vocal cord paralysis, and symptoms of distant metastasis.

Diagnosis

The first clue to thyroid cancer is usually an enlarged, palpable node in the thyroid gland, neck, lymph nodes of the neck, or vocal cords. A patient history of radiation therapy or a family history of thyroid cancer supports the diagnosis. However, tests must rule out nonmalignant thyroid enlargements, which are much more common.

Early, localized thyroid cancer

The primary sign of thyroid cancer is a painless nodule.

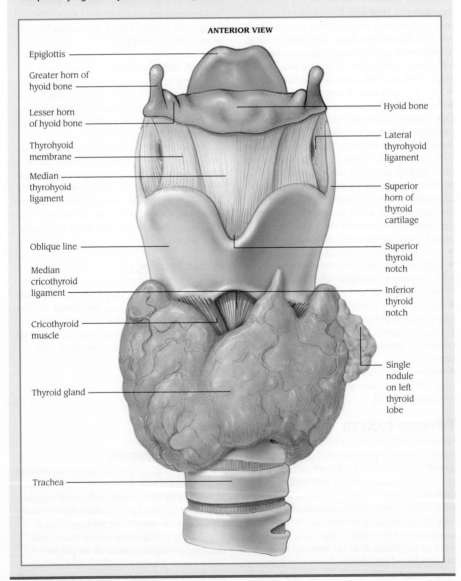

ANTERIOR VIEW

Epiglottis

Greater horn of hyoid bone

Lesser horn of hyoid bone

Thyrohyoid membrane

Median thyrohyoid ligament

Oblique line

Median cricothyroid ligament

Cricothyroid muscle

Thyroid gland

Trachea

Hyoid bone

Lateral thyrohyoid ligament

Superior horn of thyroid cartilage

Superior thyroid notch

Inferior thyroid notch

Single nodule on left thyroid lobe

Thyroid scan differentiates between functional nodes (rarely malignant) and hypofunctional nodes (commonly malignant) by measuring how readily nodules trap isotopes compared with the rest of the thyroid gland. In thyroid cancer, the scintiscan shows a "cold," nonfunctioning nodule. Other tests include needle biopsy, CT scan, ultrasonic scan, chest X-ray, serum alkaline phosphatase, and serum calcitonin assay to diagnose medullary cancer. Calcitonin assay is a reliable clue to silent medullary carcinoma.

Treatment
◆ Total or subtotal thyroidectomy, with modified node dissection (bilateral or unilateral) on the side of the primary cancer (papillary or follicular cancer)
◆ Total thyroidectomy and radical neck excision (for medullary, giant, or spindle cell cancer)
◆ Radiation (^{131}I) with external radiation (for inoperable cancer and sometimes postoperatively in lieu of radical neck excision) or alone (for metastasis)
◆ Adjunctive thyroid suppression, with exogenous thyroid hormones suppressing TSH production, and simultaneous administration of an adrenergic blocking agent such as propranolol, increasing tolerance to surgery and radiation
◆ Chemotherapy for symptom-producing, widespread metastasis is limited, but doxorubicin is sometimes beneficial

Special considerations
Before surgery, tell the patient to expect temporary voice loss or hoarseness lasting several days after surgery.
  Plan meticulous postoperative care:
◆ When the patient regains consciousness, keep him or her in semi-Fowler position, with his or her head neither hyperextended nor flexed, to avoid pressure on the suture line. Support the patient's head and neck with sandbags and pillows; when you move the patient, continue this support with your hands.

⚠ ALERT *After monitoring vital signs, check the patient's dressing, neck, and back for bleeding. If the patient complains that the dressing feels tight, loosen it and call the practitioner immediately.*
◆ Check serum calcium levels daily; hypocalcemia may develop if parathyroid glands are removed. Watch for and report other complications: hemorrhage and shock (elevated pulse rate and hypotension), tetany (carpopedal spasm, twitching, and seizures), thyroid storm (high fever, severe tachycardia, delirium, dehydration, and extreme irritability), and respiratory obstruction (dyspnea, crowing respirations, and retraction of neck tissues). (See *What happens in thyroid storm*, page 724.)

◆ Keep a tracheotomy set, suction, and oxygen equipment handy in case of respiratory obstruction. Use continuous steam inhalation in the patient's room until the chest is clear.
◆ The patient may need I.V. fluids or a soft diet, but many patients can tolerate a regular diet within 24 hours of surgery.
  Care of the patient after extensive tumor and node excision is identical to other postoperative care after radical neck surgery. Referral to a local or national support group can help relieve the patient's stress. (See *Preventing thyroid cancer*, page 724.)

MALIGNANT SPINAL NEOPLASMS
Malignant spinal neoplasms may be any one of many tumor types similar to intracranial tumors; they involve the cord or its roots and, if untreated, can eventually cause paralysis. As primary tumors, they originate in the meningeal coverings, the parenchyma of the cord or its roots, the intraspinal vasculature, or the vertebrae. Primary spinal cord tumors represent 2% to 4% of all primary tumors of the CNS. They can also occur as metastatic foci from primary tumors.

Causes and incidence
Primary tumors of the spinal cord may be extramedullary (occurring outside the spinal cord) or intramedullary (occurring within the cord itself). Extramedullary tumors may be intradural (meningiomas and schwannomas), which account for 70% to 80% of all primary malignant spinal cord neoplasms, or extradural (metastatic tumors from breasts, lungs, prostate, leukemia, or lymphomas), which account for 25% of these malignant neoplasms.
  Intramedullary tumors, or gliomas (astrocytomas or ependymomas), are comparatively rare, accounting for only about 10%. In children, they're low-grade astrocytomas.
  Spinal cord tumors are rare compared with intracranial tumors (ratio of 1:4). They occur equally in men and women, with the exception of meningiomas, which occur mostly in women. Spinal cord tumors can occur anywhere along the length of the cord or its roots.

Pathophysiology
Primary spinal tumors fall into a distinct category because their timely diagnosis and the immediate institution of treatment have an enormous impact on the patient's overall prognosis and hope for a cure. Generally, with spinal pathology, problems that arise are either chronic problems related to degenerative disease or deformity or acute manifestations of traumatic sequelae. When considering tumors of the spine,

PATHOPHYSIOLOGY
What happens in thyroid storm

Normally, the hypothalamus stimulates the release of thyrotropin-releasing hormone, which causes the anterior pituitary gland to release thyroid-stimulating hormone. The thyroid gland then secretes triiodothyronine (T_3) and thyroxine (T_4).

In thyroid storm, however, the thyroid overproduces T_3 and T_4, and systemic adrenergic activity increases. This causes epinephrine overproduction and severe hypermetabolism, leading rapidly to gastrointestinal, cardiovascular, and sympathetic nervous system decompensation.

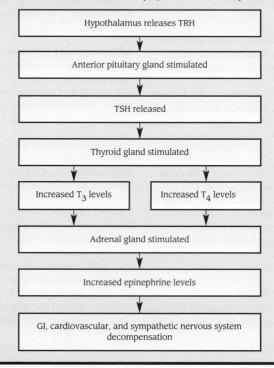

Hypothalamus releases TRH

↓

Anterior pituitary gland stimulated

↓

TSH released

↓

Thyroid gland stimulated

↓   ↓

Increased T_3 levels   Increased T_4 levels

↓   ↓

Adrenal gland stimulated

↓

Increased epinephrine levels

↓

GI, cardiovascular, and sympathetic nervous system decompensation

---

PREVENTION
Preventing thyroid cancer

Teach your patient about the following measures that may help decrease thyroid cancer risk:

Proper nutrition
To reduce the risk of not only thyroid cancer, but most types of cancer, encourage your patient to eat lots of fruits and vegetables and to eat less animal fat.

Surgery
For patients who have an inherited gene, preventive surgery may alleviate the risk of thyroid cancer; however, it will not reduce the risk of tumors affecting the adrenal or parathyroid gland.

Radioactive iodine
The federal government recommends that people living within 10 miles of a nuclear power plant be provided potassium iodide tablets. These tablets can be taken before or right after exposure to nuclear fallout. They provide protection to the thyroid gland from Iodine 131(^{131}I). Exposure to this type of radiation is especially a risk for children, and these tablets are safe for them to take. Those who have Graves disease, autoimmune thyroiditis, or a goiter shouldn't take potassium iodide tablets.

one must consider the different tissue types around the spinal column. The presence of neural tissue, meningeal tissue, bone, and cartilage makes any of these tissue types a possible nidus for neoplastic change. Also, metastatic lesions may spread to the spine from distant primary tumor sites by hematogenous or lymphatic routes.

Complications
◆ Paralysis
◆ Weakness
◆ Loss of bowel and bladder sphincter control
◆ Sensation of numbness or pain

Signs and symptoms
Extramedullary tumors produce symptoms by pressing on nerve roots, the spinal cord, and spinal vessels; intramedullary tumors, by destroying the parenchyma and compressing adjacent areas. Because intramedullary tumors may extend over several spinal cord segments, their symptoms are more variable than those of extramedullary tumors.

The following clinical effects are likely with all malignant spinal cord neoplasms:
◆ Pain—Most severe directly over the tumor, radiates around the trunk or down the limb on the affected side and is unrelieved by bed rest. It may worsen when lying down or with straining, coughing, or sneezing. Pain can be diffuse, occurring over all extremities. Generally, it progressively worsens and isn't relieved by medication.
◆ Motor symptoms—Asymmetric spastic muscle weakness, decreased muscle tone, exaggerated reflexes, and a positive Babinski sign. If the tumor is at the level of the cauda equina, muscle flaccidity, muscle wasting, weakness, and progressive diminution in tendon reflexes are characteristic.
◆ Sensory deficits—Contralateral loss of pain, temperature, and touch sensation (Brown-Séquard syndrome). These losses are less obvious to the patient than functional motor changes. Caudal lesions invariably produce paresthesia in the nerve distribution pathway of the involved roots.
◆ Bowel and bladder symptoms—Urine retention is an inevitable late sign with cord compression. Early signs include incomplete emptying or difficulty with the urine stream, which is usually unnoticed or ignored. Cauda equina tumors cause bladder and bowel incontinence due to flaccid paralysis.

Diagnosis
℞ **CONFIRMING DIAGNOSIS** *Spinal and lumbosacral MRI confirm spinal tumor.*
◆ X-rays show distortions of the intervertebral foramina; changes in the vertebrae or collapsed areas in the vertebral body; and localized enlargement of the spinal canal, indicating an adjacent block.
◆ Myelography identifies the level of the lesion by outlining it if the tumor is causing partial obstruction; it shows anatomic relationship to the cord and the dura. If obstruction is complete, the injected dye can't flow past the tumor. (This study is dangerous if cord compression is nearly complete because withdrawal or escape of CSF will allow the tumor to exert greater pressure against the cord.)
◆ Radioisotope bone scan demonstrates metastatic invasion of the vertebrae by showing a characteristic increase in osteoblastic activity.
◆ CT scan shows cord compression and tumor location.
◆ Frozen section biopsy at surgery identifies the tissue type.
◆ Lumbar puncture may be normal, abnormal, or nonspecific. It may show clear yellow CSF as a result of increased protein levels if the flow is completely blocked. If the flow is partially blocked, protein levels rise, but the fluid is only slightly yellow in proportion to the CSF protein level. Cytology of the CSF may show malignant cells of metastatic carcinoma.

Treatment
Treatment of spinal cord tumors generally includes decompression or radiation. Laminectomy is indicated for primary tumors that produce spinal cord or cauda equina compression; it *isn't* usually indicated for metastatic tumors. If the tumor is slowly progressive or if it's treated before the cord degenerates from compression, symptoms are likely to disappear, and complete restoration of function is possible. In a patient with metastatic carcinoma or lymphoma who suddenly experiences complete transverse myelitis with spinal shock, functional improvement is unlikely, even with treatment, and the outlook is ominous. If the patient has incomplete paraplegia of rapid onset, emergency surgical decompression may save cord function. Steroid therapy with dexamethasone minimizes cord edema and temporarily relieves symptoms until surgery can be performed. Partial removal of intramedullary gliomas, followed by radiation, may alleviate symptoms for a short time. Metastatic extradural tumors can be controlled with radiation, analgesics and, in the case of hormone-mediated tumors (breast and prostate), appropriate hormone therapy. Transcutaneous electrical nerve stimulation (TENS) may control radicular pain from spinal cord tumors and is a useful alternative to opioid analgesics. In TENS, an electrical charge is applied to the skin to stimulate large-diameter nerve fibers and thereby inhibit transmission of pain impulses through small-diameter

nerve fibers. Chemotherapy generally hasn't proven effective against most spinal tumors, but may be recommended as salvage therapy in the setting of surgical and radiation failure.

Special considerations

The care plan for patients with spinal cord tumors should emphasize emotional support and skilled intervention during acute and chronic phases, early recognition of recurrence, prevention and treatment of complications, and maintenance of quality of life.

◆ On your first contact with the patient, perform a complete neurologic evaluation to obtain baseline data for planning future care and evaluating changes in clinical status.

◆ Care of the patient with a spinal cord tumor is basically the same as that for the patient with spinal cord injury and requires psychologic support, rehabilitation (including bowel and bladder retraining), and prevention of infection and skin breakdown. After laminectomy, care includes checking neurologic status frequently, changing position by logrolling, administering analgesics, monitoring frequently for infection, and aiding in early walking. Physical therapy may be needed to improve muscle strength and to improve the ability to function independently when permanent neurologic losses occur.

◆ Help the patient and family to understand and cope with the diagnosis, treatment, potential disabilities, and necessary changes in lifestyle.

◆ Take safety precautions for the patient with impaired sensation and motor deficits. Use side rails if the patient is bedridden; if not, encourage the patient to wear flat shoes, and remove scatter rugs and clutter to prevent falls.

◆ Encourage the patient to be independent in performing daily activities. Avoid aggravating pain by moving the patient slowly and by making sure the body is well aligned when giving personal care. Advise the patient to use TENS to block radicular pain.

◆ Administer steroids and antacids, as ordered, for cord edema after radiation therapy. Monitor for sensory or motor dysfunction, which indicates the need for more steroids.

◆ Enforce bed rest for the patient with vertebral body involvement until the practitioner says the patient can safely walk because body weight alone can cause cord collapse and cord laceration from bone fragments.

◆ Logroll and position the patient on his or her side every 2 hours to prevent pressure ulcers and other complications of immobility.

◆ If the patient is to wear a back brace, make sure he or she wears it whenever he or she gets out of bed.

Thorax

LUNG CANCER

Even though it's largely preventable, lung cancer is the most common cause of cancer death in men and women. Lung cancer usually develops within the wall or epithelium of the bronchial tree. (See *Tumor infiltration in lung cancer*, page 727.) Its most common types are epidermoid (squamous cell) carcinoma, small cell (oat cell) carcinoma, adenocarcinoma, and large cell (anaplastic) carcinoma. Although the prognosis is usually poor, it varies with the extent of metastasis at the time of diagnosis and the cell type growth rate. Only about 13% of patients with lung cancer survive 5 years after diagnosis.

Causes and incidence

Most experts agree that lung cancer is attributable to inhalation of carcinogenic pollutants by a susceptible host. Who's most susceptible? Any smoker older than age 40, especially if they began to smoke before age 15, has smoked a whole pack or more per day for 20 years, or works with or near asbestos.

Pollutants in tobacco smoke cause progressive lung cell degeneration. Lung cancer is 10 times more common in smokers than in nonsmokers, with 85% to 95% of the cases caused by voluntary or involuntary (secondhand) smoking. Cancer risk is determined by the number of cigarettes smoked daily, the depth of inhalation, how early in life smoking began, and the nicotine content of cigarettes. Two other factors also increase susceptibility: exposure to carcinogenic industrial and air pollutants (asbestos, uranium, arsenic, nickel, iron oxides, chromium, radioactive dust, and coal dust) and familial susceptibility.

Complications

◆ Anorexia
◆ Cachexia
◆ Clubbing of fingers and toes
◆ Dysphagia
◆ Dyspnea
◆ Esophageal compression
◆ Hypertrophic osteoarthropathy
◆ Hypoxemia
◆ Phrenic nerve paralysis
◆ Pleural effusion
◆ Tracheal obstruction

Signs and symptoms

Because early-stage lung cancer usually produces no symptoms, this disease is usually in an advanced state at diagnosis. These late-stage symptoms commonly lead to diagnosis:

PATHOPHYSIOLOGY
Tumor infiltration in lung cancer

The illustrations below show tumor infiltration in lung cancer as well as a bronchoscopic view of the tumor.

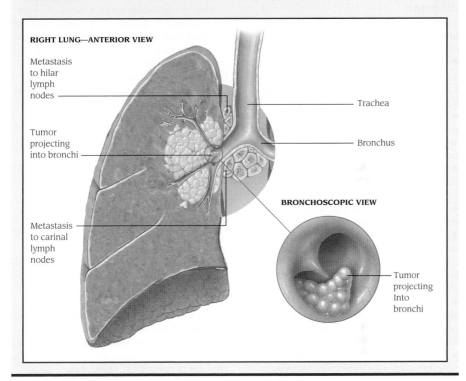

RIGHT LUNG—ANTERIOR VIEW

Metastasis to hilar lymph nodes

Tumor projecting into bronchi

Metastasis to carinal lymph nodes

Trachea

Bronchus

BRONCHOSCOPIC VIEW

Tumor projecting Into bronchi

◆ Epidermoid and small cell carcinomas—smoker's cough, hoarseness, wheezing, dyspnea, hemoptysis, and chest pain
◆ Adenocarcinoma and large cell carcinoma—fever, weakness, weight loss, anorexia, and shoulder pain

In addition to their obvious interference with respiratory function, lung tumors may also alter the production of hormones that regulate body function or homeostasis. Clinical conditions that result from such changes are known as *hormonal paraneoplastic syndromes*:
◆ Gynecomastia may result from large cell carcinoma.
◆ Hypertrophic pulmonary osteoarthropathy (bone and joint pain from cartilage erosion due to abnormal production of GH) may result from large cell carcinoma and adenocarcinoma.
◆ Cushing and carcinoid syndromes may result from small cell carcinoma.

◆ Hypercalcemia may result from epidermoid tumors.

Metastatic signs and symptoms vary greatly, depending on the effect of tumors on intrathoracic and distant structures:
◆ bronchial obstruction: hemoptysis, atelectasis, pneumonitis, dyspnea
◆ cervical thoracic sympathetic nerve involvement: miosis, ptosis, exophthalmos, reduced sweating
◆ chest wall invasion: piercing chest pain, increasing dyspnea, severe shoulder pain radiating down arm
◆ esophageal compression: dysphagia
◆ local lymphatic spread: cough, hemoptysis, stridor, pleural effusion
◆ pericardial involvement: pericardial effusion, tamponade, arrhythmias
◆ phrenic nerve involvement: dyspnea, shoulder pain, unilateral paralyzed diaphragm with paradoxical motion

♦ recurrent nerve invasion: hoarseness, vocal cord paralysis

♦ vena caval obstruction: venous distention and edema of face, neck, chest, and back

Distant metastasis may involve any part of the body, most commonly the CNS, liver, and bone.

Diagnosis

Typical clinical findings may strongly suggest lung cancer, but firm diagnosis requires further evidence.

♦ Chest X-ray usually shows an advanced lesion, but it can detect a lesion up to 2 years before symptoms appear. It also indicates tumor size and location.

♦ Sputum cytology, which is 75% reliable, requires a specimen coughed up from the lungs and tracheobronchial tree, *not* postnasal secretions or saliva.

♦ Spiral or helical CT of the chest may help to delineate the tumor's size and its relationship to surrounding structures.

♦ MRI is useful for differentiating vascular abnormalities from tumor.

♦ Bronchoscopy can locate the tumor site. Bronchoscopic washings provide material for cytologic and histologic examination. The flexible fiberoptic bronchoscope increases the test's effectiveness.

♦ Percutaneous needle biopsy of the lungs uses biplane fluoroscopic visual control to detect peripherally located tumors. This allows firm diagnosis in 80% of patients.

♦ Mediastinoscopy with tissue biopsy of accessible metastatic sites includes supraclavicular and mediastinal node and pleural biopsy. Directed needle biopsy may be performed in conjunction with CT scan.

♦ Thoracentesis allows chemical and cytologic examination of pleural fluid.

Additional studies include preoperative mediastinoscopy or mediastinotomy to rule out involvement of mediastinal lymph nodes (which would preclude curative pulmonary resection).

Other tests to detect metastasis include bone scan, bone marrow biopsy (recommended in small cell carcinoma), CT scan of the brain or abdomen, and positron emission tomography.

After histologic confirmation, staging determines the extent of the disease and helps in planning the treatment and predicting the prognosis.

Treatment

Recent treatment, which consists of combinations of surgery, radiation, and chemotherapy, may improve the prognosis and prolong survival. Nevertheless, because treatment usually begins at an advanced stage, it's largely palliative.

Surgery is the preferred treatment for stage I, stage II, or selected stage III squamous cell cancer; adenocarcinoma; and large cell carcinoma, unless the tumor is nonresectable or other conditions rule out surgery.

Surgery may include partial removal of a lung (wedge resection, segmental resection, lobectomy, or radical lobectomy) or total removal (pneumonectomy or radical pneumonectomy). A less invasive form of surgery that's used for small (1½" or less) tumors is video-assisted thoracic surgery (VATS). VATS requires small incisions and causes less pain than other types of surgery.

Preoperative radiation therapy may reduce tumor bulk to allow for surgical resection. Preradiation chemotherapy helps improve response rates. Radiation therapy is ordinarily recommended for stage I and stage II lesions, if surgery is contraindicated, and for stage III lesions when the disease is confined to the involved hemithorax and the ipsilateral supraclavicular lymph nodes.

Generally, radiation therapy is delayed until 1 month after surgery, to allow the wound to heal, and is then directed to the part of the chest most likely to develop metastasis. High-dose radiation therapy or radiation implants may also be used.

Research has shown that chemotherapy combinations of paclitaxel, gemcitabine, docetaxel, irinotecan, etoposide, and vinorelbine are more active and better tolerated when combined with cisplatin or carboplatin. Many of these drugs are also being utilized as single agents for the treatment of small cell and non-small cell lung cancers.

In laser therapy, laser energy is directed through a bronchoscope to destroy local tumors.

Special considerations

Comprehensive supportive care and patient teaching can minimize complications and speed recovery from surgery, radiation, and chemotherapy.

Before surgery:

♦ Supplement and reinforce the information given to the patient by the healthcare team about the disease and the surgical procedure.

♦ Explain expected postoperative procedures, such as insertion of an indwelling catheter, use of an endotracheal tube or chest tube (or both), dressing changes, and I.V. therapy.

♦ Teach the patient how to perform coughing, deep diaphragmatic breathing, and range-of-motion (ROM) exercises.

◆ Reassure the patient that analgesics will be provided and proper positioning will be implemented to control postoperative pain.

◆ Inform the patient that he or she may take nothing by mouth beginning after midnight the night before surgery, that he or she will shower with a soaplike antibacterial agent the night or morning before surgery, and that he or she will be given preoperative medications, such as a sedative and an anticholinergic to dry secretions.

After thoracic surgery:

◆ Maintain a patent airway, and monitor chest tubes to reestablish normal intrathoracic pressure and prevent postoperative and pulmonary complications.

◆ Check vital signs every 15 minutes during the first hour after surgery, every 30 minutes during the next 4 hours, and then every 2 hours. Watch for and report abnormal respiration and other changes.

◆ Suction the patient as needed, and encourage the patient to begin deep breathing and coughing as soon as possible. Check secretions often. Initially, sputum will be thick and dark with blood, but it should become thinner and grayish yellow within a day.

◆ Monitor and record closed chest drainage. Keep chest tubes patent and draining effectively. Fluctuation in the water seal chamber on inspiration and expiration indicates that the chest tube is patent. Watch for air leaks, and report them immediately. Position the patient on the surgical side to promote drainage and lung re-expansion.

◆ Watch for and report foul-smelling discharge and excessive drainage on dressing. Usually, the dressing is removed after 24 hours, unless the wound appears infected.

◆ Monitor intake and output. Maintain adequate hydration.

◆ Watch for and treat infection, shock, hemorrhage, atelectasis, dyspnea, mediastinal shift, and pulmonary embolus.

◆ To prevent pulmonary embolus, apply antiembolism stockings and encourage ROM exercises.

If the patient is receiving chemotherapy and radiation:

◆ Explain possible adverse effects of radiation and chemotherapy. Watch for, treat and, when possible, try to prevent them.

◆ Ask the dietary department to provide soft, nonirritating foods that are high in protein, and encourage the patient to eat high-calorie between-meal snacks.

◆ Give antiemetics and antidiarrheals, as needed.

◆ Schedule patient care activities in a way that helps the patient conserve energy.

◆ During radiation therapy, administer skin care to minimize skin breakdown. If the patient receives radiation therapy in an outpatient setting, warn the patient to avoid tight clothing, exposure to the sun, and harsh ointments on the chest. Teach the patient exercises to help prevent shoulder stiffness.

▒▒▒ **PREVENTION** *Teach high-risk patients ways to reduce their chances of developing lung cancer:*

◆ *For patients who smoke, explain the benefits of quitting and encourage them to quit.*

◆ *Refer smokers who want to quit to the American Cancer Society or smoking-cessation programs or suggest group therapy, individual counseling, or use of smoking-cessation products.*

◆ *Encourage patients with recurring or chronic respiratory infections and those with chronic lung disease who detect any change in the character of a cough to see their practitioner promptly for evaluation.*

BREAST CANCER

Breast cancer occurs more commonly in the left breast than the right and more commonly in the outer upper quadrant. Growth rates vary. Theoretically, slow-growing breast cancer may take up to 8 years to become palpable at 1 cm. It spreads by way of the lymphatic system and the bloodstream, through the right side of the heart to the lungs, and eventually to the other breast, the chest wall, liver, bone, and brain.

The estimated growth rate of breast cancer is referred to as *doubling time*, or the time it takes the malignant cells to double in number. Survival time for breast cancer is based on tumor size and spread; the number of involved nodes is the single most important factor in predicting survival time.

Breast cancer is classified by histologic appearance and location of the lesion, as follows:

◆ adenocarcinoma—arising from the epithelium

◆ intraductal—developing within the ducts (includes Paget disease)

◆ infiltrating—occurring in parenchyma of the breast

◆ inflammatory (rare)—reflecting rapid tumor growth, in which the overlying skin becomes edematous, inflamed, and indurated

◆ lobular carcinoma in situ—reflecting tumor growth involving lobes of glandular tissue

◆ medullary or circumscribed—large tumor with rapid growth rate

Breast cancer is also classified as invasive or noninvasive. Invasive tumor cells, which make up 90% of all breast cancers, break through the duct walls and encroach on other breast tissues.

Types of breast cancer

The illustrations below show ductal carcinoma in situ and infiltrating or invasive ductal carcinoma.

DUCTAL CARCINOMA IN SITU

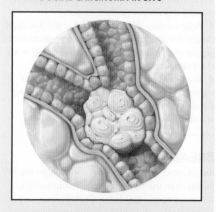

INFILTRATING (INVASIVE) DUCTAL CARCINOMA

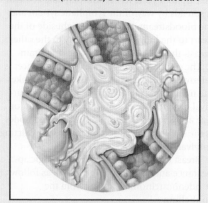

Noninvasive tumor cells remain confined to the duct in which they originated. (See *Types of breast cancer.*)

Causes and incidence

The cause of breast cancer isn't known, but its high incidence in women implicates estrogen.

Certain predisposing factors are clear; women at *high risk* include those who have a family history of breast cancer, particularly first-degree relatives (mother, sister, and maternal aunt).

Other women at high risk include those who:
♦ have long menstrual cycles or began menses early (before age 12) or menopause late (after age 55)
♦ have taken hormonal contraceptives
♦ used hormone replacement therapy for more than 5 years
♦ who took DES to prevent miscarriage
♦ have never been pregnant
♦ were first pregnant after age 30
♦ have had unilateral breast cancer
♦ have had ovarian cancer—particularly at a young age
♦ were exposed to low-level ionizing radiation
♦ have genetic mutations, such as in *BRCA1* and *BRCA2* genes

Women at *lower risk* include those who:
♦ were pregnant before age 20
♦ have had multiple pregnancies
♦ are Native American or Asian

Most breast cancer deaths occur in women age 50 and older (84% of cases), and 77% of new breast cancer cases occur in this age group. However, breast cancer may develop any time after puberty. It occurs in men, but rarely; male cases of breast cancer account for less than 1% of all cases.

The 5-year survival rate for localized breast cancer has improved because of earlier diagnosis and the variety of treatments now available. According to the most recent data, mortality rates continue to decline in White women and, for the first time, are also declining in younger Black women. Lymph node involvement is the most valuable prognostic predictor. With adjuvant therapy, 70% to 75% of women with negative nodes will survive 10 years or more compared with 20% to 25% of women with positive nodes.

Pathophysiology

A majority of breast carcinomas are invasive ductal carcinoma, followed by invasive lobular carcinomas. Invasive ductal carcinomas and invasive lobular carcinomas have distinct pathologic features. Specifically, lobular carcinomas grow as single cells arranged individually, in single file, or in sheets, and they have different molecular and genetic aberrations that distinguish them from ductal carcinomas. Ductal and lobular carcinomas may have different prognoses and treatment options, depending on all of the other features of the particular cancer. The remaining cases of invasive carcinoma are comprised of other special types of breast cancer that are characterized by unique pathologic findings. These special types include colloid (mucinous), medullary, micropapillary,

papillary, and tubular. It is important to distinguish between these various subtypes, because they can have different prognoses and treatment implications.

Complications
◆ Infection
◆ Decreased mobility
◆ Lymphedema

Signs and symptoms
Warning signals of possible breast cancer include:
◆ a lump or mass in the breast (a hard, non-tender stony mass is usually malignant)
◆ change in symmetry or size of the breast
◆ change in skin, thickening, scaly skin around the nipple, dimpling, edema (peau d'orange), or ulceration
◆ change in skin temperature (a warm, hot, or pink area; suspect cancer in a nonlactating woman older than childbearing age until proven otherwise)
◆ unusual drainage or discharge (A spontaneous discharge of any kind in a nonbreastfeeding, nonlactating woman warrants thorough investigation; so does any discharge produced by breast manipulation [greenish black, white, creamy, serous, or bloody]. If a breastfed infant rejects one breast, this may suggest possible breast cancer.)
◆ change in the nipple, such as itching, burning, erosion, or retraction
◆ pain (not usually a symptom of breast cancer unless the tumor is advanced, but it should be investigated)
◆ bone metastasis, pathologic bone fractures, and hypercalcemia
◆ edema of the arm

Diagnosis
The most reliable method of detecting breast cancer is the clinical breast examination, followed by immediate evaluation of any abnormality. Other diagnostic measures include mammography, ultrasound, needle biopsy, and surgical biopsy. Mammography is indicated for any woman whose physical examination suggests breast cancer. It should be done as a baseline on women between ages 35 and 39 and annually on all women older than age 40, on those who have a family history of breast cancer, and on those who have had unilateral breast cancer (to check for new disease).

⬡ **ELDER TIP** *Unfortunately, many older women don't receive regular mammograms, even when recommended by healthcare professionals, either because they fear radiation, discovering*

cancer, or discomfort during the procedure or because they're embarrassed about exposing their breasts.

The value of mammography is questionable for women under age 35 (because of the density of the breasts), except for those women who are strongly suspected of having breast cancer. False-negative results can occur in as many as 30% of all tests. Consequently, with a suspicious mass, a negative mammogram should be disregarded, and a fine needle aspiration or surgical biopsy should be done. Ultrasonography, which can distinguish a fluid-filled cyst from a tumor, can also be used instead of an invasive surgical biopsy.

Bone scan, brain scan, CT scan, measurement of alkaline phosphatase levels, liver function studies, and liver biopsy can detect distant metastases. A hormonal receptor assay done on the tumor can determine if the tumor is estrogen or progesterone dependent. (This test guides decisions to use therapy that blocks the action of the estrogen hormone that supports tumor growth.) (See *Understanding IVDMIA*.) Additionally, molecular testing for human epidermal growth factor receptor 2 (HER2) is recommended for determination of tumor status.

Treatment
In choosing therapy, the patient and practitioner should take into consideration the stage of the disease, the woman's age and menopausal status, and the disfiguring effects of the surgery. Treatment of breast cancer may include one or any combination of the following:
◆ Surgery involves either mastectomy or lumpectomy. A lumpectomy may be done on an outpatient basis and may be the only surgery needed, especially if the tumor is small and

---

Understanding IVDMIA

A prognostic tool for predicting breast cancer tumor recurrence recently received FDA approval. In vitro diagnostic multivariate index assay (IVDMIA) (such as MammaPrint) predicts the odds that an early-stage breast cancer will metastasize in 5 to 10 years. Using a biopsy sample taken from the tumor, the test analyzes the activity of 70 genes that affect whether or not an early-stage breast cancer will spread. It rates the patient as high risk or low risk for metastases. The test is intended for women younger than age 61 with stage I or II disease, who are lymph node-negative, and whose tumors are no larger than 5 cm.

there's no evidence of axillary node involvement. In many cases, radiation therapy is combined with this surgery.

A two-stage procedure, in which the surgeon removes the lump and confirms that it's malignant and then discusses treatment options with the patient, is desirable because it allows the patient to participate in the plan of treatment. Sometimes, if the tumor is diagnosed as clinically malignant, such planning can be done before surgery. In lumpectomy and dissection of the axillary lymph nodes, the tumor and the axillary lymph nodes are removed, leaving the breast intact. A simple mastectomy removes the breast but not the lymph nodes or pectoral muscles. Modified radical mastectomy removes the breast and the axillary lymph nodes. Radical mastectomy, the performance of which has declined, removes the breast, pectoralis major and minor muscles, and the axillary lymph nodes.

The spread of breast cancer to regional lymph nodes is considered a vital prognostic indicator. Sentinel lymph node biopsy, a reliable and minimally invasive procedure, is used to identify and sample the sentinel lymph node closest to the breast tumor. During the patient's surgery, the axillary node is injected with dye to help with identification and then sent to the pathologist to assess for cancer spread. If the node is negative, the patient can be spared an axillary node dissection, which carries its own risks and the potential for long-term complications.

Reconstructive breast surgery can be performed at the same time as mastectomy or it can be planned for a later date. Several options are available for breast reconstruction, including the insertion of breast implants or a transverse rectus abdominis musculocutaneous flap.

◆ Chemotherapy, involving various cytotoxic drug combinations, is used as either adjuvant or primary therapy, depending on several factors, including the TNM staging of the cancer, as well as estrogen receptor and HER2 status. The most commonly used antineoplastic drugs are cyclophosphamide, fluorouracil, methotrexate, doxorubicin, vincristine, and paclitaxel. A common drug combination used in both premenopausal and postmenopausal women is cyclophosphamide, doxorubicin, and paclitaxel.

Tamoxifen, an estrogen antagonist, or select aromatase inhibitors are the adjuvant treatments of choice for postmenopausal patients with positive estrogen receptor status. They have also been found to reduce the risk of breast cancer in women at high risk. For individuals with HER2-positive receptors, monoclonal antibodies such as trastuzumab are indicated for adjuvant therapy.

◆ Peripheral stem cell therapy is an option, but it's rarely used for advanced breast cancer.
◆ Primary radiation therapy before or after tumor removal is effective for small tumors in early stages with no evidence of distant metastasis; it's also used to prevent or treat local recurrence. Presurgical radiation to the breast in inflammatory breast cancer helps make tumors more surgically manageable.
◆ Estrogen, progesterone, androgen, or antiandrogen aminoglutethimide therapy may also be given to breast cancer patients. The success of these drug therapies—along with growing evidence that breast cancer is a systemic, not local, disease—has led to a decline in ablative surgery.

Special considerations

To provide good care for a patient with breast cancer, begin with a history, assess the patient's feelings about their illness, and determine what they know about it and what they expect. Preoperatively, make sure you know what kind of surgery is scheduled, so you can prepare them properly. If a mastectomy is scheduled, in addition to the usual preoperative preparation (e.g., skin preparations and not allowing the patient anything by mouth), provide the following information:

◆ Teach them how to deep-breathe and cough to prevent pulmonary complications and how to rotate their ankles to help prevent thromboembolism.
◆ Tell them they can ease their pain by lying on the affected side or by placing a hand or pillow on the incision. Preoperatively, show them where the incision will be. Inform them that they'll receive pain medication and that they need not fear addiction. Remember, adequate pain relief encourages coughing and turning and promotes general well-being. Positioning a small pillow anteriorly under the patient's arm provides comfort.
◆ Encourage them to get out of bed as soon as possible (even as soon as the anesthesia wears off or the first evening after surgery).
◆ Explain that, after mastectomy, an incisional drain or suction device will be used to remove accumulated serous or sanguineous fluid, thereby promoting healing.

Postoperative care:
◆ Inspect the dressing anteriorly and posteriorly, reporting bleeding promptly.
◆ Measure and record the amount of drainage; also note the color. Expect drainage to be bloody during the first 4 hours and afterward to become serous.
◆ Check circulatory status (blood pressure, pulse, respirations, and bleeding).
◆ Monitor intake and output for at least 48 hours after general anesthesia.

◆ Inform the patient to not let anyone draw blood, start an I.V., give an injection, or take a blood pressure on the affected side because these activities will also increase the chances of developing lymphedema.

◆ Inspect the incision. Encourage the patient and partner to look at the incision as soon as possible, perhaps when the first dressing is removed.

◆ Advise the patient to ask her practitioner about reconstructive surgery or to call the local or state medical society for the names of plastic reconstructive surgeons who regularly perform surgery to create breast mounds. In many cases, reconstructive surgery may be planned before the mastectomy.

◆ Instruct the patient about breast prostheses. The American Cancer Society's Reach to Recovery group can provide instruction, emotional support and counseling, and a list of area stores that sell prostheses.

◆ Give psychological and emotional support. Most patients fear cancer and possible disfigurement and worry about loss of sexual function. Explain that breast surgery doesn't interfere with sexual function and that the patient may resume sexual activity as soon as desired after surgery.

◆ Also explain to the patient that they may experience *phantom breast syndrome* (a phenomenon in which a tingling or a pins-and-needles sensation is felt in the area of the amputated breast tissue) or depression following mastectomy. Listen to the patient's concerns, offer support, and refer them to an appropriate organization such as the American Cancer Society's Reach to Recovery, which offers caring and sharing groups to help breast cancer patients in the hospital and at home.

▓▓▓▓▓ PREVENTION

◆ *Prevent lymphedema of the arm, which may be an eventual complication of any breast cancer treatment that involves lymph node manipulation.*

◆ *Help the patient prevent lymphedema by instructing on exercising the hand and arm regularly and to avoid activities that might cause infection or impairment in this hand or arm, which increases the chance of developing lymphedema. (See Postoperative arm and hand care.)*

Abdomen and pelvis

GASTRIC CANCER

Gastric cancer can be classified as polypoid, ulcerating, ulcerating and infiltrating, or diffuse, according to gross appearance. The parts of the stomach affected by gastric cancer, listed in order of decreasing frequency, are the pylorus and antrum, the lesser curvature, the cardia, the body of the stomach, and the greater curvature. (See *Sites of gastric cancer*, page 734.)

Postoperative arm and hand care

Hand exercises for the patient who's prone to lymphedema can begin on the day of surgery. Plan arm exercises with the provider because they can anticipate potential problems with the suture line.

◆ Have the patient open their hand and close it tightly six to eight times every 3 hours while they're awake.

◆ Elevate the arm on the affected side on a pillow above the heart level.

◆ Encourage the patient to wash their face and comb their hair—an effective exercise.

◆ Measure and record the circumference of the patient's arm 2¼" (5.7 cm) from elbow. Indicate the exact place you measured. By remeasuring a month after surgery, and at intervals during and following radiation therapy, you can determine whether lymphedema is present. The patient may complain that the arm is heavy—an early symptom of lymphedema.

◆ When the patient is home, they can elevate their arm and hand by supporting it on the back of a chair or a couch.

Gastric cancer infiltrates rapidly to regional lymph nodes, omentum, liver, and lungs by the following routes: walls of the stomach, duodenum, and esophagus; lymphatic system; adjacent organs; bloodstream; and peritoneal cavity.

Causes and incidence

The cause of gastric cancer is unknown. It's commonly associated with gastritis with gastric atrophy, which may result from gastric cancer and may not be a precursor state. Predisposing factors include environmental influences, such as smoking and high alcohol intake. Genetic factors have also been implicated because this disease occurs more commonly among people with type A blood than among those with type O; similarly, it's more common in people with a family history of gastric cancer. E-cadherin mutations have been found in approximately 25% of families with an autosomal dominant form of gastric cancer. Dietary factors also seem related, including types of food preparation, physical properties of some foods, and certain methods of food preservation (especially smoking, pickling, or salting). There's a strong correlation between infection with *Helicobacter pylori* and distal gastric cancer.

Gastric cancer is common throughout the world and affects all races; however, unexplained geographic and cultural differences in incidence

Sites of gastric cancer

The most common site of gastric cancer is the pyloric area, accounting for about 50% of cases. The next most common area is the lesser curvature of the stomach, accounting for about 25% of cases.

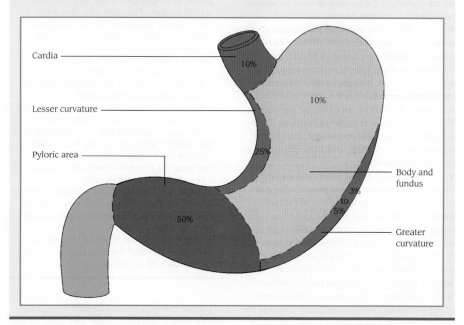

occur—for example, a higher mortality in Japan, Iceland, Chile, and Austria. In the United States, during the past 25 years, incidence has decreased by 50%; the resulting death rate is one third of what it was 30 years ago. Incidence is higher in males older than 40. Hispanic, Native, and African Americans are twice as likely to develop gastric cancer than Whites. The prognosis depends on the stage of the disease at the time of diagnosis. Gastric cancer is frequently diagnosed at an advanced stage. The overall 5-year survival rate is about 19%.

Pathophysiology

Gastric carcinomas can be divided into two major categories. These are the so-called intestinal, expanding, or differentiated type; and the diffuse, infiltrative, or undifferentiated type. The former is characterized by expansive growth and liver metastasis; whereas the latter is distinguished by infiltrative growth and peritoneal dissemination. Undifferentiated type tumors include histologically poorly differentiated adenocarcinoma, signet ring cell carcinoma, and mucinous adenocarcinoma, but some of

these tumors show biologic behavior similar to differentiated type tumors. The most important factors predicting outcomes of patients with gastric carcinoma are the depth of wall invasion and the status of lymph node metastasis.

Complications
◆ Malnutrition
◆ GI obstruction
◆ Iron deficiency anemia
◆ Metastasis

Signs and symptoms

Early clues to gastric cancer are chronic dyspepsia and epigastric discomfort, followed in later stages by weight loss, anorexia, feeling of fullness after eating, anemia, and fatigue. If the cancer is in the cardia, the first sign or symptom may be dysphagia and, later, vomiting (commonly coffee-ground vomitus). Affected patients may also have blood in their stools.

The course of gastric cancer may be insidious or fulminating. Unfortunately, the patient typically treats himself with antacids or histamine blockers until the symptoms of advanced stages appear.

Diagnosis

Diagnosis depends primarily on reinvestigations of any persistent or recurring GI changes and complaints. To rule out other conditions producing similar symptoms, diagnostic evaluation must include the testing of blood, stools, and stomach fluid samples.

Diagnosis of gastric cancer generally requires these studies:

◆ Barium X-rays of the GI tract with fluoroscopy show changes (tumor or filling defect in the outline of the stomach, loss of flexibility and distensibility, and abnormal gastric mucosa with or without ulceration).

◆ Gastroscopy with fiberoptic endoscopy helps rule out other diffuse gastric mucosal abnormalities by allowing direct visualization and gastroscopic biopsy to evaluate gastric mucosal lesions.

◆ Photography with fiberoptic endoscope provides a permanent record of gastric lesions that can later be used to determine disease progression and effect of treatment.

◆ A gastric acid stimulation test determines whether the stomach is able to properly secrete acid.

Certain other studies may rule out specific organ metastasis: CT scans, chest X-rays, liver and bone scans, and liver biopsy.

Treatment

In many cases, surgery is the treatment of choice. Excision of the lesion with appropriate margins is possible in more than one third of patients. Even in patients whose disease isn't considered surgically curable, resection offers palliation and improves potential benefits from chemotherapy and radiation.

The nature and extent of the lesion determine the kind of surgery that is most appropriate. Common surgical procedures include subtotal gastric resection (subtotal gastrectomy) and total gastric resection (total gastrectomy). When carcinoma involves the pylorus and antrum, gastric resection removes the lower stomach and duodenum (gastrojejunostomy or Billroth II). If metastasis has occurred, the omentum and spleen may also have to be removed.

If gastric cancer has spread to the liver, peritoneum, or lymph glands, palliative surgery may include gastrostomy, jejunostomy, or a gastric or partial gastric resection. Such surgery may temporarily relieve vomiting, nausea, pain, and dysphagia, while allowing enteral nutrition to continue.

Chemotherapy for GI cancers may help to control symptoms and prolong survival. Adenocarcinoma of the stomach (see *Adenocarcinoma of the stomach*, page 736.) has responded to several agents, including fluorouracil, paclitaxel, doxorubicin, cisplatin, methotrexate, etoposide, docetaxel, oxaliplatin, irinotecan, and mitomycin. Antiemetics can control nausea, which increases as the cancer advances. In the more advanced stages, sedatives and tranquilizers may be necessary to control overwhelming anxiety. Opioids are commonly necessary to relieve severe and unremitting pain.

Radiation has been particularly useful when combined with chemotherapy in patients who have unresectable or partially resectable disease. It should be given on an empty stomach and shouldn't be used preoperatively because it may damage viscera and impede healing.

Treatment with antispasmodics and antacids may help relieve GI distress. Histamine$_2$-receptor antagonists can treat GI ulcers.

Special considerations

◆ Before surgery, prepare the patient for its effects and for postsurgical procedures such as insertion of an NG tube for drainage and I.V. lines.

◆ Reassure the patient who's having a partial gastric resection that they may eventually be able to eat normally. Prepare the patient who's having a total gastrectomy for slow recovery and only partial return to a normal diet.

◆ Include the family in all phases of the patient's care.

◆ Emphasize the importance of changing position every 2 hours and of deep breathing.

◆ After surgery, give meticulous supportive care to promote recovery and prevent complications.

◆ After any type of gastrectomy, pulmonary complications may result, and oxygen may be needed. Regularly assist the patient with turning, coughing, and deep breathing. Turning the patient hourly and administering analgesic opioids, as ordered, may prevent pulmonary problems. Incentive spirometry may also be needed for complete lung expansion. Proper positioning is important as well; semi-Fowler position facilitates breathing and drainage.

◆ After gastrectomy, little (if any) drainage comes from the NG tube because no secretions form after stomach removal. Without a stomach for storage, many patients experience dumping syndrome. Intrinsic factor is absent from gastric secretions, leading to malabsorption of vitamin B$_{12}$. To prevent vitamin B$_{12}$ deficiency, the patient must take a replacement vitamin for the rest of their life as well as an iron supplement.

◆ During radiation treatment, encourage the patient to eat high-calorie, well-balanced meals.

Adenocarcinoma of the stomach

This illustration shows adenocarcinoma of the gastric mucosa.

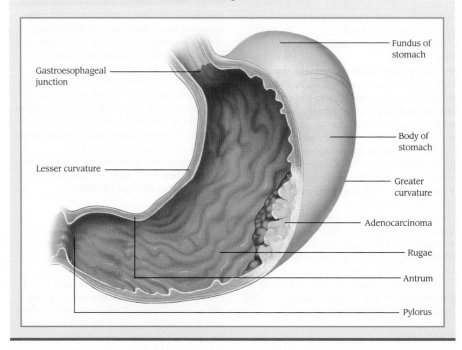

Offer fluids such as ginger ale to minimize such radiation adverse effects as nausea and vomiting.

Watch for the following complications of surgery:

♦ Patients who experience poor digestion and absorption after gastrectomy need a special diet: frequent feedings of small amounts of clear liquids, increasing to small, frequent feedings of bland food. After total gastrectomy, patients must eat small meals for the rest of their lives. (Some patients need pancreatin and sodium bicarbonate after meals to prevent or control steatorrhea and dyspepsia.)

♦ Wound dehiscence and delayed healing, stemming from decreased protein, anemia, and avitaminosis, may occur. Preoperative vitamin and protein replacement can prevent such complications. Observe the wound regularly for redness, swelling, failure to heal, or warmth. Parenteral administration of vitamin C may improve wound healing.

♦ Vitamin deficiency may result from obstruction, diarrhea, or an inadequate diet. Ascorbic acid, thiamine, riboflavin, nicotinic acid, and vitamin K supplements may be beneficial. Good nutrition promotes weight gain, strength, independence, a positive outlook, and tolerance for surgery, radiation therapy, or chemotherapy. Aside from meeting caloric needs, nutrition must provide adequate protein, fluid, and potassium intake to facilitate glycogen and protein synthesis. Anabolic agents such as methandrostenolone may induce nitrogen retention. Steroids, antidepressants, wine, or brandy may boost the appetite.

♦ When all treatments have failed, concentrate on keeping the patient comfortable and free from pain, and provide as much psychological support as possible. If the patient is going home, discuss continuing care needs with the caregiver or refer the patient to an appropriate home healthcare agency or hospice. Encourage the patient and the caregivers to express their feelings and concerns. Answer their questions honestly with tact and sensitivity. (See *Preventing gastric cancer*, page 737.)

Preventing gastric cancer

Although gastric cancer can't entirely be prevented, encourage your patient to make these lifestyles changes to reduce the risk of its occurring.

Limit nitrates
Nitrates are known to contribute to gastric cancer. They're found mainly in processed meats such as bologna, salami, and corned beef, and in cured meats, such as ham and bacon.

Limit smoked, pickled, and heavily salted foods
Smoked, pickled, and heavily salted foods have been linked to an increased risk of stomach cancer. Eating fewer of these foods may help reduce the risk of developing gastric cancer.

Stop smoking
Smoking greatly increases the risk of developing stomach cancer, especially cancer that occurs at the junction of the esophagus and the stomach.

Limit alcohol consumption
Alcohol may cause changes in cells that can lead to cancer. Limiting alcohol intake may reduce the risk of developing gastric cancer.

Limit red meat
Eating large amounts of red meat—particularly when it's barbecued or well done—increases the risk of gastric cancer. Instead, suggest eating fish or poultry.

See a physician if symptoms of an ulcer develop
Helicobacter pylori, the bacterium that causes most cases of gastric ulcers, is a leading cause of gastric cancer. Symptoms of ulcers shouldn't be ignored. Encourage your patient to report if he or she experiences a gnawing pain in the abdomen or chest that's worse at night or when the stomach is empty. Other more severe signs and symptoms of ulcers include nausea, vomiting, bleeding, and unintended weight loss.

ESOPHAGEAL CANCER
Esophageal cancer is a malignant tumor that occurs in the esophagus, the muscular tube that propels food from the mouth to the stomach. It's difficult to treat but can be cured if the cancer is confined to the esophagus. For patients whose cancer has spread beyond the esophagus, cure generally isn't possible; treatment is directed toward symptom relief.

Causes and incidence
The cause of esophageal cancer is unknown, but among predisposing factors are chronic irritation caused by heavy smoking and excessive use of alcohol, stasis-induced inflammation, nutritional deficiency, and diets high in nitrosamines. A genetic link has been proposed concerning an overexpression and mutation of the *TP63* tumor suppressor gene. Esophageal tumors are usually fungating and infiltrating. Most arise in squamous cell epithelium. However, the number of adenocarcinomas is greatly rising in the United States. (See *Common* *esophageal cancers*, page 738.) Melanomas and sarcomas are few.

Regardless of type, esophageal cancer is usually fatal, with a 5-year survival rate of about 10% and regional metastasis occurring early via submucosal lymphatics. Metastasis produces such serious complications as tracheoesophageal fistulas, mediastinitis, and aortic perforation. Common sites of distant metastasis include the liver and lungs.

Esophageal cancer most commonly develops in men older than age 50 and is nearly always fatal. This disease occurs worldwide, but incidence varies geographically. It's most common in Japan, China, the Middle East, and parts of South Africa. In the United States, it affects less than 5 in 100,000 people.

Pathophysiology
Esophageal cancer is a serious malignancy with high mortality. The two common distinctive pathologic subtypes of esophageal cancer are

Common esophageal cancers

The illustration below shows squamous cell carcinoma and adenocarcinoma of the esophagus.

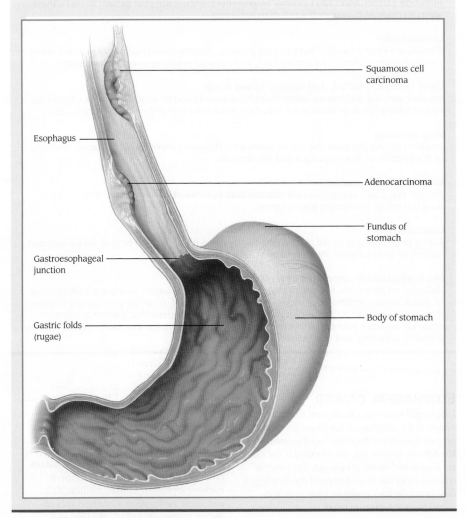

SCC and adenocarcinoma. These differ with regard to etiology, ethnic distribution, pathogenesis, and location in the esophagus.

Complications

- Mediastinitis
- Tracheoesophageal fistula
- Bronchoesophageal fistula
- Aortic perforation
- Esophageal obstruction
- Aspiration pneumonia

Signs and symptoms

Dysphagia and weight loss are the most common presenting symptoms. Dysphagia is mild and intermittent at first, but it soon becomes constant. Pain, hoarseness, coughing, and esophageal obstruction follow. Cachexia usually develops.

Diagnosis

X-rays of the esophagus, with barium swallow and motility studies, reveal structural and filling defects and reduced peristalsis.

℞ **CONFIRMING DIAGNOSIS** *Endoscopic examination of the esophagus (esophagogastroduodenoscopy), punch and brush biopsies, and exfoliative cytologic tests confirm esophageal tumors. Usually, MRI of the chest and thoracic CT are helpful in determining disease staging. Positron emission tomography is useful in determining disease staging and whether surgery is possible.*

Treatment

Multimodal therapy is usually indicated. Whenever possible, treatment includes resection to maintain a passageway for food. This may require such radical surgery as esophagogastrectomy with jejunal or colonic bypass grafts. Palliative surgery may include a feeding gastrostomy.

Cisplatin and fluorouracil are the primary chemotherapeutic agents used. Additional agents include mitomycin, bleomycin, methotrexate, doxorubicin, vindesine, irinotecan, and the taxanes. Targeted biological therapies for vascular endothelial growth factor (VEGF) receptor, and HER2 are used in combination with chemotherapy and radiation. Chemotherapy with 5-fluorouracil or cisplatin may be used. Insertion of prosthetic tubes to bridge the tumor alleviates dysphagia. Other treatments to improve the patient's ability to swallow include endoscopic dilation of the esophagus (sometimes with placement of a stent) and photodynamic therapy, which involves injecting a drug into the tumor and activating the drug by exposing it to light.

Treatment complications may be severe. Surgery may precipitate an anastomotic leak, a fistula, pneumonia, and empyema. Rarely, radiation may cause esophageal perforation, pneumonitis and pulmonary fibrosis, or myelitis of the spinal cord. Prosthetic tubes may dislodge and perforate the mediastinum or erode the tumor.

Special considerations

◆ Before surgery, answer the patient's questions and let them know what to expect after surgery, such as gastrostomy tubes, closed chest drainage, and NG suctioning.
◆ If surgery included an esophageal anastomosis, keep the patient flat on his or her back to avoid tension on the suture line.
◆ Promote adequate nutrition and assess the patient's nutritional and hydration status to determine the need for supplemental parenteral feedings.
◆ Prevent aspiration of food by placing the patient in Fowler position for meals and allowing plenty of time to eat. Provide high-calorie, high-protein, "blenderized" food, as needed.

Because the patient will probably regurgitate some food, clean the mouth carefully after each meal. Keep mouthwash handy.
◆ If the patient has a gastrostomy tube, give food slowly—by gravity—in prescribed amounts (usually 200 to 500 mL). Offer something to chew before each feeding to promote gastric secretions and a semblance of normal eating.
◆ Instruct the family in gastrostomy tube care (checking tube patency before each feeding, adequate flushing after feedings and medications, providing skin care around the tube, keeping the patient upright during and after feedings).
◆ Provide emotional support for the patient and family; refer them to appropriate organizations such as the American Cancer Society.
◆ When all treatments have failed, concentrate on keeping the patient comfortable and free from pain, providing as much psychological support as possible. If the patient is going home, discuss continuing care needs with the caregiver, or refer the patient to an appropriate home healthcare agency or hospice. Encourage the patient and caregiver to express their feelings and concerns. Answer their questions honestly, with tact and sensitivity.

PANCREATIC CANCER

A deadly GI cancer, pancreatic cancer progresses rapidly. From 75% to 80% of pancreatic cancers are metastatic at the time of diagnosis. Most pancreatic tumors are adenocarcinomas. (See *Pancreatic adenocarcinoma*, page 741.) The two main tissue types are cylinder cell and large, fatty, granular cell. (See *Types of pancreatic cancer*, page 740.)

Causes and incidence

Evidence suggests that pancreatic cancer is linked to inhalation or absorption of the following carcinogens, which are then excreted by the pancreas:
◆ cigarettes
◆ food additives
◆ industrial chemicals, such as beta-naphthalene, benzidine, and urea

Possible predisposing factors are chronic pancreatitis, diabetes mellitus, and chronic alcohol abuse (both pancreatitis and diabetes mellitus may be early manifestations of the disease as well). Genetic predisposition may be present in 5% to 10% of patients, including *CDKN2A* (p16), *BRCA2*, and *PALB2* mutations.

Pancreatic cancer incidence increases with age, peaking between ages 60 and 70. Geographically, the incidence is highest in Israel, the United States, Sweden, and Canada. From 31,000 to 32,000 new cases are diagnosed each

Types of pancreatic cancer

Type and pathology	Clinical features
Head of pancreas	
◆ Commonly obstructs ampulla of Vater and common bile duct ◆ Directly metastasizes to duodenum ◆ Adhesions anchor tumor to spine, stomach, and intestines	◆ Jaundice (late sign)—slowly progressive, unremitting; may cause skin, especially of the face and genitals, to turn olive green or black ◆ Pruritus—in many cases severe ◆ Weight loss—rapid and severe, possibly as great as 30 lb (13.6 kg); may lead to emaciation, weakness, and muscle atrophy ◆ Slowed digestion, gastric distention, nausea, diarrhea, and steatorrhea with clay-colored stools ◆ Liver and gallbladder enlargement from lymph node metastasis to biliary tract and duct wall resulting in compression and obstruction; gallbladder may be palpable (Courvoisier sign) ◆ Dull, nondescript, continuous abdominal pain radiating to right upper quadrant; relieved by bending forward ◆ GI hemorrhage and biliary infection common
Body and tail of pancreas	
◆ Large nodular masses become fixed to retropancreatic tissues and spine ◆ Direct invasion of spleen, left kidney, suprarenal gland, diaphragm ◆ Involvement of celiac plexus results in thrombosis of splenic vein and spleen infarction	**Body** ◆ Pain (predominant symptom)—usually epigastric, develops slowly and radiates to back; relieved by bending forward or sitting up; intensified by lying supine; most intense 3 to 4 hours after eating; when celiac plexus is involved, pain is more intense and lasts longer ◆ Venous thrombosis and thrombophlebitis common; may precede other symptoms by months ◆ Splenomegaly (from infarction), hepatomegaly (occasionally), and jaundice (rarely) **Tail** Symptoms result from metastasis: ◆ Abdominal tumor (most common finding) producing a palpable abdominal mass and abdominal pain radiating to the left hypochondrium and left side of the chest ◆ Anorexia leading to weight loss, emaciation, and weakness ◆ Splenomegaly and upper GI bleeding

year with about the same number of deaths occurring. It's the fourth leading cause of cancer death in the United States.

Pathophysiology

Typically, pancreatic cancer first metastasizes to regional lymph nodes, then to the liver and, less commonly, to the lungs. It can also directly invade surrounding visceral organs such as the duodenum, stomach, and colon, or it can metastasize to any surface in the abdominal cavity

via peritoneal spread. Ascites may result, and this has an ominous prognosis. Pancreatic cancer may spread to the skin as painful nodular metastases. Metastasis to bone is uncommon.

Complications

◆ Malabsorption
◆ Insulin-dependent diabetes
◆ Liver and GI problems
◆ Hemorrhage
◆ Mental status changes

Pancreatic adenocarcinoma

The illustration shows adenocarcinoma of the tail of the pancreas.

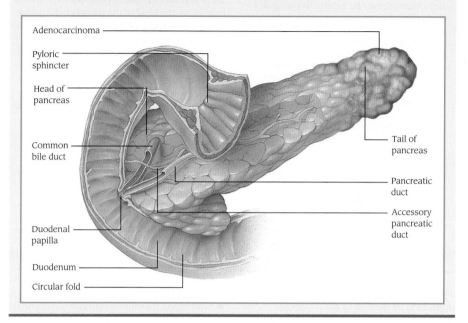

Signs and symptoms

The most common features of pancreatic cancer are weight loss, abdominal or low back pain, jaundice, and diarrhea. Other generalized effects include fever, loss of appetite, nausea, vomiting, weakness, indigestion, clay-colored stools, paleness, depression, skin lesions (usually on the legs), and fatigue.

Diagnosis

CONFIRMING DIAGNOSIS *Definitive diagnosis requires a laparotomy with a biopsy.*

Other tests used to detect pancreatic cancer include:

◆ ultrasound of the abdomen—can identify a mass but not its histology
◆ CT scan of the abdomen—similar to ultrasound but shows greater detail
◆ angiography—shows vascular supply of tumor
◆ endoscopic retrograde cholangiopancreatography—allows visualization, instillation of contrast medium, and specimen biopsy
◆ MRI of the abdomen—shows tumor size and location in great detail

Laboratory tests supporting this diagnosis include serum bilirubin (increased); serum amylase and serum lipase (sometimes elevated); prothrombin time (prolonged); aspartate aminotransferase and alanine aminotransferase (elevations indicate necrosis of liver cells); alkaline phosphatase (marked elevation occurs with biliary obstruction); plasma insulin immunoassay (shows measurable serum insulin in the presence of islet cell tumors) (see *Islet cell tumors,* page 742); hemoglobin (Hb) and hematocrit (HCT) (may show mild anemia); fasting blood glucose (may indicate hypoglycemia or hyperglycemia); and stools (occult blood may signal ulceration in GI tract or ampulla of Vater).

Treatment

Treatment of pancreatic cancer depends on tumor location and stage. Therapy consists of surgery and, possibly, radiation and chemotherapy. Standard chemotherapy for patients with locally unresectable cancer includes fluorouracil and gemcitabine. Gemcitabine has been demonstrated to improve the quality of life through better pain control, adequate performance status, decreased analgesic consumption, shrinkage of tumor, and prolonged survival.

Other medications used in pancreatic cancer include:

◆ antacids (by mouth or by NG tube)—to decrease secretion of pancreatic enzymes and

Islet cell tumors

Relatively uncommon, islet cell tumors (insulinomas) may be benign or malignant and produce signs and symptoms in three stages:
1. Slight hypoglycemia—fatigue, restlessness, malaise, and excessive weight gain
2. Compensatory secretion of epinephrine—pallor, clamminess, perspiration, palpitations, finger tremors, hunger, decreased temperature, and increased pulse and blood pressure
3. Severe hypoglycemia—ataxia, clouded sensorium, diplopia, episodes of violence, and hysteria
Usually, insulinomas metastasize to the liver alone but may metastasize to bone, brain, and lungs. Death results from a combination of hypoglycemic reactions and widespread metastasis. Treatment consists of enucleation of tumor (if benign) and chemotherapy with streptozocin or resection to include pancreatic tissue (if malignant).

to suppress peptic activity, thereby reducing stress-induced damage to gastric mucosa
◆ antibiotics (oral, I.V., or I.M.)—to prevent infection and relieve symptoms
◆ anticholinergics (particularly propantheline)—to decrease GI tract spasm and motility and reduce pain and secretions
◆ diuretics—to mobilize extracellular fluid from ascites
◆ insulin—to provide adequate exogenous insulin after pancreatic resection
◆ opioids—to relieve pain, but only after analgesics fail because morphine, meperidine, and codeine can lead to biliary tract spasm and increase common bile duct pressure
◆ pancreatic enzymes (average dose 0.5 to 1 mg with meals)—to assist in digestion of proteins, carbohydrates, and fats when pancreatic juices are insufficient because of surgery or obstruction
   Surgical resection offers the only possibility of a cure in pancreatic cancer. After resection, median survival is 12 to 18 months:
◆ Total pancreatectomy may increase survival time by resecting a localized tumor or by controlling postoperative gastric ulceration.
◆ Cholecystojejunostomy, choledochoduodenostomy, and choledochojejunostomy have partially replaced radical resection to bypass obstructing common bile duct extensions, thus decreasing the incidence of jaundice and pruritus.
◆ The Whipple procedure, or pancreatoduodenectomy, can produce wide lymphatic

clearance, except with tumors located near the portal vein, superior mesenteric vein and artery, and celiac axis. When the Whipple procedure is performed at specialized medical facilities, the 5-year survival rate approaches 40%. In this procedure, the head of the pancreas, the duodenum, and portions of the body and tail of the pancreas, stomach, jejunum, pancreatic duct, and distal portion of the bile duct are removed.
◆ Gastrojejunostomy is performed if radical resection isn't indicated and duodenal obstruction is expected to develop later.
   External beam radiation therapy is usually ineffective except as an adjunct to chemotherapy or as a palliative measure. Intraoperative electron beam radiation is a new approach in which a beam of radiation is used during surgery to allow a high dose of radiation to be focused on a tumor and avoid nearby organs.

Special considerations
Before surgery:
◆ Ensure that the patient is medically stable, particularly regarding nutrition (this may take 4 to 5 days). If the patient can't tolerate oral feedings, provide TPN and I.V. fat emulsions to correct deficiencies and maintain positive nitrogen balance.
◆ Give blood transfusions (to combat anemia), vitamin K (to overcome prothrombin deficiency), antibiotics (to prevent postoperative complications), and gastric lavage (to maintain gastric decompression), as ordered.
◆ Tell the patient about expected postoperative procedures and expected adverse effects of radiation and chemotherapy.
   After surgery:
◆ Watch for and report complications, such as fistula, pancreatitis, fluid and electrolyte imbalance, infection, hemorrhage, skin breakdown, nutritional deficiency, hepatic failure, renal insufficiency, and diabetes.
◆ If the patient is receiving chemotherapy, treat adverse effects symptomatically.
   Throughout this illness, provide meticulous supportive care:
◆ Monitor fluid balance, abdominal girth, metabolic state, and weight daily. In weight loss, replace nutrients I.V., by mouth, or by NG tube; in weight gain (due to ascites), impose dietary restrictions, such as a low-sodium or fluid-retention diet, as ordered. Maintain a 2,500-calorie diet.
◆ Serve small, frequent, nutritious meals by enlisting the dietitian's services. Administer an oral pancreatic enzyme at mealtimes if needed. Give an antacid to prevent stress ulcers as ordered.
◆ To prevent constipation, administer laxatives, stool softeners, and cathartics, as ordered; modify

diet; and increase fluid intake. To increase GI motility, position the patient properly at mealtimes, and help the patient walk when they can.

◆ Ensure adequate rest and sleep. Assist with ROM and isometric exercises, as appropriate.

◆ Administer pain medication, antibiotics, and antipyretics, as ordered. Note time, site (if injected), and response.

◆ Watch for signs of hypoglycemia or hyperglycemia; administer glucose or an antidiabetic agent, as ordered. Monitor blood glucose levels and response to treatment.

◆ Document progression of jaundice.

◆ Provide meticulous skin care to avoid pruritus and necrosis. Prevent excoriation in a pruritic patient by clipping nails and having the patient wear cotton gloves.

◆ Watch for signs of upper GI bleeding, test stools and vomitus for occult blood, and keep a flow sheet of Hb levels and HCT. To control active bleeding, promote gastric vasoconstriction with prescribed medication. Replace any fluid loss. Ease discomfort from pyloric obstruction with an NG tube.

◆ To prevent thrombosis, apply antiembolism stockings and assist in ROM exercises. If thrombosis occurs, elevate the patient's legs, and give an anticoagulant or aspirin, as ordered.

◆ When all treatments have failed, concentrate on keeping the patient comfortable and free from pain, and provide as much psychological support as possible. If the patient is going home, discuss continuing care needs with the caregiver or refer the patient to an appropriate home healthcare agency or hospice. Encourage the patient and caregiver to express their feelings and concerns. Answer their questions honestly, with tact and sensitivity.

▦▦▦ **PREVENTION** *To help prevent pancreatic cancer, teach your patient to:*

◆ *avoid or stop smoking*

◆ *eat a diet high in whole grains, fruits, and vegetables*

◆ *maintain a healthy weight and exercise regularly*

COLORECTAL CANCER

Colorectal cancer is the second most common visceral malignant neoplasm in the United States and Europe. Incidence is equally distributed between men and women. Colorectal malignant tumors are almost always adenocarcinomas. (See *Types of colorectal cancer.*) About one half of these are sessile lesions of the rectosigmoid area; the rest are polypoid lesions.

Types of colorectal cancer

Colorectal cancer can occur anywhere along the small and large intestine, as well as the return.

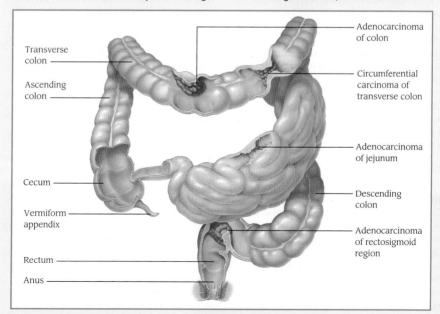

Colorectal cancer tends to progress slowly and remains localized for a long time. Consequently, it's potentially curable in about 90% of patients if early diagnosis allows resection before nodal involvement. With improved diagnosis, the overall 5-year survival rate is about 60% for adjacent organ or nodal spread, and greater than 90% for early localized disease.

Causes and incidence

The exact cause of colorectal cancer is unknown, but studies showing concentration in areas of higher economic development suggest a relationship to diet (excess saturated animal fat). Other factors that magnify the risk of developing colorectal cancer include:

◆ other diseases of the digestive tract
◆ age (older than age 40)
◆ history of ulcerative colitis (average interval before onset of cancer is 11 to 17 years)
◆ familial polyposis (cancer almost always develops by age 50)
◆ hereditary nonpolyposis (also known as *Lynch syndrome*)

There are more than 130,000 cases of colorectal cancer diagnosed in the United States each year. It's the second leading cause of cancer-related death, accounting for more than 50,000 per year. However, in almost all cases, it's treatable if caught early by colonoscopy.

Pathophysiology

The large majority of colorectal malignancies develop from adenomatous polyps. These can be defined as well demarcated masses of epithelial dysplasia, with uncontrolled crypt cell division. An adenoma can be considered malignant when neoplastic cells pass through the muscularis mucosae and infiltrate the submucosa.

Complications

◆ Abdominal distention
◆ Intestinal obstruction
◆ Anemia

Signs and symptoms

Signs and symptoms of colorectal cancer result from local obstruction and, in later stages, from direct extension to adjacent organs (bladder, prostate, ureters, vagina, sacrum) and distant metastasis (usually liver). In the early stages, signs and symptoms are typically vague and depend on the anatomic location and function of the bowel segment containing the tumor. Later signs or symptoms usually include pallor, cachexia, ascites, hepatomegaly, or lymphangiectasis.

ELDER TIP *Older patients may ignore bowel symptoms, believing that they result from constipation, poor diet, or hemorrhoids. Evaluate your older patient's responses to your questions carefully.*

On the right side of the colon (which absorbs water and electrolytes), early tumor growth causes no signs of obstruction because the tumor tends to grow along the bowel rather than surrounding the lumen, and the fecal content in this area is normally liquid. It may, however, cause black, tarry stools; anemia; and abdominal aching, pressure, or dull cramps. As the disease progresses, the patient develops weakness, fatigue, exertional dyspnea, vertigo and, eventually, diarrhea, obstipation, anorexia, weight loss, vomiting, and other signs or symptoms of intestinal obstruction. In addition, a tumor on the right side may be palpable.

On the left side, a tumor causes signs of an obstruction even in early stages because in this area stools are of a formed consistency. It commonly causes rectal bleeding (in many cases ascribed to hemorrhoids), intermittent abdominal fullness or cramping, and rectal pressure. As the disease progresses, the patient develops obstipation, diarrhea, or "ribbon" or pencil-shaped stools. Typically, the patient notices that passage of stools or flatus relieves the pain. At this stage, bleeding from the colon becomes obvious, with dark or bright red blood in the feces and mucus in or on the stools.

With a rectal tumor, the first symptom is a change in bowel habits, in many cases beginning with an urgent need to defecate on arising (morning diarrhea) or obstipation alternating with diarrhea. Other signs are blood or mucus in stools and a sense of incomplete evacuation. Late in the disease, pain begins as a feeling of rectal fullness that later becomes a dull, and sometimes constant, ache confined to the rectum or sacral region.

Diagnosis

Only a tumor biopsy can verify colorectal cancer, but other tests help detect it:

◆ Digital rectal examination can detect almost 15% of colorectal cancers.
◆ Fecal occult blood test can detect blood in stools. However, it's commonly negative in patients with colon cancer.
◆ Proctoscopy or sigmoidoscopy can detect up to 66% of colorectal cancers.
◆ Colonoscopy permits visual inspection (and photographs) of the colon up to the ileocecal valve and gives access for polypectomies and biopsies of suspected lesions.
◆ CT scan helps to detect areas affected by metastasis.

◆ Barium X-ray, using a dual contrast with air, can locate lesions that are undetectable manually or visually. Barium examination should *follow* endoscopy or excretory urography because the barium sulfate interferes with these tests.

◆ Carcinoembryonic antigen, though not specific or sensitive enough for early diagnosis, is helpful in monitoring patients before and after treatment to detect metastasis or recurrence.

Treatment

The most effective treatment of colorectal cancer is surgery to remove the malignant tumor and adjacent tissues and any lymph nodes that may contain cancer cells. The type of surgery depends on the location of the tumor:

◆ Cecum and ascending colon—right hemicolectomy (for advanced disease) may include resection of the terminal segment of the ileum, cecum, ascending colon, and right half of the transverse colon with corresponding mesentery

◆ Proximal and middle transverse colon—right colectomy to include transverse colon and mesentery corresponding to midcolic vessels, or segmental resection of transverse colon and associated midcolic vessels

◆ Sigmoid colon—surgery is usually limited to sigmoid colon and mesentery

◆ Upper rectum—anterior or low anterior resection (newer method, using a stapler, allows for resections much lower than were previously possible)

◆ Lower rectum—abdominoperineal resection and permanent sigmoid colostomy

Chemotherapy is indicated for patients with metastasis, residual disease, or a recurrent inoperable tumor. Drugs used in such treatment commonly include fluorouracil with leucovorin, irinotecan, and oxaliplatin.

Monoclonal antibody therapy helps inhibit cancer cells by binding to the protein epidermal growth factor receptors. These drugs are cetuximab and panitumumab. Bevacizumab binds with VEGF to inhibit cancer cells. These drugs are used to treat metastatic colon cancer and are usually given in conjunction with chemotherapy.

Radiation therapy induces tumor regression and may be used before or after surgery or combined with chemotherapy, especially fluorouracil.

Special considerations

Before surgery:

◆ Monitor the patient's diet modifications, laxatives, enemas, and antibiotics—all used to clean the bowel and to decrease abdominal and perineal cavity contamination during surgery.

If the patient is having a colostomy, teach the patient family about the procedure:

◆ Emphasize that the stoma will be red, moist, and swollen and that postoperative swelling will eventually subside.

◆ Show them a diagram of the intestine before and after surgery, stressing how much of the bowel will remain intact. Supplement your teaching with instructional aids. The patient can benefit from a consultation with an enterostomal therapist or wound and ostomy care nurse. Also arrange a postsurgical visit from a recovered ostomate.

◆ Prepare the patient for postoperative I.V. infusions, NG tube, and indwelling urinary catheter.

◆ Discuss the importance of performing deep-breathing and coughing exercises.

After surgery:

◆ Explain to the patient's family the importance of their positive reactions to the patient's adjustment. Consult with an enterostomal therapist, if available, to help set up a regimen for the patient.

◆ Encourage the patient to look at the stoma and participate in its care as soon as possible. Teach good hygiene and skin care. Allow the patient to shower or bathe as soon as the incision heals. If appropriate, instruct the patient with a sigmoid colostomy to do their own irrigation as soon as they can after surgery. Advise them to schedule irrigation for the time of day when they normally evacuated before surgery. Many patients find that irrigating every 1 to 3 days is necessary for regularity. If flatus, diarrhea, or constipation occurs, eliminate suspected causative foods from the patient's diet. They may be introduced again later.

◆ After several months, many patients with sigmoid colostomies establish control with irrigation and no longer need to wear a pouch. A stoma cap or gauze sponge placed over the stoma protects it and absorbs mucoid secretions.

◆ Before achieving such control, the patient can resume physical activities, including sports, provided that there's no threat of injury to the stoma or surrounding abdominal muscles. However, the patient should avoid heavy lifting because herniation or prolapse may occur through weakened muscles in the abdominal wall. A structured, gradually progressive exercise program to strengthen abdominal muscles may be instituted under medical supervision.

◆ If appropriate, refer the patient to a home health agency for follow-up care and counseling. Suggest sexual counseling for male patients; most are impotent after an abdominoperineal resection.

◆ Anyone who has had colorectal cancer is at increased risk for recurrence and should have yearly screening and testing.

▓▓▓▓ PREVENTION *Encourage the patient to have a screening colonoscopy for early detection, and to eat a diet low in fat and high in fiber.*

KIDNEY CANCER

Kidney cancer (also known as *nephrocarcinoma, renal cell carcinoma [RCC], hypernephroma,* and *Grawitz tumor*) usually occurs in older adults. Renal pelvic tumors and Wilms tumor occur primarily in children. Kidney tumors, which usually are large, firm, nodular, encapsulated, unilateral, and solitary, can be separated histologically into clear cell, granular, and spindle cell types. (See *Two forms of kidney cancer.*) The prognosis ranges from 60% to 75% for stage I to 5% to 15% for stage IV.

Causes and incidence

The causes of kidney cancer aren't known, although smokers develop more renal cell tumors than nonsmokers. However, the incidence of this malignancy is rising, possibly as a result of exposure to environmental carcinogens as well as increased longevity. Even so, this cancer accounts for only about 2% of all adult cancers. Kidney cancer is more common in men than in women and peaks in incidence between ages 50 and 70.

Pathophysiology

The tissue of origin for RCC is the proximal renal tubular epithelium. Renal cancer occurs in a sporadic (nonhereditary) and a hereditary form, and both forms are associated with structural alterations of the short arm of chromosome 3. Genetic studies of the families at high risk for developing renal cancer led to the cloning of genes whose alteration results in tumor formation. These genes are either tumor suppressors or oncogenes.

Complications

◆ Hemorrhage
◆ Respiratory problems (lung metastasis)

Two forms of kidney cancer

The illustration below shows two forms of renal cancer: transitional cell cancer and adenocarcinoma.

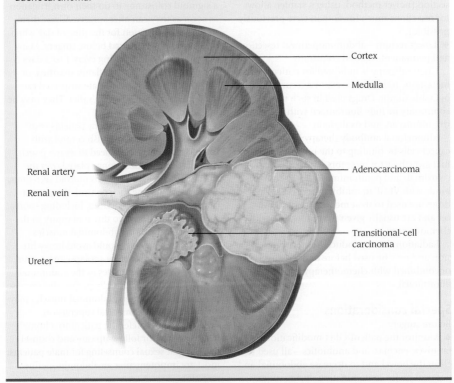

- Cortex
- Medulla
- Renal artery
- Renal vein
- Adenocarcinoma
- Transitional-cell carcinoma
- Ureter

◆ Neurologic problems (brain metastasis)
◆ GI problems (liver metastasis)

Signs and symptoms

Kidney cancer produces a classic clinical triad (hematuria, pain, and a palpable mass), but any one may be the first sign of cancer. Microscopic or gross hematuria (which may be intermittent) suggests that the cancer has spread to the renal pelvis. Constant abdominal or flank pain may be dull or, if the cancer causes bleeding or blood clots, acute and colicky. The mass is generally smooth, firm, and nontender. All three signs coexist in only about 10% of patients.

Other signs include fever (perhaps from hemorrhage or necrosis), hypertension (from compression of the renal artery with renal parenchymal ischemia), rapidly progressing hypercalcemia (possibly from ectopic parathyroid hormone production by the tumor), and urine retention. Weight loss, edema in the legs, nausea, and vomiting signal advanced disease.

Diagnosis

Studies to identify kidney cancer usually include CT scans, excretory urography, retrograde pyelography, ultrasound, cystoscopy (to rule out associated bladder cancer), and nephrotomography or renal angiography to distinguish a kidney cyst from a tumor.

Related tests include liver function studies showing increased levels of alkaline phosphatase, bilirubin, alanine aminotransferase and aspartate aminotransferase, and prolonged prothrombin time. Such results may point to liver metastasis, but if metastasis hasn't occurred, these abnormalities reverse after tumor resection.

Routine laboratory findings of hematuria, anemia (unrelated to blood loss), polycythemia, hypercalcemia, and increased erythrocyte sedimentation rate call for more testing to rule out kidney cancer.

Treatment

Radical nephrectomy, with or without regional lymph node dissection, offers the only chance of cure. Because the disease is radiation resistant, radiation is used only if the cancer spreads to the perinephric region or the lymph nodes or if the primary tumor or metastatic sites can't be fully excised. In these cases, high radiation doses are used.

Chemotherapy has been only erratically effective against kidney cancer. Fluorouracil, cyclophosphamide, vinblastine, vincristine, cisplatin, tamoxifen, teniposide, interferons, and hormones such as medroxyprogesterone and testosterone have been used, usually with poor

results. Biotherapy (interferon and interleukins), commonly used in advanced disease, has produced few durable remissions.

Several new drugs have been approved for treatment of advanced kidney cancer. Sorafenib and sunitinib target cancer cells and inhibit their growth.

Special considerations

Meticulous postoperative care, supportive treatment during other therapy, and psychological support can hasten recovery and minimize complications.

◆ Before surgery, assure the patient that the body will adapt to the loss of a kidney.
◆ Teach the patient about such expected postoperative procedures as diaphragmatic breathing, coughing properly, splinting the incision, and others.
◆ After surgery, diaphragmatic breathing and coughing, leg exercises, and frequent position changes should be encouraged.
◆ Check dressings often for excessive bleeding. Watch for signs of internal bleeding, such as restlessness, sweating, and increased pulse rate.
◆ Place the patient on the operative side to allow the pressure of adjacent organs to fill the dead space at the operative site, improving dependent drainage. If possible, the patient should be ambulated within 24 hours after surgery.
◆ Monitor intake and output. Monitor laboratory results for anemia, polycythemia, or abnormal blood values that may point to bone or liver involvement or may result from radiation or chemotherapy.
◆ Treat drug adverse effects.
◆ Stress compliance with the prescribed outpatient treatment regimen.

▓▓▓▓ **PREVENTION**
◆ *Because smoking is a key risk factor for kidney cancer, encourage your patient to quit smoking.*
◆ *Teach the patient to minimize exposure to environmental carcinogens by wearing a mask and gloves when exposed to them.*

LIVER CANCER

Liver cancer, also known as *primary* and *metastatic hepatic carcinoma*, is a rare form of cancer in the United States, with a high mortality. Most primary liver tumors (90%) originate in the parenchymal cells and are hepatomas (hepatocellular carcinoma [HCC], primary lower cell carcinoma). Some primary tumors originate in the intrahepatic bile ducts and are known as *cholangiomas* (cholangiocarcinoma, cholangiocellular carcinoma). Rarer tumors include a mixed-cell type, Kupffer cell sarcoma, and hepatoblastomas

Common sites of liver cancer

The illustration below shows metastatic liver cancer.

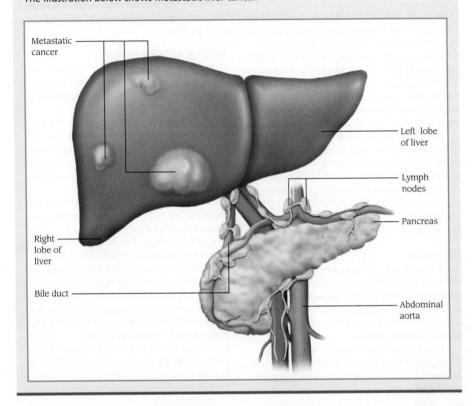

(which occur almost exclusively in children and are usually resectable and curable). The liver is one of the most common sites of metastasis from other primary cancers, particularly colon, rectum, stomach, pancreas, esophagus, lung, breast, or melanoma. In the United States, metastatic carcinoma is more than 20 times more common than primary carcinoma and, after cirrhosis, is the leading cause of liver-related death. At times, liver metastasis may appear as a solitary lesion, the first sign of recurrence after a remission. (See *Common sites of liver cancer*.)

Causes and incidence

The immediate cause of liver cancer is unknown, but it may be a congenital disease in children. Adult liver cancer may result from environmental exposure to carcinogens, such as the chemical compound aflatoxin (a mold that grows on rice and peanuts), thorium dioxide (a contrast medium formerly used in liver radiography), *Senecio* alkaloids, and possibly androgens and oral estrogens.

Roughly 30% to 70% of patients with hepatomas also have cirrhosis. (Hepatomas are 40 times more likely to develop in a cirrhotic liver than in a normal one.)

Whether cirrhosis is a premalignant state or alcohol and malnutrition predispose the liver to develop hepatomas is still unclear. Other risk factors are exposure to the hepatitis C virus and the hepatitis B virus. Nonalcoholic fatty liver, when associated with metabolic syndrome or diabetes mellitus, is associated with the development of hepatocellular cancers. (See *Preventing liver cancer*, page 749.)

Liver cancer accounts for roughly 1% of all cancers in the United States and for 10% to 50% in Africa and parts of Asia. Liver cancer is most prevalent in men (particularly men older than age 60), and incidence increases with age. It's rapidly fatal, usually within 6 months.

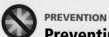

PREVENTION
Preventing liver cancer

Teach your patient the following to lessen the risk for liver cancer:

Get vaccinated for hepatitis B
Risk of developing hepatitis B can be decreased when vaccinated.

Be careful with medications
Tell your patient to use caution when taking medications known to cause liver damage, especially acetaminophen.

Limit alcohol intake
Alcohol consumption increases liver toxicity. Alcohol-induced cirrhosis is a leading cause of liver cancer.

Make healthy lifestyle choices
Risk of contracting hepatitis C is decreased by not sharing needles, by avoiding unprotected sex, and by not getting tattoos or body piercings. Also, avoid exposure to environmental carcinogens.

Pathophysiology
Liver cancer, any of several forms of disease characterized by tumors in the liver; benign liver tumors remain in the liver, whereas *malignant* tumors are, by definition, cancerous. Most malignant liver tumors are hepatomas, also called HCCs. The remaining cancers develop from blood vessels (hemangiosarcomas), small bile ducts (cholangiocarcinomas), or immature liver cells (hepatoblastomas). Hepatoblastomas occur primarily in children. Treatment and prognosis for liver cancers vary, depending on the type and stage, or degree, of advancement.

Complications
◆ GI hemorrhage
◆ Cachexia
◆ Liver failure

Signs and symptoms
Clinical effects of liver cancer include:
◆ a mass in the right upper quadrant
◆ tender, nodular liver on palpation
◆ severe pain in the epigastrium or the right upper quadrant
◆ bruit, hum, or rubbing sound if tumor involves a large part of the liver
◆ weight loss, weakness, anorexia, fever
◆ occasional jaundice or ascites
◆ occasional evidence of metastasis through venous system to lungs, from lymphatics to regional lymph nodes, or by direct invasion of portal veins
◆ dependent edema

Diagnosis
CONFIRMING DIAGNOSIS *The confirming test for liver cancer is liver biopsy by needle or open biopsy.*

Liver cancer is difficult to diagnose in the presence of cirrhosis, but several tests can help identify it:
◆ Alanine aminotransferase, aspartate aminotransferase, alkaline phosphatase, lactic dehydrogenase, and bilirubin all show abnormal liver function.
◆ Alpha-fetoprotein rises to a level above 500 μg/mL.
◆ Chest X-ray may rule out metastasis.
◆ Liver scan may show filling defects.
◆ Arteriography may define large tumors.
◆ Electrolyte studies may indicate an increased retention of sodium (resulting in functional renal failure) and hypoglycemia, leukocytosis, hypercalcemia, or hypocholesterolemia.

Treatment
Because liver cancer is commonly in an advanced stage at diagnosis, few hepatic tumors are resectable. A resectable tumor must be a single tumor in one lobe, without cirrhosis, jaundice, or ascites. Resection is done by lobectomy or partial hepatectomy. In the absence of extrahepatic disease and where the cancer is inoperable, embolization procedures may reduce blood flow to the tumor and result in tumor death.

Radiation therapy for unresectable tumors is usually palliative. Because of the liver's low tolerance for radiation, external beam radiation hasn't increased survival. However, radiolabeled antibodies have been used to selectively target cancer tissue; when used concurrently with chemotherapy, patients can convert from nonresectable to resectable.

Another method of treatment is chemotherapy with I.V. fluorouracil, mitomycin, or doxorubicin, or with regional infusion of fluorouracil or floxuridine (catheters are placed directly into the hepatic artery or left brachial artery for continuous infusion for 7 to 21 days, or permanent implantable pumps are used on an outpatient basis for long-term infusion). Sorafenib, an oral multikinase inhibitor, has proved beneficial in advanced disease.

Another treatment involves injecting pure alcohol into the tumor. This causes the cells to dry out and die.

With radiofrequency ablation, thin needles are inserted into a tumor through small abdominal incisions, and then an electric current is applied to destroy the tumor cells.

Appropriate treatment for liver metastasis may include resection by lobectomy or chemotherapy with mitomycin or fludarabine (results similar to those in hepatoma). Liver transplantation is now an alternative for a small subset of patients.

Special considerations

The patient care plan should emphasize comprehensive supportive care and emotional support.

◆ Control edema and ascites. Monitor the patient's diet throughout. Most patients need a special diet that restricts sodium, fluids (no alcohol allowed), and protein. Weigh the patient daily, and note intake and output accurately. Watch for signs of ascites (peripheral edema, orthopnea, or dyspnea on exertion). If ascites is present, measure and record abdominal girth daily. To increase venous return and prevent edema, elevate the patient's legs whenever possible.

◆ Monitor respiratory function. Note any increase in respiratory rate or shortness of breath. Bilateral pleural effusion (noted on chest X-ray) is common, as is metastasis to the lungs. Watch carefully for signs of hypoxemia from intrapulmonary arteriovenous shunting.

◆ Relieve fever. Administer sponge baths and aspirin suppositories if there are no signs of GI bleeding. Avoid acetaminophen, because the diseased liver can't metabolize it. High fever indicates infection and requires antibiotics.

◆ Give meticulous skin care. Turn the patient frequently and keep their skin clean to prevent pressure ulcers. Apply lotion to prevent chafing, and administer an antipruritic such as diphenhydramine for severe itching.

◆ **ALERT** *Watch for encephalopathy. Many patients develop end-stage signs or symptoms of ammonia intoxication, including confusion, restlessness, irritability, agitation, delirium, asterixis, lethargy, and, finally, coma. Monitor the patient's serum ammonia level, vital signs, and neurologic status. Be prepared to control ammonia accumulation with sorbitol (to induce osmotic diarrhea), neomycin (to reduce bacterial flora in the GI tract), lactulose (to control bacterial elaboration of ammonia), and sodium polystyrene sulfonate (to lower potassium level).*

◆ If a transhepatic catheter is used to relieve obstructive jaundice, irrigate it frequently with prescribed solution (normal saline or, sometimes, 5,000 units of heparin in 500 mL dextrose 5% in water). Monitor vital signs frequently for any indication of bleeding or infection.

◆ After surgery, give standard postoperative care.

◆ **ALERT** *Watch for intraperitoneal bleeding and sepsis, which may precipitate coma.*

◆ Monitor for renal failure by checking urine output, blood urea nitrogen, and creatinine levels hourly. Remember that, throughout the course of this intractable illness, your primary concern is to keep the patient as comfortable as possible.

◆ When all treatments have failed, concentrate on keeping the patient comfortable and free from pain, and provide as much psychological support as possible. If the patient is going home, discuss continuing care needs with the caregiver or refer the patient to an appropriate home healthcare agency or hospice. Encourage the patient and caregiver to express their feelings and concerns. Answer their questions honestly, with tact and sensitivity.

BLADDER CANCER

Bladder tumors can develop on the surface of the bladder wall (benign or malignant papillomas) or grow within the bladder wall (generally more virulent) and quickly invade underlying muscles. (See *Bladder tumor,* page 751.) Ninety percent of bladder tumors are transitional cell carcinomas, arising from the transitional epithelium of mucous membranes. Less common are adenocarcinomas, epidermoid carcinomas, squamous cell cancers, sarcomas, tumors in bladder diverticula, and carcinoma in situ. Cancer of the bladder is the most common cancer of the urinary tract.

Bladder tumor

The illustration below shows a cancerous tumor infiltrating the bladder wall.

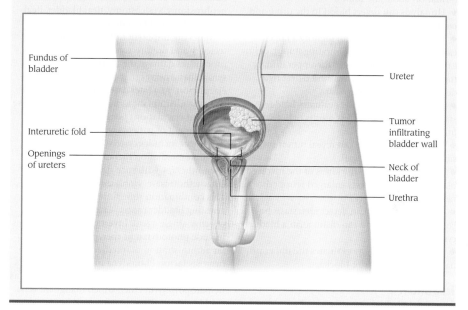

Fundus of bladder

Ureter

Interuretic fold

Tumor infiltrating bladder wall

Openings of ureters

Neck of bladder

Urethra

Causes and incidence

Certain environmental carcinogens, such as 2-naphthylamine, benzidine, tobacco, and nitrates, predispose people to transitional cell tumors. Thus, workers in certain industries (rubber workers, weavers and leather finishers, aniline dye workers, hairdressers, petroleum workers, and spray painters) are at high risk for such tumors. The period between exposure to the carcinogen and development of symptoms is about 18 years.

Squamous cell cancer of the bladder is most common in geographic areas where schistosomiasis is endemic. It's also associated with chronic bladder irritation and infection (e.g., from renal calculi, indwelling urinary catheters, and cystitis caused by cyclophosphamide).

Bladder tumors are most prevalent in men older than age 55—50% of all cases occur in patients age 73 and older—and are more common in densely populated industrial areas.

Signs and symptoms

In early stages, about 25% of patients with bladder tumors have no symptoms. Commonly, the first sign is gross, painless, intermittent hematuria (in many cases with clots in the urine). Many patients with invasive lesions have suprapubic pain after voiding. Other signs and symptoms include bladder irritability, urinary frequency, nocturia, and dribbling.

Pathophysiology

Bladder cancer, disease characterized by the growth of malignant cells within the urinary bladder, the organ responsible for storing urine prior to elimination. Bladder cancer can also be associated with cancers of the kidneys, ureters, or urethra.

Complications

◆ Anemia
◆ Hydronephrosis
◆ Metastasis
◆ Urinary incontinence
◆ Urethral stricture

Diagnosis

℞ **CONFIRMING DIAGNOSIS** *Only cystoscopy and biopsy confirm bladder cancer. Cystoscopy should be performed when hematuria first appears. When it's performed under anesthesia, a bimanual examination is usually done to determine if the bladder is fixed to the pelvic wall.*

A thorough history and physical examination may help determine whether the tumor has invaded the prostate or the lymph nodes.

The following tests can provide essential information about the tumor:

◆ Urinalysis can detect blood in the urine and malignant cytology.

◆ Excretory urography can identify a large, early-stage tumor or an infiltrating tumor, delineate functional problems in the upper urinary tract, assess hydronephrosis, and detect rigid deformity of the bladder wall.

◆ Retrograde cystography evaluates bladder structure and integrity. Test results help to confirm the diagnosis.

◆ Pelvic arteriography can reveal tumor invasion into the bladder wall.

◆ CT scan reveals the thickness of the involved bladder wall and detects enlarged retroperitoneal lymph nodes.

◆ Ultrasonography can detect metastasis beyond the bladder and can distinguish a bladder cyst from a tumor.

◆ Excretory urography evaluates the upper urinary tract for tumors or blockage.

Treatment

Superficial bladder tumors are removed by transurethral (cystoscopic) resection and fulguration (electrical destruction). This procedure is adequate when the tumor hasn't invaded the muscle.

Intravesicular chemotherapy is also used for superficial tumors (especially those that occur in many sites) and to prevent tumor recurrence. This treatment involves washing the bladder directly with antineoplastic drugs—most commonly, thiotepa, doxorubicin, mitomycin, or bacillus Calmette–Guérin immunotherapy.

If additional tumors develop, fulguration may have to be repeated every 3 months for years. However, if the tumors penetrate the muscle layer or recur frequently, cystoscopy with fulguration is no longer appropriate.

Tumors too large to be treated through a cystoscope require segmental bladder resection to remove a full-thickness section of the bladder. This procedure is feasible only if the tumor isn't near the bladder neck or ureteral orifices. Bladder instillation of thiotepa, mitomycin, or doxorubicin after transurethral resection may also help control such tumors.

For infiltrating bladder tumors, radical cystectomy is the treatment of choice. The week before cystectomy, treatment may include external beam therapy to the bladder. Surgery involves removal of the bladder with perivesical fat, lymph nodes, urethra, the prostate and seminal

vesicles (in males), and the uterus and adnexa (in females). The surgeon forms a urinary diversion, usually an ileal conduit. The patient must then wear an external pouch continuously. Other diversions include ureterostomy, nephrostomy, vesicostomy, ileal bladder, ileal loop, and sigmoid conduit.

Males are impotent following radical cystectomy and urethrectomy because these procedures damage the sympathetic and parasympathetic nerves that control erection and ejaculation. At a later date, the patient may desire a penile implant to make sexual intercourse (without ejaculation) possible.

Treatment of patients with advanced bladder cancer includes cystectomy to remove the tumor, radiation therapy, and systemic chemotherapy with such drugs as doxorubicin, methotrexate, vinblastine, and cisplatin. This combination sometimes is successful in arresting bladder cancer. Cisplatin is the most effective single agent. Investigational treatments include photodynamic therapy and intravesicular administration of interferon-alfa and tumor necrosis factor. Photodynamic therapy involves I.V. injection of a photosensitizing agent such as hematoporphyrin ether, which malignant cells readily absorb. Then a cystoscopic laser device introduces laser energy into the bladder, exposing the malignant cells to laser light, which kills them. Because this treatment also produces photosensitivity in normal cells, the patient must totally avoid sunlight for about 30 days.

Special considerations

◆ Before surgery, assist in selecting a stoma site that the patient can see (usually in the rectus muscle to minimize the risk of herniation). Do so by assessing the abdomen in various positions.

◆ After surgery, encourage the patient to look at the stoma. Provide a mirror to make viewing easier.

◆ To obtain a specimen for culture and sensitivity testing, catheterize the patient using sterile technique. Insert the lubricated tip of the catheter into the stoma about 2″ (5.1 cm). In many facilities, a double telescope-type catheter is available for ileal conduit catheterization.

◆ Advise the patient with a urinary stoma that they may participate in most activities, except for heavy lifting and contact sports.

◆ When a patient with a urinary diversion is discharged, arrange for follow-up home healthcare or refer them to an enterostomal therapist, who will help coordinate the patient's care.

◆ Teach the patient about their urinary stoma. Encourage their spouse, a friend, or a relative to attend the teaching session. Advise this person beforehand that a negative reaction to the stoma can impede the patient's adjustment.

◆ First, show the patient how to prepare and apply the pouch, which may be reusable or disposable. If they choose the reusable type, they'll need at least two.

◆ To select the right pouch size, measure the stoma and order a pouch with an opening that clears the stoma with a $\frac{1}{8}$" (3 mm) margin. Instruct the patient to remeasure the stoma after they go home, in case the size changes. The pouch should have a drainage valve at the bottom. Tell the patient to empty the pouch when it's one third full or every 2 to 3 hours.

◆ To ensure a good skin seal, select a skin barrier that contains synthetics and little or no karaya (which urine tends to destroy). Check the pouch frequently to make sure that the skin seal remains intact. A good skin seal with a skin barrier may last for 3 to 6 days, so change the pouch only that often. Tell the patient that they can wear a loose-fitting elastic belt to help secure the pouch.

◆ The ileal conduit stoma reaches its permanent size 2 to 4 months after surgery. Because the intestine normally produces mucus, mucus will appear in the draining urine.

◆ Keep the skin around the stoma clean and free from irritation. After removing the pouch, wash the skin with water and mild soap. Rinse well with clear water to remove soap residue, and then gently pat the skin dry; don't rub. Place a gauze sponge soaked with vinegar-water (1 part to 3 parts) over the stoma for a few minutes to prevent uric acid crystal buildup. While preparing the skin, place a rolled-up dry sponge over the stoma to collect draining urine. Coat the skin with skin protectant, and cover with the collection pouch. If skin irritation or breakdown occurs, apply a layer of antacid precipitate to the clean, dry skin before coating with the skin protector.

◆ The patient can level uneven surfaces on the abdomen, such as gullies, scars, or wedges, with various specially prepared products or skin barriers.

◆ All high-risk people—for example, chemical workers and people with a history of benign bladder tumors or persistent cystitis—should have periodic cytologic examinations and learn about the danger of disease-causing agents.

◆ Refer patients with ostomies to such support organizations as the American Cancer Society and the United Ostomy Association.

▓▓▓▓▓ **PREVENTION** *Encourage the patient to not smoke and to reduce exposure to environmental hazards.*

GALLBLADDER AND BILE DUCT CANCER

Gallbladder cancer is rare, accounting for fewer than 1% of all cancers. It's normally found by accident in patients with cholecystitis; 1 in 400 cholecystectomies reveals a malignant tumor. The disease is most prevalent in females older than age 60. It's rapidly progressive and usually fatal; patients seldom live a year after diagnosis. The poor prognosis is due to late diagnosis; gallbladder cancer isn't usually diagnosed until after cholecystectomy, when in many cases it's in an advanced, metastatic stage.

Causes and incidence

Gallbladder cancer may result from a complication of gallstones. However, this inference rests on circumstantial evidence from postmortem examinations: 60% to 90% of gallbladder cancer patients also have gallstones, but postmortem data from patients with gallstones show gallbladder cancer in only 0.5%.

The predominant tissue type in gallbladder cancer is adenocarcinoma, 85% to 95%; squamous cell, 5% to 15%. Mixed-tissue types are rare.

Lymph node metastasis is present in 25% to 70% of patients at diagnosis. Direct extension to the liver is common (in 46% to 89%); direct extension to both the cystic and the common bile ducts, stomach, colon, duodenum, and jejunum also occurs and produces obstructions. Metastasis also spreads by portal or hepatic veins to the peritoneum, ovaries, and lower lung lobes.

The cause of extrahepatic bile duct cancer isn't known; however, statistics report an unexplained increased incidence of this cancer in patients with ulcerative colitis. This association may be due to a common cause—perhaps an immune mechanism or chronic use of certain drugs by the colitis patient.

Extrahepatic bile duct cancer is the cause of about 3% of all cancer deaths in the United States. It occurs in both males and females (incidence is slightly higher in males) between ages 60 and 70. The usual site is at the bifurcation in the common duct. Cancer at the distal end of the common duct is commonly confused with cancer of the pancreas. Characteristically, metastatic spread occurs to local lymph nodes, the liver, lungs, and the peritoneum.

Complications

◆ Malabsorption
◆ Cholangitis
◆ Lymph node metastasis
◆ Obstruction of bile ducts, stomach, colon, duodenum, and jejunum

Signs and symptoms

Clinically, gallbladder cancer is almost indistinguishable from cholecystitis—pain in the epigastrium or right upper quadrant, weight loss, anorexia, nausea, vomiting, and jaundice. However, chronic, progressively severe pain in an afebrile patient suggests malignancy. In patients with simple gallstones, pain is sporadic. Another telling clue to malignancy is palpable gallbladder (right upper quadrant), with obstructive jaundice. Some patients may also have hepatosplenomegaly.

Progressive profound jaundice is commonly the first sign of obstruction due to extrahepatic bile duct cancer. The jaundice is usually accompanied by chronic pain in the epigastrium or the right upper quadrant, radiating to the back. Other common signs or symptoms, if associated with active cholecystitis, include pruritus, skin excoriations, anorexia, weight loss, chills, and fever.

Diagnosis

No test or procedure, by itself, can diagnose gallbladder cancer. However, the following laboratory tests support the diagnosis when they suggest hepatic dysfunction and extrahepatic biliary obstruction:
◆ baseline studies—complete blood count, routine urinalysis, electrolyte studies, enzymes
◆ liver function tests—typically reveal elevated serum bilirubin, urine bile and bilirubin, and urobilinogen levels in more than 50% of patients as well as consistently elevated serum alkaline phosphatase levels
◆ occult blood in stools—linked to the associated anemia
◆ cholecystography—may show calculi or calcification
◆ cholangiography—may locate the site of common duct obstruction
◆ MRI—detects tumors.

The following tests help compile data that confirm extrahepatic bile duct cancer:
◆ liver function studies—indicate biliary obstruction: elevated levels of bilirubin (5 to 30 mg/dL), alkaline phosphatase, and blood cholesterol as well as prolonged prothrombin time
◆ endoscopic retrograde cannulization of the pancreas—identifies the tumor site and allows access for obtaining a biopsy specimen.

Treatment

Surgical treatment of gallbladder cancer is essentially palliative and includes various procedures, such as cholecystectomy, common bile duct exploration, T-tube drainage, and wedge excision of hepatic tissue.

If the cancer invades gallbladder musculature, the survival rate is less than 5%, even with massive resection. Although some cases of long-term survival (4 to 5 years) have been reported, few patients survive longer than 6 months after surgery for gallbladder cancer.

Surgery is normally indicated to relieve obstruction and jaundice that result from extrahepatic bile duct cancer. The procedure used to relieve obstruction depends on the cancer site. Such procedures may include cholecystoduodenostomy or T-tube drainage of the common duct.

Other palliative measures for both kinds of cancer include radiation, radiation implants (mostly used for local and incisional recurrences), and chemotherapy (with combinations of fluorouracil, irinotecan, capecitabine, and gemcitabine). All of these treatment measures have limited effects.

Special considerations

After biliary resection:
◆ Monitor vital signs.
◆ Use strict sterile technique when caring for the incision and the surrounding area.
◆ Place the patient in low Fowler position.
◆ Prevent respiratory problems by encouraging deep breathing and coughing. The high incision makes the patient want to take shallow breaths; using analgesics and splinting the abdomen with a pillow or an abdominal binder may aid in greater respiratory efforts.
◆ Monitor bowel sounds and bowel movements. Observe the patient's tolerance to diet.
◆ Provide pain control.

ELDER TIP *Check intake and output carefully. Watch for electrolyte imbalance; monitor I.V. solutions to avoid overloading the cardiovascular system, especially in older patients.*
◆ Monitor the NG tube, which will be in place for 24 to 72 hours postoperatively to relieve distention, and the T tube. Record amount and color of drainage each shift. Secure the T tube to minimize tension on it and prevent its being pulled out.
◆ Help the patient and family cope with their initial fears and reactions to the diagnosis by offering information and support.
◆ Before discharge, teach the patient how to manage the biliary catheter.
◆ Advise the patient of the adverse effects of both chemotherapy and radiation therapy, and monitor the patient for these effects.
◆ When all treatments have failed, concentrate on keeping the patient comfortable and free from pain and provide as much psychological support as possible. If the patient is going home, discuss continuing care needs with the

caregiver or refer the patient to an appropriate home healthcare or hospice agency. Encourage the patient and caregiver to express their feelings and concerns. Answer their questions honestly, with tact and sensitivity.

Male and female genitalia

PROSTATE CANCER

Prostate cancer is the most common cancer in men older than age 50. (See *Prostate cancer.*) Adenocarcinoma is its most common form; sarcoma occurs only rarely. Most prostatic cancers originate in the posterior prostate gland; the rest originate near the urethra. Malignant prostatic tumors seldom result from the benign hyperplastic enlargement that commonly develops around the prostatic urethra in elderly men. Prostate cancer seldom produces symptoms until it's advanced.

Causes and incidence

Four factors have been suspected in the development of prostate cancer: family or racial predisposition, exposure to environmental elements, coexisting sexually transmitted diseases, and endogenous hormonal influence. Eating fat-containing animal products has also been implicated. Although androgens regulate prostate growth and function and may also speed tumor growth, no definite link between increased androgen levels and prostate cancer has been found. When primary prostatic lesions metastasize, they typically invade the prostatic capsule and spread along the ejaculatory ducts in the space between the seminal vesicles or perivesicular fascia.

Incidence is highest in Blacks and lowest in Asians. In fact, Black Americans have the highest prostate cancer incidence in the world and are considered at high risk for the disease. Incidence also increases with age more rapidly than any other cancer and is the most common cause of cancer death in men older than age 75.

Pathophysiology

Prostate cancer is the most common noncutaneous cancer in men, making the diagnosis and staging of this cancer of great medical and public interest. Although prostate cancer can be slow growing, the disease nonetheless accounts for almost 10% of cancer-related deaths in males, with thousands of men dying of prostate cancer each year.

Complications
◆ Spinal cord compression
◆ Deep vein thrombosis
◆ Pulmonary emboli
◆ Myelophthisis

Prostate cancer

Prostate cancer can constrict the urethra.

Signs and symptoms

Signs and symptoms of prostate cancer appear only in the advanced stages and include difficulty initiating a urine stream, dribbling, urine retention, unexplained cystitis, and, rarely, hematuria. Pain may be present in the lower back, with urination, ejaculation, and bowel movement.

Diagnosis

A digital rectal examination that reveals a small, hard nodule may help diagnose prostate cancer. The American Cancer Society advises a yearly digital examination for men older than age 40, a yearly blood test to detect PSA in men older than age 50, and ultrasound if abnormal results are found.

℞ **CONFIRMING DIAGNOSIS** *A biopsy confirms the diagnosis of prostate cancer. PSA levels will be elevated in all men with metastatic prostate cancer. Serum acid phosphatase levels will be elevated in two thirds of men with metastatic prostate cancer.*

Therapy aims to return the serum acid phosphatase level to normal; a subsequent rise points to recurrence. MRI, CT scan, and excretory urography may also aid diagnosis.

Elevated alkaline phosphatase levels and a positive bone scan point to bone metastasis.

Treatment

Management of prostate cancer depends on clinical assessment, tolerance of therapy, expected life span, and the stage of the disease. Treatment must be chosen carefully, because prostate cancer usually affects older men, who commonly have coexisting disorders, such as hypertension, diabetes, or cardiac disease.

Therapy varies with each stage of the disease and generally includes radiation, prostatectomy, orchiectomy to reduce androgen production, and hormone therapy with synthetic estrogen (DES) and antiandrogens, such as cyproterone, megestrol, and flutamide. Radical prostatectomy is usually effective for localized lesions.

External beam radiation therapy is used to cure some locally invasive lesions and to relieve pain from metastatic bone involvement. Internal radiation therapy, also known as *brachytherapy*, involves placing internally radioactive seeds directly in or near the tumor. This method reduces damage to surrounding tissue. The seeds are left in place either temporarily or permanently. A single injection of the radionuclide strontium 89 is also used to treat pain caused by bone metastasis.

If hormone therapy, surgery, and radiation therapy aren't feasible or successful, chemotherapy (using combinations of mitoxantrone with prednisone, estramustine, docetaxel, goserelin, leuprolide, and paclitaxel) may be tried. However, current drug therapy offers limited benefit. Combining several treatment methods may be most effective.

Special considerations

The care plan for the patient with prostate cancer should emphasize psychological support, postoperative care, and treatment of radiation adverse effects.

Before prostatectomy:
◆ Explain the expected after effects of surgery (such as impotence and incontinence) and radiation. Discuss tube placement and dressing changes.
◆ Teach the patient to do perineal exercises 1 to 10 times an hour. Have the patient squeeze their buttocks together, hold this position for a few seconds, then relax.

After prostatectomy or suprapubic prostatectomy:
◆ Regularly check the dressing, incision, and drainage systems for excessive bleeding; watch the patient for signs of bleeding (pallor, falling blood pressure, rising pulse rate) and infection.
◆ Maintain adequate fluid intake.
◆ Give antispasmodics, as ordered, to control postoperative bladder spasms. Give analgesics as needed.
◆ Urinary incontinence is common after surgery; keep the patient's skin clean, dry, and free from drainage and urine.
◆ Encourage perineal exercises within 24 to 48 hours after surgery.
◆ Provide meticulous catheter care—especially if a three-way catheter with a continuous irrigation system is in place. Check the tubing for kinks and blockages, especially if the patient reports pain. Warn the patient not to pull on the catheter.

After transurethral prostatic resection:
◆ Watch for signs of urethral stricture (dysuria, decreased force and caliber of urine stream, and straining to urinate) and for abdominal distention (from urethral stricture or catheter blockage). Irrigate the catheter as ordered.

After perineal prostatectomy:
◆ Avoid taking a rectal temperature or inserting any kind of rectal tube. Provide pads to absorb urine leakage, a rubber ring for the patient to sit on, and sitz baths for pain and inflammation.

After perineal and retropubic prostatectomy:
◆ Explain that urine leakage after catheter removal is normal and will subside.
◆ When a patient receives hormonal therapy, watch for adverse effects. Gynecomastia, fluid retention, nausea, and vomiting are common

with DES. Thrombophlebitis may also occur, especially with DES.

After radiation therapy:

◆ Watch for common adverse effects: proctitis, diarrhea, bladder spasms, and urinary frequency. Internal radiation usually results in cystitis in the first 2 to 3 weeks. Urge the patient to drink at least 67½ oz (2,000 mL) of fluid daily. Provide analgesics and antispasmodics, as ordered.

⫴⫴⫴⫴ PREVENTION *Although prostate cancer can't* ⫴⫴⫴⫴ *be prevented, advise your patient to take these actions to reduce risk factors:*

◆ *Eat a low-fat diet with foods high in lycopenes.*

◆ *Exercise regularly.*

TESTICULAR CANCER

Malignant testicular tumors primarily affect young to middle-aged men and are the most common solid tumor in this group. (See *Testicular cancer.*) (In children, testicular tumors are rare.) Most testicular tumors originate in gonadal cells. About 40% are seminomas—uniform, undifferentiated cells resembling primitive gonadal cells. The remainder are nonseminomas—tumor cells showing various degrees of differentiation. The prognosis varies with the cell type and disease stage, but testicular cancer is considered curable. When treated with surgery and radiation, almost all patients with localized disease survive beyond 5 years.

Causes and incidence

The cause of testicular cancer isn't known, but incidence (which peaks between ages 20 and 40) is higher in men with cryptorchidism (even when surgically corrected) and in men whose mothers used DES during pregnancy. Testicular cancer is rare in nonwhite males and accounts for fewer than 1% of male cancer deaths. Testicular cancer spreads through the lymphatic system to the iliac, para-aortic, and mediastinal lymph nodes and may metastasize to the lungs, liver, viscera, and bone.

Complications

◆ Back or abdominal pain
◆ Retroperitoneal adenopathy
◆ Dyspnea, cough
◆ Hemoptysis (lung metastasis)
◆ Urethral obstruction

Pathophysiology

The cause of testicular cancer is not known. The characteristic genetic change found is an isochromosome of the short arm of chromosome 12, which is often seen in sporadic cancers. This suggests that genes in this region are important in the development of germ cell tumors. A number of other genes that have a relatively weak effect are also involved in the development of testicular cancer.

Signs and symptoms

The first sign is usually a firm, painless, and smooth testicular mass, varying in size and sometimes producing a sense of testicular heaviness. When such a tumor causes chorionic gonadotropin or estrogen production, gynecomastia and nipple tenderness may result. In advanced stages, signs and symptoms include ureteral obstruction, abdominal mass, cough, hemoptysis, shortness of breath, weight loss, fatigue, pallor, and lethargy.

Diagnosis

Two effective means of detecting a testicular tumor are regular self-examinations and testicular palpation during a routine physical examination. Transillumination can distinguish between a tumor (which doesn't transilluminate) and a hydrocele or spermatocele (which does). Follow-up measures should include an examination for gynecomastia and abdominal masses.

Diagnostic tests include excretory urography to detect ureteral deviation resulting from para-aortic node involvement, urinary or serum luteinizing hormone levels, blood tests, lymphangiography, ultrasound, and abdominal CT scan. Serum alpha-fetoprotein and beta-human chorionic gonadotropin levels—indicators of testicular tumor activity—provide a baseline for

---

Testicular cancer

In testicular cancer, palpation may reveal a firm smooth testicular mass.

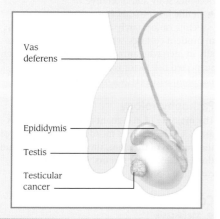

Vas deferens

Epididymis

Testis

Testicular cancer

measuring response to therapy and determining the prognosis.

Surgical excision and biopsy of the tumor and testis permits histologic verification of the tumor cell type—essential for effective treatment. Inguinal exploration determines the extent of nodal involvement.

Treatment

The extent of surgery, radiation, and chemotherapy varies with tumor cell type and stage. Surgery includes orchiectomy and retroperitoneal node dissection. Most surgeons remove the testis, not the scrotum (to allow for a prosthetic implant). Hormone replacement therapy may be needed after bilateral orchiectomy.

Radiation of the retroperitoneal and homolateral iliac nodes follows removal of a seminoma. All positive nodes receive radiation after removal of a nonseminoma. Patients with retroperitoneal extension receive prophylactic radiation to the mediastinal and supraclavicular nodes.

Essential for tumors beyond stage 0, chemotherapy combinations include bleomycin, etoposide, and cisplatin; etoposide and cisplatin; and cisplatin. Chemotherapy and radiation followed by autologous bone marrow transplantation may help unresponsive patients.

Special considerations

Develop a care plan that addresses both the patient's psychological and physical needs.

Before orchiectomy:
◆ Reassure the patient that sterility and impotence need not follow unilateral orchiectomy, that synthetic hormones can restore hormonal balance, and that most surgeons don't remove the scrotum. In many cases, a testicular prosthesis can correct anatomic disfigurement.

After orchiectomy:
◆ For the first day after surgery, apply an ice pack to the scrotum and provide analgesics, as ordered.
◆ Check for excessive bleeding, swelling, and signs of infection.
◆ Provide a scrotal athletic supporter to minimize pain during ambulation.

During chemotherapy:
◆ Give antiemetics, as needed, for nausea and vomiting. Encourage small, frequent meals to maintain oral intake despite anorexia. Establish a mouth care regimen and check for stomatitis. Watch for signs of myelosuppression. If the patient receives vinblastine, assess for neurotoxicity (peripheral paresthesia, jaw pain, and muscle cramps). If the patient receives cisplatin, check for ototoxicity. To prevent renal damage, encourage increased fluid intake and provide

I.V. fluids, a potassium supplement, and diuretics, as ordered.

PENILE CANCER

The most common form of penile cancer, epidermoid squamous cell cancer, is usually found in the glans but may also occur on the corona glandis and, rarely, in the preputial cavity. This malignancy produces ulcerative or papillary (wartlike, nodular) lesions, which may become quite large before spreading beyond the penis; such lesions may destroy the glans penis and prepuce and invade the corpora.

The prognosis varies according to staging at time of diagnosis. If begun early enough, radiation therapy increases the 5-year survival rate to over 60%; surgery only to over 55%. Unfortunately, many men delay treatment of penile cancer because they fear disfigurement and loss of sexual function.

Causes and incidence

The exact cause of penile cancer is unknown; however, it's generally associated with poor personal hygiene and with phimosis in uncircumcised men. This may account for the low incidence among Jews, Muslims, and people of other cultures that practice circumcision at birth or shortly thereafter. (Incidence isn't decreased in cultures that practice circumcision at a later date.) Early circumcision seems to prevent penile cancer by allowing for better personal hygiene and minimizing inflammatory (and commonly premalignant) lesions of the glans and prepuce. Such lesions include:
◆ leukoplakia—inflammation, with thickened patches that may fissure
◆ balanitis—inflammation of the penis associated with phimosis
◆ erythroplasia of Queyrat—squamous cell cancer in situ; velvety, erythematous lesion that becomes scaly and ulcerative
◆ penile horn—scaly, horn-shaped growth

Penile cancer rarely affects circumcised men in modern cultures; when it does occur, it's usually in men who are older than age 50. Another suspected risk factor is infection with human papillomavirus (HPV), or genital warts.

Pathophysiology

The majority of malignant tumors of the penis are SCC. The origin is mostly the inner lining of the mucosa of the glans, the coronal sulcus, and the foreskin. Other tumors, such as basal cell carcinoma, are very rare.

Complication
◆ Metastasis

Signs and symptoms

In a circumcised man, early signs of penile cancer include a small circumscribed lesion, a pimple, or a sore on the penis. In an uncircumcised man, however, such early symptoms may go unnoticed, so penile cancer first becomes apparent when it causes late-stage signs or symptoms, such as pain, hemorrhage, dysuria, purulent discharge, and obstruction of the urinary meatus. Rarely is metastasis the first sign of penile cancer.

Diagnosis

Diagnosis of penile cancer requires a tissue biopsy.

CONFIRMING DIAGNOSIS *Preoperative baseline studies include complete blood count, urinalysis, an electrocardiogram, and a chest X-ray. Enlarged inguinal lymph nodes due to infection (caused by primary lesion) make detection of nodal metastasis by preoperative CT scan difficult.*

Treatment

Depending on the stage of progression, treatment includes surgical resection of the primary tumor and, possibly, chemotherapy and radiation. Local tumors of the prepuce only require circumcision. Invasive tumors, however, require partial penectomy if there's at least a 2-cm tumor-free margin; tumors of the base of the penile shaft require total penectomy and inguinal node dissection (procedure is less common in the United States than in other countries where incidence is higher). Radiation therapy may improve treatment effectiveness after resection of localized lesions without metastasis; it may also reduce the size of lymph nodes before nodal resection. It's not adequate primary treatment for groin metastasis, however. Topical 5-fluorouracil is used for precancerous lesions. A combination of bleomycin, methotrexate, and vincristine with or without cisplatin is used for metastasis.

Special considerations

Penile cancer calls for good patient teaching, psychological support, and comprehensive postoperative care. The patient with penile cancer fears disfigurement, pain, and loss of sexual function.

Before penile surgery:
◆ Spend time with the patient, and encourage the patient talking about any fears.
◆ Supplement and reinforce what the surgeon has told the patient about the surgery and other treatment measures, and explain expected postoperative procedures, such as dressing changes and catheterization. Show the patient diagrams of the surgical procedure and pictures of the results of similar surgery to help the patient adapt to an altered body image.
◆ If the patient needs urinary diversion, refer the patient to the enterostomal therapist.

Although postpenectomy care varies with the procedure used and the surgeon's protocol, certain procedures are always applicable:
◆ Constantly monitor the patient's vital signs and record their intake and output accurately.
◆ Provide comprehensive skin care to prevent skin breakdown from urinary diversion or suprapubic catheterization. Keep the skin dry and free from urine. If the patient has a suprapubic catheter, make sure the catheter is patent at all times.
◆ Administer analgesics as ordered. Elevate the penile stump with a small towel or pillow to minimize edema.
◆ Check the surgical site often for signs of infection, such as foul odor or excessive drainage on dressing.
◆ If the patient has had inguinal node dissection, watch for and immediately report signs of lymphedema, such as decreased circulation or disproportionate swelling of a leg.
◆ After partial penectomy, reassure the patient that the penile stump should be sufficient for urination and sexual function. Refer the patient for psychological or sexual counseling if necessary.

PREVENTION *To help reduce the risk for penile cancer, teach your patient the following:*
◆ *Practice good genital hygiene, especially if he's uncircumcised.*
◆ *To prevent transmission of HPV, use condoms during sexual intercourse.*
◆ *If the patient smokes, advise about the importance of quitting.*

CERVICAL CANCER

One of the most common cancers of the female reproductive system, cervical cancer is classified as either preinvasive or invasive. (See *Cervical cancer,* page 760.)

Preinvasive cancer ranges from minimal cervical dysplasia, in which the lower third of the epithelium contains abnormal cells, to carcinoma in situ, in which the full thickness of the epithelium contains abnormally proliferating cells (also known as *cervical intraepithelial neoplasia*). Preinvasive cancer is curable 75% to 90% of the time with early detection and proper treatment. If untreated (and depending on the form in which it appears), it may progress to invasive cervical cancer.

In invasive cancer, cancer cells penetrate the basement membrane and can spread directly to

Cervical cancer

The illustrations below show cervical carcinoma in situ and squamous cell carcinoma of the cervix.

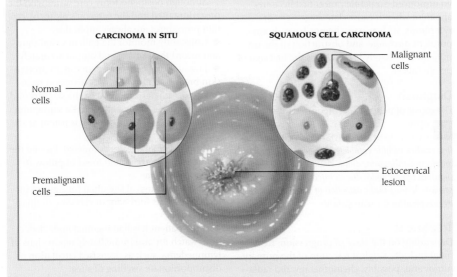

CARCINOMA IN SITU

SQUAMOUS CELL CARCINOMA

Malignant cells

Normal cells

Premalignant cells

Ectocervical lesion

contiguous pelvic structures or disseminate to distant sites by lymphatic routes.

Causes and incidence

Seventy percent of all cases of cervical cancer are caused by HPV. Although there are several types of HPV, two strains are usually responsible for causing cervical cancer. Several predisposing factors have been related to the development of cervical cancer: frequent intercourse at a young age (younger than age 16), multiple sexual partners, multiple pregnancies, exposure to sexually transmitted diseases (particularly genital HPV), and smoking. (See *Preventing cervical cancer*, page 761.)

In almost all cases of cervical cancer (95%), the histologic type is squamous cell cancer, which varies from well-differentiated cells to highly anaplastic spindle cells. Only 5% are adenocarcinomas. Usually, invasive cancer occurs between ages 30 and 50; rarely, in patients younger than age 20.

In 2010, 12,200 women were diagnosed with cervical cancer and there were 4,200 deaths from this disease.

Complications

◆ Flank pain
◆ Hematuria
◆ Renal failure

Signs and symptoms

Preinvasive cervical cancer produces no symptoms or other clinically apparent changes. Early invasive cervical cancer causes abnormal vaginal bleeding, persistent vaginal discharge, and postcoital pain and bleeding. In advanced stages, it causes pelvic pain, vaginal leakage of urine and feces from a fistula, anorexia, weight loss, and anemia.

Diagnosis

A cytologic examination (Pap smear) can detect cervical cancer before clinical evidence appears. (Systems of Pap smear classification may vary from facility to facility.) Abnormal cervical cytology routinely calls for colposcopy, which can detect the presence and extent of preclinical lesions requiring biopsy and histologic examination. Staining may identify areas for biopsy when the smear shows abnormal cells but there's no obvious lesion. Although the tests are nonspecific, they do distinguish between normal and abnormal tissues. Normal tissues absorb the iodine and turn brown; abnormal tissues are devoid of glycogen and won't change color. Additional studies, such as lymphangiography, cystography, and scans, can detect metastasis.

Treatment

Appropriate treatment depends on accurate clinical staging. Preinvasive lesions may be

PREVENTION

Preventing cervical cancer

The human papillomavirus (HPV), types 16 and 18, cause 70% of cervical cancer cases. To prevent this disorder, encourage the patient to do the following:

Get vaccinated
Since 2006, the quadrivalent HPV recombinant vaccine has been available to reduce cervical cancer. This vaccine is recommended for girls and women ages 9 to 26. The vaccine is most effective if given before the patient is sexually active. Remind the patient that Pap tests are still recommended.

Have Pap test screenings
The most effective way to screen for cervical cancer is the Papanicolaou (Pap) test. The following guidelines are recommended:
◆ Initial screening should begin within 3 years of first sexual intercourse but no later than age 21. Yearly screening should be done until age 30.
◆ Beginning at age 30, women who have had three normal Pap tests in a row may get screened every 2 to 3 years.
◆ For women age 70 and older who have had three or more normal Pap tests in the past 10 years, screening is optional.

Be careful with sexual activity
Having sexual intercourse at a young age increases risks for contracting HPV; advise your patient that delaying first intercourse may help reduce risk. Also, having fewer sexual partners may decrease risk.

Don't smoke
Chances of developing cervical cancer can be reduced by not smoking.

---

treated with total excisional biopsy, cryosurgery, laser destruction, loop electrosurgical excision procedure, conization (and frequent Pap smear follow-up) or, rarely, hysterectomy. Therapy for invasive squamous cell cancer may include radical hysterectomy and radiation therapy (internal, external, or both). Chemotherapy may be used alone or in combination with radiation therapy in treating cervical cancer. Cisplatin and fluorouracil are the agents used. Topotecan combined with cisplatin is used to treat late-stage cervical cancer.

Special considerations
Management of cervical cancer requires skilled preoperative and postoperative care, comprehensive patient teaching, and emotional and psychological support.
◆ If you assist with a biopsy, drape and prepare the patient as for routine Pap smear and pelvic examination. Have a container of formaldehyde ready to preserve the specimen during transfer to the pathology laboratory. Explain to the patient that they may feel pressure, minor abdominal cramps, or a pinch from the punch forceps. Reassure them that pain will be minimal because the cervix has few nerve endings.

◆ If you assist with cryosurgery, drape and prepare the patient as if for a routine Pap smear and pelvic examination. Explain that the procedure takes about 15 minutes, during which time the practitioner will use refrigerant to freeze the cervix. Warn the patient that they may experience abdominal cramps, headache, nausea, and sweating, but reassure that they'll feel little, if any, pain.
◆ If you assist with laser therapy, drape and prepare the patient as if for a routine Pap smear and pelvic examination. Explain that the procedure takes about 30 minutes and may cause abdominal cramps.
◆ After excisional biopsy, cryosurgery, and laser therapy, tell the patient to expect a discharge or spotting for about 1 week after these procedures, and advise the patient not to douche, use tampons, or engage in sexual intercourse during this time. Tell them to watch for and report signs of infection. Stress the need for a follow-up Pap smear and a pelvic examination within 3 to 4 months after these procedures and periodically thereafter.
◆ Tell the patient what to expect postoperatively if they'll have a hysterectomy.
◆ After surgery, monitor vital signs every 4 hours.

◆ Watch for and immediately report signs or symptoms of complications, such as bleeding, abdominal distention, severe pain, and breathing difficulties.

◆ Administer analgesics, prophylactic antibiotics, and subcutaneous heparin, as ordered.

◆ Encourage deep-breathing and coughing exercises.

For radiation therapy:

◆ Find out if the patient is to have internal or external therapy, or both. Usually, internal radiation therapy is the first procedure.

◆ Explain the internal radiation procedure, and answer the patient's questions. Internal radiation requires a 2- to 3-day hospital stay, bowel preparation, a povidone–iodine vaginal douche, a clear liquid diet, insertion of an indwelling urinary catheter, and nothing by mouth the night before the implantation.

◆ Explain to the patient that they'll have less contact with staff and visitors while the implant is in place.

◆ Tell the patient that the internal radiation applicator will be inserted in the operating room under general anesthesia and that the radioactive material (such as radium or cesium) will be loaded into it when back in their room.

◆ Remember that safety precautions—time, distance, and shielding—begin as soon as the radioactive source is in place. Inform the patient that they'll require a private room. (See *Internal radiation safety precautions*.)

◆ Strict bed rest is required for most internal radiation sources. The patient must lie on their back with the head of bed elevated to no more than 30 degrees.

◆ Check vital signs every 4 hours; watch for skin reaction, vaginal bleeding, abdominal discomfort, or evidence of dehydration. Make sure the patient can reach everything she needs without stretching or straining. Assist them in ROM *arm* exercises (leg exercises and other body movements could dislodge the implant). If ordered, administer a tranquilizer to help the patient relax and remain still. Organize the time you spend with the patient to minimize your exposure to radiation.

◆ Inform visitors of safety precautions, and hang a sign listing these precautions on the patient's door.

◆ Explain that external outpatient radiation therapy, when necessary, continues for 4 to 6 weeks.

◆ Teach the patient to watch for and report uncomfortable adverse effects. Because radiation therapy may increase susceptibility to infection by lowering the WBC count, warn the patient to avoid persons with obvious infections during therapy.

◆ Teach the patient to use a vaginal dilator to prevent vaginal stenosis and to facilitate vaginal examinations and sexual intercourse.

◆ Reassure the patient that this disease and its treatment shouldn't radically alter lifestyle or prohibit sexual intimacy.

Internal radiation safety precautions

There are three cardinal safety rules in internal radiation therapy:

◆ *Time*. Wear a radiosensitive badge. Remember, your exposure increases with time, and the effects are cumulative. Therefore, carefully plan your time with the patient to prevent overexposure. (However, don't rush procedures, ignore the patient's psychological needs, or give the impression you can't get out of the room fast enough.)

◆ *Distance*. Radiation loses its intensity with distance. Avoid standing at the foot of the patient's bed, where you're in line with the radiation.

◆ *Shield*. Lead shields reduce radiation exposure. Use them whenever possible.

In internal radiation therapy, remember that the patient is radioactive while the radiation source is in place, usually 48 to 72 hours.

◆ Pregnant women shouldn't be assigned to care for these patients.

◆ Check the position of the source applicator every 4 hours. If it appears dislodged, notify the practitioner immediately. If it's completely dislodged, remove the patient from the bed; pick up the applicator with long forceps, place it on a lead-shielded transport cart, and notify the practitioner immediately.

◆ *Never* pick up the source with your bare hands. Notify the practitioner and radiation safety officer whenever there's an accident, and keep a lead-shielded transport cart on the unit as long as the patient has a source in place.

POSITIONING OF INTERNAL RADIATION APPLICATOR FOR UTERINE CANCER

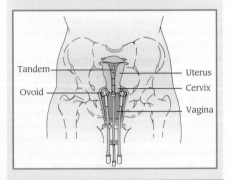

UTERINE CANCER

Uterine cancer, or endometrial cancer, involves cancerous growth of the endometrial lining. The 5-year survival rate is 75% to 95% for stage I cancers; as the stages progress, the survival rate diminishes. For stage II, there's a 50% survival rate; stage III, 30%; and there's less than a 5% survival rate for stage IV.

Causes and incidence

Uterine cancer seems linked to several predisposing factors, including:
◆ abnormal uterine bleeding
◆ diabetes
◆ familial tendency
◆ history of uterine polyps or endometrial hyperplasia
◆ hypertension
◆ low fertility index and anovulation
◆ nulliparity
◆ obesity
◆ uninterrupted estrogen stimulation

In most cases, uterine cancer is an adenocarcinoma that metastasizes late, usually from the endometrium to the cervix, ovaries, fallopian tubes, and other peritoneal structures. It may spread to distant organs, such as the lungs and the brain, through the blood or the lymphatic system. Lymph node involvement can also occur. Less common are adenoacanthoma, endometrial stromal sarcoma, lymphosarcoma, mixed mesodermal tumors (including carcinosarcoma), and leiomyosarcoma.

Uterine cancer usually affects postmenopausal women between ages 50 and 60; it's uncommon between ages 30 and 40 and extremely rare before age 30. Most premenopausal women who develop uterine cancer have a history of anovulatory menstrual cycles or other hormonal imbalance. About 40,100 new cases of uterine cancer are reported annually, with about 7,470 deaths occurring annually.

Pathophysiology

Uterine cancer, a disease characterized by the abnormal growth of cells in the uterus. Cancers affecting the lining of the uterus (endometrium) are the most common cancers of the female reproductive tract. Other uterine cancers, called uterine sarcomas, develop from underlying muscle or connective tissue; they are much rarer.

Complications

◆ Intestinal obstruction
◆ Ascites
◆ Hemorrhage

Signs and symptoms

Uterine enlargement, and persistent and unusual premenopausal bleeding, or any postmenopausal bleeding, are the most common indications of uterine cancer. The discharge may at first be watery and blood-streaked, but it gradually becomes more bloody. Other signs or symptoms, such as pain and weight loss, don't appear until the cancer is well advanced.

Diagnosis

Unfortunately, a Pap test, so useful for detecting cervical cancer, doesn't dependably predict early-stage uterine cancer. The diagnosis of uterine cancer requires endometrial, cervical, and endocervical biopsies. Negative biopsies call for a fractional dilatation and curettage to determine the diagnosis. Positive diagnosis requires the following tests for baseline data and staging:
◆ multiple cervical biopsies and endocervical curettage to pinpoint cervical involvement
◆ Schiller test, staining the cervix and vagina with an iodine solution that turns healthy tissues brown; cancerous tissues resist the stain
◆ complete physical examination
◆ MRI or CT scan to detect metastasis to the myometrium, cervix, lymph nodes, and other organs
◆ excretory urography and, possibly, cystoscopy to evaluate the urinary system
◆ complete blood studies
◆ electrocardiogram
◆ proctoscopy or barium enema studies, if bladder and rectal involvement are suspected

Treatment

Treatment varies, depending on the extent of the disease:
◆ Surgery—Rarely curative, surgery generally involves total abdominal hysterectomy, bilateral salpingo-oophorectomy, or possibly omentectomy with or without pelvic or para-aortic lymphadenectomy. Total exenteration involves removal of all pelvic organs, including the vagina, and is done only when the disease is sufficiently contained to allow surgical removal of diseased parts. (See *Managing pelvic exenteration*, page 764.)
◆ Radiation therapy—When the tumor isn't well differentiated, intracavitary or external radiation (or both), given 6 weeks before surgery, may inhibit recurrence and lengthen survival time.
◆ Hormonal therapy—Synthetic progesterones, such as medroxyprogesterone or megestrol, may be administered for systemic disease. Tamoxifen (which produces a 20% to 40% response rate) may be given as a second-line treatment for advanced-stage disease.

Managing pelvic exenteration

Before pelvic exenteration

♦ Teach the patient about ileal conduit and possible colostomy, and make sure that the patient understands the vagina will be removed.

♦ To minimize the risk of infection, supervise a rigorous bowel and skin preparation procedure. Decrease the residue in the patient's diet for 48 to 72 hours, and then maintain a diet ranging from clear liquids to nothing by mouth. Administer oral or I.V. antibiotics, as ordered, and prep skin daily with antibacterial soap.

♦ Instruct the patient about postoperative procedures: I.V. therapy, central venous pressure catheter, blood drainage system, and an unsutured perineal wound with gauze packing.

After pelvic exenteration

♦ Check the stoma, incision, and perineal wound for drainage. Be especially careful to check the perineal wound for bleeding after the packing is removed. Expect red or serosanguineous drainage, but notify the practitioner immediately if drainage is excessive, continuously bright red, foul-smelling, or purulent or if there's bleeding from the conduit.

♦ Provide excellent skin care because of draining urine and feces. Use warm water and saline solution to clean the skin, because soap may be too drying and may increase skin breakdown.

♦ Chemotherapy—Varying combinations of cisplatin, doxorubicin, carboplatin, topotecan, paclitaxel, and gemcitabine are usually tried when other treatments have failed.

Special considerations

Patients with uterine cancer require patient teaching to help them cope with surgery, radiation, and chemotherapy. Also provide good postoperative care and psychological support.

Before surgery:

♦ Explain the routine tests (e.g., repeated blood tests the morning after surgery) and postoperative care. If the patient is to have a lymphadenectomy *and* a total hysterectomy, explain that she'll probably have a wound drainage system for about 5 days after surgery. Also explain indwelling urinary catheter care. The patient should be fitted with antiembolism stockings for use during and after surgery. Make

sure the patient's blood has been typed and cross-matched. If the patient is premenopausal, instruct them that removal of the ovaries will induce menopause.

After surgery:

♦ Measure fluid contents of the wound drainage system every shift. Notify the practitioner immediately if drainage exceeds 400 mL.

♦ If the patient has received subcutaneous heparin, continue administration, as ordered, until the patient is fully ambulatory again. Give prophylactic antibiotics as ordered, and provide good indwelling urinary catheter care.

♦ Check vital signs every 4 hours. Watch for and immediately report any sign of complications, such as bleeding, abdominal distention, severe pain, wheezing, or other breathing difficulties. Provide analgesics as ordered.

♦ Regularly encourage the patient to breathe deeply and cough to help prevent complications. Promote the use of an incentive spirometer several times every waking hour to help keep lungs expanded.

For radiation therapy:

♦ Find out if the patient is to have internal or external radiation or both. Usually, internal radiation therapy is done first.

♦ Explain the internal radiation procedure, answer the patient's questions, and encourage the patient to express fears and concerns.

♦ Explain that internal radiation usually requires a 2- to 3-day hospital stay, bowel preparation, a povidone–iodine vaginal douche, a clear liquid diet, and nothing taken by mouth the night before the implantation.

♦ Mention that internal radiation also requires an indwelling urinary catheter.

♦ Tell the patient that, if the procedure is performed in the operating room, they'll receive a general anesthetic. They'll be placed in a dorsal position, with their knees and hips flexed and their heels resting in footrests.

♦ Inform the patient that the radioactive source may be implanted in the vagina by the physician, or it may be implanted by a member of the radiation team while the patient is in the room.

♦ Remember that safety precautions, including time, distance, and shielding, must be imposed immediately after the patient's radioactive source has been implanted.

♦ Tell the patient that they'll require a private room.

♦ Encourage the patient to limit movement while the source is in place. If they prefer, elevate the head of the bed slightly. Make sure the patient can reach everything they will need (call bell, telephone, water) without stretching or straining. Assist them in ROM *arm* exercises (leg exercises and other body movements could dislodge the source). If ordered, administer a tranquilizer to help the patient relax and remain still. Organize the time you spend with the patient to minimize your exposure to radiation.

◆ Check the patient's vital signs every 4 hours; watch for skin reaction, vaginal bleeding, abdominal discomfort, or evidence of dehydration.

◆ Inform visitors of safety precautions and hang a sign listing these precautions on the patient's door.

If the patient receives external radiation:

◆ Teach the patient and family about the therapy before it begins. Tell the patient that treatment is usually given 5 days a week for 6 weeks. Warn the patient not to scrub body areas marked with indelible ink for treatment because it's important to direct treatment to exactly the same area each time.

◆ Instruct the patient to maintain a high-protein, high-carbohydrate, low-residue diet to reduce bulk and yet maintain calories. Administer diphenoxylate with atropine, as ordered, to minimize diarrhea, a possible adverse effect of pelvic radiation.

◆ To minimize skin breakdown and reduce the risk of skin infection, tell the patient to keep the treatment area dry, to avoid wearing clothes that rub against the area, and to avoid using heating pads, alcohol rubs, or any skin creams.

◆ Teach the patient how to use a vaginal dilator to prevent vaginal stenosis and to facilitate vaginal examinations and sexual intercourse.

Remember, a patient with uterine cancer needs special counseling and psychological support to help cope with this disease and the necessary treatments. Fearful about survival, the patient may also be concerned that treatment will alter lifestyle and prevent sexual intimacy. Explain that except in total pelvic exenteration, the vagina remains intact and that after she recovers, sexual intercourse is possible. Your presence and interest will help the patient, even if you can't answer every question they may ask.

VAGINAL CANCER

Vaginal cancer accounts for about 2% of all gynecologic cancers. It usually appears as squamous cell cancer, but occasionally as melanoma, sarcoma, or adenocarcinoma.

Causes and incidence

The exact cause of vaginal cancer remains unknown. This cancer generally occurs in women in their early to mid-50s, but some of the rarer types occur in younger women, and rhabdomyosarcoma appears in children. (Clear cell adenocarcinoma has an increased incidence in young women whose mothers took DES.)

Vaginal cancer varies in severity according to its location and effect on lymphatic drainage. (The vagina is a thin-walled structure with a rich lymphatic drainage.) Vaginal cancer is similar to cervical cancer in that it may progress from an intraepithelial tumor to an invasive cancer. However, it spreads more slowly than cervical cancer.

A lesion in the upper third of the vagina (the most common site) usually metastasizes to the groin nodes; a lesion in the lower third (the second most common site) usually metastasizes to the hypogastric and iliac nodes; but a lesion in the middle third metastasizes erratically. A posterior lesion displaces and distends the vaginal posterior wall before spreading to deep layers. By contrast, an anterior lesion spreads more rapidly into other structures and deep layers because, unlike the posterior wall, the anterior vaginal wall isn't flexible.

Pathophysiology

Malignant diseases of the vagina are either primary vaginal cancers or metastatic cancers from adjacent or distant organs. Primary vaginal cancers are defined as arising solely from the vagina, with no involvement of the external cervical os proximally or the vulva distally. The importance of this definition lies in the different clinical approaches to the treatment of upper and lower vaginal cancer.

Signs and symptoms

Commonly, the patient with vaginal cancer has experienced abnormal bleeding and discharge. Also, she may have a small or large, in many cases firm, ulcerated lesion in any part of the vagina. As the cancer progresses, it commonly spreads to the bladder (producing frequent voiding and bladder pain), the rectum (bleeding), vulva (lesion), pubic bone (pain), or other surrounding tissues.

Diagnosis

The diagnosis of vaginal cancer is based on the presence of abnormal cells on a vaginal Pap smear. Careful examination and a biopsy rule out the cervix and vulva as the primary sites of the lesion. In many cases, however, the cervix contains the primary lesion that has metastasized to the vagina. Then, any visible lesion is biopsied and evaluated histologically. It's sometimes difficult to visualize the entire vagina because the speculum blades may hide a lesion, or the patient may be uncooperative because of discomfort. When lesions aren't visible, colposcopy is used to search out abnormalities. Painting the suspected vaginal area with Lugol solution also helps identify malignant areas by staining glycogen-containing normal tissue, while leaving abnormal tissue unstained.

Treatment

In early stages, treatment aims to preserve the normal parts of the vagina. Topical chemotherapy with 5-fluorouracil and laser surgery can be used for stages 0 and I. Radiation or surgery varies with the size, depth, and location of the lesion and the patient's desire to maintain a functional vagina. Preservation of a functional vagina is generally possible only in the early stages. Survival rates are the same for patients treated with radiation as for those treated with surgery.

Surgery is usually recommended only when the tumor is so extensive that exenteration is needed because close proximity to the bladder and rectum permits only minimal tissue margins around resected vaginal tissue.

Radiation therapy is the preferred treatment of advanced vaginal cancer. Most patients need preliminary external radiation treatment to shrink the tumor before internal radiation can begin. Then, if the tumor is localized to the vault and the cervix is present, radiation (using radium or cesium) can be given with an intrauterine tandem or ovoids; if the cervix is absent, a specially designed vaginal applicator is used instead.

To minimize complications, radioactive sources and filters are carefully placed away from radiosensitive tissues, such as the bladder and rectum. Internal radiation lasts 48 to 72 hours, depending on the dosage.

Special considerations

For internal radiation:
◆ Explain the internal radiation procedure, answer the patient's questions, and encourage them to express their fears and concerns.
◆ Because the effects of radiation are cumulative, wear a radiosensitive badge and a lead shield (if available) when you enter the patient's room, and adhere to internal radiation safety precautions.
◆ Check with the radiation therapist concerning the maximum recommended time that you can safely spend with the patient when giving direct care.
◆ While the radiation source is in place, the patient must lie flat on their back with the head of the bed elevated no more than 30 degrees. Insert an indwelling urinary catheter (usually done in the operating room), and don't change the patient's linens unless they're soiled. Give

only partial bed baths, and make sure the patient has a call bell, phone, water, or anything else she needs within easy reach. The practitioner will order a clear liquid or low-residue diet and an antidiarrheal drug to prevent bowel movements.
◆ To compensate for immobility, encourage the patient to do active ROM exercises with both arms.
◆ Before radiation treatment, explain the necessity of immobilization, and tell the patient what it entails (such as no linen changes and the use of an indwelling urinary catheter). Throughout therapy, encourage the patient to express any anxieties.
◆ Instruct the patient to use a stent or do prescribed exercises to prevent vaginal stenosis. Coitus is also helpful in preventing stenosis.

OVARIAN CANCER

Ovarian cancer is the fifth most common cancer in women and the leading cause of gynecologic deaths in the United States. (See *Ovarian cancer*, page 767.) In women with previously treated breast cancer, metastatic ovarian cancer is more common than cancer at any other site and may be linked to mutations in the *BRCA1* or *BRCA2* gene.

The prognosis varies with the histologic type and stage of the disease but is generally poor because ovarian tumors produce few early signs and are usually advanced at diagnosis. Although about 46% of women with ovarian cancer survive for 5 years, the overall survival rate hasn't improved significantly. However, early diagnosis and treatment improves the 5-year survival rate to 94%.

Three main types of ovarian cancer exist:
◆ Primary epithelial tumors account for 90% of all ovarian cancers and include serous cystadenocarcinoma, mucinous cystadenocarcinoma, and endometrioid and mesonephric malignancies. Serous cystadenocarcinoma is the most common type and accounts for 50% of all cases.
◆ Germ cell tumors include endodermal sinus malignancies, embryonal carcinoma (a rare ovarian cancer that appears in children), immature teratomas, and dysgerminoma.
◆ Sex cord (stromal) tumors include granulosa cell tumors (which produce estrogen and may have feminizing effects), granulosa-theca cell tumors, and the rare arrhenoblastomas (which produce androgen and have virilizing effects).

Causes and incidence

Exactly what causes ovarian cancer isn't known, but the greatest number of cases occurs in the fifth decade of life. However, it can occur during

Ovarian cancer

The illustration below shows carcinoma of the left ovary.

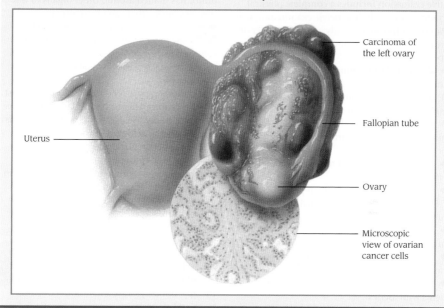

Uterus

Carcinoma of
the left ovary

Fallopian tube

Ovary

Microscopic
view of ovarian
cancer cells

childhood. Other contributing factors include infertility, nulliparity, familial tendency, ovarian dysfunction, irregular menses, hormone replacement therapy, and possible exposure to asbestos, talc, and industrial pollutants.

Primary epithelial tumors arise in the ovarian surface epithelium; germ cell tumors, in the ovum itself; and sex cord tumors, in the ovarian stroma. Ovarian tumors spread rapidly intraperitoneally by local extension or surface seeding and, occasionally, through the lymphatics and the bloodstream. Generally, extraperitoneal spread is through the diaphragm into the chest cavity, which may cause pleural effusions. Other metastasis is rare.

Pathophysiology

Historically, most theories of the pathophysiology of ovarian cancer included the concept that it begins with the dedifferentiation of the cells overlying the ovary. During ovulation, these cells can be incorporated into the ovary, where they then proliferate. However, new evidence indicates that the majority of these tumors actually originate in the fimbria of the fallopian tube. Detailed pathologic studies have pushed much of the thinking about the origin of these tumors in this direction.

Complications
- Fluid and electrolyte imbalance
- Leg edema
- Ascites
- Intestinal obstruction
- Malnutrition
- Profound cachexia
- Pleural effusions

Signs and symptoms

Typically, symptoms vary with the size of the tumor. An ovarian tumor may grow to considerable size before it produces overt symptoms. Occasionally, in the early stages, ovarian cancer causes vague abdominal discomfort, dyspepsia, and other mild GI disturbances. As it progresses, it causes urinary frequency, constipation, pelvic discomfort, distention, and weight loss. Tumor rupture, torsion, or infection may cause pain, which, in young patients, may mimic appendicitis. Granulosa cell tumors have feminizing effects (such as bleeding between periods in premenopausal women); conversely, arrhenoblastomas have virilizing effects. Advanced ovarian cancer causes ascites, rarely postmenopausal bleeding and pain, and symptoms relating to metastatic sites (most commonly pleural effusions).

Diagnosis

The diagnosis of ovarian cancer requires clinical evaluation, complete patient history, surgical exploration, and histologic studies. Preoperative evaluation includes a complete physical examination, including pelvic examination with Pap smear (positive in only a small number of women with ovarian cancer) and the following special tests:

♦ abdominal ultrasonography, CT scan, or MRI (may delineate tumor size)
♦ complete blood count, blood chemistries, and electrocardiogram
♦ excretory urography for information on renal function and possible urinary tract anomalies or obstruction
♦ chest X-ray for distant metastasis and pleural effusions
♦ barium enema (especially in patients with GI symptoms) to reveal obstruction and size of tumor
♦ lymphangiography to show lymph node involvement
♦ mammography to rule out primary breast cancer
♦ liver function studies or a liver scan in patients with ascites
♦ ascites fluid aspiration for identification of typical cells by cytology
♦ laboratory tumor marker studies, such as CA-125, carcinoembryonic antigen, and human chorionic gonadotropin

Despite extensive testing, accurate diagnosis and staging are impossible without exploratory laparotomy, including lymph node evaluation and tumor resection.

Treatment

Depending on the staging of the disease and the patient's age, the treatment of ovarian cancer requires varying combinations of surgery, chemotherapy, and, in some cases, radiation.

Occasionally, in girls or young women with a unilateral encapsulated tumor who wish to maintain fertility, the following conservative approach may be appropriate:

♦ resection of the involved ovary
♦ biopsies of the omentum and the uninvolved ovary
♦ peritoneal washings for cytologic examination of pelvic fluid
♦ careful follow-up, including periodic chest X-rays to rule out lung metastasis for the first 2 years after surgery when recurrence is most likely

Ovarian cancer usually requires more aggressive treatment, including total abdominal hysterectomy and bilateral salpingo-oophorectomy with tumor resection, omentectomy, appendectomy, lymph node biopsies with lymphadenectomy, tissue biopsies, and peritoneal washings. Complete tumor resection is impossible if the tumor has matted around other organs or if it involves organs that can't be resected.

PEDIATRIC TIP *Bilateral salpingo-oophorectomy in a prepubertal girl necessitates hormone replacement therapy, beginning at puberty, to induce the development of secondary sex characteristics.*

Chemotherapy extends survival time in most ovarian cancer patients, but it's largely palliative in advanced disease. However, prolonged remissions are being achieved in some patients.

Chemotherapeutic drugs useful in ovarian cancer include carboplatin, docetaxel, cyclophosphamide, doxorubicin, paclitaxel, cisplatin, and topotecan. These drugs are usually given in combination; they may be administered intraperitoneally.

Radiation therapy generally isn't used for ovarian cancer because the resulting myelosuppression would limit the effectiveness of chemotherapy.

Radioisotopes have been used as adjuvant therapy, but they cause small-bowel obstructions and stenosis.

Special considerations

Because the treatment of ovarian cancer varies widely, so must the patient care plan.

Before surgery:

♦ Thoroughly explain all preoperative tests, the expected course of treatment, and surgical and postoperative procedures.
♦ Reinforce what the surgeon has told the patient about the surgical procedures listed in the surgical consent form. Explain that this form lists multiple procedures because the extent of the surgery can only be determined after the surgery itself has begun.
♦ In premenopausal women, explain that bilateral salpingo-oophorectomy artificially induces early menopause, so they may experience hot flashes, headaches, palpitations, insomnia, depression, and excessive perspiration.

After surgery:

♦ Monitor vital signs frequently, and check I.V. fluids often. Monitor intake and output, while maintaining good catheter care. Check the dressing regularly for excessive drainage or bleeding, and watch for signs of infection.
♦ Provide abdominal support, and watch for abdominal distention. Encourage coughing and deep breathing. Reposition the patient often, and encourage them to walk shortly after surgery.

◆ Monitor and treat adverse effects of radiation and chemotherapy.

◆ Provide psychological support for the patient and family. Encourage open communication, while discouraging overcompensation or "smothering" of the patient by their family. If the patient is a young woman who grieves for her lost ability to bear children, help her (and the family) overcome feelings that "there's nothing else to live for."

PEDIATRIC TIP *If the patient is a child, find out whether the parents have told her the patient that they have cancer, and deal with any questions accordingly. Also, enlist the help of a social worker, chaplain, and other members of the healthcare team for additional supportive care.*

CANCER OF THE VULVA

Cancer of the vulva most commonly affects the skin folds around the vagina, called the *labia*. It isn't very common, accounting for 3% to 4% of all gynecologic cancers, but is considered serious because it makes sexual intercourse painful and difficult. If found early, it has a high cure rate, with a 70% to 75% 5-year survival rate.

Causes and incidence

Although the cause of cancer of the vulva is unknown, several factors seem to predispose women to this disease:

◆ chronic pruritus of the vulva, with friction, swelling, and dryness

◆ chronic vulvar granulomatous disease

◆ diabetes

◆ hypertension

◆ irradiation of the skin, such as nonspecific treatment for pelvic cancer

◆ leukoplakia (white epithelial hyperplasia)—in about 25% of patients

◆ obesity

◆ pigmented moles that are constantly irritated by clothing or perineal pads

◆ sexually transmitted diseases (herpes simplex, condyloma acuminatum caused by HPV)

Cancer of the vulva can occur at any age, even in infants, but its peak incidence is in the mid-60s. The most common vulvar cancer is squamous cell cancer. Early diagnosis increases the chance of effective treatment and survival. Lymph node dissection allows 5-year survival in 85% of patients if it reveals no positive nodes; otherwise, the survival rate falls to less than 75%.

Pathophysiology

Vulvar cancer is a malignant, invasive growth in the vulva, or the outer portion of the female genitals. The labia majora are the most common site involved representing about 50% of all cases, followed by the labia minora. The clitoris and Bartholin glands may rarely be involved. Vulvar cancer is separate from vulvar intraepithelial neoplasia (VIN), a superficial lesion of the epithelium that has not invaded the basement membrane—or a pre-cancer. VIN may progress to carcinoma in situ and, eventually, squamous cell cancer.

Signs and symptoms

In 50% of patients, cancer of the vulva begins with vulval pruritus, bleeding, or a small vulval mass (which may start as a small ulcer on the surface, which eventually becomes infected and painful), so such symptoms call for immediate diagnostic evaluation. Seventy percent of lesions develop on the labia, but tumors can be found on the clitoris, Bartholin glands, and perineum. Less common indications include a mass in the groin or abnormal urination or defecation.

Diagnosis

A Pap smear that reveals abnormal cells, pruritus, bleeding, or a small vulvar mass strongly suggests vulvar cancer. Firm diagnosis requires histologic examination. Abnormal tissues for biopsy are identified by colposcopic examination to pinpoint vulvar lesions or abnormal skin changes and by staining with toluidine blue dye, which, after rinsing with dilute acetic acid, is retained by diseased tissues.

Other diagnostic measures include complete blood count, chest X-ray, electrocardiogram, and thorough physical (including pelvic) examination. Occasionally, CT, MRI, or positron emission tomography may pinpoint lymph node involvement. Colonoscopy is used to rule out bowel involvement. Cystoscopy may be used to evaluate for bladder or kidney involvement.

Treatment

Depending on the stage of the disease, cancer of the vulva usually calls for radical or simple vulvectomy (or laser therapy, for some small lesions). Radical vulvectomy requires bilateral dissection of superficial and deep inguinal lymph nodes. Depending on the extent of metastasis, resection may include the urethra, vagina, and bowel, leaving an open perineal wound until healing—about 2 to 3 months. Plastic surgery, including mucocutaneous graft to reconstruct pelvic structures, may be done later.

Small, confined lesions with no lymph node involvement may require a simple vulvectomy or hemivulvectomy (without pelvic node dissection). Personal considerations (young age of patient, active sexual life) may also mandate such conservative management. However, a simple vulvectomy requires careful postoperative surveillance because it leaves the patient at higher risk for developing a new lesion.

Chemotherapy alone or in combination with radiation therapy can be used in advanced cases of vulvar cancer. Cisplatin, fluorouracil, bleomycin, and doxorubicin have shown some effectiveness as a palliative treatment option.

If extensive metastasis, advanced age, or fragile health rules out surgery, irradiation of the primary lesion can offer palliative treatment.

Special considerations
Patient teaching, preoperative and postoperative care, and psychological support can help prevent complications and speed recovery.

Before surgery:
◆ Supplement and reinforce what the practitioner has told the patient about the surgery and postoperative procedures, such as the use of an indwelling urinary catheter, preventive respiratory care, and exercises to prevent venous stasis.
◆ Encourage the patient to ask questions, and answer them honestly.

After surgery:
◆ Provide scrupulous routine gynecologic care and special care to reduce pressure at the operative site, reduce tension on suture lines, and promote healing through better air circulation.
◆ Place the patient on an air mattress or convoluted foam mattress, and use a cradle to support the top covers.
◆ Periodically reposition the patient with pillows. Make sure their bed has a half-frame trapeze bar to help the patient move.
◆ For several days after surgery, the patient will be maintained on I.V. fluids or a clear liquid diet. As ordered, give the patient an antidiarrheal drug three times daily to reduce the discomfort and possible infection caused by defecation. Later, as ordered, give stool softeners and a low-residue diet to combat constipation.
◆ Teach the patient how to clean the surgical tube thoroughly.
◆ Check the operative site regularly for bleeding, foul-smelling discharge, or other signs of infection. The wound area will look lumpy, bruised, and battered, making it difficult to detect occult bleeding. This situation calls for a physician or a primary nurse, who can more easily detect subtle changes in appearance.
◆ Within 5 to 10 days after surgery, as ordered, help the patient to walk. Encourage and assist in coughing and ROM exercises.

◆ To prevent urine contamination, the patient will have an indwelling urinary catheter in place for about 2 weeks. Record fluid intake and output, and provide standard catheter care.
◆ Counsel the patient and partner about resumption of sexual activity. Explain that sensation in the vulva will eventually return after the nerve endings heal and that they'll probably be able to have sexual intercourse 6 to 8 weeks following surgery. Explain that they may want to try different sexual techniques, especially if surgery has removed the clitoris. Help the patient adjust to the drastic change in body image.

▓▓▓ **PREVENTION** *To help a patient decrease risk factors for vulvar cancer, encourage the patient to practice safe sex and to have routine pelvic examinations.*

FALLOPIAN TUBE CANCER
Primary fallopian tube cancer is extremely rare and accounts for fewer than 0.5% of all gynecologic malignancies. Because this disease is generally well advanced before diagnosis (up to 30% of such cancers are bilateral with extratubal spread), prognosis is poor.

Causes and incidence
The causes of fallopian tube cancer aren't clear, but this disease appears to be linked with nulliparity. In fact, over one half of the women with this disease have never had children.

Fallopian tube cancer usually occurs in postmenopausal women in their 50s and 60s but occasionally is found in younger women.

Pathophysiology
Fallopian tube malignancy usually starts as a dysplasia or carcinoma in situ. Typically, transition to adenocarcinoma is observed.

Signs and symptoms
Generally, early-stage fallopian tube cancer produces no symptoms. Late-stage disease is characterized by an enlarged abdomen with a palpable mass, amber-colored vaginal discharge, excessive bleeding during menstruation or, at other times, abdominal cramps, frequent urination, bladder pressure, persistent constipation, weight loss, and unilateral colicky pain produced by hydrops tubae profluens. (This last symptom occurs when the abdominal end of the fallopian tube closes, causing the tube to become greatly distended until its accumulated secretions suddenly overflow into the uterus.) Metastasis develops by local extension or by lymphatic spread to the abdominal organs or to the pelvic, aortic, and inguinal lymph nodes. Extra-abdominal metastasis is rare.

Diagnosis

CONFIRMING DIAGNOSIS *Unexplained post-menopausal bleeding and an abnormal Pap smear (suspicious or positive in up to 50% of all cases) suggest fallopian tube cancer, but laparotomy is usually necessary to confirm this diagnosis.*

When fallopian tube cancer involves both the ovary and the fallopian tube, the primary site is difficult to identify. The preoperative workup includes:

◆ ultrasound or plain film of the abdomen to help delineate tumor mass
◆ excretory urography to assess renal function and show urinary tract anomalies and ureteral obstruction
◆ chest X-ray to rule out metastasis
◆ barium enema to rule out intestinal obstruction
◆ CT of the abdomen and pelvis
◆ routine blood studies
◆ electrocardiogram

Treatment

Treatment of fallopian tube cancer consists of total abdominal hysterectomy, bilateral salpingo-oophorectomy, and omentectomy; chemotherapy with progestogens, cyclophosphamide, and cisplatin; and external radiation for 5 to 6 weeks. All patients should receive some form of adjunctive therapy (radiation or chemotherapy), even when surgery has removed all evidence of the disease.

Special considerations

Good preoperative patient preparation and postoperative care, patient instruction, psychological support, and symptomatic measures to relieve radiation and chemotherapy adverse effects can promote a successful recovery and minimize complications.

For example, reinforce the practitioner's explanation of the diagnostic and treatment procedures. Explain the need for preoperative studies, and tell the patient what to expect: fasting from the evening before surgery, an enema to clear the bowel, insertion of an indwelling urinary catheter attached to a drainage bag, placement of an I.V. line and, possibly, sedative medication. Describe the tubes and dressings the patient can expect to have in place when she returns from surgery. Teach the patient deep-breathing and coughing techniques to prepare for postoperative exercises.

After surgery:

◆ Check vital signs every 4 hours. Report fever, tachycardia, and hypotension to the practitioner.
◆ Monitor I.V. fluids.
◆ Change dressings regularly, and check for excessive drainage and bleeding and signs of infection.
◆ Provide antiembolism stockings as ordered.
◆ Encourage regular deep breathing and coughing.
◆ If necessary, institute incentive spirometry.
◆ Turn the patient often, and help them reposition, using pillows for support.
◆ Auscultate for bowel sounds. When the patient's bowel function returns, ask the dietitian to provide a clear liquid diet; then, when tolerated, a regular diet.
◆ Encourage the patient to walk within 24 hours after surgery. Reassure them that they won't harm themselves or cause wound dehiscence by sitting up or walking.
◆ Provide psychological support. Encourage the patient to express anxieties and fears. If they seem worried about the effect of surgery on their sexual activity, reassure them that this surgery will not inhibit sexual intimacy.
◆ Before radiation therapy begins, explain that the area to be irradiated will be marked with ink to precisely locate the treatment field. Explain that radiation may cause a skin reaction, bladder irritation, myelosuppression, and other systemic reactions.
◆ During and after treatment, watch for and treat adverse effects of radiation and chemotherapy.
◆ Before discharge, to minimize adverse effects during outpatient radiation and chemotherapy, advise the patient to maintain a high-carbohydrate, high-protein, low-fat, low-bulk diet to maintain caloric intake but reduce bulk. Suggest that they eat several small meals per day instead of three large ones.
◆ Include the patient's husband or other close relatives in patient care and teaching as much as possible.

PREVENTION *Stress the importance of regular pelvic examinations to patients, and tell them to contact a practitioner promptly about any gynecologic symptom.*

Bone, skin, and soft tissue

PRIMARY MALIGNANT BONE TUMORS

Primary malignant bone tumors (also called *sarcomas of the bone* and *bone cancer*) are rare, constituting less than 1% of all malignant tumors. Most bone tumors are secondary, caused by seeding from a primary site. Primary malignant bone tumors are more common in males, especially in children and adolescents, although some types do occur in people between ages 35 and 60. They may originate in osseous or nonosseous tissue. Osseous bone tumors arise from the bony structure itself and include osteogenic sarcoma (the most common), parosteal osteogenic sarcoma, chondrosarcoma, and malignant giant cell tumor. Together they make up 60% of all malignant bone tumors. Nonosseous tumors arise from hematopoietic, vascular, and neural tissues and include Ewing sarcoma, fibrosarcoma, and chordoma. Osteogenic and Ewing sarcomas are the most common bone tumors in childhood.

Causes and incidence

Causes of primary malignant bone tumors are unknown. Some researchers suggest that primary malignant bone tumors arise in areas of rapid growth because children and young adults with such tumors seem to be much taller than average. Additional theories point to heredity, trauma, and excessive radiotherapy. Genetic mutations in *TP53* result in sarcomas, including osteosarcoma. Gene rearrangements for *EWSR1* and *ETS1* genes have been found in the Ewing sarcoma family of tumors.

For incidence information, see *Comparing primary malignant bone tumors*, pages 772 and 773.

Comparing primary malignant bone tumors

Type	Clinical features	Treatment
Osseous origin		
Chondrosarcoma	◆ Develops from cartilage ◆ Painless; grows slowly, but is locally recurrent and invasive ◆ Occurs most commonly in pelvis, proximal femur, ribs, and shoulder girdle ◆ Usually in males ages 30 to 50	◆ Chemotherapy ◆ Hemipelvectomy, surgical resection (ribs) ◆ Radiation (palliative)
Malignant giant cell tumor	◆ Arises from benign giant cell tumor ◆ Found most commonly in long bones, especially in knee area ◆ Usually in females ages 18 to 50	◆ Curettage ◆ Radiation (recurrent disease) ◆ Total excision
Osteogenic sarcoma	◆ Osteoid tumor present in specimen ◆ Tumor arises from bone-forming osteoblast and bone-digesting osteoclast ◆ Occurs most commonly in femur, but also tibia and humerus; occasionally, in fibula, ileum, vertebra, or mandible ◆ Usually in males ages 10 to 30	◆ Chemotherapy ◆ Surgery (tumor resection, high thigh amputation, hemipelvectomy)
Parosteal osteogenic sarcoma	◆ Develops on surface of bone instead of interior ◆ Progresses slowly ◆ Occurs most commonly in distal femur, but also in tibia, humerus, and ulna ◆ Usually in females ages 30 to 40	◆ Chemotherapy ◆ Surgery (tumor resection, possible amputation, hemipelvectomy) ◆ Combination of above
Nonosseous origin		
Chordoma	◆ Derived from embryonic remnants of notochord ◆ Progresses slowly ◆ Usually found at end of spinal column and in spheno-occipital, sacrococcygeal, and vertebral areas ◆ Characterized by constipation and vision disturbances ◆ Usually in males ages 50 to 60	◆ Radiation (palliative, or when surgery not applicable, as in occipital area) ◆ Surgical resection (commonly resulting in neural defects)

Comparing primary malignant bone tumors (continued)

Type	Clinical features	Treatment
Ewing sarcoma	◆ Originates in bone marrow and invades shafts of long and flat bones ◆ Usually affects lower extremities, most commonly femur, innominate bones, ribs, tibia, humerus, vertebra, and fibula; may metastasize to lungs ◆ Pain increasingly severe and persistent ◆ Usually in males ages 10 to 20	◆ Amputation (only if there's no evidence of metastasis) ◆ Chemotherapy (to slow growth) ◆ High-voltage radiation (if tumor is radiosensitive)
Fibrosarcoma	◆ Relatively rare ◆ Originates in fibrous tissue of bone ◆ Invades long or flat bones (femur, tibia, mandible) but also involves periosteum and overlying muscle ◆ Usually in males ages 30 to 40	◆ Amputation ◆ Bone grafts (with low-grade fibrosarcoma) ◆ Chemotherapy ◆ Radiation

Complications
◆ Hypercalcemia
◆ Metastasis
◆ Pain

Signs and symptoms
Bone pain is the most common indication of primary malignant bone tumors. It's generally more intense at night and isn't usually associated with mobility. The pain is dull and usually localized, although it may be referred from the hip or spine and result in weakness or a limp. Another common sign is a mass or tumor. The tumor site may be tender and may swell; the tumor itself is often palpable. Pathologic fractures are common. In late stages, the patient may be cachectic, with fever and impaired mobility.

Diagnosis
Ⓡ **CONFIRMING DIAGNOSIS** *A biopsy (by incision or by aspiration) is essential to confirm primary malignant bone tumors. Bone X-rays and radioisotope bone and CT scans show tumor size. Serum alkaline phosphatase level is usually elevated in patients with sarcoma.*

Treatment
Excision of the tumor with a 3" (7.6 cm) margin is the treatment of choice. It may be combined with preoperative chemotherapy.

In some patients, radical surgery (such as hemipelvectomy or amputation) is necessary; however, surgical resection of the tumor (commonly with preoperative *and* postoperative chemotherapy) has saved limbs from amputation.

Intensive chemotherapy includes administration of doxorubicin, vincristine, cyclophosphamide, cisplatin, dacarbazine, and etoposide in various combinations. Chemotherapy may be infused intra-arterially into the long bones of the legs.

Special considerations
◆ Be sensitive to the emotional strain caused by the threat of amputation. Encourage communication and help the patient set realistic goals. If the surgery will affect the patient's lower extremities, have a physical therapist teach the patient how to use assistive devices (such as a walker) preoperatively.
◆ Teach the patient how to readjust their body weight so that they can get in and out of the bed and wheelchair.
◆ Before surgery, start I.V. infusions to maintain fluid and electrolyte balance and to have an open vein available if blood or plasma is needed during surgery.
◆ After surgery, check vital signs every hour for the first 4 hours, every 2 hours for the next 4 hours, and then every 4 hours if the patient is stable. Check the dressing periodically for oozing. Elevate the foot of the bed or place the stump on a pillow for the first 24 hours. (Be careful not to leave the stump elevated for >48 hours because this may lead to contractures.)
◆ To ease the patient's anxiety, administer analgesics for pain before morning care. If necessary, brace the patient with pillows, keeping the affected part at rest.

◆ Urge the patient to eat foods high in protein, vitamins, and folic acid and to get plenty of rest and sleep to promote recovery. Encourage some exercise. Administer laxatives, if necessary, to maintain proper elimination.

◆ Encourage fluids to prevent dehydration. Record intake and output accurately. After a hemipelvectomy, insert an NG tube to prevent abdominal distention. Continue low gastric suction for 2 days after surgery or until the patient can tolerate a liquid diet. Administer antibiotics to prevent infection. Give transfusions, if necessary, and administer medication to control pain. Keep drains in place to facilitate wound drainage and prevent infection. Use an indwelling urinary catheter until the patient can void voluntarily.

◆ Keep in mind that rehabilitation programs after limb salvage surgery will vary, depending on the patient, the body part affected, and the type of surgery performed. For example, one patient may have a surgically implanted prosthesis (e.g., after joint surgery), whereas another may have reconstructive surgery requiring an allograft (such as bone from a bone bank) or an autograft (bone from the patient's own body).

Encourage early rehabilitation for patients with amputated limbs as follows:

◆ Start physical therapy 24 hours postoperatively. Pain is usually not severe after amputation. If it is, watch for a wound complication, such as hematoma, excessive stump edema, or infection.

◆ Be aware of the "phantom limb" syndrome, in which the patient "feels" an itch or tingling in an amputated extremity. This can last for several hours or persist for years. Explain that this sensation is normal and usually subsides.

◆ To avoid contractures and ensure the best conditions for wound healing, warn the patient not to hang the stump over the edge of the bed; sit in a wheelchair with the stump flexed; place a pillow under the hip, knee, or back or between the thighs; lie with knees flexed; or rest an above-the-knee stump on the crutch handle or abduct it.

◆ Wash the stump, massage it gently, and keep it dry until it heals. Make sure the bandage is firm and is worn day and night. Know how to reapply the bandage to shape the stump for a prosthesis.

◆ To help the patient select a prosthesis, consider their needs and the types of prostheses available. The rehabilitation staff will help the patient make the final decision, but because most patients are uninformed about choosing a prosthesis, give some guidelines. Keep in mind the patient's age and possible vision problems.

PEDIATRIC TIP *Generally, children need relatively simple devices. Children also outgrow prostheses, so advise parents to plan accordingly.*

ELDER TIP *Elderly patients may need prostheses that provide more stability. Consider finances, too.*

◆ The same points are applicable for a patient with an arm amputation, but losing an arm causes a greater cosmetic problem. Consult an occupational therapist, who can teach the patient how to perform daily activities with one arm.

◆ Try to instill a positive attitude toward recovery. Urge the patient to resume an independent lifestyle. Refer elderly patients to community health services if necessary. Suggest tutoring for children to help them keep up with schoolwork.

MULTIPLE MYELOMA

Multiple myeloma, also known as *malignant plasmacytoma, plasma cell myeloma*, and *myelomatosis*, is a disseminated malignant neoplasm of marrow plasma cells that infiltrates bone to produce osteolytic lesions throughout the skeleton (flat bones, vertebrae, skull, pelvis, ribs). In late stages, it infiltrates the body organs (liver, spleen, lymph nodes, lungs, adrenal glands, kidneys, skin, and GI tract). Prognosis is usually poor because diagnosis is commonly made after the disease has already infiltrated the vertebrae, pelvis, skull, ribs, clavicles, and sternum. By then, skeletal destruction is widespread and, without treatment, leads to vertebral collapse; 52% of patients die within 3 months of diagnosis, 90% within 2 years. Early diagnosis and treatment prolong the lives of many patients, with the 5-year survival rate being 33%. Death usually follows complications, such as infection, renal failure, hematologic imbalance, fractures, hypercalcemia, hyperuricemia, or dehydration.

Causes and incidence

Multiple myeloma mainly affects older adults, but its causes are unknown. Possible risk factors include exposure to radiation, working with petroleum-related products, being overweight, and family history. It's rare, with estimates of 19,900 new cases in 2007. Men are twice as likely as women and blacks are twice as likely as whites to develop multiple myeloma.

Pathophysiology

Multiple myeloma, also known as plasma cell myeloma, is a cancer of plasma cells, a type of WBC normally responsible for producing antibodies. Often, no symptoms are noticed initially. When advanced, bone pain, bleeding, frequent infections, and anemia may occur. The cause is unknown. Risk factors include drinking alcohol, obesity, radiation exposure, family history, and certain chemicals. The underlying mechanism involves abnormal plasma cells producing abnormal antibodies which can cause kidney problems.

Complications
◆ Pneumonia
◆ Pyelonephritis
◆ Renal calculi
◆ Renal failure
◆ Fractures
◆ Hypercalcemia
◆ Hyperuricemia
◆ Dehydration
◆ GI bleeding

Signs and symptoms
The earliest indication of multiple myeloma is severe, constant back and rib pain that increases with exercise and may be worse at night. Arthritic symptoms may also occur: achiness, joint swelling, and tenderness, possibly from vertebral compression. Other effects include fatigue, fever, malaise, slight evidence of peripheral neuropathy (such as peripheral paresthesia), and pathologic fractures. As multiple myeloma progresses, symptoms of vertebral compression may become acute, accompanied by anemia, weight loss, thoracic deformities (ballooning), and loss of body height (5″ [12.7 cm] or more) due to vertebral collapse. Renal complications such as pyelonephritis (caused by tubular damage from large amounts of Bence Jones protein, hypercalcemia, and hyperuricemia) may occur. Severe, recurrent infection such as pneumonia may follow damage to nerves associated with respiratory function.

Diagnosis
℞ CONFIRMING DIAGNOSIS *After a physical examination and a careful medical history, the following diagnostic tests and nonspecific laboratory abnormalities confirm the presence of multiple myeloma:*
◆ *Bone marrow aspiration and biopsy detects myelomatosis cells (abnormal number of immature plasma cells).*
◆ *Urine studies may show Bence Jones protein and hypercalciuria. Absence of Bence Jones protein doesn't rule out multiple myeloma; however, its presence almost invariably confirms the disease. (See Bence Jones protein.)*
◆ Complete blood count shows moderate or severe anemia. The differential may show 40%

to 50% lymphocytes but seldom more than 3% plasma cells. Rouleaux formation (usually the first clue) seen on differential smear results from elevation of the erythrocyte sedimentation rate.
◆ Serum electrophoresis shows elevated globulin spike that's electrophoretically and immunologically abnormal.
◆ X-rays during early stages may show only diffuse osteoporosis. Eventually, they show multiple, sharply circumscribed osteolytic (punched-out) lesions, particularly on the skull, pelvis, and spine—the characteristic lesions of multiple myeloma.
◆ Excretory urography can assess renal involvement. To avoid precipitation of Bence Jones protein, iothalamate or diatrizoate is used instead of the usual contrast medium and, although oral fluid restriction is usually the standard procedure before excretory urography, patients with multiple myeloma receive large quantities of fluid, generally orally but sometimes I.V., before excretory urography is done.

Treatment
Long-term treatment of multiple myeloma consists mainly of chemotherapy to suppress plasma cell growth and control pain. Commonly used combinations include cyclophosphamide, doxorubicin, and prednisone as well as carmustine, doxorubicin, and prednisone. Bortezomib, a proteasome inhibitor, has shown benefit in combination with dexamethasone and other chemotherapy agents. Adjuvant local radiation reduces acute lesions, such as collapsed vertebrae, and relieves localized pain. Other treatments usually include a melphalan-prednisone combination in high intermittent doses or low continuous daily doses

Bence Jones protein
The hallmark of multiple myeloma, the Bence Jones protein (a light chain of gamma globulin) was named for Henry Bence Jones, an English physician who in 1848 noticed that patients with a curious bone disease excreted a unique protein—unique in that it coagulated at 113° to 131° F (45° to 55° C) and then redissolved when heated to boiling.

It remained for Otto Kahler, an Austrian, to demonstrate in 1889 that Bence Jones protein was related to myeloma. Bence Jones protein isn't found in the urine of *all* multiple myeloma patients, but it's almost never found in the urine of patients without this disease.

and analgesics for pain. Oral thalidomide or lenalidomide, a thalidomide analog with immunomodulating properties (with or without steroids), has shown promise in relapsed multiple myeloma. For spinal cord compression, the patient may require a laminectomy; for renal complications, dialysis. For younger patients, bone marrow transplants may improve survival time.

Clinical trials are currently under way to evaluate the role of biological response modifiers (interferon) in the management of multiple myeloma. In addition, high-dose chemotherapy and radiotherapy with peripheral stem cell rescue have been helpful in select cases.

Because the patient may have bone demineralization and may lose large amounts of calcium into blood and urine, he's a prime candidate for renal calculi, nephrocalcinosis, and, eventually, renal failure due to hypercalcemia. Hypercalcemia is managed with hydration, diuretics, corticosteroids, oral phosphate, mithramycin I.V., or bisphosphonates I.V. (such as pamidronate or zoledronic acid) to decrease serum calcium levels.

Special considerations
◆ Push fluids; encourage the patient to drink about 100 to 135 oz (3,000 to 4,000 mL) of fluids daily, particularly before an excretory urography. Monitor fluid intake and output (daily output shouldn't be <1,500 mL).
◆ Encourage the patient to walk (immobilization increases bone demineralization and vulnerability to pneumonia), and give analgesics, as ordered, to lessen pain. Never allow the patient to walk unaccompanied; make sure that they use a walker or other supportive aid to prevent falls. Because the patient is particularly vulnerable to pathologic fractures, they may be fearful. Give reassurance, and allow the patient them to move at their own pace.
◆ Prevent complications by watching for fever or malaise, which may signal the onset of infection, and for signs of other problems, such as severe anemia and fractures. If the patient is bedridden, change position every 2 hours. Give passive ROM and deep-breathing exercises. When they can tolerate them, promote active exercises.
◆ If the patient is taking melphalan (a phenylalanine derivative of nitrogen mustard that depresses bone marrow), make sure the blood count (platelet and WBC) is taken before each treatment. If they're taking prednisone, watch closely for infection because this drug commonly masks it.

◆ Whenever possible, get the patient out of bed within 24 hours after laminectomy. Check for hemorrhage, motor or sensory deficits, and loss of bowel or bladder function. Position the patient as ordered, maintain alignment, and logroll when turning.
◆ Provide much-needed emotional support for the patient and family, as they're likely to be anxious. Help relieve their anxiety by truthfully informing them about diagnostic tests (including painful procedures, such as bone marrow aspiration and biopsy), treatment, and prognosis. If needed, refer them to an appropriate community resource for additional support.

BASAL CELL EPITHELIOMA
Basal cell epithelioma, also known as basal cell carcinoma, is a slow-growing, destructive skin tumor. (See *Basal cell carcinoma.*) It's the most common form of cancer in the United States, accounting for 75% of all skin cancers. If caught and treated early, it has a cure rate of 95%. Regular follow-up is required because new sites of basal cell epithelioma can occur. (See *Preventing basal cell carcinoma*, page 777.)

Causes and incidence
Prolonged sun exposure is the most common cause of basal cell epithelioma, but arsenic ingestion, radiation exposure, burns, and immunosuppression are other possible causes.

Basal cell carcinoma

The illustration below shows the central crater and papule characteristic of basal cell carcinoma.

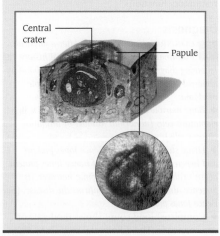

Central crater

Papule

Although the pathogenesis of basal cell epithelioma is uncertain, some experts now hypothesize that it originates when, under certain conditions, undifferentiated basal cells become carcinomatous instead of differentiating into sweat glands, sebum, and hair.

This cancer usually occurs in people older than age 40; it's more prevalent in blond, fair-skinned males and is the most common malignant tumor affecting whites.

Pathophysiology
Although the exact etiology of BCC is unknown, a well-established relationship exists between BCC and the pilosebaceous unit, as tumors are most often discovered on hair-bearing areas.

Many believe that BCCs arise from pluripotential cells in the basal layer of the epidermis or follicular structures. These cells form continuously during life and can form hair, sebaceous glands, and apocrine glands. Tumors usually arise from the epidermis and occasionally arise from the outer root sheath of a hair follicle, specifically from hair follicle stem cells residing just below the sebaceous gland duct in an area called the bulge.

Complication
♦ Disfiguring lesions of the eyes, nose, and cheeks

Signs and symptoms
Three types of basal cell epithelioma occur:
♦ Noduloulcerative lesions usually occur on the face, particularly the forehead, eyelid margins, and nasolabial folds. In early stages,

these lesions are small, smooth, pinkish, and translucent papules. Telangiectatic vessels cross the surface, and the lesions are occasionally pigmented. As the lesions enlarge, their centers become depressed and their borders become firm and elevated. Ulceration and local invasion eventually occur. These ulcerated tumors, known as *rodent ulcers*, rarely metastasize; however, if untreated, they can spread to vital areas and become infected or cause massive hemorrhage if they invade large blood vessels.

◆ Superficial basal cell epitheliomas are multiple in many cases and commonly occur on the chest and back. They're oval or irregularly shaped, lightly pigmented plaques, with sharply defined, slightly elevated threadlike borders. Due to superficial erosion, these lesions appear scaly and have small, atrophic areas in the center that resemble psoriasis or eczema. They're usually chronic and don't tend to invade other areas. Superficial basal cell epitheliomas are related to ingestion of or exposure to arsenic-containing compounds.

◆ Sclerosing basal cell epitheliomas (morphea-like epitheliomas) are waxy, sclerotic, yellow to white plaques without distinct borders. Occurring on the head and neck, sclerosing basal cell epitheliomas commonly look like small patches of scleroderma.

Diagnosis
All types of basal cell epitheliomas are diagnosed by clinical appearance, incisional or excisional biopsy, and histologic study.

Treatment
Depending on the size, location, and depth of the lesion, treatment may include curettage and electrodesiccation, chemotherapy, surgical excision, irradiation, or chemosurgery.

◆ Curettage and electrodesiccation offer good cosmetic results for small lesions.

◆ Topical 5-fluorouracil is commonly used for superficial lesions. This medication produces marked local irritation or inflammation in the involved tissue but no systemic effects.

◆ Microscopically controlled surgical excision carefully removes recurrent lesions until a tumor-free plane is achieved. After removal of large lesions, skin grafting may be required.

◆ Irradiation is used for tumor locations that require it and for elderly or debilitated patients who might not withstand surgery.

◆ Cryosurgery with liquid nitrogen freezes and kills the cells.

◆ Chemosurgery generally is necessary for persistent or recurrent lesions. Chemosurgery consists of periodic applications of a fixative paste

(such as zinc chloride) and subsequent removal of fixed pathologic tissue. Treatment continues until tumor removal is complete.

◆ Photodynamic therapy involves applying a photosensitizing agent on the lesion followed by irradiation with a light source.

Special considerations
◆ Instruct the patient to eat frequent small meals that are high in protein. Suggest "blenderized" foods or liquid protein supplements if the lesion has invaded the oral cavity and caused eating problems.

◆ Advise the patient to relieve local inflammation from topical fluorouracil with cool compresses or corticosteroid ointment.

◆ Instruct the patient with noduloulcerative basal cell epithelioma to wash the face gently when ulcerations and crusting occur; scrubbing too vigorously may cause bleeding.

SQUAMOUS CELL CARCINOMA
SCC of the skin is an invasive tumor with metastatic potential that arises from the keratinizing epidermal cells. Any change in an existing skin lesion, such as a wart or mole, or the development of a new lesion that ulcerates and doesn't heal may indicate skin cancer. If caught and treated early, there's a high cure rate. However, if SCC is allowed to spread, it can result in disability or death.

Causes and incidence
Predisposing factors associated with SCC include overexposure to the sun's ultraviolet rays, the presence of premalignant lesions (such as actinic keratosis or Bowen disease), X-ray therapy, ingestion of herbicides containing arsenic, chronic skin irritation and inflammation, exposure to local carcinogens (such as tar and oil), and hereditary diseases (such as xeroderma pigmentosum and albinism). (See *Premalignant skin lesions*, page 779.) Rarely, SCC may develop on the site of smallpox vaccination, psoriasis, or *chronic discoid lupus erythematosus*.

SCC usually occurs in fair-skinned white males older than age 60. Outdoor employment and residence in a sunny, warm climate (southwestern United States and Australia, for example) greatly increase the risk of developing SCC.

Pathophysiology
Cutaneous SCC is an invasive malignant neoplasm of epidermal keratinocytes showing squamous phenotypic differentiation (see the following image). Bowen disease is an SCC in situ with full-epidermal thickness dysplasia that has the potential for significant lateral spread before invasion.

Premalignant skin lesions

Disease	Cause	Patient	Lesion	Treatment
Actinic keratosis	Solar radiation	White men with fair skin (middle-aged to elderly)	Reddish-brown lesions 1 mm to 1 cm in size (may enlarge if untreated) on face, ears, lower lip, bald scalp, dorsa of hands and forearms	Topical 5-fluorouracil, cryosurgery using liquid nitrogen, or curettage by electrodesiccation
Bowen disease	Unknown	White men with fair skin (middle-aged to elderly)	Brown to reddish-brown lesions, with scaly surface on exposed and unexposed areas	Surgical excision, topical 5-fluorouracil
Erythroplasia of Queyrat	Bowen disease of the mucous membranes	Men (middle-aged to elderly)	Red lesions with a glistening or granular appearance on mucous membranes, particularly the glans penis in uncircumcised males	Surgical excision
Leukoplakia	Smoking, alcohol use, chronic cheek-biting, ill-fitting dentures, misaligned teeth	Men (middle-aged to elderly)	Lesions on oral, anal, and genital mucous membranes, vary in appearance from smooth and white to rough and gray	Elimination of irritating factors, surgical excision, or curettage by electrodesiccation (if lesion is still premalignant)

Complications
◆ Lymph node involvement
◆ Respiratory problems

Signs and symptoms
SCC commonly develops on the skin of the face, the ears, the dorsa of the hands and forearms, and other sun-damaged areas. Lesions on sun-damaged skin tend to be less invasive and less likely to metastasize than lesions on unexposed skin. Notable exceptions to this tendency are squamous cell lesions on the lower lip and the ears. These are almost invariably markedly invasive metastatic lesions with a generally poor prognosis.

Transformation from a premalignant lesion to SCC may begin with induration and inflammation of the preexisting lesion. When SCC arises from normal skin, the nodule grows slowly on a firm, indurated base. If untreated, this nodule eventually ulcerates and invades underlying tissues. Metastasis can occur to the regional lymph nodes, producing characteristic systemic symptoms of pain, malaise, fatigue, weakness, and anorexia.

Diagnosis
An excisional biopsy provides definitive diagnosis of SCC. Other appropriate laboratory tests depend on systemic symptoms.

Treatment
The size, shape, location, and invasiveness of a squamous cell tumor and the condition of the underlying tissue determine the treatment method used; a deeply invasive tumor may require a combination of techniques. All the major treatment methods have excellent cure rates; generally, the prognosis is better with a well-differentiated lesion than with a poorly differentiated one in an unusual location. Depending on the lesion, treatment may consist of:
◆ wide surgical excision
◆ electrodesiccation and curettage (offer good cosmetic results for small lesions)
◆ radiation therapy (generally for older or debilitated patients; especially if the lesion has substantial perineural involvement
◆ chemosurgery (reserved for resistant or recurrent lesions)

Special considerations
The care plan for patients with SCC should emphasize meticulous wound care, emotional support, and thorough patient instruction.
◆ Coordinate a consistent care plan for changing the patient's dressings. Establishing a standard routine helps the patient and family learn how to care for the wound.

♦ Keep the wound dry and clean.

♦ Try to control odor with balsam of Peru, yogurt flakes, oil of cloves, or other odor-masking substances, even though they're typically ineffective for long-term use. Topical or systemic antibiotics also temporarily control odor and eventually alter the lesion's bacterial flora.

♦ Be prepared for other problems that accompany a metastatic disease (pain, fatigue, weakness, anorexia).

♦ Help the patient and family set realistic goals and expectations.

♦ Disfiguring lesions are distressing to the patient and you. Try to accept the patient as they are and to increase their self-esteem and strengthen a caring relationship.

!!!!!! **PREVENTION** *Advise patients to do the following:*

♦ *Avoid excessive sun exposure.*

♦ *Wear protective clothing (hats, long sleeves).*

♦ *Periodically examine the skin for precancerous lesions; have any removed promptly.*

♦ *Use strong sunscreening agents containing para-aminobenzoic acid, benzophenone, and zinc oxide. These should be applied 30 to 60 minutes before sun exposure.*

♦ *Use lip sunscreen to protect the lips from sun damage.*

MALIGNANT MELANOMA

A malignant neoplasm that arises from melanocytes, malignant melanoma is relatively rare and accounts for only 1% to 2% of all malignancies. (See *Malignant melanoma*.) However, the incidence has greatly increased, with a noted 300% increase in the past 40 years. The four types of melanomas are superficial spreading melanoma, nodular malignant melanoma, lentigo maligna, and acral lentiginous melanoma.

Melanoma spreads through the lymphatic and vascular systems and metastasizes to the regional lymph nodes, skin, liver, lungs, and CNS. Its course is unpredictable, however, and recurrence and metastasis may not appear for more than 5 years after resection of the primary lesion. The prognosis varies with tumor thickness. Generally, superficial lesions are curable, whereas deeper lesions tend to metastasize. The Breslow method measures tumor depth from the granular level of the epidermis to the deepest melanoma cell. Melanoma lesions less than 1.0 mm deep have an excellent prognosis with 5-year survival rates greater than 90%, whereas deeper lesions (>1.0 mm) are at risk for metastasis. The prognosis is better for a tumor on an extremity (which is drained by one lymphatic network) than for

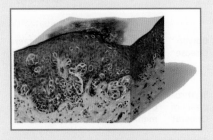

Malignant melanoma

Malignant melanoma can arise on normal skin or from an existing mole. If not treated promptly, it can spread to other areas of skin, lymph nodes, or internal organs.

one on the head, neck, or trunk (drained by several networks).

Causes and incidence

Several factors seem to influence the development of melanoma:

♦ Excessive exposure to sunlight—Melanoma is most common in sunny, warm areas and usually develops on parts of the body that are exposed to the sun.

♦ Skin type—Most persons who develop melanoma have blond or red hair, fair skin, and blue eyes; are prone to sunburn; and are of Celtic or Scandinavian ancestry. Melanoma is rare among Blacks; when it does develop, it usually arises in lightly pigmented areas (the palms, plantar surface of the feet, or mucous membranes).

♦ Hormonal factors—Pregnancy may increase risk and exacerbate growth.

♦ Family history—Melanoma is slightly more common within families.

♦ Past history of melanoma—A person who has had one melanoma is at greater risk of developing a second.

Melanoma is slightly more common in women than in men and is rare in children. Peak incidence occurs between ages 50 and 70, although the incidence in younger age groups is increasing. In the United States, 1 in 85 people will develop melanoma some time in their life.

Pathophysiology

The clinical lesion is usually an irregularly shaped, asymmetrical lesion with varying colors with a history of recent change in size, shape, color, or sensation. Melanoma may arise within an existing benign or dysplastic nevus.

Signs and symptoms

Common sites for melanoma are on the head and neck in men, on the legs in women, and on the backs of persons exposed to excessive sunlight. Up to 70% arise from a preexisting nevus. It rarely appears in the conjunctiva, choroid, pharynx, mouth, vagina, or anus.

Suspect melanoma when any skin lesion or nevus enlarges, changes color, becomes inflamed or sore, itches, ulcerates, bleeds, undergoes textural changes, or shows signs of surrounding pigment regression (halo nevus or vitiligo). (See *ABCDEs of malignant melanoma* and *Recognizing potentially malignant nevi.*)

ABCDEs of malignant melanoma

Use the ABCDE rule to assess a mole's malignant potential.
♦ Asymmetry: Is the mole irregular in shape?
♦ Border: Is the border irregular, notched, or poorly defined?
♦ Color: Does the color vary, for example, between shades of brown, red, white, blue, or black?
♦ Diameter: Is the diameter more than 6 mm?
♦ Elevation: Is the lesion elevated or enlarged?

Recognizing potentially malignant nevi

Nevi (moles) are skin lesions that are usually pigmented and may be hereditary. They begin to grow in childhood (occasionally they're congenital) and become more numerous in young adults. Up to 70% of patients with melanoma have a history of a preexisting nevus at the tumor site. Of these, about one third are reported to be congenital; the remainder develop later in life.

Changes in nevi (color, size, shape, texture, ulceration, bleeding, or itching) suggest possible malignant transformation. The presence or absence of hair within a nevus has no significance.

Types of nevi

♦ *Junctional nevi* are flat or slightly raised and light to dark brown, with melanocytes confined to the epidermis. Usually, they appear before age 40. These nevi may change into compound nevi if junctional nevus cells proliferate and penetrate into the dermis.
♦ *Compound nevi* are usually tan to dark brown and slightly raised, although size and color vary. They contain melanocytes in both the dermis and epidermis, and they rarely undergo malignant transformation. Excision is necessary only to rule out malignant transformation or for cosmetic reasons.
♦ *Dermal nevi* are elevated lesions from 2 to 10 mm in diameter and vary in color from flesh to brown. They usually develop in older adults and generally arise on the upper part of the body. Excision is necessary only to rule out malignant transformation.
♦ *Blue nevi* are flat or slightly elevated lesions from 0.5 to 1 cm in diameter. They appear on the head, neck, arms, and dorsa of the hands and are twice as common in

women as in men. Their blue color results from pigment and collagen in the dermis, which reflect blue light but absorb other wavelengths. Excision is necessary to rule out pigmented basal cell epithelioma or melanoma or for cosmetic reasons.
♦ *Dysplastic nevi* are generally greater than 5 mm in diameter, with irregularly notched or indistinct borders. Coloration is usually a variable mixture of tan and brown, sometimes with red, pink, and black pigmentation. No two lesions are exactly alike. They occur in great numbers (typically over 100 at a time), never singly, usually appearing on the back, scalp, chest, and buttocks. Dysplastic nevi are potentially malignant, especially in patients with a personal or familial history of melanoma. Skin biopsy confirms diagnosis; treatment is by surgical excision, followed by regular physical examinations (every 6 months) to detect any new lesions or changes in existing lesions.
♦ *Lentigo maligna* (melanotic freckles, Hutchinson freckles) are a precursor to malignant melanoma. (In fact, about one third of them eventually give rise to malignant melanoma.) Usually, they occur in people older than age 40, especially on exposed skin areas such as the face. At first, these lesions are flat, tan spots, but they gradually enlarge and darken and develop black speckled areas against their tan or brown background. Each lesion may simultaneously enlarge in one area and regress in another. Histologic examination shows typical and atypical melanocytes along the epidermal basement membrane. Removal by simple excision (not electrodesiccation and curettage) is recommended.

Each type of melanoma has special characteristics:

◆ Superficial spreading melanoma, the most common, usually develops between ages 40 and 50. Such a lesion arises on an area of chronic irritation. In women, it's most common between the knees and ankles; in Blacks and Asians, on the toe webs and soles (lightly pigmented areas subject to trauma). Characteristically, this melanoma has a red, white, and blue color over a brown or black background and an irregular, notched margin. Its surface is irregular, with small, elevated tumor nodules that may ulcerate and bleed. Horizontal growth may continue for many years; when vertical growth begins, prognosis worsens.

◆ Nodular melanoma usually develops between ages 40 and 50, grows vertically, invades the dermis, and metastasizes early. Such a lesion is usually a polypoidal nodule, with uniformly dark discoloration (it may be grayish), and looks like a blackberry. Occasionally, this melanoma is flesh-colored, with flecks of pigment around its base (possibly inflamed).

◆ Lentigo maligna melanoma is relatively rare. It arises from a lentigo maligna on an exposed skin surface and usually occurs between ages 60 and 70. This lesion looks like a large (3- to 6-cm) flat freckle of tan, brown, black, whitish, or slate color and has irregularly scattered black nodules on the surface. It develops slowly, usually over many years, and eventually may ulcerate. This melanoma commonly develops under the fingernails, on the face, and on the back of the hands.

Diagnosis

℞ CONFIRMING DIAGNOSIS *A skin biopsy with histologic examination can distinguish malignant melanoma from a benign nevus, seborrheic keratosis, and pigmented basal cell epithelioma; it can also determine tumor thickness. Physical examination, paying particular attention to lymph nodes, can point to metastatic involvement.*

Baseline laboratory studies include complete blood count with differential, erythrocyte sedimentation rate, platelet count, liver function studies, and urinalysis. Depending on the depth of tumor invasion and metastatic spread, baseline diagnostic studies may also include chest X-ray and a CT scan of the chest and abdomen. Signs of bone metastasis may call for a bone scan; CNS metastasis necessitates a CT scan of the brain.

Treatment

A patient with malignant melanoma requires surgical resection to remove the tumor. The extent of resection depends on the size and location of the primary lesion. Closure of a wide resection may require a skin graft. Surgical treatment may also include regional lymphadenectomy.

Deep primary lesions may merit adjuvant chemotherapy and biotherapy to eliminate or reduce the number of tumor cells. Dacarbazine, temozolomide, interferon-alfa, interleukin-2, cisplatin, vinblastine, and carmustine are used to treat melanoma. Clinical trials are currently under way to evaluate the effectiveness of isolated limb perfusion as chemotherapy for the management of malignant melanomas of extremities. Radiation therapy is usually reserved for metastatic disease. It doesn't prolong survival but may reduce tumor size and relieve pain.

Regardless of the treatment method, melanomas require close long-term follow-up to detect metastasis and recurrences. Statistics show that 13% of recurrences develop more than 5 years after primary surgery.

Special considerations

Management of the melanoma patient requires careful physical, psychological, and social assessment. Preoperative teaching, meticulous postoperative care, and psychological support can make the patient more comfortable, speed recovery, and prevent complications.

After diagnosis, review the practitioner's explanation of treatment options. Tell the patient what to expect before and after surgery, what the wound will look like, and what type of dressing he'll have. Warn the patient that the donor site for a skin graft may be as painful as the tumor excision site, if not more so. Honestly answer any questions the patient may have about surgery, chemotherapy, and radiation.

◆ After surgery, be careful to prevent infection. Check dressings often for excessive drainage, foul odor, redness, or swelling. If surgery included lymphadenectomy, minimize lymphedema by applying a compression stocking and instructing the patient to keep the extremity elevated.

◆ During chemotherapy, know what adverse effects to expect and take measures to minimize them. For instance, give an antiemetic, as ordered, to reduce nausea and vomiting.

To prepare the patient for discharge:

◆ Emphasize the need for close follow-up to detect recurrences early. Explain that recurrences and metastasis, if they occur, are commonly delayed, so follow-up must continue for years. Tell the patient how to recognize signs of recurrence.

◆ Provide psychological support. Encourage the patient to verbalize fears.

In advanced metastatic disease:
◆ Control and prevent pain with consistent, regularly scheduled administration of analgesics. *Don't* wait until after it occurs to relieve pain.
◆ Make referrals for home care, social services, and spiritual and financial assistance, as needed.
◆ If the patient is dying, identify the needs of the patient, family, and friends, and provide appropriate support and care.

▓▓▓▓ **PREVENTION** *Advise the patient of the* ☂ *following:*
◆ *Explain the detrimental effects of overexposure to the sun, especially to fair-skinned, blue-eyed patients.*
◆ *Recommend that the patient use a sunblock or sunscreen.*
◆ *In all physical examinations, especially in fair-skinned persons, look for unusual nevi or other skin lesions.*

KAPOSI SARCOMA

Initially, this cancer of the lymphatic cell wall was described as a rare blood vessel sarcoma, occurring mostly in elderly Italian and Jewish men. In recent years, the incidence of Kaposi sarcoma has risen dramatically along with the incidence of AIDS. Currently, it's the most common AIDS-related cancer.

Kaposi sarcoma causes structural and functional damage. When associated with AIDS, it progresses aggressively, involving the lymph nodes, the viscera, and possibly GI structures.

Causes and incidence

The exact cause of Kaposi sarcoma is unknown, but the disease may be related to immunosuppression. Genetic or hereditary predisposition is also suspected. In people with AIDS, Kaposi sarcoma is caused by an interaction between the human immunodeficiency virus (HIV), immune system suppression, and human herpesvirus-8 (HHV-8).

Occurrence has been linked with sexual transmission of HIV and HHV-8. About 3 out of every 100,000 people develop Kaposi sarcoma each year.

Pathophysiology

Kaposi sarcoma is a type of cancer that forms in the lining of blood and lymph vessels. The tumors (lesions) of Kaposi sarcoma typically appear as painless purplish spots on the legs, feet, or face. Lesions can also appear in the genital area, mouth, or lymph nodes. In severe Kaposi sarcoma, lesions may develop in the digestive tract and lungs. The underlying cause of Kaposi sarcoma is infection with a virus called HHV-8. In healthy people, HHV-8 infection usually causes no symptoms because the immune system keeps it under control. In people with weakened immune systems, however, HHV-8 has the potential to trigger Kaposi sarcoma.

Complications
◆ Respiratory distress
◆ GI involvement
◆ Digestive problems

Signs and symptoms

The initial sign of Kaposi sarcoma is one or more obvious lesions in various shapes, sizes, and colors (ranging from red-brown to dark purple) appearing most commonly on the skin, buccal mucosa, hard and soft palates, lips, gums, tongue, tonsils, conjunctiva, and sclera. (See *Kaposi sarcoma.*)

In advanced disease, the lesions may join, becoming one large plaque. Untreated lesions may appear as large, ulcerative masses.

Other signs and symptoms include:
◆ health history of AIDS
◆ pain (if the sarcoma advances beyond the early stages or if a lesion breaks down or impinges on nerves or organs)
◆ edema from lymphatic obstruction
◆ dyspnea (in cases of pulmonary involvement), wheezing, hypoventilation, and respiratory distress from bronchial blockage

The most common extracutaneous sites are the lungs and GI tract (esophagus, oropharynx, and epiglottis).

Signs and symptoms of disease progression and metastasis include severe pulmonary involvement and GI involvement leading to digestive problems.

Kaposi sarcoma

The illustration below shows Kaposi sarcoma.

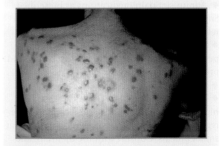

Diagnosis

℞ **CONFIRMING DIAGNOSIS** *Diagnosis is made following a tissue biopsy that identifies the lesion's type and stage. Then, a CT scan may be performed to detect and evaluate possible metastasis. Endoscopy shows Kaposi lesions.*

Treatment

Treatment isn't indicated for all patients. Indications include cosmetically offensive, painful, or obstructive lesions of rapidly progressing disease.

Radiation therapy, chemotherapy, cryotherapy, and biotherapy with biological response modifiers are treatment options. Radiation therapy alleviates symptoms, including pain from obstructing lesions in the oral cavity or extremities and edema caused by lymphatic blockage. It may also be used for cosmetic improvement.

Chemotherapy includes combinations of doxorubicin, vincristine, etoposide, paclitaxel, bleomycin, and dacarbazine.

Biotherapy with interferon-alfa-2b may be prescribed for AIDS-related Kaposi sarcoma. The treatment reduces the number of skin lesions but is ineffective in advanced disease.

Special considerations

◆ Listen to the patient's fears and concerns and answer questions honestly. Stay with the patient during periods of severe stress and anxiety.

◆ The patient who's coping poorly may need a referral for psychological counseling. Their family members may also need help in coping with the patient's disease and with any associated demands that the disorder places upon them.

◆ As appropriate, allow the patient to participate in care decisions whenever possible, and encourage the patient to participate in self-care measures as much as they can.

◆ Inspect the patient's skin every shift. Look for new lesions and skin breakdown. If the patient has painful lesions, help the patient into a more comfortable position.

◆ Follow standard precautions when caring for the patient.

◆ Administer pain medications as prescribed. Suggest distractions, and help the patient with relaxation techniques.

◆ To help the patient adjust to changes in appearance, urge the patient to share feelings, and provide encouragement.

◆ Monitor the patient's weight daily.

◆ Supply the patient with high-calorie, high-protein meals. If the patient can't tolerate regular meals, provide the patient with frequent smaller meals. Consult with the dietitian, and plan meals around the patient's treatment.

◆ If the patient can't take food by mouth, administer I.V. fluids. Also provide antiemetics and sedatives, as ordered.

◆ Be alert for adverse effects of radiation therapy or chemotherapy—such as anorexia, nausea, vomiting, and diarrhea—and take steps to prevent or alleviate them.

◆ Reinforce the practitioner's explanation of treatments. Make sure the patient understands which adverse reactions to expect and how to manage them. For example, during radiation therapy, instruct the patient to keep irradiated skin dry to avoid possible breakdown and subsequent infection.

◆ Explain all prescribed medications, including any possible adverse effects and drug interactions.

◆ Explain infection-prevention techniques and, if necessary, demonstrate basic hygiene measures to prevent infection. Advise the patient not to share their toothbrush, razor, or other items that may be contaminated with blood. These measures are especially important if the patient also has AIDS.

◆ Help the patient plan daily periods of alternating activity and rest to help the patient cope with fatigue. Teach energy-conservation techniques. Encourage the patient to set priorities, accept the help of others, and delegate nonessential tasks.

◆ Explain the proper use of assistive devices, when appropriate, to ease ambulation and promote independence.

◆ Stress the need for ongoing treatment and care.

◆ As appropriate, refer the patient to support groups offered by the social services department.

◆ If the patient's prognosis is poor (<6 months to live), suggest immediate hospice care.

◆ Explain the benefits of initiating and executing advance directives and a durable power of attorney.

▓▓▓▓ **PREVENTION** *Explain to your patient that practicing safe sex can prevent HIV and the development of Kaposi sarcoma.*

Blood and lymph

HODGKIN LYMPHOMA

HL is a neoplastic disease characterized by painless, progressive enlargement of lymph nodes, spleen, and other lymphoid tissue resulting from proliferation of lymphocytes, histiocytes, eosinophils, and Reed–Sternberg (RS) giant cells. The latter cells are its special histologic feature but aren't pathognomonic. Untreated, HL follows a variable but relentlessly progressive and ultimately fatal course. However, recent advances in therapy make HL potentially curable, even in advanced stages; appropriate treatment yields a 5-year survival rate in about 80% of patients.

Causes and incidence

Although the cause of HL is unknown, a viral etiology is suspected, with the EBV as a leading candidate. Other risk factors include a family history of infectious mononucleosis and having a compromised immune system. The disease is most common in young adults, with a higher incidence in males than in females. It occurs in all races but is slightly more common in whites. Its incidence peaks in two age groups: age 15 to 35 and after age 50—except in Japan, where it occurs exclusively among people older than age 50.

Pathophysiology

HL is a type of lymphoma which is generally believed to result from WBCs of the lymphocyte kind. Symptoms may include fever, night sweats, and weight loss. Often there will be nonpainful enlarged lymph nodes in the neck, under the arm, or in the groin. Those affected may feel tired or be itchy.

About half of cases of HL are due to EBV. Other risk factors include a family history of the condition and having HIV/AIDS. There are two major types of HL: classical HL and nodular lymphocyte-predominant HL. Diagnosis is by finding Hodgkin cells such as multinucleated RS cells in lymph nodes.

Complications

◆ Liver failure
◆ Lung problems
◆ Sterility

Signs and symptoms

The first sign of HL is usually a painless swelling of one of the cervical lymph nodes (but sometimes the axillary, mediastinal, or inguinal lymph nodes), occasionally in a patient who gives a history of recent upper respiratory infection. In older patients, the first signs and symptoms may be nonspecific—persistent fever, night sweats, fatigue, weight loss, and malaise. Rarely, if the mediastinum is initially involved, HL may produce respiratory symptoms.

Another early and characteristic indication of HL is pruritus, which, although mild at first, becomes acute as the disease progresses. Other symptoms depend on the degree and location of systemic involvement.

Lymph nodes may enlarge rapidly, producing pain and obstruction, or enlarge slowly and painlessly for months or years. It isn't unusual to see the lymph nodes "wax and wane," but they usually don't return to normal. Sooner or later, most patients develop systemic manifestations, including enlargement of retroperitoneal nodes and nodular infiltrations of the spleen, the liver, and bones. At this late stage other symptoms include edema of the face and neck, progressive anemia, possible jaundice, nerve pain, and increased susceptibility to infection.

Diagnosis

℞ **CONFIRMING DIAGNOSIS** *Diagnostic measures for confirming HL include a thorough medical history and a complete physical examination, followed by a lymph node biopsy checking for RS abnormal histiocyte proliferation and nodular fibrosis and necrosis. (See Reed–Sternberg cells.)*

Other appropriate diagnostic tests include bone marrow, liver, mediastinal, lymph node, and spleen biopsies and routine chest X-ray, abdominal CT scan, positron emission tomography, lung scan, bone scan, and lymphangiography to detect lymph node or organ involvement. Laparoscopy and lymph node biopsy are performed to complete staging.

Reed–Sternberg cells

These enlarged, abnormal histiocytes (Reed–Sternberg [RS] cells) from an excised lymph node suggest Hodgkin lymphoma (HL). Note the large, distinct nucleoli. RS cells indicate HL when they coexist with one of these four histologic patterns: lymphocyte predominance, mixed cellularity, lymphocyte depletion, or nodular sclerosis.

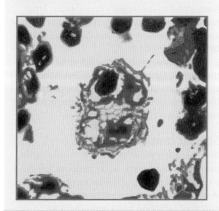

Hematologic tests show mild to severe normocytic anemia; normochromic anemia (in 50%); elevated, normal, or reduced WBC count and differential showing any combination of neutrophilia, lymphocytopenia, monocytosis, and eosinophilia. Elevated serum alkaline phosphatase indicates liver or bone involvement.

The same diagnostic tests are also used for staging. A staging laparotomy is necessary for patients younger than age 55 or without obvious stage III or stage IV disease, lymphocyte predominance subtype histology, or medical contraindications. Diagnosis must rule out other disorders that also enlarge the lymph nodes.

Treatment

Appropriate therapy (chemotherapy or radiation, or both, varying with the stage of the disease) depends on careful physical examination with accurate histologic interpretation and proper clinical staging. Correct and timely treatment allows longer survival and even induces an apparent cure in many patients. Radiation therapy is used alone for stages I and II and in combination with chemotherapy for stage III. Chemotherapy is used for stage IV, sometimes inducing a complete remission. The well-known MOPP protocol (mechlorethamine, vincristine [Oncovin], procarbazine, and prednisone) was the first to provide significant cures to patients with generalized HL; another useful combination, ABVD (doxorubicin [Adriamycin], bleomycin, vinblastine, and dacarbazine) has fewer side effects and is more effective than MOPP. Its 5-year freedom from progression is 81%. Another chemotherapy regimen—bleomycin, etoposide, cyclophosphamide, vincristine, procarbazine, and prednisone, or BEACOPP—has also shown promise in advanced HL. Stanford V, which includes doxorubicin, vinblastine, mechlorethamine, etoposide, vincristine, bleomycin, and prednisone, has also been useful in controlled clinical trials. Treatment with these drugs may require concomitant antiemetics, sedatives, or antidiarrheals to combat GI adverse effects.

New treatments include high-dose chemotherapeutic agents with autologous bone marrow transplantation or autologous peripheral blood stem cell transfusions. Biotherapy alone hasn't proven effective.

Special considerations

Because many patients with HL receive radiation or chemotherapy as outpatients, tell the patient to observe the following precautions:
♦ Watch for and promptly report adverse effects of radiation and chemotherapy (particularly anorexia, nausea, vomiting, diarrhea, fever, and bleeding).
♦ Minimize adverse effects of radiation therapy by maintaining good nutrition (aided by eating small, frequent meals of their favorite foods), drinking plenty of fluids, pacing activities to counteract therapy-induced fatigue, and keeping the skin in irradiated areas dry.
♦ Control pain and bleeding of stomatitis by using a soft toothbrush, cotton swab, or anesthetic mouthwash such as viscous lidocaine (as prescribed), by applying petroleum jelly to lips, and by avoiding astringent mouthwashes.
♦ If a female patient is of childbearing age, advise the patient to delay pregnancy until prolonged remission because radiation and chemotherapy can cause genetic mutations and spontaneous abortions.
♦ Because the patient with HL has usually been healthy up to this point, the patient is likely to be especially distressed. Provide emotional support and offer appropriate reassurance. Ease the patient's anxiety by sharing your optimism about prognosis.
♦ Make sure both the patient and the family know that the local chapter of the American Cancer Society is available for information, financial assistance, and supportive counseling.
♦ The development of further malignancies, such as acute myeloid leukemia and myelodysplastic syndrome, in patients successfully treated for HL is a concern. Patients must be educated as to the importance of long-term follow-up care following completion of treatment.

NON-HODGKIN LYMPHOMA

Non-HLs, also known as *malignant lymphomas* and *lymphosarcomas*, are a heterogeneous group of malignant diseases originating in lymph glands and other lymphoid tissue. Nodular lymphomas have a better prognosis than the diffuse form of the disease, but in both, the prognosis is worse than in HL.

Causes and incidence

The cause of non-HL is unknown, although some theories suggest a viral source. Since the early 1970s, the incidence of these lymphomas has increased more than 80%, with about 53,000 new cases appearing annually in the United States. The reason for the increase is unknown, although it has been partly attributed to AIDS. Non-HLs are two to three times more common in males than in females and occur in all age groups. Compared to HL, they occur about one to three times more often and cause twice as many deaths in children younger than age 15. Incidence rises with age (median age is 50). These lymphomas seem linked to certain races and ethnic groups, with increased incidence in whites and people of Jewish ancestry.

Pathophysiology

NHLs are tumors originating from lymphoid tissues, mainly of lymph nodes. Various neoplastic tumor cell lines correspond to each of the cellular components of antigen-stimulated lymphoid follicles.

Complications

◆ Hypercalcemia
◆ Hyperuricemia
◆ Lymphomatosis
◆ Meningitis
◆ Anemia
◆ Increased ICP

Signs and symptoms

Usually, the first indication of non-HL is swelling of the lymph glands, enlarged tonsils and adenoids, and painless, rubbery nodes in the cervical supraclavicular areas. In children, these nodes are usually in the cervical region, and the disease causes dyspnea and coughing. As the lymphoma progresses, the patient develops symptoms specific to the area involved and systemic complaints of fatigue, malaise, weight loss, fever, and night sweats.

Diagnosis

Diagnosis requires histologic evaluation of biopsied lymph nodes; of tonsils, bone marrow, liver, bowel, or skin; or of tissue removed during exploratory laparotomy. (Biopsy differentiates non-HL from HL.) (See *Classifying non-Hodgkin lymphomas.*)

Classifying non-Hodgkin lymphomas

Staging and classifying systems for non-Hodgkin lymphomas include the National Cancer Institute's (NCI) system, the Rappaport histologic classification, and Lukes classification. (*Note:* The NCI also cites a "miscellaneous" category, which includes these lymphomas: composite, mycosis fungoides, histiocytic, extramedullary plasmacytoma, and unclassifiable.)

NCI	Rappaport	Lukes
Low grade		
◆ Small lymphocytic ◆ Follicular, predominantly small cleaved cell ◆ Follicular mixed, small and large cell	◆ Diffuse well-differentiated lymphocytic ◆ Nodular poorly differentiated lymphocytic ◆ Nodular mixed lymphoma	◆ Small lymphocytic and plasmacytoid lymphocytic ◆ Small cleaved follicular center cell, follicular only, or follicular and diffuse ◆ Small cleaved follicular center cell, follicular; large cleaved follicular center cell, follicular
Intermediate		
◆ Follicular, predominantly large cell ◆ Diffuse, small cleaved cell ◆ Diffuse mixed, small and large cell ◆ Diffuse large cell, cleaved or noncleaved	◆ Nodular histiocytic lymphoma ◆ Diffuse poorly differentiated lymphoma ◆ Diffuse mixed lymphocytic-histiocytic ◆ Diffuse histiocytic lymphoma	◆ Large cleaved or noncleaved follicular center cell, or both, follicular ◆ Small cleaved follicular center cell, diffuse ◆ Small cleaved, large cleaved, or large noncleaved follicular center cell, diffuse ◆ Large cleaved or noncleaved follicular center cell, diffuse
High grade		
◆ Diffuse large cell immunoblastic ◆ Large cell, lymphoblastic ◆ Small noncleaved cell	◆ Diffuse histiocytic lymphoma ◆ Lymphoblastic, convoluted or nonconvoluted ◆ Undifferentiated, Burkitt and non-Burkitt diffuse undifferentiated lymphoma	◆ Immunoblastic sarcoma, T-cell or B-cell type ◆ Convoluted T cell ◆ Small noncleaved follicular center cell

Other tests include bone and chest X-rays; lymphangiography; liver and spleen scan; CT scan of the abdomen, chest, and pelvis; positron emission tomography; and excretory urography. Laboratory tests include complete blood count (may show anemia), uric acid (elevated or normal), serum calcium (elevated if bone lesions are present), serum protein (normal), and liver function studies.

Treatment

Radiation therapy is used mainly in the early localized stage of the disease. Total nodal irradiation is generally effective for both nodular and diffuse histologies. Combining radiation therapy and chemotherapy is an option.

Chemotherapy is most effective with multiple combinations of antineoplastic agents. For example, cyclophosphamide, vincristine, doxorubicin (Adriamycin), and prednisone (CHOP protocol) can induce a complete remission in 70% to 80% of patients with nodular histology and in 20% to 55% of patients with diffuse histology. Other combinations—such as methotrexate, bleomycin, doxorubicin (Adriamycin), cyclophosphamide (Cytoxan), vincristine (Oncovin), and prednisone (M-BACOP)—induce prolonged remission and sometimes cure the diffuse form.

In recent years, the development of monoclonal antibodies, specifically rituximab, has provided additional options for the treatment of non-HLs either alone or in combination with traditional chemotherapy regimens. Additionally, radioimmunotherapy for the treatment of these lymphomas has shown promise. Monoclonal antibodies are labeled with beta-emitting isotopes. Currently, ibritumomab tiuxetan is being used alone and in combination with rituximab. More aggressive lymphomas may require intensive therapy using a combination of the CHOP protocol and rituximab.

Special considerations

◆ Observe the patient who's receiving radiation or chemotherapy for anorexia, nausea, vomiting, or diarrhea. Plan small, frequent meals scheduled around treatment.

◆ If the patient can't tolerate oral feedings, administer I.V. fluids and, as ordered, give antiemetics and sedatives.

◆ Instruct the patient to keep irradiated skin dry.

◆ Provide emotional support by informing the patient and family about the diagnosis and prognosis and by listening to their concerns. If needed, refer them to the local chapter of the American Cancer Society for information and counseling. Stress the need for continued treatment and follow-up care.

MYCOSIS FUNGOIDES

Mycosis fungoides (MF), also known as *malignant cutaneous reticulosis* and *granuloma fungoides*, is a rare, chronic malignant cutaneous T-cell lymphoma (CTCL) of unknown cause that originates in the reticuloendothelial system of the skin, eventually affecting lymph nodes and internal organs. Unlike other lymphomas, MF allows an average life expectancy of 7 to 10 years after diagnosis. If correctly treated, particularly before it has spread beyond the skin, MF may go into remission for many years. However, after MF has reached the tumor stage, progression to severe disability or death is rapid.

Pathophysiology

Primary CTCLs are a heterogeneous group of non-HLs characterized by skin infiltration of neoplastic T lymphocytes. MF and its leukemic variant Sézary syndrome represent the most common CTCL subtypes. Current treatment for patients with MF involves topical and systemic therapies for the cutaneous manifestations.

Causes and incidence

The cause of MF is unknown. Most persons with MF have it for years and it can lead to death, but this is unusual.

In the United States, MF strikes more than 1,000 people of all races annually; most are between ages 40 and 60.

Complications

◆ Anemia
◆ Edema
◆ Infection

Signs and symptoms

The first sign of MF may be generalized erythroderma, possibly associated with itching. Eventually, MF evolves into varied combinations of infiltrated, thickened, or scaly patches, tumors, or ulcerations.

Diagnosis

CONFIRMING DIAGNOSIS *Clear diagnosis of MF depends on a history of multiple, varied, and progressively severe skin lesions associated with characteristic histologic evidence of lymphoma cell infiltration of the skin, with or without involvement of lymph nodes or visceral organs. Consequently, this diagnosis is commonly missed during the early stages until lymphoma cells are sufficiently numerous in the skin to show up in biopsy.*

Other diagnostic tests help confirm MF: complete blood count and differential; a finger-stick smear for Sézary cells (abnormal circulating lymphocytes), which may be present in the erythrodermic variants of MF (Sézary syndrome); blood chemistry studies to screen for visceral dysfunction; chest X-ray; CT scan of the abdomen and pelvis; liver–spleen isotopic scanning; lymphangiography; and lymph node biopsy to assess lymph node involvement. These tests also help to stage the disease—a necessary prerequisite to treatment.

Treatment

Depending on the stage of the disease and its rate of progression, past treatment and results, the patient's age and overall clinical status, treatment facilities available, and other factors, treatment of MF may include topical, intralesional, or systemic corticosteroid therapy; monoclonal antibody therapy; phototherapy; methoxsalen photochemotherapy; topical or oral retinoids; radiation; topical, intralesional, or systemic treatment with mechlorethamine (nitrogen mustard); and other systemic chemotherapy.

Application of topical nitrogen mustard or carmustine is the preferred treatment for inducing remission in pretumorous stages. Plaques may also be treated with sunlight and topical steroids.

Total body electron beam radiation, which is less toxic to internal organs than standard photon beam radiation, has induced remission in some patients with early-stage MF.

Chemotherapy is employed primarily for patients with advanced MF; systemic treatment with chemotherapeutic agents (cyclophosphamide, methotrexate, doxorubicin, bleomycin, etoposide, and steroids) and interferon-alfa produces transient regression.

Special considerations

♦ If the patient has difficulty applying nitrogen mustard to all involved skin surfaces, provide assistance. However, wear gloves to prevent contact sensitization and to protect yourself from exposure to chemotherapeutic agents.

♦ If the patient is receiving drug treatment, report adverse effects and infection at once.

♦ The patient who's receiving radiation therapy will probably develop alopecia and erythema. Suggest that they wear a wig to improve their self-image and protect their scalp until hair regrowth begins, and suggest or give medicated oil baths to ease erythema.

♦ Because pruritus is generally worse at night, the patient may need larger bedtime doses of antipruritics or sedatives, as ordered, to ensure adequate sleep. When the patient's symptoms have interrupted sleep, postpone early-morning care to allow the patient more sleep.

♦ The patient with intense pruritus has an overwhelming need to scratch—in many cases to the point of removing epidermis and replacing pruritus with pain, which some patients find easier to endure. Realize that you can't keep such a patient from scratching; the best you can do is help minimize the damage. Advise the patient to keep fingernails short and clean and to wear a pair of soft, white cotton gloves when itching is unbearable.

♦ The malignant skin lesions are likely to make the patient depressed, fearful, and self-conscious. Fully explain the disease and its stages to help the patient and family understand and accept the disease. Provide reassurance and support by demonstrating a positive but realistic attitude. Reinforce your verbal support by touching the patient without any hint of anxiety or distaste.

ACUTE LEUKEMIA

Acute leukemia is a malignant proliferation of WBC precursors (blasts) in bone marrow or lymph tissue and their accumulation in peripheral blood, bone marrow, and body tissues. Acute leukemias have large numbers of immature leukocytes and overproduction of cells in the blast stage of maturation. About 20% of leukemias are acute. Its most common forms are acute lymphoblastic (lymphocytic) leukemia (ALL), an abnormal growth of lymphocyte precursors (lymphoblasts); acute myeloblastic (myelogenous) leukemia (AML), the rapid accumulation of myeloid precursors (myeloblasts); and acute monoblastic (monocytic) leukemia, or Schilling type, a marked increase in monocyte precursors (monoblasts). Other variants include acute myelomonocytic leukemia and acute erythroleukemia.

Untreated, acute leukemia is invariably fatal, usually because of complications that result from leukemic cell infiltration of bone marrow or vital organs. With treatment, prognosis varies. In ALL, treatment induces remissions in 90% of children (average survival time: 5 years) and in 65% of adults (average survival time: 1 to 2 years). Children between ages 2 and 8 have the best survival rate—about 50%—with intensive therapy. In AML, the average survival time is only 1 year after diagnosis, even with aggressive treatment. In acute monoblastic leukemia, treatment induces remissions lasting 2 to 10 months in 50% of children; adults survive only about 1 year after diagnosis, even with treatment.

Predisposing factors to acute leukemia

Although the exact causes of most leukemias remain unknown, increasing evidence suggests a combination of contributing factors:

Acute lymphoblastic leukemia
◆ Congenital disorders, such as Down syndrome, Bloom syndrome, Fanconi anemia, congenital agammaglobulinemia, and ataxia-telangiectasia
◆ Familial tendency
◆ Monozygotic twins
◆ Viruses

Acute myeloblastic leukemia
◆ Congenital disorders, such as Down syndrome, Bloom syndrome, Fanconi anemia, congenital agammaglobulinemia, and ataxia-telangiectasia
◆ Exposure to the chemical benzene and cytotoxins such as alkylating agents
◆ Familial tendency
◆ Ionizing radiation
◆ Monozygotic twins
◆ Viruses

Acute monoblastic leukemia
◆ Unknown (irradiation, exposure to chemicals, heredity, and infections show little correlation with this disease)

Causes and incidence

Research into predisposing factors isn't conclusive but points to some combination of viruses (viral remnants have been found in leukemic cells), genetic and immunologic factors, and exposure to radiation and certain chemicals. (See *Predisposing factors to acute leukemia.*)

Pathogenesis isn't clearly understood, but immature, nonfunctioning WBCs appear to accumulate first in the tissue where they originate (lymphocytes in lymph tissue, granulocytes in bone marrow). These immature WBCs then spill into the bloodstream and from there infiltrate other tissues, eventually causing organ malfunction because of encroachment or hemorrhage.

Acute leukemia is more common in males than in females, in whites (especially people of Jewish descent), in children (between ages 2 and 5; 80% of all leukemias in this age group are ALL), and in people who live in urban and industrialized areas. Acute leukemia accounts for 20% of all adult leukemias. Among children, however, it's the most common form of cancer. Incidence is 6 out of every 100,000 people.

Pathophysiology

The underlying pathophysiology in AML consists of a maturational arrest of bone marrow cells in the earliest stages of development. The mechanism of this arrest is under study, but in many cases, it involves the activation or inactivation of genes through chromosomal translocations and other genetic and/or epigenetic abnormalities.

Complications
◆ Infection
◆ Organ malfunction

Signs and symptoms

Signs of acute leukemia may be gradual or abrupt; they include high fever accompanied by thrombocytopenia and abnormal bleeding (such as nosebleeds), gingival bleeding, purpura, ecchymoses, petechiae, easy bruising after minor trauma, and prolonged menses. Nonspecific signs and symptoms, such as low-grade fever, weakness, and lassitude, may persist for days or months before visible symptoms appear. Other insidious signs and symptoms include pallor, chills, and recurrent infections. In addition, ALL, AML, and acute monoblastic leukemia may cause dyspnea, anemia, fatigue, malaise, tachycardia, palpitations, systolic ejection murmur, and abdominal or bone pain. Specific AML symptoms include local infections (laryngitis, pharyngitis, meningitis) or septicemia. Joint arthralgias and abdominal fullness (from an enlarged spleen) may occur. Specific ALL symptoms include night sweats, shortness of breath, anorexia, weight loss, hepatosplenomegaly, and lymph adenopathy. When leukemic cells cross the blood–brain barrier and thereby escape the effects of systemic chemotherapy, the patient may develop meningeal leukemia (confusion, lethargy, headache).

Diagnosis

CONFIRMING DIAGNOSIS *Typical clinical findings and bone marrow aspirate showing a proliferation of immature WBCs confirm acute leukemia.*

A bone marrow biopsy, usually of the posterior superior iliac spine, is part of the diagnostic workup. Blood counts show severe anemia, thrombocytopenia, and neutropenia. Differential leukocyte count determines cell type. Lumbar puncture detects meningeal involvement. Elevated uric acid and lactic dehydrogenase levels are common.

Treatment

Systemic chemotherapy aims to eradicate leukemic cells and induce remission (<5% of blast cells in the marrow and peripheral blood are normal). Chemotherapy varies:

◆ Meningeal leukemia—intrathecal instillation of methotrexate or cytarabine with cranial radiation when clinical remission is achieved.

◆ ALL—vincristine, prednisone, high-dose cytarabine, L-asparaginase, and daunorubicin. Because there's a 40% risk of meningeal leukemia in ALL, intrathecal methotrexate or cytarabine is given. Radiation therapy is given for testicular infiltration.

◆ AML—a combination of I.V. daunorubicin and cytarabine or, if these fail to induce remission, a combination of cyclophosphamide, vincristine, prednisone, or methotrexate; high-dose cytarabine alone or with other drugs; amsacrine; etoposide; and 5-azacytidine and mitoxantrone. A subtype of AML called acute promyelocytic leukemia (APL) is treated with all-transretinoic acid (ATRA), which causes leukemic cells to mature into normal WBCs. ATRA has increased the cure rate of this type of AML. Arsenic trioxide has been approved for patients with APL who have failed ATRA as the usual chemotherapy. The monoclonal antibody gemtuzumab ozogamicin is used to treat older adults.

◆ Acute monoblastic leukemia—cytarabine and thioguanine with daunorubicin or doxorubicin.

Bone marrow transplant or a stem cell transplant may be possible. Treatment also may include antibiotic, antifungal, and antiviral drugs and granulocyte injections to control infection and transfusions of platelets to prevent bleeding and of red blood cells to prevent anemia.

Special considerations

The care plan for the leukemic patient should emphasize comfort, minimize the adverse effects of chemotherapy, promote preservation of veins, manage complications, and provide teaching and psychological support.

PEDIATRIC TIP *Because many of these patients are children, be especially sensitive to their emotional needs and those of their families.*

Before treatment:

◆ Explain the disease course, treatment, and adverse effects.

◆ Teach the patient and family how to recognize infection (fever, chills, cough, sore throat) and abnormal bleeding (bruising, petechiae) and how to stop such bleeding (pressure, ice to area).

◆ Promote good nutrition. Explain that chemotherapy may cause weight loss and anorexia, so encourage the patient to eat and drink high-calorie, high-protein foods and beverages. However, chemotherapy and adjunctive prednisone may cause weight gain, so dietary counseling and teaching are helpful.

◆ Help establish an appropriate rehabilitation program for the patient during remission.

Plan meticulous supportive care:

◆ Watch for symptoms of meningeal leukemia (confusion, lethargy, headache). If these occur, know how to manage care after intrathecal chemotherapy. After such instillation, place the patient in Trendelenburg position for 30 minutes. Force fluids, and keep the patient in the supine position for 4 to 6 hours. Check the lumbar puncture site often for bleeding. If the patient receives cranial radiation, teach the patient about potential adverse effects, and do what you can to minimize them.

◆ Prevent hyperuricemia, a possible result of rapid chemotherapy-induced leukemic cell lysis. Encourage fluids to about 2 qt (2,000 mL) daily, and give acetazolamide, sodium bicarbonate tablets, and allopurinol. Check urine pH often—it should be above 7.5. Watch for rash or other hypersensitivity reaction to allopurinol.

◆ Watch for early signs of cardiotoxicity, such as arrhythmias and signs of heart failure, if the patient receives daunorubicin or doxorubicin.

◆ Control infection by placing the patient in a private room and instituting neutropenic precautions. Coordinate patient care so the leukemic patient doesn't come in contact with staff who also care for patients with infections or infectious diseases. Avoid using indwelling urinary catheters and giving I.M. injections because they provide an avenue for infection. Screen staff and visitors for contagious diseases, and watch for and report any signs of infection.

♦ Provide thorough skin care by keeping the patient's skin and perianal area clean, applying mild lotions or creams to keep skin from drying and cracking, and thoroughly cleaning skin before all invasive skin procedures. Change I.V. tubing according to your facility's policy. Use strict sterile technique and a metal scalp vein needle (metal butterfly needle) when starting I.V. therapy. If the patient receives TPN, give scrupulous subclavian catheter care.

♦ Monitor temperature every 4 hours; patients with fever over 101° F (38.3° C) and decreased WBC counts should receive prompt antibiotic therapy.

♦ Watch for bleeding; if it occurs, apply ice compresses and pressure, and elevate the extremity. Avoid giving I.M. injections, aspirin, and aspirin-containing drugs. Also avoid taking rectal temperatures, giving rectal suppositories, and doing digital examinations.

♦ Prevent constipation by providing adequate hydration, a high-residue diet, stool softeners, and mild laxatives and by encouraging walking.

♦ Control mouth ulceration by checking often for obvious ulcers and gum swelling and by providing frequent mouth care and saline rinses. Tell the patient to use a soft toothbrush and to avoid hot, spicy foods and overuse of commercial mouthwashes.

♦ Check the rectal area daily for induration, swelling, erythema, skin discoloration, or drainage.

♦ Provide psychological support by establishing a trusting relationship to promote communication. Allow the patient and family to verbalize their anger and depression. Let the family participate in the care as much as possible.

♦ Minimize stress by providing a calm, quiet atmosphere that's conducive to rest and relaxation.

🖐 **PEDIATRIC TIP** *For children, be flexible with patient care and visiting hours to promote maximum interaction with family and friends and to allow time for schoolwork and play.*

♦ For those patients who are refractory to chemotherapy and in the terminal phase of the disease, supportive nursing care is directed to comfort; management of pain, fever, and bleeding; and patient and family support. Provide the opportunity for religious counseling. Discuss the option of home or hospice care.

CHRONIC MYELOGENOUS LEUKEMIA

Chronic myelogenous leukemia (CML), also known as *chronic granulocytic leukemia* and *chronic myelocytic leukemia*, is characterized by the abnormal overgrowth of granulocytic precursors (myeloblasts, promyelocytes, metamyelocytes, and myelocytes) in bone marrow, peripheral blood, and body tissues.

CML's clinical course proceeds in two distinct phases: the *insidious chronic phase*, with anemia and bleeding abnormalities and, eventually, the *acute phase (blastic crisis)*, in which myeloblasts, the most primitive granulocytic precursors, proliferate rapidly. This disease is invariably fatal. Average survival time is 3 to 4 years after onset of the chronic phase and 3 to 6 months after onset of the acute phase.

Causes and incidence

About 95% of patients with CML have the Philadelphia, or Ph, chromosome, an abnormality discovered in 1960 in which the long arm of chromosome 22 is translocated, usually to chromosome 9. Radiation and carcinogenic chemicals may induce this chromosome abnormality. Myeloproliferative diseases also seem to increase the incidence of CML, and some clinicians suspect that an unidentified virus causes this disease.

CML is most common in young and middle-aged adults and is slightly more common in men than in women; it's rare in children. In the United States, about 4,300 cases of CML develop annually, accounting for roughly 20% of all leukemias. The 5-year survival rate in the chronic phase is 32%.

Pathophysiology

CML, also known as chronic myeloid leukemia, is a cancer of the WBCs. It is a form of leukemia characterized by the increased and unregulated growth of predominantly myeloid cells in the bone marrow and the accumulation of these cells in the blood. CML is a clonal bone marrow stem cell disorder in which a proliferation of mature granulocytes (neutrophils, eosinophils, and basophils) and their precursors is found. It is a type of myeloproliferative neoplasm associated with a characteristic chromosomal translocation called the Philadelphia chromosome.

Complications

♦ Enlarged spleen
♦ Hemorrhage
♦ Infection
♦ Pain
♦ Stroke

Signs and symptoms

Typically, during the chronic phase, CML induces the following clinical effects:

♦ anemia (fatigue, weakness, decreased exercise tolerance, pallor, dyspnea, tachycardia, and headache)

♦ thrombocytopenia, with resulting bleeding and clotting disorders (retinal hemorrhage, ecchymoses, hematuria, melena, bleeding gums, nosebleeds, and easy bruising)

♦ hepatosplenomegaly, with abdominal discomfort and pain in splenic infarction from leukemic cell infiltration.

Other signs and symptoms include sternal and rib tenderness from leukemic infiltrations of the periosteum; low-grade fever; weight loss; anorexia; renal calculi or gouty arthritis from increased uric acid excretion; occasionally, prolonged infection and ankle edema; and, rarely, priapism and vascular insufficiency. Acceleration of the disease process results in fever, night sweats, splenomegaly, and bone pain.

Diagnosis

Rx CONFIRMING DIAGNOSIS *In patients with typical clinical changes, chromosomal analysis of peripheral blood or bone marrow showing the Philadelphia chromosome and low leukocyte alkaline phosphatase levels confirms CML.*

Other relevant laboratory results show:

♦ WBC abnormalities—leukocytosis (leukocyte count >50,000/μL, ranging as high as 250,000/μL), occasional leukopenia (leukocyte count <5,000/μL), neutropenia (neutrophil count <1,500/μL) despite high leukocyte count, and increased circulating myeloblasts

♦ Hb—commonly below 10 g/dL

♦ HCT—low (<30%)

♦ platelets—thrombocytosis (>1 million/μL) is common

♦ serum uric acid—possibly more than 8 mg/dL

♦ bone marrow aspirate or biopsy—hypercellular; characteristically shows bone marrow infiltration by significantly increased number of myeloid elements (biopsy is done only if aspirate is dry); in the acute phase, myeloblasts predominate

♦ CT scan—may identify the organs affected by leukemia

Treatment

Aggressive chemotherapy has so far failed to produce remission in CML. Consequently, the goal of treatment in the chronic phase is to control leukocytosis and thrombocytosis. Previously, the most commonly used oral agents were busulfan and hydroxyurea. Interferon-alfa–based therapy has become the new standard. However, the development and introduction of imatinib mesylate, a tyrosine kinase inhibitor, has shown significant long-term effectiveness, and has remarkably changed CML treatment.

If the patient's platelet count is more than 1 million/μL, aspirin is commonly given to prevent stroke.

Ancillary CML treatments include:

♦ local splenic radiation or splenectomy to increase platelet count and decrease adverse effects related to splenomegaly

♦ leukapheresis (selective leukocyte removal) to reduce leukocyte count

♦ allopurinol to prevent secondary hyperuricemia or colchicine to relieve gout caused by elevated serum uric acid levels

♦ prompt treatment of infections that may result from chemotherapy-induced bone marrow suppression

During the acute phase of CML, lymphoblastic or myeloblastic leukemia may develop. Treatment is similar to that for ALL. Remission, if achieved, is commonly short lived. Bone marrow transplant may produce long asymptomatic periods in the early phase of illness but has been less successful in the accelerated phase. Despite vigorous treatment, CML can progress after onset of the acute phase.

Special considerations

In patients with CML, meticulous supportive care, psychological support, and careful patient teaching help make the most of remissions and minimize complications. When the disease is diagnosed, be prepared to repeat and reinforce the practitioner's explanation of the disease and its treatment to the patient and family.

Throughout the chronic phase of CML when the patient is hospitalized:

♦ If the patient has persistent anemia, plan your care to help avoid exhausting the patient. Schedule laboratory tests and physical care with frequent rest periods in between, and assist the patient with walking, if necessary. Regularly check the patient's skin and mucous membranes for pallor, petechiae, and bruising.

♦ To minimize bleeding, suggest a soft-bristle toothbrush, an electric razor, and other safety precautions.

♦ To minimize the abdominal discomfort of splenomegaly, provide small, frequent meals. For the same reason, prevent constipation with a stool softener or laxative, as needed. Ask the dietary department to provide a high-bulk diet, and maintain adequate fluid intake.

♦ To prevent atelectasis, stress the need for coughing and deep-breathing exercises.

Because many patients with CML receive outpatient chemotherapy throughout the chronic phase, sound patient teaching is essential:

♦ Explain expected adverse effects of chemotherapy. Pay particular attention to

dangerous adverse effects such as bone marrow suppression.
◆ Tell the patient to watch for and immediately report signs and symptoms of infection: any fever over 100° F (37.8° C), chills, redness or swelling, sore throat, and cough.
◆ Instruct the patient to watch for signs of thrombocytopenia, to immediately apply ice and pressure to any external bleeding site, and to avoid aspirin and aspirin-containing compounds because of the risk of increased bleeding.
◆ Emphasize the importance of adequate rest to minimize the fatigue of anemia. To minimize the toxic effects of chemotherapy, stress the importance of a high-calorie, high-protein diet.

For more information on treatment during the acute phase, see the treatment section of *Acute leukemia* on page 789.

CHRONIC LYMPHOCYTIC LEUKEMIA

A generalized, progressive disease that's common in the elderly, chronic lymphocytic leukemia (CLL) is marked by an uncontrollable spread of abnormal, small lymphocytes in lymphoid tissue, blood, and bone marrow. Nearly all patients with CLL are older than age 50, and it's slightly more common in men than in women. According to the American Cancer Society, this disease accounts for about 25% of all new leukemia cases annually.

Causes and incidence

Although the cause of CLL is unknown, researchers suspect hereditary factors (higher incidence has been recorded within families), still-undefined chromosome abnormalities, and certain immunologic defects (such as ataxia-telangiectasia or acquired agammaglobulinemia). The disease doesn't seem to be associated with radiation exposure, carcinogenic chemicals, or viruses.

About 2 out of every 100,000 people develop CLL annually, with 90% of cases found in people who are older than age 50. Many cases go undetected by routine blood tests in people who are asymptomatic. The disease is common in Jewish people of Russian or Eastern European descent, and is uncommon in Asia.

Pathophysiology

CLL is characterized by the clonal expansion of CD5+CD23+ B cells in blood, marrow, and second lymphoid tissues. Gene-expression profiling and phenotypic studies suggest that CLL is probably derived from CD5+ B cells similar to those found in the blood of healthy adults.

Complications
◆ Anemia
◆ Infection
◆ Splenomegaly

Signs and symptoms

CLL is the most benign and the most slowly progressive form of leukemia. Clinical signs derive from the infiltration of leukemic cells in bone marrow, lymphoid tissue, and organ systems.

In early stages, patients usually complain of fatigue, malaise, fever, and nodal enlargement. They're particularly susceptible to infection.

In advanced stages, patients may experience severe fatigue and weight loss, with liver or spleen enlargement, bone tenderness, and edema from lymph node obstruction. Pulmonary infiltrates may appear when lung parenchyma is involved. Skin infiltrations, manifested by macular to nodular eruptions, occur in about one half of the cases of CLL.

As the disease progresses, bone marrow involvement may lead to anemia, pallor, weakness, dyspnea, tachycardia, palpitations, bleeding, and infection. Opportunistic fungal, viral, and bacterial infections commonly occur in late stages.

Diagnosis

Typically, CLL is an incidental finding during a routine blood test that reveals numerous abnormal lymphocytes. (See *Histologic findings*

Histologic findings in chronic lymphocytic leukemia

The illustration shows the characteristic histologic findings in chronic lymphocytic leukemia.

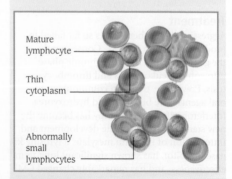

Mature lymphocyte

Thin cytoplasm

Abnormally small lymphocytes

in chronic lymphocytic leukemia.) In early stages, WBC count is mildly but persistently elevated. Granulocytopenia is the rule, but the WBC count climbs as the disease progresses. Blood studies also show Hb levels under 11 g, hypogammaglobulinemia, and depressed serum globulins. Other common developments include neutropenia (neutrophils count < 1,500/μL), lymphocytosis (lymphocytes count > 10,000/μL), and thrombocytopenia (platelets count < 150,000/μL). Bone marrow aspiration and biopsy show lymphocytic invasion.

Treatment

Systemic chemotherapy includes alkylating agents—usually chlorambucil, cyclophosphamide, vincristine, or fludarabine (singly or in combination)—and steroids (prednisone) when autoimmune hemolytic anemia or thrombocytopenia occurs.

An advance in the treatment of CLL has been the emergence of the humanized monoclonal antibodies rituximab and alemtuzumab. Alemtuzumab acts as an antibody against the surface of CLL cells and is used when fludarabine fails. Rituximab, a monoclonal antibody, acts similar to alemtuzumab; studies are ongoing.

When CLL causes obstruction or organ impairment or enlargement, local radiation treatment can be used to reduce organ size. Allopurinol can be given to prevent hyperuricemia, a relatively uncommon finding. In advanced stages, stem cell transplantation may be helpful.

Prognosis is poor if anemia, thrombocytopenia, neutropenia, bulky lymphadenopathy, and severe lymphocytosis are present.

Special considerations

◆ Plan patient care to relieve symptoms and prevent infection. Clean the patient's skin daily with mild soap and water. Frequent soaks may be ordered. Watch for signs or symptoms of infection: temperature over 100° F (37.8° C), chills, redness, or swelling of any body part.

◆ Watch for signs and symptoms of thrombocytopenia (black tarry stools, easy bruising, nosebleeds, bleeding gums) and anemia (pale skin, weakness, fatigue, dizziness, palpitations).

Advise the patient to avoid aspirin and products containing aspirin. Explain that many medications contain aspirin, even though their names don't make this clear. Teach the patient how to recognize aspirin variants on medication labels.

◆ Explain chemotherapy and its possible adverse effects. If the patient is to be discharged, tell the patient to avoid coming in contact with obviously ill people, especially children with common contagious childhood diseases. Urge the patient to eat high-protein foods and drink high-calorie beverages.

◆ Stress the importance of follow-up care, frequent blood tests, and taking all medications exactly as prescribed. Teach the patient the signs and symptoms of recurrence (swollen lymph nodes in the neck, axilla, and groin; increased abdominal size or discomfort), and tell the patient to notify their provider immediately if they detect any of these signs.

ELDER TIP *Most patients with CLL are elderly; many are frightened. Provide emotional support and be a good listener. Try to keep their spirits up by concentrating on little things, such as improving their personal appearance, providing a pleasant environment, and asking questions about their families. If possible, provide opportunities for their favorite activities.*

SELECTED REFERENCES

Ahlbom, A., et al; ICNIRP (International Commission for Non-Ionizing Radiation Protection) Standing Committee on Epidemiology. (2009). Epidemiologic evidence on mobile phones and tumor risk: A review. *Epidemiology, 20*(5), 639–652.

Albarello, L., et al. (2011). HER2 testing in gastric cancer. *Advances in Anatomic Pathology, 18*(1), 53–59.

Corradini, P., & Farina, L. (2010). Allogeneic transplantation for lymphoma: Long-term outcome. *Current Opinion in Hematology, 17*(6), 522–530.

McCorkle, R., et al. (2011). Healthcare utilization in women after abdominal surgery for ovarian cancer. *Nursing Research, 60*(1), 47–57.

Neves-E-Castro, M. (2008). Association of ovarian and uterine cancers with postmenopausal hormonal treatments. *Clinical Obstetrics and Gynecology, 51*(3), 607–617.

Rahbari, N., et al. (2011). Hepatocellular carcinoma: Current management and perspectives for the future. *Annals of Surgery, 253*(3), 453–469.

Shah, A., et al. (2010). Review and commentary on the role of radiation therapy in the adjuvant management of pancreatic cancer. *American Journal of Clinical Oncology, 33*(1), 101–106.

Suami, H., & Chang, D. (2010). Overview of surgical treatments for breast cancer-related lymphedema. *Plastic and Reconstructive Surgery, 126*(6), 1853–1863.

16

INFECTION

Introduction

Despite improved treatments and prevention including potent antibiotics, complex immunizations, and modern sanitation, infection still causes serious illness, even in highly industrialized countries. In developing countries, infection is a critical health problem.

WHAT IS INFECTION?

Infection is the invasion and multiplication of microorganisms in or on body tissues that produce signs and symptoms as well as an immune response. Such reproduction injures the host by causing cellular damage from microbal toxins or intracellular multiplication or by competing with host metabolism. The host's own immune response may increase tissue damage, which may be localized (e.g., as in infected pressure ulcers) or systemic. The severity of the infection depends on the pathogenicity and amount of the invading microorganisms and also on the strength of the hosts' defenses. The very young and the very old are most susceptible to infections.

Microorganisms that cause infectious diseases are difficult to overcome for many reasons:
- Some bacteria develop a resistance to antibiotics.
- Some microorganisms, such as human immunodeficiency virus (HIV), include many different strains, and a single vaccine cannot provide protection against all.
- Most viruses resist antiviral drugs.
- Some microorganisms localize in areas that make treatment difficult, such as the central nervous system (CNS) and bone.

Also, certain factors that normally contribute to improved health, such as availability of good nutrition, clean living conditions, and advanced medical care, can actually lead to increased risk of infection. For example, travel can expose people to diseases that they have little natural immunity against. Increased use of immunosuppressants, surgery, and other invasive procedures also increases the risk of infection.

KINDS OF INFECTIONS

A laboratory-verified infection that causes no signs and symptoms is called a *subclinical, silent,* or *asymptomatic infection.* A multiplication of microbes that produces no signs, symptoms, or immune response is called *colonization.* A person with a subclinical infection or colonization may be a carrier and transmit the infection to others. A *latent infection* occurs after a microorganism has been dormant in the host, sometimes for years. An *exogenous infection* results from environmental pathogens or sources other than the host; an *endogenous infection* results from the host's normal flora (for instance, *Escherichia coli* displaced from the colon, which causes urinary tract infection).

Microorganisms responsible for infectious diseases include bacteria, viruses, rickettsiae, chlamydiae, fungi (yeasts and molds), and protozoa; larger organisms such as helminths (parasitic worms) may also cause infectious disease.

Bacteria are single-cell microorganisms with well-defined cell walls that can grow independently on artificial media without the need for other cells. Bacteria inhabit the intestines of humans and other animals as normal flora used in the digestion of food.

Also found in soil, bacteria are vital to soil fertility. These microorganisms break down dead tissue, which allows it to then be used by other organisms.

Despite the many types of known bacteria, only a small percentage is harmful to humans. (See *How bacteria damage tissue.*) In developing countries, where poor sanitation increases the risk of infection, bacterial diseases commonly cause death and disability. In industrialized countries, bacterial infections are the most common fatal infectious diseases.

Bacteria are classified by shape. Spherical bacterial cells are called *cocci*; rod-shaped bacteria, *bacilli*; and spiral-shaped bacteria, *spirilla*. Bacteria are also classified according to their response to staining (gram-positive, gram-negative, or acid-fast bacteria); their motility (motile or nonmotile bacteria); their tendency toward encapsulation (encapsulated or nonencapsulated bacteria); and their capacity to form spores (sporulating or nonsporulating bacteria).

Spirochetes are bacteria with flexible, slender, undulating spiral rods that have cell walls. Most are anaerobic. The three forms pathogenic in humans include *Treponema*, *Leptospira*, and *Borrelia*.

Viruses are subcellular organisms made up only of a ribonucleic acid or a deoxyribonucleic acid nucleus covered with proteins. They're the smallest known organisms (so tiny they're visible only through an electron microscope). Independent of host cells, viruses can't replicate. Rather, they invade a host cell and stimulate it

---

PATHOPHYSIOLOGY
How bacteria damage tissue

The human body is constantly colonized and often infected by bacteria and other infectious organisms. Some are beneficial, such as the intestinal bacteria that produce vitamins. Others are harmful, causing illnesses ranging from the common cold to life-threatening septic shock.

To infect a host, bacteria must first enter it. They do this either by adhering to the mucosal surface and directly invading the host cell or by attaching to epithelial cells and producing toxins that eventually invade the host cells. To survive and multiply within a host, bacteria or their toxins adversely affect biochemical reactions in cells. This causes a disruption of normal cell function or cell death (see illustration below). For example, the diphtheria toxin damages heart muscle by inhibiting protein synthesis. Also, as some organisms multiply, they extend into deeper tissues and eventually gain access to the bloodstream.

Some toxins cause blood to clot in the smaller blood vessels. As a result, the tissues supplied by these vessels may become deprived of blood and subsequently damaged (see illustration below).

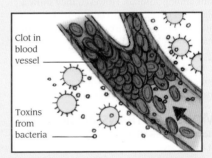

Other toxins can damage the cell walls of the smaller blood vessels, causing leakage. This fluid loss can result in decreased blood pressure, which in turn impairs the heart's ability to pump enough blood to the vital organs (see illustration below).

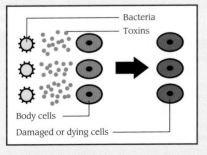

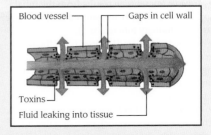

to participate in the formation of additional virus particles. The estimated 400 viruses that infect humans are classified according to their size, shape (spherical, rod shaped, or cubic), or means of transmission (respiratory, fecal, oral, or sexual).

Rickettsiae are relatively uncommon in the United States. They're small, gram-negative organisms classified as bacteria that commonly induce life-threatening infections. Like viruses, they require a host cell (such as human or insect) for replication. Three genera of rickettsiae include *Rickettsia, Coxiella,* and *Ehrlichia.*

Chlamydiae are smaller than rickettsiae and bacteria but larger than viruses. They also depend on host cells for replication but, unlike viruses, they're susceptible to antibiotics.

Fungi are single-cell organisms, with nuclei enveloped by nuclear membranes. They have rigid cell walls like plant cells but lack chlorophyll, the green matter necessary for photosynthesis; they also show relatively little cellular specialization. Fungi occur as yeasts (single-cell, oval-shaped organisms) or molds (organisms with hyphae, or branching filaments). Depending on the environment, some fungi may occur in both forms. Fungal diseases in humans are called *mycoses.*

Protozoa are the simplest single-cell organisms among animals. However, they show a high level of cellular specialization. Like other animal cells, they have cell membranes rather than cell walls, and their nuclei are surrounded by nuclear membranes.

In addition to these microorganisms, infectious diseases may also result from larger parasites, such as roundworms or flatworms.

MODES OF TRANSMISSION

Most infectious diseases are transmitted in one of four ways.

♦ In *contact transmission,* the susceptible host comes into direct contact (as in contact with blood or body fluids) or indirect contact (contaminated inanimate objects or the close-range spread of respiratory droplets) with the source. The most common method of contact transmission is contaminated hands.

♦ *Airborne transmission* results from the inhalation of contaminated aerosolized droplet nuclei (as in pulmonary tuberculosis).

♦ In *enteric (oral–fecal) transmission,* the infecting organisms are found in feces and are ingested, in many cases through fecally contaminated food or water (as in salmonella infections).

♦ *Vector-borne transmission* occurs when an intermediate carrier (vector), such as a flea, mosquito, or other animal, transfers an organism.

Many actions can be taken to prevent the transmission of infectious diseases, including:
♦ comprehensive immunization (including required immunization of travelers to, or emigrants from, endemic areas)
♦ drug prophylaxis
♦ improved nutrition, living conditions, and sanitation
♦ correction of environmental factors
♦ widespread disease tracking

Immunization can now control many diseases, including diphtheria, tetanus, pertussis, measles, rubella, some forms of meningitis, poliovirus, hepatitis B, pneumococcal pneumonia, influenza, rabies, and tetanus. Smallpox (variola)—which killed and disfigured millions—was believed to have been successfully eradicated by a comprehensive World Health Organization program of surveillance and immunization. However, in light of recent concerns regarding bioterrorism, smallpox is considered a potential agent. Healthcare personnel must recognize potential cases of smallpox and initiate appropriate precautions as well as notify health department officials. Smallpox vaccination may be appropriate for certain emergency and first-response healthcare providers.

Vaccines, which contain live but attenuated (weakened) or killed microorganisms, and toxoids, which contain modified bacterial exotoxins, induce active immunity against bacterial and viral diseases by stimulating antibody formation. Natural active immunity is produced as a patient who has the disease forms antibodies against it, thus preventing the recurrence of the disease. Immune globulins contain previously formed antibodies from hyperimmunized donors or pooled plasma and provide temporary passive immunity. Generally, passive immunization is used when active immunization is perilous or impossible or when complete protection requires both active and passive immunization. It may also be appropriate in situations requiring immediate protection such as postexposure in which active immunity from immunizations takes too long to provide the necessary and immediate protection. Maternal passive immunity crosses the placental barrier from mother to fetus and is also provided to the infant by antibodies present in breast milk.

Although preventive antibiotic therapy may prevent certain diseases, the risk of superinfection and the emergence of drug-resistant strains may outweigh the benefits. Therefore, preventive antibiotics are usually reserved for patients at high risk for exposure to dangerous infections. Antibiotic-resistant bacteria are on the rise mainly because antibiotics have been misused and overused. Some bacteria, such as enterococci, have developed mutant strains that don't respond to antibiotic therapy.

HEALTHCARE-ASSOCIATED INFECTIONS

A *healthcare-associated infection* is an infection that develops as a result of healthcare. Healthcare-associated infections were previously known as *nosocomial infections*, but the name was updated because these infections may be acquired from, or associated with, any portion of the healthcare delivery system, including such areas as outpatient care, ambulatory care, home care, or long-term care.

Healthcare-associated infections are usually transmitted by direct contact. Less commonly, transmission occurs by inhalation or by contact with contaminated equipment and solutions. Contamination of solutions during the manufacturing process is rare.

Despite facility programs of infection control that include surveillance, prevention, and education, about 1 in 25 patients who enter healthcare facilities contract a healthcare-associated infection. Staphylococcal infections, which had been declining since the 1960s, are currently a common cause of infection. Gram-negative bacilli, resistant enterococci, and fungal infections are also on the rise.

Healthcare-associated infections continue to be a difficult problem, because today's hospital patients are older and more debilitated with chronic underlying diseases than in the past. Also, the increased use of invasive and surgical procedures, immunosuppressants, and antibiotics predisposes patients to infection and superinfection. At the same time, the growing number of personnel who can come in contact with each patient makes the risk of exposure greater.

The following measures can help prevent healthcare-associated infections:
◆ Follow strict infection control procedures. (See *Standard precautions*, pages 799 and 780. See also *CDC isolation precautions*, page 801.)
◆ Document hospital infections as they occur.
◆ Identify outbreaks early, and take steps to prevent their spread.
◆ Eliminate unnecessary procedures that contribute to infection.
◆ Strictly follow necessary isolation techniques.
◆ Observe *all* patients for signs of infection, especially those patients at high risk.
◆ Always follow proper hand hygiene technique and encourage other staff members to follow these guidelines as well.
◆ Keep staff members and visitors with obvious infection and well-known carriers away from susceptible, high-risk patients.
◆ Take special precautions with vulnerable patients, such as those with indwelling urinary catheters, mechanical ventilators, or I.V. lines, and those recovering from surgery.

Standard precautions

The Centers for Disease Control and Prevention recommends that the following standard blood and body-fluid precautions be used for *all* patients. This is especially important in emergency care settings, where the risk of blood exposure is high and the patient's infection status is usually unknown.

It's important to remember that implementing standard precautions doesn't eliminate the need for maintaining other transmission-based precautions designed for specific airborne, droplet, and contact infectious diseases.

Sources of potential exposure
Standard precautions apply to blood, semen, vaginal secretions, and cerebrospinal, synovial, pleural, peritoneal, pericardial, and amniotic fluids. Standard precautions also apply to other body substances, such as feces, urine, nasal secretions, saliva, sputum, tears, vomitus, and breast milk.

Barrier precautions
◆ Wear gloves when touching blood and body fluids, mucous membranes, or the broken skin of patients; when handling items or touching surfaces soiled with blood or body fluids; and when performing venipuncture and other vascular access procedures.
◆ Change gloves and wash hands after contact with each patient.
◆ Wear a mask and protective eyewear, or a face shield, to protect the mucous membranes of the mouth, nose, and eyes during procedures that may generate the splatter of blood or other body fluids.
◆ In addition to the mask and protective eyewear or face shield, wear a gown or an apron during procedures that are likely

(continued)

Standard precautions (*continued*)

to cause splashing of blood or other body fluids.

♦ After removing gloves and other protective equipment, thoroughly wash hands and other skin surfaces that may be contaminated with blood or other body fluids.

Precautions for invasive procedures

♦ During all invasive procedures, wear gloves and a surgical mask and goggles or a face shield as appropriate.

♦ During procedures that commonly cause droplets or splashes of blood or other body fluids, or for those that generate bone chips, wear protective eyewear and a surgical mask or a face shield.

♦ During invasive procedures that are likely to cause splashing or a splattering of blood or other body fluids, wear a gown or an impervious apron.

♦ If performing or assisting in a vaginal or cesarean delivery, wear gloves and a gown when handling the placenta or the infant and during umbilical cord care.

♦ During spinal procedures (lumbar puncture, spinal and epidural anesthesia, myelogram), wear a face mask to prevent droplet spread of oral flora.

Work practice precautions

♦ To prevent needle-stick injuries, don't recap used needles, bend or break needles, remove needles from their disposable syringes or phlebotomy blood tube holders, or manipulate them.

♦ Whenever possible, use single-dose vials over multi-dose vials, especially when medications will be administered to multiple patients.

♦ Use a sterile, single-use, disposable syringe and needle for each injection.

♦ Use sharps safety devices. Activate safety mechanisms as directed.

♦ Place disposable syringes and needles, scalpel blades, and other sharps items in puncture-resistant containers for disposal. Make sure these containers are always located near the area of use.

♦ Place large-bore reusable needles in a puncture-resistant container for transport to the reprocessing area immediately after a procedure.

♦ If a glove tears or a needle-stick or other injury occurs, remove the gloves, wash your hands and the site of the needle-stick thoroughly, and put on new gloves as quickly as patient safety permits. Remove the needle or instrument involved in the incident from the sterile field. Promptly report injuries and mucous membrane exposure to the appropriate infection control practitioner per facility protocol.

Hand hygiene, either by washing with soap and water or by sanitizing with an alcohol-based sanitizer, is recognized as the most effective method of interrupting the transmission of infection. Plain soap is adequate for removing visible soil. Antimicrobial soap is encouraged for washing after contamination with blood or body fluids. Alcohol-based hand sanitizers, which reduce the number of viable microorganisms on the hands, are designed for waterless use. In the United States, these products usually contain 60% to 95% ethanol or isopropanol.

Indications for washing with either ordinary or antimicrobial soap include:

♦ when hands are visibly dirty or contaminated with proteinaceous material or visibly soiled with blood or other body fluids (even if gloves were worn)

♦ before eating and after using the restroom

♦ exposure to suspected or proven *Bacillus anthracis* (alcohol, chlorhexidine, iodophors, and other antiseptic agents have a poor potency against its spores)

♦ after caring for a patient with *Clostridium difficile* (alcohol, chlorhexidine, iodophors, and other antiseptic agents are largely ineffective against its spores)

Alcohol-based hand sanitizers may be used in all other clinical situations if the hands aren't visibly soiled.

Additional precautions

♦ Make sure mouthpieces, one-way valve masks, resuscitation bags, and other ventilation devices are available in areas where the need for resuscitation is likely. *Note:* Saliva has not been implicated in human immunodeficiency virus transmission.

♦ If you have any exudative lesions or weeping dermatitis, refrain from direct patient care and from handling patient care equipment until the condition resolves.

♦ Respiratory hygiene/cough etiquette includes covering the mouth and nose with a tissue when coughing and prompt disposal of used tissues, using surgical masks on the coughing person when tolerated, and hand hygiene before and after contact with respiratory secretions.

CDC isolation precautions

To help healthcare facilities maintain up-to-date isolation practices, the Centers for Disease Control and Prevention (CDC) and the Hospital Infection Control Practices Advisory Committee (HICPAC) have developed the *Guideline for Isolation Precautions: Preventing Transmission of Infectious Agents in Healthcare Settings.* The HICPAC/CDC guidelines contain two tiers of precautions to prevent transmission of infectious agents: standard precautions and transmission-based precautions. In addition, the guidelines also include recommendations for creating a protective environment for allogeneic hematopoietic stem cell (HSCT) patients.

Standard precautions

Standard precautions are designated for the care of all hospital patients regardless of their diagnosis or presumed infection. Standard precautions are the primary strategy for preventing nosocomial infection and take the place of universal precautions. These precautions apply to:

♦ blood
♦ all body fluids, secretions, and excretions—except sweat—regardless of whether or not they contain visible blood
♦ skin that is not intact
♦ mucous membranes

Transmission-based precautions

These precautions are instituted for patients who are known to be, or suspected of being, infected with a highly transmissible infection—one that requires precautions beyond those set forth for standard precautions. There are three types of transmission-based precautions: airborne, droplet, and contact precautions.

Airborne precautions

Airborne precautions are designed to reduce the risk of airborne transmission of infectious agents. Microorganisms carried through the air can be widely dispersed by air currents, making them available for inhalation or deposit on a susceptible host in the same room or at a longer distance from the infected patient if ventilation creates shared air space.

Airborne precautions include special air handling and ventilation procedures to prevent the spread of infection. They also require the use of respiratory protection such as a respirator (the N95 or higher disposable respirator or a powered air-purifying respirator)—in addition to standard precautions—when entering an infected patient's room.

Droplet precautions

Droplet precautions are designed to reduce the risk of transmitting infectious agents through large-particle (exceeding 5 µm) droplets. Such transmission involves the contact of infectious agents to the conjunctivae or to the nasal or oral mucous membranes of a susceptible person. Large-particle droplets don't remain in the air and generally travel short distances of 3′ (1 m) or less. They require the use of a surgical mask—in addition to standard precautions—to protect the mucous membranes.

Contact precautions

Contact precautions are designed to reduce the risk of transmitting infectious agents by direct or indirect contact. Direct-contact transmission can occur through patient care activities that require physical contact. Indirect-contact transmission involves a susceptible host coming in contact with a contaminated object, usually inanimate, in the patient's environment or with items contaminated with the patient's secretions, excretions, or blood outside of the patient's environment that may have been removed from the environment without appropriate cleaning and disinfection.

Contact precautions require the use of gloves and a gown—in addition to standard precautions—to avoid contact with the infectious agent. A mask is only required if there's a chance of splash or splatter of body fluids to the face. Stringent hand hygiene is also necessary after removal of the protective items.

Protective environment

A *protective environment* refers to isolation practices designed to decrease the risk of exposure to environmental fungal agents in allogeneic HSCT patients. Environmental controls include high-efficiency particulate air filtration of incoming air, directed room airflow, positive room air pressure relative to the corridor, well-sealed rooms that prevent infiltration of outside air, at least 12 air exchanges per hour, strategies to minimize dust (such as avoiding upholstery and carpet), and prohibiting dried and fresh flowers and potted plants in rooms of HSCT clients. In addition, during periods of construction or renovation, it is advised that severely immunocompromised patients wear a high-efficiency respiratory protection device when they are outside the protective environment.

ACCURATE ASSESSMENT VITAL

Accurate assessment helps identify infectious diseases and prevents avoidable complications. Complete assessment consists of patient history, physical examination, and laboratory data. The history should include the patient's sex, age, address, occupation, and place of work; known exposure to illness and recent medications, including antibiotics; and date of disease onset. Signs and symptoms, including their duration and whether they occurred suddenly or gradually, should be included in the history as well as precipitating factors, relief measures, and weight loss or gain. Detail information about recent hospitalization, blood transfusions, blood donation denial by the Red Cross or other agencies, recent travel or camping trips, exposure to animals, and vaccinations. (See *Immunization schedule.*) If applicable, ask about possible exposure to sexually transmitted diseases or about drug abuse. Also, try to determine the patient's resistance to infectious disease. Ask about usual dietary patterns, unusual fatigue,

and any conditions, such as neoplastic disease or alcoholism, that may predispose the patient to infection. Notice if the patient is listless or uneasy, lacks concentration, or has any obvious abnormality of mood or affect.

In suspected infection, a physical examination must assess the skin, mucous membranes, liver, spleen, and lymph nodes. Check for and make note of the location and type of drainage from any skin lesions. Record skin color, temperature, and turgor; ask if the patient has pruritus. Take the patient's temperature, using the same route consistently, and watch for a fever, which is the best indicator of many infections. Keep in mind that some patients, such as those who are immunocompromised, are unable to spike a fever. Note and record the pattern of temperature change and the effect of antipyretics. Be aware that certain analgesics may contain antipyretics. With a high fever, especially in children, watch for seizures.

Check the pulse rate. Infection commonly increases heart rate, but some infections, notably

Immunization schedule

Before immunization, ask the parents if the child is receiving corticosteroids or other drugs that suppress the immune response or if there has been a recent febrile illness. Obtain a history of allergic responses, especially to antibiotics, eggs, feathers, and past immunizations. Keep in mind that a child who's at risk for acquired immunodeficiency syndrome or who tests positive for human immunodeficiency virus infection may need special consideration.

After immunization, tell the parents to watch for and report reactions other than local swelling and pain and mild temperature elevation. Give them the child's immunization record. The following are the 2018 general vaccine recommendations approved by the Advisory Committee on Immunization Practices, the American Academy of Pediatrics, the American Academy of Family Physicians, and the American College of Obstetricians and Gynecologists.

Age	Immunization
Birth	HepB
1 to 4 months	HepB
2 months	DTaP, HIB, IPV, PCV, Rota
4 months	DTaP, HIB, IPV, PCV, Rota
6 months	DTaP, HIB, PCV, Rota
6 to 18 months	HepB, IPV
12 to 15 months	HIB, MMR, PCV, varicella
6 months to 18 years	Influenza (yearly)
12 to 23 months	HepA (×2 doses)
15 to 18 months	DTaP
4 to 6 years	DTaP, IPV, MMR, varicella
11 to 12 years	HPV, Tdap, meningococcal
16 years	Meningococcal

typhoid fever and psittacosis, may decrease it. Also observe for increased respiratory rate or a change in mental status. In severe infection or when complications are possible, watch for hypotension, hematuria, oliguria, hepatomegaly, jaundice, bleeding from gums or into joints, and an altered level of consciousness (LOC). Obtain laboratory studies and appropriate cultures as ordered.

Gram-positive cocci

STAPHYLOCOCCAL INFECTIONS

Staphylococci are gram-positive bacteria, either coagulase-negative (*Staphylococcus epidermidis*) or coagulase-positive (*Staphylococcus aureus*). Coagulase-negative staphylococci grow abundantly as normal flora on skin, but they can also cause boils, abscesses, and carbuncles. In the upper respiratory tract, they're usually nonpathogenic but can cause serious infections in some individuals such as those who are immunocompromised. Pathogenic strains of staphylococci are found in many adult carriers—usually on the nasal mucosa, axilla, or groin. Sometimes, carriers shed staphylococci, infecting themselves or other susceptible people. Coagulase-positive staphylococci tend to form pus and cause many different types of infections. (See *Comparing staphylococcal infections*, pages 804 to 808.)

METHICILLIN-RESISTANT *S. AUREUS* INFECTION
Causes and incidence

Methicillin-resistant *S. aureus* (MRSA) is a type of staphylococci that is resistant to the beta-lactam antibiotics (methicillin, oxacillin, penicillin, and amoxicillin). It is spread easily by direct person-to-person contact. Once limited to large teaching hospitals and tertiary care centers, MRSA infection is now endemic in nursing homes, long-term care facilities, and the community. In addition, community-acquired MRSA skin infections have been associated with athletic facilities, dormitories, military barracks, correctional facilities, and daycare centers.

Patients most at risk for MRSA infection include immunosuppressed patients, burn patients, intubated patients, and those with central venous catheters, surgical wounds, or dermatitis. Others at risk include those with prosthetic devices, heart valves, and postoperative wound infections. Additional risk factors include prolonged hospital stays, extended therapy with multiple or broad-spectrum antibiotics, and close proximity to those colonized or infected with MRSA. Patients with acute endocarditis, bacteremia, cervicitis, meningitis, pericarditis, and pneumonia are also at risk.

MRSA infection has become prevalent with the overuse of antibiotics. Over the years, this overuse has given once-susceptible bacteria the chance to develop defenses against antibiotics. This new capability allows resistant strains to flourish when antibiotics kill their more-sensitive cousins.

Pathophysiology

The evolution of MRSA is not well understood, but it is known that the prevalent strains today closely resemble that of the original ones. One characteristic that must be present for a strain to be considered MRSA is the antibiotic resistance gene for methicillin, called *mec*.

MRSA enters healthcare facilities through an infected or colonized patient or a colonized healthcare worker. Although MRSA has been recovered from environmental surfaces, it's transmitted mainly by healthcare workers' hands. Many colonized individuals become silent carriers. The most frequent site of colonization is the anterior nares (25% to 30% of people are colonized in the nares with *S. aureus*, <2% are colonized with MRSA). Other, less common sites are the groin, axilla, and the gut. Typically, MRSA colonization is diagnosed by isolating bacteria from nasal secretions.

In individuals in whom the natural defense system breaks down, such as after an invasive procedure, trauma, or chemotherapy, the normally benign bacteria can invade tissue, proliferate, and cause infection. Today, up to 90% of *S. aureus* isolates or strains are penicillin resistant, and about 50% of all *S. aureus* isolates are resistant to methicillin, a penicillin derivative, as well as to nafcillin and oxacillin. These strains may also resist cephalosporins, aminoglycosides, erythromycin, tetracycline, and clindamycin.

Complications
◆ Sepsis
◆ Death

Signs and symptoms

MRSA may start as small, red bumps that resemble pimples, boils, or spider bites. They can quickly turn into deep, painful abscesses. The bacteria can remain confined to the skin or they can burrow deep into the body and cause life-threatening infections in joints, bones, surgical wounds, heart valves, lungs, and the bloodstream.

Diagnosis

MRSA can be cultured from the suspected site with the appropriate method. For example, a wound can be swabbed for culture. Cultures of blood, urine, and sputum specimens will reveal sources of MRSA. Many laboratories

Comparing staphylococcal infections

Predisposing factors	Signs and symptoms	Diagnosis
Bacteremia		
◆ Infected surgical wounds ◆ Abscesses ◆ Infected I.V. or intra-arterial catheter sites or catheter tips ◆ Infected vascular grafts or prostheses ◆ Infected pressure ulcers ◆ Osteomyelitis ◆ Parenteral drug abuse ◆ Source unknown (primary bacteremia) ◆ Cellulitis ◆ Burns ◆ Immunosuppression ◆ Debilitating diseases, such as chronic renal insufficiency or diabetes ◆ Infective endocarditis (coagulase-positive staphylococci) and subacute bacterial endocarditis (coagulase-negative staphylococci) ◆ Cancer (leukemia) or neutrophil nadir after chemotherapy or radiation	◆ Fever (high fever with no obvious source in children younger than age 1), shaking chills, tachycardia ◆ Cyanosis or pallor ◆ Confusion, agitation, stupor ◆ Skin microabscesses ◆ Joint pain ◆ Complications: sepsis; shock; acute bacterial endocarditis (in prolonged infection; indicated by new or changing systolic murmur); retinal hemorrhages; splinter hemorrhages under nails and small, tender red nodes on pads of fingers and toes (Osler nodes); abscess formation in skin, bones, lungs, brain, and kidneys; pulmonary emboli if tricuspid valve is infected ◆ Prognosis depends on early diagnosis and treatment, and presence of other medical conditions	◆ Blood cultures (two to four samples from different sites at different times): growing staphylococci and leukocytosis (usually 12,000 white blood cells [WBCs]/μL), with a shift to the left of polymorphonuclear leukocytes (70% to 90% neutrophils) ◆ Urinalysis may show microscopic hematuria ◆ Erythrocyte sedimentation rate (ESR) elevated, especially in chronic or subacute bacterial endocarditis ◆ Prolonged partial thromboplastin time and prothrombin time; low fibrinogen and platelet counts, and low factor assays; possible disseminated intravascular coagulation ◆ Cultures of urine, sputum, and skin lesions with discharge may identify primary infection site; chest X-rays and scans of lungs, liver, abdomen, and brain may assist with identification ◆ Echocardiogram may show heart valve vegetation
Pneumonia		
◆ Immune deficiencies, especially in elderly and in children younger than age 2 ◆ Chronic lung diseases and cystic fibrosis ◆ Malignant tumors ◆ Antibiotics that kill normal respiratory flora but spare S. aureus ◆ Viral respiratory infections, especially influenza ◆ Hematogenous (bloodborne) bacteria spread to the lungs from primary sites of infection (such as heart valves, abscesses, and pulmonary emboli) ◆ Recent bronchial or endotracheal suctioning or intubation	◆ High temperature: adults, 103° to 105° F (39.4° to 40.6° C); children, 101° F (38.3° C) or above ◆ Cough, with purulent, yellow, or bloody sputum ◆ Dyspnea, crackles, and decreased breath sounds ◆ Pleuritic pain ◆ In infants: mild respiratory infection that suddenly worsens: irritability, anxiety, dyspnea, anorexia, vomiting, diarrhea, spasms of dry coughing, marked tachypnea, expiratory grunting, sternal retractions, and cyanosis ◆ Complications: necrosis, lung abscess, pyopneumothorax, empyema, pneumatocele, shock, hypotension, pleural effusions, respiratory failure, confusion	◆ WBC count may be elevated (15,000 to 40,000/μL in adults; 15,000 to 20,000/μL in children), with predominance of polymorphonuclear leukocytes ◆ Sputum Gram stain: mostly gram-positive cocci in clusters, with many polymorphonuclear leukocytes ◆ Sputum culture: mostly coagulase-positive staphylococci ◆ Chest X-rays: usually patchy infiltrates ◆ Arterial blood gas analysis: hypoxia and respiratory acidosis

Treatment	Special considerations
◆ Semisynthetic penicillins (oxacillin, nafcillin) or cephalosporins (cefazolin) given I.V. ◆ Vancomycin I.V. for patients with penicillin allergy or suspected methicillin-resistant organisms ◆ I.V. fluids to reverse shock ◆ Removal of infected catheter or foreign body ◆ Surgery	◆ Report infection to authorities as required. ◆ *S. aureus* bacteremia can be fatal within 12 hours. Be especially alert for it in debilitated patients with I.V. catheters or in those with a history of drug abuse. ◆ Administer antibiotics on time to maintain adequate blood levels, but give them slowly, using the prescribed amount of diluent, to prevent thrombophlebitis. ◆ Watch for signs of penicillin allergy, especially pruritic rash (anaphylaxis) and breathing difficulties. Keep epinephrine 1:1,000 and resuscitation equipment handy. Monitor the patient's vital signs, urine output, and mental state for signs of shock. ◆ Obtain cultures carefully, and observe for clues to the primary site of infection. Never refrigerate blood cultures; it delays identification of organisms by slowing their growth. ◆ If the patient has methicillin-resistant *S. aureus* (MRSA): regardless of site, place patient in contact precautions. ◆ Obtain peak and trough levels of vancomycin to determine the adequacy of treatment. ◆ Administer vancomycin I.V. slowly over 1 hour to avoid any adverse reactions.
◆ Semisynthetic penicillins (oxacillin, nafcillin) or cephalosporins (cefazolin) given I.V. ◆ Vancomycin I.V. for patients with penicillin allergy or suspected methicillin-resistant organisms ◆ Isolation for MRSA until the patient is off antibiotics and symptoms resolve (some facilities may require negative cultures)	◆ The Centers for Disease Control and Prevention's isolation guidelines require standard precautions unless MRSA, which requires contact precautions, is present. ◆ Keep the door to the patient's room closed. Don't store extra supplies in the room. Disposable suction containers are preferred. ◆ When obtaining sputum specimens, make sure to collect thick sputum, not saliva. The presence of epithelial cells (found in the mouth, not lungs) indicates a poor specimen. ◆ Administer antibiotics strictly on time, but slowly. Watch for signs of penicillin allergy and for signs of infection at the I.V. sites. Change the I.V. site every third day. ◆ Perform frequent chest physical therapy. Do chest percussion and postural drainage after intermittent positive pressure breathing treatments. Concentrate on consolidated areas (revealed by X-rays or auscultation).

(continued)

Comparing staphylococcal infections (*continued*)

Predisposing factors	Signs and symptoms	Diagnosis
Enterocolitis		
◆ Broad-spectrum antibiotics (tetracycline, chloramphenicol, or neomycin) or aminoglycosides (tobramycin, streptomycin, or kanamycin) as prophylaxis for bowel surgery or treatment of hepatic coma ◆ Usually occurs in elderly patients, but also in neonates (associated with staphylococcal skin lesions)	◆ Sudden onset of profuse, watery diarrhea usually 2 days to several weeks after start of antibiotic therapy, I.V. or by mouth (P.O.) ◆ Nausea, vomiting, abdominal pain and distention ◆ Hypovolemia and dehydration (decreased skin turgor, hypotension, fever)	◆ Stool Gram stain: many gram-positive cocci and polymorphonuclear leukocytes, with few gram-negative rods ◆ Stool culture: *S. aureus* ◆ Sigmoidoscopy: mucosal ulcerations ◆ Blood studies: leukocytosis, moderately increased blood urea nitrogen level, and decreased serum albumin level
Osteomyelitis		
◆ Hematogenous organisms ◆ Skin trauma ◆ Infection spreading from adjacent joint or other infected tissues ◆ *S. aureus* bacteremia ◆ Orthopedic surgery or trauma ◆ Cardiothoracic surgery ◆ Usually occurs in growing bones, especially femur and tibia, of children younger than age 12 ◆ More common in males	◆ Abrupt onset of fever—usually 101° F (38.3° C) or above; shaking chills; pain and swelling over infected area; restlessness; headache ◆ About 20% of children develop a chronic infection if not properly treated	◆ Possible history of prior trauma to involved area ◆ Positive bone and pus cultures (and blood cultures in about 50% of patients) ◆ X-ray changes apparent after second or third week ◆ ESR elevated with leukocyte shift to the left
Food poisoning		
◆ Enterotoxin produced by toxigenic strains of *S. aureus* in contaminated food (second most common cause of food poisoning in United States)	◆ Anorexia, nausea, vomiting, diarrhea, and abdominal cramps 1 to 6 hours after ingestion of contaminated food ◆ Symptoms usually subside within 18 hours, with complete recovery occurring in 1 to 3 days	◆ Clinical findings sufficient ◆ Stool cultures: usually negative for *S. aureus* ◆ Epidemiologic history: if others are ill and food history is a commonality; health department may be contacted for an outbreak

Treatment	Special considerations
♦ Broad-spectrum antibiotics discontinued ♦ Possibly, antistaphylococcal agents such as vancomycin P.O. ♦ Normal flora replenished with yogurt that contains live cultures	♦ Monitor vital signs frequently to detect early signs of shock. ♦ Force fluids to correct dehydration. ♦ Know serum electrolyte levels. Measure and record bowel movements when possible. Check serum chloride level for alkalosis (hypochloremia). Watch for dehydration and electrolyte imbalance. ♦ Collect serial stool specimens for Gram stain and culture to confirm diagnosis. (The effectiveness of therapy is usually measured by clinical response.) ♦ Observe standard precautions. Use contact precautions for diapered or incontinent children for duration of illness. ♦ Follow reporting requirements, especially in a group situation such as a nursing home. They may vary per facility protocol.
♦ Surgical debridement ♦ Prolonged antibiotic therapy (4 to 8 weeks) ♦ Vancomycin I.V. for patients with penicillin allergy or methicillin-resistant organisms ♦ Possibly, removal of prosthesis or hardware	♦ Identify the infected area, and mark it on the care plan. ♦ Check the penetration wound from which the organism originated for evidence of present infection. ♦ Severe pain may render the patient immobile. If so, perform passive range-of-motion exercises. Apply heat as needed, and elevate the affected part. (Extensive involvement may require casting until the infection subsides.) ♦ Before procedures such as surgical debridement, warn the patient to expect some pain. Explain that drainage is essential for healing, and that the patient will continue to receive analgesics and antibiotics after surgery.
♦ No treatment necessary unless dehydration becomes a problem (usually in infants and elderly); oral rehydrating solution or I.V. therapy may be necessary to replace fluids	♦ Monitor vital signs, fluid balance, and serum electrolyte levels. ♦ Check for dehydration if vomiting is severe or prolonged and for decreased blood pressure. ♦ Observe and report the number and color of stools. ♦ Report infection to authorities as required. ♦ Obtain a complete history of symptoms, recent meals, and other known cases of food poisoning.

(continued)

Comparing staphylococcal infections (*continued*)

Predisposing factors	Signs and symptoms	Diagnosis
Skin infections		
◆ Decreased resistance ◆ Burns or pressure ulcers ◆ Decreased blood flow ◆ Possible skin contamination from nasal discharge ◆ Foreign bodies ◆ Underlying skin diseases, such as eczema and acne ◆ Common in people with poor hygiene living in crowded quarters ◆ Insulin-dependent diabetes mellitus ◆ Hemodialysis ◆ I.V. drug injection	◆ Cellulitis—diffuse, acute inflammation of soft tissue (no discharge) ◆ Pus-producing lesions in and around hair follicles (folliculitis) ◆ Boil-like lesions (furuncles and carbuncles) extend from hair follicles to subcutaneous tissues; these painful, red, indurated lesions are 1 to 2 cm and have a purulent yellow discharge ◆ Small macules or skin blebs that may develop into vesicles containing pus (bullous impetigo); common in school-age children ◆ Mild or spiking fever ◆ Malaise	◆ Clinical findings and analysis of pus cultures if sites are draining ◆ Cultures of nondraining cellulitis taken from the margin of the reddened area by infiltration with 1 mL sterile saline solution (nonbacteriostatic saline) and immediate fluid aspiration

use oxacillin disks to check for staphylococcus sensitivity when testing culture specimens; resistance to oxacillin indicates MRSA. In addition, a rapid blood test, Staph SR Assay, can detect certain genes common in MRSA. This test, recently approved by the U.S. Food and Drug Administration (FDA), can provide results in 2 hours.

Treatment

To eradicate MRSA colonization in the nares, the physician may order topical mupirocin to be applied inside the nostrils. Other protocols involve combining a topical agent and an oral antibiotic. Most facilities keep patients in isolation until surveillance cultures are negative.

The Centers for Disease Control and Prevention (CDC) recommends incision and drainage as the first-line treatment for mild abscesses. If antibiotics are needed in the hospital setting, vancomycin or daptomycin are the drugs of choice. (See *Vancomycin-resistant infections*, page 809.) In the community setting, oral medications such as clindamycin, trimethoprim-sulfamethoxazole, or doxycycline are reasonable choices for treatment. Treatment should be tailored to susceptibility testing, however. For serious MRSA infections, an infectious disease specialist should be consulted.

Special considerations

◆ People in contact with the patient should perform hand hygiene before and after patient care.

◆ Good hand hygiene is the most effective way to prevent MRSA infection from spreading.

◆ Use an antiseptic soap such as chlorhexidine. Bacteria have been cultured from worker's hands washed with milder soap. One study showed that, without proper hand hygiene, MRSA could survive on healthcare workers' hands for up to 3 hours. Chlorhexidine has a residual antimicrobial effect on the skin.

◆ Contact isolation precautions should be used when in contact with the patient. A disinfected private room should be made available with dedicated equipment.

◆ Change gloves when contaminated or when moving from a "dirty" area of the body to a clean one.

◆ Instruct the patient's family and friends to wear protective clothing when they visit, and show them how to dispose of it properly.

◆ Provide teaching and emotional support to the patient and family members.

◆ Consider grouping infected patients together and having the same nursing staff provide care.

◆ Don't lay equipment used on the patient on the bed or bed stand. Be sure to wipe it with appropriate disinfectant before leaving the room.

◆ Ensure judicious and careful use of antibiotics. Encourage physicians to limit their use.

◆ Instruct the patient to take antibiotics for the full period prescribed, even if he or she begins to feel better.

Treatment	Special considerations
◆ Topical ointments; gentamicin or bacitracin-neomycin-polymyxin ◆ P.O. trimethoprim-sulfamethoxazole, doxycycline, minocycline, clindamycin; vancomycin or daptomycin for methicillin-resistant organisms ◆ Application of heat to reduce pain ◆ Surgical drainage ◆ Identification and treatment of sources of reinfection (nostrils, perineum) ◆ Cleaning and covering the area with moist, sterile dressings	◆ Identify the site and extent of infection. ◆ Keep lesions clean with saline solution and peroxide irrigations, as ordered. Cover infections near wounds or the genitourinary tract with gauze pads. Keep pressure off the site to facilitate healing. ◆ Be alert for the extension of skin infections. ◆ Severe infection or abscess may require surgical drainage. Explain the procedure to the patient. Determine if cultures will be taken, and be prepared to collect a specimen. ◆ Impetigo is contagious. Isolate the patient and alert the family. Use contact precautions for all draining lesions. ◆ Use contact precautions for duration of illness for major skin/wound infections where there is no dressing or dressing does not adequately contain drainage.

STREPTOCOCCAL INFECTIONS

Streptococci are small gram-positive bacteria, spherical to ovoid in shape, and linked together in pairs or chains. Several species occur as part of normal human flora in the respiratory, gastrointestinal (GI), and genitourinary tracts. Although researchers have identified a growing number of species of streptococci, three classes—groups A, B, and D—cause most of the infections. (See *Comparing streptococcal infections*, pages 810 to 815.) Organisms belonging to groups A and B beta-hemolytic streptococci are associated with a characteristic pattern of human infections. Most disorders due to group D streptococcus are caused by *Enterococcus faecalis*, formerly called *Streptococcus faecalis*, or *S. bovis*. Group C and group G streptococci have been identified as the etiologic agent in such infections as bacteremia, meningitis, pharyngitis, osteomyelitis, and neonatal sepsis.

Vancomycin-resistant infections

Some *S. aureus* organisms have developed resistance to vancomycin. In some cases, the resistance is considered intermediate-strength resistance and is known as vancomycin intermittent-resistant *S. aureus* (VISA). Another mutation, vancomycin-resistant *S. aureus* (VRSA), is fully resistant to vancomycin.

Researchers believe VISA and VRSA enter healthcare facilities through an infected or colonized patient or a colonized healthcare worker. They spread through direct contact between the patient and caregiver or between patients. They may also be spread through patient contact with contaminated surfaces.

Patients with laboratory-confirmed VISA or VRSA must be placed in a single room on contact precautions, and the number of healthcare workers involved in patient care should be limited. Other patients who shared the patient's room should be checked for VISA or VRSA colonization using an anterior nares culture. (Notify the laboratory to look specifically for *S. aureus* and to check sensitivity).

People involved in direct care of the patient before the initiation of contact precautions should be interviewed regarding the extent of their interactions. Those with extensive interaction should have an anterior nares culture. The local health department should be notified immediately. Antimicrobial treatment may include an increased dosage of vancomycin (for VISA only) and linezolid, quinupristin and dalfopristin (for life-threatening vancomycin-resistant *Enterococcus faecium*), or a combination of other antimicrobials according to the sensitivity pattern of the organism.

Comparing streptococcal infections

Streptococcus pyogenes (Group A streptococcus)

Streptococcal pharyngitis (strep throat)

◆ Accounts for 20% to 30% of pharyngitis in children and 5% to 15% in adults.
◆ Most common in children ages 5 to 15, from October to April
◆ Spread by direct person-to-person contact via droplets of saliva or nasal secretions
◆ Organism usually colonizes throats of persons with no symptoms
◆ Up to 20% of school children may be carriers

◆ After 2- to 5-day incubation period: temperature of 101° to 104° F (38.3° to 40° C), sore throat with severe pain on swallowing, beefy red pharynx, tonsillar exudate, edematous tonsils and uvula, swollen glands along the jaw line, generalized malaise and weakness, anorexia, occasional abdominal discomfort
◆ Fever abates in 3 to 5 days; nearly all symptoms subside within a week

◆ Clinically indistinguishable from viral pharyngitis
◆ Rapid antigen detection test (RADT) can be used for diagnosis
◆ Throat culture showing group A beta-hemolytic streptococci (carriers have positive throat culture). This is the gold standard test.
◆ Elevated white blood cell (WBC) count

Scarlet fever (scarlatina)

◆ Usually follows streptococcal pharyngitis; may follow wound infections or puerperal sepsis
◆ Caused by streptococcal strain that releases an erythrogenic toxin
◆ Most common in children ages 2 to 10
◆ Spread by large respiratory droplets or direct contact with items soiled with respiratory secretions

◆ Streptococcal sore throat, fever, strawberry tongue, fine erythematous rash that blanches on pressure and resembles sunburn with goose bumps
◆ Rash usually appears first on upper chest, then spreads to neck, abdomen, legs, and arms, sparing soles and palms; flushed cheeks, pallor around mouth
◆ Skin sheds during convalescence

◆ Characteristic rash and strawberry tongue
◆ RADT
◆ Positive throat culture or Gram stain showing S. pyogenes from nasopharynx
◆ Granulocytosis

Erysipelas

◆ Occurs primarily in infants and adults older than age 30
◆ Usually follows streptococcal pharyngitis
◆ Exact mode of spread to skin unknown

◆ Sudden onset, with reddened, swollen, raised lesions (skin looks like an orange peel), usually on face and scalp, bordered by areas that often contain easily ruptured blebs filled with yellow-tinged fluid; lesions sting and itch; lesions on the trunk, arms, or legs usually affect incision or wound sites
◆ Other symptoms: vomiting, fever, headache, cervical lymphadenopathy, sore throat

◆ Typical reddened lesions
◆ Culture taken from edge of lesions showing group A beta-hemolytic streptococci
◆ Throat culture almost always positive for group A beta-hemolytic streptococci

♦ Mastoiditis, peritonsillar abscess, or cervical lymphadenitis
♦ Rarely, bacteria spread and may cause arthritis, endocarditis, meningitis, osteomyelitis, or liver abscess
♦ Poststreptococcal sequelae: acute rheumatic fever or acute glomerulonephritis

♦ Penicillin or erythromycin, analgesics, and antipyretics may be ordered.
♦ Stress the need for bed rest and droplet precaution isolation from other children for 24 hours after antibiotic therapy begins; the patient should finish the prescription, even if symptoms subside; abscess, glomerulonephritis, and rheumatic fever can occur.
♦ Tell the patient not to skip doses and to properly dispose of soiled tissues.

♦ Although rare, complications are similar to those with strep throat and include peritonsillar abscesses, cervical lymphadenitis, and spread of strep

♦ Penicillin or erythromycin may be ordered.
♦ Keep the patient in isolation for the first 24 hours.
♦ Carefully dispose of purulent discharge.
♦ Stress the need for prompt and complete antibiotic treatment.

♦ Untreated lesions on trunk, arms, or legs may involve large body areas and lead to death

♦ Mild infection can be treated with oral penicillin, cephalexin, or clindamycin. More severe infections can be treated with intravenous cefazolin.
♦ Cold packs, analgesics, and topical anesthetics may be used to increase comfort.
♦ Prevention includes prompt treatment of streptococcal infections and drainage and secretion precautions.

(continued)

Comparing staphylococcal infections (*continued*)

Impetigo (streptococcal pyoderma)

♦ Common in children ages 2 to 5 in hot, humid weather; high rate of familial spread
♦ Predisposing factors: close contact in schools, overcrowded living quarters, poor skin hygiene, minor skin trauma
♦ May spread by direct contact, environmental contamination, or arthropod vector

♦ Small macules rapidly develop into vesicles, then become pustular and encrusted, causing pain, surrounding erythema, regional adenitis, cellulitis, and itching; scratching spreads infection
♦ Lesions commonly affect the face, heal slowly, and leave depigmented areas

♦ Characteristic lesions with honey-colored crust
♦ Culture and Gram stain of swabbed lesions showing *S. pyogenes*

Streptococcus agalactiae (Group B streptococcus)

Neonatal streptococcal infections

♦ Incidence of early-onset infection (age 6 days or younger): 0.23/1,000 live births
♦ Incidence of late-onset infection (age 7 days to 3 months): 0.3 to 0.4/1,000 live births
♦ Spread by vaginal delivery or hands of nursery staff
♦ Predisposing factors: maternal genital tract colonization, membrane rupture over 24 hours before delivery, crowded nursery
♦ Mortality rate is 5% of infants and adults

♦ Early onset: bacteremia, pneumonia, and meningitis
♦ Late onset: bacteremia with meningitis, fever, and bone and joint involvement
♦ Other signs and symptoms, such as skin lesions, depend on the site affected

♦ Isolation of group B streptococcus from blood, cerebrospinal fluid (CSF), or skin
♦ Chest X-ray showing massive infiltrate similar to that of respiratory distress syndrome or pneumonia

Adult group B streptococcal infection

♦ Most adult infections occur in postpartum women, usually in the form of endometritis or wound infection following cesarean section
♦ Incidence of group B streptococcal endometritis: identified in 2% to 14% of cases as single organism but also frequently as part of polymicrobial infections
♦ Group B streptococcal bacteremia and pneumonia: occur in the elderly and frequently in patients with diabetes
♦ Invasive group B streptococcal infection: occurs in patients with human immunodeficiency virus, diabetes, malignancy, or advanced hepatic or renal disease

♦ Fever, malaise, and uterine tenderness
♦ Change in lochia
♦ Bacteremia and pneumonia patients: can exhibit neurologic symptoms such as a change in mental status

♦ Isolation of group B streptococcus from blood or infection site

♦ Septicemia (rare)
♦ Ecthyma, a form of impetigo with deep ulcers

♦ Topical mupirocin if area affected is limited; if widespread, I.V. dicloxacillin or cephalexin may be ordered.
♦ Perform frequent washing of lesions with antiseptics, such as povidone-iodine or antibacterial soap, followed by thorough drying.
♦ Isolate a patient with draining wounds, using contact precautions.
♦ Prevention includes good hygiene and proper wound care.

♦ Overwhelming pneumonia, sepsis, and death

♦ Ampicillin and gentamicin may be ordered empirically (depends on site and whether early or late onset), but PCN G is the definitive treatment
♦ Patient isolation is unnecessary unless an open draining lesion is present, but proper hand hygiene is essential; for a draining lesion, take drainage and secretion precautions.
♦ Group B streptococcus prophylaxis may be ordered for women who are pregnant if vaginal or rectal cultures are positive at 35 to 37 weeks' gestation or if the patient meets other criteria, such as delivery earlier or later than 3 weeks of term, amniotic fluid rupture for 18 hours or more, or an intrapartum— temperature greater than or equal to 100.4° F [38.0° C]).

♦ Bacteremia followed by meningitis or endocarditis

♦ Ampicillin, PCN G, or cephalexin may be ordered.
♦ Perform careful observation for symptoms of infection following delivery.
♦ Follow drainage and secretion precautions.

(continued)

Comparing staphylococcal infections (*continued*)

Streptococcus pneumoniae

Pneumococcal pneumonia

♦ Accounts for 5% to 15% of bacterial pneumonia cases in the United States ♦ More common in those with HIV, cancer, diabetes, COPD, alcoholism, cochlear implants ♦ Spread by droplets and contact with infective secretions ♦ Other predisposing factors: trauma, viral infection, overcrowded living quarters, asplenia	♦ Sudden onset with severe shaking chills, temperature of 102° to 105° F (38.9° to 40.6° C), bacteremia, cough (with thick, scanty, blood-tinged sputum) accompanied by pleuritic pain ♦ Malaise, weakness, and prostration common ♦ Tachypnea, anorexia, nausea, and vomiting less common ♦ Severity of pneumonia usually caused by host's cellular defenses, not bacterial virulence	♦ Gram stain of sputum showing gram-positive diplococci; culture showing *S. pneumoniae* ♦ Chest X-ray showing lobular consolidation in adults; bronchopneumonia in children and elderly patients ♦ Elevated WBC count ♦ Blood cultures usually positive for *S. pneumoniae*

Streptococcus pneumoniae

Otitis media

♦ High incidence, with about 76% to 95% of all children having otitis media at least once (*S. pneumoniae* causes half of these cases.)	♦ Ear pain, ear drainage, hearing loss, fever, lethargy, and irritability ♦ Other possible symptoms: vertigo, nystagmus, and tinnitus	♦ Fluid in middle ear ♦ Isolation of *S. pneumoniae* from aspirated fluid if necessary

Meningitis

♦ Can follow bacteremic pneumonia, mastoiditis, sinusitis, skull fracture, or endocarditis ♦ Occurs in 17 per 100,000 children less than 5 years old ♦ Mortality rates are highest in infants and elderly people	♦ Fever, headache, nuchal rigidity, vomiting, photophobia, lethargy, coma, wide pulse pressure, and bradycardia	♦ Isolation of *S. pneumoniae* from CSF or blood culture ♦ Increased CSF cell count and protein level; decreased CSF glucose level ♦ Computed tomography scan of head ♦ EEG

Group D streptococcus

Endocarditis

♦ Group D streptococcus (enterococcus): causes 6% of all bacterial endocarditis ♦ Most common in elderly people and in those who abuse I.V. substances ♦ Typically follows bacteremia from an obvious source, such as a wound infection, urinary tract infection, or I.V. insertion site infection ♦ Most cases are subacute ♦ Also causes urinary tract infection	♦ Weakness, fatigability, weight loss, fever, night sweats, anorexia, arthralgia, splenomegaly, and new systolic murmur	♦ Anemia, increased erythrocyte sedimentation rate and serum immuno-globulin level, and positive blood culture for group D streptococcus ♦ Echocardiogram showing vegetation on valves

♦ Pleural effusion (occurs in 40% of patients)
♦ Pericarditis (rare)
♦ Lung abscess (rare)
♦ Bacteremia
♦ AMI or cardiac arrhythmias such as atrial fibrillation
♦ Death possible if bacteremia is present

♦ Penicillin or a third-generation cephalosporin
♦ Monitor and support respirations, as needed.
♦ Record sputum color and amount.
♦ Prevent dehydration.
♦ Avoid sedatives and opioids to preserve cough reflex.
♦ Carefully dispose of all purulent drainage (standard precautions); advise high-risk patients to receive a vaccine and to avoid infected people.

♦ Recurrent attacks (may cause hearing loss)

♦ Amoxicillin or ampicillin and analgesics may be ordered.
♦ Tell the patient to report a lack of response to therapy after 72 hours.

♦ Persistent hearing deficits, seizures, hemi-paresis, or other nerve deficits
♦ Encephalitis

♦ Ampicillin plus cefotaxime if <1 month; vancomycin plus third-generation cephalo-sporin in most other groups; add ampicillin if >50
♦ Monitor the patient closely for neurologic changes.
♦ Watch for symptoms of septic shock, such as acidosis and tissue hypoxia.

♦ Embolization
♦ Pulmonary infarction
♦ Osteomyelitis

♦ Penicillin G or ceftriaxone for *Streptococcus bovis* (non-enterococcal group D strepto-coccus) may be ordered.
♦ Penicillin or ampicillin *and* an aminoglyco-side for enterococcal group D streptococcus may be ordered.

Clinically, there are three states of streptococcal infection: carrier, acute, and delayed nonsuppurative complications. In the carrier state, the patient is infected with a disease-causing species of streptococci without evidence of infection. In the acute form, streptococci invade the tissues and cause physical symptoms. In the delayed nonsuppurative complication state, specific signs and symptoms associated with streptococcal infection occur. These include those associated with the inflammatory state of acute rheumatic fever, chorea, and glomerulonephritis. If further complications occur, they usually appear about 2 weeks after the acute illness, but they may be evident after a nonsymptomatic illness.

NECROTIZING FASCIITIS
Causes and incidence
Most commonly referred to as *flesh-eating bacteria*, necrotizing fasciitis is a progressive, rapidly spreading inflammatory infection located in the deep fascia that destroys fascia and fat with secondary necrosis of subcutaneous tissue. Also referred to as *hemolytic streptococcal gangrene*, *acute dermal gangrene*, *suppurative fasciitis*, and *synergistic necrotizing cellulites*, necrotizing fasciitis is most commonly caused by the pathogenic bacteria *S. pyogenes*, also known as group A *Streptococcus* (GAS), although other aerobic and anaerobic pathogens may be present.

This severe and potentially fatal infection may begin at the site of a small insignificant wound or surgical incision. It's characterized by invasive and progressive necrosis of the soft tissue and underlying blood supply. (See *Necrotizing fasciitis.*) The high mortality rates associated with it have been attributed to the emergence of more virulent strains of streptococci caused by changes in the bacteria's deoxyribonucleic acid.

This would account for an increase in the frequency and severity of the cases reported since 1985, following a 50- to 60-year span of clinical insignificance. Noted for decades and described in the medical literature since the Civil War, necrotizing fasciitis accounts for 8% of reported cases of invasive GAS infections today. The mortality rate is very high, at 70% to 80%. Mortality drops significantly and prognosis improves with early intervention and treatment. Cases treated aggressively with surgery, antibiotics, and hyperbaric oxygen therapy have seen mortality rates reduced to as low as 9% to 20%.

Men are three times more likely to develop this rare condition than women, and the disease rarely occurs in children except in countries with poor hygienic practices. The mean age of the population contracting the disease is 38 to 44 years.

Pathophysiology
More than 80 types of the causative bacteria *S. pyogenes* are in existence, making the epidemiology of GAS infections most complex. Wounds as minor as pinpricks, needle punctures, bruises, blisters, and abrasions or as serious as a traumatic injury or surgical incision can provide an opportunity for bacteria to enter the body.

In necrotizing fasciitis, group A beta-hemolytic *Streptococcus* and *S. aureus*, working alone or together, are most commonly the primary infecting bacteria. They can enter the host via local tissue injury or through a breach in the integrity of a mucous membrane barrier. Other aerobic and anaerobic pathogens, including *Bacteroides, Clostridium, Peptostreptococcus,* Enterobacteriaceae, coliforms, *Proteus, Pseudomonas,* and *Klebsiella,* may be present. They can proliferate in an environment of tissue hypoxia caused by trauma, recent surgery, or medical compromise. The end product of this invasion is necrosis of the surrounding tissue, which accelerates the disease process by creating an even more favorable environment for the organisms.

Complications
◆ Renal failure
◆ Septic shock
◆ Cardiovascular collapse
◆ Scarring
◆ Myositis
◆ Myonecrosis

Signs and symptoms
Pain, out of proportion to the size of the wound or injury it's associated with, is usually the first symptom of necrotizing fasciitis. It generally presents before all other physical findings.

Necrotizing fasciitis

Below is a picture of necrotizing fasciitis of the leg

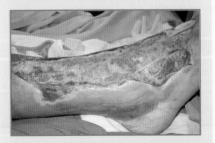

The infective process will usually begin with a mild area of erythema at the site of insult, which will quickly progress within the first 24 hours. During the first 24- to 48-hour period, the erythema changes from red to purple and then to blue, with the formation of fluid-filled blisters and bullae that indicate the rapid progression of the necrotizing process. By days 4 and 5, multiple patches of this erythema form, producing large areas of gangrenous skin. By days 7 to 10, dead skin begins to separate at the margins of the erythema, revealing extensive necrosis of the subcutaneous tissue. At this stage, fascial necrosis is typically more advanced than appearance would suggest.

Other clinical symptoms include fever and hypovolemia. In later stages, hypotension and respiratory insufficiency, which are signs of overwhelming sepsis requiring supportive care, occur. In the most severe cases, necrosis advances rapidly until several large areas of the body are involved. This may cause the patient to become mentally cloudy, delirious, or even unresponsive secondary to the intoxication rendered.

Other complications include renal failure, septic shock with cardiovascular collapse, and scarring with cosmetic deformities. Without treatment, involvement of deeper muscle layers may occur, resulting in myositis or myonecrosis.

Diagnosis

Tissue biopsy during surgical exploration is the best method of diagnosing necrotizing fasciitis. Cultures of microorganisms can be obtained locally from the periphery of the spreading infection or from deeper tissues during surgical debridement. Gram stain and culturing of biopsied tissue are useful in establishing the type of invasive organisms and the effective treatment against them.

Radiographic studies can pinpoint the presence of subcutaneous gases, and computed tomography (CT) scans can locate the anatomic site of involvement by locating the necrosis. In combination with clinical assessment, magnetic resonance imaging (MRI) determines areas of necrosis and the need for surgical debridement. While this testing may be useful, it should not delay surgical intervention.

Other supportive studies include blood cultures and laboratory values such as complete blood count with differential, electrolytes, glucose, blood urea nitrogen and creatinine, liver function tests, lactate levels, inflammatory markers, urinalysis, and arterial blood gas (ABG) levels.

Other conditions to consider in the differential diagnosis include cellulitis, testicular torsion, epididymitis and orchitis (as related to Fournier gangrene), gas gangrene, hernias, and toxic shock syndrome (TSS).

Treatment

Prompt and aggressive exploration and debridement of suspected necrotizing fasciitis is mandatory for early, definitive diagnosis and to improve prognosis. Ninety percent of patients who present with clinical signs and symptoms will need immediate surgical debridement, fasciotomy, or amputation.

Currently, empiric antibiotic regimens include a carbapenem (imipenem, meropenem) or beta-lactam-beta-lactamase inhibitor (piperacillin-tazobactam, ampicillin-sulbactam), plus vancomycin or linezolid, plus clindamycin. Blood and tissue cultures will dictate appropriate adjustment of antibiotics once these results are available.

Other treatments may include measures to ensure hemodynamic stability such as intravenous fluids, albumin administration, and vasopressors.

Special considerations

◆ Antibiotic therapy should be initiated immediately.

◆ Accurate and frequent assessment of the patient's pain level, mental status, wound status, and vital signs is essential in order to recognize the progression of the wound changes or the development of new signs and symptoms. Changes must be reported and documented immediately.

◆ The need for supportive care, such as endotracheal intubation, cardiac monitoring, fluid replacement, and supplemental oxygen, should be assessed and provided as warranted.

◆ Care of postoperative patients and patients with trauma wounds requires strict sterile technique, good hand hygiene, and barriers between healthcare providers and patients to prevent contamination.

◆ Use contact precautions for draining wounds for 24 hours after beginning appropriate antibiotic therapy. Use droplet precautions, especially for bedside wound debridement. Outbreaks of serious invasive disease have occurred secondary to transmission among patients and healthcare workers.

◆ Healthcare workers with sore throats should see their physician to determine if they have a streptococcal infection. If they are diagnosed positive, they shouldn't return to work until 24 hours after the initiation of antibiotic therapy.

◆ Risk factors for contracting necrotizing fasciitis include patients with advanced age, HIV infection, history of alcohol abuse, and varicella infection. Patients with chronic illnesses, such as cancer, diabetes, cardiopulmonary disease, and kidney disease requiring hemodialysis, as well as those using steroids are more susceptible to GAS infection due to their debilitated immune response.

▼ **ALERT** *Watch for signs and symptoms of TSS, which is associated with any streptococcal soft-tissue infection, and the development of shock, acute respiratory distress syndrome (ARDS), renal impairment, or bacteremia, any of which can lead to sudden death.*

VANCOMYCIN INTERMITTENT-RESISTANT *S. AUREUS*

Vancomycin intermittent-resistant S. *aureus* (VISA) is a mutation of a bacterium that's easily spread by direct person-to-person contact. It was first discovered in mid-1996 in a Japanese infant's surgical wound; similar isolates were later reported in Michigan and New Jersey. The U.S. patients had received multiple courses of vancomycin for MRSA infections.

Another mutation, vancomycin-resistant S. *aureus* (VRSA), is fully resistant to vancomycin.

Causes and incidence

VISA or VRSA enters a healthcare facility through an infected or colonized (symptom-free but infected) patient or colonized healthcare worker. It's spread during direct contact between the patient and caregiver or patient to patient. It may also be spread through patient contact with contaminated surfaces, such as an overbed table. It's able to live for weeks on surfaces. It has been detected on patient gowns, bed linens, and handrails.

A colonized patient is more than 10 times as likely to become infected with the organism, such as through a breach in the immune system. Patients most at risk for infection include immunosuppressed patients or those with severe underlying disease; patients with a history of taking vancomycin, third-generation cephalosporins, or antibiotics targeted at anaerobic bacteria (such as C. *difficile*); patients with indwelling urinary or central venous catheters; elderly patients, especially those with prolonged or repeated facility admissions; patients with malignancies or chronic renal failure; patients undergoing cardiothoracic or intra-abdominal surgery or organ transplants; patients with wounds with an opening to the pelvic or intra-abdominal area, such as surgical wounds, burns, and pressure ulcers; patients with enterococcal bacteremia,

often associated with endocarditis; and patients exposed to contaminated equipment or to a patient with the infecting microbe.

Complications
◆ Sepsis
◆ Multisystem organ involvement
◆ Death

Signs and symptoms

The carrier patient is commonly asymptomatic but may have signs and symptoms related to the primary diagnosis. Depending on the source of the infection and the reason for treatment, the patient may exhibit cardiac, respiratory, or other major symptoms. Assessment should focus on the affected body system.

Diagnosis

The causative agent may be found incidentally when culture results show the organism. A person with no signs or symptoms of infection is considered colonized if VISA or VRSA can be isolated from stool or a rectal swab.

Treatment

Because no single antibiotic to combat VISA or VRSA is currently available, combinations of various drugs are typically used, depending on the source of the infection. Daptomycin and ceftaroline are reasonable choices for combination therapy.

To prevent the spread of VISA and VRSA, some hospitals perform weekly surveillance cultures on at-risk patients in intensive care units or oncology units and those transferred from a long-term care facility. Any colonized patient is then placed in contact isolation until the culture is negative or at discharge. Colonization can last indefinitely; no protocol has been established for the length of time a patient should remain in isolation.

The CDC and the Hospital Infection Control Practices Advisory Committee implemented a two-level system of precautions to simplify isolation for resistant organisms. The first level calls for standard precautions. The second level calls for transmission-based precautions, implemented when a particular infection is suspected.

Special considerations

◆ Wash your hands before and after providing patient care. Good handwashing is the most effective way to prevent VISA and VRSA from spreading. Use an antiseptic soap such as chlorhexidine; bacteria have been cultured from workers' hands after washing with milder soap.

◆ Minimize the number of staff caring for the patient.

◆ Contact isolation precautions should be used when in contact with the patient. A private room should be used. Use dedicated equipment and disinfect the environment.

◆ Change gloves when contaminated or when moving from a soiled area of the body to a clean one.

◆ Wear mask/eye protection or a face shield when performing splash-generating activities, such as suctioning.

◆ Don't touch potentially contaminated surfaces, such as a bed or bed stand, after removing gown and gloves.

◆ Be particularly cautious in caring for a patient with an ileostomy, colostomy, or draining wound that isn't contained by a dressing.

◆ Equipment used on the patient shouldn't be laid on the bed or bed stand and should be wiped with appropriate disinfectant before leaving the room.

◆ Ensure judicious and careful use of antibiotics. Encourage physicians to limit the use of antibiotics.

◆ Instruct family and friends to wear protective garb when they visit the patient. Demonstrate how to dispose of it.

◆ Provide teaching and emotional support to the patient and family members.

◆ Instruct the patient to take antibiotics for the full prescription period, even if he or she begins to feel better.

◆ Contact public health authorities before transfer or discharge.

VANCOMYCIN-RESISTANT ENTEROCOCCUS INFECTION

Vancomycin-resistant enterococcus (VRE) is a mutation of a common bacterium normally found in the GI tract that is spread easily by direct person-to-person contact. VRE is common, most occurring in hospital settings.

Patients most at risk for VRE infection include:

◆ immunosuppressed patients or those with severe underlying disease

◆ patients with a history of taking vancomycin, third-generation cephalosporins, antibiotics targeted at anaerobic bacteria (such as *C. difficile*), or multiple courses of antibiotics

◆ patients with indwelling urinary or central venous catheters

◆ elderly patients, especially those with prolonged or repeated hospital admissions

◆ patients with cancer or chronic renal failure

◆ patients undergoing cardiothoracic or intra-abdominal surgery or organ transplant

◆ patients with wounds opening into the pelvic or intra-abdominal area, including surgical wounds, burns, and pressure ulcers

◆ patients with enterococcal bacteremia, typically associated with endocarditis

◆ patients exposed to contaminated equipment or to another VRE-positive patient

Causes and incidence

VRE enters healthcare facilities through an infected or colonized patient or a colonized healthcare worker. It can also develop following treatment with vancomycin. VRE spreads through direct contact between the patient and caregiver or between patients. It can also spread through patient contact with contaminated surfaces such as an overbed table, where it's capable of living for weeks. VRE has also been detected on patient gowns, bed linens, and handrails.

Complications

◆ Sepsis
◆ Multisystem dysfunction
◆ Pneumonia
◆ Meningitis
◆ Endocarditis
◆ Death (in immunocompromised patients)

Signs and symptoms

There are no specific signs and symptoms related to VRE infection. The causative agent may be found incidentally with culture results.

Diagnosis

Persons with no signs or symptoms of infection are considered colonized if VRE can be isolated from stool or a rectal swab.

Once colonized, a patient is more than 10 times as likely to become infected with VRE, for example, through a breach in the immune system.

Treatment

Antimicrobials, such as daptomycin and linezolid, are available for treatment of VRE infection if the strain is ampicillin-resistant. However, optimal treatment remains uncertain.

To prevent the spread of VRE, some facilities perform weekly surveillance cultures on at-risk patients in the intensive care or oncology units and on patients who have been transferred from a long-term care facility. Any colonized patient is then placed in contact isolation until culture-negative or until discharged. Colonization can last indefinitely; no protocol has been established for the length of time a patient should remain in isolation.

Special considerations
◆ Hand hygiene before and after care of the patient is crucial. Good hand hygiene is the most effective way to prevent VRE from spreading. Use an antiseptic soap such as chlorhexidine. Bacteria have been cultured from workers' hands after they've washed with milder soap. Alcohol-based hand sanitizers are effective as well.

◆ Use contact precautions when in contact with the patient or support equipment. Provide the patient with a private room and dedicated equipment. Disinfect the environment and the equipment frequently.

◆ Change gloves when contaminated or when moving from a "dirty" area of the body to a clean one.

◆ Don't touch potentially contaminated surfaces such as an overbed table after removing your gown and gloves.

◆ Be particularly prudent in caring for a patient with an ileostomy, colostomy, or draining wound that isn't contained by a dressing.

◆ Instruct the patient's family and friends to wear protective garb when they visit him, and teach them how to dispose of it. Instruct them on proper hand hygiene.

◆ Provide teaching and emotional support to the patient and family members.

◆ Consider grouping ("cohorting") infected or colonized patients together and assigning the same nursing staff to them.

◆ Don't lay equipment used on the patient on the bed or on the overbed table. Wipe the equipment with the appropriate disinfectant before leaving the room.

◆ Ensure judicious and careful use of antibiotics. Encourage physicians to limit their use.

◆ Instruct patients to take antibiotics for the full period prescribed, even if they begin to feel better.

◆ Report to public health authorities.

SCARLET FEVER
Causes and incidence
Although scarlet fever (scarlatina) usually follows streptococcal pharyngitis, it may also occur after other streptococcal infections, such as wound infections, urosepsis, and puerperal sepsis. It's most common in children ages 5 to 15. The incubation period commonly lasts from 2 to 4 days, but may be only 1 day or extend to 7 days.

Pathophysiology
Group A beta-hemolytic streptococci cause scarlet fever. The infecting strain produces one of three erythrogenic toxins, which triggers a local sensitivity reaction in the patient. This inflammatory reaction dilates the blood vessels and leads to the characteristic rash.

Complications
◆ Infection of the middle ear
◆ Pneumonia
◆ Acute rheumatic fever
◆ Hepatitis
◆ Glomerulonephritis

Signs and symptoms
The patient may report a sore throat, headache, chills, anorexia, abdominal pain, and malaise. A temperature of 101° to 103° F (38.3° to 39.4° C) is likely. In addition, he or she commonly has had contact with a person with a sore throat.

Inspection of the patient's mouth initially shows an inflamed and heavily coated tongue. As the disease progresses, the tongue takes on the appearance of strawberry. Eventually, the tongue begins to peel and becomes beefy red. It returns to normal by the end of the second week. The uvula, tonsils, and posterior oropharynx appear red and edematous, with mucopurulent exudate.

Inspection of the skin may reveal a fine, erythematous rash that appears first on the upper chest and back. It later spreads to the neck, abdomen, legs, and arms but doesn't appear on the soles and palms. The rash resembles sunburn with goose bumps and blanches when pressure is applied. The patient's face appears flushed, except around the mouth, which remains pale. During convalescence, desquamation of the skin occurs at the tips of the fingers and toes and, occasionally, over wide areas of the trunk and limbs. It's more pronounced where the erythematous rash was most severe.

The cervical lymph nodes feel enlarged and tender on palpation. The liver may also feel slightly enlarged and tender, and tachycardia may be noted.

Diagnosis
A pharyngeal culture is positive for group A beta-hemolytic streptococci. A complete blood count reveals granulocytosis and, possibly, a reduced red blood cell (RBC) count.

Treatment
Antibiotic therapy with penicillin or erythromycin is given for 10 days, along with antipyretics.

Special considerations
◆ Implement droplet precautions for 24 hours after starting antibiotic therapy.

◆ Keep the patient on complete bed rest while febrile to prevent complications, promote recovery, and help conserve energy.
◆ Offer frequent oral fluids and oral hygiene and give antipyretics as ordered.
◆ Apply topical anesthetics on the patient's tongue and throat to relieve pain.
◆ Provide skin care to relieve discomfort from the rash.
◆ Instruct the patient (or parents) to make sure they take oral antibiotics for the prescribed length of time.

Gram-negative cocci

MENINGOCOCCAL INFECTIONS

Causes and incidence

Two major meningococcal infections (meningitis and meningococcemia) are caused by the gram-negative bacteria *Neisseria meningitidis*, which also causes primary pneumonia, purulent conjunctivitis, endocarditis, sinusitis, and genital infection. Meningococcemia occurs as simple bacteremia, fulminating meningococcemia, and, rarely, chronic meningococcemia. It commonly accompanies meningitis. (See *Meningitis*, Chapter 3, page 174.) Meningococcal infections may occur sporadically or in epidemics; particularly virulent infections may be fatal within a matter of hours.

Meningococcal infections usually occur among children (ages 6 months to 2 years) and men, usually military recruits or those enrolled at institutions, such as colleges, because of overcrowding.

Pathophysiology

Neisseria meningitidis has seven serogroups (A, B, C, D, X, Y, and Z); group A causes most epidemics. Transmission takes place through inhalation of an infected droplet from a carrier (an estimated 2% to 38% of the population). The bacteria localize in the nasopharynx. After incubating about 3 to 4 days, they spread through the bloodstream to joints, skin, adrenal glands, lungs, and the CNS. The tissue damage that results (possibly due to the effects of bacterial endotoxins) produces symptoms and, in fulminating meningococcemia and meningococcal bacteremia, hemorrhage, thrombosis, and necrosis.

Complications

◆ Respiratory failure
◆ Disseminated intravascular coagulation (DIC)
◆ Septic arthritis
◆ Pericarditis
◆ Endophthalmitis
◆ Neurologic deterioration
◆ Death

Signs and symptoms

Features of *meningococcal bacteremia* include sudden spiking fever, headache, sore throat, cough, chills, myalgia (in back and legs), arthralgia, tachycardia, tachypnea, mild hypotension, and a petechial, nodular, or maculopapular rash. Headache and stiff neck can also occur as the infection extends to the meninges.

In about 10% to 20% of patients, the disease progresses to *fulminating meningococcemia*, with extreme prostration, enlargement of skin lesions, DIC, and shock. Without prompt treatment, death from respiratory or heart failure occurs in 6 to 24 hours.

Characteristics of the rare *chronic meningococcemia* include intermittent fever, rash, joint pain, and an enlarged spleen.

Diagnosis

CONFIRMING DIAGNOSIS *Gram-negative diplococci, on blood or cerebrospinal fluid (CSF) Gram stain, are highly suspicious for* N. meningitidis *isolation of* N. meningitidis *through a positive blood culture, CSF: culture, or lesion scraping confirms the diagnosis, except in nasopharyngeal infections because* N. meningitidis *is part of the normal nasopharyngeal flora.*

Tests that support the diagnosis include low white blood cell (WBC) count and, in patients with skin or adrenal hemorrhages, decreased platelet and clotting levels. Diagnostic evaluation must rule out Rocky Mountain spotted fever (RMSF) and vascular purpuras.

Treatment

As soon as meningococcal infection is suspected, treatment begins with a second-generation cephalosporin such as ceftriaxone along with vancomycin (due to increase in penicillin resistance) until cultures come back. Ampicillin may still be ordered in conjunction with these medications in adults >50. Some studies show that giving dexamethasone can decrease neurological effects and mortality; however, culture results should dictate continuation of this medication. Supportive measures include careful fluid and electrolyte maintenance, reducing intracranial pressure, ventilation (maintenance of a patent airway and oxygen, if necessary), insertion of an arterial or central venous pressure (CVP) line to monitor cardiovascular status, and bed rest.

Prophylaxis with ciprofloxacin, ceftriaxone, or rifampin aids healthcare personnel who work in close contact with the patient, such as those administering cardiopulmonary resuscitation or assisting with intubation or suctioning without wearing a surgical mask. In addition, anyone who has come into contact with the infected person, including family or child care providers, may need prophylactic antibiotics.

Special considerations

◆ Give I.V. antibiotics, as ordered, to maintain blood and CSF drug levels.

◆ Enforce bed rest in early stages. Provide a dark, quiet, restful environment.

◆ Maintain adequate ventilation with oxygen or a ventilator, if necessary. Suction and turn the patient frequently.

◆ Keep accurate intake and output records to maintain proper fluid and electrolyte levels. Monitor blood pressure, pulse, ABG levels, and CVP.

◆ Watch for complications, such as DIC, arthritis, endocarditis, and pneumonia.

◆ If the patient is receiving chloramphenicol, monitor complete blood count.

◆ Check the patient's drug history for allergies before giving antibiotics.

To prevent the infection's spread:

◆ Impose droplet precautions until the patient has had antibiotic therapy for 24 hours.

◆ Label all meningococcal specimens. Deliver them to the laboratory quickly because meningococci are very sensitive to changes in humidity and temperature.

◆ Report all meningococcal infections to public health department officials.

▓▓▓▓ **PREVENTION** *As a preventive measure, the meningococcal vaccine can be administered to first-year college students living in dormitories.*

Gram-positive bacilli

DIPHTHERIA
Causes and incidence

Diphtheria is an acute, highly contagious tox-in-mediated infection caused by *Corynebacterium diphtheriae*, a gram-positive rod that usually infects the respiratory tract, primarily the tonsils, nasopharynx, and larynx. The GI and urinary tracts, conjunctivae, and ears are rarely involved.

Diphtheria is more prevalent during the colder months because of closer person-to-person indoor contact; however, it may be contracted at any time during the year. Many more people carry this disease than contract active infection.

Thanks to effective immunization, diphtheria is rare in many parts of the world. In the United States, less than five cases have been reported to the CDC in the last 10 years.

Pathophysiology

Transmission usually occurs through intimate contact or by airborne respiratory droplets from asymptomatic carriers or convalescing patients. This causes inflammation in the respiratory tract and/or skin. As an exotoxin, it allows penetration into the cell membrane, where it then causes cell death.

Complications

◆ Thrombocytopenia
◆ Myocarditis
◆ Neurologic involvement (primarily affecting motor fibers but possibly also sensory neurons)
◆ Renal involvement
◆ Pulmonary involvement (bronchopneumonia) caused by *C. diphtheriae* or other superinfecting organisms

Signs and symptoms

Most infections go unrecognized, especially in partially immunized individuals. After an incubation period of less than a week, clinical cases of diphtheria characteristically show a thick, patchy, grayish green membrane over the mucous membranes of the pharynx, larynx, tonsils, soft palate, and nose; fever; sore throat; and a rasping cough, hoarseness, and other symptoms similar to croup. Attempts to remove the membrane usually cause bleeding, which is highly characteristic of diphtheria. If this membrane causes airway obstruction (particularly likely in laryngeal diphtheria), symptoms include tachypnea, stridor, possibly cyanosis, suprasternal retractions, and suffocation, if untreated. Adenopathy and cervical swelling can occur. In cutaneous diphtheria, skin lesions resemble impetigo.

Diagnosis

℞ **CONFIRMING DIAGNOSIS** *Examination showing the characteristic membrane and a throat culture, or culture of other suspect lesions growing C. diphtheriae, plus a positive toxin assay, confirm this diagnosis.*

Treatment

Treatment must not wait for confirmation by culture. Standard treatment includes diphtheria antitoxin administered I.M. or I.V.; antibiotics, such as erythromycin or penicillin G I.V. followed by penicillin V orally to eliminate the organisms from the upper respiratory tract and other sites and terminate the carrier state; measures to prevent complications; and possible tracheotomy if airway obstruction occurs.

Special considerations

Diphtheria requires comprehensive supportive care with psychological support.

◆ To prevent the spread of this disease, stress the need for droplet precautions. Teach proper disposal of nasopharyngeal secretions. Maintain infection precautions until after two consecutive negative nasopharyngeal cultures—at least 1 week after discontinuing drug therapy. Treatment of exposed individuals with antitoxin remains controversial. Suggest that the patient's family receive diphtheria toxoid if they haven't been immunized.

◆ Monitor respirations carefully, especially in laryngeal diphtheria (usually, such patients are in a high-humidity environment). Watch for signs of airway obstruction, and be ready to give immediate life support, including intubation and tracheotomy.

◆ Watch for signs of shock, which can develop suddenly.

◆ Obtain cultures as ordered.

◆ If neuritis develops, tell the patient it's usually transient. Be aware that peripheral neuritis may not develop until 2 to 3 months after the onset of illness.

⚠ ALERT *Be alert for signs of myocarditis, such as the development of heart murmurs or electrocardiogram changes. Ventricular fibrillation is a common cause of sudden death in patients with diphtheria.*

▓ PREVENTION *Stress the need for childhood immunizations to all parents. Protective immunity doesn't last longer than 10 years after the last vaccination, so it's important to get tetanus-diphtheria boosters every 10 years.*

◆ Report all cases to public health authorities.

LISTERIOSIS
Causes and incidence
Listeriosis is an infection caused by the weakly hemolytic, gram-positive bacillus *Listeria monocytogenes*. It occurs most commonly in fetuses, neonates (during the first 3 weeks of life), and in older or immunosuppressed adults. The infected fetus is usually stillborn or is born prematurely, almost always with lethal listeriosis. This infection produces milder illness in pregnant women and varying degrees of illness in older and immunosuppressed patients; their prognoses depend on the severity of underlying illness.

Pathophysiology
The primary method of person-to-person transmission is neonatal infection in utero (through the placenta) or during passage through an infected birth canal. Other modes of transmission may include inhaling contaminated dust; drinking contaminated, unpasteurized milk; eating unprocessed soft cheese or deli meats; coming in contact with infected animals, contaminated sewage or mud, or soil contaminated with feces containing *L. monocytogenes*; and, possibly, person-to-person transmission.

From 2009 to 2011, there were 0.29 cases per 100,000 people. From 2000 to 2008, the mortality rate from listeriosis was 16%.

Complications
◆ Sepsis
◆ Diffuse clotting dyscrasias
◆ Respiratory insufficiency
◆ Circulatory insufficiency
◆ Meningitis
◆ Cerebritis
◆ Nonpurulent conjunctivitis
◆ Granulomatous skin infection
◆ Long-term neurologic damage and delayed development in infants

Signs and symptoms
Contact with *L. monocytogenes* commonly causes a transient asymptomatic carrier state. But sometimes it produces bacteremia and a -febrile, generalized illness. In a pregnant woman, especially during the third trimester, listeriosis causes a mild illness with malaise, chills, fever, and back pain. However, a severe uterine infection may produce abortion, premature delivery, or stillbirth. Transplacental infection may also cause early neonatal death or granulomatosis infantiseptica, which produces organ abscesses in infants.

Infection with *L. monocytogenes* commonly causes meningitis (especially in immunocompromised patients), resulting in tense fontanels, irritability, lethargy, seizures, and coma in neonates and low-grade fever and personality changes in adults. Fulminant manifestations with coma are rare.

Diagnosis
℞ CONFIRMING DIAGNOSIS L. monocytogenes *is identified by its diagnostic tumbling motility on a wet mount of the culture of CSF or blood.*

MRI with contrast can help determine whether intracranial lesions are present when neurological symptoms are involved. Listeriosis also causes monocytosis.

Treatment
The treatment of choice is ampicillin or penicillin G with gentamicin I.V. infusion for 3 to 6 weeks. If gentamicin cannot be used, TMP-SMX is preferred.

Ampicillin or penicillin G is best for treating meningitis due to *L. monocytogenes* because they can easily cross the blood–brain barrier. Pregnant women require prompt, vigorous treatment to combat fetal infection.

Special considerations

◆ Deliver specimens to the laboratory promptly. Because few organisms may be present, take at least 10 mL of spinal fluid for culture.

◆ Use standard precautions until a series of cultures are negative. Be especially careful when handling lochia from an infected mother and secretions from her infant's eyes, nose, mouth, and rectum, including meconium.

◆ Evaluate neurologic status at least every 2 hours. In an infant, check fontanels for bulging. Maintain adequate I.V. fluid intake; measure intake and output accurately.

◆ If the patient has CNS depression and becomes apneic, provide respiratory assistance, monitor respirations, and obtain frequent ABG measurements.

◆ Provide adequate nutrition by total parenteral nutrition, nasogastric (NG) tube feedings, or a soft diet, as ordered.

◆ Allow the patient's parents to see and, if possible, hold their infant in the neonatal intensive care unit. Be flexible about visiting privileges. Keep the parents informed of the infant's status and prognosis at all times.

◆ Reassure the parents of an infected neonate who may feel guilty about the infant's illness.

◆ Report all cases to public health authorities.

▦▦▦ PREVENTION

◆ *Advise pregnant women to avoid infective materials on farms where listeriosis is endemic among livestock.*

◆ *To avoid infection, instruct the patient and his family to avoid soft cheeses and to cook such foods as hot dogs thoroughly. Immunocompromised patients should avoid soft cheeses and deli meats.*

TETANUS

Causes and incidence

Tetanus, also known as *lockjaw*, is an acute exotoxin-mediated infection caused by the anaerobic, spore-forming, gram-positive bacillus *Clostridium tetani*. This infection is usually systemic; less commonly, it is localized. Tetanus mortality has declined to about 10% of unimmunized people, usually within 10 days of onset. When symptoms develop within 3 days after exposure, the prognosis is poor.

Tetanus occurs worldwide, but is more prevalent in agricultural regions and developing countries that lack mass immunization programs. It's one of the most common causes of neonatal deaths in developing countries, where infants of unimmunized mothers are delivered under unsterile conditions. In such infants, the unhealed umbilical cord is the portal of entry.

In the United States, almost cases occur between April and September.

Pathophysiology

Normally, transmission occurs through a puncture wound that's contaminated by soil, dust, or animal excreta containing *C. tetani* or by way of burns and minor wounds. After *C. tetani* enters the body, it causes local infection and tissue necrosis. It also produces toxins that then enter the bloodstream and lymphatics and eventually spread to CNS tissue.

Complications

◆ Atelectasis
◆ Pneumonia
◆ Pulmonary emboli
◆ Acute gastric ulcers
◆ Seizures
◆ Flexion contractures
◆ Cardiac arrhythmias

Signs and symptoms

The incubation period varies from 3 to 21 days with a median of 8 days in mild tetanus to under 2 days in severe cases. When symptoms occur within 3 days after injury, death is more likely. If tetanus remains localized, signs of onset are spasm and increased muscle tone near the wound.

If tetanus is generalized (systemic), indications include marked muscle hypertonicity, hyperactive deep tendon reflexes, tachycardia, profuse sweating, low-grade fever, and painful, involuntary muscle contractions:

◆ neck and facial muscles, especially cheek muscles—locked jaw (trismus), painful spasms of masticatory muscles, difficulty opening the mouth, and *risus sardonicus*, a grotesque, grinning expression produced by spasm of facial muscles

◆ somatic muscles—arched-back rigidity (opisthotonos); board-like abdominal rigidity

◆ intermittent tonic seizures lasting several minutes, which may result in cyanosis and sudden death by asphyxiation

Despite such pronounced neuromuscular symptoms, cerebral and sensory functions remain normal. Complications can include atelectasis, pneumonia, pulmonary emboli, acute gastric ulcers, flexion contractures, and cardiac arrhythmias.

Neonatal tetanus is always generalized. The first clinical sign is difficulty in sucking, which usually appears 3 to 10 days after birth. It progresses to total inability to suck with excessive crying, irritability, and nuchal rigidity.

Diagnosis

Diagnosis must rest on clinical features, a history of trauma, and no previous tetanus immunization. Blood cultures and tetanus antibody tests are often negative; only a third of patients have a positive wound culture. CSF pressure may rise above normal. Diagnosis must also rule out meningitis, rabies, phenothiazine or strychnine toxicity, and other conditions that mimic tetanus.

Treatment

Within 72 hours after a puncture wound, a patient with no previous history of tetanus immunization first requires tetanus immune globulin (TIG) or tetanus antitoxin to neutralize the toxins and to confer temporary protection. Next, the patient needs active immunization with tetanus toxoid. If the patient hasn't received tetanus immunization within 10 years, a booster injection of tetanus toxoid is necessary. If tetanus develops despite immediate post-injury treatment, the patient will require airway maintenance and a muscle relaxant, such as diazepam, to decrease muscle rigidity and spasm. If muscle contractions aren't relieved by muscle relaxants, a neuromuscular blocker may be prescribed. The patient with tetanus needs high-dose antibiotics (metronidazole or penicillin G). The source of the toxin needs to be removed and destroyed through surgical exploration and wound debridement.

Special considerations

◆ Thoroughly debride and clean the injury site, and check the patient's immunization history. Record the cause of injury. If it's an animal bite, report the case to local public health authorities.
◆ Before giving penicillin and TIG, antitoxin, or toxoid, obtain an accurate history of allergies to immunizations or penicillin. If the patient has a history of allergies, keep epinephrine 1:1,000 and resuscitation equipment available.
◆ Stress the importance of maintaining active immunization with a booster dose of tetanus toxoid every 10 years.
After tetanus develops:
◆ Maintain an adequate airway and ventilation to prevent pneumonia and atelectasis. Suction often and watch for signs of respiratory distress. Keep emergency airway equipment on hand because the patient may require artificial ventilation or oxygen administration.
◆ Maintain an I.V. line for medications and emergency care, if necessary.
◆ Monitor the electrocardiogram frequently for arrhythmias. Record intake and output accurately, and check vital signs often.

◆ Turn the patient frequently to prevent pressure ulcers and pulmonary stasis.
◆ Because even minimal external stimulation provokes muscle spasms, keep the patient's room quiet and only dimly lighted. Warn visitors not to upset or overly stimulate the patient.
◆ If urine retention develops, insert an indwelling urinary catheter.
◆ Give muscle relaxants and sedatives, as ordered, and schedule patient care—such as passive range-of-motion exercises—to coincide with periods of heaviest sedation.
◆ Insert an artificial airway, if necessary, to prevent tongue injury and maintain airway during spasms.
◆ Provide adequate nutrition to meet the patient's increased metabolic needs. The patient may need NG feedings or total parenteral nutrition. (See *Preventing tetanus*, page 826.)

BOTULISM

Causes and incidence

Botulism, a life-threatening paralytic illness, results from an exotoxin produced by the gram-positive, anaerobic bacillus *Clostridium botulinum*. It occurs with botulism food poisoning, wound botulism, and infant botulism. The mortality from botulism is about 8%; death is usually caused by respiratory failure during the first week of illness.

Botulism is usually the result of ingesting inadequately cooked contaminated foods, especially those with low acid content, such as home-canned fruits and vegetables, sausages, and smoked or preserved fish or meat. Rarely, it's a result of wound infection with *C. botulinum*.

Botulism occurs worldwide and affects more adults than children. Recently, findings have shown that an infant's GI tract can become colonized with *C. botulinum* from some unknown source, and then the exotoxin is produced within the infant's intestine. Infant botulism is usually attributed to the ingestion of honey or corn syrup. Incidence had been declining, but the current trend toward home canning has resulted in an upswing (~250 cases per year in the United States) in recent years.

Pathophysiology

Botulism toxin can target multiple tissues, blocking cholinergic innervation of striated and smooth muscle, along with that of the tear, salivary, and sweat glands. It can also alter the release of neurotransmitters such as dopamine, serotonin, and somatostatin. These are some of the mechanisms that leads to the progressive neurologic defects seen in botulism.

PREVENTION

Preventing tetanus

Tetanus can be easily prevented through immunization against the toxin. Almost all cases of tetanus occur in people who've never been immunized or who haven't had a tetanus booster shot within the past 10 years. Having had a tetanus infection doesn't provide immunity. Following recommendations for vaccinations is necessary to prevent recurrence of tetanus.

The tetanus vaccine is usually given to children as part of the diphtheria and tetanus toxoids and pertussis (DTP) shot.

It's recommended that adolescents get a booster shot between ages 11 and 18, and that adults receive a routine tetanus booster shot every 10 years. In the event of a deep or dirty wound that occurs when more than 5 years have passed since the last booster shot, it is recommended that another booster be given. Tell your patient to follow these guidelines to help prevent tetanus infection.

Take care of a wound
Tell the patient to do the following:
♦ Rinse the wound thoroughly with clean water.
♦ Clean the wound and the area around it with soap and a washcloth.
♦ Contact a practitioner if debris is embedded in the wound.

Consider the wound source
♦ Tell the patient to contact a practitioner if the wound is deep, especially if it's dirty or is a result of an animal bite.
♦ Tell the patient to contact a practitioner if the date of the most recent tetanus shot is uncertain.

Use antibiotic ointment or cream
♦ After the wound has been cleaned, the patient should apply a thick layer of an antibiotic cream or ointment, such as the multi-ingredient antibiotics Neosporin or Polysporin.

Cover the wound
♦ Bandages can help keep the wound clean and keep harmful bacteria out. Have the patient cover blisters that are draining; they're vulnerable to infection until a scab forms.

Change the dressing
♦ To help prevent infection, tell the patient to apply a new dressing at least once per day or whenever the dressing becomes wet or dirty.

Complications
♦ Respiratory failure
♦ Paralytic ileus

Signs and symptoms
Symptoms usually appear within 18 to 36 hours (range is 6 hours to 10 days) after the ingestion of contaminated food. Severity varies with the amount of toxin ingested and the patient's degree of immunocompetence. Generally, early onset (within 24 hours) signals critical and potentially fatal illness. Initial signs and symptoms include dry mouth, sore throat, weakness, dizziness, vomiting, and diarrhea. The cardinal sign of botulism, though, is acute symmetrical cranial nerve impairment (ptosis, diplopia, and dysarthria), followed by descending weakness or paralysis of muscles in the extremities or trunk, and dyspnea from respiratory muscle paralysis. Such impairment doesn't affect mental or sensory processes and isn't associated with fever.

Infant botulism usually afflicts infants between ages 3 and 20 weeks and can produce hypotonic (floppy) infant syndrome. Signs and symptoms are constipation, feeble cry, depressed gag reflex, and inability to suck. Cranial nerve deficits also occur in infants and are manifested by a flaccid facial expression, ptosis, and ophthalmoplegia. Infants also develop generalized muscle weakness, hypotonia, and areflexia. Loss of head control may be striking. Respiratory arrest is likely.

Diagnosis
℞ CONFIRMING DIAGNOSIS *Identification of the offending toxin in the patient's serum, stool, gastric content, or the suspected food confirms the diagnosis. An electromyogram showing diminished muscle action potential after a single supramaximal nerve stimulus is also diagnostic. The decision to give antitoxin should be made based on presumptive diagnosis and should not be delayed while awaiting these results.*

Diagnosis also must rule out other diseases commonly confused with botulism, such as Guillain–Barré syndrome, myasthenia gravis, stroke, staphylococcal food poisoning, tick paralysis, chemical intoxications, carbon monoxide poisoning, fish poisoning, trichinosis, and diphtheria.

Treatment
Treatment consists of I.V. or I.M. administration of botulinum antitoxin (available through the state health department).

If breathing difficulty develops, intubation and mechanical ventilation may be required. I.V. fluids can be given if there are swallowing problems, and an NG tube can also be ordered.

Special considerations
If you suspect ingestion of contaminated food:
◆ Obtain a careful history of the patient's food intake for the past several days. See if other family members exhibit similar symptoms and share a common food history.
◆ Observe carefully for abnormal neurologic signs. Tell the patient's family to watch for signs of weakness, blurred vision, and slurred speech. If such signs appear, the patient must return to the hospital immediately.
◆ If ingestion has occurred within several hours, induce vomiting, begin gastric lavage, and give a high enema to purge any unabsorbed toxin from the bowel.

If clinical signs of botulism appear:
◆ Admit the patient to the intensive care unit, and monitor cardiac and respiratory functions carefully.
◆ Administer botulinum antitoxin, as ordered, to neutralize any circulating toxin. Before giving the antitoxin, be sure to obtain an accurate patient history of allergies, especially to horses, and perform a skin test. Afterward, watch for anaphylaxis or other hypersensitivity and serum sickness. Keep epinephrine 1:1,000 (for subcutaneous administration) and emergency airway equipment available.
◆ Assess respiratory function every 4 hours. Report decreased vital capacity on inspiratory effort and any signs of respiratory distress.
◆ Closely assess and accurately record neurologic function, including bilateral motor status (reflexes, ability to move arms and legs).
◆ Give I.V. fluids as ordered. Turn the patient often, and encourage deep-breathing exercises. Isolation isn't required.
◆ As botulism is sometimes fatal, keep the patient and family informed regarding the course of the disease.
◆ Immediately report all cases of botulism to public health authorities.

▨▨▨▨ **PREVENTION** *Encourage patients to observe*
◢◣◤ *proper techniques in processing and preserving*
foods. Warn them to avoid even tasting food from a bulging can or one with a peculiar odor and to sterilize by boiling any utensil that comes in contact with suspected food. Ingestion of even a small amount of food contaminated with botulism toxin can prove fatal. Avoid giving honey to infants younger than age 1 year.

GAS GANGRENE
Causes and incidence
Gas gangrene results from local infection with the anaerobic, spore-forming, gram-positive rod *Clostridium perfringens* (or another clostridial species). It occurs in devitalized tissues and results from compromised arterial circulation after trauma, surgery, compound fractures, or lacerations. This rare infection carries a high mortality unless therapy begins immediately; however, with prompt treatment, 80% of patients with gas gangrene of the extremities survive. The prognosis is poorer for gas gangrene in other sites, such as the abdominal wall or the bowel. The usual incubation period is 1 to 4 days but can vary from 3 hours to 6 weeks or longer.

Gas gangrene is rare, with only around 1,000 cases occurring in the United States annually.

Pathophysiology
Clostridium perfringens is a normal inhabitant of the GI and female genital tracts; it's also prevalent in soil. Transmission occurs by entry of organisms during trauma or surgery. Because *C. perfringens* is anaerobic and spore forming, gas gangrene is usually found in deep wounds, especially those in which tissue necrosis further reduces oxygen supply. Clostridium bacteria produce four different toxins (alpha, beta, epsilon, iota) that can cause potentially fatal symptoms. When *C. perfringens* invades soft tissues, it produces thrombosis of regional blood vessels, tissue necrosis, localized edema, and damage to the myocardium, liver, and kidneys. Such necrosis releases both carbon dioxide and hydrogen subcutaneously, producing interstitial gas bubbles. Gas gangrene usually occurs in the extremities and in abdominal wounds; it's less common in the uterus.

Complications
◆ Renal failure
◆ Shock
◆ Hemolytic anemia
◆ Jaundice with liver damage
◆ Tissue death
◆ Amputation

Signs and symptoms

True gas gangrene produces myositis and another form of this disease, involving only soft tissue, called *anaerobic cellulitis*. Most signs of infection develop within 72 hours of trauma or surgery. The hallmark of gas gangrene is crepitation (a crackling sensation when the skin is touched), a result of carbon dioxide and hydrogen accumulation as a metabolic by-product in necrotic tissues. Other typical indications are severe localized pain, swelling, and discoloration (usually dusky brown or reddish), with formation of bullae and necrosis within 36 hours from onset of symptoms. The skin over the wound may rupture, revealing dark red or black necrotic muscle, a foul-smelling watery or frothy discharge, intravascular hemolysis, thrombosis of blood vessels, and evidence of infection spread.

In addition to these local symptoms, gas gangrene produces early signs of toxemia and hypovolemia (tachycardia, tachypnea, and hypotension), with moderate fever usually not above 101° F (38.3° C). Although pale, prostrate, and motionless, patients with gas gangrene may exhibit toxic delirium and are extremely apprehensive. Possible sudden death is preceded by delirium and coma and is sometimes accompanied by vomiting, profuse diarrhea, and circulatory collapse.

ELDER TIP *Absence of a fever doesn't necessarily mean absence of infection in an elderly person. Many older adults develop a subnormal temperature in response to infection.*

Diagnosis

CONFIRMING DIAGNOSIS *A history of recent surgery or a deep puncture wound and the rapid onset of pain and crepitation around the wound suggest gas gangrene.*

Gas gangrene is confirmed by anaerobic cultures of wound drainage showing *C. perfringens*; a Gram stain of wound drainage showing large, gram-positive, rod-shaped bacteria; X-rays showing gas in tissues; and blood studies showing leukocytosis and, later, hemolysis. CT and MRI are also useful to determine whether infection is localized or more widespread.

Diagnosis must rule out synergistic gangrene and necrotizing fasciitis; unlike gas gangrene, both these disorders anesthetize the skin around the wound.

Treatment

Treatment includes careful observation for signs of myositis and cellulitis and *immediate treatment if these signs appear; immediate* wide surgical excision of all affected tissues and necrotic muscle in myositis (*delayed or inadequate surgical excision is a fatal mistake*); I.V. administration of high-dose penicillin plus clindamycin or tetracycline. The concurrent use of hyperbaric oxygenation is an option, as well, although it is controversial and should not be utilized in an unstable patient.

Special considerations

Careful observation may result in early diagnosis. Look for signs and symptoms of ischemia (cool skin; pallor or cyanosis; sudden, severe pain; sudden edema; and loss of pulses in involved limb).

After the diagnosis:
◆ Throughout this illness, provide adequate fluid replacement, and assess pulmonary and cardiac functions often. Maintain airway and ventilation.
◆ To prevent skin breakdown and further infection, give good skin care. After surgery, provide meticulous wound care. Use contact precautions for significant drainage.
◆ Before penicillin administration, obtain a patient history of allergies; afterward, watch closely for signs of hypersensitivity.
◆ Psychological support is critical, because these patients can remain alert until death, knowing that death is imminent and unavoidable.
◆ Deodorize the room to control foul odor from the wound. Prepare the patient emotionally for a large wound after surgical excision, and refer for physical rehabilitation, as necessary.
◆ Institute standard precautions. Use contact precautions if drainage is significant. Dispose of drainage material properly, and wear sterile gloves when changing dressings. Spore-forming bacteria aren't destroyed by ordinary disinfecting methods. Contaminated items should be cleaned and disinfected or sterilized, as appropriate.

PREVENTION
◆ *Routinely take precautions to render all wound sites unsuitable for growth of clostridia by attempting to keep granulation tissue viable; adequate debridement is imperative to reduce anaerobic growth conditions. The surgeon may delay closure of wounds.*
◆ *Be alert for devitalized tissues, and notify the surgeon promptly.*
◆ *Position the patient to facilitate drainage, and eliminate all dead spaces in closed wounds.*

ACTINOMYCOSIS
Causes and incidence
Actinomycosis is a rare infection primarily caused by the gram-positive anaerobic bacillus *Actinomyces israelii*, which produces granulomatous, suppurative lesions with abscesses. Common infection sites are the head, neck, thorax, and abdomen, but it can spread to contiguous tissues, causing multiple draining sinuses.

Actinomycosis affects twice as many males—especially those ages 15 to 35—as females. People with dental disease or HIV infection are at increased risk.

Pathophysiology
Actinomyces israelii occurs as part of the normal flora of the throat, tonsillar crypts, and mouth (particularly around carious teeth); infection results from its traumatic introduction into body tissues.

Complications
◆ Sinus and maxilla facial subcutaneous tissue involvement
◆ Abscesses and fistulas of the brain
◆ Pneumonia
◆ Empyema

Signs and symptoms
Symptoms appear from days to months after injury and may vary, depending on the site of infection.

In *cervicofacial actinomycosis* (lumpy jaw), painful, indurated swellings appear in the mouth or neck up to several weeks after dental extraction or trauma. They gradually enlarge and form fistulas that open onto the skin. Sulfur granules (yellowish gray masses that are actually colonies of *A. israelii*) appear in the exudate.

In *pulmonary actinomycosis*, aspiration of bacteria from the mouth into areas of the lungs already anaerobic from infection or atelectasis produces a fever and a cough that becomes productive and occasionally causes hemoptysis. Eventually, empyema follows, a sinus forms through the chest wall, and septicemia may occur.

In *GI actinomycosis*, ileocecal lesions are caused by swallowed bacteria, which produce abdominal discomfort, fever, sometimes a palpable mass, and an external sinus. This follows intestinal mucosa disruption, usually by surgery or an inflammatory bowel condition such as appendicitis.

Rare sites of actinomycotic infection are the bones, brain, liver, kidneys, and female reproductive organs. Symptoms reflect the organ involved.

Diagnosis
CONFIRMING DIAGNOSIS *Isolation of A. israelii in exudate or tissue confirms actinomycosis. Other tests that help identify this condition are:*
◆ *microscopic examination of sulfur granules*
◆ *Gram staining of excised tissue or exudate to reveal branching gram-positive rods*
◆ *chest X-ray to show lesions in unusual locations such as the shaft of a rib*

Treatment
Treatment is long term, with 1 to 2 months of penicillin I.V. followed by 6 to 12 months of penicillin taken by mouth. Erythromycin and clindamycin are usually acceptable alternatives. In some cases, surgical drainage of the lesion may be required.

Special considerations
◆ Dispose of all dressings in a sealed plastic bag.
◆ After surgery, provide proper sterile wound management.
◆ Administer antibiotics as ordered. Before giving the first dose, obtain an accurate patient history of allergies. Watch for hypersensitivity reactions, such as rash, fever, itching, and signs of anaphylaxis. If the patient has a history of any allergies, keep epinephrine 1:1,000 and resuscitation equipment available.

PREVENTION *Stress the importance of good oral hygiene and proper dental care.*

NOCARDIOSIS
Causes and incidence
Nocardiosis is an acute, subacute, or chronic bacterial infection caused by a weakly gram-positive species of the genus *Nocardia*—usually *Nocardia asteroides*. It's most common in men, especially those with a compromised immune system. In patients with brain infection, mortality exceeds 80%; in other forms, mortality is 10% in cases with uncomplicated pneumonia.

Pathophysiology
Nocardia are aerobic gram-positive bacteria with branching filaments resembling fungi. Normally found in soil, these organisms cause occasional sporadic disease in humans and animals throughout the world. Their incubation period is unknown but is probably several weeks. The usual mode of transmission is inhalation of organisms suspended in dust. Transmission by direct inoculation through puncture wounds or abrasions is less common.

Complications
◆ Meningitis
◆ Seizures
◆ Cardiac arrhythmias

Signs and symptoms
Nocardiosis originates as a pulmonary infection with a cough that produces thick, tenacious, purulent, mucopurulent, and possibly blood-tinged sputum. It may also cause a fever as high as 105° F (40.6° C), chills, night sweats, anorexia, malaise, and weight loss. This infection may lead to pleurisy, intrapleural effusions, and empyema. Other potential complications include tracheitis, bronchitis, pericarditis, endocarditis, peritonitis, mediastinitis, septic arthritis, and keratoconjunctivitis.

If the infection spreads through the blood to the brain, abscesses form, causing confusion, disorientation, dizziness, headache, nausea, and seizures. Rupture of a brain abscess can cause purulent meningitis. Extrapulmonary, hematogenous spread may cause endocarditis or lesions in the kidneys, liver, subcutaneous tissue, and bone.

Diagnosis
Identifying *Nocardia* by culture of sputum or discharge is difficult. In many cases, special staining techniques must be used to make the diagnosis, in conjunction with a typical clinical picture (usually progressive pneumonia, despite antibiotic therapy). Occasionally, diagnosis requires biopsy of lung or other tissue. Chest X-rays and CT may show fluffy or interstitial infiltrates, nodules, or abscesses.

In brain infection with meningitis, lumbar puncture shows nonspecific changes such as increased opening pressure. CSF shows increased WBC and protein levels and decreased glucose levels compared with serum glucose.

Treatment
Nocardiosis requires at least 6 months of treatment, preferably with trimethoprim-sulfamethoxazole. In patients who don't respond to sulfonamide treatment, other drugs, such as amikacin, ceftriaxone, or minocycline, may be added. Treatment also includes surgical drainage of abscesses and excision of necrotic tissue. The acute phase requires complete bed rest; as the patient improves, activity can increase.

Special considerations
Because it isn't transmitted from person to person, nocardiosis requires no isolation.

◆ Provide adequate nourishment through total parenteral nutrition, NG tube feedings, or a balanced diet.
◆ Give the patient tepid sponge baths and antipyretics, as ordered, to reduce fevers.
◆ Monitor for allergic reactions to antibiotics.
◆ High-dose sulfonamide therapy (especially sulfadiazine) predisposes the patient to crystalluria and oliguria; so assess frequently, encourage fluids, and alkalinize the urine with sodium bicarbonate, as ordered, to prevent these complications.
◆ In patients with pulmonary infection, administer chest physiotherapy. Auscultate the lungs daily, checking for increased crackles or consolidation. Note and record the amount, color, and thickness of sputum.
◆ In brain infection, regularly assess neurologic function. Watch for signs of increased intracranial pressure, such as a decreased LOC and respiratory abnormalities.
◆ In long-term hospitalization, turn the patient often, and assist with range-of-motion exercises.
◆ Before the patient is discharged, stress the need to follow a regular medication schedule to maintain therapeutic blood levels and to continue drugs even after symptoms subside. Explain the importance of frequent follow-up examinations.
◆ Provide support and encouragement to help the patient and family cope with this long-term illness.

CLOSTRIDIUM DIFFICILE INFECTION

Causes and incidence
Clostridium difficile is a gram-positive anaerobic bacterium that typically causes antibiotic-associated diarrhea. Symptoms may range from asymptomatic carrier states to severe pseudomembranous colitis and are caused by the exotoxins produced by the organism. Toxin A is an enterotoxin and toxin B is a cytotoxin.

Clostridium difficile colitis can be caused by almost any antibiotic that disrupts the bowel flora, but it's classically associated with clindamycin use. High-risk groups include individuals on greater numbers of antibiotics, those having abdominal surgery, patients receiving antineoplastics that have an antibiotic activity, immunocompromised individuals, pediatric patients (commonly in daycare centers), and nursing home patients.

Other factors that alter normal intestinal flora include enemas and intestinal stimulants. *C. difficile* is most often transmitted directly from patient to patient by contaminated hands of facility personnel; it may also be indirectly spread by contaminated equipment such as bedpans, urinals, call bells, rectal thermometers, NG tubes, and contaminated surfaces such as bed rails, floors, and toilet seats.

Pathophysiology

Toxins produced by the pathogen work on the gut to kill cells in the colon, decrease intestinal barrier function, and eventually lead to neutrophilic colitis.

Complications

- Electrolyte abnormalities
- Hypovolemic shock
- Anasarca (caused by hypoalbuminemia)
- Toxic megacolon
- Colonic perforation
- Peritonitis
- Sepsis
- Hemorrhage
- Death (rare)

Signs and symptoms

Risk of *C. difficile* begins 1 to 2 days after antibiotic therapy is started and extends for as long as 2 to 3 months after the last dose. The patient may be asymptomatic or may exhibit any of the following symptoms: soft, unformed, or watery diarrhea (more than three stools in a 24-hour period) that may be foul smelling or grossly bloody; abdominal pain, cramping, or tenderness; and fever. The patient's WBC count may be elevated to 20,000/μL. In severe cases, toxic megacolon, colonic perforation, and peritonitis may develop.

Diagnosis

Diagnosis is by identification of the toxin through one of these acceptable methods:
- *nucleic acid amplification test*—highly sensitive; improved over the cell cytotoxin test. Only one sample needed; results within an hour.
- *molecular tests*—the FDA has approved polymerase chain reaction (PCR) assay test for the gene encoding toxin B; this is usually completed with the nucleic acid test.
- *cell cytotoxin test*—tests for both toxin A and B. It's highly sensitive and specific for *C. difficile* but is rarely used due to the time it takes to perform—at least 2 days.
- *enzyme immunoassays (EIA)*—slightly less sensitive than the cell cytotoxin test but has a turnaround time of only a few hours. Specificity is excellent.
- *stool culture*—seldom used because of the turnaround time of 2 days to obtain results.

Non-toxin–producing strains of *C. difficile* can be easily identified; discovery of the toxin in stool requires further testing.

Treatment

After the causative antibiotic is withdrawn (if possible), symptoms resolve in patients who are mildly symptomatic. This is usually the only treatment needed. In more severe cases, vancomycin or fidaxomicin is an effective therapy; metronidazole is an acceptable alternative treatment. Retesting for *C. difficile* is unnecessary if symptoms resolve.

About 10% to 20% of patients experience recurrence with the same organism within 14 to 30 days of treatment. Beyond 30 days, a recurrence may be a relapse or reinfection of *C. difficile*. If the previous treatment was metronidazole, low-dose vancomycin may be an effective choice.

There's varying levels of evidence to support the effectiveness of eating yogurt or taking probiotics. I.V. immunoglobulin has been used successfully in children and adults with relapsing infections.

Special considerations

- Patients with known or suspected *C. difficile* diarrhea who are unable to practice good hygiene should be placed on contact precautions in a single room or in a room with other patients with similar status.
- Use contact precautions for contact with blood and body fluids and for all direct contact with the patient and immediate environment.
- Wash your hands with an antiseptic soap after direct contact with the patient or the immediate environment. Alcohol hand rubs will not inactivate *C. difficile* spores.
- A patient who is asymptomatic, without diarrhea or fecal incontinence for 72 hours, and who is able to practice good hygiene may have contact precautions discontinued.

ALERT *The spores of C. difficile are resistant to most common facility disinfectants; therefore, contamination will remain in the room even though the patient may be discharged. The immediate environment should be thoroughly cleaned and disinfected with 0.5% sodium hypochlorite.*

- Make sure reusable equipment is disinfected before it's used on another patient.
- Teach good handwashing technique to prevent the spread of the infection.
- Review proper disinfection of contaminated clothing or household items.
- Tell the patient to inform healthcare workers of condition before admission.

Gram-negative bacilli

SALMONELLOSIS

Causes and incidence

A common infection in the United States, salmonellosis is caused by gram-negative bacilli of the genus *Salmonella*, a member of the Enterobacteriaceae family. It occurs as enterocolitis, bacteremia, localized infection, typhoid, or paratyphoid fever. Nontyphoidal forms usually produce mild to moderate illness with low mortality. (See *Types of salmonellosis.*)

Typhoid, the most severe form of salmonellosis, usually lasts from 1 to 4 weeks. Mortality is about 3% in patients who are treated. In

Types of salmonellosis

Type	Cause	Clinical features
Bacteremia	Any *Salmonella* species, but most commonly *S. choleraesuis*. Incubation period: variable	Fever, chills, anorexia, weight loss (without GI symptoms), and joint pain
Enterocolitis	Any species of nontyphoidal *Salmonella*, but usually *S. enteritidis*. Incubation period: 6 to 48 hours	Mild to severe abdominal pain, diarrhea, sudden fever of up to 102° F (38.9° C), nausea, and vomiting; usually self-limiting, but may progress to enteric fever (resembling typhoid), local abscesses (usually abdominal), dehydration, and septicemia
Localized infections	Usually follows bacteremia caused by *Salmonella* species	Site of localization determines symptoms; localized abscesses may cause osteomyelitis, endocarditis, bronchopneumonia, pyelonephritis, and arthritis
Paratyphoid	*S. paratyphi* and *S. schottmuelleri* (formerly *S. paratyphi B*). Incubation period: 3 weeks or more	Fever and transient diarrhea; generally resembles typhoid but less severe
Typhoid fever	*S. typhi* enters the GI tract and invades the bloodstream via the lymphatics, setting up intracellular sites. During this phase, infection of the biliary tract leads to intestinal seeding with millions of bacilli. Involved lymphoid tissues (especially Peyer patches in the ilium) enlarge, ulcerate, and necrose, resulting in hemorrhage. Incubation period: usually 1 to 2 weeks	Symptoms of enterocolitis may develop within hours of ingestion of *S. typhi*; they usually subside before the onset of typhoid fever symptoms *First week:* gradually increasing fever, anorexia, myalgia, malaise, headache, and slow pulse *Second week:* remittent fever up to 104° F (40° C) usually in the evening, chills, diaphoresis, weakness, delirium, increasing abdominal pain and distention, diarrhea or constipation, cough, moist crackles, tender abdomen with enlarged spleen, and maculopapular rash (especially on abdomen) *Third week:* persistent fever, increasing fatigue and weakness; usually subsides by the end of third week, although relapses may occur *Complications:* intestinal perforation or hemorrhage, abscesses, thrombophlebitis, cerebral thrombosis, pneumonia, osteomyelitis, myocarditis, acute circulatory failure, and chronic carrier state

those who are untreated, 10% of cases result in fatality, usually as a result of intestinal perforation or hemorrhage, cerebral thrombosis, toxemia, pneumonia, or acute circulatory failure. An attack of typhoid confers lifelong immunity, although the patient may become a carrier. Salmonellosis is 20 times more common in patients with acquired immunodeficiency syndrome (AIDS). Features are increased incidence of bacteremia, inability to identify the infection source, and tendency of infection to recur after therapy is stopped.

Most typhoid patients are younger than age 30; most carriers are women older than age 50. There are about 5,700 cases of typhoid in the United States each year, 75% as a result of travelers returning from endemic areas.

Pathophysiology

Of an estimated 1,700 serotypes of *Salmonella*, 10 cause the diseases most common in the United States; all 10 can survive for weeks in water, ice, sewage, or food. Nontyphoidal salmonellosis generally follows the ingestion of contaminated or inadequately processed foods, especially eggs, chicken, turkey, and duck. Proper cooking reduces the risk of contracting salmonellosis. Other causes include contact with infected people or animals or ingestion of contaminated dry milk, chocolate bars, or drugs of animal origin. Salmonellosis may occur in children younger than age 5 from fecal–oral spread. Enterocolitis and bacteremia are common (and more virulent) among infants, elderly persons, and people already weakened by other infections; paratyphoid fever is rare in the United States.

Typhoid usually results from drinking water contaminated by excretions of a carrier or from ingesting contaminated shellfish. (Contamination of shellfish occurs by leakage of sewage from offshore disposal depots.)

Complications

- Intestinal perforation
- Intestinal hemorrhage
- Cerebral thrombosis
- Pneumonia
- Endocarditis
- Myocarditis
- Meningitis
- Pyelonephritis
- Osteomyelitis
- Cholecystitis
- Hepatitis
- Septicemia
- Acute circulatory failure
- Reactive arthritis

Signs and symptoms

Clinical manifestations of salmonellosis vary but usually include fever, abdominal pain, and severe diarrhea with enterocolitis. Headache, increasing fever, and constipation are more common in typhoidal infection.

Diagnosis

Generally, diagnosis depends on isolation of the organism in a culture, particularly blood (in typhoid, paratyphoid, and bacteremia) or feces (in enterocolitis, paratyphoid, and typhoid). Other appropriate culture specimens include urine, bone marrow, pus, and vomitus. In endemic areas, clinical symptoms of enterocolitis allow a working diagnosis before the cultures are positive. The presence of *Salmonella typhi* in stool 1 or more years after treatment indicates that the patient is a carrier, which is true of 3% of patients.

Widal test, an agglutination reaction against somatic and flagellar antigens, may suggest typhoid with a fourfold rise in titer. However, drug use, hepatic disease, and previous infection can also increase these titers and invalidate test results. Other supportive laboratory values may include transient leukocytosis during the first week of typhoidal salmonellosis, leukopenia during the third week, and leukocytosis in local infection.

Treatment

Antimicrobial therapy for typhoid, paratyphoid, and bacteremia depends on organism sensitivity. It may include fluoroquinolones, third-generation cephalosporins, or azithromycin. In those with severe systemic illness, concurrent treatment with dexamethasone may be considered. Localized abscesses may also need surgical drainage. Enterocolitis requires a short course of antibiotics only if it causes septicemia or prolonged fever. Other treatments include bed rest and fluid and electrolyte replacement.

Special considerations

- All infections caused by *Salmonella* must be reported to the state health department.
- Follow contact precautions if the patient is incontinent or diapered; otherwise, standard precautions are appropriate. Always wash your hands thoroughly before and after any contact with the patient, and advise other facility personnel to do the same. Teach the patient to use proper handwashing, especially after defecating and before eating or handling food. Wear gloves and a gown when disposing of feces or fecally contaminated objects. Continue precautions until three consecutive stool cultures are

negative—the first one taken 48 hours after antibiotic treatment ends, followed by two more at 24-hour intervals.

◆ Observe the patient closely for signs and symptoms of bowel perforation from erosion of intestinal ulcers: sudden pain in the lower right side of the abdomen and abdominal rigidity, possibly after one or more rectal bleeding episodes; sudden fall in temperature or blood pressure; and rising pulse rate (indicating shock).

◆ During acute infection, plan care and activities to allow the patient as much rest as possible. Raise the side rails and use other safety measures, because the patient may become delirious. Assign a room close to the nurses' station so the patient can be checked often. Use a room deodorizer to minimize odor from diarrhea and to provide a comfortable atmosphere for rest.

◆ Accurately record intake and output. Maintain adequate I.V. hydration. When the patient can tolerate oral feedings, encourage high-calorie fluids such as milkshakes. Watch for constipation.

◆ Provide good skin and mouth care. Turn the patient frequently, and perform mild passive exercises, as indicated. Apply mild heat to the abdomen to relieve cramps.

◆ *Don't* administer antipyretics. These mask fever and lead to possible hypothermia. Instead, to promote heat loss through the skin without causing shivering (which keeps fever high by vasoconstriction), apply tepid, wet towels (don't use alcohol or ice) to the patient's groin and axillae. To promote heat loss by vasodilation of peripheral blood vessels, use additional wet towels on the arms and legs, wiping with long, vigorous strokes.

◆ After draining the abscesses of a joint, provide heat, elevation, and passive range-of-motion exercises to decrease swelling and maintain mobility.

◆ If the patient has positive stool cultures on discharge, advise them to be sure to wash hands after using the bathroom and to avoid preparing uncooked foods, such as salads, for family members. The patient also shouldn't work as a food handler until cultures are negative. (See *Preventing recurrence of salmonellosis.*)

◆ Report all cases to public health authorities.

SHIGELLOSIS
Causes and incidence

Shigellosis, also known as *bacillary dysentery*, is an acute intestinal infection caused by the bacteria *Shigella*, a short, nonmotile, gram-negative rod. *Shigella* can be classified into four groups, all of which may cause shigellosis: group A (*S. dysenteriae*), which is most common in Central America and causes particularly severe infection and septicemia; group B (*S. flexneri*); group C (*S. boydii*); and group D (*S. sonnei*). Typically, shigellosis causes a high fever (especially in children), acute self-limiting diarrhea with tenesmus (ineffectual straining at stool), and, possibly, electrolyte imbalance and dehydration. It's most common in children ages 1 to 4; however, many adults acquire the illness from children.

The prognosis is good. Mild infections usually subside within 10 days; severe infections may persist for 2 to 6 weeks. With prompt

---

PREVENTION
Preventing recurrence of salmonellosis

Take the following actions to help your patient prevent a recurrence of salmonellosis:

◆ Explain the causes of salmonella infection.

◆ Show the patient how to wash hands by wetting them under running water, lathering with soap and scrubbing, rinsing under running water with fingers pointing down, and drying with a clean towel or paper towel.

◆ Tell the patient to wash hands after using the bathroom and before eating.

◆ Tell the patient to cook foods thoroughly—especially eggs and chicken—and to refrigerate them at once.

◆ Teach the patient how to avoid cross-contaminating foods by cleaning preparation surfaces with hot, soapy water and drying them thoroughly after use; cleaning surfaces between foods when preparing more than one food; and washing hands before and after handling each food.

◆ Tell the patient with a positive stool culture to avoid handling food and to use a separate bathroom or clean the bathroom after each use.

◆ Tell the patient to report dehydration, bleeding, or recurrence of signs of salmonella infection.

treatment, shigellosis is fatal in only 1% of cases, although in severe *S. dysenteriae* epidemic mortality may reach 8%.

Shigellosis is endemic in North America, Europe, and the tropics. In the United States, about 500,000 cases appear annually, usually in children or in elderly, debilitated, or malnourished people. Shigellosis commonly occurs among confined populations, such as those in mental institutions or daycare centers.

Pathophysiology

Transmission occurs through the fecal–oral route; by direct contact with contaminated objects; or through ingestion of contaminated food or water. Occasionally, the housefly is a vector. *Shigella* invades mucosal cells in the colon, triggering an inflammatory response. The result is the death of these cells and the development of ulcerations and abscesses in the colon.

Complications

- ◆ Electrolyte imbalances
- ◆ Metabolic acidosis
- ◆ Shock
- ◆ Conjunctivitis
- ◆ Urethritis
- ◆ Arthritis
- ◆ Rectal prolapse
- ◆ Bacterial infection

Signs and symptoms

After an incubation period of 1 to 7 days (3 days is the average), *Shigella* organisms invade the intestinal mucosa and cause inflammation. In children, shigellosis usually produces high fever, diarrhea with tenesmus, nausea, vomiting, irritability, drowsiness, and abdominal pain and distention. Within a few days, the child's stool may contain pus, mucus, and—from the superficial intestinal ulceration typical of this infection—blood. Without treatment, dehydration and weight loss are rapid and overwhelming.

In adults, shigellosis produces sporadic, intense abdominal pain, which may be relieved at first by passing formed stools. Eventually, however, it causes rectal irritability, tenesmus, and, in severe infection, headache and prostration. Stools may contain pus, mucus, and blood. Fever may be present.

Diagnosis

℞ CONFIRMING DIAGNOSIS *Fever (in children) and diarrhea with stools containing blood, pus, and mucus point to this diagnosis; stool culture is the preferred method of diagnosis.*

Microscopic examination of a fresh stool may reveal mucus, RBCs, and polymorphonuclear leukocytes; direct immunofluorescence with specific antisera will demonstrate *Shigella*. Severe infection increases hemagglutinating antibodies. PCR studies can be used, as well, but should be followed up with by a stool culture. Sigmoidoscopy or proctoscopy may reveal typical superficial ulcerations.

Diagnosis must rule out other causes of diarrhea, such as enteropathogenic *E. coli* infection, malabsorption diseases, and amebic or viral diseases.

Treatment

Treatment of shigellosis includes enteric precautions, low-residue diet, and, most importantly, replacement of fluids and electrolytes with I.V. infusions of normal saline solution (with electrolytes) in sufficient quantities to maintain a urine output of 40 to 50 mL/hour. Antibiotics are of questionable value but may be used in more severe cases in an attempt to eliminate the pathogen and thereby prevent further spread. A fluoroquinolone, azithromycin, and trimethoprim/sulfamethoxazole may be useful in these cases.

Antidiarrheals that slow intestinal motility are contraindicated in shigellosis because they delay fecal excretion of *Shigella* and prolong fever and diarrhea.

Special considerations

Supportive care can minimize complications and increase patient comfort.

- ◆ To prevent dehydration, administer I.V. fluids as ordered. Measure intake and output (including stools) carefully.
- ◆ Correct identification of *Shigella* requires examination and culture of fresh stool specimens. Therefore, hand carry specimens directly to the laboratory. Because shigellosis is suspected, include this information on the laboratory slip.
- ◆ Use a disposable hot-water bottle to relieve abdominal discomfort, and schedule care to conserve patient strength.

▓▓▓▓ **PREVENTION**

◆ *To help prevent spread of this disease, use contact precautions for diapered or incontinent persons for the duration of the illness or to control institutional outbreaks. Keep the patient's (and your own) nails short to avoid harboring organisms and use frequent and proper handwashing.*

◆ *During shigellosis outbreaks, obtain stool specimens from all potentially infected staff, and instruct those infected to remain away from work until two stool specimens are negative.*

♦ *Basic food safety precautions and disinfection of drinking water prevents shigellosis from food and water contamination.*

♦ *Report cases to the local health authorities.*

E. COLI AND OTHER ENTEROBACTERIACEAE INFECTIONS

Causes and incidence

The Enterobacteriaceae—a group of mostly aerobic, gram-negative bacilli—cause local and systemic infections, including an invasive diarrhea resembling shigellosis and, more commonly, a noninvasive toxin-mediated diarrhea resembling cholera. With other Enterobacteriaceae, *E. coli* causes most nosocomial infections. Noninvasive, enterotoxin-producing *E. coli* infections may be a major cause of diarrheal illness in children in the United States. (See *Enterobacterial infections.*)

The prognosis in mild to moderate infection is good. Severe infection requires immediate fluid and electrolyte replacement to avoid fatal dehydration, especially among children, in whom mortality may be quite high.

Transmission can occur directly from an infected person or indirectly by ingestion of contaminated food or water or contact with contaminated utensils. Incubation takes 12 to 72 hours.

Enterobacterial infections

The Enterobacteriaceae include *E. coli, Arizona, Citrobacter, Enterobacter, Erwinia, Hafnia, Klebsiella, Morganella, Proteus, Providencia, Salmonella, Serratia, Shigella,* and *Yersinia.*

Enterobacterial infections are exogenous (from other people or the environment), endogenous (from one part of the body to another), or a combination of both. Enterobacteriaceae infections may cause any of a long list of bacterial diseases: bacterial (gram-negative) pneumonia, empyema, endocarditis, osteomyelitis, septic arthritis, urethritis, cystitis, bacterial prostatitis, urinary tract infection, pyelonephritis, perinephric abscess, abdominal abscesses, cellulitis, skin ulcers, appendicitis, gastroenterocolitis, diverticulitis, eyelid and periorbital cellulitis, corneal conjunctivitis, meningitis, bacteremia, and intracranial abscesses.

Antibiotic therapy is generally not indicated for these infections.

Incidence of *E. coli* infection is highest among travelers returning from other countries, particularly Mexico, Southeast Asia, and South America. *E. coli* infection also induces other diseases, especially in people whose resistance is low. The strain *E. coli* 0157:H7 has been associated with undercooked hamburger and with animals and petting zoos.

Pathophysiology

Although some strains of *E. coli* exist as part of the normal GI flora, infection usually results from certain nonindigenous strains. For example, noninvasive diarrhea results from two toxins produced by strains called enterotoxic or enteropathogenic *E. coli*. Enteropathogenic *E. coli* serotype 0157:H7 is the most well-known strain in the United States. These toxins interact with intestinal juices and promote excessive loss of chloride and water. In the invasive form, *E. coli* directly invades the intestinal mucosa without producing enterotoxins, thereby causing local irritation, inflammation, and diarrhea. Normal strains can cause infection in immunocompromised patients.

Complications

♦ Bacteremia
♦ Severe dehydration
♦ Life-threatening electrolyte disturbances
♦ Acidosis
♦ Shock
♦ Hemolytic–uremic syndrome

Signs and symptoms

Effects of noninvasive diarrhea depend on the causative toxin but may include the abrupt onset of watery diarrhea with cramping abdominal pain and, in severe illness, acidosis. Invasive infection produces chills, abdominal cramps, and diarrheal stools containing blood and pus.

Infantile diarrhea from an *E. coli* infection is usually noninvasive; it begins with loose, watery stools that change from yellow to green and contain little mucus or blood. Vomiting, listlessness, irritability, and anorexia commonly precede diarrhea. This condition can progress to fever, severe dehydration, acidosis, and shock. Bloody diarrhea may occur from infection with *E. coli* 0157:H7, which has also been associated with hemolytic–uremic syndrome in children.

Diagnosis

Stool cultures are recommended to determine whether *E. coli* 0157:H7 is present. Additionally, Shiga toxin-producing strains such as *E. coli* O104:H4 can be detected with enzyme-linked immunosorbent assay (ELISA) or PCR.

Diagnosis must rule out salmonellosis and shigellosis, other common infections that produce similar signs and symptoms.

Treatment

Treatment consists of correction of fluid and electrolyte imbalances. With an increased risk of hemolytic–uremic syndrome, antibiotics are not recommended for treatment.

Special considerations

◆ Keep accurate intake and output records. Measure stool volume and note the presence of blood or pus. Replace fluids and electrolytes as needed, monitoring for decreased serum sodium and chloride levels and signs of gram-negative shock. Watch for signs of dehydration, such as poor skin turgor and dry mouth.

◆ For infants, use contact precautions, give nothing by mouth, and maintain body warmth.

To prevent spread of this infection:

◆ Prevent direct patient contact during epidemics. Report cases to local public health authorities. *E. coli* 0157:H7 is a reportable disease.

◆ Use proper handwashing technique. Teach healthcare personnel, patients, and their families to do the same.

◆ Follow standard precautions. Provide the patient with a private room, wear protective clothing as necessary, such as when handling feces or soiled linens, and perform scrupulous handwashing before entering and after leaving the patient's room.

◆ Advise travelers to foreign countries to avoid unbottled water and uncooked fruits and vegetables.

PSEUDOMONAS INFECTIONS

Causes and incidence

Pseudomonas is a small gram-negative bacillus that produces nosocomial infections, superinfections of various parts of the body, and a rare disease called melioidosis. (See *Melioidosis*.) This bacillus is also associated with bacteremia, endocarditis, and osteomyelitis in drug addicts. In local *Pseudomonas* infections, treatment is usually successful and complications rare; however, in patients with any type of lowered immunologic resistance—premature neonates; elderly patients; patients with debilitating disease, burns, or wounds; or patients receiving chemotherapy or radiation therapy—septicemic *Pseudomonas* infections are serious and commonly fatal.

Pathophysiology

The most common species of *Pseudomonas* is *P. aeruginosa*. Other species that typically cause

---

Melioidosis

Melioidosis, also called *Whitmore disease*, results from wound penetration, inhalation, or ingestion of the gram-negative bacteria produced by the *Burkholderia* species (gram-negative rods). Although it was once confined to Southeast Asia, Central America, South America, Madagascar, and Guam, incidence in the United States has risen as a result of the influx of Southeast Asians. It is also an organism that is a potential agent for biological warfare and terrorism.

Melioidosis occurs in two forms: chronic melioidosis, which causes osteomyelitis and lung abscesses, and the rare acute melioidosis, which causes pneumonia, bacteremia, and prostration. Acute melioidosis is commonly fatal; however, most melioidosis infections are chronic and asymptomatic, producing clinical symptoms only with accompanying malnutrition, major surgery, or severe burns.

Diagnostic measures consist of isolation of *P. pseudomallei* in a culture of exudate, blood, or sputum; serology tests (complement fixation, passive hemagglutination); and chest X-ray (findings resemble tuberculosis). Treatment includes intravenous antibiotics even in mild cases for at least 2 weeks, followed by an oral regimen for at least 3 months. I.V. preparations include ceftazidime, meropenem, or imipenem.

The prognosis is good because most patients have a mild infection and acquire permanent immunity; aggressive use of antibiotics has improved the prognosis in acute melioidosis.

---

disease in humans include *Xanthomonas maltophilia* (formerly known as *P. maltophilia*), *Burkholderia cepacia* (formerly known as *P. cepacia*), *P. fluorescens*, *P. testosteroni*, *P. acidovorans*, *P. alcaligenes*, *P. stutzeri*, *P. putrefaciens*, and *P. putida*. These organisms are commonly found in liquids that have been allowed to stand for a long time, such as benzalkonium chloride, saline solution, penicillin, water in flower vases, and fluids in incubators, humidifiers, and inhalation therapy equipment. *P. aeruginosa* is associated with chronic obstructive pulmonary disease. *B. cepacia* is the organism most closely associated with cystic fibrosis, although *P. aeruginosa* is also associated with it. In elderly patients, *Pseudomonas* infection usually enters through the genitourinary tract; in neonates and infants, through the umbilical cord, skin, and GI tract.

Complications
- Septic shock
- Severe mucopurulent pneumonia
- Systemic inflammatory response syndrome
- Multiple organ dysfunction
- Death

Signs and symptoms
The most common infections associated with *Pseudomonas* include skin infections (such as burns and pressure ulcers), urinary tract infections, infant epidemic diarrhea and other diarrheal illnesses, bronchitis, pneumonia, bronchiectasis, meningitis, corneal ulcers, mastoiditis, otitis externa, otitis media, endocarditis, and bacteremia.

Drainage in *Pseudomonas* infections has a distinct, sickly sweet odor and a greenish-blue pus that forms a crust on wounds. Other symptoms depend on the site of infection. For example, when it invades the lungs, *Pseudomonas* causes pneumonia with fever, chills, and a productive cough.

Diagnosis
CONFIRMING DIAGNOSIS *Diagnosis requires isolation of the* Pseudomonas *organism in blood, spinal fluid, urine, exudate, or sputum culture.*

Treatment
In the debilitated or otherwise vulnerable patient with clinical evidence of *Pseudomonas* infection, treatment should begin immediately, without waiting for results of laboratory tests. Antibiotic treatment includes aminoglycosides, such as gentamicin or tobramycin, combined with an antipseudomonal penicillin, such as ticarcillin or piperacillin. An alternative combination is amikacin and a similar penicillin or imipenem and cilastatin. Such combination therapy is necessary because *Pseudomonas* quickly becomes resistant to ticarcillin alone.

Local *Pseudomonas* infections or septicemia secondary to wound infection requires 1% acetic acid irrigations; topical applications of colistimethate, polymyxin B, and silver sulfadiazine cream; and debridement or drainage of the infected wound.

Special considerations
- Observe and record the character of wound exudate and sputum.
- Before administering antibiotics, ask the patient about a history of drug allergies, especially to penicillin. If combinations of piperacillin or ticarcillin and an aminoglycoside are ordered, schedule the doses 1 hour apart (ticarcillin may decrease the antibiotic effect of the aminoglycoside). *Don't* give both antibiotics through the same administration set.
- Monitor the patient's renal function (output, blood urea nitrogen level, specific gravity, urinalysis, and creatinine level) during treatment with aminoglycosides. Obtain drug levels to ensure effectiveness.
- Protect immunocompromised patients from exposure to this infection. Proper handwashing and sterile techniques prevent further spread. (See *Preventing Pseudomonas infection.*)

CHOLERA
Causes and incidence
Cholera (also known as *Asiatic cholera* or *epidemic cholera*) is an acute enterotoxin-mediated GI infection caused by the gram-negative bacillus *Vibrio cholerae*. It produces profuse diarrhea, vomiting, massive fluid and electrolyte loss, and, possibly, hypovolemic shock, metabolic acidosis, and death. A similar bacterium, *Vibrio parahaemolyticus*, causes food poisoning. (See *Vibrio parahaemolyticus food poisoning*, page 839.)

Cholera is most common in Africa, southern and Southeast Asia, and the Middle East, although outbreaks have occurred in Japan, Australia, and Europe. The incidence of cholera in the United States is rare. However, U.S. travelers to areas with epidemic cholera may be exposed to the bacterium.

PREVENTION
Preventing *Pseudomonas* infection

Maintain proper endotracheal and tracheostomy suctioning technique by doing the following:
- Use strict sterile technique when caring for I.V. lines, catheters, and other tubes.
- Use suction catheters only once.
- Properly dispose of suction bottle contents.
- Label and date solution bottles and change them frequently, according to policy.
- Change water for fresh flowers in the patient's room daily.
- Avoid using humidifiers in the patient's room.

Vibrio parahaemolyticus food poisoning

Vibrio parahaemolyticus is a common cause of gastroenteritis in Japan. Outbreaks also occur on American cruise ships and in the eastern and southeastern coastal areas of the United States, especially during the summer.

Vibrio parahaemolyticus, which thrives in a salty environment, is transmitted by ingesting uncooked or undercooked contaminated shellfish, particularly crab, oysters, and shrimp. After an incubation period of 2 to 48 hours, *V. parahaemolyticus* causes watery diarrhea, moderately severe cramps, nausea, vomiting, headache, weakness, chills, and fever. Food poisoning is usually self-limiting and subsides spontaneously within 2 days. Occasionally, however, it's more severe, and may even be fatal in debilitated or elderly persons.

Diagnosis requires bacteriologic examination of vomitus, blood, stool smears, or fecal specimens collected by rectal swab. Diagnosis must rule out not only other causes of food poisoning, but also other acute GI disorders.

Treatment is supportive, consisting primarily of bed rest and oral fluid replacement. I.V. replacement therapy is seldom necessary, but oral tetracycline may be prescribed. Thorough cooking of seafood prevents this infection.

Cholera occurs during the warmer months and is most prevalent among lower socioeconomic groups. In India, it's common among children ages 1 to 5, but in other endemic areas, it's equally distributed among all age groups. Susceptibility to cholera may be increased by a deficiency or an absence of hydrochloric acid.

Even with prompt diagnosis and treatment, cholera is fatal in up to 2% of children; in adults, it's fatal in less than 1%. However, untreated cholera may be fatal in as many as 50% of patients. Cholera infection confers only transient immunity.

Pathophysiology

Humans are the only hosts and victims of *V. cholerae*, a motile, aerobic organism. It's transmitted through food and water contaminated with fecal material from carriers or people with active infections. In order for it to cause symptoms, it must first survive the gut's acidic environment and then cause formation of colonies of bacteria on the surface of the small intestine.

These organisms produce cholera toxin which produce the characteristic diarrhea.

Complications

- ◆ Hypoglycemia
- ◆ Severe electrolyte depletion
- ◆ Hypovolemic shock
- ◆ Metabolic acidosis
- ◆ Renal failure
- ◆ Liver failure
- ◆ Bowel ischemia
- ◆ Bowel infarction

Signs and symptoms

After an incubation period ranging from several hours to 5 days, cholera produces acute, painless, profuse, watery diarrhea and effortless vomiting (without preceding nausea). As diarrhea worsens, the stools contain white flecks of mucus (rice-water stools). Because of massive fluid and electrolyte losses from diarrhea and vomiting (fluid loss in adults may reach 1 L/ hour), cholera causes intense thirst, weakness, loss of skin turgor, wrinkled skin, sunken eyes, pinched facial expression, muscle cramps (especially in the extremities), cyanosis, oliguria, tachycardia, tachypnea, thready or absent peripheral pulses, falling blood pressure, fever, and inaudible, hypoactive bowel sounds.

Patients usually remain oriented but apathetic, although small children may become stuporous or develop seizures. If complications don't occur, the symptoms subside and the patient recovers within a week. However, if treatment is delayed or inadequate, cholera may lead to metabolic acidosis, uremia, and, possibly, coma and death. About 3% of patients who recover continue to carry *V. cholerae* in the gallbladder; however, most patients are free from the infection after about 2 weeks.

Diagnosis

In endemic areas or during epidemics, characteristic clinical features strongly suggest cholera.

℞ CONFIRMING DIAGNOSIS *A stool culture of V. cholerae confirms the illness; however, due to the risk of severe volume depletion, treatment should be started based on clinical suspicion.*

A dark-field microscopic examination of fresh feces showing rapidly moving bacilli (like shooting stars) allows for a quick, tentative diagnosis. Immunofluorescence also allows rapid diagnosis. Diagnosis must rule out *E. coli* infection, salmonellosis, and shigellosis.

Treatment

Improved sanitation and the administration of cholera vaccine to travelers in endemic areas can control this disease. Unfortunately, the vaccine now available confers only 60% to 80% immunity and is effective for only 3 to 6 months. Consequently, vaccination is impractical for residents of endemic areas.

Treatment requires rapid I.V. infusion of large amounts (50 to 100 mL/minute) of isotonic saline solution, alternating with isotonic sodium bicarbonate or sodium lactate. Potassium replacement may be added to the I.V. solution. Antibiotic therapy using such drugs as tetracycline, doxycycline, erythromycin, and ciprofloxacin can shorten the course of infection and reduce the rehydration requirement.

When I.V. infusions have corrected hypovolemia, fluid infusion decreases to quantities sufficient to maintain normal pulse and skin turgor or to replace fluid loss through diarrhea. An oral glucose-electrolyte solution may be a substitute for I.V. infusions. In mild cholera, oral fluid replacement is adequate.

Special considerations

A cholera patient requires contact precautions, supportive care, and close observation during the acute phase.

◆ Wear gloves when handling feces-contaminated articles and wash your hands after leaving the patient's room.

◆ Use contact precautions for diapered or incontinent persons for the duration of illness or to control institutional outbreaks.

◆ Monitor output (including stool volume) and I.V. infusion accurately. To detect overhydration, carefully observe neck veins, take serial patient weights, and auscultate the lungs (fluid loss in cholera is massive, and improper replacement may cause potentially fatal renal insufficiency).

◆ Protect the patient's family by administering oral tetracycline or doxycycline, if ordered.

◆ Advise anyone traveling to an endemic area to boil all drinking water and avoid uncooked vegetables and unpeeled fruits.

◆ Report all cases to public health authorities.

SEPTIC SHOCK
Causes and incidence

Second only to cardiogenic shock as the leading cause of shock-related death, septic shock causes inadequate tissue perfusion, abnormalities of oxygen supply and demand, metabolic changes, and circulatory collapse. It typically occurs among hospitalized patients, usually as a result of bacterial infection. About 25% of patients who develop gram-negative bacteremia go into shock. Unless vigorous treatment begins promptly, preferably before symptoms

fully develop, septic shock rapidly progresses to death (in many cases within a few hours) in up to 80% of these patients. Septic shock is the most common cause of death in acute care units in the United States.

Septic shock commonly occurs in patients hospitalized for primary infection of the genitourinary, biliary, GI, or gynecologic tract. Other predisposing factors include immunodeficiency, advanced age, trauma, burns, diabetes mellitus, cirrhosis, and disseminated cancer.

Pathophysiology

In two-thirds of patients, septic shock results from infection with the gram-negative bacteria *E. coli, Klebsiella, Enterobacter, Proteus, Pseudomonas,* or *Bacteroides;* in a few, from the gram-positive bacteria *S. pneumoniae, S. pyogenes, S. aureus,* or *Actinomyces.* Infections with viruses, rickettsiae, chlamydiae, and protozoa may be complicated by shock.

These organisms produce septicemia in people whose resistance is already compromised by an existing condition; infection also results from translocation of bacteria from other areas of the body through surgery, I.V. therapy, and catheters. Septic shock occurs when cells cannot contain or control a localized infection and inflammation becomes more widespread. Proinflammatory responses that work toward eliminating the offending agent actually cause collateral tissue damage, and anti-inflammatory pathways lead to the possibility of secondary infections. Many other processes take place, such as edema caused by weakening of the vascular endothelium and cell death. Eventually, multiple organ dysfunction and failure occurs as a result of hypotension and decreased oxygen supply from mitochondrial damage.

Complications

◆ Disseminated intravascular coagulation
◆ Respiratory failure
◆ Renal failure
◆ Heart failure
◆ GI ulcers
◆ Hepatic dysfunction

Signs and symptoms

Signs and symptoms of septic shock vary according to the stage of shock, the organism causing it, and the patient's immune response and age:

◆ *early stage*—oliguria, sudden fever (over 101° F [38.3° C]), and chills; tachypnea, tachycardia, full bounding pulse, hyperglycemia, nausea, vomiting, diarrhea, and prostration

◆ *late stage*—restlessness, apprehension, irritability, thirst from decreased cerebral tissue perfusion, hypoglycemia, hypothermia, and anuria. Hypotension, altered LOC, and hyperventilation may be the *only* signs among infants and the elderly.

Diagnosis

One or more typical symptoms (fever, confusion, nausea, vomiting, and hyperventilation) in a patient suspected of having an infection suggests septic shock and necessitates immediate treatment.

In early stages, ABG levels indicate respiratory alkalosis (low partial pressure of carbon dioxide [$PaCO_2$], low or normal bicarbonate [HCO_3^-], and high pH). As shock progresses, metabolic acidosis develops with hypoxemia, indicated by decreasing $PaCO_2$ (may increase as respiratory failure ensues); partial pressure of oxygen; HCO_3^-, and pH.

The following tests support the diagnosis and determine the treatment:
◆ blood cultures to isolate the organism
◆ decreased platelet count and leukocytosis (15,000 to 30,000/µL)
◆ increased blood urea nitrogen and creatinine levels, decreased creatinine clearance
◆ abnormal prothrombin consumption and partial thromboplastin time
◆ simultaneous measurement of urine and plasma osmolalities for renal failure (urine osmolality below 400 mOsm, with a ratio of urine to plasma below 1.5)
◆ decreased CVP, pulmonary artery pressure, and pulmonary artery wedge pressure (PAWP); decreased cardiac output (in early septic shock, cardiac output increases); low systemic vascular resistance
◆ on electrocardiogram, ST-segment depression, inverted T waves, and arrhythmias resembling myocardial infarction

Treatment

The first goal of treatment is to monitor for and then reverse shock through volume expansion with I.V. fluids and insertion of a pulmonary artery catheter to check PAWP. Administration of whole blood or plasma can then raise the PAWP to a high normal to slightly elevated level of 14 to 18 mm Hg. A ventilator may be necessary to overcome hypoxia. Urinary catheterization allows accurate measurement of hourly urine output.

Treatment also requires immediate administration of I.V. antibiotics to control the infection. Depending on the organism, the antibiotic combination may include vancomycin plus piperacillin-tazobactam or a third-generation cephalosporin such as ceftriaxone. If pseudomonas is suspected, a third antibiotic such as meropenem, ciprofloxacin, or gentamicin should be added. Appropriate antibiotics for other causes of septic shock depend on the suspected organism. Other measures to combat infection include surgery to drain and excise abscesses and debridement.

If shock persists after fluid infusion, treatment with vasopressors, such as dopamine, maintains adequate blood perfusion in the brain, liver, GI tract, kidneys, and skin. Other treatment includes I.V. bicarbonate to correct acidosis and corticosteroids (if initial therapy has failed). Other treatments may include inotropic therapy such as dobutamine or epinephrine and blood transfusion as necessary.

Special considerations

Determine which of your patients are at high risk for developing septic shock. Know the signs of impending septic shock, but don't rely solely on technical aids to judge the patient's status. Consider any change in mental status and urine output as significant as a change in CVP. Report such changes promptly.
◆ Carefully maintain the pulmonary artery catheter. Check ABG levels for adequate oxygenation or gas exchange, and report any changes immediately.
◆ Record intake and output and daily weight. Maintain adequate urine output (0.5 to 1 mL/kg/hour) and systolic pressure. Avoid fluid overload.
◆ Monitor serum antibiotic levels, and administer drugs as ordered.

ALERT *Watch closely for signs of DIC (abnormal bleeding), renal failure (oliguria, increased specific gravity), heart failure (dyspnea, edema, tachycardia, distended neck veins), GI ulcers (hematemesis and melena), and hepatic abnormality (jaundice, hypoprothrombinemia, and hypoalbuminemia).*

HAEMOPHILUS INFLUENZAE INFECTION

Causes and incidence

Haemophilus influenzae causes diseases in many organ systems but usually attacks the respiratory system. It's a common cause of epiglottitis, laryngotracheobronchitis, pneumonia, bronchiolitis, otitis media, and meningitis. Less commonly, it causes bacterial endocarditis, conjunctivitis, facial cellulitis, septic arthritis, and osteomyelitis.

It infects about half of all children before age 1 and virtually all children by age 3, although a *H. influenzae* type b vaccine given at ages 2, 4, and 6 months has reduced this number.

Pathophysiology

Haemophilus influenzae, the cause of this infection, is a small, gram-negative, pleomorphic aerobic bacillus that colonizes the respiratory tract. Transmission occurs by direct contact with secretions or by respiratory droplets.

Complications

- Subdural effusions
- Permanent neurologic sequelae
- Upper airway obstruction
- Cellulitis
- Pericarditis
- Pleural effusion
- Respiratory failure

Signs and symptoms

Haemophilus influenzae provokes a characteristic tissue response—acute suppurative inflammation. When *H. influenzae* infects the larynx, trachea, or bronchial tree, it leads to irritable cough, dyspnea, mucosal edema, and thick, purulent exudate. When it invades the lungs, it leads to bronchopneumonia. In the pharynx, *H. influenzae* usually produces no remarkable changes, except when it causes epiglottitis, which generally affects both the laryngeal and pharyngeal surfaces. The pharyngeal mucosa may be reddened, rarely with soft yellow exudate. Usually, though, it appears normal or shows only slight diffuse redness, even while severe pain makes swallowing difficult or impossible. *Haemophilus influenzae* infections typically cause high fever and generalized malaise. Meningitis, the most serious infection caused by *H. influenzae*, is indicated by fever and altered mental status. In young children, nuchal rigidity may be absent.

Diagnosis

CONFIRMING DIAGNOSIS *Isolation of the organism, usually with a blood culture, confirms the diagnosis of* H. influenzae *infection. Newer diagnostic tools are being developed such as PCR and ribosomal amplification.*

Other laboratory findings include:
- polymorphonuclear leukocytosis (15,000 to 30,000/µL)
- leukopenia (2,000 to 3,000/µL) in young children with severe infection
- *Haemophilus influenzae* bacteremia, found in many patients with meningitis

Treatment

Haemophilus influenzae infections usually respond to a course of ampicillin, or a second- or third-generation cephalosporin as an initial treatment, although resistant strains are becoming more common. As an alternative, azithromycin is prescribed.

Special considerations

- Maintain adequate respiratory function through proper positioning, humidification (croup tent) in children, and suctioning, as needed. Monitor rate and type of respirations. Watch for signs of cyanosis and dyspnea, which require intubation or a tracheotomy. Monitor the patient's LOC; decreased LOC may indicate hypoxemia. For home treatment, suggest using a room humidifier or breathing moist air from a shower or bath, as necessary.
- Place patients with type b *H. influenzae* meningitis on droplet precautions until 24 hours of appropriate antibiotic therapy.
- Check the patient's history for drug allergies before administering antibiotics. Monitor his complete blood count for signs of bone marrow depression when therapy includes ampicillin or chloramphenicol.
- Monitor the patient's intake (including I.V. infusions) and output. Watch for signs of dehydration, such as decreased skin turgor, parched lips, concentrated urine, decreased urine output, and increased pulse rate.
- Organize your physical care measures beforehand, and do them quickly so as not to disrupt the patient's rest.
- Report to local and state health department.

PREVENTION *Advise your patient on preventive measures, such as vaccinating infants, maintaining droplet precautions, using proper hand hygiene technique, properly disposing of respiratory secretions, placing soiled tissues in a plastic bag, and decontaminating all equipment.*

WHOOPING COUGH

Causes and incidence

Whooping cough, also known as *pertussis*, is a highly contagious respiratory infection usually caused by the nonmotile, gram-negative coccobacillus *Bordetella pertussis* and, occasionally, by the related similar bacteria *B. parapertussis* and *B. bronchiseptica*. Characteristically, whooping cough produces an irritating and violent cough that becomes paroxysmal and commonly ends in a high-pitched inspiratory whoop.

Since the 1940s, immunization and aggressive diagnosis and treatment have significantly reduced mortality from whooping cough in the United States. Mortality in children younger than age 1 is usually a result of pneumonia and other complications. The disease is also dangerous in the elderly but tends to be less severe in older children and adults.

Whooping cough is endemic throughout the world, usually occurring in late winter and early spring. In about 50% of cases, it strikes unimmunized children younger than age 1, because the immunization series hasn't been completed and the child has had contact with an adult harboring the organisms.

Pertussis was on the rise in recent years in the United States. In 2010, the CDC recommended a single tetanus-diphtheria acellular pertussis (Tdap) vaccination dose for persons age 11 through 18 years who have completed DTP/DTap vaccination series and for all adults to improve immunity against pertussis. Because of this recommendation, there was a 37% decrease in pertussis cases in 2015 than in 2014.

Pathophysiology

Whooping cough is usually transmitted by the direct inhalation of contaminated droplets from a patient in the acute stage; it may also be spread indirectly through soiled linen and other articles contaminated by respiratory secretions.

Complications

◆ Epistaxis (nosebleed)
◆ Periorbital edema
◆ Conjunctival hemorrhage
◆ Detached retina
◆ Pneumonia
◆ Encephalopathy
◆ Atelectasis
◆ Seizures

Signs and symptoms

After an incubation period of about 7 to 10 days, *B. pertussis* enters the tracheobronchial mucosa, where it produces progressively tenacious mucus. Whooping cough follows a classic 6-week course that includes three stages, each of which lasts about 2 weeks.

First, the *catarrhal stage* characteristically produces an irritating hacking, nocturnal cough, anorexia, sneezing, listlessness, infected conjunctiva, and, occasionally, a low-grade fever. This stage is highly communicable.

After a period of 7 to 14 days, the *paroxysmal stage* produces spasmodic and recurrent coughing that may expel tenacious mucus. Each cough characteristically ends in a loud, crowing inspiratory whoop; excessive coughing; and choking on mucus, causing vomiting. (Patients with persistent cough should be evaluated for whooping cough, because not every patient will develop paroxysms or the distinctive whooping sound.) Paroxysmal coughing may induce such complications as nosebleed, increased venous pressure, periorbital edema, conjunctival

hemorrhage, hemorrhage of the anterior chamber of the eye, detached retina (and blindness), rectal prolapse, inguinal or umbilical hernia, seizures, atelectasis, and pneumonitis. In infants, choking spells may cause apnea, anoxia, and disturbed acid–base balance. During this stage, patients are highly vulnerable to fatal secondary bacterial or viral infections. Suspect such secondary infection (usually otitis media or pneumonia) in any whooping cough patient with a fever during this stage, because whooping cough itself seldom causes fever.

During the *convalescent stage*, paroxysmal coughing and vomiting gradually subside. However, for months afterward, even a mild upper respiratory tract infection may trigger paroxysmal coughing. (Paroxysmal coughing may not be present in partially immunized individuals.)

Diagnosis

Classic clinical findings, especially during the paroxysmal stage, suggest this diagnosis and is all that is technically needed for confirmation; however, laboratory studies can confirm it. Nasopharyngeal swabs and sputum cultures show *B. pertussis* only in the early stages of this disease; fluorescent antibody screening of nasopharyngeal smears provides quicker results than cultures but is less reliable. PCR and culture meet the standards for national reporting. In addition, the WBC count is usually increased, especially in children older than age 6 months and early in the paroxysmal stage. Sometimes, the WBC count may reach 175,000 to 200,000/µL, with 60% to 90% lymphocytes.

Treatment

Vigorous supportive therapy requires hospitalization of infants (commonly in the intensive care unit) and fluid and electrolyte replacement. Other measures include adequate nutrition; codeine and mild sedation to decrease coughing; oxygen therapy in apnea; and antibiotics, such as azithromycin or clarithromycin, to shorten the period of communicability and prevent secondary infections.

Because very young infants (younger than age 1) are particularly susceptible to whooping cough, immunization—most commonly with the diphtheria-tetanus acellular pertussis vaccine—begins at ages 2, 4, and 6 months. Boosters follow at age 18 months and at ages 4 to 6. The risk of pertussis is greater than the risk of vaccine complications such as neurologic damage. However, seizures or unusual and persistent crying may be a sign of a severe neurologic reaction, and the physician may not order the other doses. The vaccine has been reformulated for older children and adults. All adults age 19 years and older should receive a Tdap once.

Special considerations

Whooping cough calls for aggressive, supportive care and droplet precautions (surgical masks only) for 5 to 7 days after initiation of antibiotic therapy.

◆ Monitor acid–base, fluid, and electrolyte balances.

◆ Carefully suction secretions, and monitor oxygen therapy. *Remember:* Suctioning removes oxygen as well as secretions.

◆ Create a quiet environment to decrease coughing stimulation. Provide small, frequent meals, and treat constipation or nausea caused by codeine.

◆ Offer emotional support to the parents of children with whooping cough.

◆ To decrease exposure to organisms, empty the suction bottle and change the trash bag at least once each shift. Change soiled linens as often as needed.

◆ Administer antibiotic therapy prophylactically to close contacts within 3 weeks of exposure.

◆ Report all cases to public health authorities.

◆ Place patients on droplet precautions.

PLAGUE

Causes and incidence

Plague, also known as the *black death*, is an acute infection caused by the gram-negative, nonmotile, nonsporulating bacillus *Yersinia pestis* (formerly called *Pasteurella pestis*).

Plague occurs in several forms. *Bubonic plague*, the most common, causes the characteristic swollen, and sometimes suppurating, lymph glands (buboes) that give this infection its name. Other forms include *septicemic plague*, a severe, rapid systemic form, and *pneumonic plague*, which can be primary or secondary to the other two forms. *Primary pneumonic plague* is an acutely fulminant, highly contagious form that causes acute prostration, respiratory distress, and death—in many cases within 2 to 3 days after onset.

Without treatment, mortality is about 60% in bubonic plague and approaches 100% in both septicemic and pneumonic plagues. With treatment, mortality is approximately 15% for all forms of plague, largely due to the delay between onset and treatment and the patient's age and physical condition.

Pathophysiology

Plague is usually transmitted to humans through the bite of a flea from an infected rodent host, such as a rat, squirrel, prairie dog,

or hare. (See *Carrier of bubonic plague.*) Occasionally, transmission occurs from handling infected animals or their tissues. After transmission, plague invades the lymphatic system and travel to the regional lymph nodes, where an inflammatory response occurs and buboes are created. Left untreated, sepsis eventually occurs, which causes the release of proinflammatory mediators and results in inflammatory response syndrome and symptoms such as DIC, organ failure, necrosis and gangrene of fingertips, toes, ears, and the nose may occur. Bubonic plague is notorious for the historic pandemics in Europe and Asia during the Middle Ages, which in some areas killed up to two-thirds of the population. This form is rarely transmitted from person to person. However, the untreated bubonic form may progress to a secondary pneumonic form, which is transmitted by contaminated respiratory droplets (coughing) and is highly contagious. In the United States, the primary pneumonic form usually occurs after inhalation of *Y. pestis* in a laboratory.

Sylvatic (wild rodent) plague remains endemic in South America, the Near East, central and Southeast Asia, north central and southern Africa, Mexico, and western United States and Canada. Plague tends to occur between May and September; between October and February it usually occurs in hunters who skin wild animals. One attack confers permanent immunity.

Signs and symptoms

The incubation period, early symptoms, severity at onset, and clinical course vary in the three forms of plague. In *bubonic plague*,

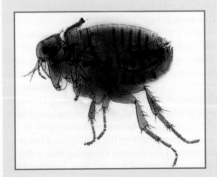

Carrier of bubonic plague

Bubonic plague is usually transmitted to humans through the bite of a flea (*Xenopsylla cheopis*), shown here.

the incubation period is 2 to 8 days. The milder form begins with malaise, fever, and pain or tenderness in regional lymph nodes, possibly associated with swelling. Lymph node damage (usually axillary or inguinal) eventually produces painful, inflamed, and possibly suppurative buboes. The classic sign of plague is an excruciatingly painful bubo. Hemorrhagic areas may become necrotic; in the skin, such areas appear dark—hence the name "black death."

This infection can progress extremely rapidly. A seemingly mildly ill person with only fever and adenitis may become moribund within hours. Plague may also begin dramatically, with a sudden high fever of 103° to 106° F (39.4° to 41.1° C), chills, myalgia, headache, prostration, restlessness, disorientation, delirium, toxemia, and staggering gait. Occasionally, it causes abdominal pain, nausea, vomiting, and constipation followed by diarrhea (frequently bloody), skin mottling, petechiae, and circulatory collapse.

In *primary pneumonic plague*, the incubation period is 2 to 3 days followed by a typically acute onset, with high fever, chills, severe headache, tachycardia, tachypnea, dyspnea, and a productive cough (first mucoid sputum, later frothy pink or red).

Secondary pneumonic plague, the pulmonary extension of the bubonic form, complicates about 5% of cases of untreated plague. A cough producing bloody sputum signals this complication. Both the primary and secondary forms of pneumonic plague rapidly cause severe prostration, respiratory distress, and, usually, death.

Septicemic plague usually develops without overt lymph node enlargement. In this form, the patient shows toxicity, hyperpyrexia, seizures, prostration, shock, and DIC. Septicemic plague causes widespread nonspecific tissue damage—such as peritoneal or pleural effusions, pericarditis, and meningitis. It's rapidly fatal unless promptly and correctly treated.

Diagnosis

Because plague is rare in the United States, it's commonly overlooked until after the patient dies or multiple cases develop. Characteristic buboes and a history of exposure to rodents in known endemic areas strongly suggest bubonic plague.

CONFIRMING DIAGNOSIS *Stained smears and cultures of* Y. pestis *obtained from a needle aspirate of a small amount of fluid from skin lesions confirm this diagnosis.*

Postmortem examination of a guinea pig inoculated with a sample of blood or purulent drainage allows isolation of the organism.

Other laboratory findings include a WBC count of over 20,000/µL with increased polymorphonuclear leukocytes and hemagglutination reaction (antibody titer) studies. Diagnosis should rule out tularemia, typhus, and typhoid.

In pneumonic plague, a chest X-ray may show fulminating pneumonia and a stained smear and culture of sputum will identify *Y. pestis*. Other bacterial pneumonias and psittacosis must be ruled out. Stained smear and blood culture containing *Y. pestis* are diagnostic in septicemic plague. However, cultures of *Y. pestis* grow slowly, so in suspected plague (especially pneumonic and septicemic plagues), treatment should begin without waiting for laboratory confirmation. For a presumptive diagnosis of plague, a fluorescent antibody test may be ordered.

Treatment

Antimicrobial treatment of suspected plague must begin immediately after blood specimens have been taken for culture and shouldn't be delayed for laboratory confirmation. Generally, treatment consists of large doses of streptomycin, the drug proven most effective against *Y. pestis*. Other effective drugs include gentamicin, doxycycline, and tetracycline. Penicillins are ineffective against plague.

In both septicemic and pneumonic plagues, life-saving antimicrobial treatment must begin within 18 hours of onset. Supportive management aims to control fever, shock, and seizures and to maintain fluid balance.

Special considerations

◆ Patients with bubonic plague require standard precautions. Place patients with pneumonic plague on droplet precautions.

◆ Use an approved insecticide to rid the patient and clothing of fleas. Carefully dispose of soiled dressings and linens, feces, and sputum. If the patient has pneumonic plague, wear a mask and follow droplet precautions. Handle all exudates, purulent discharge, and laboratory specimens with gloves. For more information, consult your infection control officer.

◆ Give drugs and treat complications as ordered.

◆ Treat buboes with hot, moist compresses. Never excise or drain them because this could spread the infection.

◆ When septicemic plague causes peripheral tissue necrosis, prevent further injury to necrotic tissue. Avoid using restraints or armboards, and pad the bed's side rails.

◆ For patients with pneumonic plague, obtain a history of patient contacts so that they can be evaluated. Administer prophylactic antibiotics, as ordered.

◆ Report suspected cases of plague to local public health department officials so they can identify the source of infection.

▧▧▧▧▧ PREVENTION *To help prevent plague, discourage contact with wild animals (especially those that are sick or dead), and support programs aimed at reducing insect and rodent populations. Recommend immunization with plague vaccine to travelers to, or residents of, endemic areas, even though the effect of immunization is transient.*

BRUCELLOSIS
Causes and incidence

Brucellosis (also known as *undulant fever, Malta fever,* or *Bang disease*) is an acute febrile illness transmitted to humans from animals. It's caused by the nonmotile, nonspore-forming, gram-negative coccobacilli of the genus *Brucella,* notably *B. suis* (found in swine), *B. melitensis* (in goats and sheep), *B. abortus* (in cattle), and *B. canis* (in dogs). Brucellosis causes fever; profuse sweating; anxiety; general aching; and bone, spleen, liver, kidney, or brain abscesses.

It's most common among farmers, stock handlers, butchers, and veterinarians. Because of such occupational risks, brucellosis infects six times more men than women, especially those between ages 20 and 50; it's less common in children. Because hydrochloric acid in gastric juices kills *Brucella* bacteria, people with achlorhydria are particularly susceptible to this disease.

Although brucellosis occurs throughout the world, it's most prevalent in the Middle East, Africa, the former Soviet Union, India, South America, and Europe; it's seldom found in the United States. The incubation period usually lasts from 5 to 60 days, but in some cases it can last for months.

The prognosis is good. With treatment, brucellosis is seldom fatal, although complications can cause permanent disability.

Pathophysiology

Brucellosis is transmitted through the consumption of unpasteurized dairy products and through contact with infected animals or their secretions or excretions. It is readily ingested by macrophages and polymorphonuclear cells and then travels to localized lymph nodes. They tend to create long-lasting infection and can become chronic.

Complications

◆ Endocarditis
◆ Orchitis
◆ Hepatosplenomegaly
◆ Arthritis
◆ Osteomyelitis
◆ Eczematous rashes
◆ Petechiae
◆ Purpura
◆ Pleural effusions
◆ Pneumothorax
◆ Abscesses in testes, ovaries, kidneys, spleen, liver, bone, and brain

Signs and symptoms

The onset of brucellosis is usually insidious, but the disease course falls into two distinct phases. Characteristically, the acute phase causes fever, chills, profuse sweating, fatigue, headache, backache, enlarged lymph nodes, hepatosplenomegaly, weight loss, and abscess and granuloma formulation in subcutaneous tissues, lymph nodes, liver, and spleen. Despite this disease's common name—undulant fever—few patients have a truly intermittent (undulant) fever; in fact, fever is commonly insignificant. It may be observed if the patient goes without treatment for a long time.

The chronic phase produces recurrent depression, sleep disturbances, fatigue, headache, sweating, and sexual impotence; hepatosplenomegaly and enlarged lymph nodes persist. In addition, abscesses may form in the testes, ovaries, kidneys, and brain (meningitis and encephalitis). About 10% to 15% of patients with such brain abscesses develop hearing and visual disorders, hemiplegia, and ataxia. Other complications include osteomyelitis, orchitis, and, rarely, subacute bacterial endocarditis, which is difficult to treat.

Diagnosis

In patients with characteristic clinical features, a history of exposure to animals, occupational exposure, or ingestion of high-risk foods suggests brucellosis. Multiple agglutination tests help to confirm the diagnosis. Approximately 90% of patients with brucellosis have agglutinin titers of 1:160 or more within 3 weeks of developing this disease. However, elevated agglutinin titers also follow vaccination against tularemia, *Yersinia* infection, or cholera; skin tests; or relapse. Agglutinin titers testing can also monitor the effectiveness of treatment.

℞ CONFIRMING DIAGNOSIS *Three to six cultures of blood and bone marrow and biopsies of infected tissue (e.g., the spleen) may provide a definite diagnosis. Culturing is best done during the acute phase.*

Hematologic studies indicate an increased erythrocyte sedimentation rate (ESR) and normal or reduced WBC count. Diagnosis must rule out infectious diseases that produce similar symptoms, such as typhoid and malaria.

Treatment

Treatment consists of bed rest during the febrile phase. Antibiotic therapy includes a combination of doxycycline and gentamicin or doxycycline and rifampin. Standard precautions are required until lesions stop draining.

Special considerations

In suspected cases of brucellosis, take a full history. Ask the patient about their occupation and if they have recently traveled or eaten unprocessed food such as dairy products (especially unpasteurized dairy products).

◆ During the acute phase, monitor and record the patient's temperature every 4 hours. Be sure to use the same route (oral or rectal) every time. Ask the dietary department to provide between-meal milk shakes and other supplemental foods to counter weight loss. Watch for heart murmurs, muscle weakness, vision loss, and joint inflammation—which may signal complications.

◆ During the chronic phase, watch for depression and disturbed sleep patterns. Administer sedatives as ordered, and plan your care to allow adequate rest.

◆ Keep suppurative granulomas and abscesses dry. Properly dispose of all secretions and soiled dressings. Reassure the patient that this infection *is* curable.

◆ Before discharge, stress the importance of continuing medication for the prescribed duration. To prevent recurrence, advise the patient to avoid using unpasteurized milk or other dairy products. Warn meat packers and other people at risk for occupational exposure to wear gloves and goggles.

◆ Laboratory technicians should handle all specimens using appropriate biosafety conditions (e.g., hoods or biological safety cabinets).

◆ Report all cases to public health authorities.

ANTHRAX
Causes and incidence

Anthrax is an acute bacterial infection that most commonly occurs in grazing animals, such as cattle, sheep, goats, and horses. It can also affect people who come in contact with contaminated animals or their hides, bones, fur, hair, or wool. It's also used as an agent for bioterrorism and biological warfare.

Anthrax occurs worldwide but is most common in developing countries. In humans, anthrax occurs in three forms, depending on the mode of transmission: cutaneous, inhalational, and GI.

Pathophysiology

Anthrax is caused by the bacteria *B. anthracis*, which exists in the soil as spores that can live for years. Transmission to humans usually occurs through exposure to, or handling of, infected animals or animal products. Anthrax spores can enter the body through abraded or broken skin (*cutaneous anthrax*), by inhalation (*inhalational anthrax*), or through ingestion of undercooked meat from an infected animal (*GI anthrax*). Anthrax isn't known to spread from person to person.

Complications

◆ Septicemia
◆ Death

Signs and symptoms

From the time of exposure, signs and symptoms of infection usually occur within 1 to 7 days but may take as long as 60 days to appear. The signs and symptoms of anthrax depend on the form acquired:

◆ *Cutaneous anthrax:* This is the most common form of anthrax. Skin infection may begin as a small, elevated, itchy lesion that resembles an insect bite, develops into a vesicle in 1 to 2 days, and finally becomes a small, painless ulcer with a necrotic center. Enlarged lymph glands in the surrounding area are common. Without treatment, mortality from cutaneous anthrax is 20%; it's less than 1% with treatment.

◆ *Inhalational anthrax:* The patient may initially report flu-like signs and symptoms, such as malaise, fever, headache, myalgia, and chills. These mild signs and symptoms may progress to severe respiratory difficulties, such as dyspnea, stridor, chest pain, and cyanosis, followed by the onset of shock. Even with treatment, inhalational anthrax is usually fatal.

◆ *GI anthrax:* Ingestion of anthrax spores can cause acute inflammation of the intestinal tract. The patient may present with nausea, vomiting, decreased appetite, and fever, which then progress to abdominal pain, vomiting blood, and severe diarrhea. With treatment, death occurs in 25% to 60% of cases.

Diagnosis

Anthrax can be diagnosed through cultures of the blood, skin lesions, or sputum of an exposed patient. If *B. anthracis* is isolated, the diagnosis is confirmed. Additionally, specific antibodies may be detected in the blood.

Treatment

Treatment that's initiated as soon as exposure to anthrax is suspected is essential to preventing anthrax infection; early treatment may also help prevent fatality. Many antibiotics are effective against anthrax and treatment depends on the complications involved. For meningitis, ciprofloxacin plus meropenem plus linezolid is used. If no meningitis is present, treatment includes ciprofloxacin plus clindamycin or linezolid. For cutaneous anthrax, ciprofloxacin, doxycycline, or levofloxacin is the appropriate treatment option.

Special considerations
◆ Any case of anthrax in either livestock or a person must be reported to the appropriate public health department.
◆ Supportive measures are geared toward the type of anthrax exposure.
◆ An anthrax vaccine is available but, due to limited supplies, it's now administered only to U.S. military personnel and isn't for routine civilian use.
◆ Anthrax isn't transmitted from person to person.
◆ Perform hand hygiene with soap and water; alcohol-based hand rubs do not inactivate spores.
◆ For large draining cutaneous lesions, use contact precautions.

CAMPYLOBACTERIOSIS
Causes and incidence
Campylobacteriosis is an intestinal infection caused by the *Campylobacter* organism, a spiral-shaped bacteria that invades and destroys the epithelial cells of the jejunum, ileum, and colon. It may spread to the bloodstream in persons with compromised immune systems, causing a life-threatening infection.

Campylobacteriosis, which is more common in the summer months, is the most common bacterial cause of diarrheal illness in the United States. Risk factors include recent family infection with *Campylobacter jejuni* and travel to an area with poor hygiene or sanitation practices.

Pathophysiology
Campylobacteriosis is transmitted by the consumption of contaminated food, such as raw poultry, fresh produce, water, or unpasteurized milk, and through contact with an infected person's stool. Transmission is also possible through contact with infected pets and wild animals. The bacteria have flagella which promote motility and secretion of proteins that aid in invasion of the digestive tract.

Complications
◆ Bacteremia
◆ Severe dehydration
◆ Electrolyte disturbances
◆ Sepsis, endocarditis, meningitis, and thrombophlebitis in immunocompromised patients
◆ Guillain–Barré syndrome

Signs and symptoms
Signs and symptoms usually develop 2 to 4 days after exposure to *Campylobacter*. The patient's history typically reveals consumption of contaminated food or water, followed by an acute onset of mild or severe diarrhea. There may also be a history of recent close contact with a person experiencing diarrhea.

On examination, the patient may complain of cramping, abdominal pain, nausea, and vomiting. Fever may be present, and there may be traces of blood in the stool. Complications associated with campylobacteriosis include bacteremia, severe dehydration and electrolyte disturbances, Guillain–Barré syndrome, and Reiter syndrome. Patients with campylobacteriosis who are immunocompromised are more susceptible to sepsis, endocarditis, meningitis, and thrombophlebitis because of the spread of the bacteria into the bloodstream.

Diagnosis
℞ **CONFIRMING DIAGNOSIS** *Stool culture identifying* Campylobacter *confirms the diagnosis of campylobacteriosis; occasionally, blood culture may be positive, as well.*

History and physical examination help in diagnosing campylobacteriosis.

Treatment
Campylobacteriosis typically resolves on its own and isn't usually treated with antibiotics unless severe signs and symptoms are present. If severe symptoms are present, antibiotics such as levofloxacin, ciprofloxacin, or azithromycin may be ordered. Fluid and electrolyte imbalances are corrected with increased fluid intake or I.V. fluid replacement, as indicated.

Special considerations
◆ Monitor the patient's intake and output and vital signs. Assess for signs of dehydration, such as tachycardia, tachypnea, and decreased urine output.
◆ Monitor the patient's electrolyte levels and assess the effects of replacement electrolyte therapy and I.V. fluids.
◆ Observe standard precautions. Use contact precautions for diapered or incontinent patients.
◆ Instruct the patient and family on handwashing techniques and preventive measures, including the proper handling and preparing of foods.
◆ Report cases to public health authorities.

TULAREMIA
Causes and incidence

Tularemia is a highly infectious disease that can be caused by as few as 10 *Francisella tularensis* organisms, a gram-negative pleomorphic bacterium. There are six forms: ulceroglandular, glandular, oculoglandular, oropharyngeal, pneumonic, and septicemic. The disease is fatal in about 5% of patients who don't receive treatment and in less than 1% of patients who do receive treatment.

Francisella tularensis is considered a potential bioterrorism agent. If dispersed in aerosol form (the most likely method of dispersion), infected persons would generally develop signs and symptoms of severe respiratory illness, including pneumonia and systemic infection.

In the United States, there are about 120 human cases of tularemia reported annually, with most occurring in the south-central and western areas of the country.

Pathophysiology

Tularemia is transmitted by the bites of infected ticks and deerflies, consuming contaminated food or water, and through contact with the blood of an infected animal (such as by skinning or handling infected carcasses), especially rabbits. The organism gains access to the host by skin or mucous membrane inoculation, inhalation, or ingestion. After inoculation, a papule and high fever develop. (The papule eventually develops into an ulcer.) The incubation period is 3 to 4 days.

Complications
◆ Pneumonia
◆ Lung abscess
◆ Respiratory failure
◆ Rhabdomyolysis
◆ Meningitis
◆ Pericarditis
◆ Osteomyelitis

Signs and symptoms

Common signs and symptoms are ulcer and fever, but signs and symptoms also vary according to the form of tularemia the patient is infected with. In the ulceroglandular form, ulcers occur at the site of inoculation and are accompanied by swollen regional lymph nodes. In the glandular form, swollen regional lymph nodes are present. In the oculoglandular form, the patient exhibits a painful, red eye with purulent exudates and swollen submandibular, preauricular, or cervical lymph nodes. In the oropharyngeal form, the patient has a sore throat, abdominal pain, nausea, vomiting, diarrhea, and, occasionally, GI bleeding. In the

pneumonic form, the patient presents with a dry cough, dyspnea, and pleuritic chest pain. In the septicemic form, the patient has fever, chills, myalgia, malaise, and weight loss.

Complications of tularemia include pneumonia, lung abscess, respiratory failure, rhabdomyolysis, meningitis, pericarditis, and osteomyelitis.

Diagnosis

Diagnosis is based on presenting signs and symptoms, as well as the patient's history, which may include a tick bite and exposure to contaminated food or water or to contaminated blood. Other results may include a WBC count that is normal or elevated and blood or sputum cultures that are positive for *F. tularensis*. Chest X-ray may show pneumonia. PCR test of a sample from an ulcer may reveal tularemia.

Treatment

General treatment involves proper skin care and increased fluid intake or supportive therapy with I.V. fluids. Medications include I.V., I.M., or oral antibiotic therapy with streptomycin or tetracycline. Antipyretics may be administered for fever.

Special considerations
◆ Monitor the patient's intake and output and vital signs.
◆ Assess the patient for signs of dehydration, such as tachycardia, tachypnea, and decreased urine output.
◆ Monitor for complications, such as meningitis, pneumonia, pericarditis, and osteomyelitis.
◆ Use standard precautions and alert laboratory personnel when tularemia is suspected because diagnostic tests should be done in a biological safety cabinet.
◆ Report cases to public health authorities.

EHRLICHIOSIS
Causes and incidence

Human ehrlichiosis, an infectious rickettsial disease that's transmitted by the bite of an infected tick, was first diagnosed in 1986. The genus *Ehrlichia* contains an emerging number of species that can transmit potentially life-threatening infections.

In the United States, most cases of ehrlichiosis are reported in the south-central and southern Atlantic areas of the country, but it has also been reported in the upper Midwest. Persons at highest risk include those who live in endemic and highly wooded areas, engage in activities in high grassy areas, and own a pet that may introduce a tick into the home.

Pathophysiology

Ehrlichiosis is caused by *Ehrlichia* organisms, specifically *E. chaffeensis* and granulocytic *Ehrlichia*. Known vectors include the lone star tick (*Amblyomma americanum*), the American dog tick (*Dermacentor variabilis*), and deer ticks (*Ixodes dammini* and *Ixodes scapularis*).

Complications

- Acute respiratory distress syndrome
- Disseminated intravascular coagulation
- Seizures
- Coma

Signs and symptoms

The incubation period for ehrlichiosis is 1 to 2 weeks from the time of the tick bite. Early symptoms include fever, chills, headache, confusion, muscle pain (myalgia), and nausea. A maculopapular or petechial rash appears in about half of the cases.

Most people infected with ehrlichiosis don't seek medical help, but it can be fatal. The fatality rate is 2% to 5%.

Diagnosis

Diagnosis of ehrlichiosis is based on evaluation of signs and symptoms and supporting laboratory data. A fluorescent antibody test may return positive for *E. chaffeensis* or granulocytic *Ehrlichia*; however, these tests will frequently be negative in the first 7 to 10 days of illness. A complete blood cell count shows decreased WBCs, indicative of leukopenia, and a low platelet count, indicative of thrombocytopenia. Granulocyte stain shows clumps of bacteria inside the WBCs. Liver enzymes show elevated levels of transaminase.

Treatment

Ehrlichiosis is treated with tetracycline, which is the first-line treatment, or other medications such as chloramphenicol, producing rapid improvement when used early in the disease's course. Death can occur if treatment is delayed.

PEDIATRIC TIP *Oral tetracycline usually isn't prescribed for children until all permanent teeth have erupted because it can permanently discolor teeth that are still forming.*

Supportive therapy is provided to help relieve signs and symptoms.

Special considerations

- Review with the patient measures to prevent tick bites when outdoors, such as wearing long-sleeve shirts and pants, tucking pants inside boots, and using insect repellent.
- Advise the patient to stick to trails and avoid dense brush when hiking. Also tell the patient to avoid standing under overhanging foliage.
- Tell the patient they should examine themselves for ticks after being outdoors and they should remove any ticks found on the body; studies suggest that a tick must be attached for at least 24 hours in order to cause ehrlichiosis.
- Report cases to public health authorities.

Spirochetes and mycobacteria

LYME DISEASE

Causes and incidence

A multisystemic disorder, Lyme disease is caused by the spirochete *Borrelia burgdorferi*, which is carried by *I. dammini*, *I. pacificus*, and other ticks in the Ixodidae family. It commonly begins in the summer with a papule that becomes red and warm but isn't painful. This classic skin lesion is called *erythema chronicum migrans* (ECM), which may be confused with a similar rash caused by Southern tick–associated rash illness. (See *Southern tick–associated rash illness*, page 851.) Weeks or months later, cardiac or neurologic abnormalities sometimes develop, possibly followed by arthritis of the large joints.

Initially, Lyme disease was identified in a group of children in Lyme, Connecticut. Now it's known to occur primarily in three parts of the United States: in the northeast, from Massachusetts to Maryland; in the Midwest, in Wisconsin and Minnesota; and in the west, in California and Oregon. Although it's endemic to these areas, cases have been reported in all 50 states and in 20 other countries, including Germany, Switzerland, France, and Australia.

Pathophysiology

Lyme disease occurs when a tick injects spirochete-laden saliva into the bloodstream. After incubating for 3 to 32 days, the spirochetes migrate out to the skin, causing ECM. Then they disseminate to other skin sites or organs via the bloodstream or lymph system. They may survive for years in the joints, or they may trigger an inflammatory response in the host and then die.

Complications

- Myocarditis
- Pericarditis
- Arrhythmias
- Heart block
- Meningitis
- Encephalitis
- Cranial or peripheral neuropathies
- Arthritis

Southern tick–associated rash illness

Southern tick–associated rash illness (STARI) is a newly recognized tick-borne disease that produces a rash similar to the rash caused by Lyme disease. STARI is associated with the bite of the lone star tick, *A. americanum*, and occurs primarily in the southeastern and south-central states of the United States. Deoxyribonucleic acid analysis of the spirochetes found in the *A. americanum* tick has indicated that they aren't *B. burgdorferi*, the agent of Lyme disease, but are a different, newly recognized species, *Borrelia lonestari*.

Individuals living or traveling to southeastern or south-central states who develop a red, expanding rash with central clearing following a tick bite should see a physician. Mild illness, characterized by such signs and symptoms as fatigue, headache, stiff neck, and, occasionally, fever, may accompany the rash.

Currently, there's no specific diagnostic test for STARI. It's suspected if diagnostic tests rule out Lyme disease, the patient's travel history is as indicated above, and a known lone star tick bite has been reported or the patient has participated in activities that may have resulted in exposure to a tick.

There are no current recommendations for treating STARI, but the rash and other accompanying signs and symptoms usually resolve with doxycycline therapy.

Signs and symptoms

Typically, Lyme disease has three stages. ECM heralds stage 1, or early localized stage, with a red macule or papule, commonly at the site of a tick bite. This lesion typically feels hot and itchy and may grow to over 20″ (50.8 cm) in diameter; it resembles a bull's eye or target. Within a few days, more lesions may erupt, and a migratory, ringlike rash, conjunctivitis, or diffuse urticaria occurs. In 3 to 4 weeks, lesions are replaced by small red blotches, which persist for several more weeks. Malaise and fatigue are constant, but other findings are intermittent: headache, neck stiffness, fever, chills, achiness, and regional lymphadenopathy. Less common effects are meningeal irritation, mild encephalopathy, migrating musculoskeletal pain, hepatitis, and splenomegaly. A persistent sore throat and dry cough may appear several days before ECM.

Weeks to months later, the second stage, or early disseminated stage, begins, and patients may develop additional symptoms depending on the system affected. Neurologic abnormalities—fluctuating meningoencephalitis with peripheral and cranial neuropathy—usually resolve after days or months. Facial palsy is especially noticeable. Cardiac abnormalities, such as a brief, fluctuating atrioventricular heart block, left ventricular dysfunction, or cardiomegaly may also develop. Cardiac involvement lasts only a few weeks but can be fatal.

Stage 3, or late disseminated stage, usually begins weeks or years later and is characterized by arthritis in about 80% of patients. Migrating musculoskeletal pain leads to frank arthritis with marked swelling, especially in the large joints. Recurrent attacks may precede chronic arthritis with severe cartilage and bone erosion.

From 10% to 20% of patients continue to have symptoms of Lyme disease that last months to years after antibiotic treatment; this condition is referred to as posttreatment Lyme disease syndrome. The causes of these symptoms are not known, but there is some evidence that it may be a result of an autoimmune response even after the infection has been cleared.

Diagnosis

Because isolation of *B. burgdorferi* is difficult in humans and serologic testing isn't standardized, diagnosis is usually based on the characteristic ECM lesion and related clinical findings, especially in endemic areas. Antibodies to *B. burgdorferi* are identified by immunofluorescence or ELISA. ELISAs are confirmed with Western blot tests. Mild anemia and an elevated ESR, leukocyte count, serum immunoglobulin M, and aspartate aminotransferase levels support the diagnosis.

Clinicians must differentiate between Lyme disease and arthritis, encephalopathy, or polyneuropathy.

Treatment

A 28-day course of an antibiotic, such as doxycycline, is the treatment of choice for nonpregnant adults. Amoxicillin is usually prescribed for children. Alternatives include cefuroxime and ceftriaxone. When given in the early stages, these drugs can minimize later complications. When given during the late stages, high-dose I.V. ceftriaxone may be successful.

Special considerations

◆ Take a detailed patient history, asking about travel to endemic areas and exposure to ticks.
◆ Check for drug allergies, and administer antibiotics carefully.

◆ For a patient with arthritis, help with range-of-motion and strengthening exercises, but avoid overexertion. Ibuprofen helps relieve joint stiffness.

◆ Assess the patient's neurologic function and LOC frequently. Watch for signs of increased intracranial pressure and cranial nerve involvement, such as ptosis, strabismus, and diplopia. Also check for cardiac abnormalities, such as arrhythmias and heart block. (See *Preventing Lyme disease.*)

◆ Report cases to public health authorities.

RELAPSING FEVER

Causes and incidence

An acute infectious disease caused by spirochetes of the genus *Borrelia*, relapsing fever (also called *tick, fowl-nest, cabin,* or *vagabond fever* or *bilious typhoid*) is transmitted to humans by lice or ticks and is characterized by relapses and remissions. Rodents and other wild animals serve as the primary reservoirs for the *Borrelia* spirochetes. Humans can become secondary reservoirs but cannot transmit this infection by ordinary contagion; however, congenital infection and transmission by contaminated blood are possible.

Louse-borne relapsing fever is most common in North and Central Africa, Europe, Asia, and South America. No cases of louse-borne relapsing fever have been reported in the United States since 1900.

Tick-borne relapsing fever, however, is found in the United States and is caused by at least 15 *Borrelia* species; the three species most commonly identified with tick carriers are *B. hermsii* (associated with *Ornithodoros hermsi*), *B. turicatae* (associated with *O. turicata*), and *B. parkeri* (associated with *O. parkeri*). This form of the disease is most prevalent in Texas and other western states, usually during the summer when ticks and their hosts (chipmunks, goats, squirrels, rabbits, mice, rats, owls, lizards, and prairie dogs) are most active. In the colder weather, outbreaks sometimes afflict people such as campers who sleep in tick-infested cabins.

Because tick bites are virtually painless and most *Ornithodoros* ticks feed at night but don't imbed themselves in the victim's skin, many people are bitten unknowingly.

PREVENTION

Preventing Lyme disease

Advise your patient to do the following to help prevent contracting Lyme disease.

Protect yourself from ticks

♦ Wear long pants and sleeves.

♦ Wear shoes, long pants with cuffs tucked into the socks, a long-sleeved shirt, a hat, and gloves when walking in wooded or grassy areas.

♦ Stay on trails and avoid walking through low bushes and long grass.

♦ Keep dogs on a leash.

♦ Use insect repellents with a 20% to 30% concentration of N,N-diethyltoluamide (DEET) on the skin and clothing.

♦ Choose an insect repellent with the concentration based on the hours of protection that's needed; for example, a 20% concentration is effective for about 2 hours, while higher concentrations protect longer.

♦ Don't use DEET on the hands of young children or on infants younger than age 2 months.

♦ According to the Centers for Disease Control and Prevention, oil of lemon eucalyptus, a more natural product, offers the same protection as DEET when used in similar concentrations.

Tick-proof your yard

♦ Clear brush and leaves where ticks live.

♦ Keep woodpiles in sunny areas.

♦ Check yourself, your children, and your pets for ticks, especially after spending time in wooded or grassy areas.

♦ Search carefully for deer ticks. Deer ticks are usually no bigger than the head of a pin, so they're difficult to find.

♦ Shower as soon as you come indoors because ticks commonly remain on the skin for hours before attaching themselves.

♦ Be aware that even if you've had Lyme disease before, you can get it again.

Carefully remove ticks on yourself or others

♦ Remove the tick with tweezers. Gently grasp the tick near its head or mouth. Don't squeeze or crush the tick; pull carefully and steadily.

♦ Once the entire tick has been removed, dispose of it and apply antiseptic to the bite area.

Untreated louse-borne relapsing fever normally carries a mortality of 5% to 10%, but during an epidemic, the mortality rate may rise to 50%. With treatment, however, the prognosis for both louse- and tick-borne relapsing fevers is excellent.

Pathophysiology

The body louse (*Pediculus humanus corporis*) carries louse-borne relapsing fever (*Borrelia recurrentis*), which typically occurs in epidemics during wars, famines, and mass migrations. Cold weather and crowded living conditions also favor the spread of body lice.

Inoculation takes place when the victim crushes the louse, causing its infected blood or body fluid to soak into the victim's bitten or abraded skin or mucous membranes.

Complications
◆ Nephritis
◆ Bronchitis
◆ Pneumonia
◆ Endocarditis
◆ Seizures
◆ Cranial nerve lesions
◆ Paralysis
◆ Coma
◆ Death

Signs and symptoms

The incubation period for relapsing fever is 5 to 15 days (the average is 7 days). Clinically, tick- and louse-borne diseases are similar. Both begin suddenly, with a temperature approaching 105° F (40.6° C), prostration, headache, severe myalgia, arthralgia, diarrhea, vomiting, coughing, and eye or chest pains. Splenomegaly is common; hepatomegaly and lymphadenopathy may occur. During febrile periods, the victim's pulse and respiratory rates rise, and a transient macular rash may develop over the torso.

The first attack usually lasts from 3 to 6 days; then the patient's temperature drops quickly and is accompanied by profuse sweating. A skin rash on the trunk lasting 1 to 2 days is common after the primary febrile episode. The rash may be petechiae, macular, or papular. About 5 to 10 days later, a second febrile, symptomatic period begins. In louse-borne infection, additional relapses are unusual, but in tick-borne cases a second or third relapse is common. As the afebrile intervals become longer, relapses become shorter and milder because of antibody accumulation. Relapses are possibly due to antigenic changes in the *Borrelia* organism.

Complications from relapsing fever include nephritis, bronchitis, pneumonia, endocarditis,

seizures, cranial nerve lesions, paralysis, and coma. Death may occur from hyperpyrexia, massive bleeding, circulatory failure, splenic rupture, or a secondary infection.

Diagnosis

CONFIRMING DIAGNOSIS *Diagnosis requires demonstration of the spirochetes in peripheral blood smears during febrile periods, using Wright or Giemsa stain. If unable to obtain, PCR testing should be performed.*

Borrelia spirochetes may be more difficult to detect in later relapses because their number declines in the blood. In such cases, injecting the patient's blood or tissue into a young rat and incubating the organism in the rat's blood for 1 to 10 days commonly allows spirochete identification.

In severe infection, spirochetes are found in the urine and CSF. Other abnormal laboratory results usually include a WBC count as high as 25,000/µL, with increases in lymphocytes and ESR; however, the WBC count may be normal. Because the *Borrelia* organism is a spirochete, relapsing fever may cause a false-positive test for syphilis in 5% to 10% of cases.

Treatment

Doxycycline or azithromycin is the treatment of choice and should continue for 4 to 5 days. In cases of drug allergy or resistance, penicillin may be administered as an alternative. However, neither drug should be given at the height of a severe febrile attack because it may cause Jarisch–Herxheimer reaction, resulting in malaise, rigors, leukopenia, flushing, fever, tachycardia, rising respiration rate, and hypotension. This reaction, which is caused by toxic by-products from massive spirochete destruction, can mimic septic shock, but usually subsides within 24 hours. This should not affect antimicrobial therapy.

Special considerations
◆ During the initial evaluation period, obtain a complete history of the patient's travels and activities.
◆ Throughout febrile periods, monitor vital signs, LOC, and temperature every 4 hours. Watch for and immediately report any signs of neurologic complications, such as decreasing LOC or seizures. To reduce fever, give tepid sponge baths and antipyretics, as ordered.
◆ Maintain adequate fluid intake to prevent dehydration. Provide I.V. fluids as ordered. Measure intake and output accurately, especially if the patient is vomiting or has diarrhea.
◆ Administer antibiotics carefully. Document and report any hypersensitive reactions (rash,

fever, anaphylaxis), especially a Jarisch–Herx-heimer reaction.

◆ Treat flushing, hypotension, or tachycardia with vasopressors or fluids, as ordered.

◆ Look for symptoms of relapsing fever in family members and in others who may have been exposed to ticks or lice along with the victim.

◆ Use proper handwashing technique, and teach it to the patient. Isolation is unnecessary because the disease isn't transmitted from person to person.

◆ Report all cases of louse- or tick-borne relapsing fever to the local public health department, as required by law.

▒▒▒▒ **PREVENTION** *To prevent relapsing fever, advise anyone traveling to tick-infested areas (Asia, North and Central Africa, and South America) to wear clothing that covers as much skin as possible and to tuck pant legs into boots or socks. Advise the use of insect repellant to reduce risk.*

LEPROSY
Causes and incidence
Leprosy, also known as *Hansen disease*, is a chronic, systemic infection characterized by progressive cutaneous lesions. It's caused by *Mycobacterium leprae*, an acid-fast bacillus that attacks cutaneous tissue and peripheral nerves, producing skin lesions, anesthesia, infection, and deformities.

With timely and correct treatment, leprosy has a good prognosis and is seldom fatal. Untreated, however, it can cause severe disability. The lepromatous type may lead to blindness and deformities.

Leprosy is most prevalent in the underdeveloped areas of Asia (especially India and China), Africa, South America, and the islands of the Caribbean and Pacific. In 2010, approximately 200,000 new cases were reported worldwide; in the United States approximately 100 per year are diagnosed, mostly in the South, California, Hawaii, and U.S. Island possessions.

Leprosy occurs in three distinct forms:

◆ *Lepromatous leprosy*, the most serious type, causes damage to the upper respiratory tract, eyes, and testes as well as to the nerves and skin.

◆ *Tuberculoid leprosy* affects peripheral nerves and sometimes the surrounding skin, especially the face, arms, legs, and buttocks.

◆ *Borderline (dimorphous) leprosy* has characteristics of both lepromatous and tuberculoid leprosies. Skin lesions in this type of leprosy are diffuse and poorly defined.

Pathophysiology
Contrary to popular belief, leprosy isn't highly contagious; it actually has a low rate of infectivity. Continuous, close contact is needed to transmit it. In fact, 9 out of 10 persons have a natural immunity to it. Susceptibility appears highest during childhood and seems to decrease with age. Presumably, transmission occurs through nasal droplets containing *M. leprae* or by inoculation through skin breaks (e.g., with a contaminated hypodermic or tattoo needle). The incubation period is unusually long—2 to 40 years with an average of 5 to 7 years.

Complications
◆ Fever
◆ Malaise
◆ Lymphadenopathy
◆ Ulceration into muscle and fascia
◆ Secondary bacterial infection

Signs and symptoms
Mycobacterium leprae attacks the peripheral nervous system, especially the ulnar, radial, facial, anterior-tibial, and posterior-popliteal nerves. The CNS appears highly resistant. When the bacilli damage the skin's fine nerves, they cause anesthesia, anhidrosis, and dryness. If they attack a large nerve trunk, motor nerve damage, weakness, and pain occur, followed by peripheral anesthesia, muscle paralysis, or atrophy. In later stages, clawhand, footdrop, and ocular complications—such as corneal insensitivity and ulceration, conjunctivitis, photophobia, and blindness—can occur. Injury, ulceration, infection, and disuse of the deformed parts cause scarring and contracture. Neurologic complications occur in both lepromatous and tuberculoid leprosy but are less extensive and develop more slowly in the lepromatous form. Lepromatous leprosy can invade tissue in virtually every organ of the body, but the organs generally remain functional.

The lepromatous and tuberculoid forms affect the skin in markedly different ways. In lepromatous disease, early lesions are multiple, symmetrical, and erythematous, sometimes appearing as macules or papules with smooth surfaces. Later, they enlarge and form plaques or nodules called *lepromas* on the earlobes, nose, eyebrows, and forehead, giving the patient a characteristic leonine appearance. In advanced stages, *M. leprae* may infiltrate the entire skin surface. Lepromatous leprosy also causes loss of eyebrows, eyelashes, and sebaceous and sweat gland function and, in advanced stages, conjunctival and scleral nodules. Upper respiratory lesions cause epistaxis, ulceration of the uvula and tonsils, septal perforation, and nasal collapse. Lepromatous leprosy can lead to hepatosplenomegaly and orchitis. Fingertips and toes deteriorate as bone resorption follows trauma and infection in these insensitive areas.

When tuberculoid leprosy affects the skin (sometimes its effect is strictly neural), it produces raised, large, erythematous plaques or macules with clearly defined borders. As they grow, they become rough, hairless, and hypopigmented and leave anesthetic scars.

In borderline leprosy, skin lesions are numerous but smaller, less anesthetic, and less sharply defined than tuberculoid lesions. Untreated, borderline leprosy may deteriorate into lepromatous disease.

Occasionally, acute episodes intensify leprosy's slowly progressing course. Whether such exacerbations are part of the disease process or a reaction to therapy remains controversial. Erythema nodosum leprosum (ENL), seen in lepromatous leprosy, produces fever, malaise, lymphadenopathy, and painful red skin nodules, usually during antimicrobial treatment, although it may occur in untreated people. In Mexico and other Central American countries, some patients with lepromatous disease develop Lucio phenomenon. This malady produces generalized punched-out ulcers that may extend into muscle and fascia. Leprosy may also lead to secondary bacterial infection of skin ulcers and to amyloidosis.

Diagnosis

Early clinical indications of skin lesions and muscular and neurologic deficits are usually sufficiently diagnostic in patients from endemic areas. Biopsies of skin lesions are also diagnostic. Peripheral nerve biopsy or smears of the skin or of ulcerated mucous membranes help confirm the diagnosis. Blood tests show increased ESR; decreased albumin, calcium, and cholesterol levels; and, possibly, anemia.

Treatment

Treatment consists of antimicrobial therapy using a combination of medications such as oral dapsone, rifampin, and clofazimine. It should be noted that sulfones may cause hypersensitivity reactions. Hepatitis and exfoliative dermatitis, although uncommon, are especially dangerous reactions. If they occur, sulfone therapy should be stopped immediately.

Failure to respond to sulfone or the occurrence of respiratory involvement or other complications requires the use of alternative therapy, such as minocycline, ofloxacin, levofloxacin, or clarithromycin. Clawhand, wristdrop, or footdrop may require surgical correction.

When a patient's disease becomes inactive, as determined by the morphologic and bacterial index, treatment is discontinued according to the following schedule: tuberculoid, 6 to 12 months and borderline, 24 months.

Because ENL is commonly considered a sign that the patient is responding to treatment, antimicrobial therapy should be continued. Thalidomide and clofazimine have been used successfully to treat ENL at the National Hansen's Disease Center (NHDC); however, this treatment requires a signed consent form and strict adherence to established NHDC protocols. Corticosteroids are also a mainstay of ENL therapy.

Special considerations

Patient care is supportive and consists of measures to control acute infection, prevent complications, speed rehabilitation and recovery, and provide psychological support.

◆ Give antipyretics, analgesics, and sedatives, as needed. Watch for and report ENL or Lucio phenomenon.

◆ Although leprosy isn't highly contagious, take precautions against the possible spread of infection. Tell patients to cover coughs or sneezes with a paper tissue and to dispose of it properly. Follow standard precautions when handling clothing or articles that have been in contact with open skin lesions.

◆ Patients with borderline or lepromatous leprosy may suffer associated eye complications, such as iridocyclitis and glaucoma. Decreased corneal sensation and lacrimation may also occur, requiring patients to use a tear substitute daily and protect their eyes to prevent corneal irritation and ulceration.

◆ Stress the importance of adequate nutrition and rest. Watch for fatigue, jaundice, and other signs of anemia and hepatitis.

◆ Tell the patient to be careful not to injure an anesthetized leg by putting too much weight on it. Advise testing bath water carefully to prevent scalding. To prevent ulcerations, suggest the use of sturdy footwear and soaking feet in warm water after any kind of exercise, even a short walk. Advise rubbing the feet with petroleum jelly, oil, or lanolin.

◆ For patients with deformities, an interdisciplinary rehabilitation program employing a physiotherapist and plastic surgeon may be necessary. Teach the patient and help with prescribed therapies.

◆ Provide emotional support throughout treatment.

◆ Report case to public health authorities.

Mycoses

CANDIDIASIS

Causes and incidence

Candidiasis (also called *candidosis* or *moniliasis*) is usually a mild, superficial fungal infection caused by the genus *Candida*. It usually infects the nails (onychomycosis), skin (diaper rash), or mucous membranes, especially the oropharynx (thrush), vagina (moniliasis), esophagus, and GI tract. Rarely, these fungi enter the bloodstream and invade the kidneys, lungs, endocardium, brain, or other structures, causing serious infections. Such systemic infection is most prevalent among drug abusers and patients already hospitalized, particularly diabetics, immunosuppressed patients, or patients receiving broad-spectrum antibiotics. The prognosis varies, depending on the patient's resistance.

Pathophysiology

Most cases of *Candida* infection result from *C. albicans*. Other infective strains include *C. parapsilosis*, *C. tropicalis*, *C. glabrata*, and *C. guilliermondii*. These fungi are part of the normal flora of the GI tract, mouth, vagina, and skin. They cause infection when some change in the body (rising glucose levels from diabetes mellitus; lowered resistance from an immunosuppressive drug, radiation, aging, or a disease, such as cancer or HIV infection) permits their sudden proliferation or when they're introduced systemically by I.V. or urinary catheters, drug abuse, hyperalimentation, or surgery. However, the most common predisposing factor remains the use of broad-spectrum antibiotics, which decrease the number of normal flora and permit an increasing number of candidal organisms to proliferate. The baby of a mother with vaginal candidiasis can contract oral thrush while passing through the birth canal. Thrush is also found in many infants who are breast-fed. The incidence of candidiasis is rising because of wider use of I.V. therapy and a greater number of immunocompromised patients, especially those with HIV infection.

Complication

♦ Candida dissemination with kidney, brain, GI tract, eyes, lungs, and heart failure.

Signs and symptoms

Symptoms of superficial candidiasis correspond to the site of infection:
♦ skin—scaly, erythematous, papular rash, sometimes covered with exudate, appearing below the breast, between fingers, and at the axillae, groin, and umbilicus; in diaper rash, papules at the edges of the rash

♦ nails—red, swollen, darkened nail bed; occasionally, purulent discharge and the separation of a pruritic nail from the nail bed
♦ oropharyngeal mucosa (thrush)—cream-colored or bluish white curdlike patches of exudate on the tongue, mouth, or pharynx that reveal bloody engorgement when scraped. They may swell, causing respiratory distress in infants, or they may be painful or cause a burning sensation in the throats and mouths of adults. (See *Recognizing candidiasis*, page 857.)
♦ esophageal mucosa—dysphagia, retrosternal pain, regurgitation, and, occasionally, scales in the mouth and throat
♦ vaginal mucosa—white or yellow discharge, with pruritus and local excoriation; white or gray raised patches on vaginal walls, with local inflammation; dyspareunia.

Systemic infection produces chills; high, spiking fever; hypotension; prostration; myalgias; arthralgias; and a rash. Specific signs and symptoms depend on the site of infection:
♦ pulmonary—hemoptysis, cough, fever
♦ renal—fever, flank pain, dysuria, hematuria, pyuria, cloudy urine
♦ brain—headache, nuchal rigidity, seizures, focal neurologic deficits
♦ endocardium—systolic or diastolic murmur, fever, chest pain, embolic phenomena
♦ eye—endophthalmitis, blurred vision, orbital or periorbital pain, scotoma, and exudate

Diagnosis

Diagnosis of superficial candidiasis depends on clinical signs and symptoms plus evidence of *Candida* on a Gram stain of skin, vaginal scrapings, pus, or sputum or on skin scrapings prepared in potassium hydroxide solution. Punch biopsies are commonly performed and sent for culture, as well. Systemic infections require obtaining a specimen for blood or tissue culture.

Treatment

Treatment first aims to improve the underlying condition that predisposes the patient to candidiasis, such as controlling diabetes or discontinuing antibiotic therapy and catheterization, if possible.

Nystatin is an effective antifungal for superficial candidiasis. Clotrimazole, fluconazole, ketoconazole, and miconazole are effective in mucous membrane and vaginal candidal infections. Ketoconazole or fluconazole is the treatment of choice for chronic candidiasis of the mucous membranes. Treatment for systemic infection consists of I.V. caspofungin, micafungin, fluconazole, or, less commonly, amphotericin B.

Recognizing candidiasis

Candidiasis of the oropharyngeal mucosa (thrush) causes cream-colored or bluish white pseudomembranous patches on the tongue, mouth, or pharynx. Fungal invasion may extend to circumoral tissues.

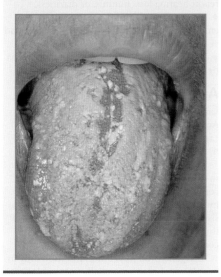

Special considerations

◆ Instruct the patient using nystatin solution to swish it around in the mouth for several minutes before swallowing it.

◆ Swab nystatin on the oral mucosa of an infant with thrush. Treat the infant after a feeding because feedings will wash the medication away. The infant's mother should also be treated to prevent the infection from being passed back and forth.

◆ Provide the patient with a nonirritating mouthwash to loosen tenacious secretions and a soft toothbrush to avoid irritation.

◆ Relieve the patient's mouth discomfort with a topical anesthetic, such as lidocaine, at least 1 hour before meals. (It may suppress the gag reflex and cause aspiration.)

◆ Provide a soft diet for the patient with severe dysphagia. Tell the patient with mild dysphagia to chew food thoroughly, to prevent choking.

◆ Use dry padding in intertriginous areas of obese patients to prevent irritation.

◆ Note dates of insertion of I.V. catheters, and replace them according to your hospital's policy to prevent phlebitis.

◆ Assess the patient with candidiasis for underlying causes such as diabetes mellitus. If the

patient is receiving amphotericin B for systemic candidiasis, they may have severe chills, fever, anorexia, nausea, and vomiting. Premedicate with acetaminophen, antihistamines, or antiemetics to help reduce adverse effects.

◆ Frequently check vital signs of patients with systemic infections. Provide appropriate supportive care. In patients with renal involvement, carefully monitor intake and output and urine blood and protein levels.

◆ Check high-risk patients daily, especially those receiving antibiotics, for patchy areas, irritation, sore throat, bleeding of the mouth or gums, or other signs of superinfection. Check for vaginal discharge; record color and amount.

◆ Encourage women in their third trimester of pregnancy to be examined for vaginal candidiasis to protect their neonate from infection at birth.

CRYPTOCOCCOSIS

Causes and incidence

Cryptococcosis, also called *torulosis* or *European blastomycosis*, is caused by the fungus *Cryptococcus neoformans*. It's most prevalent in men, usually those between ages 30 and 60, and is rare in children.

Cryptococcosis is especially likely to develop in immunocompromised patients, such as those with Hodgkin lymphoma, sarcoidosis, leukemia, or lymphoma, and in those who are receiving immunosuppressive agents. Currently, patients with AIDS are by far the most commonly affected group.

With appropriate treatment, the prognosis in pulmonary cryptococcosis is good. CNS infection, can be fatal, but treatment dramatically reduces mortality.

Pathophysiology

Because *C. neoformans* is transmitted in particles of dust contaminated by pigeon feces that harbor this organism, cryptococcosis is primarily an urban infection. Usually beginning as an asymptomatic pulmonary infection, it disseminates to extrapulmonary sites, usually to the CNS but also to the skin, bones, prostate gland, liver, or kidneys. The pathogenesis is poorly understood.

Complications

◆ Optic atrophy
◆ Ataxia
◆ Hydrocephalus
◆ Deafness
◆ Paralysis
◆ Organic mental syndrome
◆ Personality changes

Signs and symptoms

Typically, signs and symptoms of pulmonary cryptococcosis include fever, cough with pleuritic pain, weight loss, and CNS disturbances. CNS involvement occurs gradually (cryptococcal meningitis) and causes progressively severe frontal and temporal headache, diplopia, blurred vision, dizziness, ataxia, aphasia, vomiting, tinnitus, memory changes, inappropriate behavior, irritability, psychotic symptoms, seizures, and fever. If untreated, symptoms progress to coma and death, usually as a result of cerebral edema or hydrocephalus.

Skin involvement produces red facial papules and other skin abscesses, with or without ulcerations; bone involvement produces painful osseous lesions of the long bones, skull, spine, and joints.

Diagnosis

Although a routine chest X-ray showing a pulmonary lesion may point to pulmonary cryptococcosis, this infection usually escapes diagnosis until it disseminates.

CONFIRMING DIAGNOSIS *Firm diagnosis requires identification of C. neoformans by culture of sputum, urine, prostatic secretions, bone marrow aspirate or biopsy, or pleural biopsy; in CNS infection, by an India ink preparation of CSF and culture. Blood cultures are positive only in severe infection.*

Supportive values include increased antigen titer in serum and CSF in disseminated infection; increased CSF pressure, protein, and WBC count in CNS infection; and moderately decreased CSF glucose levels in about half these patients. Diagnosis must rule out cancer and tuberculosis.

Treatment

The patient with pulmonary cryptococcosis will require close medical observation for a year after diagnosis. Treatment is unnecessary unless extrapulmonary lesions develop or pulmonary lesions progress.

Treatment of disseminated infection calls for I.V. amphotericin B, flucytosine, or fluconazole. Patients with AIDS will also need long-term therapy, usually with oral fluconazole.

Special considerations

Cryptococcosis doesn't require isolation.

◆ Check the patient's vital functions, and note any changes in their mental status, orientation, pupillary response, and motor function.

◆ Watch for headache, vomiting, and nuchal rigidity.

◆ Before giving I.V. amphotericin B, check for phlebitis. Infuse slowly and dilute as ordered—rapid infusion may cause circulatory collapse.

◆ Before therapy, draw blood for a serum electrolyte analysis to determine baseline renal status.

◆ During drug therapy, watch for decreased urine output, elevated blood urea nitrogen and creatinine levels, and hypokalemia.

◆ Monitor results of complete blood count, urinalysis, magnesium and potassium levels, and hepatic function tests. Ask the patient to report hearing loss, tinnitus, or dizziness.

◆ Give analgesics, antihistamines, and antiemetics, as ordered, for fever, chills, nausea, and vomiting.

◆ Provide psychological support to help the patient cope with long-term hospitalization.

ASPERGILLOSIS

Causes and incidence

Aspergillosis is an opportunistic infection caused by fungi of the genus *Aspergillus*, usually *A. fumigatus, A. flavus,* and *A. niger.*

Aspergillus is found worldwide, commonly in decaying vegetation, such as fermenting compost piles and damp hay. It's transmitted by inhalation of fungal spores or, in aspergillosis endophthalmitis, by the invasion of spores through a wound or other tissue injury. It's a common laboratory contaminant.

Aspergillus produces clinical infection only in people who become especially vulnerable to it. Such vulnerability can result from excessive or prolonged use of antibiotics, glucocorticoids, or other immunosuppressive agents; from radiation; from such conditions as AIDS, Hodgkin disease, leukemia, azotemia, alcoholism, sarcoidosis, bronchitis, or bronchiectasis; from organ transplants; and, in aspergilloma, from tuberculosis or another cavitary lung disease.

The prognosis varies with each form. Occasionally, aspergilloma causes fatal hemoptysis.

Pathophysiology

Aspergillus occurs in four major forms: *aspergilloma,* which produces a fungus ball in the lungs (called a *mycetoma); allergic aspergillosis,* a hypersensitive asthmatic reaction to *Aspergillus* antigens; *aspergillosis endophthalmitis,* an infection of the anterior and posterior chambers of the eye that can lead to blindness; and *disseminated aspergillosis,* an acute infection that produces septicemia, thrombosis, and infarction of virtually any organ, but especially the heart, lungs, brain, and kidneys.

Aspergillus may cause infection of the ear (otomycosis), cornea (mycotic keratitis), and prosthetic heart valves (endocarditis); pneumonia (especially in patients receiving immunosuppressants, such as antineoplastic agents or high-dose steroids); sinusitis; and brain abscesses.

Complications
- Bronchiectasis
- Respiratory failure
- Death

Signs and symptoms
The incubation period in aspergillosis ranges from a few days to weeks. In aspergilloma, colonization of the bronchial tree with *Aspergillus* produces plugs and atelectasis and forms a tangled ball of hyphae (fungal filaments), fibrin, and exudate in a cavity left by a previous illness such as tuberculosis. Characteristically, aspergilloma either causes no symptoms or mimics tuberculosis, causing a productive cough and purulent or blood-tinged sputum, dyspnea, empyema, and lung abscesses.

Allergic aspergillosis causes wheezing, dyspnea, cough with some sputum production, pleural pain, and fever.

Aspergillosis endophthalmitis usually appears 2 to 3 weeks after an eye injury or surgery and accounts for half of all cases of endophthalmitis. It causes clouded vision, eye pain, and reddened conjunctiva. Eventually, *Aspergillus* infects the anterior and posterior chambers, where it produces purulent exudate.

! ALERT *In disseminated aspergillosis, Aspergillus invades blood vessels and causes thrombosis, infarctions, and the typical signs and symptoms of septicemia (chills, fever, hypotension, delirium), with azotemia, hematuria, urinary tract obstruction, headaches, seizures, bone pain and tenderness, and soft-tissue swelling. It's rapidly fatal.*

Diagnosis
In patients with aspergilloma, a chest X-ray reveals a crescent-shaped radiolucency surrounding a circular mass. This finding, along with a positive culture (usually from sputum), confirms the diagnosis.

℞ CONFIRMING DIAGNOSIS *In aspergillosis endophthalmitis, a history of ocular trauma or surgery and a culture or exudate showing* Aspergillus *is diagnostic. In disseminated aspergillosis, culture and microscopic examination of affected tissue can confirm the diagnosis, but this form is usually diagnosed at autopsy.*

In allergic aspergillosis, sputum examination shows eosinophils. Culture of mouth scrapings or sputum showing *Aspergillus* is inconclusive because even healthy people harbor this fungus.

Treatment
Aspergillosis doesn't require isolation. Treatment requires local excision of the lesion and supportive therapy, such as chest physiotherapy and coughing, to improve pulmonary function. Endocarditis caused by *Aspergillus* is treated by surgical

removal of infected heart valves and long-term voriconazole. Allergic aspergillosis requires desensitization and, possibly, steroids. Disseminated aspergillosis and aspergillosis endophthalmitis require a 2- to 3-week course of I.V. amphotericin B (as well as prompt cessation of immunosuppressive therapy). Voriconazole or itraconazole can also be used for treatment. However, the disseminated form results in an infection that's so virulent that amphotericin B therapy can't stop the systemic involvement; eventually, death ensues.

Special considerations
- Assist with chest physiotherapy and instruct the patient to cough effectively.
- Monitor the patient's vital signs, intake and output, and diagnostic test results.
- Provide emotional support for the patient and family.

HISTOPLASMOSIS
Causes and incidence
Histoplasmosis is a fungal infection caused by *Histoplasma capsulatum*. This disease may also be called *Ohio Valley, Central Mississippi Valley, Appalachian Mountain,* or *Darling disease.* In the United States, it occurs in three forms: primary acute histoplasmosis, progressive disseminated histoplasmosis (acute disseminated or chronic disseminated disease), and chronic pulmonary (cavitary) histoplasmosis, which produces cavitations in the lung similar to those in pulmonary tuberculosis.

A fourth form, African histoplasmosis, occurs only in Africa and is caused by the fungus *Histoplasma duboisii.*

The incubation period is from 5 to 18 days, although chronic pulmonary histoplasmosis may progress slowly for many years. Probably because of occupational exposure, histoplasmosis is more common in adult males. Fatal disseminated disease, however, is more common in infants and elderly men.

Histoplasmosis occurs worldwide, especially in the temperate areas of Asia, Africa, Europe, and North and South America. In the United States, it's most prevalent in the central and eastern states, especially in the Mississippi and Ohio River valleys.

The prognosis varies with each form. The primary acute disease is benign; the progressive disseminated disease is fatal in approximately 90% of patients; and, without proper chemotherapy, chronic pulmonary histoplasmosis is fatal in 50% of patients within 5 years.

Pathophysiology
Histoplasma capsulatum is found in the feces of birds and bats or in soil contaminated by their

feces, such as that near roosts, chicken coops, barns, caves, or underneath bridges. Transmission occurs through inhalation of *H. capsulatum* or *H. duboisii* spores or through the invasion of spores after minor skin trauma. Possibly, oral ingestion of spores may cause the disease.

Complications
◆ Vascular or bronchial obstruction
◆ Acute pericarditis
◆ Pleural effusion
◆ Mediastinal fibrosis or granuloma
◆ Intestinal ulceration
◆ Addison disease
◆ Endocarditis
◆ Meningitis

Signs and symptoms
Symptoms vary with each form of this disease. Primary acute histoplasmosis may be asymptomatic or may cause symptoms of a mild respiratory illness similar to a severe cold or influenza. Typical clinical effects may include fever, malaise, headache, myalgia, anorexia, cough, chest pain, anemia, leukopenia, thrombocytopenia, and oropharyngeal ulcers.

Progressive disseminated histoplasmosis causes hepatosplenomegaly, general lymphadenopathy, anorexia, weight loss, fever, and, possibly, ulceration of the tongue, palate, epiglottis, and larynx, with resulting pain, hoarseness, and dysphagia. It may also cause endocarditis, meningitis, pericarditis, and adrenal insufficiency.

Chronic pulmonary histoplasmosis mimics pulmonary tuberculosis and causes a productive cough, dyspnea, and occasional hemoptysis. Eventually, it produces weight loss, extreme weakness, breathlessness, and cyanosis.

African histoplasmosis produces cutaneous nodules, papules, and ulcers; lesions of the skull and long bones; lymphadenopathy; and visceral involvement without pulmonary lesions.

Diagnosis
A history of exposure to contaminated soil in an endemic area, miliary calcification in the lung or spleen or a positive urine antigen test indicates exposure to histoplasmosis. Rising complement fixation and agglutination titers (>1:32) strongly suggest histoplasmosis. A histoplasmosis antigen assay test can help in diagnosis.

CONFIRMING DIAGNOSIS *The diagnosis of histoplasmosis requires a morphologic examination of tissue biopsy and culture of* H. capsulatum *from sputum in acute primary and chronic pulmonary histoplasmosis and from bone marrow, lymph node, blood, and infection sites in disseminated histoplasmosis. However, cultures take*

several weeks to grow these organisms. Faster diagnosis is possible with stained biopsies. Also available is a deoxyribonucleic acid probe for Histoplasma *that can be used for difficult isolates.*

Findings must rule out tuberculosis and other diseases that produce similar symptoms. The diagnosis of histoplasmosis caused by *H. duboisii* necessitates examination of tissue biopsy and culture of the affected site.

Treatment
Treatment consists of antifungal therapy, surgery, and supportive care. Antifungal therapy is most important. Except for asymptomatic primary acute histoplasmosis (which resolves spontaneously) and the African form, histoplasmosis requires high-dose or long-term (12-week) therapy with itraconazole (for mild infection) and amphotericin B (for moderately severe infection). For a patient who also has AIDS, long-term therapy with itraconazole is indicated.

Supportive care usually includes oxygen for respiratory distress, glucocorticoids for adrenal insufficiency, and parenteral fluids for dysphagia due to oral or laryngeal ulcerations. Histoplasmosis doesn't require isolation.

Special considerations
Patient care is primarily supportive.
◆ Give medications as ordered, and teach a patient about possible adverse effects. Because amphotericin B may cause chills, fever, nausea, and vomiting, give appropriate antipyretics and antiemetics, as ordered.
◆ A patient with chronic pulmonary or disseminated histoplasmosis also needs psychological support because of long-term hospitalization. As needed, refer the patient to a social worker or occupational therapist. Help the parents of children with this disease arrange for a visiting teacher.

PREVENTION *Teach a patient in an endemic area to watch for early signs and to seek treatment promptly. Instruct a patient who's at risk for occupational exposure to contaminated soil to wear a face mask.*

BLASTOMYCOSIS
Causes and incidence
Blastomycosis (sometimes called *North American blastomycosis* or *Gilchrist disease*) is caused by the yeastlike fungus *Blastomyces dermatitidis*, which usually infects the lungs and produces bronchopneumonia. Less commonly, this fungus may disseminate through the blood and cause osteomyelitis and CNS, skin, and genital disorders.

Blastomyces dermatitidis is probably inhaled by people who are in close contact with the soil.

The incubation period may range from weeks to months. Blastomycosis is generally found in North America (where *B. dermatitidis* normally inhabits the soil), and is endemic to the southeastern United States. Sporadic cases have also been reported in Africa. Blastomycosis usually infects men ages 30 to 50, but no occupational link has been found.

Untreated blastomycosis is slowly progressive and usually fatal; however, spontaneous remissions occasionally occur. With antifungal drug therapy and supportive treatment, the prognosis for patients with blastomycosis is good.

Pathophysiology

After inhalation, *B. dermatitidis* survives phagocytosis partially because of its thick cell wall. A lipid and phospholipid layer are also believed to play a role in the virulence.

Complications

◆ Skin abscesses
◆ Skin fistulas
◆ Meningitis
◆ Cerebral abscesses
◆ Addison disease
◆ Pericarditis
◆ Arthritis

Signs and symptoms

Fifty percent of cases are asymptomatic. Initial signs and symptoms of pulmonary blastomycosis mimic those of a bacterial upper respiratory tract infection. These findings typically include a dry, hacking, or productive cough (occasionally hemoptysis), pleuritic chest pain, fever, shaking, chills, night sweats, malaise, anorexia, weight loss, and arthralgia. It can progress to pneumonia.

Cutaneous blastomycosis causes small, painless, nonpruritic, and nondistinctive macules or papules on exposed body parts. These lesions become raised and reddened and occasionally progress to draining skin abscesses or fistulas.

Dissemination to the bone causes soft-tissue swelling, tenderness, and warmth over bony lesions, which generally occur in the thoracic, lumbar, and sacral regions; long bones of the legs; and, in children, the skull.

Genital dissemination produces painful swelling of the testes, epididymis, or prostate; deep perineal pain; pyuria; and hematuria. CNS dissemination, which usually only occurs in immunocompromised hosts, causes meningitis or cerebral abscesses with resulting decreased LOC, lethargy, and change in mood or affect. Other forms of dissemination may result in Addison disease (adrenal insufficiency), pericarditis, and arthritis.

Diagnosis

Diagnosis of blastomycosis requires:
◆ culture of *B. dermatitidis* from skin lesions, pus, sputum, or pulmonary secretions
◆ microscopic examination of tissue specimens from the skin or the lungs or of bronchial washings, sputum, or pus, as the physician finds appropriate
◆ immunodiffusion testing, which detects antibodies for the A and B antigen of blastomycosis

In addition, suspected pulmonary blastomycosis requires a chest X-ray, which may show pulmonary infiltrates. Other abnormal laboratory findings include increased WBC count and ESR, slightly increased serum globulin levels, mild normochromic anemia, and, with bone lesions, increased alkaline phosphatase.

Treatment

All forms of blastomycosis respond to amphotericin B or itraconazole. Patient care is mainly supportive.

Special considerations

◆ In severe pulmonary blastomycosis, check for hemoptysis. If the patient is febrile, provide a cool room and give tepid sponge baths.
◆ If blastomycosis causes joint pain or swelling, elevate the joint and apply heat. In CNS infection, watch the patient carefully for decreasing LOC and unequal pupillary response. In men with disseminated disease, watch for hematuria.
◆ Infuse I.V. antifungal agents slowly (too rapid infusion may cause circulatory collapse). During infusion, monitor vital signs (temperature may rise but should subside within 1 to 2 hours). Watch for decreased urine output and monitor laboratory results for increased blood urea nitrogen and creatinine levels. Monitor serum potassium levels for signs of amphotericin B-induced hypokalemia, which may indicate renal toxicity. Report any hearing loss, tinnitus, or dizziness immediately. To relieve the adverse effects of amphotericin B, give antiemetics and antipyretics, as ordered.

COCCIDIOIDOMYCOSIS
Causes and incidence

Coccidioidomycosis, also called *valley fever* or *San Joaquin Valley fever*, is caused by the fungus *Coccidioides immitis* and occurs primarily as a respiratory infection. Secondary sites include the skin, bones, joints, and meninges. Generalized dissemination is also possible. The *primary* pulmonary form is usually self-limiting and seldom fatal. The rare *secondary* (progressive, disseminated) form produces abscesses throughout the body and carries a mortality of up to 60%, even with treatment.

Such dissemination is more common in dark-skinned men, pregnant women, and patients who are receiving immunosuppressants.

Coccidioidomycosis is endemic to the southwestern United States, especially between the San Joaquin Valley in California and southwestern Texas; it's also found in Mexico, Guatemala, Honduras, Venezuela, Colombia, Argentina, and Paraguay. It may result from inhalation of *C. immitis* spores found in the soil in these areas or from inhalation of spores from dressings or plaster casts of infected people. It's most prevalent during warm, dry months.

Because of population distribution and an occupational link (it's common in migrant farm laborers), coccidioidomycosis generally strikes Filipinos, Mexicans, Native Americans, and Blacks. In primary infection, the incubation period is from 1 to 3 weeks.

Pathophysiology

Coccidioidomycosis occurs by inhalation of a single arthroconidium. In the lung, its appearance changes from a barrel-shaped cell to a sphere and enlarges. It then produces endospores. Eventually, the spherule ruptures and the endospores are released to invade other tissues. These endospores can each produce an additional spherule.

Complications

◆ Bronchiectasis
◆ Osteomyelitis
◆ Meningitis
◆ Hepatosplenomegaly
◆ Liver failure

Signs and symptoms

Primary coccidioidomycosis usually produces acute or subacute respiratory signs and symptoms (dry cough, pleuritic chest pain, and pleural effusion), fever, sore throat, dyspnea, chills, malaise, headache, and an itchy macular rash. Chest pain, night sweats, and arthralgias can occur as well. Occasionally, the only sign is a fever that persists for weeks. From 3 days to several weeks after onset, some patients, particularly white women, may develop tender red nodules (erythema nodosum) on their legs, especially the shins, with joint pain in the knees and ankles. Generally, primary disease heals spontaneously within a few weeks.

In rare cases, coccidioidomycosis disseminates to other organs several weeks or months after the primary infection. Disseminated coccidioidomycosis causes fever and abscesses throughout the body, especially in skeletal, CNS, splenic, hepatic, renal, and subcutaneous tissues. Depending on the location of these abscesses, disseminated coccidioidomycosis may cause bone pain and meningitis.

Chronic pulmonary cavitation, which can occur in both the primary and the disseminated forms, causes hemoptysis with or without chest pain.

Diagnosis

CONFIRMING DIAGNOSIS *Typical clinical features and skin and serologic studies confirm this diagnosis. The primary form—and sometimes the disseminated form—produces a positive coccidioidin skin test.*

Other abnormal laboratory results include increased WBC count, eosinophilia, increased ESR, and a chest X-ray showing bilateral diffuse infiltrates.

In coccidioidal meningitis, examination of CSF shows WBC count increased to more than 500/ μL (primarily due to mononuclear leukocytes), increased protein levels, and decreased glucose levels. Ventricular fluid obtained from the brain may contain complement fixation antibodies.

After diagnosis, the results of serial skin tests, blood cultures, and serologic testing may document the therapy's effectiveness.

Treatment

Usually, mild primary coccidioidomycosis requires only bed rest and relief of symptoms. Severe primary disease and dissemination, however, also require long-term I.V. infusion (or, in CNS dissemination, intrathecal administration) of fluconazole or itraconazole for 3 to 6 months. Amphotericin B is reserved from the most severe cases due to its toxicity. Severe pulmonary lesions may require lobectomy. Patients require follow-up for at least a year regardless of the severity of the infection.

Special considerations

◆ In mild primary disease, encourage bed rest and adequate fluid intake. Record the amount and color of sputum. Watch for shortness of breath that may point to pleural effusion. In patients with arthralgia, provide analgesics as ordered.
◆ Coccidioidomycosis requires standard precautions, such as gloves for contact with drainage or broken skin, and good hand hygiene.
◆ In CNS dissemination, monitor the patient carefully for decreased LOC or change in mood or affect.
◆ Before intrathecal administration of amphotericin B, explain the procedure to the patient, and reassure that he'll receive analgesics before a lumbar puncture. If the patient is to receive I.V. amphotericin B, infuse it slowly, as ordered, because rapid infusion may cause circulatory collapse. During infusion, monitor vital signs (temperature may rise but should return to normal within 1 to 2 hours). Watch for decreased urine output, and monitor laboratory results for elevated blood urea nitrogen and creatinine levels and for

hypokalemia. Tell the patient to immediately report hearing loss, tinnitus, dizziness, and all signs of toxicity. To ease adverse effects of amphotericin B, give antiemetics and antipyretics, as ordered.

◆ Report cases for public health authorities.

SPOROTRICHOSIS

Causes and incidence

Sporotrichosis is a chronic disease caused by the fungus *Sporothrix schenckii*. It occurs in three forms: *cutaneous lymphatic*, which produces nodular erythematous primary lesions and secondary lesions along lymphatic channels; *pulmonary*, a rare form that produces a productive cough and pulmonary lesions; and *disseminated*, another rare form that may cause arthritis or osteomyelitis. The course of sporotrichosis is slow, the prognosis is good, and fatalities are rare. However, untreated skin lesions may cause secondary bacterial infection.

Sporothrix schenckii is found in soil, wood, sphagnum moss, and decaying vegetation throughout the world. Because this fungus usually enters through broken skin (the pulmonary form through inhalation), sporotrichosis is more common in horticulturists, agricultural workers, and home gardeners. Perhaps because of occupational exposure, it's more prevalent in adult men than in women and children.

Pathophysiology

Sporotrichosis usually produces a localized reaction in cutaneous and subcutaneous tissue. The pathophysiology is not well understood, but it is thought that it has the ability to hydrolyze collagen and elastin, possibly contributing to its virulence.

Complications

◆ Arthritis
◆ Osteomyelitis
◆ Meningitis

Signs and symptoms

After an incubation period that lasts from 1 week to 3 months, cutaneous lymphatic sporotrichosis produces characteristic skin lesions, usually on the hands or fingers. Each lesion begins as a small, painless, movable subcutaneous nodule but grows progressively larger, discolors, and eventually ulcerates. (See *Recognizing sporotrichosis*.) Later, additional lesions form along the adjacent lymph node chain.

Pulmonary sporotrichosis causes a productive cough, lung cavities and nodules, hilar adenopathy, pleural effusion, fibrosis, and the formation of a fungus ball. It's commonly associated with sarcoidosis and tuberculosis.

Disseminated sporotrichosis produces multifocal lesions that spread from the primary lesion in the skin or lungs. The disease begins

Recognizing sporotrichosis

Ulcerations, swelling, and crusting on the leg are characteristic of lymphocutaneous sporotrichosis.

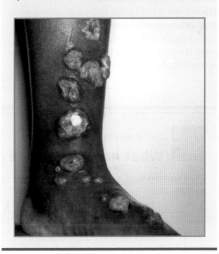

insidiously, typically causing weight loss, anorexia, synovial or bony lesions, and, possibly, arthritis or osteomyelitis.

Diagnosis

℞ **CONFIRMING DIAGNOSIS** *Typical clinical findings and a culture of* S. schenckii *in sputum, pus, or tissue biopsy confirm the diagnosis of sporotrichosis.*

Histologic identification is difficult. Diagnosis must rule out tuberculosis, sarcoidosis, and, in patients with the disseminated form of sporotrichosis, bacterial osteomyelitis and neoplasm.

Treatment

Sporotrichosis doesn't require isolation precautions. The cutaneous lymphatic form usually responds to itraconazole. Occasionally, cutaneous lesions must be excised or drained. The disseminated form responds to amphotericin B and itraconazole. Local heat application relieves pain. Cavitary pulmonary lesions may require surgery.

Special considerations

◆ Keep lesions clean, make the patient as comfortable as possible, and carefully dispose of contaminated dressings.
◆ Warn the patient about the possible adverse effects of drugs. Because amphotericin B may cause fever, chills, nausea, and vomiting, give antipyretics and antiemetics, as ordered.

PREVENTION *Advise a patient who gardens to wear gloves while working.*

Respiratory viruses

COMMON COLD
Causes and incidence
The common cold (also known as *acute coryza*) is an acute, usually afebrile viral infection that causes inflammation of the upper respiratory tract. It's the most common infectious disease, accounting for more time lost from school or work than any other cause. Although a cold is benign and self-limiting, it can lead to secondary bacterial infections.

About 90% of colds stem from a viral infection of the upper respiratory passages and consequent mucous membrane inflammation; occasionally, colds result from a mycoplasmal infection. (See *What happens in the common cold.*)

The common cold is more prevalent in children than in adults; in adolescent boys than in girls; and in women than in men. In temperate zones, it's more common in the colder months; in the tropics, during the rainy season.

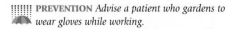

PATHOPHYSIOLOGY
What happens in the common cold

The common cold is a viral infection of the upper respiratory passages.

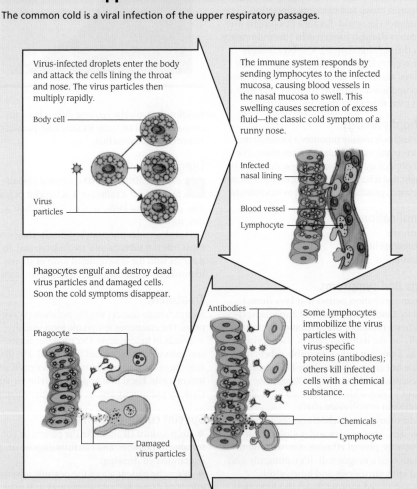

Virus-infected droplets enter the body and attack the cells lining the throat and nose. The virus particles then multiply rapidly.

Body cell

Virus particles

The immune system responds by sending lymphocytes to the infected mucosa, causing blood vessels in the nasal mucosa to swell. This swelling causes secretion of excess fluid—the classic cold symptom of a runny nose.

Infected nasal lining

Blood vessel

Lymphocyte

Phagocytes engulf and destroy dead virus particles and damaged cells. Soon the cold symptoms disappear.

Phagocyte

Damaged virus particles

Antibodies

Some lymphocytes immobilize the virus particles with virus-specific proteins (antibodies); others kill infected cells with a chemical substance.

Chemicals

Lymphocyte

Pathophysiology

More than 100 different viruses can cause the common cold. Major offenders include rhinoviruses, coronaviruses, myxoviruses, adenoviruses, coxsackieviruses, and echoviruses.

Transmission occurs through airborne respiratory droplets, contact with contaminated objects, and hand-to-hand transmission. Children acquire new strains from their schoolmates and pass them on to family members. Fatigue or drafts don't increase susceptibility.

Complications

◆ Sinusitis
◆ Otitis media
◆ Pharyngitis
◆ Lower respiratory tract infection

Signs and symptoms

After a 1- to 4-day incubation period, the common cold produces pharyngitis, nasal congestion, coryza, headache, and burning, watery eyes. Additional effects may include fever (in children), chills, myalgia, arthralgia, malaise, lethargy, and a hacking, nonproductive, or nocturnal cough.

As the cold progresses, clinical features develop more fully. After a day, symptoms include a feeling of fullness with a copious nasal discharge that commonly irritates the nose, adding to discomfort. About 3 days after onset, major signs diminish, but the "stuffed up" feeling generally persists for about a week. Reinfection (with productive cough) is common, but complications (sinusitis, otitis media, pharyngitis, and lower respiratory tract infection) are rare. A cold is communicable for 2 to 3 days after the onset of symptoms.

Diagnosis

No explicit diagnostic test exists to isolate the specific organism responsible for the common cold. Consequently, diagnosis rests on the typically mild, localized, and afebrile upper respiratory symptoms. Despite infection, WBC counts and differential are within normal limits. Diagnosis must rule out allergic rhinitis, measles, rubella, and other disorders that produce similar early symptoms. A temperature higher than 100° F (37.8° C), severe malaise, anorexia, tachycardia, exudate on the tonsils or throat, petechiae, and tender lymph glands may point to more serious disorders and require additional diagnostic tests.

Treatment

The primary treatments—acetaminophen or ibuprofen, fluids, and rest—are purely symptomatic because the common cold has no cure.

Analgesics ease myalgia and headache; fluids help loosen accumulated respiratory secretions and maintain hydration; and rest combats fatigue and weakness. In a child with a fever, acetaminophen is the drug of choice.

Decongestants can relieve congestion, and throat lozenges relieve soreness. Steam encourages expectoration. Nasal douching, sinus drainage, and antibiotics aren't necessary except when complications or chronic illness develop. Pure antitussives relieve severe coughs but are contraindicated in productive coughs, when cough suppression is harmful. The role of vitamin C and zinc remains controversial. In infants, saline nose drops and mucus aspiration with a bulb syringe may be beneficial.

In 2008, the FDA recommended that nonprescription cold medicines not be given to children younger than age 4 years, because cold medicines don't appear to be effective for these children and may not be safe, especially for those under age 2.

Special considerations

◆ Emphasize that antibiotics don't cure the common cold.
◆ Tell the patient to maintain bed rest during the first few days, to use a lubricant on the nostrils to decrease irritation, to relieve throat irritation with hard candy or cough drops, to increase fluid intake, and to eat light meals.
◆ Warm baths or heating pads can reduce aches and pains but won't hasten a cure. Suggest hot- or cold-steam vaporizers. Commercial expectorants are available, but their effectiveness is questionable.
◆ Advise against overuse of nose drops or sprays because they may cause rebound congestion.

▓▓▓▓▓ **PREVENTION** *Warn the patient to minimize contact with people who have colds. To avoid spreading colds, teach the patient to wash hands often and before touching eyes, to cover coughs and sneezes, and to avoid sharing towels and drinking glasses.*

RESPIRATORY SYNCYTIAL VIRUS INFECTION

Causes and incidence

Respiratory syncytial virus (RSV) infection results from a subgroup of the myxoviruses that resemble paramyxovirus. RSV is the leading cause of lower respiratory tract infections in infants and young children. It's the major cause of pneumonia, tracheobronchitis, and bronchiolitis in this age group and is a suspected cause of the fatal respiratory diseases of infancy.

The organism that causes RSV is transmitted from person to person by respiratory secretions and has an incubation period of 4 to 5 days. Antibody titers seem to indicate that few children younger than age 4 escape contracting some form of RSV, even if it's mild. In fact, RSV is the only viral disease that has its maximum impact during the first few months of life (incidence of RSV bronchiolitis peaks at age 2 months). School-age children, adolescents, and young adults with mild reinfections are probably the source of infection for infants and young children.

This virus occurs in annual epidemics during the late winter and early spring in temperate climates and during the rainy season in the tropics. It can also be seen in immunocompromised adults, especially patients with bone marrow transplants.

Pathophysiology

RSV replicates in the nasopharynx, travels to the bronchiolar epithelium, then to alveolar pneumocytes. Epithelial cells become necrosed and initiate an immune response. Eventually, this inflammatory response causes airway obstruction, trapping, and resistance.

Complications

◆ Pneumonia
◆ Bronchiolitis
◆ Tracheobronchitis
◆ Otitis media
◆ Apnea
◆ Respiratory failure

Signs and symptoms

Clinical features of RSV infection vary in severity from mild, coldlike symptoms to bronchiolitis or bronchopneumonia, and, in a few patients, severe, life-threatening lower respiratory tract infections. Symptoms usually include coughing, wheezing, malaise, pharyngitis, dyspnea, and inflamed mucous membranes in the nose and throat. Reinfection is common, producing milder symptoms than the primary infection.

Otitis media is a common complication of RSV in infants. RSV has also been identified in patients with a variety of CNS disorders, such as meningitis and myelitis.

Diagnosis

Diagnosis is usually based on clinical findings and epidemiologic information.
◆ Many facilities can perform rapid tests for the virus using fluid obtained from the nose.

◆ Cultures of nasal and pharyngeal secretions may show RSV; however, the virus is labile, so cultures aren't always reliable.
◆ Chest X-rays help detect pneumonia.

Treatment

Treatment aims to support respiratory function, maintain fluid balance, and relieve symptoms. Ribavirin in aerosol form may be administered to severely ill patients or those at high risk for complications.

Special considerations

Your care plan should provide support and relief of symptoms.
◆ Monitor respiratory status, including rate and pattern. Watch for nasal flaring or retraction, cyanosis, pallor, and dyspnea; listen or auscultate for wheezing, rhonchi, or other signs of respiratory distress. Monitor ABG levels and oxygen saturation.
◆ Maintain a patent airway, and be especially watchful when the patient has periods of acute dyspnea. Perform percussion and provide drainage and suction, when necessary. Use a croup tent to provide a high-humidity atmosphere. Semi-Fowler position may help prevent aspiration of secretions.
◆ Monitor intake and output carefully. Observe for signs of dehydration such as decreased skin turgor. Encourage the patient to drink plenty of high-calorie fluids. Administer I.V. fluids as needed.
◆ Promote bed rest. Plan your nursing care to allow uninterrupted rest.
◆ Hold and cuddle infants; talk to and play with toddlers. Offer diversionary activities that are appropriate for the child's condition and age. Encourage parental visits and cuddling. Restrain the child only as necessary.
◆ Impose contact and droplet precautions. Enforce strict hand hygiene, because RSV may be transmitted from fomites. Avoid hand contact with nose or eyes; wear a surgical mask and eye protection.
◆ Make sure that staff members with respiratory illnesses don't care for infants.

PARAINFLUENZA
Causes and incidence

Parainfluenza refers to any of a group of respiratory illnesses caused by paramyxoviruses, a subgroup of the myxoviruses. Affecting both the upper and lower respiratory tracts, these self-limiting diseases resemble influenza but are milder and seldom fatal. They primarily affect young children.

Parainfluenza is rare among adults but widespread among children, especially males. By age 8, most children demonstrate antibodies to Para 1 and 3. Most adults have antibodies to all four types as a result of childhood infections and subsequent multiple exposures. Incidence rises in the winter and spring.

Pathophysiology
Parainfluenza is transmitted by direct contact or by inhalation of contaminated airborne droplets. Paramyxoviruses occur in four forms—Para 1 to 4—that are linked to several diseases: croup (Para 1, 2, 3), acute febrile respiratory illnesses (1, 2, 3), the common cold (1, 3, 4), pharyngitis (1, 3, 4), bronchitis (1, 3), and bronchopneumonia (1, 3). Para 3 ranks second to RSVs as the most common cause of lower respiratory tract infections in children. Para 4 rarely causes symptomatic infections in humans.

Complications
◆ Croup
◆ Bronchiolitis
◆ Pneumonia

Signs and symptoms
After a short incubation period (usually 3 to 6 days), signs and symptoms emerge that are similar to those of other respiratory diseases: sudden fever, nasal discharge, reddened throat (with little or no exudate), chills, and muscle pain. Bacterial complications are uncommon, but in infants and very young children, parainfluenza may lead to croup or laryngotracheobronchitis. Reinfection is usually less severe and affects only the upper respiratory tract.

Diagnosis
Parainfluenza infections are usually clinically indistinguishable from similar viral infections. A swab or washing of nasal secretions is useful for rapid viral testing. Isolation of the virus and serum antibody titers differentiate parainfluenza from other respiratory illness but is rarely done. In the immunocompromised patient, PCR testing is preferred since it has the highest sensitivity.

Treatment
Parainfluenza may require no treatment or bed rest, antipyretics, analgesics, and antitussives, depending on the severity of the symptoms. Complications, such as croup and pneumonia, require appropriate treatment. No current vaccine is effective against parainfluenza, although vaccines are being developed.

Give corticosteroids and nebulization to treat respiratory symptoms and to reduce airway edema.

Special considerations
◆ Throughout the illness, monitor respiratory status and temperature, and ensure adequate fluid intake and rest.
◆ Strict attention to standard and contact precautions should decrease or prevent spread of infection in healthcare settings.

ADENOVIRUS INFECTION
Causes and incidence
Adenoviruses cause acute, self-limiting febrile infections, with inflammation of the respiratory or ocular mucous membranes, or both. (See *Major adenovirus infections*, page 868.)

Pathophysiology
Adenovirus has 51 known serotypes; it causes five major infections, all of which occur in epidemics. These organisms are common and can remain latent for years; they infect almost everyone early in life, although maternal antibodies offer some protection during the first 6 months of life.

Transmission of adenovirus can occur by direct inoculation into the eye, by the oral–fecal route (adenovirus may persist in the GI tract for years after infection), or by inhalation of an infected droplet.

Complications
◆ Acute conjunctivitis
◆ Sinusitis
◆ Pharyngitis
◆ Bronchiolitis
◆ Pneumonia

Signs and symptoms
The incubation period—usually lasting less than 1 week—is followed by acute illness lasting less than 5 days. Clinical features vary, depending on the type of infection. Prolonged asymptomatic reinfection may occur.

Diagnosis
CONFIRMING DIAGNOSIS *Definitive diagnosis requires isolation of the virus from respiratory, ocular secretions, or fecal smears. Other options include PCR testing or viral antigen assays. During epidemics, however, typical symptoms alone can confirm the diagnosis.*

Adenoviral diseases cause lymphocytosis in children. When they cause respiratory disease, chest X-ray may show pneumonitis.

Major adenovirus infections

Disease	Age group	Clinical features
Acute febrile respiratory illness	Children	Nonspecific coldlike symptoms, similar to other viral respiratory illnesses: fever, pharyngitis, tracheitis, bronchitis, and pneumonitis
Acute respiratory disease	Adults (usually military recruits)	Malaise, fever, chills, headache, pharyngitis, hoarseness, and dry cough
Viral pneumonia	Children and adults	Sudden onset of high fever, rapid infection of upper and lower respiratory tracts, rash, diarrhea, and intestinal intussusception
Acute pharyngoconjunctival fever	Children (particularly after swimming in pools or lakes)	Spiking fever lasting several days, headache, pharyngitis, conjunctivitis, rhinitis, and cervical adenitis
Acute follicular conjunctivitis	Adults	Unilateral tearing and mucoid discharge; later, milder symptoms in other eye
Epidemic keratoconjunctivitis	Adults	Unilateral or bilateral ocular redness and edema, periorbital swelling, local discomfort, and superficial opacity of the cornea without ulceration
Hemorrhagic cystitis	Children (boys)	Adenovirus in urine, hematuria, dysuria, and urinary frequency
Diarrhea	Infants	Fever and watery diarrhea

Treatment

Supportive treatment includes bed rest, antipyretics, and analgesics. Ocular infections may require corticosteroids and direct supervision by an ophthalmologist. Hospitalization is required in cases of pneumonia (in infants) to prevent death and in epidemic keratoconjunctivitis (EKC) to prevent blindness. If antiviral medication is being considered, cidofovir is the drug of choice. However, due to severe nephrotoxicity, this medication should only be given in consultation with an infectious diseases specialist.

Special considerations

◆ During acute illness, monitor respiratory status and intake and output. Give analgesics and antipyretics, as needed. Stress the need for bed rest.
◆ Strict attention to contact and droplet precautions is effective for stopping nosocomial outbreaks of adenovirus-associated disease.
◆ To help minimize the incidence of adenoviral disease, instruct all patients in proper handwashing to reduce fecal–oral transmission and eye inoculation.
◆ EKC can be prevented by sterilization of ophthalmic instruments, adequate chlorination in swimming pools, and avoidance of swimming pools during epidemics. Killed virus vaccine (not widely available) or a live oral virus vaccine can prevent adenoviral infection and are recommended for high-risk groups.

INFLUENZA
Causes and incidence

Influenza (also called the *grippe* or the *flu*), an acute, highly contagious infection of the respiratory tract, results from three different types of *Myxovirus influenzae*. It occurs sporadically or in epidemics (usually during the colder months). Epidemics tend to peak within 2 to 3 weeks after initial cases and subside within a month.

Although influenza affects all age groups, its incidence is highest in schoolchildren. However, its effects are most severe in persons who are young, elderly, or suffering from chronic disease. In these groups, influenza may even lead to death. The catastrophic pandemic of 1918 was responsible for an estimated 20 million deaths. Two of the most recent pandemics (in 1957, 1968, and 2009) began in mainland China; the latest one started in the United States.

Pathophysiology

Transmission of influenza occurs through inhalation of a respiratory droplet from an infected person or by indirect contact with a contaminated object, such as a drinking glass or other items contaminated with respiratory secretions. The influenza virus then invades the epithelium of the respiratory tract, causing inflammation and desquamation. (See *How influenza viruses multiply*.)

One of the remarkable features of the influenza virus is its capacity for *antigenic variation* into numerous distinct strains, allowing it to infect new populations that have little or no immunologic resistance. Antigenic variation is characterized as *antigenic drift* (minor changes that occur yearly or every few years) and *antigenic shift* (major changes that lead to pandemics). Influenza viruses are classified into three groups:

◆ Type A, the most prevalent, strikes every year, with new serotypes causing epidemics every 3 years.
◆ Type B also strikes annually but causes epidemics only every 4 to 6 years.
◆ Type C is endemic and causes only sporadic cases.

Each year, tens of millions of people in the United States get the flu; about 600,000 people get sick enough to be hospitalized, and about 36,000 people die.

Complications

◆ Pneumonia
◆ Myositis
◆ Bronchitis
◆ Reye syndrome
◆ Myocarditis (rare)
◆ Pericarditis (rare)
◆ Transverse myelitis (rare)
◆ Encephalitis (rare)

Signs and symptoms

After an incubation period of 24 to 48 hours, flu symptoms begin to appear: sudden onset of chills, temperature of 101° to 104° F (38.3° to 40° C), headache, malaise, myalgia (particularly in the back and limbs), a nonproductive cough, and, occasionally, laryngitis, hoarseness, conjunctivitis, rhinitis, and rhinorrhea. These symptoms usually subside in 3 to 5 days, but cough and weakness may persist. Fever is usually higher in children than in adults. Also, cervical adenopathy and croup are likely to be associated with influenza in children. In some patients (especially elderly patients), lack of energy and easy fatigability may persist for several weeks.

Fever that persists longer than 3 to 5 days signals the onset of complications. The most common complication is pneumonia, which occurs as primary influenza virus pneumonia or secondary to bacterial infection. Influenza may also cause myositis, exacerbation of chronic obstructive pulmonary disease, Reye syndrome, and, rarely, myocarditis, pericarditis, transverse myelitis, and encephalitis.

Diagnosis

At the beginning of an influenza epidemic, early cases are usually mistaken for other respiratory disorders.

℞ CONFIRMING DIAGNOSIS *Because signs and symptoms of influenza aren't pathognomonic, isolation of* M. influenzae *through nose and throat cultures and increased serum antibody titers help*

PATHOPHYSIOLOGY
How influenza viruses multiply

An influenza virus, classified as type A, B, or C, contains the genetic material ribonucleic acid (RNA), which is covered and protected by protein. RNA is arranged in genes that carry the instruction for viral replication. This genetic material has an extraordinary ability to mutate, causing the generation of new serologically distinct strains of influenza virus. Being a virus, the pathogen can't reproduce or carry out chemical reactions on its own. It needs a host cell.

After attaching to the host cell, the viral RNA enters the host cell and uses host components to replicate its genetic material and protein, which are then assembled into the new virus particles. These newly produced viruses can burst forth to invade other healthy cells.

The viral invasion destroys the host cells, impairing respiratory defenses, especially the mucociliary transport system, and predisposing the patient to secondary bacterial infection.

◆ Virus attaches to host
◆ Viral RNA enters host cell
◆ Viral RNA replicates within host cell
◆ New virus particles are assembled and released

confirm this diagnosis. Also, rapid diagnostic methods for detecting influenza are now available and help confirm this diagnosis.

After these measures confirm an influenza epidemic, diagnosis requires only observation of clinical signs and symptoms. Uncomplicated cases show a decreased WBC count with an increase in lymphocytes.

Treatment

Treatment of uncomplicated influenza includes bed rest, adequate fluid intake, aspirin or acetaminophen (in children) to relieve fever and muscle pain, and antitussives to relieve nonproductive coughing. Prophylactic antibiotics aren't recommended because they have no effect on the influenza virus.

Oseltamivir and zanamivir are effective against influenza A and B infection. In influenza complicated by pneumonia, supportive care (fluid and electrolyte supplements, oxygen, and assisted ventilation) and treatment of bacterial superinfection with appropriate antibiotics are necessary. No specific therapy exists for cardiac, CNS, or other complications.

Special considerations

Unless complications occur, influenza doesn't require hospitalization; patient care focuses on relief of symptoms:

◆ Advise the patient to increase fluid intake. Warm baths or heating pads may relieve myalgia. Give the patient nonopioid analgesics–antipyretics as ordered.

◆ Screen visitors to protect the patient from bacterial infection and the visitors from influenza. Use droplet precautions.

◆ Teach the patient proper disposal of tissues and proper handwashing technique to prevent the virus from spreading.

◆ Watch for signs and symptoms of developing pneumonia, such as crackles, another temperature rise, or coughing accompanied by purulent or bloody sputum. Assist the patient to gradually resume normal activities.

◆ Educate patients about influenza immunizations. For those age 6 months and older, the CDC recommends a yearly flu vaccine. People at high risk for serious flu complications, including young children, pregnant women, people with chronic health conditions, and those age 65 years and older should have an annual flu vaccine to decrease their risk of severe illness. Caregivers of children younger than age 6 months should be vaccinated because these children are at high risk for serious flu illness.

◆ Inform people receiving the vaccine of possible adverse effects (discomfort at the vaccination site, fever, malaise, and, rarely,

Guillain–Barré syndrome). Influenza vaccine (inactivated) is recommended for women who are pregnant and who will be in the second or third trimester during influenza season.

◆ Report flu deaths to the health department.

HANTAVIRUS PULMONARY SYNDROME

Causes and incidence

Mainly occurring in the southwestern United States, but not confined to that area, *Hantavirus* pulmonary syndrome is a viral disease first reported in May 1993. The syndrome, which rapidly progresses from flu-like symptoms to respiratory failure and, possibly, death, is known for its high mortality. The hantavirus strain that causes disease in Asia and Europe—mainly hemorrhagic fever and renal disease—is distinctly different from the one currently described in North America.

Pathophysiology

A member of the Bunyaviridae family, the genus *Hantavirus* (first isolated in 1977) is responsible for *Hantavirus* pulmonary syndrome. Disease transmission is associated with exposure to aerosols (such as dust) contaminated by urine or feces from infected rodents, the primary reservoir for this virus. Field mice cause hemorrhagic fever with renal syndrome; Puumala virus is carried by vole. Deer mice are responsible for hantavirus cardiopulmonary syndrome. Hantavirus infections have been documented in people whose activities are associated with rodent contact, such as farming, hiking or camping in rodent-infested areas, and occupying rodent-infested dwellings.

Infected rodents manifest no apparent illness but shed the virus in feces, urine, and saliva. Human infection may occur from inhalation, ingestion (of contaminated food or water, for example), contact with rodent excrement, or rodent bites. Transmission from person to person or by mosquitoes, fleas, or other arthropods hasn't been reported.

Complications

◆ Respiratory failure
◆ Death

Signs and symptoms

Noncardiogenic pulmonary edema distinguishes the syndrome. Common chief complaints include myalgia, fever, headache, nausea, vomiting, and cough. Respiratory distress typically follows the onset of a cough. Fever, hypoxia, and, in some patients, serious hypotension typify its course.

Other signs and symptoms include a rising respiratory rate (28 breaths/minute or more) and an increased heart rate (120 beats/minute or more).

Screening for *Hantavirus* pulmonary syndrome

The Centers for Disease Control and Prevention (CDC) has developed a screening procedure to track cases of *Hantavirus* pulmonary syndrome. The screening criteria identify potential and actual cases.

Potential cases

For a diagnosis of possible *Hantavirus* pulmonary syndrome, a patient must have one of the following:

♦ febrile illness (temperature equal to or above 101° F [38.3° C]) occurring in a previously healthy person and characterized by unexplained acute respiratory distress syndrome (ARDS)

♦ clinical diagnosis of ARDS

♦ an unexplained respiratory illness resulting in death and autopsy findings demonstrating noncardiogenic pulmonary edema without an identifiable specific cause of death

Exclusions

Of the patients who meet the criteria for having potential *Hantavirus* pulmonary syndrome, the CDC excludes those who have any of the following:

♦ a predisposing underlying medical condition (e.g., severe underlying pulmonary disease), solid tumors or hematologic cancers, congenital or acquired immunodeficiency disorders, or medical conditions or treatments—such as rheumatoid arthritis or organ transplantation—requiring immunosuppressive drug therapy (e.g., steroids or cytotoxic chemotherapy)

♦ an acute illness that provides a likely explanation for the respiratory illness (e.g., a recent major trauma, burn, or surgery; recent seizures or history of aspiration; bacterial sepsis; another respiratory disorder such as respiratory syncytial virus in young children; influenza; or *Legionella* pneumonia)

Confirmed cases

Cases of confirmed *Hantavirus* pulmonary syndrome must include the following:

♦ at least one serum or tissue specimen available for laboratory testing for evidence of hantavirus infection

♦ in a patient with a compatible clinical illness, serologic evidence (presence of hantavirus-specific immunoglobulin [Ig] M or rising titers of IgG), polymerase chain reaction for hantavirus ribonucleic acid, or positive immunohistochemistry for hantavirus antigen

Diagnosis

There are ongoing efforts to identify clinical and laboratory features that distinguish *Hantavirus* pulmonary syndrome from other infections with similar features, and serologic testing is the main method of diagnosis.

Laboratory tests usually reveal an elevated WBC count with a predominance of neutrophils, myeloid precursors, and atypical lymphocytes; elevated hematocrit; decreased platelet count; elevated partial thromboplastin time; and a normal fibrinogen level. Usually, laboratory findings demonstrate only minimal abnormalities in renal function, with serum creatinine levels no higher than 2.5 mg/dL.

Chest X-rays eventually show bilateral diffuse infiltrates in almost all patients (findings consistent with ARDS).

Treatment

Primarily supportive, treatment consists of maintaining adequate oxygenation, monitoring vital signs, and intervening to stabilize the patient's heart rate and blood pressure.

Drug therapy includes vasopressors, such as dopamine or epinephrine, for hypotension.

Fluid volume replacement may also be ordered (with precautions not to overhydrate the patient).

Special considerations

♦ Assess the patient's respiratory status and ABG values often.

♦ Monitor serum electrolyte levels and correct imbalances as appropriate.

♦ Maintain a patent airway by suctioning. Ensure adequate humidification, and check ventilator settings frequently.

♦ In patients with hypoxemia, assess neurologic status frequently along with heart rate and blood pressure.

♦ Administer drug therapy, and monitor the patient's response.

♦ Provide I.V. fluid therapy based on results of hemodynamic monitoring.

♦ Provide emotional support for the patient and family.

♦ Report cases of *Hantavirus* pulmonary syndrome to the appropriate state health department.

♦ Provide the patient with prevention guidelines. (Until more is known about *Hantavirus* pulmonary syndrome, preventive measures currently focus on rodent control.)

ROTAVIRUS
Causes and incidence
Rotavirus is the most common cause of severe diarrhea among children. The disease is characterized by vomiting and watery diarrhea for 3 to 8 days, commonly with fever and abdominal pain.

In the United States and other countries with a temperate climate, the disease has a winter seasonal pattern, with annual epidemics occurring from November to April. The illness occurs most often in infants and young children; most children in the United States are infected by age 2. Rotavirus is responsible for the hospitalization of about 40 to 50,000 children each year in the United States and for the death of more than 600,000 children annually worldwide.

Pathophysiology
The primary mode of transmission is fecal–oral, although some have reported low titers of virus in respiratory tract secretions and other body fluids. Because of the endurance of the virus in the environment, transmission may occur through ingestion of contaminated water or food and contact with contaminated surfaces.

Billions of rotavirus particles are passed in the stool of the infected individual. Small numbers of the rotavirus may lead to infection if a baby puts fingers or other objects contaminated with the virus into the mouth. Young children can pass it on to siblings and parents.

Immunity after infection is incomplete, but recurrent infections tend to be less severe than the original infection.

Complications
◆ Severe dehydration
◆ Shock
◆ Skin breakdown

Signs and symptoms
The incubation period for rotavirus disease is about 2 days. Rotavirus gastroenteritis commonly starts with a fever, nausea, and vomiting, followed by diarrhea. The illness can range from mild to severe and last from 3 to 9 days. Diarrhea and vomiting may cause dehydration.

Diagnosis
The diagnosis is determined by rapid antigen detection of rotavirus in stool specimens.

Rotavirus is the most common diagnosis for young children with acute diarrhea, but other causes may include bacteria (*Salmonella*, *Shigella*, and *Campylobacter* are the most common),

parasites (*Giardia* and *Cryptosporidium* are the most common), localized infection elsewhere, antibiotic-associated adverse effects (such as those related to treatment for *C. difficile*), and food poisoning. Noninfectious causes include overfeeding (particularly of fruit juices), irritable bowel syndrome, celiac disease, milk protein intolerance, lactose intolerance, cystic fibrosis, and inflammatory bowel syndrome.

Treatment
For a person with a healthy immune system, rotavirus gastroenteritis is a self-limited illness, lasting only days. Treatment is nonspecific and consists of oral rehydration therapy to prevent dehydration.

Special considerations
◆ Enforce strict handwashing and careful cleaning of all equipment, including the child's toys, to prevent the spread of rotavirus.
◆ Implement contact precautions.
◆ Help the patient maintain adequate hydration. Remember that dehydration occurs rapidly in infants and young children. Ice pops, gelatin, and ice chips may be included in the diet to maintain hydration.
◆ Breast-fed infants should continue to nurse without restrictions. Lactose-free soybean formulas may be used for infants who are bottle-fed.
◆ Carefully monitor intake and output (including stools).
◆ Clean the perineum thoroughly to prevent skin breakdown.
◆ Instruct parents about proper handwashing techniques for themselves and the infant. Provide instructions about diaper changing and cleaning all affected surfaces.
◆ Teach parents and caregivers how to measure intake and output. Tell them to notify their physician about any increased diarrhea or dehydration.

AVIAN INFLUENZA
Causes and incidence
Avian influenza (flu) mainly infects birds, but is of concern to humans, who have no immunity against it. The virus that causes this infection in birds can mutate and easily infect humans and potentially start a deadly worldwide epidemic. The first avian flu virus to infect humans directly occurred in Hong Kong in 1997 and has since spread across Asia. About 860 people have been infected with avian influenza A virus (H5N1) and the current death rate with confirmed infection is more than 50%. Prognosis depends on the severity of infection as well as the type of avian flu virus that caused it.

Those at risk include:
- farmers and other people working with poultry
- travelers visiting affected countries
- people who handle infected birds
- people who eat raw or undercooked poultry meat
- healthcare workers and others in contact with patients who have avian flu

Pathophysiology

H5N1 virus is commonly referred to as *bird flu virus*. Highly infective avian flu viruses, such as H5N1, have been shown to survive in the environment for long periods of time, and infection may be spread simply by touching contaminated surfaces. Birds who recover from flu can continue to shed the virus in their feces and saliva for as long as 10 days.

Influenza viruses are made up of enveloped RNA with a segmented genome. Over the years, antigenic drift occurs, or mutations in the genetic makeup of the viruses. The severity of human H5N1 may be related to excessive inflammatory response of the host in response to the virus, which actually worsens tissue destruction and can lead to pathogenicity.

Complications
- Conjunctivitis
- Pneumonia
- Acute respiratory distress
- Viral pneumonia
- Sepsis
- Organ failure

Signs and symptoms

Symptoms of avian flu infection in humans depend on the particular strain of virus. In the case of the H5N1 virus, infection causes more classic flu-like symptoms, which might include headache, malaise, dry or productive cough, sore throat, fever greater than 100.4° F (38° C), runny nose, difficulty breathing, diarrhea, and muscle aches.

Diagnosis

CONFIRMING DIAGNOSIS *H5N1 can be confirmed using a PCR assay. The test gives preliminary results within 4 hours; older tests required 2 to 3 days.*

Chest X-ray, nasopharyngeal culture, and blood differential can also aid in diagnosis.

Treatment

The antiviral medication oseltamivir may decrease the severity of the disease, if started within 48 hours after symptoms begin. Oseltamivir

may also be prescribed for household contacts of people diagnosed with avian flu. Provide supportive treatment with mechanical ventilation, I.V. fluids, and symptomatic treatment.

It's currently recommended that people diagnosed with H5N1 infection be put in an airborne isolation room that has negative air pressure, with 6 to 12 air changes per hour and high-efficiency particulate air filtration. Healthcare workers should wear N95 respirator masks.

Currently, there's no available vaccine against avian flu. However, a vaccine against H5N1 is being tested in clinical trials.

A flu shot may be administered to reduce the chance of an avian flu virus mixing with a human flu virus, which would create a new virus that might spread easily.

Special considerations
- Tell patients to call their healthcare provider if they develop flu-like symptoms within 10 days of handling infected birds or traveling to an area with a known avian flu outbreak.
- Travelers should avoid visits to live-bird markets in areas with an avian flu outbreak.
- Those who work with birds who might be infected should use protective clothing and special breathing masks.
- Watch for signs and symptoms of complications.
- Report cases to the public health authorities.

⫶⫶⫶⫶⫶ PREVENTION
- *Tell the patient that avoiding undercooked or uncooked meat reduces the risk of exposure to avian flu and other food-borne diseases.*
- *Teach the patient about proper disposal of tissues and proper handwashing technique.*
- *Healthcare professionals should wear eye protection within 3 feet of the patient and wear N95 respirators approved by the National Institute for Occupational Safety and Health.*
- *Maintain strict adherence to standard and contact precautions.*

Rash-producing viruses

VARICELLA
Causes and incidence

Varicella, commonly known as *chickenpox*, is a common, acute, and very contagious infection caused by the herpesvirus varicella-zoster, the same virus that, in its latent stage, causes herpes zoster (shingles).

Chickenpox can occur at any age, but it's most common in children ages 2 to 8. Congenital varicella may affect infants whose mothers had acute infections in their first or early second trimester.

Neonatal infection is rare, probably because of transient maternal immunity. However, neonates born to mothers who develop varicella 5 days before delivery or up to 2 days after delivery are at risk for developing severe generalized varicella. Second attacks are also rare.

Chickenpox occurs worldwide and is endemic in large cities. Outbreaks occur sporadically, usually in areas with large groups of susceptible children. It affects all races and both sexes equally. Seasonal distribution varies; in temperate areas, incidence is higher during late autumn, winter, and spring.

Most children recover completely. Potentially fatal complications may affect children on corticosteroids, antimetabolites, or other immunosuppressants and those with leukemia, other neoplasms, or immunodeficiency disorders. Congenital and adult varicella may also have severe effects.

Pathophysiology

This infection is transmitted by direct contact (primarily with respiratory secretions; less commonly, with skin lesions) and indirect contact (airborne). The incubation period usually lasts 14 to 17 days but can be as short as 10 days and as long as 20 days. (See *Incubation and duration of common rash-producing infections.*) Chickenpox is probably communicable from 1 day before lesions erupt to 6 days after vesicles form (it's most contagious in the early stages of eruption of skin lesions).

Complications

◆ Pneumonia
◆ Encephalitis

Signs and symptoms

Chickenpox produces distinctive signs and symptoms, notably a pruritic rash. During the prodromal phase, the patient has slight fever, malaise, and anorexia. Within 24 hours, the rash typically begins as crops of small, erythematous macules on the trunk or scalp. It progresses to papules and then clear vesicles on an erythematous base (the so-called dewdrop on a rose petal). These become cloudy and break easily; then scabs form.

The rash spreads to the face and over the trunk of the body, then to the limbs, buccal mucosa, axillae, upper respiratory tract, conjunctivae, and, occasionally, the genitalia. New vesicles continue to appear for 3 or 4 days, so the rash contains a combination of red papules, vesicles, and scabs in various stages.

Congenital varicella causes hypoplastic deformity and limb scarring, retarded growth, and CNS and eye manifestations. In progressive varicella, an immunocompromised patient may have lesions and a high fever for more than 7 days.

Severe pruritus with this rash may provoke persistent scratching, which can lead to infection, scarring, impetigo, furuncles, and cellulitis. Rare complications include pneumonia, myocarditis, fulminating encephalitis (Reye syndrome), bleeding disorders, arthritis, nephritis, hepatitis, and acute myositis.

Diagnosis

Diagnosis rests on the characteristic clinical signs and usually doesn't require laboratory tests. However, the virus can be isolated from vesicular fluid within the first 3 or 4 days of the rash (before crusting occurs); PCR is fast and sensitive. Serum contains antibodies 7 days after onset.

Treatment

Chickenpox calls for droplet and contact isolation in a negative-pressure room until all vesicles and most of the scabs are dry (no new lesions; usually 1 week after the onset of the rash). Children with only a few remaining scabs are no

---

Incubation and duration of common rash-producing infections

	Incubation	Duration
Herpes simplex	2 to 12	7 to 21
Roseola infantum	10 to 15	3 to 6
Rubella	14 to 21	3
Rubeola	8 to 14	5
Varicella	14 to 17	7 to 14

longer contagious and can return to school. Congenital chickenpox requires no isolation.

In most cases, treatment consists of local or systemic antipruritics: lukewarm oatmeal baths, calamine lotion, or diphenhydramine (or another antihistamine). Antibiotics are unnecessary unless bacterial infection develops. Salicylates are contraindicated because of their link with Reye syndrome.

Susceptible patients may need special treatment. Acyclovir and valacyclovir, antiviral agents, may slow vesicle formation, speed skin healing, and control the systemic spread of infection.

Special considerations

Care is supportive and emphasizes patient and family teaching and preventive measures.
◆ Teach the child and family how to apply topical antipruritic medications correctly. Stress the importance of good hygiene.
◆ Tell the patient not to scratch the lesions. However, because the need to scratch may be overwhelming, parents should trim the child's fingernails or tie mittens on hands.
◆ Warn parents to watch for and immediately report signs of complications. Severe skin pain

and burning may indicate a serious secondary infection and require prompt medical attention.

 PREVENTION
◆ *Varicella vaccine, part of the recommended childhood immunization schedule, effectively prevents infection.*
◆ *To help prevent chickenpox, don't admit a child exposed to chickenpox to a unit that contains children who receive immunosuppressants or who have leukemia or immunodeficiency disorders.*

HERPES SIMPLEX
Causes and incidence

Herpes simplex, a recurrent viral infection, is caused by *herpesvirus hominis* (HVH), a widespread infectious agent. Herpes simplex type 1 (HSV-1), which is transmitted by oral and respiratory secretions, affects the skin and mucous membranes, commonly producing cold sores and fever blisters. Herpes simplex type 2 (HSV-2) primarily affects the genital area and is transmitted by sexual contact. However, cross-infection may result from orogenital sex or autoinoculation from one site to another. (See *Understanding the genital herpes cycle.*)

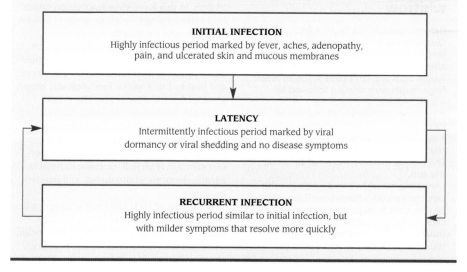

PATHOPHYSIOLOGY
Understanding the genital herpes cycle

After a patient is infected with genital herpes, a latency period follows. The virus resides permanently in the nerve cells surrounding the lesions, and intermittent viral shedding may take place.

Repeated outbreaks may develop at any time, again followed by a latent stage during which the lesions heal completely. Outbreaks may recur as often as three to eight times per year. Although the cycle continues indefinitely, some people remain asymptomatic for years.

INITIAL INFECTION
Highly infectious period marked by fever, aches, adenopathy, pain, and ulcerated skin and mucous membranes

LATENCY
Intermittently infectious period marked by viral dormancy or viral shedding and no disease symptoms

RECURRENT INFECTION
Highly infectious period similar to initial infection, but with milder symptoms that resolve more quickly

About 85% of all HVH infections are subclinical; the others produce localized lesions and systemic reactions. After the first infection, a patient is a carrier susceptible to recurrent infections, which may be provoked by fever, menses, stress, heat, and cold. However, the patient usually has no constitutional signs and symptoms in recurrent infections.

Primary HVH is the leading cause of childhood gingivostomatitis in children ages 1 to 3. It causes the most common form of nonepidemic encephalitis and is the second most common viral infection in pregnant women. It can pass to the fetus transplacentally and, in early pregnancy, may cause spontaneous abortion or premature birth. (See *Recognizing herpetic whitlow*.)

Herpes infection is equally common in males and females. Worldwide in distribution, it's most prevalent among children in lower socioeconomic groups who live in crowded environments. Saliva, stool, skin lesions, purulent eye exudate, and urine are potential sources of infection.

Pathophysiology

The acute virus acts on dermal keratinocytes and other areas of the epithelium and rapidly replicates, causing tissue destruction. This leads to activation of the immune response. The virus can also travel along axons in the nervous system, leading to infection of the ganglia within 24 hours of exposure.

Recognizing herpetic whitlow

Herpetic whitlow is a finger infection caused by the microorganism that causes herpes simplex virus (HSV). It commonly affects nurses, usually only in one finger. Typical signs and symptoms in the affected finger begin with tingling followed by:
♦ pain, redness, and swelling
♦ vesicular eruptions bordered by red halos
♦ vesicular ulceration or coalescence—related effects include satellite vesicles, fever, chills, malaise, and a red streak up the arm.

Healing occurs in 2 to 3 weeks. Health-care workers with herpetic whitlow must be restricted from patient care. In health-care workers, the infecting organism usually is HSV-1. In others, the infection usually is secondary to HSV-2 infection.

Complications
♦ Abortion
♦ Premature labor
♦ Microcephaly
♦ Uterine growth retardation
♦ Increased risk of cervical cancer
♦ Perianal ulcers
♦ Colitis
♦ Esophagitis
♦ Pneumonitis

Signs and symptoms

In neonates, HVH symptoms usually appear 1 to 2 weeks after birth. They range from localized skin lesions to a disseminated infection of organs, such as the liver, lungs, or brain. Common complications include seizures, mental retardation, blindness, chorioretinitis, deafness, microcephaly, diabetes insipidus, and spasticity. Up to 90% of infants with disseminated disease die.

Primary infection in childhood may be localized or generalized and occurs after an incubation period of 2 to 12 days. After brief prodromal tingling and itching, localized infection causes typical primary lesions. These erupt as vesicles on an erythematous base, eventually rupture and leave a painful ulcer, followed by a yellowish crust. Vesicles may form on any part of the oral mucosa, especially the tongue, gingiva, and cheeks. Healing begins 7 to 10 days after onset and is complete in 3 weeks.

Generalized infection begins with fever, pharyngitis, erythema, and edema. Vesicles occur with submaxillary lymphadenopathy, increased salivation, halitosis, anorexia, and a fever of up to 105° F (40.6° C). Herpetic stomatitis may lead to severe dehydration in children. A generalized infection usually runs its course in 4 to 10 days. In this form, virus reactivation causes cold sores—a single vesicle or group of vesicles in and around the mouth.

Genital herpes usually affects adolescents and young adults. Typically painful, the initial attack produces fluid-filled vesicles that ulcerate and heal in 1 to 3 weeks. Fever, regional lymphadenopathy, and dysuria may also occur.

Usually, herpetic keratoconjunctivitis is unilateral and causes only local signs and symptoms: conjunctivitis, regional adenopathy, blepharitis, and vesicles on the lid. Other ocular effects may include excessive lacrimation, edema, chemosis, photophobia, and purulent exudate.

Both types of HVH can cause acute sporadic encephalitis with altered LOC, personality changes, and seizures. Other effects may include smell and taste hallucinations and neurologic abnormalities such as aphasia.

Herpetic whitlow, an HVH finger infection, affects many nurses. First the finger tingles and then it becomes red, swollen, and painful. Vesicles with a red halo erupt and may ulcerate or coalesce. Other effects may include satellite vesicles, fever, chills, malaise, and a red streak up the arm.

Diagnosis

℞ CONFIRMING DIAGNOSIS *Typical lesions may suggest HVH infection. However, confirmation requires isolation of the virus from local lesions. A viral culture or PCR testing is the preferred method of diagnosis for those with active lesions.*

A rise in antibodies and moderate leukocytosis may support the diagnosis.

Treatment

No cure for herpes exists; however, recurrences tend to be milder and of shorter duration than the primary infection. Symptomatic and supportive therapy is essential. Generalized primary infection usually requires an analgesic-antipyretic to reduce fever and relieve pain. Anesthetic mouthwashes, such as viscous lidocaine, may reduce the pain of gingivostomatitis, enabling the patient to eat and preventing dehydration. (Avoid alcohol-based mouthwashes.) Drying agents, such as calamine lotion, ease the pain of labial or skin lesions. Avoid petroleum-based ointments, which promote viral spread and slow healing.

Refer patients with eye infections to an ophthalmologist.

Oral acyclovir, valacyclovir, or famciclovir may bring relief to patients with herpes. Frequent prophylactic use of acyclovir in immunosuppressed transplant patients prevents disseminated disease.

Special considerations

◆ Teach the patient with genital herpes to use warm compresses or take sitz baths several times per day, to increase fluid intake, and to avoid all sexual contact during the active stage.
◆ For pregnant women with active HVH infection at the time of delivery, a cesarean delivery is recommended to decrease the risk of infecting the neonate. Infants with neonatal herpes should be placed in contact precautions.
◆ Healthcare personnel should use standard precautions, such as gloves, for contact with mucous membranes to prevent acquisition of herpetic whitlow.
◆ Instruct patients with herpetic whitlow not to share towels or eating utensils. Educate staff members and other susceptible people about the risk of contagion. Abstain from direct patient care if you have herpetic whitlow.

◆ Tell patients with cold sores not to kiss people. (Those with genital herpes pose no risk to infants if their hygiene is meticulous.)
◆ Patients with CNS infection alone need no isolation.
◆ Place patients with severe primary or disseminated mucocutaneous herpes simplex (with lesions) on contact precautions.

HERPES ZOSTER
Causes and incidence

Herpes zoster (also called *shingles*) is an acute unilateral and segmental inflammation of the dorsal root ganglia caused by infection with the herpesvirus varicella-zoster, which also causes chickenpox. This infection usually occurs in adults. It produces localized vesicular skin lesions, confined to a dermatome, and severe neuralgic pain in peripheral areas innervated by the nerves arising in the inflamed root ganglia.

Herpes zoster occurs primarily in adults, especially those older than age 60. It seldom recurs. It's also seen in patients with HIV and other immunodeficiency disorders.

The prognosis is good unless the infection spreads to the brain. Eventually, most patients recover completely, except for possible scarring and, in corneal damage, visual impairment. Occasionally, neuralgia may persist for months or years.

Pathophysiology

Herpes zoster results from reactivation of varicella virus that has lain dormant in the cerebral ganglia (extramedullary ganglia of the cranial nerves) or the ganglia of posterior nerve roots since a previous episode of chickenpox. Exactly how or why this reactivation occurs isn't clear. Some believe that the virus multiplies as it's reactivated and that antibodies remaining from the initial infection neutralize it. However, if effective antibodies aren't present, the virus continues to multiply in the ganglia, destroy the host neuron, and spread down the sensory nerves to the skin.

Complications

◆ Postherpetic neuralgia—most common
◆ Vision loss if eye affected
◆ Pneumonia
◆ Hearing loss
◆ Encephalitis (rare)

Signs and symptoms

Herpes zoster begins with fever and malaise. Within 2 to 4 days, severe deep pain, pruritus, and paresthesia or hyperesthesia develop, usually on the trunk and occasionally on the arms and legs in a dermatomal distribution. Pain may be continuous or intermittent and usually lasts from 1 to 4 weeks. Up to 2 weeks after the first symptoms (but usually in 1 to 5 days), small red nodular skin lesions erupt on the painful areas. (These lesions typically spread unilaterally around the thorax or vertically over the arms or legs.) Sometimes nodules don't appear at all, but when they do, they quickly become vesicles filled with clear fluid or pus. About 10 days after they appear, the vesicles dry and form scabs. (See *Recognizing shingles*.) When ruptured, such lesions usually become infected and, in severe cases, may lead to the enlargement of regional lymph nodes; they may even become gangrenous. Intense pain may occur before the rash appears and after the scabs form.

Occasionally, herpes zoster involves the cranial nerves, especially the trigeminal and geniculate ganglia or the oculomotor nerve. Geniculate zoster may cause vesicle formation in the external auditory canal, ipsilateral facial palsy, hearing loss, dizziness, and loss of taste. Trigeminal ganglion involvement causes eye pain and, possibly, corneal and scleral damage and impaired vision. Rarely, oculomotor involvement causes conjunctivitis, extraocular weakness, ptosis, and paralytic mydriasis.

In rare cases, herpes zoster leads to generalized CNS infection, muscle atrophy, motor paralysis (usually transient), acute transverse myelitis, and ascending myelitis. More commonly, generalized infection causes acute urine retention and unilateral diaphragm paralysis. In postherpetic neuralgia, most common in elderly persons, intractable neurologic pain may persist for years. Scars may be permanent.

Patients with immunodeficiency disorders may develop disseminated zoster. Lesions are bilateral and not limited to dermatomal distribution.

Diagnosis

Diagnosis of herpes zoster usually isn't possible until the characteristic skin lesions develop. Before then, the pain may mimic that of appendicitis, pleurisy, or other conditions. Individuals who are susceptible to varicella may develop a varicella infection following exposure to patients with zoster. Examination of vesicular fluid and infected tissue shows eosinophilic intranuclear inclusions and varicella virus. Also, a lumbar puncture shows increased pressure; examination of CSF shows increased protein levels and, possibly, pleocytosis. Differentiation of herpes zoster from localized herpes simplex requires staining antibodies from vesicular fluid and identification under fluorescent light.

Treatment

Antiviral therapy is the mainstay of treatment. Acyclovir, valacyclovir, and famciclovir seem to stop the rash's progression and prevent visceral complications. Capsaicin, topical lidocaine, and tricyclic antidepressants such as amitriptyline, gabapentin, or pregabalin are the current treatments of choice for postherpetic neuralgia. Topical antiviral ointment is helpful if started early in the disease process.

Herpes zoster ophthalmicus is treated with oral antiviral therapy and possibly topical steroids.

Special considerations

Your care plan should emphasize keeping the patient comfortable, maintaining meticulous hygiene, and preventing further infection. During the acute phase, adequate rest and supportive care can promote proper healing of lesions.

◆ If calamine lotion has been ordered, apply it liberally to the lesions. If lesions are severe and widespread, apply a wet dressing. Drying therapies, such as oxygen or air-loss bed, and Silvadene ointment, may also be used.

◆ Instruct the patient to avoid scratching the lesions.

◆ If vesicles rupture, apply a cold compress as ordered.

◆ To decrease the pain of oral lesions, tell the patient to use a soft toothbrush, eat soft foods, and use a saline or bicarbonate mouthwash.

◆ To minimize neuralgic pain, never withhold or delay administration of analgesics. Give them exactly on schedule because the pain of herpes zoster can be severe. In postherpetic neuralgia, consult a pain specialist to maximize pain relief without risking tolerance to the analgesic.

Recognizing shingles

The characteristic skin lesions in herpes zoster (shingles) are fluid-filled vesicles that dry and form scabs after about 10 days.

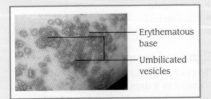

Erythematous base

Umbilicated vesicles

◆ Repeatedly reassure the patient that herpetic pain will eventually subside. Encourage diversionary or relaxation activity.
◆ Institute droplet and contact precautions. Disseminated zoster requires the same isolation precautions as primary varicella as well as negative-pressure rooms.

▌▌▌ PREVENTION *Vaccination with Shingrix is recommended to prevent the occurrence of shingles in adults older than age 50.*

RUBELLA
Causes and incidence

Rubella, commonly called *German measles*, is an acute, mildly contagious viral disease that produces a distinctive 3-day rash and lymphadenopathy. It usually occurs among children ages 5 to 9, adolescents, and young adults. Rubella flourishes worldwide during the spring (particularly in big cities), and epidemics occur sporadically. This disease is self-limiting, with an excellent prognosis.

Pathophysiology

The rubella virus is transmitted through contact with the blood, urine, stools, or nasopharyngeal secretions of infected people and, possibly, by contact with contaminated articles of clothing. Transplacental transmission, especially in the first trimester of pregnancy, can cause serious birth defects, such as microcephaly, mental retardation, patent ductus arteriosus, glaucoma, and bone defects. (See *Congenital rubella syndrome.*) Humans are the only known hosts for the rubella virus. The disease is contagious from about 10 days before the rash appears until 5 days after it has appeared.

Complications
◆ Arthritis (females)
◆ Encephalitis
◆ Myocarditis
◆ Thrombocytopenia
◆ Hepatitis

Signs and symptoms

In children, after an incubation period of 14 to 21 days, an exanthematous, maculopapular rash erupts abruptly. (See *Incubation and duration of common rash-producing infections*, page 874.) In adolescents and adults, prodromal signs and symptoms—headache, malaise, anorexia, low-grade fever, coryza, lymphadenopathy, and, sometimes, conjunctivitis—are the first to appear. Suboccipital, postauricular, and postcervical lymph node enlargement is a hallmark of this disease and precedes the rash.

Congenital rubella syndrome

Congenital rubella is by far the most serious form of the disease. Intrauterine rubella infection, especially during the first trimester, can lead to spontaneous abortion or stillbirth as well as single or multiple birth defects. (As a rule, the earlier the infection occurs during pregnancy, the greater the damage to the fetus.)

The combination of cataracts, deafness, and cardiac disease characterizes congenital rubella syndrome. Low birth weight, microcephaly, and mental retardation are other common manifestations. However, researchers now believe that congenital rubella can cause more disorders, many of which don't appear until later in life. These include dental abnormalities, thrombocytopenic purpura, hemolytic and hypoplastic anemia, encephalitis, giant cell hepatitis, seborrheic dermatitis, and diabetes mellitus. Indeed, it now appears that congenital rubella may be a lifelong disease. This theory is supported by the fact that the rubella virus has been isolated from urine 15 years after its acquisition in the uterus.

Neonates born with congenital rubella should be placed on contact precautions immediately because they excrete the virus for several months to a year after birth. Cataracts and cardiac defects may require surgery. The prognosis depends on the particular malformations that occur. The overall mortality for neonates with rubella is 6%, but it's higher for neonates born with thrombocytopenic purpura, congenital cardiac disease, or encephalitis. Parents of affected children need emotional support and guidance in finding help from community resources and organizations.

Typically, the rubella rash begins on the face and spreads rapidly, in many cases covering the trunk and extremities within hours. Small, red, petechial macules on the soft palate (Forchheimer spots) may precede or accompany the rash but aren't diagnostic of rubella. By the end of the second day, the facial rash begins to fade, but the rash on the trunk may become confluent and be mistaken for scarlet fever. The rash continues to fade downward in the order in which it appeared. It generally disappears on the third day, but it may persist for 4 or 5 days—sometimes accompanied by mild coryza and conjunctivitis. The rapid appearance and disappearance of the rubella rash distinguishes it from rubeola. In rare cases, rubella can occur without a rash. Low-grade fever may accompany the rash (99° to 101° F [37.2° to 38.3° C]), but it usually doesn't persist after the first day of the rash; rarely, temperature may reach 104° F (40° C).

Complications seldom occur in children with rubella, but when they do, they commonly appear as hemorrhagic problems such as thrombocytopenia. Many young women, however, experience transient joint pain or arthritis, usually just as the rash is fading. Fever may then recur. These complications usually subside spontaneously within 5 to 30 days.

A significant number of cases, 20% to 50%, are asymptomatic.

Diagnosis

The rubella rash, lymphadenopathy, other characteristic signs, and a history of exposure to infected people usually permit clinical diagnosis without laboratory tests.

CONFIRMING DIAGNOSIS *The rubella rash has been confused with scarlet fever, measles (rubeola), infectious mononucleosis, roseola, erythema infectiosum, and other viral exanthems. Therefore, without exposure history, laboratory confirmation is beneficial. The most common way to diagnose rubella is by detection of IgM antibodies with EIA. Cell cultures of the throat, blood, urine, and CSF can also confirm the virus' presence.*

Treatment

Because the rubella rash is self-limiting and only mildly pruritic, it doesn't require topical or systemic medication. Treatment consists of analgesics for fever and joint pain. Bed rest isn't necessary, but the patient should be on droplet precautions until 7 days after onset of the rash.

Special considerations

◆ Make the patient with active rubella as comfortable as possible. If the patient is a child, give them children's books to read or games to play to keep the patient occupied.
◆ Explain to the patient why droplet precautions are necessary. Make sure the patient understands how important it is to avoid exposing women who are pregnant to this disease.
◆ Report confirmed cases of rubella to local public health officials.

Before giving the rubella vaccine:
◆ Obtain a history of allergies, especially to neomycin. If the patient has this allergy or has had a reaction to immunization in the past, check with the physician before giving the vaccine.

◆ Ask women of childbearing age if they're pregnant. If they are or think they may be, *don't* give the vaccine or perform a pregnancy test first. Warn women who receive rubella vaccine to use an effective means of birth control for at least 28 days after immunization.
◆ Give the vaccine at least 3 months after any administration of immune globulin or blood, which could have antibodies that neutralize the vaccine.
◆ Don't vaccinate patients who are immunocompromised, patients with immunodeficiency diseases, or those receiving immunosuppressive, radiation, or corticosteroid therapy.

After giving the rubella vaccine:
◆ Observe the patient for signs of anaphylaxis for at least 30 minutes. Keep epinephrine 1:1,000 handy.
◆ Warn the patient about possible mild fever, slight rash, transient arthralgia (in adolescents), and arthritis (in elderly patients). Suggest acetaminophen for fever.
◆ If swelling persists after the initial 24 hours, suggest a cold compress to promote vasoconstriction and prevent antigenic cyst formation.

PREVENTION *Immunization with live-virus vaccine RA27/3, the only rubella vaccine available in the United States, is necessary for prevention and appears to be more immunogenic than previous vaccines. The rubella vaccine should be given with measles and mumps vaccines (MMR) between ages 12 and 15 months to decrease the cost and number of injections.*

RUBEOLA
Causes and incidence

Rubeola, also known as the *measles* or *morbilli*, is an acute, highly contagious paramyxovirus infection that may be one of the most common and most serious of all communicable childhood diseases. Use of the vaccine has reduced the occurrence of measles during childhood; as a result, measles is becoming more prevalent in adolescents and adults. (See *Administering measles vaccine*, page 881.) In the United States, the prognosis is usually excellent; however, measles is a major cause of death in children in underdeveloped countries.

Pathophysiology

Measles is spread by direct contact or by contaminated airborne respiratory droplets. The portal of entry is the upper respiratory tract. In temperate zones, incidence is highest in late winter and early spring. Before the availability of measles vaccine, epidemics occurred every 2 to 5 years in large urban areas.

Administering measles vaccine

♦ Ask the patient about known allergies, especially to neomycin (each dose contains a small amount). However, a patient who's allergic to eggs may receive the vaccine because it contains only minimal amounts of albumin and yolk components.
♦ Avoid giving the vaccine to a pregnant woman (ask for date of last menstrual period). Warn female patients to avoid pregnancy for at least 28 days following vaccination.
♦ Don't vaccinate children with untreated tuberculosis, immunodeficiencies, leukemia, or lymphoma or those receiving immunosuppressants.
♦ Delay vaccination for 8 to 12 weeks after administration of whole blood, plasma, or gamma globulin because measles antibodies in these components may neutralize the vaccine.

♦ Watch for signs of anaphylaxis for 30 minutes after vaccination. Keep epinephrine 1:1,000 handy.
♦ Warn the patient or parents that possible adverse effects are anorexia, malaise, rash, mild thrombocytopenia or leukopenia, and fever. Advise them that mild reactions may occur, usually within 7 to 10 days. If swelling occurs within 24 hours after vaccination, tell the patient to apply cold compresses to the injection site to promote vasoconstriction and to prevent antigenic cyst formation.
♦ Generally, one bout of measles provides immunity (a second infection is extremely rare and may indicate a misdiagnosis); infants younger than age 4 months may be immune because of circulating maternal antibodies. Under normal conditions, measles vaccine isn't administered to children younger than age 12 months.

Complications
♦ Otitis media
♦ Cervical adenitis
♦ Laryngitis
♦ Pneumonia
♦ Encephalitis

Signs and symptoms
Incubation is from 8 to 14 days. Initial symptoms begin and greatest communicability occurs during the prodromal phase, about 11 days after exposure to the virus. This phase lasts from 4 to 5 days; signs and symptoms include fever, photophobia, malaise, anorexia, conjunctivitis, coryza, hoarseness, and hacking cough.

Rubeola

The child shown below displays the characteristic red blotchy skin of rubeola.

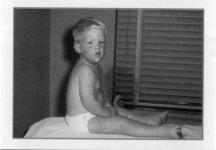

At the end of the prodrome, Koplik spots, the hallmark of the disease, appear. These spots look like tiny, bluish white specks surrounded by a red halo. They appear on the oral mucosa opposite the molars and occasionally bleed. About 5 days after Koplik spots appear, temperature rises sharply, spots slough off, and a slightly pruritic rash appears. This characteristic rash starts as faint macules behind the ears and on the neck and cheeks. The macules become papular and erythematous, rapidly spreading over the entire face, neck, eyelids, arms, chest, back, abdomen, and thighs. (See *Rubeola*.) When the rash reaches the feet (2 to 3 days later), it begins to fade in the same sequence that it appeared, leaving a brownish discoloration that disappears in 7 to 10 days. (See *Incubation and duration of common rash-producing infections*, page 874.)

The disease climax occurs 3 to 4 days after the rash appears and is marked by a fever of 103° to 105° F (39.4° to 40.6° C), severe cough, puffy red eyes, and rhinorrhea. About 5 days after the rash appears, other symptoms disappear and communicability ends. Symptoms are usually mild in patients with partial immunity (conferred by administration of gamma globulin) or infants with transplacental antibodies. More severe symptoms and complications are more likely to develop in young infants, adolescents, adults, and patients who are immunocompromised than in young children.

Atypical measles may appear in patients who received the killed measles vaccine. These patients are acutely ill with a fever and maculopapular rash that's most obvious in the arms and legs or with pulmonary involvement and no skin lesions.

Severe infection may lead to secondary bacterial infection and to autoimmune reaction or organ invasion by the virus, resulting in otitis media, pneumonia, and encephalitis. Subacute sclerosing panencephalitis, a rare and invariably fatal complication, may develop several years after measles, but it's less common in patients who have received the measles vaccine.

Diagnosis

Diagnosis rests on distinctive clinical features, especially the pathognomonic Koplik spots. Mild measles may resemble rubella, roseola infantum, enterovirus infection, toxoplasmosis, and drug eruptions; laboratory tests are required for a differential diagnosis. Serology can show positive IgM antibodies, or the virus may be isolated from the blood, nasopharyngeal secretions, and urine during the febrile period. Serum antibodies appear within 3 days after onset of the rash and reach peak titers 2 to 4 weeks later.

Treatment

Treatment for measles requires bed rest, relief of symptoms, and droplet isolation throughout the communicable period. Vaporizers and a warm environment help reduce respiratory irritation, and antipyretics can reduce fever. There is evidence that vitamin A administration may improve outcomes. Cough preparations and antibiotics are generally ineffective. Therapy must also combat complications.

Special considerations

◆ Teach the patient's parents supportive measures, and stress the need for isolation, plenty of rest, and increased fluid intake. Advise them to cope with photophobia by darkening the room or providing sunglasses and to reduce fever with antipyretics and tepid sponge baths.
◆ Warn the patient's parents to watch for and report the early signs and symptoms of complications, such as encephalitis, otitis media, and pneumonia.
◆ Airborne precautions are required for patients during the contagious phase of the illness, until 4 days after onset of rash.
◆ Report cases to the public health authorities.

VARIOLA
Causes and incidence

Variola, or *smallpox*, was an acute, highly contagious infectious disease caused by the poxvirus variola. After a global eradication program,

the World Health Organization pronounced smallpox eradicated on October 26, 1979, 2 years after the last naturally occurring case was reported in Somalia. Vaccination is no longer recommended, except for certain laboratory workers. The last known case in the United States was reported in 1949. Although naturally occurring smallpox has been eradicated, variola virus preserved in laboratories remains an unlikely source of infection. In response to bioterrorism concerns, smallpox vaccination was offered to members of the military, health department officials, first responders, and key healthcare providers. If a bioterrorism event involving smallpox is suspected or occurs, vaccination programs can be initiated.

Smallpox developed in three major forms: *variola major* (classic smallpox), which carried a high mortality; *variola minor*, a mild form that occurred in nonvaccinated people and resulted from a less virulent strain; and *varioloid*, a mild variant of smallpox that occurred in previously vaccinated people who had only partial immunity.

Smallpox affected people of all ages. In temperate zones, incidence was highest during the winter; in the tropics, during the hot, dry months. Smallpox was transmitted directly by respiratory droplets or dried scales of virus-containing lesions or indirectly through contact with contaminated linens or other objects. Variola major was contagious from onset until after the last scab was shed.

Pathophysiology

Smallpox was inhaled through the respiratory tract where the virus multiplied and eventually spread to the lymph nodes by macrophages. Eventually, lymphoid organs such as the spleen were affected. Viral replication here resulted in a secondary viremia that caused the rash. Vesicles resulted from replication of the virus in blood vessels near the dermis, and pockmark scars were a product of infection of the sebaceous glands.

Complications

◆ Arthritis
◆ Pneumonia
◆ Bronchitis
◆ Pneumonitis
◆ Encephalitis

Signs and symptoms

Characteristically, after an incubation period of 7 to 14 days, smallpox caused an abrupt onset of chills (and possible seizures in children), high fever (above 104° F [40° C]), headache, backache, severe malaise, vomiting (especially in children), marked prostration, and, occasionally, violent delirium, stupor, or coma. Two days after onset, symptoms became more severe, but by the third day the patient began to feel better.

However, the patient soon developed a sore throat and cough as well as lesions on the mucous membranes of the mouth, throat, and respiratory tract. Within days, skin lesions also appeared, progressing from macular to papular, vesicular, and pustular (pustules were as large as 8.5 mm in diameter). All skin lesions were in the same stage of development. During the pustular stage, the patient's temperature again rose, and early symptoms returned. By day 10, the pustules began to rupture and eventually dried and formed scabs. Symptoms finally subsided about 14 days after onset. Desquamation of the scabs took another 1 to 2 weeks, caused intense pruritus, and commonly left permanently disfiguring scars.

In fatal cases, a diffuse dusky appearance came over the patient's face and upper chest. Death resulted from encephalitic manifestations, extensive bleeding from any or all orifices, or secondary bacterial infections.

Diagnosis

Before the global eradication program, smallpox was readily recognizable, especially during an epidemic or after known contact. However, most of today's healthcare workers aren't familiar with the disease's telltale signs and symptoms. The most conclusive laboratory test is a culture of variola virus isolated from an aspirate of vesicles and pustules. Other laboratory tests include microscopic examination of smears from lesion scrapings and complement fixation to detect virus or antibodies to the virus in the patient's blood.

Treatment

Treatment for smallpox requires hospitalization with droplet, airborne, and contact precautions; antimicrobial therapy to treat bacterial complications; vigorous supportive measures; and symptomatic treatment of lesions with antipruritics, starting during the pustular stage. If the smallpox vaccination is given within 2 to 3 days of exposure to the disease, it may prevent illness or lessen symptoms. Treatment once the disease has started is limited.

Special considerations

◆ Give analgesics to relieve pain.
◆ I.V. infusions and gastric tube feedings provide fluids, electrolytes, and calories because pharyngeal lesions make swallowing difficult.

◆ If smallpox is suspected, the state health department should be notified immediately.
◆ Place patients on contact and airborne isolation.

MONKEYPOX
Causes and incidence

Monkeypox is a rare viral disease identified mostly in the rainforest countries of central and West Africa. The virus was originally discovered in laboratory monkeys in 1958. It was later recovered from an African squirrel, which was thought to be the natural host. It may also infect other rodents, such as rats, mice, and rabbits. The first human cases of monkeypox were reported in remote African locations in 1970. In June 2003, there was an outbreak in the United States involving people who had fell ill following contact with infected prairie dogs.

Pathophysiology

The *monkeypox virus*, belonging to the Orthopoxvirus group of viruses, causes monkeypox. It's related to variola and cowpox. People can contract monkeypox from an infected animal through a bite or direct contact with the animal's blood, body fluids, or lesions. It's spread person to person via respiratory droplets during direct and prolonged face-to-face contact. It's less infectious than smallpox, but it can also be spread through direct contact with an infected person's body fluids or with virus-contaminated objects, such as bedding or clothing.

Complications

◆ Encephalitis (rare)
◆ Death (rare)

Signs and symptoms

The signs and symptoms of monkeypox are similar to those of smallpox, but milder. After an incubation period of about 12 days, the patient may report fever, headache, muscle aches, backache, swollen lymph nodes, and a general feeling of discomfort and exhaustion. A papular rash begins on the face or other area of the body within 1 to 3 days after onset of the fever. The lesions go through several stages before crusting and falling off. The illness' duration is 2 to 4 weeks.

In Africa, monkeypox is fatal in 10% of those who contract the disease.

Diagnosis

Diagnosis is based on history and presenting signs and symptoms. The virus may be isolated from vesicular fluid to aid in diagnosis and differentiation from other rash-producing viruses.

Treatment

There is no specific treatment for monkeypox, but the smallpox vaccine appears to reduce the risk of contracting the disease. The CDC recommends that persons who are investigating monkeypox outbreaks and caring for infected individuals or animals should receive smallpox vaccination. Persons exposed to individuals or animals confirmed to have monkeypox should also receive vaccinations (up to 14 days after exposure).

Vaccinia immune globulin may be considered in some cases, such as in patients who are severely immunocompromised. There are no data available on the effectiveness of cidofovir in the treatment of human monkeypox cases.

Special considerations

◆ Notify the local health department immediately if you suspect monkeypox.

◆ A combination of airborne and contact precautions should be applied in all health-care settings. Because of the risk of airborne transmission, use an N95 (or comparable) filtering disposable respirator certified by the National Institute for Occupational Safety and Health that has been fit-tested. Surgical masks may be worn if the respirator is not available. Isolation continues until all lesions are crusted over or until the local or state health department advises that isolation is no longer necessary.

◆ Perform scrupulous handwashing after contact with an infected patient or contaminated objects. Teach the patient and family members proper handwashing as well.

◆ Eye protection should be used if splash or spray of body fluids is possible.

◆ Place the patient in a private room. Use a negative-pressure room if available.

◆ When transporting the patient, place a mask over the nose and mouth, and cover exposed skin lesions with a sheet or gown. If the patient is to remain at home, he or she should maintain the same precautions.

ROSEOLA INFANTUM

Causes and incidence

Roseola infantum (exanthema subitum), an acute, benign, presumably viral infection, usually affects infants and young children ages 6 months to 3 years. Characteristically, it first causes a high fever and then a rash that accompanies an abrupt drop to normal temperature. It's also known as *sixth disease*.

It affects boys and girls alike and occurs year-round. Overt roseola, the most common

exanthem in children younger than age 2, affects 30% of all children; inapparent roseola (febrile illness without a rash) may affect the rest. Rarely does an infected child transmit roseola to a sibling.

Pathophysiology

Human herpesvirus 6 causes roseola. The mode of transmission isn't known, but oral secretions are suspected. This double-stranded DNA virus replicates best in vitro and has been found in a wide variety of tissues and cell types, from lymph nodes to monocytes and macrophages to renal tubular cells.

Complications

◆ Febrile seizures
◆ Encephalitis (rare)
◆ Meningitis
◆ Hepatitis

Signs and symptoms

After a 5- to 15-day incubation period (average, 10 days), the infant with roseola develops an abruptly rising, unexplainable fever, and, sometimes, seizures. Temperature peaks at 103° to 105° F (39.4° to 40.6° C) for 3 to 5 days, then drops suddenly. In the early febrile period, the infant may be anorexic, irritable, and listless but doesn't appear particularly ill. Simultaneously, with an abrupt drop in temperature, the infant develops a maculopapular, nonpruritic rash that blanches on pressure. The rash is profuse on the trunk, arms, and neck and mild on the face and legs. It fades within 24 hours. Complications are extremely rare.

Diagnosis

Diagnosis requires observation of the characteristic rash that appears about 48 hours after fever subsides. Serologic evidence of primary infection can be determined by checking antibody levels in acute and convalescent sera.

Treatment

Because roseola is self-limiting, treatment is supportive and symptomatic: antipyretics to lower fever and, if necessary, anticonvulsants to relieve seizures.

Special considerations

◆ Teach parents how to reduce their infant's fever by giving tepid baths, keeping the patient in lightweight clothes, and maintaining normal room temperature. Stress the need for adequate fluid intake. Strict bed rest and isolation are unnecessary.

Enteroviruses

HERPANGINA

Causes and incidence

Herpangina is an acute infection caused by group A coxsackieviruses (usually types 1 through 10, 16, and 22) and, less commonly, by group B coxsackieviruses and echoviruses. The disease typically produces vesicular lesions on the mucous membranes of the soft palate, tonsillar pillars, and throat.

Because fecal–oral transfer is the main mode of transmission, herpangina usually affects children ages 3 to 10. It's also transmitted via contact with nose and throat discharges. It's slightly more common in late summer and fall and can be sporadic, endemic, or epidemic. It generally subsides in 4 to 7 days.

Pathophysiology

Once in the body, the virus replicates in submucosal lymphoid tissue of the intestine and also in the pharynx. These then spread to the lymph nodes which disseminates the virus throughout the body. If it reaches organ tissue and replicates, it causes cell necrosis and inflammation.

Complication

◆ Dehydration

Signs and symptoms

After a 2- to 9-day incubation period, herpangina begins abruptly with a sore throat, pain on swallowing, and a temperature of 101° to 104° F (38.3° to 40° C) that persists for 1 to 4 days and may cause seizures, headache, anorexia, malaise, and pain in the stomach, back of the neck, legs, or arms. Grayish white papulovesicles (up to 12) appear on the soft palate and, less commonly, on the tonsils, uvula, tongue, and larynx. These lesions grow from 1 to 2 mm in diameter to large, punched-out ulcers that are several millimeters in diameter and surrounded by small, inflamed margins.

Diagnosis

℞ CONFIRMING DIAGNOSIS *Characteristic oral lesions suggest this diagnosis; isolation of the virus from mouth washings or feces confirm it if necessary.*

Other routine test results are normal except for slight leukocytosis.

Diagnosis requires distinguishing the mouth lesions in herpangina from those in streptococcal tonsillitis (no ulcers; lesions confined to tonsils).

Treatment

Treatment for herpangina is entirely symptomatic, emphasizing measures to reduce fever (acetaminophen, ibuprofen) and prevent seizures and possible dehydration. Herpangina doesn't require isolation but does require careful hand hygiene and sanitary disposal of excretions. Topical anesthetic agents, such as benzocaine or lidocaine, may be applied to the mouth for discomfort.

Special considerations

◆ Teach parents to provide adequate fluids and a nonirritating diet, to enforce bed rest, and to administer tepid sponge baths and antipyretics.

POLIOMYELITIS

Causes and incidence

Poliomyelitis, also called *polio* or *infantile paralysis*, is an acute communicable disease caused by the poliovirus. It ranges in severity from inapparent infection to fatal paralytic illness. First recognized in 1840, poliomyelitis became epidemic in Norway and Sweden in 1905. Outbreaks reached pandemic proportions in Europe, North America, Australia, and New Zealand during the first half of this century. Incidence peaked during the 1940s and early 1950s, and led to the development of the Salk vaccine. (See *Polio protection.*)

Polio protection

Dr. Jonas Salk's poliomyelitis vaccine, which became available in 1955, has been rightly called one of the miracle drugs of modern medicine. The vaccine contains dead (formalin-inactivated) polioviruses that stimulate the production of circulating antibodies in the human body. This vaccine so effectively eliminated poliomyelitis that today it's difficult to appreciate how fearful people once were of this disease. Oral polio vaccine is no longer used in the United States because polio had been eliminated from the western hemisphere and there were new cases of vaccine-associated polio. Instead, inactivated poliovirus vaccine (IPV) has been the recommended form of vaccine since January 2000. Children should receive four doses of IPV at ages 2, 4, and 6 to 18 months and at age 4 to 6 years. Routine poliovirus vaccination isn't generally recommended for people ages 18 or older residing in the United States.

Minor polio outbreaks still occur, usually among nonimmunized groups such as the Amish of Pennsylvania. The disease usually strikes during the summer and fall. Once confined mainly to infants and children, poliomyelitis mostly occurs today in people older than age 15. Adults and girls are at greater risk for infection; boys, for paralysis.

Factors that increase the risk of paralysis include pregnancy; old age; localized trauma, such as a recent tonsillectomy, tooth extraction, or inoculation; and unusual physical exertion at or just before the clinical onset of poliomyelitis.

If the CNS is spared, the prognosis is excellent. However, CNS infection can cause paralysis and death. The mortality for all types of poliomyelitis is 5% to 10%.

Pathophysiology

The poliovirus has three antigenically distinct serotypes—types I, II, and III—all of which cause poliomyelitis. These viruses are found worldwide and are transmitted from person to person by direct contact with infected oropharyngeal secretions or feces. The incubation period ranges from 5 to 35 days—7 to 14 days on average.

The virus usually enters the body through the alimentary tract, multiplies in the oropharynx and lower intestinal tract, and then spreads to regional lymph nodes and the blood. How it travels to the CNS is not understood, but once it does, the virus replicates and leads to death of the motor neuron which causes paralysis. The virus can affect other neurons, as well.

Complications

◆ Respiratory failure
◆ Pulmonary edema
◆ Pulmonary embolism
◆ Urinary tract infection
◆ Urolithiasis
◆ Atelectasis
◆ Pneumonia
◆ Cor pulmonale
◆ Soft-tissue and skeletal deformities
◆ Paralytic shock
◆ Hypertension

Signs and symptoms

Manifestations of poliomyelitis follow three basic patterns. Inapparent (subclinical) infections constitute 95% of all poliovirus infections. Abortive poliomyelitis (minor illness), which accounts for 4% to 8% of all cases, causes slight fever, malaise, headache, sore throat, inflamed pharynx, and vomiting. The patient usually recovers within 72 hours. Most cases of inapparent or abortive poliomyelitis go unnoticed.

Major poliomyelitis, however, involves the CNS and takes two forms: nonparalytic and paralytic. Children commonly show a biphasic course, in which the onset of major illness occurs after recovery from the minor illness stage. *Nonparalytic poliomyelitis* produces moderate fever, headache, vomiting, lethargy, irritability, and pains in the neck, back, arms, legs, and abdomen. It also causes muscle tenderness, weakness, and spasms in the extensors of the neck and back and sometimes in the hamstring and other muscles. (These spasms may be observed during maximum range-of-motion exercises.) Nonparalytic polio usually lasts about a week, with meningeal irritation persisting for about 2 weeks.

Paralytic poliomyelitis usually develops within 5 to 7 days of the onset of fever. The patient displays symptoms similar to those of nonparalytic poliomyelitis, with asymmetrical weakness of various muscles, loss of superficial and deep reflexes, paresthesia, hypersensitivity to touch, urine retention, constipation, and abdominal distention. The extent of paralysis depends on the level of the spinal cord lesions, which may be cervical, thoracic, or lumbar.

Resistance to neck flexion is characteristic in nonparalytic and paralytic poliomyelitis. The patient will "tripod"—extend arms behind the body for support—when sitting up. He or she display Hoyne sign—the head will fall back when supine and the shoulders are elevated. From a supine position, he or she won't be able to raise legs a full 90 degrees. Paralytic poliomyelitis also causes positive Kernig and Brudzinski signs.

When the disease affects the medulla of the brain, it's called *bulbar paralytic poliomyelitis*, which is the most perilous type. This form affects the respiratory muscle nerves, leading to respiratory paralysis, and weakens the muscles supplied by the cranial nerves (particularly IX and X), producing symptoms of encephalitis. Other signs and symptoms include facial weakness, diplopia, dysphagia, difficulty chewing, inability to swallow or expel saliva, regurgitation of food through the nasal passages, and dyspnea as well as abnormal respiratory rate, depth, and rhythm, which may lead to respiratory arrest. Fatal pulmonary edema and shock are possible.

Diagnosis

CONFIRMING DIAGNOSIS *Diagnosis requires isolation of the poliovirus from throat washings during the first week or symptoms, from stools throughout the disease, and from CSF cultures in CNS infection (the gold standard).*

Coxsackievirus and echovirus infections must be ruled out. (See *Enterovirus facts*.) Convalescent serum antibody titers four times greater than acute titers support a diagnosis of poliomyelitis. Routine laboratory tests are usually within normal limits. However, CSF pressure and protein levels may be slightly increased and WBC count elevated initially, mostly due to polymorphonuclear leukocytes, which constitute 50% to 90% of the total count. Thereafter, mononuclear cells constitute most of the diminished number of cells.

Treatment

Treatment is supportive and includes analgesics to ease headache, back pain, and leg spasms. Moist heat applications may also reduce muscle spasm and pain.

Bed rest is necessary only until extreme discomfort subsides; in paralytic polio, this may take a long time. Paralytic polio also requires long-term rehabilitation using physical therapy, braces, corrective shoes, and, in some cases, orthopedic surgery.

Special considerations

Your care plan must be comprehensive to help prevent complications and to assist polio patients—physically and emotionally—during their prolonged convalescence.

◆ Observe the patient carefully for signs of paralysis and other neurologic damage, which can occur rapidly. Maintain a patent airway, and watch for respiratory weakness and difficulty in swallowing. A tracheotomy is typically done at the first sign of respiratory distress, after which the patient is placed on a mechanical ventilator. Practice strict sterile technique during suctioning, and use only sterile solutions to nebulize medications.

◆ Perform a brief neurologic assessment at least once a day, but don't demand any vigorous muscle activity. Encourage a return to mild activity as soon as the patient is able.

◆ Check blood pressure frequently, especially in bulbar poliomyelitis, which can cause hypertension or shock because of its effect on the brainstem.

◆ Watch for signs of fecal impaction due to dehydration and intestinal inactivity. To prevent this, give sufficient fluids to ensure an adequate daily output of low-specific-gravity urine (1.5 to 2 L/day for adults).

◆ Monitor the bedridden patient's food intake for an adequate, well-balanced diet. If tube feedings are required, give liquid baby foods, juices, lactose, and vitamins.

◆ Be sure to prevent pressure ulcers by providing good skin care, repositioning the patient often, and keeping the bed dry. Remember, muscle paralysis may cause bladder weakness or transient bladder paralysis.

◆ Apply high-top sneakers or use a footboard to prevent footdrop. To alleviate discomfort, use foam rubber pads and sandbags, as needed, and light splints as ordered.

◆ To control the spread of poliomyelitis, place the patient on contact precautions. Wash your hands thoroughly after contact with the patient. Instruct the ambulatory patient to wash hands after contact with secretions. (Only hospital personnel who have been vaccinated against poliomyelitis should have direct contact with the patient.)

◆ Provide emotional support to the patient and family. Reassure the nonparalytic patient chances for recovery are good. Long-term support and encouragement are essential for maximum rehabilitation.

◆ An interdisciplinary rehabilitation program should be set up for a paralytic patient. It should include physical and occupational therapists, physicians, and, if necessary, a psychiatrist to help the patient process the emotional impact of facing severe physical disabilities.

◆ Report all cases of poliomyelitis to the public health authority.

Enterovirus facts

Enteroviruses (polioviruses, coxsackieviruses, and echoviruses) infect the gastrointestinal tract. These viruses, among the smallest that affect humans, include 3 known polioviruses, 23 group A coxsackieviruses, 6 group B coxsackieviruses, and 34 echoviruses. They usually infect humans as a result of ingestion of fecally contaminated material, causing a wide range of diseases (hand, foot, and mouth disease; aseptic meningitis; myocarditis; pericarditis; gastroenteritis; and poliomyelitis). They can appear in the pharynx, feces, blood, cerebrospinal fluid, and central nervous system tissue. Enterovirus infections are more prevalent in the summer and fall.

Arbovirus

COLORADO TICK FEVER

Causes and incidence

Colorado tick fever is an acute viral infection caused by the bite of the *Dermacentor andersoni* wood tick. It occurs in the Rocky Mountain region of the United States, mostly in April and May at lower altitudes and in June and July at higher altitudes. Because of occupational or recreational exposure, it's more common in men than in women. Colorado tick fever apparently confers long-lasting immunity against reinfection.

Incidence is high in Colorado, where up to 15% of people who regularly camp show past exposure. It's much less common in the rest of the United States.

Pathophysiology

Colorado tick fever is transmitted to humans by a hard-shelled wood tick called *D. andersoni*. The adult tick acquires the virus when it bites infected rodents and remains permanently infective.

Complications

◆ Pericarditis
◆ Myocarditis
◆ Epididymitis
◆ Orchitis
◆ Atypical pneumonia
◆ Meningoencephalitis

Signs and symptoms

After a 3- to 6-day incubation period, Colorado tick fever begins abruptly with chills; temperature of 104° F (40° C); severe aching of back, arms, and legs; lethargy; and headache with eye movement such as extraocular movement. Photophobia, abdominal pain, nausea, and vomiting may occur. Rare effects include petechial or maculopapular rashes and CNS involvement. Symptoms subside after several days but return within 2 to 3 days and continue for 3 more days before slowly disappearing. Complete recovery usually follows.

Diagnosis

CONFIRMING DIAGNOSIS *A history of recent exposure to ticks along with moderate to severe leukopenia, complement fixation tests, or immunofluorescence antibody confirm the diagnosis. Keep in mind that IgM antibodies may not be positive for 2 to 3 weeks after exposure.*

Treatment

After correct removal of the tick, supportive treatment focuses on relieving symptoms, combating secondary infection, and maintaining fluid balance. Colorado tick fever needs to be differentiated from RMSF and tularemia.

Special considerations

◆ Carefully remove the tick by grasping it with forceps or gloved fingers and pulling gently. Be careful not to crush the tick's body. Keep it

for identification. Thoroughly wash the wound with soap and water. If the tick's head remains embedded, surgical removal is necessary. Give a tetanus-diphtheria booster as ordered.
◆ Be alert for secondary infection.
◆ Monitor the patient's fluid and electrolyte balance, and provide replacement therapy, as indicated.
◆ Reduce fever with antipyretics and tepid sponge baths.

PREVENTION *To prevent tick-borne infection, tell the patient to avoid tick bites by wearing long-sleeved clothing, tucking pant bottoms into the top of boots, and carefully checking the body and scalp for ticks several times a day whenever in tick-infested areas. The patient should also use insect repellant.*

Miscellaneous viruses

MUMPS

Causes and incidence

Mumps, also known as *infectious* or *epidemic parotitis*, is an acute viral disease caused by a paramyxovirus. It causes painful enlargement of the salivary or parotid glands. It may also infect other organs, such as the testes, the CNS, and the pancreas. The prognosis for complete recovery is good, although mumps sometimes causes complications.

Mumps is most prevalent in children between ages 6 and 8. Infants younger than age 1 seldom get this disease because of the passive immunity received from maternal antibodies. Peak incidence occurs during late winter and early spring.

Pathophysiology

The mumps paramyxovirus is found in the saliva of an infected person and is transmitted by droplets or by direct contact. The virus is present in the saliva 6 days before to 9 days after onset of parotid gland swelling; the 48-hour period immediately preceding onset of swelling is probably the time of highest communicability. The incubation period ranges from 14 to 25 days (the average is 18). One attack of mumps (even if unilateral) almost always confers lifelong immunity.

Complications

◆ Mumps meningitis
◆ Epididymo-orchitis, producing abrupt onset of testicular swelling and tenderness, scrotal erythema, lower abdominal pain, nausea, vomiting, fever, and chills in about 25% of postpubertal males

Signs and symptoms

The clinical features of mumps vary widely. An estimated 30% of susceptible people have sub-clinical illness.

Mumps usually begins with prodromal symptoms that last for 24 hours and include myalgia, anorexia, malaise, headache, and low-grade fever followed by an earache that's ag-gravated by chewing; parotid gland tenderness and swelling; a temperature of 101° to 104° F (38.3° to 40° C); and pain when chewing or when drinking sour or acidic liquids. Simulta-neously with the swelling of the parotid gland or several days later, one or more of the other salivary glands may become swollen.

Mumps meningitis complicates the disease in 10% of patients and affects three to five times more males than females. Signs and symptoms include fever, meningeal irritation (nuchal rigid-ity, headache, and irritability), vomiting, drowsi-ness, and a CSF lymphocyte count ranging from 500 to 2,000/μL. Recovery is usually complete. Less common effects are pancreatitis, deafness, arthritis, myocarditis, encephalitis, pericarditis, oophoritis, and nephritis. In pregnant women, contracting mumps, especially during the first trimester, may lead to miscarriage.

Diagnosis

Diagnosis is usually made after the character-istic signs and symptoms develop, especially parotid gland enlargement with a history of exposure to mumps. Serologic antibody testing can verify the diagnosis when parotid or other salivary gland enlargement is absent, as IgM can be positive for up to 4 weeks. As an alternative, an oral swab can be tested for mumps via re-verse-transcriptase PCR.

Treatment

Treatment includes analgesics for pain, anti-pyretics for fever, and adequate fluid intake to prevent dehydration from fever and anorexia. If the patient can't swallow, consider I.V. fluid replacement. Warm saltwater gargles, soft foods, and extra fluids may also help relieve symptoms.

Special considerations

◆ Stress the need for bed rest during the febrile period. Give analgesics and apply warm or cool compresses to the neck to relieve pain. Give antipyretics and tepid sponge baths for fever. To prevent dehydration, encourage the patient to drink fluids; to minimize pain and anorexia, advise them to avoid spicy, irritating foods and those that require a lot of chewing. Offer a soft, bland diet.

◆ During the acute phase, observe the patient closely for signs of CNS involvement, such as altered LOC and nuchal rigidity.
◆ Follow droplet precautions for 5 days from the onset of symptoms.
◆ Report all cases of mumps to public health authorities.

▦▦▦ **PREVENTION** *Emphasize the importance of routine immunization with live attenuated mumps virus (paramyxovirus) at age 12 to 15 months, a second dose at age 4 to 6 years and for susceptible patients (especially males) who are ap-proaching or are past puberty.*

INFECTIOUS MONONUCLEOSIS
Causes and incidence

Infectious mononucleosis is an acute infectious disease caused by the Epstein–Barr virus (EBV), a member of the herpes group. It primarily affects young adults and children, although in children it's usually so mild that it's generally overlooked. This infection characteristically pro-duces fever, sore throat, and cervical lymphade-nopathy (the hallmarks of the disease) as well as hepatic dysfunction, increased lymphocyte and monocyte counts, and development and persistence of heterophil antibodies. The prog-nosis is excellent, and major complications are uncommon.

Infectious mononucleosis is fairly common in the United States, Canada, and Europe and affects both sexes equally. Incidence varies sea-sonally among college students but not among the general population.

Pathophysiology

Apparently, the reservoir of EBV is limited to humans. Infectious mononucleosis probably spreads by the oropharyngeal route because about 80% of patients carry EBV in the throat during the acute infection and for an indefin-ite period afterward. It can also be transmitted by blood transfusions and has been reported after cardiac surgery as the post-pump perfusion syndrome. Infectious mononucleosis is proba-bly contagious from before symptoms develop until the fever subsides and oropharyngeal le-sions disappear. The virus replicates in the oro-pharynx and affects B cells. These EBV-infected cells are responsible for the spread of the virus throughout the lymphoreticular system.

Complications

◆ Splenic rupture
◆ Aseptic meningitis
◆ Encephalitis
◆ Hemolytic anemia
◆ Pericarditis

◆ Guillain–Barré syndrome
◆ Hepatitis
◆ Lymphoma (rare)

Signs and symptoms

The symptoms of mononucleosis mimic those of many other infectious diseases, including hepatitis, rubella, and toxoplasmosis. Typically, after an incubation period of about 10 days in children and from 30 to 50 days in adults, infectious mononucleosis produces prodromal symptoms, such as headache, malaise, and fatigue. After 3 to 5 days, patients typically develop a triad of symptoms: sore throat, cervical lymphadenopathy, and temperature fluctuations, with an evening peak of 101° to 102° F (38.3° to 38.9° C). Splenomegaly, hepatomegaly, stomatitis, exudative tonsillitis, or pharyngitis may also develop.

Sometimes, early in the illness, a maculopapular rash that resembles rubella develops; also, jaundice occurs in about 5% of patients. Major complications are rare but may include splenic rupture, aseptic meningitis, encephalitis, hemolytic anemia, idiopathic thrombocytopenic purpura, and Guillain–Barré syndrome. Symptoms usually subside about 6 to 10 days after onset of the disease but may persist for weeks.

Diagnosis

Physical examination demonstrating the clinical triad suggests infectious mononucleosis.

℞ CONFIRMING DIAGNOSIS *The following abnormal laboratory results confirm the diagnosis:*
◆ *Monospot test is positive for infectious mononucleosis.*
◆ *Leukocyte count increases to 10,000 to 20,000/μL during the second and third weeks of illness. Lymphocytes and monocytes account for 50% to 70% of the total WBC count; 10% of the lymphocytes are atypical.*
◆ *Heterophil antibodies (agglutinins for sheep RBCs) in serum drawn during the acute illness and at 3- to 4-week intervals rise to four times the normal number.*
◆ *Indirect immunofluorescence shows antibodies to EBV and cellular antigens. Such testing is usually more definitive than heterophil antibodies.*
◆ *Liver function studies are abnormal.*

Treatment

Infectious mononucleosis resists prevention and antimicrobial treatment. Therapy is essentially supportive: relief of symptoms; bed rest during the acute febrile period; and acetaminophen or ibuprofen for headache and

sore throat. Sore throat can also be helped with warm saltwater gargles. If severe throat inflammation causes airway obstruction, steroids can be used to relieve swelling and avoid tracheotomy. Splenic rupture, marked by sudden abdominal pain, requires splenectomy. About 20% of patients with infectious mononucleosis will also have streptococcal pharyngotonsillitis; these patients should receive antibiotic therapy.

Special considerations

Because uncomplicated infectious mononucleosis doesn't require hospitalization, patient teaching is essential. Convalescence may take several weeks, usually until the patient's WBC count returns to normal.
◆ During the acute illness, stress the need for bed rest. If the patient is a student, they may continue less demanding school assignments and see friends but should avoid long, difficult projects until after recovery.
◆ To minimize throat discomfort, encourage the patient to drink milk shakes, fruit juices, and broths and to eat cool, bland foods. Suggest gargling with saline mouthwash and taking acetaminophen, as needed.

RABIES
Causes and incidence

Rabies, also known as *hydrophobia*, is an acute CNS infection caused by a virus that's transmitted by the saliva of an infected animal (especially wild animals). If symptoms occur, rabies is almost always fatal. Treatment soon after exposure, however, may prevent fatal CNS invasion.

Rabies symptoms appear earlier if the head or face is severely bitten. If the bite is on the face, the risk of developing rabies is about 60%; on the upper extremities, 15% to 40%; and on the lower extremities, about 10%.

In the United States, dog vaccinations have reduced the incidence of rabies transmission to humans. Wild animals, such as skunks, foxes, raccoons, and bats, account for 70% of rabies cases.

Pathophysiology

The rabies virus is usually transmitted to a human through the bite of an infected animal. The virus begins to replicate in the striated muscle cells at the bite site. Then it spreads up the nerve to the CNS and replicates in the brain. Finally, it moves through the nerves into other tissues, including the salivary glands. Occasionally, airborne droplets and infected tissue transplants can transmit the virus.

Complications
◆ Confusion
◆ Agitation
◆ Hallucinations
◆ Usually fatal without prompt treatment

Signs and symptoms
After an incubation period of a few days to several years, but usually 30 to 90 days, rabies typically produces local or radiating pain or burning and a sensation of cold, pruritus, and tingling at the bite site. It also produces prodromal signs and symptoms, such as a slight fever (100° to 102° F [37.8° to 38.9° C]), malaise, headache, anorexia, nausea, sore throat, and persistent loose cough. After this, the patient begins to display nervousness, anxiety, irritability, hyperesthesia, photophobia, sensitivity to loud noises, pupillary dilation, tachycardia, shallow respirations, pain and paresthesia in the bitten area, and excessive salivation, lacrimation, and perspiration.

About 2 to 10 days after the onset of prodromal symptoms, a phase of excitation (neurologic phase) begins. It's characterized by agitation, aphasia, incoordination, marked restlessness, anxiety, and apprehension and cranial nerve dysfunction that causes ocular palsies, strabismus, asymmetrical pupillary dilation or constriction, absence of corneal reflexes, weakness of facial muscles, and hoarseness. Severe systemic symptoms include tachycardia or bradycardia, cyclic respirations, hypotension, DIC, coma, cardiac arrest, urine retention, and a temperature of about 103° F (39.4° C).

About 50% of affected patients exhibit hydrophobia (literally, "fear of water"). Forceful, painful pharyngeal muscle spasms expel liquids from the mouth and cause dehydration and, possibly, apnea, cyanosis, and death. Difficulty swallowing causes frothy saliva to drool from the patient's mouth. Eventually, even the sight, mention, or thought of water causes uncontrollable pharyngeal muscle spasms and excessive salivation. Between episodes of excitation and hydrophobia, the patient commonly is cooperative and lucid. After about 3 days, excitation and hydrophobia subside, and the progressively paralytic, terminal phase of this illness begins.

⚠️ ALERT *The patient experiences progressive, generalized, flaccid paralysis that ultimately leads to peripheral vascular collapse, coma, and death.*

Diagnosis
Because rabies is fatal unless treated promptly, always suspect rabies in any person who suffers an unprovoked animal bite until you can prove otherwise.

℞ CONFIRMING DIAGNOSIS *Virus isolation from the patient's saliva or throat and examination of blood by direct fluorescent antibody (DFA) are diagnostic. In addition, tests are performed on samples of saliva, serum, spinal fluid, and skin biopsies. Saliva is tested using reverse transcription polymerase chain reaction (RT-PCR). Serum and spinal fluid are tested for antibodies; skin biopsy examined for rabies antigen.*

Other results typically include elevated WBC count, with increased polymorphonuclear and large mononuclear cells, and elevated urinary glucose, acetone, and protein levels.

Confinement of the suspected animal for 10 days of observation by a veterinarian also helps support this diagnosis. If the animal appears rabid, it should be euthanized and its brain tissue tested for DFA and Negri bodies (oval or round masses that conclusively confirm rabies).

Treatment
Treatment consists of wound care and immunization as soon as possible after exposure. Thoroughly wash all bite wounds and scratches with soap and water to remove any infected saliva. (See *First aid for animal bites.*) Check the patient's immunization status, and administer tetanus-diphtheria prophylaxis if needed. Take measures to control bacterial infection as ordered. If the wound requires suturing, special treatment and suturing techniques must be used to allow proper drainage.

After rabies exposure, a patient who has not been immunized before must receive passive immunization with rabies immune globulin (RIG) and active immunization with human diploid cell vaccine (HDCV). If the patient has received HDCV before and has an adequate rabies antibody titer, they don't need RIG immunization, just an HDCV booster.

First aid for animal bites

Immediately wash the bite vigorously with soap and water for at least 10 minutes to remove the animal's saliva. As soon as possible, flush the wound with a virucidal agent, followed by a clear-water rinse. After cleaning the wound, apply a sterile dressing. If possible, don't suture the wound, and don't immediately stop the bleeding (unless it's massive) because blood flow helps to clean the wound.

Question the patient about the bite. Ask if the patient provoked the animal (if so, chances are it isn't rabid) and if they can identify it or its owner (because the animal may be confined for observation).

Special considerations

◆ When injecting rabies vaccine, rotate injection sites on the deltoid muscle. Watch for and symptomatically treat redness, itching, pain, and tenderness at the injection site. Half of the RIG should be infiltrated into and around the bite wound, with the remainder given I.M.

◆ Cooperate with public health authorities to determine the vaccination status of the animal. If the animal is proven rabid, help identify others at risk.

If rabies develops:

◆ Monitor cardiac and pulmonary function continuously.

◆ Transmission from person to person is rare and transmission from patient to healthcare worker has not been documented. Use standard precautions when handling body fluids. Take precautions to avoid being bitten by the patient during the excitation phase.

◆ Keep the room dark and quiet.

◆ Establish communication with the patient and family. Provide psychological support to help them cope with the patient's symptoms and probable death.

▞▞▞▞ **PREVENTION** *Take these actions to help prevent rabies:*

◆ *Stress the need for vaccination of household pets that may be exposed to rabid wild animals.*

◆ *Warn the patient not to try to touch wild animals, especially if they appear ill or overly docile (possible signs of rabies).*

◆ *Assist in the prophylactic administration of rabies vaccine to high-risk people, such as farm workers, forest rangers, spelunkers (cave explorers), and veterinarians.*

CYTOMEGALOVIRUS INFECTION

Causes and incidence

Cytomegalovirus (CMV) infection is caused by the cytomegalovirus, a deoxyribonucleic acid, ether-sensitive virus belonging to the herpes family. Also known as *generalized salivary gland disease* or *cytomegalic inclusion disease*, CMV infection occurs worldwide and is transmitted by human contact.

CMV has been found in the saliva, urine, semen, breast milk, feces, blood, and vaginal and cervical secretions of infected people. The virus is usually transmitted through contact with these infected secretions, which can harbor the virus for months or even years. It may be transmitted by sexual contact and can travel across the placenta, causing a congenital infection. Immunosuppressed patients, especially those who have received transplanted organs, run a 90% chance of contracting CMV infection. Recipients of blood transfusions from donors with positive CMV antibodies are at some risk.

About four out of five people older than age 35 have been infected with CMV, usually during childhood or early adulthood. In most of these people, the disease is so mild that it's overlooked. However, CMV infection during pregnancy can be hazardous to the fetus, possibly leading to stillbirth, brain damage, and other birth defects or to severe neonatal illness. About 1% of all neonates have CMV.

Pathophysiology

CMV probably spreads through the body in lymphocytes or mononuclear cells to the lungs, liver, GI tract, eyes, and CNS, where it commonly produces inflammatory reactions.

Complications

◆ Mononucleosis
◆ Retinitis
◆ Colitis
◆ Esophagitis
◆ Hepatitis
◆ Encephalitis
◆ Pneumonia

Signs and symptoms

Most patients with CMV infection have mild, nonspecific complaints or none at all, even though antibody titers indicate infection. In these patients, the disease usually runs a self-limiting course. However, immunodeficient patients and those receiving immunosuppressants may develop pneumonia or other secondary infections. In patients with AIDS, disseminated CMV infection may cause chorioretinitis (resulting in blindness), colitis, encephalitis, abdominal pain, diarrhea, or weight loss. Infected infants ages 3 to 6 months usually appear asymptomatic but may develop hepatic dysfunction, hepatosplenomegaly, spider angiomas, pneumonitis, and lymphadenopathy. (See *CMV infection in immunosuppressed patients,* page 893.)

Congenital CMV infection is seldom apparent at birth, although the neonate's urine contains the virus. Children with congenital CMV shed CMV for 2 years in their saliva and urine. CMV can cause brain damage that may not show up for months after birth. It also can produce a rapidly fatal neonatal illness characterized by jaundice, petechial rash, hepatosplenomegaly, thrombocytopenia, hemolytic anemia, microcephaly, psychomotor retardation, mental deficiency, and hearing loss. Occasionally, this form is rapidly fatal.

In some adults, CMV may cause cytomegalovirus mononucleosis, with 3 weeks or more of irregular, high fever. Other findings may include a normal or elevated WBC count, lymphocytosis, and increased atypical lymphocytes.

CMV infection in immunosuppressed patients

The table below lists immunosuppressed patients, their risk factors for cytomegalovirus (CMV) infection, associated disorders, and prevention tips.

Patient	Risk factors	Associated disorders	Prevention
Fetus	Primary maternal infection in early pregnancy	Cytomegalic inclusion disease	Avoidance of exposure
Organ transplant recipient	Seropositive donor, seronegative recipient; intensive immunosuppression, particularly with antilymphocyte globulins, cyclosporine	Febrile leukopenia, pneumonia, GI disease	Donor matching, CMV immunoglobulin, ganciclovir or high-dose valganciclovir
Bone marrow transplant recipient	Graft-versus-host disease, older age, seropositive recipient, viremia	Pneumonia, GI disease	Ganciclovir or high-dose valganciclovir
Patient with acquired immunodeficiency syndrome	Less than 100 CD4$^+$ cells/μL; CMV seropositivity	Retinitis, GI disease, neurologic disease	Ganciclovir or foscarnet

Diagnosis

CONFIRMING DIAGNOSIS *Molecular amplification is used for diagnosis, but it can also be made with virus isolated from saliva, throat, cervix, WBCs, or biopsy specimens. Chest X-ray typically shows bilateral, diffuse, white infiltrates.*

Other laboratory tests supporting the diagnosis include complement fixation studies, hemagglutination inhibition antibody tests, and, for congenital infections, indirect immunofluorescent tests for CMV immunoglobulin M antibody.

Treatment

Treatment aims to relieve symptoms and prevent complications. In the immunosuppressed patient, CMV may be treated with I.V. ganciclovir or oral valganciclovir. Most important, parents of children with severe congenital CMV infection need support and counseling to help them cope with the possibility of brain damage or death.

Special considerations

To help prevent CMV infection:
◆ Because many patients who excrete CMV are asymptomatic, standard precautions should be maintained at all times.
◆ Warn immunosuppressed patients and pregnant women to avoid exposure to confirmed or suspected CMV infection. (Maternal CMV infection can cause fetal abnormalities: hydrocephaly, microphthalmia, seizures, encephalitis, hepatosplenomegaly, hematologic changes, microcephaly, and blindness.)
◆ Urge patients with CMV infection to use good hand hygiene to prevent spreading it. Stress this particularly with young children.
◆ Be sure to observe standard precautions when handling body secretions.

LASSA FEVER

Causes and incidence

Lassa fever is an epidemic hemorrhagic fever caused by the Lassa virus, an extremely virulent arenavirus that occurs in West Africa. During epidemics this highly fatal disorder can kill up to 50% of its victims, but those who survive its early stages usually recover and acquire immunity to secondary attacks.

It is estimated that 100,000 to 300,000 cases of Lassa fever occur annually in western Africa.

Pathophysiology

A chronic infection in rodents, Lassa virus is transmitted to humans by contact with infected rodent urine, feces, and saliva. The virus enters the bloodstream, lymph vessels, and respiratory and digestive tracts. It then multiplies in the cells of the reticuloendothelial system. In the early stages of this illness, when the virus is in the throat, human transmission may occur through inhalation of infected droplets.

Complications
◆ Deafness
◆ Hemorrhage (gums, eyes, nose)
◆ Encephalitis
◆ Spontaneous abortion
◆ Death related to multiorgan system failure

Signs and symptoms
After a 7- to 18-day incubation period, this disease produces a fever that persists for 2 to 3 weeks, exudative pharyngitis, oral ulcers, lymphadenopathy with swelling of the face and neck, purpura, conjunctivitis, and bradycardia. Severe infection may also cause hepatitis, myocarditis, pleural infection, encephalitis, and permanent unilateral or bilateral deafness.

Virus multiplication in reticuloendothelial cells causes capillary lesions that lead to erythrocyte and platelet loss; mild to moderate thrombocytopenia (with a tendency toward bleeding); and secondary bacterial infection. These capillary lesions may also cause focal hemorrhage in the stomach, small intestine, kidneys, lungs, and brain and, possibly, hemorrhagic shock and peripheral vascular collapse.

Diagnosis
℞ **CONFIRMING DIAGNOSIS** *Lassa fever is most often diagnosed by using ELISAs, which detect IgM and IgG antibodies as well as Lassa antigen.*

Treatment
Treatment of Lassa fever includes I.V. ribavirin. It has been shown to be most effective when given early in the course of the illness. Patients should also receive supportive care, including I.V. colloids for shock, analgesics for pain, and antipyretics for fever.

Special considerations
◆ Carefully monitor fluid and electrolyte status, vital signs, and intake and output. Watch for and immediately report signs of infection or shock.
◆ Contact and droplet precautions are necessary for at least 3 weeks, until the patient's throat washings and urine are free of the virus. To prevent the spread of this contagious disease, carefully dispose of, or disinfect, all materials contaminated with the infected patient's urine, feces, respiratory secretions, or exudates. Watch known contacts closely for at least 3 weeks for signs of the disease.
◆ Provide good oral care. Remember to clean the patient's mouth with a soft-bristled toothbrush to avoid irritating any oral ulcers. Ask your facility's dietary department to supply a soft, bland, nonirritating diet.

◆ Immediately contact the Viral Diseases Division of the CDC in Atlanta to get specific guidelines for managing suspected or confirmed cases of Lassa fever.
◆ Report all cases of Lassa fever to the public health authorities.

EBOLA VIRUS INFECTION
Causes and incidence
One of the most frightening viruses to come out of the African subcontinent, the Ebola virus first appeared in 1976. More than 400 people in Zaire (now known as Democratic Republic of Congo) and the neighboring Sudan were killed by the hemorrhagic fever that it caused. Ebola virus has been responsible for several outbreaks in the years since then, including outbreaks in 2007 in Uganda and in 2014 in the Democratic Republic of the Congo.

Ebola virus is caused by a virus belonging to the family Filoviridae; it can cause headache, malaise, myalgia, and high fever, progressing to severe diarrhea, vomiting, and internal and external hemorrhage.

Five strains of the Ebola virus are known to exist: Ebola Zaire, Ebola Sudan, Ebola Ivory Coast, Ebola Bundibugyo, and Ebola Reston. All five types are structurally similar, although they have different antigenic properties. However, Ebola Reston causes illness only in monkeys, not in humans, as do the other four.

The prognosis for Ebola virus infection is extremely poor, with mortality as high as 90%. The incubation period ranges from 2 to 21 days.

Pathophysiology
Ebola virus infection is caused by Filoviridae RNA virus that's passed from person to person by direct contact with infected blood, body secretions, or organs. Nosocomial and community-acquired transmission can occur. Contaminated needles can also cause the infection. Transmission through semen may occur up to 7 weeks after clinical recovery. The virus remains contagious even after the patient has died. (See *Preventing the spread of Ebola virus*, page 895.)

The virus enters the body through mucus membranes or breaks in the skin and replicates within many different types of cells. As these cells die, more viral particles are released into the bloodstream. They also spread into the lymph nodes, allowing further rapid dissemination. Death occurs when tissues are attacked in organs such as the liver and spleen. A systemic inflammatory response also occurs which is thought to play a role in GI dysfunction and the multiorgan failure that later occurs.

Complications
◆ Liver and kidney dysfunction
◆ Dehydration
◆ Hemorrhage

Signs and symptoms
The patient's health history usually reveals contact with an infected person. However, no clear line of infection may be apparent at the beginning of an Ebola virus outbreak. The patient usually complains of flu-like signs and symptoms (such as headache, malaise, myalgia, fever, cough, and sore throat), which first appear within 3 days of infection.

As the virus spreads through the body, inspection reveals bruising as capillaries rupture and dead blood cells infiltrate the skin. A maculopapular eruption appears after the fifth day of infection. The patient may also display melena, hematemesis, epistaxis, and bleeding gums. As the infection progresses, severe complications, including liver and kidney dysfunction, dehydration, and hemorrhage, may develop. In pregnant women, the Ebola virus leads to abortion and massive hemorrhage.

In the final stages of the disease, the skin blisters and sloughs off, blood seeps from all body orifices, and the patient begins vomiting liquefied internal organs. Death usually results during the second week of illness from organ failure or hemorrhage.

Diagnosis
Specialized laboratory tests reveal specific antigens or antibodies and may show the isolated virus such as an ELISA test using EBO-2 viral antigens and immunoglobulin G ELISA. As with other types of hemorrhagic fever, tests also demonstrate neutrophil leukocytosis, hypofibrinogenemia, thrombocytopenia, and microangiopathic hemolytic anemia.

Treatment
No cure exists for Ebola virus infection; treatment consists mainly of intensive supportive care. Administration of I.V. fluids helps offset the effects of severe dehydration and electrolyte imbalance.

Throughout treatment, the patient should remain on contact and droplet precautions. If diagnostic tests indicate that the patient is free from the virus—which typically occurs 21 days after onset in those few who survive—the patient can be released.

Special considerations
◆ Follow the guidelines for standard precautions formulated by the CDC when assessing a patient who may have Ebola virus.

◆ Check the results of complete blood count and coagulation studies for signs of blood loss and coagulopathy.

◆ Assess the patient daily for petechiae, ecchymoses, and oozing blood. Note and document the size of ecchymoses at least every 24 hours.

◆ Protect all areas of petechiae and ecchymoses from further injury.

◆ Test stools, urine, and vomitus for occult blood.

◆ Watch for frank bleeding, including GI bleeding and, in women, menorrhagia. Note and document the amount of bleeding every 24 hours or more often.

◆ Monitor the patient's family and other close contacts for fever and other signs of infection.

◆ Provide emotional support for the patient and family during the course of this devastating disease. Encourage them to ask questions and discuss any concerns they have about the disease and its treatment.

◆ Report cases to public health authorities.

WEST NILE ENCEPHALITIS
Causes and incidence
West Nile encephalitis is categorized as an infectious disease that primarily causes an inflammation or "encephalitis" of the brain. West Nile virus (WNV), a flavivirus commonly found in humans, birds, and other vertebrates in Africa, west Asia, and the Middle East, causes the disease, which is a part of a family of vector-borne diseases that also includes malaria, yellow fever, and Lyme disease.

The virus had not been previously documented in the western hemisphere until late August 1999. A virus found in numerous dead birds in New York, New Jersey, and Connecticut was definitively identified by genetic sequencing as the WNV. Scientists in the United States discovered the rare strain initially in and around the Bronx Zoo and believe that infected birds may have carried the disease and that it was spread as mosquitoes fed on them.

In the temperate areas of the world, West Nile encephalitis cases occur mainly in the late summer or early fall. In the southern climates where temperatures are milder, West Nile encephalitis can occur all year-round.

The risk of contracting West Nile encephalitis is greater for all residents of areas where active cases have been identified, but persons older than age 50 or those with compromised immune systems have the greatest risk. At present, there is no documented evidence that a pregnant woman's fetus is at risk due to an infection with WNV. The mortality rate of West Nile encephalitis is measured by case-fatality rates, which range from 3% to 15% (higher in the elderly population).

Pathophysiology
The pathogenesis of WNV is not understood. WNV is transmitted to humans by the bite of a mosquito (primarily the *Culex* species) infected with the virus. It's considered the primary vector for WNV and the source of the August 1999 outbreak in New York, New Jersey, and Connecticut. Mosquitoes become infected by feeding on birds contaminated with the WNV and then transmit it to humans and animals during a blood meal or "bite." (See *Transmission routes of West Nile virus*, page 897.)

Ticks have been found infected with WNV in Africa and Asia only. The role of ticks in the transmission and maintenance of the virus remains uncertain, and to date they aren't considered vectors for WNV in the United States.

The CDC has reported that there is no evidence that a person can contract the virus from handling live or dead infected birds. However, avoid barehanded contact when handling dead animals, including birds, and use gloves or double plastic bags to dispose of a carcass. Report the finding to the local health department.

Complications
◆ Tremors
◆ Convulsions
◆ Paralysis
◆ Coma
◆ Death (rare)

Signs and symptoms
Mild infections of the virus are more common and include fever, headache, and body aches, usually accompanied by a skin rash and swollen lymph glands. Severe infections can be manifested by headache, high fever, neck stiffness, stupor, disorientation, coma, tremors, occasional convulsions, paralysis, and, rarely, death.

The incubation period for West Nile encephalitis is anywhere from 5 to 15 days after exposure. Most patients who are bitten by an infected mosquito won't develop symptoms. It's estimated that only 1 in 300 people who are bitten by an infected mosquito will actually get sick.

Diagnosis
The immunoglobulin (Ig) M antibody capture enzyme-linked immunosorbent assay (MAC-ELISA) is the test of choice for rapid definitive diagnosis. The major advantage of MAC-ELISA laboratory analysis is the high probability of accurate diagnosis of WNV infection when performed with acute serum or CSF specimens obtained while the patient is still hospitalized.

This test detects levels of IgM antibodies in a patient's serum and is intended for use in patients with clinical symptoms consistent with viral encephalitis.

Other conditions to consider include St. Louis encephalitis, which is symptomatically similar.

Encephalitis can be caused by numerous viral and bacterial infections; all data must be examined to determine a definitive diagnosis.

Treatment
There is no specific therapy utilized to treat West Nile encephalitis and no known cure. Treatment is generally aimed at controlling the specific symptoms. Supportive care, such as I.V. fluids, fever control, and respiratory support, is rendered when necessary.

There is no vaccine present to prevent the transmission of West Nile encephalitis. Research

Transmission routes of West Nile virus

Birds are the reservoir of the West Nile virus. They harbor the virus but are unable to spread it. Mosquitoes serve as the vectors, spreading it from bird to bird and from birds to people. Humans are believed to be "dead-end hosts" because the virus can live and cause illness in humans, but it isn't believed that a feeding mosquito can acquire the virus from an infected person.

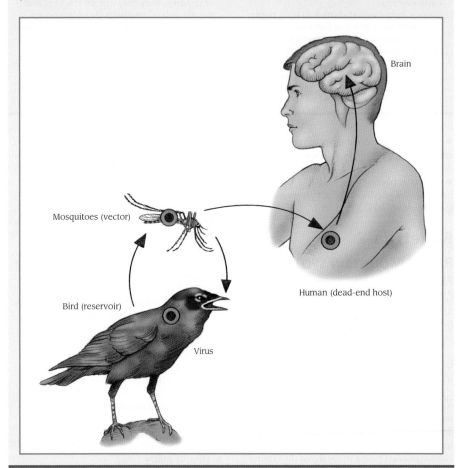

trials are underway to determine if ribavirin, an antiviral drug, interferon, or IVIG may be helpful.

Special considerations

◆ Obtain an extensive history of the patient's whereabouts within the past 2 to 3 weeks (especially around bodies of water, such as lakes and ponds), the presence of dead birds, and recent mosquito bites acquired.
◆ Perform a comprehensive physical assessment and report signs of fever, headache, lymphadenopathy, and a maculopapular rash.

◆ Perform a complete neurologic examination and report any signs of confusion, lethargy, weakness, or slurred speech.
◆ Maintain adequate hydration with I.V. fluids.
◆ Monitor strict intake and output.
◆ Use fever control methods, such as cooling blankets and acetaminophen as ordered.
◆ Provide respiratory support measures when applicable.
◆ West Nile encephalitis isn't transmitted from person to person, but use standard precautions when handling body fluids and blood.

♦ Report any suspected cases of West Nile encephalitis to the applicable state health department.

♦ Teach the patient ways to reduce the risk of becoming infected with West Nile encephalitis. (See *Preventing West Nile virus*.)

Rickettsia

ROCKY MOUNTAIN SPOTTED FEVER

Causes and incidence

RMSF is a febrile, rash-producing illness caused by *Rickettsia rickettsii*. The disease is transmitted to humans by a tick bite.

RMSF is fatal in about 5% of patients. Mortality rises when treatment is delayed and in older patients.

Rickettsia rickettsii is transmitted to a human or small animal by the prolonged bite (4 to 6 hours) of an adult tick—the wood tick (*D. andersoni*) in the west, the dog tick (*D. variabilis*) in the east, and the brown dog tick (*Rhipicephalus sanguineus*) found throughout the United States. Occasionally, it's acquired through inhalation (it can occur in laboratory settings where aerosolization of blood and specimens may occur) or through the contact of abraded skin with tick excreta or tissue juices. (This explains why people shouldn't crush ticks between their fingers when removing them from other people and animals.) In most tick-infested areas, 1% to 5% of the ticks harbor *R. rickettsii*.

Endemic throughout the continental United States, RMSF is particularly prevalent in the southeast and southwest. Because RMSF is associated with outdoor activities, such as camping and backpacking, the incidence of this illness is usually higher in the spring and summer.

Epidemiologic surveillance reports for RMSF indicate that the incidence is also higher in children ages 5 to 9, men and boys, and whites.

Pathophysiology

Rickettsia rickettsii is a bacterium that has an affinity for endothelial cells in the vascular system. Infection causes direct injury and activates the clotting cascade secondary to increased vascular permeability. Antidiuretic hormone is released in response to decreased tissue perfusion and hypovolemia which also leads to low sodium levels. Other symptoms result from the body's inflammatory response activation.

Complications

♦ Lobar pneumonia

♦ Pneumonitis

♦ Otitis media

♦ Parotitis

♦ Disseminated intravascular coagulation

♦ Shock

♦ Renal failure

♦ Meningoencephalitis

♦ Hepatic injury

Signs and symptoms

The incubation period is usually about 7 days, but it can range from 2 to 14 days. Generally, the shorter the incubation time, the more severe the infection. Signs and symptoms, which usually begin abruptly, include a persistent temperature of 102° to 104° F (38.9° to 40° C); a generalized, excruciating headache; nausea and vomiting; and aching in the bones, muscles, joints, and back. In addition, the tongue is covered with a thick white coating that gradually turns brown as the fever persists and rises.

Initially, the skin may simply appear flushed. Between days 2 and 5, eruptions begin around the wrists, ankles, or forehead; within 2 days, they cover the entire body, including the scalp, palms, and soles. The rash consists of erythematous macules 1 to 5 mm in diameter that blanch on pressure; if untreated, the rash may become petechial and maculopapular. By the third week, the skin peels off and may become gangrenous over the elbows, fingers, and toes.

The pulse is strong initially, but it gradually becomes rapid (possibly reaching 150 beats/ minute) and thready.

⚠ **ALERT** *A rapid pulse rate and hypotension (systolic pressure <90 mm Hg) herald imminent death from complete vascular collapse.*

Other signs and symptoms include a bronchial cough, a rapid respiratory rate (as high as 60 breaths/minute), anorexia, constipation, abdominal pain, hepatomegaly, splenomegaly, insomnia, restlessness, and, in extreme cases, delirium. Urine output falls to half of the normal level or less, is dark in color, and contains albumin.

Diagnosis

℞ **CONFIRMING DIAGNOSIS** *Diagnosis is usually based on a history of tick bite or travel to a tick-infested area and a positive indirect immunofluorescence assay with R. rickettsii antigen test (which shows a fourfold increase in convalescent antibody titer compared with acute titers). This test should be performed on two paired serum samples, one taken as early as possible in disease and the second taken 2 to 4 weeks later. Blood cultures or skin biopsy at the rash site should be performed to isolate the organism and confirm the diagnosis.*

Additional recommended laboratory tests consist of a platelet count for thrombocytopenia (12,000 to 150,000/µL) and a WBC count (elevated to 11,000 to 33,000/µL) during the second week of illness.

Treatment

Treatment requires careful removal of the tick and administration of antibiotics, preferably doxycycline, started in the first 5 days of symptoms, and given until 3 days after the fever subsides. Chloramphenicol may be considered as an alternate antibiotic in cases of life-threatening allergies to doxycycline. Treatment also includes symptomatic measures.

Special considerations

◆ Carefully monitor the patient's intake and output. Watch closely for decreased urine output—a possible indicator of renal failure.
◆ Be alert for signs of dehydration, such as poor skin turgor and dry mouth.
◆ Administer antipyretics as ordered, and provide tepid sponge baths to reduce fever.

◆ Monitor vital signs, and watch for profound hypotension and shock.
◆ Be prepared to administer oxygen therapy and assisted ventilation if pulmonary complications develop.
◆ Turn the patient frequently to prevent complications of immobility, such as pressure ulcers and pneumonia.
◆ Pay attention to the patient's nutritional needs; vomiting may indicate a need for parenteral nutrition or for scheduling frequent small meals.
◆ Instruct the patient to report any recurrent symptoms to the physician at once so that treatment measures may resume immediately.
◆ Report all cases to the public health authorities.

PREVENTION
◆ *Advise the patient to avoid tick-infested areas (woods, meadows, streams, and canyons) if possible.*
◆ *Teach the patient ways to reduce the risk of becoming infected with RMSF:*
   ◆ *–Encourage the patient to inspect the entire body (including scalp) every 3 to 4 hours for attached ticks.*
   ◆ *–Remind the patient to wear protective clothing, such as a long-sleeved shirt, pants securely tucked into laced boots, and a protective head covering such as a cap.*
   ◆ *–Advise the patient to apply insect repellent to exposed skin as well as to clothing.*
◆ Offer printed and illustrated instructions, if available, to teach the patient and family members or other caregivers how to correctly and safely remove a tick. Demonstrate how to use tweezers or forceps and apply steady traction to release the entire tick without leaving its mouth parts in the skin.
◆ After the patient removes the tick, caution not to handle it or its fragments.
◆ Finally, instruct the patient to clean skin with alcohol at the point of attachment.
◆ Report all cases to the appropriate health department.

Protozoa

PNEUMOCYSTIS JIROVECI PNEUMONIA

Causes and incidence

Because of its association with HIV infection, the opportunistic infection *Pneumocystis jiroveci* pneumonia, formerly called *Pneumocystis carinii*, has increased in incidence since the 1980s. Before the advent of *Pneumocystis* pneumonia preventive measures, this disease was the first clue in about 60% of patients that HIV infection was present.

Pneumocystis jiroveci pneumonia was the leading cause of death in these patients. Preventive therapy with trimethoprim/sulfamethoxazole in HIV patients with low immune function has prevented higher mortality rates from this pneumonia. Disseminated infection doesn't occur.

Pneumocystis pneumonia is also associated with other immunocompromising conditions, including organ transplantation, leukemia, lymphoma, and steroid use.

Pathophysiology

Pneumocystis jiroveci pneumonia, previously classified as a protozoan, is a fungus. The organism exists as a saprophyte in the lungs of humans and various animals as part of the normal flora in most healthy people. It becomes an aggressive pathogen in the immunocompromised patient. Impaired cell-mediated (T-cell) immunity is thought to be more important than impaired humoral (B-cell) immunity in predisposing the patient to *P. jiroveci* pneumonia, but the immune defects involved are poorly understood. *Pneumocystis jiroveci* becomes activated in immunocompromised patients when the $CD4^+$ T-cell count falls below $200/\mu L$.

Pneumocystis jiroveci invades the lungs bilaterally and multiplies extracellularly. As the infestation grows, alveoli fill with organisms and exudate, impairing gas exchange. The alveoli hypertrophy and thicken progressively, eventually leading to extensive consolidation.

The primary transmission route seems to be air, although the organism is already present in most people. The incubation period probably lasts for 4 to 8 weeks.

Complications
- Respiratory failure
- Death

Signs and symptoms

The patient typically has a history of an immunocompromising condition (such as HIV infection, leukemia, or lymphoma) or procedure (such as organ transplantation).

Pneumocystis jiroveci pneumonia begins insidiously with increasing shortness of breath and a nonproductive cough. Anorexia, generalized fatigue, and weight loss may follow. Although the patient may have hypoxemia and hypercapnia, he or she may not exhibit significant symptoms. A low-grade, intermittent fever may be present, however.

Other signs and symptoms include tachypnea, dyspnea, accessory muscle use for breathing, crackles (in about one-third of patients), marked pallor, and decreased breath sounds (in advanced pneumonia). Cyanosis may appear with acute illness; pulmonary consolidation develops later.

Diagnosis

℞ CONFIRMING DIAGNOSIS *Histologic studies confirm P. jiroveci in all patients. Fiberoptic bronchoscopy remains the most commonly used study to confirm P. jiroveci pneumonia. Invasive procedures, such as transbronchial biopsy and open-lung biopsy, are performed less commonly.*

In patients with HIV infection, initial examination of a first-morning sputum specimen (induced by inhaling an ultrasonically dispersed saline mist) may be sufficient; however, this technique usually is ineffective in patients without HIV infection.

Chest X-rays may show slowly progressing, fluffy infiltrates, and, occasionally, nodular lesions or a spontaneous pneumothorax, but these findings must be differentiated from findings in other types of pneumonia or ARDS.

ABG studies detect hypoxia and an increased A-a gradient.

Treatment

Pneumocystis jiroveci pneumonia may respond to drug therapy with trimethoprim/sulfamethoxazole. Other agents used to treat *P. jiroveci* include trimethoprim/dapsone, clindamycin-primaquine, and atovaquone. Corticosteroids are frequently used as well. However, because of immune system impairment, many patients with *P. jiroveci* pneumonia, who also have HIV, experience severe adverse reactions to drug therapy.

Supportive measures, such as oxygen therapy, mechanical ventilation, adequate nutrition, and fluid balance, are important adjunctive therapies. Oral morphine sulfate solution may reduce the respiratory rate and anxiety, thereby enhancing oxygenation.

Special considerations
- Implement standard precautions to prevent contagion.
- Frequently assess the patient's respiratory status, and monitor ABG levels every 4 hours.
- Administer oxygen therapy as ordered. Encourage the patient to ambulate as well as to perform deep-breathing exercises and incentive spirometry to facilitate effective gas exchange.
- Administer antipyretics as ordered, to relieve fever.
- Monitor the patient's intake and output and daily weight to evaluate fluid balance. Replace fluids as ordered.
- Provide diversionary activities and coordinate healthcare team activities to allow adequate rest periods between procedures.

◆ Teach the patient energy conservation techniques.

◆ Supply nutritional supplements as needed. Encourage the patient to eat a high-calorie, protein-rich diet. Offer small, frequent meals if the patient cannot tolerate large amounts of food.

◆ Reduce anxiety by providing a relaxing environment, eliminating excessive environmental stimuli, and allowing ample time for meals.

◆ Give emotional support and help the patient identify and use meaningful support systems.

◆ Instruct the patient about the medication regimen, especially about the adverse effects.

◆ Emphasize the importance of continuing chemoprophylaxis for those patients at high risk of developing *P. jiroveci* pneumonia.

◆ If the patient will require oxygen therapy at home, explain that an oxygen concentrator may be most effective.

◆ Because this infection is usually associated with AIDS, provide the patient with resources and support organizations for both AIDS and HIV.

MALARIA

Causes and incidence

Malaria, an acute infectious disease, is caused by protozoa of the genus *Plasmodium*: *P. falciparum*, *P. vivax*, *P. malariae*, and *P. ovale*, all of which are transmitted to humans by mosquito vectors. Falciparum malaria is the most severe form of the disease. When treated, malaria is rarely fatal; untreated, it's fatal in 10% of victims, usually as a result of complications such as DIC.

Untreated primary attacks last from a week to a month, or longer. Relapses are common and can recur sporadically for several years. Susceptibility to the disease is universal.

Malaria is a worldwide health problem that continues to impede the development of many countries.

Malaria is a tropical and subtropical disease. It's most prevalent in Asia, Africa, and Latin America. The CDC estimates 300 to 500 million cases occur each year, with more than 1 million resulting in death. On average, 1,500 cases of malaria are reported every year in the United States even though malaria has been eradicated in this country since the early 1950s. It's the greatest disease hazard for travelers in warm climates.

Pathophysiology

Malaria literally means "bad air" and for centuries was thought to result from the inhalation of swamp vapors. It's now known that malaria is transmitted by the bite of female *Anopheles* mosquitoes, which abound in humid, swampy areas. When an infected mosquito bites, it injects *Plasmodium* sporozoites into the wound. The infective sporozoites migrate by blood circulation

to parenchymal cells of the liver; there they form cystlike structures containing thousands of merozoites.

Upon release, each merozoite invades an erythrocyte and feeds on hemoglobin. Eventually, the erythrocyte ruptures, releasing heme (malaria pigment), cell debris, and more merozoites, which, unless destroyed by phagocytes, enter other erythrocytes. (See *What happens in malaria*, page 902.) At this point, the infected person becomes a reservoir of malaria who infects any mosquito that feeds on him, thus beginning a new cycle of transmission. Hepatic parasites (*P. vivax*, *P. ovale*, and *P. malariae*) may persist for years in the liver. These parasites are responsible for the chronic carrier state. Because blood transfusions and street-drug paraphernalia can also spread malaria, drug addicts have a higher incidence of the disease.

Complications

◆ Renal failure
◆ Liver failure
◆ Heart failure
◆ Pulmonary edema
◆ Disseminated intravascular coagulation
◆ Seizures
◆ Hypoglycemia
◆ Splenic rupture
◆ Cerebral dysfunction
◆ Death

Signs and symptoms

After an incubation period of 12 to 30 days, malaria produces chills, fever, cough, fatigue, headache, and myalgia, interspersed with periods of well-being (the hallmark of the benign form of malaria). Acute attacks (paroxysms) occur when erythrocytes rupture. There are three stages:

◆ *cold stage*, lasting 1 to 2 hours, ranging from chills to extreme shaking

◆ *hot stage*, lasting 3 to 4 hours, characterized by a high fever (up to 107° F [41.7° C])

◆ *wet stage*, lasting 2 to 4 hours and characterized by profuse sweating.

Paroxysms occur every 48 to 72 hours when malaria is caused by *P. malariae* and every 42 to 50 hours when malaria is caused by *P. vivax* or *P. ovale*. All three types have low levels of parasitosis and are self-limiting as a result of early acquired immunity.

Plasmodium vivax and *P. ovale* also produce hepatosplenomegaly. Hemolytic anemia is present in all but the mildest infections.

The most severe form of malaria, which causes the most morbidity and mortality, is caused by *P. falciparum*. This species produces persistent high fever, orthostatic hypotension, and RBC sludging that leads to capillary

PATHOPHYSIOLOGY
What happens in malaria

A female *Anopheles* mosquito bites, injecting saliva containing sporozoites, the infective form of the malaria parasite.

The sporozoites enter liver cells and multiply.

Liver cell

In the liver, the sporozoites change into merozoites, another form of the parasite.

Merozoites are released from the liver and enter the bloodstream.

Merozoites attack red blood cells (RBCs).

Red blood cell

Merozoites

Merozoites multiply in RBCs.

RBCs burst and release the merozoites, which invade other RBCs and cause recurring chills and fever.

obstruction at various sites. Signs and symptoms of obstruction include:

◆ *cerebral*—hemiplegia, seizures, delirium, and coma
◆ *pulmonary*—coughing and hemoptysis
◆ *splanchnic*—vomiting, abdominal pain, diarrhea, and melena
◆ *renal*—oliguria, anuria, and uremia

During blackwater fever (a complication of *P. falciparum* infection), massive intravascular hemolysis causes jaundice, hemoglobinuria, a tender and enlarged spleen, acute renal failure, and uremia. This complication is fatal in about 2% of patients.

Diagnosis

℞ CONFIRMING DIAGNOSIS *A history showing travel to endemic areas, recent blood transfusion, or drug abuse in a person with high fever of unknown origin strongly suggests malaria. However, because symptoms of malaria mimic other diseases, unequivocal diagnosis depends on laboratory identification of the parasites in RBCs of peripheral blood smears.*

The CDC can identify donors responsible for transfusion malaria through indirect fluorescent serum antibody tests. These tests are unreliable in the acute phase because antibodies can be undetectable for 2 weeks after onset. Rapid diagnostic tests are available and useful in areas that do not have adequate resources or training, as well.

The CDC provides a website (www.cdc.gov) to assist clinicians needing guidance on the diagnosis and management of malaria.

Supplementary laboratory values that support this diagnosis include decreased hemoglobin levels, normal to decreased leukocyte count (as low as 3,000/μL), and protein and leukocytes in urine sediment. In falciparum malaria, serum values reflect DIC: reduced number of platelets (20,000 to 50,000/μL); prolonged prothrombin time (18 to 20 seconds); prolonged partial thromboplastin time (60 to 100 seconds); and decreased plasma fibrinogen.

Treatment

Malaria is best treated with oral chloroquine in all forms except chloroquine-resistant *P. falciparum*. Symptoms and parasitemia decrease within 24 hours after such therapy begins, and the patient usually recovers within 3 to 4 days. If the patient is comatose or vomiting frequently, chloroquine is given I.M.

Malaria caused by *P. falciparum*, which is resistant to chloroquine, requires treatment with a combination medication such as artemether-lumefantrine, artesunate-amodiaquine, or artesunate-mefloquine.

The only drug effective against the hepatic stage of the disease that's available in the United States is primaquine. This drug can induce hemolytic anemia, especially in patients with glucose-6-phosphate dehydrogenase deficiency. (See *Special considerations for antimalarial drugs*.)

Special considerations for antimalarial drugs

Chloroquine
◆ Perform baseline and periodic ophthalmologic examinations, and report blurred vision, increased sensitivity to light, and muscle weakness to the physician.
◆ Consult with the physician about altering therapy if muscle weakness appears in a patient on long-term therapy.
◆ Monitor the patient for tinnitus and other signs of ototoxicity, such as nerve deafness and vertigo.
◆ Caution the patient to avoid excessive exposure to the sun to prevent exacerbating drug-induced dermatoses.

Primaquine
◆ Give with meals or antacids.
◆ Halt administration if you observe a sudden fall in hemoglobin concentration or in erythrocyte or leukocyte count or marked darkening of the urine, suggesting impending hemolytic reaction.

Pyrimethamine
◆ Administer with meals to minimize GI distress.
◆ Check blood counts (including platelets) twice per week. If signs of folic or folinic acid deficiency develop, reduce or discontinue dosage while the patient receives parenteral folinic acid until blood counts become normal.

Quinine
◆ Use with caution in patients with cardiovascular conditions. Discontinue dosage if you see any signs of idiosyncrasy or toxicity, such as headache, epigastric distress, diarrhea, rashes, and pruritus, in a mild reaction; or delirium, seizures, blindness, cardiovascular collapse, asthma, hemolytic anemia, and granulocytosis, in a severe reaction.
◆ Monitor blood pressure frequently while administering quinine I.V. infusion. Rapid administration causes marked hypotension.

PREVENTION
How to prevent malaria

Advise patients on these actions that should be taken to help prevent malaria:
◆ Drain, fill, and eliminate breeding areas of the *Anopheles* mosquito.
◆ Install screens in living and sleeping quarters in endemic areas.
◆ Use a residual insecticide on clothing and skin to prevent mosquito bites.
◆ Seek treatment for known cases.
◆ Question blood donors about a history of malaria or possible exposure to malaria. They *may* give blood if:
  ◆ they haven't taken any antimalarial drugs and are asymptomatic after 6 months outside an endemic area
  ◆ they were asymptomatic after treatment for malaria more than 3 years ago
  ◆ they were asymptomatic after receiving malaria prophylaxis more than 3 years ago.
◆ Seek preventive drug therapy before traveling to an endemic area. Agents include mefloquine, doxycycline, chloroquine, hydroxychloroquine, or malarone (a combination of atovaquone and proguanil). They're usually started 2 weeks before visiting the endemic area and continue for 6 weeks after leaving the area.

For travelers spending less than 3 weeks in areas where malaria exists, weekly prophylaxis includes oral chloroquine beginning 2 weeks before the trip and ending 6 weeks after it. (See *How to prevent malaria*.) Any traveler who develops an acute febrile illness should seek prompt medical attention, regardless of the prophylaxis taken.

Special considerations
◆ Obtain a detailed patient history, noting any recent travel, foreign residence, blood transfusion, or drug addiction. Record symptom pattern, fever, type of malaria, and any systemic signs.
◆ Assess the patient on admission and daily thereafter for fatigue, fever, orthostatic hypotension, disorientation, myalgia, and arthralgia. Enforce bed rest during periods of acute illness.
◆ Protect the patient from secondary bacterial infection by following proper handwashing and sterile techniques.
◆ Protect yourself by maintaining standard precautions.
◆ Activate safety devices, and use safety syringes in practice.
◆ Discard needles and syringes in an impervious container designated for incineration.
◆ Handle bed linens according to standard precautions.
◆ To reduce fever, administer antipyretics as ordered. Document onset, duration, and symptoms before and after episodes.
◆ Fluid balance is fragile, so keep a strict record of intake and output. Monitor I.V. fluids closely. Avoid fluid overload (especially in *P. falciparum*), because it can lead to pulmonary edema and aggravate cerebral symptoms. Observe blood chemistry levels for hyponatremia and increased blood urea nitrogen, creatinine, and bilirubin levels. Monitor urine output hourly, and maintain it at 40 to 60 mL/hour for an adult and at 15 to 30 mL/hour for a child. Immediately report any decrease in urine output or the onset of hematuria as a possible sign of renal failure; be prepared to perform peritoneal dialysis for uremia caused by renal failure.
◆ Slowly administer packed RBCs or whole blood while checking for crackles, tachycardia, and shortness of breath.
◆ If humidified oxygen is ordered, note the patient's response, particularly any changes in rate or character of respirations, or any improvement in mucous membrane color.
◆ Watch for and immediately report signs of internal bleeding, such as tachycardia, hypotension, and pallor.
◆ Encourage frequent coughing and deep breathing, especially if the patient is on bed rest or has pulmonary complications. Record the amount and color of sputum.
◆ Watch for adverse effects of drug therapy, and take measures to relieve them.
◆ If the patient is comatose, make frequent, gentle changes in position, and perform passive range-of-motion exercises every 3 to 4 hours. If the patient is unconscious or disoriented, use restraints as needed, and keep an airway available as appropriate.
◆ Provide emotional support and reassurance, especially in critical illness. Explain the procedures and treatment to the patient and family. Suggest that other family members be tested for malaria. Emphasize the need for follow-up care

to check the effectiveness of treatment and to manage residual problems.

◆ Report all cases of malaria to public health authorities.

AMEBIASIS
Causes and incidence

Amebiasis, also known as *amebic dysentery*, is an acute or chronic protozoal infection caused by *Entamoeba histolytica*. This infection produces varying degrees of illness, from no symptoms at all or mild diarrhea to fulminant dysentery. Extraintestinal amebiasis can induce hepatic abscess and infections of the lungs, pleural cavity, pericardium, peritoneum, and, rarely, the brain.

The prognosis is generally good, although complications—such as ameboma, intestinal stricture, hemorrhage or perforation, intussusception, or abscess—increase mortality. Brain abscess, a rare complication, is usually fatal.

Amebiasis occurs worldwide but is most common in the tropics, subtropics, and other areas with poor sanitation and health practices. Incidence in the United States averages between 1% and 3% but may be higher among homosexuals and institutionalized people, in whom fecal–oral contamination is common.

Pathophysiology

Entamoeba histolytica exists in two forms: a cyst (which can survive outside the body) and a trophozoite (which can't survive outside the body). Transmission occurs through ingesting feces-contaminated food or water. The ingested cysts pass through the intestine, where digestive secretions break down the cysts and liberate the motile trophozoites within. The trophozoites multiply and either invade and ulcerate the mucosa of the large intestine or simply feed on intestinal bacteria. As the trophozoites are carried slowly toward the rectum, they are encysted and then excreted in feces. Humans are the principal reservoir of infection.

Complications

◆ Chronic diarrhea
◆ Abdominal pain
◆ Liver abscesses
◆ Ameboma
◆ Megacolon
◆ Intussusception
◆ Intestinal stricture
◆ Intestinal hemorrhage
◆ Intestinal perforation

Signs and symptoms

The clinical effects of amebiasis vary with the severity of the infestation. *Acute amebic dysentery* causes a sudden high temperature of 104° to 105° F (40° to 40.6° C) accompanied by chills and abdominal cramping; profuse, bloody, mucoid diarrhea with tenesmus; and diffuse abdominal tenderness due to extensive rectosigmoid ulcers.

Chronic amebic dysentery produces intermittent diarrhea that lasts for 1 to 4 weeks and recurs several times a year. Such diarrhea produces 4 to 8 (or, in severe diarrhea, up to 18) foul-smelling mucus- and blood-tinged stools daily in a patient with a mild fever, vague abdominal cramps, possible weight loss, tenderness over the cecum and ascending colon, and, occasionally, hepatomegaly. Amebic granuloma (ameboma), commonly mistaken for cancer, can be a complication of the chronic infection. Amebic granuloma produces blood and mucus in the stool and, when granulomatous tissue covers the entire circumference of the bowel, causes partial or complete obstruction.

Parasitic and bacterial invasion of the appendix may produce typical signs of subacute appendicitis (abdominal pain and tenderness). Occasionally, *E. histolytica* perforates the intestinal wall and spreads to the liver. When it perforates the liver and diaphragm, it spreads to the lungs, pleural cavity, peritoneum, and, rarely, the brain.

Diagnosis

℞ **CONFIRMING DIAGNOSIS** *Isolating E. histolytica (cysts and trophozoites) in fresh feces or aspirates from abscesses, ulcers, or tissue confirms acute amebic dysentery.*

Diagnosis must distinguish between cancer and ameboma with X-rays, sigmoidoscopy, stool examination for amebae, and cecum palpation. In patients with amebiasis, exploratory surgery is hazardous; it can lead to peritonitis, perforation, and pericecal abscess.

Other laboratory tests that support the diagnosis of amebiasis include:
◆ antigen testing using ELISA
◆ serology testing
◆ PCR techniques (molecular testing)
◆ sigmoidoscopy—detects rectosigmoid ulceration; a biopsy may be helpful

Patients with amebiasis shouldn't have preparatory enemas because these may remove exudates and destroy the trophozoites, thus interfering with test results.

Treatment

Drugs used to treat amebic dysentery include metronidazole, tinidazole, and paromomycin, which act as amebicides at intestinal and extraintestinal sites, including the liver and lungs.

Special considerations

◆ Tell patients with amebiasis to avoid drinking alcohol when taking metronidazole. The combination may cause nausea, vomiting, and headache.

◆ Antidiarrheals should not be prescribed and can make the condition worse.

◆ After treatment, stools should be rechecked to make sure the infection has been cleared.

GIARDIASIS

Causes and incidence

Giardiasis (also called *Giardia duodenalis* or *lambliasis*) is an infection of the small bowel caused by the symmetrical flagellate protozoan *Giardia lamblia*. A mild infection may not produce intestinal symptoms. In untreated giardiasis, symptoms wax and wane; with treatment, recovery is complete.

Giardiasis occurs worldwide but is most common in developing countries and other areas where sanitation and hygiene are poor. In the United States, giardiasis is most common in travelers who have recently returned from endemic areas and in campers who drink unpurified water from contaminated streams. Probably because of frequent hand-to-mouth activity, children are more likely to become infected with *G. lamblia* than adults. Hypogammaglobulinemia also appears to predispose people to this disorder. Giardiasis doesn't confer immunity, so reinfections may occur.

Pathophysiology

Giardia lamblia has two stages: the cystic stage and the trophozoite stage. Ingestion of *G. lamblia* cysts in fecally contaminated water or the fecal–oral transfer of cysts by an infected person results in giardiasis. Giardiasis may be transmitted through sexual contact (direct or indirect fecal–oral contact). When cysts enter the small bowel, they become trophozoites and attach themselves with their sucking disks to the bowel's epithelial surface. After this, the trophozoites encyst again, travel down the colon, and are excreted. Unformed feces that pass quickly through the intestine may contain trophozoites as well as cysts.

Complications

◆ Malabsorption
◆ Dehydration
◆ Lactose intolerance

Signs and symptoms

Attachment of *G. lamblia* to the intestinal lumen causes superficial mucosal invasion and destruction, inflammation, and irritation. All of these destructive effects decrease food transit time through the small intestine and result in malabsorption. Such malabsorption produces chronic GI complaints—such as abdominal cramps—and pale, loose, greasy, malodorous, and frequent stools (from 2 to 10 daily) with concurrent nausea. Stools may contain mucus but not pus or blood. Chronic giardiasis may produce fatigue and weight loss in addition to these typical signs and symptoms.

Diagnosis

Suspect giardiasis when travelers to endemic areas or campers who may have drunk unpurified water develop symptoms.

℞ **CONFIRMING DIAGNOSIS** *Actual diagnosis requires laboratory examination of a fresh stool specimen for cysts or examination of duodenal aspirate for trophozoites. A fecal immunoassay test of the stool for giardiasis is also very effective in diagnosis. A small-bowel biopsy shows Giardia.*

Diagnosis must also rule out other causes of diarrhea and malabsorption.

Treatment

Giardiasis responds readily to a 10-day course of tinidazole or nitazoxanide. Metronidazole is used in children and infants. Severe diarrhea may require parenteral fluid replacement to prevent dehydration if oral fluid intake is inadequate.

Special considerations

◆ Inform the patient receiving metronidazole of the possible adverse effects of this drug: commonly, headache, anorexia, and nausea and, less commonly, vomiting, diarrhea, and abdominal cramps. Warn against drinking alcoholic beverages, which may provoke a disulfiram-like reaction. If the patient is a woman, ask if she's pregnant because metronidazole is contraindicated during pregnancy.

◆ When talking to family members and other suspected contacts, emphasize the importance of stool examinations for *G. lamblia* cysts.

◆ If hospitalization is required, use contact precautions. A diapered incontinent person requires a private room. Pay strict attention to hand hygiene, particularly after handling feces. Quickly dispose of fecal material. (Normal sewage systems can remove and process infected feces adequately.)

◆ Teach good personal hygiene, particularly proper handwashing technique.

◆ To help prevent giardiasis, warn travelers to endemic areas not to drink water or eat uncooked and unpeeled fruits or vegetables (they may have been rinsed in contaminated water).

Prophylactic drug therapy isn't recommended. Advise campers to purify all stream water before drinking it.

◆ Report epidemic situations to the public health authorities.

TOXOPLASMOSIS

Causes and incidence

Toxoplasmosis, one of the most common infectious diseases, is caused by the protozoa *Toxoplasma gondii.* Distributed worldwide, it's less common in cold or hot, arid climates and at high elevations. It usually causes localized infection but may produce significant generalized infection, especially in neonates and patients who are immunodeficient. Congenital toxoplasmosis, characterized by lesions in the CNS, may result in stillbirth or serious birth defects. For this reason, pregnant women are advised to avoid cleaning cat litter boxes because fecal–oral contamination from infected cats transmits toxoplasmosis.

In addition to possible fecal–oral transmission from infected cats, ingestion of tissue cysts in raw or uncooked meat (heating, drying, or freezing destroys these cysts) or eating fruits and vegetables from contaminated soil can contribute to transmission.

Congenital toxoplasmosis follows transplacental transmission from a chronically infected mother or one who acquired toxoplasmosis shortly before or during pregnancy.

Receiving an infected organ transplant or infected blood transfusion can cause toxoplasmosis, although this is rare.

Pathophysiology

Toxoplasma gondii exists in trophozoite forms in the acute stages of infection and in cystic forms (tissue cysts and oocysts) in the latent stages. Follicular hyperplasia occurs in lymph nodes and distention of sinuses occurs. Infection is typically localized.

Complications

◆ Encephalitis
◆ Myocarditis
◆ Pneumonitis
◆ Hepatitis
◆ Polymyositis

Signs and symptoms

Toxoplasmosis acquired in the first trimester of pregnancy commonly results in stillbirth. About one-third of infants who survive have congenital toxoplasmosis. The later in pregnancy that maternal infection occurs, the greater the risk of congenital infection in the infant. Obvious

Ocular toxoplasmosis

Ocular toxoplasmosis (active retinochoroiditis), characterized by focal necrotizing retinitis, accounts for about 25% of all cases of granulomatous uveitis. It's usually the result of congenital infection, but may not appear until adolescence or young adulthood, when infection is reactivated. Symptoms include blurred vision, scotoma, pain, photophobia, and impairment or loss of central vision. Vision improves as inflammation subsides but usually without recovery of lost visual acuity. Ocular toxoplasmosis may subside after treatment with prednisone and antibiotics.

signs of congenital toxoplasmosis include retinochoroiditis, hydrocephalus or microcephalus, cerebral calcification, seizures, lymphadenopathy, fever, hepatosplenomegaly, jaundice, and rash. Other defects, which may become apparent months or years later, include strabismus, blindness, epilepsy, and mental retardation. (See *Ocular toxoplasmosis.*)

Acquired toxoplasmosis may cause localized (mild lymphatic) or generalized (fulminating, disseminated) infection. Localized infection produces fever and a mononucleosis-like syndrome (malaise, myalgia, headache, fatigue, and sore throat) and lymphadenopathy. Generalized infection produces encephalitis, fever, headache, vomiting, delirium, seizures, and a diffuse maculopapular rash (except on the palms, soles, and scalp). Generalized infection may lead to myocarditis, pneumonitis, hepatitis, and polymyositis.

Diagnosis

CONFIRMING DIAGNOSIS *Identification of* T. gondii *in an appropriate tissue specimen with ELISA confirms the diagnosis of toxoplasmosis.*

Serologic tests may be useful and, in patients with toxoplasmosis encephalitis, CT scans and MRI disclose lesions.

Treatment

No treatment is typically required, as toxoplasmosis is usually self-limiting. If required, treatment of acute disease consists of drug therapy with sulfonamides, pyrimethamine, clindamycin, or trimethoprim/sulfamethoxazole. In patients who also have AIDS, treatment continues indefinitely. No safe, effective treatment exists for chronic toxoplasmosis or toxoplasmosis occurring in the first trimester of pregnancy.

Special considerations

When caring for patients with toxoplasmosis, monitor drug therapy carefully and emphasize thorough patient teaching to prevent complications and control spread of the disease.

◆ Because sulfonamides cause blood dyscrasias and pyrimethamine depresses bone marrow, closely monitor the patient's hematologic values. Also emphasize the importance of regularly scheduled follow-up care.

◆ Teach all patients to wash their hands after working with soil (because it may be contaminated with cat oocysts); to cook meat thoroughly and freeze it promptly if it isn't for immediate use; to change cat litter daily (cat oocysts don't become infective until 1 to 4 days after excretion); to cover children's sandboxes; and to keep flies away from food (flies transport oocysts).

◆ Advise all pregnant women to avoid cleaning and handling of cat litter boxes. If this can't be avoided, advise them to wear gloves.

◆ Patients who are receiving immunosuppressants are very susceptible to toxoplasmosis. Warn them of the risks and suggest having all cats that go outdoors tested for toxoplasmosis.

CRYPTOSPORIDIOSIS

Causes and incidence

Cryptosporidiosis is an intestinal infection that typically results in acute, self-limited diarrhea. However, in immunocompromised patients— who contract it more often—cryptosporidiosis causes chronic, severe, and life-threatening symptoms.

Those at greatest risk for contracting cryptosporidiosis include:

◆ Patients with hypogammaglobulinemia
◆ Patients receiving immunosuppressants for cancer therapy or organ transplantation
◆ Malnourished children

Cryptosporidiosis is especially prevalent in patients with AIDS.

In addition to immunocompromised patients, travelers to foreign countries, medical personnel caring for patients with the disease, and children are at particular risk. It's spread easily in daycare centers and among household contacts and medical providers. Contaminated water, such as in a swimming pool, is a frequent source of infection. This disease occurs worldwide.

Pathophysiology

Cryptosporidiosis is caused by the protozoan *Cryptosporidium*. These small spherules inhabit the microvillus border of the intestinal epithelium. There, the protozoa shed infected oocysts into the intestinal lumen, where they pass into the stool.

These oocysts are particularly hardy, resisting destruction by routine water chlorination. This increases the risk of infection spreading through contact with contaminated water. The disease can also be transmitted via contaminated food and person-to-person contact.

Complications

◆ Severe fluid and electrolyte depletion
◆ Malnutrition
◆ Rectal excoriation and breakdown
◆ Papillary stenosis
◆ Sclerosing cholangitis
◆ Cholecystitis

Signs and symptoms

Although asymptomatic infections can occur in both healthy and immunocompromised patients, the typical patient with cryptosporidiosis develops symptoms after an incubation period of about 7 days. (The incubation period may be shorter in an immunocompromised patient.) The patient initially complains of watery, nonbloody diarrhea. The patient may also report abdominal pain, anorexia, nausea, fever, and weight loss. In the 10% of patients who develop biliary tract involvement, right upper abdominal pain may be severe. Signs and symptoms usually subside within 2 weeks but may recur sporadically for months to years.

The history of an immunocompromised patient typically reveals a more gradual onset of symptoms. Such a patient may also develop more severe diarrhea with daily fluid losses as high as 20 L.

For all patients, auscultation of the abdomen may reveal hyperactive bowel sounds. Palpation may reveal abdominal tenderness.

Diagnosis

Cryptosporidiosis often goes undetected as the cause of profuse diarrhea because an acid-fast stain needed to detect the organism isn't routinely used. However, the acid-fast stain as well as microscopic examinations, such as DFA and EIAs, of stool samples reveal the presence of oocysts. Molecular methods such as PCR can be used to identify the species of *Cryptosporidium*.

The infecting organisms can also be detected by light and electron microscopy at the apical surfaces of intestinal epithelium obtained through biopsies of the small bowel. Although serologic tests exist, their value in diagnosing acute or chronic infections in immunocompromised patients hasn't been determined.

With biliary tract involvement, studies may reveal an elevated alkaline phosphatase level, gallbladder wall thickening, and dilated bile ducts.

Treatment

Although no treatment currently exists to eradicate the infecting organism, nitazoxanide or paromomycin has been used.

Treatment for cryptosporidiosis consists mainly of supportive measures to control symptoms. Such measures include fluid replacement to prevent dehydration as well as administration of analgesics to relieve pain and antidiarrheal and antiperistaltic agents to control diarrhea.

Special considerations

◆ Closely monitor the patient's fluid and electrolyte balance.
◆ Encourage an adequate intake of fluids, especially those rich in electrolytes.
◆ Monitor the patient's intake and output, and weigh daily to evaluate the need for fluid replacement. Watch closely for signs of dehydration and provide fluid replacement as indicated.
◆ Administer analgesics, antidiarrheal and antiperistaltic agents, and antibiotics as indicated. Watch the patient for signs of adverse reactions as well as therapeutic effects.
◆ Apply perirectal protective cream to prevent excoriation and skin breakdown.
◆ Encourage frequent small meals to help prevent nausea.
◆ Teach the patient about all medications. Make sure he or she understands how to take the drugs and what adverse reactions to watch for. Stress the importance of calling his or her healthcare provider immediately if an adverse reaction develops.
◆ Teach the patient and family to recognize the signs and symptoms of dehydration, including weight loss, poor skin turgor, oliguria, irritability, and dry flushed skin. Report such findings to the physician.
◆ Teach the patient and family about good personal hygiene, especially proper handwashing technique. Explain how to safely handle potentially infectious material, such as soiled bed sheets.
◆ Advise the patient's family members and close contacts to have their stools tested.
◆ Report cases to the public health department.

Helminths

TRICHINOSIS
Causes and incidence

Trichinosis (also known as *trichiniasis* or *trichinellosis*) is an infection caused by larvae of the intestinal roundworm *Trichinella spiralis*. It occurs worldwide, especially in populations that eat pork or bear meat. Trichinosis may produce multiple symptoms; respiratory, CNS, and cardiovascular complications; and, rarely, death.

Trichinosis, though common worldwide, is seldom seen in the United States because of regulations regarding animal feed and meat processing.

Pathophysiology

Transmission is through ingestion of uncooked or undercooked meat that contains *T. spiralis* cysts. Such cysts are found primarily in swine, less commonly in dogs, cats, bears, foxes, wolves, and marine animals. These cysts result from the animals' ingestion of similarly contaminated flesh. In swine, such infection results from eating table scraps or raw garbage.

After gastric juices free the worm from the cyst capsule, it reaches sexual maturity in a few days. The female roundworm burrows into the intestinal mucosa and reproduces. Larvae are then transported through the lymphatic system and the bloodstream. They become embedded as cysts in striated muscle, especially in the diaphragm, chest, arms, and legs. Human-to-human transmission doesn't take place.

Complications

◆ Encephalitis
◆ Myocarditis
◆ Pneumonia
◆ Respiratory failure

Signs and symptoms

In the United States, trichinosis is usually mild and seldom produces symptoms. When symptoms do occur, they vary with the stage and degree of infection:
◆ *Stage 1* (invasion) occurs 1 week after ingestion. Release of larvae and reproduction of adult *T. spiralis* may cause anorexia, nausea, vomiting, diarrhea, abdominal pain, and cramps.
◆ *Stage 2* (dissemination) occurs 7 to 10 days after ingestion. *T. spiralis* penetrates the intestinal mucosa and begins to migrate to striated muscle. Signs and symptoms include edema, especially of the eyelids or face; muscle pain, particularly in extremities; and, occasionally, itching and burning skin, sweating, skin lesions, a temperature of 102° to 104° F (38.9° to 40° C), and delirium. In severe respiratory, cardiovascular, or CNS infections, palpitations and lethargy can occur.
◆ *Stage 3* (encystment) occurs during convalescence, generally 1 week later. *T. spiralis* larvae invade muscle fiber and become encysted.

Diagnosis

A history of ingestion of raw or improperly cooked pork or pork products, with typical clinical features, suggests trichinosis, but infection may be difficult to prove. Stools may contain mature worms and larvae during the invasion stage. Diagnosis is most often made with detection of *Trichinella* antigen or antiparasite antibodies. Skeletal muscle biopsies, which are rarely performed, can show encysted larvae 10 days after ingestion; if available, analyses of contaminated meat also show larvae.

Other abnormal results include elevated aspartate aminotransferase, alanine aminotransferase, creatine kinase, and lactate dehydrogenase levels during the acute stages and an elevated eosinophil count (up to 15,000/µL). A normal or increased CSF lymphocyte count (to 300/µL) and increased protein levels indicate CNS involvement.

Treatment

Mebendazole or albendazole effectively combats this parasite during the intestinal stage (neither drug has been approved) for treatment of pregnant women or children age 2 and younger; severe infection (especially CNS invasion) may warrant glucocorticoids to combat possible inflammation. There's no treatment for trichinosis once it's in the muscles, but analgesics may be used for muscle pain.

Special considerations

◆ Question the patient about recent ingestion of pork products and the methods used to store and cook them.
◆ Reduce fever with alcohol rubs, tepid baths, cooling blankets, or antipyretics; relieve muscle pain with analgesics, enforced bed rest, and proper body alignment.
◆ To prevent pressure ulcers, frequently reposition the patient, and gently massage bony prominences.
◆ Explain the importance of bed rest. Sudden death from cardiac involvement may occur in a patient with moderate to severe infection who has resumed activity too soon. Warn the patient to continue bed rest into the convalescent stage to avoid a serious relapse and possible death.

▓▓▓ PREVENTION *To help prevent trichinosis take these actions:*

◆ *Educate the public about proper cooking and storing methods not only for pork and pork products but also for meat from other carnivores. To kill trichinae, internal meat temperatures should reach 150° F (70° C) and meat color should change from pink to gray unless the meat has been cured or frozen for at least 10 days at low temperatures.*
◆ *Warn travelers to foreign countries or to poor areas in the United States to avoid eating pork; swine in these areas are commonly fed raw garbage.*

◆ *Report all cases of trichinosis to local public health authorities.*

HOOKWORM DISEASE
Causes and incidence

Hookworm disease, also called *uncinariasis* or *ground itch,* is an infection of the upper intestine caused by *Ancylostoma duodenale* (found in the eastern hemisphere) or *Necator americanus* (in the western hemisphere). Sandy soil, high humidity, a warm climate, and failure to wear shoes all favor its transmission. In the United States, hookworm disease is most common in the southeast. Although this disease can cause cardiopulmonary complications, it's rarely fatal, except in debilitated people and infants younger than age 1.

Hookworm disease, affecting billions of people worldwide, is most common in moist tropical and subtropical regions. There's little risk of acquiring hookworm disease in the United States because of advances in sanitization and waste control.

Pathophysiology

Both forms of hookworm disease are transmitted to humans through direct skin penetration (usually in the foot) by hookworm larvae in soil contaminated with feces containing hookworm ova. These ova develop into infectious larvae in 1 to 3 days. Larvae travel through the lymphatics to the pulmonary capillaries, where they penetrate alveoli and move up the bronchial tree to the trachea and epiglottis, where they're swallowed and enter the GI tract. When they reach the small intestine, they mature, attach to the jejunal mucosa, and suck blood, oxygen, and glucose from the intestinal wall. These mature worms then deposit ova, which are excreted in the stool, starting the cycle anew. Hookworm larvae mature in approximately 5 to 6 weeks.

Complications

◆ Cardiomegaly
◆ Heart failure
◆ Massive edema

Signs and symptoms

Most cases of hookworm disease produce few symptoms and may be overlooked until worms are passed in the stool. The earliest signs and symptoms include irritation, pruritus, and edema at the site of entry, which are sometimes accompanied by secondary bacterial infection with pustule formation.

When the larvae reach the lungs, they may cause pneumonitis and hemorrhage with fever, sore throat, crackles, and cough. Finally, intestinal infection may cause fatigue, nausea, weight loss, dizziness, melena, and uncontrolled diarrhea.

In severe and chronic infection, anemia from blood loss may lead to cardiomegaly (a result of increased oxygen demands), heart failure, and generalized massive edema.

Diagnosis

℞ **CONFIRMING DIAGNOSIS** *Identification of hookworm ova in the stool confirms the diagnosis. Anemia suggests severe chronic infection.*

Treatment

Treatment of hookworm infestation includes administering mebendazole or albendazole, and providing an iron-rich diet or iron supplements to prevent or correct anemia.

Special considerations

◆ Obtain a complete history, with special attention to travel or residency in endemic areas. Note the sequence and onset of symptoms. Interview the patient's family and other close contacts to see if they have symptoms.

◆ Carefully assess the patient, noting signs of entry, lymphedema, and respiratory status.

◆ Perform meticulous hand hygiene after every patient contact.

◆ For severe anemia, administer oxygen, if ordered, at low to moderate flow. Be sure the oxygen is humidified because the patient may already have upper airway irritation from the parasites. Encourage coughing and deep breathing to stimulate removal of blood or secretions from involved lung areas and to prevent secondary infection. Plan your care to allow frequent rest periods because the patient may tire easily. If anemia causes immobility, reposition the patient often to prevent skin breakdown.

◆ Closely monitor intake and output. Note the frequency of diarrhea and the quantity of stools. Dispose of feces promptly, and wear gloves when doing so.

◆ To help assess nutritional status, weigh the patient daily. To combat malnutrition, emphasize the importance of good nutrition, with particular attention to foods high in iron and protein. If the patient receives iron supplements, explain that they will darken stools. Administer anthelmintics on an empty stomach, but without a purgative.

◆ To help prevent reinfestation, educate the patient in proper handwashing technique and sanitary disposal of feces. Tell the patient to wear shoes in endemic areas.

ASCARIASIS

Causes and incidence

Ascariasis, also known as *roundworm infestation*, is caused by *Ascaris lumbricoides*. It's the most common type of intestinal worm infestation, occurring worldwide. Most patients recover without treatment, but complications can occur when adult worms move into certain organs and multiply, resulting in blockage of the intestine.

Ascariasis is most common in tropical areas with poor sanitation and in Asia, where farmers use human feces as fertilizer. In the United States, it's more prevalent in the South, particularly among children ages 4 to 12.

Pathophysiology

Ascaris lumbricoides is a large roundworm resembling an earthworm. It's transmitted to humans by ingestion of soil contaminated with human feces that harbor *A. lumbricoides* ova. Such ingestion may occur directly (by eating contaminated soil) or indirectly (by eating poorly washed raw vegetables grown in contaminated soil).

Ascariasis never passes directly from person to person. After ingestion, *A. lumbricoides* ova hatch and release larvae, which penetrate the intestinal wall and reach the lungs through the bloodstream. After about 10 days in pulmonary capillaries and alveoli, the larvae migrate to the bronchioles, bronchi, trachea, and epiglottis. There they are swallowed and return to the intestine to mature into worms.

Complications

◆ Biliary or intestinal obstruction
◆ Pulmonary disease

Signs and symptoms

Ascariasis produces two phases: early pulmonary and prolonged intestinal. Mild intestinal infestation may cause only vague stomach discomfort. The first clue may be vomiting a worm or passing a worm in the stool. Severe infestation, however, causes stomach pain, vomiting, restlessness, disturbed sleep, and, in extreme cases, intestinal obstruction. Larvae migrating by the lymphatic and the circulatory systems cause symptoms that vary; for instance, when they invade the lungs, pneumonitis may result.

Diagnosis

℞ **CONFIRMING DIAGNOSIS** *The key to diagnosis is identifying ova in the stool or adult worms, which may be passed rectally or by mouth.*

When migrating larvae invade alveoli, other conclusive tests include X-rays that show characteristic bronchovascular markings: infiltrates, patchy areas of pneumonitis, and widening of hilar shadows. Ultrasound, CT scan, or MRI may show invasion in the pancreas or liver. In a patient with ascariasis, these findings usually accompany a complete blood count that shows eosinophilia.

Treatment

Drug therapy, the primary treatment consists of albendazole or mebendazole to kill intestinal parasitic worms, permitting peristalsis to expel them. No specific treatment exists for migratory infestation because anthelmintics affect only mature worms.

In intestinal obstruction, NG suctioning controls vomiting. If there's a blockage caused by a large number of worms, a paralyzing vermifuge (such as pyrantel pamoate or piperazine) can make the worms relax and pass through the intestine to relieve obstruction. However, ascariasis may necessitate surgery if the paralyzed worms result in intestinal blockage.

Special considerations

◆ Although isolation is unnecessary, properly dispose of feces and soiled linen, and carefully wash your hands after patient contact.
◆ If the patient is receiving NG suction, be sure to give good mouth care.
◆ Teach the patient to prevent reinfestation with good handwashing, especially before eating and after defecation.

TAENIASIS
Causes and incidence

Taeniasis, also called *tapeworm disease* or *cestodiasis*, is a parasitic infestation by *Taenia saginata* (beef tapeworm), *Taenia solium* (pork tapeworm), or *Taenia asiatica* (Asian pork tapeworm). Taeniasis is usually a chronic, benign intestinal disease; however, infestation with *T. solium* may cause dangerous systemic and CNS symptoms if larvae invade the brain and striated muscle of vital organs.

Pathophysiology

Taenia saginata, *T. solium*, and *T. asiatica* are transmitted to humans by ingestion of beef or pork that contains tapeworm cysts. Gastric acids break down these cysts in the stomach, liberating them to mature. Mature tapeworms fasten to the intestinal wall and produce ova that are passed in the feces. (See *Common tapeworm infestations*.)

Complications
◆ Dehydration
◆ Malnutrition

Signs and symptoms

Taeniasis may produce mild symptoms, such as nausea, flatulence, hunger sensations, weight loss, diarrhea, and increased appetite, or no symptoms at all. Occasionally, worm segments may exit through the anus and appear on bed clothes. (See *Taeniases*, page 913.)

Common tapeworm infestations

Type and source of infection	Incidence	Clinical features
Taenia saginata (beef tapeworm)		
Uncooked or undercooked infected beef	Worldwide, but prevalent in Europe and East Africa	Crawling sensation in the perianal area caused by worm segments that have been passed rectally; intestinal obstruction and appendicitis due to long worm segments that have twisted in the intestinal lumen
Taenia solium (pork tapeworm)		
Uncooked or undercooked infected pork	Highest in Mexico and Latin America; lowest among Muslims and Jews	Seizures, headaches, personality changes; commonly overlooked in adults
Taenia asiatica (pork tapeworm)		
Uncooked or undercooked infected pork	Limited to Asia and is mostly seen in the Republic of Korea, China, Taiwan, Indonesia, and Thailand	Mild digestive symptoms, such as abdominal pain, nausea, and loss of appetite

Taeniases

The photo shows a specimen of *T. saginata* obtained from a patient after treatment.

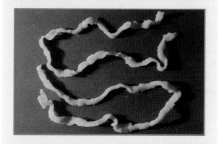

Diagnosis

Rx **CONFIRMING DIAGNOSIS** *Diagnosis of tapeworm infestations requires laboratory observation of tapeworm ova or body segments in feces.*

Because ova aren't excreted continuously, confirmation may require multiple specimens. A supporting dietary or travel history aids confirmation.

Treatment

The drugs of choice for tapeworm infestation are praziquantel and niclosamide.

Laxative use or induced vomiting is contraindicated because of the danger of autoinfection and systemic disease.

After drug treatment, tapeworm infestation requires a follow-up laboratory examination of stool specimens during the next 2 to 3 months to check for any remaining ova or worm segments. Persistent infestation typically requires a second course of medication.

Special considerations

◆ Obtain a complete history, including recent travel to endemic areas, dietary habits, and physical symptoms.
◆ Dispose of the patient's excretions carefully. Wear gloves when giving personal care and handling fecal excretions, bedpans, and bed linens; wash your hands thoroughly, and tell the patient to do the same.
◆ Use enteric precautions. Avoid procedures and drugs that may cause vomiting or gagging. If the patient is a child or is incontinent, a private room is required. Obtain a list of contacts.
◆ To prevent reinfestation, teach proper hand hygiene technique and the need to cook beef

and pork thoroughly. Stress the need for follow-up evaluations to monitor the success of therapy and to detect possible reinfestation.

ENTEROBIASIS

Causes and incidence

Enterobiasis (also called *pinworm, seatworm,* or *threadworm infection,* or *oxyuriasis*) is a benign intestinal disease caused by the nematode *Enterobius vermicularis.* Found worldwide, even in temperate regions with good sanitation, it's the most prevalent helminthic infection in the United States.

Enterobiasis infestation and reinfestation occur most commonly in children between ages 5 and 14 and in certain institutionalized groups because of poor hygiene and frequent hand-to-mouth activity. Crowded living conditions increase the likelihood of it spreading to several members of a family.

Pathophysiology

Adult pinworms live in the intestine; female worms migrate to the perianal region to deposit their ova. *Direct transmission* occurs when the patient's hands transfer infective eggs from the anus to the mouth. *Indirect transmission* occurs when the patient comes in contact with contaminated articles, such as linens and clothing.

Complications

◆ Salpingitis
◆ Appendicitis
◆ Bowel ulceration
◆ Pelvic granuloma

Signs and symptoms

Asymptomatic enterobiasis is commonly overlooked. However, intense perianal pruritus may occur, especially at night, when the female worm leaves the anus to deposit ova. Pruritus causes irritability, scratching, skin irritation, and, sometimes, vaginitis.

Diagnosis

Rx **CONFIRMING DIAGNOSIS** *A history of anal pruritus suggests enterobiasis; identification of Enterobius ova recovered from the perianal area with a cellophane tape swab taken before the patient bathes and defecates in the morning confirms it. A stool sample is usually ova- and worm-free because the worms deposit ova outside the intestine and die after return to the anus.*

Treatment

Drug therapy with pyrantel (available over-the-counter), mebendazole, or albendazole destroys the causative parasites. These drugs are to be given in one dose at first and then another single dose 2 weeks later. Effective eradication requires simultaneous treatment of the patient's family members and, in institutions, other patients.

Special considerations
◆ If the patient receives pyrantel, tell the patient and family that this drug colors the stool bright red and may cause vomiting (vomitus will also be red). The tablet form of this drug is coated with aspirin and shouldn't be given to aspirin-sensitive patients.
◆ To help prevent this disease, tell parents to bathe children daily (showers are preferable to tub baths) and to change underwear and bed linens daily.
◆ Tell the patient's family not to shake bed linens, to avoid aerosolization of eggs that may be on linens.
◆ Educate children in proper personal hygiene, and stress the need for proper handwashing after defecation and before handling food. Discourage nail biting. If the child can't stop, suggest that the patient wear gloves until the infestation clears.

◆ Report *all* outbreaks of enterobiasis to school authorities.
◆ Tell parents to strictly adhere to the prescribed drug dosage as directed by a physician.

SCHISTOSOMIASIS
Causes and incidence
Schistosomiasis, also known as *bilharziasis*, is a slowly progressive disease caused by blood flukes of the class Trematoda. There are three major types: *Schistosoma mansoni* and *S. japonicum* infect the intestinal tract; *S. haematobium* infects the urinary tract. (See *Types of schistosomes*.) The degree of infection determines the intensity of illness. Complications—such as portal hypertension, pulmonary hypertension, heart failure, ascites, hematemesis from ruptured esophageal varices, and renal failure—can be fatal.

Pathophysiology
The mode of transmission is bathing, swimming, wading, or working in water contaminated with *Schistosoma* larvae. These larvae penetrate the skin or mucous membranes and

Types of schistosomes

Species and incidence	Signs and symptoms	Treatment	Adverse effects
Schistosoma mansoni			
Western hemisphere, particularly Puerto Rico, Lesser Antilles, Brazil, and Venezuela; also Nile delta, Sudan, and central Africa	Irregular fever, malaise, weakness, abdominal distress, weight loss, diarrhea, ascites, hepatosplenomegaly, portal hypertension, fistulas, and intestinal stricture	Praziquantel: 60 mg/kg in three equally divided doses at 4- to 6-hour intervals on the same day	Abdominal discomfort, dizziness, drowsiness, fever, headache, malaise, minimal increase in liver enzyme levels, nausea, and urticaria
Schistosoma japonicum			
Affects men more than women; particularly prevalent among farmers in Japan, China, and the Philippines	Irregular fever, malaise, weakness, abdominal distress, weight loss, diarrhea, ascites, hepatosplenomegaly, portal hypertension, fistulas, and intestinal stricture	Praziquantel: 60 mg/kg in three equally divided doses at 4- to 6-hour intervals on the same day	Abdominal discomfort, dizziness, drowsiness, fever, headache, malaise, minimal increase in liver enzyme levels, nausea, and urticaria
Schistosoma haematobium			
Africa, Cyprus, Greece, and India	Terminal hematuria, dysuria, ureteral colic; with secondary infection—colicky pain, intermittent flank pain, vague GI complaints, and total renal failure	Praziquantel: 60 mg/kg in three equally divided doses at 4- to 6-hour intervals on the same day	Abdominal discomfort, dizziness, drowsiness, fever, headache, malaise, minimal increase in liver enzyme levels, nausea, and urticaria

eventually work their way to the liver's venous portal circulation. There, they mature in 1 to 3 months. The adults then migrate to other parts of the body.

The female cercariae lay spiny eggs in blood vessels surrounding the large intestine or bladder. After penetrating the mucosa of these organs, the eggs are excreted in feces or urine. If the eggs hatch in fresh water, the first-stage larvae (miracidia) penetrate freshwater snails, which act as passive intermediate hosts. Cercariae produced in snails escape into water and begin a new life cycle.

Complications
◆ Portal hypertension
◆ Hepatosplenomegaly
◆ Pulmonary hypertension
◆ Ascites
◆ Hematemesis
◆ Heart failure
◆ Renal failure

Signs and symptoms
Initial signs and symptoms of schistosomiasis depend on the site of infection and the stage of the disease. Initially, a transient, pruritic rash develops at the site of cercariae penetration, along with fever, myalgia, and cough. Later signs and symptoms may include hepatomegaly, splenomegaly, and lymphadenopathy. Worm migration and egg deposition may cause such complications as flaccid paralysis, seizures, and skin abscesses.

Diagnosis
℞ CONFIRMING DIAGNOSIS *Typical symptoms and a history of travel to endemic areas suggest the diagnosis; ova in the urine or stool or a mucosal lesion biopsy confirms it.*

The WBC count shows eosinophilia.

Treatment
The treatment of choice is the anthelmintic drug praziquantel. Between 3 and 6 months after treatment, the patient will need to be examined again. If this checkup detects any living eggs, treatment may be resumed. With acute infection, corticosteroids may be ordered.

Special considerations
◆ To help prevent schistosomiasis, teach people in endemic areas to work for a pure water supply and to avoid swimming or bathing in water that's known to be contaminated or potentially contaminated. If they must enter the water, tell them to wear protective clothing and to dry themselves afterward.

STRONGYLOIDIASIS
Causes and incidence
Strongyloidiasis, also called *threadworm infestation*, is a parasitic intestinal infestation caused by the helminth *Strongyloides stercoralis*. This worldwide infestation is endemic in the tropics and subtropics. Susceptibility to strongyloidiasis is universal. Infection doesn't confer immunity, and people who are immunocompromised may suffer overwhelming disseminated infection. Because the threadworm's reproductive cycle may continue in the untreated host for up to 45 years, autoinfection is highly probable. Most patients with strongyloidiasis recover, but debilitation from protein loss may result in death.

Pathophysiology
Transmission to humans usually occurs through contact with soil that contains infective *S. stercoralis* filariform larvae; such larvae develop from noninfective rhabdoid (rod-shaped) larvae in human feces. The filariform larvae penetrate the human skin, usually at the feet. They migrate by way of the lymphatic system to the bloodstream and the lungs.

Once they enter into pulmonary circulation, the filariform larvae break through the alveoli and migrate upward to the pharynx, where they are swallowed. They then lodge in the small intestine, where they deposit eggs that mature into noninfectious rhabdoid larvae. Next, these larvae migrate into the large intestine and are excreted in feces, starting the cycle again. The threadworm life cycle, which begins with penetration of the skin and ends with excretion of rhabdoid larvae, takes 17 days.

In autoinfection, rhabdoid larvae mature within the intestine to become infective filariform larvae.

Complications
◆ Malnutrition
◆ Secondary bacterial infection
◆ Intestinal perforation

Signs and symptoms
The patient's resistance and the extent of infection determine the severity of symptoms. Some patients have no symptoms, but many develop an erythematous maculopapular rash at the site of penetration that produces swelling and pruritus that may be confused with an insect bite. As the larvae migrate to the lungs, pulmonary signs develop, including minor hemorrhage, pneumonitis, and pneumonia; later, intestinal infection produces frequent, watery, and bloody diarrhea, accompanied by intermittent abdominal pain.

Severe infestation can cause malnutrition from substantial fat and protein loss, anemia, and lesions resembling ulcerative colitis, all of which invite secondary bacterial infection. Ulcerated intestinal mucosa may lead to perforation and, possibly, potentially fatal dissemination, especially in patients with malignancy or immunodeficiency diseases or in those who receive immunosuppressants.

Diagnosis

Diagnosis requires observation of *S. stercoralis* larvae in a fresh stool specimen (2 hours after excretion, rhabdoid larvae look like hookworm larvae). Duodenal aspirations show larvae present in duodenal fluid and an antigen test that's positive for *S. stercoralis*. During the pulmonary phase, sputum shows *S. stercoralis*; marked eosinophilia also occurs in disseminated strongyloidiasis.

Treatment

The goal of treatment is to eliminate the larvae with anthelmintics, such as ivermectin or albendazole. Patients may need protein replacement, blood transfusions, and I.V. fluids. Retreatment is necessary if *S. stercoralis* remains in stools after therapy.

Special considerations

◆ Keep accurate intake and output records. Ask the dietary department to provide a high-protein diet. The patient may need tube feedings to increase caloric intake.

◆ Use standard precautions when handling bedpans or giving perineal care, and dispose of feces promptly.

◆ Because direct person-to-person transmission doesn't occur, isolation isn't required.

◆ In pulmonary infection, reposition the patient frequently, encourage coughing and deep breathing, and administer oxygen as ordered.

◆ To prevent reinfestation, teach the patient proper handwashing technique. Stress the importance of proper hand hygiene before eating and after defecating and of wearing shoes when in endemic areas. Check the patient's family and close contacts for signs of infestation. Emphasize the need for follow-up stool examination, continuing for several weeks after treatment.

Miscellaneous infections

PSITTACOSIS

Causes and incidence

Psittacosis (also called *ornithosis* or *parrot fever*) is caused by the gram-negative intracellular parasite *Chlamydia psittaci* and is transmitted by infected birds. This disease occurs worldwide and is mainly associated with occupational exposure to birds (such as poultry farming). With adequate antimicrobial therapy, psittacosis is fatal in fewer than 4% of patients.

Incidence is higher in women and in people ages 20 to 50.

Pathophysiology

Psittacine birds (parrots, parakeets, and cockatoos), pigeons, and turkeys may harbor *C. psittaci* in their blood, feathers, tissues, nasal secretions, liver, spleen, and feces. Transmission to humans occurs primarily through inhalation of dust containing *C. psittaci* from bird droppings; less commonly, through direct contact with infected secretions or body tissues, as in laboratory personnel who work with birds. Person-to-person transmission seldom occurs but usually causes severe psittacosis.

Signs and symptoms

After an incubation period of 4 to 15 days, onset of symptoms may be insidious or sudden. Clinical effects include chills and a low-grade fever that increases to 103° to 105° F (39.4° to 40.6° C) for 7 to 10 days then, with treatment, declines during the second or third week. Other signs and symptoms include headache, myalgia, sore throat, cough (may be dry, hacking, and nonproductive or may produce blood-tinged sputum), abdominal distention and tenderness, nausea, vomiting, photophobia, decreased pulse rate, slightly increased respiratory rate, secondary purulent lung infection, and a faint macular rash. Severe infection also produces delirium, stupor, and, in extensive pulmonary infiltration, cyanosis. Psittacosis may recur but is usually milder.

Diagnosis

Characteristic symptoms and a recent history of exposure to birds suggest ornithosis.

CONFIRMING DIAGNOSIS *Firm diagnosis requires recovery of* C. psittaci *from mice, eggs, or tissue culture that has been inoculated with the patient's blood or sputum. Culture of* C. psittaci *can be dangerous for laboratory personnel, making serology the preferred method of confirming diagnosis.*

Comparison of acute and convalescent serum shows a fourfold rise in *Chlamydia* antibody titers. In addition, a patchy lobar infiltrate appears on chest X-rays or chest CT scan during the first week of illness.

Treatment

Psittacosis calls for treatment with doxycycline. If the infection is severe, doxycycline may be given via I.V. infusion until the fever subsides.

Fever and other symptoms should begin to subside 48 to 72 hours after antibiotic treatment begins, but treatment must continue for 2 weeks after temperature returns to normal. Other antibiotics used to treat psittacosis include erythromycin, azithromycin, chloramphenicol, and rifampin.

Special considerations
◆ Monitor the patient's fluid and electrolyte balance. Give I.V. fluids as needed.
◆ Carefully monitor the patient's vital signs. Watch for signs of overwhelming infection.
◆ Reduce fever with tepid sponge baths and a hypothermia blanket.
◆ Observe standard precautions. Instruct the patient to use tissues when coughing and to dispose of them in a closed plastic bag. Also instruct the patient to wash their hands afterward.
▓▓▓ **PREVENTION** *Persons who raise birds for sale should feed them tetracycline-treated birdseed and follow regulations on bird importation. However, routine use of antibiotics in animal and bird feed may contribute to antimicrobial resistance. Infected or possibly infected birds should be segregated from healthy birds, and the structures that housed the infected ones should be disinfected.*
◆ Report all cases of psittacosis to public health authorities.

TOXIC SHOCK SYNDROME
Causes and incidence
TSS is an acute bacterial infection caused by toxin-producing, penicillin-resistant strains of *S. aureus*, such as TSS toxin-1 and staphylococcal enterotoxins B and C. TSS can also be caused by toxins from GAS bacteria. Initially, the disease was thought to primarily affect menstruating women younger than age 30 and was associated with continuous use of tampons during the menstrual period; however, only about 55% of cases are associated with menses. TSS is fatal in 5% of cases.

Risk factors include recent use of barrier contraceptives (diaphragms or vaginal sponges), childbirth, and surgery.

Pathophysiology
Theoretically, tampons may contribute to the development of TSS by introducing *S. aureus* into the vagina during insertion (insertion with fingers instead of the supplied applicator increases the risk) or traumatizing the vaginal mucosa during insertion, thus leading to infection.

When TSS isn't related to menstruation, it appears to be linked to *S. aureus* infections, such as abscesses, osteomyelitis, and postsurgical infections. It's also associated with prior antibiotic use.

Complications
◆ Shock
◆ Renal failure
◆ Death

Signs and symptoms
Typically, TSS produces intense myalgias, fever over 104° F (40° C), vomiting, diarrhea, headache, decreased LOC, rigors, conjunctival hyperemia, and vaginal hyperemia and discharge. Severe hypotension occurs with hypovolemic shock. Within a few hours of onset, a deep red rash develops—especially on the palms and soles—and later desquamates.

Major complications include persistent neuropsychological abnormalities, mild renal failure, rash, and cyanotic arms and legs.

Diagnosis
Diagnosis is based on several criteria: fever, hypotension, rash that peels after 1 to 2 weeks, and at least three organs with signs of dysfunction. In some cases, blood cultures may be positive for *S. aureus* or GAS. Organs with signs of dysfunction may include:
◆ GI effects, including vomiting and profuse diarrhea
◆ muscular effects, with severe myalgias or a fivefold or greater increase in creatine kinase levels
◆ soft-tissue necrosis
◆ renal involvement with elevated blood urea nitrogen or creatinine levels (at least twice the normal levels)
◆ liver involvement with elevated bilirubin, aspartate aminotransferase, or alanine aminotransferase levels (at least twice the normal levels)
◆ blood involvement with signs of thrombocytopenia and a platelet count of less than 100,000/μL
◆ CNS effects such as disorientation without focal signs
◆ acute respiratory distress syndrome

Negative results on blood tests for RMSF, leptospirosis, and measles help rule out these disorders.

Treatment
Treatment involves examination and removal of foreign material, such as tampons, vaginal sponges, or nasal packing, and drainage of any identified site of infection such as surgical wounds. Typically, treatment includes clindamycin plus meropenem, or clindamycin plus piperacillin-tazobactam. To reverse shock, expect to replace fluids with saline solution and colloids, as ordered. Blood pressure support and dialysis may be necessary. In some cases, I.V. immunoglobulin may be required.

Special considerations

◆ Instruct women to change their tampons frequently and to always wash their hands before and after doing so.

◆ Monitor the patient's vital signs frequently.

◆ Administer antibiotics slowly and strictly on time. Be sure to watch for signs of penicillin allergy.

◆ Check the patient's fluid and electrolyte balance.

◆ Obtain specimens of vaginal and cervical secretions or other sites of TSS infection for culture of *S. aureus*, or GAS.

◆ Implement standard precautions.

◆ Report cases of TSS (other than streptococcal) to public health authorities.

SELECTED REFERENCES

Andrews-Polymenis, H., et al. (2010). Taming the elephant: Salmonella biology, pathogenesis, and prevention. *Infection and Immunity, 78*(6), 2356–2369.

Angus, D., & van der Poll, T. (2013). Severe sepsis and septic shock. *New England Journal of Medicine, 369*, 840–851. doi:10.1056/NEJMra1208623

Barrett, B., et al. (2010). Echinacea for treating the common cold: A randomized trial. *Annals of Internal Medicine, 153*(12), 769–777.

Barros, L., & Pegram, S. (2018). Clinical manifestations, diagnosis, and treatment of diphtheria. In E. Baron (Ed.), *UpToDate.* Retrieved from https://www.uptodate.com/contents/clinical-manifestations-diagnosis-and-treatment-of-diphtheria

Centers for Disease Control and Prevention. (2018). *About diphtheria.* Retrieved from https://www.cdc.gov/diphtheria/about/index.html

Centers for Disease Control and Prevention. (2018). *Bacterial meningitis.* Retrieved from https://www.cdc.gov/meningitis/bacterial.html

Centers for Disease Control and Prevention. (2018). *HAI data and statistics.* Retrieved from https://www.cdc.gov/hai/surveillance/index.html

Centers for Disease Control and Prevention. (2018). *Pharyngitis (strep throat).* Retrieved from https://www.cdc.gov/groupastrep/diseases-hcp/strep-throat.html

Centers for Disease Control and Prevention. (2018). *Tetanus.* Retrieved from https://www.cdc.gov/vaccines/pubs/pinkbook/tetanus.html

Centers for Disease Control and Prevention. (2018). *Typhoid fever.* Retrieved from https://www.cdc.gov/typhoid-fever/index.html

Centers for Disease Control and Prevention. (2018). *Vaccine recommendations and guidelines of the ACIP.* Retrieved from https://www.cdc.gov/vaccines/hcp/acip-recs/index.html

Currie, B., & Anstey, N. (2017). Treatment and prognosis of melioidosis. In A. Bloom (Ed.), *UpToDate.* Retrieved from https://www.uptodate.com/contents/treatment-and-prognosis-of-melioidosis

Davis, L., et al. (2010). Recurrent herpes simplex virus type 2 meningitis in elderly persons. *Archives of Neurology, 67*(6), 759–760.

Del Bono, V., et al. (2008). Invasive aspergillosis: Diagnosis, prophylaxis and treatment. *Current Opinion in Hematology, 15*(6), 586–593.

Friedman, H., & Isaacs, S. (2017). The epidemiology, pathogenesis, and clinical manifestations of smallpox. In J. Mitty (Ed.), *UpToDate.* Retrieved from https://www.uptodate.com/contents/the-epidemiology-pathogenesis-and-clinical-manifestations-of-smallpox

Gelfand, M. (2018). Clinical manifestations and diagnosis of *Listeria monocytogenes* infection. In J. Mitty (Ed.), *UpToDate.* Retrieved from https://www.uptodate.com/contents/clinical-manifestations-and-diagnosis-of-listeria-monocytogenes-infection

Kauffman, C. (2017). Primary coccidioidal infection. In J. Mitty (Ed.), *UpToDate.* Retrieved from https://www.uptodate.com/contents/primary-coccidioidal-infection

Kelly, C., et al. (2018). Clostridium difficile infection in adults: Treatment and prevention. In E. Baron (Ed.), *UpToDate.* Retrieved from https://www.uptodate.com/contents/clostridium-difficile-infection-in-adults-treatment-and-prevention

LaRocque, R., & Harris, J. (2018). Cholera: Clinical features, diagnosis, treatment, and prevention. In A. Bloom (Ed.), *UpToDate.* Retrieved from https://www.uptodate.com/contents/cholera-clinical-features-diagnosis-treatment-and-prevention

Lin, M., & Hayden, M. (2010). Methicillin-resistant *Staphylococcus aureus* and Vancomycin-resistant Enterococcus: Recognition and prevention in intensive care units. *Critical Care Medicine, 38*(8 Suppl), S335–S344.

Lowy, F. (2017). Methicillin-resistant *Staphylococcus aureus* (MRSA): Microbiology. In E. Baron (Ed.), *UpToDate.* Retrieved from https://www.uptodate.com/contents/methicillin-resistant-staphylococcus-aureus-mrsa-microbiology

Marrie, T., & Tuomanen, E. (2018). Pneumococcal pneumonia in adults. In S. Bond (Ed.), *UpToDate.* Retrieved from https://www.uptodate.com/contents/pneumococcal-pneumonia-in-adults

Puopolo, K., & Baker, C. (2018). Group B streptococcal infection in neonates and young infants. In C. Armsby (Ed.), *UpToDate.* Retrieved from https://www.uptodate.com/contents/group-b-streptococcal-infection-in-neonates-and-young-infants

Puopolo, K., et al. (2017). Group B streptococcal infection in pregnant women. In A. Bloom (Ed.), *UpToDate.* Retrieved from https://www.uptodate.com/contents/group-b-streptococcal-infection-in-pregnant-women

Rabinowitz, P., et al. (2010). Contact variables for exposure to avian Influenza H5N1 virus at the human–animal interface. *Zoonoses and Public Health, 57*(4), 227–238.

Scollard, D., et al. (2018). Leprosy: Treatment and prevention. In E. Baron (Ed.), *UpToDate.* Retrieved from https://www.uptodate.com/contents/leprosy-treatment-and-prevention

Sexton, D. (2018). Tetanus. In A. Bloom (Ed.), *UpToDate.* Retrieved from https://www.uptodate.com/contents/tetanus

Stephenson, I. (2017). Epidemiology, transmission, and pathogenesis of avian influenza. In A. Thorner (Ed.), *UpToDate.* Retrieved from https://www.uptodate.com/contents/epidemiology-transmission-and-pathogenesis-of-avian-influenza

Stevens, D. (2018). Treatment of streptococcal toxic shock syndrome. In E. Baron (Ed.), *UpToDate.* Retrieved from https://www.uptodate.com/contents/treatment-of-streptococcal-toxic-shock-syndrome

Stevens, D., & Baddour, L. (2018). Necrotizing soft tissue infections. In E. Baron (Ed.), *UpToDate.* Retrieved from https://www.uptodate.com/contents/necrotizing-soft-tissue-infections

Tunkel, A. (2017). Initial therapy and prognosis for bacterial meningitis in adults. In J. Mitty (Ed.), *UpToDate.* Retrieved from https://www.uptodate.com/contents/initial-therapy-and-prognosis-of-bacterial-meningitis-in-adults

Wilson, K. (2017). Treatment of anthrax. In A. Bloom (Ed.), *UpToDate.* Retrieved from https://www.uptodate.com/contents/treatment-of-anthrax

World Health Organization. (2018). *Cumulative number of confirmed human cases of avian influenza A (H5N1) reported to WHO.* Retrieved from http://www.who.int/influenza/human_animal_interface/H5N1_cumulative_table_archives/en

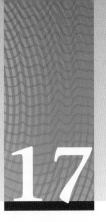

TRAUMA

Introduction

Trauma is one of the leading causes of death in the United States. Emergency trauma care basics include triage; assessing and maintaining airway, breathing, and circulation (the ABCs); protecting the cervical spine; assessing the level of consciousness (LOC); and, as needed, preparing the patient for transport and possibly surgery.

Common mechanisms of trauma include car, bicycle, vehicle crashes, car–pedestrian accidents, drowning, firearms, burns, and falls.

TRIAGE: FIRST THINGS FIRST

Triage is the setting of medical priorities for emergency care by making sound, rapid assessments. The need for triage usually arises at the scene of injury and continues in the emergency department. Following healthcare facility protocol, you'll decide which patient to treat first, which injury to treat first, how to best utilize other members of the medical team, and how to control patient and staff traffic.

In most cases, victims are assigned to the following categories and can be remembered by the acronym "D-I-M-E":

◆ *Delayed (nonurgent/minor)*—presence of minor or stable illness or injury that doesn't require treatment within 2 hours; includes patients with ear discomfort, minor or isolated soft-tissue wounds, and sore throat.

◆ *Immediate (emergent)*—life-threatening or limb-threatening injury requiring treatment within a few minutes to prevent death or further injury; includes patients with moderate-to-severe respiratory distress, cardiopulmonary arrest, compensated or uncompensated shock, limb injury with neurovascular compromise, alteration in neurologic status, and patients who have attempted suicide.

◆ *Minimal (urgent)*—serious, but not immediately life-threatening injury that should receive treatment within 2 hours; includes patients with mild wheezing and mild or no respiratory distress, mild-to-moderate dehydration, and suspected forearm fracture. (These patients require periodic assessment because they can deteriorate and become emergent.)

◆ *Expectant*—in a large mass casualty situation (or on a battlefield), there may be such an overwhelming amount of wounded that some patients cannot be saved based on supplies on hand, time, and immediate casualties present. An example could be patients with massive, open head injuries when neurosurgery is not available.

During the assessment, if the patient is discovered to have a life-threatening condition, immediate intervention is needed. It may also be necessary to prioritize patients within the same triage category based on the severity of each patient's symptoms.

Trauma care is very stressful. Often, you must deal with patients and families who are upset, angry, belligerent, intoxicated, or frightened; some may speak only a foreign language. Thus, you must work calmly and rationally, employing crisis-intervention techniques. You can help the patient a great deal by talking to they. Be sure to tell they what you're going to do before you touch they. You must also handle difficult situations diplomatically and intelligently, recognize your limitations, and ask for help when you need it.

THE ABCS

Begin your care of an injured patient with a quick primary assessment of the ABCs. Also assess for disability and neurologic status.

To assess airway patency, routinely check for respiratory distress or signs of obstruction, such as stridor, choking, conversational dyspnea, or cyanosis. Be especially alert for respiratory distress in a patient who inhaled chemicals, was in a fire, or has upper body burns. If the airway is obstructed, remove vomitus, dentures, blood clots, or foreign bodies from the mouth.

In a semiconscious or unconscious patient, open the airway using a jaw-thrust maneuver. (Don't use the head-tilt maneuver for a trauma patient. Suspect cervical spine injury until X-rays rule it out.) Then insert an oropharyngeal or nasopharyngeal airway. A nasopharyngeal airway is contraindicated in patients with massive facial trauma and those with possible basal skull fractures. Assist with endotracheal tube insertion as necessary. If rescue personnel have performed an alternate airway insertion, leave it in place until the patient has been tracheally intubated. This will prevent them from vomiting and possibly aspirating.

Next, make sure the patient's breathing is adequate. Look, listen, and feel for respirations. If the patient isn't breathing, call for help immediately, begin bag-valve-mask resuscitation, and prepare for intubation. Give supplemental oxygen; then draw samples for arterial blood gas measurement and calculate the supplemental oxygen's effects to establish a baseline for oxygen and acid–base therapy. Multiple injuries create a need for supplemental oxygen because of blood loss and significant physiologic stress. A conscious multiple-injury patient usually displays compensatory hyperventilation. If the patient doesn't, expect neurologic involvement or chest injury. Needle thoracentesis may be done to decompress tension pneumothorax.

To assess circulation, check for central and peripheral pulses, as well as capillary refill (which should be <2 seconds). If a carotid pulse is absent, institute cardiopulmonary resuscitation (CPR). If external hemorrhage is evident, apply direct pressure to the bleeding site and, if the wound is on a limb, elevate it above heart level if possible. Apply a tourniquet only if the hemorrhage is life threatening.

Monitor the patient's vital signs even if they appear stable. Because vital signs can change rapidly, taking them serially can identify subtle and overt changes. Document baseline readings, and obtain new readings every 5 to 15 minutes until the patient is stable. Assess trends in vital sign readings to detect changes. Place them on a cardiac monitor and a pulse oximeter. Remember that the patient may have from 15% to 30% volume loss before it's reflected in vital sign readings.

Draw blood for type and crossmatch, complete blood count, prothrombin time, partial thromboplastin time, platelet count, and routine blood studies, including amylase and lipase levels. Begin at least two I.V. lines with 14G or 16G catheters for fluid resuscitation with normal saline or lactated Ringer's solution. Administer tetanus prophylaxis as needed. (See *Managing tetanus prophylaxis*.)

Managing tetanus prophylaxis

History of tetanus immunization (number of doses)	Tetanus-prone wounds		Non–tetanus-prone wounds	
	T	TIG**	Tdap*	TIG
Uncertain	Yes	Yes	Yes	No
0 to 1	Yes	Yes	Yes	No
2	Yes	Yes	Yes	No
3 or more	No (*yes* if >5 years since last dose)	No	No (*yes* if >10 years since last dose)	No

*Tetanus, diphtheria, and acellular pertussis, 0.5 mL.
**Tetanus immune globulin (human), 250 units.
Note: When Tdap and TIG are given concurrently, separate syringes and separate sites should be used. For children younger than age 7, tetanus and diphtheria toxoids and pertussis vaccine, adsorbed (DPT) are preferred over tetanus toxoid alone. If pertussis vaccine is contraindicated, administer tetanus and diphtheria toxoids, adsorbed (DT).

Immobilize the patient's head and neck with a rigid cervical collar, supportive blocks, backboard, and tape, if this hasn't been done. Obtain cervical spine X-rays as appropriate and rule out cervical spine injury before moving the patient again. Presume spinal injury and take precautions to prevent further injury, such as logrolling and using adequate staff to move the patient, until spinal injury has been ruled out.

Proceed with assessment of the patient's disability; assess the patient's LOC and pupillary and motor response to check the patient's neurologic status. Attempt to establish the patient's Glasgow Coma Scale rating. Report decorticate or decerebrate responses immediately. The patient need not have a head injury to exhibit an abnormal neurologic response. Any injury that impairs ventilation or perfusion can cause cerebral edema and raise intracranial pressure (ICP).

EXPOSE THE PATIENT FOR SECONDARY ASSESSMENT

Secondary assessment includes removal of the patient's clothes to enable a more thorough examination. The clothing is placed in bags, which are labeled with the patient's name and the date and time they were brought to your facility. The bag will be given to the patient's family or to the authorities if an investigation into the circumstances of the trauma is necessary. If the clothing must be given to the authorities, document having done so. Institute environmental controls by providing warming measures, such as warming blankets and units, warmed oxygen and I.V. solutions, and increased environmental temperature.

Assess the patient's vital signs, and inform the patient's family of status. They can help to provide the history, especially the immunization status. Assess the need for comfort measures; pain medication may be given as appropriate, and other techniques may be used to make the patient comfortable.

Head-to-toe assessment

Secondary assessment also includes a thorough head-to-toe assessment of the patient. Quickly and carefully look for multiple injuries by systematically examining the patient. If you detect no spinal injury, carefully logroll the patient over to inspect the back for other wounds.

In chest trauma, assess for open wounds, tension pneumothorax, hemothorax, cardiac tamponade, bruises and hematomas, flail chest, tracheal deviation, and fractured larynx. Cover open wounds, and apply direct pressure to the wound as necessary. Be ready to assist with insertion of chest tubes, pericardiocentesis, cricothyrotomy, or tracheotomy, as appropriate.

Insert an indwelling urinary catheter and a nasogastric tube, and give prophylactic antibiotics and immunizations, as indicated. Appropriate diagnostic studies—such as X-rays, computed tomography (CT) scans, peritoneal lavage, magnetic resonance imaging (MRI), and excretory urography—may be performed based on assessment findings and patient stabilization. Notify medical or surgical specialists, as appropriate.

STABILIZE THE PATIENT

Because severe injuries commonly lead to shock, check skin temperature, color, and moisture. To control shock, administer I.V. fluids (lactated Ringer's or normal saline solution) followed by blood or blood products.

In all cases of massive external bleeding or suspected internal bleeding, watch for hypovolemia and estimate blood loss. Remember, however, that a blood loss of 500 to 1,000 mL might not change systolic blood pressure but may elevate the pulse rate. However, bradycardia may be an ominous sign and a late finding of hemorrhagic shock. Stay alert for signs of occult bleeding, which commonly occurs in the chest, abdomen, and thigh. Repeat abdominal examinations frequently to assess the patient for abdominal distention; this could be a sign of internal injuries and bleeding.

Increased diameter of the legs or abdomen usually means that blood has leaked into these tissues (as much as 4,000 mL into the abdomen, 3,000 mL into the chest, and 2,000 mL into a thigh). Such blood loss will induce signs of hypovolemic shock (tachycardia, tachypnea, hypotension, restlessness, decreased urine output, delayed capillary refill, and cold, clammy skin).

If the patient has renal injuries or a fractured pelvis, look for the classic sign of retroperitoneal hematoma—numbness or pain in the leg on the affected side as a result of pressure on the lateral femoral cutaneous nerve in L1 to L3. Retroperitoneal bleeding may not cause abdominal tenderness. If the patient shows clinical signs of hypovolemia, immediately begin I.V. therapy with two or more large-bore catheters, and regulate fluids according to the severity of the hypovolemia. Although the initial resuscitation fluids are crystalloids, significant hypovolemia caused by hemorrhage requires blood transfusion. Assist with insertion of a central venous pressure or pulmonary artery catheter to monitor circulating blood volume.

If spinal trauma is suspected, methylprednisolone may be given I.V. If head trauma is present, the patient may be given emergency medication, such as hypertonic saline, and ventilation may be controlled. The patient may also require emergency surgery—either exploratory or lifesaving—to help with stabilization, depending on the injury's type and extent.

Limb fractures can be a source of blood loss. Look for limb fractures and dislocations. Check circulation and neurovascular status distal to the injury by palpating pulses distal to the injury and looking for the classic signs of arterial insufficiency: decreased or absent pulse, pallor, paresthesia, pain, and paralysis. Splint and apply traction as needed.

The patient will require X-rays, a CT scan, or an MRI to determine the extent of injury to the limb, so prepare the patient for transport. Use special care in suspected cervical spinal injury. If necessary, after splinting the injury site, also splint the areas above and below it to prevent further soft-tissue and neurovascular damage and to minimize pain. For example, if the forearm is injured, splint the wrist and elbow, too.

Types of splints include:
◆ *air splint*—an inflatable splint
◆ *hard splint*—a rigid splint with a firm surface, such as a long or short board, an aluminum ladder splint, or a cardboard splint
◆ *soft splint*—a nonrigid splint, such as a pillow or blanket
◆ *traction splint*—a splint that uses traction to decrease angulation and reduce pain.

Tips on applying a splint
◆ Splint most injuries "as they lie," except when the patient's neurovascular status is compromised.
◆ Whenever possible, have one person support the injured part while another applies padding and the splint.
◆ Secure the splint with straps or gauze, *not* an elastic bandage.
◆ To apply an air splint, slide the splint backward over your arm and grasp the distal portion of the injured limb. Then slip the splint from your arm onto the injured limb and inflate the splint. Don't apply the splint too tightly; be sure to assess neurovascular integrity before placing the splint and then after the splint is in place.

SPECIAL CONSIDERATIONS
After the patient is stabilized, he'll need ongoing care and assessment and, possibly, rehabilitation to ensure recovery. Specialists may be consulted for certain types of trauma.

◆ Regularly evaluate the patient's ABCs, as well as the neurologic status.
◆ Keep the patient's family informed about their condition and provide support as indicated.

Depending on the type of injury, the patient may be admitted to your facility or transferred to another facility.

Head
CONCUSSION
By far the most common traumatic brain injury, a concussion results from a blow to the head—a blow hard enough to jostle the brain and make it strike the skull, causing temporary neural dysfunction, but not hard enough to cause a cerebral contusion. Most concussion patients recover completely within 24 to 48 hours. However, as many as 30% of patients who experience a concussion develop postconcussion syndrome (PCS). PCS involves persistent symptoms such as headache, dizziness, blurred vision, memory loss, swings in mood, or sleep disturbances. PCS usually lasts 2 to 4 months postinjury. Repeated concussions exact a cumulative toll on the brain.

Causes and incidence
The blow that causes a concussion is usually sudden and forceful. It occurs when the head strikes a stationary object (as in a fall to the ground) or when a moving object strikes the head (as in a punch to the head). Such blows may also result from automobile crashes, athletic injury, or child abuse. Significant jarring can lead to unconsciousness.

Pathophysiology
A concussion is defined as physiologic injury to the brain tissue without evidence of any actual structural changes. This creates neurometabolic dysfunction within the brain that does not normally appear on CAT scans or MRIs. The metabolic chemical changes that occur cause the signs and symptoms associated with this injury.

Complications
◆ Seizures
◆ Persistent vomiting
◆ Second-impact syndrome

Signs and symptoms
A concussion may produce vomiting and/or a short-term loss of consciousness. The patient may also suffer from anterograde and retrograde amnesia, in which the patient not only can't recall what happened immediately after

the injury but also has difficulty recalling events that led up to the traumatic incident. The presence of anterograde amnesia and the duration of retrograde amnesia reliably correlate with the injury's severity. The length of the unconsciousness may also relate to the concussion's severity.

This type of injury commonly causes adults to be irritable or lethargic, to behave out of character, and to complain of dizziness, nausea, or severe headache. Some children have no apparent ill effects, but many grow lethargic and somnolent in a few hours.

Diagnosis

Differentiating between a concussion and more serious head injuries requires a thorough history of the injury and a neurologic examination. Such an examination must evaluate the patient's LOC, mental status, cranial nerve and motor function, deep tendon reflexes, and orientation to time, place, and person. If no abnormalities are found and if a severe head injury appears unlikely, the patient should be observed for signs of more severe cerebral trauma. Observation provides a baseline for gauging any deterioration in the patient's condition. Whenever you suspect a severe head injury, obtain a CT scan or MRI to rule out fractures and more serious injuries. A neurosurgeon should be consulted immediately.

Treatment

Treatment for concussion varies according to the type of injury. Supportive care may include application of an ice pack to the site of injury, analgesics for mild headache, and sutures or adhesive strips for lacerations.

If the neurologic examination revealed no abnormalities, observe the patient in the emergency department. Check vital signs, LOC, and pupil size every 15 minutes. The patient who remains stable after 4 or more hours of observation can be discharged in the care of a responsible adult.

Special considerations

⚠ ALERT *Before discharge, provide a head injury instruction sheet and advise the patient to be alert for vomiting, worsening of headache, and signs of an ear bleed or cerebrospinal fluid (CSF) leak.*
◆ Instruct the family or caregiver to wake the patient every few hours at night for observation of the mental state and for medication administration. Tell them they should follow these precautions for at least 3 days. Review the head injury instruction sheet and ensure that the family or caregiver is aware of signs necessitating a return to the emergency department.

To avoid second-impact syndrome, it is important for athletes not to return to sports while they are still experiencing signs and symptoms of a concussion. Experiencing a second concussion before the first concussion has resolved may result in a rapid, possibly fatal brain swelling.

CEREBRAL CONTUSION

A cerebral contusion is a bruising of brain tissue as a result of a severe blow to the head. More serious than a concussion, a contusion is usually associated with a closed head injury, disrupts normal nerve function in the bruised area, and may cause loss of consciousness, hemorrhage, edema, and even death.

Causes and incidence

A cerebral contusion results from coup–contrecoup or acceleration–deceleration injuries. Such injuries can occur directly beneath the site of impact when the brain rebounds against the skull from the force of a blow (such as in a beating with a blunt instrument), when the force of the blow drives the brain against the opposite side of the skull, or when the head is hurled forward and stopped abruptly (as in an automobile crash when a driver's head strikes the windshield). The brain continues moving and slaps against the skull (acceleration) and then rebounds (deceleration). These injuries can also cause the brain to strike against bony prominences inside the skull (especially the sphenoidal ridges), causing intracranial hemorrhage or hematoma that may result in tentorial herniation. (See *Hemorrhage, hematoma, and tentorial herniation,* page 924.)

Signs and symptoms

The patient with a cerebral contusion may have severe scalp wounds and labored respirations. The patient may lose consciousness for a few minutes or longer. If conscious, the patient may be drowsy, confused, disoriented, agitated, or even violent. The patient may display hemiparesis, unequal pupillary response, and in late stages may even demonstrate decorticate or decerebrate posturing. Eventually, the patient should return to a relatively alert state, perhaps with temporary aphasia, slight hemiparesis, or unilateral numbness.

Diagnosis

An accurate history of the injury and a neurologic examination are the principal diagnostic tools. A CT scan or MRI shows ischemic tissue, hematomas, and fractures. Intracranial hemorrhage contraindicates lumbar puncture.

Hemorrhage, hematoma, and tentorial herniation

Among the most serious consequences of a head injury are hemorrhage, hematoma, and tentorial herniation. An epidural hematoma results from a rapid accumulation of arterial blood between the skull and the dura mater; a subdural hematoma results from a slow accumulation of venous blood between the dura mater and the subarachnoid membrane. Intracerebral hemorrhage occurs within the cerebrum itself. Tentorial herniation occurs when injured brain tissue swells and squeezes downward through the tentorial notch, constricting the brain stem.

Epidural hemorrhage or hematoma can cause immediate loss of consciousness, followed by a lucid interval lasting minutes to hours, which eventually gives way to a rapidly progressive decrease in the LOC. Other effects are contralateral hemiparesis, progressively severe headache, ipsilateral pupillary dilation, and signs of increased ICP.

With a subacute or chronic subdural hemorrhage or hematoma, blood accumulates slowly, so symptoms may not occur until days after the injury. In an acute subdural hematoma, symptoms appear within 24 hours of the injury. Loss of consciousness occurs, commonly with weakness or paralysis. Intracerebral hemorrhage usually causes nuchal rigidity, photophobia, nausea, vomiting, dizziness, seizures, decreased respiratory rate, and progressive obtundation.

Tentorial herniation causes drowsiness, confusion, dilation of one or both pupils, hyperventilation, nuchal rigidity, bradycardia, and decorticate or decerebrate posturing. Irreversible brain damage or death can occur rapidly.

Intracranial hemorrhage may require a craniotomy to locate and control bleeding and to aspirate blood. Increased ICP may be controlled with I.V. hypertonic saline, steroids, hyperventilation, or induced coma, but emergency surgery is usually required.

Treatment

Treatment of a cerebral contusion focuses on establishing a patent airway and performing regular evaluations of the patient's LOC, motor responses, and ICP. If needed, assist with a tracheotomy or endotracheal intubation. Start an I.V. fluid infusion with lactated Ringer's or normal saline solution. Hypertonic saline I.V. may be given in consultation with a neurosurgeon to reduce cerebral edema.

Special considerations

◆ Verify that a head CT scan has been performed to assess for a basilar skull fracture.
◆ Restrict total fluid intake to 1,200 to 1,500 mL/day to reduce volume and intracerebral swelling.
◆ If spinal injury is ruled out, elevate the bed's head 30 degrees. Enforce bed rest.
◆ If the patient is intubated, use mild hyperventilation until the partial pressure of arterial carbon dioxide reaches 30 to 35 mm Hg.
◆ Type and crossmatch blood for a patient suspected of having an intracerebral hemorrhage. Such a patient may need a blood transfusion, and possibly a craniotomy, to control bleeding and to aspirate blood.
◆ Insert an indwelling urinary catheter as ordered and monitor intake and output. If the patient is unconscious, insert a nasogastric tube to prevent aspiration.

◆ Observe carefully for leakage of CSF from the nostrils and ear canals. If you detect blood in the canal and aren't sure whether CSF is mixed in, place a drop on a white sheet or a piece of filter paper and check for a central spot of blood surrounded by a lighter ring (halo sign). If CSF leakage develops, raise the bed's head 30 degrees. If you detect CSF leaking from the nose, place a gauze pad under the nostrils. Be sure to tell the patient not to blow the nose, but to wipe it instead. If CSF leaks from the ear, position the patient so that the ear drains naturally, and don't pack the ear or nose.
◆ Monitor the patient's vital signs and respirations regularly (usually every 15 minutes). Abnormal respirations could indicate a breakdown in the respiratory center in the brain stem and, possibly, impending tentorial herniation—a critical neurologic emergency.
◆ Check the neurologic status frequently. Assess for restlessness, LOC, pupillary responses, and orientation.
◆ After the patient is stabilized, clean and dress any superficial scalp wounds. (If the skin has been broken, tetanus prophylaxis may be in order.) Assist with suturing if necessary.

FRACTURED SKULL

Because of possible brain damage, a skull fracture is considered a neurosurgical condition. Skull fractures may be classified as simple (closed) or compound (open) and may displace bone fragments. Skull fractures are further described as linear, comminuted, depressed, or diastatic. A linear fracture is a common hairline break, without displacement of structures; a comminuted fracture splinters or crushes the bone into several fragments; a depressed fracture pushes the bone toward the brain; a diastatic fracture causes the skull to separate at the suture (joint between two plates).

In children, the skull's thinness and elasticity allow a depression without a fracture. (A linear fracture across a suture line increases the possibility of epidural hematoma.) Skull fractures are also classified according to location, such as cranial vault fracture and basilar fractures. Because of the danger of grave cranial complications and meningitis, basilar fractures are usually far more serious than cranial vault fractures.

Causes and incidence

Skull fractures invariably result from a traumatic blow to the head. Motor vehicle crashes, falls, sports injuries, and physical assaults top the list of causes. Closed head injuries occur in 200 of every 100,000 patients. About 30% to 75% of blunt head trauma has some form of temporal skull fracture involvement.

Pathophysiology

Skull fractures may be classified as simple (closed) or compound (open) and may displace bone fragments. Skull fractures are further described as linear, comminuted, depressed, or diastatic. A linear fracture is a common hairline break, without displacement of structures; a comminuted fracture splinters or crushes the bone into several fragments; a depressed fracture pushes the bone toward the brain; a diastatic fracture causes the skull to separate at the suture (joint between two plates). The location of the actual fracture may predict other trauma injuries. Temporal bone fractures are often associated with carotid artery injures, whereas fractures of the base of the skull are also seen with injuries to cranial nerves III, IV, V, and VI.

Complications

◆ Infection
◆ Intracerebral hemorrhage
◆ Hematoma
◆ Brain abscess
◆ Increased ICP

Signs and symptoms

Many skull fractures are accompanied by scalp wounds—abrasions, contusions, lacerations, or avulsions. If the scalp has been lacerated or torn away, bleeding may be profuse because the scalp contains many blood vessels. Occasionally, bleeding may be heavy enough to induce hypovolemic shock. The patient may also be in shock from other injuries or from medullary failure in severe head injuries.

Linear fractures that are associated only with concussion don't produce loss of consciousness. They require evaluation, but not definitive treatment. A fracture that results in a cerebral contusion or laceration, however, may cause the classic signs of brain injury: agitation and irritability, loss of consciousness, changes in respiratory pattern (labored respirations), abnormal deep tendon reflexes, and altered pupillary and motor responses.

If the patient with a skull fracture remains conscious, they are apt to complain of a persistent, localized headache. A skull fracture may also result in cerebral edema, which may cause compression of the reticular activating system. This cuts off the normal flow of impulses to the brain and results in possible respiratory distress. The patient may experience alterations in LOC, progressing to unconsciousness or even death.

When jagged bone fragments pierce the dura mater or the cerebral cortex, skull fractures may cause subdural, epidural, or intracerebral hemorrhage or hematoma. With the resulting space-occupying lesions, clinical findings may include hemiparesis, unequal pupils, dizziness, seizures, projectile vomiting, progressive unresponsiveness, and decreased pulse and respiratory rates. Sphenoidal fractures may also damage the optic nerve, causing blindness, whereas temporal fractures may cause unilateral deafness or facial paralysis. Symptoms reflect the head injury's severity and extent. However, some elderly patients may have cortical brain atrophy, with more space for brain swelling under the cranium, and consequently may not show signs of increased ICP until it's very high.

Vault fractures commonly produce soft-tissue swelling near the fracture, making it difficult to detect without a CT scan.

Basilar fractures commonly produce a hemorrhage from the nose, pharynx, or ears; blood under the periorbital skin (raccoon eyes) and under the conjunctiva; and Battle's sign (supramastoid ecchymosis), sometimes with bleeding behind the eardrum (hemotympanum). This type of fracture may also cause CSF or even brain tissue to leak from the nose or ears.

Depending on the extent of brain damage, the patient with a skull fracture may suffer residual effects, such as seizures, hydrocephalus, and organic brain syndrome. Children may develop headaches, giddiness, easy fatigability, neuroses, and behavior disorders.

Diagnosis

Suspect brain injury in all patients with a skull fracture until clinical evaluation proves otherwise. Consequently, you'll need to obtain a thorough injury history and MRI or a CT scan (to locate the fracture) for every suspected skull injury. (Keep in mind that many vault fractures aren't visible or palpable.)

A fracture also requires a neurologic examination to check cerebral function (mental status and orientation to time, place, and person), LOC, pupillary response, motor function, and deep tendon reflexes.

Brain damage can be assessed by a CT scan and MRI, which reveal intracranial hemorrhage from ruptured blood vessels and swelling. Expanding lesions contraindicate a lumbar puncture.

Treatment

Although occasionally even a simple linear skull fracture can tear an underlying blood vessel or cause a CSF leak, linear fractures generally require only supportive treatment, including mild analgesics such as acetaminophen, and cleaning, debridement, and repair of any wounds after injection of a local anesthetic.

If the patient with a skull fracture hasn't lost consciousness, observe they in the emergency department for at least 4 hours. Following this observation period, if the vital signs are stable and if the neurosurgeon concurs, you can discharge them. Before discharge, give the patient an instruction sheet to follow for 24 to 48 hours of observation at home.

More severe vault fractures, especially depressed fractures, usually require a craniotomy to elevate or remove fragments that have been driven into the brain and to extract foreign bodies and necrotic tissue. This reduces the risk of infection and further brain damage. Other treatments for severe vault fractures include antibiotic therapy and, in profound hemorrhage, blood transfusions.

Currently evidence-based practice does not support the routine use of prophylactic antibiotics with basilar fractures. Close observation should be used for CSF leakage, secondary hematomas, and hemorrhages. Surgery may be necessary.

Special considerations

♦ Establish and maintain a patent airway; nasal airways are contraindicated in patients who may have a basilar skull fracture. Intubation may be necessary. Suction the patient through the mouth, not the nose, to prevent introducing bacteria if a CSF leak is present.

♦ Be sure to obtain a complete history of the traumatic injury from the patient, family members, any eyewitnesses, and emergency medical services personnel. Ask whether the patient lost consciousness and, if so, for how long.

♦ Assist with diagnostic tests, including a complete neurologic examination, CT scan, and other studies.

♦ Check for abnormal reflexes such as Babinski reflex, or lack of gag and cough.

♦ Look for CSF draining from the patient's ears, nose, or mouth. Check pillowcases and linens for CSF leaks and look for a halo sign. If the patient's nose is draining CSF, wipe it—*don't let them blow it*. If an ear is draining, cover it lightly with sterile gauze—*don't pack it*.

♦ Position the patient with a head injury so that secretions can drain properly. Elevate the bed's head 30 degrees if intracerebral injury is suspected.

♦ Cover scalp wounds carefully with a sterile dressing; control any bleeding as necessary.

♦ Take seizure precautions, but don't restrain the patient. Agitated behavior may be due to hypoxia or increased ICP, so check for these symptoms. Speak in a calm, reassuring voice, and touch the patient gently. Don't make any sudden, unexpected moves.

♦ Don't give the patient opioids or sedatives prior to evaluation by neurosurgery because they may depress respirations, increase carbon dioxide levels, lead to increased ICP, and mask changes in neurologic status. Give acetaminophen or another mild analgesic for pain as ordered.

If a skull fracture requires surgery, proceed as follows:

♦ Obtain consent, as needed, to shave the patient's head. Explain that you're performing this procedure to provide a clean area for surgery. Type and crossmatch blood. Obtain baseline laboratory studies, such as a complete blood count, serum electrolyte studies, prothrombin time, partial thromboplastin time, and urinalysis.

♦ After surgery, monitor the patient's vital signs and neurologic status frequently (usually every 5 minutes until the patient is stable and then every 15 minutes for 1 hour), and note any changes in LOC. Because skull fractures and brain injuries heal slowly, don't expect dramatic postoperative improvement.

♦ Monitor intake and output frequently, and maintain the patency of the indwelling urinary catheter. Monitor fluid intake carefully. Because hypotonic fluids (such as dextrose 5% in water) can increase cerebral edema, give fluids only as indicated.

◆ If the patient is unconscious, provide parenteral nutrition. (Remember, the patient may regurgitate and aspirate food if you use a nasogastric tube for feedings.)

If the fracture doesn't require surgery, proceed as follows:

◆ Wear sterile gloves to examine the scalp laceration. With your finger, probe the wound for foreign bodies and a palpable fracture. Gently clean lacerations and the surrounding area; cover them with sterile gauze. The wound should be sutured if necessary.

◆ Provide emotional support for the patient and family. Explain the need for procedures to reduce the risk of brain injury.

◆ Before discharge, instruct the patient's family to watch closely for changes in mental status, LOC, or respirations and to give the patient acetaminophen for a headache. Tell them to return to the hospital immediately if the LOC decreases, if the headache persists after several doses of mild analgesics, if the patient vomits more than once, or if they develop weakness in the arms or legs.

◆ Teach the patient and family how to care for the scalp wound. Emphasize the need to return for suture removal and follow-up evaluation.

FRACTURED NOSE

The most common facial fracture, a fractured nose usually results from blunt injury and may be associated with other facial fractures. The fracture's severity depends on the direction, force, and type of the blow. A severe, comminuted fracture may cause extreme swelling or bleeding that may partially obstruct the airway. Inadequate or delayed treatment may cause permanent nasal displacement, septal deviation, and obstruction.

Causes and incidence

Nasal bone fractures usually result from direct trauma. The causative injury may be relatively minor, such as a fall, or more severe, such as a car crash.

Pathophysiology

The most common facial fracture, a fractured nose usually results from blunt injury and may be associated with other facial fractures. The fracture's severity depends on the direction, force, and type of the blow. The majority of nasal fractures involve the septum, which could create problems in reducing the fracture. Determining if there is a septal hematoma early in the injury process is key to a successful recovery.

Complications

◆ Deviated septum
◆ Airway obstruction
◆ Septal hematoma
◆ CSF leakage
◆ Intracranial air penetration

Signs and symptoms

Immediately after injury, a nosebleed may occur, and soft-tissue swelling may quickly obscure the break. Nasal fractures may cause significant blood loss. After several hours, pain, edema, periorbital ecchymoses, and nasal displacement and deformity are prominent. Possible complications include septal hematoma, which may lead to abscess formation, resulting in avascular septal necrosis and saddle nose deformity.

Diagnosis

℞ **CONFIRMING DIAGNOSIS** *Palpation, X-rays, and clinical findings such as a deviated septum confirm a nasal fracture.*

Diagnosis also requires a complete patient history, including the injury's cause and the amount of nasal bleeding. Watch for clear fluid drainage, which may suggest a CSF leak and a basilar skull fracture. If facial or mandibular fractures are suspected, a CT scan is necessary.

Treatment

Treatment restores normal facial appearance and re-establishes bilateral nasal passage after swelling subsides. Reduction of the fracture corrects alignment; immobilization (intranasal packing and an external splint shaped to the nose and taped) maintains it. Reduction is best accomplished in the operating room under local anesthesia for adults and general anesthesia for children. Severe swelling may delay treatment. CSF leakage calls for close observation, a CT scan of the basilar skull, and antibiotic therapy; septal hematoma requires incision and drainage to prevent necrosis.

Start treatment immediately. While waiting for X-rays, apply ice packs to the nose to minimize swelling. Wrap the ice packs in a light towel to prevent ice from directly contacting the skin. To control anterior bleeding, gently apply local pressure. Posterior bleeding is rare and requires an internal tamponade applied in the emergency department.

Special considerations

◆ Because the patient will find breathing more difficult as swelling increases, instruct the patient to breathe slowly through the mouth. To warm the inhaled air during cold weather, tell the patient to cover their mouth with a handkerchief or scarf. To prevent subcutaneous emphysema or intracranial air penetration (and potential meningitis), warn the patient not to blow their nose.

◆ After packing and splinting, apply ice in a plastic bag.

◆ Before discharge, tell the patient that ecchymoses should fade after about 2 weeks.

DISLOCATED OR FRACTURED JAW

Dislocation of the jaw is a displacement of the temporomandibular joint. A jaw fracture is a break in one or both of the two maxillae (upper jawbones) or the mandible (lower jawbone). Treatment can usually restore jaw alignment and function.

Causes and incidence

Simple fractures or dislocations are usually caused by a manual blow along the jawline. Other causes of serious compound fractures include industrial accidents, recreational or sports injuries, assaults, and other trauma. Recurrence of a dislocated jaw is common.

Pathophysiology

Fractures of the jaw are the most common type of maxillofacial fracture. These fractures result from mechanical overload of forces to the mandible.

Complications

◆ Infection
◆ Sublingual hematoma
◆ Trauma to nerves of jaw and face

Signs and symptoms

Malocclusion is the most obvious sign of a dislocation or fracture. Other signs include mandibular pain, swelling, ecchymosis, loss of function, and asymmetry. In addition, mandibular fractures that damage the alveolar nerve produce paresthesia or anesthesia of the chin and lower lip. Maxillary fractures produce infraorbital paresthesia and commonly accompany fractures of the nasal and orbital complex.

Diagnosis

📖 CONFIRMING DIAGNOSIS *Abnormal maxillary or mandibular mobility during the physical examination and a history of traumatic injury suggest a fracture or dislocation; X-rays confirm it.*

Treatment

As in all traumatic injuries, check first for a patent airway, adequate ventilation, and pulses; then control hemorrhage and check for other injuries. As necessary, maintain a patent airway

with an oropharyngeal airway, nasotracheal intubation, or a cricothyrotomy. Relieve pain with analgesics as needed.

After the patient stabilizes, surgical reduction and fixation by wiring restores mandibular and maxillary alignment. Maxillary fractures may also require reconstruction and repair of soft-tissue injuries. Teeth and bones are never removed during surgery unless unavoidable. If the patient has lost teeth from trauma, the surgeon will decide whether they can be reimplanted. If they can, he'll reimplant them within 6 hours, while they're still viable. Viability is increased if the tooth is placed in milk, saliva, or normal saline solution. Dislocations are usually reduced manually under anesthesia.

Special considerations

After reconstructive surgery, perform the following:

◆ Position the patient on one side with the head slightly elevated. The patient will usually have a nasogastric tube in place, with low suction to remove gastric contents and prevent nausea, vomiting, and aspiration of vomitus. As necessary, suction the nasopharynx through the nose or by pulling the cheek away from the teeth and inserting a small suction catheter through any natural gap between teeth.

◆ If the patient isn't intubated, provide nourishment through a straw. After the patient can tolerate clear liquids, offer milkshakes, broth, juices, pureed foods, and nutritional supplements.

◆ If the patient can't tolerate oral fluids, I.V. therapy can maintain hydration postoperatively.

◆ Administer antiemetics as indicated to minimize nausea and prevent aspiration of vomitus (a real danger in a patient whose jaw is wired). Keep a pair of wire cutters at the bedside to snip the wires should the patient vomit.

◆ A dental water-pulsator may be used for mouth care while the wires are intact.

◆ Because the patient will have difficulty talking while the jaw is wired, provide a Magic Slate or pencil and paper and suggest appropriate diversionary activities.

PERFORATED EARDRUM

Perforation of the eardrum is a rupture of the tympanic membrane that may cause otitis media and hearing loss.

Causes and incidence

The usual cause of perforated eardrum is trauma, such as the deliberate or accidental insertion of foreign objects (cotton swabs or bobby pins) or sudden excessive changes in pressure (explosion, a blow to the head, flying, or diving). The injury may also result from untreated otitis media and, in children, from acute otitis media.

Complications
◆ Mastoiditis
◆ Meningitis
◆ Otitis media
◆ Permanent hearing loss

Pathophysiology
Perforation of the ear drum may result from mechanical, such as an instrument, or blast injuries such as the force of an explosion that cause a disruption in the integrity of the tympanic membrane.

Signs and symptoms
Sudden onset of a severe earache and bleeding, clear drainage, or drainage of pus from the ear are the first signs of a perforated eardrum. Other symptoms include hearing loss, tinnitus, and vertigo. Purulent otorrhea within 24 to 48 hours of injury signals infection.

Diagnosis
⚠ ALERT *A severe earache and bleeding from the ear with a history of trauma strongly suggest a perforated eardrum; direct visualization of the perforated tympanic membrane with an otoscope confirms it.*

Additional diagnostic measures include audiometric testing and a check of voluntary facial movements to rule out facial nerve damage.

Treatment
If you detect bleeding from the ear, use a sterile, cotton-tipped applicator to absorb the blood, and check for purulent drainage or evidence of CSF leakage. A culture of the specimen may be appropriate.

⚠ ALERT *Irrigation of the ear is absolutely contraindicated in a patient with perforation of the eardrum.*

Apply a sterile dressing over the outer ear, and refer the patient to an ear specialist. A large perforation with uncontrolled bleeding may require immediate surgery to approximate the ruptured edges. Other measures may include administration of a mild analgesic, a sedative to decrease anxiety, and an oral antibiotic.

Special considerations
◆ Before discharge, tell the patient not to blow the nose or get water in the ear canal until the perforation heals.
◆ Advise the patient to follow up with an ear specialist, as appropriate.
◆ Instruct the patient and the family to notify the physician if developing signs of infection,

such as fever, increasing discomfort, and continued or purulent drainage.
◆ Inform the authorities if child abuse is suspected as the cause of injuries.

Neck and spine

ACCELERATION–DECELERATION CERVICAL INJURIES
Acceleration–deceleration cervical injuries (commonly known as *whiplash*) result from sharp hyperextension and flexion of the neck that damages soft tissues, muscles, and ligaments. The prognosis for this type of injury is excellent; symptoms are usually self-limiting and subside with treatment.

Causes and incidence
Whiplash commonly results from rear-end automobile crashes. A seat belt keeps a person's body from being thrown forward, but the head may snap forward, then backward, causing a whiplash injury to the neck. Other causes include roller coasters or other amusement park rides, sports injuries, or punches or shoves.

Signs and symptoms
Although symptoms may develop immediately, they're often delayed 12 to 24 hours if the injury is mild. Whiplash produces moderate-to-severe anterior and posterior neck pain. Within several days, the anterior pain diminishes, but the posterior pain persists or even intensifies, causing patients to seek medical attention if they didn't do so before. Whiplash may also cause dizziness, gait disturbances, vomiting, headache, nuchal rigidity, neck muscle asymmetry, and rigidity or numbness in the arms.

Diagnosis
Full cervical spine X-rays are required to rule out cervical fractures. If the X-rays are negative, the physical examination focuses on motor ability and sensation below the cervical spine to detect signs of nerve root compression. If the patient's cervical spine continues to be tender to examination, MRI or CT scan may be required to rule out ligamentous injury.

Treatment
Treatment aims to control symptoms and includes:
◆ a mild analgesic—such as aspirin with codeine or ibuprofen—and possibly a muscle relaxant—such as diazepam, cyclobenzaprine, or chlorzoxazone with acetaminophen
◆ ice or cool compresses to the neck to relieve pain

♦ immobilization with a soft, padded cervical collar for several days or weeks
♦ in severe muscle spasms, short-term cervical traction

Most whiplash patients are discharged immediately.

Special considerations

⚠ **ALERT** *In all suspected spinal injuries, assume that the spine is injured until proven otherwise. Until an X-ray rules out a cervical fracture, move the patient as little as possible. Before the X-ray is taken, remove any ear and neck jewelry carefully. Don't undress the patient; cut clothes away if necessary. Caution them to avoid making movements that could injure the spine.*

♦ Teach the patient to watch for possible adverse drug effects; to avoid alcohol if he's taking diazepam, opioids, or muscle relaxants; and to rest for a few days and avoid lifting heavy objects.
♦ Instruct the patient to return to the hospital immediately if experiencing persistent pain or develops numbness, tingling, or weakness on one or both sides.

SPINAL INJURIES

Spinal injuries (without cord damage) include fractures, contusions, and compressions of the vertebral column, usually as a result of head or neck trauma. The real danger lies in possible spinal cord damage. Spinal fractures most commonly occur in the 5th, 6th, and 7th cervical, 12th thoracic, and 1st lumbar vertebrae.

Causes and incidence

Most serious spinal injuries result from motor vehicle crashes, falls, dives into shallow water, and gunshot wounds. Less serious injuries result from heavy object lifting and minor falls. Spinal dysfunction may also result from hyperparathyroidism, neoplastic lesions, and osteoporosis.

Spinal cord injuries occur in 12,000 to 15,000 people per year in the United States. About 10,000 of these injuries cause permanent paralysis; many other patients die as a result of these injuries. The average age at injury has changed from 29 years in the mid-1970s to 42 years in 2015; 82% are male.

Pathophysiology

The primary injury is due to the actual force applied to the bones of the spine, causing compression of the spine from bone fragments, bullet casings, or other objects. The secondary injuries are caused by edema and swelling in the area. This creates chemical changes in the electrical pattern of the neurons, leading to spinal cord shock.

Complications

♦ Spinal cord injury
♦ Autonomic dysreflexia
♦ Spinal shock
♦ Neurogenic shock

Signs and symptoms

The most obvious symptoms of spinal injury are muscle spasm and back pain that worsen with movement. In cervical fractures, pain may produce point tenderness; in dorsal and lumbar fractures, it may radiate to other body areas such as the legs. After mild injuries, symptoms may be delayed for several days or weeks. If the injury damages the spinal cord, clinical effects range from mild paresthesia to quadriplegia and shock.

Diagnosis

The diagnosis is typically based on the patient's history, physical examination, X-rays, CT scan, and MRI.

The patient history may reveal a traumatic injury, a metastatic lesion, an infection that could produce a spinal abscess, or an endocrine disorder. The physical examination (including a neurologic evaluation) locates the level of injury and detects cord damage.

Spinal X-rays, the most important diagnostic measure, locate the fracture. In spinal compression, a lumbar puncture may show increased CSF pressure from a lesion or trauma; a CT scan or MRI can locate a spinal mass.

Treatment

The primary treatment after a spinal injury is immediate immobilization to stabilize the spine and prevent cord damage; other measures are supportive. Cervical injuries require immobilization, using a type of cervical immobilization device (CID) on both sides of the patient's head, a hard cervical collar, or skeletal traction with skull tongs or a halo device.

Treatment of stable lumbar and dorsal fractures consists of bed rest on firm support (such as a bed board), analgesics, and muscle relaxants until the fracture stabilizes (usually in 10 to 12 weeks). Later measures include exercises to strengthen the back muscles and use of a back brace or other device to provide support when walking.

An unstable dorsal or lumbar fracture requires a plaster cast, a turning frame, and, in severe fracture, a laminectomy and spinal fusion.

When the spinal injury results in compression of the spinal column, neurosurgery may relieve the pressure. If the cause of compression is a metastatic lesion, chemotherapy and radiation may relieve it. Surface wounds accompanying the spinal injury require tetanus prophylaxis unless the patient has been immunized recently.

Special considerations

In all spinal injuries, suspect cord damage until proven otherwise.

◆ During the initial assessment and X-ray studies, immobilize the patient on a firm surface with CID. Tell them not to move, and avoid moving the patient yourself because hyperflexion can damage the cord. If you must move the patient, get at least three other members of the staff to help you logroll the patient to avoid disturbing body alignment.

◆ Throughout assessment, offer comfort and reassurance. Remember, the fear of possible paralysis will be overwhelming. Talk to the patient quietly and calmly. Allow a family member who isn't too distraught to accompany them.

◆ If the injury requires surgery, administer prophylactic antibiotics as ordered. Catheterize the patient as ordered to avoid urine retention, and monitor bowel elimination patterns to avoid impaction.

◆ Explain traction methods to the patient and family. Reassure them that traction devices don't penetrate the brain. If the patient has a halo or skull-tong traction device, clean pin sites daily, trim hair short, and provide analgesics for persistent headaches. During traction, turn the patient often to prevent pneumonia, embolism, and skin breakdown; perform passive range-of-motion exercises to maintain muscle tone. If available, use a CircOlectric bed or Stryker frame to facilitate turning and to avoid spinal cord injury.

◆ Turn the patient on the side during feedings to prevent aspiration. Create a relaxed atmosphere at mealtimes.

◆ Suggest appropriate diversionary activities to fill the patient's hours of immobility.

◆ Watch closely for neurologic changes. Immediately report changes in skin sensation and loss of muscle strength—either of which might indicate pressure on the spinal cord, possibly as a result of edema or shifting bone fragments.

◆ Help the patient walk as soon as the physician allows; he'll probably need to wear a back brace.

◆ Before discharge, instruct the patient about continuing analgesics or other medication, and stress the importance of regular follow-up examinations.

◆ To help prevent a spinal injury from becoming a spinal cord injury, educate firemen, policemen, paramedics, and the general public about the proper way to handle such injuries.

Thorax

BLUNT CHEST INJURIES

Chest injuries, including blunt chest injuries, consist of myocardial contusion as well as rib and sternal fractures that may be simple, multiple, displaced, or jagged. Such fractures may cause potentially fatal complications, such as hemothorax, pneumothorax, hemorrhagic shock, and diaphragmatic rupture.

Causes and incidence

Motor vehicle crashes cause two thirds of major chest injuries in the United States. Other common causes include sports and blast injuries and CPR. About 50% of these injuries affect the chest wall; 80% of those with significant blunt chest trauma also have extrathoracic injuries.

Chest and thoracic injuries account for 70% of all trauma-related deaths in the United States.

Pathophysiology

Injuries to the lung tissue frequently occur, decreasing oxygenation by increasing dead space and alveolar shunting. When blood or air occupy space in the chest cavity, blood returning to the heart and lungs are compromised. Also, inflammatory mediators are released that depress myocardial contractility, further exacerbating cardiac output.

Complications

◆ Hemothorax
◆ Hemorrhagic shock
◆ Pneumothorax
◆ Tension pneumothorax
◆ Diaphragmatic rupture
◆ Liver laceration
◆ Myocardial tears
◆ Cardiac tamponade
◆ Pulmonary artery tears
◆ Ventricular rupture
◆ Rupture of the aorta
◆ Bronchial, tracheal, or esophageal tears

Signs and symptoms

Rib fractures produce tenderness, slight edema over the fracture site, and pain that worsens with deep breathing and movement; this painful breathing causes the patient to display shallow, splinted respirations that may lead to hypoventilation. Sternal fractures, which are usually transverse and located in the middle or upper sternum, produce persistent chest pains, even at rest. If a fractured rib tears the pleura and punctures a lung, it causes pneumothorax. This usually produces severe dyspnea, cyanosis, agitation, extreme pain, and, when air escapes into chest tissue, subcutaneous emphysema.

Multiple rib fractures within two or more places may cause flail chest, in which a portion of the rib cage becomes unstable, causing a loss of chest wall integrity and preventing adequate lung inflation. (See *Flail chest: Paradoxical breathing,* page 932.)

Flail chest: Paradoxical breathing

A patient with a blunt chest injury may develop flail chest, in which a portion of the ribcage becomes unstable. This results in paradoxical breathing, described below.

Inhalation
♦ Injured chest wall collapses in.
♦ Uninjured chest wall moves out.

Exhalation
♦ Injured chest wall moves out.
♦ Uninjured chest wall moves in.

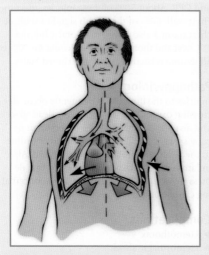
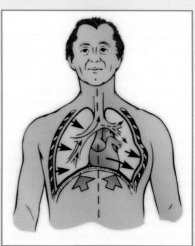

Signs and symptoms of flail chest include bruised skin, extreme pain caused by rib fracture and disfigurement, paradoxical chest movements, tachycardia, hypotension, respiratory acidosis, cyanosis, and rapid, shallow respirations. If the pleural lining is cut by the end of a fractured rib, flail chest can also cause tension pneumothorax; a condition in which air enters the chest but can't be ejected during exhalation. This life-threatening thoracic pressure buildup causes lung collapse and subsequent mediastinal shift. The cardinal symptoms of tension pneumothorax include severe dyspnea, absent breath sounds (on the affected side), agitation, jugular vein distention, tracheal deviation (away from the affected side), cyanosis, and shock.

Hemothorax occurs when a rib lacerates lung tissue or an intercostal artery, causing blood to collect in the pleural cavity, thereby compressing the lung and limiting respiratory capacity. It can also result from rupture of large or small pulmonary vessels.

Massive hemothorax is the most common cause of shock after a chest injury. Although slight bleeding occurs even with mild pneumothorax, such bleeding resolves very quickly, usually without changing the patient's condition. Rib fractures may also cause pulmonary contusion (resulting in hemoptysis, hypoxia, dyspnea, and possible obstruction), large myocardial tears (which can be rapidly fatal), and small myocardial tears (which can cause pericardial effusion).

Myocardial contusions—actual bruising of the heart muscle—produce electrocardiographic (ECG) abnormalities. Laceration or rupture of the aorta is almost always immediately fatal. Because aortic laceration may develop 24 hours after blunt injury, patient observation is critical. Diaphragmatic rupture (usually on the left side) causes severe respiratory distress. Unless treated early, abdominal viscera may herniate through the rupture into the thorax (with resulting bowel sounds in the chest), compromising both circulation and the lungs' vital capacity.

Other complications of blunt chest trauma may include cardiac tamponade, pulmonary artery tears, ventricular rupture, and bronchial, tracheal, or esophageal tears or rupture.

Diagnosis

A history of trauma with dyspnea, chest pain, and other typical clinical features suggest a blunt chest injury. To determine its extent, a physical examination and diagnostic tests are needed.

◆ In hemothorax, percussion reveals dullness. In tension pneumothorax, it reveals tympany. In a late case, auscultation may reveal a change in position of the loudest heart sound.

◆ Chest X-rays may confirm rib and sternal fractures, pneumothorax, flail chest, pulmonary contusions, lacerated or ruptured aorta, tension pneumothorax, diaphragmatic rupture, lung compression, or atelectasis with hemothorax.

◆ With cardiac damage, the ECG may show abnormalities, including unexplained tachycardias, atrial fibrillation, bundle-branch block (usually right), ST-segment changes, and ventricular arrhythmias such as multiple premature ventricular contractions.

◆ Serial aspartate aminotransferase, alanine aminotransferase, lactate dehydrogenase, creatine kinase (CK), and CK-MB levels are elevated. However, cardiac enzymes fail to detect up to 50% of patients with myocardial damage.

◆ Retrograde aortography, CT angiography, and transesophageal echocardiography reveal aortic laceration or rupture.

◆ Contrast studies and liver and spleen scans detect diaphragmatic rupture.

◆ Echocardiography, CT scans, and cardiac and lung scans show the injury's extent.

Treatment

Blunt chest injuries call for immediate physical assessment, control of bleeding, maintenance of a patent airway, adequate ventilation, and fluid and electrolyte balance.

Special considerations

◆ Check all pulses and LOC. Evaluate skin color and temperature, depth of respiration, use of accessory muscles, and length of inhalation compared to exhalation.

◆ Check pulse oximetry values for adequate oxygenation.

◆ Observe tracheal position. Look for distended jugular veins and paradoxical chest motion. Listen to heart and breath sounds carefully; palpate for subcutaneous emphysema (crepitation) or a lack of structural integrity of the ribs.

◆ Obtain a history of the injury. Unless severe dyspnea is present, have the patient locate the pain, and ask if he's having trouble breathing. Obtain laboratory studies (arterial blood gas analysis, cardiac enzyme studies, complete blood count, type, and crossmatch).

◆ For simple rib fractures, have the patient cough and breathe deeply to mobilize secretions while splinting to decrease pain. Give adequate analgesics, encourage bed rest, and apply heat. Don't strap or tape the chest.

◆ More severe fractures may require administration of intercostal nerve blocks. (Obtain X-rays before and after the nerve blocks to rule out pneumothorax.) Intubate the patient with excessive bleeding or hemopneumothorax. Chest tubes may be inserted to treat hemothorax and to assess the need for thoracotomy. To prevent atelectasis, turn the patient frequently and encourage coughing and deep-breathing exercises.

◆ Pneumothorax may require placement of a chest tube anterior to the midaxillary line at the fourth intercostal space to aspirate as much air as possible from the pleural cavity and to re-expand the lungs.

◆ For flail chest, place the patient in semi-Fowler's position. Re-expanding the lung is the first definitive care measure. Administer oxygen at a high flow rate under positive pressure. Suction the patient frequently, as completely as possible. Maintain acid–base balance. Observe carefully for signs of tension pneumothorax. Start I.V. therapy, using lactated Ringer's or normal saline solution. Beware of both excessive and insufficient fluid resuscitation.

⚠ ALERT *For hemothorax, treat shock with I.V. infusions of lactated Ringer's or normal saline solution. Administer packed red blood cells for blood losses greater than 1,500 mL or circulating blood volume losses exceeding 30%. Administer oxygen. The patient may need insertion of chest tubes in the fourth intercostal space anterior to the midaxillary line to remove blood. Monitor and document vital signs and blood loss. Watch for and respond immediately to falling blood pressure, rising pulse rate, and hemorrhage— all require a thoracotomy to stop bleeding.*

◆ For a pulmonary contusion, give limited amounts of colloids (such as albumin, whole blood, or plasma) as appropriate to replace volume and maintain oncotic pressure. Give analgesics as necessary. Monitor blood gas levels to ensure adequate ventilation; provide oxygen therapy, mechanical ventilation, and chest tube care.

◆ For suspected cardiac damage, close intensive care or telemetry may detect arrhythmias and prevent cardiogenic shock. Impose bed rest in semi-Fowler's position (unless the patient requires shock position); administer oxygen, analgesics, and supportive drugs to control heart failure or supraventricular arrhythmias as needed. Watch for cardiac tamponade, which calls for pericardiocentesis. (Provide essentially the same care as you would for a patient with a myocardial infarction.)

⚠ ALERT *For myocardial rupture, septal perforation, and other cardiac lacerations, immediate surgical repair is mandatory. Less severe ventricular wounds require use of a digital or balloon catheter; atrial wounds require a clamp or balloon catheter.*

⚠ ALERT *For patients with aortic rupture or laceration, immediate surgery is mandatory, using synthetic grafts or anastomosis to repair the damage. Give large volumes of I.V. fluids (lactated Ringer's or normal saline solution) and whole blood, along with oxygen at very high flow rates; then transport the patient promptly to the operating room.*

⚠ ALERT *For tension pneumothorax, the patient may need insertion of a 14G to 16G angiocatheter in the second intercostal space at the midclavicular line to release pressure in the chest. After this, insert a chest tube to normalize pressure and re-expand the lung. Administer oxygen under positive pressure along with I.V. fluids.*

◆ For a diaphragmatic rupture, insert a nasogastric tube to temporarily decompress the stomach, and prepare the patient for surgical repair.

PENETRATING CHEST WOUNDS

Depending on their size, penetrating chest wounds may cause varying degrees of damage to bones, soft tissue, blood vessels, and nerves. Mortality and morbidity from such wounds depend on the wound's size and severity. Gunshot wounds are usually more serious than stab wounds because they cause more severe wounds with rapid blood loss. Ricochet within a gunshot wound commonly damages large areas and multiple organs. Despite prompt, aggressive treatment, up to 90% of patients with penetrating chest wounds die.

Causes and incidence

Stab wounds from a knife or an ice pick are the most common penetrating chest wounds; gunshot wounds are a close second. Wartime explosions or firearms fired at close range are the usual sources of large, gaping wounds.

Penetrating chest injuries cause one in every four deaths in the United States. Many patients with this type of injury die after reaching the hospital.

Pathophysiology

Penetrating chest wounds are caused by such things as stab wounds, gunshot wounds, explosions, and other sharp forces to the chest. There is a disruption in vasculature in the upper neck, the diaphragm, and organs situated high in the abdominal compartment.

Complications
◆ Arrhythmias
◆ Cardiac tamponade
◆ Mediastinitis
◆ Subcutaneous emphysema

◆ Bronchopleural fistula
◆ Myocardial rupture
◆ Pneumothorax
◆ Rib and sternal fractures
◆ Shock
◆ Tears and lacerations of the tracheobronchial tree

Signs and symptoms

In addition to the obvious chest injuries, penetrating chest wounds can also cause:
◆ a sucking sound as the diaphragm contracts and air enters the chest cavity through the opening in the chest wall
◆ tachycardia because of anxiety and blood loss
◆ weak, thready pulse because of massive blood loss and hypovolemic shock
◆ varying levels of consciousness, depending on the injury's extent. If the patient is awake and alert, the severe pain may cause them to splint respirations, thereby reducing the vital capacity

Penetrating chest wounds may also cause lung lacerations (bleeding and substantial air leakage through the chest wall), arterial lacerations (loss of >100 mL blood/hour through the chest tube), exsanguination, pneumothorax (air in pleural space causes loss of negative intrathoracic pressure and lung collapse), tension pneumothorax (intrapleural air accumulation causes potentially fatal mediastinal shift), and hemothorax. Other effects may include arrhythmias, cardiac tamponade, mediastinitis, subcutaneous emphysema, esophageal perforation, bronchopleural fistula, and tracheobronchial, abdominal, or diaphragmatic injuries.

Diagnosis

℞ CONFIRMING DIAGNOSIS *An obvious chest wound and a sucking sound during breathing confirm the diagnosis of a penetrating chest wound. Consider any lower thoracic chest injury a thoracoabdominal injury until proven otherwise.*

Baseline tests include:
◆ pulse oximetry and arterial blood gas analysis to assess respiratory status
◆ chest X-rays before and after chest tube placement to evaluate the injury and tube placement (However, in an emergency, don't wait for chest X-ray results before inserting the chest tube.)
◆ complete blood count, including hemoglobin (Hb) level, hematocrit (HCT), and differential (Low Hb level and HCT reflect severe blood loss; in early blood loss, these values may be normal.)
◆ palpation and auscultation of the chest and abdomen to evaluate damage to adjacent organs and structures

Treatment

Penetrating chest wounds require immediate support of respiration and circulation, prompt surgical repair, and measures to prevent complications.

Special considerations

◆ Immediately assess ABCs. Establish a patent airway, support ventilation, and monitor pulses frequently.

◆ Place an occlusive dressing over the sucking wound. Watch for signs of tension pneumothorax (respiratory distress, tachycardia, tachypnea, and diminished or absent breath sounds on the affected side [tracheal shift]); if tension pneumothorax develops, temporarily remove the occlusive dressing to create a simple pneumothorax.

◆ Control blood loss (remember to look *under* the patient to estimate loss), type and crossmatch blood, and replace blood and fluids as necessary.

◆ Assist with chest X-ray and placement of chest tubes (using water-seal drainage) to re-establish intrathoracic pressure and to drain blood in a hemothorax. A second X-ray will evaluate the position of tubes and their function.

◆ Emergency surgery may be needed to repair the damage caused by the wound.

◆ Throughout treatment, monitor central venous pressure and blood pressure to detect hypovolemia, and assess vital signs. Provide analgesics as appropriate. Tetanus and antibiotic prophylaxis may be necessary.

◆ Reassure the patient. Report the incident to the police in accordance with local laws. Help contact the patient's family and offer them reassurance as well.

Abdomen

BLUNT AND PENETRATING ABDOMINAL INJURIES

Blunt and penetrating abdominal injuries may damage major blood vessels and internal organs. Their most immediate life-threatening consequences are hemorrhage and hypovolemic shock; later threats include infection. The prognosis depends on the extent of the injury and the specific organs damaged, but it's usually improved by prompt diagnosis and surgical repair.

Causes and incidence

Blunt (nonpenetrating) abdominal injuries usually result from automobile crashes, falls, assaults, or sports injuries; whereas penetrating abdominal injuries frequently result from stab and gunshot wounds.

The most commonly injured organs associated with penetrating abdominal trauma are the small intestine (29%), liver (28%), and colon (23%). Penetrating abdominal trauma affects 35% of those admitted to urban trauma centers and 1% to 12% of those admitted to suburban and rural centers.

Pathophysiology

Solid organs such as the liver and spleen create large areas of internal bleeding. Hollow organs such as the intestines may spill fecal material into the abdominal cavity, increasing the risk of sepsis. The retroperitoneal space is a highly vascular area and can hold up to 4 L of blood from pelvic vessel rupture.

Complications

◆ Hemorrhage
◆ Hypovolemic shock
◆ Infection
◆ Dysfunction of major organs such as liver, spleen, pancreas, and kidneys

Signs and symptoms

Symptoms vary with the degree of injury and the organs damaged. Penetrating abdominal injuries cause obvious wounds (gunshots commonly produce both entrance and exit wounds) with variable blood loss, pain, and tenderness. They commonly result in pallor, cyanosis, tachycardia, shortness of breath, and hypotension. (See *Projectile pathway*, page 936.) Blunt abdominal injuries cause severe pain (which may radiate beyond the abdomen to the shoulders), bruises, abrasions, contusions, or distention. They may also result in tenderness, abdominal splinting or rigidity, nausea, vomiting, pallor, cyanosis, tachycardia, and shortness of breath. Rib fractures commonly accompany blunt injuries. (See *Effects of blunt abdominal trauma*, page 937.)

In both blunt and penetrating injuries, massive blood loss may cause hypovolemic shock. Damage to solid abdominal organs (liver, spleen, pancreas, and kidneys) generally causes hemorrhage. Damage to hollow organs (stomach, intestine, gallbladder, and bladder) causes rupture and release of the organs' contents (including bacteria) into the abdomen, which in turn produces inflammation and, possibly, infection.

Diagnosis

℞ CONFIRMING DIAGNOSIS *A history of abdominal trauma, clinical features, and laboratory test results confirm the diagnosis of blunt or penetrating abdominal injury and determine organ damage.*

Consider any upper abdominal injury a thoracoabdominal injury until proven otherwise.

Projectile pathway

In a penetrating abdominal injury, you can estimate probable internal damage by determining the organs lying on the pathway between the entry and exit sites.

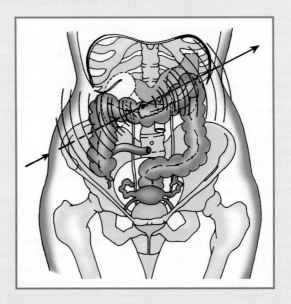

Laboratory studies vary with the patient's condition but usually include:
♦ chest X-rays (preferably done with the patient upright to show free air)
♦ CT scan may reveal solid organ injuries or vertebral or pelvic fractures
♦ examination of stools and stomach aspirate for blood
♦ blood studies (Decreased hematocrit and hemoglobin levels point to blood loss; coagulation studies evaluate hemostasis; white blood cell count is usually elevated but doesn't necessarily point to infection; type and crossmatch to prepare for a blood transfusion.)
♦ arterial blood gas analysis to evaluate respiratory status
♦ serum amylase and lipase levels, which may be elevated in pancreatic injury
♦ aspartate aminotransferase and alanine aminotransferase levels, which increase with tissue injury and cell death
♦ excretory urography and cystourethrography to detect renal and urinary tract damage
♦ angiography to detect specific injuries, especially to the kidneys
♦ exploratory laparotomy to detect specific injuries when other clinical evidence is incomplete

♦ other laboratory studies to rule out associated injuries
♦ peritoneal lavage with insertion of a lavage catheter to check for blood, gastrointestinal (GI) content, vegetable fibers, and bile. In blunt trauma with equivocal abdominal findings, this procedure helps establish the need for exploratory surgery.

Treatment

Emergency treatment of abdominal injuries controls hemorrhage and prevents hypovolemic shock through the infusion of I.V. fluids and blood components. After stabilization, most abdominal injuries require surgical repair; some patients, however, require immediate surgery. Analgesics and antibiotics increase patient comfort and prevent infection. Most patients require hospitalization; if they're asymptomatic, they may require observation for only 6 to 24 hours.

Special considerations

Emergency care in patients with abdominal injuries supports vital functions by maintaining ABCs. At admission, immediately evaluate respiratory and circulatory status and, if possible, obtain a history. Follow these guidelines:

Effects of blunt abdominal trauma

When a blunt object strikes a person's abdomen, it raises intra-abdominal pressure. Depending on the blow's force, the trauma can lacerate the liver and spleen, rupture the stomach, bruise the duodenum, and damage the kidneys.

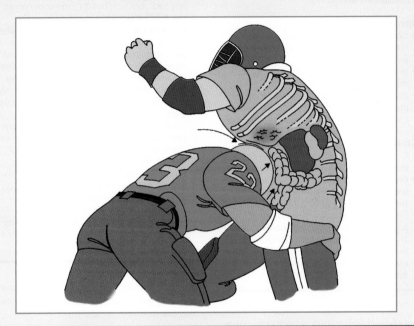

◆ To maintain airway and breathing, intubate the patient and provide mechanical ventilation as necessary; otherwise, provide supplemental oxygen.
◆ Using a large-bore needle, start two or more I.V. lines for rapid infusion of normal saline solution, lactated Ringer's solution, or blood. Then draw a blood sample for laboratory studies, and type and crossmatch blood. Also, insert a nasogastric tube and, if necessary, an indwelling urinary catheter. Monitor stomach aspirate and urine for blood.
◆ Obtain baseline vital signs, and continue to monitor them every 15 minutes.
◆ Apply a sterile dressing to open wounds. After assessing the patient, splint a suspected pelvic injury by tying the patient's legs together with a pillow between them. Mast trousers may be used to splint pelvic fractures. Try not to move the patient.
◆ Give analgesics as ordered. Opioids usually aren't recommended, but if the pain is severe, give opioids in small, titrated I.V. doses.
◆ Give tetanus prophylaxis and prophylactic I.V. antibiotics as ordered.
◆ Prepare the patient for surgery. Have the patient or a responsible relative sign a consent form. Remove dentures.

◆ If the injury was caused by a motor vehicle accident, find out if the police were notified; if not, notify them. If the patient suffered a gunshot or stab wound, notify the police. Place the patient's clothes in a paper bag, labeled with the patient's name and the date and time the patient was brought to your facility; the police will require the clothing as part of their investigation into the circumstances surrounding the patient's injury. Document the number and sites of the wounds. Contact the patient's family and offer them reassurance.

Extremities

SPRAINS AND STRAINS

A sprain is a complete or incomplete tear in the supporting ligaments surrounding a joint that usually follows a sharp twist. A strain is an injury to a muscle or tendinous attachment. Both injuries usually heal without surgical repair. (See *Classifying sprains and strains*, page 938.)

Causes and incidence

Sprains and strains may result from accidental injury, various sports-related injuries, or from

Classifying sprains and strains

This guide will help you classify the severity of sprains and strains.

Sprains
- *Grade 1 (mild):* minor or partial ligament tear with normal joint stability and function
- *Grade 2 (moderate):* partial tear with mild joint laxity and some function loss
- *Grade 3 (severe):* complete tear or incomplete separation of ligament from bone, causing total joint laxity and function loss

Strains
- *Grade 1 (mild):* microscopic muscle or tendon tear (or both) with no loss of strength
- *Grade 2 (moderate):* incomplete tear with bleeding into muscle tissue and some loss of strength
- *Grade 3 (severe):* complete rupture, usually resulting from separation of muscle from muscle, muscle from tendon, or tendon from bone (This type of strain usually stems from sudden, violent movement or direct injury.)

Muscle–tendon ruptures

Perhaps the most serious muscle–tendon injury is a rupture of the muscle–tendon junction. This type of rupture may occur at any such junction, but it's most common at the Achilles tendon, extending from the posterior calf muscle to the foot. An Achilles tendon rupture produces a sudden, sharp pain, and, until swelling begins, a palpable defect. Such a rupture typically occurs in men between ages 35 and 40, especially during physical activities such as jogging and tennis.

To distinguish an Achilles tendon rupture from other ankle injuries, the physician performs this simple test: With the patient prone and the feet hanging off the foot of the table, the physician squeezes the calf muscle. If this causes plantar flexion, the tendon is intact; if it causes ankle dorsiflexion, it's partially intact; if there's no flexion of any kind, the tendon is ruptured.

An Achilles tendon rupture usually requires surgical repair, followed first by a long leg cast for 4 weeks and then by a short cast for an additional 4 weeks.

---

simple household or work-related tasks. More than 4 of 10 injuries resulting in time absent from work are due to sprains and strains, mostly affecting the back.

Pathophysiology

Structural and chemical changes occur at the site of injury, triggering the inflammatory-immune response.

Complications

- Avulsion fracture
- Chronic strain

Signs and symptoms

A sprain causes local pain (especially during joint movement), swelling, loss of mobility (which may not occur until several hours after the injury), and a black-and-blue discoloration from blood extravasating into surrounding tissues. A sprained ankle is the most common joint injury. (See *Muscle–tendon ruptures.*)

A strain may be acute (an immediate result of vigorous muscle overuse or overstress) or chronic (a result of repeated overuse). An acute strain causes a sharp, transient pain (the patient may report having heard a snapping noise) and rapid swelling. When severe pain subsides, the muscle is tender; after several days, ecchymoses

appear. A chronic strain causes stiffness, soreness, and generalized tenderness several hours after the injury.

Diagnosis

A history of a recent injury or chronic overuse, clinical findings, and X-ray or MRI to rule out fractures establish the diagnosis. (See *Sprains and strains: An inside view,* page 939.)

Treatment

Treatment of sprains consists of controlling pain and swelling. Immediately after the injury, control swelling by elevating the joint above the level of the heart and by applying ice intermittently for 24 to 48 hours. To prevent a cold injury, place a towel between the ice pack and the skin.

Support the joint, using an elastic bandage. Place patient on weight-bearing as tolerated. Codeine or another analgesic may be necessary if the injury is severe. If the patient has a sprained ankle, they may need crutch gait training. Because patients with sprains seldom require hospitalization, provide patient teaching.

A sprain usually heals in 2 to 3 weeks, after which the patient can gradually resume normal activities. Occasionally, however, torn ligaments don't heal properly and cause recurrent dislocation, requiring surgical repair. Some athletes may request immediate surgical repair to hasten

Sprains and strains: An inside view

Except for possible swelling and discoloration, you can't see a sprain or a strain. However, these conditions are very painful. With a sprain, the patient feels the stretching or tearing of a ligament—the fibrous tissue that binds joints together. With an acute or chronic strain, the patient will feel a partial muscle tear. A strain also may affect tendons—the fibrous tissue that connects muscle to bone. The following illustrates each type of injury.

SPRAIN

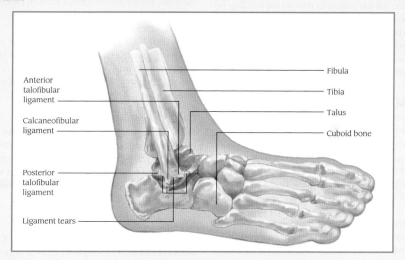

- Fibula
- Tibia
- Talus
- Cuboid bone
- Anterior talofibular ligament
- Calcaneofibular ligament
- Posterior talofibular ligament
- Ligament tears

STRAIN

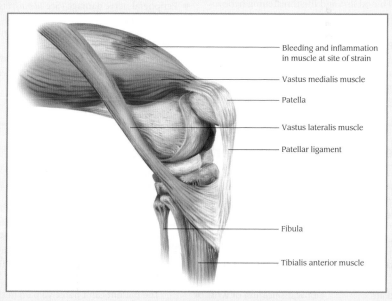

- Bleeding and inflammation in muscle at site of strain
- Vastus medialis muscle
- Patella
- Vastus lateralis muscle
- Patellar ligament
- Fibula
- Tibialis anterior muscle

healing; to prevent sprains, they may tape their wrists and ankles before sports activities.

Acute strains require analgesics and application of ice for up to 48 hours and then application of heat. Complete muscle rupture may require surgery. Chronic strains usually don't need treatment, but heat application, nonsteroidal anti-inflammatory drugs such as ibuprofen, or an analgesic-muscle relaxant can relieve discomfort.

Special considerations

◆ Tell the patient to elevate the joint for 48 to 72 hours after the injury (pillows can be used while sleeping) and to apply ice intermittently for 24 to 48 hours.

◆ If an elastic bandage has been applied, teach the patient to reapply it by wrapping from below to above the injury, forming a figure eight. For a sprained ankle, apply the bandage from the toes to midcalf. Tell the patient to remove the bandage before going to sleep and to loosen it if it causes the leg to become pale, numb, discolored, or painful.

◆ Instruct the patient to call the physician if the pain worsens or persists; if so, an additional X-ray may reveal a previously undetected fracture.

ARM AND LEG FRACTURES

Arm and leg fractures usually result from trauma and commonly cause substantial muscle, nerve, and other soft-tissue damage. The prognosis varies with the extent of disablement or deformity, the amount of tissue and vascular damage, the adequacy of reduction and immobilization, and the patient's age, health, and nutritional status. Children's bones usually heal rapidly and without deformity. Bones of adults in poor health and with impaired circulation may never heal properly. Severe open fractures, especially of the femoral shaft, may cause substantial blood loss and life-threatening hypovolemic shock.

Causes and incidence

Most arm and leg fractures result from major traumatic injury, such as a fall on an outstretched arm, a skiing accident, or child abuse (suggested by multiple or repeated episodes of fractures). However, in a person with a pathologic bone-weakening condition, such as osteoporosis, bone tumors, or metabolic disease, a mere cough or sneeze can also produce a fracture. Prolonged standing, walking, or running can cause stress fractures of the foot and ankle—usually in soldiers, nurses, postal workers, and joggers.

Fractures are among the most common orthopedic problems; about 6.8 million people seek medical attention for fractures in the United States each year.

ELDER TIP *Brittle bones make an older person especially vulnerable to fractures. A fall on an outstretched arm or hand or a direct blow to the arm or shoulder is likely to fracture the radius or humerus.*

Pathophysiology

Fractures cause a disruption in the integrity of the bone surface and structure. Usually the result of a fall or other type of injury, extreme force on the bone can cause the fracture as well as bleeding, possible nerve and other soft-tissue damage.

Complications

◆ Permanent deformity and dysfunction if bones fail to heal (nonunion) or heal improperly (malunion)

◆ Peripheral nerve damage (See *Identifying peripheral nerve damage.*)

◆ Aseptic necrosis of bone segments from impaired circulation

◆ Hypovolemic shock as a result of blood vessel damage (This is especially likely to develop in patients with a fractured femur.)

◆ Muscle contractures

Identifying peripheral nerve damage

The chart below lists signs and symptoms that can help you pinpoint where a patient has nerve damage. Keep in mind that you won't be able to rely on these signs and symptoms in a patient with severed extension tendons or severe muscle damage.

Nerve	*Associated injury*	*Sign or symptom*
Radial	Fracture of the humerus (especially the middle and distal thirds)	The patient can't extend the thumb.
Ulnar	Fracture of the medial humeral epicondyle	The patient can't perceive pain in the tip of the little finger.
Median	Elbow dislocation or wrist or forearm injury	The patient can't perceive pain in the tip of the index finger.
Peroneal	Tibia or fibula fracture or dislocation of the knee	The patient can't extend the foot (this also may indicate sciatic nerve injury).
Sciatic and tibial	Rare with fractures or dislocations	The patient can't perceive pain in the sole.

Fat embolism

A complication of long-bone fracture, fat embolism may also follow severe soft-tissue bruising and fatty liver injury. Posttraumatic embolization may occur as bone marrow releases fat into the veins. The fat can lodge in the lungs, obstructing the pulmonary vascular bed, or pass into the arteries, eventually disturbing the respiratory and circulatory systems.

Fat embolism occurs 12 to 48 hours after an injury, typically producing fever, tachycardia, tachypnea, blood-tinged sputum, cyanosis, anxiety, restlessness, altered LOC, seizures, coma, and a rash. Diagnostic test results reveal decreased hemoglobin level, increased serum lipase level, leukocytosis, thrombocytopenia, hypoxemia, and fat globules in urine and sputum. A chest X-ray may show mottled lung fields and right ventricular dilation. An electrocardiogram may reveal tachycardia and large S waves in lead I, large Q waves and an inverted T wave in lead III, and right axis deviation.

Treatment may include steroids to reduce inflammation, fluids for adequate circulatory volume, and oxygen to correct hypoxemia. Early immobilization of fractures is the best way to prevent embolism. Assist with endotracheal intubation and ventilation as ordered.

♦ Renal calculi from decalcification (because of prolonged immobility)
♦ Fat embolism (See *Fat embolism.*)
♦ Compartment syndrome (See *Recognizing compartment syndrome.*)

Signs and symptoms

Arm and leg fractures may produce any or all of the "5 Ps": pain and point tenderness, pallor, pulse loss, paresthesia, and paralysis. (The last three occur distal to the fracture site.) Other signs include deformity, swelling, discoloration, crepitus, and loss of limb function. Numbness and tingling, mottled cyanosis, cool skin at the end of the limb, and loss of pulses distal to the injury indicate possible arterial compromise or nerve damage. Open fractures also produce an obvious skin wound.

Diagnosis

A history of traumatic injury and the results of the physical examination, including gentle palpation and a cautious attempt by the patient to move parts distal to the injury, suggest an arm or leg fracture.

Note: When performing the physical examination, also check for other injuries.

℞ **CONFIRMING DIAGNOSIS** *Anteroposterior and lateral X-rays of the suspected fracture as well as X-rays of the joints above and below it confirm the diagnosis. (See Classifying fractures, pages 942 and 943.)*

Treatment

Emergency treatment consists of splinting the limb above and below the suspected fracture, applying a cold pack, and elevating the limb to reduce edema and pain.

In severe fractures that cause blood loss, apply direct pressure to control bleeding, and administer fluid replacement as soon as possible to prevent or treat hypovolemic shock.

After confirming a fracture diagnosis, begin treatment with reduction (which involves restoring displaced bone segments to their normal position).

After reduction, the fractured arm or leg must be immobilized by a splint or a cast or with traction. In closed reduction (accomplished by manual manipulation), a local anesthetic such

---

Recognizing compartment syndrome

Compartment syndrome occurs when pressure within the muscle compartment, resulting from edema or bleeding, increases to the point of interfering with circulation. Crush injuries, burns, bites, and fractures requiring casts or dressings may cause this syndrome. Compartment syndrome most commonly occurs in the lower arm, hand, lower leg, and foot. Symptoms include:
♦ increased severe pain
♦ decreased touch sensation

♦ increased weakness of the affected part
♦ increased swelling and pallor
♦ decreased pulses and capillary refill

Treatment includes:

♦ placing the limb at heart level
♦ removing constricting forces
♦ monitoring neurovascular status and compartment pressures
♦ emergency fasciotomy

PATHOPHYSIOLOGY
Classifying fractures

One of the best-known systems for classifying fractures uses a combination of general terms to describe the fracture (e.g., a simple, nondisplaced, oblique fracture).

Here are definitions of the classifications and terms used to describe fractures, along with illustrations of fragment positions and fracture lines.

General classification of fractures

Simple (closed): Bone fragments don't penetrate the skin.
Compound (open): Bone fragments penetrate the skin.
Incomplete (partial): Bone continuity isn't completely interrupted.
Complete: Bone continuity is completely interrupted.

Classification of fragment position

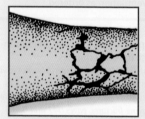

Comminuted: Bone breaks into separate small pieces.

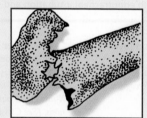

Displaced: Fracture fragments separate and are deformed.

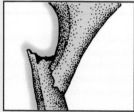

Overriding: Fragments overlap, shortening the total bone length.

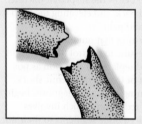

Angulated: Fragments lie at an angle to each other.

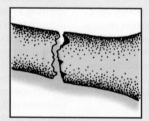

Nondisplaced: The two sections of bone maintain essentially normal alignment.

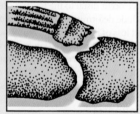

Avulsed: Fragments are pulled from normal position by muscle contractions or ligament resistance.

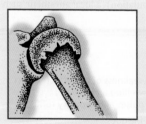

Impacted: One bone fragment is forced into another.

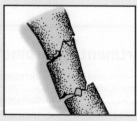

Segmental: Fractures occur in two adjacent areas with an isolated central segment.

Classifying fractures (*continued*)

Classification of fragment position

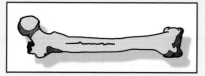

Linear: The fracture line runs parallel to the bone's axis.

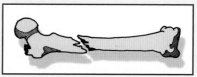

Spiral: The fracture line crosses the bone at an oblique angle, creating a spiral pattern.

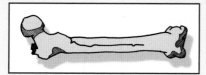

Longitudinal: The fracture line extends in a longitudinal (but not parallel) direction along the bone's axis.

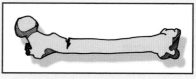

Transverse: The fracture line forms a right angle with the bone's axis.

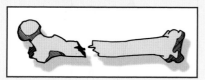

Oblique: The fracture line crosses the bone at roughly a 45-degree angle to the bone's axis.

---

as lidocaine and an analgesic such as I.V. morphine help relieve pain; a muscle relaxant such as I.V. diazepam or a sedative such as midazolam facilitates the muscle stretching necessary to realign the bone.

X-rays are ordered to confirm that the reduction was successful and that proper bone alignment was achieved.

When closed reduction is impossible, open reduction during surgery reduces and immobilizes the fracture by means of rods, plates, or screws. Afterward, a cast is usually applied.

When a splint or cast fails to maintain the reduction, immobilization requires skin or skeletal traction, using a series of weights and pulleys. In skin traction, elastic bandages and sheepskin coverings are used to attach traction devices to the patient's skin. In skeletal traction, a pin or wire inserted through the bone distal

to the fracture and attached to a weight allows more prolonged traction.

Treatment of open fractures also requires tetanus prophylaxis, prophylactic antibiotics, surgery to repair soft-tissue damage, and thorough debridement of the wound.

Special considerations

◆ Watch for signs of shock in the patient with a severe open fracture of a large bone such as the femur.

ALERT *Monitor vital signs and be especially alert for rapid pulse, decreased blood pressure, pallor, and cool, clammy skin—all of which may indicate that the patient is in shock.*

◆ Administer I.V. fluids as indicated.

◆ Offer reassurance to the patient, who's likely to be frightened and in pain.

◆ Ease pain with analgesics as needed.

◆ Help the patient set realistic goals for recovery.

◆ If the fracture requires long-term immobilization with traction, reposition the patient often to increase comfort and prevent pressure ulcers. Assist with active range-of-motion exercises to prevent muscle atrophy. Encourage deep breathing and coughing to avoid hypostatic pneumonia.

◆ Urge adequate fluid intake to prevent urinary stasis and constipation. Watch for signs of renal calculi (flank pain, nausea, and vomiting).

◆ Provide good cast care, and support the cast with pillows. Observe for skin irritation near cast edges and check for foul odors or discharge. Tell the patient to report signs of impaired circulation (skin coldness, numbness, tingling, or discoloration) immediately. Warn the patient not to get the cast wet and not to insert foreign objects under the cast.

◆ Encourage the patient to start moving around as soon as he's able. Help the patient to walk. (Remember, a patient who has been bedridden for some time may be dizzy at first.) Demonstrate how to use crutches properly.

◆ After cast removal, refer the patient to a physical therapist to restore limb mobility.

◆ If the patient is a child who sustained the fracture at or near the growth plate, have the family continue to follow up with the child's pediatrician to ensure that there are no problems as the limb grows.

DISLOCATIONS AND SUBLUXATIONS

Dislocations displace joint bones so that their articulating surfaces lose contact; subluxations partially displace the articulating surfaces. (See *Common dislocation.*) Dislocations and subluxations occur at the joints of the shoulders, elbows, wrists, digits, hips, knees, ankles, and feet. These injuries may accompany joint fractures or result in deposition of fracture fragments between joint surfaces. Prompt reduction can limit the resulting damage to soft tissue, nerves, and blood vessels.

Causes and incidence

A dislocation or subluxation may be congenital (as in congenital hip dislocation) or it may follow trauma or disease of surrounding joint tissues.

Signs and symptoms

Dislocations and subluxations produce deformity around the joint, change the involved limb's length, impair joint mobility, and cause point tenderness. When the injury results from

trauma, it's extremely painful and commonly accompanies joint surface fractures. Even in the absence of concomitant fractures, the displaced bone may damage surrounding muscles, ligaments, nerves, and blood vessels and may cause bone necrosis, especially if reduction is delayed.

Common dislocation

Children commonly dislocate elbow joints as a result of an adult pulling the child by the hand, as occurs when crossing the street; the stress on the joint causes the dislocation.

NORMAL ELBOW JOINT

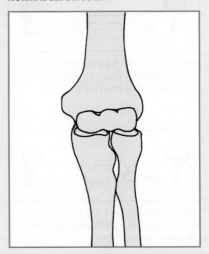

ELBOW JOINT WITH LATERAL DISLOCATION

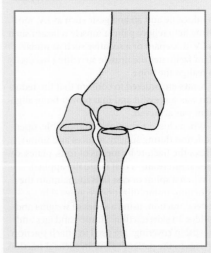

Diagnosis

Patient history, X-rays, and a physical examination rule out or confirm a fracture.

Treatment

Immediate reduction (before tissue edema and muscle spasm make reduction difficult) can prevent additional tissue damage and vascular impairment. Closed reduction consists of manual traction under general anesthesia (or local anesthesia and sedatives). During such reduction, I.V. morphine controls pain; I.V. midazolam controls muscle spasm and facilitates muscle stretching during traction. Some injuries require open reduction under regional block or general anesthesia. Such surgery may include wire fixation of the joint, skeletal traction, and ligament repair.

After reduction, a splint, a cast, or traction immobilizes the joint. In most cases, immobilizing the digits for 2 weeks, hips for 6 to 8 weeks, and other dislocated joints for 3 to 6 weeks allows surrounding ligaments to heal. Follow-up with a physical therapist is usually required to maintain optimal joint function.

Special considerations

◆ Until reduction immobilizes the dislocated joint, don't attempt manipulation. Apply ice to ease pain and edema. Splint the limb "as it lies," even if the angle is awkward. If severe vascular compromise is present or is indicated by pallor, pain, loss of pulses, paralysis, or paresthesia, an immediate orthopedic examination (and possibly immediate reduction) is necessary.

◆ Because a patient who receives opioids or benzodiazepines I.V. may develop respiratory depression or arrest, keep an airway and a bag-valve-mask in the room. Monitor respirations and pulse rate closely. Also have opioids and benzodiazepine reversal agents readily available.

◆ To avoid injury from a dressing that's too tight, instruct the patient to report numbness, pain, cyanosis, or coldness of the limb below the cast or splint.

◆ To avoid skin damage, watch for signs of pressure injury (pressure, pain, or soreness) both inside and outside the dressing.

◆ After the cast or splint is removed, inform the patient that they may gradually return to normal joint activity.

◆ A dislocated hip needs immediate reduction. At discharge, stress the need for follow-up visits to detect aseptic femoral head necrosis from vascular damage.

TRAUMATIC AMPUTATION

Traumatic amputation is the accidental loss of a body part, usually a finger, toe, arm, or leg. In a complete amputation, the extremity is totally severed; in a partial amputation, some soft-tissue connection remains. The prognosis for such injuries has improved as a result of earlier emergency and critical care management, new surgical techniques, early rehabilitation, prosthesis fitting, and new prosthesis design. New limb reimplantation techniques have been moderately successful, but incomplete nerve regeneration remains a major limiting factor.

Causes and incidence

Traumatic amputations usually result directly from accidents involving factory, farm, or power tools or motor vehicles. Natural disasters, wars, and terrorist attacks can also cause traumatic amputations.

Below-the-knee amputations account for 53% of traumatic leg amputations, with about 33% above the knee. Lower limb amputations account for 91.7% of traumatic amputations. Incidence of below-the-elbow amputation is 4.4%, and above the elbow amputations account for 2%.

Pathophysiology

When an explosion occurs, such as a terrorist bombing or upon a battlefield, gases under high pressure are produced rapidly the bomb materials. This high-pressure wave travels quickly in all directions. Research suggests that this high-pressure wave creates fractures and massive soft-tissue trauma to a limb. Hemorrhage, not injury from the shock wave of the blast, is the primary cause of death.

Complications

◆ Hypovolemic shock
◆ Sepsis
◆ Residual paralysis with reimplantation

Signs and symptoms

The obvious sign of amputation is a body part that has been cutoff. Every traumatic amputee requires careful monitoring of vital signs. If amputation involves more than a finger or toe, assessment of ABCs is also required. Because profuse bleeding is likely, watch for signs of hypovolemic shock, and draw blood for a hemoglobin level, hematocrit, and type and crossmatch. In partial amputation, check for pulses distal to the amputation site. After any traumatic amputation, assess for other traumatic injuries as well. The patient may exhibit crushed body tissue, in which the body part is badly mangled but still partially attached by muscle, bone, tendon, or skin.

Treatment

Because the greatest immediate threat after traumatic amputation is blood loss and hypovolemic shock, emergency treatment consists of local measures to control bleeding, fluid replacement with normal saline solution and colloids, and blood replacement as needed. Reimplantation remains controversial, but it's becoming more common and successful because of advances in microsurgery techniques. If reconstruction or reimplantation is possible, surgical intervention attempts to preserve usable joints.

When arm or leg amputations are done, the surgeon creates a stump to be fitted with a prosthesis. A rigid dressing permits early prosthesis fitting and rehabilitation.

⬡ **ELDER TIP** *Leg amputation can be a life-threatening procedure, especially in patients older than age 60 with peripheral vascular disease. Such patients suffer significant morbidity with above-the-knee amputations because of associated poor health, disease, or malnutrition; complications such as sepsis; and the physiologic insult of amputation.*

Special considerations

◆ During emergency treatment, monitor vital signs (especially in hypovolemic shock), clean the wound, and give tetanus prophylaxis, analgesics, and antibiotics as ordered.
◆ After a complete amputation, wrap the amputated part in wet dressings soaked in normal saline solution. Label the part, seal it in a plastic bag, and float the bag in ice water. Flush the wound with sterile saline solution, apply a sterile pressure dressing, and elevate the limb. Notify the reimplantation team.
◆ After a partial amputation, position the limb in normal alignment and drape it with towels or dressings soaked in sterile normal saline solution.
◆ Preoperatively, irrigate and debride the wound thoroughly (using a local block). Postoperatively, perform dressing changes using sterile technique to help prevent skin infection and ensure skin graft viability.
◆ Help the amputee cope with altered body image. Encourage the patient to perform prescribed exercises while taking care to prevent stump trauma.

Whole body

BURNS

A major burn is a catastrophic injury, requiring painful treatment and a long period of rehabilitation. It's commonly fatal or permanently disfiguring and incapacitating (both emotionally and physically).

Causes and incidence

Thermal burns, the most common type, are usually the result of residential fires, automobile crashes, children playing with matches, improperly stored gasoline, space heater or electrical malfunctions, or arson. Other causes include improper handling of firecrackers, scalding accidents, and kitchen accidents (such as a child climbing on top of a stove or grabbing a hot iron). Some burns in children are traced to parental abuse.

Chemical burns result from the contact, ingestion, inhalation, or injection of acids, alkalis, or vesicants. Electrical burns usually occur after contact with faulty electrical wiring or high-voltage power lines; many children sustain them by chewing on electric cords. In the United States, about 2.4 million people suffer burns annually. Fire ranks fifth among accidental injuries, after motor vehicle crashes, poisoning, falls, and drowning.

Pathophysiology

Burns that are greater than 20% total body surface area have increased capillary permeability and fluid volume deficits in the first 24 hours postinjury. Fluid resuscitation in this period is vital to prevent organ dysfunction. Trauma from a large burn creates dramatic changes in the cardiovascular system. A decrease in cardiac output, increase in peripheral vascular resistance, and fluid shifts out of the intravascular space happen immediately.

Complications

◆ Respiratory complications
◆ Sepsis
◆ Hypovolemic shock
◆ Anemia
◆ Multiorgan dysfunction syndrome

Signs and symptoms

One goal of assessment is to determine the *depth* of skin and tissue damage. A partial-thickness burn damages the epidermis and part of the dermis, whereas a full-thickness burn affects the full dermis and, possibly, subcutaneous tissue. A more traditional method gauges burn depth by degrees. However, most burns are a combination of different degrees and thicknesses. (See *Gauging burn depth,* page 947.)

Burn degrees are classified as follows:
◆ *Superficial (first-degree) burns*—Damage is limited to the epidermis, causing erythema and pain. An example is a sunburn.
◆ *Partial-thickness (second-degree) burns*—The epidermis and part of the dermis are damaged, producing blisters and mild-to-moderate edema and pain.

Gauging burn depth

One method of assessing burns is by determining the burn's depth. A partial-thickness burn damages the epidermis and part of the dermis, whereas a full-thickness burn damages the epidermis, dermis, subcutaneous tissue, and muscle, as shown below.

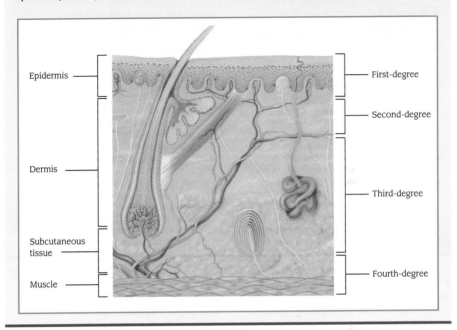

◆ *Full-thickness (third-degree) burns*—The epidermis and the dermis are damaged. No blisters appear, but white, brown, or black leathery tissue and thrombosed vessels are visible. Nerves are damaged so there is no pain or sensation within the burned area.

◆ *Fourth-degree burns*—Damage extends through deeply charred subcutaneous tissue to muscle and bone.

Another assessment goal is to estimate the *size* of a burn, which is usually expressed as the percentage of body surface area (BSA) covered by the burn. The Rule of Nines chart usually provides this estimate, but the Lund and Browder chart is more accurate because it allows for BSA changes with age.

A correlation of the burn's depth and size permits an estimate of its severity as follows:

◆ *major full-thickness (third degree)*—on more than 10% of BSA; second-degree burns on more than 25% of adult BSA (>20% in children); burns of hands, face, feet, or genitalia; burns complicated by fractures or inhalation injury; electrical burns; all burns in poor-risk patients.

◆ *moderate full-thickness (third degree)*—third-degree burns on 2% to 10% of BSA; second-degree burns on 15% to 25% of adult BSA (10% to 20% in children).

◆ *minor full-thickness (third degree)*—third-degree burns on less than 2% of BSA; second-degree burns on less than 15% of adult BSA (10% in children).

Here are other important factors in assessing burns:

◆ Location—Burns on the face, hands, feet, and genitalia are the most serious because of possible function loss.

◆ Configuration—Circumferential burns can cause total occlusion of circulation in a limb as a result of burn constriction and/or edema. Burns on the neck can produce airway obstruction, whereas burns on the chest can lead to restricted respiratory expansion.

◆ History of complicating medical problems—Note any disorders that impair peripheral circulation, especially diabetes, peripheral vascular disease, and chronic alcohol abuse.

Managing burns with skin grafts

When a patient has a limited, well-defined burn, they may need a temporary graft to minimize fluid and protein loss from the burn surface, to prevent infection, and to reduce pain. Types of temporary grafts include:

♦ *allografts (homografts)*, which are usually cadaver skin
♦ *xenografts (heterografts)*, which are typically pigskin
♦ *biosynthetic grafts*, which are a combination of collagen and synthetics
  To treat a full-thickness burn, a patient may need an *autograft*. This method uses the patient's own skin—usually a split-thickness graft—to replace the burned skin. For areas where appearance or joint movement is important, the autograft will be transplanted intact. In flat areas where appearance is less critical, the graft may be meshed (fenestrated) to cover up to three times its original size.
  When burns cover the entire body surface, epithelial cells grown in culture for autograft may provide lifesaving

treatment. In this method, a small full-thickness biopsy yields epidermal cells that are cultured into sheets and then grafted onto the burns. It takes several weeks to grow confluent sheets and the process is costly. The cells are produced in a fragile sheet that's sensitive to infection.
  Bilayer collagen matrices—porous, sponge like lattices composed of bovine collagen, chondroitin-6-sulfate, and glycosaminoglycans—are another option. These matrices serve as a dermal substitute and a scaffold to support developing fibroblasts and blood vessels, which eventually replace the matrices. A silicone membrane is sealed over the surface, becoming progressively less adherent as it's incorporated into the body. After 3 weeks, it's peeled off and replaced with cultured epithelial cells or thin, split-thickness grafts.

♦ Patient age—Victims younger than age 4 or older than age 60 have a higher incidence of complications and, consequently, a higher mortality.
♦ Smoke inhalation—This can result in pulmonary injury. Inhalation injury should be suspected if the victim was in an enclosed space, has burned nasal hairs, or is couching up carbonaceous sputum.
♦ Other injuries sustained at the time of the burn—Thermal burns sustained from a car crash or explosion may mask other traumas.

Treatment

Immediate, aggressive burn treatment increases the patient's chances of survival. Later, supportive measures and strict sterile technique can minimize infection. Because burns require such comprehensive care, good treatment can make the difference between life and death. (See *Managing burns with skin grafts*.)

Moderate or major burns

♦ Immediately assess the patient's ABCs. Be especially alert for signs of smoke inhalation and pulmonary damage: singed nasal hairs, mucosal burns, voice changes, coughing, wheezing, soot in the mouth or nose, and darkened sputum. Prepare for endotracheal intubation, and administer 100% oxygen as indicated.

♦ When you have ensured the patient's ABCs, take a brief history of the burn. Draw blood samples for complete blood count, type and crossmatch, and electrolyte, glucose, blood urea nitrogen, creatinine, and arterial blood gas levels, including a carboxyhemoglobin level.
♦ Control bleeding and remove smoldering clothing (soak it first in normal saline solution if it's stuck to the patient's skin), rings, and other constricting items. Be sure to cover burns with a clean, dry, sterile bed sheet. (Never cover large burns with saline-soaked dressings because they can drastically lower body temperature.)
♦ Begin I.V. therapy immediately to prevent hypovolemic shock and maintain cardiac output. Use lactated Ringer's solution or a fluid replacement formula as ordered. (See *Fluid replacement after a burn*, page 949.) Closely monitor intake and output and frequently check vital signs. You'll need to take the patient's blood pressure despite burned limbs.

Minor burns

For minor burns, immerse the burned area in cool normal saline solution (55° F [12.8° C]) or apply cool compresses; never place ice directly on burned skin. Administer pain medication as appropriate. Debride the devitalized tissue, taking care not to break any blisters.

Fluid replacement after a burn

Use the Parkland formula as a general guideline for the amount of fluid replacement. For an adult with a thermal burn, administer 2 mL/kg of crystalloid X% total burn surface area; give half of the solution over the first 8 hours (calculated from the time of the injury) and the balance over the next 16 hours. Vary the specific infusions according to the patient's response, especially urine output. For an adult with an electrical burn injury, use 4 mL/kg or crystalloid in the fluid calculation.

Cover the wound with an antimicrobial agent and a nonstick bulky dressing, and administer tetanus prophylaxis as indicated.

Electrical or chemical burns

◆ Tissue damage from electrical burns is difficult to assess because internal destruction along the conduction pathway is usually greater than the surface burn would indicate. Electrical burns that ignite the patient's clothes may cause thermal burns as well. If the electric shock caused ventricular fibrillation with cardiac and respiratory arrest, begin CPR at once. Get a voltage estimate. (For more details, see *Electric shock section.*)
◆ Irrigate a chemical burn with copious amounts of water or normal saline solution. Using a weak base such as sodium bicarbonate to neutralize hydrofluoric acid, hydrochloric acid, or sulfuric acid on skin or mucous membrane is contraindicated because the neutralizing agent can actually produce more heat and tissue damage.

If the chemical entered the patient's eyes, flush them with large amounts of water or normal saline solution for at least 30 minutes; in an alkali burn, irrigate until the pH of the cul-de-sacs returns to 7. Have the patient close the eyes, and cover them with a dry, sterile dressing. Note the type of chemical that caused the burn and the presence of any noxious fumes. The patient will need an emergency ophthalmologic examination.

Special considerations

◆ Don't treat the burn wound itself in the emergency department if the patient is to be transferred to a specialized burn care unit within 4 hours after the burn. Instead, prepare the patient for transport by wrapping in a sterile sheet and a blanket for warmth and elevating the burned limb to decrease edema. Then transport the patient immediately.

While the patient is hospitalized:
◆ A central venous pressure line and additional I.V. lines (using venous cutdown if necessary) and an indwelling urinary catheter may be inserted. To combat fluid evaporation through the burn and the release of fluid into interstitial spaces (possibly resulting in hypovolemic shock), continue fluid therapy as ordered.
◆ Check vital signs every 15 minutes (by arterial line if blood pressure is unobtainable with a cuff). Send a urine specimen to the laboratory to check for myoglobinuria and hemoglobinuria.
◆ Consult the nutritional therapy department to provide tube feeding, total parenteral nutrition, or a high-calorie diet, as appropriate.
◆ Insert a nasogastric tube to decompress the stomach and avoid aspiration of stomach contents.

Before the patient is released from the hospital:
◆ Ensure that the patient's immunizations are current, particularly tetanus.
◆ Arrange physical and occupational therapy consultations for the severely burned patient, as indicated.
◆ Provide referral to a reconstructive surgeon for the patient disfigured by burns. Psychological counseling may also be beneficial.
◆ Provide thorough teaching and complete aftercare instructions for the patient. Stress the importance of keeping the dressing dry and clean, elevating the burned limb for the first 24 hours, taking analgesics as ordered, and returning for a wound check in 1 to 2 days.

PEDIATRIC TIP *Consult a pediatrician if the patient is a child; consultation with a child-life therapist may also help to ensure the child's normal growth and development.*

ELECTRIC SHOCK

When an electric current passes through the body, the damage it does depends on the current's intensity (amperes, milliamperes, or microamperes), the resistance of the tissues through which it passes, the kind of current (AC, DC, or mixed), and the frequency and duration of current flow. Electric shock may cause ventricular fibrillation, respiratory paralysis, burns, and death. The prognosis depends on the site and extent of damage, the patient's health, and the speed and adequacy of treatment.

Causes and incidence

Electric shock usually follows accidental contact with exposed parts of electrical appliances or wiring, but it may also result from lightning or the flash of electric arcs from high-voltage power lines or machines. The increased use in hospitals of electrical medical devices, many of which are connected directly to the patient, has raised serious concerns about electrical safety and has led to the development of electrical safety standards. But even well-designed equipment with reliable safety features can cause electric shock if mishandled. (See *Preventing electric shock.*)

Electric current can cause injury in three ways: true electrical injury as the current passes through the body, arc or flash burns from current that doesn't pass through the body, and thermal surface burns caused by associated heat and flames.

In the United States, about 1,000 people die of electric shock each year.

Pathophysiology

Electrical burns are very deceptive. On the surface, the patient may only show signs of two burn wounds from the point of entrance and exit of the current flow. However, electricity flows along the path of least resistance. This means electrical current travels faster along wet areas (such as muscles, nerve pathways, and vascular beds) than dry areas (such as intact skin and bone). The pathway below the skin surface where the current follows creates unseen trauma, coagulation of tissue, and necrosis.

Complications

◆ Sepsis
◆ Neurologic, cardiac, or psychiatric dysfunction
◆ Renal failure
◆ Electrolyte abnormalities
◆ Peripheral nerve injuries
◆ Thrombi
◆ Cardiac arrhythmias

Signs and symptoms

Severe electric shock usually causes muscle contraction, followed by unconsciousness and loss of reflex control, sometimes with respiratory paralysis (by way of prolonged contraction of respiratory muscles or as a direct effect on the respiratory nerve center). Tissue damage may lead to rhabdomyolysis and kidney injury. After

PREVENTION
Preventing electric shock

◆ Check for cuts, cracks, or frayed insulation on electric cords, call buttons (also check for warm call buttons), and electric devices attached to the patient's bed; keep these away from hot or wet surfaces and sharp corners. Don't set glasses of water, damp towels, or other wet items on electrical equipment. Wipe up accidental spills before they leak into electrical equipment. Avoid using extension cords because they may circumvent the ground; if they're absolutely necessary, don't place them under carpeting or in areas where they'll be walked on.
◆ Make sure ground connections on electrical equipment are intact. Line cord plugs should have three prongs, which should be straight and firmly fixed. Check that the prongs fit wall outlets properly and that outlets aren't loose or broken. Don't use adapters on plugs.
◆ Promptly report faulty equipment to maintenance personnel. If a machine sparks, smokes, seems unusually hot, or gives you or your patient a slight shock, unplug it immediately, if doing so won't endanger the patient's life. Check inspection labels and report equipment overdue for inspection.

◆ Be especially careful when using electrical equipment near patients with pacemakers or direct cardiac lines because a cardiac catheter or pacemaker can create a direct, low-resistance path to the heart; even a small shock may cause ventricular fibrillation.
◆ Remember that dry, calloused, unbroken skin offers more resistance to electric current than mucous membranes, an open wound, or thin, moist skin.
◆ Make sure defibrillator paddles are free of dry, caked gel before applying fresh gel because poor electric contact can cause burns. Also, don't apply too much gel. If the gel runs over the paddle's edge and touches your hand, you'll receive some of the defibrillator shock while the patient loses some of the energy in the discharge.
◆ Tell all patients how to avoid electrical hazards at home and at work. Warn them not to use electrical appliances when they're wet, such as in the shower. Warn them never to touch electrical appliances while touching faucets or cold water pipes in the kitchen because these pipes often provide the ground for all of the house's circuits.

momentary shock, hyperventilation may follow initial muscle contraction. Passage of even the smallest electric current (if it passes through the heart) may induce ventricular fibrillation or another arrhythmia that progresses to fibrillation or myocardial infarction.

Electric shock from a high-frequency current (which generates more heat in tissues than a low-frequency current) usually causes burns, local tissue coagulation, and necrosis. Low-frequency currents can also cause serious burns if the contact with the current is concentrated in a small area (e.g., when a toddler bites into an electric cord). Contusions, fractures, and other injuries can result from violent muscle contractions, falls, or being thrown during the shock; later, the patient may develop renal shutdown. Residual hearing impairment, latent rhythm effects on the heart (such as ventricular fibrillation), cataracts, and vision loss may persist after severe electric shock.

Diagnosis

In most cases, the cause of electrical injuries is either obvious or suspected. However, an accurate history can identify the voltage and the length of contact.

In addition, several tests may be ordered to determine injuries, such as X-rays to reveal fractures; electrocardiogram to check for cardiac damage, and urine enzymes to look for severe muscle injury.

Treatment

Immediate emergency treatment consists of carefully separating the victim from the current source, quick assessment of vital functions, and emergency measures, such as CPR and defibrillation.

To separate the victim from the current source, immediately turn it off or unplug it. If this isn't possible, pull the victim free with a nonconductive device, such as a loop of dry cloth or rubber, a dry rope, or a leather belt—with metal buckle detached.

Emergency treatment then begins as follows:
◆ Quickly assess vital functions. If you don't detect a pulse or breathing, start CPR at once. Continue until vital signs return or emergency help arrives with a defibrillator and other advanced life-support equipment. Then monitor the patient's cardiac rhythm continuously and obtain a 12-lead electrocardiogram.
◆ Because internal tissue destruction may be much greater than indicated by skin damage, give I.V. lactated Ringer's solution as ordered to maintain urine output of 50 to 100 mL/ hour. Insert an indwelling urinary catheter and

send the first specimen to the laboratory. Measure intake and output hourly and watch for tea- or port wine–colored urine, which occurs when coagulation necrosis and tissue ischemia liberate myoglobin and hemoglobin. These proteins can precipitate in the renal tubules, causing tubular necrosis and renal shutdown. To prevent this, give mannitol and furosemide as indicated.
◆ Administer sodium bicarbonate as needed to counteract acidosis caused by widespread tissue destruction and anaerobic metabolism.
◆ Assess the patient's neurologic status frequently because central nervous system damage may result from ischemia or demyelination. Because a spinal cord injury may follow cord ischemia or a compression fracture, watch for sensorimotor deficits.
◆ Check for neurovascular damage in the extremities by assessing peripheral pulses and capillary refill and by asking if the patient feels numbness, tingling, or pain. Elevate any injured extremities.
◆ Apply a temporary sterile dressing, and admit the patient for surgical debridement and observation as needed. Frequent debridement and use of topical and systemic antibiotics can help reduce the risk of infection. As indicated, prepare the patient for grafting or, if the injuries are extreme, for amputation.

Special considerations

Take measures to prevent electric shock in patients.

PEDIATRIC TIP *Advise parents of small children to put safety guards on all electrical outlets and to keep children away from electrical devices.*

COLD INJURIES

Cold injuries result from overexposure to cold air or water and occur in two major forms: localized injuries such as frostbite and systemic injuries such as hypothermia. Untreated or improperly treated frostbite can lead to gangrene and may require amputation; severe hypothermia can be fatal.

Causes and incidence

Localized cold injuries occur when ice crystals form in the tissues and expand extracellular spaces. With compression of the tissue cell, the cell membrane ruptures, interrupting enzymatic and metabolic activities. Increased capillary permeability accompanies histamine release, resulting in aggregation of red blood cells and microvascular occlusion. Hypothermia effects chemical changes that slow the functions of most major organ systems, such as decreased renal blood flow and decreased glomerular filtration. Frostbite results from prolonged exposure to dry temperatures far below freezing; hypothermia, from near drowning in cold water and prolonged exposure to cold temperatures.

The risk of serious cold injuries, especially hypothermia, is increased by youth, old age, lack of insulating body fat, wet or inadequate clothing, drug abuse, cardiac disease, smoking, fatigue, hunger and depletion of caloric reserves, and excessive alcohol intake (which draws blood into capillaries and away from body organs).

> **ELDER TIP** *The following risk factors put elderly people at increased risk for cold injuries: cardiovascular disease, alcohol abuse, malnutrition, diabetes, skin diseases, scarring from major burns, inadequate fluid intake, working outdoors, wearing inappropriate clothing, and living in poor environmental conditions. The use of anticholinergics, phenothiazines, diuretics, antihistamines, antidepressants, or beta-adrenergic blockers also increases the risk.*

Pathophysiology

Hypothermia is defined as a clinical condition in which core body is less than 35° C (95° F). The adaptation of the body to cold temperatures is achieved through multiple pathways, all of which attempt to increase and conserve the generation of heat. In mild hypothermia, the body starts peripheral vasoconstriction, tachycardia, increased cardiac output (from increased sympathetic nervous system tone), increased production of catecholamine, and skeletal muscle shivering. If unchecked, severe hypothermia leads to decreased cardiac output, bradycardia, decreased oxygenation to the brain, decline in shivering, changes in blood coagulation, coma, and death.

Complications

- Renal failure
- Rhabdomyolysis
- Gangrene
- Aspiration pneumonia
- Cardiac arrhythmias
- Hypoglycemia
- Hyperglycemia
- Metabolic acidosis
- Pancreatitis

Signs and symptoms

Frostbite may be deep or superficial. Superficial frostbite affects skin and subcutaneous tissue, especially of the face, ears, extremities, and other exposed areas. Although it may go unnoticed at first, frostbite produces burning, tingling, numbness, swelling, and a mottled, blue-gray skin color when the person returns to a warm place.

Deep frostbite extends beyond subcutaneous tissue and usually affects the hands or feet. The skin becomes white until it's thawed; then it turns purplish blue. Deep frostbite also produces pain, skin blisters, tissue necrosis, and gangrene. (See *Recognizing frostbite.*)

Indications of hypothermia (a core body temperature below 95° F [35° C]) vary with severity:

- *mild hypothermia*—temperature of 89.6° to 95° F (32° to 35° C), severe shivering, slurred speech, and amnesia
- *moderate hypothermia*—temperature of 82.4° to 89.6° F (28° to 32° C), unresponsiveness or confusion, muscle rigidity, peripheral cyanosis and, with improper rewarming, signs of shock
- *severe hypothermia*—temperature of 68° to 82.4° F (20° to 28° C), loss of deep tendon reflexes, and ventricular fibrillation. The patient may appear dead (in a state of rigor mortis), with no palpable pulse or audible heart sounds. the pupils may be dilated. A temperature drop below 77° F causes cardiopulmonary arrest and death.

Diagnosis

A history of severe and prolonged exposure to cold may make this diagnosis obvious. Nevertheless, hypothermia can be overlooked if outdoor temperatures are above freezing or if the patient is comatose.

Recognizing frostbite

The illustration below shows frostbite of the toes. Note the line of demarcation and ulceration.

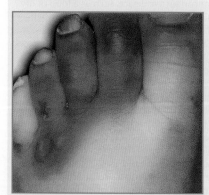

Treatment

In a localized cold injury, treatment consists of rewarming the injured part, supportive measures and, sometimes, a fasciotomy to increase circulation by lowering edematous tissue pressure. However, if gangrene occurs, amputation may be necessary. In hypothermia, therapy consists of immediate resuscitation measures, careful monitoring, and gradual rewarming of the body. If cold injuries in children suggest neglect or abuse, a thorough history should be performed.

Treat localized cold injuries as follows:
◆ Remove constrictive clothing and jewelry and slowly rewarm the affected part in warm water (100° to 108° F [37.8° to 42.2° C]). Give the patient warm fluids to drink. Never rub the injured area—this aggravates tissue damage.
◆ When the affected part begins to rewarm, the patient will feel pain, so give analgesics as ordered. Check for a pulse. Be careful not to rupture any blebs. If the injury is on the foot, place cotton or gauze sponges between the toes to prevent maceration. Instruct the patient not to walk.
◆ If the injury has caused an open skin wound, give antibiotics and tetanus prophylaxis as indicated.
◆ If a pulse fails to return, the patient may develop compartment syndrome and need a fasciotomy to restore circulation. (See *Recognizing compartment syndrome*, page 941.) If gangrene occurs, prepare the patient for amputation.
◆ Before discharge, teach the patient about possible long-term effects: increased sensitivity to cold, burning and tingling, and increased sweating. Warn the patient against smoking, which causes vasoconstriction and slows healing.

Systemic hypothermia is treated as follows:
◆ If you detect no pulse or respiration, begin CPR immediately and, if necessary, continue it for 2 to 3 hours. (Remember that hypothermia helps protect the brain from anoxia, which normally accompanies prolonged cardiopulmonary arrest. Therefore, even after the patient has been unresponsive for a long time, resuscitation may be possible, especially after cold-water near drowning.) Perform CPR until the patient is adequately rewarmed.
◆ Move the patient to a warm area, remove wet clothing, and keep dry. If the patient's conscious, give warm fluids with a high sugar content such as tea with sugar. If the patient's core temperature is above 89.6° F (32° C), use external warming techniques. Bathe the patient in water that is 104° F (40° C), cover the patient with a heating blanket set at 97.9° to 99.9° F (36.6° to 37.7° C), and cautiously apply hot water bottles at 104° F to the groin and axillae, guarding against burns.
◆ If the patient's core temperature is below 89.6° F (32° C), use internal and external warming methods. Rewarm the body core and surface 1° to 2° F (0.56° to 1.1° C) per hour concurrently. (If you rewarm the surface first, rewarming shock could cause potentially fatal ventricular fibrillation.) To warm inhalations, provide oxygen heated to 107.6° to 114.8° F (42° to 46° C). Infuse I.V. solutions that have been warmed to 98.6° F (37° C) and perform nasogastric lavage with normal saline solution that has been warmed to the same temperature. Assist with peritoneal lavage, using normal saline solution (full or half-strength) warmed to 104° to 113° F (40° to 45° C); in severe hypothermia, extracorporeal rewarming is the most rapid and efficient method.

Special considerations

◆ Throughout treatment, monitor arterial blood gas levels, intake and output, central venous pressure, temperature, and cardiac and neurologic status every 30 minutes. Also monitor laboratory test results, such as complete blood count, blood urea nitrogen and electrolyte levels, prothrombin time, and partial thromboplastin time.
◆ Cold injuries can be prevented. (See *Preventing cold injuries*.)

PREVENTION
Preventing cold injuries

To prevent cold injuries, teach patients to:
  ◆ wear mittens instead of gloves
  ◆ wear windproof, water-resistant layers of clothing
  ◆ wear two pairs of socks (cotton next to the skin and wool over the cotton socks)
  ◆ wear a scarf and a hat that covers the ears (to avoid substantial heat loss through the head)
   Before anticipated prolonged exposure to cold, advise the patient not to drink alcohol or smoke cigarettes, and to get adequate food and rest. If the patient gets caught in severe cold weather, advise them to find shelter quickly or increase physical activity to maintain body warmth.

◆ If the patient has developed a cold injury because of inadequate clothes or housing, refer to a community social service agency, if appropriate.

HEAT SYNDROME

Heat syndrome may result from environmental or internal conditions that increase heat production or impair heat dissipation. The three categories of heat syndrome are heat cramps, heat exhaustion, and heatstroke.

Causes and incidence

Normally, people adjust to excessive temperatures via complex cardiovascular and neurologic changes that are coordinated by the hypothalamus. Heat loss offsets heat production to regulate the body temperature. It does this by evaporation (sweating) or vasodilation, which cools the body's surface by radiation, conduction, and convection.

However, heat production increases with exercise, infection, and the use of certain drugs such as amphetamines, and heat loss decreases with high temperatures or humidity, lack of acclimatization, excess clothing, obesity, dehydration, cardiovascular disease, sweat gland dysfunction, and the use of such drugs as phenothiazines and anticholinergics. When heat loss mechanisms fail to offset heat production, the body retains heat and may develop heat syndrome.

Pathophysiology

The core body temperature of humans is strictly maintained at approximately 37.5° C by four mechanisms: radiation, convection, conduction, and vaporization. The pathophysiology of hyperthermia is manifested by organ dysfunction because of the abnormal heat, ischemia created by decreased blood flow to end organs, and electrolyte imbalances.

Prolonged sweating and dehydration cause decreased blood volume and increased blood viscosity. Heart rate and myocardial contractility increases, generating more energy and heat in the body. Proteins and enzymes in the body will start to denature when temperature reach 40° C (104° F).

Complications

◆ Hypovolemic shock
◆ Cardiogenic shock
◆ Cardiac arrhythmias
◆ Renal failure
◆ Rhabdomyolysis
◆ Disseminated intravascular coagulation
◆ Hepatic failure

Signs and symptoms

Signs and symptoms of heat syndrome vary-depending on the type (heat cramps, heat-exhaustion, or heatstroke) and predisposing-factors. (See *Managing heat syndrome*, page 955.)

Treatment

For specific guidelines on treating heat syndrome, see *Managing heat syndrome*.

Special considerations

Heat illnesses are easily preventable, so it's important to educate patients about the various factors that cause them. This information is especially vital for athletes, laborers, and soldiers in field training.

◆ Advise your patients to avoid heat syndrome by taking these precautions in hot weather: wearing loose-fitting, lightweight clothing; resting frequently; avoiding hot places; and drinking adequate amounts of fluid.

⬡ **ELDER TIP** *Vigorous fluid replacement in elderly people or those with underlying cardiovascular disease may cause pulmonary edema.*

◆ Advise patients who are obese, elderly, or taking drugs that impair heat regulation to avoid becoming overheated.

◆ Tell patients who have had heat cramps or heat exhaustion to exercise gradually and to increase their salt and water intake.

◆ Tell patients with heatstroke that residual hypersensitivity to high temperatures may persist for several months.

ASPHYXIA

A condition of insufficient oxygen and accumulating carbon dioxide in the blood and tissues because of interference with respiration, asphyxia results in cardiopulmonary arrest. Without prompt treatment, it's fatal.

Causes and incidence

Asphyxia results from any condition or substance that inhibits respiration, such as the following:

◆ hypoventilation because of opioid abuse, medullary disease or hemorrhage, pneumothorax, respiratory muscle paralysis, or cardiopulmonary arrest

◆ intrapulmonary obstruction, as in airway obstruction, severe asthma, foreign body aspiration, pulmonary edema, pneumonia, and near drowning

◆ extrapulmonary obstruction, as in tracheal compression from a tumor, strangulation, trauma, or suffocation

◆ inhalation of toxic agents, as in carbon monoxide poisoning, smoke inhalation, and excessive oxygen inhalation

Managing heat syndrome

Management of heat syndrome depends on the injury's severity. General treatment includes immersion or evaporative and convective cooling until core temperature is below 38° to 39° C (100.4° to 102.2° F)

Type and predisposing factors	Signs and symptoms	Management
Heat cramps		
◆ Commonly affect young adults ◆ Strenuous activity without training or acclimatization ◆ Normal to high temperature or high humidity	◆ Muscle twitching and spasms, weakness, severe muscle cramps ◆ Nausea ◆ Normal temperature or slight fever ◆ Diaphoresis	◆ Hospitalization is usually unnecessary. ◆ Replace fluids and electrolytes with clear juice or a sports beverage. ◆ Loosen the patient's clothing and have they lie down in a cool place. Massage the muscles. If muscle cramps are severe, start an I.V. infusion with normal saline solution.
Heat exhaustion		
◆ Commonly affects young people ◆ Physical activity without acclimatization ◆ Decreased heat dissipation ◆ High temperature and humidity	◆ Nausea and vomiting ◆ Decreased blood pressure ◆ Thready, rapid pulse ◆ Cool, pallid skin ◆ Headache, mental confusion, syncope, giddiness ◆ Oliguria, thirst ◆ Elevated temperature ◆ Muscle cramps	◆ Hospitalization is usually unnecessary. ◆ Immediately give a balanced electrolyte drink. ◆ Loosen the patient's clothing and put they in a shock position in a cool place. Massage the muscles. If cramps are severe, start an I.V. infusion as ordered. ◆ Give oxygen if needed.
Heatstroke		
◆ Exertional type—commonly affects young, healthy people involved in strenuous activity ◆ Classical type—commonly affects elderly, inactive people who have cardiovascular disease or who take drugs that influence temperature regulation ◆ High temperature and humidity without any wind	◆ Hypertension followed by hypotension ◆ Atrial or ventricular tachycardia ◆ Hot, dry, red skin, which later turns gray; no diaphoresis ◆ Throbbing headache, confusion, progressing to seizures and loss of consciousness ◆ Temperature higher than 104° F (40° C) ◆ Dilated pupils ◆ Slow, deep respiration; then Cheyne–Stokes respiratives	◆ Hospitalization is needed. ◆ Maintain airway, breathing, and circulation. ◆ To lower body temperature, cool the patient rapidly with ice packs on arterial pressure points and hypothermia blankets. ◆ To replace fluids and electrolytes, start an I.V. infusion. ◆ Insert a nasogastric tube to prevent aspiration. ◆ Give diazepam to control seizures. ◆ Monitor the patient's temperature, intake and output, and cardiac status. Give dobutamine, as ordered, to correct cardiogenic shock. (Vasoconstrictors are contraindicated.)

Pathophysiology

This may occur at the level of the lungs or at the cellular level. The brain cannot function without oxygen for longer than 4 minutes before large-scale problems occur. Late-stage asphyxia typically results in cardiopulmonary arrest from profound bradycardia because of depression of the cardiorespiratory centers in the brain stem.

Complications

◆ Neurologic damage
◆ Death

Signs and symptoms

Depending on the asphyxia's duration and degree, common symptoms include anxiety, dyspnea, agitation and confusion leading to coma, altered respiratory rate (apnea, bradypnea, occasional tachypnea), decreased breath sounds, central and peripheral cyanosis (cherry-red mucous membranes in late-stage carbon monoxide poisoning), seizures, and fast, slow, or absent pulse.

Diagnosis

Diagnosis is based on the patient's history and laboratory results. Arterial blood gas measurement, the most important test, indicates decreased partial pressure of oxygen (<60 mm Hg) and increased partial pressure of carbon dioxide (>50 mm Hg). Chest X-rays may show a foreign body, pulmonary edema, or atelectasis. Toxicology tests may show drugs, chemicals, or abnormal hemoglobin (carboxyhemoglobin). Pulmonary function tests may indicate respiratory muscle weakness.

Treatment

Asphyxia requires immediate respiratory support—with CPR, endotracheal intubation, and supplemental oxygen, as needed, and elimination of the underlying cause as follows: bronchoscopy for a foreign body extraction, an opioid antagonist such as naloxone for an opioid overdose, gastric lavage for poisoning, and withholding of supplemental oxygen for carbon dioxide narcosis because of excessive oxygen therapy.

Special considerations

Respiratory distress is frightening, so reassure the patient during treatment. Give prescribed drugs. Suction carefully as needed and encourage deep breathing. Closely monitor vital signs and laboratory test results. To prevent drug-induced asphyxia, warn patients about the danger of taking alcohol with other central nervous system depressants.

DROWNING

Nonfatal drowning (NFD) refers to surviving—temporarily, at least—the physiologic effects of hypoxemia and acidosis that result from submersion in fluid. Hypoxemia and acidosis are the primary problems in victims of NFD.

NFD drowning occurs in three forms: *dry*, in which the victim doesn't aspirate fluid, but suffers respiratory obstruction or asphyxia (10% to 15% of patients); *wet*, in which the victim aspirates fluid and suffers from asphyxia or secondary changes because of fluid aspiration (about 85% of patients); and *secondary*, in which the victim suffers a recurrence of respiratory distress (usually aspiration pneumonia or pulmonary edema) within minutes or 1 to 2 days after an NFD incident.

Causes and incidence

NFD results from an inability to swim or, in swimmers, from panic, a boating accident, a heart attack or blow to the head while in the water; a fall through ice; heavy drinking prior to swimming; or a suicide attempt. Children can also suffer from swimming accidents, bathing, or falling into a container of water such as a bucket or a body of water such as a pond.

Regardless of the tonicity of the fluid aspirated, hypoxemia is the most serious consequence of NFD, followed by metabolic acidosis. Other consequences depend on the kind of water aspirated. If the water is contaminated, such as water from a stagnant pool or contaminated stream, bacteria, fungus, or algae may be aspirated as well, causing infection or sepsis. After fresh water aspiration, changes in lung surfactant character result in exudation of protein-rich plasma into the alveoli. This, plus increased capillary permeability, leads to pulmonary edema and hypoxemia.

After saltwater aspiration, the hypertonicity of seawater exerts an osmotic force, which pulls fluid from pulmonary capillaries into the alveoli. The resulting intrapulmonary shunt causes hypoxemia. Also, the pulmonary capillary membrane may be injured and induce pulmonary edema. In both kinds of near drowning, pulmonary edema and hypoxemia occur secondary to aspiration.

In the United States, drowning claims nearly 6,500 lives annually. No statistics are available for NFD incidents.

Pathophysiology

When water fills the airway, hypoxia, hypercapnia, and acidosis (from anaerobic metabolism) start. Tachycardia and hypertension start with a flood of catecholamines, increasing the oxygen-debt.

Complications

◆ Neurologic impairment
◆ Seizure disorders
◆ Pulmonary edema
◆ Renal damage
◆ Bacterial aspiration
◆ Cardiac arrhythmias

Signs and symptoms

NFD victims can display a host of clinical problems: apnea, shallow or gasping respirations, substernal chest pain, asystole, tachycardia, bradycardia, restlessness, irritability, lethargy, fever, confusion, unconsciousness, vomiting, abdominal distention, and a cough that produces a pink, frothy fluid.

Diagnosis

Diagnosis requires a history of NFD, including the type of water aspirated, along with characteristic features and auscultation of crackles and rhonchi if respirations are present or the patient is being ventilated.

Arterial blood gas (ABG) analysis shows decreased oxygen content, low bicarbonate levels, and low pH. Electrolyte levels may be elevated or decreased, depending on the type of water aspirated. Leukocytosis may occur. Electrocardiogram shows arrhythmias and waveform changes.

Treatment

Emergency treatment begins with CPR and administration of 100% oxygen.

◆ Stabilize the patient's neck in case of a cervical injury.

◆ When the patient arrives at the hospital, assess for a patent airway. Establish one if necessary. Continue CPR, intubate the patient, and provide respiratory assistance such as mechanical ventilation with positive end-expiratory pressure, if needed.

◆ Assess ABG and pulse oximetry values.

◆ If the patient's abdomen is distended, insert a nasogastric tube. (Intubate the patient first if he's unconscious.) Eighty-six percent of these victims will regurgitate stomach contents during resuscitation and/or CPR.

◆ Start I.V. lines and insert an indwelling urinary catheter.

◆ Drug treatment for near drowning may include sodium bicarbonate for documented acidosis, osmotic diuretics for cerebral edema, antibiotics to prevent infections, and bronchodilators to ease bronchospasms.

Special considerations

◆ Remember that all NFD victims should be admitted for an observation period of 24 to 48 hours because of the possibility of developing delayed drowning symptoms.

◆ Observe for pulmonary complications and signs of delayed drowning (confusion, substernal pain, adventitious breath sounds). Suction often. Pulmonary artery catheters may be useful in assessing cardiopulmonary status.

◆ Monitor vital signs, intake and output, and peripheral pulses. Check for skin perfusion and watch for signs of infection.

◆ To facilitate breathing, raise the bed's head slightly.

░░░░░ **PREVENTION** *Advise swimmers to avoid drinking alcohol before swimming, to observe water safety rules, and to take a water safety course sponsored by the Red Cross or YMCA.*

DECOMPRESSION SICKNESS

Decompression sickness (the "bends") is a painful condition that results from a too-rapid change from a high- to low-pressure environment (decompression). Most victims are scuba divers who ascend too quickly from water deeper than 30′ (9.1 m) and pilots and passengers of unpressurized aircraft who ascend too quickly to high altitudes.

Causes and incidence

Decompression sickness results from an abrupt change in air or water pressure that causes inhaled gases to spill out of tissues faster than it can be diffused through respiration. It causes gas bubbles to form in blood and body tissues, which produce excruciating joint and muscle pain, neurologic and respiratory distress, and skin changes.

Pathophysiology

Gases filling hollow spaces in the body such as the intestines, as well as gases dissolved in the blood are subject to changes in pressure. Ascending too fast from an area of higher to an area of lower pressure creates nitrogen bubbles in these hollow spaces. These bubbles serve as small emboli, obstructing flow when lodged in vascular beds, nerve pathways, joints, and muscle tissue.

Complications

◆ Massive venous air embolism
◆ Intravascular volume depletion
◆ Avascular necrosis

Signs and symptoms

Symptoms usually appear during or within 30 minutes of rapid decompression, although they may be delayed up to 24 hours. Typically, decompression sickness results in:

◆ "the bends," deep and usually constant joint and muscle pain so severe that it may be incapacitating

◆ transitory neurologic disturbances, such as difficult urination (from bladder paralysis), hemiplegia, deafness, visual disturbances, dizziness, aphasia, paresthesia and hyperesthesia of the legs, unsteady gait, and, possibly, coma

◆ respiratory distress (known as the "chokes"), which includes chest pain, retrosternal burning, and a cough that may become paroxysmal and uncontrollable

Such symptoms may persist for days and result in dyspnea, cyanosis, fainting, and, occasionally, shock. Other symptoms include decreased temperature, pallor, itching, burning, mottled skin, fatigue, and, in some patients, tachypnea.

Diagnosis

℞ **CONFIRMING DIAGNOSIS** *A history of rapid decompression and a physical examination showing characteristic clinical features confirm the diagnosis.*

Treatment

Treatment consists of recompression and oxygen administration, followed by gradual decompression. In recompression, which takes place in a hyperbaric chamber (not available in all hospitals), air pressure is increased to 2.8 absolute atmospheric pressure over 1 to 2 minutes. This rapid rise in pressure reduces the size of the circulating nitrogen bubbles and relieves pain and other clinical effects. During recompression, intermittent oxygen administration, with periodic maximal exhalations, promotes gas bubble diffusion. After symptoms subside and diffusion is complete, a slow decrease of air pressure in the chamber allows for gradual, safe decompression.

Supportive measures include fluid replacement in hypovolemic shock and, sometimes, corticosteroids to reduce the risk of spinal edema. Opioids are contraindicated because they further depress impaired respiration.

Special considerations
◆ To avoid oxygen toxicity during recompression, tell the patient to alternate breathing oxygen for 5 minutes with breathing air for 5 minutes.
◆ During oxygen administration, make sure all electrical equipment is grounded. Prohibit smoking, the use of electric appliances such as razors, and the use of blankets made of wool or other materials that produce static electricity in the patient's room.
◆ If the patient with bladder paralysis needs catheterization, monitor intake and output.

▓▓▓▓▓ **PREVENTION** *Advise divers and pilots to follow the U.S. Navy's ascent guidelines.*

RADIATION EXPOSURE

Expanded use of ionized radiation (X-rays, protons, neutrons, and alpha, beta, and gamma rays) has vastly increased the incidence of radiation exposure. Cancer patients receiving radiation therapy and nuclear power plant workers are the most likely victims of this modern anomaly.

The amount of radiation absorbed by a human body is measured in radiation absorbed doses (rads), not to be confused with roentgens, which are used to measure radiation emissions. A person can absorb up to 200 rads without fatal consequences. A dose of 300 to 400 rads is fatal in about 50% of cases; more than 400 rads is nearly always fatal. (See *Effects of whole-body irradiation.*) However, when radiation is focused on a small area, the body can absorb and survive many thousands of rads if they're administered in carefully controlled doses over a long period of time. This basic principle is the key to safe and successful radiation therapy.

Causes and incidence
Exposure to radiation can occur by inhalation, ingestion, or direct contact. The existence and severity of tissue damage depend on the amount of body area exposed (the smaller, the better), length of exposure, dosage absorbed, distance from the source, and presence of protective shielding. Ionized radiation may cause

---

Effects of whole-body irradiation

Symptoms after whole-body irradiation are dose dependent. Below you'll find the effects of radiation dosages ranging from 5 to 5,000 rads.

Radiation dosage (rad)	Clinical and laboratory findings
5 to 20	Patient asymptomatic; conventional blood studies normal; chromosome aberrations detectable
20 to 100	Patient asymptomatic; minor decreases in white blood cell (WBC) and platelet counts in a few patients, especially if baseline values were established
100 to 200	Prodromal symptoms (anorexia, nausea, vomiting, fatigue) in 10% to 20% of patients within 2 days; mild decrease in WBC and platelet counts in some patients
200 to 300	Transient disability and clear hematologic changes in a majority of patients; lymphocyte count decreased by about 50% within 48 hours
300 to 400	Serious, disabling illness in most patients, with about 50% mortality if untreated; lymphocyte count decreased by 75% or more within 48 hours
400 to 1,000	Accelerated version of acute radiation syndrome with GI complications within 2 weeks; bleeding; death in most patients
1,000 to 5,000+	Fulminating course with cardiovascular, GI, and central nervous system complications, resulting in death within 24 to 72 hours

immediate cell necrosis or disturbed deoxyribonucleic acid synthesis, which impairs cell function and division. Rapidly dividing cells—bone marrow, hair follicles, gonads, and lymph tissue—are most susceptible to radiation damage; highly differentiated cells—nerve, bone, and muscle—resist radiation more successfully.

Pathophysiology
Localized exposure to high doses of radiation may cause blistering and ulceration similar to burns. The skin and the lining of the GI tract are specifically sensitive to radiation. Intestinal mucosal stem cells are quickly killed, causing symptoms such as nausea, vomiting, anorexia, fatigue, diarrhea, abdominal cramping, and dehydration. Translocation of bacteria out of the GI tract occurs, which increases the chance of sepsis. Blood cells are also involved, as lymphocytes die from radiation exposure and the bone marrow is suppressed, halting the creation of more cells.

Complications
The complications listed here are delayed.
- Leukemia
- Thyroid cancer
- Fetal growth retardation
- Genetic defects

Signs and symptoms
The effects of ionized radiation can be immediate and acute or delayed and chronic. Acute effects may be hematopoietic (after 200 to 500 rads), GI (after 400 rads or more), cerebral (after 1,000 rads or more), or cardiovascular (gross after 5,000 rads). They depend strictly on the amount of radiation absorbed.

Acute hematopoietic radiation exposure induces nausea, vomiting, diarrhea, and anorexia, which subside after 24 to 48 hours. Pancytopenia develops during the latent period that follows. Within 2 to 3 weeks, thrombocytopenia, leukopenia, lymphopenia, and anemia produce nosebleeds, hemorrhage, petechiae, pallor, weakness, oropharyngeal abscesses, and increased susceptibility to infection because of impaired immunologic response.

GI radiation exposure causes ulceration, infection, intractable nausea, vomiting, and diarrhea, resulting in severe fluid and electrolyte imbalance. Breakdown of intestinal villi later causes plasma loss, which can lead to circulatory collapse and death.

Cerebral radiation poisoning after brief exposure to large amounts of radiation causes nausea, vomiting, and diarrhea within hours. Lethargy, tremors, seizures, confusion, coma, and even death may follow within hours or days.

Repeated, prolonged exposure to small doses of radiation over a long time can seriously damage skin, causing dryness, erythema, atrophy, and malignant lesions. Such damage can also follow acute exposure. (See *Radiation dermatitis*.)

Other delayed effects include alopecia, brittle nails, hypothyroidism, amenorrhea, cataracts, decreased fertility, anemia, leukopenia, thrombocytopenia, malignant neoplasms, bone necrosis and fractures, and a shortened life span. Long-term exposure to radiation may retard fetal growth or cause genetic defects.

Diagnosis
An accurate history offers the best clues to radiation exposure. Supportive laboratory findings show decreased hematocrit; decreased white blood cell, platelet, and lymphocyte counts; and decreased hemoglobin, serum potassium, and chloride levels because of vomiting and diarrhea. Bone marrow studies show blood dyscrasia; X-rays may reveal bone necrosis. A Geiger counter may help determine the amount of radiation in open wounds.

Treatment
Treatment is essentially aimed at relieving symptoms and includes antiemetics to counter nausea and vomiting, fluid and electrolyte replacement, antibiotics, and possibly sedatives (if seizures occur). Transfusions of plasma, platelets, and red blood cells may be necessary. Bone marrow transplantation is a controversial treatment but may be the only recourse in extreme cases. When radiation exposure results from inhalation or ingestion of large amounts of radioactive iodine, potassium iodide or a strong iodine solution may be given to block thyroid uptake.

Radiation dermatitis
Repeated prolonged exposure to radiation—even small doses—often induces erythematous dermatitis and atrophy of skin at the site of radiation treatment.

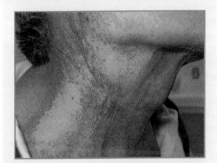

Special considerations

◆ To minimize radiation exposure, dispose of contaminated clothing properly. If the patient's skin is contaminated, wash the body thoroughly with mild soap and water. Debride and irrigate open wounds. If the patient recently ingested radioactive material, induce vomiting and start lavage.

◆ Monitor intake and output and maintain fluid and electrolyte balance. Give I.V. fluids and electrolytes as ordered. If the patient can take oral feedings, encourage a high-protein, high-calorie diet. Tell the patient to use a soft toothbrush to minimize gum bleeding. Offer lidocaine to soothe painful mouth ulcers.

◆ To prevent skin breakdown, make sure the patient avoids extreme temperatures, tight clothing, and drying soaps. Use rigid sterile technique.

◆ Prevent complications. Monitor vital signs and watch for signs of hemorrhage.

◆ Provide emotional support for the patient and family, especially after severe exposure. Suggest genetic counseling and screening as needed.

Hospital personnel can avoid exposure to radiation by wearing proper shielding devices when supervising X-ray and radiation treatments. If you work in these vulnerable areas, wear radiation detection badges and turn them in periodically for readings. (See *Preventing radiation exposure*.)

Miscellaneous injuries

POISONING

Poisoning—inhalation, ingestion, or injection of, or skin contamination with, a harmful substance—is a common problem. The prognosis depends on the amount of poison absorbed, the poison's toxicity, and the time interval between poisoning and treatment.

Causes and incidence

In the United States, about 2.5 million people are poisoned annually, 1,000 of them fatally. Because of their curiosity and ignorance, children are the primary victims of poisoning. Accidental poisoning—usually from ingestion of salicylates (aspirin), acetaminophen, cleaning agents, insecticides, paints, or cosmetics—is the fourth leading cause of death in children.

In adults, poisoning is most common among chemical company employees, particularly those in companies that use chlorine, carbon dioxide, hydrogen sulfide, nitrogen dioxide, and ammonia, and in companies that ignore safety standards. Other causes of poisoning in adults include improper cooking, canning, and storage of food; ingestion of, or skin contact with, plants (See *Common poisonous plants*, page 961.); and drug overdose (usually barbiturates or tricyclic antidepressants).

Common poisonous plants

ELEPHANT EAR PHILODENDRON

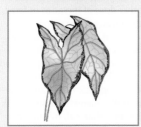

Symptoms: burning throat and GI distress
Treatment: gastric lavage or emesis; antihistamines and lime juice; symptomatic treatment

DIEFFENBACHIA

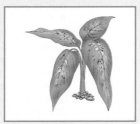

Symptoms: burning throat, edema, GI distress
Treatment: gastric lavage or emesis; antihistamines and lime juice; symptomatic treatment

POINSETTIA (MILKY JUICE)

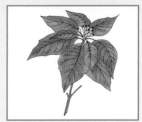

Symptoms: inflammation and blisters
Treatment: none; condition will disappear after several days

RHUBARB

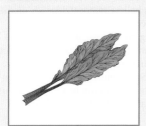

Symptoms: GI and respiratory distress, internal bleeding, coma
Treatment: gastric lavage or emesis with lime water; calcium gluconate and force fluids

MUSHROOMS

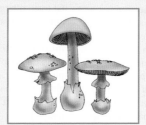

Symptoms: GI, respiratory, central nervous system, and parasympathomimetic effects
Treatment: gastric emesis with syrup of ipecac; decontamination with activated charcoal with sorbitol for catharsis; atropine

MISTLETOE

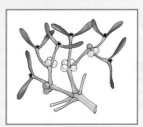

Symptoms: GI distress and slow pulse
Treatment: gastric lavage or emesis; cardiac drugs, potassium, and sodium

POISON IVY

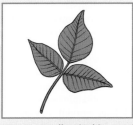

POISON OAK

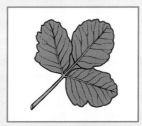

POISON SUMAC (SAP)

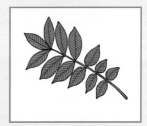

Symptoms: allergic skin reactions; if ingested, GI distress, liver and kidney damage.
Treatment: if ingested: demulcents, morphine, fluids, and high-protein, low-fat diet; for skin reactions: antihistamines and topical antipyretics

Pathophysiology

The pathophysiology of poisoning is specific to each agent. However, poisoning causes a cadre of hypotension, cardiac arrhythmias, and can lead to coma or death. Absorption can be through the lungs, skin, or GI system.

Complications

◆ Hypotension
◆ Cardiac arrhythmias
◆ Seizures
◆ Coma
◆ Death

Signs and symptoms

Signs and symptoms vary according to the type of poison.

Diagnosis

A history of ingestion, inhalation, or injection of, or skin contact with, a poisonous substance and typical clinical features suggest the diagnosis. Suspect poisoning in any unconscious patient with no history of diabetes, seizure disorders, or trauma. Odors, such as from kerosene or cleaning fluid, may be detected on the breath or clothing of some poison victims.

℞ CONFIRMING DIAGNOSIS *Toxicologic studies (including drug screens) of poison in the mouth, vomitus, urine, feces, or blood or poison on the victim's hands or clothing confirm the diagnosis.*

If possible, have the family or patient bring the container holding the poison to the emergency department for comparable study. In inhalation poisoning, chest X-rays may show pulmonary infiltrates or edema; in petroleum distillate inhalation, X-rays may show aspiration pneumonia.

Effects of some poisonous substances don't become apparent for hours or days.

Treatment

Treatment includes emergency resuscitation and support, prevention of further absorption of poison, continuing supportive or symptomatic care, and, when possible, a specific antidote. If barbiturate, or tranquilizer poisoning causes hypothermia, use a hyperthermia blanket to control the patient's temperature. Dialysis may be considered in some situations.

Special considerations

◆ Assess cardiopulmonary and respiratory function. If necessary, begin CPR. Carefully monitor vital signs and LOC.
◆ Depending on the type of poison, prevent further absorption of ingested poison by inducing vomiting using syrup of ipecac or by administering gastric lavage and cathartics. The treatment's effectiveness depends on absorption speed and the time elapsed between ingestion and removal. With syrup of ipecac, give warm water (usually <1 qt [1 L]) until vomiting occurs, or give another dose of ipecac as ordered.
◆ Never induce vomiting if you suspect corrosive acid poisoning, if the patient is unconscious or has seizures, or if the gag reflex is impaired (even in a conscious patient). Instead, neutralize the poison by instilling the appropriate antidote by nasogastric tube. Common antidotes include milk, magnesium salts (milk of magnesia), activated charcoal, or other chelating agents (deferoxamine, edetate disodium). When possible, add the antidote to water or juice.

Note: The removal of hydrocarbon poisons is controversial. For a conscious patient, gastric lavage is preferred over syrup of ipecac, especially in the emergency department. Some believe that because of poor absorption, kerosene (a hydrocarbon) doesn't require removal from the GI tract; others believe removal depends on the amount ingested.
◆ To perform gastric lavage, instill 150 to 200 mL of fluid using a large-bore gastric evacuation tube; then aspirate the liquid. Repeat until aspirate is clear. Save vomitus and aspirate for analysis. (To prevent aspiration in an unconscious patient, insert an endotracheal tube before lavage.)
◆ When you want to induce emesis and the patient has already taken syrup of ipecac, don't give activated charcoal to neutralize the poison until *after* emesis. Activated charcoal absorbs ipecac.
◆ If several hours have passed since the patient ingested the poison, administer large quantities of I.V. fluids to induce diuresis. The kind of fluid you'll use depends on the patient's acid–base balance and cardiovascular status as well as on the flow rate.
◆ Severe ingested poisoning may call for peritoneal dialysis or hemodialysis.
◆ To prevent further absorption of inhaled poison, move the patient to fresh or uncontaminated air. Alert the anesthesia department and provide supplemental oxygen. Some patients may require intubation. To prevent further absorption from skin contamination, remove clothing covering the contaminated skin and flush the area with large amounts of water.
◆ If the patient is in severe pain, give analgesics as indicated; frequently monitor fluid intake and output, vital signs, and LOC.
◆ Keep the patient warm and provide support in a quiet environment.

◆ If the poison was ingested intentionally, maintain suicide precautions and refer the patient for counseling to prevent future suicide attempts.

◆ For more specific treatment, contact your local poison center.

▓▓▓▓ PREVENTION *To prevent accidental poisoning:*

◆ *Instruct patients to read the label before they take medicine. Tell them to store all medications and household chemicals properly, to keep them out of reach of children, and to discard old medications.*

◆ *Warn patients not to take medicines prescribed for someone else, not to transfer medicines from their original bottles to other containers without labeling them properly, and never to transfer poisons to food containers.*

◆ *Tell parents not to take medicine in front of young children and not to call medicine "candy" to get children to take it.*

◆ *Stress the importance of using toxic sprays only in well-ventilated areas and of following instructions carefully.*

◆ *Tell patients to use pesticides carefully and to keep the number of their poison control center handy.*

POISONOUS SNAKEBITES

Poisonous snakebites are medical emergencies. With prompt, correct treatment, they need not be fatal. The only poisonous snakes in the United States are pit vipers (*Crotalidae*) and coral snakes (*Elapidae*). Pit vipers, such as rattlesnakes, water moccasins (cottonmouths), and copperheads, have a pitted depression between their eyes and nostrils and two fangs, ¾" to 1¼" (2 to 3 cm) long. Because fangs may break off or grow behind old ones, some snakes may have one, three, or four fangs. The fangs of coral snakes are short, but have teeth behind them. Coral snakes have distinctive red, black, and yellow bands (yellow bands always border red ones).

Causes and incidence

Of the approximately 45,000 snakebites that occur in the United States each year, 7,000 to 8,000 are from poisonous snakes, resulting in 5 to 6 deaths. Such bites are most common during summer afternoons in grassy or rocky habitats.

Pit vipers are nocturnal but active snakes that are responsible for 99% of venomous snakebites in the United States. Coral snakes are also nocturnal, but their placidity makes coral snakebites less common than pit viper bites. Coral snakes tend to bite with a chewing motion, and may leave multiple fang marks, small lacerations, and extensive tissue destruction.

Pathophysiology

The venom of poisonous snakes consists of neurotoxins and enzymatic proteins. These both disrupt proteins in cell walls, creating tissue necrosis. Some snakes possess venom with neuromuscular blocker properties, which may result in respiratory failure.

Complications
Pit viper bite
◆ Extensive vasculitis
◆ Necrosis
◆ Skin and subcutaneous tissue sloughing

Coral snakebite
◆ Respiratory arrest
◆ Cardiovascular collapse
◆ Death

Signs and symptoms

Most snakebites happen on the arms and legs, below the elbow or knee. Bites to the head or trunk are most dangerous, but any bite into a blood vessel is dangerous, regardless of location.

Most pit viper bites that result in envenomation cause immediate and progressively severe pain and edema within 30 minutes, local elevation in skin temperature, fever, skin discoloration, petechiae, ecchymoses, blebs, blisters, bloody wound discharge, and local necrosis. (See *After a snakebite.*)

Because pit viper venom is neurotoxic, pit viper bites may cause local and facial numbness and tingling, fasciculation and twitching of skeletal muscles, seizures (especially in children), extreme anxiety, difficulty speaking, fainting, weakness, dizziness, excessive sweating,

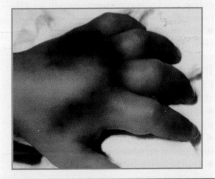

After a snakebite

Severe edema of the affected limb, as shown below, occurs within hours after a snakebite.

occasional paralysis, mild to severe respiratory distress, headache, blurred vision, marked thirst, and, in severe envenomation, coma and death. Pit viper venom may also impair coagulation and cause hematemesis, hematuria, melena, bleeding gums, and internal bleeding. Other symptoms of pit viper bites include tachycardia, lymphadenopathy, nausea, vomiting, diarrhea, hypotension, and shock.

The reaction to coral snakebite is usually delayed—sometimes up to several hours. These snakebites cause little or no local tissue reaction (local pain, swelling, or necrosis). However, because coral snake venom is neurotoxic, a reaction can progress swiftly, producing such effects as local paresthesia, drowsiness, nausea, vomiting, difficulty swallowing, marked saliva-tion, dysphonia, ptosis, blurred vision, miosis, respiratory distress and possible respiratory fail-ure, loss of muscle coordination, and, possibly, shock with cardiovascular collapse and death.

Diagnosis

The patient's history and account of the injury, observation of fang marks, snake identification (when possible), and progressive symptoms of envenomation all point to poisonous snakebite. Laboratory test results help identify the extent of envenomation and provide guidelines for supportive treatment.

Abnormal test results in poisonous snake-bites may include:
♦ prolonged bleeding time and partial throm-boplastin time
♦ decreased hemoglobin level and hematocrit
♦ sharply decreased platelet count ($<200,000/\mu L$)
♦ urinalysis disclosing hematuria
♦ increased white blood cell count in victims who develop an infection (A snake's mouth typ-ically contains gram-negative bacteria.)
♦ pulmonary edema or emboli as shown on chest X-ray
♦ possibly tachycardia and ectopic heartbeats on the electrocardiogram (usually necessary only in cases of severe envenomation for a pa-tient older than age 40)
♦ possibly abnormal Electroencephalogram (EEG) findings in cases of severe envenomation.

Treatment

Prompt, appropriate first aid can reduce venom absorption and prevent severe symptoms.
♦ If possible, identify the snake, but don't waste time trying to find it.
♦ Place the victim in the supine position to slow venom metabolism and absorption.
♦ Don't give the victim any food, beverage, or medication orally.

♦ Authorities disagree about what constitutes appropriate prehospital care. Some recommend against placing a constrictive tourniquet (band) on the affected limb.
♦ Whether you apply a tourniquet or not, im-mediately immobilize the victim's affected limb below heart level, and instruct the victim to remain as quiet as possible.
♦ If a tourniquet is applied, the victim or the person applying the tourniquet should check the victim's distal pulses regularly and loosen the tourniquet slightly as needed to maintain circulation. Remember that the goal of applying a tourniquet is to obstruct lymphatic drainage, not blood flow.
♦ When indicated, apply the tourniquet so that it's slightly constrictive, obstructing only lym-phatic and superficial venous blood flow. Apply the band about 4″ (10 cm) above the fang marks or just above the first joint proximal to the bite. The tourniquet should be loose enough to allow a finger between the band and the skin. After the tourniquet is in place, don't remove it until a physician has examined the victim.

ALERT *Don't apply a tourniquet if more than 30 minutes have elapsed since the bite. Keep in mind also that total tourniquet time shouldn't exceed 2 hours and that the use of a tourniquet shouldn't delay antivenin administration. Loss of a limb is possible if a tourniquet is too tight or if tour-niquet time is too long.*

Using a bulb syringe—or, if no other means is available, mouth suction—apply suction for up to 1 hour in the absence of antivenin administration.

ALERT *Remember, an incision and suction are effective only in pit viper bites and only within 1 hour of the bite. Suction is also indicated if trans-port time to an emergency facility would exceed 30 minutes.*

ALERT *Never give the victim alcoholic drinks or stimulants because they speed venom ab-sorption. Never apply ice to a snakebite because it will increase tissue damage.*

♦ Record the signs and symptoms of progressive envenomation and when they develop. Most snakebite victims are hospitalized for only 24 to 48 hours. Treatment usually consists of antivenin administration, but minor snakebites may not require antivenin. Other treatments include teta-nus toxoid or tetanus immune globulin; various broad-spectrum antibiotics; and, depending on respiratory status, severity of pain, and the type of snakebite, acetaminophen, codeine, mor-phine, or meperidine. (Opioids are contraindi-cated for the treatment of coral snakebites.)

Necrotic snakebites usually need surgical debridement after 3 or 4 days. Intense, rapidly progressive edema requires fasciotomy within 2 or 3 hours of the bite; extreme envenomation may require amputation of the limb and subsequent reconstructive surgery, rehabilitation, and physical therapy.

Special considerations

When the patient arrives at the hospital, immobilize the limb if this hasn't already been done. If a tight tourniquet has been applied within the past hour, apply a loose tourniquet proximally and remove the first tourniquet. Release the second tourniquet gradually during antivenin administration as ordered. A sudden release of venom into the bloodstream can cause cardiorespiratory collapse, so keep emergency equipment handy.

◆ On a flow sheet, document vital signs, LOC, skin color, swelling, respiratory status, a description of the bite and surrounding area, and symptoms. Monitor vital signs every 15 minutes and check for a pulse in the affected limb.

◆ Start an I.V. line with a large-bore needle for antivenin administration. Severe bites that result in coagulotoxic signs and symptoms may require two I.V. lines: one for antivenin and one for blood products.

◆ Before antivenin administration, obtain a patient history of allergies and other medical problems. Perform hypersensitivity tests as appropriate and desensitization as needed. During antivenin administration, keep epinephrine, oxygen, and vasopressors available to combat anaphylaxis from horse serum.

◆ Give packed red blood cells, I.V. fluids, and, possibly, fresh frozen plasma or platelets, as indicated, to counteract coagulotoxicity and maintain blood pressure.

◆ If the patient develops respiratory distress and requires endotracheal intubation or a tracheotomy, provide good tracheostomy care.

◆ Give analgesics as needed. Don't give opioids to coral snakebite victims. Clean the snakebite using sterile technique. Open, debride, and drain any blebs and blisters because they may contain venom. Change dressings daily.

◆ If the patient requires hospitalization for more than 48 hours, position carefully to avoid contractures. Perform passive exercises until the fourth day after the bite; after that, perform active exercises and give whirlpool treatments as ordered.

INSECT BITES AND STINGS

Among the most common traumatic complaints are insect bites and stings, the more serious of which include those of ticks, brown recluse spiders, black widow spiders, scorpions, bees, wasps, and yellow jackets. (See *Comparing insect bites and stings*, page 966.)

OPEN TRAUMA WOUNDS

Open trauma wounds (abrasions, avulsions, crush wounds, lacerations, missile injuries, and punctures) are injuries that commonly result from home, work, or motor vehicle accidents and from acts of violence.

Causes and incidence

Open wounds most commonly result from an accidental injury at home or work, or from a car crash. Other open wounds, such as stab and gunshot wounds, may be intentionally inflicted by the victim or by someone else. Open wounds are occasionally self-inflicted by patients with psychiatric disorders or suicidal ideations.

Pathophysiology

Infection, soft-tissue damage, direct injury to neurovascular structures normally protected by muscle. Crushing injury creates ischemia to the area as well.

Complications

◆ Infection
◆ Organ tissue damage
◆ Scarring

Signs and symptoms

In all open wounds, assess the extent of injury, vital signs, LOC, obvious skeletal damage, local neurologic deficits, and general patient condition. Obtain an accurate history of the injury from the patient or witnesses, including such details as the mechanism and time of injury and any treatment already provided. If the injury involved a weapon, notify the police.

Also assess for peripheral nerve damage—a common complication in lacerations and other open trauma wounds—as well as for fractures and dislocations. Signs of peripheral nerve damage vary with location:

◆ *radial nerve*—weak forearm dorsiflexion, inability to extend thumb in a hitchhiker's sign
◆ *median nerve*—numbness in tip of index finger; inability to place forearm in prone position; weak forearm, thumb, and index finger flexion
◆ *ulnar nerve*—numbness in tip of little finger, clawing of hand
◆ *peroneal nerve*—footdrop, inability to extend the foot or big toe
◆ *sciatic and tibial nerves*—paralysis of ankles and toes, footdrop, leg weakness, numbness in sole.

Most open wounds require emergency treatment. In those with suspected nerve involvement, however, electromyography, nerve conduction, and electrical stimulation tests can provide more detailed information about possible peripheral nerve damage.

Comparing insect bites and stings

In addition to maintaining ABCs and assessing neurologic function, treatment varies according to the type of bite or sting.

General information	*Clinical features*
Tick	
♦ Common in woods and fields throughout the United States ♦ Attaches to host in any of its life stages (larva, nymph, or adult); fastens to host with its teeth, then secretes a cementlike material to reinforce attachment ♦ Flat, brown, speckled body about ¼" (6.4 mm) long; has eight legs ♦ Also transmits Rocky Mountain spotted fever and Lyme disease	♦ Itching may be the sole symptom or, after several days, the host may develop tick paralysis (acute flaccid paralysis, starting as paresthesia and leg pain and resulting in respiratory failure from bulbar paralysis).
Brown recluse (violin) spider	
♦ Common to south-central United States; usually found in dark areas (outdoor privy, barn, or woodshed) ♦ Dark brown violin on its back; three pairs of eyes; female more dangerous than male ♦ Most bites occur between April and October	♦ Venom is coagulotoxic. Reaction begins within 2 to 8 hours after bite. ♦ Localized vasoconstriction causes ischemic necrosis at bite site. A small, reddened puncture wound forms a bleb and becomes ischemic. In 3 to 4 days, the center becomes dark and hard. Within 2 to 3 weeks, an ulcer forms. ♦ Minimal initial pain increases over time. ♦ Other symptoms include fever, chills, malaise, weakness, nausea, vomiting, edema, seizures, joint pain, petechiae, cyanosis, and phlebitis. ♦ Rarely, thrombocytopenia and hemolytic anemia develop, leading to death within the first 24 to 48 hours (usually in a child or a patient with a previous history of cardiac disease). Prompt and appropriate treatment results in recovery.
Black widow spider	
♦ Common throughout the United States, particularly in warmer climates; usually found in dark areas (outdoor privy, barn, or woodshed) ♦ Female: coal black with red or orange hourglass on ventral side; larger than male (male doesn't bite) ♦ Mortality <1% (increased risk among elderly people, infants, and those with allergies)	♦ Venom is neurotoxic. Age, size, and sensitivity of the patient determine the severity and progression of symptoms. ♦ Pinprick sensation, followed by dull, numbing pain (may go unnoticed). ♦ Edema and tiny, red bite marks appear. ♦ Rigidity of stomach muscles and severe abdominal pain occur (10 to 40 minutes after bite). ♦ Muscle spasms occur in the extremities. ♦ Ascending paralysis develops, causing difficulty swallowing and labored, grunting respirations. ♦ Other symptoms include extreme restlessness, vertigo, sweating, chills, pallor, seizures (especially in children), hyperactive reflexes, hypertension, tachycardia, thready pulse, circulatory collapse, nausea, vomiting, headache, ptosis, eyelid edema, urticaria, pruritus, and fever.

Treatment	Special considerations
♦ Removal of tick ♦ Local antipruritics for itching papule ♦ Mechanical ventilation for respiratory failure	♦ To remove a tick, cover it with a tissue or gauze pad soaked in mineral, salad, or machine oil or alcohol. This blocks the tick's breathing pores and causes it to withdraw from the skin. If the tick doesn't disengage after the pad has been in place for a half hour, carefully remove it with tweezers, taking care to remove all parts. ♦ To reduce the risk of being bitten, teach the patient to keep away from wooded areas, to wear protective clothes, and to carefully examine the body for ticks after being outdoors. ♦ Teach patients how to safely remove ticks.
♦ No known specific treatment ♦ Combination therapy with corticosteroids, antibiotics, antihistamines, tranquilizers, I.V. fluids, and tetanus prophylaxis ♦ Dapsone 100 mg b.i.d. to suppress the leukocyte response ♦ Surgical debridement and skin grafting (large ulcerative lesions) ♦ Skin grafting (large chronic ulcer)	♦ Clean the lesion with a 1:20 Burow's aluminum acetate solution, and apply antibiotic ointment as ordered. ♦ Take a complete patient history, including allergies and other preexisting medical problems. ♦ Monitor vital signs, general appearance, and any changes at bite site. ♦ Reassure the patient with a disfiguring ulcer that skin grafting can improve the appearance. ♦ To prevent brown recluse spider bites, tell the patient to spray areas of infestation with creosote at least every 2 months, to wear gloves and heavy clothing when working around woodpiles or sheds, to inspect outdoor work clothing for spiders before use, and to discourage children from playing near infested areas.
♦ Neutralization of venom using antivenin I.V., preceded by desensitization when skin or eye tests show sensitivity to horse serum ♦ Calcium gluconate I.V. to control muscle spasms ♦ Muscle relaxants such as diazepam for severe muscle spasms ♦ Adrenaline or antihistamines ♦ Oxygen by nasal cannula or mask ♦ Tetanus immunization ♦ Antibiotics to prevent infection	♦ Take a complete patient history, including allergies and other preexisting medical problems. ♦ Have epinephrine and emergency resuscitation equipment on hand in case of anaphylactic reaction to antivenin. ♦ Keep the patient quiet and warm and the affected part immobile. ♦ Clean the bite site with an antiseptic; apply ice to relieve pain and swelling and to slow circulation. ♦ Check vital signs frequently during the first 12 hours after the bite. Report any changes to the physician. Symptoms usually subside in 3 to 4 hours. ♦ When giving analgesics, monitor respiratory status. ♦ To prevent black widow spider bites, tell the patient to spray areas of infestation with creosote at least every 2 months, to wear gloves and heavy clothing when working around woodpiles or sheds, to inspect outdoor work clothing for spiders before use, and to discourage children from playing near infested areas.

(continued)

Comparing insect bites and stings (*continued*)

General information	*Clinical features*
Scorpion	
◆ Common throughout the United States (30 different species); two deadly species in southwestern states ◆ Curled tail with stinger on end; eight legs; 3" (7.6 cm) long ◆ Most stings occur during warmer months ◆ Mortality <1% (increased risk among elderly people and children)	*Local reaction* ◆ Local swelling and tenderness, sharp burning sensation, skin discoloration, paresthesia, and lymphangitis with regional gland swelling occur. *Systemic reaction (neurotoxic)* ◆ Immediate sharp pain; hyperesthesia; drowsiness; itching of the nose, throat, and mouth; impaired speech (because of sluggish tongue); generalized muscle spasms (including jaw muscle spasms, laryngospasms, incontinence, and seizures) nausea, vomiting, and drooling occur. ◆ Symptoms last from 24 to 78 hours; the bite site recovers last. ◆ Anaphylaxis is rare. ◆ Death may follow cardiovascular or respiratory failure. ◆ The prognosis is poor if symptoms progress rapidly in the first few hours.
Bee, wasp, and yellow jacket	
◆ Honeybee (rounded abdomen) or bumblebee (over 1" [2.5 cm] long; furry, rounded abdomen)—stinger remains in the victim; bee flies away and dies ◆ Wasp or yellow jacket (slender body with elongated abdomen)—retains stinger and can sting repeatedly	*Local reaction* ◆ Painful wound (protruding stinger from bees), edema, urticaria, and pruritus can occur. *Systemic reaction (anaphylaxis)* ◆ Symptoms of hypersensitivity usually appear within 20 minutes and may include weakness, chest tightness, dizziness, nausea, vomiting, abdominal cramps, and throat constriction. The shorter the interval between the sting and systemic symptoms, the worse the prognosis. Without prompt treatment, symptoms may progress to cyanosis, coma, and death.

Diagnosis

A thorough physical examination of the patient will reveal traumatic wounds. They may be seen during the primary and secondary assessment of the patient.

Treatment

If hemorrhage occurs, stop bleeding by applying direct pressure on the wound and, if necessary, on arterial pressure points. If the wound is on a limb, elevate it if possible. Don't apply a tourniquet except in a life-threatening hemorrhage. If you must do so, be aware that resulting lack of perfusion to tissue could require limb amputation. (For a description of types of wounds and specific management, see *Managing open trauma wounds*, pages 970 to 972.)

Special considerations

◆ Frequently assess vital signs in patients with major wounds. Be alert for a 20-beat increase in pulse and 20 mm Hg drop in blood pressure (compare the patient's pulse and blood pressure taken when he's sitting with those taken when he's lying down), increased respiratory rate, decreased LOC, thirst, and cool, clammy skin—all indicate blood loss and hypovolemic shock.

◆ Administer oxygen as needed.

Treatment	Special considerations
♦ Antivenin (made from goat serum) if available, to neutralize toxins ♦ Calcium gluconate I.V. for muscle spasm ♦ Anticonvulsants for seizures ♦ Emetine subcutaneously to relieve pain (opioids, such as morphine and codeine, contraindicated because they enhance the venom's effects)	♦ Take a complete patient history, including allergies and other preexisting medical conditions. ♦ Immobilize the patient, and apply a tourniquet proximal to the sting. ♦ Pack the area extending beyond the tourniquet in ice. After 5 minutes of ice pack, remove the tourniquet. ♦ Monitor vital signs. Watch closely for signs of respiratory distress. (Keep emergency resuscitation equipment available.)
♦ Antihistamines and corticosteroids (in urticaria) ♦ Tetanus prophylaxis ♦ In anaphylaxis, oxygen by nasal cannula or mask and epinephrine 1:1,000 subcutaneously or I.M. ♦ In bronchospasm, albuterol and corticosteroids ♦ In hypotension, epinephrine and isoproterenol	♦ If the stinger is in place, scrape it off. Don't pull it; this action releases more toxin. ♦ Clean the site and apply ice. ♦ Watch the patient carefully for signs of anaphylaxis. Keep emergency resuscitation equipment available. ♦ Tell a patient who's allergic to bee stings to wear a medical identification bracelet or carry a card and to carry an anaphylaxis kit. Teach they how to use the kit, and refer they to an allergist for hyposensitization. ♦ To prevent bee stings, tell the patient to avoid wearing fragrant cosmetics during insect season, to avoid wearing bright colors and going barefoot, to avoid flowers and fruit that attract bees, and to use insect repellent.

♦ Send blood samples to the laboratory for type and crossmatch, complete blood count (including hematocrit and hemoglobin level), and prothrombin and partial thromboplastin times.
♦ Prepare the patient for surgery if needed.
♦ As much as possible, tell the patient about the procedures that he'll undergo (even if he's unconscious) and provide reassurance.
♦ Start I.V. lines, using two large-bore catheters, and infuse lactated Ringer's solution, normal saline solution, or whole blood as ordered.
♦ Insert a central venous pressure line and place the patient in a modified V position (with head flat and legs elevated). If the modified V

position doesn't help, Trendelenburg's position may be an alternative.

RAPE TRAUMA SYNDROME
The term *rape* refers to sexual intercourse without consent. It's a violent assault in which sex is used as a weapon. Rape inflicts varying degrees of physical and psychological trauma. Rape trauma syndrome occurs during the period following the rape or attempted rape; it refers to the victim's short-term and long-term reactions and to the methods the victim uses to cope with this trauma.

In most cases, the rapist is a male and the victim is a female. However, rapes do occur

Managing open trauma wounds

After securing ABCs, and neurologic status, specific treatment of the wound will depend on its severity.

Type	Clinical action
Abrasion	
✦ Open surface wounds (scrapes) of epidermis and possibly the dermis, resulting from friction; nerve endings exposed ✦ Diagnosis based on scratches, reddish welts, bruises, pain, and history of friction injury	✦ Obtain a history to distinguish injury from second-degree burn. ✦ Clean the wound gently with topical germicide, and irrigate it. Too vigorous scrubbing of abrasions will increase tissue damage. ✦ Remove all imbedded foreign objects. Apply a local anesthetic if cleaning is very painful. ✦ Apply a light, water-soluble antibiotic cream to prevent infection. ✦ If the wound is severe, apply a loose protective dressing that allows air to circulate. ✦ Administer tetanus prophylaxis if necessary.
Avulsion	
✦ Complete tissue loss that prevents approximation of wound edges, resulting from cutting, gouging, or complete tearing of skin; frequently affects nose tip, earlobe, fingertip, and penis ✦ Diagnosis based on full-thickness skin loss, hemorrhage, pain, history of trauma; X-ray required to rule out bone damage	✦ Check the patient's history for bleeding tendencies and use of anticoagulants. ✦ Record the time of injury to help determine if tissue is salvageable. Preserve tissue (if available) in cool normal saline solution for a possible split-thickness graft or flap. ✦ Control hemorrhage with pressure, an absorbable gelatin sponge, or topical thrombin. ✦ Clean the wound gently, irrigate it with normal saline solution, and debride it if necessary. Cover with a bulky dressing. ✦ Tell the patient to leave the dressing in place until the return visit, to keep the area dry, and to watch for signs of infection (pain, fever, redness, and swelling). ✦ Administer analgesics and tetanus prophylaxis, if necessary.
Crush wound	
✦ Heavy falling object splits skin, causes necrosis along split margins, and damages tissue underneath; may look like a laceration ✦ Diagnosis based on history of trauma, edema, hemorrhage, massive hematomas, damage to surrounding tissues (fractures, nerve injuries, or loss of tendon function), shock, and pain; X-rays required to determine extent of injury to surrounding structures; complete blood count (CBC) and differential and electrolyte count also required	✦ Check the patient's history for bleeding tendencies and use of anticoagulants. ✦ Clean open areas gently with soap and water. ✦ Control hemorrhage with pressure and a cold pack. ✦ Apply a dry, sterile bulky dressing; wrap the entire extremity in a compression dressing. ✦ Immobilize the injured extremity, and encourage the patient to rest. Monitor vital signs, and check peripheral pulses and circulation often. ✦ Administer tetanus prophylaxis if necessary. ✦ A severe injury may require I.V. infusion of lactated Ringer's or normal saline solution with a large-bore catheter as well as surgical exploration, debridement, and repair.

Managing open trauma wounds (*continued*)

Type	Clinical action

Laceration

♦ Open wound, possibly extending into deep epithelium, resulting from penetration with knife or other sharp object or from a severe blow with a blunt object

♦ Diagnosis based on hemorrhage, torn or destroyed tissues, pain, and history of trauma

In a laceration <8 hours old and in all lacerations of the face and areas of possible functional disability (such as the elbow):

♦ Apply pressure and elevate the injured extremity to control hemorrhage.

♦ Clean the wound gently with normal saline solution or water; irrigate with normal saline solution.

♦ As necessary, debride necrotic margins and close the wound, using strips of tape or sutures.

♦ A severe laceration with underlying structural damage may require surgery.

In grossly contaminated lacerations or lacerations >8 hours old (except lacerations of the face and areas of possible functional disability):

♦ Administer a broad-spectrum antibiotic for at least a 5-day course.

♦ Don't close the wound immediately.

♦ Instruct the patient to elevate the injured extremity for 24 hours after the injury to reduce swelling.

♦ Tell they to keep the dressing clean and dry and to watch for signs of infection.

♦ If, after 5 to 7 days, the wound appears uninfected with healthy granulated tissue, you may close it with sutures or a butterfly dressing or allow it to heal by itself.

♦ Apply a sterile dressing and splint.

In all lacerations:

♦ Check the patient's history for bleeding tendencies and anticoagulant use.

♦ Determine the approximate time of injury, and estimate the amount of blood lost.

♦ Assess for neuromuscular, tendon, and circulatory damage.

♦ Administer tetanus prophylaxis as needed.

♦ Stress the need for follow-up and suture removal.

♦ If sutures become infected, culture the wound and scrub with surgical soap preparation. Remove some or all sutures, and give a broad-spectrum antibiotic as appropriate. Instruct the patient to soak the wound in warm, soapy water for 15 minutes, three times daily, and to return for a follow-up visit every 2 to 3 days until the wound heals.

♦ If the injury is the result of foul play, report it to the police department.

(*continued*)

Managing open trauma wounds (*continued*)

Type	Clinical action
Missile injury	
◆ High-velocity tissue penetration, such as a gunshot wound ◆ Diagnosis based on entry and possibly exit wounds, signs of hemorrhage, shock, pain, and history of trauma; X-rays, CBC and differential, and electrolyte levels required to assess extent of injury and estimate blood loss	◆ Check the patient's history for bleeding tendencies and use of anticoagulants. ◆ Control hemorrhage with pressure if possible. If the injury is near vital organs, use large-bore catheters to start two I.V. lines, using lactated Ringer's or normal saline solution for volume replacement. Prepare for possible exploratory surgery. ◆ Maintain a patent airway, and monitor for signs of hypovolemia, shock, and cardiac arrhythmias. Check vital signs and neurovascular response often. ◆ Cover a sucking chest wound during exhalation with an occlusive dressing. ◆ Clean the wound gently with normal saline solution or water; debride as necessary. ◆ If damage is minor, apply a dry, sterile dressing. ◆ Administer tetanus prophylaxis if necessary. ◆ Obtain X-rays to detect retained fragments. ◆ If possible, determine the caliber of the weapon. ◆ Report the injury to the police department.
Puncture wound	
◆ Small-entry wounds that probably damage underlying structures, resulting from sharp, pointed objects ◆ Diagnosis based on hemorrhage (rare), deep hematomas (in chest or abdominal wounds), ragged wound edges (in bites), small-entry wound (in very sharp object), pain, and history of trauma; X-rays can detect retention of injuring object	◆ Check the patient's history for bleeding tendencies and use of anticoagulants. ◆ Obtain a description of the injury, including force of entry. ◆ Assess the extent of the injury. ◆ Don't remove impaling objects until the injury has been completely evaluated. (If the eye is injured, call an ophthalmologist immediately.) ◆ Thoroughly clean the injured area with soap and water. Irrigate all minor wounds with normal saline solution after removing a foreign object. ◆ Unless they're on the face, very large, or gaping, leave human and animal bite wounds open. Apply a dry, sterile dressing to other minor puncture wounds. ◆ Tell the patient to apply warm soaks daily. ◆ Administer tetanus prophylaxis and, if necessary, a rabies vaccine. ◆ Deep wounds that damage underlying tissues may require exploratory surgery; retention of the injuring object requires surgical removal.

between persons of the same sex. The prognosis is good if the rape victim receives physical and emotional support and counseling to help the patient deal with their feelings. Victims who articulate their feelings are able to cope with fears, interact with others, and return to normal routines faster than those who don't.

Causes and incidence

Rape isn't primarily about sex. It's a violent crime linked to feelings of rage or hatred in the assailant. Some of the cultural, sociologic, and psychological factors that contribute to rape are increased exposure to sex, permissiveness, cynicism about relationships, feelings of anger, and powerlessness amid social pressures. Many rapists have feelings of violence or hatred toward women, or sexual problems such as impotence or premature ejaculation. They may feel socially isolated and be unable to form warm, loving relationships. Some rapists may be psychopaths who need violence for physical pleasure, no matter how it affects their victims; others rape to satisfy a need for power. Some were abused as children.

In the United States, a rape is reported every 6 to 7 minutes. The incidence of reported rape is highest in large cities and continues to rise. However, many rapes—possibly even most—are never reported.

Known victims of rape range in age from 2 months to 97 years. The age group most affected is 18- to 34-year-olds. About one in seven reported rapes involves a prepubertal child; most of these cases involve manual, oral, or genital contact with the child's genitals by a member of the child's family. More than 50% of rapes occur in the home; about one third of these involve a male intruder who forces their way into a home. In about half the cases, the victim has some casual acquaintance with the attacker. Most alleged rapists are between ages 25 and 44 and have planned the attack. Alcohol is involved in one third of cases.

Pathophysiology
Sexual assault creates both psychological and physical trauma. In women, tears are often seen to the vaginal vault and labia. In both men and women forcible anal penetration may create tears, fissures, and bleeding in the rectum.

Complications
◆ Depression
◆ Guilt
◆ Anxiety
◆ Suicide

Signs and symptoms
When a rape victim arrives in the emergency department, assess physical injuries. If the patient isn't seriously injured, allow the patient to remain clothed and take them to a private room where the patient can talk with you or a counselor before the necessary physical examination. (See *If the rape victim is a child*.) Remember, immediate reactions to rape differ and can include crying, laughing, hostility, confusion, withdrawal, or outward calm; anger and rage may not surface until later. During the attack, the victim may have felt demeaned, helpless, and afraid fort their life; afterward, the patient may feel ashamed, guilty, shocked, and vulnerable and have a sense of disbelief and

If the rape victim is a child

Carefully interview the child to assess how well she'll be able to deal with the situation after going home. Interview the child alone, away from the parents. Tell the parents that this is being done for the child's comfort, not to keep secrets from them. Ask them what words the child is comfortable with when referring to parts of the anatomy.

History and examination
A young child will place only as much importance on an experience as others do, unless there's physical pain. A good question to ask is, "Did someone touch you when you didn't want to be touched?" As with other rape victims, record information in the child's own words. A complete pelvic examination is necessary only if penetration has occurred; such an examination requires parental consent and an analgesic or a local anesthetic.

Need for counseling
The child and the parents will need counseling to minimize possible emotional disturbances. Encourage the child to talk about the experience, and try to alleviate any confusion. After a rape, a young child may regress; an older child may become fearful about being left alone. The child's behavior may change at school or at home.

Help the parents understand that it's normal for them to feel angry and guilty, but warn them against displacing or projecting these feelings onto the child. Instruct them to assure the child that they aren't angry with her; that the child is good and didn't cause the incident; that they're sorry it happened, but glad the child is all right; and that the family will work the problems out together.

lowered self-esteem. Offer support and reassurance. Help the patient explore feelings; listen, convey trust and respect, and remain nonjudgmental. Don't leave the patient alone unless they ask you to do so.

Being careful to upset the victim as little as possible, obtain an accurate history of the rape, pertinent to physical assessment. (Remember, your notes may be used as evidence if the rapist is tried.) Record the victim's statements in the first person, using quotation marks. Also, document objective information provided by others. Never speculate as to what may have happened or record subjective impressions or thoughts. Include in your notes the time the victim arrived at the facility, the date and time of the alleged rape, and the time that the victim was examined. Ask the victim if she's allergic to penicillin or other drugs, if the patient has had recent illnesses (especially venereal disease), and if the patient was pregnant before the attack. Find out the date of the last menstrual period and details of the obstetric and gynecologic history.

Thoroughly explain the examination the patient will have, and tell the patient it's necessary to rule out internal injuries and obtain a specimen for venereal disease testing. Obtain informed consent for treatment and for the police report. Allow the patient some control if possible; for instance, ask the patient if they are ready to be examined or if they would rather wait a bit.

Before the examination, ask the victim whether they douched, bathed, or washed before coming to the hospital. Note this on the chart. Have the patient change into a hospital gown, and place clothing in paper bags. Label each bag and its contents.

⚠ **ALERT** *Never use plastic bags because secretions and semen stains will mold, destroying valuable evidence.*

Tell the victim they may urinate, but warn the patient not to wipe or otherwise clean the perineal area. Stay with her, or ask a counselor to stay with her, throughout the examination.

Diagnosis
Even if the victim wasn't beaten, the physical examination (including a pelvic examination by a gynecologist) will probably show signs of physical trauma, especially if the attack was prolonged. Depending on specific body areas attacked, a patient may have a sore throat, mouth irritation, difficulty swallowing, ecchymoses, or rectal pain and bleeding.

If additional physical violence accompanied the rape, the victim may have hematomas, lacerations, bleeding, severe internal injuries, and hemorrhage; if the rape occurred outdoors, they may suffer from exposure. X-rays may reveal fractures. If severe injuries require hospitalization, introduce the victim to the primary nurse if possible.

Throughout the examination, carefully label all possible evidence. Before the victim's pelvic area is examined, take vital signs; if she's wearing a tampon, remove it, wrap it, and label it as evidence. The pelvic examination is typically very distressing for the victim. Reassure the

patient and allow the patient as much control as possible. During the examination, specimens should be collected, including those for semen and gonorrhea. Carefully label all specimens with the patient's name, the physician's name, and the location from which the specimen was obtained. List all specimens in your notes. If the case comes to trial, specimens will be used for evidence, so accuracy is essential. (See *Legal considerations.*) Most emergency departments have "rape kits" that include containers for specimens.

Carefully collect and label fingernail scrapings and foreign material obtained by combing the victim's pubic hair; these also provide valuable evidence. Note to whom you give these specimens.

For a male victim, be especially alert for injury to the mouth, perineum, and anus. As ordered, obtain a pharyngeal specimen for a gonorrhea culture and rectal aspirate for acid phosphatase or sperm analysis.

Assist in photographing the patient's injuries (this may be delayed for 1 day or repeated when bruises and ecchymoses are more apparent).

Most states require medical facilities to report rape. The patient may choose not to press charges or assist the police. If the patient doesn't go to a facility, they may choose not to report the rape.

If the police interview the patient in the facility, be supportive and encourage the patient to recall details of the rape. Your kindness and empathy are invaluable.

The patient may also want you to call the family. Help the patient to verbalize anticipation of the family's response.

Treatment
Treatment consists of supportive measures and protection against venereal disease, human immunodeficiency virus (HIV) testing and, if the patient wishes, testing for pregnancy.

Special considerations
◆ Give antibiotics, as ordered, to prevent venereal disease.

Legal considerations
If your facility observes a protocol for emergency care of rape victims, it may include a rape evidence kit. If it does, follow the kit's instructions carefully. Include only medically relevant information in your notes.

Because cultures can't detect gonorrhea or syphilis for 5 to 6 days after the rape, stress the importance of returning for follow-up venereal disease testing.

◆ To prevent pregnancy as a result of the rape, the patient may be given either Plan B One Step, which is a single tablet that contains 1.5 mg of levonorgestrel, or Next Choice, which is two doses of 0.75 mg of levonorgestrel taken at the same time or 12 hours apart. An alternative emergency contraception relies on insertion of a copper-releasing intrauterine device within 5 days (120 hours) after unprotected intercourse. It can be removed after the patient's next menstrual period or may be left in place to provide ongoing contraception.

◆ If the patient has vulvar lacerations, the physician will clean the area and repair the lacerations after all the evidence is obtained. Topical use of ice packs may reduce vulvar swelling.

◆ Offer all victims of rape testing for HIV infection as well as medical counseling and follow-up. If there's a chance that the rapist was infected with HIV, postexposure prophylaxis may be done to reduce the odds of infection by the immediate use of antiretroviral medications.

◆ Refer the patient for psychological counseling, if needed, to cope with the aftereffects of the attack. Recovery from rape, which may be prolonged, consists of the acute phase (immediate reaction) and the reorganization phase. During the acute phase, physical effects include pain, loss of appetite, and wound healing; emotional reactions typically include shaking, crying, and mood swings. Feelings of grief, anger, fear, or revenge may color the victim's social interactions. Counseling helps the victim identify coping mechanisms. The patient may relate more easily to a counselor of the same gender.

During the reorganization phase, which usually begins 1 to 3 weeks after the rape and may last months or years, the victim is concerned with restructuring their life. Initially, they often have nightmares in which they are powerless; later dreams involve gradually gaining more control. When the patient is alone, they may also suffer from "daymares"—frightening thoughts about the rape. They may have reduced sexual desire or may develop fear of intercourse or mistrust.

◆ If the patient is engaged in legal proceedings during this time, they will be forced to relive the trauma, leaving them feeling lonely and isolated, perhaps even temporarily halting emotional recovery. To help the patient cope, encourage the patient to write thoughts, feelings, and reactions in a daily diary, and refer to organizations such as a local rape crisis center for empathy and advice.

SELECTED REFERENCES

Buggia, M., et al. (2014). Drowning and adult respiratory distress syndrome. *The Journal of Emergency Medicine, 46*(6), 821–825.

Ciomartan, T. (2014). What is the best fluid for volume resuscitation in critically ill adults with sepsis? The jury is still out, but a verdict is urgently needed. *Critical Care Medicine, 42,* 1722–1723. doi:10.1097/CCM.0000000000000375

Dellinger, R. P., et al. (2013). Surviving sepsis campaign: International guidelines for management of severe sepsis and septic shock. *Critical Care Medicine, 41*(2), 580–637. doi:10.1097/CCM.0b013e31827e83af

Dellinger, R. P., et al. (2017). A user's guide to the 2016 surviving sepsis guidelines. *Intensive Care Medicine, 43*(3), 299–303. doi:10.1007/s00134-017-4681-8

Evans, D., & Nelson, L. W. (2013). Treating venomous snakebites in the United States: A guide for nurse practitioners. *The Nurse Practitioner, 10*(38), 13–22. doi:10.1097/01.NPR.0000431181.95053.89

Faulds, M., & Meekings, T. (2013). Temperature management in critically ill patients. *Continuing Education in Anaesthesia, Critical Care & Pain, 13*(3), 75–79. doi:10.1093/bjaceaccp/mks063

Foster, K. (2014). Clinical guidelines in the management of burn injury: A review and recommendations from the organization and delivery of burn care committee. *Journal of Burn Care, 35*(4), 271–283. doi:10.1097/BCR.0000000000000088

Gaudio, F., & Grissom, C. K. (2015). Cooling methods in hear stroke. *The Journal of Emergency Medicine, 50*(4), 607–616. doi:10.1016/j.jemermed.2015.09.014

Goodwin, C., ed. (2011). *Advanced burn life support manual.* Chicago: American Burn Association.

Jin, Z., et al. (2017). Assessment and spontaneous healing outcomes of traumatic eardrum perforation with bleeding. *American Journal of Otolaryngology—Head and Neck Medicine and Surgery, 38*(4), 479–783. doi:10.1016/j.amjoto.2017.04.014

Johnson, G. (2016). Trauma triage and trauma system performance. *Western Journal of Emergency Medicine, 17*(3), 331–332. doi:10.5811/westjem.2016.2.29900

Kamiya, K., et al. (2015). From Hiroshima and Nagasaki to Fukushima 1: Long-term effects of radiation exposure on health. *The Lancet, 386*(9992), 469–478. doi:10.1016/S0140-6736(15)61167-9

Lee, J., et al. (2015). Factors associated with residual symptoms after recompression in type 1 decompression sickness. *American Journal of Emergency Medicine, 33*(3), 363–366. doi:10.1016/j.ajem.2014.12.011

Lou, Z. (2014). Natural evolution of an eardrum bridge in patients with a traumatic eardrum perforation. *European Archives of Otorhinolaryngology, 271*(5), 993–996. doi:10.1007/s00405-013-2499-8

Mathews, Z., & Koyfman, A. (2015). Blast injuries. *The Journal of Emergency Medicine, 49*(4), 573–587. doi:10.1016/j.jemermed.2015.03.013

Russo, R. M., et al. (2015). Mass casualty disasters: Who should run the show? *The Journal of Emergency Medicine, 48*(6), 685–692. doi:10.1016/j.jemermed.2014.12.069

Sacks, C. A. (2017). Decompression sickness. *The New England Journal of Medicine, 377*(16), 1568. doi:10.1056/NEJMicm1615505

Scheske, L., et al. (2015). Needs and availability of snake antivenoms: Relevance and application of international guidelines. *International Journal of Health*

Policy and Management, 4(7), 447–457. doi:10.15171. ijhpm.2015.75

Szpilman, D., et al. (2012). Drowning. *The New England Journal of Medicine, 366,* 2102–2110. doi:10.1056/NEJMra1013317

Thomas, G. A., & Symonds, P. (2016). Radiation exposure and health effects—Is it time to reassess the real consequences? *Clinical Oncology, 28*(8), 231–236. doi:10.1016/j.clon.2016.01.007

Walters, B. C. (2013). Methodology of the Guidelines for the management of acute cervical spine and spinal cord injuries. *Neurosurgery, 72*(3), 17–21. doi:10.1227/NEU.0b013e318276ed9a

Walters, B. C., et al. (2013). Guidelines for the management of acute cervical spine and spinal cord injuries: 2013 update. *Clinical Neurosurgery, 60*(Suppl 1), 82–91. doi:10.1227/01.neu.0000430319.32247.7f

Wheeler, K., et al. (2013). Heat illness and deaths, New York City, 2000–2011. *Morbidity and Mortality Weekly Report, 62*(31), 617–621.

Yang, M., et al. (2017). Outcome and risk factors association with extent of central nervous system injury due to evectional heat stroke. *Medicine, 96*(44), 1–7. doi:10.1097/MD.0000000000008417

18

GENETIC DISORDERS

Introduction

Genetic diseases result from single-gene (Mendelian) alterations, chromosomal abnormalities, or multifactorial errors. Over 6,000 such abnormalities have been identified in humans, ranging from mild differences (as in certain hemoglobin [Hb] abnormalities) to fatal or overwhelmingly disabling conditions, such as trisomy 18 (Edwards syndrome) and trisomy 13 (Patau syndrome). The risk of single-gene disorders is estimated at 1 in 200 births.

Although genetic disorders are determined mainly by genetic makeup, they can also interact with environmental factors. For example, albinism (an inherited inability to generate the protective pigment melanin) greatly increases susceptibility to skin cancer with excessive exposure to sunlight.

GENETIC ANALYSIS

Genetics, the study of heredity, involves analysis of defects in chromosomal reproduction or disease processes that can be passed from one generation to the next. Various tests are used to unravel the effects of altered genes and the patterns of inheritance. As heredity becomes better understood, genetic influences are likely to assume greater importance in healthcare delivery.

The essential ingredient of heredity is *deoxyribonucleic acid* (DNA), which makes up *genes*, basic units of hereditary material that are arranged into threadlike organelles called *chromosomes* in the cell nucleus. (See *DNA and how it works*, page 978 and *DNA replication*, page 979.) Together, these elements contribute to a person's *genotype* (gene composition) and *phenotype* (outward appearance).

In humans, each body cell (except ova and sperm) has 46 chromosomes consisting of 22 pairs of autosomes and 1 pair of sex chromosomes. Females have a matched (homologous) pair of sex chromosomes (X); males have an unmatched (heterologous) pair of sex chromosomes—an X and a Y. Thus, the normal human chromosome complement is 46,XX in females and 46,XY in males. The 22 autosomes are all homologous. Each chromosome has a short arm (p) and a long arm (q) joined at the centromere.

The position that the gene for a given trait occupies on a chromosome is called a *locus*. Different loci exist for hair color, blood group, and so on. The number and arrangement of the loci on homologous chromosomes are the same. When the two genes are identical, the individual is homozygous at that locus. When the genes aren't identical, the individual is heterozygous at that locus. A different form of the same gene that occupies a corresponding locus on a homologous chromosome is called an *allele*; it determines alternative (and inheritable) forms of the same characteristic. Some alleles control normal trait variation such as hair color; other defective alleles may cause a congenital defect or even induce a spontaneous abortion. Both heterologous (codominant) alleles may express their own effects, or one (the dominant allele) may be expressed and the other (the recessive) suppressed.

A mutation is a permanent change in a DNA sequence. When a mutation occurs in a gene's DNA sequence it may cause serious, even lethal defects or it may be relatively benign. Mutations can occur spontaneously or can be caused by exposure to teratogenic agents, such as

DNA and how it works

DNA is a double helix polymer (macromolecule) made up of individual units called nucleotides. Each nucleotide is composed of one sugar (deoxyribose), one phosphate, and one nitrogen-containing base—either a purine or a pyrimidine. The purine bases are adenine (A) and guanine (G). The pyrimidine bases are thymine (T) and cytosine (Q). The two polynucleotide chains of each DNA macromolecule are attached by hydrogen bonds between the bases (see illustration). The base pairing is very specific: adenine pairs only with thymine and cytosine pairs only with guanine. The DNA within the human genome (22 different autosomes and 2 different sex chromosomes) is made up of about 3 billion base pairs.

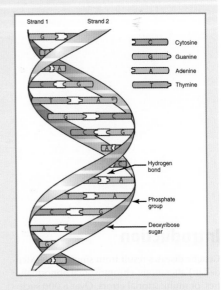

Genes make up approximately 2% of the human genome. A gene is a segment of DNA that ultimately determines the linear sequence of an amino acid chain. Through a complex process, a gene is transcribed into messenger ribonucleic acid (mRNA), which eventually is translated into an amino acid chain. A sequence of three mRNA nucleotides is called a *codon*. An mRNA codon can mark the beginning of translation, the end of translation, or a specific amino acid. Our genetic code is made up of 64 different codons, 61 of which actually code for amino acids. The eventual translated strand of amino acids must undergo further modification within the cell before it becomes a functional protein. The Human Genome Project is an international effort that officially began in 1990 and was completed in 2003 with the sequencing of the entire human genome. Emphasis is now on determining how the environment influences gene and protein function. With this information, treatment of genetic-based conditions is occurring at the molecular and cellular levels.

radiation, drugs, viruses, and synthetic chemicals. Paternal and maternal age also have effects on genetics.

TYPES OF GENETIC DISORDERS

Genetic disorders occur in several different forms. (See *Patterns of transmission in genetic disorders*, page 979.)

◆ *Mendelian or single-gene disorders* are inherited in clearly identifiable patterns.
◆ *Chromosomal aberrations or abnormalities* include structural defects within a chromosome, such as deletion and translocation, plus absence or addition of complete chromosomes.
◆ *Multifactorial disorders* reflect the interaction of at least two abnormal genes and environmental factors to produce a defect.

SINGLE-GENE DISORDERS

Single-gene disorders may be autosomal (resulting from a single altered gene or a pair of altered genes on one of the 22 pairs of autosomes) or X-linked (resulting from an altered gene on the X chromosome). Single-gene disorders may be further classified as dominant or recessive, depending on whether the altered gene is a dominant or a recessive allele.

SINGLE-GENE INHERITANCE PATTERNS

A dominant allele produces its effect in heterozygotes (people who also carry a normal gene for the same trait) because the dominant allele masks the effects of the normal paired gene (*autosomal dominant inheritance*). Because a person with an autosomal dominant disease is usually a heterozygote and carries one dominant gene as well as one normal gene, the individual's children have a 50% chance of inheriting the dominant gene and the disease. This probability remains the same for each pregnancy. Unaffected people (homozygote for the normal gene) don't carry the altered gene and therefore can't transmit it, except as a new mutation. (See *Inheritance patterns*, page 980.)

DNA replication

The body grows and replaces all dividing cells other than germ cells (sperm and ova) by *mitosis*. In mitosis, the cell's DNA replicates itself exactly and leads to the creation of a new daughter cell with the identical genetic makeup as the parent cell. Each new cell has a diploid number of chromosomes (in humans, 46).

Germ cells, however, form by *meiosis*. In meiosis, DNA first replicates. Then, through a complicated process, two cell divisions create four daughter cells (a sperm or ovum) from each parent cell, each of which has a haploid number of chromosomes (in humans, 23).

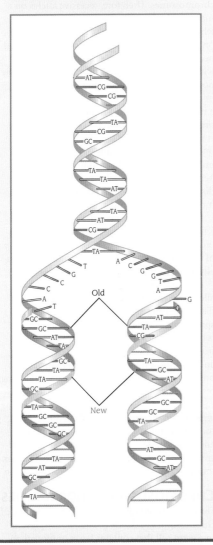

Patterns of transmission in genetic disorders

Autosomal dominant
Achondroplasia (dwarfism)
Colorectal polyposis
Hereditary hemorrhagic telangiectasia
Huntington disease
Hyperlipidemias (some types)
Hypoparathyroidism
Marfan syndrome
Neurofibromatosis (most cases)
Osteogenesis imperfecta (most cases)
Pituitary diabetes insipidus
Polycystic kidney disease
Retinoblastoma
Spherocytosis
Von Willebrand disease

Autosomal recessive
Albinism (some cases)
Congenital adrenal hyperplasia
Cretinism
Cystic fibrosis
Cystinuria
Fabry disease
Fanconi anemia
Galactosemia
Niemann–Pick disease
Osteogenesis imperfecta (some cases)
Phenylketonuria
Polycystic kidney disease
Retinitis pigmentosa (some cases)
Sickle cell anemia
Tay–Sachs disease
Thalassemia (alpha and beta)
Xeroderma pigmentosum (most cases)

X-linked
Duchenne muscular dystrophy
Fragile X mental retardation
Glucose-6-phosphate dehydrogenase
 deficiency
Hemophilia (most types)
Pseudohypoparathyroidism
Some immunodeficiencies

Chromosomal
Cri du chat syndrome
Down syndrome (trisomy 21)
Edwards syndrome (trisomy 18)
Klinefelter syndrome (XXY)
Patau syndrome (trisomy 13)
Turner syndrome (XO)

Multifactorial
Cleft lip or palate (some cases)
Congenital heart defects (some cases)
Diabetes mellitus (some cases)
Mental retardation (some cases)
Neural tube defects

Inheritance patterns

AUTOSOMAL DOMINANT DISORDERS

One heterozygous affected parent | Both heterozygous affected parents

 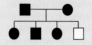

50% recurrence risk, regardless of sex | 75% recurrence risk, regardless of sex

AUTOSOMAL RECESSIVE DISORDERS

One parent affected | Both parents carriers

0% offspring affected, 100% carriers | 25% risk for being affected; 50% risk for being a carrier, regardless of sex

SEX-LINKED RECESSIVE DISORDERS

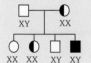 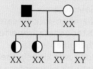

50% risk with every pregnancy with a male fetus; 50% carrier risk with every pregnancy with a female fetus | 100% sons normal; 100% daughters carriers

KEY

☐ Male

○ Female

■ ◐ Carrier

● ■ Persons affected by disease

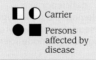

Sex doesn't influence transmission of an autosomal dominant allele. However, in some autosomal dominant diseases (such as Huntington disease), the severity of symptoms can vary in the offspring, depending on which parent transmits the dominant allele. Unless the dominant allele has arisen as a new mutation or is non-penetrant in an individual, every affected person has an affected parent. Thus, autosomal dominant traits don't skip generations. However, the severity of symptoms can range from very mild to severe among persons who inherit the allele. This variation of severity is known as *expressivity*.

Because a recessive allele can produce a disorder only when paired with another disease-causing allele (*autosomal recessive inheritance*), the offspring must receive one copy of the disease-causing allele from each parent to inherit the recessive trait. A carrier has a diseased gene, but is phenotypically normal. Autosomal recessive disorders affect males and females equally. Because both parents must be heterozygous carriers, autosomal recessive disorders are more common in children of consanguineous parents (blood relatives).

In *X-linked recessive inheritance*, nearly all affected persons are males because females have two X chromosomes and males have an X and a Y chromosome. There's very little DNA sequence in common between the X and the Y chromosomes. Therefore, recessive alleles on a male's X chromosome are expressed. Females who carry a disease-causing recessive allele on only one X chromosome are usually unaffected because they have two X chromosomes—one with the disease-causing allele and one with the normal dominant allele. However, every cell in the female, except the oocytes, undergoes a normal process called *X inactivation* where one X chromosome is turned off. This process is random. Therefore, females who carry only one copy of a disease-causing allele may have mild symptoms if a disproportionate number of cells have the X chromosome with the disease-causing allele turned on and the X chromosome with the normal allele turned off.

In *X-linked dominant inheritance*, which is rare, females are affected to varying degrees. These disorders tend to be lethal in males. A family history of multiple male miscarriages or stillbirths is usually a clue to an X-linked dominant disorder.

Sex does influence transmission of X-linked alleles. An affected male transmits the disease-causing allele to all of his female offspring, but to none of his male offspring. This is because males receive their X chromosome from their mother. When a sperm containing an X chromosome joins an ovum (which can only have an X chromosome), a female offspring results. When the X chromosome contains a disease-causing recessive allele, female offspring are typically unaffected carriers. When the X chromosome contains a disease-causing dominant allele, all female offspring are affected. Male offspring receive a Y chromosome from their father, therefore not receiving the disease-causing allele.

CHROMOSOMAL ABNORMALITIES

During germ cell formation by meiosis, failure of chromosomes to divide (*nondisjunction*) results in a germ cell that contains fewer or more than the normal 23 chromosomes. Usually, such abnormal germ cells fail to unite at conception; if fertilization does take place, the embryo is usually miscarried early in the pregnancy. Experts believe that up to 60% of spontaneous abortions at less than 90 days' gestation result from an abnormal number of fetal chromosomes; offspring with some chromosomal abnormalities are probably never even implanted. Absence of an autosomal chromosome is incompatible with life, but absence of a sex chromosome, as in Turner syndrome, is better tolerated. The presence of an extra chromosome (*trisomy*), as in Down syndrome, commonly produces physical malformation, mental retardation, or both.

Chromosomal disorders may also result from structural changes within chromosomes. For instance, in *deletion*, loss of part of a chromosome during cell division produces varying effects in the offspring, depending on the type and amount of genetic material lost. An example is velocardiofacial syndrome (VCFS), in which part of the long arm of chromosome 22 is missing.

In *translocation*, part of a chromosome attaches itself to another chromosome. If little or no genetic material is lost, the translocation is balanced (symmetrical) and the person displays no effects but may have reproductive problems, such as miscarriage, infertility, or children with malformations, cognitive effects, or both. The person may produce unaffected children, each of whom has a 50% chance of being a balanced translocation carrier, like the parent.

Another abnormality, *ring chromosomes*, results when a chromosome loses a section of genetic material from each end and the remaining stumps join together to form a ring. The effect varies, depending on the type of genetic material lost and on the specific chromosome that's involved.

In *mosaicism*, abnormal chromosomal division in the zygote results in two or more cell lines with different chromosomes. (One cell line may be normal and the other abnormal.) The patient's phenotype depends on the percentage of normal cells and on the varying effects of the abnormal cell line, which depend on the percentage of abnormal cells in each type of tissue.

Originally, Gregor Mendel's theories of heredity pointed to the understanding that an individual's phenotype is the same no matter which parent donates the allele. Now, it's known that this isn't always true. When a deletion on 15q11-13 is inherited from the father, the child will have Prader–Willi syndrome (obesity, short structure, hypogonadism). If the deletion is inherited from the mother, the child will have Angelman syndrome (mental retardation, no verbal language, seizures). This indicates that different genes are active on chromosome 15 depending on which parent provided the chromosome.

MULTIFACTORIAL DISORDERS

Multifactorial disorders are abnormalities that result from the interaction of at least two inherited abnormal genes and environmental factors. They include common malformations, such as neural tube defects (NTDs), cleft lip, and cleft palate, as well as disorders that may not appear until later in life such as diabetes mellitus. Such disorders don't follow the Mendelian patterns of inheritance, but the increased incidence of specific birth defects within families suggests familial transmission.

DETECTING GENETIC DISORDERS

Genetic testing and counseling can help prevent genetic disorders and help patients and their families deal with them when they do develop. Genetic diagnosis relies primarily on pedigree (family tree) analysis, karyotype (chromosomal) analysis, and biochemical analysis of blood, urine, or body tissues (including tissues obtained by amniocentesis or chorionic villus sampling [CVS]) to detect abnormal gene products. Neonatal screening for inherited metabolic disorders such as phenylketonuria has become standard, and prompt treatment of such disorders can prevent or minimize their effects.

Simple blood tests can detect carriers of recessive-gene disorders, such as Tay–Sachs disease and sickle cell anemia. DNA testing can detect some autosomal recessive, autosomal dominant, and X-linked recessive disorders. This gives a couple at risk the option of prenatal diagnosis (by amniocentesis or possibly CVS) for some disorders, to detect affected offspring.

A *pedigree*, a diagram of family relationships and diseases and cause of death of individual family members, helps determine a disorder's inheritance pattern, including the probability of occurrence. The pedigree chart begins with the patient (proband or index case) and traces all living and deceased blood relatives in order of their birth, listing:

♦ current age or age at death
♦ health status of all relatives, including miscarriages and stillbirths (and the reasons for them), the site and nature of congenital anomalies, and the presence of mental and growth retardation
♦ relationships (if the patient is a twin, involved in a consanguineous marriage, or divorced)

This information can be obtained from the patient's memory, autopsy and pathology reports, photographs, and medical records. The pedigree chart is analyzed in relation to the clinical features of the suspected genetic disorder and appropriate laboratory tests or medical records. In one such test, the *karyotype*, white blood cells obtained from a venous blood sample are grown in a special culture until a specific stage of mitosis, when chromosomes are most easily seen with a microscope. Then the cells are broken open and stained to show specific bands on the chromosomes. Staining techniques can be varied to help identify each chromosome and the bands it contains.

Amniocentesis, needle aspiration of amniotic fluid after transabdominal puncture of the uterus under ultrasound guidance, can now detect more than 600 genetic disorders before birth by:
◆ karyotyping cultured amniocytes
◆ using fluorescent in situ hybridization on cultured amniocytes to detect submicroscopic chromosome deletions, duplications, or translocations
◆ measuring enzyme levels or activity on cultured amniocytes
◆ performing DNA mutation or linkage analysis on cultured amniocytes
◆ measuring proteins (e.g., alpha-fetoprotein [AFP]) or biochemical substrates in amniotic fluid.

Amniocentesis allows parents to make informed decisions for a pregnancy before the birth of a child with a genetic disorder. It's recommended to patients with:
◆ maternal age over 34 at delivery
◆ family history of chromosomal abnormalities
◆ history of previous children or a first- or second-degree relative with an open or closed NTD or scoliosis with spinal dysraphism
◆ history of multiple reproductive losses
◆ parents who are known carriers of a genetic disorder that's detectable by biochemical or DNA testing

The benefits of amniocentesis must be carefully weighed against the potential complications, which may include amniotic fluid leakage, miscarriage, and (rarely) infection. The risk of complications is estimated to be 0.5% (1 in 200) or less. Genetic counseling is done to help the patient and family weigh the risks against the benefits so they can make an informed decision about testing. For some patients, CVS, another method of collecting genetic information from the fetus, may be an alternative. Using a vaginal or abdominal approach, with ultrasound as a guide, the physician collects a small amount of chorionic tissue, which is then analyzed in much the same way as the amniocentesis. Biochemical tests that are typically done on amniotic fluid can't be done on CVS tissue.

Researchers are currently studying new methods of earlier prenatal diagnosis, such as amniocyte filtration and karyotyping of fetal cells in maternal blood.

Prenatal diagnosis may be considered even when a couple would continue an affected pregnancy because knowing the diagnosis ahead of time can help the healthcare team provide the optimal timing and method of delivery, thus improving the neonate's outcome. It also gives the couple more time to look into financial, educational, and psychological support services to prepare for the birth of a child with special needs.

Healthcare providers may recommend genetic testing for selected children and adolescents; it's indicated for prevention, decreasing the need for surveillance, and examining treatment availability.

HELPING THE FAMILY COPE
Genetic counseling helps a family to understand its risk for a particular genetic disorder and to cope with the disorder if that risk becomes reality. Counseling sessions make it easier for the family to comprehend:
◆ medical facts (diagnosis, prognosis, treatment)
◆ how heredity works (risks to other relatives)
◆ options for dealing with the problem
◆ consequences of their decision

Psychological support to relieve stress and improve the child's or parents' self-concept is as important as obtaining the correct information. The birth of a child with a genetic defect may provoke parental feelings of guilt, anxiety, isolation, insecurity, and helplessness and may place undue stress on all members of the family. Family members may experience a period of shock and denial, followed by grief and mourning. Following acceptance of the diagnosis, parents may continue to experience periods of denial, guilt, and chronic sorrow, a phenomenon that manifests as episodes of sadness, particularly around developmental milestones. These feelings are a normal response to having a child with a disability.

When testing confirms a genetic disorder, here's how you can provide psychological support:
◆ Refer the family for genetic counseling. The following organizations can be contacted to obtain a list of qualified health professionals throughout the United States who can provide genetic evaluation, diagnosis, counseling, and management services:
  ◆ American College of Medical Genetics
  ◆ International Society of Nurses in Genetics
  ◆ March of Dimes Birth Defects Foundation
  ◆ National Society of Genetic Counselors
◆ Find out the services that are offered by the counseling center so you can tell the family what to expect.
◆ Provide the genetic professional with pertinent medical records and information about the family's special concerns, such as religious beliefs and social preferences.

◆ After counseling sessions, make sure family members understand the new information presented to them and reinforce the information provided. Communicate with them in an unhurried and nontechnical manner and make sure your facts are accurate.

◆ Inform the family about community resources, agencies, and available support groups to help them deal with genetic disorders. If they're interested, help them get in touch with the families of other patients with the same disorder. The Alliance of Genetic Support Groups or the National Organization for Rare Disorders are valuable resources for locating support groups and parent networking opportunities.

◆ Coordinate the assistance needed from other members of the healthcare team, such as physicians, psychologists, and social workers.

◆ Recognize the parents' stresses in caring for their child, and allow them to express their feelings.

Autosomal dominant inheritance

NEUROFIBROMATOSIS

Neurofibromatosis is a group of inherited developmental disorders of the nervous system, muscles, bones, and skin that causes formation of multiple, pedunculated, soft tumors (neurofibromas), and café-au-lait spots. The most common types are NF-1 (von Recklinghausen disease) and NF-2 (bilateral acoustic neurofibromatosis). About 80,000 Americans are known to have neurofibromatosis; in many others, the disorder is overlooked because symptoms are mild. The prognosis varies; however, spinal or intracranial tumors can shorten the patient's life span.

Causes and incidence

NF-1 is an autosomal dominant disorder of chromosome 17 that occurs in about 1 in 3,000 births. About 50% of affected families have a negative family history; in many of these families, the father is older, suggesting that advanced paternal age may influence the NF-1 mutation. NF-2 is an autosomal dominant disorder of chromosome 22; however, many patients have a negative family history.

Pathophysiology

The manifestations of NF-1 result from a mutation in or deletion of the *NF1* gene. The gene product neurofibromin serves as a tumor suppressor; decreased production of this protein results in the myriad of clinical features.

Complications

◆ Neurologic problems
◆ Skeletal problems—abnormally formed bones
◆ Vision problems—optic glioma can form
◆ Cardiovascular problems—high blood pressure and more rarely vessel abnormalities
◆ Adrenal gland tumor (pheochromocytoma)

Signs and symptoms

Signs and symptoms of NF-1 vary greatly from one family to another and within members of the same family. A patient who initially seems to have mild symptoms may develop more severe problems later.

An infant with this form may present with only café-au-lait spots or may also have congenital glaucoma, plexiform neurofibromas, or pseudoarthrosis. About 90% of patients have Lisch nodules on the iris; as many as 15% develop optic pathway gliomas, which may cause a significant loss of vision.

Cutaneous and other neurofibromas may begin to develop or become more prominent at puberty; pregnancy may exacerbate tumor growth. Some tumors become malignant; about 8% of patients develop neurofibrosarcoma (cancer of the nerve sheath). Other less-specific features may include other types of tumors (such as meningiomas), short stature, seizures, speech and learning disabilities, mental retardation (occasionally), and abnormalities of the cerebral, gastrointestinal (GI), and renal arteries.

The first sign of NF-2 is usually a central nervous system (CNS) tumor, such as a spinal or intracranial meningioma, an acoustic neuroma, and occasionally a schwannoma or spinal astrocytoma. Cutaneous neurofibromas may be less conspicuous in this form, and café-au-lait spots may be minimal or even absent. Learning disabilities and other less-specific features characteristic of NF-1 aren't typically seen in NF-2.

Diagnosis

Diagnosis rests on typical clinical findings, especially neurofibromas and café-au-lait spots. Diagnostic criteria for NF-1 include two or more of the following:

◆ first-degree relative (parent, sibling, child) with known NF-1
◆ six or more café-au-lait spots over 5 mm in diameter in a prepubertal patient and 15 mm or more in a postpubertal patient
◆ freckling in the axillary or inguinal region
◆ optic pathway glioma
◆ two or more Lisch nodules on the iris
◆ osseous lesion, such as sphenoid dysplasia or thinning long-bone cortex

Diagnostic criteria for NF-2 include a first-degree relative with NF-2 and two of the following:

♦ neurofibroma, meningioma, schwannoma, glioma, juvenile posterior subcapsular lenticular opacity
♦ unilateral eighth cranial nerve mass
♦ bilateral eighth cranial nerve masses seen on magnetic resonance imaging (MRI) or computed tomography (CT) scan

X-rays, MRI, and CT scan may be indicated to determine the presence of widening internal auditory meatus and intervertebral foramen. An eye examination to look for Lisch nodules should be done on patients suspected of having NF-1. Myelography may be used to identify spinal cord tumors, and lumbar puncture with cerebrospinal fluid (CSF) analysis will reveal elevated protein concentration in the presence of spinal neurofibromas and acoustic tumors. DNA analysis and prenatal diagnosis may also be done in some families.

Treatment

Neurofibromatosis has no specific treatment. Management consists of surgical removal of intracerebral or intraspinal tumors (when possible) and correction of kyphoscoliosis. Tumors that cause pain and loss of function are removed on an individual basis. If the entire tumor can't be removed during surgery, radiation may also be used to help relieve symptoms.

⚠ ALERT *Tumors that grow rapidly should be removed promptly because they may become malignant.*

Cosmetic surgery for disfiguring or disabling growths may be done; however, regrowth is likely. Special schooling for individuals with learning disorders or attention deficit hyperactivity disorder may be required. Annual eye examinations should be performed.

Researchers are currently investigating experimental treatments for severe tumors.

Special considerations

♦ Disfigurement may cause overwhelming embarrassment and social regression. By showing acceptance, you can help the patient adjust to this condition.
♦ Advise the patient to choose attractive clothing that covers nodules; suggest special cosmetics to cover skin lesions.
♦ Refer the patient for genetic counseling to discuss the 50% risk of transmitting this disorder to offspring. Recommend contacting the National Neurofibromatosis Foundation.

OSTEOGENESIS IMPERFECTA

Osteogenesis imperfecta (brittle bones) is a hereditary disease of bones and connective tissue that may cause varying degrees of skeletal fragility, thin skin, blue sclerae, poor teeth, hypermobility of joints, and progressive deafness. This disease occurs in many forms. In the rare congenital form, fractures are present at birth. This form is usually fatal within the first few days or weeks of life. In the late-appearing form, the child appears normal at birth but develops recurring fractures (mostly of the extremities) after the first year of life.

Causes and incidence

Osteogenesis imperfecta can result from autosomal dominant inheritance of a defect in the amount of type I collagen, an important part of the bone matrix.

Type I, the most common form of osteogenesis imperfecta, occurs in about 1 in 30,000 live births. Both types I and IV are thought to be inherited as an autosomal dominant trait. Types II and III are believed to be inherited as an autosomal recessive trait.

Pathophysiology

It occurs from defective osteoblastic activity and a defect of mesenchymal collagen (embryonic connective tissue) and its derivatives (sclerae, bones, and ligaments). The reticulum fails to differentiate into mature collagen or causes abnormal collagen development, leading to immature and coarse bone formation. Cortical bone thinning also occurs.

Complications

♦ Deafness (caused by otosclerosis)
♦ Scoliosis
♦ Multiple deformities
♦ Short stature

Signs and symptoms

Clinical severity varies, depending on the type. In type I, fractures characteristically occur from minimal trauma. The sclerae are a deep blue-black color, and the teeth may be yellow or even grayish blue from opalescent dentin. Patients with dental abnormalities are shorter and have more fractures at birth, more frequent fractures, and more severe skeletal deformities than type I patients with normal teeth.

Bowing of the lower limbs is common in this type, as is kyphosis in adults. About 40% of all adults with type I have severely impaired hearing, and virtually all adults have some degree of hearing impairment by age 50. The number of fractures may spontaneously decrease in adolescence.

Type II is characterized by intrauterine fractures because of extreme bone fragility, leading to intrauterine or early infant death. Death usually results from complications of bone fragility, heart failure, pulmonary hypertension, or respiratory failure. Therapeutic intervention doesn't usually increase survival.

Type III is generally nonlethal. Fractures are usually present at birth and occur frequently in childhood; they typically lead to progressive skeletal deformity and, eventually, impaired mobility. Patients have a poor growth rate; most fall below the third percentile in height for their age. Their sclerae are usually normal or light blue, and their teeth aren't usually opalescent.

Type IV is characterized by osteoporosis, which leads to increased bone fragility. The sclerae may be light blue at birth but appear normal in adolescents and adults. Bowed limbs may be present at birth, but only 25% of patients have fractures at birth. The number of fractures may decrease spontaneously at puberty, but the majority of patients are short. A few have a skull deformity.

Diagnosis

Family history and characteristic features, such as blue sclerae or deafness, establish the diagnosis. Whenever possible, collagen biochemical studies of cultured skin fibroblasts should be performed. Prenatal diagnosis may be available for certain families with an identified mutation. Prenatal ultrasound performed as early as 16 weeks' gestation may show evidence of severe osteogenesis imperfecta. X-rays showing evidence of multiple old fractures and skeletal deformities and a skull X-ray showing wide sutures with small, irregularly shaped islands of bone (wormian bones) between them support the diagnosis. These findings can help differentiate osteogenesis imperfecta from child abuse or from other disorders such as juvenile idiopathic osteoporosis.

In a family with a history of type II osteogenesis imperfecta, diagnostic serial ultrasound should be considered for future pregnancies to detect limb shortening, in utero fractures, and polyhydramnios.

Treatment

Treatment aims to prevent deformities by traction, immobilization, or both and to aid normal development and rehabilitation. Fractures must be repaired quickly to avoid deformities.

Surgical procedures such as inserting metal rods through bones can help strengthen bones and prevent deformity.

The use of bisphosphonates in children with osteogenesis imperfecta, such as pamidronate (Aredia) and zoledronate (Reclast) help to increase bone mass. Starting bisphosphonates after diagnosis at birth decreases fracture rates and helps spur growth. Vitamin D and calcium are supplemented as needed.

Growth hormone—studies indicate that some children respond to a daily injection with an initial increase in growth. Responders show changes in bone architecture and small increased bone mineral density. No data on the fracture rate are reported.

Research is being done on gene therapies, benefits of bone marrow transplant, and increasing the density in the trabecular bone formation.

Supportive measures include:

◆ checking the patient's circulatory, motor, and sensory abilities
◆ encouraging the patient to walk when possible (Children with osteogenesis imperfecta develop a fear of walking.)
◆ teaching preventive measures, such as avoiding contact sports or strenuous activities or wearing knee pads, helmets, or other protective devices when engaging in sports
◆ assessing for and treating scoliosis, a common complication
◆ promoting preventive dental care and repair of dental caries

Special considerations

◆ Educate the family about the disorder. Teach the parents and child how to recognize fractures and how to correctly splint them. Also teach the parents how to protect the child during diapering, dressing, and other activities of daily living.
◆ Advise the parents to encourage their child to develop interests that don't require strenuous physical activity and to develop fine motor skills. These actions will promote the child's self-esteem.
◆ Advise the parents that physical and rehabilitation therapy is beneficial. Swimming is an excellent conditioning exercise.
◆ Teach the child to assume some responsibility for precautions during physical activity to help foster independence.
◆ Stress the importance of good nutrition to heal bones and optimize muscle strength.
◆ Refer the parents and child for genetic counseling to assess the recurrence risk.

◆ Administer analgesics, as ordered, to relieve pain from frequent fractures, a hallmark of this disease.

◆ Monitor dental and hearing needs. Stress the need for regular dental care and immunizations.

◆ Instruct the parents to provide a medical identification bracelet for the child.

MARFAN SYNDROME

Marfan syndrome is a rare, predominantly inherited, degenerative, generalized disease of the connective tissue that causes ocular, skeletal, and cardiovascular anomalies. It probably results from elastin and collagen abnormalities. Death is usually attributed to cardiovascular complications and may occur any time from early infancy to adulthood, depending on the severity of the symptoms. Marfan syndrome affects males and females equally.

Causes and incidence

Marfan syndrome is inherited as an autosomal dominant trait of chromosome 15. In 85% of patients with this disease, the family history confirms Marfan syndrome in one parent as well. In the remaining 15%, a negative family history suggests a fresh mutation, possibly from advanced paternal age.

Pathophysiology

It's caused by mutations in the *fibrillin-1* gene, producing changes in elastic tissues, especially of the aorta, eye, and skin. Mutations of the *fibrillin-1* gene also cause overgrowth of long bones.

Complications

◆ Mitral valve insufficiency
◆ Endocarditis
◆ Dislocated lens

Signs and symptoms

The most common signs and symptoms of this disorder are skeletal abnormalities, particularly excessively long tubular bones and an arm span that exceeds the patient's height. The patient is usually taller than average for the family (in the 95th percentile for age), with the upper half of the body shorter than average and the lower half, longer. The patient's fingers are long and slender (arachnodactyly). Weakness of ligaments, tendons, and joint capsules results in joints that are loose, hyperextensible, and habitually dislocated. Excessive growth of the rib bones gives rise to chest deformities such as pectus excavatum (funnel chest).

Eye problems are also common; 75% of patients have crystalline lens displacement (ectopia lentis), the ocular hallmark of Marfan syndrome. Quivering of the iris with eye movement (iridodonesis) typically suggests this disorder. Most patients are severely myopic, many have retinal detachment, and some have glaucoma.

The most serious complications occur in the cardiovascular system and include weakness of the aortic media, which leads to progressive dilation or dissecting aneurysm of the ascending aorta. Such dilation appears first in the coronary sinuses and is commonly preceded by aortic insufficiency. Less common cardiovascular complications include mitral valve prolapse and endocarditis.

Other associated problems include sparsity of subcutaneous fat, frequent hernias, cystic lung disease, recurrent spontaneous pneumothorax, and scoliosis or kyphosis.

Diagnosis

Because no specific test confirms Marfan syndrome, diagnosis is based on typical clinical features (particularly skeletal deformities and ectopia lentis) and a history of the disease in close relatives. Useful supplementary procedures, though not definitive for diagnosis, include X-rays for skeletal abnormalities and an echocardiogram to detect aortic root dilation. Eye examination with slit-lamp may be used to diagnose a dislocated lens.

Treatment

Attempts to stop the degenerative process have met with little success. Therefore, treatment of Marfan syndrome is basically aimed at relieving symptoms—for example, surgical repair of aneurysms and ocular deformities. In young patients with early dilation of the aorta, prompt treatment with beta-adrenergic blockers may decrease ventricular ejection and protect the aorta; extreme dilation requires surgical replacement of the aorta and the aortic valve. Renin–angiotensin system (angiotensin receptor blockers such as losartan [Cozaar]) can be helpful in protecting the aorta. Steroids and sex hormones have been successful (especially in girls) in inducing precocious puberty and early epiphyseal closure to prevent abnormal adult height. Genetic counseling is important, particularly because pregnancy and resultant increased cardiovascular workload can produce aortic rupture.

Special considerations

◆ High school and college athletes (particularly basketball players) who fit the criteria for Marfan syndrome should undergo a careful clinical and cardiac examination before being allowed to play, to avoid sudden death because of dissecting aortic aneurysm or other cardiac complications.

◆ Provide the patient with supportive care, as appropriate for their clinical status.

◆ Educate the patient and family about the course of the disease and its potential complications.

◆ Stress the need for frequent checkups to detect and treat degenerative changes early.

◆ Emphasize the importance of taking prescribed medications and of avoiding contact sports and isometric exercise.

PEDIATRIC TIP *To encourage normal adolescent development, advise the parents to avoid unrealistic expectations for their child simply because he's tall and looks older than their years.*

◆ Refer the patient and family to the National Marfan Foundation for additional information.

STICKLER SYNDROME

Stickler syndrome also called (*arthro-ophthalmopathy*) is characterized by ocular, skeletal, auditory, and craniofacial abnormalities. Expression of clinical features is highly variable from one individual to another.

Causes and incidence

At least 19 different types of collagen have been identified. Collagen is an essential component of connective tissues. Genetic studies have identified a few families who carry the clinical diagnosis of Stickler syndrome yet don't demonstrate linkage to any of the three aforementioned collagen genes, suggesting further genetic heterogeneity (a pattern of traits caused by genetic factors in some cases and nongenetic factors in others).

About 1 in 10,000 people is affected with Stickler syndrome. However, this incidence rate is considered conservative because persons with very mild symptoms may never be diagnosed with the syndrome.

Pathophysiology

Stickler syndrome is an autosomal dominant chondrodysplasia caused by structural defects in collagen. The collagen defect in most families with Stickler syndrome is caused by a mutation in the type II collagen gene (*COL2A1*) located on chromosome 12q13. Other families demonstrate linkage to the *COL11A2* gene located on chromosome 6p21.3 and others to the *COL11A1* gene located on chromosome 1p21. *COL2A1* and *COL11A1* are expressed in the hyaline cartilage, vitreous, intervertebral disk, and inner ear. *COL11A2* isn't expressed in the vitreous.

Complications

◆ Glaucoma
◆ Retinal detachment
◆ Deafness
◆ Osteoarthritis
◆ Ear infections
◆ Difficulty breathing or feeding

Signs and symptoms

The clinical phenotype can consist of ocular, auditory, craniofacial, and skeletal abnormalities. The number of organ systems involved and the specific phenotypic features expressed can vary significantly between affected family members and, in particular, between unrelated affected persons.

Ocular symptoms, particularly high myopia, are common in persons with Sticklers syndrome, with the exception of those who have *COL11A2* mutations. Vitreal abnormalities are considered a hallmark of Stickler syndrome, although the abnormalities in the vitreous differ in persons with a *COL2A1* mutation from those with a *COL11A1* mutation. Retinal detachment resulting in blindness is the most serious ocular complication.

The vitreoretinal degeneration that leads to retinal detachment is much more common in persons with a *COL2A1* mutation. Persons with Stickler syndrome can also have congenital cataracts and develop glaucoma. Ocular symptoms are typically absent in persons with linkage to *COL11A2*.

Auditory symptoms include conductive hearing loss secondary to Eustachian tube dysfunction in children with cleft palate or collagen defects in the inner ear apparatus. Sensorineural hearing loss has an earlier onset and tends to be more progressive in persons with a *COL11A1* mutation.

Craniofacial features may include micrognathia (small lower jaw) and a flattened midface and nasal bridge. Micrognathia may be associated with some degree of cleft palate (bifid uvula to complete cleft of the palate). Micrognathia associated with glossoptosis places neonates and infants with Stickler syndrome at significant risk for episodic obstructive apnea during feeding and when lying flat.

Skeletal symptoms can include joint hypermobility in young children, spondyloepiphyseal dysplasia, and, later, degenerative arthropathy during early adult years. Also related to the collagen defect, scoliosis and mitral valve prolapse can develop in some persons with Stickler syndrome.

Diagnosis

Diagnosis is based on the recognition of clinical features consistent with Stickler syndrome. The number of genes involved in Stickler syndrome and the complexity of sequencing large genes currently preclude the clinical utility of routine genetic testing for diagnostic purposes. Therefore, diagnosis must rely on the dysmorphology skills of the practitioner performing the physical examination.

Stickler syndrome should be considered in neonates with the triad of micrognathia, cleft of the soft palate, and glossoptosis. This triad of features is known as *Pierre Robin syndrome*.

Severe myopia in infants and young children should be considered a possible symptom of Stickler syndrome. The diagnosis should also be considered in persons with a family history of cleft palate and significant myopia, deafness, or spondyloepiphyseal dysplasia. A slit-lamp examination of the vitreous is necessary to determine the presence of vitreal abnormalities that are considered pathognomonic of Stickler syndrome.

Treatment

Beginning with the first 6 months after birth, annual ophthalmology evaluation must be obtained to assess for myopia, vitreal abnormalities, and retinal degeneration and detachment. Persons who experience floaters or shadows in their vision require immediate assessment.

Persons with vitreoretinal degeneration need to avoid contact sports and other physical activity that can jar and detach the retina.

A brain stem auditory evoked response evaluation should be done during the first month after birth. The schedule for regular follow-up needs to be determined based on the results of the initial evaluation, frequency of otitis media episodes, and progress in language development.

Early use of corrective lenses and hearing aids is recommended to enable developmental progression at the infant or young child's full potential.

Depending on the infant's weight and health, surgical correction of the cleft palate can occur around age 9 months. With few exceptions, surgical closure of the palate should occur before age 2 to maximize speech and language development.

Special considerations

◆ To assess for obstructive apnea, neonates with the Pierre Robin syndrome triad need oxygen and carbon dioxide measurements while lying in different positions and while feeding.
◆ Neonates and infants with cleft palate may need a specialized cleft palate nurser to obtain adequate caloric intake.

◆ Screening for cardiac valvular disease should be considered in the older child and adult with Stickler syndrome.
◆ Genetic counseling by a person trained in genetics should be offered to adults with Stickler syndrome.
◆ Referral to appropriate support groups or networking groups should be offered to help with coping skills and to provide anticipatory guidance related to day-to-day needs of a person with Stickler syndrome.

Autosomal recessive inheritance

CYSTIC FIBROSIS

Cystic fibrosis is a generalized dysfunction of the exocrine glands that affects multiple organ systems. Transmitted as an autosomal recessive trait, it's the most common fatal genetic disease in White children.

Cystic fibrosis is a chronic disease. With improvements in treatment over the past decade, the average life expectancy has risen from age 16 to 40 and older.

Causes and incidence

A defect in the *CFTR* gene causes cystic fibrosis. Cystic fibrosis accounts for almost all cases of pancreatic enzyme deficiency in children.

In the United States, the incidence of cystic fibrosis is highest in Whites of northern European ancestry (1 in 2,000 live births) and lowest in Blacks (1 in 17,000 live births), Native Americans, and people of Asian ancestry. The disease occurs equally in both sexes.

Pathophysiology

The gene responsible for cystic fibrosis (located on chromosome 7) encodes a protein that involves chloride transport across epithelial membranes; more than 100 specific mutations of the gene are known. (See *Cystic fibrosis transmission risk*, page 989.) The immediate causes of symptoms in cystic fibrosis are increased viscosity of bronchial, pancreatic, and other mucous gland secretions and consequent obstruction of glandular ducts.

Complications

◆ Bronchiectasis
◆ Pneumonia
◆ Atelectasis
◆ Hemoptysis
◆ Dehydration
◆ Distal intestinal obstruction syndrome
◆ Malnutrition

Cystic fibrosis transmission risk

The chance that a relative of a person with cystic fibrosis or a person with no family history will carry the cystic fibrosis gene appears in the chart below.

Relative of affected person	Carrier chance
Brother or sister	2 in 3 (67%)
Niece or nephew	1 in 2 (50%)
Aunt or uncle	1 in 3 (33%)
First cousin	1 in 4 (25%)
No known family history	**Carrier chance**
Whites	1 in 25 (4%)
Blacks	1 in 65 (1.5%)
Asians	1 in 150 (0.67%)

- ◆ Nasal polyps
- ◆ Gastroesophageal reflux
- ◆ Rectal prolapse
- ◆ Cor pulmonale
- ◆ Diabetes
- ◆ Pancreatitis
- ◆ Cholecystitis

Signs and symptoms

The clinical effects of cystic fibrosis may become apparent soon after birth or may take years to develop. They include major aberrations in sweat gland, respiratory, and GI function. Sweat gland dysfunction is the most consistent abnormality. Increased concentrations of sodium and chloride in the sweat lead to hyponatremia and hypochloremia and can eventually induce fatal shock and arrhythmias, especially in hot weather.

Respiratory symptoms reflect obstructive changes in the lungs: wheezy respirations; a dry, nonproductive paroxysmal cough; dyspnea; and tachypnea. These changes stem from thick, tenacious secretions in the bronchioles and alveoli and eventually lead to severe atelectasis and emphysema. Children with cystic fibrosis display a barrel chest, cyanosis, and clubbing of the fingers and toes. They suffer recurring bronchitis and pneumonia as well as associated nasal polyps and sinusitis. Death typically results from pneumonia, emphysema, or atelectasis.

The GI effects of cystic fibrosis occur mainly in the intestines, pancreas, and liver. One early symptom is meconium ileus; the neonate with cystic fibrosis doesn't excrete meconium, a dark green mucilaginous material found in the intestine at birth. The patient develops symptoms of intestinal obstruction, such as abdominal distention, vomiting, constipation, dehydration, and electrolyte imbalance. As the child gets older, obstruction of the pancreatic ducts and resulting deficiency of trypsin, amylase, and lipase prevent the conversion and absorption of fat and protein in the GI tract. The undigested food is then excreted in frequent, bulky, foul-smelling, pale stools with a high fat content. This malabsorption induces poor weight gain, poor growth, ravenous appetite, distended abdomen, thin extremities, and sallow skin with poor turgor. The inability to absorb fats results in a deficiency of fat-soluble vitamins (A, D, E, and K), leading to clotting problems, retarded bone growth, and delayed sexual development. Males may experience azoospermia and sterility; females may experience secondary amenorrhea but can reproduce. A common complication in infants and children is rectal prolapse secondary to malnutrition and wasting of perirectal supporting tissues.

In the pancreas, fibrotic tissue, multiple cysts, thick mucus, and eventually fat replace the acini (small, saclike cluster of cells normally found in this gland), producing symptoms of pancreatic insufficiency: altered pancreatic enzymes and insufficient insulin production, abnormal glucose tolerance, and glycosuria. About 15% of patients have adequate pancreatic exocrine function for normal digestion and, therefore, have a better prognosis. Biliary obstruction and fibrosis may prolong neonatal jaundice. In some patients, cirrhosis and portal hypertension may lead to esophageal varices, episodes of hematemesis and, occasionally, hepatomegaly.

Diagnosis

℞ **CONFIRMING DIAGNOSIS** *The Cystic Fibrosis Foundation has developed certain criteria for a definitive diagnosis: two sweat tests using a pilocarpine solution (a sweat inducer) and either obstructive pulmonary disease, confirmed pancreatic insufficiency or failure to thrive, and a family history of cystic fibrosis.*

The following test results may support the diagnosis:

◆ Chest X-rays indicate early signs of obstructive lung disease.

◆ Stool specimen analysis indicates the absence of trypsin, suggesting pancreatic insufficiency.

◆ DNA testing can now locate the presence of the deltaF508 deletion (found in about 70% of cystic fibrosis patients, although the disease can cause >100 other mutations). It allows prenatal diagnosis in families with a previously affected child.

◆ Pulmonary function tests reveal decreased vital capacity, elevated residual volume because of air entrapments, and decreased forced expiratory volume in 1 second. This test is used if pulmonary exacerbation already exists.

◆ Liver enzyme tests may reveal hepatic insufficiency.

◆ Sputum culture reveals organisms that cystic fibrosis patients typically and chronically colonize, such as *Staphylococcus* and *Pseudomonas*.

◆ Serum albumin measurement helps assess nutritional status.

◆ Electrolyte analysis assesses hydration status.

Treatment

The aim of treatment is to help the child lead as normal a life as possible. The type of treatment depends on the organ systems involved.

To combat electrolyte losses in sweat, salt foods generously and, in hot weather, administer sodium supplements.

To offset pancreatic enzyme deficiencies, give oral pancreatic enzymes with meals and snacks, as ordered. Maintain a diet that's low in fat, but high in protein and calories, and provide supplements of water-miscible, fat-soluble vitamins (A, D, E, and K).

Management of pulmonary dysfunction includes chest physiotherapy, mechanical vest, postural drainage, pulmonary rehab, and breathing exercises several times daily to aid removal of secretions from lungs. Antihistamines are contraindicated because they have a drying effect on mucous membranes, making expectoration of mucus difficult or impossible. Aerosol therapy includes intermittent nebulizer treatments before postural drainage to loosen secretions.

Dornase alfa or DNase (recombinant human deoxyribonuclease), genetically engineered pulmonary enzymes given by aerosol nebulizer, help thin airway mucus, improving lung function, and reducing the risk of pulmonary infection.

Ivacaftor (Kalydeco) may improve lung function, weight, and decrease salt in sweat.

Treatment of pulmonary infection requires:

◆ broad-spectrum antimicrobials

◆ oxygen therapy as needed

◆ loosening and removal of mucopurulent secretions, using an intermittent nebulizer and postural drainage to relieve obstruction. Use of a mist tent is controversial because mist particles may become trapped in the esophagus and stomach and never reach the lungs.

Lung transplantation may be considered in some cases. Genetic research on curing cystic fibrosis by artificially inserting a "healthy" gene into a person through gene therapy is ongoing. The gene would be inserted by using an intranasal form. Research on correcting the disorder before birth is promising. Other areas of research include restoring salt transport in the cell, and use of mucus-thinning drugs and nutritional supplementation.

Special considerations

◆ Throughout this illness, teach the patient and family about the disease and its treatment. The Cystic Fibrosis Foundation can provide educational and support services.

◆ Although many males with cystic fibrosis are infertile, females may become pregnant (because of increased life expectancies). As a result, more cystic fibrosis patients are now facing difficult reproductive decisions. Refer such patients (or the parents of an affected child) for genetic counseling so they can discuss family planning issues or prenatal diagnosis options if they're considering having more children.

◆ Be aware that some patients have recently undergone lung transplants to reduce the effects of the disease. Also, aerosol gene therapy shows promise in reducing pulmonary symptoms.

◆ Research indicates that the genetic defect responsible for cystic fibrosis has also been identified in individuals experiencing some forms of unexplained pancreatitis.

TAY–SACHS DISEASE

The most common of the lipid storage diseases, Tay–Sachs disease results from a congenital deficiency of the enzyme hexosaminidase A. It's characterized by progressive mental and motor deterioration and is usually fatal before age 5, although some adolescents and adults with variations of hexosaminidase A deficiency have been noted. These individuals have significantly reduced levels of hexosaminidase A, rather than a complete absence of the enzyme.

Causes and incidence

Tay–Sachs disease appears in fewer than 100 neonates born each year in the United States. However, it's about 100 times more common in persons of Eastern European Jewish (Ashkenazi) ancestry than in the general population, occurring in about 1 in 3,600 live births in this ethnic group. About 1 in 30 Ashkenazi Jews, French Canadians, and American Cajuns are heterozygous carriers. If two such carriers have children, each of their offspring has a 25% chance of having Tay–Sachs disease.

Pathophysiology

Tay–Sachs disease (also known as GM_2 gangliosidosis) is an autosomal recessive disorder of chromosome 15 in which the enzyme hexosaminidase A is virtually absent or deficient. This enzyme is necessary for metabolism of gangliosides, water-soluble glycolipids found primarily in CNS tissues. Without hexosaminidase A, accumulating lipid pigments distend and progressively destroy and demyelinate CNS cells.

Complications

◆ Bronchopneumonia
◆ Death

Signs and symptoms

A neonate with classic Tay–Sachs disease appears normal at birth, although the patient may have an exaggerated Moro reflex. By age 3 to 6 months, the patient becomes apathetic and responds only to loud sounds. Neck, trunk, arm, and leg muscles grow weaker, and soon the patient can't sit up or lift their head. The patient has difficulty turning over, can't grasp objects, and has progressive vision loss.

By age 18 months, the infant is usually deaf and blind and has seizures, generalized paralysis, and spasticity. The pupils are dilated and don't react to light. Decerebrate rigidity and a vegetative state follow. The child suffers recurrent bronchopneumonia after age 2 and usually dies before age 5. A child who survives may develop ataxia and progressive motor retardation between ages 2 and 8.

The "juvenile" form of Tay–Sachs disease generally appears between ages 2 and 5 as a progressive deterioration of psychomotor skills and gait. Patients with this type can survive to adulthood.

Diagnosis

℞ **CONFIRMING DIAGNOSIS** *Typical clinical features point to Tay–Sachs disease, but serum analysis showing deficient hexosaminidase A is the key to diagnosis. An ophthalmologic examination showing optic nerve atrophy and a distinctive cherry-red spot on the retina supports the diagnosis. (The cherry-red spot may be absent in the juvenile form.)*

Diagnostic screening is essential for all couples when at least one partner is of Ashkenazi Jewish, French Canadian, or Cajun ancestry and for others with a family history of the disease. A blood test evaluating hexosaminidase A levels can identify carriers. Amniocentesis or CVS can detect hexosaminidase A deficiency in the fetus.

Treatment

Tay–Sachs disease has no known cure. Supportive treatment includes tube feedings of nutritional supplements, suctioning and postural drainage to remove pharyngeal secretions, skin care to prevent pressure ulcers in bedridden children, and mild laxatives to relieve neurogenic constipation. Anticonvulsants usually fail to prevent seizures. Because these children need constant physical care, many parents have full-time skilled home nursing care or place them in long-term special care facilities.

Special considerations

Your most important job is to help the family deal with inevitably progressive illness and death.

◆ Offer carrier testing to all couples from high-risk ethnic groups.
◆ Refer the parents for genetic counseling, and stress the importance of considering an amniocentesis in future pregnancies. Refer siblings for screening to determine if they're carriers. If they're carriers and are adults, refer them for genetic counseling, but stress that there's no danger of transmitting the disease to offspring if they do not bear children with another carrier.
◆ Some in vitro fertilization centers have recently started offering preimplantation genetics. Refer the couple to an appropriate center if they express interest in assisted reproductive technology.
◆ Because the parents of an affected child may feel excessive stress or guilt because of the child's illness and the emotional and financial burden it places on them, refer them for counseling if indicated.
◆ If the parents care for their child at home, teach them how to do suctioning, postural drainage, and tube feeding. Also teach them how to provide good skin care to prevent pressure ulcers.

For more information on this disease, refer parents to the National Tay–Sachs and Allied Diseases Association.

PHENYLKETONURIA

Phenylketonuria (PKU) is an inborn error in phenylalanine metabolism that results in the accumulation of high serum levels of the enzyme phenylalanine in the blood. When left untreated, it results in cerebral damage and mental retardation.

Causes and incidence

PKU is caused by a gene mutation. In the United States, this disorder occurs in 1 in about 14,000 births. (About 1 person in 60 is an asymptomatic carrier.) The gene is most common in Ireland, Scotland, Belgium, and West Germany and is rare in Blacks, Asians, Native Americans, Finns, and Ashkenazi Jews.

Pathophysiology

PKU is transmitted by an autosomal recessive gene on chromosome 12. Patients with this disorder have insufficient hepatic phenylalanine hydroxylase, an enzyme that acts as a catalyst in the conversion of phenylalanine to tyrosine. As a result, phenylalanine and its metabolites accumulate in the blood, eventually causing mental retardation if left untreated. The exact biochemical mechanism that causes this retardation is unclear.

Signs and symptoms

An infant with undiagnosed and untreated PKU appears normal at birth but by age 4 months begins to show signs of arrested brain development, including mental retardation and, later, personality disturbances (schizoid and antisocial personality patterns and uncontrollable temper). Such a child may have a lighter complexion than unaffected siblings and typically has blue eyes. The patient may also have microcephaly; eczematous skin lesions or dry, rough skin; and a musty (mousy) odor because of skin and urinary excretion of phenylacetic acid. About 80% of these children have abnormal electroencephalographic patterns, and about one-third have seizures, usually beginning between ages 6 and 12 months.

Children with PKU show a precipitous decrease in IQ in their first year, are usually hyperactive and irritable, and exhibit purposeless, repetitive motions. They have increased muscle tone and an awkward gait.

Although blood phenylalanine levels are near normal at birth, they begin to rise within a few days. By the time they reach significant levels (about 30 mg/dL), cerebral damage has begun. Such irreversible damage probably is complete by age 2 or 3. However, early detection and treatment can minimize cerebral damage, and children under strict dietary control can lead normal lives.

Diagnosis

All states require screening for PKU at birth; the Guthrie screening test on a capillary blood sample (bacterial inhibition assay) reliably detects PKU. However, because phenylalanine levels may be normal at birth, the neonate should be reevaluated after receiving dietary protein for 24 to 48 hours. The common practice of discharging new mothers from the hospital within 24 hours of delivery has resulted in failure to detect some neonates with PKU. For this reason, some states now require a minimum hospital stay of 48 hours after childbirth.

Adding a few drops of 10% ferric chloride solution to a wet diaper is another method of detecting PKU. If the area turns a deep, bluish green, phenylpyruvic acid is present in the urine.

℞ **CONFIRMING DIAGNOSIS** *Detection of elevated blood levels of phenylalanine and the presence of phenylpyruvic acid in the infant's urine confirm the diagnosis. (Urine should also be tested 4 to 6 weeks after birth because urinary levels of phenylpyruvic acid vary with the amount of protein ingested.)*

CVS can be used to detect fetal PKU as a prenatal diagnosis. Enzyme assay can be used to detect the carrier state in parents.

Treatment

Treatment consists of restricting dietary intake of the amino acid phenylalanine to keep phenylalanine blood levels between 3 and 9 mg/dL. Because most natural proteins contain 5% phenylalanine, they must be limited in the child's diet. An enzymatic hydrolysate of casein, such as Lofenalac powder or Pregestimil powder, is substituted for milk in the diets of affected infants. This milk substitute contains a minimal amount of phenylalanine, normal amounts of other amino acids, and added amounts of carbohydrate and fat. Dietary restrictions continue throughout life.

The special diet for PKU calls for careful monitoring. Because the body doesn't make phenylalanine, overzealous dietary restriction can induce phenylalanine deficiency, producing lethargy, anorexia, anemia, rashes, and diarrhea.

Special considerations

In caring for a child with PKU, it's especially important to teach both the parents and child about this disease and to provide emotional support and counseling. (Psychological and emotional problems may result from the difficult dietary restrictions.)

◆ Emphasize to the child and parents the critical importance of adhering to the special diet. The child must avoid breads, cheese, eggs, flour, meat, poultry, fish, nuts, milk, legumes, and phenylalanine sugar substitutes.

◆ Inform the parents that the child will need frequent tests for urine phenylpyruvic acid and blood phenylalanine levels to evaluate the diet's effectiveness.

◆ As the child grows older and is supervised less closely, the patient's parents will have less control over what the child eats. As a result, deviation from the restricted diet becomes more likely, as does the risk of brain damage. Encourage the parents to allow the child some choices in the kinds of low-protein foods they want to eat; this will help make the patient feel trusted and more responsible.

◆ Teach the parents about normal physical and mental growth and development so that they can recognize any developmental delay that may point to excessive phenylalanine intake.

PEDIATRIC TIP *Infants should be routinely screened for PKU because detection of the disorder and control of phenylalanine intake soon after birth can prevent severe mental retardation.*

◆ Refer females with PKU who reach reproductive age for genetic counseling because recent research indicates that their offspring may have a higher-than-normal incidence of brain damage, mental retardation, microcephaly, and major congenital malformations, especially of the heart and CNS. Such damage may be minimized with a low-phenylalanine diet before conception and during pregnancy. Even patients under good control remain at increased risk for offspring with this defect. During pregnancy, weekly blood tests should be done to make sure phenylalanine levels don't get too high.

ALBINISM

Albinism is a rare inherited defect in melanin metabolism of the skin and eyes (oculocutaneous albinism) or just the eyes (ocular albinism). Ocular albinism impairs visual acuity. Oculocutaneous albinism also causes severe intolerance to sunlight and increases susceptibility to skin cancer. Other forms are associated with deafness. About 1 in 17,000 people have one of the types of albinism.

Causes and incidence

Oculocutaneous albinism results from autosomal recessive inheritance; ocular albinism, from an X-linked recessive trait that causes hypopigmentation only in the iris and the ocular fundus.

In the United States, both types of albinism are more common in Blacks than in Whites. Native Americans have a high incidence of the tyrosinase-positive form.

Pathophysiology

Normally, melanocytes synthesize melanin. Melanosomes, melanin-containing granules within melanocytes, diffuse and absorb the sun's ultraviolet light, thus protecting the skin and eyes from its dangerous effects. In *tyrosinase-negative albinism* (the most common type), melanosomes don't contain melanin because they lack tyrosinase, the enzyme that stimulates melanin production. In *tyrosinase-positive albinism*, melanosomes contain tyrosine, a tyrosinase substrate, but a defect in the tyrosine transport system impairs melanin production.

In *tyrosinase-variable albinism* (rare), an unidentified enzyme defect probably impairs synthesis of a melanin precursor. Other rare forms of albinism are *Chédiak–Higashi syndrome* (tyrosinase-negative albinism with hematologic and neurologic manifestations); *Hermansky–Pudlak syndrome* (tyrosinase-positive albinism with platelet dysfunction, bleeding abnormalities, and inclusions in many organs); and *Cross–McKusick–Breen syndrome* (tyrosinase-positive albinism with neurologic involvement).

Complications

◆ Nystagmus
◆ Photosensitivity
◆ Errors of refraction
◆ Pigmented nevi
◆ Actinic keratoses
◆ Increased skin cancer risk

Signs and symptoms

Light-skinned Whites with tyrosinase-negative albinism have pale skin and hair color ranging from white to yellow; their pupils appear red because of translucent irides. Blacks with the same disorder have hair that may be white, faintly tinged with yellow, or yellow-brown. Both Whites and Blacks with tyrosinase-positive albinism grow darker as they age. For instance, their hair may become straw-colored or light brown and their skin cream-colored or pink. People with tyrosinase-positive albinism may also have freckles and pigmented nevi that may require excision.

In tyrosinase-variable albinism, at birth the child's hair is white, skin is pink, and the eyes are gray. As the patient grows older, though, the hair becomes yellow, irides may become darker, and the skin may even tan slightly.

The skin of a person with albinism is easily damaged by the sun. It may look weather-beaten and is highly susceptible to precancerous and cancerous growths. The patient may also have photophobia, myopia, strabismus, and congenital horizontal nystagmus.

Diagnosis

Diagnosis is based on clinical observation and the patient's family history. Microscopic examination of the skin and of hair follicles determines the amount of pigment present. Testing plucked hair roots for pigmentation when incubated in tyrosine distinguishes tyrosinase-negative albinism from tyrosinase-positive albinism. Tyrosinase-positive hair bulbs will develop color.

Treatment

No specific treatment for albinism exists.

Special considerations

◆ To help the parents work through any feelings of guilt or depression, encourage early infant–parent bonding. Also inform the parents about cosmetic measures (glasses with tinted lenses, makeup) that can lessen the child's disfigurement when he's older.

◆ Teach the child and parents what measures best protect the patient from solar radiation, and inform them of its danger signals (excessive drying of skin, crusty lesions on exposed skin, changes in skin color).

◆ Advise the patient to wear full-spectrum sunblocks, dark glasses, and appropriate protective clothing.

◆ If the patient's appearance causes social and emotional problems, they may need psychological counseling. Such counseling may also be in order for the family, if they too find it difficult to accept the disorder.

◆ Stress the need for frequent refractions and eye examinations to correct visual defects.

◆ Refer the adult patient or the parents of an affected child for genetic counseling to learn about the probability of recurrence in future offspring.

SICKLE CELL ANEMIA

A congenital hemolytic anemia that occurs primarily but not exclusively in Blacks, sickle cell anemia results from a defective Hb molecule (HbS) that causes red blood cells (RBCs)

Sickle cell trait

Sickle cell trait is a relatively benign condition that results from heterozygous inheritance of the abnormal *HbS-producing* gene. Like sickle cell anemia, this condition is most common in Blacks. Sickle cell trait never progresses to sickle cell anemia.

In persons with sickle cell trait (known as *carriers*), 20% to 40% of their total Hb is HbS; the rest is normal.

Such persons usually have no symptoms. They have normal Hb and hematocrit values and can expect a normal life span. Nevertheless, they must avoid situations that provoke hypoxia, which can occasionally cause a sickling crisis similar to that in sickle cell anemia.

Genetic counseling is essential for sickle cell carriers. If two sickle cell carriers produce offspring, each of their children has a 25% chance of inheriting sickle cell anemia.

---

to roughen and become sickle-shaped. Such cells impair circulation, resulting in chronic ill health (fatigue, dyspnea on exertion, swollen joints), periodic crises, long-term complications, and premature death.

Penicillin prophylaxis can decrease morbidity and mortality from bacterial infections. Fifty percent of patients with sickle cell anemia survive past their fifth decade.

Causes and incidence

Sickle cell is caused by a gene mutation. Sickle cell anemia is most common in tropical Africans and in people of African descent; about 1 in 10 American Blacks carries the abnormal gene. However, sickle cell anemia also appears in other ethnic populations, including people of Mediterranean or East Indian ancestry.

If two parents who are both carriers of sickle cell trait (or another hemoglobinopathy) have offspring, each child has a 25% chance of developing sickle cell anemia. (See *Inheritance patterns in sickle cell anemia*, page 995.) Overall, 1 in every 400 to 600 Black children has sickle cell anemia. The defective *HbS-producing* gene may have persisted because, in areas where malaria is endemic, the heterozygous sickle cell trait provides resistance to malaria and is actually beneficial.

Inheritance patterns in sickle cell anemia

When both parents are carriers of sickle cell trait, each child has a 25% chance of developing sickle cell anemia, a 25% chance of being a normal (unaffected) noncarrier, and a 50% chance of being a carrier of sickle cell trait.

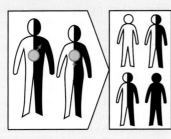

When one parent has sickle cell anemia and one is normal, all offspring will be carriers of sickle cell trait.

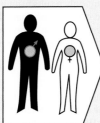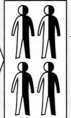

KEY

☐ Normal, noncarrier

▮ Normal, carrier of sickle cell trait

■ Sickle cell anemia (affected with sickle cell disease)

Comparing normal and sickled red blood cells

When a person with sickle cell anemia develops hypoxia, the abnormal HbS found in the RBCs becomes insoluble. This causes the RBCs to become rigid, rough, and elongated, forming the characteristic sickle shape.

NORMAL RBCs

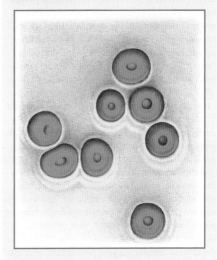

SICKLE CELLS

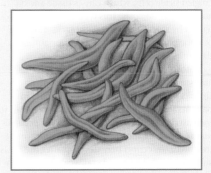

The abnormal HbS found in patients' RBCs becomes insoluble whenever hypoxia occurs. As a result, these RBCs become rigid, rough, and elongated, forming a crescent or sickle shape. (See *Comparing normal and sickled red blood cells.*) Such sickling can produce hemolysis (cell destruction). In addition, these altered cells tend to pile up in capillaries and smaller blood vessels, making blood more viscous. Normal circulation is impaired, causing pain, tissue infarctions, and swelling. Such blockage causes anoxic changes that lead to further sickling and obstruction.

Pathophysiology

Sickle cell anemia results from homozygous inheritance of the gene located on chromosome II that produces HbS. It's inherited as an autosomal recessive trait. Heterozygous inheritance of this gene results in sickle cell trait, a condition that usually produces no symptoms. (See *Sickle cell trait,* page 994.)

Complications
◆ Chronic obstructive pulmonary disease
◆ Heart failure
◆ Organ infarction
◆ Splenomegaly
◆ Stroke
◆ Premature death

Signs and symptoms
Characteristically, sickle cell anemia produces tachycardia, cardiomegaly, systolic and diastolic murmurs, pulmonary infarctions (which may result in cor pulmonale), chronic fatigue, unexplained dyspnea or dyspnea on exertion, hepatomegaly, jaundice, pallor, joint swelling, aching bones, chest pains, ischemic leg ulcers (especially around the ankles), and increased susceptibility to infection. Such symptoms usually don't develop until after age 6 months because large amounts of fetal Hb protect infants for the first few months after birth. Low socioeconomic status and related problems, such as poor nutrition and education, may delay diagnosis and supportive treatment.

Infection, stress, dehydration, and conditions that provoke hypoxia—strenuous exercise, high altitude, unpressurized aircraft, cold, and vasoconstrictive drugs—may all provoke periodic crises. A painful crisis (vaso-occlusive crisis, infarctive crisis), the most common crisis and the hallmark of the disease, usually appears periodically after age 5. It results from blood vessel obstruction by rigid, tangled sickle cells, which causes tissue anoxia and possible necrosis. This type of crisis is characterized by severe abdominal, thoracic, muscular, or bone pain and possibly worsening jaundice, dark urine, and a low-grade fever.

Autosplenectomy, in which splenic damage and scarring is so extensive that the spleen shrinks and becomes impalpable, occurs in patients with long-term disease. This can lead to increased susceptibility to *Streptococcus pneumoniae* sepsis, which can be fatal without prompt treatment. Infection may develop after the crisis subsides (in 4 days to several weeks), so watch for lethargy, sleepiness, fever, or apathy.

An aplastic crisis (megaloblastic crisis) results from bone marrow depression and is associated with infection, usually viral. It's characterized by pallor, lethargy, sleepiness, dyspnea, possible coma, markedly decreased bone marrow activity, and RBC hemolysis.

In infants between ages 8 months and 2 years, an acute sequestration crisis may cause sudden massive entrapment of RBCs in the spleen and liver. This rare crisis causes lethargy and pallor and, if untreated, commonly progresses to hypovolemic shock and death.

A hemolytic crisis is quite rare and usually occurs in patients who also have glucose-6-phosphate dehydrogenase deficiency. It probably results from complications of sickle cell anemia, such as infection, rather than from the disorder itself. Hemolytic crisis causes liver congestion and hepatomegaly as a result of degenerative changes. It worsens chronic jaundice, although increased jaundice doesn't always point to a hemolytic crisis.

Suspect any of these crises in a sickle cell anemia patient with pale lips, tongue, palms, or nail beds; lethargy; listlessness; sleepiness with difficulty awakening; irritability; severe pain; a fever over 104° F (40° C); or a fever of 100° F (37.8° C) that persists for 2 days.

Sickle cell anemia also causes long-term complications. Typically, the child is small for their age and has delayed puberty. (However, fertility isn't impaired.) If they reach adulthood, the body build tends to be spiderlike—narrow shoulders and hips, long extremities, curved spine, barrel chest, and elongated skull. An adult usually has complications from organ infarction, such as retinopathy and nephropathy. Premature death commonly results from infection or from repeated occlusion of small blood vessels and consequent infarction or necrosis of major organs (such as cerebral blood vessel occlusion causing stroke).

Diagnosis
A positive family history and typical clinical features suggest sickle cell anemia. Hb electrophoresis showing HbS or other hemoglobinopathies can also confirm it. Electrophoresis should be done on umbilical cord blood samples at birth to provide sickle cell disease screening for all neonates at risk.

Additional laboratory studies may show a low RBC count, elevated white blood cell and platelet counts, decreased erythrocyte sedimentation rate, increased serum iron, decreased RBC survival, and reticulocytosis. Hb levels may be low or normal. During early childhood, palpation may reveal splenomegaly, but, as the child grows older, the spleen shrinks.

Treatment
Treatment begins before age 4 months with prophylactic penicillin. If the patient's Hb drops suddenly or if the condition deteriorates rapidly, the patient will need to be hospitalized for a transfusion of packed RBCs. In a sequestration crisis, treatment may include sedation, administration of analgesics, a blood transfusion, oxygen administration, and large amounts of oral or I.V. fluids.

Daily folic acid supplementation is recommended to prevent megaloblastic crisis. Hydroxyurea, which causes an increase in the synthesis of fetal Hb and a significant reduction in crises, is being used for some patients with sickle cell anemia. Researchers have found it helpful for some patients because it reduces the frequency of painful crises and episodes of acute chest syndrome and decreases the need for blood transfusions.

Newer drugs are being developed to manage sickle cell anemia. Some of these agents try to induce the body to produce more fetal Hb, which helps decrease the amount of sickling. Others work by increasing the binding of oxygen to sickle cells. Currently, bone marrow transplantation offers the only cure for sickle cell anemia. Gene therapy (replacing HbS with normal HbA) may be the ideal treatment, but it's difficult to perform.

Nitric oxide gas helps blood vessels open and reduces the stickiness of RBCs.

Special considerations

Supportive measures during crises and precautions to avoid them are important. Here are some actions you can take during a painful crisis:

◆ Apply warm compresses to painful areas, and cover the child with a blanket. (Never use cold compresses because they aggravate the condition.)

◆ Administer an analgesic–antipyretic, such as aspirin or acetaminophen. (Additional pain relief may be required during an acute crisis.)

◆ Encourage fluids and bed rest, and place the patient in a sitting position. If dehydration or severe pain occurs, hospitalization may be necessary.

◆ When cultures indicate, give antibiotics as appropriate.

During remissions:

◆ Advise the patient to avoid tight clothing that restricts circulation.

◆ Warn against strenuous exercise, vasoconstricting medications, cold temperatures (including drinking large amounts of ice water and swimming), unpressurized aircraft, high altitude, and other conditions that provoke hypoxia.

PEDIATRIC TIP *Stress the importance of normal childhood immunizations, meticulous wound care, good oral hygiene, regular dental checkups, and a balanced diet as safeguards against infection.*

◆ Emphasize the need for prompt treatment of infection.

◆ Inform the patient of the need to increase fluid intake to prevent dehydration because of impaired ability to concentrate urine properly.

Tell parents to encourage the child to drink more fluids, especially in the summer, by offering fluids such as milkshakes and ice pops.

During pregnancy or surgery:

◆ Warn women with sickle cell anemia that they may have increased obstetrical risks. However, use of hormonal contraceptives may also be risky; refer them for birth control counseling to a qualified obstetric or gynecologic healthcare provider.

◆ If such women *do* become pregnant, they should maintain a balanced diet and may benefit from a folic acid supplement.

◆ During general anesthesia, a patient who has sickle cell anemia requires optimal ventilation to prevent hypoxic crisis. Make sure the surgeon and the anesthesiologist know that the patient has sickle cell anemia. Provide a preoperative transfusion of packed RBCs, as needed.

General tips:

◆ To encourage normal mental and social development, warn parents against being overprotective. Although the child must avoid strenuous exercise, the patient can enjoy most everyday activities.

◆ Refer parents of children with sickle cell anemia for genetic counseling to answer their questions about the risk to future offspring. Recommend screening of other family members to determine if they're heterozygote carriers. These parents may also need psychological counseling to cope with guilt feelings. In addition, suggest they join an appropriate community support group.

◆ Adolescent or adult males with sickle cell anemia may develop sudden, painful episodes of priapism. Such episodes are common and, if prolonged, can have serious reproductive consequences. Advise the patient to contact the physician when these episodes occur.

X-linked inheritance

HEMOPHILIA

Hemophilia is a hereditary bleeding disorder resulting from a deficiency of specific clotting factors.

Advances in treatment have greatly improved the prognosis for patients with hemophilia, many of whom live normal life spans. Surgical procedures can be done safely at special treatment centers under the guidance of a hematologist.

Causes and incidence

Both hemophilia A and B are inherited as X-linked recessive traits.

A large number of disease-causing mutations have been identified in both genes. A specific inversion mutation in the noncoding region of the *factor VIII gene* is present in about 45% of families with severe hemophilia A. Hemophilia A is a common X-linked genetic disease, occurring in about 1 in 10,000 live male births. It is five times more common than hemophilia B.

Pathophysiology

After a person with hemophilia forms a platelet plug at a bleeding site, the clotting factor deficiency impairs the blood's capacity to form a stable fibrin clot. Bleeding occurs primarily into large joints, especially after trauma or surgery. Spontaneous intracranial bleeding can occur and may be fatal.

Hemophilia A and B are inherited X-linked recessive traits. This means that female carriers have a 50% chance of transmitting the gene to each daughter, who would then be a carrier, and a 50% chance of transmitting the gene to each son, who would be born with hemophilia. Hemophilia A (classic hemophilia), which affects more than 80% of patients with hemophilia, results from a deficiency of factor VIII-C; hemophilia B (Christmas disease), which affects about 15% of patients with hemophilia, results from a deficiency of factor IX-C. The factor VIII gene is located within the *Xq28* region, and the factor IX gene is located within *Xq27*. Females with one defective *factor VIII* gene are carriers of hemophilia.

Complications

◆ Internal bleeding
◆ Arthritis caused by chronic pressure put on joints
◆ Potential for infection from blood transfusions

Signs and symptoms

Hemophilia produces abnormal bleeding, which may be mild, moderate, or severe, depending on the degree of factor deficiency.

Mild hemophilia commonly goes undiagnosed until adulthood because the patient doesn't bleed spontaneously or after minor trauma but has prolonged bleeding if challenged by major trauma or surgery. Postoperative bleeding continues as a slow ooze or ceases and starts again, up to 8 days after surgery.

Severe hemophilia causes spontaneous bleeding. In many cases, the first sign of severe hemophilia is excessive bleeding after circumcision. Later, spontaneous bleeding or severe bleeding after minor trauma may produce large subcutaneous and deep intramuscular hematomas. Bleeding into joints (hemarthrosis) and muscles causes pain, swelling, extreme tenderness, and, possibly, permanent deformity.

Moderate hemophilia causes symptoms similar to severe hemophilia but produces only occasional spontaneous bleeding episodes.

Bleeding near peripheral nerves may cause peripheral neuropathy, pain, paresthesia, and muscle atrophy. If bleeding impairs blood flow through a major vessel, it can cause ischemia and gangrene. Pharyngeal, lingual, intracardial, intracerebral, and intracranial bleeding may all lead to shock and death.

Diagnosis

Development of a large cephalohematoma or intracranial hemorrhage after prolonged labor or delivery by forceps or vacuum extraction may be the first indication of a bleeding problem. After the neonatal period, a history of prolonged bleeding after surgery (including dental extractions) or trauma or of episodes of spontaneous bleeding into muscles or joints usually indicates some defect in the hemostatic mechanism. Hemophilia A and B may be clinically indistinguishable, but specific coagulation factor assays can diagnose the type and severity of the disease. A positive family history, prenatal diagnosis, and carrier testing can also help diagnose hemophilia, but nearly one-third of all patients have no family history.

Characteristic findings in hemophilia A include:
◆ *factor VIII-C* assay 0% to 30% of normal
◆ prolonged partial thromboplastin time (PTT)
◆ normal platelet count and function, bleeding time, and prothrombin time

Characteristics of hemophilia B include:
◆ deficient factor IX-C
◆ baseline coagulation results similar to hemophilia A, with normal factor VIII

In both types of hemophilia, the degree of factor deficiency determines severity:
◆ mild hemophilia—factor levels 5% to 40% of normal
◆ moderate hemophilia—factor levels 1% to 5% of normal
◆ severe hemophilia—factor levels less than 1% of normal

Treatment

Hemophilia isn't curable, but treatment can prevent crippling deformities and prolong life expectancy. Correct treatment quickly stops bleeding by increasing plasma levels of deficient clotting factors to help prevent disabling deformities that result from repeated bleeding into muscles and joints. (See *Factor replacement products*, page 999.)

Desmopressin (DDAVP—1-deamino-8-D-arginine vasopressin), which is a synthetic hormone that stimulates the release of factor VIII, is administered I.V. or intranasally is usually

Factor replacement products

Cryoprecipitate

◆ Contains factor VIII (70 to 100 units/bag); doesn't contain factor IX

◆ Can be stored frozen up to 12 months but must be used within 6 hours after it thaws

◆ Given through a blood filter; compatible with normal saline solution only

◆ No longer treatment of choice because of the risk of human immunodeficiency virus (HIV) and hepatitis infection; can still contain viruses despite greatly improved screening and purification procedures for viral inactivation in blood products

Lyophilized factor VIII or IX

◆ Freeze-dried

◆ Can be stored up to 2 years at about 36° to 46° F (2° to 8° C), up to 6 months at room temperature not exceeding 88° F (31.1° C)

◆ Labeled with exact units of factor VIII or IX contained in vial

◆ 200 to 1,500 units of factor VIII or IX per vial; 20 to 40 mL after reconstitution with diluent

◆ No blood filter needed; usually given by slow I.V. push through a butterfly infusion set

Fresh frozen plasma

◆ Contains approximately 0.75 unit/mL of factor VII and approximately 1 unit/mL of factor IX; not practical for most people with hemophilia because a large volume is needed to raise factors to hemostatic levels.

◆ Can be stored frozen up to 12 months but must be used within 2 hours after it thaws.

◆ Given through a blood filter; compatible with normal saline solution only.

---

sufficient to manage bleeding episodes of children and adolescents with mild hemophilia A. Persons with moderate to severe hemophilia A require commercially prepared factor VIII concentrates to treat bleeding episodes. Concentrates derived from human plasma are virally attenuated by one or more available methods, significantly minimizing the risk for HIV-1, HIV-2, hepatitis B, and hepatitis C contamination. However, no currently available method has been successful in eradicating parvovirus B19 from blood products. Factor VIII concentrate derived from recombinant technology (rFVIII) has been shown in multiple clinical trials to be as effective as virally attenuated plasma-derived concentrate. Risk for viral contamination is essentially nonexistent in preparations of rFVIII that avoid human serum albumin as a stabilizer.

In hemophilia B, administration of factor IX concentrate during bleeding episodes increases factor IX levels.

The U.S. National Hemophilia Foundation first recommended prophylaxis with factor concentrates in 1994 after investigators in Sweden demonstrated repeated success with this approach. The ultimate goal is to prevent irreversible destructive arthritis that results from repeated hemarthrosis and synovial hypertrophy. Prophylaxis of persons with hemophilia A or B may begin as early as age 1 or 2.

A person with hemophilia who undergoes surgery needs careful management by a hematologist with expertise in hemophilia care. The patient will require replacement of the deficient factor before and after surgery, possibly even for minor surgery such as a dental extraction. (DDAVP may be given before dental extractions and surgery to prevent bleeding.) In addition, epsilon-aminocaproic acid is commonly used for oral bleeding to inhibit the active fibrinolytic system present in the oral mucosa.

Development of factor VIII or factor XI inhibitors occurs in up to 3.5% of children with severe hemophilia A and up to 3% of those with hemophilia B. Studies indicate that certain gene mutations predispose to an increased risk for inhibitor development. Patients with hemophilia who can't achieve hemostasis after use of previously effective factor concentrate doses should be evaluated for factor inhibitors.

Preventive measures include teaching the patient how to avoid trauma, manage minor bleeding, and recognize bleeding that requires immediate medical intervention. Genetic counseling helps carriers understand how this disease is transmitted. (See *Managing hemophilia*, page 1000.)

Special considerations

During bleeding episodes:

◆ Give clotting agents as ordered. The body uses up factor VIII in 48 to 72 hours, so repeat infusions, as indicated, until bleeding stops.

◆ Apply cold compresses or ice bags and raise the injured part.

◆ To prevent recurrence of bleeding, restrict activity for 48 hours after bleeding is under control.

Managing hemophilia

The following guidelines can help parents care for their child with hemophilia.

♦ Instruct parents to notify the physician immediately after even a minor injury, but especially after an injury to the head, neck, or abdomen. Such injuries may require special blood factor replacement. Also, tell them to check with the physician before allowing dental extractions or any other surgery.

♦ Educate the patient and parents on the early signs and symptoms of hemarthrosis: stiffness, tingling, or ache in joint, followed by decreased range of motion. If signs and symptoms are recognized early, treatment can begin earlier, potentially decreasing the possibility of long-term disability.

♦ Stress the importance of regular, careful toothbrushing with a soft-bristled toothbrush to prevent the need for dental surgery.

♦ Teach parents to be alert for signs of severe internal bleeding, such as severe pain or swelling in a joint or muscle, stiffness, decreased joint movement, severe abdominal pain, blood in urine, black tarry stools, and severe headache.

♦ Advise parents that the child is at risk for hepatitis from blood components. Early signs—headache, fever, decreased appetite, nausea, vomiting, abdominal tenderness, and pain over the liver—may appear 3 weeks to 6 months after treatment with blood components. Tell them to discuss with their physician the possibility of hepatitis vaccination.

♦ Discuss the increased risk of HIV infection. Tell parents to ask the physician about periodic testing for HIV.

♦ Urge parents to make sure their child wears a medical identification bracelet at all times.

♦ Teach parents never to give their child aspirin, which can aggravate the tendency to bleed. Advise them to give acetaminophen instead.

♦ Instruct parents to protect their child from injury, but to avoid unnecessary restrictions that impair normal development. For example, they can sew padded patches into the knees and elbows of a toddler's clothing to protect these joints during falls. They shouldn't allow an older child to participate in contact sports such as football but can encourage the patient to swim or to play golf.

♦ Teach parents to elevate and apply cold compresses or ice bags to an injured area and to apply light pressure to a bleeding site. To prevent recurrence of bleeding, advise parents to restrict the child's activity for 48 hours after bleeding is under control.

♦ If parents have been trained to administer blood factor components at home to avoid frequent hospitalization, make sure they know proper venipuncture and infusion techniques and don't delay treatment during bleeding episodes.

♦ Instruct parents to keep blood factor concentrate and infusion equipment on hand at all times, even on vacation.

♦ Emphasize the importance of having the child keep routine medical appointments at the local hemophilia center.

♦ Daughters of individuals with hemophilia should undergo genetic screening to determine if they're hemophilia carriers. Affected males should undergo counseling as well. If they produce offspring with a noncarrier, all of their daughters will be carriers; if they produce offspring with a carrier, each child has a 25% chance of being affected.

♦ For more information, refer parents to the National Hemophilia Foundation.

♦ Control pain with an analgesic, such as acetaminophen, propoxyphene, codeine, or meperidine, as appropriate. Avoid I.M. injections because of possible hematoma formation at the injection site. Aspirin and aspirin-containing medications are contraindicated because they decrease platelet adherence and may increase the bleeding. Caution should be used when trying other nonsteroidal anti-inflammatory drugs, for example, ibuprofen or ketoprofen.

If the patient has bled into a joint:
♦ Immediately elevate the joint.

♦ To restore joint mobility, begin range-of-motion exercises, if ordered, at least 48 hours after the bleeding is controlled. Tell the patient to avoid weight-bearing until bleeding stops and swelling subsides.

After bleeding episodes and surgery:
♦ Watch closely for signs of further bleeding, such as increased pain and swelling, fever, or symptoms of shock.
♦ Closely monitor PTT.
♦ Teach parents special precautions to prevent bleeding episodes.

◆ Refer new patients to a hemophilia treatment center for evaluation. The center will devise a treatment plan for such patients' primary physicians and is a resource for other medical and school personnel, dentists, and others involved in their care.

◆ Persons who have been exposed to HIV through contaminated blood products need special support.

◆ Refer patients and carriers for genetic counseling.

FRAGILE X SYNDROME

Fragile X syndrome is the most common inherited cause of mental retardation. The condition is typically caused by a well-defined mutation at a specific locus of the fragile X mental retardation 1 (FMR1) gene on the X chromosome. About 85% of males and 50% of females who inherit the FMR1 mutation will demonstrate clinical features of the syndrome. Postpubescent males with fragile X syndrome usually have distinct physical features, behavioral difficulties, and cognitive impairment. Females with fragile X syndrome tend to have more subtle symptoms.

Causes and incidence

Fragile X syndrome is an X-linked condition that doesn't follow a simple X-linked inheritance pattern.

Fragile X syndrome is estimated to occur in about 1 in 1,500 males and 1 in 2,500 females. It has been reported in almost all races and ethnic populations.

Pathophysiology

The normal sequence of the FMR1 gene was identified at Xq27.3 in 1991. The unique mutation that results in fragile X syndrome consists of an expanding region of a specific triplet of nitrogenous bases: cytosine, guanine, guanine (CGG) within the gene's DNA sequence. Normally, FMR1 contains 6 to 50 sequential copies of the CGG triplet. When the number of CGG triplets expands to the range of 50 to 200 repeats, the region of DNA becomes unstable and is referred to as a premutation. A full mutation consists of more than 200 CGG triplet repeats.

The full mutation typically causes abnormal methylation (methyl groups attach to components of the gene) of FMR1. Methylation inhibits gene transcription and thus protein production. The reduced or absent protein product (FNIRP) is responsible for the clinical features of fragile X syndrome. Of males with full mutation, 15% to 20% don't have fragile X syndrome. This may be explained by either the

ability of unmethylated portions (of the mutated FMR1) to be transcribed for eventual protein production, or that these males are mosaic for the FMR1 premutation. In asymptomatic mosaic males it's believed that the cells with a premutation can produce enough protein to compensate for the cells that contain a full mutation and consequently produce no protein.

About 50% of females who inherit a full mutation from their mother have clinical features of fragile X syndrome. This is primarily due to the normal process of random X inactivation. At the time of meiosis, both X chromosomes must be activated. However, shortly after the zygote stage, an X chromosome is inactivated in every cell. Clinically measurable effects of the full FMR1 mutation will be more likely in relevant tissues or organs that have a disproportionate number of cells in which the normal X chromosome has been inactivated.

Males with a premutation don't have fragile X syndrome. They're considered unaffected or normal-transmitting males. Because males have only one X chromosome, all daughters of a transmitting male will inherit their father's X chromosome with the premutation. None of the male's sons will inherit the premutation because they inherit their father's Y chromosome rather than the X chromosome.

Females with the premutation don't have fragile X syndrome. However, the premutation can expand into the full mutation range (>200 CGG triplets) when it's transmitted from a premutation carrier mother to her offspring. This expansion can occur during or after maternal meiosis. Therefore, the following possibilities exist for every pregnancy of a mother with a premutation.

◆ A female conceptus receives the mother's X chromosome with the nonmutated FMR1 gene. She won't be affected with fragile X syndrome. None of her future offspring will be at risk for inheriting the syndrome from her.

◆ A male conceptus receives the mother's X with the nonmutated FMR1 gene. They won't be affected with fragile X syndrome. None of his future offspring will be at risk for inheriting the syndrome from him.

◆ A female conceptus receives the mother's X chromosome with the FMR1 premutation. She'll be a carrier like her mother but won't have fragile X syndrome. Her future offspring will be at risk for inheriting a full mutation from her.

◆ A male conceptus receives the mother's X with the FMR1 premutation. They won't be affected with fragile X syndrome. All of his future daughters but none of his future sons will inherit the premutation from him.

◆ A female conceptus receives the mother's X chromosome with the *FMR1* gene whose premutation expanded into a full mutation during or after maternal meiosis. Depending on the outcome of random X inactivation, the daughter may have clinically definable fragile X syndrome. Her future offspring will be at risk for inheriting the full mutation and, thus, the syndrome from her.

◆ A male conceptus receives the mother's X chromosome with the *FMR1* gene whose premutation has expanded into a full mutation during or after maternal meiosis. In 85% of cases, the son in this situation will have fragile X syndrome. Evidence indicates, however, that the *FMR1* gene in the son's gametes will have the CGG triplet repeat within the premutation range, not the full mutation range like his somatic cells. Therefore, his future daughters wouldn't be expected to have fragile X syndrome.

It should be noted that most commonly the *FMR1* status of a mother is subsequently determined after her son is clinically and later molecularly diagnosed with fragile X syndrome. Healthcare professionals need to be sensitive to the fact that the mother could find out that either she is a carrier of a premutation or that she has a full mutation. Consequently, not only will she learn her son's diagnosis but she herself could also be diagnosed with fragile X syndrome if she has a full mutation and clinical symptoms.

Complications

◆ Birth defects—cleft lip/palate, club foot, congenital hip dislocation, hernias
◆ Urinary tract infections (UTIs)
◆ Eye disorders—strabismus, ptosis, nystagmus
◆ Connective tissue problems—scoliosis, flat feet, hernias, heart murmur, hyperflexible joints, macroorchidism

Signs and symptoms

Small children may have relatively few identifiable physical characteristics; behavioral or learning difficulties may be the initial presenting features.

Many adult male patients display a prominent jaw and forehead and a head circumference exceeding the 90th percentile. A long, narrow face with long or large ears that may be posteriorly rotated can be a helpful finding at all ages. Connective tissue abnormalities—including hyperextension of the fingers, a floppy mitral valve (in 80% of adults), and mild to severe pectus excavatum—have also been reported. Unusually large testes, found in most affected males after

puberty, are an important identifying factor of the disorder.

Behavioral characteristics such as hyperactivity, speech difficulties, language delay, and autistic-like behaviors may be attributed to other disorders, such as attention deficit hyperactivity disorder, and thus delay the diagnosis.

About 50% of females with the *FMR1* full mutation will have clinical symptoms, although the degree of severity and number of symptoms vary widely among females with fragile X syndrome. Those who are symptomatic typically have a much milder clinical presentation than males because of having an unaffected X chromosome in addition to the one with an *FMR1* full mutation. Some degree of cognitive impairment is usually present in symptomatic females. Learning disabilities—math difficulties, language deficits, and attentional problems—are most common. Some females can have IQ scores in the mental retardation range. Although affected females can have autistic-like features, excessive shyness and social anxiety are the more common behavioral symptoms. Prominent ears and connective tissue manifestations may be as significant as in males. Although males with the *FMR1* permutation are asymptomatic, some female carriers of an *FMR1* premutation can have associated symptoms. These symptoms include significantly earlier menopause and a low normal performance IQ.

Diagnosis

℞ CONFIRMING DIAGNOSIS *Diagnosis of fragile X syndrome requires identification of clinical symptoms and a positive genetic test. DNA analysis of blood or buccal samples is used to detect the size of the CGG repeat and the methylation status of FMR1.*

A specific genetic test (polymerase chain reaction) can also be performed to diagnose this disease. This test looks for an expanded mutation (called a triplet repeat) in the FRAXA gene.

Before identification of the *FMR1* mutation, a special cytogenetic (chromosome) blood test was used to microscopically detect the fragile site on the long arm of the affected X chromosome. It's now common knowledge that a full *FMR1* mutation doesn't always result in a cytogenetically detectable fragile site. Therefore, chromosome analysis alone can provide false-negative results. Chromosome analysis still has utility together with *FMR1* mutation analysis when performing a genetic evaluation on a male with mental retardation of unknown etiology.

In addition to diagnosing fragile X syndrome, genetic testing can determine whether the mother of a diagnosed individual is a carrier of the *FMR1* premutation or has a full mutation. This information can be used for preconceptional genetic counseling by a trained professional and prenatal testing if the woman so chooses. *FMR1* mutation analysis can also be subsequently performed on at-risk family members. It should be noted, however, that communication of genetic test results to at-risk family members constitutes a breach of patient confidentiality and privacy unless prior written permission to communicate results has been obtained from the previously tested patients.

Treatment

Fragile X syndrome has no known cure. Treatment is aimed at controlling individual symptoms. Surgery may be needed to repair a defective mitral valve.

Special considerations

◆ Individuals who have been identified as carriers may experience guilt and grief; provide support to help the carrier and family members accept the diagnosis.

◆ Parents of an affected child may need help to deal with their grief over unmet expectations for the child; refer them for appropriate counseling if necessary.

◆ Refer the family (and possibly the extended family) to a professional trained in genetics to discuss the diagnosis, testing, and the risk of recurrence in future offspring.

◆ Recurrent otitis media is common. To maximize the affected child's potential for language development, early diagnosis and aggressive treatment of otitis media are essential.

PEDIATRIC TIP *Encourage parents to enroll infants and toddlers in early intervention programs. Advocate for special education services and individualized speech, language, and occupational therapy services for this child during school years.*

◆ Assess and refer for hyperactivity, attention deficit, or both.

◆ The patient and family can contact the National Fragile X Foundation for additional information and support.

Chromosomal abnormalities

DOWN SYNDROME

The first disorder attributed to a chromosome aberration, Down syndrome (trisomy 21) characteristically produces mental retardation, dysmorphic facial features, and other distinctive physical abnormalities. It's commonly associated with congenital heart defects (in about 60% of patients) and other abnormalities.

Life expectancy for patients with Down syndrome has increased significantly because of improved treatment for related complications (heart defects, respiratory and other infections, acute leukemia). Nevertheless, 5% to 30% of patients who have congenital heart defects die before age 1.

Causes and incidence

Down syndrome usually results from trisomy 21, a spontaneous chromosomal abnormality.

Down syndrome occurs in 1 in 660 live births, but the incidence increases with advanced parental age, especially when the mother is age 34 or older at delivery or the father is older than age 42. At age 20, a woman has about 1 chance in 2,000 of having a child with Down syndrome; by age 49, she has 1 chance in 12. However, if a woman has had one child with Down syndrome, the risk of recurrence is 1% to 2% unless the trisomy results from translocation.

Pathophysiology

Down syndrome occurs when chromosome 21 has three copies instead of the normal two because of faulty meiosis (nondisjunction) of the ovum or, sometimes, the sperm. This results in a karyotype of 47 chromosomes instead of the normal 46. In about 4% of patients, Down syndrome results from an unbalanced translocation in which the long arm of chromosome 21 breaks and attaches to another chromosome. Most commonly, this is a Robertsonian translocation and results in an increased risk of having multiple children with Down syndrome. The disorder may also be due to chromosomal mosaicism with two cell lines—one with a normal number of chromosomes (46) and one with 47 (an extra chromosome 21).

Complications

◆ Congenital heart defects
◆ Premature dementia
◆ Increased incidence of leukemia, acute and chronic infections, diabetes mellitus, and thyroid disorders

Signs and symptoms

The physical signs of Down syndrome (especially hypotonia) as well as some dysmorphic facial features and heart defects may be apparent at birth. The degree of mental retardation may not become apparent until the infant grows older. People with Down syndrome typically have craniofacial anomalies, such as slanting, almond-shaped eyes with epicanthic folds; a flat face; a protruding tongue; a small mouth and chin; a single transverse palmar crease (simian crease); small white spots (Brushfield spots) on the iris; strabismus; a small skull; a flat bridge across the nose; slow dental development, with abnormal or absent teeth; small ears; a short neck; and cataracts.

Other physical effects may include dry, sensitive skin with decreased elasticity; umbilical hernia; short stature; short extremities, with broad, flat, and squarish hands and feet; clinodactyly (small little finger that curves inward); a wide space between the first and second toe; and abnormal fingerprints and footprints. Hypotonic limb muscles impair reflex development, posture, coordination, and balance.

Congenital heart disease (septal defects or pulmonary or aortic stenosis), duodenal atresia, megacolon, and pelvic bone abnormalities are common. The incidence of leukemia and thyroid disorders (particularly hypothyroidism) may be increased. Frequent upper respiratory infections can be a serious problem. Genitalia may be poorly developed and puberty delayed. Females may menstruate and be fertile. Males are infertile with low serum testosterone levels; many have undescended testicles.

Patients with Down syndrome may have an IQ between 30 and 70; however, social performance is usually beyond that expected for mental age and fewer than 10% will have severe mental retardation. The level of intellectual function depends greatly on the environment and the amount of early stimulation received in addition to the IQ.

Diagnosis
Physical findings at birth, especially hypotonia, may suggest this diagnosis, but no physical feature is diagnostic in itself.

CONFIRMING DIAGNOSIS *A karyotype showing the specific chromosomal abnormality provides a definitive diagnosis. Amniocentesis allows prenatal diagnosis and is recommended for pregnant women older than age 34 even if the family history is negative. Amniocentesis is also recommended for a pregnant woman of any age when either she or the father carries a translocated chromosome.*

Treatment
Down syndrome has no known cure. Surgery to correct heart defects and other related congenital abnormalities and antibiotic therapy for recurrent infections have improved life expectancy considerably. Plastic surgery is occasionally done to correct the characteristic facial traits, especially the protruding tongue. Benefits beyond improved appearance may include improved speech, reduced susceptibility to dental caries, and fewer orthodontic problems later. Most patients with Down syndrome are now cared for at home and attend special education classes. As adults, some may work in a sheltered workshop or the community and may live in a group home facility.

Special considerations
Support for the parents of a child with Down syndrome is vital. By following the guidelines listed below, you can help them meet their child's physical and emotional needs.

◆ Establish a trusting relationship with the parents, and encourage communication during the difficult period soon after diagnosis. Recognize signs of grieving.

◆ Teach parents the importance of a balanced diet for the child. Stress the need for patience while feeding the child, who may have difficulty sucking and may be less demanding and seem less eager to eat than normal babies.

◆ Encourage the parents to hold and nurture their child.

◆ Emphasize the importance of adequate exercise and maximum environmental stimulation; refer the parents for early intervention as soon as the diagnosis of Down syndrome is made.

PEDIATRIC TIP *Balanced nutrition and exercise gain increased importance as the child ages. Obesity commonly becomes problematic.*

PEDIATRIC TIP *All children with Down syndrome need to be checked for atlantoaxial instability before they engage in exercise or sports.*

◆ Refer the parents and older siblings for genetic and psychological counseling, as appropriate, to help them evaluate future reproductive risks. Discuss options for prenatal testing.

◆ Encourage the parents to remember the emotional needs of other children in the family.

◆ Refer the parents to national or local Down syndrome organizations and support groups such as the National Down Syndrome Congress.

TRISOMY 18 SYNDROME
Trisomy 18 syndrome (also known as *Edwards syndrome*) is the second most common multiple malformation syndrome. Most affected infants have *full trisomy 18*, involving an extra (third) copy of chromosome 18 in each cell, but *partial trisomy 18* (with varying phenotypes) and *translocation types* have also been reported. Most infants with this disorder present with intrauterine growth retardation, congenital heart defects, microcephaly, and other malformations.

Full trisomy 18 syndrome is generally fatal or has an extremely poor prognosis; 30% to 50%

of infants with full trisomy 18 syndrome die within the first 2 months after birth; 90% die within the first year. Most patients who survive exhibit profound mental retardation.

Causes and incidence

Most cases of trisomy 18 syndrome are caused by spontaneous meiotic nondisjunction. The risk of chromosomal abnormalities typically increases with maternal age; however, the mean maternal age for this disorder is 32½. Incidence is 1 in 3,000 neonates, with females three times more likely to be affected than males.

Pathophysiology

Most cases of trisomy 18 result from having three copies of chromosome 18 in each cell in the body instead of the usual two copies. The extra genetic material disrupts the normal course of development, causing the characteristic features of trisomy 18.

Approximately 5% of people with trisomy 18 have an extra copy of chromosome 18 in only some of the body's cells. In these people, the condition is called mosaic trisomy 18. The severity of mosaic trisomy 18 depends on the type and number of cells that have the extra chromosome. The development of individuals with this form of trisomy 18 may range from normal to severely affected.

Very rarely, part of the long (q) arm of chromosome 18 becomes attached (translocated) to another chromosome during the formation of reproductive cells (eggs and sperm) or very early in embryonic development. Affected individuals have two copies of chromosome 18, plus the extra material from chromosome 18 attached to another chromosome. People with this genetic change are said to have partial trisomy 18. If only part of the q arm is present in three copies, the physical signs of partial trisomy 18 may be less severe than those typically seen in trisomy 18. If the entire q arm is present in three copies, individuals may be as severely affected as if they had three full copies of chromosome 18.

Complications

◆ Heart defects or abnormalities of other organs
◆ Intrauterine growth retardation
◆ Low birth weight
◆ Many die before birth or within the first month, only 5% to 10% live beyond their first birthday

Signs and symptoms

Growth retardation begins in utero and remains significant after birth. Initial hypotonia may soon give way to hypertonia. Common findings include microcephaly and dolichocephaly, micrognathia, genital and perineal abnormalities (including imperforate anus), diaphragmatic hernia, and various renal defects. Congenital heart defects, such as ventricular septal defect, tetralogy of Fallot, transposition of the great vessels, and coarctation of the aorta, occur in 80% to 90% of patients and may be the cause of death in many infants.

Other findings may include a short and narrow nose with upturned nares; unilateral or bilateral cleft lip and palate; low-set, slightly pointed ears; a short neck; a conspicuous clenched hand with overlapping fingers (usually seen on ultrasound as well); NTDs; omphalocele; cystic hygroma; choroid plexus cysts (also seen in some healthy infants); and oligohydramnios.

Diagnosis

Multiple marker maternal serum screening tests involving different combinations of AFP, human chorionic gonadotropin (hCG), and unconjugated estriol may be abnormal in many pregnant women with an affected fetus; however, these tests aren't diagnostic. Fetal ultrasound may reveal varying degrees of abnormalities, but many fetuses have few detectable defects. Diagnosis should be based on karyotype, done either prenatally or using peripheral blood or skin fibroblasts after birth.

Treatment

Treatment is aimed at providing comfort for the infant and emotional support for the parents. Because the infant's sucking reflex is poor, nutrition is maintained using gavage feedings. Teach parents about home care and feeding techniques.

Special considerations

◆ Allow adequate time for the parents to bond with and hold their child.
◆ Refer the parents to early intervention if the infant is medically stable.
◆ Refer the parents of an affected child for genetic counseling to explore the cause of the disorder and discuss the risk of recurrence in a future pregnancy.
◆ Refer the parents to a social worker or grief counselor for additional support if needed.
◆ Refer the parents to the Support Organization for Trisomy 18, 13, and Related Disorders (SOFT) national support group to allow them interaction with other parents of infants with trisomy 18 and 13.

TRISOMY 13 SYNDROME

Trisomy 13 syndrome (also known as *Patau syndrome*) is the third most common multiple malformation syndrome. Most affected infants have *full trisomy 13* at birth; a few have the rare *mosaic partial trisomy 13* syndrome (with varying phenotypes) or *translocation types*. Infants with this disorder typically have brain and facial abnormalities as well as major cardiac, GI, and limb malformations. Full trisomy 13 syndrome is fatal. Many trisomic zygotes are sponta- neously aborted; 50% to 70% of infants with full trisomy 13 syndrome die within 1 month after birth and 75% by the first year. Only iso- lated cases of survival beyond 5 years have been reported in full trisomy 13 patients. All surviv- ors have profound mental retardation.

Causes and incidence

About 75% of all cases of trisomy 13 syndrome are caused by chromosomal nondisjunction. About 20% of cases are due to chromosomal translocation involving a rearrangement of chromosomes 13 and 14. About 5% of cases are estimated to be mosaics; the clinical effects in these cases may be less severe.

Incidence is estimated to be 1 in every 5,000 neonates. The risk of chromosomal abnormali- ties typically increases with advanced maternal age; however, the mean maternal age for this abnormality is about 31 years.

Pathophysiology

Most cases of trisomy 13 result from having three copies of chromosome 13 in each cell in the body instead of the usual two copies. The extra genetic material disrupts the normal course of development, causing the characteris- tic features of trisomy 13.

Trisomy 13 can also occur when part of chro- mosome 13 becomes attached (translocated) to another chromosome during the formation of reproductive cells (eggs and sperm) or very early in fetal development. Affected people have two normal copies of chromosome 13, plus an extra copy of chromosome 13 attached to another chromosome. In rare cases, only part of chromosome 13 is present in three copies. The physical signs and symptoms in these cases may be different than those found in full trisomy 13.

A small percentage of people with trisomy 13 have an extra copy of chromosome 13 in only some of the body's cells. In these people, the con- dition is called mosaic trisomy 13. The severity of mosaic trisomy 13 depends on the type and num- ber of cells that have the extra chromosome. The physical features of mosaic trisomy 13 are often milder than those of full trisomy 13.

Complications

◆ Vision problems
◆ Breathing difficulties
◆ Feeding problems
◆ Heart failure
◆ Seizures
◆ More than 90% die within the first year

Signs and symptoms

Infants with trisomy 13 syndrome may present with microcephaly, varying degrees of holopros- encephaly, sloping forehead with wide sutures and fontanelle, and a scalp defect at the vertex. Micro-ophthalmia, cataracts, and other eye ab- normalities are seen in most patients with full trisomy 13. Bilateral cleft lip with associated cleft palate is seen in at least 45% of patients. Most are born with a congenital heart defect, especially hypoplastic left heart, ventricular septal defect, patent ductus arteriosus, or dex- troposition, which may significantly contribute significantly to the cause of death.

Other possible findings include a flat and broad nose, low-set ears and inner ear abnor- malities, polydactyly of the hands and feet, club feet, omphaloceles, NTDs, cystic hygroma, gen- ital abnormalities, cystic kidneys, hydronephro- sis, and musculoskeletal abnormalities. Affected infants may also experience failure to thrive, seizures, apnea, and feeding difficulties.

Diagnosis

Multiple marker maternal serum screening tests, involving different combinations of AFP, hCG or free beta-hCG in some laboratories, and un- conjugated estriol, may be abnormal in some pregnant women with an affected fetus; how- ever, these tests aren't diagnostic.

Ultrasound commonly reveals multiple abnormalities in the fetus; however, because many multiple malformation syndromes have similar features, the diagnosis should be based on karyotype, done either prenatally or on peripheral blood lymphocytes or skin fibro- blasts in a neonate or an aborted fetus. The neonate may have a single umbilical artery at birth. MRI or a CT scan of the head may reveal a structural abnormality of the brain (holopros- encephaly) where the two cerebral hemispheres are fused.

Treatment

Supportive care is the only treatment for the infant with trisomy 13 syndrome.

Special considerations

◆ Maintain the infant's fluid balance, and posi- tion for comfort.

◆ Refer the parents to early intervention if the infant is medically stable.

◆ Provide the family with emotional support.

◆ Allow adequate time for the parents to bond with and hold their child.

◆ Refer the parents of an affected infant for genetic counseling to explore the cause of the disorder and to discuss the risk of recurrence in future pregnancies.

◆ Refer the parents to a social worker or grief counselor for additional support if needed.

◆ Refer the parents to the SOFT national support group to allow them interaction with other parents of infants with trisomy 18 and 13.

TURNER SYNDROME

Turner syndrome is the most common disorder of gonadal dysgenesis in females.

Causes and incidence

Turner syndrome occurs in about 1 per 2,000 births; 95% of fetuses with this syndrome are spontaneously aborted. The syndrome produces characteristic signs, which are irreversible.

Pathophysiology

Turner syndrome occurs when an X chromosome (or part of the second X chromosome) is missing from either the ovum or the sperm through nondisjunction or chromosome lag. Mixed aneuploidy may result from mitotic nondisjunction.

Complications

◆ Diabetes mellitus
◆ Thyroid disease
◆ Osteoarthritis
◆ Osteoporosis
◆ Cardiomyopathy
◆ Renal dysfunction
◆ Precocious aging
◆ Sterility

Signs and symptoms

Turner syndrome produces obvious characteristic signs. At birth, 50% of infants with this syndrome measure below the third percentile in length. Commonly, they have swollen hands and feet, a wide chest, and a low hairline that becomes more obvious as they grow. They may have severe webbing of the neck, and some have coarse, enlarged, prominent ears. Gonadal dysgenesis is seen at birth. Other signs and symptoms include pigmented nevi, lymphedema, hypoplasia, or malformed nails.

As the child grows, short stature is common. The patient may exhibit average to slightly below-average intelligence. Developmental problems include right–left disorientation for extrapersonal space and defective figure drawing. The patient is typically immature and socially naive.

Auscultation of the infant's chest indicates cardiovascular malformations, such as coarctation of the aorta and ventricular septal defects.

Pathophysiology

Turner syndrome is caused by the absence of one set of genes from the short arm of one X chromosome. In patients with 45,X karyotype, about two-thirds are missing the paternal X chromosome. In addition to monosomy X, a similar clinical picture is found with a 46,XXiq karyotype and in some individuals with mosaic karyotypes. A deletion of the *SHOX* gene can cause a similar skeletal phenotype known as Leri–Weill dyschondrosteosis.

Diagnosis

Turner syndrome can be diagnosed by chromosome analysis. Differential diagnosis should rule out mixed gonadal dysgenesis, Noonan syndrome, and other similar disorders.

Treatment

Cardiovascular malformations must be corrected surgically. Hormonal replacement should begin in childhood and includes androgen, human growth hormone and, possibly, small doses of estrogen. Later, progesterone and estrogen can induce sexual maturation.

Special considerations

◆ Encourage the patient and family to verbalize feelings about the patient's condition and to discuss fear of rejection by others. Offer emotional support and a realistic assessment of the patient's condition.

◆ Help the patient and family to develop coping strategies. Refer them for sexual or genetic counseling as necessary.

◆ Provide appropriate preoperative and postoperative care for the infant with cardiovascular malformations.

◆ Explain the surgical procedure and its expected outcomes to the parents of the infant with cardiovascular malformations. Help them participate in the child's care and make informed decisions about treatment options. Explain all procedures and provide ongoing information about the infant's condition.

◆ Teach the parents about normal growth and development and how their child may differ. Clarify any misconceptions and explain the treatment. Suggest strategies to help the child achieve age-related skills.

◆ Teach family members and, if appropriate, the patient about long-term hormone replacement therapy. Stress the importance of strictly complying with therapy.

KLINEFELTER SYNDROME

Klinefelter syndrome is a relatively common genetic abnormality that results when a male has an extra X chromosome. It becomes apparent at puberty, when the secondary sex characteristics develop; the testicles fail to mature, and degenerative testicular changes begin that eventually result in irreversible infertility. It commonly causes gynecomastia and is also associated with a tendency toward learning disabilities. From 25% to 85% have difficulties with language development.

Klinefelter syndrome is unlike Turner syndrome, which results from the loss of an X chromosome in a female.

Causes and incidence

Klinefelter syndrome, probably the most common cause of hypogonadism, appears in about 1 in every 500 males.

The incidence of meiotic nondisjunction increases with maternal age.

Pathophysiology

This disorder usually results from one extra X chromosome, giving such patients a 47,XXY complement instead of the normal 46,XY. (See *Fertilization in Klinefelter syndrome.*) In the rare mosaic form of this syndrome, some cells contain the extra X chromosomes, whereas others contain the normal XY complement.

Fertilization in Klinefelter syndrome

Fertilization by a sperm with X and Y chromosomes produces an XXY zygote.

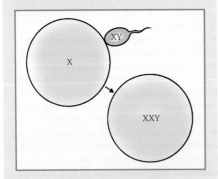

The extra chromosome responsible for Klinefelter syndrome probably results either from meiotic nondisjunction during parental gametogenesis or from meiotic nondisjunction in the zygote.

Complications
◆ Autoimmune disorders
◆ Breast cancer in men
◆ Learning disabilities
◆ Extragonadal germ cell tumor
◆ Pulmonary disorders
◆ Osteoporosis

Signs and symptoms

Klinefelter syndrome may not be apparent until puberty or later in mild cases. Because many of these patients aren't mentally retarded, behavioral problems in adolescence or infertility may be the only presenting features initially.

The syndrome's characteristic features include a small penis and prostate gland, small testicles, sparse facial and abdominal hair, feminine distribution of pubic hair (triangular shape), sexual dysfunction (impotence, lack of libido), and, in fewer than 50% of patients, gynecomastia. Aspermatogenesis and infertility result from progressive sclerosis and hyalinization of the seminiferous tubules in the testicles and from testicular fibrosis during and after puberty. In the mosaic form of Klinefelter syndrome, such pathologic changes and resulting infertility may be delayed.

Klinefelter syndrome may also be associated with osteoporosis, abnormal body build (long legs with short, obese trunk), tall stature, learning disabilities characterized by poor verbal skills, and, in some individuals, behavioral problems beginning in adolescence. It's also associated with an increased incidence of pulmonary disease and varicose veins and a significantly increased rate of breast cancer because of the extra X chromosome.

Diagnosis

℞ **CONFIRMING DIAGNOSIS** *Typical clinical features suggest Klinefelter syndrome, but only a karyotype (chromosome analysis) determined by culturing lymphocytes from the patient's peripheral blood can unequivocally confirm the disorder.*

Characteristically, Klinefelter syndrome decreases urinary 17-ketosteroid levels, increases the excretion of follicle-stimulating hormone, and decreases the levels of plasma testosterone after puberty.

Treatment

Depending on the severity of symptoms, treatment may include mastectomy in patients with persistent gynecomastia and supplemental testosterone to induce secondary sexual characteristics of puberty.

Special considerations

◆ Psychological counseling may be indicated for body image problems or emotional maladjustment due to sexual dysfunction.

◆ Genetic counseling is essential for patients with the mosaic form of the syndrome who are fertile; they may transmit this chromosomal abnormality.

◆ Improve compliance with hormone replacement therapy by making sure patients understand the potential benefits and adverse effects of testosterone administration.

VELOCARDIOFACIAL SYNDROME

VCFS is considered a chromosomal microdeletion syndrome. Most persons with VCFS have a de novo submicroscopic deletion. However, the deletion is dominantly inherited from an affected parent in up to one-third of reported cases. The phenotype demonstrates interfamilial variability consisting of more than 150 possible clinical features.

Causes and incidence

VCFS occurs in at least 1 in 5,000 live births.

Neonates or infants clinically diagnosed with DiGeorge syndrome (a similar disorder) commonly test positive for a 22q11.2 deletion. Therefore, in most cases, persons with DiGeorge syndrome represent the severe end of the VCFS clinical spectrum.

Pathophysiology

The syndrome is caused by a submicroscopic deletion of chromosome 22q11.2. In most persons with VCFS, the chromosome deletion is too small to be detected by routine chromosome analysis. Although small, the deleted region, containing 1.5 to 3 Mb, is thought to contain several genes.

Complications

◆ Cardiac complications
◆ Palatal abnormalities can cause speech and feeding difficulties
◆ Increased risk of infection
◆ Autoimmune disorders
◆ Ophthalmologic abnormalities

Signs and symptoms

Clinical features of VCFS vary greatly among affected persons. Neonates with complex heart malformations, dysmorphic features, hypocalcemia, missing thymus, and renal anomalies represent the severe end of the VCFS clinical presentation. On the other hand, the clinical features can be so mild that an affected parent isn't identified until an offspring is diagnosed and genetic testing is subsequently done on the parents. Symptoms have been reported in the cardiac, craniofacial, neuropsychological, renal, ocular, neurologic, skeletal, endocrine, immune, and hematologic systems. The most common symptoms can be classified as cardiac, craniofacial, and neuropsychological.

Clinical studies indicate that 70% to 85% of persons with VCFS have cardiac anomalies, of which conotruncal defects (e.g., tetralogy of Fallot, interrupted aortic arch, truncus arteriosus) are the most common. This incidence may decrease over time as persons with only mild symptoms, such as learning difficulties in school or subtle dysmorphic features, are tested and found to be deletion positive.

Craniofacial features include palatal abnormalities, dysmorphic facial features, and dysphagia usually because of velopharyngeal incompetence with or without pharyngoesophageal dysmotility. Therefore, feeding difficulties during infancy are common. The palate may be hypotonic and hypoplastic or have a midline cleft (ranging from bifid uvula to complete clefts of the palate). Related to palate problems are speech delays and abnormalities—particularly hypernasal speech and dyspraxia. Typical dysmorphic features include malformed ears, narrow palpebral fissures, hooded upper eyelids, ptosis, a broad square nasal root, a bulbous nasal tip (typically with a midline vertical crease), and micrognathia.

Neuropsychological symptoms are present to some degree in most persons with VCFS. Hypotonia during the neonatal stage through the early childhood period has been reported in more than 75% of cases. Even as hypotonia resolves with maturation, coordination and balance remain problematic. Cognitive symptoms, which can range from learning difficulties to varying levels of mental retardation, have been reported in more than 80% of persons with VCFS. Children with VCFS typically have difficulties in visual–spatial activities, planning, attention, and concentration. Their strengths tend to be in rote verbal memory skills. Reading skills usually exceed math skills; however, reading comprehension tends to be problematic. The behavior of children with VCFS can be either shy and withdrawn or disinhibited and impulsive. Thought problems can be recognized during childhood and adolescence. Adults with VCFS are at risk for psychiatric disorders, particularly schizophrenia.

Diagnosis

Fluorescence in situ hybridization (FISH) using *22q11.2* specific and chromosome 22 control probes is the preferred diagnostic test for VCFS and DiGeorge syndrome. Chromosome analysis with high-resolution banding detects only about one-third of affected persons. However, high-resolution chromosome analysis may be ordered in conjunction with FISH analysis for patients whose clinical presentation suggests a chromosome abnormality and *22q11.2* deletion is only one of several possible diagnoses in the differential.

Prenatal diagnosis is possible by performing a *22q11.2* FISH analysis on chorionic villi or cultured amniocytes. Prenatal diagnosis may be considered when a biologic parent is known to have a *22q11.2* deletion or when a level 2 prenatal ultrasound reveals anomalies that can be present in persons with VCFS. A *22q11.2* FISH analysis is recommended in neonates with cardiac anomalies and any one or more of the other clinical features of VCFS.

Treatment

Treatment is aimed at preventing, ameliorating, or managing symptoms.

Special considerations

♦ Infants with palatal abnormalities and suck and swallow coordination difficulties will likely require feeding interventions, such as the use of cleft palate nursers and, in some cases, nasogastric or gastric tube feedings.
♦ Infants with heart malformations may require increased caloric intake.
♦ Management of heart malformations ranges from careful monitoring to multiple surgical interventions.
♦ Repair of cleft or abnormally functioning palate may improve hypernasal speech.
♦ Referral of the patient to speech pathology for evaluation of language delays or speech problems can be helpful.
♦ Infants may require occupational and physical therapy to minimize the developmental effects of hypotonia.

🦷 **PEDIATRIC TIP** *Encourage the parents to have the child participate in early intervention programs and educational services to optimize learning abilities.*

♦ Designate a case manager to optimize care given by professionals from multiple disciplines and specialty areas.
♦ Refer the parents of an infant diagnosed with VCFS for genetic testing and counseling services.
♦ When providing patient and family teaching, assess for parental cognitive impairments and adjust teaching interventions accordingly.

♦ Anticipate, assess, and provide support for shock, denial, anger, and guilt reactions by parents discovered to have VCFS after their child's diagnosis.
♦ Help parents to identify and use effective coping strategies, and make referrals to mental health professionals as needed.
♦ Refer parents to appropriate support groups.
♦ Provide anticipatory guidance related to the physical, emotional, and neuropsychological effects of VCFS.

Multifactorial abnormalities

NEURAL TUBE DEFECTS

NTDs are serious birth defects that involve the spine or brain; they result from failure of the neural tube to close at about 28 days after conception. The most common forms of NTDs are spina bifida (50% of cases), anencephaly (40%), and encephalocele (10%).

However, in more severe forms of spina bifida, incomplete closure of one or more vertebrae causes protrusion of the spinal contents in an external sac or cystic lesion (spina bifida cystica). *Spina bifida cystica* has two classifications: *myelomeningocele (meningomyelocele)* and *meningocele*. In meningocele, less severe than myelomeningocele, the sac contains only meninges and CSF. Meningocele may produce no neurologic symptoms. (See *Types of neural tube defects*, page 1011.)

In *encephalocele*, a saclike portion of the meninges and brain protrudes through a defective opening in the skull. Usually, it's in the occipital area, but it may occur in the parietal, nasopharyngeal, or frontal area.

In *anencephaly*, the most severe form of NTD, the closure defect occurs at the cranial end of the neuroaxis and, as a result, part or the entire top of the skull is missing, severely damaging the brain. Portions of the brain stem and spinal cord may be missing. No diagnostic or therapeutic efforts are helpful; this condition is invariably fatal.

Causes and incidence

NTDs may be isolated birth defects, may result from exposure to a teratogen, or may be part of a multiple malformation syndrome (e.g., chromosomal abnormalities such as trisomy 18 or 13 syndrome). Isolated NTDs (those not because of a specific teratogen or associated with other malformations) are believed to be caused by a combination of genetic and environmental factors. Although most of the specific

Types of NTDs

The three major types of NTDs are illustrated below. Spina bifida occulta is characterized by a depression or raised area and a tuft of hair over the defect. In myelomeningocele, an external sac contains meninges, CSF, and a portion of the spinal cord or nerve roots. In meningocele, an external sac contains only meninges and CSF.

SPINA BIFIDA OCCULTA

Vertebrae are incompletely fused; no external sac is present

MYELOMENINGOCELE

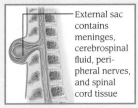

External sac contains meninges, cerebrospinal fluid, peripheral nerves, and spinal cord tissue

MENINGOCELE

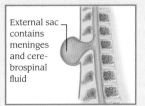

External sac contains meninges and cerebrospinal fluid

environmental triggers are unknown, recent research has identified a lack of folic acid in the mother's diet as one of the risk factors.

The incidence of NTDs varies greatly among countries and by region in the United States. For example, the incidence is significantly higher in the British Isles and low in southern China and Japan. In the United States, North and South Carolina have at least twice the incidence of NTDs as most other parts of the country. These birth defects are also less common in Blacks than in Whites.

Pathophysiology

Spina bifida occulta is the most common and least severe spinal cord defect. It's characterized by incomplete closure of one or more vertebrae without protrusion of the spinal cord or meninges. In myelomeningocele, the external sac contains meninges, CSF, and a portion of the spinal cord or nerve roots distal to the conus medullaris. When the spinal nerve roots end at the sac, motor and sensory functions below the sac are terminated.

Complications

◆ Infection
◆ Paralysis
◆ Hydrocephalus

Signs and symptoms

Spina bifida occulta is usually accompanied by a depression or dimple, tuft of hair, soft fatty deposits, port wine nevi, or a combination of these abnormalities on the skin over the spinal defect; however, such signs may be absent. Spina bifida occulta doesn't usually cause neurologic dysfunction but occasionally

is associated with foot weakness or bowel and bladder disturbances. Such disturbances are especially likely during rapid growth phases, when the spinal cord's ascent within the vertebral column may be impaired by its abnormal adherence to other tissues.

In both myelomeningocele and meningocele, a saclike structure protrudes over the spine. Like spina bifida occulta, meningocele seldom causes neurologic deficit. But myelomeningocele, depending on the level of the defect, causes permanent neurologic dysfunction, such as flaccid or spastic paralysis and bowel and bladder incontinence. Associated disorders include trophic skin disturbances (ulcerations, cyanosis), clubfoot, knee contractures, hydrocephalus (in about 90% of patients), and possibly mental retardation, Arnold–Chiari syndrome (in which part of the brain protrudes into the spinal canal), and curvature of the spine.

Clinical effects of encephalocele vary with the degree of tissue involvement and location of the defect. Paralysis and hydrocephalus are common. Infants with this defect have a better chance of survival than anencephalic infants and usually suffer less paralysis; however, surviving infants are usually severely mentally retarded.

Diagnosis

℞ **CONFIRMING DIAGNOSIS** *Amniocentesis can detect elevated AFP levels in amniotic fluid, which indicates the presence of an open NTD. Measuring acetylcholinesterase levels can confirm the diagnosis. (Biochemical testing will usually miss closed NTDs.) Because 5% to 7% of NTDs are associated with chromosomal abnormalities, a fetal* *karyotype should be done in addition to the bio-chemical tests.*

Maternal serum AFP screening in combination with other serum markers, such as hCG, free beta-hCG, or unconjugated estriol, may be offered to some patients who aren't scheduled for amniocentesis, such as those with a lower risk of NTDs and those who will be younger than 34½ years old at the time of delivery. Although this screening test can't diagnose either an open NTD or a chromosomal abnormality, it can estimate a fetus's risk of such a defect. Most patients with abnormal maternal serum AFP levels won't have an affected child; however, they may be at increased risk for perinatal complications, such as premature rupture of the membranes, abruptio placentae, or fetal death.

Ultrasound may be used when the fetus has an increased risk of an open NTD based on either the family history or the abnormal serum screening results; however, this test alone can't identify all open NTDs or ventral wall defects.

If the NTD isn't diagnosed before birth, other tests are used to make the diagnosis. For example, spina bifida occulta is commonly overlooked, although it's occasionally palpable and spinal X-ray can show the bone defect. Myelography can differentiate it from other spinal abnormalities, especially spinal cord tumors.

Myelomeningocele and meningocele are obvious on examination; transillumination of the protruding sac can sometimes distinguish between them. (In meningocele, it typically transilluminates; in myelomeningocele, it doesn't.) In myelomeningocele, a pinprick examination of the legs and trunk shows the level of sensory and motor involvement; skull X-rays, cephalic measurements, and CT scan demonstrate associated hydrocephalus. Other appropriate laboratory tests in patients with myelomeningocele include urinalysis, urine cultures, and tests for renal function starting in the neonatal period and continuing at regular intervals.

In encephalocele, X-rays show a basilar bony skull defect. CT scan and ultrasonography further define the defect.

Treatment

Prompt neurosurgical repair and aggressive management may improve the condition of children with some NTDs, but serious and permanent disability is likely.

Spina bifida occulta usually requires no treatment. Treatment of meningocele consists of surgical closure of the protruding sac and continual assessment of growth and development. Treatment of myelomeningocele requires repair of the sac and supportive measures to promote independence and prevent further complications. Surgery doesn't reverse neurologic deficits. A shunt may be needed to relieve associated hydrocephalus.

Treatment of encephalocele includes surgery during infancy to place protruding tissues back in the skull, excise the sac, and correct associated craniofacial abnormalities.

Special considerations

◆ When an NTD has been diagnosed prenatally, refer the prospective parents to a genetic counselor, who can provide information and support the couple's decisions on how to manage the pregnancy.

◆ Recent research sponsored by the March of Dimes and others has indicated that the risk of an open NTD may be reduced 50% to 70% in pregnant women who take a daily multivitamin with folic acid. Urge all women of childbearing age to take such a vitamin supplement until menopause or the end of childbearing potential. (See *Folic acid supplement recommendations.*)

 PREVENTION

Folic acid supplement recommendations

The following recommendations for folic acid supplement dosages have been endorsed by the Centers for Disease Control and Prevention, the American Academy of Pediatrics, and the Spina Bifida Association of America, among other groups.

All women of childbearing age
All women who can become pregnant should consume 0.4 mg of folic acid daily to reduce their risk of having a child with spina bifida or another NTD.

Women at high risk
Women with a previous pregnancy affected by an NTD should:
◆ receive genetic counseling before their next pregnancy
◆ consume 4 to 5 mg of folic acid daily when pregnant
◆ when actively trying to become pregnant (at least 1 month before conception), increase their intake of folic acid to 4 mg daily and continue to take 4 to 5 mg of folic acid daily through the first 3 months of pregnancy.

🔔 **PEDIATRIC TIP** *The parents of a child with an NTD will need assistance from physicians, nurses, surgeons, rehabilitation providers, and social workers. Help to coordinate such assistance as needed. Obviously, care is most complex when the neurologic deficit is severe. Immediate goals include psychological support to help parents accept the diagnosis and preoperative and postoperative care. Long-term goals include patient and family teaching, as well as measures to prevent contractures, pressure ulcers, UTIs, and other complications.*

Before surgery:
◆ Prevent local infection by cleaning the defect gently with sterile saline solution or other solutions, as ordered. Inspect the defect often for signs of infection, and cover it with sterile dressings moistened with sterile saline solution. Prevent skin breakdown by placing sheepskin or a foam pad under the infant. Keep skin clean, and apply lotion to knees, elbows, chin, and other pressure areas. Give antibiotics as needed.
◆ Handle the infant carefully, and don't apply pressure to the defect. Usually, the infant can't wear a diaper or a shirt until after surgical correction because it will irritate the sac, so keep the infant warm in an infant isolette. Hold and cuddle the infant; on your lap, position on the abdomen; teach parents to do the same.
◆ Provide adequate time for parent–child bonding if possible.
◆ Measure head circumference daily, and watch for signs of hydrocephalus and meningeal irritation, such as fever or nuchal rigidity. Be sure to mark the spot so you get accurate readings.
◆ Contractures can be minimized by passive range-of-motion exercises and casting. To prevent hip dislocation, moderately abduct hips with a pad between the knees or with sandbags and ankle rolls.
◆ Monitor intake and output. Watch for decreased skin turgor, dryness, or other signs of dehydration. Provide meticulous skin care to genitals and buttocks to prevent infection.
◆ Ensure adequate nutrition.

After surgery:
◆ Watch for hydrocephalus, which commonly follows surgery. Measure the infant's head circumference as indicated.
◆ Monitor vital signs often. Watch for signs of shock, infection, and increased intracranial pressure (ICP) such as projectile vomiting. Frequently assess the infant's fontanelles. Remember that, before age 2, infants don't show typical signs of increased ICP because suture lines aren't fully closed. In infants, the most telling sign is bulging fontanelles.
◆ Change the dressing regularly as ordered, and check for any signs of drainage, wound rupture, and infection.

◆ Place the infant in the prone position to protect and assess the site.
◆ If leg casts have been applied to treat deformities, watch for signs that the child is outgrowing the cast. Regularly check distal pulses to ensure adequate circulation.

To help parents cope with their infant's physical problems and successfully meet long-term treatment goals:
◆ Teach them to recognize early signs of complications, such as hydrocephalus, pressure ulcers, and UTIs.
◆ Provide psychological support and encourage a positive attitude. Help parents work through their feelings of guilt, anger, and helplessness.
◆ Encourage parents to begin training their child in a bladder routine by age 3. Emphasize the need for increased fluid intake to prevent UTIs. Teach intermittent catheterization and conduit hygiene, as ordered.
◆ To prevent constipation and bowel obstruction, stress the need for increased fluid intake, a high-bulk diet, exercise, and a stool softener, as ordered. If possible, teach parents to help empty their child's bowel by telling the child to bear down, and giving a glycerin suppository as needed.
◆ Urge early recognition of developmental lags (a possible result of hydrocephalus). The child may need to attend a school with special facilities. Also, stress the need for stimulation to ensure maximum mental development. Help parents plan activities appropriate to their child's age and abilities. Refer to early intervention.
◆ Refer parents for genetic counseling and suggest that parents consider an amniocentesis in future pregnancies. Also refer parents to the Spina Bifida Association of America.

CLEFT LIP AND CLEFT PALATE

Cleft lip and cleft palate—an opening in the lip or palate—may occur separately or in combination.

Cleft lip and cleft palate occur in twice as many males as females; isolated cleft palate is more common in females.

Causes and incidence

Cleft lip or palate most commonly occurs as an isolated birth defect.

Cleft lip with or without cleft palate occurs in about 1 in 1,000 births among Whites; the incidence is higher in Asians (1.7 in 1,000) and Native Americans (>3.6 in 1,000) but lower in Blacks (1 in 2,500).

A family history of cleft defects increases the risk of a couple having a child with a cleft defect. Likewise, an individual with a cleft defect is at an increased risk for having a child with a cleft defect. Children with cleft defects and their parents or adult individuals should be referred for genetic counseling for accurate diagnosis of cleft type and recurrence risk counseling. Recurrence risk information is based on family history, the presence or absence of other physical or cognitive traits within a family, and prenatal exposure information.

Pathophysiology

Cleft lip and cleft palate deformities originate in the second month of pregnancy, when the front and sides of the face and the palatine shelves fuse imperfectly. Cleft deformities usually occur unilaterally or bilaterally, rarely midline. Only the lip may be involved, or the defect may extend into the upper jaw or nasal cavity.

Isolated cleft lip with or without cleft palate and cleft palate only are the result of a disruption in the normal development of the orofacial structures. This disruption in development is thought to be the result of a combination of genetic and environmental factors, including drugs, viruses, and environmental toxins. Cleft lip or cleft palate may also occur as part of a chromosomal or Mendelian syndrome (cleft defects are associated with >300 syndromes). Exposures to specific teratogens during fetal development may also produce these defects.

Complications

- ◆ Difficulty feeding
- ◆ Ear infections which could lead to hearing loss
- ◆ Difficulty with speech or delayed speech

Signs and symptoms

Orofacial cleft defects are divided into two major groups: cleft lip with or without cleft palate or cleft palate only. Cleft of the lip may involve the alveolus (premaxilla) and may extend through the palate (hard and soft). Congenital clefts of the face occur most commonly in the upper lip. They can range from a simple notch to a complete cleft from the lip edge, through the floor of the nostril and through the alveolus. Cleft lip can occur on either one or both sides of the midline but rarely along the midline itself. A cleft lip involving only one side is a *unilateral* cleft lip, and a cleft on both sides of the midline is a *bilateral* cleft lip. When a bilateral cleft lip involves clefting of the alveolus on both sides of the premaxilla, the premaxilla is separated from the maxilla into a freely moving segment.

A cleft of the palate only may be partial or complete, involving only the soft palate or extending from the soft palate completely through the hard palate. A cleft palate can occur alone or with a cleft lip. Isolated cleft palate is more commonly associated with congenital defects other than isolated cleft lip with or without cleft palate. (See *Variations of cleft lip and cleft palate,* page 1015.) The constellation of U-shaped cleft palate, mandibular hypoplasia, and glossoptosis is known as *Pierre Robin syndrome,* or *Robin syndrome.* Robin syndrome can occur as an isolated defect or one feature of many different syndromes; therefore, a comprehensive genetic evaluation is suggested for infants with Robin syndrome. Because of the mandibular hypoplasia and glossoptosis, careful evaluation and management of the airway are mandatory for infants with Robin syndrome.

Diagnosis

A typical clinical picture confirms the diagnosis. Cleft lip with or without cleft palate is obvious at birth; occasionally, more severe defects may be seen with diagnostic prenatal ultrasonography. Cleft palate without cleft lip may not be detected until a mouth examination is done or until feeding difficulties develop.

Treatment

Treatment consists of surgical correction, but the timing of surgery varies. Some plastic surgeons repair cleft lips within the first few days of life to make feeding the baby easier. However, many surgeons delay lip repairs for 8 to 10 weeks (sometimes as long as 6 to 8 months) to allow the infant to grow and mature, thereby minimizing surgical and anesthesia risks, ruling out associated congenital anomalies, and allowing time for parental bonding. Cleft palate repair is usually completed by the 12th to 18th month. Still other surgeons repair cleft palates in two steps, repairing the soft palate between ages 6 and 18 months and the hard palate as late as age 5. In any case, surgery is performed only after the infant is gaining weight and infection free.

Surgery must be coupled with speech therapy. Because the palate is essential to speech formation, structural changes, even in a repaired cleft, can permanently affect speech patterns. To compound the problem, children with cleft palates commonly have hearing difficulties because of middle ear damage or infections.

Special considerations

- ◆ Recent research has indicated that ingestion of 0.4 mg of folic acid twice daily before conception may decrease the risk of isolated cleft defects.

Variations of cleft lip and cleft palate

The illustration below shows the four variations of cleft lip and cleft palate.

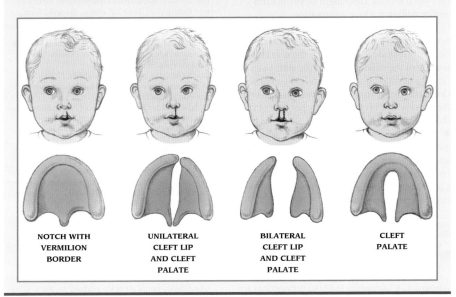

| NOTCH WITH VERMILION BORDER | UNILATERAL CLEFT LIP AND CLEFT PALATE | BILATERAL CLEFT LIP AND CLEFT PALATE | CLEFT PALATE |

! **ALERT** *Never place a child with Robin syndrome on their back because the tongue could fall back and obstruct the airway. Place these infants on their side for sleeping. Most other infants with a cleft palate can sleep on their backs without difficulty.*

◆ Maintain adequate nutrition to ensure normal growth and development. Experiment with feeding devices. A baby with a cleft palate has an excellent appetite but often has trouble feeding because of air leaks around the cleft and nasal regurgitation. The patient usually feeds better from a bottle and nipple designed specifically for feeding infants with cleft defects. These bottles come with special nipples or regular nipples with enlarged holes and may be used with cleft palate bottles.

Teach the parents how best to feed the infant. Advise them to hold the infant in a near-sitting position, with the flow directed to the side or back of the baby's tongue. Tell them to burp the baby frequently because they will tend to swallow a lot of air. If the underside of the nasal septum becomes ulcerated and the child refuses to suck because of the pain, instruct the parents to direct the nipple to the side of the mouth to give the mucosa time to heal. Tell them to gently clean the palatal cleft with a cotton-tipped applicator dipped in half-strength hydrogen peroxide or water after each feeding.

◆ Encourage the mother of a baby with cleft lip to breastfeed if the cleft doesn't prevent effective sucking. Breastfeeding an infant with a cleft palate or one who has just had corrective surgery usually isn't possible. (Postoperatively, the infant can't suck for 6 to 10 weeks.) However, if the mother desires, suggest that she use a breast pump to express breast milk and then feed it to her baby from a bottle.

◆ Following surgery, record intake and output and maintain good nutrition. To prevent atelectasis and pneumonia, the physician may gently suction the nasopharynx (this may be necessary before surgery, too). Restrain the infant to prevent the infant from self-harm. Elbow restraints allow the baby to move their hands while keeping them away from the mouth. When necessary, use an infant seat to keep the child in a comfortable sitting position. Hang toys within reach of restrained hands.

◆ Surgeons sometimes place a curved metal bow over a repaired cleft lip to minimize tension on the suture line. Remove the gauze before feedings, and replace it often. Moisten it with normal saline solution until the sutures are removed. Check your hospital policy to confirm this procedure.

◆ Help the parents deal with their feelings about the child's disability. Start by telling them about it and showing them their baby as soon as possible. Because society places undue importance on physical appearance, many parents feel shock, disappointment, and guilt when they see the child. Help them by being calm and providing positive information.

Direct the parents' attention to their child's assets. Stress the fact that surgical repairs can be made. Include the parents in the care and feeding of the child right from the start to encourage normal bonding. Provide the instructions, emotional support, and reassurance that the parents will need to take proper care of the child at home.

◆ Refer the parents to a social worker who can guide them to community resources, if needed, and to a genetic counselor to determine the recurrence risk. Refer the family to the American Cleft Palate-Craniofacial Association for information and support.

SELECTED REFERENCES

Daniel, M. (2017). *Turner syndrome.* Retrieved from https://emedicine.medscape.com/article/949681-overview#a6

De Sanctis, V., & Ciccone, S. (2010). Fertility preservation in adolescents with Klinefelter's syndrome. *Pediatric Endocrinology Reviews, 8*(Suppl 1), 178–181.

Goutagny, S., & Kalamarides, M. (2010). Meningiomas and neurofibromatosis. *Journal of Neuro-Oncology, 99*(3), 341–347.

Hsleh, D. (2017). *Neurofibromatosis type 1.* Retrieved from https://emedicine.medscape.com/article/1177266-overview#a6

Mayo Clinic. (2018). *Cystic fibrosis.* Retrieved from https://www.mayoclinic.org/diseases-conditions/cystic-fibrosis/diagnosis-treatment/drc-20353706

Mayo Clinic. (2018). *Marfan syndrome.* Retrieved from https://www.mayoclinic.org/diseases-conditions/marfan-syndrome/diagnosis-treatment/drc-20350787

Mayo Clinic. (2018). *Sickle cell anemia.* Retrieved from https://www.mayoclinic.org/diseases-conditions/sickle-cell-anemia/diagnosis-treatment/drc-20355882

Michel, S., et al. (2009). Nutrition management of pediatric patients who have cystic fibrosis. *Pediatric Clinics of North America, 56*(5), 1123–1141.

National Organization for Rare Disorders. (2018). *Stickler syndrome.* Retrieved from https://rarediseases.org/rare-diseases/stickler-syndrome

Osteogenesis Imperfecta Foundation. (2015). *Treatments for osteogenesis imperfecta.* Retrieved from http://www.oif.org/site/PageNavigator/oif_mc_treatments.html

Ross, J., et al. (2011). Growth hormone plus childhood low-dose estrogen in Turner's syndrome. *New England Journal of Medicine, 364*(13), 1230–1242.

Skotko, B., et al. (2009). Postnatal diagnosis of Down syndrome: Synthesis of the evidence on how best to deliver the news. *Pediatrics, 124*(4), e751–e758.

U.S. National Library of Medicine. (2018). *Trisomy 13.* Retrieved from https://ghr.nlm.nih.gov/condition/trisomy-13#genes

U.S. National Library of Medicine. (2018). *Trisomy 18.* Retrieved from https://ghr.nlm.nih.gov/condition/trisomy-18#genes

Wolff, T., & U.S. Preventive Services Task Force. (2009). Folic acid supplementation for the prevention of neural tube defects: An update of the evidence for the U.S. Preventive Services Task Force. *Annals of Internal Medicine, 150*(9), 632–639.

World Federation of Hemophilia. (2018). *WFH guidelines for the management of hemophilia.* Retrieved from https://www.wfh.org/en/resources/wfh-treatment-guidelines

19

OBSTETRIC AND GYNECOLOGIC DISORDERS

Introduction

Medical care of the obstetric or gynecologic patient reflects a growing interest in improving the quality of healthcare for female-bodied persons. Skills are needed to assess, counsel, teach, and refer patients, while weighing such relevant factors as the patient's desire to have children, sexual adjustment problems, and self-image. Often, this care is complicated by multiple obstetric and gynecologic abnormalities occurring simultaneously. For example, a patient with dysmenorrhea may also have trichomonal vaginitis, dysuria, and unsuspected infertility. Their condition may be further complicated by associated urologic disorders, because of the proximity of the urinary and reproductive systems. This tendency for multiple and complex disorders is readily understandable upon review of the female genitalia's anatomic structure. (See *External and internal female-bodied genitalia*, page 1018.)

EXTERNAL STRUCTURES

Female genitalia include the following external structures, collectively known as the *vulva:* mons pubis (or mons veneris), labia majora, labia minora, clitoral head, and the vestibule. The perineum is the external region between the vulva and the anus. The size, shape, and color of these structures—as well as pubic hair distribution and skin texture and pigmentation—vary greatly among individuals. Furthermore, these external structures undergo distinct changes during the life cycle.

The mons pubis is the pad of fat over the symphysis pubis (pubic bone), which is usually covered by the base of the inverted triangular patch of pubic hair that grows over the vulva after puberty.

The labia majora are the two thick, longitudinal folds of fatty tissue that extend from the mons pubis to the posterior aspect of the perineum. The labia majora protect the perineum and contain large sebaceous glands that help maintain lubrication. Virtually absent in the young child, their development is a characteristic sign of puberty's onset. The skin of the more prominent parts of the labia majora is pigmented and darkens after puberty.

The labia minora are the two thin, longitudinal folds of skin that border the vestibule. Firmer than the labia majora, they extend from the clitoral head to the fourchette.

The clitoral head and hood are the external parts of the clitoris; the majority of the clitoris is internal. The clitoris contains erectile tissue, venous cavernous spaces, and specialized sensory corpuscles that are stimulated during coitus. (See *Understanding-the-Clitoris*, page 1018.)

External and internal female-bodied genitalia

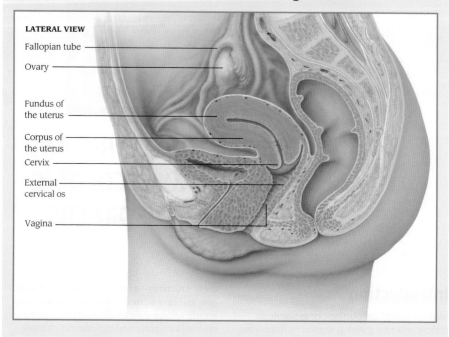

LATERAL VIEW

- Fallopian tube
- Ovary
- Fundus of the uterus
- Corpus of the uterus
- Cervix
- External cervical os
- Vagina

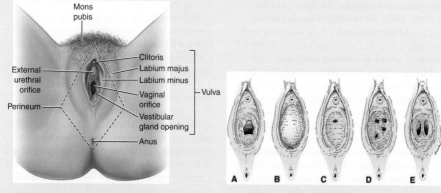

Mons pubis

- Clitoris
- Labium majus
- Labium minus
- External urethral orifice
- Vaginal orifice
- Perineum
- Vestibular gland opening
- Anus

— Vulva

Understanding-the-Clitoris

Types of hymens. (A) Normal, (B) imperforate, (C) microperforate, (D) cribriform, and (E) septate. (Used with permission from Emans, S. J., et al., eds. (2004). *Pediatric and adolescent gynecology*. 5th ed. Philadelphia: Lippincott Williams & Wilkins.)

The vestibule is the oval space bordered by the clitoris, labia minora, and fourchette. The urethral meatus is located in the anterior portion of the vestibule; the vaginal meatus, in the posterior portion. The hymen is an elastic membrane that varies in size, shape, and rigidity per individual. (See *Types of hymens.*)

Several glands lubricate the vestibule. Skene's glands open on both sides of the urethral meatus; Bartholin's glands, on both sides of the vaginal meatus.

The fourchette is the posterior junction of the labia majora and labia minora. The perineum, which includes the underlying muscles and fascia, is the external surface of the floor of the pelvis, extending from the fourchette to the anus.

INTERNAL STRUCTURES

The following internal structures are included in the female genitalia: vagina, cervix, uterus, fallopian tubes (or oviducts), ovaries, and clitoris (see above).

The vagina occupies the space between the bladder and the rectum. A muscular, membranous tube that's about 3" (7.5 cm) long, the vagina connects the uterus and the vestibule of the external genitalia. It serves as a passageway for sperm to the fallopian tubes, for the discharge of menstrual fluid, and for childbirth.

The cervix, or neck of the uterus, protrudes at least ¾" (2 cm) into the proximal end of the vagina. A rounded, conical structure, the cervix joins the uterus and the vagina at a 45- to 90-degree angle.

The uterus is the hollow, pear-shaped organ in which the conceptus grows during pregnancy. The part of the uterus above the junction of the fallopian tubes is called the *fundus*; the part below this junction is called the *corpus*. The junction of the corpus and cervix forms the lower uterine segment.

The thick uterine wall consists of mucosal, muscular, and serous layers. The inner mucosal lining—the endometrium—undergoes cyclic changes designed facilitate and maintain pregnancy.

The smooth muscular middle layer—the myometrium—interlaces the uterine and ovarian arteries and veins that circulate blood through the uterus. During pregnancy, this vascular system expands dramatically. After abortion or childbirth, the myometrium contracts to constrict the vasculature and control blood loss.

The outer serous layer—the parietal peritoneum—covers all of the fundus, part of the corpus, but none of the cervix. If surgery is necessary this incompleteness facilitates surgical entry into the uterus without incision of the peritoneum, thereby reducing the risk of peritonitis.

The fallopian tubes extend from the sides of the fundus and terminate near the ovaries. Through ciliary and muscular action, these small tubes (3¼" to 5½" [8 to 14 cm] long) carry ova from the ovaries to the uterus and facilitate the movement of sperm from the uterus toward the ovaries. Fertilization of the ovum normally occurs in a fallopian tube. The same ciliary and muscular action helps move a zygote (fertilized ovum) down to the uterus, where it implants in the blood-rich inner uterine lining, the endometrium.

The ovaries are two almond-shaped organs, one on either side of the fundus, that are situated behind and below the fallopian tubes. The ovaries produce ova and two primary hormones—estrogen and progesterone—in addition to small amounts of androgen. These hormones, in turn, produce and maintain secondary sex characteristics, prepare the uterus for pregnancy, and stimulate mammary gland development.

The ovaries are connected to the uterus by the utero-ovarian ligament and are divided into two parts: the cortex, which contains primordial and graafian follicles in various stages of development, and the medulla, which consists primarily of vasculature and loose connective tissue.

A healthy female-bodied person is born with at least 400,000 primordial follicles in her ovaries. At puberty, these ova precursors become graafian follicles, in response to the effects of pituitary gonadotropic hormones—follicle-stimulating hormone (FSH) and luteinizing hormone (LH). In the life cycle of a female, however, less than 500 ova eventually mature and develop the potential for fertilization.

THE MENSTRUAL CYCLE

Maturation of the hypothalamus and the resultant increase in hormone levels initiate puberty. In the young female-bodied person, breast development—the first sign of puberty—is followed by the appearance of pubic and axillary hair and the characteristic adolescent growth spurt. The reproductive system begins to undergo a series of hormone-induced changes that result in menarche, onset of menstruation (or menses). In North American females, menarche usually occurs at about age 12 but may occur between ages 9 and 18. Menstrual periods initially are irregular and anovulatory, but after a year or so, they become more regular. (See *Menstrual cycle*, page 1020.)

The menstrual cycle consists of three different phases: menstrual, proliferative (estrogen-dominated), and secretory (progesterone-dominated). These phases correspond to the phases of ovarian function. The menstrual and proliferative phases correspond to the follicular ovarian phase; the secretory phase corresponds to the luteal ovarian phase.

The *menstrual phase* begins with day 1 of menstruation. During this phase, low estrogen and progesterone levels stimulate the hypothalamus to secrete gonadotropin-releasing hormone (GnRH). This substance, in turn, stimulates pituitary secretion of FSH and LH. When the FSH level rises, LH output increases.

Menstrual cycle

The menstrual cycle is divided into three distinct phases:

The *menstrual phase* starts on the first day of menstruation. The top layer of the endometrium (the material lining the uterus) breaks down and flows out of the body. This flow, called the *menses*, consists of blood, mucus, and unneeded tissue.

During *the proliferative phase*, the endometrium begins to thicken, and the estrogen level in the blood rises.

In the *secretory phase*, the endometrium continues to thicken to nourish an embryo should fertilization occur. Without fertilization, the top layer of the endometrium breaks down, and the menstrual phase of the cycle begins again.

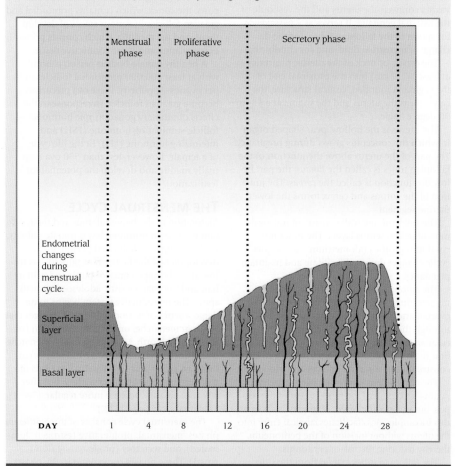

The *proliferative (follicular) phase* lasts from cycle day 6 to day 14. During this phase, LH and FSH act on the ovarian follicle, causing estrogen secretion, which in turn stimulates the buildup of the endometrium. Late in this phase, estrogen levels peak, FSH secretion declines, and LH secretion increases, surging at midcycle (around day 14). Then estrogen production decreases, the follicle matures, and ovulation occurs.

During the *secretory phase*, FSH and LH levels drop. Estrogen levels decline initially, then increase along with progesterone levels as the corpus luteum begins functioning. During this phase, the endometrium responds to progesterone stimulation by becoming thick and secretory in preparation for implantation of a fertilized ovum. About 10 to 12 days after ovulation, the corpus luteum begins to diminish, as do estrogen and progesterone levels, until hormone levels are insufficient to sustain the endometrium in a fully developed secretory state. Then the endometrial lining is shed (menses). Subsequently decreasing estrogen and progesterone levels stimulate the hypothalamus to produce GnRH, which in turn begins the cycle again.

In the nonpregnant female, LH controls the secretions of the corpus luteum; in the pregnant female, human chorionic gonadotropin (hCG) controls them. At the end of the secretory phase, the uterine lining is ready to receive and nourish a zygote. If fertilization doesn't occur, increasing estrogen and progesterone levels decrease LH and FSH production. Because LH is necessary to maintain the corpus luteum, a decrease in LH production causes the corpus luteum to atrophy and stop secreting estrogen and progesterone. The thickened uterine lining then begins to slough off, and menstruation begins again.

If fertilization and pregnancy do occur, the endometrium grows even thicker. After implantation of the zygote (about 5 or 6 days after fertilization), the endometrium becomes the decidua. Chorionic villi produce hCG soon after implantation, stimulating the corpus luteum to continue secreting estrogen and progesterone, which prevents further ovulation and menstruation.

hCG continues to stimulate the corpus luteum until the placenta—the vascular organ that develops to transport materials to and from the fetus—forms and starts producing its own estrogen and progesterone. After the placenta takes over hormonal production, secretions of the corpus luteum are no longer needed to maintain the pregnancy, and the corpus luteum gradually decreases its function and begins to degenerate.

PREGNANCY

Cell multiplication and differentiation begin in the zygote at the moment of conception. By about 17 days after conception, the placenta has established circulation to what is now an *embryo* (the term used for the conceptus between the second and seventh weeks of pregnancy). By the end of the embryonic stage, fetal structures are formed. Further development now consists primarily of growth and maturation of already formed structures. From this point until birth, the conceptus is called a *fetus*.

FIRST TRIMESTER

Normal pregnancies last an average of 280 days. Although pregnancies vary in duration, they're conveniently divided into three trimesters.

During the first trimester, a female-bodied person usually experiences physical changes, such as amenorrhea, urinary frequency, nausea and vomiting (more severe in the morning or when the stomach is empty), breast swelling and tenderness, fatigue, increased vaginal secretions, and constipation.

Within 7 to 10 days after conception, pregnancy tests, which detect hCG in the urine and serum, are usually positive. A pelvic examination at this stage can yield various findings, such as Hegar's sign (cervical and uterine softening), Chadwick's sign (a bluish coloration of the vagina and cervix resulting from increased venous circulation), and enlargement of the uterus. A pelvic examination may help estimate gestational age, but vaginal sonography is more accurate.

The first trimester is an important time for fetal development during pregnancy. Rapid cell differentiation makes the developing embryo or fetus highly susceptible to the teratogenic effects of viruses, alcohol, cigarettes, caffeine, and other drugs.

SECOND TRIMESTER

From the 13th to the 28th week of pregnancy, uterine and fetal size increases substantially, causing weight gain, a thickening waistline, abdominal enlargement and, possibly, reddish streaks as abdominal skin stretches (striation). In addition, pigment changes may cause skin alterations, such as linea nigra, melasma (mask of pregnancy), and a darkening of the areolae of the nipples.

Other physical changes may include diaphoresis, increased salivation, indigestion, continuing constipation, hemorrhoids, nosebleeds, and some dependent edema. The breasts become larger and heavier, and about 19 weeks after the last menstrual period, they may secrete colostrum. By about the 18th to the 20th week of pregnancy, the fetus is large enough for the pregnant person to feel it move (quickening). Anterior placement of the placenta may inhibit or decrease the pregnant person's sensation of fetal movement.

THIRD TRIMESTER

During this period, from the 28th week to term, the pregnant person may feel Braxton Hicks contractions—sporadic episodes of painless uterine tightening—which help strengthen uterine muscles in preparation for labor. It is more common for pregnant persons to sense Braxton Hicks in subsequent pregnancies than during their first. Increasing uterine size may displace pelvic and intestinal structures, causing indigestion, protrusion of the umbilicus, shortness of breath, and insomnia. The pregnant person may experience backaches because they walk with a swaybacked posture to counteract her frontal weight. By lying down, they can help minimize the development of varicose veins, hemorrhoids, and ankle edema.

LABOR AND DELIVERY

About 2 to 4 weeks before birth, lightening—the descent of the fetal head into the pelvis—shifts the uterine position. This relieves pressure on the diaphragm and enables the pregnant person to breathe more easily.

Onset of labor characteristically produces low back pain and passage of a small amount of bloody "show." A brownish or blood-tinged plug of cervical mucus may be passed up to 2 weeks before labor. As labor progresses, the cervix becomes soft, then effaces, and dilates; the amniotic membranes may rupture spontaneously, causing a gush or leakage of amniotic fluid. Uterine contractions typically become increasingly regular, frequent, intense, and long.

Labor is usually divided into four stages:
◆ *Stage I*, the longest stage, lasts from onset of regular contractions until full cervical dilation (4″ [10 cm]). Average duration of this stage is about 12 hours for a primigravida and 6 hours for a multigravida.
    ◆ *Stage I can be broken into two phases*: latent and active. Latent phase, during which the cervix typically dilates from 0 to 6 cm is typically longer, especially in primigravidas. Active phase is considered to begin at 6 cm dilated, when contractions are regular and last at least 1 minute.
◆ *Stage II* lasts from full cervical dilation until delivery of the infant—about 1 to 3 hours for a primigravida, 30 to 60 minutes for a multigravida.
◆ *Stage III*, the time between delivery and expulsion of the placenta, usually lasts several minutes (duration varies widely) but may last up to 30 minutes.
◆ *Stage IV* is a period of recovery during which homeostasis is re-established. This final stage lasts 1 to 4 hours after the placenta is expelled.

SOURCES OF PATHOLOGY

In no other body part do so many interrelated physiologic functions occur so close together as in the area of the female reproductive tract. Besides the internal genitalia, the female pelvis contains the organs of the urinary and the gastrointestinal (GI) systems (bladder, ureters, urethra, sigmoid colon, and rectum). The reproductive tract and its surrounding area are thus the site of urination, defecation, menstruation, ovulation, copulation, impregnation, and parturition. It's easy to understand how an abnormality in one pelvic organ can readily induce abnormality in another.

When conducting a pelvic examination, therefore, you must consider all possible sources of pathology. Remember that some serious abnormalities of the pelvic organs can be asymptomatic. Remember, too, that some abnormal findings in the pelvic area may result from pathologic changes in other organ systems, such as the upper urinary and GI tracts, the endocrine glands, and the neuromusculoskeletal system. Pain symptoms are often associated with the menstrual cycle; therefore, in many common diseases of the female reproductive tract, such pain follows a cyclic pattern. A patient with pelvic inflammatory disease (PID), for example, may complain of increasing premenstrual pain that's relieved by onset of menstruation.

PELVIC EXAMINATION

A pelvic examination and a thorough patient history are essential for any patient with symptoms related to the reproductive tract or adjacent body systems. Document any history of pregnancy, miscarriage, and abortion. Ask the patient if they have experienced any recent changes in their urinary habits or menstrual cycle. If they practice birth control, find out what method they use and whether they have experienced any adverse effects.

Then prepare the patient for the pelvic examination as follows:
◆ Ask the patient if they have douched within the past 24 hours. Explain that douching is not recommend as it washes away cells or organisms that the examination is designed and can change the pH of the vagina and cause it to be susceptible to infection.
◆ Check weight and blood pressure.
◆ For the patient's comfort, instruct them to empty their bladder before the examination. Provide a urine specimen container if needed.
◆ To help the patient relax, which is essential for a thorough pelvic examination, explain what the examination entails and why it's necessary prior to performing the exam. Explain what you will do before you do it. Encourage them to communicate if anything becomes uncomfortable or if they want you to stop the exam at any time. Stop if the patient asks you to stop. Ask them if they need a break or would like to be done completely. It is essential that you treat the patient with a calm, supportive manner as this is a sensitive exam.

◆ If the patient is scheduled for a Papanicolaou (Pap) test, inform them that another smear may have to be taken later if there are abnormal findings with the first test. Reassure them that this is done to confirm the first test's results. If they have never had a Pap test before, tell them it may be uncomfortable, they may experience some spotting and/or cramping during and/or after the procedure.

◆ After the Pap test, a bimanual examination is performed to assess the size and location of the ovaries and uterus.

◆ After the examination, offer the patient pre-moistened tissues to clean the vulva.

OTHER DIAGNOSTIC TESTS

Diagnostic measures for gynecologic disorders also include the following tests, which can be performed in the provider's office:

◆ Wet smear to examine vaginal secretions for specific organisms, such as *Trichomonas vaginalis*, bacterial vaginosis, and *Candida albicans*, or to evaluate semen specimens collected in connection with rape or infertility cases.

◆ Endometrial biopsy to assess hormonal secretions of the corpus luteum, to determine whether normal ovulation is occurring, and to check for neoplasia.

◆ Dilatation and curettage with hysteroscopy to evaluate atypical bleeding and to detect carcinoma.

◆ Laparoscopy, used to evaluate infertility, dysmenorrhea, and pelvic pain, and as a means of sterilization, is usually performed in a healthcare facility while the patient is under anesthesia. Increasingly, however, it's being performed as a less invasive procedure under conscious sedation in an office setting using microlaparoscopic technique.

Gynecologic disorders

PREMENSTRUAL SYNDROME

Also designated *late luteal phase dysphoric disorder* in *the Diagnostic and Statistical Manual of Mental Disorders*, Fifth Edition, Text Revision, premenstrual syndrome (PMS) is characterized by varying symptoms that appear 7 to 14 days before menses and usually subside with its onset. The effects of PMS range from minimal discomfort to severe, disruptive symptoms and can include nervousness, irritability, depression, and multiple somatic complaints.

Pathophysiology

The list of biologic theories offered to explain the cause of PMS is impressive. It includes conditions such as a progesterone deficiency in the menstrual cycle's luteal phase and vitamin deficiencies. Although there's no evidence that PMS is hormonally mediated, failure to identify a specific disorder with a specific mechanism suggests that PMS represents a variety of manifestations triggered by normal physiologic hormonal changes.

Causes and incidence

Researchers believe that 70% to 90% of female-bodied persons experience PMS at some time during their childbearing years, usually between ages 25 and 45.

Complications

◆ Depression
◆ Inability to function at home, work, or school

Signs and symptoms

Clinical effects vary widely among patients and may include any combination of the following:

◆ *behavioral*—mild to severe personality changes, nervousness, hostility, irritability, agitation, sleep disturbances, fatigue, lethargy, and depression

◆ *somatic*—breast tenderness or swelling, abdominal tenderness or bloating, joint pain, headache, edema, diarrhea or constipation, and exacerbations of skin problems (such as acne or rashes), respiratory problems (such as asthma), or neurologic problems (such as seizures)

PMS may need to be differentiated from premenstrual dysphoric disorder, which is a more severe form of PMS that's marked by severe depression, irritability, and tension before menstruation. (See *Premenstrual dysphoric disorder*, page 1024.)

DIAGNOSIS

The patient history shows typical symptoms related to the menstrual cycle. To help ensure an accurate history, the patient may be asked to record menstrual symptoms, mood, intake, movement, and body temperature on a calendar for 2 to 3 months prior to diagnosis. Estrogen and progesterone serum and/or urine levels may be evaluated to help rule out hormonal imbalance. A psychological evaluation is also recommended to rule out or detect an underlying or comorbid psychiatric disorder.

TREATMENT

Educating and reassuring patients that PMS is a real physiologic syndrome are important parts of treatment. Because treatment is

Premenstrual dysphoric disorder

Premenstrual dysphoric disorder (PMDD) is a severe form of PMS that has a cyclical occurrence of psychiatric symptoms that starts after ovulation (usually the week before the onset of menstruation) and ends within the first day or two of menses. Its underlying cause and pathophysiology remain unclear. However, researchers theorize that normal cyclic changes in the body cause abnormal responses to neurotransmitters, such as serotonin, resulting in physical and behavioral signs and symptoms.

PMDD affects as many as 1 in 20 American female-bodied persons who have regular menstrual periods. It's unclear why some female-bodied persons are affected while others aren't.

How PMDD and PMS differ

PMDD is characterized by severe monthly mood swings and physical signs and symptoms that interfere with everyday life. Compared with PMS, its signs and symptoms are abnormal and unmanageable. Although depression, anxiety, and sadness are common with PMS, in PMDD, these symptoms are extreme. Some female-bodied persons may feel the urge to hurt or kill themselves or others.

The Diagnostic and Statistical Manual of Mental Disorders, Fifth Edition, Text Revision, sets these criteria for diagnosing PMDD:
♦ functional impairment
♦ predominant mood symptoms, with one being affective
♦ symptoms beginning 1 week before the onset of menstruation
♦ symptoms that aren't due to any underlying primary mood disorder.

In addition, at least five of the following symptoms must be present:
♦ appetite changes
♦ decreased interests
♦ difficulty concentrating
♦ fatigue
♦ feelings of being overwhelmed
♦ insomnia or hypersomnia
♦ irritability
♦ "low mood"
♦ mood swings
♦ physical symptoms
♦ tension

predominantly symptomatic, each patient must learn to cope with their own individual set of symptoms. Treatment may include calcium and magnesium supplementation, vitamins (such as B complex), dietary changes, prostaglandin inhibitors, and nonsteroidal anti-inflammatory drugs (NSAIDs). Diuretics may be prescribed for patients who experience significant weight gain due to fluid retention. Psychiatric medications and therapy may be prescribed for female-bodied persons who develop anxiety, irritability, or depression. Hormonal therapy may include the use of progesterone cream or vaginal suppository or a trial on hormonal contraceptives, which may either decrease or increase PMS symptoms.

For treatment to be effective, the patient may have to maintain a diet that's low in simple sugars, caffeine, and salt.

Special considerations
♦ Inform the patient that self-help groups exist for female-bodied persons with PMS; help them contact such a group if appropriate.
♦ Obtain a complete patient history to help identify any emotional problems that may

contribute to PMS. Refer the patient for psychological counseling if necessary.
♦ Suggest that the patient seek further medical consultation if symptoms are severe and interfere with their normal lifestyle.

▦▦▦ PREVENTION
♦ *If possible, discuss with your patient ways they can modify their lifestyle, such as making changes in their diet, and avoiding stimulants and alcohol.*
♦ *Encourage your patient to get regular exercise and adequate rest.*

DYSMENORRHEA
Dysmenorrhea—painful menstruation—is the most common gynecologic complaint and a leading cause of absenteeism from school (affecting 10% of high school female-bodied persons each month) and work (causing about 140 million lost work hours annually). Dysmenorrhea can occur as a primary disorder or secondary to an underlying disease. Because primary dysmenorrhea is self-limiting, the prognosis is generally good. The prognosis for secondary dysmenorrhea depends on the underlying disorder.

Causes and incidence

Causes of pelvic pain

The characteristic pelvic pain of dysmenorrhea must be distinguished from the acute pain caused by many other disorders, such as:

♦ *GI disorders:* appendicitis, acute diverticulitis, acute or chronic cholecystitis, chronic cholelithiasis, acute pancreatitis, peptic ulcer perforation, intestinal obstruction

♦ *pregnancy disorders:* impending abortion (pain and bleeding early in pregnancy), ectopic pregnancy, abruptio placentae, uterine rupture, leiomyoma degeneration, toxemia

♦ *reproductive disorders:* acute salpingitis, chronic inflammation, degenerating fibroid, ovarian cyst torsion

♦ *urinary tract disorders:* cystitis, renal calculi

♦ Other conditions that may mimic dysmenorrhea include ovulation and normal uterine contractions experienced in pregnancy. Emotional conflicts can cause psychogenic (functional) pain.

Pathophysiology

Although primary dysmenorrhea has no known single cause, possible contributing factors include hormonal imbalances and psychogenic factors. The pain of dysmenorrhea probably results from increased prostaglandin secretion, which intensifies normal uterine contractions.

Dysmenorrhea may also be secondary to such gynecologic disorders as endometriosis, cervical stenosis, uterine leiomyomas, uterine malposition, PID, pelvic tumors, or adenomyosis.

Because dysmenorrhea almost always follows an ovulatory cycle, both the primary and secondary forms are rare during the anovulatory cycles of menses. After age 20, dysmenorrhea is generally secondary.

Complications

♦ mood disorders; anxiety, depression
♦ relationship difficulties
♦ inability to function in daily life, at school, at work, etc.

Signs and symptoms

Dysmenorrhea produces sharp, intermittent, cramping lower abdominal pain, which usually radiates to the back, thighs, groin, and vulva.

Such pain—sometimes compared with labor pains—typically starts with or immediately before menstrual flow and peaks within 24 hours. Dysmenorrhea may also be associated with the characteristic signs and symptoms of PMS (urinary frequency, nausea, vomiting, diarrhea, headache, chills, abdominal bloating, painful breasts, depression, and irritability).

Diagnosis

Pelvic examination and a detailed patient history may help suggest the cause of dysmenorrhea.

Primary dysmenorrhea is diagnosed when secondary causes are ruled out. Appropriate tests (such as laparoscopy, dilatation and curettage, and pelvic ultrasound) are used to diagnose underlying disorders in secondary dysmenorrhea.

Treatment

Initial treatment aims to relieve pain. Pain-relief measures may include:

♦ analgesics (such as aspirin) for mild to moderate pain (most effective when taken 24 to 48 hours before onset of menses; are especially effective for treating dysmenorrhea because they also inhibit prostaglandin synthesis; stronger anti-inflammatories may be used).

♦ opioids if pain is severe (infrequently used).

♦ prostaglandin inhibitors (such as naproxen and ibuprofen) to relieve pain by decreasing the severity of uterine contractions.

♦ heat applied locally to the lower abdomen (may relieve discomfort in mature female-bodied persons but isn't recommended in young adolescents because appendicitis may mimic dysmenorrhea).

For primary dysmenorrhea, administration of sex steroids is an effective alternative to treatment with antiprostaglandins or analgesics. Such therapy usually consists of hormonal contraceptives to relieve pain by suppressing ovulation. However, patients who are attempting pregnancy should rely on antiprostaglandin therapy instead of hormonal contraceptives to relieve symptoms of primary dysmenorrhea.

Because persistently severe dysmenorrhea may have a psychogenic cause, psychological evaluation and appropriate counseling may be helpful.

In secondary dysmenorrhea, treatment is designed to identify and correct the underlying cause. This may include surgical treatment of underlying disorders, such as endometriosis or uterine leiomyomas. However, surgical treatment is recommended only after conservative therapy fails.

Special considerations

Effective management of the patient with dysmenorrhea focuses on relief of symptoms, emotional support, and appropriate patient teaching, especially for the adolescent.

◆ Obtain a complete history, focusing on the patient's gynecologic complaints, including detailed information on any signs and symptoms of pelvic disease, such as excessive bleeding, changes in bleeding pattern, vaginal discharge, and dyspareunia.

◆ Provide thorough patient teaching. Explain normal female anatomy and physiology to the patient, as well as the nature of dysmenorrhea. This may be a good opportunity, depending on circumstances, to provide the adolescent patient with information on pregnancy and contraception.

◆ Encourage the patient to keep a detailed record of their menstrual symptoms and to seek medical care if their symptoms persist.

◆ Instruct the patient on some home care remedies that may be helpful in relieving discomfort, such as applying a heating pad to the lower abdomen, taking warm showers or baths, drinking warm beverages, and performing circular massage with the fingertips around the lower abdomen.

◆ Encourage the patient to walk or exercise regularly. Recommend pelvic rocking exercises and relaxation techniques, such as meditation or yoga. Let them know that keeping their legs elevated while lying down or lying on their side with their knees bent may also increase comfort.

◆ Instruct the patient to eat light but frequent meals and to follow a diet rich in foods high in complex carbohydrates, such as whole grains, fruits, and vegetables. Advise them to avoid alcohol and foods high in salt, sugar, and caffeine.

VULVOVAGINITIS

Vulvovaginitis is inflammation of the vulva (vulvitis) and vagina (vaginitis). Because of the proximity of these two structures, inflammation of one occasionally causes inflammation of the other. Vulvovaginitis may occur at any age and affects most female-bodied persons at some time. The prognosis is excellent with treatment.

Causes and incidence

Common causes include:

◆ Infection with *T. vaginalis*, a protozoan flagellate usually transmitted through sexual intercourse.

◆ Infection with *C. albicans*, a fungus that requires glucose for growth. Incidence rises during the menstrual cycle's secretory phase. (Such infection occurs twice as often in pregnant females as in nonpregnant females. It also commonly affects users of hormonal contraceptives, patients who are diabetic, and patients receiving systemic therapy with broad-spectrum antibiotics [incidence may reach 75%].)

◆ Excess of nonspecific vaginal bacteria with little or absent inflammation, commonly referred to as *Gardnerella vaginalis* or nonspecific vaginitis.

◆ Parasitic infection (*Phthirus pubis* [crab louse]).

◆ Trauma (skin breakdown may lead to secondary infection).

◆ Poor personal hygiene.

◆ Chemical irritations, or allergic reactions to hygiene sprays, douches, detergents, soaps, bubble baths, feminine hygiene products, clothing, or toilet paper.

◆ Vulval atrophy in menopausal female-bodied persons due to decreasing estrogen levels.

◆ Retention of a foreign body, such as a tampon or diaphragm.

Pathophysiology

Often this problem is caused by or related to an infection such as *T. vaginalis*, *C. albicans*, or *G. vaginalis*. It can also be caused by irritants such as laundry detergents, bubble bath, soaps, feminine hygiene products, and lubricants.

Complications

◆ Infection

◆ Perineal inflammation and edema

◆ Skin breakdown

Signs and symptoms

In trichomonal vaginitis, vaginal discharge is thin, bubbly, green-tinged, and malodorous. This infection causes marked irritation and itching, and urinary symptoms, such as burning and frequency. Candidal vaginitis produces a thick, white, cottage cheese-like discharge and red, edematous mucous membranes, with white flecks adhering to the vaginal wall and is often accompanied by intense itching. (See *Candida infection*, page 1027.) *G. vaginalis* produces a gray, foul, "fishy" smelling discharge.

Acute vulvitis causes a mild to severe inflammatory reaction, including edema, erythema, burning, and pruritus. Severe pain on urination and dyspareunia may necessitate immediate treatment. Herpes infection may cause painful ulceration or vesicle formation during the active phase.

Diagnosis

Diagnosis of vulvovaginitis requires identification of the infectious organism during microscopic examination of vaginal discharge

Candida infection

This illustration shows the thick, white vaginal discharge of a *Candida* infection.

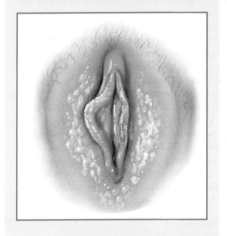

oral and topical acyclovir decreases the duration and symptoms of active lesions.

If an STD is diagnosed, it's very important that sexual partners also receive treatment, even if there are no symptoms. Failure of partners to receive treatment can lead to continual reinfection, which may eventually lead to infertility and affect the patient's overall health.

Special considerations

◆ Ask the patient if they have any drug allergies. Stress the importance of taking the medication for the length of time prescribed, even if symptoms subside.

◆ Teach the patient how to insert vaginal ointments and suppositories. Advise them to remain prone for at least 30 minutes after insertion to promote absorption (insertion at bedtime is ideal). Suggest they wear a pad to prevent staining their underclothing.

◆ Report notifiable cases of STD to local public health authorities.

◆ Advise the patient that persistent, recurring candidiasis may suggest diabetes, undiagnosed pregnancy, or immunologic issues.

PREVENTION
◆ *Encourage good hygiene.*
◆ *Advise the patient with a history of recurrent vulvovaginitis to wear all-cotton underpants. Advise them to avoid wearing tight-fitting pants and panty hose, which encourage the growth of the infecting organisms. Removing underpants at night is also helpful.*
◆ *Advise them to avoid shaving or waxing the pubic region.*
◆ *Encourage the use of condoms to avoid contracting an STD. Ensure folks with latex allergy are using nonlatex condoms.*
◆ *Advise the patient to avoid the use of irritants such as scented soaps and feminine hygiene products.*
◆ *Advise the patient to avoid baths, douching, and the use of hot tubs.*

on a wet slide preparation (a drop of vaginal discharge placed in normal saline solution) or identification of irritant after with thorough history. In some cases, a culture of the vaginal discharge may identify the organism causing the infection.

Diagnosis of vulvitis or suspected sexually transmitted disease (STD) may require complete blood count, urinalysis, cytology screening, biopsy of chronic lesions to rule out malignancy, culture of exudate from acute lesions, and possible human immunodeficiency virus testing.

Treatment

The cause of vulvovaginitis determines the appropriate treatment. It may include oral or topical antibiotics, antifungal creams, antibacterial creams, or similar medications. An antihistamine may be prescribed for allergic reactions. Cold compresses or cool sitz baths may provide relief from pruritus in acute vulvitis; severe inflammation may require warm compresses. Other therapy includes avoiding drying soaps, wearing loose clothing to promote air circulation, and applying topical corticosteroids to reduce inflammation. Chronic vulvitis may respond to topical hydrocortisone or antipruritics and good hygiene (especially in elderly or incontinent patients). Topical estrogen ointments may be used to treat atrophic vulvovaginitis. No cure exists for herpesvirus infections; however,

OVARIAN CYSTS

Ovarian cysts are usually nonneoplastic sacs on an ovary that contain fluid or semisolid material. Although these cysts are usually small and produce no symptoms, they generally require thorough investigation as possible sites of malignant change. Common ovarian cysts include follicular cysts, lutein cysts (granulosa-lutein [corpus luteum] and theca-lutein cysts), and polycystic ovarian disease. Ovarian cysts can develop at any time between puberty and menopause, including during pregnancy. Granulosa-lutein cysts occur infrequently, usually during early pregnancy. The prognosis for non-neoplastic ovarian cysts is excellent.

Causes and incidence

Follicular cysts are generally very small and arise from follicles that over-distend. When such cysts persist into menopause, they secrete excessive amounts of estrogen in response to the hypersecretion of FSH and LH that normally occurs during menopause. (See *Follicular cyst.*)

Pathophysiology

When such cysts persist into menopause, they secrete excessive amounts of estrogen in response to the hypersecretion of FSH and LH that normally occurs during menopause. (See *Follicular cyst.*)

Granulosa-lutein cysts, which occur within the corpus luteum, are functional, nonneoplastic enlargements of the ovaries caused by excessive accumulation of blood during the hemorrhagic phase of the menstrual cycle. Theca-lutein cysts are commonly bilateral and filled with clear, straw-colored fluid; they're often associated with hydatidiform mole, choriocarcinoma, or hormone therapy (with hCG or clomiphene citrate).

Complications

- Amenorrhea
- Infertility
- Oligomenorrhea
- Secondary dysmenorrhea

Follicular cyst

A common type of ovarian cyst, a follicular cyst is usually semitransparent and overdistended with watery fluid that's visible through its thin walls.

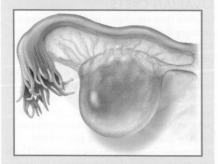

Signs and symptoms

Small ovarian cysts (such as follicular cysts) usually don't produce symptoms unless torsion or rupture causes signs of an acute abdomen (vomiting, abdominal tenderness, distention, and rigidity). Large or multiple cysts may induce mild pelvic discomfort, low back pain, dyspareunia, or abnormal uterine bleeding secondary to a disturbed ovulatory pattern. Ovarian cysts with torsion induce acute abdominal pain similar to that of appendicitis.

Granulosa-lutein cysts that appear early in pregnancy may grow as large as 2″ to 2½″ (5 to 6 cm) in diameter and produce unilateral pelvic discomfort and, if rupture occurs, massive intraperitoneal hemorrhage. In nonpregnant female-bodied persons, these cysts may cause delayed menses, followed by prolonged or irregular bleeding. Polycystic ovary syndrome (PCOS) may also produce secondary amenorrhea, oligomenorrhea, or infertility.

Diagnosis

Generally, characteristic clinical features suggest ovarian cysts.

℞ **CONFIRMING DIAGNOSIS** *Visualization of the ovary through ultrasound, computed tomography scan, magnetic resonance imaging, laparoscopy, or surgery (often for another condition) confirms ovarian cysts.*

Extremely elevated hCG titers strongly suggest theca-lutein cysts. Pregnancy, including molar pregnancy, must be ruled out.

Treatment

Follicular cysts generally don't require treatment because they tend to disappear spontaneously within 60 to 90 days. However, if they interfere with daily activities, clomiphene citrate by mouth for 5 days or progesterone I.M. (also for 5 days) re-establishes the ovarian hormonal cycle and induces ovulation. Hormonal contraceptives haven't been proven to accelerate involution of functional cysts (including both types of lutein cysts and follicular cysts).

Treatment for granulosa-lutein cysts that occur during pregnancy is aimed at relieving symptoms because these cysts diminish during the third trimester and rarely require surgery. Theca-lutein cysts disappear spontaneously after elimination of the hydatidiform mole, destruction of choriocarcinoma, or discontinuation of hCG or clomiphene citrate therapy.

Surgery, in the form of laparoscopy or exploratory laparotomy with possible ovarian cystectomy or oophorectomy, may become necessary if an ovarian cyst is found to be persistent or suspicious.

Special considerations

Thorough patient teaching is a primary consideration. Carefully explain the cyst's nature, the type of discomfort the patient may experience, and how long the condition is expected to last.
◆ Preoperatively, watch for signs of cyst rupture, such as increasing abdominal pain, distention, and rigidity. Monitor vital signs for fever, tachypnea, or hypotension, which may indicate peritonitis or intraperitoneal hemorrhage. Administer sedatives, as ordered, to ensure adequate rest before surgery.
◆ Postoperatively, encourage frequent movement in bed and early ambulation, as ordered. Early ambulation helps to prevent pulmonary embolism.
◆ Provide emotional support. Offer appropriate reassurance if the patient fears cancer or infertility.
◆ Before discharge, advise the patient to increase their activities at home gradually—preferably over 4 to 6 weeks. Advise them to abstain from sexual intercourse and not to use tampons and douches during this period.

POLYCYSTIC OVARY SYNDROME

PCOS is a metabolic syndrome characterized by multiple ovarian cysts. It produces a syndrome of hormonal disturbances that includes insulin resistance, obesity, hirsutism, acne, and ovulation and fertility problems. With proper treatment, the prognosis for ovulation and fertility is good.

As with all anovulation syndromes, the pulsatile release of GnRH is lacking. This allows for the initial ovarian follicle development to be normal, but many small follicles begin to accumulate because there's no selection of a dominant follicle. These follicles then respond abnormally to hormonal stimulation, causing an abnormal estrogen secretion during the menstrual cycle.

Insulin, along with other hormones, plays a role in regulating ovary function. Insulin resistance results in high levels of circulating insulin. The high levels of insulin affect the function of cells, including ovary cells. This can lead to anovulation and infertility.

Causes and incidence

It's most common in female-bodied persons under age 30. In the United States, it affects 4% to 12% of female-bodied persons of childbearing age.

Pathophysiology

The precise cause of PCOS isn't known. There are several theories regarding the cause, including abnormal enzyme activity triggering excess androgen secretion from the ovaries and adrenal glands, as well as endocrine abnormalities or genetic links.

Complications

◆ Hypertension
◆ Increased risk of breast or endometrial cancer
◆ Infertility
◆ Type 2 diabetes mellitus

Signs and symptoms

Signs and symptoms of PCOS include mild pelvic discomfort, lower back pain, and dyspareunia caused by multiple ovarian cysts, abnormal uterine bleeding secondary to disturbed ovulatory pattern, hirsutism and male-pattern hair loss that result from abnormal patterns of estrogen secretion, obesity caused by abnormal hormone regulation, and acne caused by excess sebum production that results from disturbed androgen secretion.

Diagnosis

In PCOS, bilaterally enlarged polycystic ovaries can be seen on ultrasound examination. Tests reveal slight elevation of urinary 17-ketosteroids and anovulation (shown by basal body temperature graphs and endometrial biopsy). Blood testing reveals an elevated LH to FSH ratio (usually 3:1 or greater), and elevated testosterone, androstenedione, and glucose levels. Direct observation must rule out paraovarian cysts of the broad ligaments, salpingitis, endometriosis, and neoplastic cysts. Ultrasonography, abdominal magnetic imaging, or surgery (commonly done for another condition) allows visualization of the ovary, which may confirm the presence of ovarian cysts.

Treatment

Treatment of PCOS may include use of such drugs as clomiphene citrate to induce ovulation or medroxyprogesterone acetate for 10 days of every month for the patient who doesn't want to become pregnant. For the patient who needs reliable contraception, a low-dose hormonal contraceptive is used to treat abnormal bleeding. Surgical treatment may involve a hysterectomy with bilateral salpingo-oophorectomy for refractory pain and bleeding.

Drugs such as metformin, pioglitazone, or rosiglitazone can be used to make cells more insulin sensitive.

Special considerations

Provide appropriate postoperative care, including the following:
◆ Watch for signs of cyst rupture, such as increasing abdominal pain, distention, and rigidity.
◆ Monitor the patient's vital signs for fever, tachypnea, or hypotension (possibly indicating peritonitis or intraperitoneal hemorrhage).

◆ Encourage frequent movement in bed and early ambulation, as ordered, to prevent pulmonary embolism.

◆ Provide emotional support, offering appropriate reassurance if the patient fears cancer or infertility.

◆ Before discharge, if the patient is overweight, discuss the importance of weight reduction and the role it may play in reducing insulin resistance.

ENDOMETRIOSIS
Causes and incidence
The mechanisms by which endometriosis causes symptoms, including infertility, are unknown. The main theories to explain this disorder are:

◆ transtubal regurgitation of endometrial cells and implantation at ectopic sites

◆ coelomic metaplasia (repeated inflammation may induce metaplasia of mesothelial cells to the endometrial epithelium)

◆ lymphatic or hematogenous spread to explain extraperitoneal disease

Endometriosis occurs in 10% of female-bodied persons during the reproductive years. Prevalence may be as high as 25% to 35% among infertile female-bodied persons. A female-bodied person with a mother or sister with endometriosis is six times more likely to develop endometriosis than a female-bodied person without this familial history.

Pathophysiology
Endometriosis is the presence of endometrial tissue outside the lining of the uterine cavity. Such ectopic tissue is generally confined to the pelvic area, most commonly around the ovaries, uterovesical peritoneum, uterosacral ligaments, and cul-de-sac, but it can appear anywhere in the body. This ectopic endometrial tissue responds to normal stimulation in the same way that the endometrium does. During menstruation, the ectopic tissue bleeds, which causes inflammation of the surrounding tissues. This inflammation causes fibrosis, leading to adhesions that produce pain and infertility.

Active endometriosis usually occurs between ages 20 and 40; it's uncommon before age 20. Severe symptoms of endometriosis may have an abrupt onset or may develop over many years. This disorder usually becomes progressively severe during the menstrual years; after menopause, it may subside.

Complications
◆ Anemia
◆ Infertility
◆ Spontaneous abortion

Signs and symptoms
The classic symptom of endometriosis is acquired dysmenorrhea, which may produce constant pain in the lower abdomen and in the vagina, posterior pelvis, and back. This pain usually begins from 5 to 7 days before menses reaches its peak and lasts for 2 to 3 days. It differs from primary dysmenorrheal pain, which is more cramplike and concentrated in the abdominal midline. However, the pain's severity doesn't necessarily indicate the extent of the disease.

Other clinical features depend on the location of the ectopic tissue:

◆ ovaries and oviducts: infertility and profuse menses

◆ ovaries or cul-de-sac: deep-thrust dyspareunia

◆ bladder: suprapubic pain, dysuria, hematuria

◆ small bowel and appendix: nausea and vomiting, which worsen before menses, and abdominal cramps

◆ cervix, vagina, and perineum: bleeding from endometrial deposits in these areas during menses

The primary complications of endometriosis are infertility and chronic pelvic pain.

Diagnosis
Pelvic examination may suggest endometriosis. Palpation may detect multiple tender nodules on uterosacral ligaments or in the rectovaginal septum in one-third of patients. These nodules enlarge and become more tender during menses. Palpation may also uncover ovarian enlargement in the presence of endometrial cysts on the ovaries or thickened, nodular adnexa (as in PID). Laparoscopy must confirm the diagnosis and determine the disease's stage before treatment is started. Endometriosis is classified in stages: Stage I, mild; Stage II, moderate; Stage III, severe; and Stage IV, extensive.

Treatment
Treatment varies according to the disease's stage and the patient's age and desire to have children. Conservative therapy for young female-bodied persons who want to have children includes androgens, such as danazol, which produce a temporary remission in Stages I and II. Progestins and hormonal contraceptives also relieve symptoms. GnRH agonists, by inducing a pseudomenopause and, thus, a "medical oophorectomy," may cause a remission of disease and are commonly used. However, medical therapy remains inadequate.

When ovarian masses are present, surgery must rule out cancer. Conservative surgery includes laparoscopic removal of endometrial implants with conventional or laser techniques and presacral neurectomy for severe dysmenorrhea. The treatment of choice for female-bodied persons who don't want to bear children or for extensive disease is a total abdominal hysterectomy with bilateral salpingo-oophorectomy.

Special considerations
◆ Because infertility is a possible complication, advise the patient who wants children not to postpone childbearing.
◆ Recommend an annual pelvic examination and Pap test to all patients.

UTERINE LEIOMYOMAS
Causes and incidence
The cause of uterine leiomyomas is unknown, but steroid hormones, including estrogen and progesterone, and several growth factors, including epidermal growth factor, have been implicated as regulators of leiomyoma growth. Leiomyomas typically arise after menarche and regress after menopause, implicating estrogen as a promoter of leiomyoma growth.

Uterine leiomyomas occur in 20% to 25% of female-bodied persons of reproductive age and reportedly affect three times as many Black female-bodied persons as White female-bodied persons. The tumors become malignant (leiomyosarcoma) in only 0.1% or less of patients.

Pathophysiology
The most common benign tumors in female-bodied persons, uterine leiomyomas, also known as *myomas*, *fibromyomas*, or *fibroids*, are smooth-muscle tumors. They usually occur in multiples in the uterine corpus, although they may appear on the cervix or on the round or broad ligament. Though uterine leiomyomas are often called *fibroids*, this term is misleading because they consist of muscle cells and not fibrous tissue.

Complications
◆ Anemia
◆ Dystocia
◆ Infertility
◆ Intestinal obstruction
◆ Preterm labor
◆ Spontaneous abortion

Signs and symptoms
Leiomyomas may be located within the uterine wall or may protrude into the endometrial cavity or from the serosal surface of the uterus. (See *Uterine fibroids*, page 1032.) Most leiomyomas produce no symptoms. The most common symptom is abnormal bleeding, which typically presents clinically as menorrhagia. Uterine leiomyomas probably don't cause pain directly except when associated with torsion of a pedunculated subserous tumor. Pelvic pressure and impingement on adjacent viscera are common indications for treatment. Other symptoms may include urine retention, constipation, or dyspareunia.

Diagnosis
Clinical findings and patient history may suggest uterine leiomyomas. Bimanual examination may reveal an enlarged, firm, nontender, and irregularly contoured uterus. Ultrasound (transvaginal or pelvic) or magnetic resonance imaging allows accurate assessment of the dimensions, number, and location of tumors. Other diagnostic procedures include hysterosalpingography, dilatation and curettage, endometrial biopsy, and laparoscopy.

Treatment
Treatment depends on the symptoms' severity, the tumors' size and location, and the patient's age, parity, pregnancy status, desire to have children, and general health.

Treatment options include nonsurgical as well as surgical procedures. Nonsurgical methods include taking serial histories and performing physical assessments at clinically indicated intervals and administering GnRH analogues, which are capable of rapidly suppressing pituitary gonadotropin release, leading to profound hypoestrogenemia and a 50% reduction in uterine volume. The peak effects of these GnRH analogues occur in the 12th week of therapy. The benefits are reduction in tumor size before surgery, reduction in intraoperative blood loss, and an increase in preoperative hematocrit. GnRH analogues aren't curative.

Surgical procedures include abdominal, laparoscopic, or hysteroscopic myomectomy—for patients who want to preserve fertility. Myolysis and uterine artery embolization can successfully treat fibroids without hysterectomy or major surgery. Performed on an outpatient basis, this laparoscopic procedure coagulates the fibroids and preserves the uterus and the patient's childbearing potential. Hysterectomy is the definitive treatment for symptomatic female-bodied persons who have completed childbearing, but uterine artery embolization may be an alternative in some situations.

Special considerations
◆ Tell the patient to report any abnormal bleeding or pelvic pain immediately.
◆ If a hysterectomy or oophorectomy is indicated, explain the operation's effects on

Uterine fibroids

The various sites for uterine fibroids.

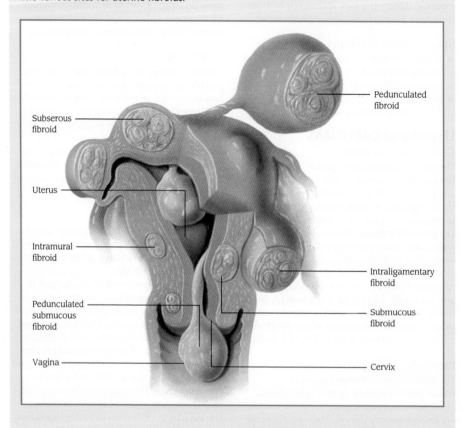

Pedunculated fibroid

Subserous fibroid

Uterus

Intramural fibroid

Pedunculated submucous fibroid

Vagina

Intraligamentary fibroid

Submucous fibroid

Cervix

menstruation, menopause, and sexual activity to the patient.

◆ Reassure the patient that they most likely won't experience premature menopause if their ovaries are left intact.

◆ If it's necessary for the patient to have a multiple myomectomy, make sure they understand pregnancy is still possible. Explain that a cesarean delivery may be indicated.

PRECOCIOUS PUBERTY

Causes and incidence

About 85% of all cases of true precocious puberty in female-bodied persons are constitutional, resulting from early development and activation of the endocrine glands without corresponding abnormality. Other causes of true precocious puberty are pathologic and include central nervous system (CNS) disorders

resulting from tumors, trauma, infection, or other lesions. These CNS disorders include hypothalamic tumors, intracranial tumors (pinealoma, granuloma, hamartoma), hydrocephaly, degenerative encephalopathy, tuberous sclerosis, neurofibromatosis, encephalitis, skull injuries, meningitis, and peptic arachnoiditis. McCune–Albright syndrome, Silver syndrome, and juvenile hypothyroidism are conditions often associated with female precocity.

Pathophysiology

In female-bodied persons, precocious puberty is the early onset of pubertal changes: breast development, pubic and axillary hair development, and menarche before age 9. (Normally, the mean age for menarche is 12.) In true precocious puberty, the ovaries mature and pubertal changes progress in an orderly manner. In pseudoprecocious puberty, pubertal changes occur without corresponding ovarian maturation.

Pseudoprecocious puberty may result from increased levels of sex hormones due to ovarian and adrenocortical tumors, adrenocortical virilizing hyperplasia, or ingestion of estrogens or androgens. It may also result from increased end-organ sensitivity to low levels of circulating sex hormones, whereby estrogens promote premature breast development and androgens promote premature pubic and axillary hair growth.

Risk factors include race (more Blacks are affected than Whites), sex (more female-bodied persons are affected than male-bodied persons), and obesity.

Other signs may include underarm hair growth, acne, and adult-type body odor.

Complications
◆ PCOS
◆ Short stature

Signs and symptoms
The usual pattern of precocious puberty in female-bodied persons is a rapid growth spurt, thelarche (breast development), pubarche (pubic hair development), and menarche—all before age 9. These changes may occur independently or simultaneously.

Diagnosis
Diagnosis requires a complete patient history, a thorough physical examination, and special tests to differentiate between true and pseudoprecocious puberty and to indicate what treatment may be necessary. X-rays of the hands, wrists, knees, and hips determine bone age and possible premature epiphyseal closure. Other tests detect abnormally high hormonal levels for the patient's age: vaginal smear for estrogen secretion, urinary tests for gonadotropic activity and excretion of 17-ketosteroids, and radioimmunoassay (RIA) for both LH and FSH.

As indicated, ultrasound, laparoscopy, or exploratory laparotomy may verify a suspected abdominal lesion; electroencephalography, ventriculography, pneumoencephalography, computed tomography scan, or angiography can detect CNS disorders.

Treatment
Treatment of constitutional true precocious puberty may include medroxyprogesterone to reduce secretion of gonadotropins and prevent menstruation. Other therapy depends on the cause of precocious puberty and its stage of development:
◆ Adrenogenital syndrome necessitates cortical or adrenocortical steroid replacement.

◆ Abdominal tumors necessitate surgery to remove ovarian and adrenal tumors. Regression of secondary sex characteristics may follow such surgery, especially in young children.
◆ Choriocarcinomas require surgery and chemotherapy.
◆ Hypothyroidism requires thyroid extract or levothyroxine to decrease gonadotropic secretions.
◆ Drug ingestion requires that the medication be discontinued.

In precocious thelarche and pubarche, no treatment is necessary.

Special considerations
The dramatic physical changes produced by precocious puberty can be upsetting and alarming for the child and their family. Provide a calm, supportive atmosphere, and encourage the patient and their family to express their feelings about these changes. Explain all diagnostic procedures and tell the patient and their family that surgery may be necessary.
◆ Explain the condition to the child in terms they can understand to prevent feelings of shame and loss of self-esteem. Provide appropriate sex education, including information on menstruation and related hygiene.
◆ Tell parents that, although their child seems physically mature, they are not psychologically mature, and the discrepancy between physical appearance and psychological and psychosexual maturation may create problems. Warn them against expecting more of them than they would expect of other children their age.
◆ Suggest that parents continue to dress their child in clothes that are appropriate for their age and that don't call attention to their physical development.
◆ Reassure parents that precocious puberty doesn't usually precipitate precocious sexual behavior.

MENOPAUSE
Causes and incidence
◆ Physiologic menopause, the normal decline in ovarian function due to aging, begins in most female-bodied persons between ages 45 and 55, on average 51, and results in infrequent ovulation, decreased menstrual function and, eventually, cessation of menstruation.
◆ Pathologic (premature) menopause, the gradual or abrupt cessation of menstruation before age 40, occurs idiopathically in about 1% of female-bodied persons in the United States. However, certain diseases, especially severe infections and reproductive tract tumors, may cause pathologic menopause by seriously impairing ovarian

function. Other factors that may precipitate pathologic menopause include malnutrition, chemotherapy, debilitation, extreme emotional stress, excessive radiation exposure, and surgical procedures that impair ovarian blood supply.

Pathophysiology

Menopause is the cessation of menstruation. It results from a complex syndrome of physiologic changes—the climacteric—caused by declining ovarian function. The climacteric produces various body changes, the most dramatic being menopause.

Complications

- Atherosclerosis
- Osteoporosis
- Urinary incontinence
- Weight gain

Signs and symptoms

Many menopausal female-bodied persons are asymptomatic but some have severe symptoms. The decline in ovarian function and consequent decreased estrogen level produce menstrual irregularities: a decrease in the amount and duration of menstrual flow, spotting, and episodes of amenorrhea and polymenorrhea (possibly with hypermenorrhea). Irregularities may last a few months or persist for several years before menstruation ceases permanently.

The following body system changes may occur (usually after the permanent cessation of menstruation):

- Reproductive system—Menopause may cause shrinkage of vulval structures and loss of subcutaneous fat, possibly leading to atrophic vulvitis; atrophy of vaginal mucosa and flattening of vaginal rugae, possibly causing bleeding after coitus or douching; vaginal itching and discharge from bacterial invasion; and loss of capillaries in the atrophying vaginal wall, causing the pink, rugal lining to become smooth and white. Menopause may also produce excessive vaginal dryness and dyspareunia due to decreased lubrication from the vaginal walls and decreased secretion from Bartholin's glands; smaller ovaries and oviducts; and progressive pelvic relaxation as the supporting structures lose their tone due to the absence of estrogen.

ELDER TIP *As a female-bodied person ages, atrophy causes the vagina to shorten and the mucous lining to become thin, dry, less elastic, and pale as a result of decreased vascularity. In addition, the pH of vaginal secretions increases, making the vaginal environment more alkaline. The type of flora also changes, increasing the older female-bodied person's chance of vaginal infections.*

- Urinary system—Atrophic cystitis due to the effects of decreased estrogen levels on bladder mucosa and related structures may cause pyuria, dysuria, and urinary frequency, urgency, and incontinence. Urethral carbuncles from loss of urethral tone and mucosal thinning may cause dysuria, meatal tenderness, and hematuria.
- Mammary system—Breast size decreases.
- Integumentary system—The patient may experience loss of skin elasticity and turgor due to estrogen deprivation, loss of pubic and axillary hair, and, occasionally, slight alopecia.
- Autonomic nervous system—The patient may exhibit hot flashes and night sweats (in 75% of female-bodied persons), vertigo, syncope, tachycardia, dyspnea, tinnitus, emotional disturbances (irritability, nervousness, crying spells, fits of anger), and exacerbation of pre-existing depression, anxiety, and compulsive, manic, or schizoid behavior.

Menopause may also induce atherosclerosis, and a decrease in estrogen level contributes to osteoporosis.

Ovarian activity in younger female-bodied persons is believed to provide a protective effect on the cardiovascular system, and the loss of this function at menopause may partly explain the increased death rate from myocardial infarction in older female-bodied persons. Also, estrogen has been found to increase levels of high-density lipoprotein cholesterol.

Diagnosis

Patient history and typical clinical features suggest menopause. Menopause is a retrospective diagnosis and can only be determined after 12 consecutive months of amenorrhea. A Pap test may show the influence of estrogen deficiency on vaginal mucosa. RIA may be performed, but because of the expense involved, it isn't necessary to confirm a diagnosis of menopause. If done, RIA shows the following blood hormone levels:

- estrogen: 0 to 14 ng/dL
- plasma estradiol: 15 to 40 pg/mL
- estrone: 25 to 50 pg/mL

RIA also shows the following urine values:

- estrogen: 6 to 28 μg/24 hours
- pregnanediol (urinary secretion of progesterone): 0.3 to 0.9 mg/24 hours

FSH production may increase as much as 15 times its normal level; LH production, as much as five times.

Pelvic examination, endometrial biopsy, and dilatation and curettage may rule out organic disease in patients with abnormal menstrual bleeding.

Treatment

Menopause is a natural process that doesn't require treatment unless menopausal symptoms, such as hot flashes or vaginal dryness, are particularly bothersome. Hormonal agents for patients with a uterus include estrogen with progesterone to prevent endometrial cancer. If the patient doesn't have a uterus, progesterone isn't necessary.

The North American Menopause Society revised its guidelines for use of hormone replacement therapy (HRT) for menopausal vasomotor symptoms (VMS) in 2017. Treatment with HRT should be individualized based on personal health history and risks/benefits should both be weighed clinically. For female-bodied persons younger than 60 years who are within 10 years of menopause and do not have contraindications, HRT benefits may outweigh risks. HRT remains the most effective treatment for VMS.

Medications may be prescribed to help with mood swings, hot flashes, and other symptoms. These include low doses of antidepressants, such as paroxetine, venlafaxine, and fluoxetine, or clonidine, which is normally used to control high blood pressure.

Special considerations

◆ Provide the patient with all the facts about HRT, if used. Make sure she realizes the need for regular monitoring.

◆ Before HRT begins, have the patient undergo a baseline physical examination, Pap test, and mammogram.

◆ Advise the patient not to discontinue contraceptive measures until cessation of menstruation has been confirmed.

◆ Tell the patient to immediately report vaginal bleeding or spotting after menstruation has ceased.

◆ Discuss alternatives to HRT, which can help with the discomforting symptoms of menopause:

  ◆ Advise the patient to dress lightly and in layers.

  ◆ Tell the patient to avoid caffeine, alcohol, and spicy foods. Encourage soy-based foods.

  ◆ Instruct the patient to practice slow, deep breathing whenever a hot flash starts to come on, or to try other relaxation techniques, such as yoga, tai chi, or meditation. Advise them that acupuncture may also be helpful.

  ◆ If the patient is sexually active, encourage them to remain sexually active to preserve vaginal elasticity. Water-based lubricants can be used during sexual intercourse to decrease dryness.

  ◆ Instruct the patient that Kegel exercises may be performed daily to strengthen the vaginal and pelvic muscles.

FEMALE INFERTILITY

Causes and incidence

About 30% to 40% of all infertility is attributed to the male-bodied person, and 40% to 50% to the female-bodied person; about 10% to 30% is due to a combination of male-bodied and female-bodied factors. Following extensive investigation and treatment, about 50% of these infertile couples achieve pregnancy. Of the 50% who don't, 10% have no pathologic basis for infertility; the prognosis for this group becomes extremely poor if pregnancy isn't achieved within 3 years. The causes of female-bodied infertility may be functional, anatomic, or psychosocial:

◆ Functional causes: complex hormonal interactions determine the normal function of the female reproductive tract and require an intact hypothalamic–pituitary–ovarian axis—the system that stimulates and regulates the hormone production necessary for normal sexual development and function. Any defect or malfunction of this axis can cause infertility due to insufficient gonadotropin secretions (both LH and FSH). The ovary controls, and is controlled by, the hypothalamus through a system of negative and positive feedback mediated by estrogen production. Insufficient gonadotropin levels may result from infections, tumors, or neurologic disease of the hypothalamus or pituitary gland. Thyroid dysfunction/disease may also impair fertility.

Pathophysiology

Primary infertility is the inability to conceive after regular intercourse for at least 1 year without contraception. Secondary infertility occurs in those who have previously been pregnant at least once, but are unable to achieve another pregnancy.

Anatomic causes include the following:

◆ Ovarian factors are related to anovulation and oligo-ovulation (infrequent ovulation) and are a major cause of infertility. Pregnancy or direct visualization provides irrefutable evidence of ovulation. Presumptive signs of ovulation include regular menses, cyclic changes reflected in basal body temperature readings, postovulatory progesterone levels, and endometrial changes due to the presence of progesterone. Absence of presumptive signs suggests anovulation. Ovarian failure, in which no ova are produced by the ovaries, may result from ovarian dysgenesis or premature menopause. Amenorrhea is often associated with ovarian failure. Oligo-ovulation may be due to a mild hormonal imbalance in gonadotropin production and regulation and may be caused by PCOS or abnormalities in the adrenal or thyroid gland that adversely affect hypothalamic–pituitary functioning.

◆ Uterine fibroids or uterine abnormalities rarely cause infertility; however, uterine abnormalities may include congenitally absent uterus, bicornuate or double uterus, leiomyomas, or Asherman syndrome, in which the anterior and posterior uterine walls adhere because of scar tissue formation.

◆ Tubal and peritoneal factors are due to faulty tubal transport mechanisms and unfavorable environmental influences affecting the sperm, ova, or recently fertilized ovum. Tubal loss or impairment may occur secondary to ectopic pregnancy.

Frequently, tubal and peritoneal factors result from anatomic abnormalities: bilateral occlusion of the tubes due to salpingitis (resulting from gonorrhea, tuberculosis, or puerperal sepsis), peritubal adhesions (resulting from endometriosis, PID, diverticulosis, or childhood rupture of the appendix), and uterotubal obstruction (due to tubal spasm).

◆ Cervical factors may include malfunctioning cervix that produces deficient or excessively viscous mucus and is impervious to sperm, preventing entry into the uterus. In cervical infection, viscous mucus may contain spermicidal macrophages. Cervical antibodies have also been found to immobilize sperm.

◆ Psychosocial problems probably account for relatively few cases of infertility. Occasionally, ovulation may stop under stress due to failure of LH release. The frequency of intercourse may be related. More often, however, psychosocial problems result from, rather than cause, infertility.

About 10% to 20% of those attempting pregnancy will be unable to conceive after 1 year. Healthy people who are younger than age 30 and having intercourse regularly only have a 25% to 30% chance of getting pregnant each month. A female-bodied person's peak fertility is in their early twenties. As a female-bodied person ages beyond 35 (and particularly beyond 40), the likelihood of conception is less than 10% per month.

Complication
◆ Depression

Diagnosis
Inability to achieve pregnancy after having regular intercourse without contraception for at least 1 year suggests infertility. (In female-bodied persons older than age 35, many clinicians use 6 months rather than 1 year as a cutoff point.)

Diagnosis requires a complete physical examination and health history, including specific questions on the patient's reproductive and sexual function, past diseases, mental state, previous surgery, types of contraception used in the past, and family history. Irregular, painless menses may indicate anovulation. A history of PID may suggest fallopian tube blockage. Sometimes PID is silent, and no history may be known.

The following tests assess ovulation:
◆ Basal body temperature graph shows a sustained elevation in body temperature postovulation until just before the onset of menses, indicating the approximate time of ovulation.

◆ Endometrial biopsy, done on or about day 26, provides histologic evidence that ovulation has occurred. However, endometrial biopsy is retrospective, which diminishes its utility.

◆ Progesterone blood levels, measured when they should be highest, can show a luteal phase deficiency or presumptive evidence of ovulation.

The following procedures assess structural integrity of the fallopian tubes, the ovaries, and the uterus:
◆ Urinary LH kits, available without a prescription, can sensitively detect the LH surge about 24 hours preovulation, allowing coitus to be timed with ovulation.

◆ Hysterosalpingography provides radiologic evidence of tubal obstruction and uterine cavity abnormalities by injecting radiopaque contrast fluid through the cervix.

Male-bodied–female-bodied interaction studies include the following:
◆ Postcoital test (Sims–Huhner test) examines the cervical mucus for motile sperm cells following intercourse that takes place at midcycle (as close to ovulation as possible).

◆ Immunologic or antibody testing detects spermicidal antibodies in the female-bodied persons sera.

Treatment
Treatment depends on identifying the underlying abnormality or dysfunction within the hypothalamic–pituitary–ovarian axis. In hyperactivity or hypoactivity of the adrenal or thyroid gland, hormone therapy is necessary; progesterone deficiency requires progesterone replacement. Anovulation necessitates treatment with clomiphene, human menopausal gonadotropins, or hCG; ovulation usually occurs several days after such administration. If mucus production decreases (an adverse effect of clomiphene), small doses of estrogen to improve

the quality of cervical mucus may be given concomitantly; however, such intervention remains unproven.

Surgical restoration may correct certain anatomic causes of infertility such as fallopian tube obstruction. Surgery may also be necessary to remove tumors located within or near the hypothalamus or pituitary gland. Endometriosis requires drug therapy (danazol or medroxy-progesterone, GnRH analogues or noncyclic administration of hormonal contraceptives), surgical removal of areas of endometriosis, or a combination of both.

Other options, sometimes controversial and involving emotional and financial cost, include surrogate mothering, frozen embryos, or in vitro fertilization (IVF). In view of the good success rate of IVF (about 20%), IVF may be used instead of surgery in many cases.

Special considerations

Management includes providing the infertile persons with emotional support and information about diagnostic and treatment techniques. (See *Preventing infertility.*)

◆ Infertile persons may suffer loss of self-esteem; they may feel angry, guilty, or inadequate, and the diagnostic procedures for this disorder may intensify their fear and anxiety. You can help by explaining these procedures thoroughly. Above all, encourage the patient and their partner to talk about their feelings, and listen to what they have to say with a non-judgmental attitude.

◆ If the patient requires surgery, tell them what to expect postoperatively; this, of course, depends on which procedure is to be performed.

PELVIC INFLAMMATORY DISEASE
Causes and incidence

PID can result from infection with aerobic or anaerobic organisms. The organisms *Neisseria gonorrhoeae* and *Chlamydia trachomatis* are the most common cause because they most readily penetrate the bacteriostatic barrier of cervical mucus.

In the United States, nearly 1 million people develop PID each year; many cases go undiagnosed. About 1 in 8 active adolescents will develop PID before age 21.

Pathophysiology

PID is any acute, subacute, recurrent, or chronic infection of the oviducts and ovaries, with adjacent tissue involvement. It includes inflammation of the fallopian tubes (salpingitis) and ovaries (oophoritis), which can extend to the connective tissue lying between the broad ligaments (parametritis). Early diagnosis and treatment prevent damage to the reproductive system. Untreated PID may cause infertility and may lead to potentially fatal septicemia and shock.

Normally, cervical secretions have a protective and defensive function. Therefore, conditions or procedures that alter or destroy cervical mucus impair this bacteriostatic mechanism and allow bacteria present in the cervix

---

 PREVENTION
Preventing infertility

Several things can be done to help prevent infertility. Advise your patient about the following:

Sexually transmitted infections (STIs)
Gonorrhea and chlamydia are the two most common STI-related causes of infertility. These STIs can lead to ectopic pregnancy and scarring of the fallopian tubes. Practicing safe sex can help prevent STIs.

Endometriosis
The early detection and treatment of endometriosis can eliminate the scarring that leads to infertility.

Lifestyle changes
Advise your patient to get regular moderate exercise, not intense exercise, which can lead to amenorrhea. Advise them to maintain adequate weight. Being underweight or overweight can affect hormones. Advise them to avoid using alcohol and illegal drugs, and if they smoke, suggest that they quit; these substances may have an effect on fertility. Suggest that they discuss with their practitioner the use of prescription over-the-counter drugs and the possible effects they may have on fertility.

or vagina to ascend into the uterine cavity; such procedures include conization or cauterization of the cervix.

Uterine infection can also follow the transfer of contaminated cervical mucus into the endometrial cavity by instrumentation. Consequently, PID can follow insertion of an intrauterine device, use of a biopsy curet or an irrigation catheter, or tubal insufflation. Other predisposing factors include abortion, pelvic surgery, and infection during or after pregnancy.

Bacteria may also enter the uterine cavity through the bloodstream or from drainage from a chronically infected fallopian tube, a pelvic abscess, a ruptured appendix, diverticulitis of the sigmoid colon, or other infectious foci.

Common bacteria found in cervical mucus are staphylococci, streptococci, diphtheroids, chlamydiae, and coliforms, including *Pseudomonas* and *Escherichia coli*. Uterine infection can result from any one or several of these organisms or may follow the multiplication of normally nonpathogenic bacteria in an altered endometrial environment. Bacterial multiplication is most common during parturition because the endometrium is atrophic, quiescent, and not stimulated by estrogen.

Complications
◆ Infertility
◆ Pulmonary emboli
◆ Septicemia
◆ Shock

Signs and symptoms
Clinical features of PID vary with the affected area but generally include a profuse, purulent vaginal discharge, sometimes accompanied by low-grade fever and malaise (particularly if gonorrhea is the cause). The patient experiences lower abdomen pain; movement of the cervix or palpation of the adnexa may be extremely painful. Frequent, painful urination is also commonly reported. Additional signs and symptoms include irregular or absent menstruation, dyspareunia, low back pain, and nausea and vomiting.

Diagnosis
Diagnostic tests generally include:
◆ Gram stain of secretions from the endocervix or cul-de-sac. Culture and sensitivity testing aids selection of the appropriate antibiotic. Urethral and rectal secretions may also be cultured.
◆ White blood cell count may reveal leukocytosis.
◆ Pelvic ultrasonography or computed tomography scan to identify an adnexal or uterine mass.

In addition, patient history is significant. In general, PID is associated with recent sexual intercourse, insertion of an intrauterine device, childbirth, abortion, or a sexually transmitted infection.

Treatment
To prevent progression of PID, antibiotic therapy begins immediately after culture specimens are obtained. Such therapy can be re-evaluated as soon as laboratory results are available (usually after 24 to 48 hours). Infection may become chronic if treated inadequately.

Development of a pelvic abscess necessitates adequate drainage. A ruptured abscess is life threatening. If this complication develops, the patient may need a total abdominal hysterectomy with bilateral salpingo-oophorectomy. Alternatively, laparoscopic drainage with preservation of the ovaries and uterus may be done.

Concurrent treatment of sexual partners and condom use throughout the course of treatment are necessary.

Special considerations
◆ After establishing that the patient has no drug allergies, administer antibiotics and analgesics, as ordered.
◆ Check for fever. If it persists, carefully monitor fluid intake and output for signs of dehydration.
◆ Watch for abdominal rigidity and distention, possible signs of developing peritonitis. Provide frequent perineal care if vaginal drainage occurs.
◆ Stress the need for the patient's sexual partners to be examined and, if necessary, treated for infection.
◆ Because PID may cause painful intercourse, advise the patient to consult with their physician about sexual activity.

PREVENTION
◆ *To prevent a recurrence, explain the nature and seriousness of PID, and encourage the patient to comply with the treatment regimen.*
◆ *To prevent infection after minor gynecologic procedures such as dilatation and curettage, tell the patient to immediately report fever, increased vaginal discharge, or pain, and advise them to avoid douching and intercourse for at least 7 days.*

Uterine bleeding disorders

AMENORRHEA
Causes and incidence
Amenorrhea may result from the absence of a uterus, endometrial damage, or from ovarian, adrenal, or pituitary tumors. It's also linked to emotional disorders and is common in patients

with severe disorders, such as depression and anorexia nervosa. Mild emotional disturbances tend merely to distort the ovulatory cycle, although severe psychic trauma may abruptly change the bleeding pattern or may completely suppress one or more full ovulatory cycles. Amenorrhea may also result from malnutrition, obesity, intense exercise, and prolonged hormonal contraceptive use. The incidence of primary amenorrhea in the United States is less than 0.1%. The incidence of secondary amenorrhea (caused by something other than pregnancy) is about 4%.

Pathophysiology

Amenorrhea is the abnormal absence or suppression of menstruation. Primary amenorrhea is the absence of menarche in an adolescent (by age 18). Secondary amenorrhea is the failure of menstruation for at least 3 months after normal onset of menarche.

Amenorrhea is normal before puberty, after menopause, or during pregnancy and lactation; it's pathologic at any other time. It usually results from anovulation due to hormonal abnormalities, such as decreased secretion of estrogen, gonadotropins, LH, and FSH; lack of ovarian response to gonadotropins; or constant presence of progesterone or other endocrine abnormalities.

Diagnosis

CONFIRMING DIAGNOSIS *A history of failure to menstruate in a female-bodied person older than age 18 confirms primary amenorrhea.*

Secondary amenorrhea can be diagnosed when a change is noted in a previously established menstrual pattern (absence of menstruation for 3 months). A thorough physical and pelvic examination rules out pregnancy, as well as anatomic abnormalities such as cervical stenosis that may cause false amenorrhea (cryptomenorrhea), in which menstruation occurs without external bleeding.

Onset of menstruation within 1 week after administration of pure progestational agents, such as medroxyprogesterone and progesterone, indicates a functioning uterus. If menstruation doesn't occur, special diagnostic studies are appropriate.

Blood and urine studies may reveal hormonal imbalances, such as lack of ovarian response to gonadotropins (elevated pituitary gonadotropins), failure of gonadotropin secretion (low pituitary gonadotropin levels), and abnormal thyroid levels. Tests for identification of dominant or missing hormones include cervical mucus ferning, vaginal cytologic

examinations, basal body temperature, endometrial biopsy (during dilatation and curettage), urinary 17-ketosteroids, and plasma progesterone, testosterone, and androgen levels. A complete medical workup, including X-rays, laparoscopy, and a biopsy, may detect ovarian, adrenal, and pituitary tumors. (See *Diagnosing amenorrhea*, page 1040.)

Treatment

Appropriate hormone replacement re-establishes menstruation. Treatment of amenorrhea not related to hormone deficiency depends on the cause. For example, amenorrhea that results from a tumor usually requires surgery.

Special considerations

◆ Explain all diagnostic procedures.
◆ Provide reassurance and emotional support. Psychiatric counseling may be necessary if amenorrhea results from emotional disturbances.
◆ After treatment, teach the patient how to keep an accurate record of their menstrual cycles to aid early detection of recurrent amenorrhea.

ABNORMAL PREMENOPAUSAL BLEEDING

Causes and incidence

Causes of abnormal premenopausal bleeding vary with the type of bleeding:
◆ Oligomenorrhea and polymenorrhea usually result from anovulation due to an endocrine or systemic disorder.
◆ Menorrhagia usually results from local lesions, such as uterine leiomyomas, endometrial polyps, and endometrial hyperplasia. It may also result from endometritis, salpingitis, and anovulation.
◆ Hypomenorrhea results from local, endocrine, or systemic disorders, or from blockage due to partial obstruction by the hymen or to cervical obstruction.
◆ Cryptomenorrhea may result from an imperforate hymen or cervical stenosis.
◆ Metrorrhagia usually results from slight physiologic bleeding from the endometrium during ovulation but may also result from local disorders, such as uterine malignancy, cervical erosions, polyps (which tend to bleed after intercourse), or inappropriate estrogen therapy. Complications of pregnancy can also cause premenopausal bleeding. Such bleeding may be as mild as spotting or as severe as menorrhagia. (See *Causes of abnormal premenopausal bleeding*, page 1041.)

Diagnosing amenorrhea

The flowchart lists possible diagnostic findings and interpretations to assist with the treatment of the patient with amenorrhea.

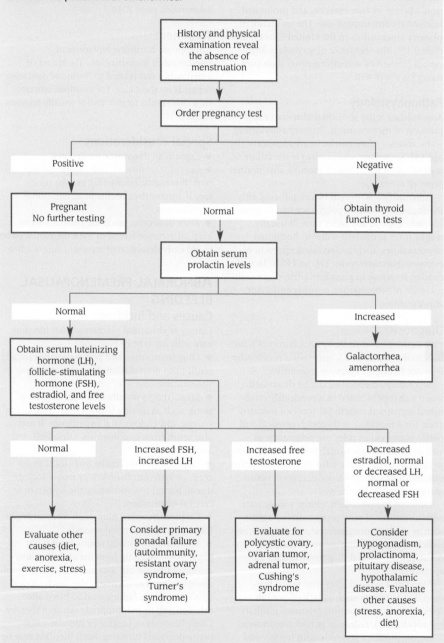

Pathophysiology

Abnormal premenopausal bleeding refers to any bleeding that deviates from the normal menstrual cycle before menopause. These deviations include menstrual bleeding that's abnormally infrequent (oligomenorrhea), abnormally frequent (polymenorrhea), excessive (menorrhagia or hypermenorrhea), deficient (hypomenorrhea), or irregular (metrorrhagia [uterine bleeding between menses]). Rarely, menstrual symptoms aren't accompanied by external bleeding (cryptomenorrhea). Premenopausal bleeding may merely be troublesome or can result in severe hemorrhage; the prognosis depends on the underlying cause. Abnormal bleeding patterns often respond to hormonal or other therapy.

Signs and symptoms

Bleeding not associated with abnormal pregnancy is usually painless, but it may be severely painful. When bleeding is associated with abnormal pregnancy, other symptoms include nausea, breast tenderness, bloating, and fluid retention. Severe or prolonged bleeding causes anemia, especially in patients with underlying disease such as blood dyscrasia and in patients receiving anticoagulants.

Diagnosis

The typical clinical picture confirms abnormal premenopausal bleeding. Special tests identify the underlying cause:
◆ Serum hormone levels reflect adrenal, pituitary, or thyroid dysfunction.
◆ Urinary 17-ketosteroids reveal adrenal hyperplasia, hypopituitarism, or PCOS.
◆ Endometrial sampling rules out malignant tumors and should be performed in all patients with premenopausal bleeding who are older than age 35.
◆ Pelvic examination, Pap test, and patient history rule out local or malignant causes.
◆ Complete blood count rules out anemia.
   If testing rules out pelvic and hormonal causes of abnormal bleeding, a complete hematologic survey (including platelet count and bleeding time) is appropriate to determine clotting abnormalities.

Treatment

Treatment depends on the type of bleeding abnormality and its cause. Menstrual irregularity alone may not require therapy unless it interferes with the patient's attempt to achieve or avoid conception or leads to anemia. When it requires treatment, clomiphene induces ovulation. Electrocautery, chemical cautery, or cryosurgery can remove cervical polyps; dilatation and curettage, uterine polyps. Organic disorders (such as cervical or uterine malignancy) may necessitate hysterectomy, radium or X-ray therapy, or both of these treatments, depending on the disease's site and extent. Anemia and infections require appropriate treatment.

Special considerations

◆ If the patient complains of abnormal bleeding, tell them to record the dates of the bleeding and the number of tampons and/or pads used per day and/or frequency of emptying menstrual cups and level of fill of cups. This helps to assess the cyclic pattern and the amount of bleeding.
◆ Instruct the patient to report abnormal bleeding immediately to help rule out major hemorrhagic disorders.
◆ Offer reassurance and support. The patient may be particularly anxious about excessive or frequent blood loss and passage of clots.

Causes of abnormal premenopausal bleeding

Premenopausal bleeding can take several forms and may be due to a number of causes.

	Hypomenorrhea	Oligomenorrhea	Metrorrhagia	Polymenorrhea	Menorrhagia
Malnutrition	◆	◆			
Hyperthyroidism	◆	◆			
Hypothyroidism				◆	◆
Severe psychic trauma	◆	◆			◆
Blood dyscrasias			◆	◆	◆
Severe infections	◆	◆			
Endometritis			◆		
Drugs (such as cardiac glycosides, corticosteroids, anticoagulants)			◆		
Uterine tumors			◆		◆

Suggest that they minimize blood flow by avoiding strenuous activity and occasionally lying down with their feet elevated.

◆ NSAIDs, such as ibuprofen, may also reduce amount of bleeding.

⫶⫶⫶⫶ PREVENTION *To prevent abnormal bleeding due to organic causes, and for early detection of malignancy, encourage the patient to have a Pap smear and a pelvic examination at least every 3 years, or more frequently if needed.*

DYSFUNCTIONAL UTERINE BLEEDING

Causes and incidence

In most cases of dysfunctional uterine bleeding (DUB), the endometrium shows no pathologic changes. However, in chronic unopposed estrogen stimulation (as from a hormone-producing ovarian tumor), the endometrium may show hyperplastic or malignant changes. DUB occurs in 20% of adolescents and in 40% of female-bodied persons older than age 40.

Pathophysiology

DUB refers to abnormal endometrial bleeding without recognizable organic lesions. The prognosis varies with the cause. DUB is the indication for almost 25% of gynecologic surgical procedures and for nearly half of all hysterectomies in the United States.

DUB usually results from an imbalance in the hormonal–endometrial relationship, where persistent and unopposed stimulation of the endometrium by estrogen occurs. Disorders that cause sustained high estrogen levels are PCOS, obesity, immaturity of the hypothalamic–pituitary–ovarian axis (in postpubertal teenagers), and anovulation (in female-bodied persons in their late thirties or early forties).

Complications

◆ Anemia
◆ Infertility

Signs and symptoms

DUB usually occurs as metrorrhagia (episodes of vaginal bleeding between menses); it may also occur as hypermenorrhea (heavy or prolonged menses, longer than 8 days) or chronic polymenorrhea (menstrual cycle of <18 days). Such bleeding is unpredictable and can cause anemia.

Diagnosis

Diagnostic studies must rule out other causes of excessive vaginal bleeding, such as organic, systemic, psychogenic, and endocrine causes, including certain cancers, polyps, incomplete abortion, pregnancy, and infection.

℞ CONFIRMING DIAGNOSIS *Dilatation and curettage (D&C) and biopsy results confirm the diagnosis by revealing endometrial hyperplasia.*

Hemoglobin levels and hematocrit determine the need for blood or iron replacement. Coagulation factors indicate coagulopathies. hCG is measured to determine if an ectopic pregnancy or a threatened or incomplete abortion is occurring. Thyroid function tests are done to check for hyperthyroidism, which can indicate an ovulation dysfunction. Pelvic ultrasound is done to check the endometrium for fibroids.

Treatment

High-dose estrogen–progestogen combination therapy (hormonal contraceptives), the primary treatment, is designed to control endometrial growth and re-establish a normal cyclic pattern of menstruation. (The patient's age and the cause of bleeding help determine the drug choice and dosage.) In patients older than age 35, endometrial biopsy is necessary before the start of estrogen therapy to rule out endometrial adenocarcinoma. Progestogen therapy is a necessary alternative in some female-bodied persons, such as those susceptible to estrogen's adverse effects (e.g., thrombophlebitis).

If drug therapy is ineffective, D&C serves as a supplementary treatment, through removal of a large portion of the bleeding endometrium. Also, D&C can help determine the original cause of hormonal imbalance and can aid in planning further therapy. Endometrial ablation may also be used as treatment if fertility is no longer desired. Regardless of the primary treatment, the patient may need iron replacement or transfusions of packed cells or whole blood, as indicated, because of anemia caused by recurrent bleeding.

Special considerations

◆ Explain the importance of adhering to the prescribed hormonal therapy. If D&C or ablation are ordered, explain the procedure and its purpose.

◆ Stress the need for regular checkups to assess the effectiveness of treatment.

POSTMENOPAUSAL BLEEDING

Causes and incidence

Postmenopausal bleeding may result from:

◆ exogenous estrogen, when administration is excessive or prolonged or when small amounts are given in the presence of a hypersensitive endometrium

◆ endogenous estrogen production, especially when levels are high, as in persons with estrogen-producing ovarian tumor; however, in some persons, even a slight fluctuation in estrogen levels may cause bleeding

◆ atrophic endometrium due to low estrogen levels

◆ atrophic vaginitis, usually triggered by trauma during coitus in the absence of estrogen production

◆ aging, which increases vascular vulnerability by thinning epithelial surfaces, increasing vascular fragility, producing degenerative tissue changes, and decreasing resistance to infections

◆ cervical or endometrial cancer (more common after age 60)

◆ adenomatous hyperplasia or atypical adenomatous hyperplasia (usually considered a premalignant lesion)

Pathophysiology

Postmenopausal bleeding is defined as bleeding from the reproductive tract that occurs 1 year or more after cessation of menses. Sites of bleeding include the vulva, vagina, cervix, and endometrium. The prognosis varies with the cause.

Complications

◆ Mood disorder; anxiety, depression
◆ Anemia
◆ Hemorrhage
◆ Infection
◆ Dyspareunia

Signs and symptoms

Vaginal bleeding, the primary symptom, ranges from spotting to outright hemorrhage; its duration also varies. Other symptoms depend on the cause. Excessive estrogen stimulation, for example, may also produce copious cervical mucus; estrogen deficiency may cause vaginal mucosa to atrophy.

Diagnosis

Diagnostic evaluation of the patient with postmenopausal bleeding should include physical examination (especially pelvic examination), a detailed history, standard laboratory tests (such as complete blood count), and cytologic examination of smears from the cervix and the endocervical canal. An endometrial biopsy or D&C with hysteroscopy reveals pathologic findings in the endometrium.

Diagnosis must rule out underlying degenerative or systemic disease. For instance, evidence of elevated levels of endogenous estrogen may suggest an ovarian tumor. Before testing for estrogen levels, the patient must stop all sources of exogenous estrogen intake—including face and body creams that contain estrogen—to rule out excessive exogenous estrogen as a cause.

Treatment

Emergency treatment to control massive hemorrhage is rarely necessary, except in advanced cancer. Treatment may include D&C to relieve bleeding. Other therapy varies according to the underlying cause. Estrogen creams and suppositories are usually effective in correcting estrogen deficiency because they're rapidly absorbed. Hysterectomy is indicated for repeated episodes of postmenopausal bleeding from the endometrial cavity. Such bleeding may indicate endometrial cancer.

Special considerations

Obtain a detailed patient history to rule out excessive exogenous estrogen as a cause of bleeding. Ask the patient about use of cosmetics (especially face and body creams), drugs, and other products that may contain estrogen. Discuss the risks and benefits of estrogen replacement therapy with them.

◆ Provide emotional support. The patient will probably be afraid that the bleeding indicates cancer.

▦▦▦ PREVENTION *To prevent disorders that cause postmenopausal bleeding, stress that periodic gynecologic examinations are as important after menopause as they were before.*

Disorders of pregnancy

ABORTION

Causes and incidence

Abortion is the spontaneous or induced (therapeutic) expulsion of the products of conception from the uterus. Up to 15% of all pregnancies and about 30% of first pregnancies end in spontaneous abortion (miscarriage). At least 75% of miscarriages occur during the first trimester. (See *Types of spontaneous abortion,* page 1044.)

Pathophysiology

Spontaneous abortion may result from fetal, placental, or maternal factors. Fetal factors, which usually cause such abortions up to 12 weeks' gestation, include the following:

◆ defective embryologic development resulting from abnormal chromosome division (most common cause of fetal death)

◆ faulty implantation of the fertilized ovum

◆ failure of the endometrium to accept the fertilized ovum.

Placental factors usually cause abortion around the 14th week of gestation, when the placenta takes over the hormone production necessary to maintain the pregnancy. These factors include:

Types of spontaneous abortion

♦ *Threatened abortion:* Bloody vaginal discharge occurs during the first half of pregnancy. Approximately 20% of pregnant female-bodied persons have vaginal spotting or actual bleeding early in pregnancy; of these, about 50% abort.

♦ *Inevitable abortion:* Membranes rupture and the cervix dilates. As labor continues, the uterus expels the products of conception.

♦ *Incomplete abortion:* The uterus retains part or all of the placenta. Before the 10th week of gestation, the fetus and placenta usually are expelled together; after the 10th week, separately. Because part of the placenta may adhere to the uterine wall, bleeding continues. Hemorrhage is possible because the uterus doesn't contract and seal the large vessels that fed the placenta.

♦ *Complete abortion:* The uterus passes all the products of conception. Minimal bleeding usually accompanies complete abortion because the uterus contracts and compresses maternal blood vessels that feed the placenta.

♦ *Missed abortion:* The uterus retains the products of conception for 2 months or more after the fetus' death. Uterine growth ceases; uterine size may even seem to decrease. Prolonged retention of the dead products of conception may cause coagulation defects, such as disseminated intravascular coagulation, usually after at least 1 month in utero.

♦ *Habitual abortion:* Spontaneous loss of three or more consecutive pregnancies constitutes habitual abortion.

♦ *Septic abortion:* Infection accompanies abortion. This may occur with spontaneous abortion but usually results from an illegal abortion.

♦ premature separation of the normally implanted placenta
♦ abnormal placental implantation
Maternal factors usually cause abortion between the 11th and 19th week of gestation and include:
♦ maternal infection, abnormalities of the reproductive organs (especially an incompetent cervix, in which the cervix dilates painlessly in the second trimester)
♦ endocrine problems, such as thyroid dysfunction or a luteal phase defect

♦ trauma
♦ phospholipid antibody disorder
♦ blood group incompatibility
♦ drug ingestion (particularly uterotonic agents)

The goal of therapeutic abortion is to preserve the pregnant person's mental or physical health in cases of rape, unplanned pregnancy, or medical conditions such as moderate or severe cardiac dysfunction.

Complications
♦ Anemia
♦ Disseminated intravascular coagulation
♦ Hemorrhage
♦ Infection

Signs and symptoms
Prodromal signs of spontaneous abortion may include a pink discharge for several days or a scant brown discharge for several weeks before the onset of cramps and increased vaginal bleeding. For a few hours, the cramps intensify and occur more frequently; then the cervix dilates to expel uterine contents. If the entire contents are expelled, cramps and bleeding subside. However, if any contents remain, cramps and bleeding continue.

Diagnosis
Diagnosis of spontaneous abortion is based on clinical evidence of expulsion of uterine contents, pelvic examination, and laboratory studies. hCG in the blood or urine confirms pregnancy; decreased hCG levels suggest spontaneous abortion or tubal pregnancy. Pelvic examination determines the uterus' size and whether this size is consistent with the pregnancy's duration. Tissue histology indicates evidence of products of conception. Laboratory tests reflect decreased hemoglobin levels and hematocrit due to blood loss. However, blood loss is rarely excessive in spontaneous abortion. It's critical that ectopic pregnancy be ruled out in a pregnant person with vaginal bleeding.

Treatment
An accurate evaluation of uterine contents is needed before a plan of treatment can be formulated. The progression of spontaneous abortion can't be prevented, except possibly in cases caused by an incompetent cervix. The patient must be hospitalized to control severe hemorrhage. If bleeding is severe, a transfusion with packed red blood cells (RBCs) or whole blood is required. Initially, I.V. administration of oxytocin stimulates uterine contractions (if given after 20 weeks' gestation—receptors are

absent before this gestational age). If any remnants remain in the uterus, D&C or dilatation and evacuation (D&E) should be performed.

D&E is also performed in first- and second-trimester therapeutic abortions. In second-trimester therapeutic abortions, the insertion of a prostaglandin vaginal suppository induces labor and the expulsion of uterine contents. When performed competently, second-trimester D&E is a very safe procedure and allows for termination of pregnancy without the need for a lengthy induction of labor. Early first-trimester abortion may also be accomplished pharmacologically with mifepristone (RU-486) an antiprogestin, followed by a dose of a prostaglandin analogue 2 days later, or surgically, using vacuum aspiration.

After an abortion, spontaneous or induced, an Rh-negative female-bodied person with a negative indirect Coombs' test should receive $Rh_o(D)$ immune globulin (human) to prevent future Rh isoimmunization.

In a habitual abortion, spontaneous abortion can result from an incompetent cervix (a clinical retrospective diagnosis suggested by a history of previous second-trimester losses accompanied by membrane rupture or painless cervical dilation). Treatment involves surgical reinforcement of the cervix (cerclage) 12 to 24 weeks after the last menstrual period. A few weeks before the estimated delivery date, the sutures are removed, and the patient awaits the onset of labor. An alternative procedure is to leave the sutures in place and to deliver the infant by cesarean birth. Cerclage hasn't been shown to be more effective than bed rest.

Special considerations

Elective abortion is a controversial issue. The decision to have an elective abortion is a personal decision that requires competent counseling. Many female-bodied persons believe they can't share their feelings with others; therefore, it's important for a female-bodied person contemplating an abortion to examine their existing support system and identify those people capable of helping them through a difficult time. A reputable provider or clinic where the female-bodied person can obtain adequate counseling regarding all options for pregnancy resolution, have the procedure performed, and obtain support and follow-up care should be identified during the decision-making process.

Before possible abortion:
◆ Be sure to inform the patient who desires an elective abortion of all the available alternatives. They need to know what the procedure involves, what the risks are, and what to expect

during and after the procedure, both emotionally and physically. Be sure to ascertain whether the patient is comfortable with their decision to have an elective abortion.
◆ The patient experiencing a spontaneous abortion *should be informed that* they may expel uterine contents without knowing it. Recommend use of a bedpan or toilet "hat" if at home have them or someone they trust inspect the contents carefully for intrauterine material.

After spontaneous or elective abortion:
◆ Note the amount, color, and odor of vaginal bleeding. If in hospital/clinic save all the pads the patient uses, for evaluation. If patient is at home have them inspect pads clearly, educate them on what to look for and when to call.
◆ Administer or prescribe analgesics and oxytocin, as needed.
◆ Educate on good perineal care.
◆ Obtain vital signs as indicated.
◆ Monitor urine output.

Care of the patient who has had a spontaneous abortion includes emotional support and counseling during the grieving process. Stress to the patient that they aren't responsible for a spontaneous abortion, as this generally can't be prevented. Encourage the patient and any family/partner to express their feelings. Some people may want to talk to a clergy member or, depending on their religion, may wish to have the fetus baptized.

The patient who has had a therapeutic abortion also benefits from support. Encourage them to verbalize their feelings. Remember, they may feel ambivalent about the procedure; intellectual and emotional acceptance of abortion aren't the same. If you identify an inappropriate coping response, refer the patient for professional counseling.

To prepare the patient for discharge:
◆ Tell the patient to expect vaginal bleeding or spotting and to report bleeding that lasts longer than 8 to 10 days or excessive, bright-red blood immediately.
◆ Advise the patient to watch for signs of infection, such as a temperature higher than $100.5°$ F ($38°$ C) and foul-smelling vaginal discharge.
◆ Encourage the gradual increase of daily activities to include whatever tasks the patient feels comfortable doing, as long as these activities don't increase vaginal bleeding or cause fatigue. Most patients return to work after 24 hours.
◆ Urge 1 to 2 weeks' abstinence from intercourse, and encourage the use of a contraceptive.
◆ Instruct the patient to avoid using tampons for 1 to 2 weeks.

◆ Tell the patient to see their provider in 2 to 4 weeks for a follow-up examination.

⁞⁞⁞⁞⁞ PREVENTION

◆ *Contraceptive counseling should meet the individual needs of the patient. Ask about access to contraception, finances, etc. Help patient to access contraception if desired.*

◆ *To minimize the risk of future spontaneous abortions, emphasize to the pregnant person the importance of good nutrition and the need to avoid alcohol, cigarettes, and drugs. If the patient has a history of habitual spontaneous abortions, suggest that they and their partner have thorough examinations. For the female-bodied person, this includes premenstrual endometrial biopsy, a hormone assessment (estrogen; progesterone; and thyroid, FSH, and LH), and hysterosalpingography and laparoscopy to detect anatomic abnormalities. Genetic counseling may also be advised.*

ECTOPIC PREGNANCY

Causes and incidence

Ectopic pregnancy may result from congenital defects in the reproductive tract or ectopic endometrial implants in the tubal mucosa. The increased prevalence of sexually transmitted tubal infection may also be a factor. Other risk factors include intrauterine device use, multiple previous elective abortions, smoking, and advanced age. It occurs in 1 in 40 to 100 pregnancies.

Pathophysiology

Ectopic pregnancy is the implantation of the fertilized ovum outside the uterine cavity. The most common site is the fallopian tube (>95% of ectopic implantations occur in the fimbria, ampulla, or isthmus), but other possible sites include the interstitium, tubo-ovarian ligament, ovary, abdominal viscera, and internal cervical os. (See *Implantation sites of ectopic pregnancy*.) The prognosis is good with prompt diagnosis, appropriate surgical intervention, and control of bleeding; rarely, in cases of abdominal implantation, the fetus may survive to term. Usually, a subsequent intrauterine pregnancy is achieved.

Conditions that prevent or retard the fertilized ovum's passage through the fallopian tube and into the uterine cavity include:

◆ diverticula, the formation of blind pouches that cause tubal abnormalities

◆ endometriosis, the presence of endometrial tissue outside the lining of the uterine cavity

◆ endosalpingitis, an inflammatory reaction that causes folds of the tubal mucosa to agglutinate, narrowing the tube

Implantation sites of ectopic pregnancy

In 90% of patients with ectopic pregnancy, the ovum implants in the fallopian tube, either in the fimbria, ampulla, or isthmus. Other possible sites include the interstitium, tubo-ovarian ligament, ovary, abdominal viscera, and internal cervical os.

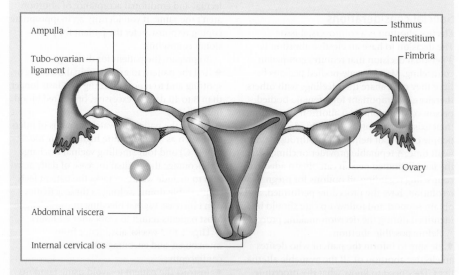

◆ PID, an infection of the oviducts and ovaries with adjacent tissue involvement
◆ previous surgery (tubal ligation or resection, or adhesions from previous abdominal or pelvic surgery)
◆ tumors pressing against the tube

Complications
◆ Hemorrhage
◆ Infertility
◆ Peritonitis
◆ Shock

Signs and symptoms
Ectopic pregnancy sometimes produces symptoms of normal pregnancy or no symptoms other than mild abdominal pain, making diagnosis difficult. Characteristic clinical effects after fallopian tube implantation include amenorrhea or abnormal menses, followed by slight vaginal bleeding, and unilateral pelvic pain over the mass. Rupture of the tube causes life—threatening complications, including hemorrhage, shock, and peritonitis. The patient experiences sharp lower abdominal pain, possibly radiating to the shoulders and neck, often precipitated by activities that increase abdominal pressure, such as a bowel movement; they feel extreme pain on motion of the cervix and palpation of the adnexa during a pelvic examination.

Diagnosis
Clinical features, patient history, and the results of a pelvic examination suggest ectopic pregnancy. The following tests help confirm it:
◆ Serum pregnancy test shows presence of hCG.
◆ Real-time ultrasonography determines extrauterine pregnancy (performed if serum pregnancy test is positive). Magnetic resonance imaging is a useful adjunct to ultrasound if an unusual ectopic location is suspected.
◆ In culdocentesis, fluid is aspirated from the pouch of Douglas through the posterior vaginal fornix to detect free or nonclotting blood in the peritoneum (sometimes performed if ultrasonography fails to detect a gestational sac in the uterus).
◆ Laparoscopy or laparotomy is used to diagnose as well as to treat an ectopic pregnancy by either removal of the tube (salpingectomy) or removal of the pregnancy with preservation of the tube (salpingostomy).

Decreased hemoglobin levels and hematocrit due to blood loss support the diagnosis. Differential diagnosis must rule out uterine abortion, appendicitis, ruptured corpus luteum cyst, salpingitis, and torsion of the ovary.

Treatment
If culdocentesis is positive or the patient has peritoneal signs consistent with a surgical abdomen, laparoscopy and laparotomy are indicated. The ovary is preserved as a rule; however, ovarian pregnancy may necessitate oophorectomy. Interstitial pregnancy may rarely require hysterectomy; abdominal pregnancy requires a laparotomy to remove the fetus, except in rare cases, when the fetus survives to term or calcifies undetected in the abdominal cavity.

Supportive treatment includes transfusion with whole blood or packed red cells to replace excessive blood loss, administration of broad-spectrum antibiotics I.V. for septic infection, and administration of supplemental iron by mouth or I.M.

Methotrexate I.M. is also a therapeutic option in stable patients, avoiding surgery in most cases.

Special considerations
Patient care measures include careful monitoring and assessment of vital signs and vaginal bleeding, preparing the patient with excessive blood loss for emergency surgery, and providing blood replacement and emotional support and reassurance.
◆ Record the pain's location and character, and administer analgesics as ordered. (Remember, however, that analgesics may mask the symptoms of intraperitoneal rupture of the ectopic pregnancy.)
◆ Check the amount, color, and odor of vaginal bleeding. Ask the patient the date of their last menstrual period and to describe this period's character.
◆ Observe for signs of pregnancy (enlarged breasts, soft cervix).
◆ Provide a quiet, relaxing environment, and encourage the patient to freely express their feelings of fear, loss, and grief.

::::::: **PREVENTION**
◆ *To prevent diseases of the fallopian tube, advise prompt treatment of pelvic infections. Tell patients who have undergone surgery involving the fallopian tubes or those with confirmed PID that they're at increased risk for ectopic pregnancy.*
◆ *Advise the patient who's vulnerable to ectopic pregnancy to delay using an intrauterine device until they decide not to have more children.*

HYPEREMESIS GRAVIDARUM
Causes and incidence
Unlike the transient nausea and vomiting normally experienced between the 6th and 12th weeks of pregnancy, hyperemesis gravidarum

is severe and unremitting nausea and vomiting that persists after the first trimester. If untreated, it produces substantial weight loss; starvation; dehydration, with subsequent fluid and electrolyte imbalance (hypokalemia); and acid–base disturbances (acidosis and alkalosis). This syndrome occurs in about 1 in 200 pregnancies. The prognosis is good with appropriate treatment. The incidence increases in molar and multiple pregnancies.

Pathophysiology

Although its cause is unknown, hyperemesis gravidarum often affects pregnant people with conditions that produce high levels of hCG, such as hydatidiform mole or multiple pregnancies. Its other possible causes include pancreatitis (elevated serum amylase levels are common), biliary tract disease, drug toxicity, inflammatory obstructive bowel disease, and vitamin deficiency (especially of B_6). In some patients, it may be related to psychological factors such as ambivalence toward pregnancy.

Complications

◆ Acid–base disturbances
◆ Dehydration
◆ Hypokalemia
◆ Weight loss

Signs and symptoms

The cardinal symptoms of hyperemesis gravidarum are unremitting nausea and vomiting. The vomitus initially contains undigested food and mucus as well as small amounts of bile; later, only bile and mucus; and finally, blood and material that resembles coffee grounds. Persistent vomiting causes substantial weight loss and eventual emaciation. Associated effects may include pale, dry, waxy, and possibly jaundiced skin; subnormal or elevated temperature; rapid pulse; a fetid, fruity breath odor from acidosis; and CNS symptoms, such as confusion, delirium, headache, lassitude, stupor and, possibly, coma.

Diagnosis

Diagnosis depends on a history of uncontrolled nausea and vomiting that persists beyond the first trimester, evidence of substantial weight loss, and other characteristic clinical features. Serum analysis shows decreased protein, chloride, sodium, and potassium levels, and increased blood urea nitrogen levels. Other laboratory tests reveal ketonuria, slight proteinuria, and elevated hemoglobin and white blood cell levels. Diagnosis must rule out other conditions with similar clinical effects.

Treatment

Hyperemesis gravidarum may necessitate hospitalization to correct electrolyte imbalance and prevent starvation. I.V. infusions maintain nutrition until the patient can tolerate oral feedings. They progress slowly to a clear liquid diet, then a full liquid diet and, finally, small, frequent meals of high-protein solid foods. A midnight snack helps stabilize blood glucose levels; vitamin B supplements help correct vitamin deficiency.

When vomiting stops and electrolyte balance has been restored, the pregnancy usually continues without recurrence of hyperemesis gravidarum. Most patients feel better as they begin to regain normal weight, but some continue to vomit throughout the pregnancy, requiring extended treatment. If appropriate, some patients may benefit from consultations with clinical nurse specialists, psychologists, or psychiatrists.

Special considerations

◆ Encourage the patient to eat. Suggest dry foods and decreased liquid intake during meals.
◆ Instruct the patient to remain upright for 45 minutes after eating to decrease reflux.
◆ Provide reassurance and a calm, restful atmosphere. Encourage the patient to discuss their feelings regarding their pregnancy.
◆ Before discharge, provide good nutritional counseling.

GESTATIONAL HYPERTENSION
Causes and incidence

The cause of gestational hypertension isn't known, but geographic, ethnic, racial, nutritional, immunologic, and familial factors and pre-existing vascular disease may contribute to its development. Age is also a factor. Primiparas who are older than age 35 are at higher risk for preeclampsia.

Preeclampsia develops in about 7% of pregnancies. Incidence is significantly higher in low socioeconomic groups. About 5% of females with preeclampsia develop eclampsia; of these, about 15% die from eclampsia or its complications. Fetal mortality is high because of the increased incidence of premature delivery and uteroplacental insufficiency.

Pathophysiology

Gestational hypertension, also known as *pregnancy-induced hypertension*, is a potentially life-threatening disorder that usually develops late in the second trimester or in the third trimester. *Preeclampsia*, the nonconvulsive form of gestational hypertension, may be mild or severe. *Eclampsia* is the convulsive form of gestational hypertension.

Complications

◆ Abruptio placentae
◆ Intrauterine growth retardation
◆ Placental infarcts

Signs and symptoms

Mild preeclampsia generally produces the following clinical effects: hypertension, proteinuria (<5 g/24 hours), generalized edema, and sudden weight gain of more than 3 lb (1.4 kg) per week during the second trimester or more than 1 lb (0.5 kg) a week during the third trimester.

Severe preeclampsia is marked by increased hypertension and proteinuria, eventually leading to the development of oliguria. The HELLP syndrome—hemolysis, elevated liver enzymes, and low platelets—is a severe variant. Other symptoms that may indicate worsening preeclampsia include blurred vision due to retinal arteriolar spasms, epigastric pain or heartburn, and severe frontal headache.

In eclampsia, all the clinical manifestations of preeclampsia are magnified and are associated with seizures and, possibly, coma, premature labor, stillbirth, renal failure, and hepatic damage.

Diagnosis

The following findings suggest preeclampsia:
◆ elevated blood pressure readings—140 mm Hg systolic, measured on two occasions, 6 hours apart; 90 mm Hg diastolic, measured on two occasions, 6 hours apart
◆ proteinuria—at least 300 mg/24 hours
◆ elevated liver enzyme and uric acid levels

The following findings suggest severe preeclampsia:
◆ elevated blood pressure readings—160/110 mm Hg or higher on two occasions, 6 hours apart, on bed rest
◆ increased proteinuria—5 g/24 hours or more
◆ presence of pulmonary edema
◆ ultrasound—may reveal oligohydramnios
◆ oliguria—urine output less than or equal to 400 mL/24 hours
◆ elevated liver enzyme and uric acid levels
◆ decreased platelet levels

Seizures strongly suggest eclampsia. Rarely, ophthalmoscopic examination may reveal vascular spasm, papilledema, retinal edema or detachment, and arteriovenous nicking or hemorrhage.

Real-time ultrasonography, stress and non-stress tests, and biophysical profiles evaluate fetal status. In the stress test, oxytocin stimulates contractions; fetal heart tones are then monitored electronically. In the nonstress test,

fetal heart tones are monitored electronically during periods of fetal activity, without oxytocin stimulation. Electronic monitoring reveals stable or increased fetal heart tones during periods of fetal activity.

Ultrasonography aids evaluation of fetal health by assessing fetal breathing movements, gross body movements, fetal tone, reactive fetal heart rate, and qualitative amniotic fluid volume.

Treatment

Therapy for preeclampsia is designed to halt the disorder's progress—specifically, the early effects of eclampsia, such as seizures, residual hypertension, and renal shutdown—and to ensure fetal survival. Some physicians advocate the prompt induction of labor, especially if the patient is near term; others follow a more conservative approach. Therapy may include complete bed rest to increase placental perfusion, reduce hypertension, and evaluate response to therapy. Antihypertensive therapy doesn't alter the potential for developing eclampsia. Diuretics aren't appropriate during pregnancy.

If the patient's blood pressure fails to respond to bed rest and sedation and persistently rises above 160/100 mm Hg, or if CNS irritability increases, magnesium sulfate may produce general sedation, promote diuresis, and prevent seizures. Cesarean birth or oxytocin induction may be required to terminate the pregnancy.

⚠ **ALERT** *Emergency treatment of eclamptic seizures consists of immediate administration of magnesium sulfate (I.V. drip), oxygen administration, and electronic fetal monitoring.*

After the seizures subside and the patient's condition stabilizes, delivery should proceed with induction of labor or cesarean birth, depending on the circumstances.

Adequate nutrition, good prenatal care, and control of pre-existing hypertension during pregnancy decrease the incidence and severity of preeclampsia. Early recognition and prompt treatment of preeclampsia can prevent progression to eclampsia.

Special considerations

◆ Monitor regularly for changes in blood pressure, pulse rate, respiration, fetal heart tones, vision, level of consciousness, and deep tendon reflexes and for headache unrelieved by medication. Report changes immediately. Assess these signs before administering medications. Absence of patellar reflexes may indicate magnesium sulfate toxicity.
◆ Assess fluid balance by measuring intake and output and by checking daily weight.

♦ Observe for signs of fetal hypoxemia by closely monitoring the results of stress and non-stress tests.

♦ Instruct the patient to lie in a left lateral position to increase venous return, cardiac output, and renal blood flow.

⚠ **ALERT** *Keep emergency resuscitative equipment and drugs available in case of seizures and cardiac or respiratory arrest. Also keep calcium gluconate at the bedside because it counteracts magnesium sulfate's toxic effects.*

♦ To protect the patient from injury, maintain seizure precautions. Don't leave an unstable patient unattended.

♦ Assist with emergency medical treatment for the convulsive patient. Provide a quiet, darkened room until the patient's condition stabilizes, and enforce absolute bed rest. Monitor administration of magnesium sulfate; give oxygen as ordered. Don't administer anything by mouth. Insert an indwelling urinary catheter for accurate measurement of intake and output.

♦ Inform the patient about the tests that are done to evaluate fetal status. The baby's welfare is of prime concern to the parents.

♦ Provide emotional support for the patient and their family. If the patient's condition necessitates premature delivery, point out that infants of pregnant persons with gestational hypertension are usually small for gestational age but sometimes fare better than other premature babies of the same weight, possibly because they have developed adaptive responses to stress in utero.

HYDATIDIFORM MOLE
Causes and incidence

The cause of hydatidiform mole is unknown. Abnormal genetic events upon fusion of the oocyte with one or more sperm play a role. It occurs in 1 in 1,500 to 2,000 pregnancies, most commonly in female-bodied persons older than age 45. Incidence is highest in Asian female-bodied persons.

Pathophysiology

Hydatidiform mole is an uncommon chorionic tumor of the placenta. Its early signs—amenorrhea and uterine enlargement—mimic normal pregnancy; however, it eventually causes vaginal bleeding. With prompt diagnosis and appropriate treatment, the prognosis is excellent; however, about 15% of patients with hydatidiform mole develop gestational trophoblastic neoplasm. Recurrence is possible in about 2% of cases.

Complications
♦ Anemia
♦ Hemorrhage
♦ Infection
♦ Spontaneous abortion
♦ Uterine rupture

Signs and symptoms

The early stages of a pregnancy in which a hydatidiform mole develops typically seem normal, except that the uterus may grow more rapidly than usual. The first obvious signs of trouble—absence of fetal heart tones, vaginal bleeding (from spotting to hemorrhage), and lower abdominal cramps—mimic those of spontaneous abortion. The blood may contain hydatid vesicles; hyperemesis is possible, and signs and symptoms of preeclampsia are also possible. Other complications of hydatidiform mole may include anemia, infection, trophoblast embolism, uterine rupture, and choriocarcinoma.

Diagnosis

Persistent bleeding and an abnormally enlarged uterus suggest hydatidiform mole. Diagnosis is based on a typical sonographic "snowstorm" pattern. Confirmation of hydatidiform mole requires D&C.

The following findings also support a diagnosis of hydatidiform mole:

♦ absence of a gestational sac, by ultrasound assessment, or absence of fetal heart tones, by Doppler, after 12 weeks

♦ pregnancy test showing elevated hCG serum levels greater than 100,000 IU

♦ development of preeclampsia prior to 20 weeks' gestation

♦ uterine size greater than estimated gestational size

♦ vaginal bleeding

Treatment

Hydatidiform mole necessitates uterine evacuation via suction curettage. Oxytocin I.V. may be used to promote uterine contractions.

Postoperative treatment varies, depending on the amount of blood lost and complications. If no complications develop, hospitalization is usually brief, and normal activities can be resumed quickly, as tolerated.

Because of the possibility of choriocarcinoma development following hydatidiform mole, scrupulous follow-up care is essential. hCG levels initially are checked on a weekly basis, until they're repeatedly negative; then on a monthly basis for 1 year. A baseline chest X-ray is used to rule out pulmonary involvement, and a head computed tomography scan may be performed to rule out cranial metastases. Another pregnancy should be postponed until at least 1 year after hCG levels return to normal.

Special considerations

◆ Preoperatively, observe for signs of complications, such as hemorrhage and uterine infection, and vaginal passage of hydatid vesicles. Save any expelled tissue for laboratory analysis.
◆ Postoperatively, monitor vital signs, especially blood pressure, and check blood loss.
◆ Provide teaching and emotional support to the patient and their family. Encourage the patient to express their feelings, and help them through the grieving process for their lost infant.
◆ Instruct the patient to promptly report new symptoms (e.g., hemoptysis, cough, suspected pregnancy, nausea, vomiting, and vaginal bleeding).
◆ Stress the need for regular follow-up by hCG and chest X-ray monitoring, for early detection of possible malignant changes.
◆ Explain to the patient that they must use contraceptives to prevent pregnancy for at least 1 year after hCG levels return to normal and regular ovulation and menstrual cycles are re-established.

PLACENTA PREVIA

Causes and incidence

In placenta previa, the placenta may cover all (total, complete, or central), part (partial or incomplete), or a fraction (marginal or low-lying) of the internal cervical os. The degree of placenta previa depends largely on the extent of cervical dilation at the time of examination because the dilating cervix gradually uncovers the placenta. (See *Three types of placenta previa*.) Although the specific cause of placenta previa is unknown, factors that may affect the site of the placenta's attachment to the uterine wall include:
◆ defective vascularization of the decidua
◆ multiple pregnancy (the placenta requires a larger surface for attachment)
◆ previous uterine surgery
◆ multiparity
◆ advanced maternal age

This disorder, one of the most common causes of bleeding during the second half of pregnancy, occurs in about 1 in 500 pregnancies, and more commonly in multigravidas than in primigravidas.

Pathophysiology

In placenta previa, the placenta is implanted in the lower uterine segment, where it encroaches

Three types of placenta previa

Low marginal implantation—A small placental edge can be felt through the internal os.

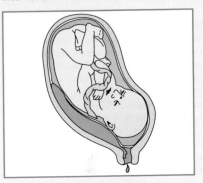

Partial placenta previa—The placenta partially caps the internal os.

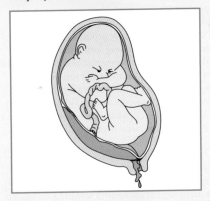

Total placenta previa—The internal os is covered entirely.

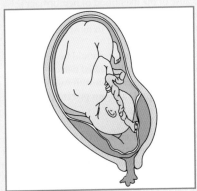

on the internal cervical os. Placenta previa with life-threatening maternal bleeding typically necessitates termination of the pregnancy. Maternal prognosis is good if hemorrhage can be controlled; fetal prognosis depends on gestational age and amount of blood lost. Anemia may be managed by blood transfusion to permit the pregnancy to continue in utero.

In placenta previa, the uterus' lower segment fails to provide as much nourishment as the fundus. The placenta tends to spread out, seeking the blood supply it needs, and becomes larger and thinner than normal. Eccentric insertion of the umbilical cord often develops, for unknown reasons. Hemorrhage occurs as the internal cervical os effaces and dilates, tearing the uterine vessels.

Complications
♦ Hemorrhage
♦ Infection
♦ Premature birth
♦ Shock
♦ Thromboembolism

Signs and symptoms
Placenta previa usually produces painless third-trimester bleeding (often the first complaint). Various malpresentations occur because of the placenta's location and interfere with proper descent of the fetal head. (The fetus remains active, however, with good heart tones.) Complications of placenta previa include shock or maternal and fetal death.

Diagnosis
Special diagnostic measures that confirm placenta previa include:
♦ transvaginal ultrasound scanning for placental position
♦ pelvic examination (under a double setup because of the likelihood of hemorrhage), performed only immediately before delivery to confirm the diagnosis. In most cases, only the cervix is visualized.

Digital examination should be deferred in any pregnant female-bodied person at or beyond 20 weeks' gestation with vaginal bleeding, until ultrasound rules out placenta previa.

Treatment
Treatment of placenta previa is designed to assess, control, and restore blood loss; to deliver a viable infant; and to prevent coagulation disorders. Immediate therapy includes starting an I.V. line using a large-bore catheter; drawing blood for hemoglobin levels and hematocrit as well as type and crossmatching; initiating external

electronic fetal monitoring; monitoring maternal blood pressure, pulse rate, and respirations; and assessing the amount of vaginal bleeding.

If the fetus is premature, following determination of the degree of placenta previa and necessary fluid and blood replacement, treatment consists of careful observation to allow the fetus more time to mature. If clinical evaluation confirms complete placenta previa, the patient may be hospitalized because of the increased risk of hemorrhage. As soon as the fetus is sufficiently mature, or in case of intervening severe hemorrhage, immediate delivery by cesarean birth may be necessary. Vaginal delivery is considered only when the bleeding is minimal and the placenta previa is marginal, or when the labor is rapid. Because of the possibility of fetal blood loss through the placenta, a pediatric team should be on hand during such delivery to immediately assess and treat neonatal shock, blood loss, and hypoxia.

Complications of placenta previa necessitate appropriate and immediate intervention.

Special considerations
♦ If the patient shows active bleeding because of placenta previa, a primary nurse should be assigned for continuous monitoring of maternal blood pressure, pulse rate, respirations, central venous pressure, intake and output, amount of vaginal bleeding, and fetal heart tones. Electronic monitoring of fetal heart tones is recommended.
♦ Prepare the patient and their family for a possible cesarean birth and the birth of a premature infant. Thoroughly explain postpartum care, so the patient and their family know what measures to expect.
♦ Provide emotional support during labor. Because of the infant's prematurity, the patient may not be given analgesics, so labor pain may be intense. Reassure them of their progress throughout labor and keep them informed of the fetus' condition. Although neonatal death is a possibility, continued monitoring and prompt management reduce this prospect.
♦ Placenta previa, especially in female-bodied persons who have had one or more cesarean births, is associated with placenta accreta, a dangerous condition in which the placenta grows into the myometrium.

ABRUPTIO PLACENTAE
Causes and incidence
The cause of abruptio placentae is often unknown. Predisposing factors include trauma, such as a direct blow to the uterus, placental site bleeding from a needle puncture during

amniocentesis, diabetes, chronic or gestational hypertension (which raises pressure on the placenta's maternal side), multiparity, smoking, and cocaine abuse. If abruptio placentae occurred in previous pregnancies, the chance for recurrence is 10% to 20%.

In abruptio placentae, blood vessels at the placental bed rupture spontaneously owing to a lack of resiliency or to abnormal changes in uterine vasculature. Hypertension complicates the situation, as does an enlarged uterus, which can't contract sufficiently to seal off the torn vessels. Consequently, bleeding continues unchecked, possibly shearing off the placenta partially or completely. Typically, such bleeding is external or marginal (in about 80% of patients) if a peripheral portion of the placenta separates from the uterine wall; it is internal or concealed (in about 20% of patients) if the central portion of the placenta becomes detached and the still-intact peripheral portions trap the blood. As blood enters the muscle fibers, complete relaxation of the uterus becomes impossible, increasing uterine tone and irritability. If bleeding into the muscle fibers is profuse, the uterus turns blue or purple, and the accumulated blood prevents its normal contractions after delivery (Couvelaire uterus, or uteroplacental apoplexy).

Pathophysiology

In abruptio placentae, also called *placental abruption*, the placenta separates from the uterine wall prematurely, usually after the 20th week of gestation, producing hemorrhage. Abruptio placentae is a common cause of bleeding during the second half of pregnancy. Firm diagnosis, in the presence of heavy maternal bleeding, may necessitate termination of pregnancy. Fetal prognosis depends on the gestational age and amount of blood lost; maternal prognosis is good if hemorrhage can be controlled.

Complications

◆ Disseminated intravascular coagulopathy (DIC)
◆ Fetal hypoxia
◆ Shock

Signs and symptoms

Abruptio placentae produces a wide range of clinical effects, depending on the extent of placental separation and the amount of blood lost from maternal circulation. (See *Degrees of placental separation in abruptio placentae.*) Mild abruptio placentae (marginal separation) develops gradually and produces mild to moderate

Degrees of placental separation in abruptio placentae

Mild separation with internal bleeding between the placenta and uterine wall

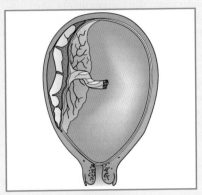

Moderate separation with external hemorrhage through the vagina

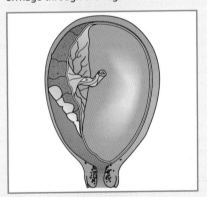

Severe separation

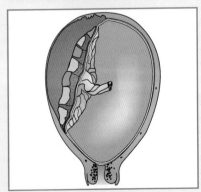

bleeding, vague lower abdominal discomfort, mild to moderate abdominal tenderness, and uterine irritability. Fetal heart tones remain strong and regular.

Moderate abruptio placentae (about 50% placental separation) may develop gradually or abruptly and produces continuous abdominal pain, moderate dark red vaginal bleeding, a tender uterus that remains firm between contractions, barely audible or irregular and bradycardiac fetal heart tones and, possibly, signs of shock. Labor usually starts within 2 hours and often proceeds rapidly.

Severe abruptio placentae (70% placental separation) develops abruptly and causes agonizing, unremitting uterine pain (described as tearing or knifelike); a boardlike, tender uterus; moderate vaginal bleeding; rapidly progressive shock; and absence of fetal heart tones.

In addition to hemorrhage and shock, complications of abruptio placentae may include renal failure, DIC, and maternal and fetal death.

Diagnosis

Diagnostic measures for abruptio placentae include observation of clinical features, speculum examination, and ultrasonography to rule out placenta previa. Decreased hemoglobin (Hb) levels and platelet counts support the diagnosis. Periodic assays for fibrin split products aid in monitoring the progression of abruptio placentae and detect the development of DIC.

Treatment

Treatment of abruptio placentae is designed to assess, control, and restore the amount of blood lost; to deliver a viable infant; and to prevent coagulation disorders. Immediate measures for abruptio placentae include starting I.V. infusion (via large-bore catheter) of appropriate fluids (lactated Ringer's solution) to combat hypovolemia; placement of a central venous pressure line and urinary catheter to monitor fluid status; drawing blood for Hb levels and hematocrit determination, for coagulation studies, and for type and crossmatching; external electronic fetal monitoring; and monitoring of maternal vital signs and vaginal bleeding.

ALERT *After determination of the severity of abruption and appropriate fluid and blood replacement, prompt delivery by cesarean birth is necessary if the fetus is in distress.*

If the fetus isn't in distress, monitoring continues; delivery is usually performed at the first sign of fetal distress. Because of possible fetal blood loss through the placenta, a pediatric team should be ready at delivery to assess and treat the neonate for shock, blood loss, and hypoxia. If placental separation is severe and there are no signs of fetal life, vaginal delivery may be performed unless uncontrolled hemorrhage or other complications contraindicate it.

Complications of abruptio placentae require appropriate treatment. For example, DIC requires immediate intervention with heparin, platelets, and whole blood to prevent exsanguination.

Special considerations

◆ Check maternal blood pressure, pulse rate, respirations, central venous pressure, intake and output, and amount of vaginal bleeding every 10 to 15 minutes. Monitor fetal heart tones electronically.

◆ Prepare the patient and their family for cesarean birth. Thoroughly explain postpartum care so the patient and their family will know what to expect.

◆ If vaginal delivery is elected, provide emotional support during labor. Because of the infant's prematurity, the pregnant person may not receive analgesics during labor and may experience intense pain. Reassure the patient of their progress through labor and keep them informed of the fetus' condition.

◆ Provide emotional support. In the case of fetal demise, encourage the patient to seek counseling as appropriate.

PREVENTION
◆ *Encourage the patient to participate in prenatal care throughout their pregnancy, especially if they're diabetic or hypertensive.*
◆ *Discuss the importance of avoiding alcohol and illegal drugs during pregnancy.*

CARDIOVASCULAR DISEASE IN PREGNANCY

Causes and incidence

About 1% to 2% of pregnant females have cardiac disease, but the incidence is rising because medical treatment today allows more females with rheumatic heart disease (present in >80% of patients who develop cardiovascular complications) and congenital defects (present in 10% to 15% of patients) to reach childbearing age. Coronary artery disease accounts for about 2% of cardiovascular complications.

Pathophysiology

Cardiovascular disease ranks fourth (after infection, gestational hypertension, and hemorrhage) among the leading causes of maternal death. The physiologic stress of pregnancy and delivery is often more than a compromised heart can tolerate and often leads to maternal and fetal mortality.

The prognosis for the pregnant patient with cardiovascular disease is good, with careful management. Decompensation is the leading cause of maternal death. Infant mortality increases with decompensation because uterine congestion, insufficient oxygenation, and the elevated carbon dioxide content of the blood not only compromise the fetus but also commonly cause premature labor and delivery.

The diseased heart is sometimes unable to meet the normal demands of pregnancy: 25% increase in cardiac output, 40% to 50% increase in plasma volume, increased oxygen requirements, retention of salt and water, weight gain, and alterations in hemodynamics during delivery. This physiologic stress often leads to the heart's failure to maintain adequate circulation (decompensation). The degree of decompensation depends on the patient's age, the duration of cardiac disease, and the heart's functional capacity at the pregnancy's outset.

Complications
◆ Endocarditis
◆ Miscarriage
◆ Preterm delivery
◆ Stillbirth

Signs and symptoms
Typical clinical features of cardiovascular disease during pregnancy include distended jugular veins, diastolic murmurs, moist basilar pulmonary crackles, cardiac enlargement (discernible on percussion or as a cardiac shadow on chest X-ray), and cardiac arrhythmias (other than sinus or paroxysmal atrial tachycardia). Other characteristic abnormalities may include cyanosis, pericardial friction rub, pulse delay, and pulsus alternans.

Decompensation may develop suddenly or gradually, with persistent crackles at the lung bases. As it progresses, edema, increasing dyspnea on exertion, palpitations, a smothering sensation, and hemoptysis may occur.

Diagnosis
A diastolic murmur, cardiac enlargement, a systolic murmur of grade $^3/_6$ intensity, and severe arrhythmia suggest cardiovascular disease. Determination of the disease's extent and cause may necessitate electrocardiography, echocardiography (for valvular disorders such as rheumatic heart disease), or other studies. X-rays show cardiac enlargement and pulmonary congestion. Cardiac catheterization should be postponed until after delivery, unless surgery is necessary.

Treatment
The goal of antepartum management is to prevent complications and minimize the strain on the pregnant person's heart, primarily through rest. This may require periodic hospitalization for patients with moderate cardiac dysfunction or with symptoms of decompensation, toxemia, or infection. Older female-bodied persons or those with previous decompensation may require hospitalization and bed rest throughout the pregnancy.

Drug therapy is often necessary and should always include the safest possible drug in the lowest possible dosage to minimize harmful effects to the fetus. Diuretics and drugs that increase blood pressure, blood volume, or cardiac output should be used with extreme caution. If an anticoagulant is needed, heparin is the drug of choice. Cardiac glycosides and common antiarrhythmics, such as quinidine and procainamide, are often required. The prophylactic use of antibiotics is reserved for patients who are susceptible to endocarditis.

A therapeutic abortion should be considered for patients with severe cardiac dysfunction, especially if decompensation occurs during the first trimester. Patients hospitalized with heart failure usually follow a regimen of cardiac glycosides, oxygen, rest, sedation, diuretics, and restricted intake of sodium and fluids. Patients in whom symptoms of heart failure don't improve after treatment with bed rest and cardiac glycosides may require cardiac surgery, such as valvotomy and commissurotomy. During labor, the patient may require oxygen and an analgesic, such as meperidine or morphine, for relief of pain and apprehension without undue depression of the fetus or themselves. Depending on which procedure promises to be less stressful for the patient's heart, delivery may be vaginal or by cesarean birth. Forceps may augment vaginal delivery to minimize the need to push, which strains the heart.

Bed rest and medications already instituted should continue for at least 1 week after delivery because of a high incidence of decompensation, cardiovascular collapse, and maternal death during the early puerperal period. These complications may result from the sudden release of intra-abdominal pressure at delivery and the mobilization of extracellular fluid for excretion, which increase the strain on the heart, especially if excessive interstitial fluid has accumulated. Breastfeeding is undesirable for patients with severely compromised cardiac dysfunction because it increases fluid and metabolic demands on the heart.

Special considerations

◆ During pregnancy, stress the importance of rest and weight control to decrease the strain on the heart. Suggest a diet of limited fluid and sodium intake to prevent vascular congestion. Encourage the patient to take supplementary folic acid and iron to prevent anemia.

! **ALERT** *During labor, watch for signs of decompensation, such as dyspnea and palpitations. Monitor pulse rate, respirations, and blood pressure.*

Auscultate for crackles every 30 minutes during the first phase of labor and every 10 minutes during the active and transition phases. Check carefully for edema and cyanosis, and assess intake and output. Administer oxygen for respiratory difficulty.

◆ Use electronic fetal monitoring to watch for the earliest signs of fetal distress.

◆ Keep the patient in a semirecumbent position. Limit their efforts to bear down during labor, which significantly raise blood pressure and stress the heart.

◆ After delivery, provide reassurance and encourage the patient to adhere to their program of treatment. Emphasize the need to rest during their hospital stay.

PREVENTION *To help prevent complications during pregnancy, teach the patient with cardiovascular disease the following:*

◆ *Advise them to follow the practitioner's recommendations for rest, which may include bed rest.*

◆ *If appropriate, encourage a practitioner-approved exercise regimen.*

◆ *Advise them to avoid stress during pregnancy by becoming informed about what to expect during pregnancy.*

◆ *Suggest that they maintain a healthy diet and avoid gaining more weight than is recommended. Extra weight may place added stress on the heart.*

◆ *Advise them to avoid heat and humidity, which can cause vasodilation and divert blood from the uterus.*

◆ *Have them report signs of infection to the practitioner, and advise that they avoid persons with upper respiratory infections.*

◆ *Tell them to change positions frequently and avoid crossing their legs. If on bed rest, have them wear anti-embolism stockings to prevent blood clots.*

ADOLESCENT PREGNANCY

As a rule, the younger the pregnant person the greater the health risk for both pregnant person and infant. Adolescents account for one-third of all abortions performed in the United States.

Causes and incidence

Adolescent pregnancy is prevalent in all socioeconomic levels, and its contributing factors vary. Such factors may include ignorance about sexuality and contraception, increasing sexual activity at a young age, rebellion against parental influence, and a desire to escape an unhappy family situation and to fulfill emotional needs unmet by the family.

In the United States, an estimated 750,000 adolescents become pregnant each year.

Pathophysiology

Adolescent pregnancy can pose a major health risk to both the mother and the child because up to 70% of adolescents who become pregnant don't receive adequate prenatal care. Pregnant adolescents develop special problems and are known to have a significantly higher incidence of anemia, pregnancy-induced hypertension, and perinatal mortality. For example, they're more likely to have babies who are premature or of low birth weight, with a higher neonatal mortality, and who are predisposed to injury at birth, childhood illness, and have mental handicaps or other neurologic defects. These risks are aggravated if the mother has abused drugs during the pregnancy. (See *How maternal drug use affects infants*, page 1057.)

Complications

◆ Anemia
◆ Gestational hypertension
◆ Intrauterine growth retardation
◆ Low birth weight
◆ Placentae previa
◆ Prematurity
◆ Toxemia

Signs and symptoms

Clinical manifestations of adolescent pregnancy are the same as those of adult pregnancy (amenorrhea, nausea, vomiting, breast tenderness, fatigue). However, the pregnant adolescent is much more likely to develop complications, such as poor weight gain during pregnancy, premature labor, and pregnancy-induced hypertension. In addition, the neonate is more likely to be of low birth weight. Some of these complications are related to the pregnant adolescent's physical immaturity, rapid growth, interest in fad diets, and generally poor nutrition; other complications may stem from the adolescent's need to deny their condition or to their ignorance of early signs of pregnancy, which often delays initiation of prenatal care.

Diagnosis

Rx **CONFIRMING DIAGNOSIS** *A positive pregnancy test that shows hCG in the blood or urine and a pelvic examination confirm pregnancy.*

PATHOPHYSIOLOGY
How maternal drug use affects infants

An infant born to a drug-dependent person risks developing certain medical problems during the first 8 months of life. These problems range from mild to severe withdrawal symptoms, to a host of complications that affect virtually every body system.

The onset and severity of adverse reactions vary with the type and amount of drugs the pregnant person has been taking and for how long. However, *any* drug the pregnant person takes, including over-the-counter products, alcohol, and illicit drugs, may cross the placenta and enter the fetal circulation, where its concentration is 50% to 100% higher than the maternal drug concentration. This chart lists fetal body systems affected by drugs and some common adverse reactions that may result.

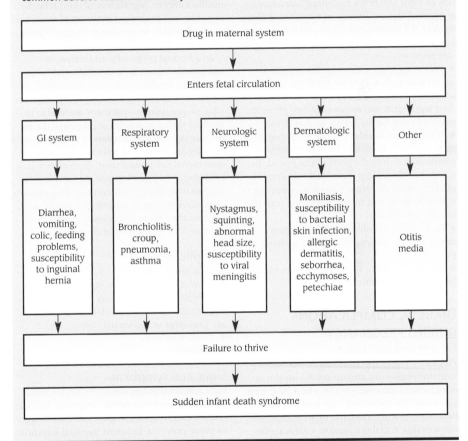

Auscultation of fetal heart sounds with a Doppler ultrasonic flowmeter or fetoscope and ultrasonography assess fetal gestational age.

Treatment

The pregnant adolescent requires the standard prenatal care that's appropriate for an adult. However, they also need psychological support and close observation for signs of complications.

Special considerations

◆ Because you may be the first healthcare professional the pregnant adolescent encounters, you must help motivate them to follow sound medical advice without being judgmental, condescending, or threatening. Emphasize the importance of adhering to the prescribed diet, getting plenty of rest, and taking prescribed vitamin and iron supplements. Your understanding and support can ensure proper healthcare during the pregnancy for both pregnant person and infant. Encourage them to ask questions and to express their feelings about the pregnancy. Answer their questions fully. It's also important to ascertain if the patient wishes to place the child for adoption or is considering abortion. Any decision should be accepted in a nonjudgmental way.

◆ Try to help the pregnant adolescent identify their own strengths and support systems for coping with pregnancy, birth, and parenting.

◆ Prepare the patient and their partner and/or family for the physical and psychological process of labor and birth. Encourage attendance at prenatal classes: The use of educational films, tours of the healthcare facility, and role-playing techniques will facilitate their cooperation with care providers.

◆ Following birth, encourage the patient to set realistic goals for the future. If they opt for adoption, make sure they clearly understand their legal rights and responsibilities. Allow the patient to care for the infant, as they desire.

◆ If the patient decides to raise the infant, help them make the transition from pregnancy to parenthood during the postpartum period. Facilitate bonding. Help them establish a realistic plan regarding childcare, parenting, returning to school or work, and their relationship with the infant's other parent.

◆ In the event of stillbirth or the neonate's death, help the patient through the grieving process.

◆ Before the patient is discharged, provide information on contraception.

DIABETIC COMPLICATIONS DURING PREGNANCY
Causes and incidence
Pregnancy places special demands on carbohydrate metabolism and causes the insulin requirement to increase, even in a healthy female. Consequently, pregnancy may lead to a prediabetic state, to the conversion of an asymptomatic subclinical diabetic state to a clinical one (gestational diabetes occurs in about 1% to 2% of all pregnancies), or to complications in a previously stable diabetic state.

The incidence of diabetes mellitus increases with age. Maternal and fetal prognoses can be equivalent to those in nondiabetic female-bodied persons if maternal blood glucose is well controlled and ketosis and other complications are prevented. Infant morbidity and mortality depend on recognizing and successfully controlling hypoglycemia, which may develop within hours after delivery.

Preconceptual counseling is helpful in optimizing pregnancy outcomes.

Pathophysiology
In diabetes mellitus, glucose is inadequately utilized either because insulin isn't synthesized or because tissues are resistant to the hormonal action of endogenous insulin. During pregnancy, the fetus relies on maternal glucose as a primary fuel source. Pregnancy triggers protective mechanisms that have anti-insulin effects: increased hormone production (placental lactogen, estrogen, and progesterone), which antagonizes insulin's effects; degradation of insulin by the placenta; and prolonged elevation of stress hormones (cortisol, epinephrine, and glucagon), which raise blood glucose levels.

In a normal pregnancy, an increase in anti-insulin factors is counterbalanced by an increase in insulin production to maintain normal blood glucose levels. However, females who are prediabetic or diabetic are unable to produce sufficient insulin to overcome the insulin antagonist mechanisms of pregnancy, or their tissues are insulin-resistant. As insulin requirements rise toward term, the patient who's prediabetic may develop gestational diabetes, necessitating dietary management and, possibly, exogenous insulin to achieve glycemic control, whereas the patient who's insulin-dependent may need increased insulin dosage.

Complications
◆ Fetal anomalies
◆ Neonatal hypoglycemia, hypocalcemia, hyperbilirubinemia, respiratory distress syndrome
◆ Neonatal size inappropriate for gestational age (too large or too small)
◆ Preterm delivery
◆ Stillbirth

Signs and symptoms
Indications for diagnostic screening for maternal diabetes mellitus during pregnancy include obesity, excessive weight gain, excessive hunger or thirst, polyuria, recurrent monilial infections, glycosuria, previous delivery of a large neonate, polyhydramnios, maternal hypertension, and a family history of diabetes.

Diagnosis
The prevalence of gestational diabetes makes careful screening for hyperglycemia appropriate in all pregnancies. A screening 50-g 1-hour glucose tolerance test is normally performed at 24 to 28 weeks' gestation. In addition, female-bodied persons with a history of fetal macrosomia or who may have nongestational

diabetes should be formally tested for diabetes with a 3-hour glucose tolerance test.

℞ CONFIRMING DIAGNOSIS *A 100-g 3-hour glucose tolerance test confirms diabetes mellitus when two or more values are above normal.*

Procedures to assess fetal status include stress and nonstress tests; ultrasonography to determine fetal age and growth; measurement of phosphatidyl-glycerol; and determination of the lecithin–sphingomyelin (L/S) ratio from amniotic fluid to predict pulmonary maturity. The L/S ratio is less useful in diabetic pregnancies; generally a ratio of 3.5:1 is required to confirm fetal lung maturity.

Treatment

Treatment of both the newly diagnosed and the established diabetic is designed to maintain blood glucose levels within acceptable limits through dietary management and insulin administration. Some female-bodied persons with overt diabetes mellitus require hospitalization at the beginning of pregnancy to assess physical status, check for cardiac and renal disease, and regulate diabetes.

For pregnant patients with diabetes, therapy includes:

◆ bimonthly visits to the obstetrician and the internist during the first 6 months of pregnancy; weekly visits may be necessary during the third trimester
◆ maintenance of fasting blood glucose levels at or below 100 mg/dL and 2-hour postprandial blood glucose levels at or below 120 mg/dL during the pregnancy
◆ frequent monitoring for glycosuria and ketonuria (ketosis presents a grave threat to the fetal CNS)
◆ weight control (gain not to exceed 3 to 3½ lb [1.4 to 1.6 kg] per month during the last 6 months of pregnancy)
◆ high-protein diet of 2 g/day/kg of body weight, or a minimum of 80 g/day during the second half of pregnancy; daily calorie intake of 30 to 40 calories/kg of body weight; daily carbohydrate intake of 200 g; and enough fat to provide 36% of total calories (however, vigorous calorie restriction can cause starvation ketosis)
◆ exogenous insulin if diet doesn't control blood glucose levels. Be alert for changes in insulin requirements from one trimester to the next and immediately postpartum. Oral antidiabetic drugs are contraindicated during pregnancy because they may cause fetal hypoglycemia and congenital anomalies

Generally, the optimal time for delivery is between 37 and 39 weeks' gestation, although with reassuring antenatal testing and no evidence of macrosomia, 40 weeks or later is also feasible. The insulin-dependent diabetic may require hospitalization before delivery for frequent monitoring of blood glucose levels and prompt intervention if complications develop.

Depending on fetal status and maternal history, the obstetrician may induce labor or perform a cesarean delivery. During labor and delivery, the patient with diabetes should receive continuous I.V. infusion of dextrose with regular insulin in water. Maternal and fetal status must be monitored closely throughout labor. The patient may benefit from half their prepregnancy dosage of insulin before a cesarean delivery. Their insulin requirement will fall markedly after delivery.

Special considerations

◆ Teach the newly diagnosed patient about diabetes, including dietary management, insulin administration, home monitoring of blood glucose or urine testing for glucose and ketones, and skin and foot care. Instruct them to report ketonuria immediately.
◆ Evaluate the patient who's diabetic for their knowledge about this disease and provide supplementary patient teaching, as they require. Inform the patient that frequent monitoring and adjustment of insulin dosage are necessary throughout the course of their pregnancy.
◆ Give reassurance that strict compliance with prescribed therapy should ensure a favorable outcome.
◆ Refer the patient to appropriate social service agencies if financial assistance is necessary because of prolonged hospitalization.
◆ Encourage medical counseling regarding the prognosis of future pregnancies.

Abnormalities of parturition

PRETERM LABOR

Causes and incidence

The possible causes of premature labor are many; they may include premature rupture of the membranes (occurs in 30% to 50% of preterm labors), preeclampsia, chronic hypertensive vascular disease, hydramnios, multiple pregnancy, placenta previa, abruptio placentae, incompetent cervix, abdominal surgery, trauma, structural anomalies of the uterus, infections (such as rubella or toxoplasmosis), congenital adrenal hyperplasia, and fetal death.

Pathophysiology

Preterm labor, also called *premature labor*, is the onset of rhythmic uterine contractions that produce cervical change after fetal viability but before fetal maturity. It usually occurs between the 20th and 37th weeks of gestation. About 5% to 10% of pregnancies end preterm; about 75% of neonatal deaths and a great many birth defects stem from this disorder. Fetal prognosis depends on birth weight and length of gestation: Neonates weighing less than 1 lb 10 oz (737 g) and of less than 26 weeks' gestation have a survival rate of 40% to 50%; neonates weighing 1 lb 10 oz to 2 lb 3 oz (737 to 992 g) and of 27 to 28 weeks' gestation have a survival rate of 70% to 80%; those weighing 2 lb 3 oz to 2 lb 11 oz (992 to 1,219 g) and of 28 weeks' gestation have an 85% to 97% survival rate.

Other important provocative factors include:
◆ fetal stimulation—Genetically imprinted information tells the fetus that nutrition is inadequate and that a change in environment is required for well-being; this provokes onset of labor.
◆ oxytocin sensitivity—Labor begins because the myometrium becomes hypersensitive to oxytocin, the hormone that normally induces uterine contractions.
◆ myometrial oxygen deficiency—The fetus becomes increasingly proficient in obtaining oxygen, depriving the myometrium of the oxygen and energy it needs to function normally, thus making the myometrium irritable.
◆ maternal genetics—A genetic defect in the mother shortens gestation and precipitates premature labor.

Complications
◆ Cerebral palsy
◆ Intracranial bleeding
◆ Infection
◆ Visual impairment

Signs and symptoms
Like labor at term, preterm labor produces rhythmic uterine contractions, cervical dilation and effacement, possible rupture of the membranes, expulsion of the cervical mucus plug, and a bloody discharge.

Diagnosis
Preterm labor is confirmed by the combined results of prenatal history, physical examination, presenting signs and symptoms, and ultrasonography (if available) showing the fetus' position in relation to the mother's pelvis. Vaginal examination confirms progressive cervical effacement and dilation.

Treatment
Treatment is intended to suppress preterm labor when tests show immature fetal pulmonary development, cervical dilation is less than 1½″ (4 cm), and the absence of factors that contraindicate continuation of pregnancy. Such treatment consists of bed rest and, when necessary, drug therapy, but neither has been proven beneficial in all patients.

The following pharmacologic agents can suppress preterm labor for up to 48 hours:
◆ beta-adrenergic stimulants (terbutaline, isoxsuprine, or ritodrine)—Stimulation of the beta$_2$-adrenergic receptors inhibits contractility of uterine smooth muscle. Adverse effects include maternal tachycardia and hypotension, and fetal tachycardia.
◆ magnesium sulfate—Direct action on the myometrium relaxes the muscle. It also produces maternal adverse effects, such as drowsiness, slurred speech, flushing, decreased reflexes, decreased GI motility, and decreased respirations. Fetal and neonatal adverse effects may include CNS depression, decreased respirations, and decreased sucking reflex.

Maternal factors that jeopardize the fetus, making preterm delivery the lesser risk, include intrauterine infection, abruptio placentae, placental insufficiency, and severe preeclampsia. Among the fetal problems that become more perilous as pregnancy nears term are severe isoimmunization and congenital anomalies.

Ideally, treatment for active premature labor should take place in a regional perinatal intensive care center, where the staff is specially trained to handle this situation. In such settings, the neonate can remain close to his parents. (Community healthcare facilities commonly lack the equipment necessary for special neonatal care and transfer the neonate alone to a perinatal center.)

Treatment and delivery require an intensive team effort, focusing on:
◆ continuous assessment of the neonate's health through fetal monitoring
◆ administration of antenatal steroids to assist fetal lung development, unless contraindicated
◆ maintenance of adequate hydration through I.V. fluids

Special considerations
A patient in preterm labor requires close observation for signs of fetal or maternal distress, as well as comprehensive supportive care.
◆ During attempts to suppress preterm labor, maintain bed rest and administer medications, as ordered. Give sedatives and analgesics sparingly, because they can have potentially harmful effects on the fetus. Minimize the need for these drugs by providing comfort measures, such as frequent repositioning and good perineal and back care.

◆ When administering beta-adrenergic stimulants, sedatives, and opioids, monitor blood pressure, pulse rate, respirations, fetal heart rate, and uterine contraction pattern. Minimize adverse effects by keeping the patient in a lateral recumbent position as much as possible. Provide adequate hydration.

◆ Tocolytic therapy has never been shown to benefit fetal morbidity and mortality; it's best used to delay delivery for 48 hours while allowing antenatal steroids to effect lung development in the fetus.

◆ When administering magnesium sulfate, monitor neurologic reflexes. Watch the neonate for signs of magnesium toxicity, including neuromuscular and respiratory depression.

◆ Offer emotional support to the patient and their family. Encourage the parents to express their fears concerning the neonate's survival and health.

◆ During active preterm labor, remember that the premature neonate has a lower tolerance for the stress of labor and is much more likely to become hypoxic than the term neonate. If necessary, administer oxygen to the patient through a nasal cannula. Encourage the patient to lie on their left side or sit up during labor; this position prevents caval compression, which can cause supine hypotension and subsequent fetal hypoxia. Observe fetal response to labor through continuous fetal monitoring. Prevent maternal hyperventilation; a rebreathing bag may be necessary. Continually reassure the patient throughout labor to help ease their anxiety.

⚠ ALERT *Help the patient get through labor with as little analgesic medication and anesthetic as possible. To minimize fetal CNS depression, avoid administering analgesics when delivery seems imminent. Monitor fetal and maternal response to local and regional anesthetics.*

◆ Explain all procedures. Throughout labor, keep the patient informed of their progress and the fetus' condition. If the other parent is present during labor, allow the parents some time together to share their feelings.

◆ A prepared resuscitation team, consisting of a physician, nurse, respiratory therapist, and an anesthesiologist or anesthetist, should be in attendance to take care of the neonate immediately. Have resuscitative equipment available in case of neonatal respiratory distress.

◆ Inform the parents of their child's condition. Describe their appearance and explain the purpose of any supportive equipment. Help them gain confidence in their ability to care for their child. Provide privacy and encourage them to hold and feed the neonate, when possible.

◆ As necessary, before the parents leave the facility with the neonate, refer them to a community health nurse who can help them adjust to caring for a premature neonate.

▒▒▒ **PREVENTION**
◆ *Advise the patient to get good prenatal care, adequate nutrition, and proper rest.*
◆ *Insertion of a purse-string suture (cerclage) to reinforce an incompetent cervix at 14 to 18 weeks' gestation may prevent preterm labor in patients with histories of this disorder. However, this can be dangerous if an incompetent cervix is misdiagnosed and preterm labor is the true cause.*

PREMATURE RUPTURE OF MEMBRANES
Causes and incidence
Premature rupture of membranes (PROM) is a spontaneous break or tear in the amniochorial sac before onset of regular contractions, resulting in progressive cervical dilation. Labor usually starts within 24 hours; more than 80% of these neonates are mature. The latent period (between membrane rupture and onset of labor) is generally brief when the membranes rupture near term; when the neonate is premature, this period is prolonged, which increases the risk of mortality from maternal infection (amnionitis, endometritis), fetal infection (pneumonia, septicemia), and prematurity.

PROM occurs in nearly 10% of all pregnancies over 20 weeks' gestation.

Pathophysiology
Although the cause of PROM is unknown, malpresentation and contracted pelvis commonly accompany the rupture. Predisposing factors may include:
◆ poor nutrition and hygiene, and lack of proper prenatal care
◆ incompetent cervix
◆ increased intrauterine tension due to hydramnios or multiple pregnancies
◆ defects in the amniochorial membranes' tensile strength
◆ uterine infection

Complications
Maternal
◆ Amnionitis
◆ Cesarean delivery
◆ Endometritis

Neonatal
◆ Asphyxia
◆ Congenital anomalies
◆ Cord prolapse

◆ Fetal distress
◆ Malpresentation
◆ Pulmonary hypoplasia
◆ Respiratory distress syndrome

Signs and symptoms

Typically, PROM causes blood-tinged amniotic fluid containing vernix particles to gush or leak from the vagina. Maternal fever, fetal tachycardia, and foul-smelling vaginal discharge indicate infection.

Diagnosis

Characteristic passage of amniotic fluid confirms PROM. Physical examination shows amniotic fluid in the vagina. Examination of this fluid helps determine appropriate management. For example, aerobic and anaerobic cultures and a Gram stain from the cervix reveal pathogenic organisms and indicate uterine or systemic infection.

℞ CONFIRMING DIAGNOSIS *Alkaline pH of fluid collected from the posterior fornix turns Nitrazine paper deep blue. (The presence of blood can give a false-positive result.) If a smear of fluid is placed on a slide and allowed to dry, it takes on a fernlike pattern due to the high sodium and protein content of amniotic fluid.*

Staining the fluid with Nile blue sulfate reveals two categories of cell bodies. Blue-stained bodies represent shed fetal epithelial cells, whereas orange-stained bodies originate in sebaceous glands. Incidence of prematurity is low when more than 20% of cells stain orange.

Physical examination also determines the presence of multiple pregnancies. Fetal presentation and size should be assessed by abdominal palpation (Leopold's maneuvers).

Other data determine the fetus's gestational age:

◆ historical: date of last menstrual period, quickening
◆ physical: initial detection of unamplified fetal heart sound, measurement of fundal height above the symphysis, ultrasound measurements of fetal biparietal diameter
◆ chemical: tests on amniotic fluid, such as the lecithin–sphingomyelin (L/S) ratio (an L/S ratio > 2 indicates pulmonary maturity); foam stability (shake test) also indicates fetal pulmonary maturity. Presence of phosphatidylglycerol (PG) in the fluid indicates that respiratory distress is unlikely.

Treatment

Treatment for PROM depends on fetal age and the risk of infection. In a term pregnancy, if spontaneous labor and vaginal delivery aren't achieved within a relatively short time (usually within 24 hours after the membranes rupture), induction of labor with oxytocin is usually required; if induction fails, cesarean delivery is usually necessary. Cesarean hysterectomy is recommended with gross uterine infection.

Management of a preterm pregnancy of less than 34 weeks is controversial. However, with advances in technology, a conservative approach to PROM has now been proven effective. With a preterm pregnancy of 28 to 34 weeks, treatment includes hospitalization and observation for signs of infection (maternal leukocytosis or fever, and fetal tachycardia) while awaiting fetal maturation. If clinical status suggests infection, baseline cultures and sensitivity tests are appropriate. If these tests confirm infection, labor must be induced, followed by I.V. administration of antibiotics. A culture should also be made of gastric aspirate or a swabbing from the neonate's ear because antibiotic therapy may be indicated for him as well. At such delivery, have resuscitative equipment available to treat neonatal distress.

Special considerations

◆ Teach the patient in the early stages of pregnancy how to recognize PROM. Make sure they understand that amniotic fluid doesn't always gush; it may leak slowly.
◆ Stress that the patient *must* report PROM immediately because prompt treatment may prevent dangerous infection.
◆ Warn the patient not to engage in sexual intercourse or to douche after the membranes rupture.
◆ Before physical examination in suspected PROM, explain all diagnostic tests and clarify any misunderstandings the patient may have. During the examination, stay with the patient and provide reassurance. Such examination requires sterile gloves and sterile lubricating jelly. Don't use iodophor antiseptic solution, because it discolors Nitrazine paper and makes pH determination impossible.
◆ After the examination, provide proper perineal care. Send fluid samples to the laboratory promptly because bacteriologic studies need immediate evaluation to be valid. If labor starts, observe the mother's contractions and monitor vital signs every 2 hours. Watch for signs of maternal infection (fever, abdominal tenderness, and changes in amniotic fluid, such as foul odor or purulence) and fetal tachycardia. (Fetal tachycardia may precede maternal fever.) Report such signs immediately.
◆ The L/S ratio isn't useful if obtained from a vaginal pool of amniotic fluid, because vaginal

epithelium secretes lecithin. The PG level is accurate, however.

CESAREAN BIRTH

Cesarean birth, also known as *cesarean section*, is delivery of a neonate by surgical incision through the abdomen and uterus. It can be performed as elective surgery or as an emergency procedure when conditions prohibit vaginal delivery.

Causes and incidence

The most common reasons for cesarean birth are malpresentation (such as shoulder or face presentation), fetal intolerance of labor distress, cephalopelvic disproportion (CPD; the pelvis is too small to accommodate the fetal head), certain cases of toxemia, previous cesarean birth, and inadequate progress in labor (failure of induction).

Conditions causing fetal distress that indicate a need for cesarean birth include prolapsed cord with a live fetus, fetal hypoxia, abnormal fetal heart rate patterns, unfavorable intrauterine environment (from infection), and moderate to severe Rh isoimmunization. Less common maternal conditions that may necessitate cesarean birth include complete placenta previa, abruptio placentae, placenta accreta, malignant tumors, and chronic diseases in which delivery is indicated before term.

Cesarean birth may also be necessary if induction is contraindicated or difficult or if advanced labor increases the risk of morbidity and mortality.

In the case of a previous cesarean delivery, some providers encourage a subsequent vaginal delivery if the cesarean wasn't classic or if the original reason for the cesarean no longer exists. Vaginal delivery has a small risk of uterine rupture if the uterus is scarred.

The rising incidence of cesarean birth coincides with recent medical and technologic advances in fetal and placental surveillance and care. In the United States, 32% of all pregnancies terminate in cesarean births.

Pathophysiology

Cesarean birth, also known as *cesarean section*, is delivery of a neonate by surgical incision through the abdomen and uterus. It can be performed as elective surgery or as an emergency procedure when conditions prohibit vaginal delivery.

Complications

- Infection
- Hemorrhage
- Injury to organs
- Injury to fetus

- Blood clots; deep vein thrombosis, pulmonary embolism, stroke, etc.
- Maternal death
- Fetal death

Signs and symptoms

Indications that a cesarean birth may be necessary are:

- Lack of labor progress
- Infant in distress
- Abnormal position of infant
- Multiple birth
- Prolapsed umbilical cord
- Previous cesarean birth
- Problem with placenta such as placenta previa

Diagnosis

Special tests and monitoring procedures provide early indications of the need for cesarean birth:

- Magnetic resonance imaging or clinical pelvimetry reveals CPD and malpresentation.
- Ultrasonography shows pelvic masses that interfere with vaginal delivery and fetal position.
- Auscultation of fetal heart rate (by fetoscope, Doppler unit, or electronic fetal monitor) determines acute fetal intolerance of labor.

Treatment

The most common type of cesarean birth is the *lower segment cesarean*, in which a transverse incision across the lower abdomen opens the visceral peritoneum over the uterus. The lower anterior uterine wall is then incised (transversely or longitudinally) behind the bladder.

The *classic cesarean*—in which a longitudinal incision is made into the body of the uterus, extending into the fundus and opening the top of the uterus—is rarely performed because it exaggerates the risk of infection and of uterine rupture in subsequent pregnancies. *Cesarean hysterectomy* removes the entire uterus and is reserved for such cases as malignant tumors, severe infection, and placenta accreta.

Patients may have general or regional anesthetic for surgery, depending on the extent of maternal or fetal distress. Possible maternal complications of cesarean delivery include respiratory tract infection, wound dehiscence, thromboembolism, paralytic ileus, hemorrhage, and genitourinary tract infection.

Special considerations

Before cesarean delivery:

- Explain cesarean birth to the patient and their partner, and answer any questions they may have. Provide reassurance and emotional support. Cesarean birth is often performed after hours of labor have exhausted the patient.

◆ Administer preoperative medications as ordered.

◆ Prepare the patient by shaving them from below the umbilicus to the pubic region and the upper quarter of the anterior thighs. Make sure their bladder is empty, using an indwelling urinary catheter as ordered. Insert an I.V. line for fluid replacement therapy as ordered. Assess maternal temperature, pulse rate, respirations, and blood pressure and fetal heart rate.

◆ In the operating room, place the patient in a slight lateral position. Use of a 15-degree wedge reduces caval compression (supine hypotension) and subsequent fetal hypoxia.

After cesarean delivery:

◆ Check vital signs every 15 minutes until they stabilize. Maintain a patent airway. If general anesthetic was used, remain with the patient until they're responsive. If regional anesthetic was used, monitor the return of sensation to the legs.

◆ Encourage parent–infant bonding as soon as practical.

◆ Gently assess the fundus. Check the incision and lochia for signs of infection such as a foul odor. Check frequently for bleeding and report it immediately. Keep the incision clean and dry.

◆ Observe the neonate for signs of respiratory distress (tachypnea, retractions, and cyanosis) until there's evidence of physiologic stability. Keep resuscitative equipment available.

◆ Assess intake and output (some patients have indwelling urinary catheters in place up to 48 hours postoperative). Observe the patient closely for indications of bladder fullness or urinary tract infection.

◆ Administer pain medication, as ordered, and provide comfort measures for breast engorgement as appropriate. Offer reassurance and reduce anxiety by answering any questions. If the mother wishes to breastfeed, offer encouragement and help. Recognize afterpains in multiparas.

◆ Promote early ambulation to prevent cardiovascular and pulmonary complications.

◆ Provide psychological support. If the patient seems anxious about having had a cesarean delivery, encourage them to share their feelings with you. If appropriate, suggest that they participate in a cesarean birthsharing group. Encourage support from their family members as well.

Postpartum disorders

PUERPERAL INFECTION

A common cause of childbirth-related death, puerperal infection is a postpartum infection of the uterus and higher structures, with a characteristic fever pattern. It can result in endometritis, parametritis, pelvic and femoral thrombophlebitis, and peritonitis. The prognosis is good with treatment.

Causes and incidence

In the United States, puerperal infection develops in about 5% to 7% of maternity patients.

Pathophysiology

Microorganisms that commonly cause puerperal infection include group B streptococci, coagulase-negative staphylococci, *Clostridium perfringens*, *Bacteroides fragilis*, and *E. coli*. Most of these organisms are considered normal vaginal flora but are known to cause puerperal infection in the presence of certain predisposing factors:

◆ prolonged and premature rupture of the membranes

◆ prolonged (>24 hours) labor

◆ frequent or unsanitary vaginal examinations or unsanitary delivery

◆ retained products of conception

◆ hemorrhage

◆ maternal conditions, such as anemia or debilitation from malnutrition

◆ cesarean birth (20-fold increase in risk for puerperal infection)

Complications

◆ Infertility
◆ Pulmonary embolism
◆ Septic shock
◆ Stroke

Signs and symptoms

A characteristic sign of puerperal infection is fever (at least 100.4° F [38° C]) that occurs in the first 24 hours in the first 9 days postpartum. This fever can spike as high as 105° F (40.6° C) and is commonly associated with chills, headache, malaise, restlessness, and anxiety. Abortion or miscarriage isn't usually associated with this infection and fever.

Accompanying signs and symptoms depend on the infection's extent and site and may include:

◆ endometritis: heavy, sometimes foul-smelling lochia; tender, enlarged uterus; backache; severe uterine contractions persisting after childbirth

◆ parametritis (pelvic cellulitis): vaginal tenderness and abdominal pain and tenderness (pain may become more intense as infection spreads)

The inflammation may remain localized, may lead to abscess formation, or may spread through the blood or lymphatic system. Widespread inflammation may cause:

◆ pelvic thrombophlebitis: severe, repeated chills and dramatic swings in body temperature; lower abdominal or flank pain; and, possibly, a palpable tender mass over the affected area, which usually develops near the second postpartum week

◆ femoral thrombophlebitis: pain, stiffness, or swelling in a leg or the groin; inflammation or shiny, white appearance of the affected leg; malaise; fever; and chills, usually beginning 10 to 20 days postpartum (these signs may precipitate pulmonary embolism)

◆ peritonitis: body temperature usually elevated, accompanied by tachycardia (>140 beats/minute), weak pulse, hiccups, nausea, vomiting, and diarrhea; constant and possibly excruciating abdominal pain

Diagnosis

Development of the typical clinical features, especially fever within 48 hours after delivery, suggests a diagnosis of puerperal infection. Uterine tenderness is also highly suggestive.

A culture of lochia, incisional exudate (from cesarean incision or episiotomy), uterine tissue, or material collected from the vaginal cuff that reveals the causative organism may confirm the diagnosis, but such cultures are generally contaminated with vaginal flora and aren't considered helpful.

Within 36 to 48 hours, white blood cell count usually demonstrates leukocytosis (15,000 to 30,000/µL).

Typical clinical features usually suffice for diagnosis of endometritis and peritonitis. In parametritis, pelvic examination shows induration without purulent discharge.

Diagnosis of pelvic or femoral thrombophlebitis is suggested by characteristic clinical signs, venography, Doppler ultrasonography, palpable veins inside the thigh and calf, pain in the calf when pressure is applied on the inside of the foot, and pain on passive dorsiflexion of the foot with the knee extended (Homans' sign). Homans' sign should be elicited passively by asking the patient to dorsiflex the foot. Active dorsiflexion could lead to embolization of a clot.

Treatment

Treatment of puerperal infection usually begins with I.V. infusion of a broad-spectrum antibiotic to control the infection and prevent its spread while awaiting culture results. After identification of the infecting organism, a more specific antibiotic should be administered. (An oral antibiotic may be prescribed after hospital discharge.)

Ancillary measures include analgesics for pain; antiseptics for local lesions; and antiemetics for nausea and vomiting from peritonitis. Isolation or transfer from the maternity unit generally isn't appropriate.

Supportive care includes bed rest, adequate fluid intake, I.V. fluids when necessary, and measures to reduce fever. Sitz baths and heat lamps may relieve discomfort from local lesions.

Surgery may be necessary to remove any remaining products of conception or to drain local lesions such as an abscess in parametritis.

Management of septic pelvic thrombophlebitis consists of heparinization for about 10 days in conjunction with broad-spectrum antibiotic therapy.

Special considerations

◆ Monitor vital signs every 4 hours (more frequently if peritonitis has developed) and intake and output. Enforce strict bed rest.

◆ Frequently inspect the perineum. Assess the fundus and palpate for tenderness (subinvolution may indicate endometritis). Note the amount, color, and odor of vaginal drainage, and document your observations.

◆ Administer antibiotics and analgesics, as ordered. Assess and document the type, degree, and location of pain as well as the patient's response to analgesics. Give the patient an antiemetic to relieve nausea and vomiting, as necessary.

◆ Provide sitz baths and a heat lamp for local lesions. Change bed linen and perineal pads and under pads frequently. Keep the patient warm.

◆ Elevate the thrombophlebitic leg about 30 degrees. Provide warm soaks. Watch for signs of pulmonary embolism, such as cyanosis, dyspnea, and chest pain.

⚠ **ALERT** *Don't rub or manipulate the thrombophlebitic leg or compress it with bed linen.*

◆ Offer reassurance and emotional support. Thoroughly explain all procedures to the patient and their family.

◆ If the postpartum person is separated from their neonate, provide them with frequent reassurance about his progress. Encourage the other parent to reassure the postpartum person about the neonate's condition as well.

◆ *Maintain sterile technique when performing a vaginal examination. Limit the number of vaginal examinations done during labor. Wash your hands thoroughly after each patient contact.*

◆ *Tell a pregnant patient to call their practitioner immediately when their membranes rupture. Warn them to avoid intercourse after rupture or leaking of the amniotic sac.*

◆ *Keep the episiotomy site clean and teach the patient how to maintain good perineal hygiene.*

◆ *Screen personnel and visitors to keep persons with active infections away from maternity patients.*

MASTITIS AND BREAST ENGORGEMENT

Mastitis (parenchymatous inflammation of the mammary glands) and breast engorgement (congestion) are disorders that may affect lactating females. The prognosis for both disorders is good.

Causes and incidence

Mastitis occurs postpartum in about 1% of postpartum persons, mainly in primiparas who are breastfeeding. It occurs occasionally in non-lactating female-bodied persons and rarely in male-bodied persons All breastfeeding postpartum persons develop some degree of engorgement, which isn't an infectious process.

Pathophysiology

Mastitis develops when a pathogen that typically originates in the nursing infant's nose or pharynx invades breast tissue through a fissured or cracked nipple and disrupts normal lactation. The most common pathogen of this type is *Staphylococcus aureus*; less frequently, it's *S. epidermidis* or beta-hemolytic streptococci. Rarely, mastitis may result from disseminated tuberculosis or the mumps virus. Predisposing factors include a fissure or abrasion on the nipple; blocked milk ducts; and an incomplete let-down reflex, usually due to emotional trauma. Blocked milk ducts can result from a tight bra or prolonged intervals between breastfeedings. Causes of breast engorgement include venous and lymphatic stasis, and alveolar milk accumulation. (See *Physiology of lactation,* page 1067.)

Complication

◆ Abscess

Signs and symptoms

Mastitis may develop anytime during lactation but usually begins 1 to 2 weeks postpartum with fever (101° F [38.3° C] or higher in acute mastitis), malaise, and flulike symptoms.

The breast (or, occasionally, both breasts) becomes tender, hard, swollen, and warm. Unless mastitis is treated adequately, it may progress to breast abscess.

Breast engorgement generally starts with onset of lactation (day 2 to day 5 postpartum). The breasts undergo changes similar to those in mastitis, and body temperature may be elevated. Engorgement may be mild, causing only slight discomfort, or severe, causing considerable pain. A severely engorged breast can interfere with the infant's capacity to feed because of their inability to position their mouth properly on the swollen, rigid breast.

Diagnosis

℞ **CONFIRMING DIAGNOSIS** *Diagnosis is usually easily made if pus is expressed from the nipple; culture may be helpful in confirming mastitis.*

Treatment

Antibiotic therapy, the primary treatment for mastitis, generally consists of oral cephalosporins, cloxacillin, or dicloxacillin to combat staphylococcus; azithromycin may be used in patients allergic to penicillin. Although symptoms usually subside 2 to 3 days after treatment begins, antibiotic therapy should continue for 10 days. Other appropriate measures include analgesics for pain and, rarely, when antibiotics fail to control the infection and mastitis progresses to breast abscess, incision and drainage of the abscess.

The goal of treatment of breast engorgement is to relieve discomfort and control swelling and may include analgesics to alleviate pain, and ice packs and an uplift support bra to minimize edema. Rarely, oxytocin nasal spray may be necessary to release milk from the alveoli into the ducts. To facilitate breastfeeding, the mother may manually express excess milk before a feeding so the infant can grasp the nipple properly.

Special considerations

If the patient has mastitis:

◆ Isolate the patient and their infant to prevent the spread of infection to other nursing mothers. Explain mastitis to the patient and why isolation is necessary.

◆ Obtain a complete patient history, including a drug history, especially allergy to penicillin.

◆ Assess and record the cause and amount of discomfort. Give analgesics as needed.

◆ Reassure the postpartum person that breastfeeding during mastitis won't harm their infant. However, if an open abscess develops, they must

Physiology of lactation

During pregnancy, progesterone and estrogen normally interact to suppress milk secretion while developing the breasts for lactation. Estrogen causes the breasts to grow by increasing their fat content; progesterone causes lobule growth and develops the alveolar cells' secretory capacity.

After childbirth, the postpartum person's anterior pituitary gland secretes prolactin (suppressed during pregnancy), which helps the alveolar epithelium produce and release colostrum. Usually, within 3 days of prolactin release, the breasts secrete large amounts of milk rather than colostrum. The infant's sucking stimulates nerve endings at the nipple, initiating the let-down reflex that allows the expression of milk from the postpartum person's breasts. Sucking also stimulates the release of another pituitary hormone, oxytocin, into the postpartum person's bloodstream. This hormone causes alveolar contraction, which forces milk into the ducts and the lactiferous sinuses beneath the alveolar surface, making milk available to the infant. (It also promotes normal involution of the uterus.)

The infant's suckling provides the stimulus for both milk production and milk expression. As a result, the more the infant breast-feeds, the more milk the breast produces. Conversely, the less sucking stimulation the breast receives, the less milk it produces.

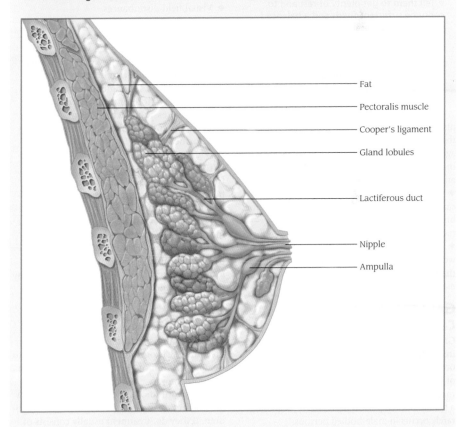

Fat

Pectoralis muscle

Cooper's ligament

Gland lobules

Lactiferous duct

Nipple

Ampulla

stop breastfeeding with this breast and use a breast pump until the abscess heals. They should continue to breastfeed on the unaffected side.
◆ Instruct the patient to combat fever by getting plenty of rest, drinking sufficient fluids, and following the prescribed antibiotic therapy.

If the patient has breast engorgement:
◆ Assess and record the level of discomfort. Give analgesics, and apply ice packs and a compression binder, as needed.
◆ Teach the patient how to express excess breast milk manually. They should do this

just before nursing to enable the infant to get the swollen areola into their mouth. Caution against excessive milk expression between feedings because this stimulates milk production and prolongs engorgement.
♦ Explain that because breast engorgement is caused by the physiologic processes of lactation, breastfeeding is the best remedy for engorgement. Suggest breastfeeding every 2 to 3 hours.
♦ Ensure that the postpartum person wears a well-fitted nursing bra, usually a size larger than they normally wear. (See *Preventing mastitis*.)

GALACTORRHEA
Causes and incidence
Galactorrhea, also known as *hyperprolactinemia*, is inappropriate breast milk secretion. It generally occurs 3 to 6 months after the discontinuation of breastfeeding (usually after a first delivery). It may also follow an abortion or may develop in a female-bodied person hasn't been pregnant; it rarely occurs in male-bodied persons.

Pathophysiology
Galactorrhea usually develops in a person with increased prolactin secretion from the anterior pituitary gland, with possible abnormal patterns of secretion of growth, thyroid, and adrenocorticotropic hormones. However, increased prolactin serum concentration doesn't always cause galactorrhea.

Additional factors that may precipitate this disorder include the following:
♦ endogenous: pituitary (high incidence with chromophobe adenoma), ovarian, or adrenal tumors and hypothyroidism; in male-bodied persons, pituitary, testicular, or pineal gland tumors
♦ idiopathic: possibly from stress or anxiety, which causes neurogenic depression of the prolactin-inhibiting factor
♦ exogenous: breast stimulation, genital stimulation, or drugs (such as hormonal contraceptives, meprobamate, and phenothiazines)

Complications
♦ CNS disturbances
♦ Increased intracranial pressure
♦ Visual field disturbances

Signs and symptoms
In the female-bodied person with galactorrhea, milk continues to flow after the 21-day period that's normal after weaning. Galactorrhea may also be spontaneous and unrelated to normal lactation, or it may be caused by manual expression. Such abnormal flow is usually bilateral and may be accompanied by amenorrhea.

Diagnosis
Characteristic clinical features and the patient history (including drug and sex histories) confirm galactorrhea.

Laboratory tests to help determine the cause include measurement of serum levels of prolactin, cortisol, thyroid-stimulating hormone, triiodothyronine, and thyroxine. A computed tomography scan and, possibly, mammography may also be indicated.

Treatment
Treatment varies according to the underlying cause and ranges from simple avoidance of precipitating exogenous factors such as drugs to treatment of tumors with surgery, radiation, or chemotherapy.

Therapy for idiopathic galactorrhea depends on whether the patient plans to have more children. If they do, treatment usually consists of bromocriptine or cabergoline; if they don't oral estrogens such as ethinyl estradiol and progestins such as progesterone effectively treat this disorder. Idiopathic galactorrhea may recur after discontinuation of drug therapy.

Special considerations
♦ Watch for CNS abnormalities, such as headache, failing vision, and dizziness.

◆ Maintain adequate fluid intake, especially if the patient has a fever. However, advise the patient to avoid tea, coffee, and certain tranquilizers that may aggravate engorgement.

◆ Instruct the patient to keep their breasts and nipples clean.

◆ Tell the patient who's taking bromocriptine to report nausea, vomiting, dyspepsia, appetite loss, dizziness, fatigue, numbness, and hypotension. To prevent GI upset, advise them to eat small meals frequently and to take this drug with dry toast or crackers. After treatment with bromocriptine, milk secretion usually stops in 1 to 2 months, and menstruation recurs after 6 to 24 weeks.

Hemolytic diseases of the neonate

HYPERBILIRUBINEMIA

Untreated, severe hyperbilirubinemia may result in kernicterus, a neurologic syndrome resulting from deposition of unconjugated bilirubin in the brain cells and characterized by severe neurologic symptoms. Survivors may develop cerebral palsy, epilepsy, or mental retardation or have only minor sequelae, such as perceptual-motor handicaps and learning disorders.

Causes and incidence (See *Causes of hyperbilirubinemia.*)

◆ Prematurity
◆ Rh factor hemolytic disease
◆ ABO incompatibility
◆ Jaundice associated with G6PD deficiency
◆ Birth injury

About 60% to 70% of neonates will develop hyperbilirubinemia during the first week of life. About 8% to 9% will develop severe hyperbilirubinemia (total serum bilirubin > 95th percentile). Incidence is higher in East Asians and American-Indians, and lower in African Americans. The risk for neonatal hyperbilirubinemia is higher in males.

Pathophysiology

Hyperbilirubinemia, also called *neonatal jaundice*, is the result of hemolytic processes in the neonate. It's marked by elevated serum bilirubin levels and mild jaundice and can be physiologic (with jaundice the only symptom) or pathologic (resulting from an underlying disease). Physiologic jaundice tends to be more common and more severe in certain ethnic groups (Chinese, Japanese, Koreans, Native Americans), whose mean peak of unconjugated bilirubin is about twice that of the rest of the population. Physiologic jaundice is self-limiting; the prognosis for pathologic jaundice varies, depending on the cause.

As erythrocytes break down at the end of their neonatal life cycle, hemoglobin (Hb) separates into globin (protein) and heme (iron) fragments. Heme fragments form unconjugated (indirect) bilirubin, which binds with albumin for transport to liver cells to conjugate with glucuronide, forming direct bilirubin. Because unconjugated bilirubin is fat-soluble and can't be excreted in the urine or bile, it may escape to extravascular tissue, especially fatty tissue and the brain, resulting in hyperbilirubinemia.

This pathophysiologic process may develop when:

◆ certain factors disrupt conjugation and usurp albumin-binding sites, including drugs (such as aspirin, tranquilizers, and sulfonamides) and conditions (such as hypothermia, anoxia, hypoglycemia, and hypoalbuminemia)

◆ decreased hepatic function results in reduced bilirubin conjugation

◆ increased erythrocyte production or breakdown results from hemolytic disorders, or Rh or ABO incompatibility

◆ biliary obstruction or hepatitis results in blockage of normal bile flow

◆ maternal enzymes present in breast milk inhibit the neonate's glucuronyl-transferase conjugating activity (See *Causes of hyperbilirubinemia*, page 1070.)

Complications

◆ Cerebral palsy
◆ Deafness
◆ Kernicterus

Signs and symptoms

The primary sign of hyperbilirubinemia is jaundice, which doesn't become clinically apparent until serum bilirubin levels reach about 7 mg/dL. Physiologic jaundice develops 24 hours after delivery in 50% of term neonates (usually day 2 to day 3) and 48 hours after delivery in 80% of premature neonates (usually day 3 to day 5). It generally disappears by day 7 in term neonates and by day 10 in premature neonates. Throughout physiologic jaundice, serum unconjugated bilirubin levels don't exceed 12 mg/dL. Pathologic jaundice may appear anytime after the first day of life and persists beyond 7 days with serum bilirubin levels greater than 12 mg/dL in a term neonate, 15 mg/dL in a premature neonate, or increasing more than 5 mg/dL in 24 hours.

Diagnosis

℞ **CONFIRMING DIAGNOSIS** *Jaundice and elevated levels of serum bilirubin confirm the diagnosis of hyperbilirubinemia.*

Causes of hyperbilirubinemia

The neonate's age at onset of hyperbilirubinemia may provide clues to the sources of this jaundice-causing disorder.

Day 1
♦ Blood type incompatibility (Rh, ABO, other minor blood groups)
♦ Intrauterine infection (rubella, cytomegalic inclusion body disease, toxoplasmosis, syphilis and, occasionally, bacteria such as *E. coli, Staphylococcus, Pseudomonas, Klebsiella, Proteus,* and *Streptococcus*)

Day 2 or 3
♦ Infection (usually from gram-negative bacteria)
♦ Polycythemia
♦ Enclosed hemorrhage (skin bruises, subdural hematoma)
♦ Respiratory distress syndrome (hyaline membrane disease)
♦ Heinz body anemia from drugs and toxins (vitamin K_3, sodium nitrate)
♦ Transient neonatal hyperbilirubinemia

♦ Abnormal RBC morphology
♦ Red cell enzyme deficiencies (glucose-6-phosphate dehydrogenase, hexokinase)
♦ Physiologic jaundice
♦ Blood group incompatibilities

Days 4 and 5
♦ Breastfeeding, respiratory distress syndrome, maternal diabetes
♦ Crigler–Najjar syndrome (congenital nonhemolytic icterus)
♦ Gilbert syndrome

Days 7 and later
♦ Herpes simplex
♦ Pyloric stenosis
♦ Hypothyroidism
♦ Neonatal giant cell hepatitis
♦ Infection (usually acquired in neonatal period)
♦ Bile duct atresia
♦ Galactosemia
♦ Choledochal cyst

Inspection of the neonate in a well-lit room (without yellow or gold lighting) reveals yellowish skin coloration, particularly in the sclerae. Jaundice can be verified by pressing the skin on the cheek or abdomen lightly with one finger, then releasing pressure and observing skin color immediately. Signs of jaundice necessitate measuring and charting serum bilirubin levels every 4 hours. Testing may include direct and indirect bilirubin levels, particularly for pathologic jaundice. Bilirubin levels that are excessively elevated or vary daily suggest a pathologic process.

Identifying the underlying cause of hyperbilirubinemia requires a detailed patient history (including prenatal history), family history (paternal Rh factor, inherited red cell defects), present neonate status (immaturity, infection), and blood testing of the neonate and mother (blood group incompatibilities, Hb levels, direct Coombs' test, hematocrit).

Treatment

Depending on the underlying cause, treatment may include phototherapy, exchange transfusions, albumin infusion and, possibly, drug therapy. Phototherapy is the treatment of choice for physiologic jaundice, and pathologic jaundice due to erythroblastosis fetalis (after the initial exchange transfusion). Phototherapy uses fluorescent light to decompose bilirubin in the skin by oxidation and is usually discontinued after bilirubin levels

fall below 10 mg/dL and continue to decrease for 24 hours. However, phototherapy is rarely the only treatment for jaundice due to a pathologic cause.

An exchange transfusion replaces the neonate's blood with fresh blood (<48 hours old), removing some of the unconjugated bilirubin in serum. Possible indications for exchange transfusions include hydrops fetalis, polycythemia, erythroblastosis fetalis, marked reticulocytosis, drug toxicity, and jaundice that develops within the first 6 hours after birth.

Other therapy for excessive bilirubin levels may include albumin administration (1 g/kg of 25% salt-poor albumin), which provides additional albumin for binding unconjugated bilirubin. This may be done 1 to 2 hours before exchange or as a substitute for a portion of the plasma in the transfused blood.

Drug therapy, which is rare, usually consists of phenobarbital administered to the pregnant person before delivery and to the neonate several days after delivery. This drug stimulates the hepatic glucuronide-conjugating system.

Special considerations

♦ Assess and record the neonate's jaundice, and note the time it began. Report the jaundice and serum bilirubin levels immediately.
♦ Reassure parents that most neonates experience some degree of jaundice. Explain hyperbilirubinemia, its causes, diagnostic

tests, and treatment. Also, explain that the neonate's stool contains some bile and may be greenish.

For the neonate receiving phototherapy:

◆ Keep a record of how long each bilirubin light bulb is in use because these bulbs require frequent changing for optimum effectiveness.

◆ Undress the neonate, so their entire body surface is exposed to the light rays. Keep them 18″ to 30″ (46 to 76 cm) from the light source. Protect their eyes with shields that filter the light.

◆ Monitor and maintain the neonate's body temperature; high and low temperatures predispose him to kernicterus. Remove the neonate from the light source every 3 to 4 hours and take off the eye shields. Allow their parents to visit and feed them.

◆ The neonate usually shows a decrease in serum bilirubin level 1 to 12 hours after the start of phototherapy. When the neonate's bilirubin level is less than 10 mg/dL and has been decreasing for 24 hours, discontinue phototherapy as ordered. Resume therapy, as ordered, if serum bilirubin increases several milligrams per deciliter, as it often does because of a rebound effect.

For the exchange transfusions:

◆ Prepare the neonate warmer and tray before the transfusion. Try to keep the neonate quiet. Give them nothing by mouth for 3 to 4 hours before the procedure.

◆ Check the blood to be used for the exchange—type, Rh, age. Keep emergency equipment (resuscitative and intubation equipment, and oxygen) available. During the procedure, monitor respiratory and heart rates every 15 minutes; check the neonate's temperature every 30 minutes. Continue to monitor vital signs every 15 to 30 minutes for 2 hours.

◆ Measure intake and output. Observe for cord bleeding and complications, such as hemorrhage, hypocalcemia, sepsis, and shock. Report serum bilirubin and Hb levels. Bilirubin levels may rise, as a result of a rebound effect, within 30 minutes after transfusion, necessitating repeat transfusions.

▓▓▓▓ PREVENTION

◆ *Advise your patient to maintain oral intake and to not skip meals, because fasting stimulates the conversion of heme to bilirubin.*

◆ *Administer Rh$_o$(D) immunoglobulin (human), as indicated, to an Rh-negative person after amniocentesis, or—to prevent hemolytic disease in subsequent children—to an Rh-negative person during the third trimester, after the birth of an Rh-positive neonate, or after spontaneous or elective abortion.*

ERYTHROBLASTOSIS FETALIS

Causes and incidence

Although more than 60 red cell antigens can stimulate antibody formation, erythroblastosis fetalis usually results from Rh isoimmunization—a condition that develops in about 7% of all pregnancies in the United States. Before the development of Rh$_o$(D) immunoglobulin, this condition was an important cause of kernicterus and neonatal death. (See *ABO incompatibility*, page 1072.)

Pathophysiology

Erythroblastosis fetalis, a hemolytic disease of the fetus and neonate, stems from an incompatibility of fetal and maternal blood, resulting in maternal antibody activity against fetal red cells. Intrauterine transfusions can save 40% of fetuses with erythroblastosis. However, in severe, untreated erythroblastosis fetalis, the prognosis is poor, especially if kernicterus develops. About 70% of these neonates die, usually within the first week of life; survivors inevitably develop pronounced neurologic damage—sensory impairment, mental deficiencies, and cerebral palsy. Severely affected fetuses that develop hydrops fetalis (the most severe form of this disorder, associated with profound anemia and edema) are commonly stillborn; even if they're delivered live, they rarely survive longer than a few hours.

During their first pregnancy, an Rh-negative female-bodied person becomes sensitized (during delivery or abortion) by exposure to Rh-positive fetal blood antigens inherited from the sperm-donating parent. A female-bodied person may also become sensitized from receiving blood transfusions with alien Rh antigens, causing agglutinins to develop; from inadequate doses of Rh$_o$(D); or from failure to receive Rh$_o$(D) after significant fetal–maternal leakage from abruptio placentae. Subsequent pregnancy with an Rh-positive fetus provokes increasing amounts of maternal agglutinating antibodies to cross the placental barrier, attach to Rh-positive cells in the fetus, and cause hemolysis and anemia. To compensate for this, the fetus steps up the production of RBCs, and erythroblasts (immature RBCs) appear in the fetal circulation. Extensive hemolysis results in the release of large amounts of unconjugated bilirubin, which the liver is unable to conjugate and excrete, causing hyperbilirubinemia and hemolytic anemia. (See *What happens in Rh isoimmunization*, page 1073.)

Complications

◆ Cerebral palsy
◆ Kernicterus
◆ Mental deficiencies
◆ Sensory impairment

ABO incompatibility

ABO incompatibility, a form of fetomaternal incompatibility, occurs between pregnant person and fetus in about 25% of all pregnancies, with highest incidence among Blacks. In about 1% of this number, it leads to hemolytic disease of the neonate. Although ABO incompatibility is more common than Rh isoimmunization, it's less severe. Low antigenicity of fetal or neonatal ABO factors may account for the milder clinical effects.

Each blood group has specific antigens on RBCs and specific antibodies in serum. Maternal antibodies form against fetal cells when blood groups differ. Neonates with group A blood, born of group O mothers, account for approximately 50% of all ABO incompatibilities. Unlike Rh isoimmunization, which always follows sensitization in a previous pregnancy, ABO incompatibility is likely to develop in a firstborn neonate.

Blood group	Antigens on RBCs	Antibodies in serum	Most common incompatible groups
A	A	Anti-B	Mother A, neonate B or AB
B	B	Anti-A	Mother B, neonate A or AB
AB	A and B	No antibodies	Mother AB, neonate (no incompatibility)
O	No antigens	Anti-A and anti-B	Mother O, neonate A or B

Clinical effects of ABO incompatibility include jaundice, which usually appears in the neonate in 24 to 48 hours, mild anemia, and mild hepatosplenomegaly.

Diagnosis is based on clinical symptoms in the neonate, the presence of ABO incompatibility, a weak to moderate positive Coombs' test, and elevated serum bilirubin levels. Cord hemoglobin and indirect bilirubin levels indicate the need for an exchange transfusion. This type of transfusion is done with blood of the same group and Rh type as that of the postpartum person. Because infants with ABO incompatibility respond so well to phototherapy, an exchange transfusion is seldom necessary.

Signs and symptoms

Jaundice usually isn't present at birth but may appear as soon as 30 minutes later or within 24 hours. The mildly affected neonate shows mild to moderate hepatosplenomegaly and pallor. In severely affected neonates who survive birth, erythroblastosis fetalis usually produces pallor, edema, petechiae, hepatosplenomegaly, grunting respirations, pulmonary crackles, poor muscle tone, neurologic unresponsiveness, possible heart murmurs, a bile-stained umbilical cord, and yellow or meconium-stained amniotic fluid. About 10% of untreated neonates develop kernicterus from hemolytic disease and show symptoms such as anemia, lethargy, poor sucking ability, retracted head, stiff limbs, squinting, a high-pitched cry, and seizures.

Hydrops fetalis causes extreme hemolysis, fetal hypoxia, heart failure (with possible pericardial effusion and circulatory collapse), edema (ranging from mild peripheral edema to anasarca), peritoneal and pleural effusions (with dyspnea and pulmonary crackles), and green- or brown-tinged amniotic fluid (usually indicating a stillbirth).

Other distinctive characteristics of the neonate with hydrops fetalis include enlarged placenta, marked pallor, hepatosplenomegaly, cardiomegaly, and ascites. Petechiae and widespread ecchymoses are present in severe cases, indicating concurrent disseminated intravascular coagulation. This disorder retards intrauterine growth, so the neonate's lungs, kidneys, brain, and thymus are small, and despite edema, their body size is smaller than that of neonates of comparable gestational age.

Diagnosis

Diagnostic evaluation takes into account both prenatal and neonatal findings:
♦ maternal history (for erythroblastosis stillbirths, abortions, previously affected children, previous anti-Rh titers)
♦ blood typing and screening (titers should be taken frequently to determine changes in the degree of maternal immunization)
♦ paternal blood test (for Rh, blood group, and Rh zygosity)
♦ history of blood transfusion

In addition, amniotic fluid analysis may show an increase in bilirubin (indicating possible hemolysis) and anti-Rh titers. Radiologic studies may show edema and, in hydrops fetalis, the halo sign (edematous, elevated,

PATHOPHYSIOLOGY
What happens in Rh isoimmunization

Rh isoimmunization occurs when a pregnant person who's Rh-negative develops antibodies against an Rh-positive fetus, as shown below.

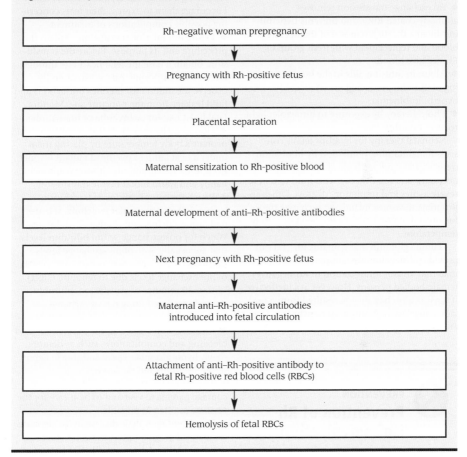

subcutaneous fat layers) and the Buddha position (fetus' legs are crossed).

Neonatal findings indicating erythroblastosis fetalis include:
◆ direct Coombs' test of umbilical cord blood to measure RBC (Rh-positive) antibodies in the neonate (positive only when the mother is Rh-negative and the fetus is Rh-positive)
◆ decreased cord hemoglobin (Hb) level (<10 g), signaling severe disease
◆ many nucleated peripheral RBCs

Treatment
Treatment depends on the degree of maternal sensitization and hemolytic disease's effects on the fetus or neonate.

◆ Percutaneous umbilical cord sampling allows for assessment of fetal well-being and direct transfusion, if necessary.
◆ An intrauterine-intraperitoneal transfusion is performed when amniotic fluid analysis suggests the fetus is severely affected and delivery is inappropriate because of fetal immaturity. A transabdominal puncture under fluoroscopy into the fetal peritoneal cavity allows infusion of group O, Rh-negative blood. This may be repeated every 2 weeks until the fetus is mature enough for delivery. Some facilities can perform percutaneous umbilical blood sampling to provide transfusion.
◆ Planned delivery is usually done 2 to 4 weeks before term date, depending on maternal

history, serologic tests, and amniocentesis; labor may be induced from the 34th to 38th week of gestation. During labor, the fetus should be monitored electronically; capillary blood scalp sampling determines acid–base balance. Any indication of fetal distress necessitates immediate cesarean delivery.

◆ An exchange transfusion removes antibody-coated RBCs and prevents hyperbilirubinemia through removal of the neonate's blood and replacement with fresh group O, Rh-negative blood.

◆ Albumin infusion aids in the binding of bilirubin, reducing the chances of hyperbilirubinemia.

◆ Phototherapy by exposure to ultraviolet light reduces bilirubin levels.

Neonatal therapy for hydrops fetalis consists of maintaining ventilation by intubation, oxygenation, and mechanical assistance, when necessary, and removal of excess fluid to relieve severe ascites and respiratory distress. Other appropriate measures include an exchange transfusion and maintenance of the neonate's body temperature.

Gamma globulin that contains $Rh_o(D)$ can provide passive immunization, which prevents maternal Rh isoimmunization in Rh-negative female-bodied persons. However, it's ineffective if sensitization has already resulted from a previous pregnancy, abortion, or transfusion. (See *Prevention of Rh isoimmunization.*)

PREVENTION

Prevention of Rh isoimmunization

Administering $Rh_o(D)$ immune human globulin to an unsensitized Rh-negative pregnant person at 28 weeks' gestation and immediately after the birth of an Rh-positive neonate or after a spontaneous or elective abortion prevents complications in later pregnancies.

The following patients should be screened for Rh isoimmunization or irregular antibodies:

◆ all Rh-negative pregnant persons during their first prenatal visit and at 28 weeks' gestation

◆ all Rh-positive pregnant persons with histories of transfusion, a jaundiced baby, stillbirth, cesarean birth, induced abortion, placenta previa, or abruptio placentae

Special considerations

Structure the care plan around close maternal and fetal observation, explanations of diagnostic tests and therapeutic measures, and emotional support.

◆ Reassure the parents that they aren't to blame for having a child with erythroblastosis fetalis. Encourage them to express their fears concerning possible complications of treatment.

◆ Before intrauterine transfusion, explain the procedure and its purpose. Before the transfusion, obtain a baseline fetal heart rate through electronic monitoring. Afterward, carefully observe the mother for uterine contractions and fluid leakage from the puncture site. Monitor fetal heart rate for tachycardia or bradycardia.

◆ During exchange transfusion, maintain the neonate's body temperature by placing them under a heat lamp or overhead radiant warmer. Keep resuscitative and monitoring equipment handy and warm blood before transfusion.

◆ Watch for complications of transfusion, such as lethargy, muscular twitching, seizures, dark urine, edema, and change in vital signs. Watch for postexchange serum bilirubin levels that are usually 50% of pre-exchange levels (although these levels may rise to 70% to 80% of pre-exchange levels due to rebound effect). Within 30 minutes of transfusion, bilirubin may rebound, requiring repeat exchange transfusions.

◆ Measure intake and output. Observe for cord bleeding and complications, such as hemorrhage, hypocalcemia, sepsis, and shock. Report serum bilirubin and Hb levels.

◆ To promote normal parental bonding, encourage parents to visit and to help care for the neonate as often as possible.

◆ To prevent hemolytic disease in the neonate, evaluate all pregnant persons for possible Rh incompatibility. Administer $Rh_o(D)$ I.M., as ordered, to all Rh-negative, antibody-negative females following transfusion reaction or ectopic pregnancy, or during the second and third trimesters to patients with abruptio placentae, placenta previa, or amniocentesis.

SELECTED REFERENCES

American Psychiatric Association. (2013). *Diagnostic and statistical manual of mental disorders* (5th ed.). Arlington, VA: Author.

Brander, E. A., & McQuillan, S. K. (2018). Prepubertal vulvovaginitis. *CMAJ: Canadian Medical Association Journal, 190*(26), E800. doi:10.1503/cmaj.180004

Davey, M. A., & Gibson, K. L. (2018). Intrapartum care factors associated with adverse early breastfeeding problems. *Journal of Paediatrics & Child Health, 54*, 16. doi:10.1111/jpc.13882_35

Holloway, D. (2014). Causes of post-menopausal bleeding. *Practice Nursing, 25*(12), 602–605.

Sandler, S. G., & Queenan, J. T. (2017). A guide to terminology for Rh immunoprophylaxis. *Obstetrics & Gynecology, 130*(3), 633–635.

Simmons, D. P., & Savage, W. J. (2015). Hemolysis from ABO incompatibility. *Hematology/Oncology Clinics of North America, 29*(3), 429–443. doi:10.1016/j .hoc.2015.01.003

The North American Menopause Society. (2017). *The 2017 hormone therapy position statement of The North American Menopause Society.* Retrieved from https://www .menopause.org/docs/default-source/2017/ nams-2017-hormone-therapy-position-statement.pdf

Zhang, Y., et al. (2018). "The Therapy of Elimination First" for early acute mastitis: A systematic review and meta-analysis. *Evidence-Based Complementary & Alternative Medicine (Ecam), 2018,* 1–12. doi:10.1155/2018/8059256

20

SEXUAL DISORDERS

Introduction

Sexuality is an integral human function that's inevitably affected by many interrelated factors. Its expression reflects the interaction of the biologic, psychological, and sociologic ingredients that affect a person's self-image and behavior.

Depending on these complex factors, human sexuality can be healthy and enriching, or it can be the source of mental and physical distress. A sexually healthy person is commonly defined as a person who:
◆ exhibits behavior that agrees with gender identity can participate in mutually consensual and emotionally mature relationships
◆ finds erotic stimulation pleasurable
◆ can make decisions about sexual behavior that are compatible with their values and beliefs

HAZARDS TO SEXUAL HEALTH

An important group of sex-related disorders results from infection that's transmitted through sexual contact. These disorders include human immunodeficiency virus (HIV) infection, gonorrhea, syphilis, chlamydial infections, genital herpes, genital warts, trichomoniasis, chancroid, and lymphogranuloma venereum (LGV). Sexually transmitted infections (STIs) are among the most prevalent infections around the world; gonorrhea, chlamydial infections, and genital warts are approaching epidemic proportions in the United States.

Sexual dysfunction disorders, including arousal disorders, orgasmic disorders, erectile dysfunction, and sexual pain disorders (dyspareunia and vaginismus), may be caused by a general medical condition, psychological factors, or a combination of factors, or they may be substance induced. Other disorders have a definite physical etiology.

Gender identity disorders and paraphilias are sexual disorders whose diagnostic criteria are found in the *Diagnostic and Statistical Manual of Mental Disorders*, Fifth Edition, Text Revision.

PHYSICAL ASSESSMENT

Physical assessment, primarily a diagnostic tool, can also serve as an excellent opportunity for patient teaching.
◆ During examination of the female-bodied person, evaluate breast development, pubic hair distribution, and the development of external genitalia. With gloved hands, use a speculum to examine internal genitalia, including the cervix and vagina. Palpate the uterus and ovaries.

⬡ **ELDER TIP** *Take special care when examining an older female-bodied person because atrophic changes of the vaginal mucosa may increase their discomfort during a pelvic examination. Use a small speculum because of the decreased vaginal size. To ease insertion, dampen the speculum with warm water or use a small amount of lubricant; copious lubricant may alter Papanicolaou test results. Proceed slowly; abrupt insertion of the speculum may damage sensitive degenerating tissue.*
◆ During examination of the male-bodied persons, check pubic and axillary hair distribution. With a gloved hand, palpate the penis, scrotum,

prostate gland, and rectum. Inspect the penis (shaft, glans, and urethral meatus) for lesions, swelling, inflammation, scars, or discharge. In the uncircumcised male-bodied persons, retract the foreskin to visualize the glans. Examine the scrotum for size, shape, and abnormalities, such as nodules or inflammation. Check for the presence of both testes (the left testis is typically lower than the right) and testicular volume.

ELDER TIP *The testes of an older male-bodied persons may be slightly smaller than those of a younger male-bodied persons, but they should be equal in size, smooth, freely moveable, and soft without nodules.*

◆ Inspect and palpate the inguinal canal; you shouldn't observe any bulging of tissues or organs. (See *Male sexual anatomy.*)

SEXUAL HISTORY

Careful assessment helps identify the cause of a sexual problem as psychological or physical. A sexual history provides the basis for prevention, diagnosis, and treatment.

◆ Ensure privacy, as for physical assessment. Allow sufficient time so that the patient doesn't feel rushed.

◆ Approach a sexual history objectively. Remember, sexual health is relative; avoid making assumptions or judgments about the patient's sexual activities.

◆ After listening to the patient, determine their level of sexual understanding and phrase your questions in language that they can understand. Avoid technical terms.

◆ Begin with the least threatening questions. Usually, a menstrual or urologic history helps lead into a sexual history.

◆ Inquire about what the patient accepts as normal sexual behavior. Ask about sexual needs and priorities and whether the patient can discuss them with sex partners.

◆ Assess risk behavior concerning selection of sex partners and specific sexual practices.

◆ Ask about homosexual activity, which can influence the risk and treatment of some sexually transmitted diseases (STDs).

◆ Ask about history of sexual abuse or trauma, including rape and incest.

◆ Ask the female-bodied person patient if they have adequate lubrication during intercourse and if they have ever experienced orgasm or pain with sexual contact. Ask the male-bodied person patient if they have ever had difficulties with erection or ejaculation.

◆ Ask about desire for pregnancy within the next 12 months.

Male sexual anatomy

Pelvic structures of a male-bodied person.

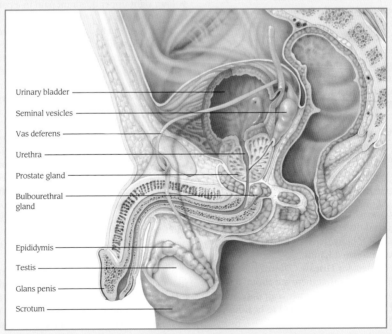

- Urinary bladder
- Seminal vesicles
- Vas deferens
- Urethra
- Prostate gland
- Bulbourethral gland
- Epididymis
- Testis
- Glans penis
- Scrotum

♦ Ask about current or past contraceptive practices.
♦ Try to use the history therapeutically by encouraging the patient to express anxiety. Such fears may be alleviated simply by providing factual information and answering questions.

TYPES OF SEX THERAPY

Sex therapy can be a vital therapeutic tool for treating sexual dysfunction. Before therapy begins, a history, a physical examination, and appropriate treatment must rule out organic causes of sexual dysfunction. The major forms of sex therapy include psychoanalysis, behavioral therapy, group therapy, classic (Masters and Johnson) therapy, and Kaplan's sex therapy. The type of therapy appropriate for the patient depends on their problems, needs, and finances.

Sexually transmitted diseases/infections

GONORRHEA

A common STD, gonorrhea is an infection of the genitourinary (GU) tract (especially the urethra and cervix) and, occasionally, the rectum, pharynx, and eyes. Untreated gonorrhea can spread through the blood to the joints, tendons, meninges, and endocardium; in female-bodied persons, it can also lead to chronic pelvic inflammatory disease (PID) and sterility. After adequate treatment, the prognosis for both male-bodied persons and female-bodied persons is excellent, although reinfection is common. Gonorrhea is especially prevalent among young people and people with multiple partners, particularly those between ages 15 and 29. In these patients concomitant chlamydia infection is likely.

Causes and incidence

Transmission of *Neisseria gonorrhoeae*, the organism that causes gonorrhea, usually follows sexual contact with an infected person. Children born of infected pregnant persons can contract gonococcal ophthalmia neonatorum during passage through the birth canal. Children and adults with gonorrhea can contract gonococcal conjunctivitis by touching their eyes with contaminated hands.

The Centers for Disease Control and Prevention estimates that there are about 700,000 new cases of gonorrhea each year; only about half of these cases are reported to healthcare officials.

Complications
♦ Conjunctivitis
♦ Dermatitis
♦ Epididymitis
♦ Perihepatitis
♦ Proctitis
♦ Salpingitis
♦ Septic arthritis

Signs and symptoms

Although many infected male-bodied persons may be asymptomatic, after a 3- to 6-day incubation period, some develop symptoms of urethritis, including dysuria and purulent urethral discharge, with redness and swelling at the infection site. Most infected female-bodied persons remain asymptomatic but may develop inflammation and a greenish-yellow discharge from the cervix—the most common gonorrheal symptoms in female-bodied persons. (See *What happens in gonorrhea*, page 1079.)

Other clinical features vary according to the site involved:
♦ *urethra*: dysuria, urinary frequency and incontinence, purulent discharge, itching, and red and edematous meatus
♦ *vulva*: occasional itching, burning, and pain due to exudate from an adjacent infected area (symptoms tend to be more severe before puberty or after menopause)
♦ *vagina* (most common site in children older than age 1): engorgement, redness, swelling, and profuse purulent discharge
♦ *liver*: right upper quadrant pain in a patient with perihepatitis
♦ *pelvis*: severe pelvic and lower abdominal pain, muscle rigidity, tenderness, and abdominal distention. As the infection spreads, nausea, vomiting, fever, and tachycardia may develop in a patient with salpingitis or PID

Other possible symptoms include pharyngitis, tonsillitis, rectal burning and itching, and bloody mucopurulent discharge.

Gonococcal septicemia is more common in female-bodied persons than in male-bodied persons. Its characteristic signs include tender papillary skin lesions on the hands and feet; these lesions may be pustular, hemorrhagic, or necrotic. Gonococcal septicemia may also produce migratory polyarthralgia and polyarthritis and tenosynovitis of the wrists, fingers, knees, or ankles. Untreated septic arthritis leads to progressive joint destruction.

Signs of gonococcal ophthalmia neonatorum include lid edema, bilateral conjunctival infection, and abundant purulent discharge 2 to 3 days after birth. Adult conjunctivitis, most common in men, causes unilateral conjunctival

PATHOPHYSIOLOGY
What happens in gonorrhea

After exposure to *N. gonorrhoeae*, the epithelial cells at the infection site become infected; then the disease begins to spread locally. The disease pattern depends on the individual infected and the infection site.

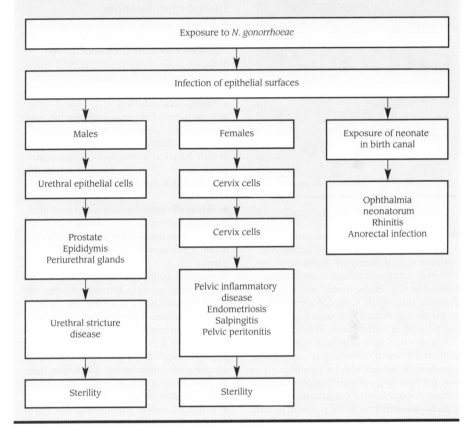

redness and swelling. Untreated gonococcal conjunctivitis can progress to corneal ulceration and blindness.

Diagnosis

CONFIRMING DIAGNOSIS *A culture from the infection site (urethra, cervix, rectum, or pharynx), grown on a Thayer–Martin or Transgrow medium, usually establishes the diagnosis by isolating* N. gonorrhoeae. *(See* Neisseria gonorrhoeae, *page 1080.) A Gram stain showing gram-negative diplococci supports the diagnosis and may be sufficient to confirm gonorrhea in male-bodied persons.*

Ligase chain reaction is an assay that can detect *N. gonorrhoeae* and *Chlamydia trachomatis*

from urethral or cervical swabs. It allows for rapid diagnosis and offers improved sensitivity and specificity compared with swab specimen cultures.

Confirmation of gonococcal arthritis requires identification of gram-negative diplococci on smears made from joint fluid and skin lesions. Complement fixation and immunofluorescent assays of serum reveal antibody titers four times the normal rate. Culture of conjunctival scrapings confirms gonococcal conjunctivitis.

Treatment

For adults and adolescents, the recommended treatment for uncomplicated gonorrhea caused

Neisseria gonorrhoeae

In gonorrhea, microscopic examination reveals gram-negative diplococcus— *N. gonorrhoeae*, the causative organism.

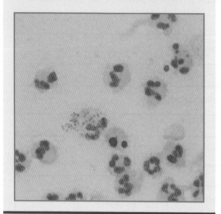

by susceptible non–penicillinase-producing *N. gonorrhoeae* is a single dose of ceftriaxone or cefixime; for presumptive treatment of concurrent *C. trachomatis* infection, doxycycline. Gonorrhea may also be treated with a single dose of azithromycin. Common alternative prescriptions may include cefuroxime, cefpodoxime proxetil, or erythromycin. A follow-up visit 7 days after treatment to recheck cultures and confirm the cure of infection is recommended, especially for women who are asymptomatic or may not have symptoms associated with the infection. A single dose of ceftriaxone and erythromycin is recommended for pregnant patients and those allergic to penicillin.

Treatment of gonococcal conjunctivitis requires a single dose of ceftriaxone, and lavage of the infected eye with saline solution once.

Routine instillation of erythromycin ointment into the neonate's eyes soon after delivery has greatly reduced the incidence of gonococcal ophthalmia neonatorum.

Special considerations

◆ Before treatment, establish whether the patient has any drug sensitivities, and watch closely for adverse drug reactions during therapy.

◆ Warn the patient that, until cultures prove negative, they are still infectious and can transmit gonococcal infection.

◆ If the patient has gonococcal arthritis, apply moist heat to ease pain in affected joints.

◆ Urge the patient to inform sexual contacts of their infection so that they can seek treatment, even if cultures are negative. Advise them to avoid sexual intercourse until treatment is complete.

◆ Report all cases of gonorrhea to local public health authorities for follow-up on sexual contacts. Examine and test all people exposed to gonorrhea as well as children of infected parents.

◆ Routinely instill erythromycin ointment in the eyes of all neonates immediately after birth. Check the neonate of an infected parent for signs of infection. Take specimens for culture from the neonate's eyes, pharynx, and rectum.

◆ To prevent gonorrhea, tell patients to avoid anyone *suspected* of being infected. Encourage use of barrier contraceptives and inform them that abstinence is the only sure way to prevent gonorrhea. (See *Preventing gonorrhea*.)

◆ Report all cases of gonorrhea in children to child abuse authorities.

PREVENTION

Preventing gonorrhea

To prevent gonorrhea, teach your patient the following:

◆ Tell the patient to avoid sexual contact until test cultures are negative and infection is gone.

◆ Advise partners of an infected person to be treated even if partners don't have a positive culture. Recommend that partners avoid sexual contact with anyone until treatment is complete because reinfection is very common.

◆ Advise the patient and all sexual partners to be tested for HIV and hepatitis B infection.

◆ Tell the patient to take anti-infective drugs for the length of time prescribed.

◆ To prevent reinfection, tell the patient to avoid sexual contact with anyone suspected of being infected, to use condoms during intercourse, to wash genitalia with soap and water before and after intercourse, and to avoid sharing washcloths or using douches.

◆ Advise the patient to return for follow-up testing.

Lymphogranuloma venereum

A rare disease in the United States, lymphogranuloma venereum (LGV) is caused by serovars L_1, L_2, or L_3 of C. trachomatis. The most common clinical manifestation of LGV among heterosexuals, especially male-bodied persons is enlarged inguinal lymph nodes (usually unilateral). These nodes may become fluctuant, tender masses. Regional nodes draining the initial lesion may enlarge and appear as a series of bilateral buboes. Untreated buboes may rupture and form sinus tracts that discharge a thick, yellow, granular secretion.

Female-bodied persons and homosexually active male-bodied persons may have proctocolitis or inflammatory involvement of perirectal or perianal lymphatic tissues, resulting in fistulas and strictures.

By the time most patients seek treatment, the self-limited genital ulcer that sometimes occurs at the inoculation site is no longer present. The diagnosis usually is made serologically and by excluding other causes of inguinal lymphadenopathy or genital ulcers.

The treatment of choice is doxycycline. Treatment cures infection and prevents ongoing tissue damage, although the patient may develop a scar or an indurated inguinal mass. Buboes may require aspiration or incision and drainage through intact skin.

CHLAMYDIAL INFECTIONS

Untreated, chlamydial infections can lead to complications such as acute epididymitis, salpingitis, PID and, eventually, sterility. Some studies show that a chlamydial infection in a pregnant person is associated with spontaneous abortion and premature delivery.

Causes and incidence

Transmission of C. trachomatis primarily follows vaginal or rectal intercourse or orogenital contact with an infected person. Because symptoms of chlamydial infections commonly appear late in the disease's course, sexual transmission of the organism typically occurs unknowingly. Children born of mothers who have chlamydial infections may contract associated conjunctivitis, otitis media, and pneumonia during passage through the birth canal.

Chlamydial infections are the most common STDs in the United States, affecting an estimated 4 million people in the United States each year.

Pathophysiology

Chlamydial infections—including urethritis in male-bodied persons and urethritis and cervicitis in female-bodied persons—are a group of infections that are linked to one organism: C. trachomatis. Trachoma inclusion conjunctivitis, a chlamydial infection that seldom occurs in the United States, is a leading cause of blindness in Third World countries. LGV, a rare disease in the United States, is also caused by C. trachomatis. (See *Lymphogranuloma venereum*.)

Complications
- Epididymitis
- Neonatal death
- Pelvic inflammatory disease
- Premature rupture of membranes
- Preterm delivery
- Salpingitis
- Spontaneous abortion
- Sterility

Signs and symptoms

Both male-bodied persons and female-bodied persons with chlamydial infections may be asymptomatic or may show signs of infection on physical examination. Individual signs and symptoms vary with the specific type of chlamydial infection and are determined by the organism's route of transmission to susceptible tissue.

A person with cervicitis may develop cervical erosion, mucopurulent discharge, pelvic pain, and dyspareunia.

A person with endometritis or salpingitis may experience signs of PID, such as pain and tenderness of the abdomen, cervix, uterus, and lymph nodes; chills; fever; breakthrough bleeding; bleeding after intercourse; and vaginal discharge. They may also have dysuria.

A person with urethral syndrome may experience dysuria, pyuria, and urinary frequency.

A person with urethritis may experience dysuria, erythema, tenderness of the urethral meatus, urinary frequency, pruritus, and clear urethral discharge. In urethritis, such discharge may be copious and purulent or scant and clear or mucoid.

A person with epididymitis may experience painful scrotal swelling and urethral discharge.

A person with prostatitis may have lower back pain, urinary frequency, dysuria, nocturia, and painful ejaculation.

A person with proctitis may have diarrhea, tenesmus, pruritus, bloody or mucopurulent discharge, and diffuse or discrete ulceration in the rectosigmoid colon.

Diagnosis

A swab from the site of infection (urethra, cervix, or rectum) establishes a diagnosis of urethritis, cervicitis, salpingitis, endometritis, or proctitis. A culture of aspirated material establishes a diagnosis of epididymitis.

Antigen detection methods, including the enzyme-linked immunosorbent assay and the direct fluorescent antibody test, have long been used for identifying chlamydial infection. Tissue cell cultures, however, are more sensitive and specific. Newer nucleic acid probes using polymerase chain reactions are also commercially available and have become the diagnostic tests of choice.

Treatment

The recommended first-line treatment for adults and adolescents who have chlamydial infections is drug therapy with tetracycline, erythromycin, or azithromycin.

For pregnant people with chlamydial infections, erythromycin (stearate base) or azithromycin may be used.

Special considerations

◆ Practice standard precautions when caring for a patient with a chlamydial infection.
◆ Make sure that the patient fully understands the dosage requirements of prescribed medications for this infection.
◆ Stress the importance of completing the entire course of drug therapy even after the symptoms subside.
◆ Teach the patient to follow meticulous personal hygiene measures as recommended.
◆ Urge the patient to inform sexual contacts of their infection so that they can receive appropriate treatment.
◆ If required in your state, report all cases of chlamydial infection to the appropriate local public health authorities, who will then conduct follow-up notification of the patient's sexual contacts.
◆ Suggest that the patient and their sex partners receive testing for the HIV.
◆ Ask the patient to return for follow-up testing.
◆ Check the neonate of an infected parent for signs of chlamydial infection. Obtain appropriate specimens for diagnostic testing.

PREVENTION
◆ *To prevent eye contamination, tell the patient to avoid touching any discharge and to wash and dry their hands thoroughly before touching their eyes.*
◆ *To prevent reinfection during treatment, urge the patient to abstain from sexual intercourse until they and their partners are free of infection.*

GENITAL HERPES

Causes and incidence

Genital herpes is usually caused by infection with herpes simplex virus type 2, but some studies report increasing incidence of infection with herpes simplex virus type 1. This disease is typically transmitted through sexual intercourse, orogenital sexual activity, kissing, and hand-to-body contact. Pregnant people may transmit the infection to neonates during vaginal delivery if an active infection is present. Such transmitted infection may be localized (for instance, in the eyes) or disseminated and may be associated with central nervous system involvement.

An estimated 86 million people worldwide are thought to have genital herpes.

Pathophysiology

Genital herpes is an acute inflammatory disease of the genitalia. The prognosis varies, depending on the patient's age, the strength of their immune defenses, and the infection site. Primary genital herpes is usually self-limiting but may cause painful local or systemic disease. (See *Understanding the genital herpes cycle*, page 1083.) In neonates and patients who are immunocompromised, such as those with acquired immunodeficiency syndrome, genital herpes is usually severe, resulting in complications and a high mortality rate.

Complications

General
◆ Increased risk of contracting other STDs

During pregnancy
◆ Neonatal brain damage
◆ Neonatal blindness

Signs and symptoms

After a 3- to 7-day incubation period, fluid-filled vesicles appear, usually on the cervix (the primary infection site) and possibly on the labia, perianal skin, vulva, or vagina of the female-bodied persons and on the glans penis, foreskin, or penile shaft of the male-bodied person. Extragenital lesions may appear on the mouth or anus. In both male and female-bodied persons the vesicles, usually painless at first, will rupture and develop into extensive, shallow, painful ulcers, with redness, marked edema, tender inguinal lymph nodes, and the characteristic yellow, oozing centers.

Other features of initial mucocutaneous infection include fever, malaise, dysuria, and, in female-bodied persons, leukorrhea. Rare complications (generally from extragenital

PATHOPHYSIOLOGY
Understanding the genital herpes cycle

After a patient is infected with genital herpes, a latency period follows. The virus takes up permanent residence in the nerve cells surrounding the lesions, and intermittent viral shedding may take place.

Repeated outbreaks may develop at any time, again followed by a latent stage during which the lesions heal completely. Outbreaks may recur as often as three to eight times yearly.

Although the cycle continues indefinitely, some people remain symptom-free for years.

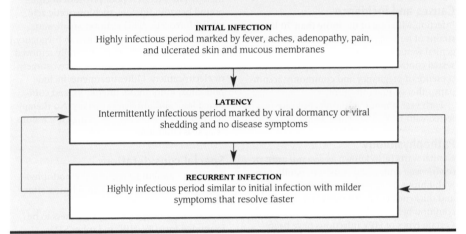

lesions) include herpetic keratitis, which may lead to blindness, and potentially fatal herpetic encephalitis.

Diagnosis

Diagnosis is based on the physical examination and patient history. Helpful (but nondiagnostic) measures include laboratory data showing increased antibody titers, smears of genital lesions showing atypical cells, and cytologic preparations (Tzanck test) that reveal giant cells.

CONFIRMING DIAGNOSIS *Diagnosis can be confirmed by demonstration of the herpes simplex virus in vesicular fluid, using tissue culture techniques, or by antigen tests that identify specific antigens.*

Treatment

Acyclovir has proved to be an effective treatment for genital herpes. I.V. administration may be required for patients who are hospitalized with severe genital herpes or for those who are immunocompromised and have a potentially life-threatening herpes infection. Oral acyclovir may be prescribed for the patient with a first-time infection or recurrent outbreak. Other agents include famciclovir, valacyclovir, and penciclovir. Antiviral medications suppress symptoms but don't cure the infection. Daily prophylaxis with acyclovir reduces the frequency of recurrences by at least 50%, but this is only appropriate for a patient with frequent outbreaks and may not decrease the transmission rate of the disease.

Foscarnet, a powerful antiviral agent, is the treatment of choice for herpes strains that are severe in nature or have become resistant to acyclovir and similar drugs. Administered I.V., foscarnet can have several toxic effects, such as reversible impairment of kidney function or induction of seizures. As with other antiviral drugs, this drug doesn't cure herpes.

Special considerations

◆ Encourage the patient to get adequate rest and nutrition and to keep the lesions dry.

◆ Tell the patient that warm baths may relieve the pain associated with genital lesions.

◆ Recommend gentle cleaning of the lesions with soap and water.

◆ Secondary infections of skin lesions by bacteria require a topical or oral antibiotic. Tell the patient to report worsening of lesions, indicating possible secondary infection, to the healthcare provider.

◆ Advise the patient to avoid sexual intercourse during the active stage of this disease (while lesions are present) and to use condoms during all sexual exposures. Urge them to have their sex partners seek medical examination.

◆ Advise the female-bodied patient to have a Papanicolaou test every 6 months.

◆ Refer patients to the Herpes Resource Center, which has local chapters nationwide, for support.

GENITAL WARTS
Causes and incidence
Infection with one of the more than 70 known strains of human papillomavirus (HPV) causes genital warts, which are transmitted through sexual contact. The warts grow rapidly in the presence of pregnancy and commonly accompany other genital infections.

Each year, about 6 million people are infected with HPV in the United States.

Pathophysiology
Genital warts (also known as *venereal warts* or *condylomata acuminata*) consist of papillomas with fibrous tissue overgrowth from the dermis and thickened epithelial coverings. They're uncommon before puberty or after menopause. Certain types of HPV infections have been strongly associated with genital dysplasia and, over a period of years (depending on the viral strain), with cervical neoplasia.

Complication
◆ Genital tract dysplasia or cancer

Signs and symptoms
After a 1- to 6-month incubation period (usually 2 months), genital warts develop on moist surfaces: in male-bodied persons on the subpreputial sac, within the urethral meatus and on the penile shaft; in female-bodied persons on the vulva and on vaginal and cervical walls. In both sexes, papillomas spread to the perineum and the perianal area. These painless warts start as tiny red or pink swellings that grow (sometimes up to 10 cm) and become pedunculated. Typically, multiple swellings give them a cauliflower-like appearance. If infected, the warts become malodorous.

Most patients report no symptoms; a few complain of itching or pain.

Diagnosis
℞ CONFIRMING DIAGNOSIS *Dark-field examination of scrapings from wart cells shows marked vascularization of epidermal cells, which helps to differentiate genital warts from condylomata lata associated with second-stage syphilis.*

Applying 5% acetic acid (white vinegar) to the warts turns them white. Warts usually are diagnosed early by visual inspection; biopsy is indicated only when neoplasia is strongly suspected.

Treatment
Treatment is mostly for cosmetic reasons and should be guided by the patient's preference. Treatment aims to remove exophytic warts and to ameliorate signs and symptoms. Topical drug therapy (10% to 25% podophyllum in compound benzoin tincture, trichloroacetic acid, or dichloroacetic acid) removes small warts. (Podophyllum is contraindicated in pregnancy.) Warts larger than 2.5 cm are generally removed by carbon dioxide laser treatment, cryosurgery, or electrocautery. Other treatments include podofilox, imiquimod, interferon, and combined laser and interferon therapy. No therapy has proved effective in eradicating HPV lesions; relapse is common.

Special considerations
◆ Tell the patient to remove the podophyllum with soap and water 4 to 6 hours after applying it.

◆ Encourage the patient's sex partners to be examined for HPV, HIV, and other STDs.

◆ Advise the female-bodied person to have a Papanicolaou test according to guidelines.

◆ An HPV vaccine is available that helps to protect against four types of HPV. In female-bodied persons age 9 to 26, the HPV vaccine helps protect against two types of HPV that cause approximately 75% of cervical cancer cases, in addition to two more types that cause 90% of genital warts cases. In male-bodied persons age 9 to 26, the vaccine helps protect against 90% of genital warts cases.

▥▥▥ PREVENTION *Recommend the use of condoms, and tell the patient that abstinence is the only sure way to avoid genital warts and other STDs.*

SYPHILIS
Causes and incidence
Infection from the spirochete *Treponema pallidum* causes syphilis. Transmission occurs primarily through sexual contact during the primary, secondary, and early latent stages of infection. Prenatal transmission from an infected pregnant person to the fetus is also possible. (See *Prenatal syphilis*, page 1085.)

Incidence is highest in people ages 20 to 29. In 2014, there were 6 new cases per every 100,000 people.

Prenatal syphilis

A pregnant person can transmit syphilis transplacentally to the fetus throughout pregnancy. This type of syphilis is often called congenital, but prenatal is a more accurate term. About 50% of infected fetuses die before or shortly after birth. The prognosis is better for infants who develop overt infection after age 2.

Signs and symptoms
The neonate with prenatal syphilis may appear healthy at birth, but usually develops characteristic lesions—vesicular, bullous eruptions, often on the palms and soles approximately 3 weeks later. Shortly afterward, a maculopapular rash similar to that in secondary syphilis may erupt on the face, mouth, genitalia, palms, or soles. Condylomata lata typically occur around the anus. Lesions may erupt on the mucous membranes of the mouth, pharynx, and nose. When the infant's larynx is affected, their cry becomes weak and forced. If nasal mucous membranes are involved, they may also develop nasal discharge, which can be slight and mucopurulent or copious with blood-tinged pus. Visceral and bone lesions, liver or spleen enlargement with ascites, and nephrotic syndrome may also occur.

Late prenatal syphilis becomes apparent after age 2; it may be identifiable only through blood studies or may cause unmistakable syphilitic changes: screwdriver-shaped central incisors, deformed molars or cusps, thick clavicles, saber shins, bowed tibias, nasal septum perforation, eighth nerve deafness, and neurosyphilis.

Diagnosis and treatment
In the neonate with prenatal syphilis, the Venereal Disease Research Laboratory titer, if reactive at birth, stays the same or rises, indicating active disease. The infant's titer drops in 3 months if the gestating parent has received effective prenatal treatment. Absolute diagnosis necessitates dark-field examination of umbilical vein blood or lesion drainage.

An infant with abnormal cerebrospinal fluid (CSF) may be treated with aqueous crystalline penicillin G. An infant with normal CSF may be treated with a single injection of penicillin G.

When caring for a child with prenatal syphilis, record the extent of the rash and watch for signs of systemic involvement, especially laryngeal swelling, jaundice, and decreasing urine output.

Pathophysiology
A chronic, infectious, STD, syphilis begins in the mucous membranes and quickly becomes systemic, spreading to nearby lymph nodes and the bloodstream. This disease, when untreated, is characterized by progressive stages: primary, secondary, latent, and late (formerly called *tertiary*). Untreated syphilis leads to long-term health problems, but the prognosis is excellent with early treatment.

Complications
◆ Aortic regurgitation
◆ Aneurysm
◆ Central nervous system damage
◆ Meningitis

Signs and symptoms
Primary syphilis develops after an incubation period that generally lasts about 3 weeks. Initially, one or more chancres (small, fluid-filled lesions) erupt on the genitalia; others may erupt on the anus, fingers, lips, tongue, nipples, tonsils, or eyelids. These chancres, which are usually painless, start as papules and then erode; they have indurated, raised edges and clear bases. Chancres typically disappear after 3 to 6 weeks, even when untreated. They're usually associated with regional lymphadenopathy (unilateral or bilateral). In female-bodied persons chancres are commonly overlooked because they usually develop on internal structures—the cervix or the vaginal wall.

The development of symmetrical mucocutaneous lesions and general lymphadenopathy signals the onset of *secondary syphilis*, which may develop within a few days or up to 8 weeks after onset of initial chancres. The rash of secondary syphilis can be macular, papular, pustular, or nodular. Lesions are of uniform size, well defined, and generalized. Macules typically erupt between rolls of fat on the trunk and, proximally, on the arms, palms, soles, face, and scalp. In warm, moist areas (perineum, scrotum, vulva, and between rolls of fat), the lesions enlarge and erode, producing highly contagious, pink or grayish white lesions (condylomata lata).

Mild constitutional symptoms of syphilis appear in the second stage and may include headache, malaise, anorexia, weight loss, nausea, vomiting, sore throat, and, possibly, slight fever. Alopecia may occur, with or without treatment, and is usually temporary. Nails become brittle and pitted.

Latent syphilis is characterized by an absence of clinical symptoms but a reactive serologic test for syphilis. Because infectious mucocutaneous lesions may reappear when infection is of less than 4 years' duration, early latent syphilis is considered contagious. About two-thirds of patients remain asymptomatic in the late latent stage; the rest develop characteristic late-stage symptoms.

Late syphilis is the final, destructive but noninfectious stage of the disease. It has three subtypes, any or all of which may affect the patient: late benign syphilis, cardiovascular syphilis, and neurosyphilis. The lesions of *late benign syphilis* develop on the skin, bones, mucous membranes, upper respiratory tract, liver, or stomach between 1 and 10 years after infection. The typical lesion is a gumma—a chronic, superficial nodule or deep, granulomatous lesion that's solitary, asymmetrical, painless, and indurated. Gummas can be found on any bone—particularly the long bones of the legs—and in any organ. If late syphilis involves the liver, it can cause epigastric pain, tenderness, enlarged spleen, and anemia; if it involves the upper respiratory tract, it can cause perforation of the nasal septum or the palate. In severe cases, late benign syphilis results in destruction of bones or organs, which eventually causes death.

Cardiovascular syphilis develops about 10 years after the initial infection in about 10% of patients with late, untreated syphilis. It causes fibrosis of elastic tissue of the aorta and leads to aortitis, usually in the ascending and transverse sections of the aortic arch. Cardiovascular syphilis may be asymptomatic or may cause aortic insufficiency or aneurysm.

Symptoms of *neurosyphilis* develop in about 8% of patients with late, untreated syphilis and appear from 5 to 35 years after infection. These clinical effects consist of meningitis and widespread central nervous system damage that may include general paresis, personality changes, and arm and leg weakness.

Diagnosis

CONFIRMING DIAGNOSIS *Identifying T. pallidum from a lesion on dark-field examination confirms the diagnosis of syphilis. This method is most effective when moist lesions are present, as in primary, secondary, and prenatal syphilis. (See Treponema pallidum.)*

Treponema pallidum

In syphilis, a dark-field examination that shows spiral-shaped bacterial organisms—*T. pallidum*—confirms the diagnosis.

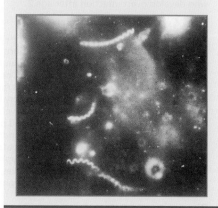

The fluorescent treponemal antibody-absorption test identifies antigens of *T. pallidum* in tissue, ocular fluid, CSF, tracheobronchial secretions, and exudates from lesions. This is the most sensitive test available for detecting syphilis in all stages. Once reactive, it remains so permanently.

Other appropriate procedures include the following:

◆ Venereal Disease Research Laboratory (VDRL) slide test and rapid plasma reagin (RPR) test detect nonspecific antibodies. Both tests, if positive, become reactive within 1 to 2 weeks after the primary lesion appears or 4 to 5 weeks after the infection begins.

◆ CSF examination identifies neurosyphilis when the total protein level is above 40 mg/dL, the VDRL slide test is reactive, and the cell count exceeds 5 mononuclear cells/μL.

Treatment

Treatment of choice is administration of penicillin I.M. or I.V. depending on the infection's stage. After therapy, follow-up RPR tests are usually done to check for adequacy of treatment. The nonpregnant patient who is allergic to penicillin may be treated with tetracycline or doxycycline. Nonpenicillin therapy for latent or late syphilis should be used only after neurosyphilis has been excluded. Tetracycline is contraindicated in the pregnant person because it causes discoloration of the infant's teeth. If a pregnant person with syphilis is allergic to penicillin, desensitization is recommended to permit the use of penicillin.

Special considerations

◆ Stress the importance of completing the full course of antibiotic therapy even after symptoms subside.

◆ Check for a history of drug sensitivity before administering the first dose.

◆ In secondary syphilis, keep lesions clean and dry. If they're draining, dispose of contaminated materials properly.

◆ In late syphilis, provide symptomatic care during prolonged treatment.

◆ In cardiovascular syphilis, check for signs of decreased cardiac output (decreased urine output, hypoxia, and decreased sensorium) and pulmonary congestion.

◆ In neurosyphilis, regularly check level of consciousness and monitor vital signs. Watch for signs of ataxia.

◆ Urge the patient to seek testing after treatment to determine the treatment's effectiveness. A patient treated for latent or late syphilis should be encouraged to continue follow-up care after treatment to determine its effectiveness.

◆ Be sure to report all cases of syphilis to local public health authorities. Urge the patient to inform sex partners of their infection so that they can also receive treatment.

◆ Refer the patient and their sex partners for HIV testing as appropriate.

PREVENTION

◆ *Advise the patient to practice safe sex and consistently use condoms.*

◆ *Screen people who are pregnant for syphilis to lessen the risk of infection for an unborn baby.*

TRICHOMONIASIS

Causes and incidence

Trichomonas vaginalis—a tetra flagellated, motile protozoan—causes trichomoniasis in female-bodied persons by infecting the vagina, the urethra and, possibly, the endocervix, bladder, Bartholin's glands, or Skene's glands; in male-bodied person it infects the lower urethra and, possibly, the prostate gland, seminal vesicles, or epididymis.

Trichomonas vaginalis grows best when the vaginal mucosa is more alkaline than normal (pH about 5.5 to 5.8). Therefore, factors that raise the vaginal pH—use of hormonal contraceptives, pregnancy, bacterial overgrowth, exudative cervical or vaginal lesions, or frequent douching, which disturbs lactobacilli that normally live in the vagina and maintain acidity—may predispose a person to trichomoniasis.

Trichomoniasis is usually transmitted by intercourse; less commonly, by contaminated douche equipment or moist washcloths. In the United States, incidence is highest in women ages 16 to 35.

Complications

◆ Pelvic inflammatory disease
◆ Vaginal erosion

Signs and symptoms

About 70% of female-bodied persons—including those with chronic infections—and most male-bodied persons with trichomoniasis are asymptomatic. In female-bodied persons acute infection may produce variable signs, such as a gray or greenish-yellow and possibly profuse and frothy, malodorous vaginal discharge. Its other effects include severe itching, redness, swelling, tenderness, dyspareunia, dysuria, urinary frequency, and, occasionally, postcoital spotting, menorrhagia, or dysmenorrhea.

Such symptoms may persist for 1 week to several months and may be more pronounced just after menstruation or during pregnancy. If trichomoniasis is untreated, symptoms may subside, although *T. vaginalis* infection persists, possibly associated with an abnormal cytologic smear of the cervix.

In male-bodied persons, trichomoniasis may produce mild to severe transient urethritis, possibly with dysuria and frequency.

Diagnosis

CONFIRMING DIAGNOSIS *Direct microscopic examination of vaginal or seminal discharge is decisive when it reveals* T. vaginalis *(a motile, pear-shaped organism) on wet prep. A Papanicolaou test may also detect the organism. Examination of clear urine specimens may also reveal* T. vaginalis.

Physical examination of symptomatic female-bodied persons shows vaginal erythema; edema; frank excoriation; a frothy, malodorous, greenish-yellow vaginal discharge and, rarely, a thin, gray pseudomembrane over the vagina. Cervical examination demonstrates punctate cervical hemorrhages, giving the cervix a strawberry appearance that's almost pathognomonic for this disorder.

Treatment

The treatment of choice for trichomoniasis is metronidazole given to all sex partners. Oral metronidazole hasn't been proven safe during the first trimester of pregnancy but can be considered for use if symptoms are severe. In general, treatment during the first trimester should be avoided if possible. Effective alternatives aren't available for patients who are allergic to metronidazole. Sitz baths may be used to help relieve symptoms.

Special considerations

◆ Instruct the patient to refrain from douching before being examined for trichomoniasis.

◆ Warn the patient to abstain from alcoholic beverages while taking metronidazole because alcohol consumption may provoke a disulfiram-type reaction (confusion, headache, cramps, vomiting, and seizures). Also, tell them this drug may turn urine dark brown.

◆ Caution the patient to avoid over-the-counter douches and vaginal sprays because chronic use can alter vaginal pH.

◆ Advise the patient to scrub the bathtub with a disinfecting cleaner before and after sitz baths.

◆ Tell the patient they can reduce the risk of GU bacterial growth by wearing loose-fitting, cotton underpants, which allow ventilation; bacteria flourish in a warm, dark, moist environment.

░░░░ PREVENTION *Advise abstinence from intercourse until treatment is completed. Refer partners for treatment. Advise female-bodied persons to avoid using tampons.*

CHANCROID

Causes and incidence

Chancroid results from *Haemophilus ducreyi*, a gram-negative *Streptobacillus*, and is transmitted through sexual contact. Poor hygiene may predispose male-bodied persons to this disease.

This infection occurs worldwide but is particularly common in tropical countries; it affects more male-bodied than female-bodied persons.

Pathophysiology

Chancroid, also known as *soft chancre*, is a STD characterized by painful genital ulcers and inguinal adenitis. Chancroidal lesions may heal spontaneously and usually respond well to treatment in the absence of secondary infections. A high rate of HIV infection has been reported among patients with chancroid.

Complications

◆ Phimosis
◆ Secondary infections
◆ Urethral fistulas

Signs and symptoms

After a 3- to 5-day incubation period, a small papule appears at the entry site, usually the groin or inner thigh; in the male-bodied person, it may appear on the penis; in female-bodied person, on the vulva, vagina, or cervix. (See *Chancroidal lesion.*) Occasionally, this papule may erupt on the tongue, lip, breast, or navel. The papule rapidly ulcerates, becoming painful, soft, and malodorous; it bleeds easily

Chancroidal lesion

Chancroid produces a soft, painful chancre, similar to that of syphilis. Without treatment, it may progress to inguinal adenitis and formation of buboes (enlarged, inflamed lymph nodes).

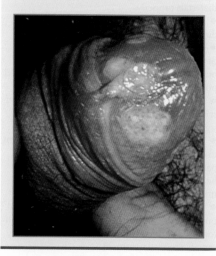

and produces pus. It's gray and shallow, with irregular edges, and measures up to 2.5 cm in diameter. Within 2 to 3 weeks, inguinal adenitis develops, creating suppurated, inflamed nodes that may rupture into large ulcers or buboes. Headache and malaise occur in 50% of patients. During the healing stage, phimosis may develop.

Diagnosis

Gram stain smears of ulcer exudate or bubo aspirate are 50% reliable; blood agar cultures are 75% reliable. Biopsy confirms the diagnosis but is reserved for resistant cases or cases in which cancer is suspected. Dark-field examination and serologic testing rule out other STDs that cause similar ulcers. Testing for HIV infection should be done at the time of diagnosis.

Treatment

The treatment of choice is azithromycin, erythromycin, ceftriaxone, or ciprofloxacin. The safety of azithromycin for pregnant or lactating people hasn't been established. Aspiration of fluid-filled nodes may be indicated as well.

Special considerations

◆ Make sure the patient isn't allergic to any drug before giving the first dose.

◆ Instruct the patient not to apply lotions, creams, or oils on or near the genitalia or on other lesion sites.

◆ Tell the patient to abstain from sexual contact until healing is complete (usually about 2 weeks after treatment begins) and to wash the genitalia daily with soap and water. Instruct uncircumcised male-bodied persons to retract the foreskin for thorough cleaning.

:::::::: PREVENTION *Advise the patient to avoid sexual contact with infected people, to use condoms during sexual activity, and to wash the genitalia with soap and water after sexual activity. Tell the patient that abstinence is the only sure way to prevent chancroid.*

NONSPECIFIC GU INFECTIONS
Causes and incidence
Nonspecific GU infections are spread primarily through sexual intercourse. In male-bodied persons, nongonococcal urethritis (NGU) commonly results from infection with *C. trachomatis* or *Ureaplasma urealyticum*. Less commonly, infection may be related to pre-existing strictures, neoplasms, and chemical or traumatic inflammation. Some cases remain unexplained.

Although less is known about nonspecific GU infections in female-bodied persons, chlamydial organisms may also cause these infections. A thin vaginal epithelium may predispose prepubertal and postmenopausal female-bodied persons to nonspecific vaginitis.

Pathophysiology
Nonspecific GU infections, including NGU in male-bodied persons and mild vaginitis or cervicitis in female-bodied persons are a group of infections with similar manifestations that aren't linked to a single organism. These STI's have become more prevalent since the mid-1960s. They're more widespread than gonorrhea and may be the most common STDs in the United States. The prognosis is good if sex partners are treated simultaneously.

Complications
◆ Concurrent STI's
◆ Increased risk of other STI infection

Signs and symptoms
NGU occurs 1 week to 1 month after coitus, with scant or moderate mucopurulent urethral discharge, variable dysuria, and occasional hematuria. If untreated, NGU may lead to acute epididymitis. Subclinical urethritis may be found on physical examination, especially if sex partners have a positive diagnosis.

Female-bodied persons with nonspecific GU infections may experience persistent vaginal discharge, acute or recurrent cystitis for which no underlying cause can be found, or cervicitis with inflammatory erosion.

Both male and female-bodied persons with nonspecific GU infections may be asymptomatic but show signs of urethral, vaginal, or cervical infection on physical examination.

Diagnosis
In male-bodied persons, microscopic examination of smears of prostatic or urethral secretions shows excess polymorphonuclear leukocytes but few, if any, specific organisms.

In female-bodied persons cervical or urethral smears also reveal excess leukocytes and no specific organisms. "Clue cells" (normal epithelial cells covered with bacteria that appear stippled) are diagnostic.

Treatment
Therapy for both sexes consists of azithromycin or doxycycline. If the infection recurs or persists, metronidazole with erythromycin is recommended.

Special considerations
◆ Tell the female-bodied persons patient to clean the pubic area before applying vaginal medication and to avoid using tampons during treatment.

◆ Make sure the patient clearly understands and strictly follows the dosage schedule for prescribed medications.

PREVENTION
:::::::: ◆ *Advise the patient to abstain from sexual contact with infected partners. Tell the patient to use condoms during sexual activity and to practice good hygiene afterward. Encourage the patient to maintain adequate fluid intake.*
◆ *Advise female-bodied person to avoid routinely using douches and feminine hygiene sprays, wearing tight-fitting pants or pantyhose, and inserting foreign objects into the vagina.*
◆ *Suggest that the female-bodied person patient wear cotton underpants and remove them before going to bed.*

Male-bodied persons reproductive disorders

HYPOGONADISM
Causes and incidence
Primary hypogonadism results directly from interstitial (Leydig's cell) cellular or seminiferous tubular damage because of faulty development

or damage from gonadotoxins or radiation. This causes increased secretion of gonadotropins by the pituitary in an attempt to increase the testicular functional state and is therefore termed *hypergonadotropic hypogonadism*. This form of hypogonadism includes Klinefelter syndrome, Reifenstein syndrome, Turner syndrome, Sertoli cell–only syndrome, anorchism, orchitis, and sequelae of irradiation.

Secondary hypogonadism is because of faulty interaction within the hypothalamic–pituitary axis, resulting in failure to secrete normal levels of gonadotropins, and is therefore termed *hypogonadotropic hypogonadism*. This form of hypogonadism includes hypopituitarism, isolated follicle-stimulating hormone deficiency, isolated luteinizing hormone (LH) deficiency, Kallmann syndrome, and Prader–Willi syndrome. Depending on the patient's age at onset, hypogonadism may cause eunuchism (complete gonadal failure) or eunuchoidism (partial failure).

Medications, such as exogenous testosterone or anabolic steroids, can also cause hypogonadism, resulting in infertility.

Hypogonadism is rare, and it has no racial predilection.

Pathophysiology

Hypogonadism is a condition resulting from decreased androgen production in male-bodied persons, which may impair spermatogenesis (causing infertility) and inhibit the development of normal secondary sex characteristics. (See *Production of sperm*.) The clinical effects of androgen deficiency depend on the patient's age at onset.

Complications

◆ Impotence
◆ Infertility
◆ Loss of sex drive
◆ Osteoporosis

Signs and symptoms

Although symptoms vary, depending on the specific cause of hypogonadism, some characteristic findings in prepubescent male-bodied persons may include delayed closure of epiphyses and immature bone age; delayed puberty; infantile penis and small, soft testes; below-average muscle development and strength; fine, sparse facial hair; scant or absent axillary, pubic, and body hair; and a high-pitched, effeminate voice. In an adult, hypogonadism diminishes sex drive and potency and causes regression of secondary sex characteristics.

Production of sperm

Spermatogenesis, the production of male-bodied persons gametes within the seminiferous tubules of the testes, is basically a five-step process:
1. Diploid spermatogonia, the cells forming the tubule's outer layer, divide mitotically to generate new cells used in spermatozoa production.
2. Some of the spermatogonia move toward the lumen of the tubule and enlarge to primary spermatocytes.
3. Each primary spermatocyte divides meiotically, forming two secondary spermatocytes, one retaining the X chromosome and the other the Y chromosome.
4. Each secondary spermatocyte also divides meiotically, becoming spermatids.
5. After a series of structural changes, the spermatids develop into mature spermatozoa.

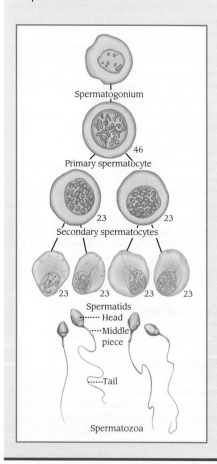

Spermatogonium

46

Primary spermatocyte

23   23

Secondary spermatocytes

23   23   23   23

Spermatids
····· Head
·····Middle piece

····Tail

Spermatozoa

Diagnosis

Accurate diagnosis necessitates a detailed patient history, physical examination, and hormonal studies. Serum gonadotropic levels increase in primary (hypergonadotropic) hypogonadism but decrease in secondary (hypogonadotropic) hypogonadism. Other relevant hormonal studies include assessment of neuroendocrine functions, such as thyrotropin, corticotropin, growth hormone, and vasopressin levels. Chromosomal analysis may determine the specific causative syndrome. Testicular biopsy and semen analysis determine sperm production, identify impaired spermatogenesis, and assess low levels of testosterone.

Treatment

Treatment depends on the underlying cause and may consist of hormonal replacement, especially with testosterone, estrogen, progesterone, or human chorionic gonadotropin (hCG) for primary hypogonadism, and with hCG for secondary hypogonadism. Fertility can't be restored after permanent testicular damage. However, eunuchism that results from hypothalamic–pituitary lesions can be corrected when administration of gonadotropins stimulates normal testicular function.

Special considerations

Because the patient with hypogonadism tends to have multiple associated physical problems, the care plan should be tailored to meet their specific needs.

◆ When caring for an adolescent with hypogonadism, make every possible effort to promote their self-confidence. If they feel sensitive about their underdeveloped body, provide access to a private bathroom. Explain hypogonadism to their parents. Encourage them to express their concerns about their child's delayed development. Reassure them and the patient that effective treatment is available.

◆ Make sure the parents and the patient understand hormone replacement therapy fully, including expected adverse effects, such as acne and water retention.

◆ Encourage counseling as appropriate.

UNDESCENDED TESTES

Causes and incidence

The mechanism whereby the testes descend into the scrotum is still unexplained. Some evidence is available to implicate hormonal factors—most likely androgenic hormones from the placenta, maternal or fetal adrenals, or the immature fetal testis and, possibly, maternal progesterone or gonadotropic hormones from the maternal pituitary.

Researchers have linked undescended testes to the development of the gubernaculum, a fibromuscular band that connects the testes to the scrotal floor. In the normal male-bodied fetus, testosterone stimulates the formation of the gubernaculum. This band probably helps direct the testes into the scrotum by shortening as the fetus grows. Thus, cryptorchidism may result from inadequate testosterone levels or a defect in the testes or the gubernaculum.

Because the testes normally descend into the scrotum during the eighth month of gestation, cryptorchidism most commonly affects premature neonates. (It occurs in 30% of premature male-bodied neonates but in only 3% to 4% of those born at term.) In about 80% of affected infants, the testes descend spontaneously during the first year; in the rest, the testes may descend later.

Pathophysiology

Undescended testes is a congenital disorder in which one or both testes fail to descend into the scrotum, remaining in the abdomen or inguinal canal or at the external ring. Although this condition, also known as *cryptorchidism*, may be bilateral, it more commonly affects the right testis. True undescended testes remain along the path of normal descent, whereas ectopic testes deviate from that path. If bilateral cryptorchidism persists untreated into adolescence, it may result in sterility, make the testes more vulnerable to trauma, and significantly increase the risk of testicular cancer, presumably because of the higher temperature of the abdominal cavity.

Complications

◆ Infertility
◆ Testicular cancer

Signs and symptoms

In the young male-bodied person with unilateral cryptorchidism, the testis on the affected side isn't palpable in the scrotum, and the scrotum may appear underdeveloped. On the unaffected side, the scrotum occasionally appears enlarged as a result of compensatory hypertrophy. After puberty, uncorrected bilateral cryptorchidism prevents spermatogenesis and results in infertility, although testosterone levels remain normal.

Diagnosis

CONFIRMING DIAGNOSIS *Physical examination confirms cryptorchidism after the following laboratory tests determine sex:*
◆ *Buccal smear determines genetic sex by showing a male-bodied sex chromatin pattern.*
◆ *Serum gonadotropin confirms the presence of testes by assessing the level of circulating hormone.*

Treatment

If the testes don't descend spontaneously by age 1 year, surgical correction may be indicated. Orchiopexy secures the testes in the scrotum and is commonly performed before the male-bodied person reaches age 4 (optimum age is 1 to 2). Orchiopexy reduces the incidence of subfertility and prevents excessive trauma from abnormal positioning. It also prevents harmful psychological effects. hCG or testosterone may be given to stimulate descent. However, hormonal therapy with hCG is ineffective if the testes are located in the abdomen.

Special considerations

◆ Encourage parents of the child with undescended testes to express their concern about their condition. Provide information about causes, available treatments, and the ultimate effect on reproduction. Emphasize that, especially in premature neonates, the testes may descend spontaneously.

◆ If orchiopexy is necessary, explain the surgery to the child, using terms they understand. Explain that their scrotum may swell but shouldn't be painful.

After orchiopexy:

◆ Monitor vital signs and intake and output. Check dressings. Encourage coughing and deep breathing. Watch for urine retention.

◆ Keep the operative site clean. Tell the child to wipe from front to back after defecating.

◆ Encourage parents to participate in postoperative care, such as bathing or feeding the child. Also urge the child to do as much for themselves as possible.

TESTICULAR TORSION

Causes and incidence

Normally, the tunica vaginalis envelops the testis and attaches to the epididymis and spermatic cord. In *intravaginal torsion* (the most common type of testicular torsion in adolescents), testicular twisting may result from an abnormality of the tunica, in which the testis is abnormally positioned, or from a narrowing of the mesentery support. In extravaginal torsion (most common in neonates), loose attachment of the tunica vaginalis to the scrotal lining causes spermatic cord rotation above the testis. Typically, there's no history of trauma, and the pain occurs suddenly. A sudden forceful contraction of the cremaster muscle may precipitate this condition. (See *Extravaginal torsion*.)

Pathophysiology

Testicular torsion is an abnormal twisting of the spermatic cord due to rotation of a testis or the mesorchium (a fold in the area between the

Extravaginal torsion

In extravaginal torsion, rotation of the spermatic cord above the testis causes strangulation and, eventually, infarction of the testis.

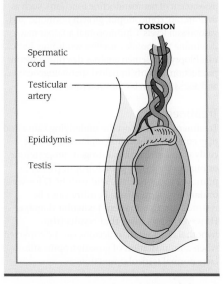

testis and epididymis), which causes strangulation and, if untreated, eventual infarction of the testis. This condition is almost always (90%) unilateral in presentation, but the defect is bilateral, requiring both testicles to be surgically treated. Testicular torsion is most common between ages 12 and 18, but it may occur at any age. The prognosis is good with early detection and prompt treatment.

Complications

◆ Complete testicular infarction
◆ Testicular atrophy

Signs and symptoms

Torsion produces excruciating pain in the affected testis or iliac fossa. Nausea, vomiting, and light-headedness may also occur.

Diagnosis

Physical examination reveals tense, tender swelling in the scrotum or inguinal canal and hyperemia of the overlying skin. Doppler ultrasonography helps distinguish testicular torsion from strangulated hernia, undescended testes, or epididymitis.

Treatment

Treatment consists of untwisting the testes and immediate surgical repair by orchiopexy (fixation of a viable testis to the scrotum) or orchiectomy (excision of a nonviable testis). Both testes are usually anchored to the scrotum as a preventive measure. As with ovarian torsion in the female-bodied person, preservation of the organ is the preferred option. If surgery is performed within 6 hours, most testicles can be saved.

Special considerations
◆ Promote the patient's comfort before and after surgery.
◆ After surgery, administer pain medication as ordered. Monitor voiding, and apply an ice bag with a cover to reduce edema. Protect the wound from contamination. Otherwise, allow the patient to perform as many normal daily activities as possible.

MALE-BODIED INFERTILITY
Causes and incidence
Some factors associated with male-bodied infertility include:
◆ varicocele, a mass of dilated and tortuous varicose veins in the spermatic cord
◆ semen disorders, such as volume or motility disturbances and inadequate sperm density
◆ proliferation of abnormal or immature sperm, with variations in the head's size and shape
◆ systemic disease, such as diabetes mellitus, neoplasms, hepatic and renal diseases, and viral disturbances, especially mumps-related orchitis
◆ genital infections, such as gonorrhea, tuberculosis, and herpes
◆ disorders of the testes, such as cryptorchidism, Sertoli cell–only syndrome, and ductal obstruction (caused by absence or ligation of vas deferens or infection)
◆ genetic defects, such as Klinefelter and Reifenstein syndromes
◆ immunologic disorders, such as autoimmune infertility and allergic orchitis
◆ endocrine imbalances that disrupt pituitary gonadotropins, inhibiting spermatogenesis, testosterone production, or both (as in Kallmann syndrome, panhypopituitarism, hypothyroidism, and congenital adrenal hyperplasia)
◆ chemicals and drugs that can inhibit gonadotropins or interfere with spermatogenesis, such as arsenic, methotrexate, medroxyprogesterone, nitrofurantoin, monoamine oxidase inhibitors, and some antihypertensives
◆ sexual problems, such as erectile dysfunction, ejaculatory incompetence, and low libido
Age, occupation, and traumatic injury to the testes can also contribute to male-bodied infertility. About 30% to 40% of infertility problems in the United States are attributed to male-bodied persons.

Complication
◆ Emotional or psychological distress

Signs and symptoms
The obvious indication of male-bodied infertility is failure to impregnate a fertile female-bodied person. Clinical features may include atrophied testes; empty scrotum; scrotal edema; varicocele or anteversion of the epididymis; inflamed seminal vesicles; beading or abnormal nodes on the spermatic cord and vas; penile nodes, warts, plaques, or hypospadias; prostatitis, which may be acute or chronic; and prostatic enlargement, nodules, swelling, or tenderness. In addition, male-bodied infertility commonly induces troublesome negative emotions—anger, hurt, disgust, guilt, and loss of self-esteem.

Diagnosis
A detailed patient history may reveal abnormal sexual development, delayed puberty, infertility in previous relationships, and a medical history of prolonged fever, mumps, impaired nutritional status, previous surgery, or trauma to genitalia. After a thorough patient history and physical examination, the most conclusive test for male-bodied infertility is semen analysis. The specimen is collected after 2 to 3 days of complete abstinence to determine volume and viscosity as well as sperm count, motility, swimming speed, and shape. One month later, a second specimen is obtained for analysis.

Other laboratory tests include gonadotropin assay to determine the integrity of the pituitary gonadal axis, and serum testosterone levels to determine end organ response to LH. A transrectal ultrasound or scrotal ultrasound may be needed to evaluate the infertile male-bodied person.

Treatment
When anatomic dysfunction or infection causes infertility, treatment consists of correcting the underlying problem. A varicocele requires surgical repair or removal. For patients with sexual dysfunction, treatment includes education, counseling or therapy (on sexual techniques, coital frequency, and reproductive physiology), and proper nutrition with vitamin supplements. Decreased follicle-stimulating hormone levels may respond to vitamin B therapy (although clinical studies have shown this to be ineffective); decreased LH levels, to hCG therapy. Normal or elevated LH level requires low dosages of testosterone. Decreased testosterone levels,

decreased semen motility, and volume distur- bances may respond to hCG.

A patient with oligospermia who has a normal history and physical examination, normal hormonal assays, and no signs of sys- temic disease requires emotional support and counseling, adequate nutrition, multivitamins, and selective therapeutic agents, such as clomi- phene, hCG, and low dosages of testosterone. Alternatives to such treatment are adoption and artificial insemination.

Special considerations

◆ Educate, as necessary, about reproductive and sexual function and about factors that may in- terfere with fertility such as the use of lubricants and douches.

◆ Urge people with oligospermia to avoid hab- its that may interfere with normal spermato- genesis by elevating scrotal temperature, such as wearing tight underwear and athletic support- ers, taking hot tub baths, or habitually riding a bicycle. Explain that cool scrotal temperature is essential for normal spermatogenesis.

◆ When possible, advise those with infertility to join group programs to share their feelings and concerns with others who have the same problem.

PREVENTION

▓▓▓ ◆ *Encourage the aging patient to have regu- lar physical examinations.*
◆ *Advise the patient to protect their gonads during athletic activity.*
◆ *Advise the patient to receive early treatment for STDs and surgical correction for anatomic defects.*

PRECOCIOUS PUBERTY IN MALE-BODIED PERSONS
Causes and incidence

True precocious puberty may be idiopathic (constitutional) or cerebral (neurogenic). In some patients, idiopathic precocity may be genetically transmitted as a dominant trait. Cerebral precocity results from pituitary or hy- pothalamic intracranial lesions that cause exces- sive secretion of gonadotropin.

Pseudoprecocious puberty may result from testicular tumors (hyperplasia, adenoma, or carcinoma) or from congenital adrenogenital syndrome. Testicular tumors produce excessive testosterone levels; adrenogenital syndrome produces high levels of adrenocortical steroids.

Pathophysiology

In precocious puberty, male-bodied persons begin to mature sexually before age 10. This disorder can occur as *true precocious puberty,*

which is most common, with early maturation of the hypothalamic–pituitary–gonadal axis, development of secondary sex characteristics, gonadal development, and spermatogenesis, or as *pseudoprecocious puberty*, with develop- ment of secondary sex characteristics without gonadal development. Male-bodied persons with true precocious puberty reportedly have impregnated sexual partners as early as age 7.

In most male-bodied persons with preco- cious puberty, sexual characteristics develop in essentially normal sequence; these children function normally when they reach adulthood.

Complications

◆ Emotional disturbances
◆ Increased intracranial pressure
◆ Pituitary tumors
◆ Stunted adult stature
◆ Vision disturbances

Signs and symptoms

All male-bodied persons with precocious puberty experience early bone development, causing an initial growth spurt, early muscle development, and premature closure of the epiphyses, which results in stunted adult stat- ure. Other features are adult hair pattern, penile growth, and bilateral enlarged testes. Symptoms of precocity due to cerebral lesions include nau- sea, vomiting, headache, vision disturbances, and internal hydrocephalus.

In pseudoprecocity caused by testicular tu- mors, adult hair patterns and acne develop. A discrepancy in testis size also occurs; the enlarged testis may be hard or may contain a palpable, isolated nodule. Scrotal ultrasound can evaluate the structure of the testes. Adrenogenital syndrome produces adult skin tone, excessive hair (including beard), and deepened voice. A male-bodied person with this syndrome appears stocky and muscular; their penis, scrotal sac, and prostate are enlarged (but not the testes).

Diagnosis

Assessing the cause of precocious puberty requires a complete physical examination. A detailed patient history can help evaluate the patient's recent growth pattern, behav- ior changes, a family history of precocious puberty, or ingestion of hormones. Scrotal ultrasound should be performed to evaluate possible testicular tumors.

In true precocity, laboratory results include the following:
◆ Serum levels of luteinizing and follicle-stimulating hormones and corticotropin are elevated.

◆ Plasma tests for testosterone demonstrate elevated levels (equal to those of an adult male-bodied person).

◆ Evaluation of ejaculate reveals the presence of live spermatozoa.

◆ Brain scan, skull X-rays, and electroencephalogram can detect possible central nervous system tumors. Abdominal scans can detect testicular tumors.

A child with an initial diagnosis of idiopathic precocious puberty should be reassessed regularly for possible tumors.

In pseudoprecocity, chromosomal karyotype analysis demonstrates an abnormal pattern of autosomes and sex chromosomes. Elevated levels of 24-hour urinary 17-ketosteroids and other steroids also indicate pseudoprecocity.

Treatment

Male-bodied persons with idiopathic precocious puberty generally require no medical treatment and suffer no physical complications in adulthood. Supportive psychological counseling is the most important therapy.

When precocious puberty is caused by tumors, the outlook is less encouraging. Brain tumors necessitate neurosurgery but may resist treatment and prove fatal. Testicular tumors may be treated by removing the affected testis (orchiectomy). Malignant tumors require chemotherapy and lymphatic radiation therapy. The prognosis is generally good, depending on tumor histology and degree of differentiation.

Adrenogenital syndrome that causes precocious puberty may respond to lifelong therapy with maintenance doses of glucocorticoids (cortisol) to inhibit corticotropin production.

Special considerations

◆ Emphasize to parents that the child's social and emotional development should remain consistent with their chronological age, not with their physical development. Advise parents not to place unrealistic demands on them.

◆ Reassure the child that, although their body is changing more rapidly than those of others, eventually they will experience the same changes. Help them feel less self-conscious about their changing body. Suggest clothing that de-emphasizes sexual development.

◆ Provide sex education for the child with true precocity.

◆ If the child must take glucocorticoids for the rest of their life, explain the medication's adverse effects (Cushingoid symptoms) to the family.

SELECTED REFERENCES

Bennett, N. J. (2018). Sexual dysfunction: Behavioral, medical, and surgical treatment. *The Medical Clinics of North America, 102*(2), 349–360. doi:10.1016/j.mcna.2017.10.016

Bouchemal, K., et al. (2017). Strategies for prevention and treatment of trichomonas vaginalis infections. *Clinical Microbiology Reviews, 30*(3), 811–825. doi:10.1128/CMR.00109-16

Dickson, C., et al. (2017). A systematic review and appraisal of the quality of practice guidelines for the management of Neisseria gonorrhoeae infections. *Sexually Transmitted Infections, 93*(7), 487–492. doi:10.1136/sextrans-2016-052939

Foster, L. R., & Byers, E. S. (2016). Predictors of the sexual well-being of individuals diagnosed with herpes and human papillomavirus. *Archives of Sexual Behavior, 45*(2), 403–414. doi:10.1007/s10508-014-0388-x

Park, I. U., et al. (2015). Human papillomavirus and genital warts: A review of the evidence for the 2015 Centers for Disease Control and Prevention Sexually Transmitted Diseases Treatment Guidelines. *Clinical Infectious Diseases: An Official Publication of the Infectious Diseases Society of America, 61* Suppl 8, S849–S855. doi:10.1093/cid/civ813

Patoulias, D., et al. (2017). Transient testicular torsion: From early diagnosis to appropriate therapeutic intervention (a prospective clinical study). *Folia Medica Cracoviensia, 57*(2), 53–62.

21

PSYCHIATRIC DISORDERS

Introduction

Social, economic, and professional developments have continued to dramatically change the mental health field. Community and professional organizations have established family advocacy programs, substance abuse rehabilitation programs, stress management workshops, bereavement groups, victim assistance programs, and violence shelters. The public education system has established widespread information programs about mental health issues, and more effective drugs are available to treat many of these illnesses. Efforts continue to reduce the stigma associated with mental illness.

SOCIAL CHANGES

Today, more people than ever experience mental health concerns. The loss of effective support systems strains a person's ability to cope with even minor problems. For example, a working parent may lack the needed support to meet the demands of job, home, partner, and children. The person may view themselves as ineffective in these roles, which causes self-esteem to falter and the level of stress to intensify.

Alcohol and substance abuse are also increasing, particularly among younger people. Despite underage drinking laws in the United States, individuals between the ages of 12 and 20 drink 11% of all alcohol consumed in the country. In 2016, an estimated 3.1 million U.S. teens between 12 and 17 had experienced at least one major depressive episode, with females being affected more frequently than males. Fear of violent crime and

loneliness have contributed to a similar rise in depression among older adults. Victims of violence, abuse, and social discord struggle to cope with the trauma they have experienced.

ECONOMIC FORCES

Continued cuts in Federal funding of mental health programs may place future control of mental health services in the hands of state and local authorities, drastically reducing the funds available for training and care. This places a need on increased collaboration between community psychiatric facilities (short-term inpatient, outpatient, and auxiliary services) and long-term inpatient state facilities, especially as availability of long-term care and lengths of stay for acute patient care decrease.

PROFESSIONAL PERSPECTIVE, FOCUS, AND DIRECTION

Mental health professionals gain perspective, focus, and direction from the American Psychiatric Association's *Diagnostic and Statistical Manual of Mental Disorders*, Fifth Edition, Text Revision (*DSM-5*). With this system of identifying mental disorders, clinicians must consider many aspects of a patient's behavior, mental performance, and history, emphasizing observable data rather than subjective and theoretical impressions.

RELATED PROFESSIONAL FORCES

An increased emphasis on holistic care has brought a closer relationship between psychiatry and the rest of medicine. More hospitalized patients benefit from psychiatric consultations, reflecting a growing recognition of the emotional accompaniment to physical disorders. Advances in neurobiology have increased our understanding of the physiologic basis of mental function. This has resulted in better diagnosis and treatment of mental disorders. Integrative therapies such as acupuncture, massage, and aromatherapy are also available to accompany traditional treatment.

BIOPSYCHOSOCIAL ASSESSMENT

The biopsychosocial model of health and illness assessment stresses an integrated approach to human behavior or disease. The *biological system* refers to evaluating the anatomy, structure, and function of an illness at a chemical or molecular level. *Psychosocial* refers to looking at the psychodynamic factors such as motivation, personality, social issues, and reaction to illness. This model of assessment examines how cultural influences and the environment interact to affect the development of disease. The goal of use of this model is to promote a more comprehensive understanding of illness and treatment.

PSYCHOSOCIAL ASSESSMENT

You will encounter patients with mental and emotional problems in all clinical areas and settings. Begin your care of these patients with a psychosocial assessment.

For this assessment to be effective, you need to establish a therapeutic relationship with the patient that's based on trust. You must communicate to the patient that his or her thoughts and behaviors are valued and important. Effective communication involves sending and receiving clear messages through eye contact, posture, facial expressions, gestures, clothing, affect, and even silence. (For *Communication barriers*, see page 1098.)

Choose a quiet, private setting for the assessment interview. Interruptions and distractions threaten confidentiality and interfere with effective listening. If you're meeting the patient for the first time, introduce yourself and explain the interview's purpose. Sit at a comfortable distance, and give the patient your undivided attention.

During the interview, adopt a professional yet open, nonjudgmental attitude, and maintain eye contact to the level that the patient can tolerate. A calm, nonthreatening tone of voice will encourage the patient to talk more openly. Avoid value judgments. Don't rush through the interview; building a trusting therapeutic relationship takes time.

PATIENT HISTORY

A patient history establishes a baseline and gives clues to the underlying or precipitating causes of the current problem. The patient may not be a reliable source of information, particularly if there is a significant mental illness that affects functioning. If possible, verify the patient's responses with family members, friends, or healthcare personnel. Also check facility records from previous admissions, if possible, and compare the patient's past behavior, symptoms, and circumstances with the current situation.

Explore the reason for the evaluation, current symptoms, psychiatric history, demographic data, socioeconomic data, cultural and religious beliefs, medication history, and physical illnesses. Identify the patient's strengths and coping mechanisms, as well as concerns.

◆ *Reason for evaluation.* The patient may not voice a chief complaint directly. Instead, you or others may note that he or she is having difficulty coping, or is exhibiting unusual behavior. If this occurs, determine whether the patient is aware of the problem. When documenting the patient's response, write it verbatim and enclose it in quotation marks.

◆ *Current symptoms.* Ask about the onset of symptoms, their severity and persistence, and whether they occurred abruptly or insidiously. Compare the patient's condition with his or her normal level of functioning.

◆ *Psychiatric history.* Discuss past psychiatric disturbances, such as episodes of delusions, violence, depression, attempted suicides, drug or alcohol abuse, previous psychiatric treatment, and the patient's adherence to past recommended treatments.

◆ *Demographic data.* Determine the patient's age, sex, ethnic origin, primary language, birthplace, religion, and marital status. Use this information to establish a baseline and confirm the patient's record.

◆ *Socioeconomic data.* Obtain information about the patient's educational level, housing conditions, income, current employment status, and family, because these data may provide information about the current problem and may aid in the development of a treatment plan. Determine current stressors from a holistic perspective.

◆ *Cultural and spiritual beliefs.* A patient's background and values affect response to illness and adaptation to care. Certain questions and behaviors considered acceptable in one culture may be inappropriate in another. Determine the extent to which the patient may utilize or desire cultural rituals, treatments, and healing practices.

Communication barriers

Ineffective communication can prevent a successful interview.

Language difficulties or differences

If the patient speaks English, try to use language that's appropriate to the individual's educational level and culture. Avoid medical terms that may not be understood.

If the patient speaks a foreign language or an unfamiliar dialect, contact an interpreter.

Be aware of words that can have more than one meaning. For instance, the word *bad* also can be used as slang to mean "good."

Inappropriate responses

Your responses to the patient can inadvertently suggest disinterest, anxiety, or annoyance, or they can imply value judgments. Examples include abruptly changing the subject or discounting the patient's feelings.

Hearing loss

If the patient can't hear you clearly, your responses may be misinterpreted. If you're interviewing a patient with impaired hearing, check for the presence of a hearing aid. If so, is it turned on? If not, can the patient read lips? If possible, face the patient and speak clearly and slowly, using common words and keeping your questions short, simple, and direct.

For older adult patients, use a low tone of voice. With aging, the ability to hear high-pitched tones deteriorates first. If the hearing impairment is severe, the patient may have to communicate by writing, or you may need to collect information from the family or caregivers.

Thought disorders

If the patient's thought patterns are incoherent or irrelevant, he or she may be unable to interpret messages correctly, focus on the interview, or provide appropriate responses.

When assessing such a patient, ask simple questions about concrete topics and clarify responses. Encourage the patient to self-express clearly.

Paranoid thinking

Interact with a patient with paranoia in a nonthreatening way. Avoid touching the patient as this may be misinterpreted

as an attempt to bring harm. Restrict hand motions and maintain physical distance. Accept the patient's statements of paranoid thoughts in a nonjudgmental manner.

Hallucinations

A hallucinating patient experiences imaginary sensory perceptions with no basis in reality. These distortions prevent the patient from hearing and responding appropriately.

Show concern if the patient is hallucinating, but don't reinforce misperceptions. Be as specific as possible when giving directions. For instance, if the patient is hearing voices, instruct the patient to stop listening to the voices and to listen to you instead.

Delusions

A patient experiencing delusions defends irrational beliefs or ideas despite factual evidence to the contrary. Some delusions may be so bizarre that you'll immediately recognize them; others may be difficult to identify.

Don't condemn or agree with a patient's delusional beliefs and don't dismiss a statement because you think it's delusional. Instead, gently emphasize reality without being argumentative.

Delirium

A patient with delirium experiences a disturbance in awareness and cognition that develops rapidly. Misinterpretation and inappropriate responses commonly result. Talk directly to such a patient and ask simple questions. Offer frequent reassurance. Provide protection and appropriate physical care to address the underlying cause of the delirium.

Dementia

The patient who suffers dementia—an irreversible deterioration of mental capacity—may experience changes in memory and thought patterns, and language may become distorted or slurred.

When interviewing a patient with dementia, use simple, concise language and minimize distractions. Don't make statements that may easily be misinterpreted. Maintain calm and establish a routine.

◆ *Medication history*. Certain drugs can cause symptoms of mental illness. Review any medications the patient may be taking, including over-the-counter drugs and herbal supplements or remedies, and check for interactions. If the patient is taking an antipsychotic, antidepressant, anxiolytic, or antimanic drug, ask if symptoms have improved, if the medication is being taken as prescribed, and if there have been any adverse reactions.

◆ *Physical illnesses*. Find out if the patient has a history of medical disorders that may cause distorted thought processes, disorientation, depression, or other symptoms of mental illness. For instance, is there a history of renal or hepatic failure, infection, thyroid disease, increased intracranial pressure, or a metabolic disorder? Additionally, has the patient suffered recent head trauma, infection, or physical illness?

PATIENT APPEARANCE, BEHAVIOR, AND MENTAL STATUS

Assess the patient's appearance, behavior, mood, thought processes, cognitive function, coping mechanisms, and potential for self-destructive behavior, and record your assessment.

◆ *General appearance*. The patient's appearance helps to indicate emotional and mental status. Specifically, note dress and grooming. Is the patient's appearance clean and appropriate for age, sex, and situation?

Is the patient's posture erect or slouched? Is the head lowered? Is the gait brisk, slow, shuffling, or unsteady? Note facial expression for alertness or blank stares. Does the patient appear sad or angry, and maintain direct eye contact?

◆ *Behavior*. Note the patient's demeanor and overall attitude as well as any extraordinary behavior such as speaking to a person who isn't present. Also record mannerisms. Does the patient bite nails, fidget, or pace? Are tics or tremors present? How does the patient respond to the interviewer? Would you describe the patient's interaction as cooperative, friendly, hostile, or indifferent?

Behavior should be evaluated also in light of the patient's culture. For instance, making eye contact is considered respectful and attentive behavior in many Western cultures. However, avoiding eye contact is considerate and respectful in other cultures.

◆ *Mood*. Does the patient appear excited or depressed? Do you notice sweating, breathing heavily, crying, or trembling? Does his or her mood change with little provocation? Ask the patient to describe current feelings in concrete terms and to suggest possible reasons for these feelings. Note inconsistencies between body language and mood (such as smiling when discussing an anger-provoking situation).

◆ *Thought processes and cognitive function*. Evaluate the patient's orientation to time, place, and person, noting any confusion or disorientation. Look for delusions, hallucinations, obsessions, compulsions, fantasies, and daydreams.

Assess the patient's attention span and ability to recall events in the distant and recent past. For example, to assess immediate recall, ask to repeat a series of five or six names of objects. Test intellectual functioning by asking the patient to add a series of numbers. Evaluate sensory perception and coordination by having the patient copy a simple drawing. Inappropriate responses to a hypothetical situation ("What would you do if you won the lottery?") can indicate impaired judgment. Keep in mind that the patient's cultural background and personal values will influence answers.

Note speech characteristics that may indicate altered thought processes, including monosyllabic responses; irrelevant or illogical replies to questions; convoluted or excessively detailed speech; repetitious, accelerated, or slowed speech patterns; flight of ideas; and sudden silence with an obvious reason.

Finally, assess the patient's insight by asking about understanding of the significance of illness, the plan of treatment, and the effect it will have on daily life.

◆ *Coping mechanisms*. The patient who's faced with a stressful situation will utilize coping, or defense, mechanisms—behaviors that operate on an unconscious level to protect the ego. Examples include denial, regression, displacement, projection, reaction formation, and fantasy. Look for an excessive reliance on these coping mechanisms. (See *Coping mechanisms defined*, page 1100.)

◆ *Potential for self-destructive behavior*. Mentally healthy people may intentionally take death-defying risks such as participating in dangerous sports. The risks taken by self-destructive patients, however, aren't death-defying but rather death-seeking.

Not all self-destructive behavior is suicidal in intent. The patient may engage in self-destructive behavior to feel "alive." A patient who has lost touch with reality may cut or mutilate body parts to focus on physical pain, which may be less overwhelming than emotional distress.

Assess patients for suicidal tendencies, particularly if they report signs and symptoms of depression. (See *Warning signs associated with suicide*, page 1100.) Not all such patients want

Coping mechanisms defined

Coping, or defense, mechanisms help to relieve anxiety. Common ones include:
* *denial*—avoiding awareness of truth or reality
* *displacement*—shifting of an emotion from its original object to a substitute
* *fantasy*—creation of unrealistic or improbable images to escape from daily pressures and responsibilities
* *identification*—unconscious adoption of the personality characteristics, attitudes, values, and behavior of another person
* *projection*—displacement of negative feelings onto another person
* *rationalization*—substitution of acceptable reasons for the real or actual reasons motivating behavior
* *reaction formation*—conduct in a manner opposite from the way the person feels
* *regression*—return to behavior of an earlier, less worrisome time in life
* *repression*—exclusion of unacceptable thoughts and feelings from the conscious mind, leaving them to operate in the subconscious

Warning signs associated with suicide

* Withdrawal and social isolation
* Signs and symptoms of depression, which may include crying, fatigue, sadness, helplessness, poor concentration, reduced interest in sex and other activities, constipation, and weight loss. Note that a patient is more likely to attempt suicide if he gains more energy. This may occur in the early stages of treatment with antidepressants, so be alert for mood shifts that may indicate the patient feels better.
* Farewells to friends and family
* Putting affairs in order
* Giving away prized possessions
* Covert suicide messages and death wishes
* Hoarding medication or purchasing a lethal item (e.g., a gun)
* Obvious suicide messages ("I'd be better off dead; no one would miss me if I was gone.")

to die; however, the risk for suicide in depressed patients should not be underestimated.

DIAGNOSTIC TESTS
The laboratory tests, psychological tests, and electroencephalogram (EEG) and brain imaging studies summarized here provide information about the patient's mental status and possible physical causes of signs and symptoms.

LABORATORY TESTS
Urinalysis, hemoglobin level, hematocrit, serum electrolyte and serum glucose levels, and liver, kidney, and thyroid function tests screen for physical disorders that can cause or contribute to psychiatric signs and symptoms. Toxicology studies of blood and urine can detect the presence of many drugs, and current laboratory methods can quantify the blood levels of these drugs. Patients on psychoactive drugs may need routine toxicology screening to ensure that they aren't receiving a toxic dose. (See *Toxicology screening*.)

PSYCHOLOGICAL AND MENTAL STATUS TESTS
These tests evaluate the patient's mood, personality, and mental status. Commonly used tests include the following:
◆ The Mini–Mental Status Examination measures orientation, registration, recall, calculation, language, and graphomotor function.
◆ The Mini Cog screens for cognitive impairment in older adults.
◆ The Global Deterioration Scale assesses and stages primary degenerative dementia, based on orientation, memory, and neurologic function.
◆ The Beck Depression Inventory helps diagnose depression, determine its severity, and monitor the patient's response during treatment.

Toxicology screening

Toxic levels of certain drugs can be detected in blood, urine, or both.

Blood
* Alcohol (ethyl, isopropyl, and methyl)
* Ethchlorvynol

Urine (most common in the United States)
* Amphetamine
* Cocaine
* Marijuana
* Opioids
* Phencyclidine (PCP)

◆ The Eating Attitudes Test (EAT-26) detects patterns that suggest an eating disorder.
◆ The Montreal Cognitive Assessment tool assesses for mild cognitive impairment.
◆ The Minnesota Multiphasic Personality Inventory helps assess personality traits and ego function in adolescents and adults. Test results include information on coping strategies, defenses, strengths, gender identification, and self-esteem. The test pattern may strongly suggest a diagnostic category, point to a suicide risk, or indicate the potential for violence.

EEG AND BRAIN IMAGING STUDIES

To screen for brain abnormalities, the physician may order tests that visualize electrical brain-wave pattern disturbances or anatomic alterations.

◆ An EEG graphically records the brain's electrical activity. Abnormal results may indicate organic disease, psychotropic drug use, or certain psychological disorders.
◆ A computed tomography (CT) scan combines radiologic and computer analysis of tissue density to produce images of intracranial structures not readily seen on standard X-rays. This test can help detect brain contusions or calcifications, cerebral atrophy, hydrocephalus, inflammation, space-occupying lesions, and vascular abnormalities.
◆ A magnetic resonance imaging (MRI) scan is a noninvasive imaging technique. MRI localizes atomic nuclei that magnetically align and then fall out of alignment in response to a radio frequency pulse. The MRI scanner records signals from nuclei as they realign; it then translates the signals into detailed pictures of anatomic structures. Compared with conventional X-rays and CT scans, the MRI scan provides superior contrast of soft tissues and sharper differentiation of normal and abnormal tissues. It also provides images of multiple planes, including sagittal and coronal views, in regions where bones usually interface.
◆ A functional MRI (fMRI) detects blood flow in the brain. It is useful to localize neuronal activity to a particular lobe or subcortical nucleus and even to a single gyrus. No radioactive isotopes are used. fMRI has recently been used to evaluate details about the organization of language in the brain. This imaging technique is used to study brain abnormality related to cognitive dysfunction.
◆ A positron emission tomography (PET) scan provides colorimetric information about the brain's metabolic activity by detecting how quickly tissues consume radioactive isotopes. PET scanning is used mainly for diagnosing

neuropsychiatric problems, such as Alzheimer disease, and some mental illnesses.

Disorders of infancy, childhood, and adolescence

INTELLECTUAL DISABILITY (INTELLECTUAL DEVELOPMENTAL DISORDER)

The American Association on Intellectual and Developmental Disabilities (AAIDD) defines *intellectual disability* as "a disability characterized by significant limitations in both **intellectual functioning** and in **adaptive behavior**, which covers many everyday social and practical skills. This disability originates **before the age of 18.**"

Intellectual disability commonly is accompanied by other physical and emotional disorders that may constitute disabilities in themselves. Intellectual disability can place a significant burden on patients and their families, resulting in stress, frustration, and family problems.

Causes and incidence

A specific cause is identifiable in only a small percentage of people who are intellectually disabled, and, of these, very few have the potential for cure. (See *Causes of intellectual disability*.)

Causes of intellectual disability

◆ Chromosomal abnormalities (Down syndrome, Klinefelter syndrome)
◆ Disorders resulting from unknown prenatal influences (hydrocephalus, hydrencephaly, microcephaly)
◆ Disorders of metabolism or nutrition (phenylketonuria, hypothyroidism, Hurler syndrome, galactosemia, Tay–Sachs disease)
◆ Environmental influences (cultural–familial retardation, poor nutrition, lack of medical care)
◆ Gestational disorders (prematurity)
◆ Gross brain disorders that develop after birth (neurofibromatosis, intracranial neoplasm)
◆ Infection and intoxication (congenital rubella, syphilis, lead poisoning, meningitis, encephalitis, insecticides, drugs, maternal viral infection, toxins)
◆ Psychiatric disorders (autism)
◆ Trauma or physical conditions (mechanical injury, asphyxia, hyperpyrexia)

In the remaining population, predisposing factors, such as deficient prenatal or perinatal care, inadequate nutrition, poor social environment, and poor child-rearing practices, contribute significantly to intellectual disability.

Prenatal screening for genetic defects (such as Tay–Sachs disease) and counseling for families at risk for specific defects have reduced the incidence of genetically transmitted intellectual disabilities.

An estimated 1% to 3% of the population has intellectual disabilities, demonstrating an IQ below 70 and associated difficulty in carrying out tasks required for personal independence.

The AAIDD criteria promote a threshold IQ of 75 rather than 70 to be considered in the mild intellectual disability range to enable many more persons to receive social services.

Pathophysiology
The pathophysiology of intellectual disability, like many other psychiatric and psychological conditions, is not fully understood. This condition can occur independently, or in combination with other neurologic abnormalities such as structural brain anomaly, congenital abnormality, or epilepsy. Researchers continue to investigate biologic, psychiatric, and psychosocial factors that contribute to this condition. For the causes of intellectual disability that are understood, the majority include genetic abnormalities. Other pre-, peri-, and postnatal causes thought to contribute to intellectual disability include metabolic disorders, teratogens, toxins, infections, trauma, birth asphyxia, and nutrition deficiency.

Complications
◆ Delay or inability to meet developmental milestones
◆ Impaired social interaction
◆ Other comorbid conditions
◆ Slight or significant delay in intellectual and/or motor processing

Signs and symptoms
The observable effects of intellectual disabilities range from learning disabilities and uncontrollable behavior to severe cognitive and motor skill impairment. The earlier a child's adaptive needs are recognized and placement can be made into a special learning program, the more likely the child is to achieve age-appropriate adaptive behaviors. If the patient is older, review environmental adaptation to date.

The family of a patient who's intellectually disabled may report many problems stemming from frustration, fear, and exhaustion. These problems, such as financial difficulties, abuse, and divorce, can compromise the child's care. Physical examination may reveal signs of abuse or neglect.

People who are intellectually disabled may exhibit signs and symptoms of other disorders, such as cleft lip, congenital heart defects, and cerebral palsy as well as a lowered resistance to infection.

Diagnosis
℞ **CONFIRMING DIAGNOSIS** *A score of less than 70 on a standardized IQ test confirms the diagnosis of intellectual disability.*

The IQ test primarily predicts school performance and must be supplemented by other diagnostic evaluations.

For example, the AAIDD's Diagnostic Adaptive Behavior Scale deals with behaviors important to activities of daily living. This test evaluates self-help skills (toileting and eating), physical and social development, language, socialization, and time and number concepts. It also examines inappropriate behaviors, such as violent or destructive acts, withdrawal, and self-abusive or sexually aberrant behavior.

Age-appropriate adaptive behaviors are assessed by using developmental screening tests such as the Denver Developmental Activities and Denver II test forms. These tests compare the subject's functional level with the normal level for the same chronologic age. The greater the discrepancy between chronologic and developmental age, the more severe the intellectual disability. In most European and North American cultures, the Vineland Adaptive Behavior Scale Third Edition, a tool used to determine social competence, is recommended for use when appropriate.

In children, the functional level is based on sensorimotor skills, self-help skills, and socialization. In adolescents and adults, it's based on academic skills, reasoning and judgment skills, and social skills.

Treatment
Effective management requires an interprofessional team approach, which continues to assist the patient and his family on primary, secondary, and tertiary levels. A major goal is to develop the patient's strengths. Another important goal is the development of social adaptive skills.

Children with an intellectual developmental disorder require special education and training, ideally beginning in infancy. An individualized, effective education program can optimize the quality of life for even those with profound disability.

The prognosis for people with intellectual disability is related as much to timing and aggressive treatment, personal motivation, training opportunities, and associated conditions as to the degree of intellectual disability itself. With good support systems, many people with intellectual disability can succeed in many avenues of life. Successful management leads to independent functioning and occupational skills for some and a sheltered environment for others.

Special considerations

◆ Support the parents of a child diagnosed with an intellectual disability. They may be overwhelmed by caretaking and financial concerns. They may be grieving for their child, or may have difficulty accepting and/or bonding with their child.

◆ Remember that a child with intellectual disability has all the ordinary needs of a healthy child plus those associated with the disability. The child especially needs affection, acceptance, stimulation, and prudent, consistent discipline; the child is less able to cope if rejected, overprotected, or forced beyond appropriate abilities.

◆ When caring for a hospitalized patient who's intellectually disabled, promote continuity of care by acting as a liaison for parents and other healthcare professionals.

◆ During hospitalization, continue behavioral training programs already in place, but remember that illness may bring on some regression.

◆ For the parents of a child with severe intellectual disability, suggest ways to cope with the guilt, frustration, and exhaustion that commonly accompany caregiving for this population. The parents may need an extensive teaching and discharge planning program, including physical care procedures, stress reduction techniques, support services, and referral to developmental programs. Ask the social services department to recommend community resources.

◆ Teach parents how to care for the special needs of a child with intellectual disability. Suggest that they contact the AAIDD.

◆ Teach adolescents with intellectual disability how to deal with physical changes and sexual maturation. Encourage them to participate in appropriate sex education classes. People with intellectual disability may have difficulty expressing sexual concerns because of limited verbal skills.

TIC DISORDERS

Tic disorders, which include Tourette disorder, chronic motor or vocal tic disorder, and transient tic disorder, are similar pathophysiologically but differ in severity and prognosis. All tic disorders, commonly known simply as *tics*, are involuntary, spasmodic, recurrent, and purposeless motor movements or vocalizations. These disorders are classified as motor or vocal and as simple or complex. (See *Classifying tics.*) Tics usually begin before age 18. Transient tics are usually self-limiting, but Tourette syndrome follows a chronic course with remissions and exacerbations. Some people who have very mild tics don't seek treatment.

Causes and incidence

Although their exact cause is unknown, tic disorders occur more in certain families, suggesting a genetic cause. Tics commonly develop when a child experiences overwhelming anxiety, usually associated with normal maturation. There is evidence that the dopamine system is involved in the causation of tic disorders. Medications that suppress dopamine (haloperidol—Haldol,

---

Classifying tics

According to the *DSM-5*, tic disorders comprise four categories: Tourette disorder, persistent (chronic) motor or vocal tic disorder, provisional tic disorder, and other specified and unspecified tic disorders. Tics may be motor or vocal in origin.

Motor tics
Simple motor tics include eye blinking, neck jerking, shoulder shrugging, head banging, head turning, tongue protrusion, lip or tongue biting, nail biting, hair pulling, and facial grimacing.

Some examples of complex motor tics are facial gestures, grooming behaviors, hitting or biting oneself, jumping, hopping, touching, squatting, deep knee bends, retracing steps, twirling when walking, stamping, smelling an object, and imitating the movements of someone who is being observed (echopraxia).

Vocal tics
Examples of simple vocal tics include coughing, throat clearing, grunting, sniffing, snorting, hissing, clicking, yelping, and barking.

Complex vocal tics may involve repeating words out of context; using socially unacceptable words, many of which are obscene (coprolalia); or repeating the last-heard sound, word, or phrase of another person (echolalia).

fluphenazine) suppress tics, and medications that increase central dopamine levels (amphetamines, cocaine) increase tics. Immunologic and postinfectious processes may also be involved.

Obsessive-compulsive disorder (OCD), a condition that often includes tics in 29% of affected individuals, is more common in boys than in girls in childhood, and more common in adult females than in males. About 2% of the population has Tourette disorder.

Pathophysiology

Current research indicates that tic disorder involves multiple brain areas and complex pathways; some of these areas and pathways contribute to tic expression, while others house or contribute to the premonitory urge associated with this disorder. At this time, it is thought that the corticobasal ganglia pathway; its interaction with motor, sensory, limbic, and executive networks; and neuromodulators are involved.

Complications

◆ Physical injury
◆ Impaired social interaction
◆ Impaired self-esteem
◆ Depression
◆ Self-mutilation

Signs and symptoms

Assessment findings vary according to the type of tic disorder. Inspection, coupled with the patient's history, may reveal the specific motor or vocal patterns that characterize the tic as well as the frequency, complexity, and precipitating factors. The patient or his family may report that the tics occur sporadically many times per day. (See *Stress disorders with physical signs*, page 1105.)

Note whether certain situations worsen the tics. All tic disorders may be worsened by stress, and they usually diminish markedly during sleep. The patient also may report that they occur during activities that require concentration, such as reading or taking part in a hobby.

Determine whether the patient can control the tics. Most patients can do so, with conscious effort, for short periods of time.

Psychosocial assessment may reveal underlying stressful factors, such as problems with social adjustment, lack of self-esteem, and depression, resulting from tics.

Diagnosis

For very specific diagnostic criteria, see the *DSM-5*.

Treatment

Medications are not recommended unless the tics are severely disabling. Studies have shown that behavioral therapy such as habit reversal treatments is effective in treating transient tics. Psychotherapy may help with secondary emotional problems caused by tics.

Haloperidol (Haldol) is the drug of choice for treating Tourette syndrome. Pimozide (Orap, an oral dopamine-blocking drug) and clonidine (Catapres) are alternative choices. Tetrabenazine (Xenazine) has been used but is associated with depression of movement. Anxiolytics may be useful in dealing with secondary anxiety, but they don't reduce the severity or frequency of the tics.

Special considerations

◆ Offer emotional support and help the patient prevent emotional fatigue.
◆ Suggest that the patient with Tourette syndrome contact the Tourette Association of America or the Tourette Syndrome Association to obtain information and support.
◆ Help the patient identify and eliminate any avoidable stress and learn positive new ways to deal with anxiety.
◆ Encourage the patient to verbalize feelings about this disorder. Help the patient to understand that the movements are involuntary, and that he or she should not feel guilt or blame for such.

AUTISTIC SPECTRUM DISORDER

A severe, pervasive developmental disorder, autistic spectrum disorder is marked by characteristics such as persistent social communication and interaction deficits, and restrictive repetitive patterns of behavior, interest, or activities. These characteristics can range from mild to severe, with the most severe symptoms including unresponsiveness to social contact, gross deficits in language development, ritualistic and compulsive behaviors, restricted capacity for developmentally appropriate activities and interests, and abnormal responses to the environment. Autistic spectrum disorder may be complicated by epileptic seizures, depression, and, during periods of stress, catatonic phenomena. Autism usually becomes apparent before the child reaches age 36 months but, in some children, the actual onset is difficult to determine. Occasionally, autistic spectrum disorder isn't recognized until the child enters school.

The prognosis for autistic spectrum disorder varies based on the severity of presentation; most patients require a structured environment

Stress disorders with physical signs

Besides tic disorders, stress-related disorders that produce physical signs in children include stuttering, functional enuresis, functional encopresis, sleepwalking, and sleep terrors.

Stuttering
Characterized by abnormal speech rhythms with repetitions and hesitations at the beginning of words, stuttering may involve movements of the respiratory muscles, shoulders, and face. There is no evidence to indicate that psychiatric problems cause stuttering or that people who stutter have more psychiatric disturbances than those with other forms of speech disorders. However, this disorder most commonly occurs in children of average or superior intelligence who fear they can't meet expectations. Related problems may include low self-esteem, tension, anxiety, humiliation, and withdrawal from social situations.

Evaluation and treatment by a speech pathologist teaches patients who stutter to place equal weight on each syllable in a sentence, how to breathe properly, and how to control anxiety.

Enuresis
This disorder is characterized by intentional or involuntary voiding of urine, usually during the night (nocturnal enuresis). Enuresis occurs somewhat frequently in children; prevalence is 5% to 10% in children under the age of 10, with up to 75% of children affected having a familial component.

Causes may be related to stress, such as the birth of a sibling, the move to a new home, divorce, separation, hospitalization, faulty toilet training (inconsistent, demanding, or punitive), and unrealistic responsibilities. Associated problems include low self-esteem, social withdrawal or isolation from peers because of ostracism and ridicule, and anger, rejection, and punishment by caregivers.

Teach parents or caregivers that an objective, nonjudgmental attitude helps the child learn bladder control without undue stress. If enuresis persists into late childhood, treatment with imipramine (Tofranil) may help. Dry-bed therapy may include the use of an alarm (wet bell pad), social motivation, self-correction of accidents, and positive reinforcement.

Encopresis
Encopresis is denoted by voluntary or involuntary passage of feces into the child's clothes or other inappropriate receptacles, such as closets or floors. This condition is more common in boys than in girls, and must occur at least once monthly for 3 or more months to meet diagnostic criteria. This condition may be related to constipation or impaction, or due to psychological stressors such as repressed anger, withdrawal from peer relationships, and loss of self-esteem.

Treatment involves encouraging the child to be open with parents or caregivers when he or she has an "accident." Teach parents or caregivers to give the child clean clothes without criticism or punishment. Medical examination should rule out any physical disorder. Child, adult, and family therapy may help reduce anger and disappointment over the child's development and improve parenting techniques. Supportive psychotherapy and relaxation therapy techniques may be useful in reducing anxiety and improving self-esteem.

Sleepwalking and sleep terrors
In sleepwalking, the child calmly rises from bed in a state of altered consciousness and walks around with no subsequent recollection of any dreams. In sleep terrors, the child awakens terrified, in a state of clouded consciousness, usually unable to recognize parents and familiar surroundings. Visual hallucinations are common.

Sleepwalking is usually a response to an emotional concern. Tell parents to gently "talk" the child back to bed. If the child wakes, he or she should be comforted and supported.

Sleep terrors are a normal developmental event in very young children, usually occurring within 30 minutes to 3½ hours of sleep onset. Tachycardia, tachypnea, diaphoresis, dilated pupils, and piloerection are associated with sleep terrors. The child may also fear being alone.

Teach parents to make sure that the child has access to them at night. Sleep terrors usually are self-limiting and subside within a few weeks.

throughout life. Prognosis improves in a supportive environment.

Causes and incidence

The causes of autistic spectrum disorder remain unclear; however, studies show a biological basis for this disorder. Genetic, biological, immunologic, perinatal, and biochemical causes have been proposed.

Some children with autism show abnormal but nonspecific EEG findings that suggest brain dysfunction, possibly resulting from trauma, disease, or a structural abnormality. Autism spectrum disorder has also been associated with numerous other conditions involving intellectual and/or language impairment, motor deficits, and macrocephaly, with conditions such as Rett syndrome and Fragile X syndrome, and with history of environmental exposure (e.g., valproate, fetal alcohol syndrome, and/or very low birth weight). Autism spectrum disorder has become much more common in the past decades, with 1 in 40 to 1 in 500 children affected in the United States. It affects three to four times more boys than girls, and appears to have a genetic component.

Pathophysiology

The pathophysiology of autism spectrum disorder is not fully understood. Research suggests that there are genetic, neurobiologic, environmental, and perinatal factors that contribute.

Complications

◆ Social isolation
◆ Failure to meet developmental milestones
◆ Need for ongoing care, into adulthood

Signs and symptoms

A primary characteristic of autism spectrum disorder is unresponsiveness to people. Infants with this disorder won't cuddle, avoid eye contact and facial expressions, and are indifferent to affection and physical contact. Parents may report that the child becomes rigid or flaccid when held, cries when touched, and shows little or no interest in human contact.

As the infant grows older, the smiling response is delayed or absent. This child doesn't lift his or her arms in anticipation of being picked up or form an attachment to a specific caregiver. Furthermore, stranger anxiety that's typical in the 8-month-old infant is often absent.

A child with autism spectrum disorder fails to learn the usual socialization games (peek-a-boo, pat-a-cake, or bye-bye). The child is likely to relate to others only to fill a physical need and even then it may be without eye contact or speech. The end result may be mutual withdrawal between parents and child.

Severe language impairment and lack of imaginative play are characteristic. The child may be mute or may use immature speech patterns. For example, the child may use a single word to express a series of activities; the word "ground" may be used when referring to any step in using a playground slide.

The child's speech commonly shows echolalia (meaningless repetition of words or phrases) and pronoun reversal ("you go walk" when he means, "I want to go for a walk"). When answering a question, the child may simply repeat the question to mean yes and remain silent to mean no.

The child may show little imagination, seldom acting out adult roles or engaging in fantasy play. Lining up an exact number of toys in the same manner over and over is common, as is repetitively mimicking someone else's actions.

A child with severe autism spectrum disorder may show characteristically abnormal behavior patterns, such as engaging in screaming fits, rituals, rhythmic rocking, arm flapping, crying without tears, head banging, and disturbed sleeping and eating patterns. Behavior may be self-destructive (hand biting, eye gouging, hair pulling, or head banging) or self-stimulating (playing with own saliva, feces, and urine). These responses to the environment include an extreme compulsion for sameness.

In response to sensory stimuli, the child may underreact or overreact, and may ignore objects—dropping those given or not looking at them—or may become excessively absorbed in them—continually watching the objects or the movement of his or her own fingers over the objects. The child commonly responds to stimuli by head banging, rocking, whirling, and hand flapping, and may avoid using sight and hearing to interact with the environment.

A child with autism spectrum disorder may exhibit additional behavioral abnormalities, such as:
◆ eating, drinking, and sleeping problems, for example, limiting the diet to just a few foods, excessive drinking, or repeatedly waking during the night and rocking
◆ mood disorders, including labile mood, giggling or crying without reason, lack of emotional responses, no fear of real danger but excessive fear of harmless objects, and generalized anxiety

Diagnosis

For very specific diagnostic criteria, see the *DSM-5*.

Treatment

The difficult and prolonged treatment of autism spectrum disorder must begin early, continue for years (through adolescence or adulthood), and coordinate efforts to encourage social adjustment and speech development and to reduce self-destructive behavior.

Behavioral techniques are used to decrease symptoms and increase the child's ability to respond. Positive reinforcement, using food and other rewards, can enhance language and social skills. Providing pleasurable sensory and motor stimulation (such as jogging or playing with a ball) encourages appropriate behavior and helps discourage inappropriate behavior. Drug therapy with an agent, such as haloperidol (Haldol), may be helpful. Risperidone (Risperdal) has been used successfully to diminish aggressiveness and hyperactivity.

Treatment may take place in the home, in a psychiatric institution, in a specialized school, or in a day-care program depending on the severity of symptoms. Family members may benefit from counseling, respite services, and interprofessional team coordination of care. Until the causes of infantile autism are known, prevention isn't possible.

Special considerations

◆ Reduce self-destructive behaviors. Physically stop the child from self-harm, while firmly saying "no." When the child responds to your voice, first give a primary reward (such as food); later, substitute verbal or physical reinforcement as tolerated (such as saying "good" or giving the child a hug or a pat on the back). Work to identify positive ways for the child to channel energy.

◆ Foster appropriate use of language. Provide positive reinforcement when the child indicates needs correctly. Give verbal reinforcement at first (e.g., by saying "good" or "great"); later, give physical reinforcement as tolerated (such as a hug or a pat on the hand or shoulder).

◆ Encourage development of self-esteem.

◆ Encourage self-care. For example, place a brush in the child's hand and guide the hand to brush hair. Similarly, teach the child to wash hands and face.

◆ Encourage acceptance of minor environmental changes. Prepare the child for the change by explaining it beforehand. Make initial changes minor; for example, change the color of a bedspread or the placement of food on a plate. When the child has accepted minor changes, provide positive reinforcement, and move on to bigger ones.

◆ Provide emotional support to the parents and caregivers, and refer them to the Autism Society.

◆ Teach the parents or caregivers how to physically care for the child's needs.

◆ Teach the parents or caregivers how to identify signs of excessive stress and the coping skills to use under these circumstances. Emphasize that they'll be ineffective caregivers if they don't take the time to meet their own needs in addition to those of their child.

◆ Help the parents understand that they aren't responsible for their child's condition and shouldn't feel guilty about it.

ATTENTION DEFICIT HYPERACTIVITY DISORDER

The patient with attention deficit hyperactivity disorder (ADHD) has difficulty focusing attention; engaging in quiet, passive activities; or both. In some cases, the patient isn't diagnosed until adulthood.

Causes and incidence

ADHD is thought to be caused by a physiologic brain disorder with a familial tendency. Some studies indicate that it may result from disturbances in neurotransmitter levels in the brain caused by reduced blood flow in the striated area of the brain. It affects approximately 5% of school-age children. Adults with ADHD often experience comorbid conditions such as mood or anxiety disorders, substance user disorder, or intermittent explosive disorder.

Pathophysiology

The pathophysiology of ADHD is not fully understood. It is thought that there is dysfunction of the frontal-subcortical and parietal circuits; smaller volume in the frontal cortex, cerebellum, and subcorticoid structures; and possible genetic connection.

Complications

◆ Emotional and social complications

◆ Poor nutrition

◆ Academic or workplace difficulty

Signs and symptoms

The principal sign of ADHD is hyperactivity that's present over a long period, in at least two settings (such as school and home), and is accompanied by easy distractibility. The patient may be impulsive, emotionally labile, explosive, or irritable. Although the patient may be highly intelligent, school or work performance patterns are sporadic and may not represent the patient's actual ability. The patient may jump from one partly completed project, thought, or task to another. The patient may have an attention deficit without hyperactivity, which is less likely to be diagnosed and treated.

In a younger child, signs and symptoms include an inability to wait in line, remain seated, wait for a turn, or concentrate on one activity until its completion. An older child or an adult may be described as impulsive and easily distracted by irrelevant thoughts, sounds, or sights. The patient may also be characterized as emotionally labile, inattentive, or prone to daydreaming. Disorganization becomes apparent as the patient has difficulty meeting deadlines and keeping track of school or work tools and materials.

Diagnosis
For very specific diagnostic criteria, see the *DSM-5*. The child with ADHD is often referred for evaluation by the school. Diagnosis of ADHD usually begins by obtaining data from several sources, including the parents, teachers, and the child personally. Complete psychological, medical, and neurologic evaluations should be completed to rule out other problems. Then the child undergoes tests that measure impulsiveness, attention, and the ability to sustain a task. The combined findings portray a clear picture of the disorder and of the areas of support the child will need.

Treatment
Education is the first step in effective treatment. The entire treatment team (which ideally includes parents, teachers, and therapists as well as the patient and the healthcare provider) must understand the disorder and its effect on the individual's functioning.

Treatment varies, depending on the severity of symptoms and their effects on the child's ability to function. Behavior modification, coaching, external structure, use of planning and organizing systems, and supportive psychotherapy help the patient cope with the disorder.

The patient may benefit from medication to relieve symptoms. Ideally, the treatment team identifies the symptoms to be managed, selects appropriate medication, and then tracks the patient's symptoms carefully to determine the drug's effectiveness. Stimulants are the most commonly used drugs. Antipsychotics may sometimes be used in combination with stimulants. However, other drugs, including tricyclic

antidepressants (TCAs), mood stabilizers, and beta-adrenergic blockers, sometimes help control symptoms.

Special considerations
◆ Work with the patient and parents or caregivers to develop external structure and controls.
◆ Set realistic expectations and limits because the patient with ADHD can become easily frustrated (which leads to decreased self-control).
◆ Remain calm and consistent.
◆ Keep instructions short and simple.
◆ Provide praise, rewards, and positive feedback whenever possible.

CONDUCT DISORDER
Aggressive behavior is the hallmark of conduct disorder. A child with this disorder fights, bullies, intimidates, and assaults others physically or sexually, and is truant from school at an early age. Typically, the patient has poor relationships with peers and adults and violates others' rights and society's rules. Conduct disorder evolves slowly over time until a consistent pattern of behavior is established.

Causes and incidence
Studies have suggested that the disorder has biological (including genetic) and psychosocial components. Social risk factors that may predispose a child to conduct disorder include socioeconomic deprivation; harsh, punitive parenting with verbal or physical aggression; separation from parents; early institutionalization; family neglect, abuse, or violence; frequent verbal abuse from parents, teachers, or other authority figures; parental psychiatric illness, substance abuse, or marital discord; large family size, crowding, and poverty; and divorce with persistent hostility between the parents. The prevalence of conduct disorder is between 2% and 10%, with prevalence rates rising from childhood to adolescence. The prognosis is worse in children with an earlier onset; these children are more likely to develop antisocial personality disorder as adults.

Pathophysiology
The pathophysiology of conduct disorder is not fully understood. In addition to psychosocial components, it is thought that neurologic damage caused by low birth weight or birth complications, underarousal of the autonomic nervous system, learning impairments, insensitivity to physical pain and punishment, and impaired functioning of the nonadrenergic system may contribute.

Complications
- Poor performance in school
- Substance abuse
- Higher incidence of other psychosocial disorders such as ADHD, oppositional defiant disorder, mood disorders, anxiety disorders, depression, and learning disabilities

Signs and symptoms
- Physical and/or sexual abuse of others
- Cheating in school
- Cruelty to animals
- Engaging in precocious sexual activity
- Fighting with family members and peers
- Skipping classes
- Smoking cigarettes
- Speaking to others in a hostile manner
- Stealing or shoplifting
- Using drugs or alcohol
- Vandalizing or destroying property

Diagnosis
Medical and psychiatric evaluations, feedback from parents, a school consultant's recommendations, case manager plan, and probation officer reports can assist in a team approach to diagnosis. For very specific diagnostic criteria, see the *DSM-5*.

Treatment
Treatment focuses on coordinating the child's psychological, physiologic, and educational needs. A structured living environment with consistent rules and consequences can help reduce many symptoms. Parents need to be taught how to deal with the child's behavior. Juvenile justice interventions may also be used. Medication can be useful as an adjunct to treatment. Overt aggression may be managed with antipsychotics, lithium (Lithobid) or selective serotonin reuptake inhibitors (SSRIs). Comorbid conditions should also be addressed.

Special considerations
- Work to establish a trusting relationship with the child.
- Provide clear behavioral guidelines, including consequences for disruptive and manipulative behavior.
- Teach the child effective coping skills, social skills, and problem-solving skills, and ask for return demonstration.
- Teach the child to express anger appropriately through constructive methods to release negative feelings and frustrations.
- Help the child accept responsibility for behavior rather than blaming others, becoming defensive, and wanting revenge.

- Use role-playing to help the child practice handling stress and gain skill and confidence in managing difficult situations.
- Support the parents in setting firm, appropriate limits for the child.

Substance-related and addictive disorders

ALCOHOL USE DISORDER
The patient with alcohol use disorder experiences a need for the daily intake of large amounts of alcohol for day-to-day functioning. A regular pattern of heavy drinking limited to weekends, with periods of sobriety between weekends, also suggests a pattern of abuse. People with these patterns of drinking may show impaired social and occupational functioning.

Causes and incidence
Numerous biological, psychological, and sociocultural factors appear to be involved in alcohol addiction. An offspring of one parent with alcohol use disorder is many times more likely to become an alcoholic than is a peer without such a parent.

Psychological factors may include the urge to drink alcohol to reduce anxiety or symptoms of mental illness; the desire to avoid responsibility in familial, social, and work relationships; and the need to improve self-esteem.

Sociocultural factors include the availability of alcoholic beverages, group or peer pressure, an excessively stressful lifestyle, and social attitudes that approve of frequent drinking.

More than 8.5% of American adults have a problem with alcohol use. Research shows that one in six Americans binge drink weekly. Alcohol use disorder cuts across all social and economic groups, involves both sexes, and occurs at all stages of the life cycle, beginning as early as elementary school.

Pathophysiology
The pathophysiology of alcohol use disorder is not fully understood. Biological factors that contribute to this disorder are thought to include genetic or biochemical abnormalities, nutritional deficiencies, endocrine imbalances, and allergic responses.

Complications (Also see *Complications of alcohol use.*)
- Malnutrition
- Cirrhosis of the liver
- Peripheral neuropathy
- Brain damage
- Cardiomyopathy
- Financial difficulty
- Strained familial relationships

Complications of alcohol use

Alcohol can damage body tissues by its direct irritating effects, by changes that take place in the body during its metabolism, by aggravation of existing disease, by accidents occurring during intoxication, and by interactions between the substance and drugs. Such tissue damage can cause these complications.

Cardiopulmonary complications
♦ Cardiac arrhythmias
♦ Cardiomyopathy
♦ Chronic obstructive pulmonary disease
♦ Essential hypertension
♦ Increased risk of tuberculosis
♦ Pneumonia

Gastrointestinal (GI) complications
♦ Chronic diarrhea
♦ Esophageal cancer
♦ Esophageal varices
♦ Esophagitis
♦ Gastric ulcers
♦ Gastritis
♦ GI bleeding
♦ Malabsorption
♦ Pancreatitis

Hematologic complications
♦ Anemia
♦ Leukopenia
♦ Reduced number of phagocytes

Hepatic complications
♦ Alcoholic hepatitis
♦ Cirrhosis
♦ Fatty liver

Neurologic complications
♦ Alcoholic dementia
♦ Alcoholic hallucinosis
♦ Alcohol withdrawal delirium
♦ Korsakoff syndrome
♦ Peripheral neuropathy
♦ Seizure disorders
♦ Subdural hematoma
♦ Wernicke encephalopathy

Psychiatric complications
♦ Amotivational syndrome
♦ Depression
♦ Fetal alcohol syndrome
♦ Impaired social and occupational functioning
♦ Multiple substance abuse
♦ Suicide

Other complications
♦ Beriberi
♦ Hypoglycemia
♦ Infertility
♦ Leg and foot ulcers
♦ Impaired respiratory diffusion
♦ Increased incidence of pulmonary infections
♦ Myopathies
♦ Prostatitis
♦ Sexual performance difficulties

Signs and symptoms

Because the person with alcohol dependence may hide or deny addiction, and may temporarily manage to maintain a functional life, assessing for alcohol use disorder can be difficult. Note physical and psychosocial symptoms that suggest alcohol use disorder. For example, the patient's history may suggest a need for daily or episodic alcohol use to maintain adequate functioning, an inability to discontinue or reduce alcohol intake, episodes of anesthesia or amnesia (blackouts) during intoxication, episodes of violence during intoxication, and interference with social and familial relationships and occupational responsibilities. Many minor complaints may be alcohol-related. The patient may report malaise, dyspepsia, mood swings or depression, and an increased incidence of infection. Observe the patient for poor personal hygiene and untreated injuries, such as cigarette burns, fractures, and bruises, that can't be fully explained. Note any evidence of an unusually high tolerance of sedatives and opioids.

Secretive or manipulative behavior may be a manifestation of the patient's denial of the severity of addiction. Suspect alcohol use disorder if the patient uses inordinate amounts of aftershave or mouthwash. When confronted, the patient may deny or rationalize the problem, or be guarded or hostile in response. He or she may project anger or feelings of guilt or inadequacy onto others to avoid confronting the illness. This patient may even sign out of the hospital against medical advice.

After abstinence or reduction in alcohol intake, signs and symptoms of withdrawal—which begin shortly after drinking has stopped and last for 5 to 7 days—may vary. The patient initially experiences anorexia, nausea, anxiety, fever, insomnia, diaphoresis, and tremor, progressing to severe tremulousness, agitation and, possibly, hallucinations and violent behavior. Major motor seizures (alcohol withdrawal seizures) can occur during withdrawal. Suspect alcohol use disorder in any patient with unexplained seizures. (See *Signs and symptoms of alcohol withdrawal,* page 1111.)

Signs and symptoms of alcohol withdrawal

Alcohol withdrawal signs and symptoms may vary in degree from mild (morning hangover) to severe (alcohol withdrawal delirium). Alcohol withdrawal delirium is marked by acute distress following abrupt withdrawal after prolonged or massive use.

Signs and symptoms	Mild	Moderate	Severe
Anxiety	Mild restlessness	Obvious motor restlessness and anxiety	Extreme restlessness and agitation with intense fearfulness
Appetite	Impaired appetite	Marked anorexia	Rejection of all food and fluid except alcohol
Blood pressure	Normal or slightly elevated systolic	Usually elevated systolic	Elevated systolic and diastolic
Confusion	None	Variable	Marked confusion and disorientation
GI symptoms	Nausea	Nausea and vomiting	Dry heaves and vomiting
Hallucinations	None	Vague, transient visual and auditory hallucinations and illusions (commonly nocturnal)	Visual and occasionally auditory hallucinations, usually of fearful or threatening content; misidentification of people and frightening delusions related to hallucinatory experiences
Seizures	None	Possible	Common
Sleep disturbance	Restless sleep or insomnia	Marked insomnia and nightmares	Total wakefulness
Sweating	Slight	Obvious	Marked hyperhidrosis

 ELDER TIP *Remember to consider the possibility of alcohol use when evaluating older patients.*

Diagnosis

For very specific diagnostic criteria, see the *DSM-5*.

Clinical findings may help support the diagnosis of alcohol use disorder. For example, laboratory tests can confirm alcohol use and complications and document recent alcohol ingestion. A blood alcohol level ranging from 0.08% to 0.10% weight/volume (200 mg/dL) is accepted as the level of intoxication, depending on the state or country. The blood alcohol level in a physically dependent and tolerant drinker may exceed levels that would cause severe dysfunction or death in a nontolerant drinker. For example, a tolerant drinker might have a blood alcohol level of more than 0.5 mg (the usual lethal level) and still be alive, talking, and moving.

In severe hepatic disease, the blood urea nitrogen level is increased, and the serum glucose level is decreased. Further testing may reveal increased serum ammonia and amylase levels. Urine toxicology studies may help determine if the patient with alcohol withdrawal delirium or another acute complication abuses other drugs as well.

Liver function studies revealing increased levels of serum cholesterol, lactate dehydrogenase, alanine aminotransferase, aspartate aminotransferase, and creatine kinase may point to liver damage, and elevated serum amylase and lipase levels point to acute pancreatitis. A hematologic workup can identify anemia, thrombocytopenia, prolonged prothrombin time, and prolonged partial thromboplastin time.

Treatment

Total abstinence from alcohol is the only effective treatment. Supportive programs that offer detoxification, rehabilitation, and aftercare, including continued involvement in Alcoholics Anonymous (AA), may produce good long-term results.

Acute intoxication is treated symptomatically by supporting respiration, preventing aspiration of vomitus, replacing fluids, administering I.V. glucose to prevent hypoglycemia, correcting hypothermia or acidosis, and initiating emergency treatment for trauma, infection, or gastrointestinal (GI) bleeding.

Treatment of chronic alcohol use requires a varied approach that may include medications to deter alcohol use and treat effects of withdrawal; psychotherapy, consisting of behavior modification techniques, group therapy, and family therapy; and appropriate measures to relieve associated physical problems.

Aversion, or deterrent, therapy involves a daily oral dose of disulfiram (Antabuse) to prevent compulsive drinking. This drug interferes with alcohol metabolism and allows toxic levels of acetaldehyde to accumulate in the patient's blood, producing immediate and potentially fatal distress in the event that he or she consumes alcohol up to 2 weeks after taking it. Disulfiram (Antabuse) is contraindicated during pregnancy and in the patient with diabetes, heart disease, severe hepatic disease, or any disorder in which such a reaction could be especially dangerous. Another form of aversion therapy attempts to induce aversion by administering alcohol with an emetic.

The first drug approved by the U.S. Food and Drug Administration (FDA) for the treatment of alcohol use disorder since disulfiram (Antabuse) is naltrexone (Vivitrol), an opiate antagonist that effectively reduces the amount of intake, severity of craving, and relapse incidence. It's believed to work by preventing the effects of increased endorphins produced as a product of increased alcohol intake.

For long-term success, the recovering individual must learn to fill the place alcohol once occupied in life with something constructive. Therapy using disulfiram (Antabuse) or naltrexone (Vivitrol) may only substitute one drug dependence for another, so it should be used prudently.

Benzodiazepines aren't recommended during rehabilitation due to their addictive nature and the potential for reinforcing the substance abuse behavior.

✦ **ELDER TIP** *Because the older patient may be more sensitive to these drugs, withdrawal may take longer (weeks or months) and be more severe than what a younger adult experiences.*

Supportive counseling or individual, group, or family psychotherapy may help. Ongoing support groups are helpful. In AA, a self-help group with over a million members worldwide, the patient with alcohol use disorder finds emotional support from others with similar problems. Many of AA's members stay sober as long as 5 years or more.

Special considerations
✦ During acute intoxication or withdrawal, carefully monitor the patient's mental status, heart rate, breath sounds, blood pressure, and temperature every 30 minutes to 6 hours.
✦ Assess the patient for signs of inadequate nutrition and dehydration. Start seizure precautions and administer drugs prescribed to treat the signs and symptoms of withdrawal in chronic alcohol abuse.

✦ During withdrawal, orient the patient to reality. Hallucinations may occur which predisposes the patient to harm self or others. Maintain a calm environment, minimizing noise and shadows to reduce the incidence of delusions and hallucinations. Avoid restraining the patient unless necessary; follow agency policy for restraint application and monitoring.
✦ Approach the patient in a nonthreatening way. Limit sustained eye contact. Listen attentively and respond with empathy. Explain all procedures.
✦ Monitor the patient for signs of depression or impending suicide.
✦ In chronic alcohol use disorder, help the patient accept the drinking problem and the necessity for abstinence. Confront the patient about behaviors.
✦ If the patient is taking disulfiram (Antabuse) (or has taken it within the past 2 weeks), teach about the effects of alcohol ingestion, which may last from 30 minutes to 3 hours or longer. The reaction includes nausea, vomiting, facial flushing, headache, shortness of breath, red eyes, blurred vision, sweating, tachycardia, hypotension, and fainting. Emphasize that even a small amount of alcohol will induce this adverse reaction and that the longer the patient takes the drug, the greater the sensitivity to alcohol will be. Even medicinal sources of alcohol, such as mouthwash, cough syrups, liquid vitamins, and cold remedies, must be avoided.
✦ Refer the patient to AA and offer to arrange a visit from an AA member. Stress the effectiveness of this organization.
✦ For the individual who has lost all contact with family and friends and who has a long history of unemployment, trouble with the law, or other problems associated with alcohol use disorder, rehabilitation may involve job training, sheltered workshops, halfway houses, and other supervised facilities.
✦ Refer the spouse of an alcoholic to Al-Anon and children of an alcoholic to Alateen. By participating in these self-help groups, family members learn to relinquish responsibility for the individual's drinking. Point out that family involvement in rehabilitation can reduce family tensions.
✦ Refer adult children of an alcoholic to the National Association for Children of Alcoholics.

SUBSTANCE USE DISORDER
Substance use and dependence causes physical, mental, emotional, and/or social harm. Examples of abused drugs include opioids, stimulants, depressants, anxiolytics, and hallucinogens. (See *Understanding commonly abused substances*, pages 1113 to 1117.) Chronic drug abuse, especially I.V. use, can lead to life-threatening complications, such as cardiac and respiratory arrest,

Understanding commonly abused substances

Substance	Signs and symptoms	Interventions
Cannabinoids		

Marijuana

Street names: 420, Aunt Mary, BC bud, blunt (cannabis within tobacco), boom, chronic, dope, gangster, ganja, grass, hash, herb, hydro, indo, joint (cannabis cigarette), kif, Mary Jane, mota, pot, reefer, roach, sinsemilla, skunk, smoke, weed, and yerba. Street names of synthetic cannabinoids include synthetic weed, legal high, spice, K2, Blaze, RedX Dawn, Paradise, Demon, Black Magic, Spike, Mr. Nice Guy, Ninja, Zohai, Dream, Genie, Sence, Smoke, Skunk, Serenity, Yucatan, Fire, and Crazy Clown. ♦ *Routes:* ingestion, smoking ♦ *Dependence:* psychological ♦ *Duration of effect:* 2 to 3 hours ♦ *Medical uses:* antiemetic for chemotherapy	♦ *Of use:* acute psychosis; agitation; amotivational syndrome; anxiety; asthma; bronchitis; conjunctival reddening; decreased muscle strength; delusions; distorted sense of time and self-perception; dry mouth; euphoria; hallucinations; impaired cognition, short-term memory, and mood; incoordination; increased hunger; increased systolic pressure when supine; orthostatic hypotension; paranoia; spontaneous laughter; tachycardia; and vivid visual imagery ♦ *Of withdrawal:* chills, decreased appetite, increased rapid eye movement sleep, insomnia, irritability, nervousness, restlessness, tremors, and weight loss	♦ Place the patient in a quiet room. ♦ Monitor vital signs. ♦ Give supplemental oxygen for respiratory depression and I.V. fluids for hypotension. ♦ Give diazepam (Valium), as ordered, for extreme agitation and acute psychosis.
Depressants		

Alcohol

♦ *Found in:* beer, wine, and distilled spirits; also contained in cough syrup, aftershave, and mouthwash ♦ *Route:* ingestion ♦ *Dependence:* physical and psychological ♦ *Duration of effect:* varies according to individual and amount ingested; metabolized at rate of 10 mL/hour ♦ *Medical uses:* neurolysis (absolute alcohol); emergency tocolytic; and treatment of ethylene glycol and methanol poisoning	♦ *Of acute use:* coma, decreased inhibitions, euphoria followed by depression or hostility, impaired judgment, incoordination, respiratory depression, slurred speech, unconsciousness, and vomiting ♦ *Of withdrawal:* delirium, hallucinations, seizures, and tremors	♦ Place the patient in a quiet room. ♦ If alcohol was ingested within 4 hours, induce vomiting or perform gastric lavage; give activated charcoal and a saline cathartic. ♦ Monitor vital signs. ♦ Treat withdrawal seizures, tremors, diaphoresis, anxiety, tachycardia, and hypertension. Diazepam (Valium) may be used if an I.V. route needs to be used. ♦ Institute seizure precautions. ♦ Provide I.V. fluid replacement as well as dextrose, thiamine, B-complex vitamins, and vitamin C to treat dehydration, hypoglycemia, and nutritional deficiencies. ♦ Assess for aspiration pneumonia. ♦ Prepare for dialysis if patient's vital functions are severely depressed.

(continued)

Understanding commonly abused substances (continued)

Substance	Signs and symptoms	Interventions

Barbiturates (amobarbital—Amytal Sodium, phenobarbital—Phenobarb, secobarbital—Seconal)

♦ *Street names:* for barbiturates—barbs and downers; for amobarbital—blue angels, blue devils, blue heavens; for phenobarbital—goofballs and purple hearts; and for secobarbital—reds, red birds, red devils, lilly, F-40s, pinks, pink ladies, seggy ♦ *Routes:* ingestion and injection ♦ *Dependence:* physical and psychological ♦ *Duration:* 1 to 16 hours ♦ *Medical uses:* anesthetic, anticonvulsant, sedative, hypnotic	♦ *Of use:* absent reflexes, blisters or bullous lesions, cyanosis, depressed level of consciousness (LOC) (from confusion to coma), fever, flaccid muscles, hypotension, hypothermia, nystagmus, paradoxical reaction in children and elderly people, poor pupil reaction to light, and respiratory depression ♦ *Of withdrawal:* agitation, anxiety, fever, insomnia, orthostatic hypotension, tachycardia, and tremors ♦ *Of rapid withdrawal:* anorexia, apprehension, hallucinations, orthostatic hypotension, tonic–clonic seizures, tremors, and weakness	♦ If ingestion was recent, induce vomiting or perform gastric lavage. Follow with activated charcoal. ♦ Monitor the patient's vital signs and perform frequent neurologic assessments. ♦ As ordered, give an I.V. fluid bolus for hypotension and alkalinized urine. ♦ Institute seizure precautions. ♦ Relieve withdrawal symptoms as ordered. ♦ Use a hypothermia or hyperthermia blanket for temperature alterations.

Benzodiazepines (alprazolam—Xanax, chlordiazepoxide—Librium, clonazepam—Klonopin, clorazepate—Tranxene, diazepam—Valium, flurazepam, lorazepam—Ativan, midazolam—Midazolam + SyrSpend SF PH4, oxazepam, quazepam—Doral, temazepam—Restoril, triazolam—Halcion)

♦ *Street names:* dolls and yellow jackets ♦ *Routes:* ingestion and injection ♦ *Dependence:* physical and psychological ♦ *Duration of effect:* 4 to 8 hours ♦ *Medical uses:* anxiolytic, anticonvulsant, sedative, hypnotic	♦ *Of use:* ataxia, drowsiness, hypotension, increased self-confidence, relaxation, and slurred speech ♦ *Of overdose:* confusion, coma, drowsiness, and respiratory depression ♦ *Of withdrawal:* abdominal cramps, agitation, anxiety, diaphoresis, hypertension, tachycardia, tonic–clonic seizures, tremors, and vomiting	♦ If the drug was ingested, induce vomiting or perform gastric lavage. Follow with activated charcoal and a cathartic. ♦ Monitor the patient's vital signs. ♦ Give supplemental oxygen for hypoxia-induced seizures. ♦ As ordered, give I.V. fluids for hypertension, and physostigmine salicylate for respiratory or central nervous system (CNS) depression. Flumazenil, a specific benzodiazepine antagonist, can be used in cases of overdose to reverse the effects of the benzodiazepine.

Understanding commonly abused substances (continued)

Substance	Signs and symptoms	Interventions

Opiates (codeine, heroin, morphine—MS Contin, meperidine—Demerol, and opium)

◆ *Street names:* for heroin—junk, white horse, white lady, white girl, white boy, white stuff, boy, H, smack, China White, Mexican mud, Mexican brown, snow, snowball, skunk; for morphine—morph, M, and microdots, salt and sugar, Miss Emma ◆ *Routes:* for codeine, meperidine, and morphine—ingestion, injection, and smoking; for heroin—ingestion, injection, inhalation, and smoking; for opium—ingestion and smoking ◆ *Dependence:* physical and psychological ◆ *Duration of effect:* 3 to 6 hours ◆ *Medical uses:* for codeine—analgesia and antitussive; for heroin—none; for morphine and meperidine—analgesia; for opium—analgesia and antidiarrheal	◆ *Of use:* anorexia, arrhythmias, clammy skin, constipation, constricted pupils, decreased LOC, detachment from reality, drowsiness, euphoria, hypotension, impaired judgment, increased pigmentation over veins, lack of concern, lethargy, nausea, needle marks, respiratory depression, seizures, shallow or slow respirations, skin lesions or abscesses, slurred speech, swollen or perforated nasal mucosa, thrombotic veins, urine retention, and vomiting ◆ *Of withdrawal:* abdominal cramps, anorexia, chills, diaphoresis, dilated pupils, hyperactive bowel sounds, irritability, nausea, panic, piloerection, runny nose, sweating, tremors, watery eyes, and yawning	◆ If the drug was ingested, induce vomiting or perform gastric lavage. ◆ As ordered, give naloxone (Narcan) until CNS effects are reversed. ◆ Give I.V. fluids to increase circulatory volume. ◆ Use extra blankets for hypothermia; if ineffective, use a hyperthermia blanket. ◆ Reorient the patient to time, place, and person. ◆ Assess breath sounds to monitor for pulmonary edema. ◆ Monitor for signs and symptoms of withdrawal. ◆ Naltrexone (Vivitrol) is an opiate antagonist that reverses the effects of the opiate.

Hallucinogens

Lysergic acid diethylamide

◆ *Street names:* LSD, acid, blotters, blue heaven, cube, dots, mellow yellow, window pane, yellow sunshine, and microdot ◆ *Routes:* ingestion, smoking ◆ *Dependence:* possibly psychological ◆ *Duration of effect:* 8 to 12 hours ◆ *Medical uses:* none	◆ *Of use:* abdominal cramps, arrhythmias, chills, depersonalization, diaphoresis, diarrhea, distorted visual perception and perception of time and space, dizziness, dry mouth, fever, grandiosity, hallucinations, heightened sense of awareness, hyperpnea, hypertension, illusions, increased salivation, muscle aches, mystical experiences, nausea, palpitations, seizures, tachycardia, and vomiting ◆ *Of withdrawal:* none	◆ Place the patient in a quiet room. ◆ If the drug was ingested, induce vomiting or perform gastric lavage. Follow with activated charcoal and a cathartic. ◆ Monitor vital signs, and give diazepam (Valium) for seizures as ordered. ◆ Reorient the patient to time, place, and person, and restrain per facility policy as needed.

(continued)

Understanding commonly abused substances (continued)

Substance	Signs and symptoms	Interventions
Phencyclidine		
♦ *Street names:* PCP, hog, angel dust, boat, love boat, peace pill, sherm, zombie weed (when mixed with marijuana) ♦ *Routes:* ingestion, injection, and smoking ♦ *Dependence:* possibly psychological ♦ *Duration of effect:* 30 minutes to several days ♦ *Medical uses:* veterinary anesthetic	♦ *Of use:* amnesia; blank stare; cardiac arrest; decreased awareness of surroundings; delusions; distorted body image; distorted sense of sight, hearing, and touch; drooling; euphoria; excitation and psychoses; fever; gait ataxia; hallucinations; hyperactivity; hypertensive crisis; individualized unpredictable effects; muscle rigidity; nystagmus; panic; poor perception of time and distance; possible chromosomal damage; psychotic behavior; recurrent coma; renal failure; seizures; sudden behavioral changes; tachycardia; and violent behavior ♦ *Of withdrawal:* none	♦ Place the patient in a quiet room. ♦ If the drug was ingested, induce vomiting or perform gastric lavage. Follow with activated charcoal. ♦ Add ascorbic acid to I.V. solution to acidify urine. ♦ Monitor the patient's vital signs and urine output. ♦ If ordered, give a diuretic; propranolol (Inderal) for hypertension or tachycardia; nitroprusside (Nipride) for severe hypertensive crisis; diazepam (Valium) for seizures; diazepam (Valium) or haloperidol (Haldol) for agitation or psychotic behavior; and physostigmine, diazepam (Valium), chlordiazepoxide (Librium), or chlorpromazine (Thorazine) for a "bad trip."
Stimulants		
Amphetamines (amphetamine sulfate, methamphetamine, dextroamphetamine)		
♦ *Street names:* for amphetamine sulfate—bennies, cartwheels, and grennies; for methamphetamine—speed, meth, and crystal; and for dextroamphetamine sulfate—dexies, hearts, and oranges ♦ *Routes:* ingestion and injection ♦ *Dependence:* psychological ♦ *Duration of effect:* 1 to 4 hours ♦ *Medical uses:* hyperkinesis, narcolepsy, and weight control	♦ *Of use:* altered mental status (from confusion to paranoia), coma, diaphoresis, dilated reactive pupils, dry mouth, exhaustion, hallucinations, hyperactive deep tendon reflexes, hypertension, hyperthermia, paradoxical reaction in children, psychotic behavior with prolonged use, seizures, shallow respirations, tachycardia, and tremors ♦ *Of withdrawal:* abdominal tenderness, apathy, depression, disorientation, irritability, long periods of sleep, and muscle aches, or suicide (with sudden withdrawal)	♦ Place the patient in a quiet room. ♦ If the drug was ingested, induce vomiting or perform gastric lavage; give activated charcoal and a saline or magnesium sulfate cathartic. ♦ Add ammonium chloride or ascorbic acid to I.V. solution to acidify urine to a pH of 5. Also, administer mannitol (Osmitrol) to induce diuresis, as ordered. ♦ Monitor the patent's vital signs. ♦ As ordered, give a short-acting barbiturate, such as pentobarbital (Nembutal), for seizures; haloperidol (Haldol) for assaultive behavior; phentolamine for hypertension; propranolol (Inderal) for tachyarrhythmias; and lidocaine (Xylocaine) for ventricular arrhythmias. ♦ Restrain the patient if hallucinations or paranoia are exhibited. ♦ Give a tepid sponge bath for fever. ♦ Institute suicide precautions.

Understanding commonly abused substances (continued)

Substance	Signs and symptoms	Interventions
Cocaine		
♦ *Street names:* blow, bump, C, Charlie, coke, Coca, snow, nose candy, soda cot, toot, crack (hardened form), rock, and crank ♦ *Routes:* ingestion, injection, sniffing, and smoking ♦ *Dependence:* psychological ♦ *Duration of effect:* 15 minutes to 2 hours; with crack, rapid high of short duration followed by down feeling ♦ *Medical uses:* local anesthetic	♦ *Of use:* abdominal pain; alternating euphoria and fear; anorexia; cardiotoxicity, such as ventricular fibrillation or cardiac arrest; coma; confusion; diaphoresis; dilated pupils; excitability; fever; grandiosity; hyperpnea; hypotension or hypertension; insomnia; irritability; nausea and vomiting; pallor or cyanosis; perforated nasal septum with prolonged use; pressured speech; psychotic behavior with large doses; respiratory arrest; seizures; spasms; tachycardia; tachypnea; visual, auditory, and olfactory hallucinations; and weight loss ♦ *Of withdrawal:* anxiety, depression, and fatigue	♦ Place the patient in a quiet room. ♦ If cocaine was ingested, induce vomiting or perform gastric lavage. Follow with activated charcoal and a saline cathartic. ♦ If cocaine was sniffed, remove residual drug from mucous membranes. ♦ Monitor the patient's vital signs. ♦ Give propranolol (Inderal) for tachycardia. ♦ Perform cardiopulmonary resuscitation for ventricular fibrillation and cardiac arrest, as indicated. ♦ Give a tepid sponge bath for fever. ♦ Administer an anticonvulsant, as ordered, for seizures.

intracranial hemorrhage, acquired immunodeficiency syndrome, tetanus, subacute infective endocarditis, hepatitis, vasculitis, septicemia, thrombophlebitis, pulmonary emboli, gangrene, malnutrition and GI disturbances, respiratory infections, musculoskeletal dysfunction, trauma, depression, increased risk of suicide, and psychosis. Materials used to "cut" street drugs also can cause toxic or allergic reactions.

Psychoactive substance abuse can occur at any age. Experimentation with drugs commonly begins in adolescence or even earlier. In many cases, drug abuse leads to addiction, which may involve physical or psychological dependence or both. The most dangerous form of abuse occurs when users mix several drugs simultaneously—including alcohol.

Causes and incidence

Psychoactive drug abuse commonly results from a combination of low self-esteem, peer pressure, inadequate coping skills, and curiosity. Taking drugs gives people pleasure by relieving tension, abolishing loneliness, allowing them to achieve a temporarily peaceful or euphoric state, or simply relieving boredom.

Drug dependence may follow experimentation with drugs in response to peer pressure.

It also may follow the use of drugs to relieve physical pain, which is an underlying cause for the current opioid crisis in the United States.

Pathophysiology

Pathophysiology is very specific to the substance utilized.

Complications

- ◆ Financial difficulty
- ◆ Impaired relationships
- ◆ Cardiac and respiratory arrest
- ◆ Intracranial hemorrhage
- ◆ Acquired immunodeficiency syndrome
- ◆ Subacute bacterial endocarditis
- ◆ Hepatitis
- ◆ Septicemia
- ◆ Pulmonary emboli
- ◆ Gangrene
- ◆ Death

Signs and symptoms

The signs and symptoms of acute intoxication vary, depending on the drug. The drug user seldom may not desire treatment specifically for the drug problem, yet may seek care for drug-related injuries or complications, such as a motor vehicle accident, burns from freebasing, an overdose, physical deterioration from illness or malnutrition, or symptoms of withdrawal. Friends, family members, or law enforcement officials may bring the patient to the hospital because of respiratory depression, unconsciousness, acute injury, or a psychiatric crisis.

Examine the patient for signs and symptoms of drug use or drug-related complications as well as for clues to the type of drug ingested. For example, fever can result from stimulant or hallucinogen intoxication, from withdrawal, or from infection caused by I.V. drug use.

Inspect the eyes for lacrimation from opiate withdrawal, nystagmus from central nervous system (CNS) depressants or phencyclidine intoxication, and drooping eyelids from opiate or CNS depressant use. Constricted pupils occur with opiate use or withdrawal; dilated pupils, with the use of hallucinogens or amphetamines.

Examine the nose for rhinorrhea from opiate withdrawal and the oral and nasal mucosa for signs of drug-induced irritation. Drug sniffing can result in inflammation, atrophy, or perforation of the nasal mucosa. Dental conditions commonly result from the poor oral hygiene associated with chronic drug use. Also inspect under the tongue for evidence of I.V. drug injection.

Inspect the skin. Sweating, a common sign of intoxication associated with opiates or CNS stimulants, also accompanies most drug withdrawal syndromes. Drug use sometimes induces a sensation of bugs crawling on the skin, known as *formication*; as a result, the patient's skin may be excoriated from scratching.

Needle marks or tracks are an obvious sign of I.V. drug abuse. Keep in mind that the patient may attempt to conceal or disguise injection sites by selecting an inconspicuous site such as under the nails or in areas normally covered by clothing. Self-injection can sometimes cause cellulitis or abscesses. Edematous hands can be a late sign of thrombophlebitis or of fascial infection due to self-injection on the hands or arms.

Auscultation may disclose bilateral crackles and rhonchi caused by smoking and inhaling drugs or by opiate overdose. Other cardiopulmonary signs of overdose include pulmonary edema, respiratory depression, aspiration pneumonia, and hypotension. CNS stimulants and some hallucinogens may cause refractory acute-onset hypertension or cardiac arrhythmias. Withdrawal from opiates or depressants also can provoke arrhythmias and, occasionally, hypotension.

During opiate withdrawal, the patient may report abdominal pain, nausea, or vomiting.

He may also complain of hemorrhoids, a consequence of the constipating effects of these drugs. Palpation of an enlarged liver, with or without tenderness, may indicate hepatitis.

Neurologic symptoms of drug abuse include tremors, hyperreflexia, hyporeflexia, and seizures. Abrupt withdrawal may precipitate signs of CNS depression (ranging from lethargy to coma), hallucinations, or signs of overstimulation, including euphoria and violent behavior.

Carefully review the patient's medical history. Suspect drug abuse if a painful injury or chronic illness is reported, yet the patient refuses a diagnostic workup. In an attempt to obtain drugs, the dependent patient may feign illnesses, such as migraine headaches, myocardial infarction, and renal colic; claim an allergy to over-the-counter analgesics; or even request a specific medication. Also be alert for a history of overdose or a high tolerance for potentially addictive drugs. A patient who is an I.V. drug user may have a history of hepatitis or human immunodeficiency virus (HIV) infection from sharing dirty needles.

A patient who uses substances may give you a fictitious name and address, be reluctant to discuss previous hospitalizations, or seek treatment at a medical facility across town rather than in a close neighborhood. If possible, obtain the patient's previous medical records and interview family members to verify responses. Many electronic health records have a function that ties facility records together; monitor to see whether the patient has been seen and treated at other neighboring facilities.

If the patient admits to drug use, try to determine the extent to which this behavior interferes with normal functioning. Note whether he expresses a desire to overcome dependence on drugs. If possible, obtain a drug history consisting of substances ingested, amount, frequency, and last dose. Expect incomplete or inaccurate responses. Drug-induced amnesia, a depressed level of consciousness, or ignorance may distort the patient's recollection of the facts; the patient also may fabricate answers to avoid arrest or to conceal a suicide attempt.

The abuse of psychoactive substances may cause a need for dosage adjustments to prescribed medications. Cross-tolerance occurs when one drug that has particular properties results in tolerance of another drug. Drugs with similar pharmacologic properties, such as CNS depressants, will cause the need for more of a similar class of drug to get the same response. This may occur, for example, when a patient on an opiate goes to surgery. More anesthesia may be needed for this patient than is needed for a patient who has not used opiates.

The hospitalized patient who uses substances may be uncooperative, disruptive, or even violent. Mood swings, anxiety, impaired memory, sleep disturbances, flashbacks, slurred speech, depression, and thought disorders may be experienced. The patient may make different attempts to obtain drugs, including attempts to triangulate staff.

Be aware that psychoactive substances may be used in cultural practices. For instance, some cultures use hallucinatory drugs to help achieve spiritual experiences. Therefore, delineation between use and abuse must be carefully distinguished.

Diagnosis

For very specific diagnostic criteria, see the *DSM-5*. Various tests can confirm drug use, determine the amount and type of drug taken, and reveal complications. A serum or urine drug screen can detect recently ingested substances.

Characteristic findings in other tests include elevated serum globulin levels, hypoglycemia, leukocytosis, liver function abnormalities, positive Venereal Disease Research Laboratory test results, positive rapid plasma reagin test results due to elevated protein fractions, an elevated mean corpuscular hemoglobin level, elevated uric acid levels, and reduced blood urea nitrogen levels.

Treatment

The patient with acute drug intoxication should receive symptomatic treatment based on the drug ingested. Measures include fluid replacement therapy and nutritional and vitamin supplements, if indicated; detoxification processes will vary based on substance taken and route of use. Careful use of sedatives may be considered to induce sleep; anticholinergics and antidiarrheals can be used to relieve GI distress; anxiolytics may be indicated for severe agitation; and symptomatic treatment of complications should be addressed. Depending on the dosage and time elapsed before admission, additional treatment may include gastric lavage, induced emesis, activated charcoal, forced diuresis, and, possibly, hemoperfusion or hemodialysis.

Treatment of drug dependence commonly involves a triad of care: detoxification, short- and long-term rehabilitation, and aftercare; the latter means a lifetime of abstinence, usually aided by participation in Narcotics Anonymous (NA) or a similar self-help group.

Detoxification, the controlled and gradual withdrawal of an abused drug, is achieved through substituting a drug with a similar action. Such gradual replacement of the abused drug controls the effects of withdrawal, thereby reducing the patient's discomfort and associated risks.

Depending on which drug the patient has used, detoxification may take place on an inpatient or outpatient basis. For example, withdrawal from depressants can produce hazardous adverse reactions, such as generalized tonic–clonic seizures, status epilepticus, and hypotension. The severity of these reactions determines whether the patient can be safely treated as an outpatient or if hospitalization is required. Withdrawal from depressants usually requires detoxification because abrupt or poorly managed withdrawal from barbiturates can cause death.

Opioid withdrawal causes severe physical discomfort and can be life threatening. To minimize these effects, patients who chronically use opioids may be detoxified with methadone (Methadose).

To ease withdrawal from opioids, depressants, and other drugs, useful nonchemical measures may include psychotherapy, exercise, relaxation techniques, and nutritional support. Sedatives and tranquilizers may be administered temporarily to help the patient cope with insomnia, anxiety, and depression.

Buprenorphine with naloxone (Suboxone) is another drug that's being used to lessen craving in opiate-addicted patients. Naloxone is an opiate antagonist; it blocks opiate receptors. A person taking buprenorphine with naloxone (Suboxone) won't respond to the effects of other opioids.

After withdrawal, the patient needs to participate in a rehabilitation program to prevent a recurrence. Rehabilitation programs are available for inpatients and outpatients; they usually last a month or longer and may include individual, group, and family psychotherapy. During and after rehabilitation, participation in a drug-oriented self-help group may be helpful. The largest such group is NA.

Special considerations

Focus on restoring the patient's physical health, teaching about drug abuse and dependence, providing support, and encouraging participation in drug treatment programs and self-help groups.

During an acute episode:

◆ Continuously monitor the patient's vital signs, and observe for complications of overdose and withdrawal, such as cardiopulmonary arrest, seizures, and aspiration.

♦ Based on standard hospital policy, institute appropriate measures to prevent suicide attempts.

♦ Give medications, as ordered, to decrease withdrawal symptoms; monitor and record their effectiveness.

♦ Maintain a quiet, safe environment during withdrawal from any drug because excessive noise may agitate the patient.

♦ Remove harmful objects from the patient's room, and use restraints only if you suspect that the patent might harm himself or others. Follow agency requirements carefully. Institute seizure precautions.

After an acute episode:

♦ Learn to control your reactions to the patient's undesirable behaviors—commonly, psychological dependency, manipulation, anger, frustration, and alienation.

♦ Set limits for dealing with demanding, manipulative behavior.

♦ Promote adequate nutrition and monitor the patient's nutritional intake.

♦ Administer medications carefully to prevent hoarding by the patient. Check the patient's mouth to ensure that medication has been swallowed. Closely monitor visitors who might supply the patient with drugs.

♦ Refer the patient for detoxification and rehabilitation, as appropriate. Provide a list of available resources.

♦ Encourage family members to seek help whether or not the patient seeks it. You can suggest private therapy or community mental health clinics.

If the patient refuses to participate in a rehabilitation program, teach how to minimize the risk of drug-related complications:

♦ Review measures for preventing HIV infection and hepatitis. Stress that these infections are readily transmitted by sharing needles with other drug users and by having unprotected sexual intercourse.

♦ Advise the patient to use a new needle for every injection.

♦ Emphasize the importance of using a condom during intercourse to prevent disease transmission and pregnancy. Teach about other reliable methods of birth control also, such as birth control pills, and injectable forms of contraception (although these do not prevent disease transmission). Explain the devastating effects of drugs on the developing fetus.

Psychotic disorders

SCHIZOPHRENIA

Schizophrenia is characterized by disturbances (for at least 6 months), with or without catatonia, in thought content and form, perception, affect, sense of self, volition, interpersonal relationships, and psychomotor behavior that impairs functioning. (See *Phases of schizophrenia*.) The onset of symptoms usually occurs during adolescence or early adulthood. The disorder produces varying degrees of impairment. Some patients with schizophrenia have just one psychotic episode and no more. Some patients have no disability between periods of exacerbation; others need continuous institutional care. The prognosis worsens with each episode.

Causes and incidence

Schizophrenia affects 0.3% to 0.7% of the population in the United States; gender incidence varies depending on geographic origin. The condition is thought to result from a combination of biological, cultural, psychological, and genetic factors. Close relatives of people with schizophrenia have a greater likelihood of developing schizophrenia; the closer the degree of biological relatedness, the higher the risk.

Numerous psychological and sociocultural causes, such as disturbed family and interpersonal patterns, also have been proposed. Schizophrenia is more common in children raised in urban environments. Incidence is also linked to season of birth—late winter/early

Phases of schizophrenia

Phase	Characteristics
Prodromal	The time span from the onset of first symptoms leading up to psychosis
Acute (or active)	The active phase of the condition characterized by hallucinations, delusions, disorganized thinking and speech
Residual	Period following the active phase; often accompanied by negative symptoms such as withdrawal, emotional bluntness, and fatigue

spring in some locations and summer (for the deficit form of schizophrenia).

Pathophysiology

The most widely accepted biochemical theory holds that schizophrenia results from excessive activity at dopaminergic synapses. Other neurotransmitter alterations, such as serotonin increases, may also contribute to schizophrenic symptoms. In addition, patients with schizophrenia have structural abnormalities of the frontal and temporolimbic systems. CT scans and MRI studies show various structural brain abnormalities, including frontal lobe atrophy and increased lateral and third ventricles. PET scans substantiate frontal lobe hypometabolism.

Complications

◆ Impaired social relationships
◆ Difficulty or inability to function occupationally
◆ Nutrition deficit
◆ Self-care deficit

Signs and symptoms

Schizophrenia is associated with many abnormal behaviors; therefore, signs and symptoms vary widely, depending on the type and phase (prodromal, active, or residual) of the illness.

Watch for these signs and symptoms:
◆ ambivalence—coexisting strong positive and negative feelings, leading to emotional conflict
◆ apathy and other affective abnormalities
◆ clang associations—words that rhyme or sound alike used in an illogical, nonsensical manner—for instance, "It's the rain, train, pain"
◆ concrete associations—inability to form or understand abstract thoughts
◆ delusions—false ideas or beliefs accepted as real by the patient; delusions of grandeur, persecution, and reference (distorted belief regarding the relation between events and one's self—e.g., a belief that television programs address the patient on a personal level); feelings of being controlled, somatic illness, and depersonalization
◆ echolalia—automatic and meaningless repetition of another's words or phrases
◆ echopraxia—involuntary repetition of movements observed in others
◆ flight of ideas—rapid succession of incomplete and loosely connected ideas
◆ hallucinations—false sensory perceptions with no basis in reality; usually visual or auditory, but may also be olfactory (smell), gustatory (taste), or tactile (touch)
◆ loose associations—rapid shifts among unrelated ideas

◆ magical thinking—belief that thoughts or wishes can control others or events
◆ neologisms—bizarre words that have meaning only for the patient
◆ poor interpersonal relationships
◆ regression—return to an earlier developmental stage
◆ thought blocking—sudden interruption in the patient's train of thought
◆ withdrawal—disinterest in objects, people, or surroundings
◆ word salad—illogical word groupings, such as "She had a star, barn, plant"

Diagnosis

After a complete physical and psychiatric examinations rule out an organic cause of symptoms such as an amphetamine-induced psychosis, a diagnosis of schizophrenia may be considered. For very specific diagnostic criteria, see the *DSM-5*.

Treatment

In schizophrenia, treatment focuses on meeting the physical and psychosocial needs of the patient, based on his previous level of adjustment and his response to medical and nursing interventions. Treatment may combine drug therapy, long-term psychotherapy for the patient and family or caregivers, psychosocial rehabilitation, vocational counseling, and the use of community resources.

The primary treatment for more than 50 years, first-generation antipsychotic drugs (also called neuroleptic drugs) appear to work by blocking postsynaptic dopamine receptors. These drugs reduce the incidence of positive psychotic symptoms, such as hallucinations and delusions, and relieve anxiety and agitation. Second-generation antipsychotics are effective in relieving positive and negative symptoms of schizophrenia. Other psychiatric drugs, such as antidepressants and anxiolytics, may control associated signs and symptoms.

Certain antipsychotic drugs are associated with numerous adverse reactions, some of which are irreversible. (See *Reviewing adverse effects of antipsychotic drugs*, page 1122.) Second-generation antipsychotic drugs appear to be effective in treating the negative symptoms of schizophrenia (withdrawal, apathy, or blunted affect). However, these drugs have problematic adverse effects. Antipsychotic drugs are broken down into two major classes: dopamine receptor antagonists (haloperidol—Haldol and chlorpromazine—Thorazine) and dopamine–serotonin antagonists, also called *atypical antipsychotics* (risperidone—Risperdal

Reviewing adverse effects of antipsychotic drugs

Second-generation antipsychotic drugs (known as atypical antipsychotics) produce fewer extrapyramidal symptoms than the first, older class of antipsychotics. Risperidone (Risperdal) is associated with increases in serum prolactin. Olanzapine (Zyprexa), in moderate doses, induces few extrapyramidal symptoms, but has been associated with weight gain and blood glucose abnormalities. Quetiapine (Seroquel) can cause weight gain, hypotension, and sedation.

First-generation antipsychotic drugs like chlorpromazine can cause sedative, anticholinergic, or extrapyramidal effects; orthostatic hypotension; and, rarely, neuroleptic malignant syndrome.

Sedative, anticholinergic, and extrapyramidal effects

High-potency drugs (such as haloperidol) are minimally sedative and anticholinergic but cause a high incidence of extrapyramidal adverse effects. Intermediate-potency drugs (such as molindone—Moban) are associated with a moderate incidence of adverse effects, whereas low-potency drugs (such as chlorpromazine) are highly sedative and anticholinergic but produce few extrapyramidal adverse effects.

The most common extrapyramidal effects are dystonia, parkinsonism, and akathisia. Dystonia usually occurs in young male patients within the first few days of treatment. Characterized by severe tonic contractions of the muscles in the neck, mouth, and tongue, dystonia may be misdiagnosed as a psychotic symptom. Diphenhydramine (Benadryl) or benztropine (Cogentin) administered I.M. or I.V. provides rapid relief from this symptom.

Drug-induced parkinsonism results in bradykinesia, muscle rigidity, shuffling or propulsive gait, stooped posture, flat facial affect, tremors, and drooling. Parkinsonism may occur from 1 week to several months after the initiation of drug treatment. Drugs prescribed to reverse or prevent this syndrome include benztropine (Cogentin), trihexyphenidyl (Inderal), and amantadine (Osmolex ER).

Tardive dyskinesia can occur after only several months of continuous therapy and is usually irreversible. No effective treatment is available for this disorder, which is characterized by various involuntary movements of the mouth and jaw; flapping or writhing; purposeless, rapid, and jerky movements of the arms and legs; and dystonic posture of the neck and trunk.

Signs and symptoms of akathisia include restlessness, pacing, and an inability to rest or sit still. Akathisia may be misinterpreted as agitation or a worsening of psychotic behavior. Propranolol (Inderal) relieves this adverse effect.

Orthostatic hypotension

Low-potency neuroleptics can cause orthostatic hypotension because they block alpha-adrenergic receptors. If hypotension is severe, the patient is placed in the supine position and given I.V. fluids for hypovolemia. If further treatment is needed, an alpha-adrenergic agonist, such as norepinephrine (Levophed), may be ordered to relieve hypotension. Mixed alpha- and beta-adrenergic drugs (such as epinephrine) or beta-adrenergic drugs (such as isoproterenol—Isuprel) shouldn't be given because they can further reduce blood pressure.

Neuroleptic malignant syndrome

Neuroleptic malignant syndrome is a life-threatening syndrome that occurs in up to 1% of patients taking antipsychotic drugs. Signs and symptoms include fever, muscle rigidity, and altered level of consciousness occurring hours to months after initiating drug therapy or increasing the dose. Treatment is symptomatic, largely consisting of dantrolene (Dantrium) and other measures to counter muscle rigidity associated with hyperthermia. You'll need to monitor vital signs and mental status continuously.

and clozapine—Clozaril). The long-acting drugs haloperidol (Haldol) and fluphenazine may be given I.M. every 3 to 4 weeks to improve compliance.

Clozapine (Clozaril) may be prescribed for severely ill patients who fail to respond to standard treatment. This drug effectively controls more psychotic signs and symptoms without the usual adverse effects. However, clozapine (Clozaril) can cause drowsiness, sedation, excessive salivation, tachycardia, dizziness, and seizures. Agranulocytosis, a potentially fatal blood disorder characterized by a low white blood cell count and pronounced neutropenia, may also occur; therefore, patients on clozapine (Clozaril) must be monitored closely with frequent complete blood counts. Risperidone (Risperdal) and olanzapine (Zyprexa), like clozapine (Clozaril), have reduced the incidence of adverse effects, including extrapyramidal symptoms and anticholinergic adverse effects. These new antipsychotics may cause weight gain, hormone irregularities, and diabetes.

Routine blood monitoring is essential to detect patients taking clozapine (Clozaril) who develop agranulocytosis. If caught in the early stages, this disorder is reversible.

Research is mixed regarding the efficacy of psychotherapy in treating the patient with schizophrenia. Some studies show it is a useful adjunct to drug therapy. Other studies suggest that psychosocial rehabilitation, education, and social skills training are more effective for chronic schizophrenia. In addition to improving understanding of the disorder, these methods teach the patient and family members or caregivers coping strategies, effective communication techniques, and social skills.

Because schizophrenia typically disrupts the family, family therapy may be helpful to reduce guilt and disappointment as well as improve acceptance of the patient and behaviors.

Special considerations

◆ Assess the patient's ability to carry out activities of daily living, paying special attention to nutrition status. Monitor the patient's weight regularly. For patients who are paranoid about food poisoning by others, provide food in closed containers or allow the patient to prepare his or her own food, if safe to do so. Allow the patient to open liquid medication in a unit-dose container that has already been dose-verified.

◆ Maintain a safe environment, minimizing stimuli. Administer prescribed medications to decrease symptoms and anxiety. Use physical restraints only when necessary, and carefully follow agency policy.

◆ Adopt an accepting and consistent approach with the patient. Short, repeated contacts are best until trust has been established.

◆ Avoid promoting dependence. Reward positive behavior to help the patient improve level of functioning.

◆ Engage the patient in reality-oriented activities that involve human contact, such as inpatient social skills training groups, outpatient day care, and sheltered workshops. Provide reality-based explanations for distorted body images or hypochondriacal complaints. Explain

to the patient that private language or neologisms aren't understood. Set limits on inappropriate behavior.

◆ If the patient is hallucinating, explore the content of the hallucinations. Assess whether the patient who hears voices believes that he or she must do what the voices command. Explore the emotions connected with the hallucinations, but don't argue about them.

◆ Assist the patient to recognize the nonreality of hallucinatory experience.

◆ Teach the patient techniques that interrupt the hallucinations (listening to an audiocassette player, singing out loud, or reading out loud).

◆ Don't tease or joke with a patient with schizophrenia. Choose words and phrases that are unambiguous and clearly understood. For instance, a patient who's told, "That procedure will be done on the floor," may become frightened, thinking he'll need to lie down on the floor.

◆ If the patient expresses suicidal thoughts or is assessed to be a suicide risk, institute suicide precautions. Document behavior and your actions.

◆ If the patient homicidal thoughts (e.g., "I have to kill my mother"), institute homicidal precautions. Notify the healthcare provider, appropriate authorities, and the potential victim. Document the patient's comments and the names of those who were notified.

◆ Don't touch the patient without first explaining exactly what you're going to do—for example, "I'm going to put this cuff on your arm so I can take your blood pressure."

◆ If necessary, postpone procedures that require physical contact with hospital personnel until the patient is less suspicious or agitated.

◆ Remember, institutionalization may produce symptoms and disabilities that aren't part of the patient's illness, so evaluate symptoms carefully.

◆ Mobilize community resources to provide a support system for the patient. Ongoing support is essential to the patient's adaptation of social skills.

◆ Encourage adherence to the medication regimen to prevent a relapse. Also, monitor the patient carefully for adverse reactions to drug therapy, including acute dystonia, drug-induced parkinsonism, akathisia, tardive dyskinesia, and neuroleptic malignant syndrome. Document and report such reactions promptly.

◆ Help the patient explore possible connections between anxiety and stress and the exacerbation of symptoms.

For patients with schizophrenia with catatonia:

◆ Assess for physical illness. Remember that the mute patient won't report pain or physical

symptoms; if the patient assumes an uncomfortable posture, there is risk for pressure ulcers or decreased circulation to a body area.
◆ Meet the patient's physical needs for adequate food, fluid, exercise, and elimination; follow orders with respect to nutrition, urinary catheterization, and enema.
◆ Provide range-of-motion exercises for the patient or assist with ambulation every 2 hours.
◆ Prevent physical exhaustion and injury during periods of hyperactivity.
◆ Tell the patient directly, specifically, and concisely which procedures need to be done. For example, you might say to the patient, "It's time to go for a walk. Let's go."
◆ Spend some time with the patient even if he or she is mute and unresponsive. The patient is acutely aware of the environment even though it appears otherwise. Your presence can be reassuring and supportive.
◆ Verbalize for the patient the message that nonverbal behavior seems to convey; encourage the patient to do so as well.
◆ Offer reality orientation. You might say, "The leaves on the trees are turning colors and the air is cooler. It's fall!" Emphasize reality in all contacts to reduce distorted perceptions.
◆ Stay alert for violent outbursts; if they occur, get help promptly to ensure the patient's safety and your own.

For the patient with paranoid schizophrenia:
◆ When the patient is newly admitted, minimize contact with the hospital staff.
◆ Don't crowd the patient physically or psychologically; this may induce physical responses as the patient attempts to protect himself or herself.
◆ Be flexible; allow the patient some control. Approach the patient in a calm and unhurried manner. Let the patient talk about anything initially, but keep the conversation light. Avoid entering into power struggles.
◆ Respond to the patient's condescending attitudes (arrogance, put-downs, sarcasm, or open hostility) with neutral remarks.
◆ Don't let the patient put you on the defensive, and don't take remarks personally. If the patient tells you to leave him or her alone, do leave (if safe to do so) but return soon. Brief contacts with the patient may be most useful at first.
◆ Don't make attempts to combat the patient's delusions with logic. Instead, respond to feelings, themes, or underlying needs—for example, "It seems you feel you've been treated unfairly."
◆ Be honest and dependable. Don't threaten the patient or make promises that you can't fulfill.

◆ If the patient is taking clozapine (Clozaril), stress the importance of returning weekly or biweekly to the hospital or an outpatient setting to have bloodwork monitored.
◆ Teach the patient the importance of adhering to the medication regimen. Tell the patient to report any adverse reactions instead of discontinuing the drug. If prescribed a slow-release formulation, make sure the patient understands when to return to the physician for the next dose.
◆ Involve the patient's family or caregivers in treatment, when appropriate. Teach them how to recognize an impending relapse, and suggest ways to manage symptoms, such as tension, nervousness, insomnia, decreased ability to concentrate, and apathy.

DELUSIONAL DISORDER

Delusional disorder is characterized by false beliefs with a plausible basis in reality. Subtypes include erotomanic, grandiose, jealous, somatic, or persecutory themes. (See *Delusional themes*, page 1125.) Some patients experience several types of delusions, whereas others experience unspecified delusions with no dominant theme. Typically chronic, these disorders commonly interfere with interpersonal and social relationships, but may not impair intellectual or occupational functioning significantly.

Causes and incidence

Delusional disorder, which usually occurs in middle or late adulthood, has been associated with a family history of paranoid personality disorder and sensory impairment. These uncommon illnesses affect less than 1% of the population; the incidence is thought to be equal in men and women, although quantification is difficult because many cases are thought to be underreported.

Pathophysiology

The pathophysiology of delusion disorder is unknown. Research has studied sensory impairment (particularly vision and hearing), those with family history of suspiciousness or jealousy, those with differences in reasoning biases, and those with medical diseases, yet a clear connection has not been made. There is some evidence to a genetic predisposition to a selective D2 receptor-related hyperdopaminergia, and to dopamine neurotransmitter dysfunction, although further research is necessary.

Complications
◆ Violent behavior
◆ Suicide
◆ Impaired interpersonal relationships

Delusional themes

In a patient with a delusional disorder, delusions usually are well systematized and follow a predominant theme. Common delusional themes are discussed below.

Erotomanic delusions
This prevalent delusional theme concerns romantic or spiritual love. The patient believes that he or she shares an idealized (rather than sexual) relationship with someone of higher status—a superior at work, a celebrity, or an anonymous stranger.

The patient may keep this delusion secret, but more commonly will try to contact the object of the delusion by phone calls, letters (including e-mail), gifts, or even stalking. The patient may attempt to rescue the beloved from imagined danger. Many patients with erotomanic delusions harass public figures and come to the attention of the police.

Grandiose delusions
The patient with grandiose delusions believes that he or she has great, unrecognized talent, special insights, prophetic power, or has made an important discovery. To achieve recognition, the patient may contact government agencies or authorities. The patient with a religious-oriented delusion of grandeur may become a cult leader. Less commonly, the patient may believe that he or she shares a special relationship with some well-known personality, such as a rock star or a world leader, or that he or she is famous.

Jealous delusions
Jealous delusions focus on infidelity. For example, a patient may insist that his or her partner has been unfaithful, and may search for evidence to justify the delusion such as looking for text messages that substantiate the delusion. The patient may confront the partner, try to control the partner's movements, follow the partner, or try to track down a perceived romantic rival. The patient may resort to physical altercation with the partner, or with the perceived romantic rival.

Somatic delusions
Somatic delusions center on an imagined physical defect or deformity. The patient may perceive a foul odor coming from his skin, mouth, rectum, or another body part. Other delusions involve skin-crawling insects, internal parasites, or physical illness.

Persecutory delusions
The patient suffering from persecutory delusions, the most common type of delusion, believes that he or she is being followed, harassed, plotted against, poisoned, mocked, or deliberately prevented from achieving personal long-term goals. These delusions may evolve into a simple or complex persecution scheme, in which even the slightest injustice is interpreted as part of the scheme.

Such a patient may file numerous lawsuits or seek redress from government agencies (querulous paranoia). A patient who becomes resentful and angry may lash out violently against the alleged offender.

Signs and symptoms

The psychiatric history of a patient with delusion disorder may be unremarkable, aside from behavior related to the delusions. The patient is likely to report problems with social and interpersonal relationships, including depression or sexual dysfunction. He or she may describe a life marked by social isolation or hostility. The patient may deny feeling lonely, relentlessly criticizing or placing unreasonable demands on others.

Gathering accurate information from a delusional patient may prove difficult. The patient may deny feelings, disregard the circumstances that led to hospitalization, and refuse treatment. However, patient responses and behavior during the assessment interview provide clues that can help to identify this disorder. Family members may confirm your observations—for example, by reporting that the patient is chronically jealous or suspicious.

Note how well the patient communicates; he or she may be evasive or reluctant to answer questions. Conversely, the patient may be overly talkative, explaining events in great detail and emphasizing achievements, prominent people he or she knows, or places traveled. Statements that first seem logical may later prove irrelevant.

Some of the patient's answers may be contradictory, jumbled, or irrational.

Be alert for expressions of denial, projection, and rationalization. Once delusions become firmly entrenched, the patient will no longer seek to justify beliefs. However, if the patient is still struggling to maintain delusional defenses, statements such as "People at work won't talk to me because I'm smarter than them" can provide important diagnostic information. Accusatory statements are also characteristic of the delusional patient. Record pervasive delusional themes (e.g., grandiose or persecutory).

Monitor for nonverbal cues, such as excessive vigilance or obvious apprehension on entering the room. During questions, the patient may listen intently, reacting defensively to imagined slights or insults. The patient may sit at the edge of the seat or fold arms as if to shielding. If the patient carries papers or money, these may be clutched firmly.

Diagnosis

For very specific diagnostic criteria, see the *DSM-5*.

Blood and urine tests, psychological tests, and neurologic evaluation can rule out organic causes of the delusions, such as amphetamine-induced psychoses and Alzheimer disease. Endocrine function tests rule out hyperadrenalism, pernicious anemia, and thyroid disorders.

Treatment

Effective treatment of delusional disorder, consisting of a combination of drug therapy and psychotherapy, must correct the behavior and mood disturbances that result from the patient's mistaken beliefs. Treatment may also include mobilizing a support system for the isolated elderly patient.

Drug treatment with antipsychotics is similar to that used in schizophrenic disorders. Antipsychotics appear to work by blocking postsynaptic dopamine receptors. These drugs reduce the incidence of psychotic symptoms, such as hallucinations and delusions, and relieve anxiety and agitation. Other psychiatric drugs, such as antidepressants and cautious use of anxiolytics, may be prescribed to control associated symptoms.

A patient's history of medication response is the best guide when selecting treatment. The lowest dose should be started initially and increased slowly based on the patient's response. If the symptoms don't improve during a 6-week trial, other classes of antipsychotics may be tried. Haloperidol (Haldol) and fluphenazine decanoate are depot formulations that are implanted I.M. to release the drug gradually over a 30-day period, improving compliance. Usually, however, this type of treatment isn't needed. Pimozide (Orap) may be particularly effective in patients with somatic delusions.

Clozapine (Clozaril) can cause drowsiness, sedation, excessive salivation, tachycardia, dizziness, and seizures. Agranulocytosis, a potentially fatal blood disorder characterized by a low white blood cell count and pronounced neutropenia, may also occur. Routine blood monitoring is essential to detect patients taking clozapine (Clozaril) who develop agranulocytosis. If caught in the early stages, this disorder is reversible.

Special considerations

◆ In dealing with the delusional patient, be direct, straightforward, and dependable. Whenever possible, elicit the patient's feedback. Move slowly and matter-of-factly and respond without anger or defensiveness to hostile remarks.

◆ Respect the patient's privacy and space needs. Don't touch him unnecessarily.

◆ Take steps to reduce social isolation, if the patient allows. Gradually increase social contacts after a comfort level with staff has been achieved.

◆ Watch for refusal of medication or food, resulting from the patient's irrational fear of poisoning.

◆ Monitor the patient carefully for the adverse effects of antipsychotic drugs: drug-induced parkinsonism, acute dystonia, akathisia, tardive dyskinesia, and malignant neuroleptic syndrome.

◆ If the patient is taking clozapine (Clozaril), stress the importance of returning weekly to the hospital or an outpatient setting to have bloodwork monitored.

◆ Involve the patient's family in treatment. Teach them how to recognize an impending relapse, and suggest ways to manage symptoms. These include tension, nervousness, insomnia, decreased concentration ability, and apathy.

◆ Remember to consider cultural beliefs.

Mood disorders

BIPOLAR DISORDERS

Marked by severe pathologic mood swings from hyperactivity and euphoria to sadness and depression, bipolar disorders involve various symptom combinations. Type I bipolar disorder is characterized by alternating episodes of mania and depression, whereas type II is characterized by recurrent depressive episodes and occasional mild manic (hypomanic) episodes.

Causes and incidence

The cause of bipolar disorder is unclear, but biological, psychological, and genetic factors may play a part. The prevalence of bipolar depends on population and geographic location being studied; in the United States, lifetime prevalence is estimated to be 1% for bipolar I disorder and 1.3% for bipolar II disorder.

The American Psychiatric Association estimates that 0.6% of adults experience bipolar disorder. This disorder affects women more frequently than men and is more common in higher socioeconomic groups. It can begin any time after adolescence, but onset usually occurs between ages 18 and 20. This illness is associated with a significant mortality; patients with bipolar disorder are 15 times more likely to commit suicide than the general population, many just as the depression lifts.

Pathophysiology

The pathophysiology of bipolar disorder is not fully known. Although certain biochemical changes accompany mood swings, it isn't clear whether these changes cause the mood swings or result from them. In mania and depression, intracellular sodium concentration increases during illness and returns to normal with recovery.

Patients with mood disorders have a defect in the way the brain handles certain neurotransmitters—chemical messengers that shuttle nerve impulses between neurons. Low levels of the chemicals dopamine and norepinephrine, for example, have been linked to depression, whereas excessively high levels of these chemicals are associated with mania.

Changes in the concentration of acetylcholine and serotonin may also play a role. Although neurobiologists have yet to establish that these chemical shifts cause bipolar disorder, it's widely assumed that most antidepressant medications work by modifying these neurotransmitter systems.

New data suggest that changes in the circadian rhythms that control hormone secretion, body temperature, and appetite may contribute to the development of bipolar disorder.

Emotional or physical trauma, such as bereavement, disruption of an important relationship, or a serious accidental injury, may precede the onset of bipolar disorder; however, bipolar disorder commonly appears without identifiable predisposing factors.

Manic episodes may follow a stressful event, but they're also associated with antidepressant therapy and childbirth. Major depressive episodes may be caused by chronic physical illness, psychoactive drug dependence, psychosocial stressors, and childbirth. Other familial influences, especially the early loss of a parent, parental depression, incest, or abuse, may predispose a person to depressive illness.

Complications

- Impaired social relationships
- Compromise in self-esteem
- Financial concerns
- Sexually risky behaviors
- Suicide risk

Signs and symptoms

Signs and symptoms vary widely, depending on whether the patient is experiencing a manic or a depressive episode.

During the assessment interview, the patient with *mania* typically appears grandiose, euphoric, expansive, or irritable with little control over activities and responses. The patient may describe or exhibit hyperactive or excessive behavior, including making elaborate plans for numerous social events, attempting to renew old acquaintances by telephoning friends at all hours of the night, going on buying sprees, or exhibiting promiscuous sexual activity.

The patient's activities may have a strange quality, such as dressing in colorful or strange garments, wearing excessive makeup, or giving advice to passing strangers. There is commonly an inflated sense of self-esteem, ranging from uncritical self-confidence to marked grandiosity, which may be delusional.

Note the patient's speech patterns and concentration level. Accelerated and pressured speech, frequent changes of topic, and flight of ideas are common features of the manic phase. The patient is easily distracted and responds rapidly to external stimuli, such as background noise or a ringing telephone.

Physical examination of the manic patient may reveal signs of malnutrition and poor personal hygiene. The patient may report sleeping and eating less as well as being more physically active than usual.

Hypomania, more common than acute mania, can be recognized during the assessment interview by three classic symptoms: euphoric but unstable mood, pressured speech, and increased motor activity. The patient with hypomania may appear elated, hyperactive, easily distracted, talkative, irritable, impatient, impulsive, and full of energy but seldom exhibits flight of ideas. Delusions and other symptoms of psychotic intensity are never present.

The patient who experiences a *depressive episode* may report a loss of self-esteem, overwhelming inertia, social withdrawal, and feelings of hopelessness, apathy, or self-reproach. The patient may believe that he or she deserves to be punished. Growing sadness, guilt, negativity, and fatigue place extraordinary burdens on the family.

During the assessment interview, the depressed patient may speak and respond slowly. He or she may report difficulty concentrating or thinking clearly but is usually not obviously disoriented or intellectually impaired.

Physical examination may reveal reduced psychomotor activity, lethargy, low muscle tonus, weight loss, slowed gait, and constipation. The patient may also report sleep disturbances (falling asleep, staying asleep, or early-morning awakening), sexual dysfunction, headaches, chest pains, and a heaviness in the limbs. Typically, symptoms are worse in the morning and gradually subside as the day goes on.

Health concerns may become hypochondriacal; the patient may worry excessively about having cancer or some other serious illness. In an older adult, physical symptoms may be the only clues to depression.

Suicide is an ever-present risk, especially as the depression begins to lift. At that point, a rising energy level may strengthen the patient's resolve to carry out suicidal plans.

The suicidal patient may also harbor homicidal ideas—for example, thinking of killing family either in anger or to spare them pain and disgrace.

Diagnosis

For very specific diagnostic criteria, see the *DSM-5*.

Physical examination and laboratory tests, such as endocrine function studies, rule out medical causes of the mood disturbances, including intra-abdominal neoplasm, hypothyroidism, hyperthyroidism, heart failure, cerebral arteriosclerosis, parkinsonism, psychoactive drug abuse, brain tumor, and uremia. Moreover, a review of the medications prescribed for other disorders may point to drug-induced depression or mania.

Treatment

Widely used to treat bipolar disorders, lithium has proved to be highly effective in relieving and preventing manic episodes. It curbs the accelerated thought processes and hyperactive behavior without producing the sedating effect of antipsychotic drugs. In addition, it may prevent the recurrence of depressive episodes; however, it's ineffective in treating acute depression.

Because lithium (Lithobid) has a narrow therapeutic range, treatment must be started cautiously and the dosage must be adjusted slowly. Therapeutic blood levels must be closely monitored and maintained for 7 to 10 days before the drug's beneficial effects appear; for this reason, antipsychotic drugs commonly are used in the interim to provide sedation and symptomatic relief. Because lithium (Lithobid) is excreted by the kidneys, any renal impairment necessitates withdrawal of the drug. Long-term use of lithium (Lithobid) may affect thyroid function.

Anticonvulsants, such as carbamazepine (Tegretol), valproic acid (Depakote), and clonazepam (Klonopin), are used either alone or with lithium (Lithobid) to treat mood disorders. Carbamazepine (Tegretol) and divalproex (Depakote) are effective in many patients who are lithium (Lithobid) resistant. Other anticonvulsant drugs have also been used. Electroconvulsive therapy (ECT) is also effective.

Antidepressants are used to treat depressive symptoms, but they may trigger a manic episode.

Quetiapine (Seroquel) has been used to treat both the manic and depressive phases of bipolar disorder. It may also be used with lithium (Lithobid) or divalproex (Depakote) for acute manic episodes.

Special considerations

For the patient with mania:

◆ Remember the manic patient's physical needs. Encourage nutrition intake. Alter the diet so that it's high in calories, carbohydrates, and liquids if necessary.

◆ As the patient's symptoms subside, encourage assumption of responsibility for personal care.

◆ Provide emotional support, maintain a calm environment, and set realistic goals for behavior.

◆ Provide diversionary activities suited to a short attention span; firmly discourage the patient if he or she attempted to overextend. Provide structured activities involving large motor movements to expend surplus energy. Reduce or eliminate group activities during acute manic episodes.

◆ When necessary, reorient the patient to reality. Tactfully divert conversations when they become intimately concerned with other patients or staff members.

◆ Set limits in a calm, clear, and self-confident manner for the patient's demanding, hyperactive, manipulative, and acting-out behaviors that accompany a manic episode. Setting limits tells the patient that you'll provide security and protection by refusing inappropriate and possibly harmful requests. Avoid leaving an opening for the patient to test or argue.

◆ Listen to requests attentively and with a neutral attitude. Avoid power struggles. Explain that you'll seriously consider the request and will respond later.

◆ Encourage solitary activities such as writing out one's thoughts.

◆ Collaborate with other staff members to provide consistent responses to the patient's manipulative or acting-out behaviors.

◆ Watch for early signs of frustration (when the patient's anger escalates from verbal threats to hitting an object). Tell the patient firmly that threats and hitting are unacceptable. Inform that the patient will be moved to a quiet area to protect himself or herself and others. Staff members who have practiced as a team can work effectively to prevent acting-out behavior or to remove and confine a patient.

◆ Alert the staff promptly when acting-out behavior escalates. It's safer to have help available before you need it than to try controlling an anxious or frightened patient by yourself.

◆ After the incident is over and the patient is calm and in control, allow expression of feelings and offer suggestions on how to prevent a recurrence.

◆ If the patient is taking lithium (Lithobid), teach the patient and family to immediately notify the healthcare provider if signs or symptoms of toxicity, such as diarrhea, abdominal cramps, vomiting, unsteadiness, drowsiness, muscle weakness, polyuria, and tremors, occur.

For the patient with depression:

◆ The patient with depression needs ongoing positive reinforcement to improve self-esteem. Provide a structured routine, including activities to boost self-confidence and promote interaction with others (for instance, group therapy). Reassure that the depression will lift.

◆ Encourage the patient to talk or to write down feelings. Listen attentively and respectfully; allow the patient time to formulate thoughts. Record your observations and conversations.

◆ To prevent possible self-injury or suicide, remove harmful objects (such as glass, belts, rope, or bobby pins) from the patient's environment, observe closely, and strictly supervise medication administration. Institute suicide precautions as dictated by facility policy.

◆ Be attentive to the patient's physical needs. If the patient is too depressed to take care of himself or herself, assist with personal hygiene measures. Encourage eating, and help to feed if necessary. For constipation, add high-fiber foods to the diet; offer small, frequent meals; and encourage physical activity. Recommend good sleep hygiene measures to improve sleep.

◆ If the patient is taking an antidepressant, watch for signs of mania.

MAJOR DEPRESSIVE DISORDER

Major depressive disorder is a syndrome of persistently sad, dysphoric mood, accompanied by disturbances in sleep and appetite, lethargy, and an inability to experience pleasure (anhedonia).

Many patients with major depressive disorder experience a single episode and recover completely; the rest have at least one recurrence. Major depressive disorder can profoundly alter social, family, and occupational functioning. However, suicide is the most serious consequence of major depression—feelings of worthlessness, guilt, and hopelessness are so overwhelming that patients no longer consider life worth living. Nearly twice as many women as men attempt suicide, but men are far more likely to complete suicide.

Causes and incidence

The multiple causes of depression aren't completely understood. Depression occurs in up to 18 million Americans, affecting all racial, ethnic, and socioeconomic groups. It affects both sexes, but is more common in women.

Pathophysiology

The pathophysiology of depression is not fully understood. Research suggests possible genetic, familial, biochemical, physical, psychological, and social causes. Psychological causes (the focus of many nursing interventions) may include feelings of helplessness and vulnerability, anger, hopelessness and pessimism, and low self-esteem. They may be related to abnormal character and behavior patterns and troubled personal relationships. In many cases, the history identifies a specific personal loss or severe stressor that probably interacts with the person's predisposition to provoke major depression.

Depression may be secondary to a specific medical condition—for example, metabolic disturbances, such as hypoxia and hypercalcemia; endocrine disorders, such as diabetes and Cushing syndrome; neurologic diseases, such as Parkinson and Alzheimer diseases; cancer (especially of the pancreas); viral and bacterial infections, such as influenza and pneumonia; cardiovascular disorders, such as heart failure; pulmonary disorders, such as chronic obstructive lung disease; musculoskeletal disorders, such as degenerative arthritis; GI disorders, such as irritable bowel syndrome; genitourinary problems, such as incontinence; collagen vascular diseases, such as lupus; and anemias.

Drugs prescribed for medical and psychiatric conditions as well as many commonly abused substances can also cause depression. Examples include antihypertensives, psychotropics, opioid and nonopioid analgesics, antiparkinsonian drugs, numerous cardiovascular medications, oral antidiabetic agents, antimicrobials, steroids, chemotherapeutic agents, cimetidine, and alcohol.

Complications

♦ Self-esteem compromise
♦ Loss of pleasure in regular life activities
♦ Occupational and social dysfunction
♦ Self-care deficit
♦ Suicide risk

Signs and symptoms

The primary features of major depression are a predominantly sad mood and a loss of interest or pleasure in daily activities. The patient may report feeling "down in the dumps," express doubts about self-worth or ability to cope, or simply appear unhappy and apathetic. The patient may also report feeling angry or anxious. Symptoms tend to be more severe than those caused by persistent depressive disorder (dysthymia), which is a milder, chronic form of depression. Other common signs include difficulty concentrating or thinking clearly, distractibility, and indecisiveness. In some patients, physiologic and psychological processes are slowed. Anergia and fatigue are common, as are anhedonia (inability to experience pleasure) and insomnia. Other patients may show signs of agitated depression with irritability and anxiety. Note if the patient reveals suicidal thoughts, a preoccupation with death, or has made previous suicide attempts.

The psychosocial history may reveal life problems or losses that contribute to depression. Or, the patient's medical history may implicate a physical disorder or the use of prescription, nonprescription, or illegal drugs that can contribute to depression. Note that many of the characteristics of depression, such as changes in eating and sleeping patterns, fatigue, and problems with concentration, may also occur in chronic medical conditions.

The patient may report an increase or a decrease in appetite, sleep disturbances (e.g., insomnia or early awakening), a lack of interest in sexual activity, constipation, or diarrhea. Other signs that you may note during a physical examination include agitation (such as hand-wringing or restlessness) and reduced psychomotor activity (e.g., slowed speech).

Diagnosis

For very specific diagnostic criteria, see the *DSM-5*.

The diagnosis is supported by psychological tests, such as the Beck Depression Inventory, which may help determine the onset, severity, duration, and progression of depressive symptoms. A toxicology screening may suggest drug-induced depression.

Treatment

Depression is treatable, although successful treatment may take time. The primary treatment methods are drug therapy and psychotherapy, particularly cognitive behavioral therapy. Research shows that better outcomes are realized when the patient engages in both approaches.

Drug therapy includes TCAs such as amitriptyline (Elavil), monoamine oxidase inhibitors (MAOIs) such as isocarboxazid (Marplan), maprotiline, and trazodone. SSRIs, such as fluoxetine (Prozac), paroxetine (Paxil), sertraline (Zoloft), bupropion (Wellbutrin), venlafaxine (Effexor XR), and mirtazapine (Remeron) are equally effective and have more tolerable adverse effect profiles.

Other drugs target serotonin as well as dopamine (bupropion—Wellbutrin) and norepinephrine (venlafaxine—Effexor XR and duloxetine—Cymbalta). These varied psychopharmacologic drugs allow for increased specificity of action. So, for example, a patient who shows neurovegetative signs of depression may benefit from bupropion (Wellbutrin), and another patient who's experiencing co-occurring anxiety and depression may benefit more from venlafaxine (Effexor XR).

TCAs, the oldest class of antidepressants, prevent the reuptake of norepinephrine or serotonin (or both) into the presynaptic nerve endings, resulting in increased synaptic concentrations of these neurotransmitters. Although often effective, these drugs have significant side effects. Because of their effect on cardiac conduction, TCAs may be lethal in overdoses. They also cause a gradual loss in the number of beta-adrenergic receptors.

MAOIs block the enzymatic degradation of norepinephrine and serotonin. These drugs commonly are prescribed for patients with atypical depression (e.g., depression marked by an increased appetite and need for sleep, rather than anorexia and insomnia) and for some patients who fail to respond to other classes of antidepressant drugs. MAOIs are associated with a high risk of toxicity; patients treated with one of these drugs must be able to comply with the necessary dietary restrictions.

Maprotiline is a potent blocker of norepinephrine uptake, whereas trazodone is an SSRI. The mechanism of action of bupropion (Wellbutrin) is not fully understood.

ECT may be considered in particularly severe or drug-resistant depression. Six to 12 treatments are typically needed, although in many cases improvement is evident after only a few treatments. However, ECT has been associated with later short-term memory loss, heart arrhythmias, and seizure activity. Researchers hypothesize that ECT affects the same receptor sites as antidepressants.

Short-term psychotherapy is also effective in treating major depression. Many psychiatrists believe that the best results are achieved with a combination of individual, family, or group psychotherapy and medication. After resolution of the acute episode, patients with a history of recurrent depression may be maintained on low doses of antidepressants as a preventive measure.

Depression may be experienced differently by members of different cultures, so assess for cultural beliefs and implications.

Special considerations

◆ Share your observations of the patient's behavior. For instance, you might say, "You're sitting all by yourself, looking very sad. Is that how you feel?" Because the patient may think and react sluggishly, speak slowly and allow ample time for response. Avoid feigned cheerfulness. However, don't hesitate to laugh with the patient and point out the value of humor.

◆ Value the patient by listening attentively and respectfully, preventing interruptions, and avoiding judgmental responses.

◆ Provide a structured routine, including noncompetitive activities, to build the patient's self-confidence and encourage interaction with others. Urge the patient to join group activities and to socialize.

◆ Inform the patient that depression can be eased by expressing feelings, participating in pleasurable activities, and improving grooming and hygiene.

◆ Ask the patient if he or she thinks of death or suicide. Such thoughts signal an immediate need for consultation and assessment. The risk of suicide increases as the depression lifts, typically in the early stages of treatment with antidepressants. The FDA has issued "black box" warnings on antidepressants because of this increased risk. (See *Suicide prevention guidelines*.)

Suicide prevention guidelines

When the patient is diagnosed with major depression, keep in mind these guidelines.

Assess for clues to suicide
Watch for the patient's suicidal thoughts, threats, and messages—describing a suicide plan, hoarding medication, purchasing a lethal item like a gun, talking about death and feelings of futility, giving away prized possessions, and changing behavior—especially as depression begins to lift.

Provide a safe environment
Check patient areas and correct dangerous conditions, such as exposed pipes, windows without safety glass, and access to the roof or balconies.

Remove dangerous objects
Take away potentially dangerous objects, such as belts, razors, suspenders, light cords, glass, knives, nail files and clippers, and metal and hard plastic objects.

Consult with staff
Recognize and document verbal and nonverbal suicidal behaviors, keep the healthcare provider informed, share data with all staff members, clarify the patient's specific restrictions, assess risk and plan for observation, and clarify day and night staff responsibilities and the frequency of consultations.

Observe the suicidal patient
Be alert when the patient is using a sharp object (such as a razor), taking medication, or using the bathroom (to prevent hanging or other injury). Assign the patient to a room near the nurses' station and with another patient. Continuously observe the acutely suicidal patient.

Maintain personal contact
Help the suicidal patient feel that he or she isn't alone or without resources or hope. Encourage continuity of care and consistency of primary nurses. Building therapeutic relationships with others is an important technique for preventing suicide.

⬡ ELDER TIP *The older adult at highest risk for suicide is at least age 85, is depressed, has high self-esteem, and needs to control his or her own life.*

◆ To prevent possible drug interactions, tell the patient to inform the healthcare provider about taking antidepressants.

◆ While tending to the patient's psychological needs, don't forget physical needs. Help with personal hygiene and encourage nutrition intake. Help with feeding if necessary. If the patient is constipated, add high-fiber foods to the diet; offer small, frequent meals; and encourage physical activity and fluid intake. Create a quiet environment at bedtime to improve sleep.

◆ Inform the patient that antidepressants may take several weeks to produce an effect.

◆ Teach the patient about depression. Emphasize that effective methods are available to relieve symptoms. Help the patient to recognize distorted perceptions that may contribute to depression. After the patient learns to recognize depressive thought patterns, he or she can consciously begin to substitute self-affirming thoughts.

◆ Instruct the patient about prescribed medications. Stress the need for compliance and review adverse effects. For drugs that produce strong anticholinergic effects, such as amitriptyline (Elavil), suggest sugarless gum or hard candy to relieve dry mouth. Many antidepressants are sedating (e.g., amitriptyline—Elavil and trazodone); teach the patient to avoid activities that require alertness, including driving and operating mechanical equipment until the CNS effects of the drug are known.

◆ Caution the patient taking a TCA to avoid drinking alcoholic beverages or taking other CNS depressants during therapy.

◆ If the patient is taking an MAOI, emphasize that certain foods that contain tyramine, caffeine, or tryptophan must be avoided. The ingestion of tyramine can cause a hypertensive crisis. Examples of foods that contain these substances include cheese, sour cream, pickled herring, liver, canned figs, raisins, bananas, avocados, chocolate, soy sauce, fava beans, yeast extracts, meat tenderizers, coffee, cola drinks, and beer, Chianti, or sherry.

◆ Because alcohol acts as a CNS depressant, recommend avoiding alcohol to a patient who's experiencing depression.

◆ During assessment, ask if the patient is taking herbal remedies for depression. A common herbal remedy, St. John's wort, can interact with many other antidepressants.

Anxiety disorders

PHOBIAS

Defined as a persistent and irrational fear of a specific object, activity, or situation, a phobia results in a compelling desire to avoid the perceived hazard. The patient recognizes that the fear is out of proportion to any actual danger, but he or she can't control it or explain it away. Agoraphobia is a specific type of phobia that involves the fear of being alone or of open space.

Social anxiety disorder, or social phobia, typically begins in late childhood or early adolescence; a specific phobia usually begins in childhood. Many phobic patients have no family history of psychiatric illness, including phobias.

Agoraphobia and social anxiety disorder tend to be chronic, but new treatments are improving the prognosis. A specific phobia usually resolves spontaneously as the child matures.

Causes and incidence

A phobia develops when anxiety about an object or a situation compels the patient to avoid it. The precise cause of most phobias is unknown. Psychoanalytic theory holds that the phobia is actually repression and displacement of an internal conflict. Behavior theorists view phobia as a stimulus–response reflex, avoiding a situation or object that causes anxiety.

Phobias are more common in women than in men; lifetime prevalence in the United States for a specific phobia range from 3.5% to 8.7%.

Pathophysiology

Genetic, neurobiological, personality, cognitive, and social and environmental factors must be taken into consideration when considering the pathophysiology of phobias, which is not fully understood. Specific phobias appear to have a genetic connection.

Complications

◆ Impaired self-esteem
◆ Depression

Signs and symptoms

The phobic patient typically reports signs of severe anxiety when confronted with the feared object or situation. A patient with agoraphobia, for example, may report dizziness, a sensation of falling, a feeling of unreality (depersonalization), vomiting, or cardiac distress when leaving home or crossing a bridge. Similarly, a patient who fears flying may report sweating, the sensation of a pounding heart, and panicky when on an airplane.

A patient who routinely avoids the object of phobia may report a loss of self-esteem and feelings of weakness, cowardice, depression, or ineffectiveness. Avoidance behavior reinforces the fear related to a phobia.

Diagnosis
For very specific diagnostic criteria, see the *DSM-5*.

Treatment
The effectiveness of treatment depends on the severity of the patient's phobia. Because phobic behavior may never be completely cured, the goal of treatment is to help the patient function effectively.

Anxiolytics, TCAs, MAOIs, and SSRIs may help relieve symptoms in patients with agoraphobia or social phobias. Gabapentin (Neurontin) has been used to treat social phobia. Performance anxiety may be lessened by beta-adrenergic blockers, such as propranolol (Inderal), used 1 to 2 hours before the performance.

Systematic desensitization, a type of behavioral therapy, may be more effective than drugs, especially if it includes encouragement, instruction, and suggestion.

In some areas, phobia clinics and group therapy are available. People who have recovered from phobias can usually help other patients who have similar phobias.

Special considerations
◆ Provide for the patient's safety and comfort, and monitor fluid and food intake, as needed. Certain phobias may inhibit food or fluid intake, disturb hygiene, and disrupt the patient's ability to rest.
◆ No matter how illogical the patient's phobia seems, avoid the urge to trivialize those fears. Remember that this behavior represents an essential coping mechanism.
◆ Ask the patient about normal coping mechanisms that have been helpful in the past. When the patient is able to face the fear, encourage verbalization of personal strengths and recourses.
◆ Don't let the patient withdraw completely. If a patient with agoraphobia is being treated as an outpatient, suggest small steps to overcome fears such as planning a brief shopping trip with a supportive family member or friend.
◆ In social phobias, the patient fears criticism. Encourage interaction with others and provide continuous support and positive reinforcement.
◆ Support participation in psychotherapy, including desensitization therapy. However, don't force insight. Challenging the patient may aggravate anxiety or lead to panic attacks.
◆ Teach the patient specific relaxation techniques, such as listening to music and meditating.
◆ Suggest ways to channel the patient's energy and relieve stress (such as running and creative activities).

GENERALIZED ANXIETY DISORDER
Anxiety is a feeling of apprehension that some describe as an exaggerated feeling of impending doom, dread, or uneasiness. Unlike fear—a reaction to danger from a specific external source—anxiety is a reaction to an internal threat, such as an unacceptable impulse or a repressed thought that's straining to reach a conscious level.

A rational response to a real threat, occasional anxiety is a normal part of life. Overwhelming anxiety, however, can result in generalized anxiety disorder (GAD)—uncontrollable, unreasonable worry that persists for at least 6 months and narrows perceptions or interferes with normal functioning. Evidence indicates that the prevalence of GAD is greater than previously thought and may rival even that of depression.

Causes and incidence
Theorists share a common premise: Conflict, whether intrapsychic, sociopersonal, or interpersonal, promotes an anxiety state.

GAD has a 1-year prevalence range of 2.9% in the adult population of the United States. It's more common in women than in men, and many cases begin in childhood or adolescence.

Pathophysiology
The pathophysiology of GAD is not fully understood. Genetic, developmental, and personality factors continue to be studied. PET scans of patients with GAD seem to indicate a relative increase in glucose metabolism in parts of the occipital, right posterior temporal lobe, inferior gyrus, cerebellum and right frontal gyrus, and an absolute decrease in the basal ganglia: benzodiazepine administration was associated with decreases in absolute metabolic rates for cortical surface, limbic system, and basal ganglia.

Complications
◆ Impaired self-worth
◆ Inability to engage in activities desired due to the anxiety
◆ Physical concerns that mimic other medical conditions

Signs and symptoms

GAD can begin at any age but typically has an onset at around 30 years old. Psychological or physiologic symptoms of anxiety states vary with the degree of anxiety. Mild anxiety mainly causes psychological symptoms, with unusual self-awareness and alertness to the environment. Moderate anxiety leads to selective inattention but with the ability to concentrate on a single task. Severe anxiety causes an inability to concentrate on more than scattered details of a task. A panic state with acute anxiety causes a complete loss of concentration, typically with unintelligible speech.

Physical examination of the patient with GAD may reveal signs or symptoms of motor tension, including trembling, muscle aches and spasms, headaches, and an inability to relax. Autonomic signs and symptoms include shortness of breath, tachycardia, sweating, and abdominal complaints.

In addition, the patient may startle easily and report feeling apprehensive, fearful, or angry. There may also be difficulty concentrating, eating, and sleeping. The medical, psychiatric, and psychosocial histories fail to identify a specific physical or environmental cause of the anxiety.

Diagnosis

For very specific diagnostic criteria, see the *DSM-5*.

Laboratory tests must exclude organic causes of the patient's signs and symptoms, such as hyperthyroidism, pheochromocytoma, coronary artery disease, supraventricular tachycardia, and Ménière disease. For example, an electrocardiogram can rule out myocardial ischemia in a patient who reports chest pain. Blood tests, including complete blood count, white blood cell count and differential, and serum lactate and calcium levels, can rule out hypocalcemia.

Because anxiety accompanies other psychiatric disorders, psychiatric evaluation must rule out phobias, OCD, depression, and acute schizophrenia.

Behaviors commonly associated with a diagnosis of anxiety may have cultural origins or acceptance. Be sure to thoroughly address cultural implications when conducting an assessment.

Treatment

A combination of drug therapy and psychotherapy may help a patient with GAD. Judicial use of benzodiazepines may relieve mild anxiety and improve the patient's ability to cope.

ELDER TIP *A benzodiazepine with a long half-life tends to accumulate in an older adult's system and may cause oversedation. Benzodiazepines are sometimes given along with opioids to add to the analgesic effect or as a preanesthetic. Remember, if an older adult is scheduled for surgery, it may take longer to recover from anesthesia if these combinations are used.*

TCAs or higher doses of short-acting benzodiazepines may relieve severe anxiety and panic attacks. Buspirone, an anxiolytic, causes the patient less sedation and poses less risk of physical and psychological dependence than the benzodiazepines. Venlafaxine (Effexor XR), a serotonin and norepinephrine reuptake inhibitor, is FDA-approved for the treatment of GAD.

Psychotherapy for GAD has two goals: helping the patient identify and deal with the cause of the anxiety and eliminating environmental factors that precipitate an anxious reaction. In addition, the patient can learn relaxation techniques, such as deep breathing, progressive muscle relaxation, focused relaxation, and visualization.

Special considerations

◆ Stay with the patient during times of anxiety, and encourage discussion of feelings. Reduce environmental stimuli and remain calm.

◆ Administer anxiolytics or antidepressants as prescribed, and evaluate the patient's response. Teach the patient about prescribed medications, including the need for adherence with the medication regimen. Review adverse reactions.

◆ Teach the patient effective coping strategies and relaxation techniques. Help to identify stressful situations that trigger anxiety, and provide positive reinforcement when appropriate alternative coping strategies are used.

PANIC DISORDER

Characterized by recurrent episodes of intense apprehension, terror, and impending doom, panic disorder represents anxiety in its most severe form. Initially unpredictable, panic attacks may become associated with specific situations or tasks. The disorder commonly exists concurrently with agoraphobia.

Panic disorder typically has an onset in late adolescence or early adulthood, typically in response to a sudden loss. It may also be triggered by severe separation anxiety experienced during early childhood. Without treatment, panic disorder can persist for years, with alternating exacerbations and remissions. The patient with panic disorder is at high risk for a psychoactive substance abuse disorder, resorting to alcohol or anxiolytics in an attempt to relieve extreme anxiety.

Causes and incidence

Like other anxiety disorders, panic disorder may stem from a combination of physical and psychological factors. For example, some theorists emphasize the role of stressful events or unconscious conflicts that occur early in childhood.

Panic disorder affects about 2% to 3% of the population, with females being affected more than males. Symptoms develop around the age of 14.

Pathophysiology

The most recent evidence indicates that a hyperexcitable amygdala or hypothalamus may contribute to panic disorder. Research shows that there may be genetic implications, while anxious temperament places patients at higher risk for the development of panic disorder.

Complications

◆ Compromised self-esteem
◆ Inability to participate in activities of interest due to panic
◆ Physical concerns that mimic other medical disorders

Signs and symptoms

The patient with panic disorder typically reports repeated episodes of unexpected apprehension, fear or, rarely, intense discomfort. These panic attacks may last for minutes or hours and leave the patient shaken, fearful, and exhausted. They may occur several times a week, sometimes even daily. Because the attacks occur spontaneously, without exposure to a known anxiety-producing situation, the patient generally worries between attacks about when the next episode will occur. This is referred to as *anticipatory anxiety*.

Physical examination of the patient during a panic attack may reveal signs of intense anxiety, such as hyperventilation, tachycardia, trembling, and profuse sweating. The patient may also report difficulty breathing, digestive disturbances, and chest pain.

Diagnosis

For very specific diagnostic criteria, see the *DSM-5*.

Because many medical conditions can mimic panic disorder, additional tests may be ordered to rule out an organic basis for the symptoms. For example, tests for serum glucose levels rule out hypoglycemia; studies of urine catecholamines and vanillylmandelic acid rule out pheochromocytoma; and thyroid function tests rule out hyperthyroidism.

Urine and serum toxicology tests may reveal the presence of psychoactive substances that can cause panic attacks, including barbiturates, caffeine, and amphetamines.

Treatment

Panic disorder may respond to behavioral therapy, supportive psychotherapy, or drug therapy, alone or in combination. Behavioral therapy works best when agoraphobia accompanies panic disorder because the identification of anxiety-inducing situations is easier.

Psychotherapy commonly uses cognitive techniques to enable the patient to view anxiety-provoking situations more realistically and to recognize panic symptoms as a misinterpretation of essentially harmless physical sensations.

Drug therapy includes anxiolytics, such as diazepam (Valium), alprazolam (Xanax), and clonazepam (Klonopin), and beta blockers, such as propranolol (Inderal), to provide symptomatic relief. Antidepressants, including TCAs, SSRIs, and MAOIs, are also effective.

Special considerations

◆ Stay with the patient until the attack subsides. If left alone, the patient may become even more anxious.
◆ Maintain a calm, serene approach. Statements such as "I won't let anything here hurt you" and "I'll stay with you" can assure the patient that you're in control of the immediate situation. Avoid giving insincere expressions of reassurance.
◆ The patient's perceptual field may be narrowed, and excessive stimuli may cause feelings of being overwhelmed. Dim bright lights or raise dim lights as needed.
◆ If the patient loses control, relocate to a smaller, quieter space.
◆ The patient may be so overwhelmed that he or she can't follow lengthy or complicated instructions. Speak in short, simple sentences, and slowly give one direction at a time. Avoid giving lengthy explanations and asking too many questions.
◆ Allow the patient to pace around the room to help expend energy. Demonstrate taking slow, deep breaths in the presence of hyperventilation.
◆ Avoid touching the patient until you've established a rapport. Until trust is established, the patient may be too stimulated or frightened to find touch reassuring.
◆ Administer medication as prescribed.
◆ During and after a panic attack, encourage the patient to express feelings. Discuss fears and help the patient identify situations or events that trigger the attacks.
◆ Teach the patient relaxation techniques, and explain how these can be used to relieve stress or avoid a panic attack.

◆ Review with the patient any adverse effects of the drugs prescribed. Caution the patient and notify the healthcare provider before discontinuing the medication because abrupt withdrawal could cause severe symptoms.

◆ Encourage the patient and family to use community resources such as the Anxiety Disorders Association of America.

OBSESSIVE-COMPULSIVE DISORDER

Obsessive thoughts and compulsive behaviors represent recurring efforts to control overwhelming anxiety, guilt, or unacceptable impulses that persistently enter the consciousness. The word *obsession* refers to a recurrent idea, thought, impulse, or image that's intrusive and inappropriate, causing marked anxiety or distress. A *compulsion* is a ritualistic, repetitive, and involuntary defensive behavior. Performing a compulsive behavior reduces the patient's anxiety and increases the probability that the behavior will recur. Compulsions are commonly associated with obsessions.

Patients with OCD are prone to use psychoactive substances, such as alcohol and anxiolytics, in an attempt to relieve their anxiety. In addition, other anxiety disorders and major depression commonly coexist with OCD.

OCD is typically a chronic condition with remissions and flare-ups. Mild forms of the disorder are relatively common in the population at large.

Causes and incidence

The cause of OCD is unknown. OCD affects 1.2% of Americans, and adult females are affected slightly more than males.

Pathophysiology

The pathophysiology of OCD is not fully understood. Some studies suggest that neuroanatomical abnormalities in Cortico-Striato-Thalamo-Cortical (CSTC) circuits of patients with OCD exist. Other studies base an explanation on psychological theories. In addition, major depression, organic brain syndrome, and schizophrenia may contribute to the onset of OCD. Some authorities think that OCD is closely related to some eating disorders. Genetic and environmental factors continue to be studied.

Complications

◆ Impaired self-esteem
◆ Impaired social interactions due to need to carry out rituals
◆ Impairment in occupational function due to need to carry out rituals

◆ Self-care deficit, if ritual completion supersedes self-care

Signs and symptoms

The psychiatric history of a patient with OCD may reveal the presence of obsessive thoughts, words, or mental images that persistently and involuntarily invade the consciousness. Some common obsessions include thoughts of violence (such as stabbing, shooting, maiming, or hitting), thoughts of contamination (images of dirt, germs, or feces), repetitive doubts and worries about a tragic event, and repeating or counting images, words, or objects in the environment. The patient recognizes that the obsessions are a product of his or her own mind and that they interfere with normal daily activities.

The patient's history may also reveal the presence of compulsions, irrational and recurring impulses to repeat a certain behavior. Common compulsions include repetitive touching, sometimes combined with counting; doing and undoing (for instance, opening and closing doors or rearranging things); washing (especially hands); and checking (to be sure no tragedy has occurred since the last time he checked). In many cases, the patient's anxiety is so strong that he or she will avoid the situation or the object that evokes the impulse.

When the obsessive-compulsive phenomena are mental, observation may reveal no behavioral abnormalities. However, compulsive acts may be observed. Feelings of shame, nervousness, or embarrassment may prompt the patient to try limiting these acts to personal, private time.

Also evaluate the impact of obsessive-compulsive phenomena on the patient's normal routine. He'll typically report moderate to severe impairment of social and occupational functioning.

Diagnosis

For very specific diagnostic criteria, see the *DSM-5*.

Treatment

OCD is tenacious, but improvement occurs in many patients who obtain treatment. Current treatment usually involves a combination of medication and cognitive behavioral therapy. Other types of psychotherapy may also be helpful.

Effective medications include clomipramine (Anafranil), a TCA; SSRIs, such as fluoxetine (Prozac), paroxetine (Paxil), sertraline (Zoloft), and fluvoxamine; and the benzodiazepine clonazepam (Klonopin).

Behavioral therapies—aversion therapy, thought stopping, thought switching, flooding, implosion therapy, and response prevention—have also been effective. (See *Behavioral therapies for obsessive-compulsive disorder*.)

Special considerations

◆ Approach the patient unhurriedly.

◆ Provide an accepting atmosphere; don't appear shocked, amused, or critical of the ritualistic behavior.

◆ Keep the patient's physical health in mind. For example, compulsive hand washing may cause skin breakdown; rituals or preoccupations may cause inadequate food and fluid intake and exhaustion. Provide for basic needs, such as rest, nutrition, and grooming, if the patient becomes involved in ritualistic thoughts and behaviors to the point of self-neglect.

◆ Let the patient know that you're aware of the behavior. For example, you might say, "I noticed you've made your bed three times today; that must be very tiring for you." Help the patient explore feelings associated with the behavior. For example, ask, "What do you think about while you're performing your chores?"

◆ Make reasonable demands and set reasonable limits, explaining their purpose clearly. Avoid creating situations that increase frustration and provoke anger, which may interfere with treatment.

◆ Explore patterns leading to the behavior or recurring problems.

◆ Listen attentively, offering feedback.

◆ Encourage the use of appropriate defenses to relieve loneliness and isolation.

◆ Engage the patient in activities to create positive accomplishments and raise self-esteem and confidence.

◆ Encourage active diversionary activities, such as whistling or humming a tune, to divert attention from the unwanted thoughts and to promote a pleasurable experience.

◆ Help the patient develop new ways to solve problems and cultivate more effective coping skills by setting limits on unacceptable behavior (e.g., by limiting the number of times per day he or she may indulge in compulsive behavior). Gradually shorten the time allowed for compulsive behavior. Help the patient focus on other feelings or problems for the remainder of the time.

Behavioral therapies for obsessive-compulsive disorder

The following behavioral therapies are used to treat the patient with obsessive-compulsive disorder.

Aversion therapy
Application of a painful stimulus creates an aversion to the obsession that leads to undesirable behavior (compulsion).

Flooding
Flooding is frequent, full-intensity exposure (through the use of imagery) to an object that triggers a symptom. It must be used with caution because it produces extreme discomfort.

Implosion therapy
A form of desensitization, implosion therapy calls for repeated exposure to a highly feared object.

Response prevention
Preventing compulsive behavior by distraction, persuasion, or redirection of activity, response prevention may require hospitalization or involvement of the patient's family to be effective.

Thought stopping
Thought stopping breaks the habit of fear-inducing anticipatory thoughts. The patient learns to stop unwanted thoughts by actually saying the word "stop" and then focusing attention on achieving calmness and muscle relaxation.

Thought switching
To replace fear-inducing self-instructions with competent self-instructions, the patient learns to replace negative thoughts with positive ones until the positive thoughts become strong enough to overcome the anxiety-provoking ones.

◆ Identify insight and improved behavior (reduced compulsive behavior and fewer obsessive thoughts). Evaluate behavioral changes by your own observations and the patient's reports.

◆ Identify disturbing topics of conversation that reflect underlying anxiety or terror.

◆ When interventions don't work, reevaluate them and recommend alternative strategies.

◆ Help the patient identify progress and set realistic expectations of self and others.

◆ Explain how to channel emotional energy to relieve stress (e.g., through sports and creative endeavors). In addition, teach the patient relaxation and breathing techniques to help reduce anxiety.

◆ Work with the patient and other treatment team members to establish behavioral goals and to help the patient tolerate anxiety in pursuing these goals.

POSTTRAUMATIC STRESS DISORDER

Characteristic psychological consequences that persist for at least 1 month after a traumatic event are classified as posttraumatic stress disorder (PTSD). This disorder can follow almost any distressing event, including a natural or man-made disaster, physical or sexual abuse, or an assault or a rape. Psychological trauma, which accompanies the physical trauma, is characterized by intense fear and feelings of helplessness and loss of control. PTSD can be acute, chronic, or delayed. When the precipitating event is of human design, the disorder is more severe and more persistent. Onset can occur at any age, even during childhood.

Causes and incidence

PTSD occurs in response to an extremely distressing event, including a serious threat of harm to the patient or family, such as war, abuse, or violent crime. It may be triggered by sudden destruction of his or her home or community by a bombing, fire, flood, tornado, earthquake, or similar disaster. It may also follow witnessing the death or serious injury of another person by torture, in a death camp, by natural disaster, in a mass shooting, or by a motor vehicle or airplane crash.

Any person who has experienced traumatic relocation due to such events as rioting or other civil strife, extreme natural disasters, or war should be assessed for signs of PTSD.

PTSD can occur at any age. Some cases resolve in the months following the traumatic event, while other cases can last for years. The 12-month prevalence of PTSD in Americans is approximately 3.5%.

Pathophysiology

Preexisting psychopathology can predispose some patients to this disorder, but anyone can develop it, especially if the stressor is extreme. Genetic and environmental contributors continue to be studied. MRI scans of patients with PTSD show a decreased volume of the hippocampus, left amygdala, and anterior cingulate cortex in patients with PTSD compared with matched controls.

Complications

◆ Impaired social and occupational function
◆ Risk for harm to self or others
◆ Risk for substance use

Signs and symptoms

The psychosocial history of a patient with PTSD may reveal early life experiences, interpersonal factors, military experiences, or other incidents that suggest the precipitating event. Typically, the patient may report that the symptoms began immediately or soon after the trauma, although they may not develop until months or years later. In such a case, avoidance symptoms usually have been present during the latency period.

Symptoms include pangs of painful emotion and unwelcome thoughts; intrusive memories; dissociative episodes (flashbacks); a traumatic re-experiencing of the event; difficulty falling or staying asleep, frequent nightmares of the traumatic event, and aggressive outbursts on awakening; emotional numbing (diminished or constricted response); and chronic anxiety or panic attacks (with physical signs and symptoms).

The patient may display rage and/or survivor guilt, use of violence to solve problems, depression and suicidal thoughts, phobic avoidance of situations that arouse memories of the traumatic event (such as hot weather and tall grasses for the Vietnam veteran), memory impairment or difficulty concentrating, and feelings of detachment or estrangement that destroy interpersonal relationships. Some have physical symptoms, fantasies of retaliation, and engage in substance use.

Diagnosis

For very specific diagnostic criteria, see the *DSM-5*.

Treatment

Treatment of PTSD aims to reduce the target symptoms, prevent chronic disability, and promote occupational and social rehabilitation. Specific treatments may emphasize behavioral techniques (such as relaxation therapy to decrease anxiety and induce sleep or progressive desensitization). SSRIs, such as sertraline (Zoloft) and paroxetine (Paxil), are considered first-line treatments for PTSD. SSRIs reduce all symptoms associated with PTSD. Patients who respond to an SSRI should remain on the drug for at least 1 year before an attempt is made to withdraw it. Other drugs shown to be helpful include anticonvulsants (divalproex sodium—Depakote) and MAOIs such as phenelzine (Nardil).

Behavior, cognitive, and hypnosis therapy must be individualized because re-experiencing the trauma overwhelms some patients. Two major therapeutic approaches have been recommended: exposure therapy, which is re-experiencing the traumatic event through imaging techniques or in vivo exposure, and stress management and relaxation techniques. Group and family therapy have been reported to be helpful in some cases of PTSD.

Many patients need treatment for depression, alcohol or drug abuse, or medical conditions before psychological healing can take place. Treatment of this disorder may be complex, and the prognosis varies.

Special considerations
◆ Encourage the patient with PTSD to express grief, complete the mourning process, and develop coping skills to relieve anxiety and desensitize memories of the traumatic event.
◆ Know and practice crisis intervention techniques as appropriate in PTSD.
◆ Establish trust by accepting the patient's current level of functioning and assuming a positive, consistent, honest, and nonjudgmental attitude toward the patient.
◆ Provide encouragement as the patient shows a commitment to work on symptoms associated with this condition.
◆ Deal constructively with the patient's displays of anger.
◆ Encourage joint assessment of angry outbursts (identify how anger escalates and explore preventive measures that family members can take to regain control).
◆ Provide a safe, staff-monitored room in which the patient can safely deal with urges to commit physical violence or self-abuse through displacement (such as pounding clay or destroying selected items).
◆ Encourage the patient to move from physical to verbal expressions of anger.
◆ Help the patient relieve shame and guilt precipitated by real actions (such as killing or mutilation) that violated a consciously held moral code. Help the patient put the behavior into perspective, recognize isolation and self-destructive behavior as forms of atonement, learn to forgive himself or herself, and accept forgiveness from others.
◆ Refer the patient to a member of the clergy, as appropriate.
◆ Provide for group therapy with other victims for peer support and forgiveness, or refer the patient to such a support group.
◆ Refer the patient to appropriate community resources.

Somatic symptom and related disorders

SOMATIC SYMPTOM DISORDER
When multiple recurrent signs and symptoms of several years' duration suggest that physical disorders exist without a verifiable disease or pathophysiologic condition to account for them, somatization disorder is present. The patient with somatic symptom disorder usually undergoes repeated medical examinations and diagnostic testing that—unlike the symptoms themselves—can be potentially dangerous or debilitating.

Somatic symptom disorder is usually chronic, with exacerbations occurring during times of stress. The patient's signs and symptoms are involuntary, and he or she consciously wants to feel better. Nonetheless, the patient is seldom entirely symptom-free.

Pathophysiology
The pathophysiology of somatic symptom disorder is not understood. Genetic, temperamental, cultural, and environmental factors are thought to contribute to the development of somatization disorder.

Causes and incidence
Causes are not fully understood. This disorder appears to be more frequent in individuals with few years of education and those of lower socioeconomic status. Signs and symptoms often begin in adolescence, and females tend to be affected more than males. The presentation of this disorder varies across cultures, depending on the cultural norm of the group studied. Actual prevalence is not known.

Complications
◆ Impaired self-esteem
◆ Impaired social or occupational function
◆ Comorbidity with other conditions such as depression increases suicide risk

Signs and symptoms

Examination of a patient with somatic symptom disorder is characterized by physical concerns presented in a dramatic, vague, or exaggerated way, typically as part of a complicated medical history in which many medical diagnoses have been considered. An important clue to this disorder is a history of multiple medical evaluations by different healthcare providers at different institutions—sometimes simultaneously—without significant findings.

The patient may appear anxious and depressed. Common physical concerns include:
◆ conversion or pseudoneurologic signs and symptoms (e.g., paralysis or blindness)
◆ GI discomfort (abdominal pain, nausea, or vomiting)
◆ chronic pain (e.g., back pain)
◆ headaches
◆ cardiopulmonary symptoms (chest pain, dizziness, or palpitations)

The patient may relate current concerns and previous evaluations in great detail. He or she may be quite knowledgeable about tests, procedures, and medical jargon. Attempts to explore areas other than his or her medical history may cause noticeable anxiety. The patient may disparage previous healthcare professionals and previous treatments, and states, "Everyone thinks I'm imagining these things."

Ongoing assessment should focus on new signs or symptoms or any change in old ones to avoid missing a developing physical disorder.

Diagnosis

For very specific diagnostic criteria, see the *DSM-5*.

Diagnostic tests rule out physical disorders that cause vague and confusing symptoms, such as hyperparathyroidism, porphyria, multiple sclerosis, chronic fatigue syndrome, and systemic lupus erythematosus. In addition, multiple physical signs and symptoms that appear for the first time late in life are usually due to physical disease rather than somatization disorder.

Treatment

The goal of treatment is to help the patient learn to live with signs and symptoms. After diagnostic evaluation has ruled out organic causes, the patient should be told that there is no serious illness currently but that he or she will receive care for genuine distress and ongoing medical attention for symptoms.

The most important aspect of treatment is a continuing supportive relationship with a healthcare provider who acknowledges the patient's signs and symptoms and is willing to help him or her live with them. The patient should have visits that emphasize coping strategies. The patient with somatic symptom disorder seldom may not acknowledge any psychological aspect of the illness and may reject psychiatric treatment.

Special considerations

◆ Acknowledge the patient's symptoms and efforts to cope despite distress. Don't characterize symptoms as imaginary. Explain test results and their significance.
◆ Emphasize strengths, for example, "It's good that you can still work with this pain." Gently point out the time relationship between stress and symptoms.
◆ Help the patient manage stress. Typically, relationships are linked to symptoms; relieving symptoms may change the patient's interactions with others.
◆ Negotiate a plan of care with input from the patient and, if possible, the family. Help them to understand the patient's condition.

CONVERSION DISORDER (FUNCTIONAL NEUROLOGIC SYMPTOM DISORDER)

Conversion disorder allows a patient to resolve a psychological conflict through the loss of a specific physical function—for example, by paralysis, blindness, or inability to swallow. Conversion disorder results in an involuntary loss of physical function. However, laboratory tests and diagnostic procedures fail to disclose an organic cause. The conversion symptom itself isn't life threatening and usually has a short duration.

Causes and incidence

The patient suddenly develops the conversion symptom soon after experiencing a traumatic conflict.

Conversion disorder can occur in either sex at any age. An uncommon disorder, it usually is first seen in the patient's 40s.

Pathophysiology

The pathophysiology of conversion disorder is not fully understood. Genetic, environmental, and temperamental research continues. Two theories may explain why conversion disorder occurs. According to the first, the patient achieves a "primary gain" when the symptom keeps a psychological conflict out of conscious awareness. For example, a person may experience blindness after witnessing a violent crime. In this case, anxiety relating to witnessing a violent crime is converted into a physical symptom.

The second theory suggests that the patient achieves "secondary gain" from the symptom by avoiding a traumatic activity. For example, a soldier may develop a "paralyzed" hand that prevents him or her from entering into combat.

Complication
◆ Difficulty discerning between the condition and an actual physical concern

Signs and symptoms
The history of a patient with conversion disorder may reveal the sudden onset of a single, debilitating sign or symptom that prevents normal function of the affected body part, such as paralysis of a leg. The patient may describe a psychologically stressful event that recently preceded the symptom. However, the patient doesn't display the affect and concern that such a severe symptom usually elicits.

Assessment findings obtained during a physical examination are inconsistent with the primary symptom. For instance, tendon reflexes may be normal in a "paralyzed" part of the body, loss of function fails to follow anatomic patterns of innervation, or pupillary responses and evoked potentials are normal in a patient who complains of blindness.

Diagnosis
For very specific diagnostic criteria, see the *DSM-5*.

A thorough physical evaluation must rule out a physical cause, especially diseases that typically produce vague physical symptoms (such as multiple sclerosis or systemic lupus erythematosus).

Treatment
Psychotherapy, family therapy, relaxation therapy, behavioral therapy, or hypnosis may be used alone or in combination (two or more).

Special considerations
◆ Help the patient maintain integrity of the affected system. Regularly exercise paralyzed limbs to prevent muscle wasting and contractures.
◆ Frequently change the bedridden patient's position to prevent pressure ulcers.
◆ Ensure adequate nutrition.
◆ Provide a supportive environment, and encourage the patient to discuss the stressful event that may have contributed to this disorder.
◆ Don't force the patient to talk, but convey a caring attitude to help the patient share feelings.
◆ Don't insist that the patient use the affected system. This may hinder the therapeutic relationship.

◆ Add your support to the recommendation for psychiatric care.
◆ Include the patient's family in all care. They may be contributing to the patient's stress, and they're essential to help him regain normal functioning.

Dissociative disorders
DISSOCIATIVE IDENTITY DISORDER
A complex disturbance of identity and memory, dissociative identity disorder is characterized by the existence of two or more distinct, fully integrated personalities (sometimes called "alters") in the same person. The personalities alternate in dominance. Each comprises unique memories, behavior patterns, and social relationships; in many cases, rigid and flamboyant personalities are combined. Usually, one personality is unaware of the existence of the others.

Causes and incidence
The cause isn't known. The patient may have experienced abuse, commonly sexual, or another form of emotional trauma in childhood. A child may evolve multiple personalities to dissociate himself or herself from the traumatic situation. The dissociated contents become linked with one of many possible shaping influences for personality organization.

Dissociative identity disorder usually begins in childhood, but patients seldom seek treatment until much later in life. The disorder, with a prevalence of 1.5%, is almost equal between males and females.

Pathophysiology
The pathophysiology of dissociative identity disorder is unknown, largely because the diagnosis is controversial. The trauma model, as well as childhood trauma, has been investigated as contributory to this condition.

Complications
◆ Impaired self-esteem
◆ Impaired social or occupational function
◆ Increased suicide risk, depending on the "persona" of the different "alters"
◆ Increased risk for violence toward others, depending on the "persona" of the different "alters"

Signs and symptoms
The patient may seek treatment for a concurrent psychiatric disorder present in one of the personalities. He or she may have a history

of unsuccessful psychiatric treatment, or the patient may report periods of amnesia and disturbances in time perception. Family members may describe incidents that the patient can't recall as well as alterations in facial presentation, voice, and behavior.

Stress or idiosyncratically meaningful social or environmental cues commonly trigger the transition from one personality to another. Although usually sudden, the transition can occur over hours or days. Hypnosis and amobarbital may facilitate transition.

Diagnosis
For very specific diagnostic criteria, see the *DSM-5*.

Treatment
Insight-oriented psychotherapy and hypnotherapy may be helpful in uniting the personalities and preventing the personality from splitting again. Treatment is usually intensive and prolonged, with success linked to the strength of the patient–therapist relationship with each of the personalities, all of which require equal respect and concern.

Special considerations
◆ Establish an empathetic relationship with each emerging personality.
◆ Monitor the patient's actions for evidence of self-directed violence or violence directed at others.
◆ Recognize even small gains.
◆ Stress the importance of continuing psychotherapy. Point out that the therapy can be prolonged, with alternating successes and failures, and that one or more of the personalities may resist treatment.

DISSOCIATIVE AMNESIA
The essential feature of dissociative amnesia is a sudden inability to recall important personal information that can't be explained by ordinary forgetfulness. The patient typically is unable to recall all events that occurred during a specific period, but other types of recall disturbance are also possible.

This disorder has been known to occur during war and natural disasters. The amnesic event typically ends abruptly, and recovery is complete, with rare recurrences.

Causes and incidence
Dissociative amnesia follows severe psychosocial stress, commonly involving a threat of physical injury or death. It has been observed across the life span. Prevalence in American adults has been reported at 1.8%.

Pathophysiology
The pathophysiology of dissociative amnesia is unknown. The most widely accepted conceptual model for this disorder is an epigenetic model showing the disorder resulting from genes and other neurobiological and environmental factors that influence gene expression.

Complications
◆ Inability to locate family or caregivers
◆ Risk for suicide or self-destructive behavior once memory returns

Signs and symptoms
During the assessment interview, the patient with dissociative amnesia may appear perplexed and disoriented, wandering aimlessly. The patient won't be able to remember the event that precipitated the episode and probably won't recognize his or her inability to recall information.

After the episode has ended, the patient is usually unaware that he or she has suffered a disturbance in recall.

Diagnosis
For very specific diagnostic criteria, see the *DSM-5*.

Treatment
Psychotherapy aims to help the patient recognize the traumatic event that triggered the amnesia and the anxiety it produced. A trusting, therapeutic relationship is essential to achieving this goal. The therapist subsequently attempts to teach the patient reality-based coping strategies.

Special considerations
◆ Establish a therapeutic, nonjudgmental relationship with the patient.
◆ When providing care in this disorder, teach the patient effective coping strategies to use in stressful situations rather than those strategies that distort reality.
◆ Help the patient with dissociative amnesia recognize and deal with experiences that produce anxiety.

DEPERSONALIZATION/ DEREALIZATION DISORDER
Persistent or recurrent episodes of detachment characterize depersonalization/derealization disorder. During these episodes, self-awareness is temporarily altered or lost; the patient, in many cases, perceives this alteration in consciousness as a barrier

between self and the outside world. The sense of depersonalization may be restricted to a single body part, such as a limb, or it may encompass the whole self. The patient with this disorder may feel mechanical, in a dream, or detached from the body.

Although the patient seldom loses touch with reality completely, the episodes of depersonalization/derealization may cause severe distress. Depersonalization/derealization disorder usually has a sudden onset in adolescence around the age of 16. It follows a chronic course, with periodic exacerbations and remissions, and resolves gradually. Onset in the 20s is uncommon, and even less common as the patient ages.

Causes and incidence
Depersonalization disorder typically stems from severe stress, including war experiences, accidents, and natural disasters. It may also be due to neurologic or systemic disease.

Pathophysiology
The pathophysiology of depersonalization/derealization disorder is unknown. However, studies have shown that patients with this disorder have physiological hyporeactivity to emotional stimuli. Head injuries, seizures, and substance use have been shown to be organic risk factors. Several neurotransmitter systems, brain regions, and functional circuits have also been shown to be connected to this disorder, as well, although the clearest association is with childhood interpersonal trauma.

Complications
◆ Inability to maintain connectivity with reality, even if only situationally or for a short period of time
◆ Risk for suicide or self-destructive behavior once function returns

Signs and symptoms
The patient with depersonalization disorder may complain of feeling detached from his entire being and body, as if he were watching himself from a distance or living in a dream. He may also report sensory anesthesia, a loss of self-control, difficulty speaking, and feelings of derealization and losing touch with reality.

Common findings during the assessment interview include symptoms of depression, obsessive rumination, somatic concerns, anxiety, fear of going insane, a disturbed sense of time, and a prolonged recall time as well as physical complaints such as dizziness.

Diagnosis
For very specific diagnostic criteria, see the *DSM-5*.

Treatment
Psychotherapy aims to establish a trusting, therapeutic relationship in which the patient recognizes the traumatic event that triggered the disorder and the anxiety it evoked. The therapist subsequently teaches the patient to use reality-based coping strategies rather than to detach from the situation.

Special considerations
◆ Establish a therapeutic, nonjudgmental relationship with the patient.
◆ When providing care in this disorder, assist the patient in using reality-based coping strategies under stress rather than those strategies that distort reality.
◆ Help the patient who has depersonalization/derealization disorder recognize and deal with experiences that produce anxiety.

PERSONALITY DISORDERS
Defined as individual traits that reflect chronic, inflexible, and maladaptive patterns of behavior, personality disorders cause social discomfort and impair social and occupational functioning. The *DSM-5* groups personality disorders into three clusters:
◆ Cluster A—paranoid, schizoid, and schizotypal personality disorders. These disorders share odd or eccentric behavior.
◆ Cluster B—antisocial, borderline, histrionic, and narcissistic personality disorders. Dramatic, emotional, or erratic behavior highlights these disorders.
◆ Cluster C—avoidant, dependent, and obsessive-compulsive personality disorders. These disorders are marked by anxious or fearful behavior.

Each disorder produces characteristic signs and symptoms, which may vary among patients and even with the same patient at different times.

Personality disorders are lifelong conditions with an onset in adolescence or early adulthood. Cluster A and B disorders tend to grow less intense in middle age and late life, whereas cluster C disorders tend to become exaggerated. Patients with cluster B disorders are susceptible to substance use, poor impulse control, and suicidal behavior.

Personality disorders often overlap with other psychiatric disorders, such as substance use disorder, mood disorders, and/or anxiety disorders.

Causes and incidence

Various theories attempt to explain the origin of personality disorders. Personality structure affects how a person responds to life experiences and interacts with the social environment. Over time, each person develops distinctive ways of perceiving the world and of feeling, thinking, and behaving.

Social theories hold that disorders reflect learned responses, having much to do with reinforcement, modeling, and aversive stimuli as contributing factors. According to psychodynamic theories, personality disorders reflect deficiencies in ego and superego development and are related to poor mother–child relationships characterized by unresponsiveness, overprotectiveness, or early separation.

Personality disorders are common and affect approximately 16.5% of the population in the United States. Gender influences presence; for example, antisocial and obsessive-compulsive personality disorders are more common in men, whereas borderline, dependent, and histrionic personality disorders are more prevalent in women.

Pathophysiology

The pathophysiology of personality disorders is not fully understood. Genetic factors influence the biological basis of brain function as well as basic personality structure. Some researchers suspect that poor regulation of the areas controlling emotion within the brain increases the risk of a personality disorder, especially when combined with such factors as abuse, neglect, or separation. For a biologically predisposed person, the major developmental challenges of adolescence and early adulthood may trigger a personality disorder.

Complications

Complications are dependent upon the type of personality disorder. Complications that are common to most personality disorders include:
◆ Low self-esteem
◆ Inability to recognize personal responsibility for behaviors
◆ Impaired social and/or occupational function

Signs and symptoms

Each specific personality disorder produces characteristic signs and symptoms, which may vary among patients and within the same patient at different times. In general, the history of the patient with a personality disorder will reveal long-standing difficulties in interpersonal relationships, ranging from dependency to withdrawal, and problems in occupational functioning, with effects ranging from compulsive perfectionism to intentional sabotage.

The patient with a personality disorder may show any degree of self-confidence, ranging from no self-esteem to arrogance. Convinced that his or her behavior is normal, the patient avoids responsibility for its consequences, commonly resorting to projections and blame.

Diagnosis

For very specific diagnostic criteria, see the *DSM-5*.

Treatment

Personality disorders are difficult to treat. Successful therapy requires a trusting relationship in which the therapist can use a direct approach. The type of therapy chosen depends on the patient's symptoms. Family and group therapies can be effective. Cognitive and self-help groups have also been beneficial. Dialectical behavioral therapy is commonly used to treat patients with personality disorders.

Drug therapy is effective in some types of personality disorders; for example, pimozide (Orap) has been successfully used to reduce paranoia ideation in some patients with paranoid personality disorder. Antipsychotic drugs (olanzapine—Zyprexa, or risperidone—Risperdal) may be used to treat severe agitation or delusional thinking. SSRIs, such as fluoxetine (Prozac), may be used to treat irritability, anger, and obsessional thinking. Careful use of anxiolytics may be used to treat severe anxiety that interferes with normal thinking.

Hospital inpatient milieu therapy can be effective in crisis situations and possibly for long-term treatment of some disorders. Inpatient treatment is controversial, however, because some patients with personality disorders don't comply with extended therapeutic regimens; for such patients, outpatient therapy may be more helpful.

Special considerations

◆ Provide consistent care. Take a direct, consistent approach to ensure trust. Keep in mind that many of these patients don't respond well to interviews, whereas others are charming and convincing.
◆ Teach the patient social skills, and reinforce appropriate behavior.
◆ Encourage expression of feelings, self-analysis of behavior, and accountability for actions.

◆ Set appropriate boundaries with the patient who may push limits and blame others for his or her feelings and behaviors.

Specific care measures vary with the particular personality disorder.

For *antisocial personality disorder:*

◆ Be clear about your expectations and the consequences of failing to meet them.

◆ Use a straightforward, matter-of-fact approach to set limits on unacceptable behavior. Encourage and reinforce positive behavior.

◆ Expect the patient to refuse to cooperate so that the patient can gain control.

◆ Avoid power struggles and confrontations to maintain the opportunity for therapeutic communication.

◆ Avoid defensiveness and arguing.

◆ Observe for physical and verbal signs of agitation.

◆ Help the patient manage anger.

◆ Teach the patient social skills and reinforce appropriate behavior.

For *avoidant personality disorder:*

◆ Assess for signs of depression. Impaired social interaction increases the risk of affective disorders.

◆ Establish a trusting relationship with the patient. Be aware that the patient may become dependent on the few staff members whom he or she believes can be trusted.

◆ Make sure that the patient has plenty of time to prepare for all upcoming procedures. This patient has difficulty with surprises.

◆ Inform the patient when you will and won't be available if assistance is needed.

For *borderline personality disorder:*

◆ Deliberate self-harm is different from a suicide attempt. Self-harm involves such activities as cutting oneself, burning oneself, hitting one's head or other body part, or inserting objects into the body with the intent of causing pain. Self-harm is often used as a way to modulate affect or to control uncomfortable feelings. Although some patients do die from serious self-harm, the patient's intent when engaging in self-harm isn't to die, but rather to decrease emotional pain.

◆ Encourage the patient to take self-responsibility. Don't attempt to rescue the patient from the consequences of his or her actions (except for suicidal and self-mutilating behaviors).

◆ Don't try to solve problems that the patient can personally solve.

◆ Maintain a consistent approach in all interactions with the patient, and ensure that other staff members do so as well.

◆ Recognize behaviors that the patient uses to manipulate people so that you can avoid unconsciously reinforcing them.

◆ Set appropriate expectations for social interactions, and praise the patient when expectations are met.

◆ To promote trust, respect the patient's personal space.

◆ Recognize that the patient may idolize some staff members and devalue others.

◆ Don't take sides in the patient's disputes with other staff members.

For *dependent personality disorder:*

◆ Encourage the patient to make decisions. Continue to provide support and reassurance as the patient's decision-making ability improves.

◆ Give the patient as much opportunity to control treatment as possible. Offer options and allow choice, even if all are chosen.

◆ Encourage activities that require decision-making to promote autonomy.

For *histrionic personality disorder:*

◆ Give the patient choices in care strategies, and incorporate his or her wishes into the plan of treatment as much as possible. By increasing the patient's sense of self-control, anxiety will be reduced.

◆ Be aware that the patient will want to "win over" caregivers and, at least initially, will be responsive and cooperative.

For *narcissistic personality disorder:*

◆ Convey respect and acknowledge the patient's sense of self-importance so that a coherent sense of self can be reestablished. Don't reinforce either pathologic grandiosity or weakness.

◆ If the patient makes unreasonable demands or has unreasonable expectations, explain in a matter-of-fact way that he or she is being unreasonable. Remain nonjudgmental because a critical attitude may make the patient more demanding and difficult. Don't avoid the patient as this could increase maladaptive attention-seeking behavior.

◆ Focus on positive traits, or on feelings of pain, loss, or rejection.

For *obsessive-compulsive personality disorder:*

◆ Allow the patient to participate in his or her own treatment plan by offering choices whenever possible.

◆ Adopt a professional approach in your interactions with the patient. Avoid informality; this patient expects strict attention to detail.

For *paranoid personality disorder:*

◆ Avoid situations that threaten or challenge the patient's autonomy or beliefs.

◆ Approach the patient in a straightforward and candid manner, adopting a professional, rather than a casual or friendly, attitude. Remember that the patient with paranoid personality disorder easily misinterprets remarks intended to be humorous.

◆ Encourage the patient to take part in social interactions to gain exposure to others' perceptions and realities and to promote social skills development.

◆ Help the patient identify negative behaviors that interfere with relationships so that he or she can see how his or her behavior affects others.

◆ Provide a supportive and nonjudgmental environment in which the patient can safely explore and verbalize his feelings.

For *schizoid personality disorder:*

◆ Remember that the patient with schizoid personality disorder needs close human contact but is easily overwhelmed. Respect the patient's need for privacy, and slowly build a trusting, therapeutic relationship, so that he or she finds more pleasure than fear in relating to you.

◆ Give the patient plenty of time to express feelings. Keep in mind that the patient will retreat if pushed too soon.

For *schizotypal personality disorder:*

◆ Recognize that the patient with this disorder is easily overwhelmed by stress. Allow the patient plenty of time to make difficult decisions.

◆ Avoid defensiveness and arguing.

◆ Recognize the patient's need for physical and emotional distance.

◆ Be aware that the patient may relate unusually well to certain staff members and not at all to others.

Eating disorders

BULIMIA NERVOSA

The essential features of bulimia nervosa include eating binges followed by feelings of guilt, humiliation, and self-deprecation. These feelings cause the patient to engage in self-induced vomiting, use laxatives or diuretics, follow a strict diet, or fast to overcome the effects of the binges. Unless the patient spends an excessive amount of time bingeing and purging, bulimia nervosa seldom is incapacitating. However, electrolyte imbalances (metabolic alkalosis, hypochloremia, and hypokalemia) and dehydration can occur, increasing the risk of life-threatening physical complications.

Causes and incidence

The cause of bulimia is unknown, but psychosocial factors may contribute to its development.

Eating disorders are most prevalent in affluent cultural groups and are essentially unknown in cultural groups where poverty and malnutrition are prevalent. In developing countries, almost no cases of eating disorders have been recognized. Cultural forces that influence body image are major factors in the development of eating disorders. In most cultures in the United States, thinness is valued and being overweight is denigrated. However, media messages are mixed. A commercial for fast food may be seen right after a commercial for a weight loss program. Young girls especially are at risk for these mixed messages, although boys may be influenced as well. Certain sports or activities such as ballet, wrestling, and gymnastics may unintentionally encourage potentially unhealthy weight loss.

Bulimia nervosa usually begins in adolescence and peaks in early adulthood and can occur simultaneously with anorexia nervosa. It affects 10 females for every male. Between 1% and 1.5% of adult women meet the diagnostic criteria for bulimia nervosa.

Pathophysiology

The pathophysiology of bulimia nervosa is not fully understood, but is thought to be related to psychosocial factors. These factors include family disturbance or conflict, sexual abuse, maladaptive learned behavior, struggle for control or self-identity, cultural overemphasis on physical appearance, and parental obesity. Bulimia nervosa is associated with depression, anxiety, phobias, and OCD.

Complications

◆ Impulse control concerns

◆ Physical illnesses that develop as a result of behaviors associated with bulimia (e.g., GI symptoms such as esophageal tears, dental caries, etc.)

Signs and symptoms

The history of a patient with bulimia nervosa is characterized by episodes of binge eating that may occur up to several times per day. The patient commonly reports a binge-eating episode during which eating continues until abdominal pain, sleep, or the presence of another person interrupts it. The preferred food is usually sweet, soft, and high in calories and carbohydrate content.

The patient with bulimia usually stays within normal weight limits through the use of diuretics, laxatives, vomiting, and exercise. So, unlike the patient with anorexia, the patient with bulimia can usually hide the eating disorder.

Overt clues to this disorder include hyperactivity, peculiar eating habits or rituals, frequent weighing, and a distorted body image. (See *Characteristics of patients with bulimia*.)

The patient may report abdominal and epigastric pain caused by acute gastric dilation. The female patient may have amenorrhea. Repetitive vomiting may cause painless swelling of the salivary glands, hoarseness, throat irritation or lacerations, and dental erosion. The patient may also exhibit calluses on the knuckles or abrasions and scars on the dorsum of the hand, resulting from tooth injury during self-induced vomiting, although it's common for the patient with bulimia to induce vomiting chemically, such as with ipecac.

The patient's psychosocial history may reveal an exaggerated sense of guilt, symptoms of depression, childhood trauma (especially sexual abuse), parental obesity, or a history of unsatisfactory sexual relationships.

Diagnosis

For very specific diagnostic criteria, see the *DSM-5*.

Additional diagnostic tools include the Beck Depression Inventory, which may identify coexisting depression, and laboratory tests to help determine the presence and severity of complications. Serum electrolyte studies may show elevated bicarbonate, decreased potassium, and decreased sodium levels.

A baseline electrocardiogram may be done if TCAs will be prescribed for the patient.

Characteristics of patients with bulimia

Recognizing patients with bulimia isn't always easy. Unlike patients with anorexia, patients with bulimia don't deny that their eating habits are abnormal, but they commonly conceal their behavior out of shame. If you suspect bulimia nervosa, watch for these features:
♦ difficulty with impulse control
♦ chronic depression
♦ exaggerated sense of guilt
♦ low tolerance for frustration
♦ recurrent anxiety
♦ feelings of alienation
♦ self-consciousness
♦ difficulty expressing feelings such as anger
♦ impaired social or occupational adjustment

Treatment

Treatment of bulimia nervosa may continue for years. Interrelated physical and psychological symptoms must be treated simultaneously. Cognitive behavioral therapy is the first-line psychotherapeutic treatment for bulimia nervosa. Psychodynamic psychotherapy assists with uncovering maladaptive defense mechanisms.

Psychotherapy concentrates on interrupting the binge-purge cycle and helping the patient regain control over eating behavior. Inpatient or outpatient treatment includes behavior modification therapy, which may take place in highly structured psychoeducational group meetings. Cognitive behavioral therapy, group therapy, and family therapy, which address the eating disorder as a symptom of unresolved conflict, may help the patient understand the basis of behavior and teach self-control strategies. Antidepressants such as SSRIs (e.g., sertraline—Zoloft and paroxetine—Paxil), as well as TCAs and MAOIs, have been shown to be helpful in bulimia.

The patient may also benefit from participation in self-help groups, such as Overeaters Anonymous, or in a drug rehabilitation program if there is a concurrent substance use problem.

Special considerations

♦ Supervise the patient during mealtimes and for a specified period after meals (usually 1 hour). Set a time limit for each meal. Provide a pleasant, relaxed environment for eating.
♦ Use behavior modification techniques, and reward the patient for satisfactory weight maintenance or gain.
♦ Establish a contract with the patient, specifying the amount and type of food to be eaten at each meal.
♦ Encourage the patient to recognize and express feelings about eating behaviors. Maintain an accepting and nonjudgmental attitude.
♦ Encourage the patient to talk about stressful issues, such as achievement, independence, socialization, sexuality, family problems, and control.
♦ Identify the patient's elimination patterns.
♦ Assess suicide potential.
♦ Refer the patient and her family to the American Anorexia and Bulimia Association for additional information and support.
♦ Teach the patient how to keep a food journal to monitor treatment progress.
♦ Outline the risks of laxative, emetic, and diuretic abuse for the patient.
♦ Provide assertiveness training to help the patient gain control over behaviors and achieve a realistic and positive self-image.

ANOREXIA NERVOSA

The key feature of anorexia nervosa is self-imposed starvation, resulting from a distorted body image and an intense, irrational fear of gaining weight, even when the patient is obviously emaciated. A patient with anorexia is preoccupied with body size, describes himself or herself as "fat," and commonly expresses dissatisfaction with a particular aspect of his or her physical appearance. Although the term *anorexia* suggests that the patient's weight loss is associated with a loss of appetite, this is rare. Anorexia nervosa and bulimia nervosa can occur simultaneously. In anorexia nervosa, the refusal to eat may be accompanied by compulsive exercising, self-induced vomiting, or laxative or diuretic abuse.

Causes and incidence

No causes of anorexia nervosa have been identified. About 95% of those affected by anorexia nervosa are women. This disorder occurs primarily in adolescents and young adults but may also affect older women. The occurrence among males is rising. The prognosis varies but improves if the patient is diagnosed early, or if he or she wants to overcome the disorder and seeks help voluntarily.

Pathophysiology

Genetic, social, and psychological factors have been studied in terms of their connection to pathophysiology of anorexia nervosa. Researchers in neuroendocrinology are seeking a physiologic cause, but have found nothing definite. Different brain abnormalities seen using fMRI and PET scans have been seen in patients with anorexia nervosa; however, the degree to which these abnormalities contribute to the condition is still unknown. Clearly, social attitudes that equate slimness with beauty play some role in provoking this disorder; family factors are also implicated. Most theorists believe that refusing to eat is a subconscious effort to exert personal control over one's life. Anorexia nervosa has been associated with other psychiatric disorders, such as OCD, depression, and anxiety.

Complications

◆ Impaired social function
◆ Cardiac arrhythmia
◆ Risk for suicide
◆ Death

Signs and symptoms

The patient's history usually reveals a 25% or greater weight loss for no organic reason, coupled with a morbid dread of being fat and a compulsion to be thin. Such a patient tends to be angry and ritualistic. The patient may report infertility, loss of libido, fatigue, sleep alterations, intolerance to cold, and constipation. Female patients may report amenorrhea.

Hypotension and bradycardia may be present. Inspection may reveal an emaciated appearance, with skeletal muscle atrophy, loss of fatty tissue, atrophy of breast tissue, blotchy or sallow skin, lanugo on the face and body, and dryness or loss of scalp hair. If also bulimic, calluses on the knuckles and abrasions and scars on the dorsum of the hand may result from tooth injury during self-induced vomiting. Other signs of vomiting include dental caries and oral or pharyngeal abrasions. (See *Complications of anorexia nervosa*, page 1149.)

Palpation may disclose painless salivary gland enlargement and bowel distention. Slowed reflexes may occur on percussion. Oddly, the patient usually demonstrates hyperactivity and vigor (despite malnourishment). The patient may exercise avidly without apparent fatigue.

During psychosocial assessment, the patient with anorexia may express a morbid fear of gaining weight and an obsession with physical appearance. Paradoxically, the patient may also be obsessed with food, preparing elaborate meals for others. Social regression, including poor sexual adjustment and fear of failure, is common. Like bulimia nervosa, anorexia nervosa is commonly associated with depression. The patient may report feelings of despair, hopelessness, and worthlessness as well as suicidal thoughts.

Diagnosis

For very specific diagnostic criteria, see the *DSM-5*.

Laboratory tests help to identify various disorders and deficiencies and help to rule out endocrine, metabolic, and CNS abnormalities; cancer; malabsorption syndrome; and other disorders that cause physical wasting.

Abnormal findings that may accompany a weight loss exceeding 30% of normal body weight include:
◆ low hemoglobin level, platelet count, and white blood cell count
◆ prolonged bleeding time due to thrombocytopenia
◆ decreased erythrocyte sedimentation rate
◆ decreased levels of serum creatinine, blood urea nitrogen, uric acid, cholesterol, total protein, albumin, sodium, potassium, chloride, calcium, and fasting blood glucose (resulting from malnutrition)

Complications of anorexia nervosa

Serious medical complications can result from the malnutrition, dehydration, and electrolyte imbalances caused by prolonged starvation, frequent vomiting, or laxative abuse that's typical in anorexia nervosa.

Malnutrition and related problems
Malnutrition may cause hypoalbuminemia and subsequent edema or hypokalemia, leading to ventricular arrhythmias and renal failure.

Poor nutrition and dehydration, coupled with laxative abuse, produce changes in the bowel similar to those in chronic inflammatory bowel disease. Frequent vomiting can cause esophageal erosion, ulcers, tears, and bleeding as well as tooth and gum erosion and dental caries.

Cardiovascular consequences
Cardiovascular complications, which can be life threatening, include decreased left ventricular muscle mass, chamber size, and myocardial oxygen uptake; reduced cardiac output; hypotension; bradycardia; electrocardiographic changes, such as a nonspecific ST interval, T-wave changes, and a prolonged PR interval; heart failure; and sudden death, possibly caused by ventricular arrhythmias.

Infection and amenorrhea
Anorexia nervosa may increase the patient's susceptibility to infection.

In addition, amenorrhea, which may occur when the female patient loses about 25% of her normal body weight, usually is associated with anemia. Possible complications of prolonged amenorrhea include estrogen deficiency (increasing the risk of calcium deficiency and osteoporosis) and infertility. Menses usually returns to normal when the patient weighs at least 95% of her normal weight.

◆ elevated levels of alanine aminotransferase and aspartate aminotransferase in severe starvation states
◆ elevated serum amylase levels when pancreatitis isn't present
◆ in females, decreased levels of serum luteinizing hormone and follicle-stimulating hormone
◆ decreased triiodothyronine levels resulting from a lower basal metabolic rate
◆ dilute urine caused by the kidneys' impaired ability to concentrate urine
◆ nonspecific ST interval, prolonged PR interval, and T-wave changes on the electrocardiogram. Ventricular arrhythmias may also be present

Treatment

Appropriate treatment aims to promote weight gain or control the patient's compulsive binge eating and purging. Malnutrition and the underlying psychological dysfunction must be corrected. Hospitalization in a medical or psychiatric unit may be required to improve the patient's compromised physical condition. The hospital stay may be as brief as 2 weeks or may stretch from a few months to 2 years or longer.

A team approach to care—combining aggressive medical management, nutrition counseling, and individual, group, or family psychotherapy or behavior modification therapy—is most effective in treating anorexia. Many clinical centers are now developing inpatient and outpatient programs specifically aimed at managing eating disorders.

Treatment may include cognitive behavioral therapy, either in the inpatient or in the outpatient setting. This has been found effective for weight gain. Monitoring of food intake and linking this to feelings and emotions is taught to patients. Cognitive restructuring is also taught to identify automatic thoughts. Problem-solving and coping skills are learned. Medications are not generally used to directly treat anorexia nervosa, although they may be considered for comorbid conditions after risks versus benefits of drug therapy are considered.

Special considerations
◆ During hospitalization, regularly monitor the patient's vital signs, nutritional status, and intake and output. Weigh the patient daily—before breakfast if possible. Because she fears being weighed, vary the weighing routine.

Keep in mind that weight should increase from morning to night.

◆ Help the patient establish a target weight and support efforts to achieve this goal.

◆ Negotiate an adequate food intake with the patient. Make sure the patient understands the need for compliance with this contract or that privileges will be lost. Frequently offer small portions of food or drinks if the patient wants them. Allow the patient to maintain control over the types and amounts of food eaten, if possible.

◆ Maintain one-on-one supervision of the patient during meals and for 1 hour afterward to ensure compliance with the dietary treatment program. For the hospitalized patient with anorexia, food is considered a medication.

◆ During an acute anorexic episode, nutritionally complete liquids are more acceptable than solid food because they eliminate the need to choose between foods—something the patient with anorexia may find difficult. If tube feedings or other special feeding measures become necessary, fully explain these measures to the patient and be ready to discuss fears or reluctance; limit the discussion about food itself.

◆ Expect a weight gain of about 1 lb (0.5 kg) per week.

◆ If edema or bloating occurs after the patient has returned to normal eating behavior, reassure that this phenomenon is temporary. The patient may fear gaining weight and stop complying with the plan of treatment.

◆ Encourage the patient to recognize and express feelings freely.

◆ If a patient receiving outpatient treatment must be hospitalized, maintain contact with the treatment team to facilitate a smooth return to the outpatient setting.

◆ Remember that the patient with anorexia uses exercise, preoccupation with food, ritualism, manipulation, and lying as mechanisms to preserve control.

◆ Because the patient and family may need therapy to uncover and correct dysfunctional patterns, refer them to Anorexia Nervosa and Related Eating Disorders, a national information and support organization. This organization may help them understand what anorexia is, explain how they can help, and assist them to find a psychotherapist or healthcare provider who's experienced in treating this disorder.

◆ Teach the patient how to keep a food journal, including the types of food eaten, eating frequency, and feelings associated with eating and exercise.

◆ Advise family members to avoid discussing food with the patient.

Gender dysphoria

Gender dysphoria is a descriptive term used to explain an individual's affective and cognitive discontent with their assigned gender. Gender identity is defined as a category of social identity reflecting a sense of being male, female, or some other category. It's based culturally on determined sets of attitude behavior patterns and other attributes usually associated with masculinity or femininity. When an individual experiences distress with the incongruence between what he or she experiences or expresses, and what was assigned at birth (their natal gender), gender dysphoria results.

Causes and incidence

Research regarding cause for gender dysphoria is ongoing. Gender dysphoria may occur in children and adults. Actual incidence is unknown since many individuals do not reveal their gender identity until later in life, for personal and psychosocial reasons.

Pathophysiology

The pathophysiology of gender dysphoria is not fully understood. Research suggests a biologic basis based on neuroanatomical differences and possible influence of prenatal androgen exposure.

Complications

◆ Social isolation
◆ Self-identity crisis
◆ Risk for suicide and/or self-mutilation

Signs and symptoms

Gender dysphoria may emerge at an early age. A child may express the desire to be—or insist that he or she is—the opposite sex. For example, a male child may express disgust with his genitalia; a female child may wish to be a man when she grows up.

Men with gender dysphoria may describe a lifelong history of feeling feminine and pursuing feminine activities. Women report similar propensities for opposite-sex activities and discomfort with the female role. For both sexes, the crisis often intensifies during puberty.

Diagnosis

For very specific diagnostic criteria, see the *DSM-5.*

Treatment

Individual and family therapy is indicated for patients with gender dysphoria and their families.

Sex reassignment through hormonal and surgical treatment may be an option for some individuals. These treatments are expensive and carry additional risks for cancer (related to hormones) and infection (related to surgery). Psychological concerns may persist after gender confirmation surgery.

Appropriate psychiatric management, including hospitalization, may be needed if the patient displays the potential for violent behavior, such as suicide or self-mutilation.

Special considerations

◆ Convey a nonjudgmental approach in facial expression, tone of voice, and choice of words to convey your acceptance of the person's choices.

◆ Respect the patient's privacy and sense of modesty, particularly during procedures or examinations.

◆ Monitor the patient for related or compounded problems, such as suicidal thought or intent, depression, and anxiety.

◆ As needed, refer the patient to a counselor.

◆ As a helpful guideline, inform the patient to seek a therapist who is certified and specializes in gender dysphoria to increase the chance of quality treatment.

Sexual disorders

PARAPHILIAS

Characterized by a dependence on unusual behaviors or fantasies to achieve sexual excitement, paraphilias are complex psychosexual disorders. Paraphilias are considered sex offenses or crimes because they violate social mores or norms. However, everyone has sexual fantasies, and sexual behavior between consenting adults that isn't physically or psychologically harmful isn't considered a paraphilia. A patient with a paraphilia has ongoing, intense, sexually arousing fantasies, urges, or behaviors involving various aberrant sexual expressions that cause clinically significant distress or impairment in social, occupational, or other important areas of functioning.

Causes and incidence

The cause of paraphilias is unknown, but multiple contributing factors have been identified. Numerous people with these disorders come from dysfunctional families characterized by isolation and sexual, emotional, or physical abuse. Others suffer from personality or psychoactive substance use disorders. Incidence is unknown, as many cases go unreported.

Pathophysiology

The pathophysiological associated with paraphilias is not fully understood. Abnormal hormonal values, neurologic disorders, chromosomal abnormalities, seizure disorders, and dyslexia have been identified as contributing factors.

Complications

◆ Inappropriate sexual behaviors
◆ Criminal sexual behaviors

Signs and symptoms

The patient's history often reveals the particular pattern of abnormal sexual behaviors associated with one of the eight recognized paraphilias.

Diagnosis

For very specific diagnostic criteria, see the *DSM-5*.

Treatment

Paraphilias require mandatory treatment when the patient's sexual behaviors result in socially unacceptable, harmful, or criminal behavior. Depending on the paraphilia, treatment may include combinations of psychotherapy, behavior therapy, surgery, or pharmacotherapy.

Special considerations

◆ Use a nonjudgmental approach when dealing with the patient.

◆ Realize that treating such a patient with empathy doesn't threaten your own sexuality.

◆ Encourage the patient to express emotions in an appropriate manner.

◆ As needed, refer the patient to a counselor trained in sex therapy.

◆ As a helpful guideline, inform the patient that a therapist's certification by the American Association of Sexuality Educators, Counselors, and Therapists or by the Society for Sex Therapy and Research increases the chance of quality treatment.

SELECTED REFERENCES

American Association of Intellectual and Developmental Disabilities. (2018). *Definition of intellectual disability.* Retrieved from http://aaidd.org/intellectual-disability/definition#.WxBeTlMvwU0

American Psychiatric Association. (2013). *Diagnostic and statistical manual of mental disorders* (5th ed.). Arlington, VA: Author.

Baldwin, D. (2018). *Generalized anxiety disorder in adults: Epidemiology, pathogenesis, clinical manifestations, course, assessment, and diagnosis.* Retrieved from https://www.uptodate.com/contents/generalized-anxiety-disorder-in-adults-epidemiology-pathogenesis-clinical-manifestations-course-assessment-and-diagnosis

Bukstein, O. (2018). *Attention deficit hyperactivity disorder in adults: Epidemiology, pathogenesis, clinical features, course, assessment, and diagnosis.* Retrieved from https://www.uptodate.com/contents/attention-deficit-hyperactivity-disorder-in-adults-epidemiology-pathogenesis-clinical-features-course-assessment-and-diagnosis

Burger-Kaplan, R., et al. (2017). *Vineland adaptive behavior scales. Encyclopedia of clinical neuropsychology.* Retrieved from https://link.springer.com/referenceworkentry/10.10 07%2F978-3-319-56782-2_1602-4

Centers for Disease Control and Prevention. (2018a). *During binges, U.S. adults have 17 billion drinks a year.* Retrieved from https://www.cdc.gov/media/releases/2018/ p0316-binge-drinking.html

Centers for Disease Control and Prevention. (2018b). *Fact sheets—Underage drinking.* Retrieved from https://www .cdc.gov/alcohol/fact-sheets/underage-drinking.htm

Hoffman, R. (2017). *Testing for drugs of abuse (DOA).* Retrieved from https://www.uptodate.com/contents/ testing-for-drugs-of-abuse-doa

Loewenstein, R. (2018). *Dissociative amnesia: Epidemiology, pathogenesis, clinical manifestations, course, and diagnosis.* Retrieved from https://www.uptodate.com/contents/ dissociative-amnesia-epidemiology-pathogenesis-clinical-manifestations-course-and-diagnosis

Manschreck, T. (2017). *Delusional disorder.* Retrieved from https://www.uptodate.com/contents/delusional-disorder

Mitchell, D. (2018). *Bulimia nervosa in adults: Cognitive-behavioral therapy (CBT).* Retrieved from https://www.uptodate.com/contents/bulimia-nervosa-in-adults-cognitive-behavioral-therapy-cbt

National Institute of Mental Health Information Resource Center. (2017). *Major depression.* Retrieved from https:// www.nimh.nih.gov/health/statistics/major-depression .shtml

Pivalizza, P., & Lalani, S. (2016). *Intellectual disability in children: Evaluation for a cause.* Retrieved from https://www.uptodate.com/contents/ intellectual-disability-in-children-evaluation-for-a-cause

Roy-Burnes, P. (2018). *Panic disorder in adults: Epidemiology, pathogenesis, clinical manifestations, course, assessment, and diagnosis.* Retrieved from https://www.uptodate.com/contents/panic-disorder-in-adults-epidemiology-pathogenesis-clinical-manifestations-course-assessment-and-diagnosis

Sareen, J. (2018). *Posttraumatic stress disorder in adults: Epidemiology, pathophysiology, clinical manifestations, course, assessment, and diagnosis.* Retrieved from https:// www.uptodate.com/contents/posttraumatic-stress-disorder-in-adults-epidemiology-pathophysiology-clinical-manifestations-course-assessment-and-diagnosis

Simeon, D. (2018). *Depersonalization/derealization disorder in adults: Epidemiology, pathogenesis, clinical manifestations, course, and diagnosis.* Retrieved from https://www .uptodate.com/contents/depersonalization-derealization-disorder-epidemiology-pathogenesis-clinical-manifestations-course-and-diagnosis

Simpson, H. (2017). *Obsessive-compulsive disorder in adults: Epidemiology, pathogenesis, clinical manifestations, course, and diagnosis.* Retrieved from https://www .uptodate.com/contents/obsessive-compulsive-disorder-in-adults-epidemiology-pathogenesis-clinical-manifestations-course-and-diagnosis

Special Olympics. (2018). *What is intellectual disability?* Retrieved from https://www.specialolympics.org/Sections/ Who_We_Are/What_Is_Intellectual_Disability.aspx

Stovall, J. (2018). *Bipolar disorder in adults: Epidemiology and pathogenesis.* Retrieved from https://www.uptodate .com/contents/bipolar-disorder-in-adults-epidemiology-gy-and-pathogenesis

Tangpricha, V., & Safer, J. (2018). *Transgender women: Evaluation and management.* Retrieved from https://www.uptodate.com/contents/ transgender-women-evaluation-and-management

Yael, D., et al. (2015). Pathophysiology of tic disorders. *Movement Disorders, 30*(9), 1171-1178.

1 APPENDIX

Rare Diseases

Potential Agents of Bioterrorism

Complementary and Integrative Therapies for Specific Conditions

Care of LGBTQ Patient

Acknowledgments

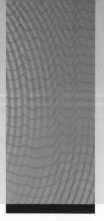

RARE DISEASES

Disease	Description
Addison–Schilder disease: adrenoleukodystrophy	Adrenal atrophy and diffuse degeneration of the brain characterized by loss of myelin and increasing cognitive and behavioral abnormalities, blindness, and quadriparesis. Presents usually between 4 and 8 years old (Wanders & Eichler, 2017)
African trypanosomiasis: sleeping sickness	Febrile illness followed months or years later by progressive neurologic impairment and death; the Gambian form, found in west and central Africa, causes daytime drowsiness and nighttime insomnia and progresses to coma (human African trypanosomiasis); the Rhodesian form, found in east Africa, is more virulent
Alport syndrome	Hereditary nephritis characterized by recurrent gross or microscopic hematuria; associated with bilateral sensorineural hearing loss, albuminuria, and progressive azotemia
American trypanosomiasis: Chagas disease	Febrile parasitic illness prevalent in Central and South America; cardiomyopathy may occur; megaesophagus and megacolon may develop many years later; can be severe in children
Amyloidosis	Rare, chronic disorders that result in the accumulation of an abnormal fibrillar scleroprotein (amyloid), which infiltrates body organs and soft tissues
Anorectal stricture	Also known as anorectal stenosis or contracture, the anorectal lumen size decreases and stenosis prevents dilation of the sphincter
Arc welders' disease: siderosis	Benign pneumoconiosis that can occur in iron ore miners, welders, metal grinders, and polishers from the inhalation and retention of iron

Cause	Treatment
Transmitted as X-linked disorder	Allogenic hematopoietic cell transplantation; gene therapy (Wanders & Eichler, 2017)
Trypanosoma brucei rhodesiense and *T. brucei gambiense* transmitted by tsetse fly bite	Melarsoprol or pentamidine
Transmitted as X-linked autosomal trait	Supportive and symptomatic; antibiotic therapy for infection; antihypertensive therapy (angiotensin-converting enzyme [ACE] inhibitor or angiotensin receptor blocker); protein-restricted diet; dialysis or renal transplant; avoidance of ototoxic drugs
Trypanosoma cruzi transmitted by insect; can also be transmitted through the transfusion of blood donated by a person who's infected	Nifurtimox or benznidazole in acute phase (pills crushed for infants); supportive treatment in chronic phase
Sometimes familial, especially in people of Portuguese ancestry. It may also occur with tuberculosis, chronic infection, rheumatoid arthritis, multiple myeloma, Hodgkin lymphoma, paraplegia, brucellosis, and Alzheimer disease.	Elimination of underlying cause; mainly supportive
Results from scarring after anorectal surgery or inflammation, inadequate postoperative care, or laxative abuse	Surgical removal of scar tissue; digital or instrumental dilation may be beneficial, but it may need to be repeated frequently and may cause additional tears and fissures
Inhalation and retention of iron after exposure to iron oxide fumes and dust	Supportive and symptomatic treatment; limiting or preventing exposure to iron dust or fumes with approved industrial respirators prevents progression of this disease

(continued)

Disease	Description
Aseptic meningitis: lymphocytic meningitis (incidence 8 to 11 patients per 100,000)	Meningitis, usually occurring in adults; asymptomatic or mild, although severe end organ damage can occur
Ataxia telangiectasia: Louis–Bar syndrome	Progressive, severe ataxia with telangiectasia of the face, earlobes, and conjunctivae; chronic recurrent sinopulmonary infections occur; ataxia usually occurs before age 2 but may not develop until as late as age 9; degree of immunodeficiency determines rate of deterioration
Barometer-maker's disease: chronic mercury poisoning	Soreness of gums, loosening of teeth, salivation, fetid breath, abdominal cramping and diarrhea, weakness, ataxia, intention tremors, irritability and depression, reproductive failures, birth defects (especially developmental neurologic damage), and death
Bauxite workers' disease: bauxite pneumoconiosis, Shaver disease	Occupational disorder causing rapid and progressive pneumoconiosis and leading to empyema; may be accompanied by pneumothorax; puts patient at increased risk for blood and bladder cancers
Berylliosis: Beryllium poisoning and beryllium disease	Systemic granulomatous disorder that's a form of pneumoconiosis with dominant pulmonary manifestations; two forms: acute nonspecific pneumonitis and chronic noncaseating granulomatous disease with interstitial fibrosis; death may result from respiratory failure and cor pulmonale
Blinding filarial disease: onchocerciasis, river blindness	Invasion of eye tissues by the filarial worm, which is enclosed in fibrous cysts or nodules; lesions also develop on the skin and, in severe infection, lead to chronic pruritus and disfiguring skin lesions
Bouillaud syndrome: rheumatic endocarditis	Manifests as a heart murmur of either mitral or aortic insufficiency; pericarditis and heart failure are seen in severe cases
Brill disease: Brill–Zinsser disease, latent or recrudescent typhus	Relapse of typhus, which can occur years after the primary attack
Brown–Symmers disease: Acute serous encephalitis in children	Viral pathogens (rabies, measles, mumps, rubella, influenza)
Budd–Chiari syndrome: Hepatic vein obstruction that impairs blood flow out of the liver, producing massive ascites and hepatomegaly; may be acute or chronic	Any condition or medication that obstructs blood flow from hepatic veins; acute form due to acute thrombosis of main hepatic vein or inferior vena cava; chronic form due to fibrosis of intrahepatic veins
Burkitt tumor: Burkitt lymphoma	Undifferentiated malignant lymphoma that usually begins as a large mass in the jaw (African Burkitt) or as an abdominal mass (American Burkitt)

Cause	Treatment
Infection caused by several viruses (enteroviruses, human immunodeficiency virus [HIV], West Nile virus, varicella-zoster virus, mumps, and lymphocytic choriomeningitis virus)	Supportive and symptomatic treatment; infection can be prevented by careful handwashing (although mode of transmission may be airborne); presumptive antibiotics for first 48 hours; identification of those with HIV
Transmitted as autosomal recessive disorder; a genetic mutation found in the *ATM* gene	Supportive treatment with early, aggressive antibiotic therapy to prevent or control recurrent infections; immune globulin; fetal thymus transplant or histocompatible bone marrow transplant
Mercury poisoning resulting from chronic exposure to mercury or its vapors (possibly from batteries, thermometers, or dental amalgams) or to contaminated fish or fungicides used on seeds	Induce emesis or evacuate stomach, lavage with milk or sodium bicarbonate, and administer polythiol resins; penicillamine is the chelating agent of choice but dimercaprol is also effective; neurologic toxicity isn't considered reversible, although some practitioners recommend a trial dose of penicillamine
Inhalation of dust particles of alumina and silica (bauxite), the chief source of aluminum	Elimination of exposure to bauxite
Inhalation or absorption of beryllium; severity depends on amount inhaled or absorbed	Beryllium ulcer requires excision or curettage; acute form requires prompt corticosteroid therapy, oxygen, and, possibly, mechanical ventilation; chronic form is treated with corticosteroids
Onchocerca volvulus transmitted by the blackfly (*Simulium* and *Eusimulium*)	Microfilaricidal or macrofilaricidal agents, such as ivermectin and diethylcarbamazine
Delayed sequel to pharyngeal infection by group B streptococci	Although no specific cure is available, a course of penicillin should still be given to eliminate group A streptococci; additionally, supportive therapy to reduce morbidity and mortality should be provided
Rickettsia prowazekii	Tetracycline, chloramphenicol, analgesics, antipyretics
	Supportive care; control of intracranial pressure; correction of metabolic problems, disseminated intravascular coagulation, bleeding, renal failure, pulmonary emboli, and pneumonia; invariably fatal
	Surgery to shunt hepatic blood flow and remove obstruction; if congenital, transcardiac membranectomy or percutaneous stent placement for patients with inferior vena cava web; liver transplant may be recommended for patients with marked hepatocellular dysfunction; anticoagulation
Unknown, but Epstein–Barr virus suspected in some cases	Chemotherapy; radiation therapy; surgical resection in extensive local disease; in patients with a relapse, autologous bone marrow transplantation

(continued)

Disease	Description
Cat-scratch fever: cat-scratch disease	Subacute self-limiting disease characterized by a primary local lesion and regional lymphadenopathy; more common in children and young adults in contact with cats (90% of cases); disseminated form, bacillary angiomatosis, found in people who are immunocompromised, such as those infected with the HIV
Charcot–Marie–Tooth disease	Neuropathic (peroneal) muscular atrophy characterized by progressive weakness of the distal muscles of the arms and feet; most common form of the muscular dystrophies
Chédiak–Higashi syndrome	Characterized by morphologic changes in granulocytes that impair the ability to respond to chemotaxis and to digest or kill invading organisms; associated with partial albinism
Chester disease: cerebrotendinous xanthomatosis	Form of leukodystrophy indicated by excessive accumulation of lipids in the long bones; results in progressive cerebellar ataxia, dementia, mental retardation, spinal cord paresis, tendon xanthomas, and cataracts
Choriocarcinoma: Rapidly metastasizing malignant tumor of placental tissue that typically causes profuse vaginal and intra-abdominal bleeding	Possibly hydatidiform mole, abortion, fetal–maternal histoincompatibility, inherited factors, or infections; more common with complete molar pregnancy
Chromomycosis: Chromoblastomycosis	Slowly spreading fungal infection of the skin and subcutaneous tissues; produces cauliflower-like lesions on the legs or arms and may spread to the brain, causing an abscess
Cockayne syndrome	Hereditary syndrome consisting of dwarfism with retinal atrophy and deafness; associated with progeria, prognathism, mental retardation, photosensitivity, and accelerated atherosclerosis
Concato disease	Progressive malignant polyserositis with large effusions into the pericardium, pleura, and peritoneum; associated with tuberculosis
Contact ulcers	Erosions on the laryngeal mucosa over the vocal cords, producing hoarseness, mild dysphagia, and gradual tissue necrosis
Copper deficiency anemia: hypocupremia	Nutritional deficiency that impairs hemoglobin synthesis and causes shortness of breath, pallor, fatigue, edema, poor wound healing, and anorexia; if prolonged, can cause poor mental development in infants and mental deterioration in adults
Csillag disease: lichen sclerosus et atrophicus	Acute inflammatory dermatitis, such as heat rash, prickly heat, miliaria rubra; chronic atrophic and lichenoid dermatitis
Cystinuria	Inborn error of amino acid transport in the kidneys and intestine that allows excessive urinary excretion of cystine and other dibasic amino acids; results in recurrent cystine renal calculi

Cause	Treatment
Bartonella henselae; flea-borne transmission to kittens creates a feline reservoir for the disease	Symptomatic treatment; if patient is ill, can use ciprofloxacin, doxycycline, trimethoprim and sulfamethoxazole, erythromycin, cefoxitin, cefotaxime, mezlocillin, aminoglycosides, or antimycobacterials
Transmitted as autosomal dominant trait	Supportive treatment, including counseling, braces for foot drop, or orthopedic surgery to stabilize the foot and treat fractures
Transmitted as autosomal recessive trait; mutations found in *CHS1* gene	Vigorous early treatment with antimicrobials and surgical drainage; large doses of vitamin C
Transmitted as autosomal recessive trait that causes disturbances of lipid metabolism	Chenodeoxycholic acid to arrest and reverse progression of disease
	Chemotherapy, suction to empty uterine contents, hysterectomy; serial chest X-rays; monitoring for progressively decreasing beta-human chorionic gonadotropin levels
Phialophora verrucosa, Fonsecaea pedrosoi, F. compacta, and *Cladosporium carrionii*; found in warm climates, especially in South America; usually introduced through an injury, such as a splinter or a thorn in the skin	Cryosurgery with liquid nitrogen; oral itraconazole (alone or with flucytosine); heat therapy; terbinafine has been shown to be effective, but posaconazole may be slightly superior
Transmitted as autosomal recessive trait	Effective treatment unknown; symptomatic treatment, establishment of protective environment
Mycobacterium tuberculosis	Thoracentesis; parenteral or oral antitubercular antibiotics, such as aminosalicylic acid and ethionamide
Vocal strain, laryngeal trauma, or emotional stress; prolonged alteration may lead to granulomas	Supportive treatment with absolute voice rest, adequate humidification, and aerosol therapy; granulomas tend to recur after surgical removal
Diseases associated with low protein levels; substantial protein loss; decreased gastrointestinal (GI) absorption of copper; total parenteral nutrition without copper supplement; or Wilson disease	Copper sulfate; supportive treatment of associated symptoms; treatment of underlying cause
Keratin obstruction of sweat ducts	Symptomatic treatment, including cool environment, application of calamine lotion, and desquamation by ultraviolet rays
Transmitted as autosomal recessive trait	Supportive treatment, including increasing fluid intake, sodium bicarbonate administration, alkaline-ash diet, and penicillamine; surgical removal of calculi

(continued)

Disease	Description
Dengue: breakbone or dandy fever	Acute febrile disease with myalgia and arthralgia; endemic during the warmer months in the tropics and subtropics; rarely fatal unless it progresses to hemorrhagic shock syndrome
Duhring disease: dermatitis herpetiformis	Chronic inflammatory disease marked by erythematous, papular, vesicular, bulbous, or pustular lesions, with tendency toward grouping and associated with itching and burning; usually symmetrical, with eruptions in elbows, knees, sacrum, buttocks, and occiput
Dukes disease: fourth disease, Filatov–Dukes disease	Marked by myalgia, headache, fever, pharyngitis, conjunctivitis, generalized adenopathy, and desquamation following confluent raised erythema
Duroziez disease: congenital mitral stenosis	Narrowing of the mitral valve orifice that obstructs blood flow from atrium to ventricle
Eales disease: peripheral neovascular retinopathy	Condition marked by recurrent hemorrhages into the retina and vitreous; mainly affects males in the second and third decades of life; most cases spontaneous and unilateral; some cases associated with trauma or stress, but also occurs after awakening
Economo disease: lethargic encephalitis	Epidemic encephalitis marked by increasing languor, apathy, and drowsiness, progressing to lethargy; accompanied by ophthalmoplegia; usually occurs in winter
Elevator disease	Form of occupational pneumoconiosis affecting people who work in grain elevators
Eosinophilic endomyocardial disease: Loeffler endocarditis	Form of progressive endocarditis denoted by a highly increased number of eosinophilic granulocytes in the blood; fibrosis and thickening of the endocardium occur; cardiomegaly and heart failure may be present
Erysipeloid	Acute, self-limiting skin infection most common in butchers, farmers, cooks, fishermen, and others who handle infected material; may progress to infective endocarditis or affect other body systems if primary lesions aren't treated
Erythrasma	Superficial, bacterial skin infection that usually affects the skin folds, especially in the groin, axillae, and toe webs
Fabry disease	Renal disorder that produces malfunctions of the proximal renal tubules, leading to hyperkalemia, hypernatremia, glycosuria, phosphaturia, aminoaciduria, uricosuria, bicarbonate wasting, retarded growth and development, and rickets
Fanconi syndrome: de Toni–Fanconi syndrome	Disorder of fat storage related to a deficiency of enzyme alpha-galactosidase A; characterized by glycolipid accumulation in body tissues; results in clouding of the cornea, burning sensations of hands and feet, small raised purple blemishes on the skin, impaired arterial circulation, and renal and GI involvement

Cause	Treatment
Group B arboviruses transmitted by the female *Aedes* mosquito	Symptomatic treatment; nonaspirin analgesics; I.V. fluid replacement; complete bed rest
Associated with intestinal sensitivity to dietary gluten (celiac sprue)	Sulfa-based antibiotics; strict gluten-free diet
Most likely a viral exanthema of the coxsackievirus or echovirus group	Symptomatic and supportive treatment
Congenital	Surgery, if possible; otherwise, supportive treatment, including medications to increase blood flow
Etiology unknown	Treatment of underlying causes
Pathogen not clearly identified, but may be arthropod-borne virus or sequela of influenza, rubella, varicella, or vaccinia	Symptomatic treatment, including appropriate antibiotics for secondary infection
Inhalation of dust particles, causing irritation and inflammation of respiratory tract	Avoidance of exposure to dust
Unknown	Suppression of eosinophilia with prednisolone or hydroxyurea; digoxin; diuretics; medical and surgical therapy for cardiac complications as indicated
Erysipelothrix rhusiopathiae (insidiosa) transmitted by contact with infected animals	Penicillin or erythromycin in combination with rifampin if the patient has penicillin allergy; the patient with the systemic form may need valve replacement surgery or other surgery depending on the organ involved
Corynebacterium minutissimum	Topical antibiotics; treatment with oral erythromycin or tetracycline often produces quick resolution; antibacterial soap to prevent recurrence
Transmitted as X-linked recessive trait	Symptomatic treatment with low-dose phenytoin or carbamazepine for pain in hands and feet; metoclopramide or nutritional supplement for GI hyperactivity; enzyme replacement therapy
If diagnosed as a child, may be congenital; if diagnosed as an adult, considered acquired and may be secondary to Wilson disease, cystinosis, galactosemia, or exposure to toxins, as in heavy metal poisoning	Symptomatic treatment with replacement therapy, vitamin D for rickets, and aluminum hydroxide for hyperphosphatemia; treatment of underlying cause for acquired form; dialysis as necessary

(continued)

Disease	Description
Fifth disease: erythema infectiosum	Contagious disease characterized by rose-colored eruptions diffused over the skin, usually starting on the cheeks; mainly affects children ages 4 to 10; infection in a patient who's pregnant can cause fetal hydrops and increase the risk of fetal death in the first half of pregnancy
File-cutter's disease: Lead poisoning from inhalation of lead particles that arise during file cutting	
Fish skin disease: ichthyosis vulgaris	Condition of dry and scaly skin resembling fish skin; several forms, including vulgaris and lamellar
Flax-dresser's disease: byssinosis	Pulmonary disorder of flax-dressers or textile workers
Flecked retina syndrome	Group of retinal disorders, including fundus flavimaculatus, fundus albipunctatus, drusen, and congenital macular degeneration, all of which may be primary abnormalities of retinal pigment epithelium
Fleischner disease	Inflammation of bone and cartilage affecting the middle phalanges of the hand
Friedländer disease: endarteritis obliterans	Chronic, progressive thickening of the intima, an artery leading to stenosis or obstruction of the lumen
Friedrich disease: paramyoclonus multiplex, Friedrich ataxia	Ataxic gait, cerebellar dysfunction, leg weakness, sensory disturbances in the limbs, and depressed tendon reflexes
Geotrichosis	Fungal infection affecting the mouth, throat, lungs, or intestines
Gerlier disease: endemic paralytic vertigo, paralyzing vertigo	Nervous system disorder marked by pain, vertigo, paresis, and muscle contractions
Glioma of the optic nerve	Slow-growing tumor that causes progressive vision loss
Glossopharyngeal neuralgia	Disease of the ninth cranial (glossopharyngeal) nerve that produces paroxysms of pain in the ear, posterior pharynx, base of the tongue, or jaws; sometimes accompanied by syncope
Glucose-6-phosphate dehydrogenase (G6PD) deficiency	Deficiency of the red blood cell enzyme G6PD, which causes anemia; common in people of African or Mediterranean descent
Grinder's disease: pneumoconiosis	Permanent deposition of particles in the lungs
Hand–foot–mouth syndrome	Infectious disease that most often occurs in young children and is characterized by a rash of small blister-like lesions on the palms of the hands, soles of the feet, and in the mouth

Cause	Treatment
Human parvovirus B19, probably transmitted by respiratory tract secretions	Symptomatic treatment; screening of donated blood, which might prevent transfusion-related transmission; transfusion if aplastic crisis; immune globulin I.V. if immunocompromised; intra-arterial blood transfusion if fetal hydrops present
Inhalation of lead particles	Avoidance of exposure to lead; chelates should be used for moderate to high-level poisoning
Hereditary form is an autosomal dominant genetic disorder; acquired form seen in adulthood usually associated with internal disease such as malignancy	Alpha hydroxy acids (lactic, glycolic, or pyruvic acids) to help hydrate the skin; removal of scales by keratolytics; propylene glycol; topical retinoids; treatment of underlying systemic condition for acquired form
Inhalation of dust from cotton or other vegetable fibers, such as flax or hemp	Avoidance of exposure to source; bronchodilators to manage symptoms (corticosteroids in severe cases)
Congenital	Supportive and symptomatic treatment such as drugs for pain, anxiety, and depression
Unknown	Anti-inflammatory drugs (including steroids in severe cases); analgesics
Trauma, pyogenic bacterial infection, infective thrombi, or syphilis	Endarterectomy
Central nervous system damage secondary to trauma or infection; may be hereditary	Treatment of underlying disease; no specific treatment for hereditary form
Geotrichum candidum	Gentian violet for oral, throat, or intestinal infections; oral potassium iodide for pulmonary infections
Disease of the internal ear from pressure of cerumen on the drum membrane	Symptomatic treatment, including scopolamine to combat nausea
Unknown	Surgical excision; radiation therapy
Unknown	Surgery; carbamazepine, phenytoin
Transmitted as an X-linked trait	Avoidance of known oxidant drugs, including primaquine, salicylates, sulfonamides, nitrofurans, phenacetin, naphthalene
Inhalation of dust particles	Irreversible pulmonary disease; eliminating exposure to dust particles can prevent further irritation of tissues
In most cases, caused by coxsackievirus A16	Supportive treatment, which may include antipyretics for fever and acetaminophen and ibuprofen for mouth pain

(continued)

Disease	Description
Heavy chain disease: Neoplasms of the lymphoplasma-cytes, in which abnormal prolif-eration occurs among cells that produce immunoglobulins, causing incomplete heavy chains and no light chains in their molecular structure	Possibly microorganisms and immune deficiency syndrome due to malnutrition or genetic predisposition
Heerfordt syndrome: Uveoparotid fever	Variant of sarcoidosis manifested by parotid swelling and single or multiple palsies of cranial nerves
Hemangioma of the eye	In children, tumors not encapsulated, grow quickly in the first year, and then regress by about age 7; in adults, tu-mors encapsulated
Hemochromatosis: bronze diabe-tes, Recklinghausen–Applebaum disease	Disorder characterized by iron overload in parenchymal cells, leading to cirrhosis, diabetes, cardiomegaly with heart failure and arrhythmias, and increased skin pigmentation
Hemoglobin C–thalassemia disease	Simultaneous heterozygosity for hemoglobin C and thal-assemia; characterized by mild hemolytic anemia and per-sistent splenomegaly
Henderson–Jones disease: osteochondromatosis	Presence of numerous benign cartilaginous tumors in the joint cavity or in the bursa of a tendon sheath
Hereditary spherocytosis	Anemia resulting in increased red blood cell membrane per-meability and intracellular hypertonicity; characterized by slight jaundice, splenomegaly, and cholelithiasis
Heubner disease	Syphilitic inflammation of tunica intima of cerebral arteries
Hoffa disease	Proliferation of fatty tissue (solitary lipoma) in the knee joint
Hutchinson–Gifford disease: progeria	Premature old age marked by small stature, wrinkled skin, and gray hair, with attitude and appearance of old age in very young children
Hutinel disease	Tuberculous pericarditis, with cirrhosis of the liver in children
Hydatid disease, alveolar	Infestation characterized by invasion and destruction of tis-sue by cysts, which undergo endogenous budding and form an aggregate of innumerable small cysts that honeycomb the affected organ—usually the liver—and may metastasize
Hydatid disease, unilocu-lar: *Echinococcus granulosus*, hydatidosis	Infestation causing marked formation of single or multiple unilocular cysts
Intestinal lymphangiectasia: Dila-tion and possible rupture of intes-tinal lymphatic vessels, resulting in hypoproteinemia and steatorrhea due to loss of fat and albumin into the intestinal lumen	Congenital or may be acquired when obstruction, valvular heart disease, or constrictive pericarditis increases pressure on the lymphatics

Cause	Treatment
Supportive and palliative treatment with chemotherapy, radiation therapy, antibiotics, and steroids	
Impaired regulation of thymus-derived lymphocytes (T cells) and bone-marrow–derived lymphocytes (B cells)	Adrenocorticosteroids to suppress inflammation and control symptoms
Unknown	Surgical excision for adults; no treatment for children
Erythropoietic disorders, hepatic disorders that increase iron absorption, autosomal recessive inheritance	Phlebotomy to remove excess iron; chelates such as deferoxamine
Hereditary and congenital	Supportive treatment, including transfusions for severe anemia and folate therapy
Irritation and trauma	Resection of tumor with curettage and bone grafts
Transmitted as autosomal dominant trait	Splenectomy; supplementation with folic acid
Treponema pallidum	Supportive treatment, including antibiotic therapy
Tissue trauma	Aspiration or surgery
Unknown	No known treatment
M. tuberculosis	Tuberculostatic agents
Infestation by *Echinococcus multilocularis* (larvae)	Symptomatic treatment and surgery; usually fatal; high-dose mebendazole may be used in patients with medical problems that preclude surgery, or in cases where surgery wouldn't be indicated
Infestation by *E. granulosus* (larvae); hydatid tapeworm in dogs and cats	Surgery; drug therapy with an anthelmintic, such as albendazole or mebendazole
No-fat diet; replacement of dietary sources of long-chain triglycerides with medium-chain triglycerides	

(continued)

Disease	Description
Isambert disease: tuberculosis laryngitis	Acute miliary tuberculosis of the larynx and pharynx
Jansen disease: metaphyseal dysostosis	Skeletal abnormality with nearly normal epiphyses in which the metaphyseal tissues are replaced by masses of cartilage
Jensen disease: retinochoroiditis juxtapapillaris	Inflammation of the retina and choroid marked by small inflammatory areas on the fundus close to the papilla
Juvenile angiofibroma: benign nasal tumor	Highly vascular, nasopharyngeal tumor that causes nasal obstruction and severe recurrent epistaxis; capable of eroding bone
Keratoconus	Degenerative eye disorder typified by thinning and anterior protrusion of the cornea, causing major changes in the refractive power of the eye and requiring frequent eyeglass changes
Keratosis pilaris: keratosis follicularis, Darier disease	Skin condition marked by formation of horny plugs in the orifices of hair follicles; lesions appearing primarily on the lateral aspects of the upper arms, thighs, and buttocks; may also occur on face; more severe in the winter months
Kienböck disease: lunatomalacia	Slowly progressive osteochondrosis of the semilunar (carpal lunate) bone from avascular necrosis
Köhler bone disease: tarsal scaphoiditis, epiphysitis juvenilis	Osteochondrosis of the tarsal navicular bone in children, occurring at about age 5
Krabbe disease: globoid cell leukodystrophy	Rapidly progressive cerebral demyelination with large globoid bodies in the white matter; associated with irritability, rigidity, tonic–clonic seizures, blindness, deafness, and progressive mental deterioration
Kümmell disease: posttraumatic spondylitis	Intercostal neuralgia with spinal pain and motor disturbances in the legs
Kuru: Chronic, progressive, and fatal neurologic disease found only in New Guinea	
Laron syndrome	A rare genetic disorder characterized by short stature and delayed bone age, as well as high levels of circulating growth hormone (GH). The defective GH-receptor gene prevents the proper binding of the GH molecule, leaving high levels of unbound GH in the plasma.
Larsen disease: Sinding–Larsen and Johansson syndrome, Larsen–Johansson disease, patellar chondropathy	Accessory center of ossification within the patella, associated with flat facies and short metacarpals
Lenégre disease	Acquired complete heart block

Cause	Treatment
M. tuberculosis	Tuberculostatic drugs
Unknown	Surgery in an effort to remove the skeletal abnormality
Unknown; probably an autoimmune process	Steroids may induce improvements
Unknown	Surgery in an effort to remove the tumor
Possibly genetic inheritance and systemic and ocular associations; risk factors include eye rubbing, ocular allergies, and use of contact lenses	Hard contact lenses or glasses with high astigmatic correction; possibly, corneal graft or transplantation
Genetic follicular disease but may be transmitted as an autosomal dominant trait	No specific therapy; keratolytic lotions to prevent cracking, drying, and skin breakdown possibly useful
Degenerative process precipitated by trauma	Anti-inflammatories and immobilization of wrist for several months (if ineffective, surgery)
Unknown but trauma suspected	Protection of foot from excessive use or trauma; if pain is severe, plaster cast may be required for 6 to 8 weeks; oral analgesics as needed; complete spontaneous recovery may occur
Genetic deficiency of galactosylceramidase, an enzyme for myelin metabolism	Symptomatic treatment; bone marrow transplantation improves diagnosis, but death usually occurs before age 2
Compression fracture of the vertebrae	Treatment of fracture; extension of spine; pain relief
Caused by a prion, a naturally occurring protein considered the infectious agent and cause of spongiform encephalopathy; thought to be associated with cannibalism of Fore culture in New Guinea	No effective treatment; invariably fatal
Autosomal recessive inheritance	Administration of recombinant human insulin-like growth factor-1
Unknown	Supportive treatment such as drugs for pain, anxiety, or depression; surgery
Primary sclerodegeneration of the conduction system	Artificial pacemaker; supportive treatment

(continued)

Disease	Description
Leptospirosis	Infectious disease that causes meningitis, hepatitis, nephritis, or febrile disease; may be mild (anicteric) or severe (icteric, or Weil disease)
Lesch–Nyhan syndrome	Disorder of purine metabolism marked by behavioral problems that include cognitive dysfunction and aggressive and impulsive behaviors; also includes self-injurious behaviors, spasticity, hyperuricemia, and excessive uricaciduria
Letterer–Siwe disease: nonlipid reticuloendotheliosis; disseminated histiocytosis X	Hemorrhagic tendency with eczematoid skin eruptions, lymph node enlargement, hepatosplenomegaly, and progressive anemia; occurs mainly in infants
Lewandowsky–Lutz disease: epidermodysplasia verruciformis	May manifest as flat-topped papules that vary in color from pink to brown, resembling verruca plana; have a tendency to become malignant; they increase in number and coalesce to form large plaques or scales on the knees, elbows, and trunk; often associated with mental retardation
Lichen planus	Benign pruritic skin eruption that usually produces scaling and purple papules marked by white lines or spots
Lichtheim disease: Lichtheim syndrome	Subacute degeneration of the spinal cord associated with pernicious anemia
Li–Fraumeni syndrome	Inherited syndrome predisposing patient to lung, breast, and soft-tissue cancers
Little disease: cerebral palsy	Form of cerebral spastic paralysis and stiffness of the limbs associated with muscle weakness, seizures, bilateral athetosis, and mental deficiencies
Ludwig angina	Infection of the sublingual and submandibular spaces characterized by brawny induration of the submaxillary region, edema of the sublingual floor of the mouth, and elevation of the tongue
Lung fluke disease: *Paragonimus westermani, P. heterotremus*	Parasitic hemoptysis, or oriental hemoptysis from pulmonary cysts
Macroglobulinemia: Waldenström macroglobulinemia	Malignant neoplastic disease of plasma and lymphoid cells that produces immunoglobulin M antibodies; may produce no symptoms or diverse signs and symptoms
Malignant melanoma of the eye	Malignant tumor stemming from the melanocytes in the uvea, retina, or iris
Maple syrup urine disease	Enzyme defect in the metabolism of the branched-chain amino acids, resulting in mental and physical retardation, reflex changes, feeding difficulties, characteristic odor of urine and perspiration, seizures, and death; four clinical phenotypes: classic, intermediate, intermittent, and thiamine-responsive

Cause	Treatment
Bacteria of genus *Leptospira* transmitted by contact with water, soil, food, or vegetation contaminated with urine from an infected lower mammal	Doxycycline or ampicillin
Defective enzyme transmitted by female carriers as X-linked recessive trait	Allopurinol to control urine and sedimentation; baclofen and benzodiazepines for spasticity; symptomatic and supportive treatment, such as behavioral modification and medications for behavior treatment; few patients live beyond age 40 and most die suddenly
Acute, disseminated form of histiocytosis X, an intense proliferation of reticulohistiocytic cells	Symptomatic and supportive treatment of anemia; local radiation is effective for osseous lesions; corticosteroids should be used to treat lung involvement
Autosomal recessive trait with impaired cell immunity; about 15 human papillomaviruses are implicated	No effective treatment
Unknown, but may be induced by arsenic, bismuth, gold, quinidine, propranolol, statins, and naproxen	Symptomatic; oatmeal baths, antihistamines, prednisone
Vitamin B_{12} deficiency	Correction of vitamin B_{12} deficiency
Inherited family trait, deletion of tumor-suppression gene (chromosome 17)	Treatment specific to cancer
Congenital, resulting from birth trauma, fetal anoxia, or maternal illness during pregnancy	Preventive measures; symptomatic treatment
Causative bacteria include many gram-negative and anaerobic organisms, streptococci, and staphylococci	Significant airway obstruction may require tracheotomy; high doses of penicillin G given I.V., sometimes in combination with other drugs; incision and drainage to relieve pressure in affected tissues
Infestation by trematodes or flukes (Flukes may be classified as blood flukes, liver flukes, lung flukes, or intestinal flukes depending on location in the infected host)	Praziquantel is the drug of choice; symptomatic and supportive treatment of hemoptysis is usually necessary; surgery may be needed for complications
Unknown but genetic predisposition suspected	Plasmapheresis for hyperviscosity; chemotherapy; interferon-alfa; asymptomatic patients need no specific therapy
Unknown, but excessive exposure to sunlight is a risk factor	Laser or radiation therapy; chemotherapy; surgical excision; eye enucleation
Decarboxylation of the corresponding alpha-keto acids by the branched-chain alpha-keto acid dehydrogenase components; transmitted as an autosomal recessive trait	Supportive treatment; controlled intake of branched-chain amino acids; peritoneal dialysis, hemodialysis, or both; one form is responsive to early initiation of thiamine

(continued)

Disease	Description
Marburg disease: Marburg virus disease; Marburg hemorrhagic fever	Severe viral disease characterized by fever, malaise, myalgia, headache, pharyngitis, vomiting, diarrhea, and rash, often accompanied by hepatic damage and renal failure, encephalitis, and multiorgan dysfunction
Medullary cystic disease: familial juvenile nephronophthisis	Congenital renal disorder marked by cyst formation, primarily in the medulla and the corticomedullary junction, with insidious onset of uremia that causes death between ages 4 and 14
Megaloblastic anemia	Folic acid or vitamin B_{12} deficiency that alters the nucleic acid production needed for erythrocyte maturation in bone marrow
Meyer–Betz disease: idiopathic or familial myoglobinuria	Myoglobinuria that may be precipitated by strenuous exertion or possibly by infection; marked by tenderness, swelling, and muscle weakness
Microdrepanocytic disease: sickle cell thalassemia	Anemia involving simultaneous heterozygosity for hemoglobin and thalassemia
Milroy disease: congenital lymphedema	Chronic lymphatic obstruction causing lymphedema of the legs; sometimes associated with edema of the arms, trunk, and face
Minamata disease	Severe neurologic disorder characterized by peripheral and circumoral paresthesia, ataxia, mental disabilities, and loss of peripheral vision
Minor disease: tremor familiaris	Hematomyelia (hemorrhage into the spinal cord) involving the central parts of the spinal cord; marked by sudden onset of flaccid paralysis, with sensory disturbances
Mule-spinner's disease	Warts or ulcers, especially on the scrotum, that tend to become malignant; common among operators of spinning mules in cotton mills
Mushroom picker's disease: farmer's lung, bird breeder's lung, extrinsic allergic alveolitis	Allergic respiratory disease of persons working with moldy compost prepared for growing mushrooms; chronic form leads to pulmonary fibrosis
Mycetoma: maduromycosis, Madura foot, watering can foot	Chronic infection of the skin, subcutaneous tissues, and bone, usually affecting the foot; results in sinus tracts of the foot; deformity may occur
Myelosclerosis	Sclerosis of the spinal cord; obliteration of the normal marrow cavity by the formation of small spicules of bone
Niemann–Pick disease: sphingomyelin lipidosis	Lipid storage disorder resulting in abnormal accumulation of sphingomyelin in reticuloendothelial cells; most common in people of Ashkenazi Jewish ancestry; occurs in five different phenotypes, each with slightly different symptoms but characterized by pulmonary infiltrates, brownish skin, and sea blue histiocytes

Cause	Treatment
Zoonotic (animal-borne) ribonucleic acid virus of the filovirus family; initially discovered in exposure to African green monkeys	Symptomatic and supportive treatment; usually fatal
Transmitted as an autosomal recessive or dominant trait	Symptomatic treatment: erythropoietin for anemia, recombinant GH for growth retardation, peritoneal dialysis or hemodialysis; transplantation
Cobalamin (vitamin B_{12}) deficiency, secondary to pernicious anemia and folate deficiency, resulting from poor diet, sprue, pregnancy, or antifolate medication	Folic acid or vitamin B_{12} supplementation
Unknown; familial tendencies possible	Bed rest; anti-inflammatory agents, steroids in extreme cases, analgesics for pain
Hereditary transmission	Management of anemia
Congenital and hereditary; transmitted as an autosomal dominant trait	Microsurgery to rechannel lymph flow; supportive care; compression stockings
Alkyl mercury poisoning	Avoidance of causative agents; supportive and symptomatic treatment; chelation therapy with dimercaprol or 2,3-dimercaptosuccinic acid for acute cases; exchange transfusions; usually fatal
Usually seen with vascular malformation, blood dyscrasia, and in people on anticoagulants; possibly inheritable	Treatment of underlying disease; supportive treatment, which may include medication for pain, anxiety, or depression
Found in cotton textile workers who had frequent scrotal contact with mineral oils on a long-term basis while working on a machine called the *mule*	Chemotherapy; radiotherapy; bone marrow transplantation; surgery if needed
Airborne irritant, usually mold spores: *Micropolyspora faeni* or *Thermoactinomyces vulgaris*	Surgery; chemotherapy as indicated
Actinomycetes or fungi found in soil and plant material of tropical region	Supportive and symptomatic treatment; avoidance of exposure to allergen; glucocorticosteroids in chronic forms
Unknown	Antibiotics for actinomycetoma (streptomycin, trimethoprim and sulfamethoxazole, amikacin, rifampin, minocycline); itraconazole or ketoconazole for eumycetoma from fungi; surgery for affected tissue or amputation if bone is involved
Transmitted as an autosomal recessive trait	Supportive and symptomatic treatment; possibly liver transplantation in an infant with type A

(continued)

Disease	Description
Nystagmus	Recurring, involuntary eyeball movement that may be jerking or pendular
Olivopontocerebellar atrophy	Progressively deteriorating neurologic disease marked by ataxia, dysarthria, and an action tremor that develops late in middle life; usually normal deep tendon reflexes; associated with occasional rigidity and other extrapyramidal signs
Opitz disease	Thrombophlebitic splenomegaly
Osteitis pubis	Inflammation of the pubic symphysis and surrounding muscle insertions; painful condition characterized by bony resorption and spontaneous reossification; excruciating pain radiating along the adductor aspect of both thighs; pain intensified by movement, especially abduction
Paracoccidioidomycosis: South American blastomycosis	Fungal infection of the skin, lungs, mucous membranes, lymphatics, and viscera, seen primarily in the tropical forests of South America and Mexico
Paroxysmal nocturnal hemoglobinuria	Red cell breakdown with release of hemoglobin in the urine, resulting in dark-colored urine in the morning; symptoms include hemolytic anemia, thrombosis of large vessels, and a deficiency of hematopoiesis resulting in anemia (pancytopenia)
Pelizaeus–Merzbacher disease: sudanophilic leukodystrophy	Hyperplastic centrolobular sclerosis marked by nystagmus, ataxia, tremors, choreoathetotic movements, parkinsonian facies, and mental deterioration; begins early in life and occurs primarily in males
Pellegrini disease: Pellegrini–Stieda disease, Köhler–Stieda–Pellegrini disease	Ossification of the superior portion of the medial collateral ligament of the knee with pain, swelling, tenderness, and limited motion; a calcified mass develops within weeks
Pemphigus	Chronic blistering disease that causes superficial and deep lesions; pemphigus vulgaris, most common form of this disease, can be fatal
Perrin–Ferraton disease: snapping hip; iliotibial band syndrome	Condition marked by slippage of the hip joint; sometimes occurs with an audible snap (due to slipping of a tendinous band over the greater trochanter)
Pick disease	Very rare progressive disease that affects certain areas of the brain such as the temporal and frontal lobes and includes a loss of intellectual abilities and changes in behavior and personality

Cause	Treatment
May be congenital or acquired; jerking nystagmus results from excessive stimulation of the vestibular apparatus in the inner ear, lesions of the brainstem or cerebellum, drug and alcohol toxicity, and congenital neurologic disorder; pendular nystagmus results from improper transmission of visual impulses to the brain in the presence of corneal opacification, high astigmatism, congenital cataract, or congenital anomalies of optic disk or bilateral macular lesions	Correction of the underlying cause if possible; eyeglasses for vision disturbances
Transmitted as an autosomal dominant trait	No definitive therapy; death usually follows aspiration pneumonia secondary to loss of cough reflex
Thrombosis of the splenic vein	Symptomatic and supportive treatment, including anticoagulation
Cause unknown; repetitive microtrauma or shearing force to the pubic symphysis, which can happen while participating in sports involving running and kicking, may be a contributing factor	Symptomatic treatment; nonsteroidal anti-inflammatory drugs or cyclooxygenase-2 inhibitors, corticosteroids
Paracoccidioides brasiliensis	Ketoconazole, itraconazole, fluconazole; amphotericin B given I.V. for extremely ill patients
Unknown; possibly acquired clonal stem cell disorder	Symptomatic treatment with corticosteroids; androgen therapy; oral iron supplements and folic acid; transfusions; treatment of thrombotic complications
Familial transmission as an X-linked recessive trait, caused by mutations of the *PLP* gene located on the long arm of the X chromosome (Xq22)	No specific treatment; supportive care, such as physical therapy, orthotics, and antispasticity agents; severely affected patients need airway protection and anticonvulsant therapy
Trauma, such as a complication of athletic injuries	Surgical correction; supportive treatment
Autoimmune disorder; occasionally caused by reaction to such medications as penicillamine, captopril, carbidopa, and levodopa	Corticosteroids, immunosuppressants; antibiotics for secondary skin infections; plasmapheresis; dapsone for pemphigus foliaceus
Unknown	No effective treatment
Unknown, but thought to be an inherited autosomal dominant genetic trait	Supportive therapy such as medications to manage symptoms and care to maximize quality of life

(continued)

Disease	Description
Progressive multifocal leukoencephalopathy	Demyelination of the white substance of the brain, producing sensory aphasia, cortical blindness, deafness, weakness, spasticity of the limbs, and, eventually, complete paralysis, dementia, and coma; primarily affects patients who are immunosuppressed
Pulseless disease: Takayasu arteritis	Progressive changes of the aorta and its branches resulting in decreased or absent radial pulse bilaterally with pain in arm and forearm; inflammation of carotid arteries cause vision problems, dizziness, or stroke; aneurysms and hypertension occur
Purtscher disease: Purtscher-like angiopathic retinopathy	Retinal hemorrhagic and vaso-occlusive vasculopathy with edema, white retinal patches, and severe vision loss
Q fever	Rickettsial disease with acute and chronic stages, affecting respiratory as well as GI and cardiac systems
Rat-bite fever: sodoku	Gram-negative bacterial infection that occurs 1 to 3 weeks after contact with secretions (urine, oral, or conjunctival) or bite from an infected animal (rat, squirrel, weasel, gerbil), causing chills, fever, headache, muscle pain, maculopapular rash on extremities, and painful joints
Refsum disease: type IV hereditary sensorimotor neuropathy	Defect in metabolism of phytanic acid, marked by chronic polyneuritis, retinitis pigmentosa, and cerebellar signs (mild ataxia) with persistent elevation of protein levels in cerebrospinal fluid
Retinoblastoma	Most common intraocular cancer in children, arising from retinal gum cells; white pupil (leukokoria), poorly aligned eyes (strabismus), or a red and painful eye may be first indications
Rhabdomyosarcoma	Malignant tumors of muscle; areas affected include genitourinary tract, extremities, trunk, and retroperitoneum; in children, head and neck soft-tissue sarcoma most common
Richter syndrome	Chronic lymphocytic leukemia that evolves into an aggressive lymphoma
Rickettsialpox	Mild self-limiting zoonotic febrile illness characterized by a papulovesicular skin rash at the location of a tick bite
Robles disease: onchocerciasis	Onchocerciasis of the fibroid nodules, lymph, subcutaneous connective tissue (severe dermatitis and depigmentation), and eyes (river blindness)
Rosai–Dorfman disease: sinus histiocytosis with massive lymphadenopathy	A rare disorder characterized by massive, painless, bilateral lymph node enlargement in the neck with fever

Cause	Treatment
Common human polyomavirus, JC virus	Symptomatic and supportive treatment
Unknown, but appears to be related to autoimmunity	Steroids, immunosuppressants, surgery, angioplasty; ACE inhibitors for hypertension
Trauma—usually blunt thoracic or head trauma—and such nontraumatic diseases as pancreatitis, embolization, and vasculitis; amniotic fluid aneurysm also a cause	Supportive treatment, which may include medication for pain, anxiety, or depression; treatment of underlying condition
Inhalation of infected particles by *Coxiella burnetii*; considered category B agent for biologic warfare	Appropriate antibiotic therapy (doxycycline or chloramphenicol); possibly valve replacement
Streptobacillus moniliformis or *Spirillum minus*	Penicillin or tetracycline
Transmitted as an autosomal recessive trait	Symptomatic and supportive treatment; therapeutic plasma exchange; transplantation of alpha-hydroxylase–containing tissue
Transmitted as an autosomal dominant trait (deletion of q14 band of chromosome 13)	Radiotherapy, chemotherapy-based multimodality therapy, or cryotherapy; enucleation
Unknown	Radiation therapy; surgical excision
Clonal evolution of original leukemia	Chemotherapy for the lymphoma
Rickettsia akari transmitted by bites of mites carried by infected rodents	Chloramphenicol, doxycycline, ciprofloxacin, levofloxacin; supportive care
O. volvulus transmitted by the black fly	Ivermectin or diethylcarbamazine, albendazole or mebendazole; corticosteroids or antihistamines to relieve allergic reactions from microfilariae
Unknown	Surgery for life-threatening obstruction, chemotherapy, or radiation treatment

(continued)

Disease	Description
Rubinstein–Taybi syndrome: broad-thumb-hallux syndrome	A rare genetic multisystem disorder characterized by growth retardation and delayed bone age; mental retardation; craniofacial dysmorphism (widely spaced eyes, a broad nasal bridge, and an abnormally large or "beak-shaped" nose); abnormally broad thumbs and great toes; breathing and swallowing difficulties; microcephaly; a highly arched palate; micrognathia; strabismus; ptosis; downwardly slanting palpebral fissures; and epicanthal folds. Many individuals may have malformations of the heart, kidneys, urogenital system, and skeletal system.
Sever disease	Epiphysitis of the calcaneus in children when the growth plate is injured
Silo-filler's disease	Pulmonary inflammation often associated with acute pulmonary edema
Smith–Strang disease: methionine malabsorption syndrome, oasthouse urine disease	Defective methionine absorption, resulting in white hair, mental retardation, seizures, attacks of hyperpnea, and characteristic urine odor
Soft-tissue sarcoma	Soft-tissue malignancy of muscle, fat, connective tissue, blood vessels, and synovium; composed of tightly packed cells similar to embryonic connective tissue
Sponge-divers disease: sponge dermatitis, Skevas–Zerfus disease	Burning, itching, erythema, necrosis, and ulceration of skin; common in Mediterranean divers
Tangier disease	Deficiency of high-density lipoproteins in the serum with storage of cholesterol esters in the tonsils causing orange-yellow tonsillar hyperplasia, and in the liver and spleen, causing hepatosplenomegaly
Toxocariasis: visceral larva migrans	Chronic, frequently mild syndrome common in children involving roundworm migration from the intestine to various organs and tissues (visceral larva migrans); characterized by hepatosplenomegaly, eosinophilia, cough, difficulty sleeping, abdominal pain, and behavioral problems; ocular larva migrans can also occur, resulting in decreased vision, red eye or leukokoria (white pupil), retinal detachment, and vision loss
Trench fever: Wolhynia fever, shin bone fever, His–Werner disease, quintan fever	Fever with bone pain of the tibia, neck, and back, worsening with attacks; conjunctivitis, rash, splenomegaly, and hepatomegaly may also occur
Trevor disease: dysplasia epiphysealis hemimelica	Rare developmental disorder affecting epiphyses in which the lesions increase until skeletal maturity; painless swelling occurs on the side of the joint (usually the knee), limiting movement
Trichuriasis: whipworm disease	Nematode infection of the cecum and the anterior parts of the large intestine, producing various GI effects

Cause	Treatment
A genetic defect or mutation in chromosome 16	Supportive therapy during infancy, including physical, speech, and feeding therapy; and special education
Inflammation secondary to trauma or irritation	Treatment of underlying cause; orthotics, arch supports, or heel cups; stretching exercises
Inhalation of oxides of nitrogen and other gases that collect in silos	Corticosteroids; supportive respiratory treatment; volume expanders; oxygen may be required; methylene blue if methemoglobin exceeds 30%; avoidance of exposure to silo gases
Transmitted as an autosomal recessive trait	No effective treatment
Unknown	Surgical resection; radiation therapy; chemotherapy with doxorubicin or dacarbazine
Irritation by toxins of sea anemones of the *Sagartia* and *Actinia* genera	Symptomatic treatment; dilute acetic acid; administration of antihistamines for hives and itching; oral and topical steroids
Transmitted as an autosomal recessive metabolic disorder	Dependent on symptoms; may include heart surgery, removal of organs, or gene therapy
Ingestion of *Toxocara* larvae, usually from dirt or sand; risk factors include eating without handwashing and living with or raising dogs and cats	Thiabendazole or mebendazole; albendazole; ocular surgery
Bartonella quintana transmitted by body lice	Doxycycline, ceftriaxone, tetracycline, analgesics, antipyretics; delousing with lindane or other pediculicides; valve surgery if endocarditis occurs
Unknown	No known treatment
Ingestion of food contaminated with *Trichuris*	Mebendazole or albendazole

(continued)

Disease	Description
Tropical sprue	GI disorder that causes atrophy of the small intestine, resulting in malabsorption, malnutrition, and folic acid deficiency; characterized by bulky, pale, frothy stools with increased fecal fat and macrocytic anemia; occurs mainly in Puerto Rico, Cuba, Haiti, Dominican Republic, and India
Turcot syndrome	Characterized by adenomatous polyps in the mucous lining of the GI tract with tumors of the central nervous system; symptoms may include diarrhea, bleeding from the end portion of the large intestine (rectum), fatigue, abdominal pain, and weight loss; affected individuals may also experience neurologic symptoms, depending on the type, size, and location of the associated brain tumor
Typhus, endemic: murine, rat, or flea typhus	Mild form of typhus causing systemic illness characterized by fever, headache, rash, and myalgia
Typhus, epidemic: European, classic, or louse-borne typhus	Acute systemic illness that may lead to death; signs and symptoms include severe headache, high fever, myalgia, chills, hypotension, delirium, and rash
Typhus, scrub: Japanese river or flood fever, tsutsugamushi fever	Acute systemic disease occurring almost exclusively in the western Pacific, Japan, and Southeast Asia
Tyrosinemia *Hereditary form:* results in liver failure and renal tubular failure, hypoglycemia, rickets, darkening of the skin, and mild mental retardation; occasionally causes liver cancer *Transient form:* usually occurs in premature neonates; marked by elevation of blood tyrosine levels	
Valinemia: hypervalinemia, valine transaminase deficiency	Rare metabolic disorder characterized by elevated levels of amino acid valine in the blood and urine caused by a deficiency of the enzyme valine transaminase, which is needed in the metabolism of valine; infants with valinemia usually have a lack of appetite, frequent vomiting, and failure to thrive; hypotonia and hyperactivity also occur
Verneuil disease: hidradenitis suppurativa	Disorder of the terminal follicular epithelium in skin with apocrine glands; characterized by comedo-like follicular occlusions, inflammation, mucopurulent discharge, and scarring
Vibrio vulnificus septicemia	Overwhelming sepsis in a cirrhotic patient who has ingested oysters; typically affects men older than age 40 in coastal states between May and October
Volkmann disease: Volkmann deformity	Deformity of the hand, fingers, or wrist caused by injury to the muscles of the forearm
von Hippel–Lindau disease: cerebroretinal angiomatosis	Phakomatosis characterized by angiomatosis of the retina, cerebellum, spinal cord, and, less commonly, cysts of the pancreas, kidneys, and other viscera; onset usually in third decade and marked by symptoms of retinal or cerebral tumors

Cause	Treatment
Unknown	Tetracycline or oxytetracycline; folic acid and vitamin B_{12}
Inherited as an autosomal recessive trait	Surgery, chemotherapy, and radiation as indicated
Rickettsia typhi transmitted by bites of infected fleas or lice or by inhalation of contaminated flea feces	Tetracycline, doxycycline, or chloramphenicol; analgesics; antipyretics
R. prowazekii transmitted by *Pediculus humanus*	Tetracycline, doxycycline, or chloramphenicol; analgesics; antipyretics; delousing with lindane or other pediculicide
Rickettsia tsutsugamushi transmitted by mite larvae	Chloramphenicol or tetracycline (Resistance to doxycycline and chloramphenicol has appeared in northern Thailand.)
Autosomal recessive trait resulting in excess of tyrosine in blood and urine; gene maps to band 15q23-q25 identify 30 distinct mutations	Tyrosine and phenylalanine restriction; nitisinone (a tyrosine degradation inhibitor); genetic counseling; liver transplantation is last resort
Unknown	A diet low in valine introduced during early infancy usually improves symptoms
Unknown	Supportive treatment; antiseptics, warm compresses with sodium chloride or Burow solution; irradiation; surgery; tetracycline, doxycycline; clindamycin, erythromycin, retinoids, sulfonamides, corticosteroids; hormone therapy
V. vulnificus	Tetracycline or chloramphenicol
Trauma	Surgery to fix deformity
Transmitted as an autosomal dominant trait	Early surgical intervention may include cyst removal in every stage before growth acceleration

(continued)

Disease	Description
Wegner disease: Bednar–Parrot disease, Parrot pseudoparalysis	Pseudoparalysis from osteochondrotic separation of the epiphyses; onset most common in first weeks of life and seldom after 3 months
Werdnig–Hoffmann disease: spinal muscular atrophy	Progressive degeneration of anterior horn cells and bulbar motor nuclei in a fetus or neonate; type 1 is most severe, as neonates are born with weak, thin muscles and breathing problems; type 2 has less severe symptoms during early infancy, but becomes progressively weaker until the infant's death; type 3 is the least severe form, with signs and symptoms appearing after age 2 (weakening becomes more profound as the patient ages, but survival may be into early adulthood)
Whipple disease: intestinal lipodystrophy, lipophagia granulomatosis	GI malabsorption disorder characterized by chronic diarrhea and progressive wasting, with skin pigmentation and polyarthralgia
Wilms tumor: congenital nephroblastoma, embryonal adenomyosarcoma	Malignant mixed tumors of the kidneys, primarily affecting children; major signs—abdominal mass, enlarged abdomen, hypertension, vomiting, and hematuria
Wilson disease	Also called hepatolenticular degeneration; a metabolic disorder characterized by excessive copper retention in the liver, kidneys, brain, and corneas
Wiskott–Aldrich syndrome	Also called immunodeficiency with eczema and thrombocytopenia; an X-linked, recessive immunodeficiency disorder characterized by defective B-cell and T-cell function
Wolman disease: infantile form of acid lipase deficiency	A lysosomal storage disorder; hepatosplenomegaly, steatorrhea, and adrenal calcification manifested in the first weeks of life; results from accumulation of large amounts of lipids (especially cholesteryl esters and glycerides) in the liver, spleen, lymph nodes, and other tissues
Yaws: frambesia tropica	Chronic relapsing infection characterized by highly contagious primary and secondary cutaneous lesions and noncontagious tertiary lesions, as well as systemic signs and symptoms; primarily occurs in Africa, Asia, South America, and Oceania—where overcrowding and poor sanitation prevail in warm, humid tropical regions
Yellow fever	Flavivirus infection that causes sudden illness accompanied by fever, slow pulse rate, and headache, nausea, and vomiting; endemic in tropical Africa and Central and South America
Zygomycosis: phycomycosis, mucormycosis	Fungal infection most often seen in patients who are immunocompromised; several forms, including rhinocerebral, GI, pulmonary, and disseminated mucormycosis

Cause	*Treatment*
Congenital syphilis	Effective treatment of syphilis during pregnancy; after delivery, neonate is also treated for syphilis
Transmitted as an autosomal recessive trait	Symptomatic and supportive treatment, including physiotherapy and bracing; airway clearance is a priority due to secretions
Tropheryma whippelii	Appropriate antibiotic therapy; supportive therapy with fluid and electrolyte replacement; iron, folate, vitamin D, and magnesium supplementation
Wilms tumor recessive oncogene WT_1 at 11p15 locus	Nephrectomy, radiation therapy, chemotherapy
Inherited as an autosomal recessive trait	Lifetime therapy with pyridoxine (vitamin B_6) in conjunction with penicillamine, a copper chelating agent
Inherited as an X-linked, recessive trait	Limit bleeding through use of fresh, crossmatched platelet transfusions, antibiotics to control infection, topical corticosteroids to treat eczema; bone marrow transplant has been successful in some patients
Transmitted as an autosomal recessive trait; transmission caused by mutations of a specific gene located on chromosome 10	No specific therapy; usually fatal by age 6 months
Treponema pertenue	Penicillin G benzathine, tetracycline, or erythromycin; after single penicillin injection, early lesions become noninfectious in 24 hours; tissue damage occurring later in yaws is irreversible
Flavivirus transmitted by *Haemagogus* mosquitoes in South America and *Aedes africanus* in Africa; the mosquitoes bite monkeys, which act as hosts for the virus, then the mosquitoes bite humans, transmitting the disease	Supportive treatment for fluid volume and maintenance of normothermia; yellow fever vaccine; prevention of gastric bleeding with histamine-2 antagonists
Zygomycetes	Treatment of the underlying condition; amphotericin B; surgical removal of necrotic tissue

POTENTIAL AGENTS OF BIOTERRORISM

Listed below are examples of biologic agents that may be used as biologic weapons, as well as major signs and symptoms for each. This table has been created using information found via the Centers for Disease Control and Prevention (2017) regarding specific biologic agents.

Major associated signs and symptoms

Potential agents	Abdominal pain	Back pain	Blood pressure, decreased	Chest pain	Chills	Cough	Diarrhea, bloody	Diarrhea, watery	Diplopia	Dysarthria	Dysphagia	Dyspnea	Fever	Headache	Hematemesis
Anthrax (cutaneous)															
Anthrax (GI)	●				●		●	●			●		●	●	●
Anthrax (inhalation)	●			●	●	●						●	●	●	
Botulism									●	●	●				
Cholera			●					●							
Plague (bubonic and septicemic)	●				●								●	●	
Plague (pneumonic)				●	●	●							●	●	
Smallpox													●	●	
Tularemia				●		●							●	●	

Hemoptysis	Lymphadenopathy	Malaise	Muscle spasms (muscle cramps)	Myalgias	Nausea	Oliguria	Papular rash (skin lesions)	Ptosis	Skin turgor, decreased	Stridor	Tachycardia	Tachypnea	Vomiting	Weakness	
							●								
	●				●								●		Sore throat hoarseness
		●		●	●								●		Confusion and dizziness sweating
								●						●	
			●			●			●		●		●	●	Dehydration
	●													●	
●												●		●	Pneumonia
				●			●						●		
	●														

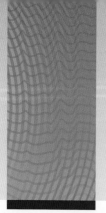

COMPLEMENTARY AND INTEGRATIVE THERAPIES FOR SPECIFIC CONDITIONS

Here are examples of complementary and integrative therapies that practitioners may consider for specific conditions, diseases, and signs and symptoms. In many cases, these therapies are used as adjuncts to conventional therapies. Because many of these therapies remain experimental, help your patient research any therapy under consideration before beginning it. Advise the patient to discuss any complementary or integrative therapies with a practitioner before beginning therapy.

Allergies, hay fever
◆ Nasal lavage (Neti pot)
◆ Steam inhalation

Alzheimer disease
◆ Aromatherapy
◆ Art therapy
◆ Dance therapy
◆ Massage therapy
◆ Music therapy

Anxiety
◆ Acupressure
◆ Acupuncture
◆ Aromatherapy
◆ Art therapy
◆ Biofeedback
◆ Guided imagery
◆ Massage therapy
◆ Meditation
◆ Music therapy
◆ Tai chi
◆ Yoga

Arthritis and osteoporosis
◆ Glucosamine, chondroitin supplements
◆ Tai chi
◆ Yoga

Asthma
◆ Biofeedback
◆ Breathing therapy

Atherosclerosis and cardiovascular conditions
◆ Meditation
◆ Garlic
◆ CoQ10

Autism
◆ Aromatherapy
◆ Art therapy
◆ Music therapy

Back pain
◆ Acupressure
◆ Acupuncture

◆ Guided imagery
◆ Massage therapy
◆ Meditation
◆ Tai chi
◆ Warm or cold compresses
◆ Yoga

Benign prostatic hyperplasia
◆ Saw palmetto

Bone fractures
◆ Calcium and calcium salt blend (calcium citrate, calcium triphosphate, calcium carbonate)
◆ Vitamin D
◆ Phosphorus

Cancer (all types)
◆ Acupressure
◆ Acupuncture
◆ Antioxidant supplementation

- Aromatherapy
- Art therapy
- Dance therapy
- Fiber (for colon cancer)
- Guided imagery
- Immunotherapy
- Massage
- Meditation
- Music therapy
- Tai chi
- Yoga

Childbirth
- Guided imagery
- Hypnotherapy
- Massage
- Music therapy

Colds and flu
- Echinacea
- Nasal lavage (Neti pot)
- Warm or cold compresses
- Steam inhalation
- Vitamin C

Constipation
- Diet (high fiber, drink plenty of water)

Dental disorders
- Hypnotherapy

Depression
- Acupuncture
- Aromatherapy
- Art therapy
- Guided imagery
- Massage
- Meditation
- Music therapy
- St. John's wort
- Tai chi
- Yoga

Diabetes mellitus
- Chromium picolinate

Drug and alcohol addiction
- B vitamin complex
- Omega-3 fatty acids

Emphysema
- Diet (avoid mucus-producing foods, such as dairy products, salt, and "junk" food)

Fatigue syndrome, chronic
- B vitamin complex
- Tai chi
- Yoga

Fibromyalgia
- Guided imagery
- Meditation
- Omega-3 fatty acids
- Tai chi
- Yoga

Gout
- Diet (low purine diet)

Headaches (including migraine)
- Acupressure
- Biofeedback
- Feverfew (*Tanacetum parthenium*)
- Guided imagery
- Magnesium
- Massage
- Meditation
- Warm or cold compresses

Hemorrhoids
- Fiber
- Hydrotherapy

Human immunodeficiency virus infection
- Antioxidants

Ichthyosis
- Omega-3 fatty acids

Insomnia
- Acupressure
- Acupuncture
- Aromatherapy
- Art therapy
- Biofeedback
- Guided imagery

- Massage
- Meditation
- Melatonin
- Music therapy
- Relaxation therapy
- Tai chi
- Yoga

Menopause
- Soy isoflavones

Multiple sclerosis
- Apitherapy

Pain
- Acupressure
- Acupuncture
- Aromatherapy
- Art therapy
- Biofeedback
- Guided imagery
- Hypnotherapy
- Massage
- Meditation
- Music therapy
- Relaxation therapy
- Tai chi
- Transcutaneous electrical nerve stimulation
- Yoga

Sinusitis
- Nasal lavage (Neti pot)
- Steam inhalation

Sore throat
- Herbal therapy (soothing and astringent gargles)
- Nasal lavage (Neti pot)
- Steam inhalation

Urinary problems (chronic)
- Cranberry (*Vaccinium macrocarpon*)

CARE OF LGBTQ PATIENT

Patients who identify as LGBTQ (lesbian, gay, bisexual, transgender, queer) should be treated with the same care, compassion, dignity, and quality that is afforded to any other patient. Providers of care must be educated to use appropriate terminology and dialogue, and committed to broadening access to this population, in order to decrease, and eventually eradicate, health disparities, stigma, and bias.

The first step in providing culturally appropriate care is to understand terminology. For the purposes of this resource, the acronym of LGBTQ has been chosen, as it is one of the most commonly recognized abbreviations. It is important to note that other acronyms do exist that are inclusive of others, such as LGBTAIQQ (which includes the A for asexual or allies; the I for intersex, and two Qs: one for queer, and one for questioning) or LGBTQIA (with the same representation for the I as intersex and A as ally or asexual). It is also important to note that it is inappropriate for others to identify someone as "queer"; this is a noun that is used internally by an individual or group of individuals who identify as such.

Healthcare providers must understand the difference between sex and gender. Sex is the physical or biologic characteristics that are noted at birth when a child is declared to be male or female. Sex includes chromosomes, genitalia and reproductive organs, and hormones. Gender, however, is a social construct, one in which an individual's self-concept identifies as male, female, gender fluid, nonbinary, or otherwise. Gender expression may be noted in an infinite variety of ways ranging from attire to posture to interests (Eliason & Chinn, 2018).

To provide culturally appropriate care, it is important that the healthcare provider speaks with the patient about sex and gender in an open, nonjudgmental capacity. It is entirely appropriate to ask the patient how they would like to be addressed, and which pronouns they prefer. This is possibly the most important step in establishing a therapeutic and trusting provider and patient relationship.

Depending on the patient's identity, care from this point forward will be personalized according to the needs of their specific health status. For example, a patient who is transitioning via hormone therapy or gender-affirming surgery will need care and teaching that is specific to those interventions. A patient who identifies as a different gender, yet has reproductive organs of another gender, will need information about how to best care for self based on the current state of their reproductive organs (e.g., a patient who identifies as male, yet has female reproductive organs, can benefit from information on Pap smears to screen for cervical cancer).

REFERENCES

Centers for Disease Control and Prevention. (2017). *Bioterrorism*. Retrieved from https://emergency.cdc.gov/bioterrorism/index.asp

Eliason, M., & Chinn, P. (2018). *LGBTQ cultures: What health care professionals need to know about sexual and gender diversity*. Philadelphia: Wolters Kluwer.

Wanders, R., & Eichler, F. (2017). *Adrenoleukodystrophy*. Retrieved from www.uptodate.com

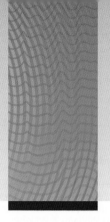

ACKNOWLEDGMENTS

We thank the following people, companies, and sources for contributing the photographs and artwork:

Marc S. Lapayowker, MD, Temple University Hospital, Philadelphia	p. 236, *The "string sign"*
Consultant Magazine, Cliggot Publishing Company, Greenwich, Connecticut	p. 493, *Recognizing pellagra*
Ron Hurst, Photographer, Little Brown & Co., Boston, Massachusetts	p. 528, *Trousseau sign*
John Murphy, Photographer	p. 785, *Reed–Sternberg cells*
Stedman's pediatric book. (2001). Baltimore: Lippincott Williams & Wilkins.	p. 262, *Types of rectal prolapse*
Berg, D., & Worzala, K. (2006). *Atlas of adult physical diagnosis.* Philadelphia: Lippincott Williams & Wilkins.	p. 602, *Recognizing chalazion*
Bickley, L. S. (2003). *Bates' guide to physical examination and history* (8th ed.). Philadelphia: Lippincott Williams & Wilkins.	p. 603, *Recognizing a stye*
McConnell, T. M. (2003). *The nature of diseases: Pathology for the health professions.* Philadelphia: Lippincott Williams & Wilkins.	p. 612, *The uveal tract and causes of uveitis*
Anatomical Chart Company	p. 648, *Locate the paranasal sinuses*
	p. 658, *Vocal cord nodules*
	p. 672, *Scabies: Cause and effect*
	p. 947, *Gauging burn depth*
	p. 1011, *Types of neural tube defects*
Goodheart, H .P. (2003). *Goodheart's photoguide of common skin disorders* (2nd ed.). Philadelphia: Lippincott Williams & Wilkins.	p. 665, *Recognizing impetigo*
	p. 680, *Alopecia areata*

	p. 682, *Recognizing vitiligo*
	p. 693, *Psoriatic plaques*
	p. 857, *Recognizing candidiasis*
	p. 1088, *Chancroidal lesion*
Gary Marshall, MD	p. 668, *Identifying staphylococcal scalded skin syndrome*
Weber, J., & Kelley, J. (2003). *Health assessment in nursing* (2nd ed.). Philadelphia: Lippincott Williams & Wilkins.	p. 670, *Athlete's foot*
LifeART	p. 674, *Types of lice*
Parish, L. C., et al., eds. (1983). *Cutaneous infestations of man and animals.* New York: Praeger, with permission.	p. 674, *Types of lice*
Mills, S. E. (2007). *Histology for pathologists* (3rd ed.). Philadelphia: Lippincott Williams & Wilkins.	p. 718, *MRI image of the pituitary*
Devita, V. T., Jr., et al. (1997). *AIDS: Etiology, diagnosis, treatment, and prevention* (4th ed.). Philadelphia: Lippincott-Raven.	p. 783, *Kaposi sarcoma*
Rubin, E., & Farber, J. L. (1999). *Pathology* (3rd ed.). Philadelphia: Lippincott Williams & Wilkins.	p. 863, *Recognizing sporotrichosis*
Centers for Disease Control and Prevention Public Health Image Library	p. 881, *Rubeola*
Stedman's medical dictionary (28th ed.). (2006). Philadelphia: Lippincott Williams & Wilkins.	p. 959, *Radiation dermatitis*
Premkumar, K. (2004). *The massage connection: Anatomy and physiology.* Baltimore: Lippincott Williams & Wilkins.	p. 978, *DNA and how it works*
Engelkirk, P. G., & Burton, G. R. W. (2007). *Burton's microbiology for the health sciences* (8th ed.). Philadelphia: Lippincott Williams & Wilkins.	p. 979, *DNA replication*
Pillitteri, A. (2003). *Maternal & child nursing, care of the childbearing and childrearing family* (4th ed.). Philadelphia: Lippincott Williams & Wilkins.	p. 1051, *Three types of placenta previa*
Pillitteri, A. (1999). *Maternal & child nursing: Care of the childbearing and childrearing family* (3rd ed.). Philadelphia: Lippincott-Raven.	p. 1053, *Degrees of placental separation in abruptio placentae*
Koneman, W. E., et al. (1992). *Color atlas and textbook of diagnostic microbiology* (5th ed.). Philadelphia: Lippincott.	p. 1086, *Treponema pallidum*
Porth, C. M. (2005). *Pathophysiology: Concepts of altered health states* (7th ed.). Philadelphia: Lippincott Williams & Wilkins.	p. 1092, *Extravaginal torsion*

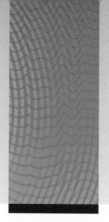

INDEX

Note: Page numbers followed by i indicate illustration; those followed by t indicate table.